Pearson's

Comprehensive

Medical
Assisting

Fourth Edition

Pearson's

Comprehensive

Medical
Assisting

Administrative and Clinical Competencies

Nina Beaman, Ed.D., MSN, CMA (AAMA), CNE (NLN), RN-BC (PMH), RNC-AWHC
Aspen University, Independence University, Fortis College • Richmond, VA

Kristiana D. Routh, RMA (AMT)
Allied Health Consulting Services • Girard, PA
Managing Editor, *Pearson's Comprehensive Medical Assisting*, Fourth Edition

Lorraine M. Papazian-Boyce, MS, CPC
AHIMA-Approved ICD-10-CM/PCS Trainer/Ambassador, PB Resources, Inc. • Belfair, WA

Ron Maly, MA, RMA (AMT), CPhT (PTCB)
CHI/St. Elizabeth Hospital • Lincoln, NE

Jaime Nguyen, MD, MPH, MS
Medical Editing and Compliance Consulting

Laree J. Schoolmeesters, Ph.D., RN, CNL
Medical Editor

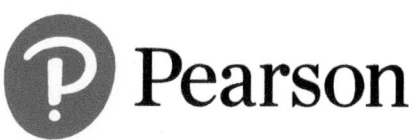

330 Hudson Street, NY, NY 10013

Vice President, Health Science and TED: Julie Levin Alexander
Director of Portfolio Management: Marlene McHugh Pratt
Development Editor: Sandra Breuer
Portfolio Management Assistant: Emily Edling
Vice President, Content Production and Digital Studio:
  Paul DeLuca
Managing Producer, Health Science: Melissa Bashe
Content Producer: Faye Gemmellaro
Operations Specialist: Mary Ann Gloriande
Creative Director: Blair Brown
Creative Digital Lead: Mary Siener
Managing Producer, Digital Studio, Health Science:
  Amy Peltier
Digital Studio Producer, REVEL and e-text 2.0:
  Ellen Viganola

Digital Content Team Lead: Brian Prybella
Digital Content Project Lead: William Johnson
Vice President, Product Marketing: David Gesell
Field Marketing Manager: Brittany Hammond
Full-Service Project Management and Composition:
  iEnergizer Aptara®, Ltd.
Inventory Manager: Vatche Demirdjian
Interior and Cover Design: Studio Montage
Cover Art: Main photo: JGI/Tom Grill/Blend Images/Getty Images;
  Bottom images, left to right: Sturti/E+/Getty Images;
  Hero Images/Getty Images; Ariel Skelley/Blend
  Images/Getty Images; Hero Images/Getty Images;
  Monkey Business Images/Shutterstock
Printer/Binder: LSC Communications, Inc.
Cover Printer: Phoenix Color/Hagerstown

Credits and acknowledgments for material borrowed from other sources and reproduced, with permission, in this textbook appear on pages 1495–1498.

Library of Congress Cataloging-in-Publication Data

Names: Beaman, Nina, author. | Routh, Kristiana D., author. | Papazian-Boyce, Lorraine, author. | Maly, Ron (Registered medical
  assistant), author. | Nguyen, Jaime, author.
Title: Pearson's comprehensive medical assisting: administrative and clinical competencies / Nina Beaman, Kristiana D. Routh,
  Lorraine M. Papazian-Boyce, Ron Maly, Jaime Nguyen.
Other titles: Comprehensive medical assisting
Description: Fourth edition. | Boston: Pearson, [2018] | Includes index.
Identifiers: LCCN 2017000538 | ISBN 9780134420202 | ISBN 0134420209 (case)
Subjects: | MESH: Physician Assistants | Medical Secretaries | Practice Management, Medical
Classification: LCC R728.8 | NLM W 21.5 | DDC 610.73/7—dc23 LC record available at https://lccn.loc.gov/2017000538

21 2023

Pearson

ISBN 13: 978-0-13-442020-2
ISBN 10:   0-13-442020-9

Brief Contents

Contents

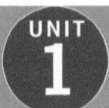

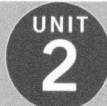

UNIT 2   Administrative Medical Assisting

UNIT 3   Anatomy and Physiology

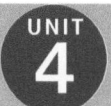

UNIT 4   Clinical Medical Assisting

UNIT 5 Career Assistance

Procedures

Preface

Medical assistants connect with people every hour of every day. They are the first line of medical care for many patients. To assist the physician with examining and treating patients, medical assistants must have a thorough knowledge of the structure and systems of the human body as well as a thorough knowledge of the procedures the physician performs and the procedures the medical assistant performs. At the same time, medical assistants must make every patient in a physician's office feel secure. They must comfort. They must listen. They must explain. They must demonstrate. Medical assistants help every patient feel like the only patient.

In addition to these clinical skills, the medical assistant must also be able to perform the administrative functions that keep the medical practice operating as a business, including such skills as telephone techniques, written communication, scheduling, billing, coding, filing claims with insurance companies, banking, ordering supplies, controlling inventory, and maintaining electronic health records.

Medical assistants must be able to work as part of a team, maintaining good working relationships with other employees of the medical practice and being flexible and willing to take on any of the variety of tasks that need to be done to keep a medical practice operating smoothly. They must also be able to work collaboratively with other health care professionals.

Because of the variety of skills and tasks medical assistants perform, medical assisting is a uniquely challenging profession and one that is seldom, if ever, boring.

FOCUS ON THE MEDICAL ASSISTANT

In this fourth edition of *Pearson's Comprehensive Medical Assisting*, the authors have made a special effort to focus on and speak directly to the student who is preparing to become a medical assistant. Extraneous information that is beyond the scope of practice of the medical assistant has been omitted. The text concentrates on explaining information and tasks that are appropriate for the medical assistant.

PROFESSIONALISM

As in prior editions, but with even greater intensity, *Pearson's Comprehensive Medical Assisting*, fourth edition, focuses on the concept of professionalism. Throughout the text, special "Professionalism" features discuss how to display a professional demeanor, how to perform various aspects of medical assisting in a professional manner, and how to aspire at all times to the highest professional standards.

ORGANIZATION

The text is organized into 5 units. **Unit 1, Introduction to Health Care**, covers the history of health care, the professional medical assistant, medical law and ethics, medical terminology, and communications. **Unit 2, Administrative Medical Assisting**, addresses front office topics such as medical billing and coding, reception, scheduling, electronic health records, and more. **Unit 3, Anatomy and Physiology**, covers body structure and function and each of the systems of the human body. **Unit 4, Clinical Medical Assisting**, deals with the medical functions of the practice, including examinations, measuring vital signs, administering medications, drawing blood, lab techniques, testing, and patient education. **Unit 5, Career Assistance**, focuses on professionalism and the skills the new medical assistant will need to obtain a position in a medical office, such as writing a résumé, having an interview, and participating in an externship program.

MEETING THE NEW CAAHEP AND ABHES STANDARDS

This fourth edition of *Pearson's Comprehensive Medical Assisting* has been revised throughout to meet all of the new standards and guidelines published by the Commission on Accreditation of Allied Health Education Programs (CAAHEP). These new standards and guidelines include the first major changes to CAAHEP curriculum since 2008.

The CAAHEP lists three kinds of standards—cognitive, psychomotor, and affective—in each of 12 content areas (for example, Anatomy and Physiology, Applied Mathematics, Infection Control, Administrative Functions, Procedural and Diagnostic Coding, and Legal Implications). (You can review the complete list in Appendix B at the CAAHEP website: www.caahep.org/documents/file/Publications-And-Governing-Documents/MedicalAssistingStandards.pdf.)

- **How we meet the Cognitive (Knowledge) Standards:** In the fourth edition of *Pearson's Comprehensive Medical Assisting*, the learning objectives have been carefully created to meet all of the CAAHEP cognitive standards, including concepts such as the patient navigator, patient coaching, new legal terminology, and patient-centered medical homes, to name a few.

- **How we meet the Psychomotor (Skills) Standards:** The psychomotor skills are addressed in 227 "Procedures" throughout the text (which include the 32 new "Procedures" listed below).

- **How we meet the Affective (Behaviors) Standards:** In the textbook, the "Professionalism" features (discussed above), as well as the "Judgment Call" and "Guidelines" features, focus on the affective standards. The workbook is also heavily focused on addressing the affective standards as they are related to the cognitive concepts discussed in the textbook.

In addition to ensuring that all of the CAAHEP standards are addressed in this edition, *Pearson's Comprehensive Medical Assisting* also addresses the new and revised curriculum changes set forth by the Accrediting Bureau of Health Education Schools (ABHES) effective January 2017. ABHES includes 10 main content areas (for example, General Orientation, Medical Terminology, Human Relations, Clinical Procedures, and Career Development). These main content areas are further broken down into entry-level competencies and sub-concepts (including credentialing of the medical assistant, Interprofessional Collaborative Practice, health laws and litigation, and many more). Complete information related to ABHES curriculum for medical assistants can be found in the accreditation manual available online at www.abhes.org/accreditationmanual.

CAAHEP and ABHES standards are mapped in each chapter of the Instructor Resource Manual. The Instructor Resource Manual also includes chapter-by-chapter mapping of the textbook to five national certification exams for medical assistants that are administered by the American Association of Medical Assistants, American Medical Technologists, National Center for Competency Testing, and National Healthcareer Association.

New Procedures in this Edition

Every chapter of this edition has been thoroughly reviewed and revised, with numerous new "Procedures" created. Listed below are the 32 "Procedures" that are new to the fourth edition.

Chapter 1, Medical Assisting: The Profession: Locating a State's Scope of Practice for Medical Assisting

Chapter 3, Medical Law and Ethics: Performing Compliance Reporting Based on Public Health Statutes; Reporting Illegal Activity in the Health Care Setting; Separating Personal and Professional Ethics

Chapter 5, Communication: Verbal and Nonverbal: Communicating with a Patient When There Is a Language Barrier

Chapter 6, The Office Environment: Completing an Incident Report

Chapter 7, Telephone Techniques: Calling the Pharmacy for a Prescription Refill

Chapter 11, Written Communication: Creating and Sending a Business Letter Using E-mail

Chapter 12, Computers in the Medical Office: Performing Data Backup

Chapter 13, The Medical Record: Completing a Request to Release Medical Records

Chapter 14, Medical Insurance: Interpreting Information on an Insurance Card

Chapter 16, Procedure Coding: Using Medical Necessity Guidelines

Chapter 17, Patient Billing and Collections: Obtaining Accurate Patient Billing Information

Chapter 36, Assisting with Medical Specialties: Performing and Educating the Patient Regarding Blood Glucose Monitoring; Instructing and Preparing a Patient for a Colonoscopy

Chapter 42, Assisting with Medical Emergencies/Emergency Preparedness: Performing First Aid for a Person in Shock; Performing First Aid for Diabetic Shock/Diabetic Coma; Performing First Aid for a Patient Having a Seizure

Chapter 44, Microbiology: Performing CLIA-Waived Microbiology Testing

Chapter 47, Hematology: Differentiating Between Normal and Abnormal Test Values

Chapter 52, Math for Pharmacology: Preparing Proper Medication Dosage: Applying Mathematic Computations to Solve Equations; Preparing Proper Medication Dosage: Converting from One Measurement System to Another; Preparing Proper Medication Dosage: Calculating Correct Dosage for an Injectable Medication; Applying Mathematic Computations to Solve Equations: Calculating Correct Pediatric Dosage Using Body Surface Area; Applying Mathematic Computations to Solve Equations: Calculating Correct Pediatric Dosage Using Body Weight

Chapter 54, Administering Medications: Administering Medication Safely; Reviewing Parenteral Medication Injection Sites
Chapter 55, Patient Education: Providing Patient Education on Disease Prevention: Smoking Cessation; Coaching Patients with Consideration of Communication Barriers: A Hearing-Impaired Patient; Creating an Office Policies Brochure; Working as a Patient Navigator: Facilitating a Referral for Community Resources
Chapter 57, Mental Health: Assisting a Terminally Ill Patient

Successful Connections

CHAPTER OPENER FEATURES

The chapter opener highlights some of the most important aspects of the chapter.

Case Studies give brief scenarios that help students understand how the chapter information relates to their careers. Questions at the end of the chapter refer back to the case study, providing a critical thinking opportunity.

Learning Objectives focus students on what they should get out of the chapter.

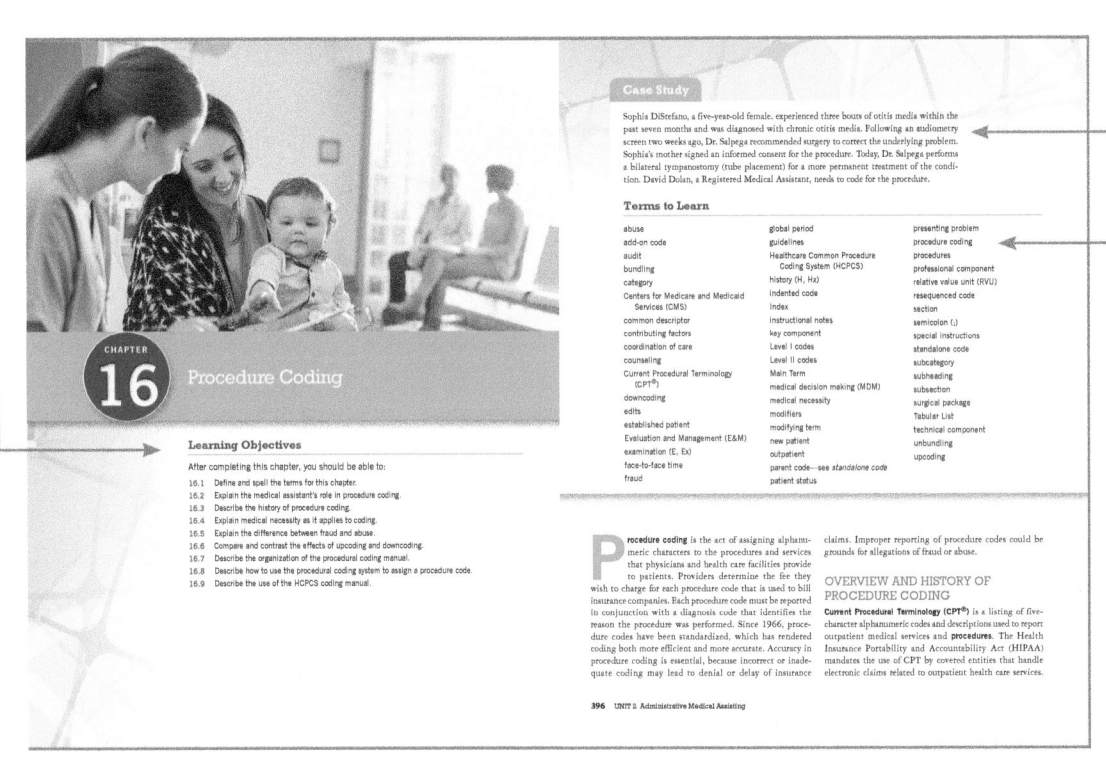

CHAPTER 16 — Procedure Coding

Case Study

Sophia DiStefano, a five-year-old female, experienced three bouts of otitis media within the past seven months and was diagnosed with chronic otitis media. Following an audiometry screen two weeks ago, Dr. Salpega recommended surgery to correct the underlying problem. Sophia's mother signed an informed consent for the procedure. Today, Dr. Salpega performs a bilateral tympanostomy (tube placement) for a more permanent treatment of the condition. David Dolan, a Registered Medical Assistant, needs to code for the procedure.

Terms to Learn

abuse
add-on code
audit
bundling
category
Centers for Medicare and Medicaid Services (CMS)
common descriptor
contributing factors
coordination of care
counseling
Current Procedural Terminology (CPT®)
downcoding
edits
established patient
Evaluation and Management (E&M)
examination (E, Ex)
face-to-face time
fraud

global period
guidelines
Healthcare Common Procedure Coding System (HCPCS)
history (H, Hx)
indented code
index
instructional notes
key component
Level I codes
Level II codes
Main Term
medical decision making (MDM)
medical necessity
modifiers
modifying term
new patient
outpatient
parent code—see standalone code
patient status

presenting problem
procedure coding
procedures
professional component
relative value unit (RVU)
resequenced code
section
semicolon (;)
special instructions
standalone code
subcategory
subheading
subsection
surgical package
Tabular List
technical component
unbundling
upcoding

Learning Objectives

After completing this chapter, you should be able to:

16.1 Define and spell the terms for this chapter.
16.2 Explain the medical assistant's role in procedure coding.
16.3 Describe the history of procedure coding.
16.4 Explain medical necessity as it applies to coding.
16.5 Explain the difference between fraud and abuse.
16.6 Compare and contrast the effects of upcoding and downcoding.
16.7 Describe the organization of the procedural coding manual.
16.8 Describe how to use the procedural coding system to assign a procedure code.
16.9 Describe the use of the HCPCS coding manual.

Procedure coding is the act of assigning alphanumeric characters to the procedures and services that physicians and health care facilities provide to patients. Providers determine the fee they wish to charge for each procedure code that is used to bill insurance companies. Each procedure code must be reported in conjunction with a diagnosis code that identifies the reason the procedure was performed. Since 1966, procedure codes have been standardized, which has rendered coding both more efficient and more accurate. Accuracy in procedure coding is essential, because incorrect or inadequate coding may lead to denial or delay of insurance claims. Improper reporting of procedure codes could be grounds for allegations of fraud or abuse.

OVERVIEW AND HISTORY OF PROCEDURE CODING

Current Procedural Terminology (CPT®) is a listing of five-character alphanumeric codes and descriptions used to report outpatient medical services and procedures. The Health Insurance Portability and Accountability Act (HIPAA) mandates the use of CPT by covered entities that handle electronic claims related to outpatient health care services.

396 UNIT 2 Administrative Medical Assisting

Terms to Learn present key words and concepts that are highlighted the first time they appear in the chapter.

SPECIAL FEATURES

The features in this book focus on professionalism and highlight special topics for students. These help students connect the importance of adopting and maintaining a professional demeanor with success on the job.

Professionalism provides tips for how to be professional in the medical office.

Professionalism

Lifelong learning is an important responsibility for all professionals. After completion of a formal education program and successful completion of a national certification examination, the professional medical assistant will continue to search for opportunities to maintain his or her credential through continuing education. The health care industry is constantly changing, and it is imperative that professionals keep abreast of these changes by participating in continuing education activities.

Professionalism: The Law tells students how to act like a professional when dealing with legal issues.

Professionalism   The Law

Imagine that, on January 3, you are coding services for patients seen during the past week. For patients seen on December 31, you must use the CPT manual for the old year. For patients seen on January 2, you must use the CPT manual for the new year. Also remember that the effective date for CPT manuals is January 1. This differs from the effective date for ICD-10-CM diagnosis coding manuals, which is October 1.

Professionalism: The Life Span helps students develop the skills to relate to patients of all ages.

Professionalism   The Life Span

Some medical clinics and physicians' offices provide care to patients within a specific age range or stage of life. Pediatric offices treat young children, adolescents, and teens. A physician who specializes in gerontology or geriatrics provides care to a population of older adults. Each age group is unique in its stage of physical and emotional development; therefore, each group has different needs and considerations. It is not realistic to think you would communicate with a 5-year-old patient and a 45-year-old patient in the same manner. In your interactions with patients, you must consider their developmental stage and provide age-appropriate care and instruction.

Professionalism: The Workplace explores topics and issues students may encounter during participation in an externship program.

Professionalism   The Workplace

Reporting incorrect procedure codes on an insurance claim can create problems such as improper reimbursement, fraud, and inaccurate patient medical history. When uncertain of the best code, it may be tempting to "guesstimate" and assign an approximate code. This practice may result in upcoding, which is coding for a higher level of service than what was actually provided to gain higher reimbursement. Guessing could also result in downcoding, which is coding for a lower level of service than what was actually provided, to avoid potential fraud or abuse. Downcoding may seem prudent to avoid fraud, but it deprives the medical office of reimbursement to which it is legally entitled.

Professionalism: Cultural Considerations gives students the skills to connect with both patients and other health professionals from diverse backgrounds.

Professionalism   Cultural Considerations

Medical assistants must consider their moral and ethical beliefs before accepting a job. These beliefs often are derived from religious views. Some offices may perform procedures or treatments that go against your views. It is always necessary to keep personal opinions and beliefs to yourself and not impose these beliefs on patients. Examples of possible conflicts may include an office that performs an abortion or an office that performs extensive research in genetic engineering.

Judgment Call provides critical thinking opportunities for students throughout the chapters.

JUDGMENT CALL

When you are working with others in the office, you should also be aware of their interactions with patients. Let's say you observe another medical assistant talking with a patient, and you hear the patient talking about the recent loss of her husband. The medical assistant responds to the patient, stating, "You poor thing." The medical assistant also starts to cry with the patient. What would you do, if anything, to intervene in this situation? Think about the differences between empathy, sympathy, and pity—and how these attitudes may affect the patient—to help you decide on your action.

VISUAL LEARNING

The open design of this book is ideal for visual learners.

Tables present topics in an at-a-glance format.

TABLE 16-1	Radiological Modalities (Methods)
Method	**Description**
Computerized tomography (CT)	A 3-D image created using X-rays to make a series of cross-sectional images in an area of the body.
Fluoroscopy	A real-time, moving X-ray image, usually viewed on a monitor.
Magnetic resonance imaging (MRI)	An image created using powerful magnets and radio waves.
Mammography	An image of the breasts, or mammary glands, created using low-dose X-rays.
Positron emission tomography (PET)	An image created using a radioactive substance called a tracer to show how organs and tissues are functioning.
Radiation Oncology	A form of cancer treatment that uses high-energy ionizing radiation to shrink or kill tumors. Also called radiation therapy.
Ultrasound (US)	An image created using sound waves, useful to view soft structures within the body.
X-ray	A picture created using radiation particles, used primarily for solid structures within the body.

TABLE 16-2	Types of Laboratory Tests
Type of Test	**Description**
Chemistry	Quantitative tests for the amount of asubstance contained in a specimen
Microbiology	Tests that identify the presence and type of microorganisms in a specimen
Hematology	Blood tests to determine cell counts of various types of blood cells
Immunology	Tests on antigens, allergens, or antibodies
Cytopathology	The microscopic examination of cells from anywhere in the body to detect conditions and determine if neoplasms are benign or malignant
Pathology	The visual examination of body structures or tissue, with or without a microscope

Boxes separate and highlight special information.

BOX 3-5	Code of Ethics of the American Association of Medical Assistants

PREAMBLE

The Code of Ethics of the AAMA shall set forth principles of ethical and moral conduct as they relate to the medical profession and the particular practice of medical assisting.

Members of the AAMA dedicated to the conscientious pursuit of their profession, and thus desiring to merit the high regard of the entire medical profession and the respect of the general public which they serve, do hereby pledge themselves to strive always to:

Human Dignity

I. Render service with full respect for the dignity of humanity;

Confidentiality

II. Respect confidential information obtained through employment unless legally authorized or required by responsible performance of duty to divulge such information;

Honor

III. Uphold the honor and high principles of the profession and accept its disciplines;

Continued Study

IV. Seek to continually improve the knowledge and skills of medical assistants for the benefit of patients and professional colleagues;

Responsibility for Improved Community

V. Participate in additional service activities aimed toward improving the health and well-being of the community.

Note: *Copyright by the American Association of Medical Assistants, Inc. Reprinted with permission.*

Color **Drawings** and **Photographs** bring the world of medical assisting to life. They illustrate key procedures, important concepts, equipment, and interactions among MAs, patients, and other staff.

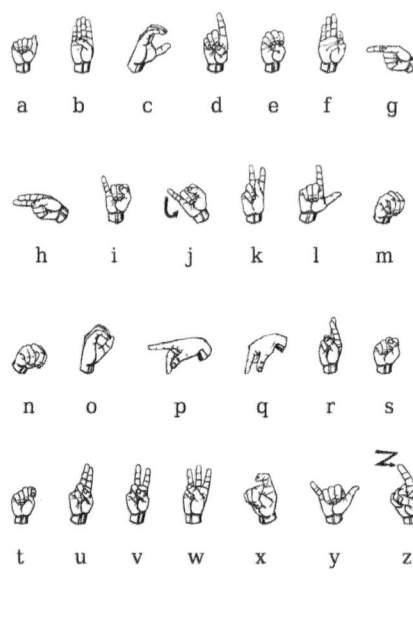
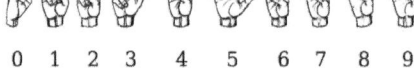

FIGURE 5-11 The American Sign Language alphabet.

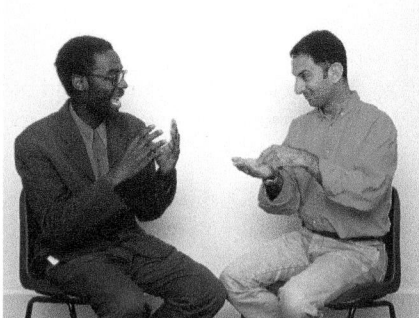

FIGURE 5-12 A hearing-impaired patient using an interpreter.

PROCEDURES

More than 225 procedures give students all they need to know to perform medical assisting skills.

The **Objective** helps students focus on the purpose of completing the procedure.

Equipment and Supplies lists what is needed for the procedure.

Charting Example shows students how to document the procedure.

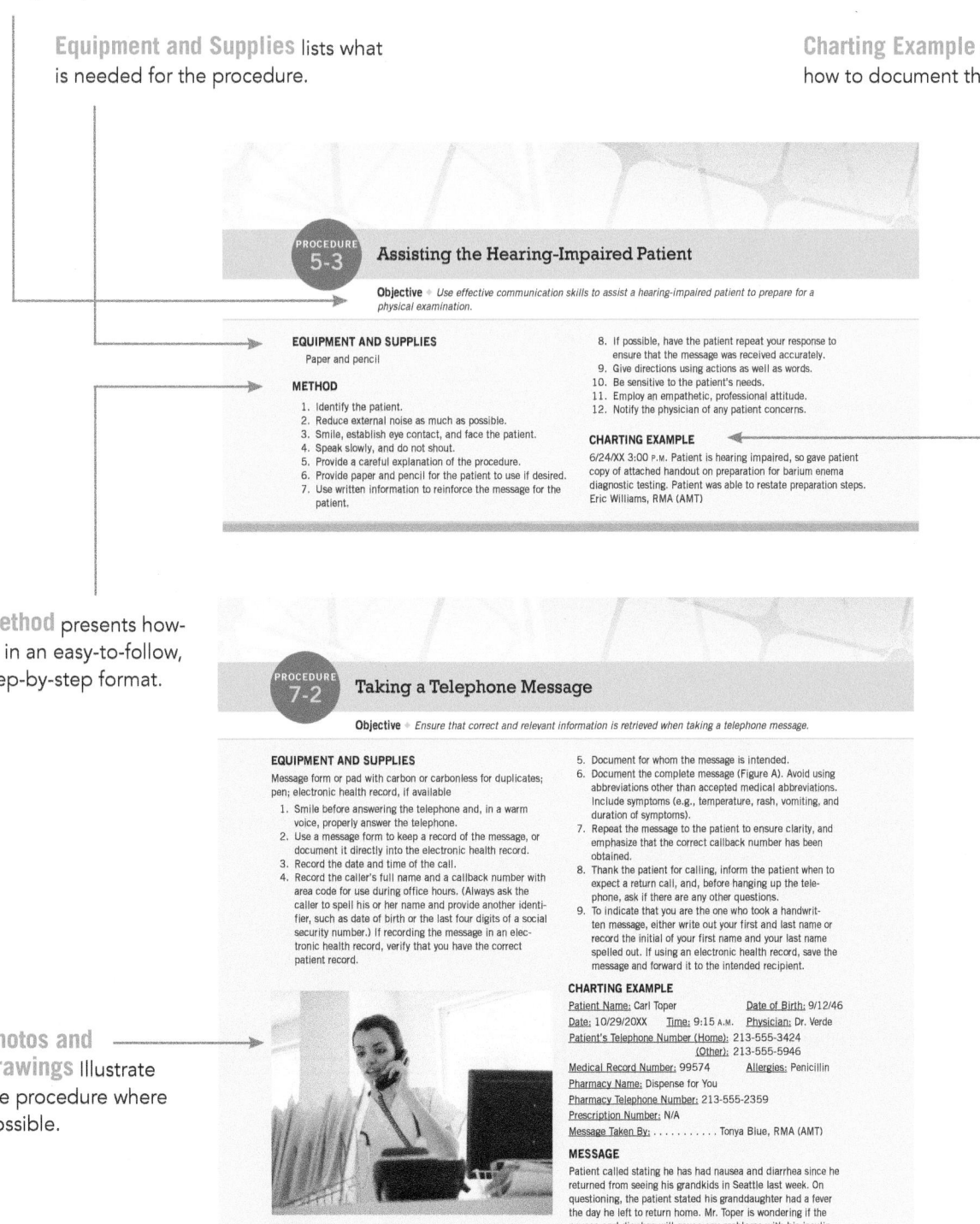

PROCEDURE 5-3

Assisting the Hearing-Impaired Patient

Objective ◆ *Use effective communication skills to assist a hearing-impaired patient to prepare for a physical examination.*

EQUIPMENT AND SUPPLIES
Paper and pencil

METHOD
1. Identify the patient.
2. Reduce external noise as much as possible.
3. Smile, establish eye contact, and face the patient.
4. Speak slowly, and do not shout.
5. Provide a careful explanation of the procedure.
6. Provide paper and pencil for the patient to use if desired.
7. Use written information to reinforce the message for the patient.
8. If possible, have the patient repeat your response to ensure that the message was received accurately.
9. Give directions using actions as well as words.
10. Be sensitive to the patient's needs.
11. Employ an empathetic, professional attitude.
12. Notify the physician of any patient concerns.

CHARTING EXAMPLE
6/24/XX 3:00 P.M. Patient is hearing impaired, so gave patient copy of attached handout on preparation for barium enema diagnostic testing. Patient was able to restate preparation steps. Eric Williams, RMA (AMT)

Method presents how-to in an easy-to-follow, step-by-step format.

PROCEDURE 7-2

Taking a Telephone Message

Objective ◆ *Ensure that correct and relevant information is retrieved when taking a telephone message.*

EQUIPMENT AND SUPPLIES
Message form or pad with carbon or carbonless for duplicates; pen; electronic health record, if available

1. Smile before answering the telephone and, in a warm voice, properly answer the telephone.
2. Use a message form to keep a record of the message, or document it directly into the electronic health record.
3. Record the date and time of the call.
4. Record the caller's full name and a callback number with area code for use during office hours. (Always ask the caller to spell his or her name and provide another identifier, such as date of birth or the last four digits of a social security number.) If recording the message in an electronic health record, verify that you have the correct patient record.
5. Document for whom the message is intended.
6. Document the complete message (Figure A). Avoid using abbreviations other than accepted medical abbreviations. Include symptoms (e.g., temperature, rash, vomiting, and duration of symptoms).
7. Repeat the message to the patient to ensure clarity, and emphasize that the correct callback number has been obtained.
8. Thank the patient for calling, inform the patient when to expect a return call, and, before hanging up the telephone, ask if there are any other questions.
9. To indicate that you are the one who took a handwritten message, either write out your first and last name or record the initial of your first name and your last name spelled out. If using an electronic health record, save the message and forward it to the intended recipient.

Photos and Drawings Illustrate the procedure where possible.

FIGURE A All messages must be documented and placed in the patient's record.

CHARTING EXAMPLE
Patient Name: Carl Toper   Date of Birth: 9/12/46
Date: 10/29/20XX   Time: 9:15 A.M.   Physician: Dr. Verde
Patient's Telephone Number (Home): 213-555-3424
(Other): 213-555-5946
Medical Record Number: 99574   Allergies: Penicillin
Pharmacy Name: Dispense for You
Pharmacy Telephone Number: 213-555-2359
Prescription Number: N/A
Message Taken By: . . . . Tonya Blue, RMA (AMT)

MESSAGE
Patient called stating he has had nausea and diarrhea since he returned from seeing his grandkids in Seattle last week. On questioning, the patient stated his granddaughter had a fever the day he left to return home. Mr. Toper is wondering if the nausea and diarrhea will cause any problems with his insulin dosing. Per the patient, he will be home all day.

END OF CHAPTER

The section at the end of the chapter highlights the importance of the chapter using a variety of learning styles.

Summary of the important topics from the chapter.

Critical Thinking questions refer back to the case study at the beginning of the chapter.

Competency Review tests student retention of key concepts.

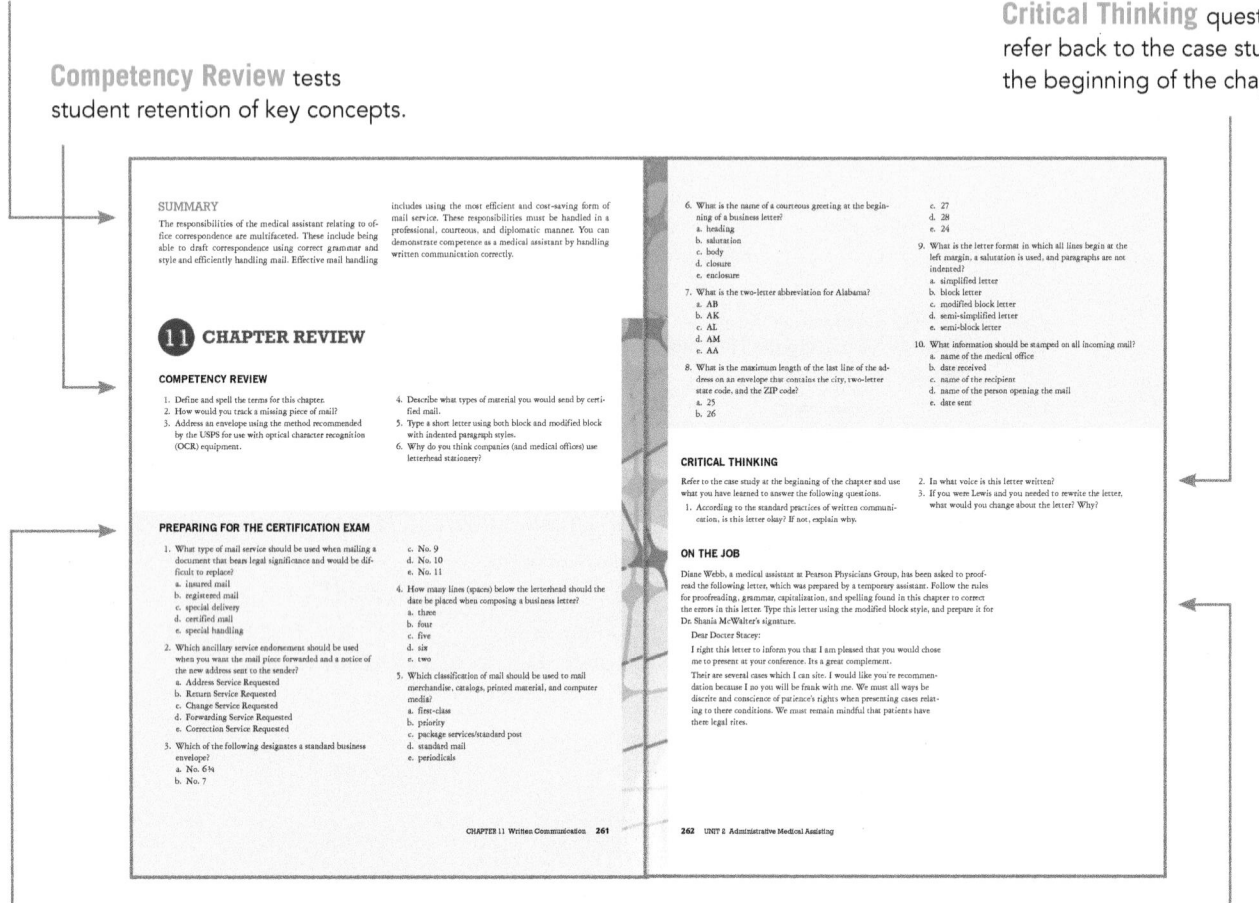

SUMMARY

The responsibilities of the medical assistant relating to office correspondence are multifaceted. These include being able to draft correspondence using correct grammar and style and efficiently handling mail. Effective mail handling includes using the most efficient and cost-saving form of mail service. These responsibilities must be handled in a professional, courteous, and diplomatic manner. You can demonstrate competence as a medical assistant by handling written communication correctly.

11 CHAPTER REVIEW

COMPETENCY REVIEW

1. Define and spell the terms for this chapter.
2. How would you track a missing piece of mail?
3. Address an envelope using the method recommended by the USPS for use with optical character recognition (OCR) equipment.
4. Describe what types of material you would send by certified mail.
5. Type a short letter using both block and modified block with indented paragraph styles.
6. Why do you think companies (and medical offices) use letterhead stationery?

PREPARING FOR THE CERTIFICATION EXAM

1. What type of mail service should be used when mailing a document that bears legal significance and would be difficult to replace?
   a. insured mail
   b. registered mail
   c. special delivery
   d. certified mail
   e. special handling
2. Which ancillary service endorsement should be used when you want the mail piece forwarded and a notice of the new address sent to the sender?
   a. Address Service Requested
   b. Return Service Requested
   c. Change Service Requested
   d. Forwarding Service Requested
   e. Correction Service Requested
3. Which of the following designates a standard business envelope?
   a. No. 6¾
   b. No. 7
   c. No. 9
   d. No. 10
   e. No. 11
4. How many lines (spaces) below the letterhead should the date be placed when composing a business letter?
   a. three
   b. four
   c. five
   d. six
   e. two
5. Which classification of mail should be used to mail merchandise, catalogs, printed material, and computer media?
   a. first-class
   b. priority
   c. package services/standard post
   d. standard mail
   e. periodicals
6. What is the name of a courteous greeting at the beginning of a business letter?
   a. heading
   b. salutation
   c. body
   d. closure
   e. enclosure
7. What is the two-letter abbreviation for Alabama?
   a. AB
   b. AK
   c. AL
   d. AM
   e. AA
8. What is the maximum length of the last line of the address on an envelope that contains the city, two-letter state code, and the ZIP code?
   a. 25
   b. 26
   c. 27
   d. 28
   e. 24
9. What is the letter format in which all lines begin at the left margin, a salutation is used, and paragraphs are not indented?
   a. simplified letter
   b. block letter
   c. modified block letter
   d. semi-simplified letter
   e. semi-block letter
10. What information should be stamped on all incoming mail?
    a. name of the medical office
    b. date received
    c. name of the recipient
    d. name of the person opening the mail
    e. date sent

CRITICAL THINKING

Refer to the case study at the beginning of the chapter and use what you have learned to answer the following questions.

1. According to the standard practices of written communication, is this letter okay? If not, explain why.
2. In what voice is this letter written?
3. If you were Lewis and you needed to rewrite the letter, what would you change about the letter? Why?

ON THE JOB

Diane Webb, a medical assistant at Pearson Physicians Group, has been asked to proofread the following letter, which was prepared by a temporary assistant. Follow the rules for proofreading, grammar, capitalization, and spelling found in this chapter to correct the errors in this letter. Type this letter using the modified block style, and prepare it for Dr. Shania McWalter's signature.

Dear Docter Stacey:

I right this letter to inform you that I am pleased that you would chose me to present at your conference. Its a great complement.

Their are several cases which I can site. I would like you're recommendation because I no you will be frank with me. We must all ways be discrete and conscience of patience's rights when presenting cases relating to there conditions. We must remain mindful that patients have there legal rites.

Preparing for the Certification Exam is a self-assessment and practice tool to help students build exam confidence.

On the Job helps students increase retention and success by linking concepts to their job functions.

Internet Activity challenges students to complete activities by using the World Wide Web.

INTERNET ACTIVITY

Access the Internet, and locate information on how to write professional medical letters. Research other information you may need, such as your extended ZIP code, an online dictionary, a medical dictionary, a thesaurus, and e-mail etiquette guidelines.

Reviewers

The invaluable editorial advice and direction provided by the following educators and health care professionals is deeply appreciated:

Cindy Abel, BS, CMA (AAMA), Pbt
Program Chair
Ivy Tech Community College
Lafayette, IN

Kendra Allen, LPN
Program Manager Healthcare Office
    Technologies
Ohio Institute of Health Careers
Columbus, OH

**Michaelann M. Allen, MA. Ed, CMA
    (AAMA)**
Medical Assisting Program Director
North Seattle Community College
Seattle, WA

Peter F. Andrus, MD
Instructor
Bryant and Stratton College
Albany, NY

**Yvonne Denise Arnold-Jenkins,
NRCMA**
Instructor
Remington College
Garland, TX

James Baird, MBA, CAHI
Medical Program Director
Computer Career Center
El Paso, TX

Jennifer Barr, MT, M.Ed., CMA (AAMA)
Chairperson, Medical Assisting
    Technology
Sinclair Community College
Dayton, OH

Sue Beaman, RN
Wayne Community College
Goldsboro, NC

Julie A. Benson, AAS, RMA, R.Phbt
Medical Assistant and Phlebotomy
    Program Chair
Oklahoma Health Academy
Tulsa, OK

Tricia Berry, MATL, OTR/L
Assistant Dean of Clinical Placement
Kaplan University
Ft. Lauderdale, FL

Suzanne Bitters, RMA-NCPT/NCICS
Program Manager
Harris School of Business
Wilmington, DE

Emily Brooks, NCMA
Medical Manager
Dorsey Schools
Saginaw, MI

**Lou Brown, MT (ASCP), CMA
    (AAMA)**
Medical Assisting Program Director
Wayne Community College
Goldsboro, NC

Minda Brown, RMA
Pima Medical Institute
Colorado Springs, CO

Beth A. Buchholz, CMA (AAMA), BS
Medical Assistant Program Director
Wichita Area Technical College
Wichita, KS

**Caren Burford-Henry, NRCMA,
    CMBS, CCA**
Medical Insurance and Coding Program
Chair
Remington College
Garland, TX

**Cara Carreon, BS, RRT, CMA (AAMA),
    CPC**
Faculty
Ivy Tech Community College
Lafayette, IN

Denise Carsillo, MS, BS, RMA
Associate Dean
Lincoln College of Technology
West Palm Beach, FL

**Ursula Cole, Med, CMA (AAMA),
    RMA, RPbt**
Instructor
Platt College
Oklahoma City, OK

Lisa Cook, CMA (AAMA)
Medical Assisting Education Program
    Chair
Bryman College
Port Orchard, WA

Janie Corbitt, RN, BSL
Central Georgia Technical College
Milledgeville, GA

**Bernadette Cox, AAS, RMA, AHI, BLS
    Instructor**
Administrative and Clinical Instructor
Ross Medical Education Center
Flint, MI

Bonnie J. Crist, BS, AAS, CMA (AAMA)
Medical Program Chair and Coordinator
Harrison College
Indianapolis, IN

Rosana Darang, MD
Department Chair, Health Studies
Bay State College
Boston, MA

**Susan DeGirolamo, AAH, RMA,
    NCPT, NCICS, NCMHT**
Instructor
Pennsylvania Institute of Technology
Media, PA

Anita Denson, CMA (AAMA)
Director of Health Care Education
National College of Business &
    Technology
Danville, KY

Hany Eissa, MD
Medical Assisting Program Director
South University
Savannah, GA

Dawn Eitel, BAS, CMA (AAMA)
Instructor
Kirkwood Community College
Cedar Rapids, IA

George Fakhoury, MD, DORCP, CMA
  (AAMA)
Academic Program Manager Healthcare
Heald College's Central Administrative
  Office
San Francisco, CA

Cassandra R. Farris, BS, RMA
Former Director of Medical Programs
Vatterott College
Joplin, MO

Suzanne Feathers, CMA (AAMA), EMT
Medical Program Coordinator
YTI Career Institute
Altoona, PA

Pamela Fleming, RN, CMA (AAMA),
  MPA
Professor
Quinsigamond Community College
Worcester, MA

Cheryl Garman, RN
Assistant Academic Dean
Berks Technical Institute
Wyomissing, PA

Beverley Giteles, CPC, CMM
Instructor
Gibbs College
Livingston, NJ

Lisa Graese, CMT, CIW Associate
Instructor
Spokane Community College
Spokane, WA

Wendy Hall-Campbell, ADN
Medical Assisting Program Director
Concorde Career Institute
Portland, OR

Carrie Hammond, CMA (AAMA)
Medical Assisting Program Director
Utah Career College
West Jordan, UT

Jessica Hart, CMA (AAMA)
Director of Healthcare Education
National College
Lexington, KY

Marsha Perkins Hemby, RN, CMA
  (AAMA)
Medical Assisting Department Chair
Pitt Community College
Greenville, NC

Elizabeth Henisse, BAS, MA
Allied Health Program Director
Florida Metropolitan University
Orlando, FL

Kimberly Hockaday, NCMA, NCET,
  NCICS
Instructor
Carrington College
Reno, NV

Jessica Holtsberry
HIT Program Instructor
Ohio Institute of Health Careers
Columbus, OH

Marsha M. Holtsberry, CMA (AAMA)
HOT Program Director
Ohio Institute of Health Careers
Columbus, OH

Susan Horn, AAS, CMA (AAMA)
Medical Program Coordinator
Harrison College
Lafayette, IN

Dolly Horton, CMA, BS, M.Ed., Ed.D.
Instructor
Asheville Buncombe Technical
  Community College
Asheville, NC

Demetria Jackson
Former Program Director
Virginia College
Birmingham, AL

Deborah E. Jacobs, RN, ENA, PCT
Medical Instructor
Dorsey Schools
Pontiac, MI

Shirley Jelmo, CMA (AAMA)
Faculty Coordinator
Pima Medical Institute
Colorado Springs, CO

Linda L. Kennedy, MBA, CMA
  (AAMA)
Program Director Medical Assisting
Everest University
Largo, FL

Deborah Kenney, BS, NCMA, NCPT,
  NCBCS
Instructor
Harris School of Business
Trenton, NJ

Amy Knight, CMA (AAMA)
Allied Health Instructor
Remington College
Largo, FL

Holly A. Lincoln, BA
Academic Coordinator
St. Louis College of Health Careers
Fenton, MO

Marta Lopez, LM, CPM
Medical Assisting Program Coordinator
Miami Dade College
Miami, FL

Marie Lorincz, LPN, CCMA
Medical Assistant Clinical Instructor
Ross Medical Education Center
Madison Heights, MI

Paul Lucas, CMA (AAMA), CPbt, PN, AS
Program Director Medical Assisting
Brown Mackie College
Fort Wayne, IN

Tabitha Lyons, AS, NCMA
Corporate Medical Assistant Program
  Manager
High-Tech Institute
Phoenix, AZ

Alice Macomber, RN, RMA, RPT,
  BXP, AHI, CPI
Medical Assisting Program Coordinator
Keiser University
Port Saint Lucie, FL

Mary M. Marks, MSN, RN-BC, Pbt
  (ASCP)
Program Coordinator
Mitchell Community College
Mooresville, NC

Natalie McBride, CMA (AAMA)
Instructor
ICM School of Business & Medical Careers
  Pittsburgh, PA

DeLeesa G. Meashintubby, BS, CMA
  (AAMA), RMA
MOA/HRT Program Coordinator
Lane Community College
Eugene, OR

Tanya Mercer, BS, RN, RMA
Curriculum Specialist
KAPLAN Higher Education
Rowell, GA

Kelly Miller, MPH, CHES, CST, RMA
Allied Health Department Chair
Remington College
Nashville, TN

Lisa Nagle, BS.Ed., CMA (AAMA)
Medical Assisting Program Director
Augusta Technical College
Augusta, GA

Kay Nave, CMA (AAMA), MRT
Medical Assisting Program Director
Kaplan University
Hagerstown, MD

Michelle Newman, LPN
Instructor
Florida Career College
Riverview, FL

Lisa K. Nicewarner
Program Director Medical Office
    Administration
Vatterott College
O'Fallon, MO

Marion D. Odom, NCMA
Medical Assisting Department
Chairperson
Illinois School of Health Careers
Chicago, IL

Kathleen M. Olewinski, MS, RHIA,
    NHA, FACHE
Medical Assisting Program Director
Bryant and Stratton College
East Milwaukee, WI

Everlee O'Nan, RMA
Director of Health Care Education
National College
Florence, KY

Karen Patrick, NCMA, CPI
Director
CAPPS College
Dothan, AL

Diane Peavy, RN, ASN, AHI
Director of Educational Services
Capps College
Foley, AL

Sonya Phipps, BA, MBA
Instructor
Everest College
Fort Worth, TX

Ellen Pinkston, CMAA
Administrative Medical Assistant
    Instructor
Ross Medical Education Center
Madison Heights, MI

Christina Rauberts-Conklin, AA, RMA
Medical Department Chair
Everest University
Tampa, FL

Kelli Revard, CMA (AAMA)
Clinical Instructor
Ross Medical Education Center
Saginaw, MI

Deanna T. Rieke, BSRN, MSHA
Program Director
Montana State University—Billings
    College of Technology
Billings, MT

Christian G. Rivera, DC, MS
Adjunct Faculty
Daytona State College, School of
    Biological & Physical Sciences
Daytona Beach, FL
Adjunct Instructor (online)
Florida Technical College, Allied Health
    Programs
Deland, FL

Jim Rocco, MS, CAHI, RMA, COLT,
    RPT, CPI, CEI, CPCI, CPhT
PCT Program Chair
Illinois School of Health Careers
Chicago, IL

Susan Saullo, RN, MS, MT (ASCP)
Medical Assisting Program Coordinator
Webster College
Ocala, FL

Kristen Schoville, RN/BSN
Medical Assistant Instructor
Southwest Wisconsin Technical College
Fennimore, WI

Wandagayle Sciambi, LPN, CMA
    (AAMA)
National Director of Medical Programs
Educational Affiliates
Baltimore, MD

Lory Lee Serrato, CCS-P
Everest College
Springfield, MO

Janet Sesser, RMA, CMA (AAMA), BS
    Ed. Admin.
Corporate Director of Education
Chubb Institute
Phoenix, AZ

Gary Shandrew, MSIA
Campus Director
Certified Careers Institute
Clearfield, UT

Lana Sherwin, BS, RMA, AHI
Medical Program Manager
Dorsey Schools
Madison Heights, MI

Maria L. Simard, LVN
Director of Allied Health Programs
Kaplan College
San Diego, CA

Lynn Slack, BS, CMA (AAMA)
Medical Programs Director
Kaplan Career Institute
Pittsburgh, PA

Peggy Smith, MEd
Medical Assisting Program Director
Marion Technical College
Marion, OH

Richard Snyder
Director of Medical Assisting Program
Kaplan University
Hagerstown, MD

Sherry Stanfield, RN, BSN, MS
Assistant Program Director, Medical
    Assisting
Miller-Motte Technical College
North Charleston, SC

Lisa Stephens, CMA (AAMA), AAS
Medical Assisting Program Director
Kaplan College
Indianapolis, IN

Donna Lee Stevenson, LPN, BA
Allied Health Department Chair
Remington College
Largo, FL

Pollyanna Strunk, RN, BSN
Lead Medical Instructor
Daymar College
Louisville, KY

Deborah Sulkowski, CMA (AAMA)
Medical Department Chair
Pittsburgh Technical Institute
Oakdale, PA

Pamela H. Swann, RN
Assistant Program Director, Medical
    Assisting Department
Virginia College
Pensacola, FL

Dr. Ruth Torres, MD, MA
Medical Instructor
Harrison College
Terre Haute, IN

Drew D. Totten, BA, NRCMA
Director of Education
Charter College
Canyon Country, CA

Wendi Walker, RN, MSN
Medical Assisting Lead Instructor
Draughons Junior College
Murfreesboro, TN

Angela Woodson, RMA
Medical Assistant Program Director
Virginia College
Montgomery, AL

Lisa Wright, MS, CMA (AAMA), MT
    (ASCP), SH
Medical Assisting Program Coordinator
Bristol Community College
Fall River, MA

Petra York, CMA (AAMA), AHI, CPT,
    CET, CphT, AAS, NRCMA
Program Director
Western Technical College
El Paso, TX

Carole A. Zeglin, MS, BS, RMA
Director of Medical Assisting Program
Westmoreland County Community College
Youngwood, PA

About the Authors

NINA BEAMAN, ED.D., MSN, CMA (AAMA), CNE (NLN), RN-BC (PMH), RNC-AWHC

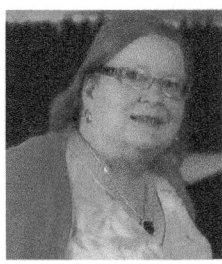

Nina Beaman earned a Doctorate of Education, a Master's Degree in Nursing, and a Master's Degree in Health Psychology in addition to an Associate Degree in Nursing, an Associate Degree in Business, a Bachelor's Degree with Honors, and the Diplôme d'Études Françaises from the University of Nice. She has been a Certified Medical Assistant (AAMA) since 1994 and participated actively on the local, state, and national levels of the American Association of Medical Assistants. She is also a triply certified Registered Nurse with certifications in Nursing Education, Psychiatric/Mental Health, and Ambulatory Women's Health. She completed her doctoral dissertation on "Using Disaster Simulation to Promote Volunteerism in Medical Assisting Students." Nina is Dean of Nursing at Aspen University, but also teaches health care courses for Independence University and Fortis College. She owns a consulting firm, Positive Transitions, through which she provides crisis intervention, education, curriculum development, continuing education review, and violence prevention training. A popular speaker and author, she writes at her farm in the Shenandoah Valley of Virginia. In her spare time, she works as a forensic nurse consultant and disaster expert.

KRISTIANA D. ROUTH, RMA (AMT)

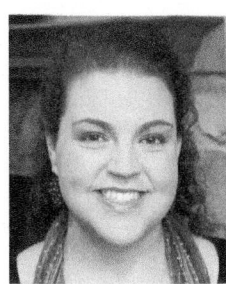

Kristiana D. Routh is a Registered Medical Assistant through American Medical Technologists. She has worked in the health care field for over 16 years and has a passion for watching the field of medical assisting grow and develop. Her experience in medical assisting education includes teaching, curriculum development, working closely with accrediting bodies, and writing multiple textbook and supplemental resources for both instructors and students. Kristiana also owns her own business, Allied Health Cousulting Services. Her business focuses on accreditation trends throughout health care, writing and developing educational content in the field of medical assisting, and project management services for physicians and health care facilities. Kristiana and her family live in Girard, Pennsylvania, near beautiful Lake Erie.

LORRAINE M. PAPAZIAN-BOYCE, MS, CPC

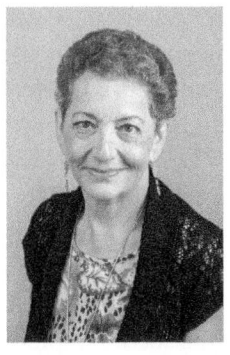

Lorraine Papazian-Boyce is an award-winning author and instructor. She holds a Master's Degree in Health Systems Management and the Certified Professional Coder (CPC) credential from AAPC. She authored *Pearson's Comprehensive Medical Coding: A Path to Success*, which received the Most Promising New Textbook Award—2016 from the Textbook and Academic Authors Association. She won the same award in 2014 for her text *ICD-10-CM/PCS Coding: A Map to Success*. She teaches health information management at the College for Health Care Professions. She was named Educator of the Year, Instruction—2011 by Career Education Corporation (CEC). Lorraine has over 30 years of experience in health care administration as a college instructor, office manager, owner of a medical billing and coding service, and management consultant to physicians, hospitals, and nursing homes. She has contributed to numerous textbooks and journals in the health professions and is a nationally known speaker. In her spare time, she enjoys boating, RVing, hiking, and working out.

RON MALY, MA, RMA (AMT), CPhT (PTCB)

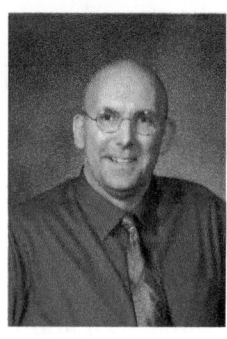

Ron Maly currently holds certifications as an RMA (AMT) and CPhT (PTCB). He obtained his Bachelor's of Science degree in Biology, Natural Science, and Pre-Med with a minor in Chemistry from Midland Lutheran College in Fremont, Nebraska, in 1989. In 1991, he received his Master's of Science degree (with thesis) in Biology from the University of Nebraska at Omaha. The abstract from his thesis has been nationally published. In 1992, Ron was employed with Harris Laboratories (currently Celerion) in Lincoln, NE, as a chemist and later as a validation scientist. In his seven years with Harris Laboratories, Ron had numerous scientific papers on LC/MS/MS pharmaceutical-based research presented at national conferences. In 1999, Ron began working as a medical assistant and histotechnologist for a Moh's micrographic surgeon in Omaha. During this time, he also began working part-time as a pharmacy technician. From 2005 to 2016, Ron held positions as a Pharmacy Technician Program Coordinator for Hamilton College/Kaplan University, Council Bluffs, IA; Medical Assisting Program Coordinator and Medical Billing and Coding Coordinator at the Omaha School of Massage and Healthcare of Herzing University, Omaha, NE; and Medical Assisting Program Coordinator and Interim Pharmacy Technician Program Coordinator for National American University, Bellevue, NE. Ron is currently employed with St. Elizabeth Hospital/CHI in Lincoln as a pharmacy technician.

JAIME NGUYEN, MD, MPH, MS

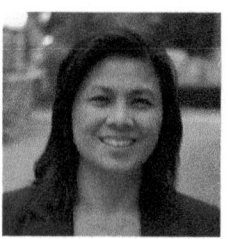

Jaime Nguyen has more than 20 years of experience in education management, health care research and analysis, compliance, and medicine. She has managed several allied health care programs, including medical assistant, pharmacy technician, and patient care technician. Before entering the education field, she was Medical Director and Chief Compliance Officer for a biopharmaceutical marketing and research company. Jaime was also a Public Health Analyst/Fellow in the Division of Medicine and Dentistry in the Department of Health and Human Services (HHS), where she conducted research and analysis on physician workforce issues. During this time, she also served on two federal advisory boards, Council on Graduate Medical Education (COGME) and the Advisory Committee on Training in Primary Care Medicine and Dentistry (ACTPCMD). Jaime has a medical degree, a Master of Public Health, and a Master of Science in Medicinal Chemistry. Her focus is on global health and medicine and public health, and she spent several years working in Israel, Ethiopia, and Indonesia on health care initiatives. Jaime worked in family medicine in Madison, Tennessee, and at the Allegheny County Health Department's STD Clinic in Pittsburgh, Pennsylvania. She is currently editing a textbook on health care administration.

UNIT 1 Introduction to Health Care

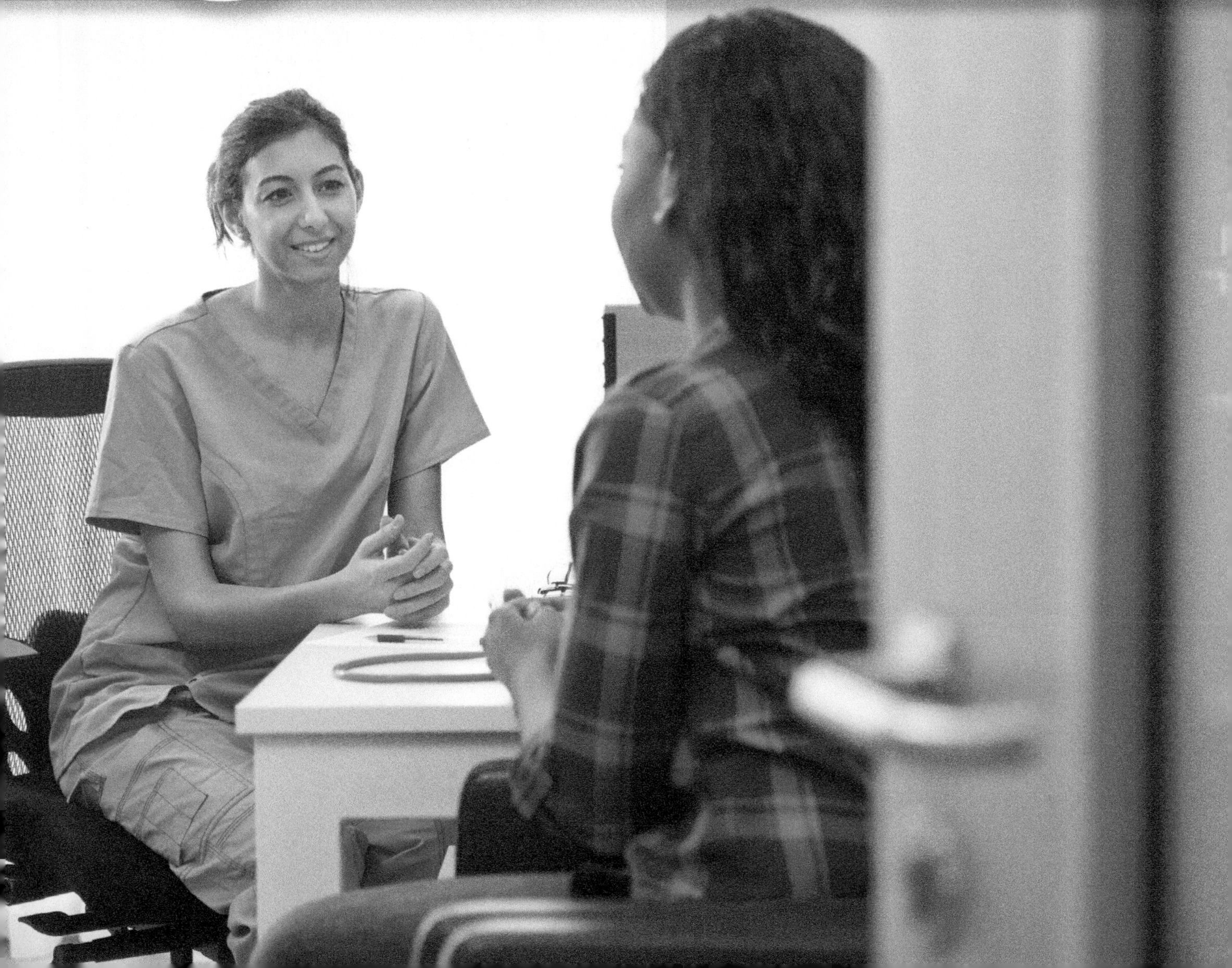

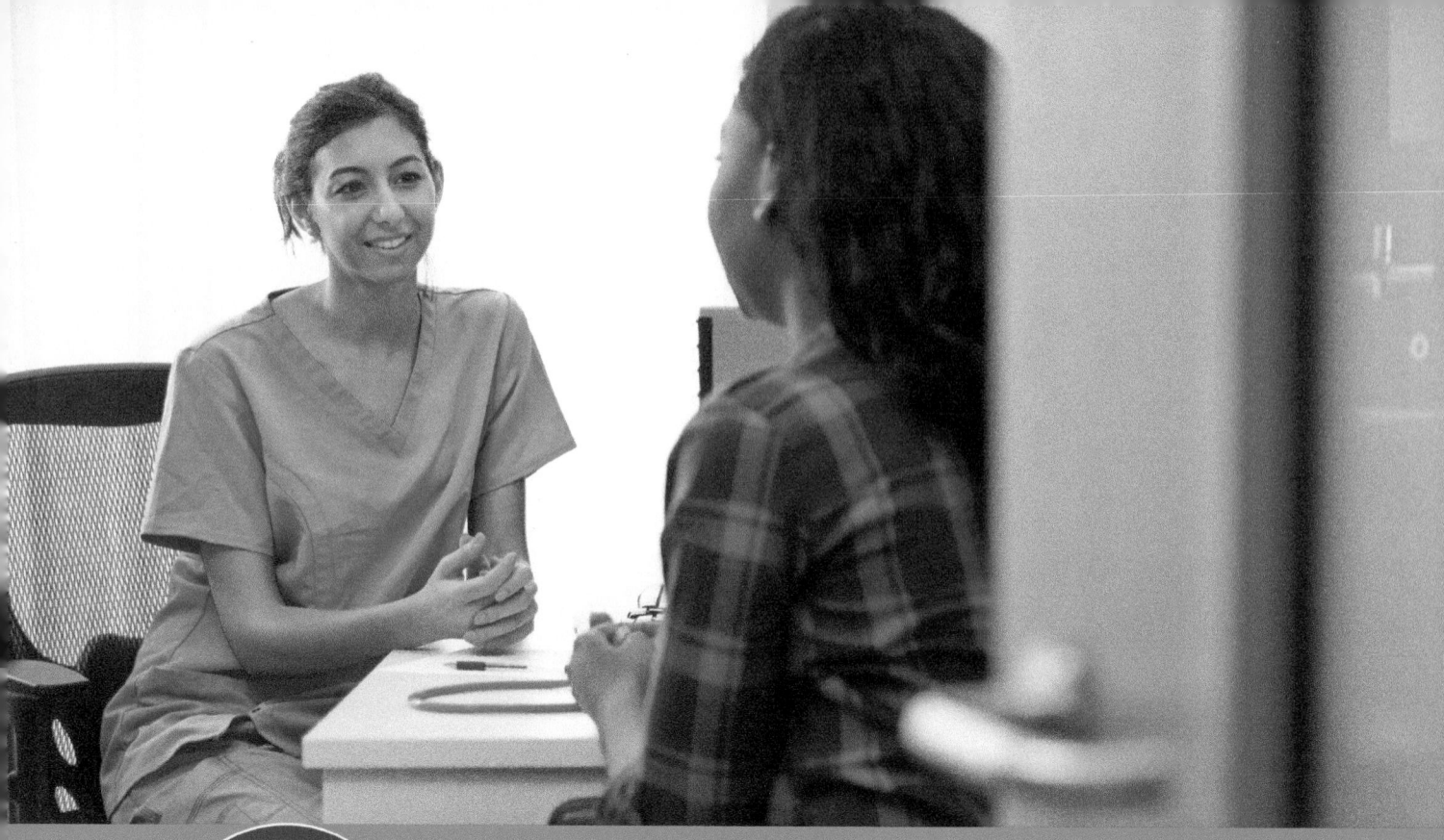

Medical Assisting: The Profession

Learning Objectives

After completing this chapter, you should be able to:

1.1 Define and spell the terms for this chapter.

1.2 Outline the history of the medical assisting profession.

1.3 Identify educational opportunities available for medical assisting students.

1.4 Explain the importance of accreditation for medical assisting programs.

1.5 List responsibilities that may be included in the medical assistant's scope of practice.

1.6 Identify health care professionals who are able to delegate duties to a medical assistant.

1.7 List professional qualities of a medical assistant.

1.8 Identify the benefits of obtaining a medical assisting credential.

1.9 List credentials available to medical assistants that are awarded by various national organizations.

1.10 Explain the current employment outlook for medical assistants.

1.11 Describe the role of a patient navigator.

Lucy Guttierez has been working a full-time job since graduating from high school three years ago. Lucy has always been interested in the health care field and wants to begin an education in a health care profession. After weeks of research, she has decided to enroll in a medical assistant program. Valley Heights Community College offers an associate degree for medical assisting, and Valley Heights Business School offers a nine-month certificate program. Lucy has not decided which program she will enroll in.

Terms to Learn

accreditation

Accrediting Bureau of Health Education Schools (ABHES)

American Association of Medical Assistants (AAMA)

American Medical Technologists (AMT)

certification

Certified Clinical Medical Assistant (CCMA)

Certified Medical Administrative Assistant (CMAA)

Certified Medical Assistant CMA (AAMA)

Commission on Accreditation of Allied Health Education Programs (CAAHEP)

continuing education unit (CEU)

delegate

externship

National Certified Medical Assistant (NCMA)

patient navigator

practicum

Registered Medical Assistant (RMA)

scope of practice

The rapidly changing health care environment requires health care providers to rely more heavily on assistive personnel. As a result, medical assistants (MAs) have become an important part of the health care team. No matter the setting, these multifunctional team members provide valuable services and support. Medical assistants are employed in a variety of settings from pediatric to chiropractic offices. No matter how varied the roles or duties of the medical assistant, the essential skills and personal qualities required of all good medical assistants are similar.

As a well-trained, multiskilled health care professional, the medical assistant fulfills many roles in the allied health field, where the everyday challenges are balanced by opportunities for advancement, personal growth, and satisfaction. Professional organizations that oversee or regulate the education, training, and certification of medical assistants are also discussed in this chapter, as well as current career opportunities and the future of the medical assisting field.

HISTORY OF MEDICAL ASSISTING

Historically, medical assistants were trained on the job by a physician. They became skilled through the day-to-day education and training provided in the medical office. Because of increasing responsibilities and liability issues, most physician offices and clinics today will employ only individuals who have received some type of formal training. Many physicians became familiar with the clinical skills of nurses while working closely with nurses in the hospital setting, so, as the need for formally trained staff arose, they chose to hire registered nurses to work in their offices. However, when a shortage of nursing personnel occurred, they had to look elsewhere for professionally trained office personnel who were specifically trained to perform both the administrative and the clinical responsibilities of a medical office (Figure 1-1). Physicians began to hire medical assistants.

The **American Association of Medical Assistants (AAMA)** was formed as a national professional organization in 1955 after previously being the Kansas Medical Assistant Society.

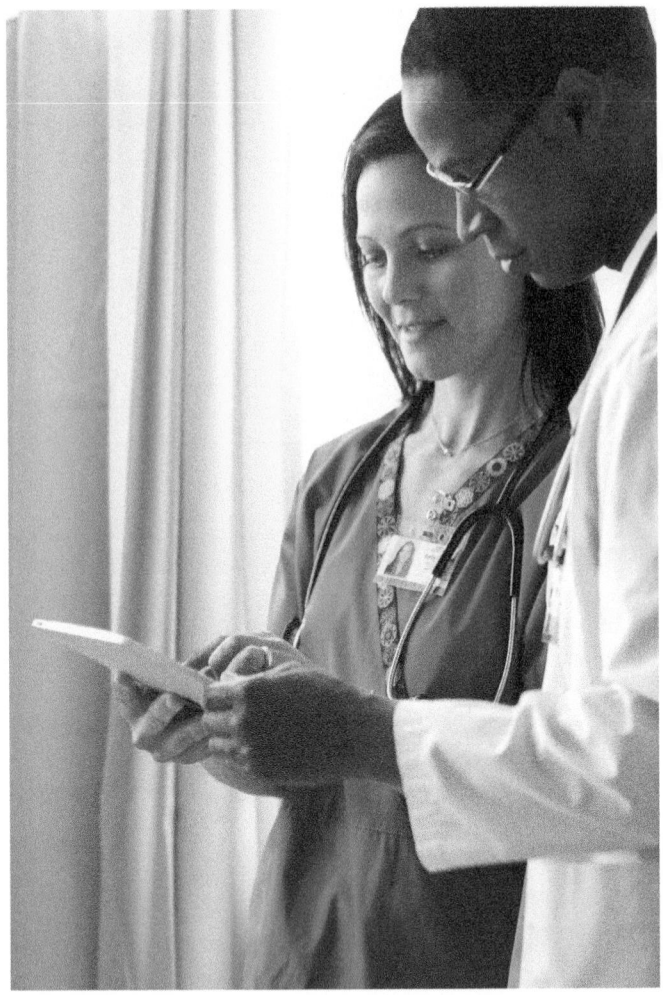

FIGURE 1-1 Medical assistants perform many functions in a physician's office or a clinic.

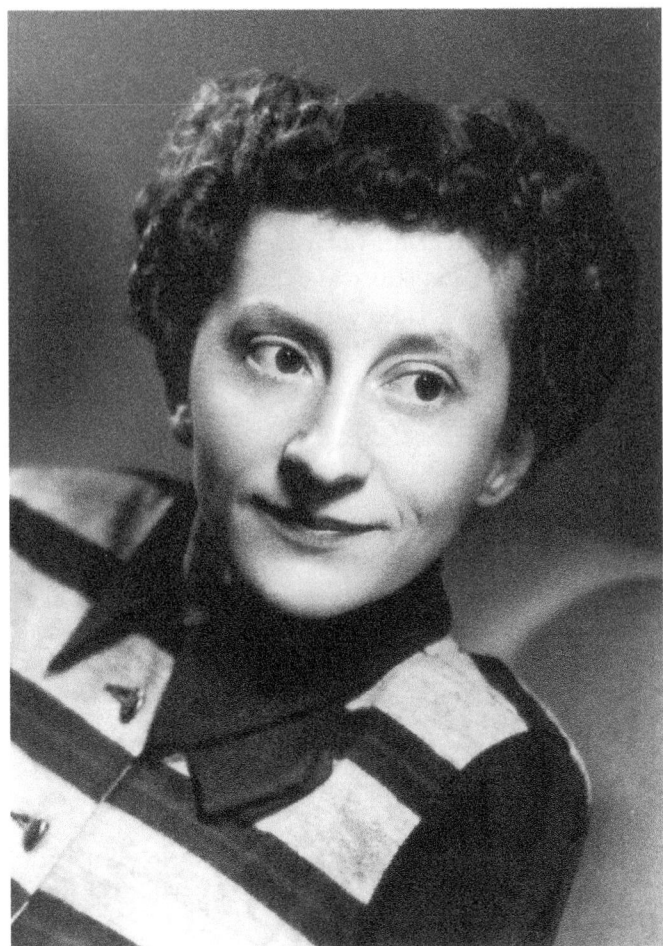

FIGURE 1-2 Maxine Williams was the first president of the AAMA.

In 1957, the first annual meeting of the AAMA was held, and Maxine Williams, who is considered the founder of the AAMA, was selected to serve as the first president (Figure 1-2). The AAMA was the first organization to place an emphasis on the educational objectives of medical assisting.

The Commission on Accreditation of Allied Health Educational Programs (CAAHEP) offers the following definition of the medical assisting profession:

> Medical assistants are multiskilled health professionals specifically educated to work in ambulatory settings performing administrative and clinical duties. The practice of medical assisting directly influences the public's health and well-being, and requires mastery of a complex body of knowledge and specialized skills requiring both formal education and practical experience that serve as standards for entry into the profession.
>
> *Source:* CAAHEP Standards and Guidelines for Medical Assistants, 2015.

EDUCATION AND TRAINING FOR THE MEDICAL ASSISTANT

Over the years, the education and training of medical assistants has undergone many changes. Today's medical assistants are well trained and respected practitioners in the allied health field. Students may obtain a certificate, diploma, or associate degree in the field of medical assisting.

- **Certificate programs**—The length of the course of study varies from one institution to the next. Some certificate programs are six weeks in length, whereas others may take up to a year to complete. These programs are typically offered in vocational schools or career colleges. Certificate programs often focus only on the development of either clinical skills or administrative skills. Students may choose the traditional classroom setting or may opt for distance learning (online). Most certificate programs require a hands-on externship to complete the program. Depending on the type of program offered, graduates of certificate programs may be eligible to sit for a national certification examination. Students who choose this training option may be supplementing prior training or may simply want an introductory career in the health care field.

- **Diploma programs**—These programs tend to be similar to certificate programs. Most diploma programs are six months to one year in length. Career and community colleges most often offer this course of study. Students selecting this option may be interested in a career as a medical assistant or may want to use this as a stepping stone to other health care careers.

- **Degree programs**—Degree programs vary widely in length. Courses of study can range from as little as eight months to approximately two years. Degree programs may be occupational or academic. Occupational programs focus more on coursework related to the actual occupation of medical assisting, whereas academic programs require more coursework in general education. A degree program is usually offered in a traditional classroom setting at a career or community college. Students complete clinical and administrative courses as well as courses in professional development and general education. Degree programs are preferred by those who want a career as a medical assistant and who have a desire to advance into supervisory or management positions.

Accreditation

Accreditation is the review an institution voluntarily undergoes to determine whether its school meets or exceeds standards set forth by an accrediting body. Accreditation ensures that a school meets established criteria. It is important to understand that schools and programs are accredited—people are not.

In addition to accreditation for the institution as a whole, a school may also seek accreditation for its medical assisting program. The learning outcomes for these programs are competency-based; that is, the desired outcomes are stated in terms of the ability to perform concrete tasks that may be required of a medical assistant rather than in terms of abstract knowledge. The U.S. Department of Education recognizes two agencies that may accredit programs in medical assisting:

- **Commission on Accreditation of Allied Health Education Programs (CAAHEP)**

- **Accrediting Bureau of Health Education Schools (ABHES)**

The CAAHEP Standards and Guidelines state that to provide for student attainment of "Entry-Level Competencies for the Medical Assistant," the curriculum "must

Professionalism

Lifelong learning is an important responsibility for all professionals. After completion of a formal education program and successful completion of a national certification examination, the professional medical assistant will continue to search for opportunities to maintain his or her credential through continuing education. The health care industry is constantly changing, and it is imperative that professionals keep abreast of these changes by participating in continuing education activities.

include anatomy and physiology, medical terminology, medical law and ethics, psychology, communications (oral and written), medical assisting administrative procedures, and medical assisting clinical procedures." The curriculum for a medical assisting program is designed so that a student meets cognitive, psychomotor, and affective skills in the following content areas:

Anatomy and Physiology

Applied Mathematics

Infection Control

Nutrition

Concepts of Effective Communication

Administrative Functions

Basic Practice Finances

Third-Party Reimbursement

Procedural and Diagnostic Coding

Legal Implications

Ethical Considerations

Protective Practices

ABHES states the following in its discussion of medical assisting programmatic curriculum standards: "Competencies required for successful completion of the program are delineated, and the curriculum ensures achievement of these entry-level competencies through mastery of coursework and skill achievement. Focus is placed on credentialing requirements and opportunities to obtain employment and to increase employability." Content areas outlined by ABHES include:

General Orientation (to the profession of medical assisting)

Anatomy and Physiology

Medical Terminology

Medical Law and Ethics

Human Relations

Pharmacology

Administrative Procedures

Clinical Procedures

Medical Laboratory Procedures

Career Development

All of these content areas have identified specific sub-concepts and skills that must be mastered by the graduates of ABHES-accredited medical assisting programs. In January of 2017, ABHES included a sub-concept under the Human Relations content area that identifies the importance of the medical assistant being able to "Demonstrate an understanding of the core competencies for Interprofessional Collaborative Practice." The Interprofessional Education Collaborative published a report outlining these core competencies. It states, "This report is inspired by a vision of interprofessional collaborative practice as key to the safe, high quality, accessible, patient-centered care desired by all. Achieving that vision for the future requires the continuous development of interprofessional competencies by health profession students as part of the learning process, so that they enter the workforce ready to practice effective teamwork and team-based care." The four main content areas identified by the ICP are:

- Values/Ethics for Interprofessional Practice
- Roles/Responsibilities
- Interprofessional Communication
- Teams and Teamwork

Concepts and ideas related to these content areas are discussed in the later chapters of this textbook.

An **externship** or **practicum** experience is a required component of the medical assistant's education. During the extern course, the student is scheduled to work unpaid in a physician's office, clinic, or possibly a hospital setting under the direct supervision of a preceptor or supervisor. Most externship courses are 160 to 200 clock hours in length.

ROLE OF THE MEDICAL ASSISTANT

The medical assistant's main responsibility is to assist the physician or health care practitioner in providing patient care. Central to a medical assistant's responsibilities are sound clinical skills. He must be able to obtain vital signs, collect specimens, administer medications, and run basic laboratory tests. It is not unusual to find medical assistants who conduct cardiac stress tests and assist with minor office surgeries. Administrative duties may also be part of the job description. In small clinics or physicians' offices, the medical assistant may function as the receptionist or insurance clerk.

The field of medical assisting is open to both men and women in a variety of work settings, such as physicians' offices, ambulatory care (outpatient) clinics, government agencies, and free-standing facilities. Although traditionally medical assistants worked only in physicians' offices, increasingly they are being employed in urgent care facilities. These facilities are typically open beyond the traditional hours—at night and on weekends.

Responsibilities of the Medical Assistant

The list of responsibilities that medical assistants perform is extensive. For this reason, the education and training for this field is carefully designed and must involve both theory and hands-on experience. The actual duties of the medical assistant vary from office to office. A good medical assistant, who has received a well-rounded education, will be able to adjust to different work environments. However, never perform duties that are beyond your level of responsibility, education, and training.

Medical assistant responsibilities will also vary according to the size and type of setting and state laws that apply. Always familiarize yourself with federal and state regulations and guidelines governing the procedures that medical assistants are allowed to perform in whatever environment you work. Most state regulations refer to this as the medical assistant **scope of practice**. Procedure 1-1 outlines how to locate a medical assistant's scope of practice in your state. Generally, medical assistant duties are grouped into two categories—administrative and clinical—and include the following competencies:

Administrative Competencies: Business and Front Office

- Scheduling patients, including referrals to specialists
- Greeting and receiving patients
- Screening nonpatients and visitors
- Arranging for patient admissions to hospitals, patient tests, and procedures such as X-rays and laboratory tests
- Providing patient instruction regarding procedures and tests performed in the physician's office and hospitals
- Updating and filing patient medical records
- Coding diagnoses and procedures for insurance purposes
- Computer skills and use of new technologies (Figure 1-3)
- Handling financial arrangements with patients

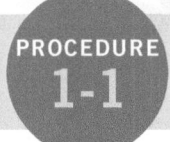

Locating a State's Scope of Practice for Medical Assisting

Objective ◆ *Locate the scope of practice for medical assisting in the state where you live.*

EQUIPMENT AND SUPPLIES
Pen and paper; highlighter; computer with Internet access and word processing software; printer

METHOD

1. Using the Internet, conduct a search to locate the legal scope of practice for medical assistants in the state where you live. For instance, you might type "Scope of practice for medical assisting in Ohio" in your preferred search engine.
2. Review the search results and select information to review from reputable websites and resources.
3. Once you have chosen a document that outlines the medical assistant's scope of practice in your state, print the document. If printing is not an option in your classroom, take detailed notes while reading the information on the computer.
4. Review the scope of practice for medical assistants in your state. Highlight any information that details exceptions to the medical assistant's scope of practice. For instance, does your state restrict medical assistants from performing phlebotomy, radiographic procedures, medication administration, etc.?
5. Either type or handwrite a summary paragraph that details your findings.
6. Review your paragraph, checking for spelling and grammatical errors. Make any corrections as necessary, and turn in your paragraph to your instructor for grading.

- Managing the telephone, reports, correspondence, and filing
- Handling mail, billing, insurance claims, credit, and collections
- Operating office equipment
- Preparing and maintaining employee records
- Handling petty cash
- Reconciling bank statements
- Maintaining records for license renewals, membership fees, and insurance premiums
- Assisting the physician with articles, lectures, and manuscripts
- Utilization review of necessary procedures and referrals
- Coordinating managed-care coverage for patients and physicians
- Ensuring compliance with the Health Insurance Portability and Accountability Act (HIPAA) guidelines (HIPAA will be discussed in the chapter on medical law and ethics.)

Clinical Competencies: Care and Treatment of Patients

- Assisting patients in preparation for physical examinations and procedures

- Obtaining a medical history
- Performing routine clinical and laboratory procedures under the supervision of a physician

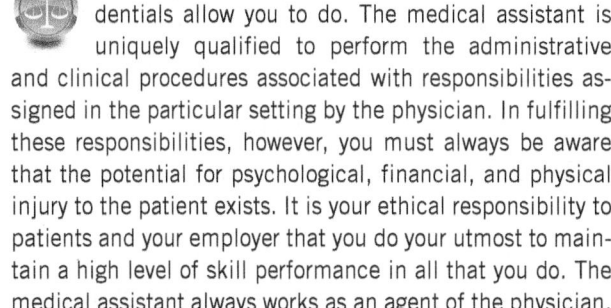

Professionalism The Law

It is important to fully understand what your credentials allow you to do. The medical assistant is uniquely qualified to perform the administrative and clinical procedures associated with responsibilities assigned in the particular setting by the physician. In fulfilling these responsibilities, however, you must always be aware that the potential for psychological, financial, and physical injury to the patient exists. It is your ethical responsibility to patients and your employer that you do your utmost to maintain a high level of skill performance in all that you do. The medical assistant always works as an agent of the physician.

It is also important that you work only within the scope of practice for medical assisting. It is a crime to perform procedures that only nurses or physicians are licensed to do. Although most duties can be performed in all states, each state may have a different scope of practice for medical assisting. It is your responsibility to become familiar with the law or qualification in your state. Be sure to understand your role as a medical assistant, and do not deviate from it.

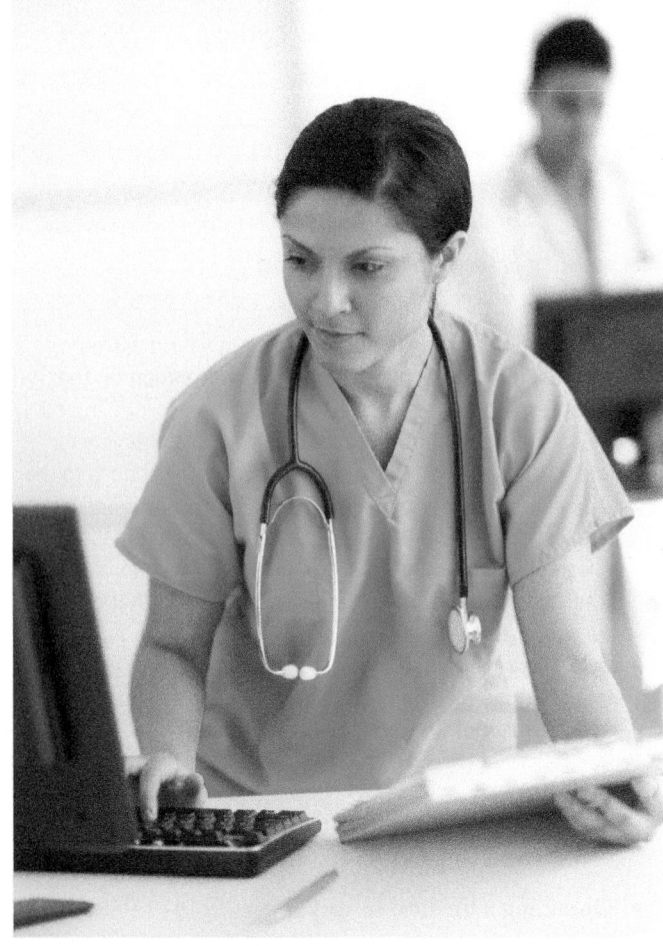

FIGURE 1-3 Good computer skills are required to be a successful member of the health care team.

- Collecting, preparing, and transporting laboratory specimens
- Performing venipuncture, where permitted
- Assisting the physician with procedures
- Instructing and educating patients on treatments and procedures (Figure 1-4)
- Cleaning and sterilizing equipment
- Obtaining patient's height, weight, and vital signs
- Preparing and maintaining examination and treatment rooms
- Inventory control—ordering and storing of supplies
- Disposing of hazardous waste and other materials
- Administering medications under the supervision and orders of the physician, where permitted
- Changing bandages and dressings, as well as suture removal, where permitted
- Handling drug refills as directed by the physician
- Performing electrocardiograms (ECGs)

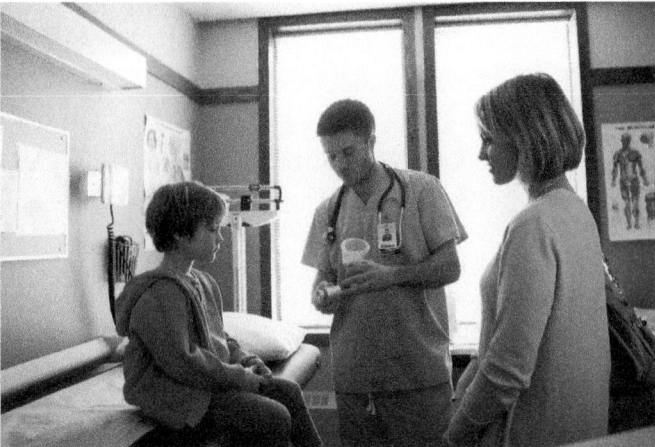

FIGURE 1-4 Proper patient instruction regarding new medications or treatments is part of the medical assistant's duties.

- Complying with Occupational Safety and Health Administration (OSHA) guidelines and employee instruction
- Performing skills relevant to a particular practice (for example, audiometry, spirometry, and Holter monitor)
- Disposing of contaminated supplies
- Sterilizing medical instruments
- Preparing patients for X-rays

Medical assistants who work in specialty offices, such as pediatric or ophthalmic offices, will have additional duties for which they will be trained by appropriate personnel.

Delegation of Duties

Medical assistants are unlicensed personnel who often perform clinical skills and assist in the clinical setting alongside the physician. Because medical assistants are unlicensed, their physician-employer is responsible for the work they perform. They must display competence in a skill or duty before they are given the full responsibility of completing the task unsupervised. A physician is allowed to **delegate**

Professionalism Cultural Considerations

Medical assistants must consider their moral and ethical beliefs before accepting a job. These beliefs often are derived from religious views. Some offices may perform procedures or treatments that go against your views. It is always necessary to keep personal opinions and beliefs to yourself and not impose these beliefs on patients. Examples of possible conflicts may include an office that performs an abortion or an office that performs extensive research in genetic engineering.

duties to a medical assistant. Delegating duties refers to assigning work-related tasks for which the medical assistant is both responsible and competent to complete. A physician may never delegate duties that could be construed as a medical assistant practicing medicine.

Other licensed health care practitioners are also able to delegate duties to a medical assistant. These may include physician assistants, nurse practitioners, and even registered nurses. It is important to note that state laws vary regarding who can delegate duties to a medical assistant, and it is important that you know the laws for your state. These laws, often found within a state's medical practice act, may be amended and changed frequently. For instance, in July 2015, the Ohio State Senate passed a bill allowing those who hold a certificate to prescribe medicine, including physician assistants and nurse practitioners, the ability to delegate the administration of medication to unlicensed allied health personnel. This ruling essentially expanded the duties that can be delegated to medical assistants in the area of medication administration.

Keeping abreast of laws and changes that affect the scope of practice for medical assisting is a vital component of being a responsible member of a health care team.

PROFESSIONAL QUALITIES OF A GOOD MEDICAL ASSISTANT

A medical assistant must have general knowledge of the medical field and understand medical terminology. It is essential that the medical assistant accurately and appropriately perform assigned administrative and clinical skills.

One of the most important qualities that a medical assistant must have is a genuine desire to help others and care about them. The nature of the patient and health care worker relationship demands that medical assistants be able to communicate effectively and get along with others.

Qualities or characteristics required of a professional medical assistant include integrity, empathy, discretion, the ability to safeguard the patient's right to confidentiality, thoroughness, punctuality, congeniality, proactivity, and competence.

- **Integrity**—Integrity includes the qualities of honesty and truthfulness. Someone with integrity is dependable, dedicated to high standards, and adheres to a code of values.

- **Empathy**—The ability to work with the sick and the infirm depends on the ability and willingness to show compassion, understanding, and sympathy. A medical assistant with empathy has the ability to be sensitive to or understand the feelings of another individual. An empathic person is able to stand in the shoes of another and identify with what that person is experiencing. For example, when a medical assistant has some insight or understanding of the pain or distress a patient is feeling, she acts in a kind and caring way that expresses sensitivity to the patient's feelings.

- **Discretion**—Discretion is the ability to make sound judgments. A medical assistant who uses discretion is able to make decisions responsibly. Someone who uses discretion is tactful in communicating with others. It is important to be able to be fair and to be familiar with policies and regulations so they can be properly applied. Discretion is important when interacting with patients and coworkers.

- **Confidentiality**—The ability to maintain privacy and safeguard patient confidences—particularly information in the medical record regarding family history, past or current diseases or illnesses, test results, and medications—is vital to the patient and health care professional relationship. No information about the patient is to be disclosed without the written permission of the patient. This is a legal and ethical issue with penalties for violating patient confidentiality. Without this trust, there can be no relationship. As the person with most frequent access to patient records and verbal confidences, the medical assistant has a serious professional responsibility to safeguard the patient's right to confidentiality (Figure 1-5).

- **Thoroughness**—The role of the medical assistant is varied and often requires multitasking. Even with so many responsibilities to attend to, attention to detail is critical to the performance of assigned tasks in the medical facility. Medical assistants should show pride in their work by thoroughly completing every task the physician orders. If a medical assistant is not thorough, errors can jeopardize patient health.

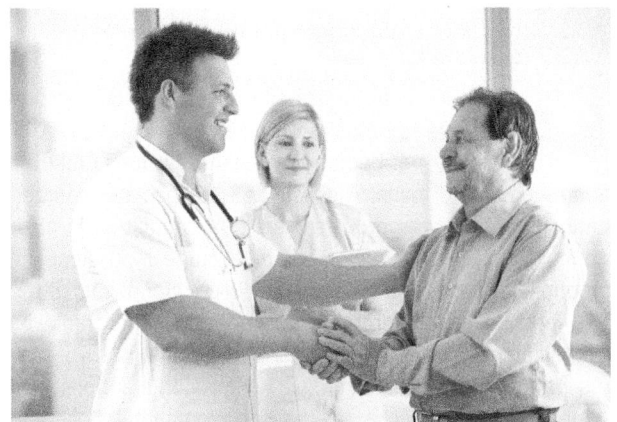

FIGURE 1-5 Medical assistants are often involved in confidential conversations between the physician and the patient.

- **Punctuality**—If a medical assistant is frequently absent, the office not only loses a valuable asset, but also the physician must pay extra for temporary help. Employee absenteeism also places an extra burden of work on other team members. The same burden occurs when a person is frequently late for a shift. It is a workplace expectation that medical assistants arrive at the office early and stay until the last patient leaves.

- **Congeniality**—A good medical assistant must get along with a diverse group of people. The ability to get along with all patients is an asset for the medical assistant. Sometimes patients may be hostile or aggressive, but a wise medical assistant will be friendly and helpful at all times to patients as well as to coworkers.

- **Proactivity**—The medical assistant must anticipate the needs of the physician and patients. Supplies should be laid out before procedures, medical records made readily available, and the physician should be briefed before the patient is even seen. Proactivity is sometimes called being a "self-starter," which means seeing what needs to be done and doing it without having to be asked.

- **Competence**—As the practice of medical assisting changes, it is important for medical assistants to keep their skills and knowledge current. Continuing education should be an expectation of the lifelong learner.

In many cases, the medical assistant is the first person a patient has interaction with in a health care facility. Patients may develop a perception of the physician and the practice, good or bad, based on how the medical assistant has interacted with them. It is important to present a confident, professional image that helps put the patient at ease. A calm, pleasant speaking voice conveys a professional attitude.

Professionalism | The Life Span

 Some medical clinics and physicians' offices provide care to patients within a specific age range or stage of life. Pediatric offices treat young children, adolescents, and teens. A physician who specializes in gerontology or geriatrics provides care to a population of older adults. Each age group is unique in its stage of physical and emotional development; therefore, each group has different needs and considerations. It is not realistic to think you would communicate with a 5-year-old patient and a 45-year-old patient in the same manner. In your interactions with patients, you must consider their developmental stage and provide age-appropriate care and instruction.

Remember that eating, drinking, or chewing gum while on the job are not appropriate in areas open to the public. Along with a basic understanding of human behavior and good communication skills—written, spoken, and nonverbal—the medical assistant must be able to handle tasks requiring basic mathematics, grammar, and spelling skills.

Medical assistants should provide the same quality of care that they would like to receive for themselves or their family members. The medical assistant must have the ability to see beyond the gruff or complaining manner of the patient who is not feeling well and project a professional, pleasant, and caring attitude.

PROFESSIONAL CERTIFYING ORGANIZATIONS

Several professional organizations certify and represent medical assistants. Obtaining a certification and aligning with a professional organization is an unparalleled level of professionalism. These organizations provide medical assistants with a network of career professionals who promote their profession and serve as a source of ongoing education. **Certification** is the process by which a recognized credentialing agency or professional organization determines that an individual has met the required education or experience criteria.

Obtaining professional credentials also has a great impact on employability. Although in the past holding credentials was simply an added benefit for a medical assistant in the field, today more and more employers are requiring credentials as a condition for employment. In fact, in October 2015, the Centers for Medicare and Medicaid Services (CMS) issued a final ruling mandating that only credentialed medical assistants are able to enter orders for a physician in a computerized order entry system. This ruling is a component of the U.S. government's Electronic Health Records Incentive Program, part of the Health Information Technology for Economic and Clinical Health Act (HITECH) that provides financial incentives to encourage the use of electronic health records (EHR). Because of this ruling, the need for credentialed medical assistants is expected to soar.

American Association of Medical Assistants

The AAMA is a national certifying agency with headquarters in Chicago, Illinois. The AAMA offers the **Certified Medical Assistant CMA (AAMA)** credential.

The AAMA certification examination is offered to graduates of programs accredited by the CAAHEP or by the ABHES. Those who meet this eligibility requirement must complete an application process and then successfully

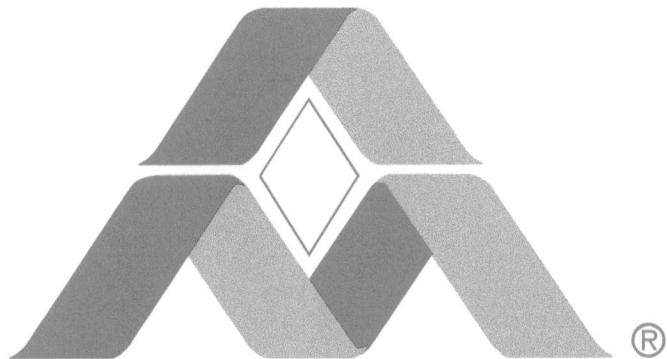

FIGURE 1-6 The American Association of Medical Assisting offers the CMA (AAMA) credential.

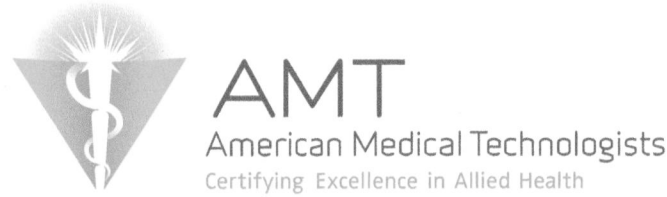

FIGURE 1-7 The AMT provides certification exams for a number of allied health professions.

complete the certification examination. Upon successful completion of the certification examination, candidates receive a CMA (AAMA) certificate, which confirms them as certified medical assistants.

To maintain certification, a CMA (AAMA) must show evidence of 60 recertification points, which are similar to continuing education units. **Continuing education units (CEUs)** represent measured increments of training and education that are obtained in order to keep abreast of current trends in health care and promote professional development. Of these 60 points, at least 30 must be AAMA-approved continuing education units. The remaining 30 CEUs may be obtained by sources other than the AAMA. If you have not completed the 60 hours of continuing education within five years, you must retake and pass the CMA (AAMA) exam to maintain your certification (Figure 1-6).

The AAMA sponsors continuing education workshops; seminars; online activities; and county, state, and national conferences for medical assistants to earn CEUs and maintain current knowledge in the field. Those medical assistants who are not eligible to sit for the CMA (AAMA) credential through the AAMA may still choose to become an associate member of the organization.

American Medical Technologists

American Medical Technologists (AMT), with national offices located in Rosemont (Chicago), Illinois, is a certifying agency for medical assistants, phlebotomists, medical technologists, medical administrative specialists, and dental assistants (Figure 1-7). AMT requires continuing education in order to maintain certification for all the disciplines. CEUs can be obtained through attending state and national conferences, completing online activities, and furthering education in the medical field.

The **Registered Medical Assistant RMA (AMT)** credential is awarded to candidates who pass the AMT certification examination. The RMA certification examination is developed around the following parameters (see also Table 1-1):

I. General Medical Assisting Knowledge
  a. Anatomy and Physiology
  b. Medical Terminology
  c. Medical Law
  d. Medical Ethics
  e. Human Rights
  f. Patient Education

II. Administrative Medical Assisting
  a. Insurance
  b. Financial Bookkeeping
  c. Medical Secretarial—Receptionist

III. Clinical Medical Assisting
  a. Asepsis
  b. Sterilization
  c. Instruments
  d. Vital Signs
  e. Physical Examinations
  f. Clinical Pharmacology
  g. Minor Surgery
  h. Therapeutic Modalities
  i. Laboratory Procedures
  j. Electrocardiography
  k. First Aid

Qualified applicants can take computerized examinations at Pearson VUE centers throughout the United States.

National Center for Competency Testing

The **National Certified Medical Assistant (NCMA)** credential is issued by the National Center for Competency Testing (NCCT) (Figure 1-8). There are three ways to meet eligibility requirements to sit for the NCMA examination. In addition to having a high school diploma or equivalent, a candidate is required to meet one of the following requirements:

- Current student of a medical assisting program of a NCCT-authorized school

- Graduate (within the last five years) of a medical assisting program of a NCCT-authorized school

Qualifications

To qualify for RMA certification:

1. Applicant shall be of good moral character.
2. Applicant shall meet one of the following requirements:
   A. Applicant shall be a recent graduate of, or scheduled to graduate from:
      1. A medical assistant program that holds programmatic accreditation by (or is in a postsecondary school or college that holds institutional accreditation by) the Accrediting Bureau of Health Education Schools (ABHES) or the Commission on Accreditation of Allied Health Education Programs (CAAHEP).
      2. A medical assistant program in a postsecondary school or college that has institutional accreditation by a Regional Accrediting Commission or by a national accrediting organization approved by the U.S. Department of Education, for which the program includes a minimum of 720 clock-hours (or equivalent) of training in medical assisting skills (including a clinical externship).
      3. A formal medical services training program of the United States Armed Forces.

      *If you graduated within the last three years, proof of work experience is not required. If you graduated over three years ago, you will be required to show proof of current work experience.
   B. Applicant shall have been employed in the profession of medical assisting for a minimum of five years, no more than two years of which may have been as an instructor in the postsecondary medical assistant program (proof of current work experience and high school education or equivalent is needed). Employment dates must be within the last five years.
   C. The AMT Board of Directors has further determined that applicants who have passed a generalist medical assistant certification examination offered by another medical assisting certification body (provided that exam has been approved for this purpose by the AMT Board of Directors) and who have been working in the medical assisting field for the past three out of five years and who have met all other AMT training and experience requirements may be considered for RMA certification without further examination.

If you have any questions, visit the AMT website at www.americanmedtech.org.

Source: Adapted from American Medical Technologists, Rosemont, IL.

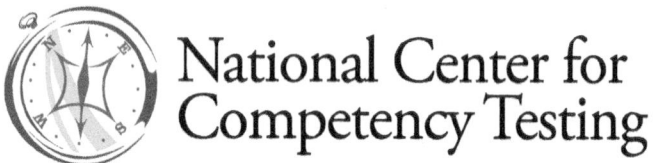

FIGURE 1-8 The National Center for Competency Testing offers the National Certified Medical Assistant credential (NCMA).

- Two years of full-time work as a medical assistant within the last five years (work must be able to be verified)
- Completion of U.S. military service training as a medical assistant (or equivalent) within the last five years

In order to maintain certification, individuals must obtain 14 hours of continuing education and pay a recertification fee each year.

Other credentials offered by the NCCT include Medical Office Assistant (NCMOA), Insurance and Coding Specialists (NCICS), ECG Technicians (NCET), Phlebotomy Technicians (NCPT), Patient Care Technicians (NCPCT), Surgical Technologists (Certified TS-C NCCT), and Certified Postsecondary Instructors (CPI).

National Healthcareer Association

Since 1989, the National Healthcareer Association (NHA) (Figure 1-9) has been partnering with allied health education programs, organizations, and employers across the nation to award more than 500,000 allied health certifications. NHA offers eight nationally accredited exams, certification preparation, and study materials. NHA also offers industry-leading outcomes-based data analytics as well as ongoing professional development and continuing education for its certification holders.

NHA grants two medical assisting credentials, the **Certified Clinical Medical Assistant (CCMA)** and the **Certified Medical Administrative Assistant (CMAA)**. A CCMA will work in the clinical or back office areas of health care settings. A CMAA will work in the administrative or front

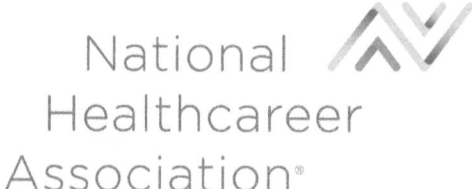

FIGURE 1-9 The NHA has been credentialing allied health professionals since 1989.

office areas of health care settings. To qualify for either of these credentials, the applicant must be over 18 years of age, have a high school diploma or GED equivalent, have completed a training program in the field of health care covered by the certification exam, or have at least one year of verifiable, full-time, supervised work experience in the field.

CAREER OPPORTUNITIES

According to the U.S. Department of Labor Statistics regarding medical assistants, "employment is expected to grow much faster than average, ranking medical assistants among the fastest growing occupations over the 2012–2022 decade. Job opportunities should be excellent, particularly for those with formal training or experience, and certification." In fact, the employment of medical assistants is projected by the U.S. Department of Labor to grow 29 percent in those 10 years. Technological advances in medicine and the growth in numbers of aging members of the U.S. population will necessitate more medical assistants. This boom in job growth is helped by the increasing number of medical settings where medical assistants work. Health care facilities will need support personnel, particularly medical assistants who can handle both administrative and clinical duties. Medical assistants work primarily in outpatient settings, a rapidly growing sector of the health care industry.

The anticipated need for more health professionals is based on the expected increase in the number of older adults who will require the care of a physician and the tremendous growth in the number of outpatient facilities. The wide range of health care settings presents many opportunities for the medical assistant who is trained in both clinical and administrative duties. Table 1-2 lists several inpatient and ambulatory care facilities or settings with descriptions of some possible job opportunities for medical assistants in each setting. Table 1-3 lists departments or specialties in which medical assistants may seek employment in either inpatient or ambulatory care settings. In some states and settings, additional education training and certification may be required for medical assistants to fulfill certain responsibilities. Although the general category "medical assistant" may be used in some career ads, some of the job title opportunities may include the following:

- Data processing clerk
- Billing or collections assistant
- Insurance claims processor
- Clinic aide
- Unit clerk
- Patient care technician
- Insurance claims coder
- Medical records clerk
- Clinical assistant
- Medical receptionist
- Multifunctional technician

TABLE 1-2 | Job Opportunities for Medical Assistants in Inpatient and Ambulatory Care Settings

Ambulatory Care Setting	Description of Job
Clinic	Use clinical and administrative skills to schedule and assist with patients who require special medical attention (e.g., eye clinic, orthopedic clinic, mental health clinic).
Urgent Care Facility	Care for patients who require immediate medical treatment.
Physician's Office	Use clinical and administrative skills in the private office setting for physicians of all specialties.
Rehabilitation Center	Provide care for patients recovering from illness or injury.
Patient-Centered Medical Home	An outpatient setting for comprehensive health care services that allows the patient to meet a variety of their health care needs in one convenient location.

TABLE 1-3 | Job Opportunities for Medical Assistants in Health Care Departments and Specialties

Department/Specialty	Description of Job
Admissions	Perform preadmission interviews, schedule laboratory testing, and document insurance coverage.
Billing and Insurance	Work with patients, third-party payers, and insurance companies to process insurance forms; claims forms; and DRG, ICD, CPT, and HCPC coding.
ECG/EKG Technician	Perform electrocardiogram studies on patients.
Medical Records	Perform administrative skills, and understand medical terminology and insurance coding; requires use of the computer.
Phlebotomy	Perform clinical skills to draw blood samples for testing.
Surgery	Perform clinical skills to sterilize surgical instruments and set up surgical trays; assist when needed.
Treatment/Procedure/ Emergency Department	Assist with minor surgeries and procedures performed in physicians' offices, hospitals, rehabilitation centers, and emergency departments.

With additional education and credentials, you may even respond to ads for the following:

- Medical laboratory assistant
- Electrocardiography (ECG) technician
- Phlebotomist
- Medical administrative specialist

Experienced medical assistants may find work as office managers, medical records managers, hospital unit secretaries, and instructors for medical assistant programs. With additional schooling, medical assistants can enter other health care occupations, such as nursing, occupational therapy, physical therapy, and medical and X-ray technologists.

The Patient Navigator

A medical assistant may work as a **patient navigator**. A patient navigator helps patients by facilitating their health care needs, encouraging adherence to care plans, and encouraging and coaching the patient regarding self-management skills. The navigator will be the primary source of communication between the patients and their providers, including primary care providers and specialists. All forms of diagnostic and laboratory testing may be scheduled by the navigator on behalf of the patient. The navigator will also work in conjunction with community organizations to help facilitate the use of community-based resources. The goal of patient navigation is to streamline the usage of health care services, improve communication, and ensure that the patients are well educated regarding their health care plans.

The ideal patient navigator will be a medical assistant who has both clinical and administrative experience, superb communication skills, and the ability to prioritize tasks and responsibilities.

SUMMARY

The field of medical assisting is rapidly growing in response to increasing health care needs of consumers. The profession of medical assistant offers many opportunities, roles, responsibilities, and settings for employment. Most medical assistants work in ambulatory settings such as physicians' offices, where they fulfill the administrative and clinical responsibilities associated with operating medical offices. The size and nature of the medical office practice will determine the number of medical assistants and tasks assigned.

Caring individuals, who are dedicated professionals with a commitment to maintain their skills through continuing education, make the best medical assistants. Qualities or characteristics regularly found in good medical assistants are integrity, discretion, empathy, the ability to safeguard the patient's right to confidentiality, thoroughness, punctuality, congeniality, proactivity, and competence.

It is most important to remember that the opportunities presented are many and the future of medical assisting looks promising. A career in medical assisting is emotionally and professionally challenging. Certification and membership with a professional organization are essential for professional development, and lifelong learning is expected in the medical assisting profession.

1 CHAPTER REVIEW

COMPETENCY REVIEW

1. Define and spell the terms for this chapter.
2. List several health care facilities or specialties to work at as a medical assistant.
3. Explain the difference between the administrative and clinical functions of medical assisting.
4. Name professional certifying organizations for the medical assistant profession.
5. Explain some professional qualities that are regularly found in good medical assistants.
6. What topics are often included in the curriculum for a medical assistant program?
7. List the job titles for which a medical assistant may qualify.
8. List the educational options available to an individual who is interested in medical assisting.

PREPARING FOR THE CERTIFICATION EXAM

1. What is the AAMA?
   a. American Medical Association
   b. American Allied Medical Association
   c. Alliance of the American Medical Association
   d. American Association of Medical Assistants
   e. American Association of Medical Assistance

2. What are two general categories that *best* describe the responsibilities of a medical assistant?
   a. phlebotomy and laboratory
   b. secretarial and direct patient care
   c. assisting the physician and paperwork
   d. clinical and secretarial
   e. administrative and clinical

3. Which organization awards the Registered Medical Assistant credential?
   a. AAMA
   b. NCCT
   c. AMT
   d. AMA
   e. DOE

4. Which administrative task would be outside the scope of practice for a medical assistant?
   a. coordinating managed care coverage
   b. handling petty cash
   c. assisting the physician with a journal article
   d. utilization review of necessary procedures
   e. signing prescriptions

5. Which of the following clinical tasks is outside the scope of practice for a medical assistant?
   a. vital signs
   b. suturing
   c. phlebotomy
   d. handling prescription refill requests
   e. patient education

6. Which of the following accurately describes the CMA (AAMA) minimum requirement for obtaining continuing education?
   a. 10 CEUs over two years
   b. 30 CEUs over five years
   c. 60 CEUs over five years
   d. 45 CEUs over five years
   e. 50 CEUs over five years

7. Which of the following statements is *true*?
   a. A medical assistant is equivalent to a nurse.
   b. A medical assistant must become licensed.
   c. A medical assistant is equivalent to a pharmacy technician.
   d. A medical assistant will never need to obtain continuing education units.
   e. A medical assistant might be qualified for a "medical records clerk" job advertisement.

8. Which of the the following statements is *true* regarding a medical assistant's scope of practice?
   a. The federal government issues a nationwide medical assisting scope of practice.
   b. The scope of practice for medical assisting varies by state.
   c. The scope of practice for a medical assistant is the same as that of a home health aide.
   d. Clinical skills are never included in a medical assistant's scope of practice.
   e. The scope of practice for a medical assistant is reviewed and amended every five years.

9. Characteristics of a professional medical assistant should include all the following *except*
   a. confidentiality.
   b. sympathy.
   c. thoroughness.
   d. integrity.
   e. discretion.
10. Which of the following statements is *true*?
   a. Medical assistants work only in physicians' offices.
   b. All medical assistant programs are diploma programs.
   c. With additional training, medical assistants may work as ECG technicians.
   d. Medical assistants can perform minor surgeries without physicians present.
   e. Medical assistants do not need good communication skills.

CRITICAL THINKING

Refer to the case study at the beginning of the chapter and use what you have learned to answer the following questions.

1. Lucy would like to have a career as a medical assistant, not simply a job. What decisions might Lucy make to support her goals?

2. Lucy is told that the medical assistant program at Valley Heights Community College is accredited by the ABHES. What does this mean for Lucy?

3. Rosa, Lucy's mother, has asked Lucy what type of jobs will be available to Lucy after she graduates from a medical assistant program. What might Lucy tell her mother?

ON THE JOB

Kayla Christianson, CMA, has been employed six years by the cardiology practice of three physicians. She is a graduate of a CAAHEP-accredited school. Furthermore, Kayla received extensive hands-on training performing ECGs while doing her required externship.

Kayla has completed an ECG ordered by Dr. Hsu for Mrs. Warner, a 76-year-old patient. Dr. Hsu, Kayla's boss, telephoned her explaining that he was behind schedule doing rounds at the hospital. He asked her to do him a favor and interpret Mrs. Warner's ECG, sign his name, and fax the report to Mrs. Warner's referring internist, who is expecting the results.

1. Given the scope of Kayla's education, training, and years of experience as a CMA, would this "favor" fall within the AAMA guidelines of her responsibilities?

2. Would any portion of Dr. Hsu's request fall within the guidelines? If so, which portion(s)? Is an exception to these guidelines ever allowed?

3. How should Kayla respond to Dr. Hsu?

INTERNET ACTIVITY

Conduct an Internet search for local medical assistant positions. How many positions require certification? What other job titles would a medical assistant be qualified to take?

Internet Resources

American Association of Medical Assistants
   www.aama-ntl.org

American Medical Technologists
   https://www.americanmedtech.org/

United States Department of Labor
   www.dol.gov

Commission on Accreditation of Allied Health Education Programs
   www.caahep.org

Accrediting Bureau of Health Education Schools
   www.abhes.org

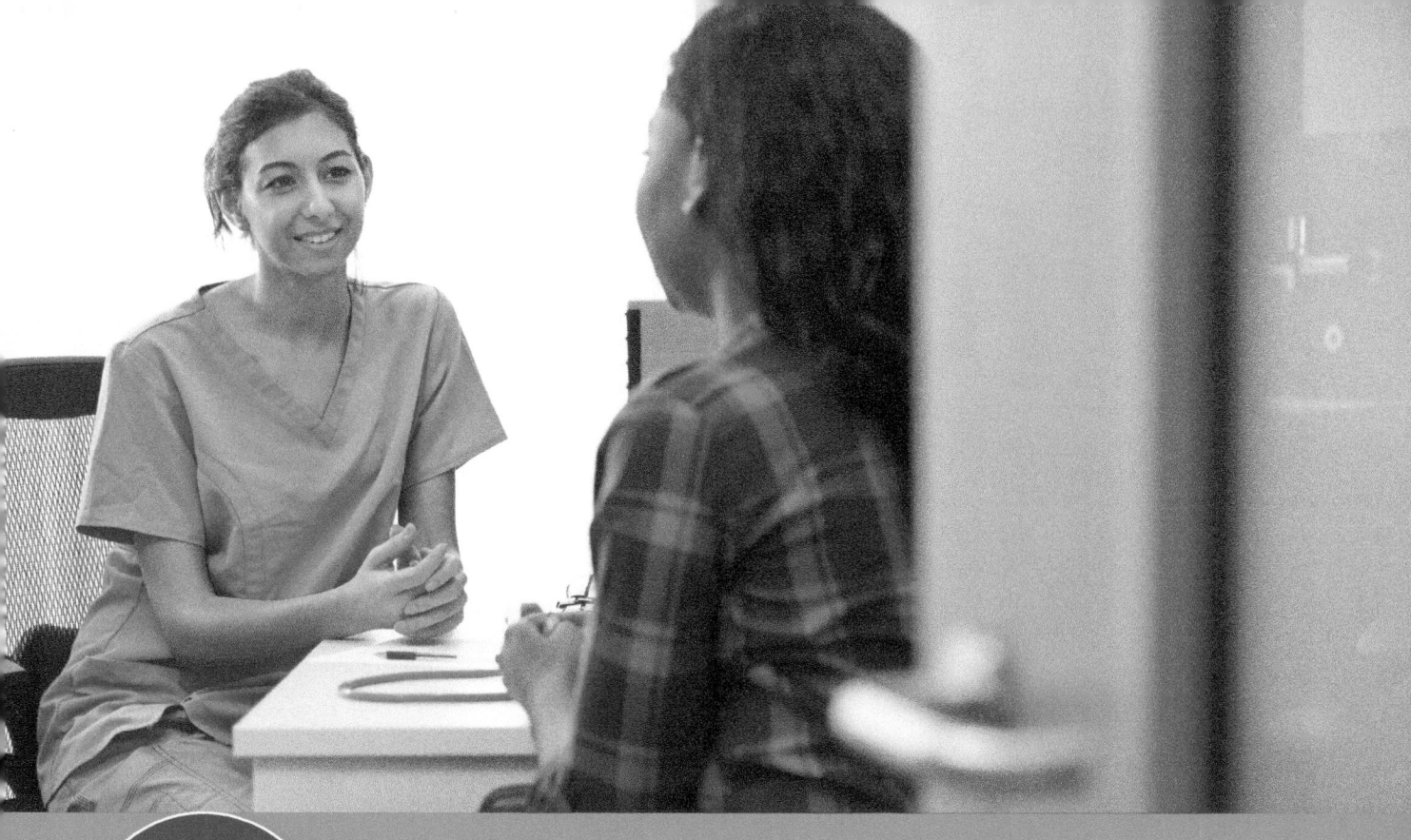

Medical Science: History and Practice

Learning Objectives

After completing this chapter, you should be able to:

2.1 Define and spell the terms for this chapter.

2.2 List contributions to medicine by ancient civilizations that are still used today.

2.3 Explain the impact Hippocrates had on health care and medicine.

2.4 Identify advances made in health care before the eighteenth century.

2.5 Outline the advances made in medicine between the eighteenth and twentieth centuries.

2.6 Identify the important roles women had in the history of medicine.

2.7 List recent advancements in modern medicine.

2.8 Explain what the title "doctor" means in various circumstances.

2.9 Identify how medical practice acts impact a physician's license.

2.10 Differentiate between the various types of medical practice settings.

2.11 Describe a variety of medical and surgical specialties.

2.12 Identify the roles of various types of health care facilities.

2.13 Compare the duties and licensure requirements of allied health providers.

2.14 Explain how the medical assistant will work alongside various types of allied health professionals.

Tania Washington has been the office manager for Pearson Physicians Group for the past eight years. The patient load has continued to increase, so Dr. Bahjat, one of the managing partners of the group, has asked Tania to help the practice locate an additional physician to add to the practice and assist with the patient load.

Terms to Learn

acquired immunodeficiency syndrome (AIDS)

anesthesia

anthrax

autopsy

bariatrics

cadavers

caduceus

certification

chemotherapy

endocrinology

hospice

human genome project

immune function

immunology

inpatient

licensure

medical privilege

microbes

morbidity

mortality

nutrition

oncology

osteopath

outpatient

pasteurization

patient-centered medical home (PCMH)

registration

stem cell

syphilis

The healing art of medicine was taught and practiced before written records were kept. This chapter describes the science and practice of medicine from the earliest evidence of healing, when disease was considered to be of supernatural origin, to the present—a time of astounding research, discovery, and healing. Contributions of many ancient peoples still influence medicine today. The discussion of present-day medical codes of ethics, rules pertaining to sanitization, personal hygiene, herbal cures, acupuncture, and other medical and surgical practices highlights the specific contributions of early medicine and those whose accomplishments catapulted the science of medicine into the amazing field that it is today.

This chapter provides a picture of today's medical practitioners—issues of licensure, including evaluations, credentials, reciprocity, renewals, suspensions, and doctors' titles. In addition, types of practices, medical and surgical specialties, and roles and educational requirements of a variety of health care team members are covered.

HISTORY OF MEDICINE

Drawings, bony remains, and archaic surgical tools are evidence of early human attempts to practice medicine.

Folk medicine, which incorporated plants, adopted a trial-and-error method to distinguish between those that were poisonous and those that had medicinal value. Early humans attributed supernatural origins to some ailments. In early medicine, some diseases were considered the work of a demon, an evil spirit, or an offended god who had placed some object, such as a worm, into the body of the patient. Treatment consisted of trying to remove the evil intruder.

The first doctors—considered "medicine men" and "medicine women"—were shamans, witch doctors, or sorcerers. In 3000 BC, Babylonian physicians practiced medicine using the written Code of Hammurabi, named for an early king of Babylon. This code had laws relating to the practice of medicine, which included severe penalties for errors. For example, according to the code, a doctor who killed a patient while opening an abscess would have his hands cut off.

Contributions of Ancient Civilizations

A study of medical practices in early Egypt offers greater insight into the basis of modern medicine. The Egyptians left behind lists of remedies, surgical treatments of wounds and injuries, and records for rules of sanitation. The Jewish religion and culture pioneered practices relating to personal

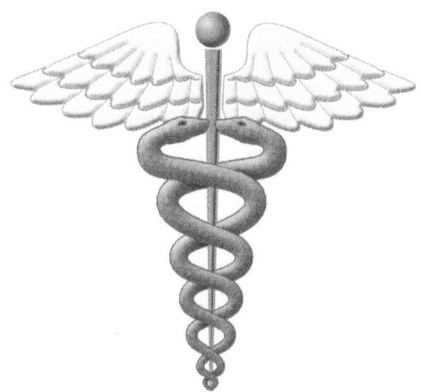

FIGURE 2-1 A caduceus, the emblem of the medical profession.

hygiene, the sanitary preparation of food, and other matters of public health.

Some records of early Greek practitioners illustrate the use of nonpoisonous snakes to treat the wounds of patients. The **caduceus**, which has become the recognized symbol for medicine, depicts a healing staff with two snakes coiled around it (Figure 2-1).

Herbal medical remedies originating in ancient India were recorded as early as 800 BC. The Chinese culture wrote about human blood pulses around 250 BC. Both early Japanese and Chinese cultures successfully practiced acupuncture.

Ancient Cures Are Today's Legacy

Early medicine, although often based on superstition, provided medicinal remedies that are still in use today. Opium, a product of the poppy plant, was known in ancient times to relieve severe pain. Today opium derivatives are used in the medication morphine. The following are other early remedies still used today:

- Nitroglycerin to treat heart patients
- Digitalis from the foxglove plant to regulate and strengthen the heartbeat
- Sulfur and cayenne pepper to stop bleeding
- Chamomile and licorice to aid digestion
- Cranberry to treat urinary tract infections

Early Medicine

Early medicine is considered to have begun in the fifth century BC with the Greek physician Hippocrates, who is credited with pioneering the scientific study of the causes of disease. (There is more about Hippocrates in the next section.)

Advances in all branches of learning came to a near halt during medieval times. This is why medieval times are often called "the dark ages." The period from the fifth to the sixteenth century was a time of little to no progress in medical practices. Poor personal hygiene, poor nutrition, and the lack of sanitation led to many epidemics. (An epidemic is a disease that infects a large part of a population in one region or location at the same time.)

Hippocrates: Father of Western Medicine

The first scientific system of medicine in the Western world originated in ancient Greece. It is usually associated with Hippocrates (460–377 BC), who is known as the Father of Western Medicine. Hippocrates took medicine from the realm of mysticism and philosophy and transformed it into an area of scientific discovery and practice. He stressed the body's healing nature, formed clinical descriptions of diseases, and discovered the ability to identify some diseases by listening to the chest. He practiced medicine at a time in history when little was known about anatomy and physiology. Nevertheless, his writings and descriptions of symptoms remain accurate today. A bust of Hippocrates appears in Figure 2-2.

The Hippocratic Oath (Box 2-1) is part of the writings of this ancient physician. The oath serves as a widely used

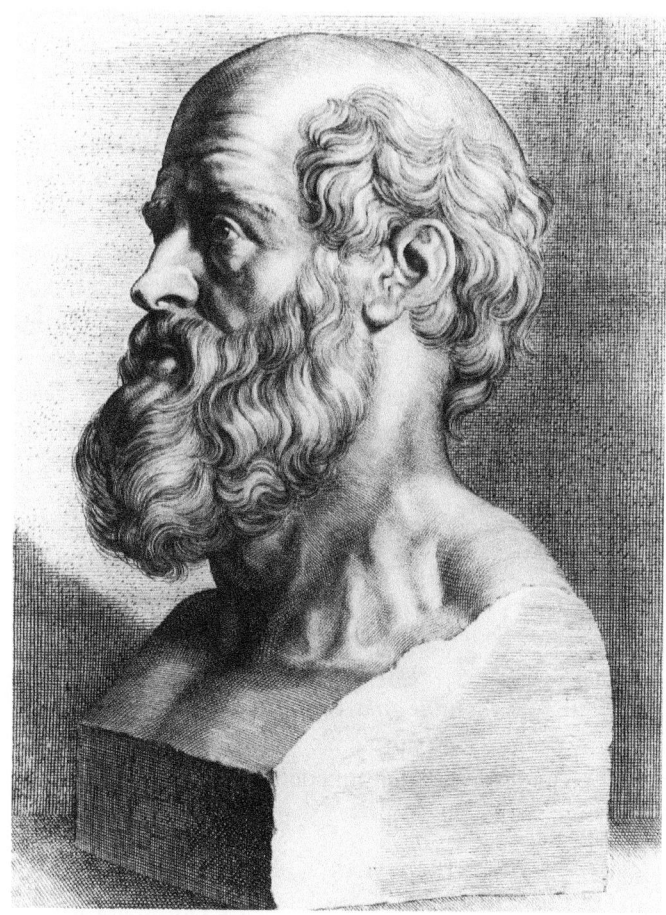

FIGURE 2-2 Hippocrates.

ethical guide for physicians who pledge to work for the good of the patient, to do the patient no harm, to prescribe no deadly drugs, to give no advice that could cause death, and to keep confidential medical information regarding the patient. The oath is still often cited as part of graduation ceremonies in medical schools.

Galen

Galen (130–201 AD), a Greek physician who practiced in Rome (Figure 2-3), initially followed the Hippocratic method. He stressed the value of anatomy and founded experimental physiology. He stated that arteries contained blood and not air as previously believed. Because the dissection of humans was illegal during Galen's time, he based his theories on the examination of pigs and apes. Although some of his work is inaccurate because of the lack of human **cadavers**, or dead bodies used to study human anatomy, he is still known as the Prince of Physicians.

William Harvey

In England during the seventeenth century, William Harvey (1578–1657) first theorized about the circulation of blood in the human body. He performed many experiments to test his theory of a single system of circulation. Before Harvey's theory, it was thought that the body had two circulation systems, one carrying purple blood and one carrying scarlet blood, to perform different functions.

Zacharias Janssen

Zacharias Janssen (1580–1638) was a Dutch eyeglass maker who invented the microscope by placing two lenses within a tube.

Anton van Leeuwenhoek

Anton van Leeuwenhoek (1632–1723) of Holland devoted his life to microscopic studies. He is known as the first person to observe and describe bacteria, which he referred to as

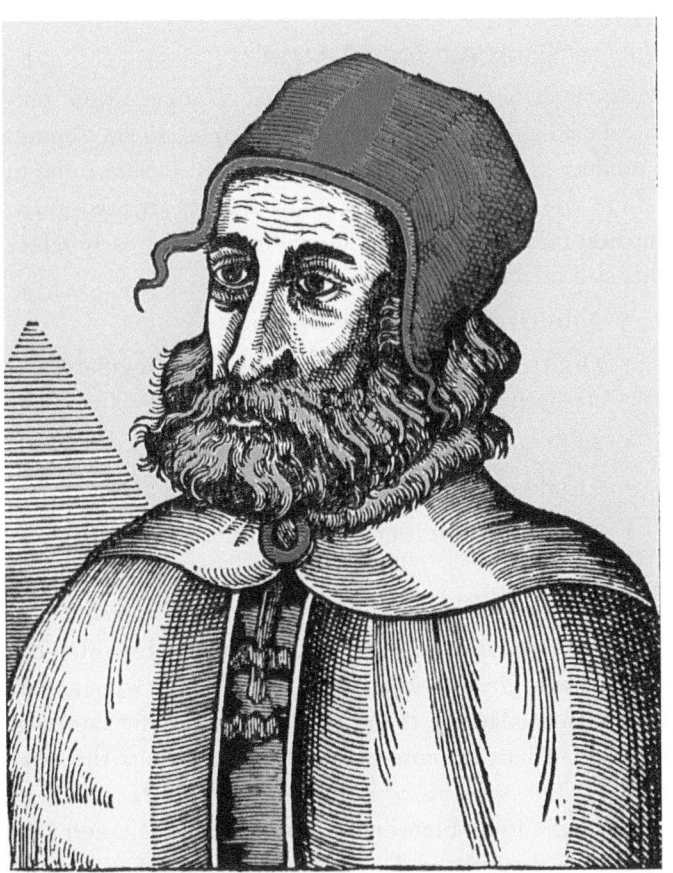

FIGURE 2-3 Galen.

"tiny little beasties." He is also responsible for describing protozoa—the simplest forms, usually one cell, of animals—and spermatozoa (mature male sex cells).

Medicine During the Eighteenth Century

In England, formal medical training began when it was required that anyone wishing to become a doctor must first become an apprentice. Medical schools in Scotland—Edinburgh and Glasgow—were developed during this era.

John Hunter

John Hunter (1728–1793) developed surgery and surgical pathology into a science. He is noted as the Founder of Scientific Surgery. Some of his contributions to medical science include the introduction of a flexible feeding tube into the stomach.

Edward Jenner

Public health and hygiene began to attract attention during the eighteenth century. A country doctor, Edward Jenner (1749–1823), a pupil of John Hunter, observed that dairy maids who had become infected with the disease cowpox would not become infected with the deadly disease smallpox. Jenner overcame ridicule from the medical community and went on to perform the first vaccination using the cowpox vaccine to combat smallpox.

The term *vaccination* comes from the Latin word *vacca*, meaning "cow." Cowpox was referred to as *vaccinia*. Today the term *vaccine* means "live or attenuated material given to a person to establish resistance to disease." Today's vaccines come from animals other than cows and from synthetic sources.

Rene Laennec

Another major advancement in medicine was made by Rene Laennec (1781–1826), who invented the stethoscope. His invention, the precursor of today's modern instrument, was the result of trial and error after three years of experimentation. His final design used a hollow wood tube that was approximately 1.4 inches in diameter and nearly 10 inches long.

Medicine During the Nineteenth Century

During the nineteenth century, the practice of medicine advanced rapidly. The documentation of accurate anatomy and physiology allowed physicians to better understand the human body. The use of sophisticated microscopes, injection materials, and instruments such as the ophthalmoscope (an instrument used to view the internal structures of the eye) all moved the practice of medicine forward.

The cell was one of the most enlightening discoveries of this era. Many believe that the greatest achievement of the nineteenth century was the knowledge that certain diseases, as well as surgical wound infections, were caused by microorganisms. The practice of surgery changed as a result of this knowledge along with advances in the use of anesthetics.

Louis Pasteur

Louis Pasteur (1822–1895) (Figure 2-4) is credited with establishing the science of bacteriology. His experiments proved that putrefaction, or decay, was caused by living organisms known as bacteria. His work solved many medical problems during his day, including rabies, anthrax in sheep and cattle, and chicken cholera. **Anthrax** is a deadly infectious disease caused by *Bacillus anthracisis.* Humans can contract the disease from infected animal hair, hides, or waste. Cholera, an acute infection of the small bowel causing severe diarrhea, was determined to be caused by a bacillus transmitted through water, milk, or food contaminated with excreta of carriers.

The process of **pasteurization** is named for Pasteur. It is the process of heating substances such as milk and cheese to a certain temperature to destroy harmful, disease-causing bacteria.

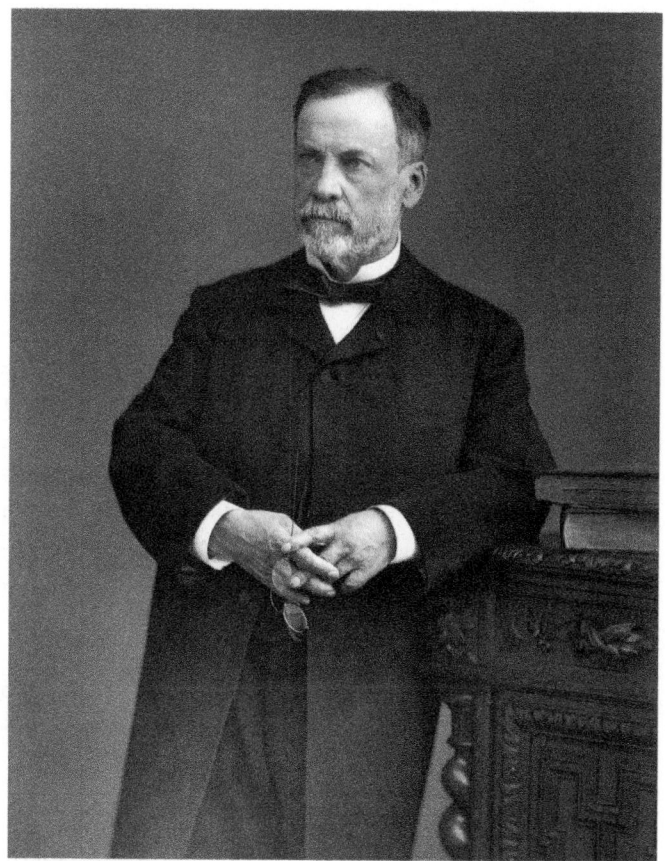

FIGURE 2-4 Louis Pasteur.

Joseph Lister

Joseph Lister (1827–1912) borrowed Pasteur's theories and eventually introduced the antiseptic system in surgery. Until that time, surgeons and obstetricians did not wash their hands between patients, so disease was spread from one patient to another. Lister advised placing an antiseptic barrier between the wound and the germ-containing atmosphere. Present-day aseptic techniques can be attributed to Lister's work.

Ignaz Semmelweiss

Ignaz Semmelweiss (1818–1865) was an obstetrician in Vienna. During the early practice of obstetrics, a physician would wear the same "butcher's coat" for all deliveries in the hospital. There was a high death rate from puerperal sepsis or childbed fever. (The term *puerperal* comes from the Latin words *puer*, meaning "child," and *pario*, meaning "to bring forth." The term *puerperium* is now used to denote a period of time after childbirth.) Women avoided having a baby in the hospital because of the high **mortality** (death) rate.

Eventually, thanks to Dr. Semmelweiss, the spread of puerperal sepsis was traced to the use of contaminated clothing and contaminated hands. Semmelweiss noted that medical students would attend a mother in childbirth immediately after having participated in an **autopsy**, an examination of the organs and tissues of a deceased body to determine the cause of death. After he advised students to disinfect their hands and put on uncontaminated clothing before attending childbirth, the incidence of disease went down dramatically. In the 1800s, however, the men who advocated disinfection were ridiculed and, in Semmelweiss's case, considered insane.

Paul Ehrlich

Paul Ehrlich (1854–1915) was a pioneer in the study of microbiology. He was also a pioneer in the fields of immunology, bacteriology, and the use of chemotherapy. **Immunology** is the study of immunity, the resistance to or protection from disease. **Chemotherapy** is the use of chemicals, including drugs, to treat or control infections and disease such as cancer. Ehrlich developed a method for staining bacteria and cells, which eventually led to a means for providing a differential diagnosis based on classifying organisms. He was one of the original "microbe hunters," **microbes** being one-celled forms of life, such as bacteria. His greatest achievement was the discovery, on his 606th attempt, of the "magic bullet" to treat **syphilis**, an infectious and chronic venereal disease.

Other Major Advances During This Period

William Roentgen (1845–1923) discovered X-rays, Pierre Curie (1859–1906) and Marie Curie (1867–1934) discovered radium, and Sigmund Freud (1856–1939) worked in the field of psychiatry.

American Medicine During This Period

William Norton, Crawford Long, and Walter Reed made significant contributions to medicine.

William Morton and Crawford Long. An important American contribution to the practice of medicine during this period was the discovery of anesthesia. William Morton (1819–1868), a dentist at Massachusetts General Hospital, and Crawford Long (1815–1878), a Georgia physician, are generally credited with having first demonstrated the use of ether as a general anesthetic. **Anesthesia** refers to the partial or complete absence of sensation. An anesthetic is a substance used to produce anesthesia. Morton and Long, working independently of each other, made possible lifesaving operations that previously, without anesthetics, could not be performed.

Walter Reed. Walter Reed (1851–1902) and others helped to conquer yellow fever, which allowed for completion of the construction of the Panama Canal by reducing the death rate for the workers. Dr. Reed, a U.S. Army physician, gathered volunteers who allowed him to inject them with yellow fever in order to find a cure.

Medicine During the Twentieth Century

Major medical advances occurred during the first half of the twentieth century. Death rates from diseases such as tuberculosis and diphtheria dropped dramatically. Overall mortality rates decreased because of improved medical care, and new emphasis was placed on **morbidity** rates (rates of disease and illness). Four major developments dominate this period:

- The specialty of **oncology**, the study and treatment of cancer, with the development of chemotherapy
- The development of immunology, the study of the **immune function**
- Progress in **endocrinology**, the study of glands and their functions
- Progress in **nutrition**, understanding the requirements of vitamins, minerals, and food in the body

Alexander Fleming

One of the most dramatic episodes of the modern era was the discovery of antibiotics. In 1928, Sir Alexander Fleming (1881–1955) (Figure 2-5) accidentally discovered that a stray mold on his culture plate of staphylococci would cause the bacteria to stop growing. He called this mold

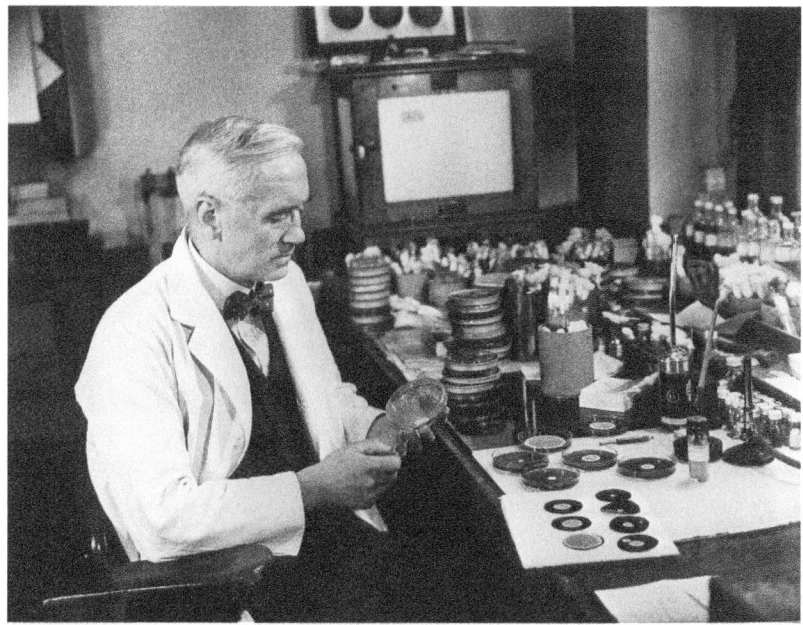
FIGURE 2-5 Alexander Fleming.

penicillium, and it has become known throughout the world as penicillin.

Fleming and two other scientists won the Nobel Prize for their work with penicillin. It was one of the first chemicals used to treat infections. Originally, the term *chemotherapy* referred to using chemicals to treat infections, so the use of penicillin to kill bacteria was considered to be chemotherapy. Today, the term *chemotherapy* generally refers to using drugs to treat forms of cancer.

Jonas Salk and Albert Sabin

The study of immunology advanced with the discovery of vaccines against typhoid, tetanus, diphtheria, tuberculosis, yellow fever, influenza, and measles. During the 1950s, Drs. Jonas Salk (1914–1996) and Albert Sabin (1906–1993) developed vaccines that eradicated the crippling disease polio.

Women in Medicine

Few women were allowed to practice medicine in the early years. In part, this was due to social constraints on women appearing in public. However, many women did practice as midwives and became skilled at delivering babies. Some remarkable female physicians and nurses overcame great odds to practice in their profession.

Elizabeth Blackwell

Elizabeth Blackwell (1821–1910) (Figure 2-6) was the first female physician in the United States. After being turned down by several medical schools, she was finally awarded a degree in 1849 from Geneva Medical College in New York. She opened the New York Infirmary for Women and Children in 1857 alongside her colleague Dr. Marie Zakrewska. This same facility, in 1867, also began functioning as a women's medical college.

Florence Nightingale

Florence Nightingale (1820–1910) is considered the founder of modern nursing. She studied nursing in Europe and cared for wounded soldiers during the Crimean War (1850–1853). Nightingale and her fellow nurses were treated poorly by the doctors at that time.

Nightingale's attention to detail, record keeping, and compassionate nursing care changed the way nursing was practiced. She advocated the use of the nursing process and elevated nursing to an honored profession. She is referred to as "The Lady with the Lamp" because of her tireless work night and day to supervise the nursing care of wounded soldiers. She started the first school of nursing in 1860 at St. Thomas Hospital in London.

Clara Barton

Clara Barton (1821–1912) was a contemporary of Florence Nightingale who nursed soldiers in a different war, the Civil

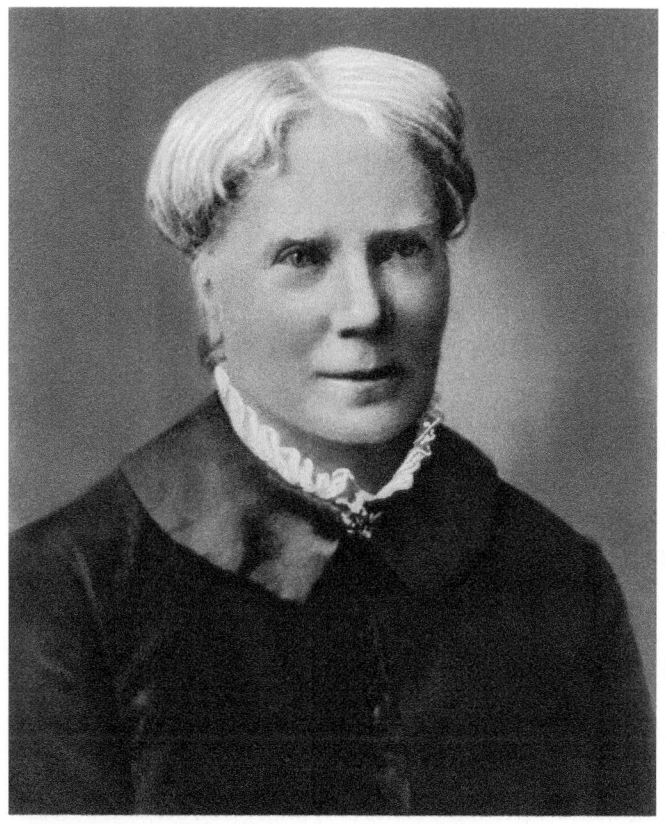
FIGURE 2-6 Elizabeth Blackwell.

War in the United States. She established the American Red Cross when she became aware of the need for support services for the soldiers. She also established the Federal Bureau of Records to help track injured and dead soldiers.

Modern Medicine and the Future

In the past 25 years, technological discoveries have permitted medical science to advance faster than in the previous 100 years. The twenty-first century holds the potential for even greater advances. The average life span of ancient humans was 30 years. According to the U.S. Census Bureau in 2001, a person born in 1900 had the life expectancy of 47 years, and someone born in 1991 had the life expectancy of 76 years. In 2008, the census bureau estimated that by the year 2020 the projected life expectancy will average 79.5. With rapid medical advancements, some estimate a life expectancy of 100 years will be possible.

Recent advances include the following:

- Improved communication techniques now allow patients' results to be examined by physicians across the country.

- Robotics is routinely used during forms of surgery.

- It is common to have patients undergo surgery to successfully replace knees, hips, kidneys, and corneas; procedures that were unheard of and inconceivable less than 100 years ago.

The future of medical science in the twenty-first century is vast.

Medical Firsts

Doctors at Brigham Hospital in Boston performed the first successful kidney transplant in 1954. In earlier attempts, patients died because physicians did not know that organs had to be compatible from the donor to the recipient for a successful transplant. In this first successful transplant, an organ was used from the patient's twin.

In 1960, Dr. Michael DeBakey (Figure 2-7) invented the heart pump, which made open-heart surgery possible for millions of heart patients. In 1962, doctors in Boston successfully reattached a young boy's severed arm. In 1967, Dr. Christian Barnard completed the first heart transplant. In 2001, a surgical team composed of 14 surgeons placed a totally implantable artificial heart in the chest of a patient. The team was led by Dr. Lamas Gray and Dr. Robert Dowling.

The discovery of the human immunodeficiency virus (HIV) as the cause of **acquired immunodeficiency syndrome (AIDS)** in 1984 was a major breakthrough in understanding this disease. AIDS is a series of illnesses that occur as a result of infection by HIV, which causes the immune system to

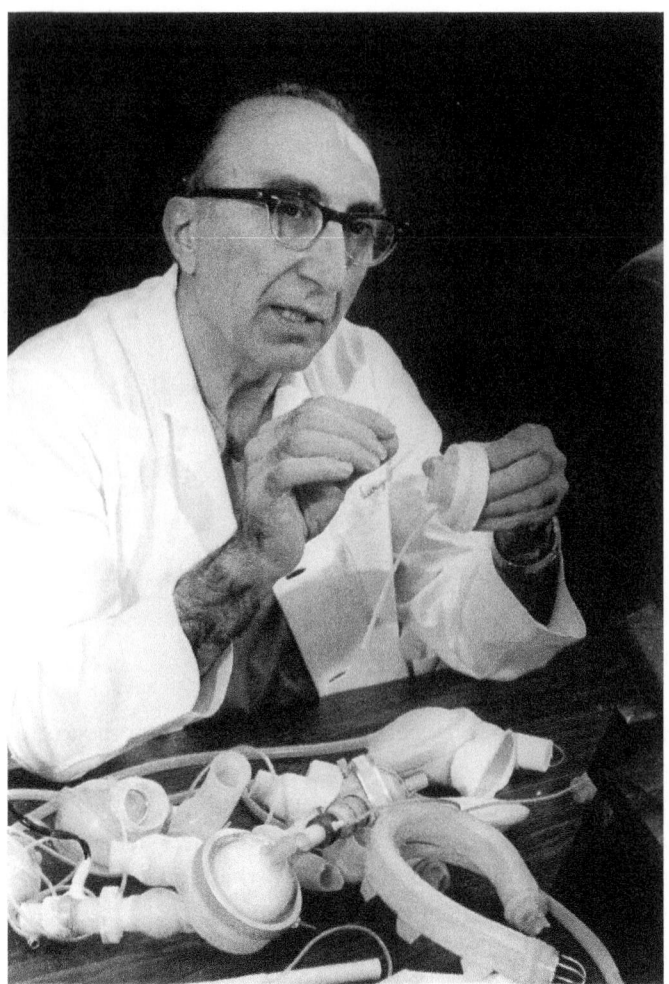

FIGURE 2-7 Dr. Michael DeBakey.

break down. Although there is as yet no cure for AIDS, a combination of drugs has stopped HIV replication to the extent that the virus is undetectable in some people. AIDS patients who start taking these antiretroviral (ARV) drugs early in the disease and continue taking them may lead greatly prolonged lives. Treatment of pregnant women with AZT and a combination of other drugs has greatly reduced the number of HIV-positive babies. Medical scientists are optimistic that a cure for HIV and better treatments for AIDS will be forthcoming.

The development of genetic engineering during the 1980s was a breakthrough that has permitted greater production of vaccines, the birth of the first test-tube baby in England in 1978, and the cloning of the first sheep in 1997.

The Medical Frontier

The **human genome project**, a publicly funded international research project to sequence and identify human genes and record their positions on chromosomes, was completed in 2001. Information from the project enables doctors to routinely screen donor eggs for many inherited diseases.

Mapping human genes has allowed for DNA testing to identify criminals, provide genetic counseling for prospective parents, and design treatments for diseases. With identification of the gene that causes Alzheimer's disease, certain types of breast cancer, and cystic fibrosis, better treatments and potential cures may be possible.

A **stem cell** is an undifferentiated cell that can give rise to other cells of the same type or from which specialized cells can develop. Stem cell research will play an important part in medical science over the next 20 years and beyond. It is already being used to induce cells in the diseased pancreas of a diabetic to produce insulin.

Hope for the future includes the following:

- A cure for AIDS
- A vaccine to prevent HIV
- Cloning organs to overcome the shortage of donors
- Better treatment and outcomes for mental illness
- Cures for heart disease, cancer, and obesity
- Methods to slow aging
- Regeneration of brain and nerve cells to overcome paralysis
- Development of antibiotics that do not allow bacteria to develop a resistant strain

MEDICAL PRACTITIONERS

The medical-assistant training and skills that you receive will enable you to work for physicians who practice in a variety of specializations. As a medical assistant, you will also encounter many allied health professionals from a wide range of fields. It is important that you understand and respect the role and educational requirements of others as you work alongside them in the field of health care.

In this section, we discuss different types of credentials for those practicing medicine. Areas covered include fields of practice as well as educational requirements for medical doctors, osteopaths, and chiropractors.

Title of Doctor

The title of doctor designates a person who holds a doctoral degree. Commonly "doctor" refers to a medical doctor (an MD) or a doctor of osteopathic medicine (DO). The practice of medicine, which is the science of diagnosis, treatment, and prevention of disease, requires a minimum of nine to ten years of education and training, which generally includes a four-year college degree in premedical studies, four years of medical school, and a period of residency. During the first year of residency, the medical student obtains vital practical

experience under the supervision of a licensed physician. (The first year of residency is sometimes called internship.) At the end of the residency, which usually lasts three years, the medical student takes a state medical board examination. If the candidate passes the state examination, she then becomes licensed to practice medicine in that state.

If the new physician wishes, she may seek graduate training in a specialty area or residency. This is a paid, on-the-job training position lasting from two to six years, depending on the specialty chosen. After the additional training is complete, the resident/doctor must sit for an American Board of Medical Specialties (ABMS) examination in his or her area of study. For example, a physician who specializes in obstetrics and passes the examination would be board certified by the American Board of Obstetrics and Gynecology. At this point, the new physician chooses how and where she would like to practice medicine. Types of medical practices are discussed later in this chapter.

Others with the Title of Doctor

The designation "doctor" is also used as a proper way of addressing—verbally or in writing—someone who holds a doctoral degree of any kind. The abbreviation for doctor is "Dr." In the medical field, the title Doctor (Dr.) indicates that a person is qualified to practice medicine. In other fields, the title Doctor (Dr.) means that a person has attained the highest educational degree in his or her field. Several designations for doctor are listed in Table 2-1 with the corresponding initials.

A Doctor of Osteopathy (DO) degree has educational requirements similar to those for the medical doctor. Both MDs and DOs are licensed physicians. Both categories of physicians use similar approaches to medicine, including

TABLE 2-1 | Designations and Initials for Doctors

Term	Initials
Doctor of Chiropractic	DC
Doctor of Dental Medicine	DMD
Doctor of Dental Surgery	DDS
Doctor of Education	EdD
Doctor of Medicine	MD
Doctor of Naturopathy	ND
Doctor of Optometry	OD
Doctor of Osteopathy	DO
Doctor of Philosophy	PhD
Doctor of Podiatric Medicine	DPM

the use of drugs, therapy, and radiation. Both groups must pass state board examinations to become licensed in their states. Doctors of Osteopathy learn the skill of manipulation therapy in schools of osteopathy. The **osteopath** places great emphasis on the relationship between the musculoskeletal system and the organs of the body. In most states, the osteopath is able to perform the same procedures as a medical doctor.

A chiropractor (DC) is trained in manipulation of the spinal column and other areas of the body. This field requires two years of premedical studies and four years of training in a licensed chiropractic school. Most states license chiropractors.

A naturopathic doctor (ND) focuses on holistic, proactive prevention and comprehensive diagnosis and treatment. The emphasis of naturopathic medicine is the use of natural healing agents. Naturopaths practice throughout the United States.

MEDICAL PRACTICE ACTS

Each state has regulations that direct the practice of medicine within that state. Although slight differences are found from state to state, in general, medical practice acts uphold who must be licensed to perform certain procedures. These acts also maintain the requirements for licensure (granting of a license); duties associated with that license; grounds on which the license can be revoked, or taken away; and reports that must be made to the government. Medical practice acts also cover the penalties for practicing without a valid license.

If a physician moves to another state, he must obtain a license to practice in that state. This may require taking and passing another state medical examination. Some states allow reciprocity of physician licenses, which is discussed later in this chapter.

Generally, physicians in different states may consult with each other without being licensed in each other's states. Physicians who practice in governmental institutions, such as Department of Veterans Affairs hospitals or military service, may practice medicine without local licensure.

Licensure

The Board of Medical Examiners in each state grants a license to practice medicine. Licensure may be granted in any of three ways: examination, endorsement, or reciprocity.

Examination

Each state offers its own examination for licensure. This examination is usually taken before the end of medical school. Within the United States, the official medical

licensing examination is called the Federation Licensing Examination (FLEX). The license is then issued after an internship is completed. Successful performance on this examination entitles the licensee to set up private practice as a general practitioner. The United States Medical Licensing Examination (USMLE), which was first administered in 1992, provides a single three-step licensing examination for graduates from accredited medical schools that can facilitate the process of obtaining reciprocity.

Endorsement

Endorsement, meaning an approval or sanction, is granted to applicants who have successfully passed the National Board of Medical Examiners (NBME). In fact, most physicians in the United States are licensed by endorsement. Any medical school graduate who is not licensed by endorsement is required to pass the state board examination (FLEX).

Graduates of foreign medical schools must pass the Certification from the Educational Commission for Foreign Medical Graduates (ECFMG). Once this examination is passed, the foreign graduate is able to apply for a residency program. The physician must complete an accredited residency training program in the United States regardless of their prior experience in another country. Once the residency period is complete, they must pass a state licensure examination exactly like their U.S.-born colleagues.

Reciprocity

In some cases, the state to which the physician is applying for a license will accept the state license that the physician already holds in another state so that the physician will not have to take another examination. This practice is known as reciprocity.

Registration

It is necessary for a physician to maintain his or her license by periodic reregistration either annually or biannually. The physician is notified by mail when to reregister and must submit the reregistration fee within a designated time period. In addition to payment of a fee to reregister, 75 hours of continuing medical education (CME) units in a three-year period are required to ensure that the physician remains current in the field of practice.

Suspension and Revocation

A physician's license may be revoked in cases of severe misconduct, which include unprofessional conduct, committing a crime, or personal incapacity to perform one's duties. Unprofessional conduct relates to behavior that fails to meet the ethical standards of the profession, such as inappropriate use of drugs or alcohol. Crimes include rape, murder, larceny, and narcotics convictions. The physician, however, does not automatically lose the license in case of a felony or malpractice conviction. Due process requires a trial by the state board of medicine before a physician's license is revoked. Personal incapacity relates to the physician's inability to perform due to physical or mental disability that renders him unable to safely and effectively perform the job.

TYPES OF MEDICAL PRACTICES

In the early twentieth century, the main form of medical practice was the solo practice in which a family practitioner set up a medical practice within a designated town or geographic area. Solo practices are becoming less popular as a result of increased costs, changes associated with practicing medicine, and the legal environment associated with managing a solo practice. Other forms of medical practice that can meet patients' needs for around-the-clock medical coverage have become popular. Alternative types of medical practices also provide the opportunity for a group of physicians to share insurance premium costs, staff, and investments in facilities.

Solo Practice

In a solo practice, a physician practices alone and is responsible for all administrative decisions associated with the practice. Solo practitioners generally enter into agreements with each other to establish coverage for patient care during off-duty times. It is also common for two solo-practice physicians to work out of the same building or office to share office expenses.

Sole Proprietorship

In a sole proprietorship, one physician is still responsible for making all the administrative decisions. However, this physician may employ other physicians and pay them a salary. The physician-owner will pay all expenses and retain all assets. In the sole proprietorship form of practice, the owner is responsible and liable for the actions of all the employees.

Partnership

A partnership established between two or more physicians is a legal agreement to share in the business operation of a medical practice. In this legal arrangement, each of the partners becomes responsible for the actions of all the partners. These include debts and all legal actions, unless otherwise stipulated in the legal partnership agreement.

Associate Practice

The associate practice is a legal arrangement in which physicians agree to share a facility and staff. They do not, as a general rule, share responsibility for the legal actions of each other as in a partnership. The legal contract of agreement stipulates the responsibilities of each party. The physicians act as if each practice is a sole proprietorship. The legal arrangement must be carefully described and discussed with patients. In some cases, patients have mistakenly believed that there was a shared responsibility by all the physicians in the practice.

Group Practice

A group practice consists of three or more physicians who share the same facility (office or clinic) and practice medicine together. In this model of medical practice, physicians share all expenses, income, personnel, equipment, and records. Some areas of medicine frequently found in group practice are anesthesiology, rehabilitative or obstetrical services, radiology, and pathology.

A group practice can also be designated as a health maintenance organization (HMO) or as an independent practice association (IPA). Group practices have grown rapidly during the past decade. Large group practices with over a hundred doctors are not uncommon. A large group practice will often form a legal corporation.

Professional Corporation

During the 1960s, state legislatures passed laws (statutes) allowing professionals (e.g., physicians, lawyers, accountants) to incorporate. A corporation is managed by a board of directors. Both legal and financial benefits result from incorporating.

Professional corporation members are known as shareholders. Therefore, the physician-members become the shareholders in the corporation. Some of the benefits that can be offered to employees of a corporation include reimbursement for medical expenses, profit sharing, pension plans, and disability insurance. These fringe benefits would not be taxable to the employee and are generally tax deductible to the employer. Although a corporation can be sued, the individual assets of the members cannot be touched. This is not the case in solo practices or sole proprietorships. A corporation will remain intact after a member leaves or dies. Other forms of practice, such as the sole proprietorship, may end with the death of the owner.

MEDICAL AND SURGICAL SPECIALTIES

Because of the dramatic advances in medicine over the past two decades, physicians continue to be interested in specialization. As mentioned earlier in the chapter, doctors who specialize in specific areas of medicine are required to have additional education. Generally, medical specialists earn a much higher income than a general physician.

A medical assistant who is employed by a medical specialty practice has the opportunity to become highly skilled and knowledgeable regarding the diseases, treatments, and procedures related to that specialty.

Medical Specialties

Common medical specialties include those described in the next sections.

Allergy and Immunology

An allergist treats abnormal responses or acquired hypersensitivity to substances with medical methods that include testing and desensitization. Pediatricians and internists may sit for the board examination in allergy and immunology after taking several years of additional training.

Anesthesiology

An anesthesiologist is trained to administer drugs both locally and generally to induce a partial or complete loss of feeling (anesthesia) during a surgical procedure. This specialist also provides respiratory and cardiovascular support during surgery. The anesthesiologist meets with the patient before the surgical procedure to explain the type of anesthetic that will be used. Certified registered nurse anesthesiologists (CRNA) also may administer anesthetics.

Bariatrics

This relatively new specialty was created in response to the obesity epidemic. Physicians specializing in **bariatrics** treat patients who are obese. Their offices usually have extra-large chairs, doors, scales, and examining tables. Nutritional counseling and weight reduction therapy are key components of bariatric care.

Bariatric surgeries are more popular now than ever. Gastric bypass, vertical sleeve gastrectomy, and the duodenal switch are different forms of bariatric surgeries that help morbidly obese patients lose drastic amounts of weight in a relatively short amount of time. These surgeries have been known to reduce or eliminate comorbidities associated with obesity, including type 2 diabetes, high blood pressure, and sleep apnea. As with all major surgeries, there are potential risks as well as benefits to bariatric surgery.

Cardiology

A cardiologist specializes in the treatment of cardiovascular disease. This physician has received additional training in the diseases and disorders of the heart and blood vessels. A cardiologist specializing in the treatment of children's heart disease would receive special training as a pediatric cardiologist.

Dermatology

A dermatologist treats injuries, growths, and infections relating to the skin, hair, and nails, either medically or surgically. A dermatologist may remove growths such as warts, moles, benign cysts, birthmarks, and skin cancers.

Emergency Medicine

The physician who specializes in emergency medicine has received additional training as an emergency medicine resident. Emergency medicine specialists typically work in hospital emergency rooms and freestanding, walk-in emergency centers. They acquire the ability and skills to quickly recognize and prioritize (triage) acute injuries, trauma, and illnesses. They also supervise paramedic prehospital care. Figure 2-8 shows an emergency department physician at work.

Endocrinology

The endocrinologist ensures that the endocrine system (glands and hormones secreted) properly communicates throughout body systems. When that system fails to work properly, an endocrinologist may be called to diagnose, treat, and coordinate the complex therapies necessary to help the patient. The patients most frequently treated by the endocrinologist are those with diabetes mellitus and thyroid disorders.

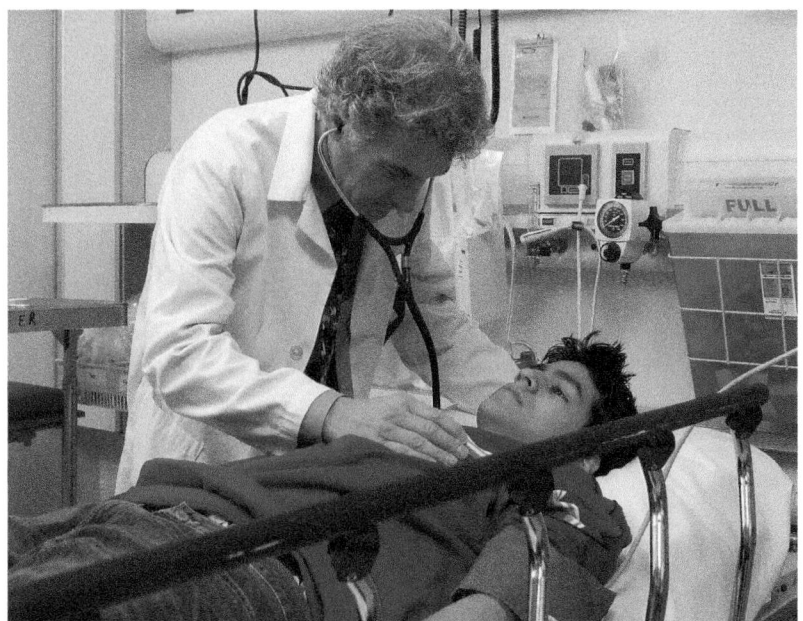
FIGURE 2-8 An emergency department physician at work.

Family Practice

Family practice physicians treat the entire family regardless of age and gender. In some cases, they will refer patients with specific medical conditions to specialists. Often, a family practice physician may also be referred to as a primary care physician.

Gastroenterology

The gastroenterologist diagnoses and treats illnesses of the gastrointestinal system. This specialty includes treatment of ulcers, digestive problems, and obesity. The gastroenterologist may need to work closely with the bariatric specialist when obesity leads to gastrointestinal diseases and disorders. Gastroenterologists perform examinations of the gastrointestinal tract, including endoscopy and colonoscopy, in outpatient settings.

Geriatric Medicine

The practice of geriatrics is focused on the care of diseases and disorders of older adults, generally those aged 65 and older. Geriatrics is a relatively new medical specialty (related to gerontology, the scientific study of aging) that has developed as a direct result of the increase in the aging population.

Hematology

Hematology is the study of blood and blood-forming tissues. Hematologists specialize in laboratory research and in the care and treatment of patients with hematological diseases such as anemia, lymphoma, leukemia, and hemophilia.

Hospitalist

A physician who specializes in the practice of hospital medicine, a hospitalist will typically complete a residency in general internal medicine, general pediatrics, or family practice. The growing trend of employing hospitalists to supervise the care of hospital patients has alleviated the need for some physicians, particularly family medicine and primary care physicians, to make hospital rounds.

Internal Medicine

Internists are physicians who specialize in internal medicine, which is similar to family medicine but the patient population is restricted to adults aged 18 and over. An internist may be considered a primary care physician for an adult patient, but they are never considered family medicine physicians because of patient age restrictions. This physician is skilled in diagnosis and treatment of nonsurgical problems. Subspecialties include cardiology, endocrinology, gastroenterology, hematology, immunology, nephrology, oncology, and pulmonary medicine, among others.

Nephrology

A nephrologist specializes in kidney disorders and diseases. A nephrologist is skilled in both surgical and medical treatments, including kidney dialysis.

Neurology

The neurologist provides nonsurgical treatment of patients who have a disorder or disease of the nervous system, which includes the brain, spinal cord, and nerves. When surgery is needed, a neurologist will refer the patient to a neurosurgeon for consultation and a review of surgical options.

Nuclear Medicine

The physician specializing in this field uses radioactive substances to diagnose and treat diseases such as cancer.

Obstetrics and Gynecology

An obstetrician treats the pregnant female from prenatal care through labor, childbirth, and the postpartum period (Figure 2-9). A gynecologist provides both medical and surgical treatment of diseases and disorders of the female reproductive system. Gynecology also deals with infertility, which is the study of a diminished capacity or inability to produce offspring.

Oncology

Oncology is the study of cancer and cancer-related tumors, and oncologists diagnose and treat patients with such diseases.

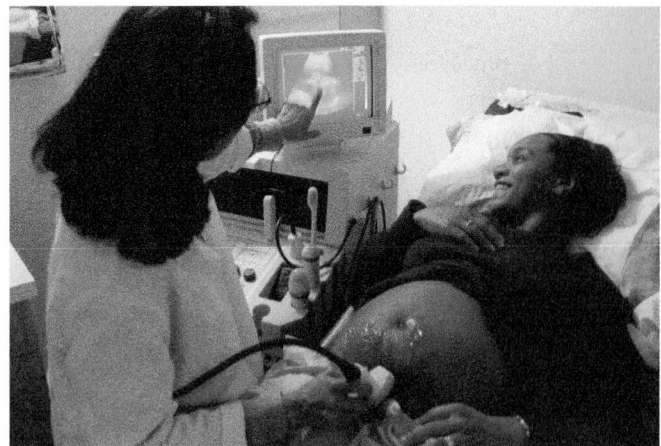

FIGURE 2-9 An obstetrician at work.

Ophthalmology

An ophthalmologist treats diseases and disorders of the eye. The study of ophthalmology includes the diagnosis of problems associated with the structures of the eye, as well as vision disorders. An ophthalmologist may use both medical and surgical treatment options.

Orthopedics

An orthopedist, or orthopod, specializes in the branch of medicine that deals with the prevention and correction of disorders of the musculoskeletal system. An orthopedic surgeon focuses on surgical procedures relating to this specialty.

Otorhinolaryngology

Otorhinolaryngology includes the study of otology (ear), rhinology (nose), and laryngology (throat). Thus, the otorhinolaryngologist specializes in the medical and surgical treatment of ear, nose, and throat (ENT) disorders. A physician with this specialty is often called just an ENT.

Pathology

A pathologist specializes in diagnosing abnormal changes in tissues that are removed during a surgical operation and in postmortem examinations. A forensic pathologist is an expert in determining the identity of a dead person based on such evidence as body parts, dental records, and tissue samples.

Pediatrics

The pediatrician specializes in the development and care of children from birth to maturity (Figure 2-10). Most patients will transition out of the care of a pediatrician when they reach 18 years of age.

Physical Medicine and Rehabilitative Medicine

Physical medicine and rehabilitative medicine specialists (physiatrists) treat patients after they have suffered an injury

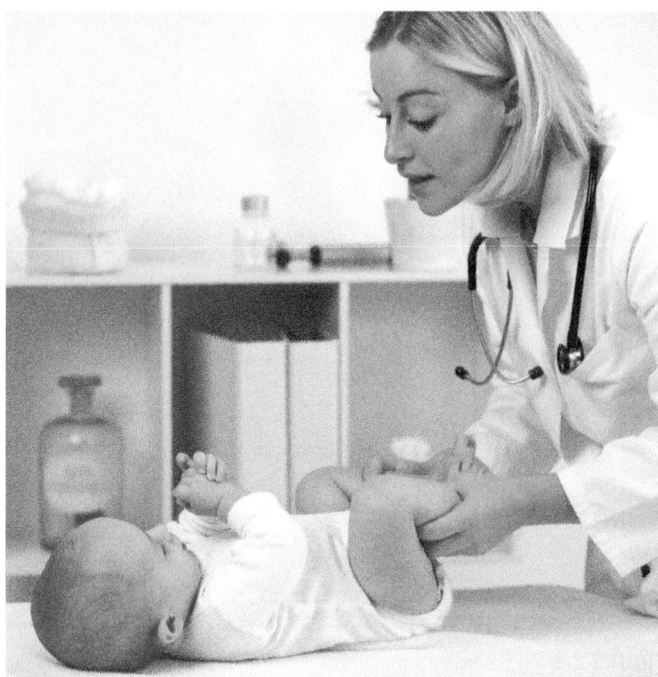

FIGURE 2-10 A pediatrician with a baby.

or disability. The purpose of treatment is to return patients to their former state of physical health if possible. This rapidly growing field is closely associated with sports medicine, in which the physician treats athletes using preventive and diagnostic medicine.

Podiatry

A podiatrist is a physician or surgeon who diagnoses and treats conditions of the foot, ankle, and related structures of the lower leg.

Psychiatry

The psychiatrist specializes in the diagnosis and treatment of patients with mental, behavioral, or emotional disorders and may also practice psychotherapy. A psychiatrist is qualified to prescribe and administer medications.

Pulmonology

This respiratory specialist treats lung problems. The pulmonologist works to ensure maximum oxygenation of patients who have respiratory disorders, such as pneumonia or chronic obstructive pulmonary disease. The pulmonologist may work closely with respiratory therapists and internists in order to achieve the best results for their patients.

Radiology

A radiologist specializes in the diagnosis and treatment of disease by using various forms of medical imaging. Examples of medical imaging include X-rays, magnetic resonance imaging (MRI), computed tomography (CT), and ultrasound, to name a few. Radiologists are tested and approved by the American Board of Radiology.

Rheumatology

A rheumatologist treats disorders and conditions of the bones, joints, and muscles, including arthritis and joint inflammation.

Urology

Urologists help patients with urinary system problems. Further, because the urological and reproductive systems are intimately entwined in the male, the urologist provides reproductive health initiatives for men. Urologists treat illnesses such as incontinence and erectile dysfunction.

Surgery

Surgery is any invasive procedure that requires entering the body by making an incision or passing instruments through the skin and organs. Surgeons correct illness, trauma, and deformities using such procedures.

Surgical Specialties

General surgery includes all areas of surgery. General surgeons may restrict their practices to abdominal surgical procedures. However, many surgeons specialize in specific areas, such as neurosurgery, cardiovascular surgery, and orthopedic surgery. Some of the more common surgical specialties are described in Table 2-2.

HEALTH CARE FACILITIES

Hospitals are the largest employers in the United States. In recent years, the public, government, and insurance companies have voiced increasing demands to curb hospital expenses. The average length of stay in the hospital has been decreasing steadily over the past decade. The result has been an increased emphasis on outpatient rather than inpatient care, especially in the area of minor surgery. **Outpatient** care refers to services provided to patients on a walk-in basis where no overnight stay is required. **Inpatient** care refers to services provided to patients who are in a facility overnight or on a long-term basis.

Same-day surgery sites, home health agencies, and physical therapy/rehabilitative and sports medicine clinics are becoming more prevalent. Also, home health care is encouraged for older adults who are homebound or unable to conveniently travel to health care facilities.

Hospitals

The hospital is still considered the key resource for health care in the United States. Although acute care is primarily performed in a physician's office, a hospital is the site of care for major surgical procedures and other major health care services. Hospitals also serve as institutions where health care professionals are trained and educated, research is conducted, and educational resources are provided to the public. Hospital sizes (measured by the number of patient beds) vary depending on the needs within the community where the hospital is located.

TABLE 2-2 | Surgical Specialties and Their Descriptions

Surgical Specialty	Description
Cardiovascular	Cardiovascular surgery is the surgical treatment of the heart and blood vessels.
Colorectal	Colorectal surgery involves the surgical treatment of the lower intestinal tract (colon and rectum).
Cosmetic/Plastic	Cosmetic, or plastic, surgery involves the reconstruction of underlying tissues. This surgical intervention is used to correct structural defects or remove scars and signs of aging.
Hand	Hand surgery is orthopedic surgery that involves surgical treatment of defects, traumas, and disorders of the hand. Hand surgeons may employ a physical therapy staff and have X-ray equipment at their disposal.
Neurosurgery	Neurosurgery involves surgical intervention for diseases and disorders of the central nervous system (brain and spinal cord).
Orthopedic	Orthopedic surgery treats musculoskeletal injuries and disorders, congenital deformities, and spinal curvatures through surgical means.
Oral (Periodontics, Orthodontics)	Oral surgery involves treatment of disorders of the jaws and teeth by means of incision and surgery as well as extraction of teeth.
Thoracic	Thoracic surgery involves treatment of disorders and diseases of the chest with surgical intervention.

To ensure quality health care, many hospitals seek accreditation. The Joint Commission (TJC), formerly the Joint Commission on the Accreditation of Healthcare Organizations (JCAHO), is a private nonprofit organization that encourages high standards of medical care. Strict guidelines must be met by the institution seeking accreditation.

Hospitals are divided into four categories:

- General hospitals (Figure 2-11) provide both routine and specialized care, such as intensive care units and emergency departments. They range in size from 50 to several hundred beds and are found in most towns and communities.

- Teaching hospitals provide the same type of care as in a general hospital. Generally, teaching hospitals are located near a university medical school, and medical students, interns, and residents treat patients under the supervision of staff physicians. More specialists may be on staff to educate and train interns and residents.

- Research hospitals provide patient care and conduct research to combat disease. Examples include Department of Veterans Affairs hospitals throughout the United States and Shriners hospitals for crippled children.

- Specialty hospitals provide specialized care for certain types of patients, such as children, psychiatric patients, or burn victims.

Many larger hospitals provide all three services: general patient care, teaching, and research. The hospital organization contains many departments that interact to provide comprehensive health care for the patient. Hospital departments include admissions, emergency services, trauma center, laboratory, radiology (diagnostic imaging), oncology, nuclear medicine, psychiatry, pathology, immunology, respiratory therapy, physical and occupational therapy, surgery services, nursing, dietary services, pharmacy, central supply, housekeeping, engineering, health information, social services (to assist in locating medical care, treatment, or placement for the patient after discharge from the hospital), human resources, and medical records. Physicians generally serve on the staff of more than one hospital but seldom more than three. They refer their patients to one of the hospitals in which they have medical privileges. **Medical privilege** refers to the physician's right to practice medicine in a particular hospital or other health care facility. A physician may also have courtesy or visiting privileges at a hospital where she may be called to see a patient on a referral basis but does not have admitting privileges.

Outpatient Surgical Centers

Historically, all surgeries were performed in hospitals, but the modern trend is for minor surgical procedures to be performed in freestanding or hospital-based outpatient surgical centers. Surgical procedures performed in outpatient centers generally require very little recovery time. In this setting the medical assistant can assist the patient with scheduling and preparing for surgery, receive and admit the patient, assist with some surgeries, and discharge the patient with postoperative instructions.

Urgent Care Centers

Because of a need for quick care in nonemergent situations, a variety of freestanding and hospital-based urgent care centers have been established. The urgent care center treats nonemergent but urgent situations, such as performing sports physical examinations, setting fractures, drawing blood for blood tests, treating infections, and providing care at times other than during the usual physician office hours. Some of these centers are also designated as primary care facilities in a specific managed care system. Because of the quick assessment and treatment they provide, these centers are popular for workers' compensation cases and occupational medicine coverage for many companies.

Patient-Centered Medical Homes

An emerging trend in health care is the development of **patient-centered medical homes (PCMH)**. These facilities help to streamline the health care needs of patients by providing a cooperative team of health care specialists in one

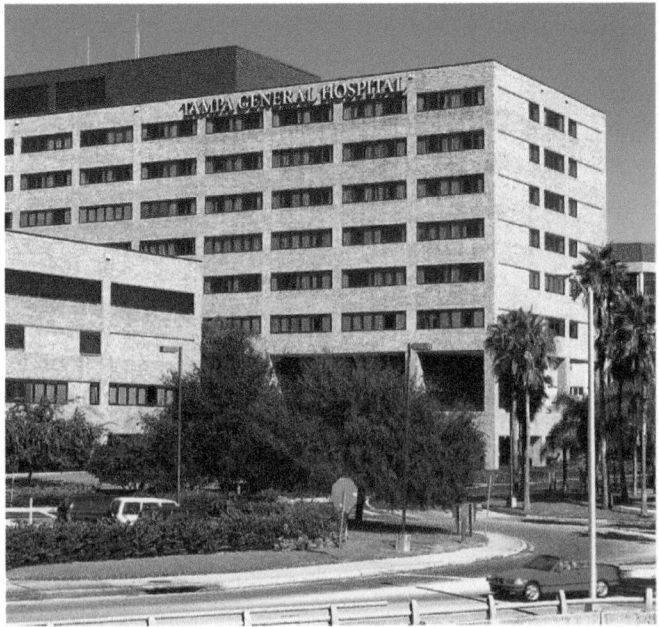

FIGURE 2-11 A general hospital.

convenient location. Concepts of overall wellness and disease prevention are the foundation of these centers, and the focus is to provide efficient, effective, and safe quality care to patients. The following is a list of types of health care specialists and service providers that may be found in a PCMH:

- Primary care physicians
- Behavioral health specialists
- Nutritionists and registered dieticians
- Obstetrics and gynecological services
- Prenatal classes
- Outpatient laboratory services
- Diagnostic imaging centers

The comprehensive and patient-centered approach of this model of health care delivery increases patient participation in their health care. It improves the quality of the patient's care and experience. In fact, a key principle of the PCMH is to create an accessible, pleasing, welcoming, and safe environment for the patient. By building a trusting rapport and establishing positive experiences and interactions, patients will be more inclined to take positive steps in their overall health and wellness.

Nursing Homes

Nursing homes were established in the nineteenth century to provide food, clothing, and shelter for older adults so that those who could not care for themselves would not be forced into an almshouse (poorhouse) with the destitute and the insane. Over the past century, the quality of care in nursing homes has improved.

Many nursing homes are owned and operated by church groups, but the majority of homes are for-profit establishments run by nursing-home corporations. Control over the quality of care is much more rigorous than in years past because of stricter regulations established by state public health departments and Medicare. Because of the increased costs of nursing home care, some patients have to convert to Medicaid (state-regulated health insurance for low-income individuals) when their funds are depleted.

For some patients, a brief nursing home stay serves as a rehabilitative bridge between hospital care and going home. For others, nursing-home care may be long-term. The present-day nursing home is primarily a long-term facility, most of whose patients are older adults who are sick or unable to care for themselves. Often these patients have no other source of care. According to the U.S. Department of Medicare and Medicaid Services (CMS), approximately 70 percent of people over 65 years of age will need long-term services at some point in their life.

Types of Long-Term Care Institutions

Long-term care institutions are classified by federal regulations either as skilled nursing facilities (SNF), intermediate care facilities (ICF), or extended care facilities (ECF). A description of these facilities and of assisted living follows.

- **Skilled nursing facility (SNF)** (Figure 2-12)—Intended for patients who require skilled nursing care around the clock. Patients must be recertified every 100 days to allow them to remain in an SNF.

- **Intermediate care facility (ICF)**—Intended for patients who are no longer able to live alone and care for themselves but do not require skilled nursing care on a 24-hour basis. Many ICFs also have occupational and rehabilitative therapists on their staff. ICFs must meet federal guidelines in order to receive federal funds for services provided to Medicare patients.

- **Extended care facility (ECF)**—Provides services to patients who no longer need the skilled nursing care of a hospital but are still too ill or incapacitated to return home. Many hospitals have opened extended care facilities for such patients (Figure 2-13). ECFs provide custodial care, and thus do not employ skilled personnel.

- **Assisted-living facility**—Offers living arrangements for the older adult in which each resident or couple has a separate apartment and pays a fixed fee to have some meals and services provided. Older adults who are able to care for themselves and require minimum assistance live in this relatively new type of environment.

Hospice

Hospice is an interdisciplinary program of care and supportive services that facilitates the care of the terminally ill patient. Hospice care can be provided in the privacy of the patient's home or in a hospice facility.

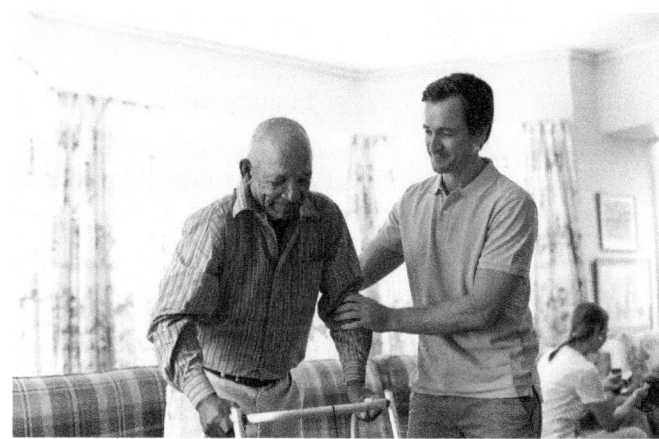

FIGURE 2-12 Skilled nursing facilities provide care for patients requiring longer stays than hospitals allow.

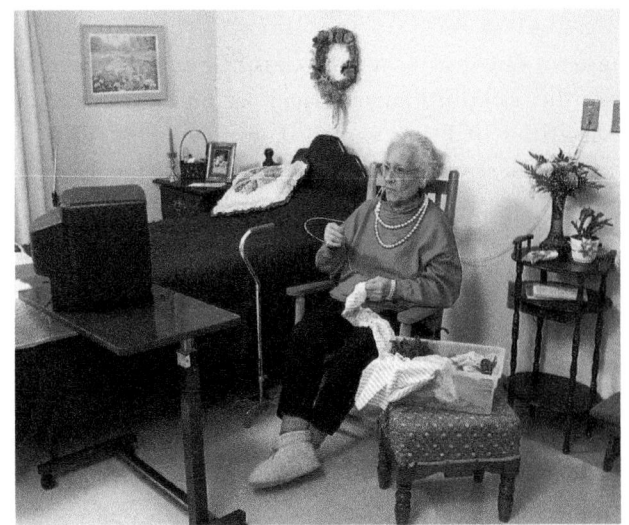

FIGURE 2-13 An extended care facility.

Hospice patients are suffering from the end stages of terminal illnesses, such as cancer, and Medicare currently covers part of end-stage care in a hospice setting. Medicare (Part B) covers part of home care with a qualifying diagnosis. During home visits, hospice personnel provide nursing care for the special needs of the dying patient, including personal care, such as help with bathing, shaving, and nail care. Pain management may be provided, but hospice generally does not provide treatment for the terminal illness itself. Visits from hospice personnel often provide great emotional support to the patient and the patient's family. The visiting health care worker will often offer suggestions for making the patient more comfortable.

ALLIED HEALTH PROFESSIONALS

It would be impossible in this single chapter to cover all of the many health care professions. Yet as a member of the health care team, it is essential that you understand the roles and educational requirements of other health care professionals. It is also important to understand how, specifically, a medical assistant will work alongside and relate to other professionals in the field.

Before we consider some specific professions, you will need an understanding of the terms *certification, registration,* and *licensure* as well as levels of education and degree titles as they relate to allied health professionals.

Education and Credentials

Educational requirements for health careers vary from state to state. In all cases, a high school diploma or equivalency is necessary. Postsecondary education in a vocational/technical school, community college, or university may be required. Table 2-3 illustrates a career ladder in health care, educational requirements, degree designations, and some examples of professions in each category. Health care institutions may require the applicant to pass a national registration or certification examination in his or her field of study as a condition of hire.

Certification involves the issuing of a certificate and credentials by a professional organization to an individual who has met the educational and experience standards of that organization, and has passed a certification exam. Certifying agencies for the field of medical assisting are discussed in the chapter titled "Medical Assisting: The Profession." **Registration** means that a professional organization in a specific health care field administers examinations, maintains a list of qualified individuals, or both. **Licensure** means that a government agency, usually a state agency, authorizes individuals to work in a given occupation, such as registered nurses (RN), licensed practical nurses (LPN), and physical therapists (PT).

Careers in the health care field involve many types of duties or responsibilities. They are categorized into National Health Care Skills Standards (NHCSS) career clusters. The

TABLE 2-3	Career Titles and Educational Levels		
Professional	**Educational Requirement**	**Diploma/Degree**	**Examples**
Professional	Four-year degree, advanced degree, and clinical training	Bachelor's (BA, BS), master's, or doctorate	Medical Doctor (MD), Pathologist
Technologist	Four-year college program	Bachelor's (BA, BS)	Medical Technologist (MT)
Technician	Two-year community college or vocational program	Associate's degree (AS)	Medical Laboratory Technician (MLT)
Assistant	Up to one-year classroom and clinical preparation	Diploma	Laboratory Assistant
Aide	On-the-job training	High school diploma or GED	Laboratory Aide

Professionalism

Physicians must obtain continuing education to retain their license. Medical assistants also need to keep abreast of new medical information. The AAMA requires Certified Medical Assistants (CMAs) to earn 60 continuing education credits (CEUs) in five years to maintain their certification. Registered Medical Assistants (RMAs) who earn certification by passing the American Medical Technologists' examination must also comply with the continuing education requirements outlined in the AMT Certification Continuation Program (CCP). The CCP program requires acquiring a certain number of points, which can be obtained through continuing education or other acceptable avenues.

Being a lifelong learner should be the goal of every medical assistant. The body of knowledge in health care is growing tremendously each year, and you will need to be vigilant about keeping up with new information. The following are a few ideas to help you become a well-informed, lifelong learner:

- Read *CMA Today*, the AAMA medical assisting journal, or *AMT Events*, the RMA professional publication, and complete the continuing education articles and tests provided in each publication.
- Select an interesting condition or disease each month to research on the Internet or at your local library. Keep this research information in a binder for future reference.
- Subscribe to other medical publications, or ask your physician employer if you may read some periodicals that she receives.
- Attend seminars provided by the local hospital, HMO, and state or local chapters of medical assisting groups.

NHCSS were developed to define the body of knowledge and specific skills health care workers are expected to possess for entry-level and technical-level positions. These core standards are used by schools, colleges, and health care facilities to establish curriculum and competencies for a wide variety of fields. The health care careers discussed next are categorized according to NHCSS career clusters, and a few examples from each category are examined. Examples of how these careers specifically relate to medical assistants are also indicated.

Therapeutic Cluster Careers

Careers in this therapeutic cluster include those that relate to the health care status of patients, including treatment, evaluation, collection of patient data, and evaluation of patient status. Medical assistants often have a direct relationship with professionals in the therapeutic cluster.

Nurse

The term *nurse* refers to a diversified group of health care professionals with a range of qualifications. Medical assistants work alongside nurses in a variety of health care settings. In some cases, a nurse may work as a direct clinical supervisor to a medical assistant. However, it is important to understand your state laws regarding the delegation of specific duties to a medical assistant. Descriptions of a certified nursing assistant (CNA), licensed practical nurse (LPN), registered nurse (RN), and nurse practitioner (NP) follow.

Certified Nursing Assistant (CNA). A certified nursing assistant is a member of the health care team who has completed a training program and has passed a state-issued examination, which allows the individual to assist nurses in nursing homes, hospitals, and other health care facilities. The CNA provides such patient care as bed baths, measuring vital signs, feeding, and ambulation. Cross-training of employees has led to positions such as patient care technician (PCT). The PCT may have a CNA or medical assisting background and perform more technical tasks, such as drawing blood and performing ECGs. The nursing assistant may also be referred to as a nurses' aide or orderly.

Licensed Practical Nurse (LPN). A licensed practical nurse performs some, but not all, of the same clinical nursing tasks a registered nurse does. The LPN must have graduated from a recognized one-year program and become licensed by the National Federation of Licensed Practical Nurses. In some states, the LPN is known as a licensed vocational nurse (LVN).

Registered Nurse (RN). A career as a registered nurse is ideal for the person who wishes to provide hands-on patient care. Nurses work in hospitals, physicians' offices, industry, governmental agencies, ambulatory care units, emergency services, and schools. Their work ranges from managed care organizations providing direct patient care, to teaching and supervising other staff, performing research, and managing agencies. Nurses receive their education and training in either a two-year or a four-year program.

To become licensed as an RN requires successful completion of the National Council Licensure Examination (NCLEX), a national licensure examination. A nurse practitioner (NP) is a registered nurse who has a master's degree and has received additional training to provide basic patient care that includes diagnosing and prescribing medications and treatments for common illnesses.

It is illegal for the medical assistant to be called a nurse; nurses have a higher level of education and training than a medical assistant. If patients or physicians refer to the medical assistant as their nurse, the medical assistant should correct the information by politely explaining that he is a medical assistant and not a nurse.

Occupational Therapist (OT)

Occupational therapy provides treatment to people who are physically, mentally, developmentally, or emotionally disabled. Occupational therapists evaluate the patient's skills for self-care, work, and leisure. The goal of the occupational therapist is to develop programs that will help to restore the patient's ability to manage activities of daily living (ADL). Occupational therapists require a bachelor's degree from an approved program in occupational therapy, plus certification by the American Occupational Therapy Association (AOTA) and six months of on-the-job training.

An *occupational therapy assistant* must complete a two-year vocational training program and be certified by AOTA. This assistant works under the supervision of an OT and implements patient treatments designated by the OT.

A medical assistant may work as an occupational therapy aide, assisting the OT and helping the occupational therapy assistant. In many cases, a medical assistant will interact with occupational therapy by scheduling referral services for patients that are ordered by physicians. The MA may also have the responsibility of obtaining therapy notes and updates related to a patient's care.

Physical Therapist (PT)

Physical therapy is the treatment of diseases or disabilities of the joints, bones, and nerves by massage, therapeutic exercises, and heat and cold treatments. Examples of conditions treated by means of physical therapy include multiple sclerosis, cerebral palsy, arthritis, fractures, spinal cord injuries, and heart disease. Practitioners work in a variety of facilities including hospitals, ambulatory care centers, rehabilitation centers, private practice, and schools for the physically challenged. A PT is required to hold a four-year degree in physical therapy, participate in a four-month clinical internship, and successfully pass the state licensure examination. After obtaining a master's degree, some PTs set up private practices and provide services on a contract basis.

A *physical therapy assistant* may be required in some states to have a degree from an accredited two-year college and pass a written licensure examination. He works under the supervision of a physical therapist and implements treatments designated by the PT.

A medical assistant may interact and work with physical therapists and physical therapy assistants in the same manner in which he would work alongside those in occupational therapy, mentioned previously.

Physician Assistant (PA)

The field of physician assistant is relatively new, emerging only since the 1970s. The goal of this professional is to assist the physician in the primary care of patients. The job description for a PA includes evaluation, monitoring, diagnosis, therapeutics, counseling, and referral skills. In nearly all states, the PA can prescribe medications. The profession has expanded to include surgeon's, pathologist's, anesthesiologist's, and radiologist's assistants, among others. The general educational program is similar to a master's-level program with two years of education after a bachelor's degree. In most programs, the student must have some combination of work or internship experience and pass an accreditation examination.

A medical assistant often works very closely with a physician's assistant in a medical practice setting. Based on the physician's direction, a medical assistant may perform the same duties for a physician assistant as they would for a physician. Again, it is important for you to understand your state laws regarding the delegation of duties. Many states recognize physician assistants as licensed personnel able to delegate duties to a medical assistant, whereas others do not.

Respiratory Therapist (RT)

A respiratory therapist evaluates, treats, and cares for patients with breathing problems. A respiratory therapist tests lung capacity, administers breathing treatments, teaches self-care to patients, and provides emergency care. An RT can be employed in hospitals, cardiopulmonary laboratories, nursing homes, health maintenance organizations (HMOs), and ambulatory care facilities. To become a certified respiratory therapy technician (CRTT), the candidate must complete a one-year internship and pass a written examination given by the National Board of Respiratory Therapy.

Becoming a registered respiratory therapist (RRT) requires successful completion of a college program, an approved training program, one year's experience in the field, and a written examination given by the National Board of Respiratory Therapy.

Medical assistants who work for a pulmonology practice are likely to have more interaction with respiratory therapists than other MAs. Because of the highly specialized nature of respiratory therapy, however, a medical assistant wouldn't have duties that overlap those of the respiratory therapist. Therefore, interaction with members of this field may be limited to communication related to patient care and the coordination of health care services.

Dietitian

Dietitians are skilled in applying the principles of good nutrition to food selection and meal preparation. They work closely with a patient's physician to coordinate the patient's diet with such other treatments as medications. Dietitians also provide consulting services, offer seminars, author books, counsel patients, plan food service systems, and design nutrition plans within fitness programs for athletes. A dietitian must have a bachelor's degree with a major in foods and nutrition. In addition, an internship in a dietary department is required. To become registered requires successful completion of an examination. Dietitians work in a variety of settings including hospitals, long-term care facilities, schools, and prisons. The employment opportunities for dietitians are currently excellent.

Medical assistants will often set up referral services for patients in need of a dietician's care, including diabetic patients, those with gastrointestinal disorders, and cancer patients. Although clinical options for an MA may be limited in a dietician's office, an administrative medical assistant may work in the front office performing a variety of administrative duties.

Dental Hygienist

A dental hygienist (Figure 2-14) works directly with the patient to clean teeth, takes oral X-rays, teaches oral health, and discusses results of dental examinations with the dentist. The dental hygienist must graduate from a two-year

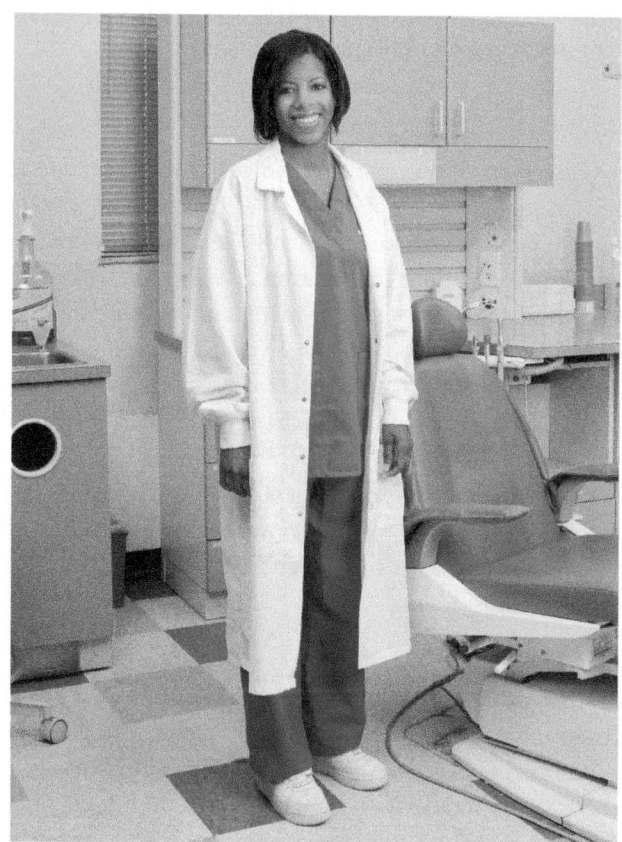

FIGURE 2-14 A dental hygienist.

community college program or a four-year bachelor's program and pass both a state written and clinical examination.

In general, a medical assistant is not likely to have much interaction with a dental hygienist in a clinical capacity. A medical assistant may be employed by a dental practice to perform administrative duties and in that capacity would have daily interaction with the clinical staff of a dental office.

Emergency Medical Responder (EMR), Emergency Medical Technician (EMT), Advanced Emergency Medical Technician (AEMT), and Paramedic

There are four levels of Emergency Medical Services (EMS) training and certification as designated by the U.S. Department of Transportation. EMS providers are skilled in recognizing and responding to trauma and medical emergencies and providing emergency care and transport to a medical facility. Each state has its own laws governing EMS. EMTs and paramedics work under the license and supervision of a physician.

The levels of EMS training and certification are:

- **Emergency Medical Responder (EMR).** The EMR is the person who is often first at the scene. Many police officers, firefighters, and industrial health personnel are trained as EMRs. The emphasis is on activating the EMS system, providing immediate care for life-threatening injuries, and preparing for the arrival of the ambulance.

- **Emergency Medical Technician (EMT).** In most areas, EMT is the minimum level of certification for ambulance personnel. EMTs provide basic-level medical and trauma care and transportation to a medical facility.

- **Advanced Emergency Medical Technician (AEMT).** The AEMT, like the EMT, provides basic-level care and transportation, and additionally provides some advanced-level care, including use of advanced airway devices and administration of some medications.

- **Paramedic.** The paramedic performs all the skills of the EMT and AEMT plus additional advanced-level skills. Paramedic is the most advanced level of prehospital emergency care.

EMS professionals receive certification after completion of an approved training program. They must be recertified every two years and receive ongoing education and training in their field.

Most often, the medical assistant will work with those in the emergency medical services by means of initiating EMS services. A medical assistant may be called upon to initiate emergency services for a patient in distress during a medical office visit. The MA may have the responsibility of printing off pertinent medical records that would accompany the patient to the hospital and providing current medical information to the EMS responders.

Pharmacist

The field of pharmacy deals with the ordering, maintenance, preparation, and distribution of prescription medications. A pharmacist (Figure 2-15) must complete five years of education in an accredited pharmacy program. In addition, a pharmacy student must serve a one-year internship and become licensed in the state where she is employed. A registered pharmacist can work in a variety of institutions including hospitals, drugstores, and nursing homes. Some pharmacists may choose to open their own pharmacy.

Pharmacy technicians attend a community college or private vocational program. They are able to assist the pharmacist in preparing medications either in a hospital or in a retail pharmacy setting. In some states, they are issued a Pharmacy Technician Certificate upon completion of an examination. A *pharmacy clerk*, a position for which a high school diploma is necessary, assists the pharmacist with typing prescription labels, assigning prescription numbers, and maintaining supplies and records.

Medical assistants work very closely with pharmacy staff, particularly via telephone interactions. Depending on the state, a medical assistant may be allowed to call in a prescription refill order; however, this task is becoming less necessary with the use of electronic prescription services. Other interactions with the pharmacy staff may include verifying a patient's prescription benefits or verifying allowed medications as determined by the patient's medical insurance. (This is referred to as a drug formulary.)

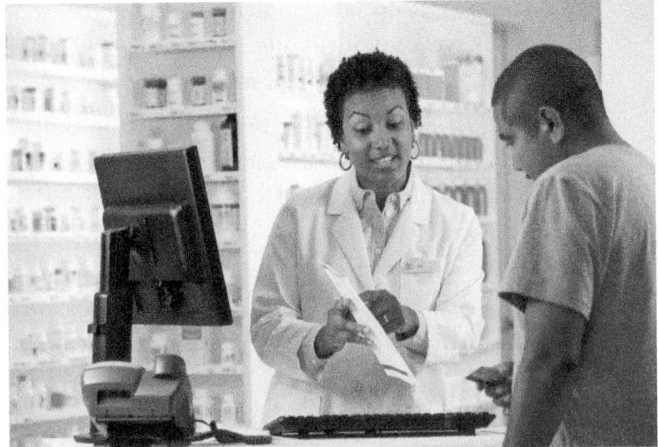

FIGURE 2-15 Pharmacists often consult with patients regarding new medications and other issues related to prescriptions and drug interactions.

Medical Social Worker

Social work involves programs and services that are developed to meet the special needs of the ill, the physically and mentally challenged, and older adults. A medical social worker cares for the total person, including the emotional, cultural, social, and physical needs of the patient.

Medical social workers assist patients and their families in handling problems associated with a long-term illness or disability. Social workers need a thorough understanding of a community's resources for the disabled. A medical social worker requires a bachelor's degree. Many states require licensing or registration for social workers and a master's degree.

Medical assistants may interact with social workers by helping to coordinate the needs of patients and their families. They will also often set up appointments with social workers on behalf of their patients.

Surgical Technologist

Also called an operating room technician, the surgical technologist assists in surgical operations. They prepare the operating rooms, arrange equipment, and help doctors and nurses during surgery. Most surgical technologists work in hospitals; however, they are also employed in outpatient surgery centers.

Unless directly employed in a surgical setting, medical assistants may have limited interactions with surgical technologists because of the specialized nature of their field.

Diagnostic Cluster Careers

The careers in this cluster are involved with procedures that create a picture of the patient's health status at a specific point in time. These careers involve measuring, evaluating, and reporting patient information.

Depending on the employment setting, medical assistants may have limited interactions with professionals in the diagnostic cluster of careers. In some states, medical assistants have the opportunity to take additional classes in order to become a general X-ray machine operator (GXMO) or a limited X-ray machine operator (LXMO). These MAs could have the opportunity to work closely alongside some of the following professionals in diagnostic imaging facilities or clinics and hospitals.

Ultrasound Technologist

An ultrasound technologist receives training in the use of ultrasound equipment, which uses inaudible sound waves to outline shapes of tissues and organs. Ultrasound equipment produces an image of the shapes. Ultrasound images of fetal development in the uterus are commonly used to assist with fetal monitoring.

X-ray Technologist (Radiologic Technologist)

An X-ray, or radiologic, technologist must hold a bachelor's degree in radiologic technology, have experience in two or more radiologic disciplines, such as nuclear medicine and radiation therapy, and be a registered radiologic technologist (ARRT).

Electroencephalograph Technician

Electroencephalography (EEG) is the field devoted to recording and studying the electrical activity of the brain. An EEG technician operates an electroencephalograph, which records the activity of the brain with a written tracing of the brain's electrical impulses. EEG technologists work primarily in hospitals.

Diagnostic Imaging Technician

Diagnostic imaging technicians are trained in the operation of X-ray equipment such as ultrasound, computerized tomography (CT), and magnetic resonance imaging (MRI) equipment. Radiology practitioners include darkroom attendants, who require only a minimum amount of education or training; radiologic technicians, who are graduates of an accredited postsecondary education program and have passed a certification exam in their field; and radiologists, who are licensed physicians who have graduated from an accredited medical school with specialized training in radiology. Employment opportunities are available in physicians' offices, hospitals, trauma centers, and other ambulatory care facilities.

Medical Laboratory Careers

A medical laboratory is a facility that is equipped for testing, research, scientific experimentation, or clinical studies of materials, fluids, or tissues taken from patients. Independent laboratories provide routine analysis of patients' blood, urine, tissue, and other materials. Hospital laboratories perform tests for both inpatients and outpatients. In some instances, a physician's office will contain a small physician office laboratory (POL) where routine tests can be conducted.

Medical assistants may interact quite often with medical laboratory professionals. Some states allow medical assistants to work as phlebotomists. These medical assistants will work directly with many of the professionals listed next. We will start the discussion by expanding on the role of the phlebotomist.

Phlebotomist or Venipuncture Technician. A phlebotomist is skilled in drawing blood from patients. This requires the ability to adhere to standard precautions, aseptic technique, excellent venipuncture technique, and good communication skills. Training in a vocational education

Professionalism   The Workplace

Because continuing education is necessary to keep skills current and to follow changes in the practice of medical assisting, the wise medical assistant will ask the employer to include continuing education in the benefits package. When a medical assistant goes to a conference and returns to the office, it is professional practice to share what was learned. In that way, the employer gets the maximum benefit for the investment.

program is required. Phlebotomy training courses at colleges or career schools vary in length but should prepare the student for certification. Every state decides licensing requirements, but most states do not require licensure for phlebotomists. California, on the other hand, requires both certification and licensure for phlebotomy technicians. Many employers prefer to hire workers with prior experience and may require certification through a national examination, indicating that the phlebotomy technician meets standards of competence. Louisiana is one state that recently passed legislation requiring phlebotomists to be certified before they are eligible for employment.

The American Society for Clinical Pathology (ASCP) has a certification program for phlebotomy technicians (ASCPPBT) that requires proof of phlebotomy skills and successful completion of a rigorous examination. The route to certification includes high school graduation or equivalency and completion of a National Accrediting Agency for Clinical Laboratory Science (NAACLS)–approved phlebotomy program, one approved by The Joint Commission, or one approved by the California Department of Health, or one year of experience as a full-time phlebotomy technician in a laboratory that is accredited and regulated by the Clinical Laboratory Improvement Amendments (CLIA) within five years of application. Completion of an RN, LPN, or another acceptable accredited allied health professional or occupational education program can also qualify an applicant. The American Medical Technologists (AMT) organization has a certification program for phlebotomy; the credential awarded is registered phlebotomy technician (AMT-RPT). Before taking the AMT's certification exam, an applicant for phlebotomy technician must have a high school diploma or GED and acceptable training. Other organizations that offer phlebotomy certification include the National Center for Competency Testing (NCCT) and the National Healthcareer Association (NHA).

Laboratory Technician (MLT and CLT). The medical laboratory technician (MLT) (Figure 2-16) is a certification

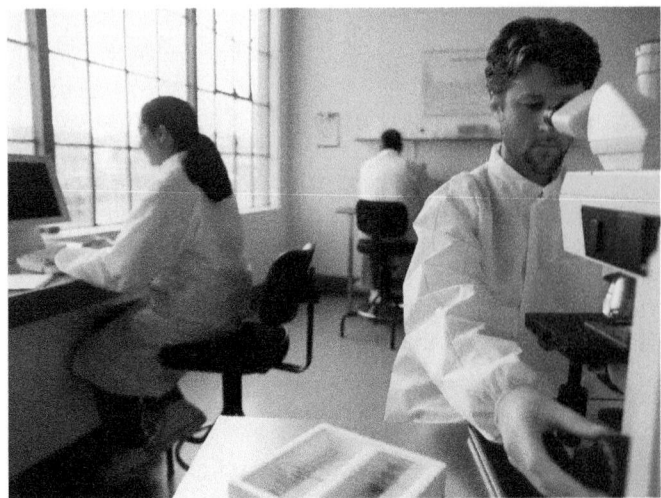

FIGURE 2-16 A medical lab technician.

obtained from the American Society of Clinical Pathology (ASCP). The American Society for Clinical Laboratory Sciences (ASCLS) is another highly regarded professional organization that promotes the Clinical Laboratory Technician (CLT) and Clinical Laboratory Scientist (CLS) certifications, which are administered through the National Credentialing Association. Both of these highly regarded credentials are awarded to laboratory technicians skilled in testing blood, urine, lymph, and body tissues. This career requires two years of training in a vocational education program before certification. The AMT also certifies medical laboratory technicians.

Medical Technologist (MT) or Clinical Laboratory Scientist (CLS). A laboratory or medical technologist must complete a four-year medical technology program in a college or university to become a certified medical technologist (CMT) or certified laboratory scientist (CLS). This person directs the work of other laboratory staff, is responsible for maintaining quality assurance standards for all equipment, and performs laboratory analysis. The examination for this profession is prepared by the Board of Registry of the ASCP. The AMT also certifies medical technologists.

Information Services Cluster Careers

Careers in this cluster are involved with documenting client information, including managing, coding, analyzing, maintaining, and retrieving information.

Medical assistants will work very closely with professionals in this career cluster. A medical assistant will contact a medical records technician many times throughout the work week in order to obtain the most up-to-date records for their patients. A physician may ask a medical assistant to work closely with a medical transcriptionist by providing appropriate audio files or reviewing transcribed documents for errors.

Many times, a medical assistant may work as an office manager for a medical practice, or become employed as a unit clerk at a hospital or clinic. All of these careers are discussed next.

Health Information Technology (Medical Records Technician)

Health information technology refers to the massive database known as medical records. Every person seen by a health care professional has a medical record. Medical records technicians, now more commonly referred to as health information technologists, maintain the permanent records relating to a patient's condition and treatment. The medical record is a legal document that can be used in a court of law.

A medical records technician must graduate from an accredited program that offers a two-year associate's degree. Successful completion of the accredited record technical examination offered by the American Medical Record Association allows the technician to use the initials ART after his or her name. The American Health Information Management Association (AHIMA) offers the Registered Health Information Technician (RHIT) examination. A registered medical records administrator (RRA) requires a bachelor's degree in health information technology and the successful completion of an examination administered by the American Medical Record Association.

Medical Transcription

A medical transcriptionist types or enters into a computer dictation that is taken from a recording machine or an audiotape. This dictation consists of medical reports from physicians and surgeons. Skills required for this profession include proficient typing ability, good spelling, understanding of medical terminology, and the ability to operate data processing equipment. The field of medical transcription may be replaced in the future by software programs that use voice recognition.

Office Management

The role of office manager is a choice open to some allied health professionals, including medical assistants and nurses. Office managers supervise the entire support staff. The position requires someone with a sound knowledge of the type of work performed in the office or institution, strong supervisory skills, and the ability to work closely with upper-level management, including physicians and directors. Excellent time-management and communication skills are a must for office managers.

Unit Clerk/Communications Clerk

The unit clerk, or ward secretary, is responsible for clerical duties, reception work, and other communication duties in hospitals, long-term care facilities, and clinics. The unit clerk in a hospital performs varied tasks, for example, taking physicians' orders from charts, dispatching those orders to various hospital departments, and assisting the nursing staff. Extensive knowledge of medical terminology is required.

SUMMARY

The medical profession has a rich history of achievement and progress. The history of medicine can be broken into four categories: early medicine going back to 3000 BC, the eighteenth century, the nineteenth century, and the twentieth century. Major advancements include the eradication of many deadly diseases with the advent of vaccines, the decrease of infections due to the discovery of aseptic technique and antibiotics, the harnessing of radium to treat disease, the inventions of the microscope and surgical instruments, the discovery of anesthesia, and a better understanding of anatomy and physiology.

Today licensed physicians must maintain their knowledge base by completing 75 continuing medical education (CME) units over a period of three years. The medical assistant will have the opportunity to pursue a career working for physicians in all areas of specialization.

The health care environment can be confusing and intimidating to the patient. It is important to have an understanding of the health care system and the diversity of institutions that deliver health care services. The descriptions provided in this chapter of inpatient facilities, including hospitals, nursing homes, hospices, and ambulatory care settings and services, provide a basic explanation of a rather complex structure. The medical assistant's understanding of the system is key to providing clear explanations to the patient.

There are numerous medical specialties. Physicians decide after rotations in medical school which area of medicine they prefer. After a residency in a specialty, a physician can practice in that specialty. Board certification in a specialty requires completing an approved residency, passing a challenging examination, and practicing in the field for years. New specialties, such as bariatrics to treat obesity problems, are created when a subspecialty is needed. Physicians can complete additional training and do another residency to change to a different area of medical interest after an initial residency. For example, a board-certified obstetrician may decide to become a pathologist or a surgeon. This would require another residency in that discipline.

Varied and numerous allied health professionals are enlisted to support physicians with patient care. Some of these professions include therapeutic cluster careers (such as nurses and dietitians), diagnostic cluster careers (such as X-ray and ultrasound technologists), laboratory cluster careers (such as phlebotomists and clinical laboratory scientists), information services cluster careers (such as unit clerks and office managers), and environmental cluster careers (such as biomedical equipment technicians). The medical assistant is a key part of the allied health team, and understanding how the medical assistant will work with various team members is helpful in understanding the overall function of the working team.

2 CHAPTER REVIEW

COMPETENCY REVIEW

1. Define and spell the terms for this chapter.
2. State at least three of the major achievements in medicine during each of these periods: early medicine, eighteenth century, nineteenth century, and twentieth century (or modern medicine).
3. List the three methods by which a physician can become licensed.
4. Explain three circumstances that would justify the suspension or revocation of a physician's license.
5. Compare and contrast three types of medical practices.
6. Find examples of four board-certified physicians in your city or town, using a local telephone or Internet directory.
7. Using the Internet or a local telephone directory, identify the names and addresses of at least five different health care facilities and describe the types of services each facility offers to the general public.
8. Consider the various types of health care cluster careers. Thinking about your future as a medical assistant, which cluster career do you look forward to working with the most? Explain what intrigues you about this cluster career.

PREPARING FOR THE CERTIFICATION EXAM

1. Which of the following is *not* an ancient remedy?
   a. digitalis
   b. ibuprofen
   c. chamomile
   d. nitroglycerine
   e. sulfur

2. Who is considered the Father of Medicine?
   a. Galen
   b. Galileo
   c. Hippocrates
   d. Socrates
   e. Curie

3. Who discovered the cure for smallpox?
   a. Harvey
   b. Hippocrates
   c. Galen
   d. Jenner
   e. Pasteur

4. Who established the science of bacteriology?
   a. Nightingale
   b. Pasteur
   c. Jenner
   d. Galileo
   e. Lister

5. The science of treating obese patients is
   a. geriatrics
   b. gynecology
   c. dermatology
   d. bariatrics
   e. radiology

6. Which allied health professional performs phlebotomy as a career?
   a. unit clerk
   b. medical transcriptionist
   c. venipuncture technician
   d. dietitian
   e. respiratory therapist

7. Which allied health professional would help a patient find an appropriate nursing home?
   a. clinical laboratory scientist
   b. certified nursing assistant
   c. physical therapist
   d. occupational therapist
   e. medical social worker

8. Which type of practice is managed by a board of directors?
   a. solo practice
   b. corporation
   c. group practice
   d. sole proprietorship
   e. partnership

9. Where should a patient go with a stomach infection?
   a. urgent care facility
   b. long-term care facility
   c. hospice
   d. nursing home
   e. outpatient surgical center

10. Which of the following medical specialties would treat a patient with hearing loss?
    a. bariatrics
    b. ophthalmology
    c. otorhinolaryngology
    d. orthopedics
    e. obstetrics

CRITICAL THINKING

Refer to the case study at the beginning of the chapter and use what you have learned to answer the following questions.

1. During a meeting about finding a new physician, Dr. Bahjat informs Tania that the new physician will not be a partner in the practice. What will this mean for the new physician the group decides to hire?

2. Pearson Physicians Group decides to hire Dr. Shania McWalter. Dr. McWalter is a DO. Tania has been receiving many phone calls from patients inquiring about the difference between an MD and a DO. What should Tania tell these patients?

3. More than 30 percent of the patients seen by Pearson Physicians Group are between the ages of 68 and 93. Dr. Bahjat has asked that Tania create an informational sheet for patients and their family members regarding the differences between skilled nursing facilities and assisted living facilities. What information should Tania include in the brochure?

ON THE JOB

One of the important characteristics of a medical assistant is to have a concrete foundation in the practice of medicine. This includes a complete understanding of the many medical and surgical specialties and subspecialties in which a physician can be board certified.

An important responsibility for the medical assistant is to have the ability to convey information about the treating physician to the anxious patient and the patient's family. This is part of patient education.

Bonnie is employed as a medical assistant for a physician who is a pediatric cardiovascular surgeon. She is taking a history of the patient, a newborn, by interviewing the parents, Mr. and Mrs. Appleby. They are extremely upset and anxious over the condition of their newborn, who was diagnosed shortly after birth with a serious, yet quite treatable, heart defect. The prognosis, should the parents agree to the corrective surgery, is quite good. However, the parents are having a difficult time understanding how the physician could help their newborn. They are not even quite sure why they were referred to this specialist and why their pediatrician could not treat the infant.

1. How could Bonnie comfort and reassure these parents?
2. What could Bonnie say about the physician that might help the parents understand why they were referred and how their newborn could be helped?

INTERNET ACTIVITY

Research ethical arguments for and against the use of fetal stem cells for medical treatment.

Research information about the main features and benefits of the Affordable Care Act of 2009.

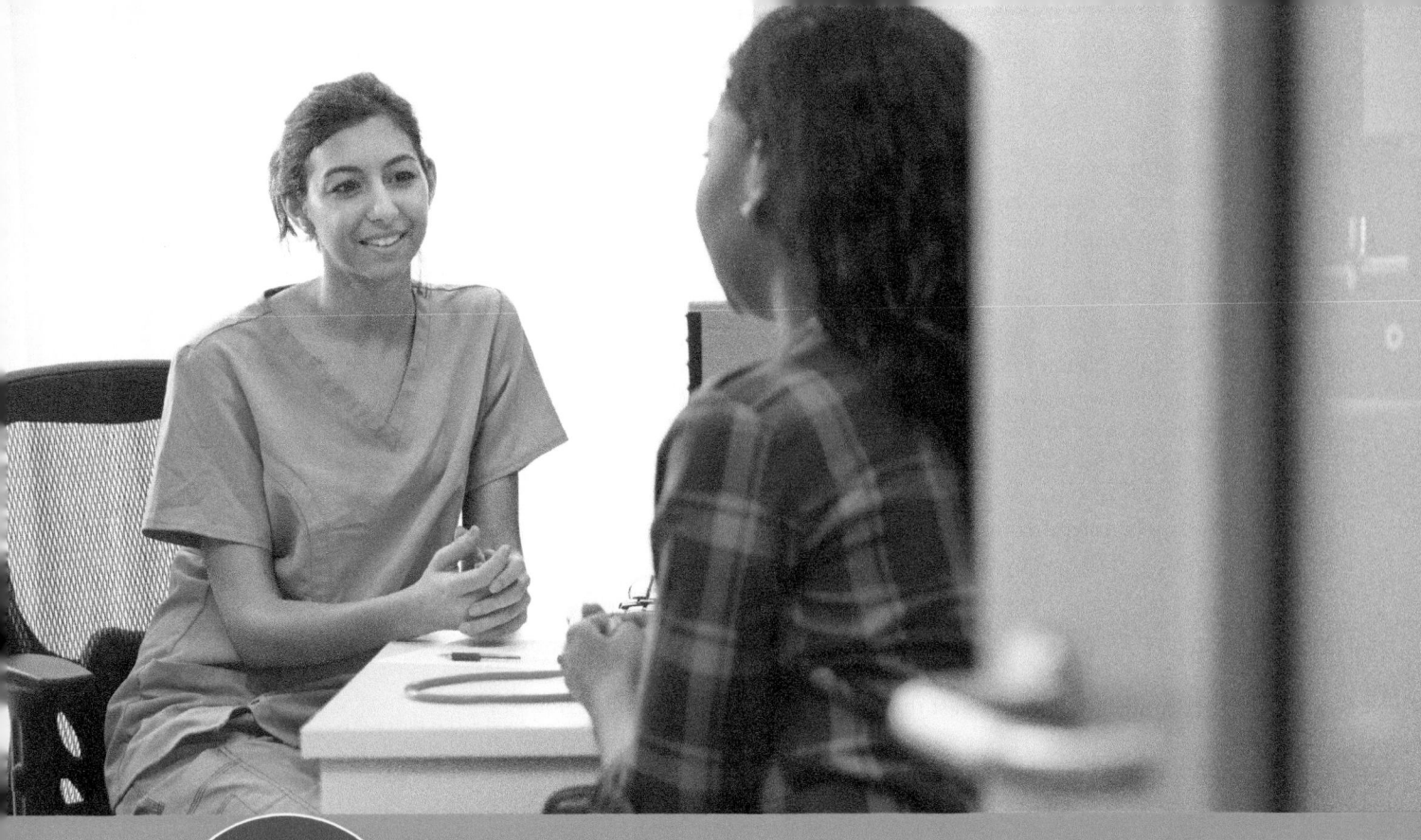

Medical Law and Ethics

Learning Objectives

After completing this chapter, you should be able to:

3.1 Define and spell the terms for this chapter.

3.2 Explain differences between criminal and civil law specifically as they pertain to the medical assistant.

3.3 Describe the four parts of a legal contract.

3.4 Identify the four Ds of negligence.

3.5 Describe the differences between the standards of care for a provider and a medical assistant.

3.6 Explain the difference between the medical assistant's scope of practice and standard of care.

3.7 Describe the three classifications for malpractice claims.

3.8 Explain the importance of insurance coverage for health care professionals.

3.9 Identify the rights of both the physician and the patient in the physician–patient relationship.

3.10 Summarize the Patient Care Partnership.

3.11 List the components of the Doctrine of Informed Consent.

3.12 Explain how a medical assistant may participate in litigation surrounding a medical malpractice case.

3.13 Identify steps to compliance reporting regarding public health statutes.

3.14 List areas that pertain to risk management in the medical office.

3.15 Describe how an individual's personal morals may affect professional performance.

3.16 Describe components of the Health Insurance Portability and Accountability Act (HIPAA).

Shandra Wilkinson is a registered medical assistant (RMA). On her way to work, she witnesses a severe multivehicle accident. Shandra stops to provide assistance. She performs CPR on a victim at the scene of the accident. The victim is revived and is transported to the emergency room by emergency medical technicians, who arrived later on the scene. Unfortunately, two of the other victims did not survive the injuries they sustained and died hours later at the local hospital. Shandra provides the police with a full account of her actions. Two months after the accident, she receives notification that the victim she assisted during the accident is planning to sue her because she broke a rib while performing CPR. He is suing for damages sustained from the result of the broken bone.

Terms to Learn

- abandonment
- administrative law
- advance directive
- arbitration
- bioethics
- breach of contract
- civil law
- contract law
- contributory negligence
- defamation of character
- defendant
- deposition
- emancipated minor
- ethics
- exploitation
- expressed consent
- Good Samaritan acts

- *guardian ad litem*
- Health Insurance Portability and Accountability Act (HIPAA)
- implied consent
- informed consent
- liable
- living will
- malfeasance
- malpractice
- mature minor
- medical durable power of attorney (MDPOA)
- misfeasance
- morals
- negligence
- nonfeasance
- patient incompetence

- Patient Self-Determination Act (PSDA)
- plaintiff
- practice of medicine
- proximate cause
- reasonable person standard
- *res ipsa loquitur*
- *respondeat superior*
- risk management
- rule of discovery
- subpoena
- *subpoena duces tecum*
- standard of care
- statute of limitations
- tort
- tortfeasor
- Uniform Anatomical Gift Act
- veracity

Today's health care consumers want to partner with the physician and the rest of the health care team in the management of their health needs. They want to be a part of the decision-making process regarding their care and treatment. The relationship between the patient, the patient's doctor, and others who participate in the patient's health care involves both legal and ethical considerations.

This chapter discusses issues such as malpractice, informed consent, and litigation, as well as specific regulations and documents that protect the patient, the patient's family, physicians, and medical staff involved in care and treatment. Other topics presented include the public duties of the physician, documentation in medical records and electronic health records, and the role of risk management in the medical office. The ethics of medical practice are also discussed. Later chapters will detail legal issues that relate to staffing and business operations.

CLASSIFICATION OF THE LAW

Laws may be considered to fall into four classifications:

- Criminal
- Civil
- International
- Military

Only criminal and civil law are discussed in this chapter because they can directly impact medical assistants. A medical assistant should be able to identify illegal actions that break either civil or criminal laws. This knowledge will enable the medical assistant to avoid or identify illegal activity, which unfortunately may occur, and, if it is observed, to report it to the appropriate authority.

Criminal Law

Criminal laws are made to protect individuals and the public as a whole from the harmful acts of others. Criminal acts fall into two categories: felony and misdemeanor. Conviction of a felony can carry a punishment of imprisonment in a state or federal prison or a death sentence. Murder, rape, robbery, and practicing medicine without a license are examples of felonious crimes. Misdemeanors are less serious offenses and carry a punishment of fines or imprisonment in jail for up to a year. They include traffic violations, disturbing the peace, and theft.

A physician's license may be revoked, or taken away, if that physician is convicted of a crime. Sexual misconduct, murder, and violating narcotics laws are all criminal convictions that have resulted in the revocation of a license to practice medicine.

The **practice of medicine** is defined as diagnosing and prescribing treatment or medication. As a medical assistant, you are not licensed to practice medicine and must make sure that you always assist the physician and do not try to diagnose or treat a patient's condition. A medical assistant who attempts to diagnose or treat a patient could be prosecuted for practicing medicine without a license.

Civil Law

Civil law concerns relationships between individuals or between individuals and the government. Civil law includes tort law, contract law, and administrative law. Tort law covers acts that result in harm to another person or another person's property. **Contract law** includes enforceable promises and agreements between two or more persons. **Administrative law** covers regulations that are set by governmental agencies. Health care employees are most frequently involved in cases of civil law, particularly tort and contract law.

Tort Law

A **tort** is a wrongful act, resulting in harm, that is committed by one person against another person or property. In medical law, to meet the definition of a tort, an individual must be able to prove damage or injury to the patient was caused by the physician or the physician's employee. A person who commits a tort is known as a **tortfeasor**.

Torts are classified as either unintentional or intentional. Intentional torts include assault, battery, false imprisonment, defamation of character, fraud, and invasion of privacy. Table 3-1 provides descriptions and examples of intentional torts.

TABLE 3-1 | Intentional Torts

Tort	Description	Example
Assault	The threat of bodily harm to another. Actual touching (battery) or injury does not have to occur for assault to take place.	Threatening to harm a patient or to perform a procedure for which the patient does not consent.
Battery	Actual bodily harm to another person without permission. This is also referred to as unlawful touching or touching without consent.	Performing surgery or a procedure without the informed consent (permission) of the patient.
False Imprisonment	A violation of the personal liberty of another person through unlawful restraint.	Refusing to allow a patient to leave an office, hospital, or medical facility when the patient requests.
Defamation of Character	Damage caused to a person's reputation through spoken or written word.	Making a negative statement about another physician's ability.
Fraud	Deceitful practice.	Promising a miracle cure.
Invasion of Privacy	The unauthorized publicizing of information about a patient.	Allowing personal information, such as test results for HIV, to become public without the patient's permission.
Slander	When a defaming statement about another person is spoken.	Implying or claiming that a physician is involved in illegal business practices or fraudulent billing where this is no basis for the claims.
Libel	When a defaming statement about another person is made in writing.	Stating that a physician has been unfaithful to her marriage partner and is having an affair with a coworker.

The most common unintentional tort in the health care arena is **negligence**. Negligence is the failure to do or perform a specific action, which results in injury to another person. A health care professional must exercise the type of care that a "reasonable" person with similar training would use in a similar circumstance. This is known as the **reasonable person standard**.

Negligence is often the key factor in a medical malpractice lawsuit. To obtain a judgment for negligence against a physician or other health care professional, the patient must be able to show proof of what is referred to as the "four Ds of negligence" as listed here. (Box 3-1 defines the four Ds with regard to a physician.)

- Duty
- Dereliction or neglect of duty
- Direct cause
- Damages

When negligence is charged, the **plaintiff** (the person who files the lawsuit) must prove **proximate cause**. This means that the plaintiff must prove that the defendant's act(s) (or failure to act) directly caused the injury. The **defendant** is the person who has been charged with wrongdoing, and as the term implies, he must defend himself. For example, if a patient returns home after having prostate surgery and experiences persistent and severe leg pains that were not present before having the surgery, the patient must prove that the physician's performance of the prostate surgery was the cause of the leg pains. **Contributory negligence** relates to the patient's contribution to the injury. If it has been proven that the patient contributed to the deterioration of medical status (e.g., the patient did not keep follow-up appointments, causing an undetected infection to advance), the physician could be released of either a portion or all of the damages that are being sought by the patient.

Negligence is easier to prevent than it is to defend. Physicians and other health care professionals can take steps to avoid negligence suits by:

- Fostering a mutually respectful and honorable relationship with the patient
- Being above reproach (blame, disgrace) in the performance of their medical duties

CONTRACT LAW

Contract law is generally concerned with a breach or the neglect of an understanding between two parties.

A contract is a voluntary agreement that two parties enter into with the intent of mutual benefit for both parties. A contract can be implied from the behavior or action of a person (implied contract), or the contract can be expressed in writing or verbally (expressed contract). A contract between two parties is composed of four parts:

- **Offer**—An individual makes the effort to provide services. For example, a physician opens a medical practice to offer medical services to patients in the local community.
- **Acceptance**—Another individual accepts the first person's offer. For example, the patient makes an appointment to see a physician. The patient agrees to see the physician in a certain office at a certain time.
- **Consideration**—This occurs when something of value is exchanged. A physician provides the service, and the patient pays for the service.
- **Competence**—Both parties involved in the contract must be competent individuals, able to fully understand that they are entering into a contractual agreement. **Patient incompetence** refers to a patient's lack of decision-making ability. Those who would be

BOX 3-2 | Premature Termination of the Physician–Patient Contract

Proper documentation is key to avoiding lawsuits, and having proper documentation is essential when defending a lawsuit. The following situations should always be clearly documented in the patient's medical record. It is important to always include the date and time of the incident and discussions with the patient related to the incident.

- Failure to pay for service.
- Missed appointments.

- Failure to follow instructions or a prescribed course of treatment, which causes harm to the patient's health.
- The patient states (orally or in writing) that he is seeking the care of another physician. There are many reasons that a patient might switch physicians, including a change in the patient's insurance whereby the patient's physician is no longer covered, or the patient may move and not be able to travel to the physician's office.

considered incompetent to enter into an agreement include minors, mentally incapacitated adults, or those who do not speak the native language of the other party. For example, a person who does not speak English would not be held **liable** (legally responsible) for entering a contract agreement that was either written or verbally discussed in English because they would not be able to understand what was being agreed upon.

For a contract to be legal, several considerations are relevant. For one, the concerned party (e.g., the patient) must be mentally competent at the time the contract is made. For example, the patient must not be under the influence of drugs or alcohol at the time the contract is entered. A **breach of contract** occurs when either party fails to comply with the terms of the agreement. In the previous example, a breach of contract would occur if the patient failed to pay the agreed-upon fee.

Abandonment. **Abandonment** occurs if a physician has agreed to take care of a patient but improperly terminates the contract. A physician may choose to end the physician–patient contract for legitimate reasons, including failure to pay medical bills or failure to comply with a prescribed course of treatment. However, if the proper steps are not followed in ending the physician–patient contract, the physician may be charged with patient abandonment. A physician choosing to discontinue the treatment of a patient should notify the patient in writing. This is usually done by sending a certified letter with return receipt via the U.S. Postal Service. The letter should indicate that the physician is willing to continue treatment, generally for a period of 30 days, in order to allow the patient to seek the services of another physician. A copy of the certified letter and the return receipt should be saved in the patient's medical record.

Termination of contract. The termination of the contract between a physician and a patient generally occurs when the treatment has ended and the fee has been paid. However,

serious issues may arise around premature termination of a physician–patient contract. It should be noted that both physicians and patients have the right to terminate the contractual relationship. Letters from the physician should indicate the date the physician's services will be terminated. The medical assistant needs to understand these situations and handle them correctly (Box 3-2).

PROFESSIONAL LIABILITY

Lawsuits related to health care have greatly increased during the past decade, and the average liability award granted to a plaintiff who prevails in a medical malpractice case is now over $1 million. Professional liability is determined by the federal, state, and local laws governing the physician–patient relationship and relates to the standard of care, legal contracts, and informed consent. An important issue in the question of liability is the physician–employee relationship. Some factors impacting this relationship are discussed here. They include *respondeat superior*, standard of care, malpractice, *res ipsa loquitur*, statute of limitations, Good Samaritan laws, and defamation of character.

Respondeat Superior

Physician-employers are especially concerned that their employees have a complete understanding of the law. The Latin term **respondeat superior** literally means "Let the master answer." This means that the physician is liable for negligent actions committed by that physician's employees. In some cases and in some states, both the physician and the employee may be held liable.

In effect, under *respondeat superior*, the physician delegates certain duties to you, the medical assistant, and if you perform them incorrectly, the ultimate liability rests with the physician-employer. However, medical assistants and other health care workers can also be named in malpractice suits. For example, if you are authorized by your employer to draw a sample of blood from a patient and you inadvertently enter a nerve, causing permanent damage to the patient's arm, then you may also be liable for that patient's injury.

Because the physician's medical license is jeopardized when errors are made, and because you, as a medical assistant, can also be held liable, it is vital that you have an understanding of the laws in your state.

Originally, malpractice insurance was purchased only by physicians. Now, however, many medical assistants purchase professional (malpractice) insurance as well. This is discussed later in the chapter in the section on medical malpractice insurance.

Physician's Standard of Care

Although a physician is under no obligation to treat everyone, once a patient is accepted for treatment, the physician has then entered into the physician–patient relationship and must provide a certain standard of care. This **standard of care** asserts that the physician must provide the same knowledge, care, and skill that a similarly trained physician would provide under the same circumstances in the same locality. The law requires only reasonable, ordinary care and skill.

The physician is expected to perform the same acts that a "reasonable and prudent" physician would. This standard also states that a physician will not perform any acts that a "reasonable and prudent" physician would not. Physicians are expected to exhaust all the resources available when they are treating a patient. These would include the following:

- Taking a thorough medical history
- Performing a complete physical examination
- Ordering and evaluating the necessary laboratory tests and imaging procedures

Physicians are not expected to expose their patients to undue risk. If this standard of care is violated, the physician is liable for negligence.

Medical Assistant's Standard of Care

As a medical assistant, you must remember that your actions can have legal consequences for the physician who employs you. If you work outside the scope of practice for medical assistants in your state, you are at risk of being sued by a patient or the patient's family. You are not held to the same standard of care as a physician, because of differing credentials, licensure, and education. However, you will carry out your duties under the direction of a physician, and therefore, you must use the same approved methods that a physician would use. For example, you must uphold the same standard of quality as any physician would when taking an electrocardiogram, drawing blood, and collecting specimens.

A medical assistant is not allowed to diagnose medical conditions, interpret electrocardiograms, or prescribe medications, because these are all within the area of the physician's scope of practice (the normal range of duties and activities of a physician). In fact, medical assistants must continually use caution and be careful not to take on any tasks or duties for which they are not trained and that do not lie within the scope of practice of a medical assistant in the state where they are employed.

The actions of medical assistants reflect on their physician-employers. Many duties performed by medical assistants could result in harm to the patient if not done properly. In some lawsuits, the physician has been found guilty of negligence because of improper performance of the medical assistant.

Malpractice

Professional misconduct or demonstration of an unreasonable lack of skill that results in injury, loss, or damage to the patient is considered **malpractice**.

Malpractice claims are classified according to the manner in which the wrongful act was committed. The classifications include:

- **Malfeasance**—Performing a wrongful or illegal act
- **Misfeasance**—Performing a lawful act but not in the proper way
- **Nonfeasance**—Being negligent or ignoring performance of a necessary lawful act

Table 3-2 lists the types of damages that may be awarded to patients in medical malpractice suits.

Not every mistake or error, however, is considered malpractice. When a treatment or diagnosis does not turn out well, the physician is not necessarily liable. The physician would not be liable for a poor outcome if it can be shown that he treated the patient according to the standard of care and scope of practice for a physician and that he is not guilty of malfeasance, misfeasance, or nonfeasance. The physician-employer and all staff must each act within the standard of care appropriate for their particular practice of medicine. All health care providers are held to this same standard.

Malpractice Insurance

In modern times, all physicians are expected to carry malpractice insurance. The cost of malpractice insurance varies based on the following considerations:

- How much coverage is the physician requesting? A physician who wants a $5,000,000 coverage policy pays more than a physician who purchases a $2,500,000 policy.

TABLE 3-2 | Penalties in Malpractice Suits

Type of Damages	Purpose	Example
Punitive Damages	Meant to punish the person for behavior.	A manufacturer dumps toxins into the water supply and might be given a high fine to prevent further occurrence.
Nominal Damages	A penalty that is not a high monetary value is given to punish.	A behavior leads to a loss of life. The defendant may be sentenced to write a letter weekly to the family to remind the person of the damage caused.
Compensatory Damages	A penalty, usually monetary, to compensate the person for damage.	A physician might be ordered to pay for the medical and rehabilitation bills of a patient the physician has injured.

- Where is the physician practicing medicine? The cost of malpractice insurance is greater in certain states or in highly populated metropolitan areas.

- What type of medicine is practiced by the physician? A general practitioner pays less for an insurance policy than an obstetrician (a physician who specializes in treating pregnant women and delivering babies) because obstetrics is considered a high-risk specialty.

Physicians can decide which type of insurance they would like to carry. The type of insurance that they choose also impacts the cost. The types of coverage include:

- **Occurrence coverage**—This covers the physician for any claim for an incident that occurred while the insurance policy was in effect, even if the physician has different coverage when the claim is filed.

- **Claims-made coverage**—This covers the physician only if the company that insured the physician at the time of the incident is the same company that insures the physician when the claim is made. If a claim is made for an alleged incident that took place before the physician's claims-made coverage, the claim would not be covered. Because of this risk, a physician may purchase additional insurance termed "tail-coverage."

- **Tail-coverage**—If a physician cancels a claims-made policy, she may choose to purchase tail-coverage, which will cover any claims that allege actions occurred during the time the physician was covered under claims-made coverage.

- **Prior-acts coverage**—This covers any claims made before the time that the physician had a claims-made policy.

To be sure that physicians are covered for occurrences before and after the insured years, complete coverage from beginning to end of career is also available. In most cases, employers carry insurance to cover acts of their employees while performing their duties. This is termed *general liability coverage*. Employees should request to see their employer's certificate of insurance to determine policy coverage.

To cover any negligence on the part of their staff, including medical assistants, some physicians carry a rider, an additional clause to their professional liability or malpractice policy. Once again, it is important for the medical assistant to determine the type of coverage the physician-employer carries and to clarify coverage. Medical assistants who are not covered by the employer's malpractice policy may choose to purchase professional liability coverage from an insurance carrier who specializes in this type of coverage. By purchasing liability coverage, the medical assistant minimizes personal liability and risk. Ultimately, the employer is responsible for the actions of the employee (*respondeat superior*). However, it is important to be sure you have insurance coverage because, as noted earlier, both the employer and the employee may be sued for the action of the employee.

Res Ipsa Loquitur

The doctrine of **res ipsa loquitur**, which translated from Latin means "the thing speaks for itself," applies to the law of negligence. This doctrine defines a breach (neglect) of duty that is so obvious that it does not need further explanation, or "it speaks for itself." For instance, leaving a sponge in the patient's abdomen during abdominal surgery or operating on the wrong body part are examples of *res ipsa loquitur*. None of these examples would have occurred without the negligence of someone involved in the procedure. It is difficult, if not impossible, to defend against a suit in which *res ipsa loquitur* applies.

Statute of Limitations

A **statute of limitations** defines the period of time during which a patient may file a lawsuit. The court will not hear a case that is filed after the time limit has run out. Statutes of limitations vary from state to state; the time periods within which a suit may be brought vary from one to six years in different states.

The time period within which a suit may be brought does not always start when the treatment is administered. It may begin when the problem is discovered, which may be some time after the actual treatment. This is known as the **rule of discovery**.

Here is a true example. A physician accidentally left a surgical sponge in a patient's abdomen during an operation. After 16 years of abdominal discomfort, the patient required more surgery, but the physician who had performed the original operation had died. Another surgeon performed the second surgery, found the sponge, and removed it. The patient then sued the estate of the original surgeon for malpractice and won because the allowable period of time for a suit under the statute of limitations, which was two years in that state, started when the sponge was discovered, not when the original medical error was committed.

Occasionally, a state's statute of limitations is prevented from coming into play. This occurs when the injury is to a minor child. Generally, the court will appoint a **guardian ad litem**, an adult who will act in court on behalf of the child. However, the child does not have to sue through a *guardian ad litem* as a minor but may wait until reaching adulthood. In such a case, an obstetrician and the medical assistants can be sued 21 years and 9 months (plus the statute of limitations period in that state) after a birth injury occurred.

Good Samaritan Acts

Good Samaritan acts are state laws that help to protect a health care professional from liability while that professional is giving emergency care to an accident victim. Such laws are in effect in all states to encourage physicians and other health care professionals to offer cardiopulmonary resuscitation (CPR) and first aid, as needed, at the scene of an accident. Persons responding in an emergency situation are only required to act within the limits of their skill and training. A medical assistant would be neither expected, nor advised, to perform emergency treatment that is within the area practiced by physicians and nurses.

Providing care at the scene of an accident is generally voluntary. No one is required to provide aid in the event of an emergency, except in the state of Vermont, where "a person who knows another is exposed to grave physical harm" is required to give reasonable assistance if it is safe to do so.

Defamation of Character

Defamation of character is a scandalous statement about someone that can injure the person's reputation. Defamation can occur even when the statement is true if *malice* is proven,

meaning if it can be shown that the true statement was made with the intention of causing injury to someone.

As a medical assistant, you will have access to privileged information about patients that may seem harmless, but in reality, the information could be very damaging to their reputations. For instance, a patient who undergoes a test for an infectious disease, such as hepatitis or AIDS, may not wish an employer to know the test took place, even if the test result is negative. If you call the patient's place of employment and leave a message regarding a test result of this nature, the action could be considered a breach of confidentiality and defamation.

The simple act of a physician seeing a patient for an appointment must also be kept confidential. The medical assistant should not fax such information or leave messages of this kind on answering machines unless specifically instructed to do so in writing by the patient. Specific instructions, including what types of messages are allowed, should be documented in the patient's medical record.

To protect yourself and avoid involvement in a lawsuit, you must practice your skills with care, be concerned about maintaining good public relations with patients and other staff members, and understand the law. Always ask your supervisor for guidance on the appropriate action to take.

PATIENT AND PHYSICIAN RELATIONSHIP

Both the physician and the patient must agree to form a relationship if there is to be a contract for service and treatment. To receive proper treatment, the patient must confide truthfully in the physician regarding all aspects of his or her health. Failure to state all the facts may result in serious consequences for the patient. The physician is not liable if the patient has withheld critical information that directly affects medical care.

Physician Rights

Physicians have the right to select the patients they wish to treat. They also have the right to refuse service to patients. From an ethical standpoint, most physicians do treat patients who need their skills. This is particularly true in cases of emergency.

Physicians also have the right to decide the type of services they provide, where their offices are located, and their open hours of operation. The physician has the right to expect payment for treatment given.

Physicians have a right to take vacations and time off from their practices. Care must be taken to inform patients if their physician will be unavailable. In most cases, another physician will cover or take care of a colleague's patients.

Patient Rights

The patient has the right to give consent, or permission, for all treatment. Consent is either expressed or implied. **Expressed consent** occurs when the patient consents to a procedure or treatment either verbally or in writing, as with the case of informed consent, which is discussed next. **Implied consent** is based on the patient's action and is not expressed verbally or in writing. For example, when a patient comes in for a routine examination for medical treatment, there is implied consent that the physician will touch the person during the examination. Generally, touching someone without the person's consent is referred to as battery. Therefore, the touching required for the examination would not be considered a crime of battery because consent for the action is implied by the nature of the appointment.

In giving consent for treatment, the patient reasonably expects that the physician will use the appropriate standard of care in providing care and treatment. Patients also expect that all information and records about their cases will be kept confidential by the physician and staff. The patient's right to privacy prohibits the presence of unauthorized persons during physical examinations or treatments.

In addition to these rights, the patient also has certain obligations. For example, the patient is expected to follow the instructions given by the physician. In addition, the patient is expected to pay the physician for medical services.

The Right to Refuse Treatment

Patients have the right to refuse treatment. Different cultural and religious groups must be accommodated, if necessary. Members of some religious groups, such as Jehovah's Witnesses and Christian Scientists, do not wish to receive blood transfusions or certain types of medical treatment. If they are adults, they should not receive the treatment against their wishes. In the case of a minor child, the court may appoint a guardian who can then give consent for the procedure if it is deemed to be in the child's best interest.

A patient might also refuse a treatment because that patient views the side effects associated with treatment to be more harmful or worse to deal with than the condition that requires treatment. It is not uncommon for some patients in advanced stages of cancer with metastasis to refuse chemotherapy and radiation treatments because they believe the quality of their remaining life would be diminished. A common belief is that the quality of one's life is more valuable than the quantity (length in years) of life.

Patients in hospital settings may often be discouraged about their treatment or prognosis or may simply hate being in the hospital. Those patients may choose to leave the hospital of their own free will. To hold someone against their will is considered false imprisonment. If a patient leaves the hospital against physician's orders, the patient is considered to be leaving AMA, against medical advice. Such patients are required to sign a document stating that they are aware of the risks associated with leaving and that they will not hold the hospital or physicians liable for any repercussions that may arise from their decision to leave.

The Patient Care Partnership

The Patient Care Partnership (formerly called the Patients' Bill of Rights) is a concept that details what you, as a patient, should expect during your hospital stay, principally:

- High-quality hospital care
- A clean and safe environment
- Your involvement in your care (This includes involvement surrounding treatment options; you must understand that you have a right to choose your treatment options, the right to consent to treatment, and, as discussed earlier, the right to refuse treatment.)
- Protection of your privacy
- Help when leaving the hospital
- Help with your billing claims

Although the Patient Care Partnership concepts pertain specifically to hospitalization, physician offices should operate on the understanding that their patients have similar rights. In fact, most medical practices adopt these rights for their patient population. As a medical assistant, you should be able to discuss with a patient, before hospitalization, what that patient has a right to expect during the hospital stay.

Informed Consent

The patient should expect to receive information concerning the advantages and potential risks of all treatments and procedures. **Informed consent** means that the patient is instructed about the possible consequences both of having and of not having certain procedures and treatments. The physician must carefully explain that in some cases, the treatment may even make the patient's condition worse.

The Doctrine of Informed Consent (Figure 3-1) includes the following:

- Explanation of advantages and risks to the treatment
- Alternatives available to the patient
- Potential outcomes to the treatment
- What might occur without treatment
- The use of understandable language

PEARSON GENERAL HOSPITAL

COMPLETE ORIGINAL IN INK FOR HOSPITAL CHART
PATIENT MUST BE AWAKE, ALERT AND ORIENTED WHEN SIGNING

DATE: _____ TIME: _____ ☐ AM ☐ PM

I AUTHORIZE THE PERFORMANCE UPON _____

OF THE FOLLOWING OPERATION (state nature and extent): _____

_____

_____

TO BE PERFORMED UNDER THE DIRECTION OF DR. _____

1. I HAVE BEEN ADVISED THAT THERE IS A FAVORABLE LIKELIHOOD OF SUCCESS, BUT I UNDERSTAND THAT A COMPLETELY SUCCESSFUL OUTCOME MAY NOT BE ACHIEVABLE, AND THERE ARE NO GUARANTEES REGARDING THE OUTCOME. I ALSO UNDERSTAND THAT CERTAIN ADVERSE EVENTS COULD OCCUR AS A RESULT OF THE PERFORMANCE OF THE PROCEDURE OR TREATMENT, INCLUDING PAIN, INFECTION, LACERATION OR PUNCTURE OF INTERNAL ORGANS, BLEEDING, NERVE DAMAGE OR EVEN IN RARE CASES, DEATH. I UNDERSTAND THAT HOSPITALIZATION OR OTHER INSTITUTIONAL CARE, HOME CARE OR CARE BY HEALTH PROFESSIONALS MAY BE NEEDED FOLLOWING THE PROCEDURE OR TREATMENT, RELATED TO FULL RECOVERY, RECUPERATION OR CONVALESCENCE. I UNDERSTAND THE ALTERNATIVES TO THIS PROCEDURE, INCLUDING MY RIGHT TO REFUSE TO CONSENT TO IT, AND I NEVERTHELESS HAVE DECIDED TO CONSENT TO PERFORMANCE OF THE PROCEDURE OR TREATMENT.

2. I CONSENT TO THE PERFORMANCE OF OPERATIONS AND PROCEDURES IN ADDITION TO OR DIFFERENT FROM THOSE NOW CONTEMPLATED, WHETHER OR NOT ARISING FROM PRESENTLY UNFORESEEN CONDITIONS WHICH THE ABOVE NAMED DOCTOR OR HIS/HER ASSOCIATES OR ASSISTANTS MAY CONSIDER NECESSARY OR ADVISABLE IN THE COURSE OF THE OPERATION.

3. I CONSENT TO THE DISPOSAL BY HOSPITAL AUTHORITIES OF ANY TISSUES OR PARTS WHICH MAY BE REMOVED.

4. THE NATURE AND PURPOSE OF THE OPERATION/PROCEDURE, POSSIBLE ALTERNATIVE METHODS OF TREATMENT, THE RISK AND BENEFITS INVOLVED, AND THE COURSE OF RECUPERATION HAVE BEEN FULLY EXPLAINED TO ME. NO GUARANTEE OR ASSURANCE HAS BEEN GIVEN BY ANYONE AS TO THE RESULTS THAT MAY BE OBTAINED.

5. I UNDERSTAND AND AGREE WITH THE ABOVE INFORMATION. I HAVE NO QUESTIONS WHICH HAVE NOT BEEN ANSWERED TO MY FULL SATISFACTION. I UNDERSTAND THAT I HAVE THE RIGHT TO ASK FOR FURTHER INFORMATION BEFORE SIGNING THIS CONSENT.

I have crossed out any paragraph above which does not apply or to which I do not give consent.

PATIENT SIGNATURE: _____   WITNESS SIGNATURE: _____
(OR PARENT OR GUARDIAN IF PATIENT IS UNDER 18 YEARS OF AGE)   *(OF PATIENT, PARENT OR GUARDIAN SIGNATURE)*

RELATIONSHIP: _____   WITNESS SIGNATURE: _____
                                          ☐ **TELEPHONE CONSENT** *(2ND WITNESS NEEDED FOR TELEPHONE CONSENT)*

FIGURE 3-1 Sample of an informed consent to perform an operation, sedation, anesthesia, and other medical services.

It is very difficult to fully inform a patient about all the things that can go wrong with a treatment. In an emergency situation, during which the patient is not able to understand the explanation or sign a consent form, a physician is protected by law to provide care. A physician cannot delegate the duty of obtaining informed consent to another person except in emergency situations. Even then, after the emergency is under control, it is important to find a responsible party with whom to discuss patient issues if the patient is unable to give consent. Sometimes consent for procedures is given by relatives or those holding medical proxies, which allow the person to act in the best interests of the patient if the patient is unable to give an informed consent. (See "Durable Power of Attorney" later in this chapter for more information.) Frequently, patients are asked at office visits to declare names of relatives or friends with whom the physician can discuss patient care. This is an important document

not only for determining with whom the physician can share information on an ongoing basis but also for identifying whom to consult in an emergency situation (Figure 3-2).

Does a signed informed-consent form protect both the physician and the staff from lawsuits? The answer generally is yes. As long as the physician has carefully explained the treatment or procedure and the patient acknowledges the risks involved by signing the consent form, some protection from lawsuits is usually in place. Here, the assumption-of-risk defense is often applied. This means that if a patient signs an informed-consent form but tries later to sue the physician for something that was clearly discussed before the procedure, the patient is considered to have assumed the risk of something going wrong. This takes a lot of the burden off the physician when making a case in court. However, this doesn't always win the case for the physician. There have been instances when patients who had been presented

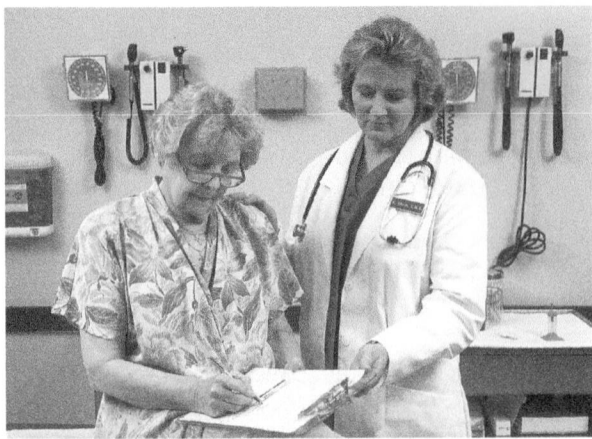

FIGURE 3-2 The patient's signature on the informed consent form indicates that the patient understands the limits and risks involved in the treatment or surgical procedure as explained by the physician.

the risks of a procedure and signed the form nevertheless sued and won a case against the physician when the treatment failed.

Informed-consent forms used in outpatient surgical and procedural facilities may be shorter in length and content than those used in physicians' offices. However, each state mandates unique exceptions to the informed consent doctrine. The following are the more general exceptions:

- A physician does not have to inform a patient about risks that are commonly known—for example, that a patient could choke while swallowing a pill.

- A physician who feels the disclosure of risks may be detrimental to the patient is not responsible for disclosing them. This might occur if a patient has a severe heart condition that may be worsened by an announcement of risks from a needed treatment.

- If the patient requests the physician not to disclose the risks, then the physician is not responsible for failing to do so.

Medical Assistant's Responsibility with Informed Consent

The medical assistant has the following responsibilities with regard to informed consent.

- The physician must thoroughly explain all procedures to the patient. The medical assistant is responsible for making sure a signed consent form has been obtained and placed in the patient chart. Never have the patient sign a document that she does not understand.

- Obtain a parent's or guardian's signature before any procedure is performed on a minor. The only exception is in a case of emergency, when the parent or guardian cannot be reached. File the signed consent form immediately.

Rights of Minors

A minor is considered a person who has not reached the age of majority. The age of majority varies from state to state but usually is 18. In most states, minors are unable to give consent for treatment. Exceptions are special cases involving pregnancy, request for birth control information, abortion, testing and treatment for sexually transmitted diseases, problems with substance abuse, and a need for psychiatric care. Two types of minors can give consent for treatment:

A **mature minor** is a young person, generally under the age of 18, who possesses the maturity to understand the nature and consequences of the treatment. **Emancipated minors** are those who have the same legal capacity as an adult under any of the following five conditions:

- They live on their own.

- They are married.

- They are self-supporting.

- They are in the armed forces.

- Any combination of these conditions.

Because not all states recognize the categories of mature minors and emancipated minors, it is wise to be familiar with the laws of your state and to handle consent on a case-by-case basis. The following are some legal implications to consider when treating a minor.

- **Right to confidentiality**—A 16-year-old girl who is seeking birth control information has a right to have her records remain confidential.

- **Financial responsibility**—The 16-year-old girl seeking birth control information may not be able to pay for the office visit. Contacting her parents for payment may breach confidentiality.

- **Minor's legal guardian**—Legal guardianship is sometimes difficult to determine if the child lives with the mother but the father is financially responsible for care and treatment, or vice versa. However, the legal guardian must always be determined and documented in the patient's medical record. In the case of divorce, the legal guardian is the individual a court has declared to be responsible. Sometimes both parents share custody in a divorce; sometimes there is only one legal guardian. If there is one legal guardian, the other parent may be informed of some kinds of information regarding the patient but not others. The physician may choose to speak with an attorney about how to handle complex issues that may arise when one parent has custody and the other wants information.

Patient Self-Determination Act

The **Patient Self-Determination Act (PSDA)**, enacted in 1990, mandates that health care institutions encourage patients to make advance decisions regarding the type of care and services they wish to have (or deny) in the event, in the future, that they are unable to make health care decisions because of illness. Several documents, recognized by the PSDA, when executed by the patient provide protection for both the patient and physician. These documents include the living will, the durable power of attorney, and the Uniform Anatomical Gift Act card.

Living Will

The **living will** (Figure 3-3) allows patients to designate, in advance, which forms of treatments and nutritional support intended to prolong the patient's life either may be used or may not be used. This document gives patients the legal right to direct the type of care they wish to receive or wish not to receive when their death is imminent. The document provides protection for physicians and hospitals when they follow the patient's wishes. This process is often discussed in the physician's office with patients when they are capable of making the decision. Other family members or significant others can also be part of the discussion and decision. One copy of the living will should be kept with the patient's record. A living will is very similar to an **advance directive**, but the advance directive generally includes not only the living will but also the durable power of attorney. A sample of an advance directive and additional information are provided in the chapter titled "Assisting with Life Span Specialties: Geriatrics."

Durable Power of Attorney

The durable power of attorney (DPOA), when signed by the patient, names an agent or representative who may act on behalf of the patient. If the patient wishes to assign an agent for health care only, then that agent may make only health-care-related decisions on behalf of the patient and is termed a **medical durable power of attorney (MDPOA)**. This agent may be a spouse, grown child, friend, or, in some cases, an attorney.

The DPOA or MDPOA is a safeguard that someone will be able to act on the patient's behalf if the patient becomes physically or mentally incapacitated. This document is in effect until the patient cancels it. A copy of the signed document should be kept with the patient's record. The DPOA or MDPOA acts on behalf of the patient until the patient is again capable of making his or her own decisions. Figure 3-4 shows a medical durable power of attorney.

Uniform Anatomical Gift Act

The **Uniform Anatomical Gift Act** allows persons 18 years or older and of sound mind to make a gift of any or all parts of their body for purposes of organ transplantation or medical research at the time of death. Two regulations that are held within this act include:

- The physician performing the transplant operation cannot be the same physician to determine death or the time of death.
- Money is not allowed to change hands for the purpose of organ donation.

The donor carries a card that has been signed in the presence of two witnesses (Figure 3-5). In some states the driver's license has an option to indicate the desire to be an organ donor with space for a signature.

In some cases, the family will make the decision for organ donation if a formal decision was not made while the donor was alive. It is generally agreed that if a member of the family opposes the donation of organs, then the physician and hospital do not insist on it.

DOCUMENTATION

The medical record, either electronic or paper, is considered a legal document. Therefore, complete and accurate documentation is absolutely necessary. There's a useful saying many health care professionals keep in mind: *If it isn't written, it wasn't done.* Carefully document all calls, visits, treatments, no-shows, appointment cancellations, medications, prescription refills, vital signs, and other pertinent information in the patient's medical record. If an action is not recorded in the medical record, then it is considered by most courts not to have been performed.

Use of Records in Litigation

Litigation is the term for a lawsuit tried in court. For purposes of litigation, a court of law may subpoena a medical record. A **subpoena** is an order to appear in court. Should you or your employing physician receive a *subpoena duces tecum* (an order to appear in court and to bring with you certain medical records or materials for trial), remember that only the records specifically stated in the subpoena are required; the entire medical record does not need to be sent.

Unless the original record is subpoenaed, a certified photocopy may be sent. A receipt for the subpoenaed record should then be placed in the patient's medical record. The patient should also be notified that the record has been subpoenaed. Both the subpoenaed record and the notification to the patient should be sent by certified mail.

LIVING WILL OF _____

I, _____, a resident of the City of _____,

_____ County, State of _____, being of sound and dispos-
ing mind, memory and understanding, do hereby willfully and voluntarily make, publish, and declare this to
be my LIVING WILL, making known my desire that my life shall not be artificially prolonged under the
circumstances set forth below, and do hereby declare:

1. This instrument is directed to my family, my physician(s), my attorney, my clergyman, any medical facility in
   whose care I happen to be, and to any individual who may become responsible for my health, welfare, or
   affairs.

2. Death is as much a reality as birth, growth, maturity, and old age. It is the one certainty of life. Let this
   statement stand as an expression of my wishes now that I am still of sound mind, for the time when I may
   no longer take part in decisions for my own future.

3. If at any time I should have a terminal condition and my attending physician has determined that there can
   be no recovery from such condition and my death is imminent, where the application of life-prolonging
   procedures and "heroic measures" would serve only to artificially prolong the dying process, I direct that
   such procedures be withheld or withdrawn, and that I be permitted to die naturally. I do not fear death
   itself as much as the indignities of deterioration, dependence, and hopeless pain. I therefore ask that
   medication be mercifully administered to me and that any medical procedures be performed on me which
   are deemed necessary to provide me with comfort or care or to alleviate pain.

4. In the absence of my ability to give directions regarding the use of such life-prolonging procedures, it is my
   intention that this declaration shall be honored by my family and physician as the final expression of my
   legal right to refuse medical or surgical treatment and accept the consequences for such refusal.

5. In the event that I am diagnosed as comatose, incompetent, or otherwise mentally or physically incapable of
   communication, I appoint _____ to
   make binding decisions concerning my medical treatment.

6. If I have been diagnosed as pregnant and my physician knows that diagnosis, this declaration shall have no
   force or effect during the course of my pregnancy.

7. I understand the full import of this declaration and I am emotionally and mentally competent to make this
   declaration. I hope you, who care for me, will feel morally bound to follow its mandate. I recognize that this
   appears to place a heavy responsibility on you, but it is with the intention of relieving you of such responsibility and of placing it on myself, in accordance with my strong convictions, that this statement is made.

IN WITNESS WHEREOF, I have hereunto subscribed my name and affixed my seal at _____,

_____, this _____ day of _____, 20 _____, in the presence of the
subscribing witnesses whom I have requested to become attesting witnesses hereto. _____

                                                                              Declarant

The declarant is known to me and I believe him/her to be of sound mind.

_____

_____Witness   Address

_____

_____Witness   Address

Subscribed and acknowledged, before me by _____, and subscribed and sworn

    to before the witnesses, on the _____ day of _____, 20_____.

_____

(SEAL)

NOTARY PUBLIC State of _____ My Commission
    Expires:_____

Copies of this instrument have been given to:

Receipt and acknowledged & date:

FIGURE 3-3 Living will.

MEDICAL DURABLE POWER OF ATTORNEY

I, _____,
(Printed or typed full name)
am of sound mind, and I voluntarily make this designation. I designate _____,
(insert name of patient advocate) my _____, (Spouse, child, friend . . .) living at _____
(Address of patient advocate) as my patient advocate to make care, custody and medical treatment decisions for me
in the event I become unable to participate in medical treatment decisions. If my first choice cannot serve, I
designate
_____ (Name of successor) living at _____
_____
_____ (Address of successor) to serve as patient advocate.

The determination of when I am unable to participate in medical treatment decisions shall be made by my attending
physician and another physician or licensed psychologist.

In making decisions for me, my patient advocate shall follow my wishes of which he or she is aware, whether
expressed orally, in a living will, or in this designation.

My patient advocate has authority to consent to or refuse treatment on my behalf, to arrange medical services for
me, including admission to a hospital or nursing care facility, and to pay for such services with my funds. My patient
advocate shall have access to any of my medical records to which I have a right.

My specific wishes concerning health care are the following: (if none, write "none")
_____
_____
_____
_____
_____
_____

I may change my mind at any time by communicating in any manner that this designation does not reflect my
wishes.

It is my intent that my family, the medical facility, and any doctors, nurses and other medical personnel involved in
my care shall have no civil or criminal liability for honoring my wishes as expressed in this designation or for
implementing the decisions of my patient advocate.

Photostatic copies of this document, after it is signed and witnessed, shall have the same legal force as the original
document.

I sign this document after careful consideration. I understand its meaning and I accept its consequences.

Signed: _____ Date: _____
Address: _____

NOTICE REGARDING WITNESSES

You must have two adult witnesses who will not receive your assets when you die (whether you die with or without a
will), and who are not your spouse, child, grandchild, brother or sister, an employee of a company through which
you have life or health insurance, or an employee at the health care facility where you are a patient.

STATEMENT OF WITNESSES

We sign below as witnesses. This declaration was signed in our presence.

The declarant appears to be of sound mind, and to be making this designation voluntarily, without duress, fraud or
undue influence.

Signed by witness: _____
(Print or type full name)
Address: _____
Signed by witness: _____
(Print or type full name)
Address: _____

FIGURE 3-4 Medical durable power of attorney.

```
┌─────────────────────────────────────────────────────────┐
│                    Uniform Donor Card                     │
│                                                           │
│  I,_____ , have spoken to my      │
│  family about organ and tissue donation. The following   │
│  people have witnessed my commitment to be a donor. I     │
│  wish to donate the following:                            │
│  ◯ any needed organs and tissue                           │
│  ◯ only the following organs and tissue:_____     │
│  Donor Signature:_____ Date:_____   │
│  Witness:_____  │
│  Witness:_____  │
│  Next of Kin:_____  │
│  Telephone:(___)_____  │
└─────────────────────────────────────────────────────────┘
```

FIGURE 3-5 Organ donor card.

Court Testimony

Not everyone who has information relating to a case will be called into court to testify. An attorney may interrogate, or ask questions, of a witness. Another means of obtaining information from a witness to be used during a court case is to submit a **deposition**. In this case, a written statement is taken of oral testimony given in front of a court officer. The person who gives the oral testimony and then signs a deposition is not required to actually appear in court. An attorney submits the deposition during the court case. Arraignment occurs when a defendant is called before the court to answer a charge.

An expert witness is a person called on to testify in court regarding the proper standard of care for a patient in a similar community. An expert witness in a medical malpractice suit is generally a physician.

In the event that you are called on to appear in court, you will want to be as comfortable as you can when giving testimony. Remember the following pointers:

- **Be professional**—You will be judged by your appearance and behavior as well as by what you say. Your attorney will advise you on how to dress and behave when preparing you for your court appearance.

- **Remain calm, dignified, and serious at all times**—The opposing attorney may try to make you nervous. Keep your mind focused on the questions being asked, and take deep breaths to help remain calm.

- **Do not answer questions you do not understand**—Simply ask the attorney to repeat the question or state, "I don't know."

- **Only present facts surrounding the case**—Do not give any additional information. Do not insert your opinion. Stating, "He was angry," is stating your opinion. "The patient was shouting" is stating a fact.

- **Do not memorize your testimony ahead of time**—You will generally be allowed to take some notes with you to refresh your memory concerning dates or other specifics surrounding the court case.

- **Always tell the truth**—A medical assistant must demonstrate **veracity** at all times (truthfulness; truth in speech or statement)

Giving testimony in court is a crucial and sensitive matter. It is best to consult an attorney if you have any questions.

In some instances, the parties involved may not want to pursue the case in court and may decide to submit to arbitration. **Arbitration** is a hearing in which a neutral third party or parties determines the outcome of a dispute or settle a difference between parties. Before arbitration, both parties must agree to abide by the decision made by the arbitrator.

PUBLIC DUTIES OF PHYSICIANS

Physicians have responsibilities to the general public. Some of these duties include reporting births, stillbirths, deaths, communicable illnesses or diseases, drug abuse, certain injuries such as rape, abuse of children or older adults, gunshot and knife wounds, and animal bites. Table 3-3 outlines the public duties of the physician.

When abuse is suspected, you must share your concerns immediately with the physician. It is best not to make assumptions or accusations in front of the patient; rather, discuss your observations privately with the physician. The physician can help determine the best way to deal with your concerns and help the patient.

TABLE 3-3 | Public Duties of the Physician

Duty	Description
Births	Issuing of a legal certificate, which will be maintained during a person's life as proof of age. Many benefits and documents, including Social Security, passport, and driver's license, depend on having a valid birth certificate.
Deaths	Physicians sign a certificate indicating the cause of a natural death. Check with your state public health department to determine specific requirements. For example, in the case of a stillbirth before the 20th week of gestation, the medical assistant will have to determine if both a birth and death certificate are required. A coroner or health official will have to sign a certificate in the following cases: • No physician present at the time of death • Violent death, unlawful death • Death as a result of criminal action • Death from an undetermined cause
Reportable Communicable Diseases	Physicians must report all diseases that can be transmitted from one person to another and are considered a general threat to the public. Some common diseases that must be reported to the CDC include: • AIDS/HIV • Chickenpox • Chlamydia trachomatis • Cholera • Diphtheria • Gonorrhea • Hepatitis A, B, and C • Lyme disease • Malaria • Measles • Mumps • Rabies (human and animal cases) • Rubella (including congenital syndrome) • Salmonellosis • Severe acute respiratory syndrome (SARS) • Smallpox • Syphilis, including congenital syphilis • Tetanus • Trichinosis
Reportable Injuries	Certain injuries are reportable, according to state requirements. These injuries include gun or knife wounds, rape and battered persons injuries, and spousal, child, and elder abuse.
Child Abuse	Questionable injuries of children, including bruises, fractured bones, and burns, must be reported. Signs of neglect, such as malnutrition, poor growth, and lack of hygiene, are reportable in some states.
Elder Abuse	Physical abuse, neglect, and abandonment of older adults is reportable in most states. The reporting agency varies by state but generally includes social service agencies.
Drug Abuse	Abuse of prescription drugs is reportable, according to the law. Such abuse can be difficult to determine because the abuser may seek prescriptions for the same drug from several different physicians. A physician will want to see a patient before prescribing a medication.

Physical abuse or neglect of children and older adults must be immediately reported to the proper authorities. Every state has child welfare departments and child abuse and neglect reporting telephone numbers. More information, including how to report child abuse, can be found at www.childwelfare.gov. Each state also has adult protection services (APS). The reporting phone number for elder abuse in each state can be found on the National Center on Elder Abuse website, https://ncea.acl.gov. When dealing with older adults, signs of possible exploitation by caregivers must also be recognized. **Exploitation** is the improper use of someone else's money or assets. Unfortunately, sometimes those who are charged with taking care of an older relative or friend become greedy and can manipulate the victim out of money

Abuse of older adults by family members or caregivers may occur at home and in institutions. Elder abuse has many forms, including:

- Stealing a patient's belongings
- Inflicting injury and pain
- Mishandling monetary funds
- Withholding care such as food, drink, or medication
- Sexual abuse
- Threatening or confining a patient

As a medical assistant, you must be alert to all signs of abuse. In some cases, especially when the abuser is a caregiver or family member, the patient may be reluctant to admit to abuse because of fear the caregiver will become angry or retaliate. Any concerns or suspicions of abuse should be immediately discussed, in private, with the treating physician.

or personal property. Like abuse, exploitation is a reportable incident. Box 3-3 provides additional information pertaining to identifying elder abuse.

The subject of domestic abuse is trickier, because sometimes the victim doesn't want to press charges against the abuser. These situations must be handled with great care and delicacy.

Compliance Reporting of Communicable Diseases

Federal, state, and local government agencies require medical laboratories and physicians to report when certain diagnoses are made (refer again to Table 3-3). These reports help in the identification of trends and possible disease outbreaks in specific locations. Office personnel, including the medical assistant, carry out many of the duties that relate to these responsibilities. Exact reporting requirements vary from state to state, so be familiar with the requirements of both your state and local county health departments.

Many of the diseases that must be reported to local and state agencies must also be reported to the U.S. Centers for Disease Control and Prevention (CDC). There are four classes of mandatory compliance reporting:

- **Total Number of Cases Report**—A physician's office is required to document the total number of cases for a disease over a predetermined period of time. Influenza and chickenpox are examples of diseases for which the total number of cases is reported.

- **Mandatory telephone reporting**—Some diseases, such as measles and whooping cough, must be reported via a telephone call to the appropriate agency. Again, state requirements vary. Although some diseases may be reported within five days of diagnosis, other diseases must be reported within hours of a diagnosis being made.

- **Mandatory written reporting**—A written report must be submitted when certain diseases, such as gonorrhea, are diagnosed.

- **Cancer**—Each state has a cancer registry. When a diagnosis of cancer is made, it must be reported to the cancer registry.

Figure 3-6 shows the State of New York's Communicable Disease Reporting Requirements, and Figure 3-7 shows the State of New York's report that must be completed when reporting communicable diseases. Procedure 3-1 outlines an example of the steps to complete compliance reporting.

RISK MANAGEMENT IN THE MEDICAL OFFICE

The term **risk management** refers to planning and implementing strategies for reducing the physician's risk of a lawsuit in the medical setting. As a medical assistant, dealing so closely with patients, you are in a position to help reduce those risks. Communicating effectively with the patient is certainly one of the primary ways to reduce the risk of being sued. Remember that in many cases you are the only one in the office who will hear a patient's complaint. Your ability to handle the complaint professionally and efficiently may eliminate a potential lawsuit for the physician. On the other hand, any promise or commitment that you make to a patient can be legally binding to the physician who employs you. This means that the physician can be held responsible for something you have said or implied to the patient with regard to how the physician might improve the patient's condition.

In addition to the information presented earlier in this chapter, you can further help your employer and protect yourself by remembering the recommendations and cautions that follow.

NEW YORK STATE DEPARTMENT OF HEALTH
Communicable Disease Reporting Requirements

Reporting of suspected or confirmed communicable diseases is mandated under the New York State Sanitary Code (10NYCRR 2.10,2.14). The primary responsibility for reporting rests with the physician; moreover, laboratories (PHL 2102), school nurses (10NYCRR 2.12), day care center directors, nursing homes/hospitals (10NYCRR 405.3d) and state institutions (10NYCRR 2.10a) or other locations providing health services (10NYCRR 2.12) are also required to report the diseases listed below.

Anaplasmosis
Amebiasis
(Animal bites for which
    rabies prophylaxis is
    given[1]
(Anthrax[2]
(Arboviral infection[3]
Babesiosis
(Botulism[2]
(Brucellosis[2]
Campylobacteriosis
Chancroid
Chlamydia trachomatis
    infection
(Cholera
Cryptosporidiosis
Cyclosporiasis
(Diphtheria
E.coli O157:H7 infection[4]
Ehrlichiosis
(Encephalitis

(Foodborne Illness
Giardiasis
(Glanders[2]
Gonococcal infection
Haemophilus influenzae[5]
    (invasive disease)
(Hantavirus disease
Hemolytic uremic syndrome
Hepatitis A
(Hepatitis A in a food
    handler
Hepatitis B (specify acute or
    chronic)
Hepatitis C (specify acute or
    chronic)
Pregnant hepatitis B carrier
Herpes infection, infants
    aged 60 days or younger
Hospital associated
    infections (as defined in
    section 2.2 10NYCRR)

Influenza,
    laboratory-confirmed
Legionellosis
Listeriosis
Lyme disease
Lymphogranuloma venereum
Malaria
(Measles
(Melioidosis[2]
Meningitis
    Aseptic or viral
    (Haemophilus
    (Meningococcal
    Other (specify type)
(Meningococcemia
(Monkeypox
Mumps
Pertussis
(Plague[2]
(Poliomyelitis

Psittacosis
(Q Fever[2]
(Rabies[1]
Rocky Mountain spotted fever
(Rubella
    (including congenital
    rubella syndrome)
Salmonellosis
(Severe Acute Respiratory
    Syndrome (SARS)
Shigatoxin-producing E.coli[4]
    (STEC)
Shigellosis[4]
(Smallpox[2]
Staphylococcus aureus[6] (due
    to strains showing reduced
    susceptibility or resistance
    to vancomycin)
(Staphylococcal
    enterotoxin B poisoning[2]

Streptococcal infection
    (invasive disease)[5]
    Group A beta-hemolytic
    strep
    Group B strep
    Streptococcus pneumoniae
(Syphilis, specify stage[7]
Tetanus
Toxic shock syndrome
Transmissable spongiform
    encephalopathies[8] (TSE)
Trichinosis
(Tuberculosis current
    disease (specify site)
(Tularemia[2]
(Typhoid
(Vaccinia disease[9]
Vibriosis[6]
(Viral hemorrhagic fever[2]
Yersiniosis

WHO SHOULD REPORT?

Physicians, nurses, laboratory directors, infection control practitioners, health care facilities, state institutions, schools.

WHERE SHOULD REPORT BE MADE?

Report to local health department where patient resides.

Contact Person _____

Name _____

Address _____

_____

Phone _____ Fax _____

WHEN SHOULD REPORT BE MADE?

Within 24 hours of diagnosis:
- Phone diseases in bold type,
- Mail case report, DOH-389, for all other diseases.
- In New York City use form PD-16.

SPECIAL NOTES

- Diseases listed in **bold type** (warrant prompt action and should be reported **immediately** to local health departments by phone followed by submission of the confidential case report form (DOH-389). In NYC use case report form PD-16.
- In addition to the diseases listed above, any unusual disease (defined as a newly apparent or emerging disease or syndrome that could possibly be caused by a transmissible infectious agent or microbial toxin) is reportable.
- Outbreaks: while individual cases of some diseases (e.g., streptococcal sore throat, head lice, impetigo, scabies and pneumonia) are not reportable, a cluster or outbreak of cases of any communicable disease is a reportable event.
- **Cases of HIV infection, HIV-related illness and AIDS are reportable on form DOH-4189 which may be obtained by contacting:**
    Division of Epidemiology, Evaluation and Research
    P.O. Box 2073, ESP Station
    Albany, NY 12220-2073
    (518) 474-4284
  In NYC: New York City Department of Health and Mental Hygiene
    For HIV/AIDS reporting, call:
    (212) 442-3388

1. Local health department must be notified prior to initiating rabies prophylaxis.
2. Diseases that are possible indicators of bioterrorism.
3. Including, but not limited to, infections caused by eastern equine encephalitis virus, western equine encephalitis virus, West Nile virus, St. Louis encephalitis virus, La Crosse virus, Powassan virus, Jamestown Canyon virus, dengue and yellow fever.
4. Positive shigatoxin test results should be reported as presumptive evidence of disease.
5. Only report cases with positive cultures from blood, CSF, joint, peritoneal or pleural fluid. Do not report cases with positive cultures from skin, saliva, sputum or throat.
6. Proposed addition to list.
7. Any non-treponemal test ≥1:16 or any positive prenatal or delivery test regardless of titer or any primary or secondary stage disease, should be reported by phone; all others may be reported by mail.
8. Including Creutzfeldt-Jakob disease. Cases should be reported directly to the New York State Department of Health Alzheimer's Disease and Other Dementias Registry at (518) 473-7817 upon suspicion of disease. In NYC, cases should also be reported to the NYCDOHMH.
9. Persons with vaccinia infection due to contact transmission and persons with the following complications from vaccination; eczema vaccinatum, erythema multiforme major or Stevens-Johnson syndrome, fetal vaccinia, generalized vaccinia, inadvertent inoculation, ocular vaccinia, post-vaccinial encephalitis or encephalomyelitis, progressive vaccinia, pyogenic infection of the infection site, and any other serious adverse events.

ADDITIONAL INFORMATION

For more information on disease reporting, call your local health department or the
    New York State Department of Health
    Bureau of Communicable Disease Control at
    (518) 473-4439
    or (866) 881-2809 after hours.
In New York City, 1 (866) NYC-DOH1.
To obtain reporting forms (DOH-389), call (518) 474-0548.

PLEASE POST THIS CONSPICUOUSLY

DOH-389 (2/11) p2 of 2

FIGURE 3-6 New York State requirements for filing a communicable disease report.

NEW YORK STATE DEPARTMENT OF HEALTH
Division of Epidemiology

Confidential Case Report

County of Residence ____________ Serial # ____________ Date of Report ____/____/____

Patient Information

Patient's Name ______________________________________
Last First MI Maiden

Patient's Alias ______________________________________
Last First MI

Guardian's Name ______________________________________
Last First MI

Patient's Date of Birth ____/____/____ Patient's Age ______ Patient's Country of Birth ____________

Patient's Primary Phone No. (____) ____-______ Patient's Secondary Phone No. (____) ____-______

Patient's Physical Address ______________________________________
Number & Street City Zip Code

Patient's Mailing Address (if different) ______________________________________
City Zip Code

Occupation (works at)	Setting (resides/attends)	Sex	Race (Check all that apply)	Ethnicity
☐ Food Service	☐ Day Care Facility	☐ Male	☐ White	☐ Hispanic
☐ Day Care	☐ Health Care Facility	☐ Female	☐ Black	☐ Non-Hispanic
☐ Health Care	☐ School	☐ Unknown	☐ Amer. Indian /Alaskan	☐ Unknown
☐ Student/School	☐ Jail/Prison		☐ Asian	
☐ Inmate	☐ Camp	Pregnant	____________	
☐ Correction Worker	☐ Homeless	☐ Yes	☐ Native Hawaiian/ Pacific Islander	
☐ Unemployed	☐ Other ______	☐ No	____________	
☐ Retired	☐ Unknown	☐ Unknown	☐ Other	
☐ Other ______		If Pregnant Due Date: ____/____/____	☐ Unknown	
☐ Unknown				

Is Patient Alive? ☐ Yes ☐ No ☐ Unknown If No, Date of Death ____/____/____

Disease ____________________ Site of Infection ____________

Date of First Symptom: ____/____/____ Date of Diagnosis ____/____/____

Hospitalized? ☐ Yes ☐ No ☐ Unknown

Name of Hospital ____________________ Medical Record No. ____________

Admission Date ____/____/____ Discharge Date ____/____/____

Reporter Information

Reporting Individual ____________________ Telephone (____) ____-____

Address ______________________________________

____

Reporting Source ☐ MD ☐ Lab ☐ Hospital ICN ☐ School Nurse ☐ Public Health Nurse ☐ Other Local Health Department ☐ Other State Health Dept ☐ Other ____________ ☐ Unknown

Provider Name ____________________ Provider Telephone (____) ____-____

Testing Laboratory ____________________ Laboratory Telephone (____) ____-____

Comments

Include applicable laboratory data, treatment, recent travel, etc. ______________________________________

____

____

For Local Health Department Use

Outbreak Related	Case Status	Local Health Department Signature	Was Patient Notified?
☐ Sporadic	☐ Confirmed	____________________	☐ Yes
☐ Cluster	☐ Probable	Date Form Received ____/____/____	☐ No
☐ Outbreak	☐ Suspect	Investigation Start Date ____/____/____	☐ Unknown
☐ Unknown	☐ Unknown		

DOH-389 (2/11) p1 of 2

FIGURE 3-7 Sample document for reporting a communicable disease.

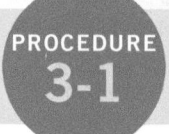

PROCEDURE 3-1

Performing Compliance Reporting Based on Public Health Statutes

Objective ◆ *Report the diagnosis of a communicable disease to the appropriate authorities.*

EQUIPMENT AND SUPPLIES

Patient medical record; black ink pen, if completing the form manually; computer and printer, if completing the form electronically; contact information for appropriate health agencies or departments; reporting form, either electronic version or printed document

METHOD

Scenario: Your patient has been diagnosed with Lyme disease. He recognized his first symptom on September 18, 20xx. The diagnosis was made one week later. The patient has not been hospitalized in relation to this diagnosis.

1. Use the Internet to determine if the disease in question requires immediate reporting via telephone, or if a case report documenting the disease can simply be mailed.*

2. Using the patient's medical record, complete the "Patient Information" section of the report form. If you are unaware of the answers to some of the questions, contact the patient to verify the correct information.
3. Accurately fill out the "Reporter Information" section of the form.
4. Review the form to ensure all information is complete and accurate.
5. Give the form to the physician for review and signature.
6. Upload a copy of the report to the patient's medical record.**
7. Mail the original, signed report to the Department of Health.

*Remember to check the requirements for your specific state. Otherwise, you may choose to reference information from Figure 3-6 in your textbook.

**If using paper records, make a copy of the record and file the document appropriately.

Office Management

Follow these office management guidelines:

- Treat all patients with the same courtesy and dignity you would expect to receive. Log and return telephone calls promptly. Explain any delays to patients who are waiting to see the physician. Offer to set up another appointment if the delay will be very long.

- Never make promises regarding what the physician can do for the patient. As mentioned before, they can be misconstrued and have the potential to hold the physician liable for your promises.

- Carefully explain to the patient all fees and responsibilities related to billing, and relay any concerns to office management or the physician.

- Relay any dissatisfied patient's comments to the physician and practice manager.

- If the physician will be out of town or absent from the office, inform patients by posting the dates in the medical office, making telephone calls, or sending patients

Professionalism

Be respectful of the sexual orientations and preferences of all patients, including those who are lesbian, gay, bisexual, or transgender (LGBT). And, although laws about what constitutes a "legal" relationship vary from state-to-state, also respect the patient's choice of friends and companions. Severe penalties can be imposed by the Centers for Medicare and Medicaid Services (CMS) for discriminating against patients based on gender expression or self-identification. The Joint Commission established a standard of providing nonbiased care to LGBT patients as a requirement for accreditation of health care facilities. Remember that transgender people may need to have tests or procedures (such a PSA or pap-smear) for a gender other than the one with which they have self-identified. They may still have genetic predisposition for illness based on their original physical gender assignment. As a medical assistant, you may need to advocate for a patient, for example when an insurance company refuses to pay for a necessary test that is not usually done for the gender the patient claims.

letters. Each specific situation will dictate the best method of informing patients. Also provide the name and telephone number of the on-call physician who will be managing patient care in the other physician's stead.

Documentation

These guidelines for documentation must be followed.

- Carefully sign or initial every entry in a medical record, whether it is electronic or paper. *Remember:* Medical documents are legal documents and may be used in a court of law.

- If the patient did not keep an appointment, be sure to document the fact as a no-show. Document canceled appointments and follow-up attempts to determine why the patient missed the appointment. This type of record keeping is especially important if a physician decides to withdraw from a patient case. It will be used to establish patient noncompliance.

- Document when a patient is referred to another physician, and follow up to make sure the patient did see the referral physician.

- Document all patient contacts, including telephone prescription refills, diagnostic tests, and procedures that have been ordered. Call all patients the day after surgery to check on their progress; document this call.

- Record all care and treatment given as soon as possible after the patient's visit. This will keep patient records current and ensure appropriate follow-up treatment if it is required.

- Be sure the physician reviews and initials all diagnostic reports in a timely fashion before they are filed.

- Provide all instructions to patients in writing explaining as necessary for complete understanding.

Certification and Licensing

The following considerations pertain to risk management because they help prevent potential liability issues for your employing physician. Keep these guidelines in mind when working in the field.

- Have a thorough understanding of the limits of certification and standards of care for the medical assisting profession. Never perform any procedure for which you are not trained or qualified to do or that the state medical practice laws do not permit.

- Do not diagnose or prescribe, including over the telephone. This applies to all drugs, even those that can be obtained over the counter. You could be charged with practicing medicine without a license.

Professionalism — The Workplace

It is important that all members of the office staff understand their respective roles. No one should pressure medical assistants to practice outside their role or scope of practice. If a medical assistant is pressured to perform tasks that are outside the legal scope, according to state guidelines or even the company policy, the medical assistant must notify a supervisor that she cannot practice outside the scope of responsibility and training.

- Do not call yourself a nurse or allow anyone else to refer to you as the nurse. You must be held to your own standard of care as a medical assistant and not that of a nurse.

- Participate in continuing education and training programs to maintain your skill levels and to stay abreast of the changes in the medical field.

Safety

Office safety is critically important to risk management in the medical office. Be sure to keep these safety guidelines in mind:

- Maintain a safe environment in the office or work site for the patients and staff. Promptly handle requests for maintenance repairs. Report any unsafe activities or hazards at once.

- Carefully check and document medical waste disposal. Be concerned about the safety of maintenance personnel who must handle the waste containers. Always correctly dispose of syringes and needles as well as contaminated medical waste in designated hazardous waste containers.

- Carefully maintain and document quality checks on laboratory testing equipment.

Box 3-4 highlights examples of unsafe activities and hazards in the medical office.

Compliance Reporting

Compliance is defined as conforming to a specific rule or acting in accordance with established guidelines to ensure that specific procedures are performed correctly. Compliance is an important component of risk management, because it takes the entire team to understand the importance of avoiding potential liability and work together toward that measure. Unfortunately, compliance with procedures and regulations is not always observed; sometimes accidentally and other times on purpose. When there is a break in compliance, it must be reported to the appropriate individuals.

The following are hazards and unsafe activities that may occur in a medical office.

- Slippery floors
- Area rugs that are out of place or not lying flat
- Overloaded electrical outlets
- Extension cords that are located in heavy traffic areas
- Frayed wires

- Shelving that is holding items that are too heavy
- Improper cleaning and disinfection procedures
- Improper disposal of hazardous waste
- Over-filled sharps containers, or sharps containers that are mounted too high for everyone's reach
- Becoming lax in handwashing and hand hygiene

Consider the following instances that would mandate compliance reporting.

Errors in Patient Care

Acting under a code of ethics that compels you to safeguard any patient whose care and safety are affected by the negligent action of someone else, you must follow the chain of command and report to your immediate supervisor any negligent action you observe. This is discussed later in the chapter. However, it goes without saying that if you accidentally make an error, you must bring this to your supervisor's attention so that it can be corrected immediately. The chapter titled "The Office Environment" outlines how to complete an incident report related to an error in patient care.

Unsafe or Illegal Activities

Unsafe activities have already been discussed in this section. The prudent medical assistant will understand the importance of safety and minimizing potential hazards in the medical office. If you knowingly overlook a hazard that a reasonable person would report and eliminate, you can be guilty of negligence.

Illegal activity, unfortunately, may also occur in the medical practice setting. Examples of illegal activities in the medical office may include:

- Fraudulent billing and coding procedures to obtain higher reimbursement for services that were or were not performed
- Stealing prescription pads and writing illegal prescriptions
- Sexual harassment
- Practicing medicine with an expired license

Any illegal activity that occurs in the health care setting must be reported to the appropriate authorities, following protocol. This may include first reporting the issue to an office manager. If the office manager fails to properly address the situation, you may need to contact authorities (for example, law enforcement) to report the illegal activity directly. This should be done in a private location where the utmost level of confidentiality can be employed. Procedure 3-2 provides an overview regarding how to handle illegal activity in the health care setting.

CODE OF ETHICS

Ethics is the branch of philosophy related to **morals** or moral principles. Morals are what a person believes to be the acceptable or right way to live. Morals govern a person's behavior. The study of ethics involves the examination of human character and conduct, the distinction between right and wrong, and a person's moral duty and obligations to the community. Ethics have been part of the medical profession since the earliest days of the profession.

The earliest code of ethics or principles to govern conduct for those in medicine dates back to around 1800 BC, to the Code of Hammurabi. In 400 BC, Hippocrates, a Greek physician referred to as the "Father of Western Medicine," wrote a statement of principles for his medical students to follow. This statement of principles is known as the Hippocratic Oath (Box 2-1 in the chapter titled "Medical Science: History and Practice") and it remains important today. This oath reminds medical students of the importance of their profession, the need to teach others, and the obligation they have to act in such a way as to never knowingly harm a patient or divulge a confidence. The Hippocratic Oath is recited at medical school graduation ceremonies, and has been for centuries, as it carries an important ethical message for physicians. Modern codes of ethics have been developed as medical science has continued to advance.

MEDICAL ETHICS

Medical ethics refer to the moral conduct of people in medical professions. This moral conduct of medical professionals is governed by the high principles and standards that these professionals set for themselves and willingly choose to follow through personal dedication. Every

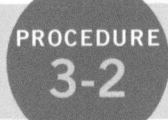

PROCEDURE 3-2

Reporting Illegal Activity in the Health Care Setting

Objective ◆ *Identify examples of illegal activity, and recognize appropriate governing authorities and proper protocol to be followed when reporting illegal activity in the health care setting.*

EQUIPMENT AND SUPPLIES

Pen and paper; phone book; computer with Internet access and word processing software; printer

METHOD

1. Create a list that identifies examples of illegal activity that may occur in the health care setting.
2. Next to each example, identify the proper authority or governing agency that would be contacted in order to report the illegal behavior (e.g., local police department, Drug Enforcement Agency).
3. Using a phone book or an Internet search engine, locate the contact information for each governing authority identified in the step above.
4. Create a document using word processing software that could be used in the medical office as an informative reference guide that summarizes the information in steps 1–3.
5. On a separate sheet of paper, write a paragraph describing the steps you would take if you found out the medical office where you worked was committing insurance fraud by billing insurance companies for services that were not performed on patients.

medical profession has a code of ethics that sets the moral standards to which members of that profession are expected to adhere.

Ethical Standards of Behavior

Ethical standards are generally more severe than standards required by law. In many cases, ethical standards are more demanding than the law. A violation of an ethical standard could mean the loss of the physician's reputation.

Ethical behavior, according to the American Medical Association (AMA), refers to moral principles or practices, the customs of the medical profession, and matters of medical policy. Any actions that do not follow these ethical standards constitute unethical behavior. When a physician is accused of unethical behavior or conduct in violation of these standards, the AMA can issue a warning or censure. The AMA Board of Examiners may recommend the expulsion or suspension of a physician from membership in the association. Expulsion, or being forced out of the association, is a severe penalty for physicians because it limits the physician's ability to practice medicine.

Not all physicians are members of the AMA, and the AMA does not have authority to bring legal action against nonmembers for unethical conduct. However, the state

medical board that issued the physician's license may limit the physician's practice or revoke the license altogether for ethical misconduct. If it is alleged (asserted or declared without proof) that a physician has committed a criminal act, the medical society is required to report it to the state board or governmental agency. A violation of the law that is followed by a conviction for the crime may result in a fine, imprisonment, or both. The state medical board can then revoke (cancel) the physician's license to practice medicine.

Professionalism   The Law

As an agent or representative of the physician, the medical assistant is responsible for understanding ethical standards related to any office issue. It is important to remember that the medical assistant cannot diagnose or treat illnesses, although educating the patient about information the physician has given is expected. Patient confidentiality cannot be breached for any reason. Staff members should not access or open any chart for which they do not have a specific, work-related need.

AMA Principles of Medical Ethics

In the United States, the American Medical Association (AMA) has taken a leadership role in setting standards for the ethical behavior of physicians. The AMA was organized in New York City in 1846, and its first code of ethics was formed shortly after that in 1847.

The AMA Principles of Medical Ethics encompass human dignity, honesty, responsibility to society, confidentiality, the need for continued study, freedom of choice, and a responsibility of the physician to improve the community. For more information about the AMA Principles of Medical Ethics, visit the AMA's website at www.ama-assn.org.

MEDICAL ASSISTANTS' PRINCIPLES OF PERSONAL AND PROFESSIONAL ETHICS

Medical assistants may not be involved with the life-and-death ethical decisions that face the physician. However, they do face many dilemmas regarding right or wrong behavior on an almost daily basis. Examples include a coworker violating patient confidentiality, a medical assistant using foul language in front of a patient, or a team of care givers treating a patient disrespectfully because of the patient's body odor. More severely, a medical assistant may be asked to perform unethical or even illegal actions by their physician-employers. It is important to remember that medical assistants, by law and scope of practice, are required to treat patients lawfully and ethically. A medical assistant may question whether an order from a physician crosses legal or ethical lines. The Blanchard and Peale Ethical Model can help the medical assistant distinguish and recognize legal and ethical issues. The model is based on applying a set of questions to determine issues of ethics and legality to given situations.

The Blanchard and Peale Ethical Model

1. Is it legal?
2. Is it ethical?
3. How will the action make me feel?
4. How would I feel if the action and my participation were to be published in a local newspaper? (This is often referred to as the Front Page of the Newspaper Test.)

As each situation varies, so will the appropriate response regarding how it should be handled.

Ethics, Morals, and Your Profession

Ethics differ from laws in key ways. Laws are legally enforceable and carry penalties (fines or imprisonment), whereas ethics are valued by professional organizations and rarely result in severe penalties for ethical violations. If an ethical violation occurs, the guilty party may be shunned professionally or have a certification revoked, but no severe penalties exist for ethical violations.

Moral decisions are different from legal and ethical decisions. For instance, it isn't illegal for two consenting adults to engage in sexual relations. However, it is considered unethical to have a sexually intimate relationship with a patient. Similarly, many people hold the moral belief that it is not appropriate to have sexual affairs before or outside a marriage. Although some acts that are considered immoral do not have a civil or professional penalty, an individual might be socially shunned by those who don't approve of certain moral choices.

In some cases, the medical assistant may have a personal moral, religious, or ethical reason for wishing not to be involved in particular procedures, such as abortions or artificial insemination. These preferences should be stated to the employer before employment, allowing them to be considered when making a hiring decision. In the event that the situation arises after employment begins, all concerns should be communicated to the employer immediately. If there is a moral or ethical disagreement, it is very important not to judge the physician's interpretation of ethical guidelines. However, you may request to be excused from participating in any procedures about which you have ethical doubts.

Bioethics is a term that refers to ethical decisions regarding life issues. For example, stem cell research, in vitro fertilization, and abortion rights are sometimes controversial issues that concern human life. The medical assistant must reflect on bioethical decisions but support the patient in the patient's own decision making. Working as a medical assistant, you must never impose your personal ethics or morals on a patient. Regardless of their personal decisions, you must always treat them with dignity and the utmost respect.

If a medical assistant's choice to not assist the physician in a specific procedure jeopardizes the health and safety of a patient, or interferes with the physician's ability to do the procedures, it may be necessary for that medical assistant to seek other employment.

Scientific Discovery and Ethical Issues

Many areas of medical ethics—When should life support be withdrawn? When does a life begin? Is euthanasia ever permissible? Should the unborn baby's life be sacrificed to save the mother? and more—have no conclusive answers. Scientific discoveries present new medical possibilities and choices every day. With these possibilities, more complicated ethical issues

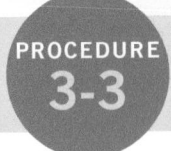

Separating Personal and Professional Ethics

Objective ◆ *Identify and recognize an individual's stance on ethical situations that impact health care; identity how to professionally address the topics.*

EQUIPMENT AND SUPPLIES

Pen and paper

METHOD

1. Consider at least two ethical topics common to the health care setting, such as abortion, stem cell research, and physician-assisted suicide, to name a few.
2. Review and apply the Blanchard and Peale Ethical Model presented in the text to the ethical topics of your choice.
3. Create and document a personal stance on each issue, and provide a brief explanation of your ethical beliefs.
4. Identify how each of your chosen issues should be approached professionally.
5. Consider if there any instances where, if presented with an ethical issue, it would impede your ability to perform your job.
6. Discuss the issues with a partner. When listening to opposing points of view, be sure to maintain professional communication and respect for the individual.

often need to be addressed before choices can be made. The medical assistant has a responsibility to keep current on medical advances and form opinions based on sound medical ethics and practice. Procedure 3-3 will help the medical assistant understand how to separate personal and professional ethics.

AAMA Code of Ethics

The Code of Ethics of the American Association of Medical Assistants (AAMA) is a professional standard that medical assistants are expected to follow. The code, which describes

ethical and moral conduct for the medical assistant, is similar to the AMA's Principles of Medical Ethics. Box 3-5 lists the code of ethics of the AAMA. Medical assistants assume a position of trust and must try to live up to the standards of the profession as stated in the code.

AAMA Creed

The Creed of the AAMA can be best followed by the medical assistant who spends time reading about and discussing ethical problems, such as transplants, artificial insemination,

---

BOX 3-5 | Code of Ethics of the American Association of Medical Assistants

PREAMBLE

The Code of Ethics of the AAMA shall set forth principles of ethical and moral conduct as they relate to the medical profession and the particular practice of medical assisting.

Members of the AAMA dedicated to the conscientious pursuit of their profession, and thus desiring to merit the high regard of the entire medical profession and the respect of the general public which they serve, do hereby pledge themselves to strive always to:

Human Dignity

I. Render service with full respect for the dignity of humanity;

Confidentiality

II. Respect confidential information obtained through employment unless legally authorized or required by responsible performance of duty to divulge such information;

Honor

III. Uphold the honor and high principles of the profession and accept its disciplines;

Continued Study

IV. Seek to continually improve the knowledge and skills of medical assistants for the benefit of patients and professional colleagues;

Responsibility for Improved Community

V. Participate in additional service activities aimed toward improving the health and well-being of the community.

Note: *Copyright by the American Association of Medical Assistants, Inc. Reprinted with permission.*

abortion, and the right to die with dignity. To be true to this creed, the medical assistant must know about the ethical issues the patient faces and be committed to treating the patient with respectful care regardless of the patient's religious beliefs or cultural practices.

Creed of the American Association of Medical Assistants

I believe in the principles and purposes of the profession of medical assisting.

I endeavor to be more effective.

I aspire to render greater service.

I protect the confidence entrusted to me.

I am dedicated to the care and well-being of all people.

I am loyal to my employer.

I am true to the ethics of my profession.

I am strengthened by compassion, courage, and faith.

AMT Standards of Practice

The American Medical Technologists (AMT) has standards of practice that reflect the ethical expectations for those with the Registered Medical Assistant (RMA) credential. Similar to the AAMA creed, the AMT Standards of Practice call for ethical behavior by medical assistants. AMT seeks to encourage, establish, and maintain the highest standards, traditions, and principles of the practices that constitute the profession of the registry. Members of the AMT certification agency and the registry must recognize their responsibilities, not only to their patients but also to society, to other health care professionals, and to themselves.

The following standards of practice are principles adopted by the AMT Board of Directors, which defines the essence of honorable and ethical behavior for a health care professional. AMT requires that any known violations of the standards are reported so they can be referred to the Judiciary Committee of AMT for consideration of revocation of the individual's certification or other disciplinary sanctions.

AMT Standards of Practice

I. While engaged in the Arts and Sciences, which constitute the practice of their profession, AMT professionals shall be dedicated to the provision of competent and compassionate service and shall always meet or exceed the applicable standard of care.

II. The AMT professional shall place the welfare of the patient above all else.

III. When performing clinical duties and procedures, the AMT professional shall act within the lawful limits of any applicable scope of practice, and when so required shall act under and in accordance with appropriate supervision by an attending physician, dentist, or other licensed practitioner.

IV. The AMT professional shall always respect the rights of patients and of fellow health care providers, shall comply with all applicable laws and regulations governing the privacy and confidentiality of protected health care information, and shall safeguard patient confidences unless legally authorized or compelled to divulge protected health care information to an authorized individual, law enforcement officer, or other legal or governmental entity.

V. AMT professionals shall strive to increase their technical knowledge, shall continue to learn, and shall continue to apply and share scientific advances in their fields of professional specialization.

VI. The AMT professional shall respect the law and will pledge to avoid dishonest, unethical or illegal practices, breaches of fiduciary duty, or abuses of the position of trust into which the professional has been placed as a certified health care professional.

VII. AMT professionals understand that they shall not make or offer a diagnosis or dispense medical advice unless they are duly licensed practitioners or unless specifically authorized to do so by an attending licensed practitioner acting in accordance with applicable law.

VIII. The AMT professional shall observe and value the judgment of the attending physician, dentist, or other attending licensed practitioner, provided that so doing does not clearly constitute a violation of law or pose an immediate threat to the welfare of the patient.

IX. AMT professionals recognize that they are responsible for any personal wrongdoing, and that they have an obligation to report to the proper authorities any knowledge of professional abuse or unlawful behavior by any party involved in the patient's diagnosis, care, and treatment.

X. The AMT professional pledges personal honor and integrity and to cooperate in protecting and advancing, by every lawful means, the interests of the American Medical Technologists and its Members.

HIPAA AND CONFIDENTIALITY

According to the federal law, all patients have the right to have their personal privacy respected and their medical records handled with confidentiality.

No information—including test results, patient histories, and even the fact that the patient is a patient—can be told to another person without the patient's permission. Therefore, it is important that a medical assistant adhere to the following guidelines:

- Never make any statements about your employing physician that could be interpreted as an admission of fault. On the other hand, as a medical assistant, you cannot remain silent if you are aware that your employing physician is doing something illegal. You can be held liable for remaining silent.

- Do not participate in negative or critical discussions of the physician(s) or other practitioners in your office with your patients. Do not comment on a patient's negative criticism of a current or former physician.

- Never discuss anything about a patient outside the office or with office staff unless they have a need to know specific information.

- Make sure that a female medical assistant is present when the physician (male or female) examines a female patient.

- Treat all patients with dignity and respect.

This is not just a matter of ethics or professionalism; as already noted, it is the law. After numerous complaints from patients unable to continue to pay premiums to the same insurance company when they changed jobs, Congress passed the **Health Insurance Portability and Accountability Act (HIPAA)** of 1996. HIPAA, also known as Public Law 104-191, seeks to improve the efficiency and effectiveness of the health care system through insurance reform and administrative simplification. Although some of the information in this section may have been already mentioned earlier in the chapter, it is important to review it in relationship to HIPAA guidelines.

Many citizens feared that certain information about their health might prevent them from getting insurance coverage, and Congress responded by legislating rigorous standards of privacy for protected health information. The U.S. Department of Health and Human Services was charged with setting privacy and security standards for health information. Covered entities include health plans, health care clearinghouses, and providers who conduct certain health care transactions electronically. Medical practices are required to notify patients about the uses, disclosures, and rights of their protected information.

These protocols, although sharing common concerns for the patient, are not standardized by the government. Each practice should have policies and procedures for handling confidential information, including privacy officers who guard the security of identifiable health information. All employees and business associates who will have access to identifiable health information must give written assurances that they will protect patient information before they may access it. Patients also must be informed about how their information might be shared with others.

HIPAA gives patients more control over their health information than they had before, sets boundaries and safeguards for release of information, and holds personnel accountable to protect the information. Patients can find out who had access to their private information, and HIPAA gives them the right to examine and copy their records. They also can request corrections to records. Penalties for the improper release of information are very expensive. There are few exceptions to this rule, such as government access, worker's compensation laws, research, and matters relating to public health and law enforcement. Medical assistants must always be vigilant about protecting patient information and following the safeguards established in their office.

Complaints under HIPAA should be addressed to the U.S. Department of Health and Human Services. However, the medical assistant and office team should make every effort to personally address and rectify any patient complaints.

All medical office employees must undergo HIPAA training during their orientation. HIPAA is organized into three parts:

- Privacy regulations
- Transaction standards
- Security regulations

To adhere to HIPAA regulations, the medical office must have an appointed privacy official, draft privacy policies and procedures, and implement a program to educate and train all employees and physicians on the mandates of HIPAA. These polices should be included in the office policy and procedures manual. Acknowledgment of receiving a copy of the privacy practices of the medical office should be signed by all new patients. This policy should be clearly posted in the waiting area of the medical office. Patients must sign an authorization to release any medical information, including information released to a spouse or adult children. Without a signed consent, the medical assistant is prohibited from disclosing any medical information.

HIPAA extends its rules to making sure that computers with confidential patient information cannot be seen or accessed by unauthorized individuals. All faxes and e-mails that contain private patient information must have a disclaimer stating that the information is confidential, and if the information is accidentally transmitted to someone without clearance to read it, the recipient must immediately notify the office and destroy the information.

Health care professionals should refrain from discussing patients' private information where it can be overheard by others. Even when the medical assistant reaches a patient's voice mail, it is important to leave only the minimal information that contains return-call information. The use of speakerphones should be avoided when discussing patient information.

Although HIPAA is the law that protects the patient and promotes the portability of insurance, massive amounts of health care data must be controlled to ensure not only privacy but also efficiency. To simplify data use, the HIPAA transactions standard requires unique identification numbers for health care providers, individuals, health care plans, and employers. With these numbers, it is clear (even if names are similar) who the interested parties are in a transaction.

HIPAA further seeks to protect the transmission of data relating to health care. To improve the efficiency and effectiveness of the health care system, Congress, the public, and the health care industry have mutually agreed that standards are needed for the electronic exchange of administrative and financial health care transactions. HIPAA designates the Secretary of Health and Human Services to adopt protective and secure standards.

National standards for electronic health care transactions ultimately sought to simplify the processes involved in transmitting information required for quality patient care. Following these standards should promote savings resulting from the reduction in administrative burdens on health care providers and health plans. A standardized national electronic claim format replaced over 400 different formats that existed before the HIPAA transactions standard. Health plans now accept one standard format for electronic claims as well as other transactions such as remittance advices and referral authorizations to health care providers. The Secretary of Health and Human Services has adopted the standards for the following administrative and financial health care transactions:

1. Health claims and equivalent encounter information

2. Enrollment and disenrollment in a health plan

3. Eligibility for a health plan

4. Health care payment and remittance advice

5. Health plan premium payments

6. Health claim status

7. Referral certification and authorization

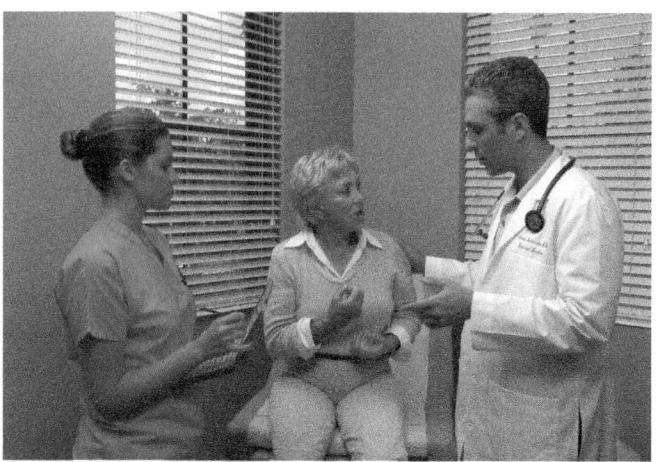

FIGURE 3-8 A medical assistant listening to the patient and physician discuss the patient's care.

The medical assistant's treatment of and concern for the patient reflects the physician's high standards of care. The human dignity of each patient must be preserved regardless of the patient's socioeconomic background, race, age, nationality, sexual orientation, or gender.

Any information that is given to a physician by a patient is considered confidential, and it may not be given to an unauthorized person (Figure 3-8). The physician's medical assistant is considered to be an authorized person with access to the patient's file and information. This information may not be divulged to anyone without permission of the doctor or patient. The physician must be notified of any information the patient gives the medical assistant, such as if the patient is not taking prescribed medications or complying with treatment.

Professionalism

 Telling the truth is one of the most important parts of being a medical professional. Every human makes mistakes; it is part of being human. However, the most important thing any professional can do is admit having made a mistake and seek to correct it. Do not offer extra information to the patient. You should only state that there is a correction to be made. Be sure to speak with the supervising physician, and document clearly in the chart the mistake that was made and how it was corrected. Honesty goes a very long way in preventing litigation and providing good, quality care to all patients. Be sure to notify the physician if there is a task you are not proficient to do. For example, if you did a procedure early in your training but have not done it for a long time, you need to notify the physician rather than perform the task without proficiency. Veracity, or speaking the truth at all times, is a professional quality that all medical assistants must have.

SUMMARY

In the United States, law is based on inalienable rights set forth in the U.S. Constitution. Laws are either criminal (against the state), civil (against people), military (involving military personnel), or international (between nations).

The medical and legal issues governing the medical profession and medical assistants are multifaceted. The medical assistant must be knowledgeable in many areas of the law. Laws governing medicine are different from those governing criminal behavior. Medicine is covered by civil law, often referred to as torts. It is the responsibility of both the physician and the medical assistant to be aware of these guidelines.

Because health care providers can harm the public, they can be held liable for damages done to patients. The physician–patient relationship is actually a contract, with rights granted to both parties. Care must be taken when terminating a relationship with a patient, or the physician can be charged with abandonment. The physician must obtain informed consent from the patient before performing invasive procedures on patients. Under the doctrine of *respondeat superior*, the physician is held liable for the medical assistant's actions while working under the physician's direction and supervision. To prove malpractice the physician must have had duty to a patient, been derelict in the duty, and caused damages that were directly related to the dereliction of duty. Standard of care is determined to be what a reasonable person of the same education and training would probably have done.

Medical ethics is based on the Hippocratic Oath. Patients must be treated equally, using the best possible standards of care. Medical assistants should understand the difference between morals and ethics. Additionally, it is important to understand how to separate personal and professional ethics. The American Medical Association (AMA), American Association of Medical Assistants (AAMA), and American Medical Technologists (AMT) have professional standards and values known as ethics. The Health Insurance Portability and Accountability Act (HIPAA) was enacted to encourage portability of insurance when citizens changed jobs, but it also includes strict provisions for maintaining confidentiality of patient information. Medical assistants have a professional duty to protect patient information.

③ CHAPTER REVIEW

COMPETENCY REVIEW

1. Define and spell the terms for this chapter.
2. What are the elements of a contract?
3. Compare the Code of Ethics of the AAMA with the AMT Standards of Practice.
4. What is informed consent?
5. Describe the medical assistant's responsibilities concerning medical ethics.
6. What is the difference between criminal and civil law?
7. List and describe the four Ds of negligence.
8. What are Good Samaritan laws, and how do they apply to you?
9. Why do you need thorough understanding of the law as it impacts your employer's practice?
10. Consider HIPAA. What do you think is the most important impact of this law on health care?

PREPARING FOR THE CERTIFICATION EXAM

1. When a physician abandons a patient, it is an offense under which type of law?
   a. criminal
   b. civil
   c. military
   d. international
   e. corporate

2. Patients of which religious preference would probably refuse a blood transfusion?
   a. Catholic
   b. Christian Scientist
   c. Jewish
   d. Muslim
   e. Hindu

3. Which of the following lists the ethics of a medical assistant?
   a. Hippocratic Oath
   b. AMA Code of Ethics
   c. state laws
   d. AAMA Code of Ethics
   e. Patient Care Partnership

4. HIPAA protects which patient right?
   a. self-determination
   b. liberty
   c. beneficence
   d. confidentiality
   e. informed consent

5. Which expression means that the physician is liable for the actions of the medical assistant?
   a. *res ipsa loquitur*
   b. *respondeat superior*
   c. *quid pro quo*
   d. *guardian ad litem*
   e. rule of discovery

6. A medical assistant who is sued in court would be judged by the standards of care that apply to a
   a. medical student.
   b. prudent medical assistant.
   c. seasoned medical assistant.
   d. nurse.
   e. medical assisting student.

7. Which must be documented in writing before undergoing surgery?
   a. informed consent
   b. check for payment
   c. knowledge of the Patient Care Partnership
   d. AMA Code of Ethics
   e. collection notice

8. Which of the following does *not* emancipate minors?
   a. living on their own
   b. being married
   c. being self-supporting
   d. being in the armed forces
   e. having sexual relations

9. Which of the following is *not* one of the four Ds of negligence?
   a. direct cause
   b. drug abuse
   c. damages
   d. duty
   e. dereliction of duty

10. Injecting medication into someone without their consent is an example of
    a. assault.
    b. battery.
    c. defamation.
    d. fraud.
    e. abandonment.

CRITICAL THINKING

Refer to the case study at the beginning of the chapter and use what you have learned to answer the following questions.

1. Does Shandra have protection from liability in this case?
2. One of the victims who did not survive the accident was an organ donor. What specific limitation has been placed on the physician who declared this individual's time of death?
3. The organ donor had a signed organ donation card. If someone wishes to be an organ donor, what other actions may be prudent to express her wishes in addition to having an organ donor card?

ON THE JOB

Dr. Spring, a board-certified obstetrician and gynecologist, has been in practice for more than 10 years. He is licensed to practice medicine in both New York and Pennsylvania. Dr. Spring employs a staff that includes two medical assistants.

On Monday one of the medical assistants, Nancy Watts, took a history on a new patient who was referred to Dr. Spring. The 40-year-old, married patient has had vaginal spotting for more than six weeks.

As part of the history, Nancy learned that the patient has been under the care and supervision of a fertility specialist for more than two years. In fact, although not always compliant, the patient has been on a medication treatment regimen for fertility problems.

After examining the patient, Dr. Spring ordered a uterine biopsy to be performed in the office. The patient returned the following week, underwent the biopsy, and was sent home.

Soon after, the patient's husband telephoned the office, requesting to speak to Dr. Spring immediately. His wife had just been admitted to the hospital because of intense vaginal bleeding.

1. Was there anything in the patient's history that the physician would take into consideration regarding performing the uterine biopsy?
2. Who would have had the responsibility to obtain an informed consent from the patient before her uterine biopsy: Nancy or the physician?
3. How should Nancy have handled the husband's telephone call?
4. Would it violate patient confidentiality to fax the patient's records to the emergency room physician, if requested?
5. Is this a potential case of medical negligence and malpractice? Could Nancy, as the medical assistant, have complicity (being an accomplice in wrongdoing) in this particular case?

INTERNET ACTIVITY

Do an Internet search for your local state health laws. Report what you find to the class.

Search the Internet for information regarding the scope of practice for medical assistants in your state. This information is typically located with the state board of medical examiners regulations.

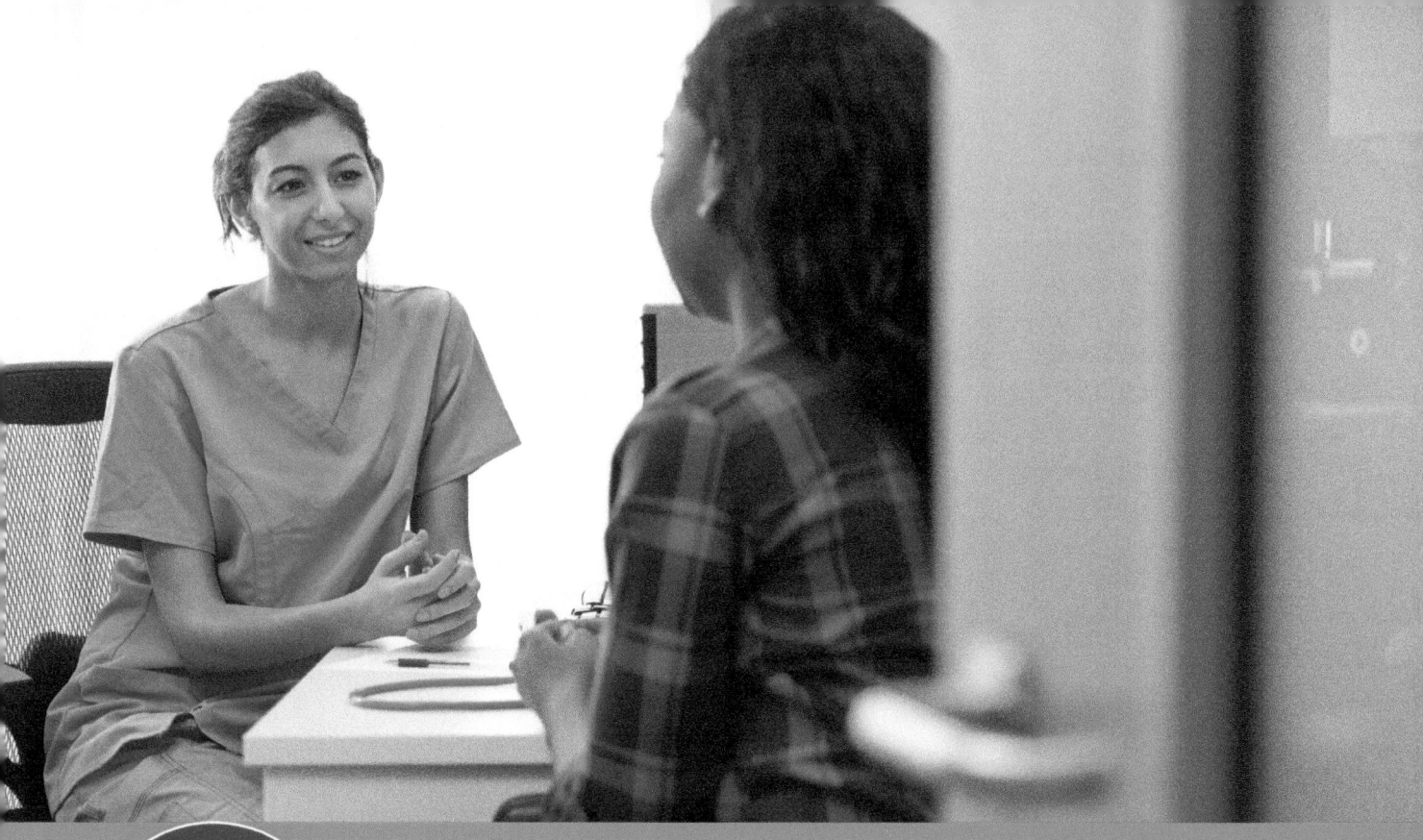

CHAPTER 4

Medical Terminology

Learning Objectives

After completing this chapter, you should be able to:

4.1	Define and spell the terms for this chapter.
4.2	Identify the components that create the structure of medical terms.
4.3	Dissect and label the word parts of medical terms.
4.4	Describe the rules related to pluralizing medical terms.
4.5	Identify medical abbreviations commonly used.
4.6	List body planes and directional terms.
4.7	Describe the cavities of the body.
4.8	Explain the difference between abdominopelvic regions and abdominal quadrants.
4.9	Identify medical terms specific to medical specialties and body systems.

Dr. McWalter saw Mickey Schultz in the office for abdominal pain. The pain Mr. Schultz described was located several centimeters above the navel, and Dr. McWalter needed to determine if the pain was cardiac or gastrointestinal in origin. She ordered a variety of tests to ensure that no chemical changes, musculoskeletal origins, or blockages in the soft tissue were causing the pain. Eventually, the cause of the pain was determined to be a peptic ulcer.

Terms to Learn

anatomy	physiology	word root
combining form	prefix	
combining vowel	suffix	

Because accurate communication among health professionals is important, medical terminology is frequently used in conversations in the medical office as well as in medical reports and patient documents. For this reason, as a medical assistant, you will need to have a solid, basic understanding of medical terminology. Of course, it is impossible to know every medical term, but you can quickly become familiar with the most common word parts and terms. Many resources are available to assist with learning new ones, including reputable Internet sites and medical dictionaries.

This chapter will help you get acquainted with the basics of medical terminology and with many of the terms you will encounter and use in your everyday work as a medical assistant. You will learn about the structure of medical terms, commonly used medical abbreviations, terms used to describe body planes and directions, and terminology used with medical specialties.

THE STRUCTURE OF MEDICAL TERMS

Learning medical terms is similar to putting a puzzle together. Medical terms are made up of word parts, each of which has a specific purpose. The parts of a medical term are the word root, prefix, suffix, and combining vowel.

The **word root** is the part that carries the main meaning, such as *cardi* for heart or *neur* for nerve. A **prefix** appears before a word root to modify its meaning and may be directional, such as *inter-* for between, or to indicate quantity, such as *poly-* for many. A **suffix** appears after a word root to describe the type of condition or procedure of the root, such as *-itis* for inflammation or *-ectomy* for excision. A **combining vowel** is usually added after the root when joining it to a suffix or combining it with another root. For example, in *cardiovascular* the letter *o* is inserted between the roots *cardi* (heart) and *vascul* (blood vessels). (The cardiovascular system is the body's system of heart and blood vessels.) The combining vowel is usually an *o* but is sometimes a different vowel, such as *a* or *i*. A combining vowel might not be added to a root if a vowel is already present in the suffix. The only purpose of the combining vowel is to make the word easier to pronounce. An example of a root joined to a suffix with a combining vowel in the middle is shown in Figure 4-1.

A medical term can contain more than one word root, and may or may not have both a suffix and a prefix.

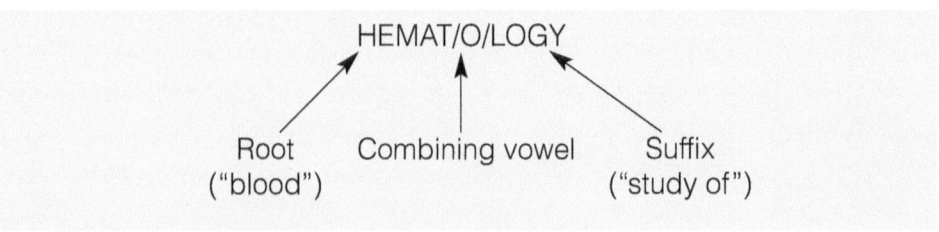

FIGURE 4-1 Analyzing a medical term.

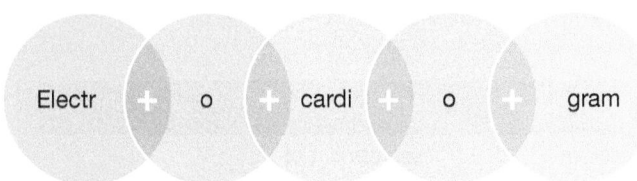

FIGURE 4-2 Word building.

Roots and Combining Forms

Most medical terms are formed from a word root to which other parts—such as additional roots, prefixes, suffixes, and/or combining vowels—are attached. For example, in Figure 4-2, the word root *cardi* is shown. As already mentioned, *cardi* means heart so, as a medical assistant, when you see this word you will immediately know it must have something to do with the heart. Another word root, *electr*, refers to electricity. When the roots *electr* and *cardi* are joined together with the combining vowel *o* after each root and the suffix *-gram* (record), the medical term *electrocardiogram* is formed. An *electrocardiogram* is a written record of the electrical activity of the heart.

As we just noted, the vowel *o* is used in two places in *electrocardiogram*, after *electr* and after *cardi*, to connect the two roots and the suffix. When a word root has a vowel attached so it can be combined with another element, the root + vowel is termed a **combining form**, such as *electr/o* or *cardi/o*. In *electrocardiogram*, the combining forms are *electro* and *cardio*.

Sometimes two combining forms are placed together to create a more complex word. An inflammation of the stomach is *gastritis*, and an inflammation of the intestines is *enteritis*. If both areas are inflamed, the term is *gastroenteritis*. The letter *o* is added after the root *gastr*, but note that *o* is not added after the root *enter* because the suffix *-itis* already begins with a vowel. An extra vowel was not needed to make the word pronounceable. Combining letters are usually used only when adding a suffix would otherwise place two consonants together or just to make the word easier to pronounce. Here are some helpful guidelines:

1. If the suffix begins with a vowel, drop the combining vowel from the combining form and add the suffix. For example, *lip/o* (fat) + *oma* (tumor) becomes *lipoma* when the *o* from *lipo* is deleted. A lipoma is a tumor composed of fat.

2. If the suffix begins with a consonant, keep the combining vowel when you add the suffix. For example, *lip/o* (fat) + *lysis* (destruction) becomes *lipolysis*, and the *o* on that combining form is retained. Lipolysis is the destruction of fat.

Because English medical terminology is based on both Greek and Latin, sometimes there are two roots that mean the same thing. For example, both *pneum* from Greek and *pulmon* from Latin mean *lung*. Sometimes the roots can be used interchangeably, and other times tradition determines which root is used. For example, *pulmonologist* describes a physician specializing in the study of the lungs, whereas *pneumonia* describes a condition of the lungs.

Table 4-1 lists some word roots commonly used in medical terminology. Table 4-2 lists common combining forms in which a combining vowel is added to the root.

TABLE 4-1 | Commonly Used Word Roots

Word Root	Meaning	Word Root	Meaning
abdomin	abdomen	aur	ear
aden	gland	aut	self
adren	adrenal gland	bil	bile
adrenal	adrenal gland	bio	life
aer	air, oxygen, gas	blephar	eyelid
alveoli	alveolus	bronch	airway, bronchus
angi	(blood) vessel, (lymph) vessel	bronchiol	bronchiole
ankyl	crooked, stiff, bent	burs	bursa
appendic	appendix	carcin	cancer
arteri, arter	artery	cardi	heart
arteriol	arteriole (small artery)	caud	tail, toward lower part of the body
arthr	joint	caus	burning sensation, capable of burning
ather	yellowish, fatty plaque	cephal	head

(continued)

TABLE 4-1 | Commonly Used Word Roots (*continued*)

Word Root	Meaning	Word Root	Meaning
cerebell	cerebellum	exocrin	secrete out of
cerebr	cerebrum, brain	faci	face
cervic	neck, cervix	fasci	fascia, fibrous band
cheil	lip	flexion	bending
chiro	hand	fract	break, broken
cholangi	bile duct	galact	milk
chole	gall, bile	gastr	stomach
chondr	cartilage	genital	pertaining to birth
coccyg	coccyx, tailbone	ger	old age, aged
col	colon, large intestine	geront	old age, aged
conjunctiv	conjunctiva	gingiv	gums
corne	cornea	glauc	gray
coron	heart, crown of the head	gloss	tongue
cost	rib	gluc	sweetness, sugar
crani	cranium, skull	glyc	sugar, glucose
cusp	point, cusp	glycos	sugar, glucose
cutane	skin	gnos	knowledge, a knowing
cyan	blue	gonad	gonad, sex glands
cyst	bladder, sac	gyn	woman
cyt, cyte	cell	gynec	woman
dacry	tears, tear duct	gyr	turning, folding
dactyl	fingers or toes	hem	blood
dent	tooth	hemat	blood
derm	skin	hepat	liver
dermat	skin	hidr	sweat
dipl	two, double	hist	tissue
diverticul	diverticulum	hom	same
dors	back (of the body)	home	sameness, unchanging
duoden	duodenum	hydr	water
ectop	located away from usual place	hyster	uterus
edema	swelling	ile	ileum
electr	electricity, electrical activity	ili	ilium
encephal	brain	immun	immune
endocrine	endocrine	irid	iris
enter	intestines (usually small intestine)	kerat	horny tissue, hard
epiglott	epiglottis	kin	movement
epitheli	epithelium	kinesi	movement, motion
erythr	red	labi	lips
esophagi	esophagus	lacrim	tear duct, tear
esthesi	sensation, feeling, sensitivity	lact	milk
eti	cause (of disease)	lapar	abdomen

TABLE 4-1 | Commonly Used Word Roots (*continued*)

Word Root	Meaning	Word Root	Meaning
laryng	larynx	or	mouth
later	side	orth	straight
lei	smooth	oste	bone
leuk	white	ot	ear
lingu	tongue	ox	oxygen
lip	fat	palpat	touch, feel, stroke
lith	stone, calculus	pancreat	pancreas
lob	lobe	par, part	bear, give birth to, labor
lumb	lumbar, loin region	parathyroid	parathyroid
lymph	lymph	path	disease, suffering
macr	abnormal largeness	pector	chest, muscle
mamm	breast	ped	child, foot
mast	breast	pelv	pelvis, pelvic bone
meat	opening or passageway	pen	penis
mediastin	mediastinum	perine	perineum
melan	black	peritone	peritoneum
men	menstruation	petr	stone, portion of temporal bone
mening	meninges	phac, phak	lens of the eye
ment	mind	phag	eat, swallow
mes, meso	middle	phalang	finger or toe bone
metr	uterus	pharyng	pharynx, throat
mon	one	phas	speech
morbid	disease, sickness	phleb	vein
muc	mucus	phot	light
my, myos	muscle	phren	mind
myc	fungus	physi	nature
myel	bone marrow, spinal cord	pleur	pleura
myelon	bone marrow	pneum	lung, air
myring	eardrum	pneumat	lung, air
narc	stupor, numbness	pneumon	lung, air
nas	nose	pod	foot
nat	birth	poli	gray matter
necr	death (cells, body)	polyp	polyp, small growth
nephr	kidney	poster	back (of body)
neur	nerve	prim	first
noct	night	proct	rectum
nyct	night	pseud	fake, false
nyctal	night	psych	mind
ocul	eye	pulmon	lung
onc	tumor	py	pus
onych	nail	pyel	renal pelvis
oophor	ovary	pylor	pylorus
ophthalm	eye	pyr	fever, heat

(continued)

TABLE 4-1 | Commonly Used Word Roots (*continued*)

Word Root	Meaning
quadr	four
rect	rectum
ren	kidney
retin	retina
rhin	nose
sacr	sacrum
salping	fallopian (uterine) tube
sanit	soundness, health
sarc	flesh, connective tissue
scler	sclera, white of eye, hard
scoli	crooked, curved
seb	sebum, oil
seps	infection
sept	infection, partition, septum
sial	saliva
somat	body
somn	sleep
son	sound
sopor	sleep
sperm	sperm, spermatozoa, seed
spermat	sperm, spermatozoa, seed
spher	round, sphere, ball
sphygm	pulse
spin	spine, backbone to
spir	breathe
splen	spleen
spondyl	vertebra, spinal or vertebral column
staphyl	grapelike clusters
stern	breastbone
steth	chest (muscles)
stoma	mouth, opening
stomat	mouth, opening
strab	squint, squint-eyed
synovi	synovia, synovial membrane
system	system
ten, tend	tendon
tendin	tendon
tens, tensi	pressure, force, stretching
test	testis, testicle
therm	heat
thorac	thorax, chest
thromb	clot
thym	thymus gland, soul

Word Root	Meaning
thyr	thyroid gland
thyroid	thyroid gland
tom	cut, section
ton	tension, pressure
tone	to stretch
tonsil	tonsils
top	place, position, location
tox, toxic	poison, poisonous
trach, trache	trachea, windpipe
trachel	neck, necklike
trich	hair
tubercul	little knot, swelling
tympan	eardrum, middle ear
ulcer	sore, ulcer
ungu	nail
ur	urine, urinary tract
ureter	ureter
urethr	urethra
uria	urination, urine
urin	urine, urinary organs
uter	uterus
uvul	uvula, little grape
vagin	vagina
valv	valve
valvul	valve
vas	vessel, duct
vascul	blood vessel, little vessel
ven	vein
versicul	seminal vesicles, blister
vertebr	vertebra, backbone
vesic	urinary bladder
vir	poison, virus
viril	masculine, manly
vis	seeing, sight
visc	sticky
viscer	viscera, internal organism
viscos	sticky
vit	life
xanth	yellow
xen	strange, foreign
xer	dry
zygot	joined together

TABLE 4-2 | Commonly Used Combining Forms

Combining Form	Meaning	Combining Form	Meaning
arter/o	artery	ophthalm/o	eye
arthr/o	joint	ot/o	ear
balan/o	penis	oste/o	bone
cardi/o	heart	pharyng/o	throat
cephal/o	head	phleb/o	vein
derm/o	skin	pulmon/o	lung
enter/o	intestines	ren/o	kidney
erythr/o	red	rhin/o	nose
gastr/o	stomach	stomat/o	mouth
hyster/o	uterus	thromb/o	clot
laryng/o	voice box	thyroid/o	thyroid
leuk/o	white	ureter/o	ureter
mamm/o, mast/o	breast	urethr/o	urethra
my/o	muscle	urin/o	urine
nas/o, rhin/o	nose	ven/o	vein

Prefixes

Prefixes are placed at the beginnings of words to alter or modify their meanings or to create new words. Table 4-3 is a list of commonly used prefixes. Prefixes are usually written with a hyphen at the end, such as *hypo-* (meaning low), to indicate that another word part would follow. It is important to study the prefix *in context* to fully understand how it impacts the word meaning. In Figure 4-3, note how the use of the prefix *hypo-*, meaning "low," significantly changes the meaning of a word when replaced with the prefix *hyper-*, meaning "high."

TABLE 4-3 | Commonly Used Prefixes

Prefix	Meaning	Prefix	Meaning
a-	without or absence of	dys-	difficult, labored, painful, abnormal
ab-	from, away from	ec-	out
ad-	to, toward	ecto-	outside
an-	without or absence of	endo-	within
ante-	before	epi-	on, upon, over
anti-	against	eso-	inward
bi-	two	eu-	normal, good
bin-	two	ex-	outside, outward
brady-	slow	exo-	outside, outward
con-	together	extra-	outside of, beyond
contra-	against	hemi-	half
de-	from, down from, lack of	hyper-	above, excessive
dia-	through, complete, between, apart	hypo-	below, incomplete, deficient
dis-	to undo, free from	in-	in, into, not

(continued)

TABLE 4-3 | Commonly Used Prefixes (*continued*)

Prefix	Meaning	Prefix	Meaning
infra-	under, below	pro-	before
inter-	between	quadri-	four
intra-	within	re-	back
mal-	bad	retro-	back, behind
meso-	middle	semi-	half
meta-	after, beyond, change	sub-	under, below
micro-	small	super-	over, above
multi-	many	supra-	above, beyond, on top
neo-	new	sym-	together, joined
nulli-	none	syn-	together, joined
pan-	all, total	tachy-	fast, rapid
para-	outside, beyond, around	tetra-	four
per-	through	trans-	through, across, beyond
peri-	surrounding (outer)	tri-	three
poly-	many, much	ultra-	beyond, excess
post-	after	uni-	one
pre-	before, in front of		

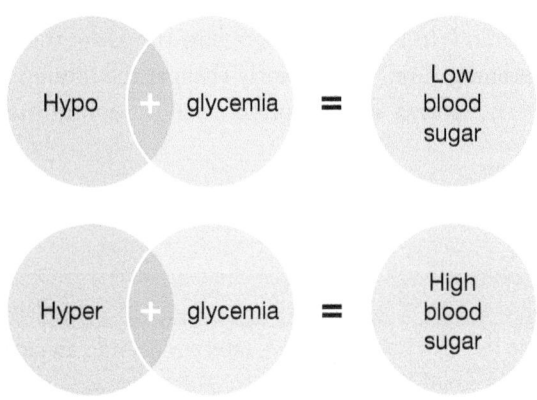

FIGURE 4-3 Exchanging word parts to change meaning.

Be aware that some prefixes can have several meanings. Table 4-4 lists some prefixes that have more than one meaning.

Suffixes

A suffix is a syllable or group of syllables attached to the end of a word to alter or modify its meaning or to create a new word. A suffix is usually written with a hyphen in front of it, such as *-algia* (meaning pain or suffering), to indicate that another word part would come before. In the word in Figure 4-1, for example, the suffix *-logy* means "the study of." The word *hematology* means "the study of blood." Simply changing the suffix can alter the entire meaning of a word.

If, as in Figure 4-1, the suffix is changed to *-uria*, which means "urine," the word would be *hematuria*, meaning "blood in the urine." Table 4-5 lists suffixes commonly used in medical terminology.

Taking Words Apart

As a medical assistant, you can apply the same skills to medical terminology that you use to understand everyday English. For example, if you know that *tele* means far away and *-gram* means record, you can take the word apart to figure out that *telegram* means "a written record from far away." In your work as a medical assistant, you can use the same skill to take apart *electrocardiogram* and understand that it means "an electrical record of the heart." After you learn the meaning of a suffix, you can apply it to a variety of medical terms. If you know that *appendicitis* means "inflammation of the appendix," and you see the same suffix, *-itis*, in the word *tonsillitis*, you can take the word apart and figure out that it means "inflammation of the tonsils." Developing the habit of taking words apart will help you understand the word-building patterns and meanings in medical terminology.

To take words apart, follow these steps:

1. Divide the medical term into each of its word parts. Example: The medical term *amenorrhea* breaks down into *a/men/o/rrhea*.

TABLE 4-4 | Selected Prefixes with More Than One Meaning

Prefix	Meaning	Prefix	Meaning
a-, an-	no, not, without, lack of, apart	extra-	outside, beyond
ad-	toward, near, to	hyper-	above, beyond, excessive
bi-	two, double	hypo-	below, under, deficient
de-	down, away from	in-	into, not
di-	two, double	mega-	large, great
dia-	through, between, complete	meta-	beyond, over, between, change
dif-, dis-	apart, free from, separate	para-	beside, alongside, abnormal
dys-	bad, difficult, painful, abnormal	poly-	many, much, excessive
ec-, ecto-	out, outside, outer	post-	after, behind
end-, endo-	within, inner	pre-	before, in front of
ep-, epi-	upon, over, above	pro-	before, in front of
eu-	good, normal	super-	upper, above
ex-, exo-	out, away from	supra-	above, beyond

TABLE 4-5 | Commonly Used Suffixes

Suffix	Meaning	Suffix	Meaning
-algia	pain, suffering	-gen	producing, forming
-asthenia	weakness	-genesis	producing, forming
-cele	hernia, protrusion	-genic	producing, forming
-centesis	surgical puncture to remove fluid	-gnosis	a knowing
-cidal	killing	-gram	record, X-ray
-clasia	break	-graph	instrument used to record
-clasis	break	-graphy	process of recording, X-ray filming
-clast	break	-ictal	seizure, attack
-clysis	irrigating, washing	-ism	state of
-coccus	berry shaped (a form of bacterium)	-itis	inflammation
-crine	separate, secrete	-lepsy	seizure
-crit	to separate	-logist	specialist
-cyte	cell	-logy	study of
-desis	fusion, to bind, tie together	-lysis	destruction, reduce, separation
-drome	run, running	-malacia	softening
-dctor	to lead or pull	-mani	madness, insane desire
-dynia	pain	-megaly	enlargement
-ectasis	stretching out, dilation, expansion	-meter	instrument used to measure
-ectomy	excision or surgical removal	-metry	measurement
-ectopia	displacement	-morph	form, shape
-emesis	vomiting	-oid, ode	resembling
-emia	blood, blood condition	-oma	tumor, mass

(*continued*)

TABLE 4-5 | Commonly Used Suffixes (*continued*)

Suffix	Meaning
-opia	vision (condition)
-opsy	to view
-oxia	oxygen
-paresis	slight paralysis
-pathy	disease
-penia	abnormal reduction in number, lack of
-peps, pepsia	digestion
-pexy	surgical fixation, suspension
-phagia	eating, swallowing
-philia	love
-phily	love
-phobia	abnormal fear of, or aversion to, specific objects or things
-phonia	sound or voice
-phoria	feeling
-physis	growth
-plasia	formation, development, a growth
-plasm	growth, formation, substance
-plasty	plastic or surgical repair
-plegia	paralysis, stroke
-pnea	breathing
-porosis	lessening in density, porous condition
-praxia	in front of, before
-ptosis	drooping, sagging, prolapse
-ptysis	spitting
-rrhage	bursting forth, an abnormal excessive discharge or bleeding

Suffix	Meaning
-rrhagia	bursting forth, an abnormal excessive discharge or bleeding
-rrhaphy	to suture or stitch
-rrhea	flow or discharge
-rrhexis	rupture
-schisis	split, fissure
-sclerosis	hardening
-scope	instrument used for visual exam
-scopic	visual exam
-scopy	visual exam with an instrument
-sepsis	infection
-sis	state of
-spasm	sudden involuntary muscle contraction
-stalsis	contraction, constriction
-stasis	control, stop, standing still
-stat	to stop
-stenosis	narrowing, constriction
-stomy	new artificial opening
-therapy	treatment
-tome	instrument used to cut
-tomy	cutting into, surgical incision
-tripsy	crushing
-trophy	nourishment
-ule	little
-uria	urine, urination

2. Identify the suffix and its meaning. Example: In the medical term *amenorrhea*, the suffix is *-rrhea*, meaning flow or discharge.

3. Identify the root and its meaning. Example: In the medical term *amenorrhea*, the root is *men*, meaning menses or menstrual.

4. Identify the combining vowel. Example: In the medical term *amenorrhea*, the combining vowel is *o*. The combining vowel has no meaning of its own but makes the word easier to pronounce.

5. Identify the prefix and its meaning. Example: In the medical term *amenorrhea*, the prefix is *a-*, meaning lack of or without.

6. Combine the meanings of the word parts to determine the meaning of the word. Example: The medical term *amenorrhea* means lack of menstrual flow.

Rules for Plurals

Medical terms that are nouns can be singular—referring to one—or plural, referring to more than one. Plurals are formed in a variety of ways, just as in English not all plurals end in "s." For example, more than one hand is *hands*, but more than one foot is *feet*. Medical terms do not end in "s" because they are based on Greek and Latin, not English. Table 4-6 shows the patterns of forming plurals for Latin-based medical terms.

Writing and Pronouncing Medical Terms

You need to be able to write and pronounce medical terms correctly because they are a key part of communication in the medical office. Spelling is important in any language, but it is especially important in medical terminology. Careful reading and spelling accuracy are important to identify

TABLE 4-6 | Forming Plurals of Medical Terms

To change each singular word listed on the left to its plural form listed on the right, replace the singular ending with the plural ending as illustrated.

Singular Ending	Plural Ending
a as in burs**a**	to **ae** as in burs**ae**
ax as in thor**ax**	to **aces** as in thor**aces** or **es** as in thor**axes**
en as in foram**en**	to **ina** as in foram**ina**
is as in cris**is**	to **es** as in cris**es**
is as in ir**is**	to **ides** as in ir**ides**
is as in femor**is**	to **a** as in femor**a**
ix as in append**ix**	to **ices** as in append**ices**
nx as in phala**nx**	to **ges** as in phalan**ges**
on as in spermatozo**on**	to **a** as in spermatozo**a**
um as in ov**um**	to **a** as in ov**a**
us as in nucle**us**	to **i** as in nucle**i**
y as in arter**y**	to **i** and add **es** as in arter**ies**

example, *ilium* refers to the pelvic or hip bone, whereas *ileum* refers to a portion of the small intestine. Table 4-7 lists prefixes and suffixes that are frequently misspelled.

The pronunciation of medical terms is important to ensure clear communication. A medical assistant must learn how to properly pronounce medical terms when speaking with patients and other health care professionals. Many medical dictionaries available on the Internet include an audio feature that allows you to hear how the word is pronounced.

MEDICAL ABBREVIATIONS

Abbreviations are a type of shorthand that saves time and space. However, health care professionals must share a common understanding of the meanings of abbreviations and use only official and common abbreviations. Do not make up your own abbreviations "on the fly" just for convenience. Every medical facility should keep a list of abbreviations that are acceptable to use in documentation and other communication. Ask for this list when you begin a new job, and keep it handy for reference. Table 4-8 provides a list of commonly used abbreviations.

Although medical abbreviations are helpful and widely used in patient charting, some abbreviations can be easily misinterpreted or misread, particularly when the abbreviations are handwritten. The Joint Commission (TJC), which

the correct meaning of a word part and, consequently, a medical term. Simple mistakes can result in serious medical errors. You have already seen how changing the prefix can cause a word to have an opposite meaning. Sometimes one letter can result in a word with a different meaning. For

TABLE 4-7 | Prefixes and Suffixes That Are Frequently Misspelled

Prefix	Meaning	Suffix	Meaning
ante-	before, forward	-poiesis	formation
anti-	against	-ptosis	prolapse, drooping, sagging, falling down
ecto-	out, outside, outer	-ptysis	spitting
endo-	within, inner	-rrhage	to burst forth, bursting forth
hyper-	above, beyond, excessive	-rrhagia	to burst forth, bursting forth
hypo-	below, under, deficient	-rrhaphy	suture
inter-	between	-rrhea	flow, discharge
intra-	within	-rrhexis	rupture
para-	beside, alongside, abnormal	-scope	instrument for examining
per-	through	-scopy	visual examination, to view, examine
supra-	above, beyond	-stomy	to form a mouth, new opening
peri-	around	-tome	instrument to cut
pre-	before, in front of	-tomy	incision
pro-	before	-tripsy	crushing
super-	above, beyond	-trophy	nourishment, development

TABLE 4-8 | Commonly Used Medical Abbreviations

Abbreviation	Meaning	Abbreviation	Meaning
AD	Alzheimer's disease	I&D	incision and drainage
AIDS	acquired immunodeficiency syndrome	ICU	intensive care unit
APAP	acetaminophen (Tylenol)	ID	intradermal
ARC	AIDS-related complex	IM	intramuscular
BE	barium enema	inj	injection
BK	below knee	IV	intravenous
BP	blood pressure	K⁺	potassium
Bx	biopsy	kg	kilogram
C1, C2, etc.	first cervical vertebra, second cervical vertebra, etc.	L	left, liter
		L1, L2, etc.	first lumbar vertebra, second lumbar vertebra, etc.
CAT	computerized axial tomography	LLQ	left lower quadrant
cc	cubic centimeter	LUQ	left upper quadrant
CC	clean catch urine specimen, chief complaint, cardiac catheterization	mcg	microgram
		mg	milligram
CV	cardiovascular	MI	myocardial infarction, mitral insufficiency
CXR	chest X-ray		
D&C	dilation and curettage	mL	milliliter
D/c, d/c	discontinue	MS	musculoskeletal, mitral stenosis, multiple sclerosis
DM	diabetes mellitus		
Dx	diagnosis	n & v	nausea and vomiting
ECC	echocardiogram, extracorporeal circulation	NG	nasogastric
		NSAID	nonsteroidal antiinflammatory drug
ECG	electrocardiogram	O₂	oxygen
ED	emergency department	OA	osteoarthritis
EDD	estimated date of delivery	OM	otitis media
EEG	electroencephalogram	OR	operating room
ENT	ear, nose, and throat	OTC	over the counter
FBOT	fecal occult blood test	oz	ounce
FBS	fasting blood sugar	P	pulse
Fx	fracture	PERRLA	pupils equal, round, reactive to light and accommodation
GB	gallbladder		
GI	gastrointestinal	pH	acidity or alkalinity of urine
gm	gram	PNS	peripheral nervous system
gr	grain	PO, po	by mouth
GTT	glucose tolerance test	prn	as needed
GU	genitourinary	pt	patient
GYN	gynecology	PT	physical therapy
HA	headache	q	every
HCT	hematocrit	R	respiration, right, roentgen
HD	Hodgkin's disease	RBC	red blood cell
HTN	hypertension		

TABLE 4-8 | Commonly Used Medical Abbreviations (*continued*)

Abbreviation	Meaning
RLQ	right lower quadrant
ROM	range of motion
RUQ	right upper quadrant
Rx	take, prescription
SC	subcutaneous
Sig	label as follows
sl	sublingual, under the tongue
sp. gr.	specific gravity
stat, STAT	immediately
T	tablespoon, temperature
t	teaspoon
T1, T2, etc.	first thoracic vertebra, second thoracic vertebra, etc.

Abbreviation	Meaning
tab	tablet
tbsp	tablespoon
TO	telephone order
tsp	teaspoon
Tx	traction, treatment
UA	urinalysis
URI	upper respiratory infection
UTI	urinary tract infection
VO	verbal order
VS	vital signs
WBC	white blood cell
wt	weight
x	times

Professionalism   The Law

In a court of law, misspelled and improperly used medical terminology can be inferred to indicate sloppy patient care. Imagine misspelled words or words used inappropriately being flashed onto a wall in a courtroom. A medical assistant's writing reflects the professionalism of care. Equally important is to pronounce medical terms properly. The medical assistant needs both to spell terms correctly and to be able to pronounce them correctly.

Professionalism   The Workplace

Although abbreviations may save time in writing, they are frequently a source of misunderstandings in the workplace. Unless a list of approved abbreviations is established for the office, expand writing whenever possible.

accredits hospitals and other health care institutions, has created a list of abbreviations that should be avoided in order to reduce the risk of medical errors. This list is referred to as the "Do Not Use" list and is further discussed in the chapter titled "Pharmacology."

GROSS ANATOMY

Specific terminology is used to describe the body's overall structure—also known as gross anatomy—in terms of directions, body planes, cavities, and regions.

Directions and Body Planes

Directional terms describe the location of a body part or organ in relation to the center of the body. When the body is visually sliced down a *coronal* or *frontal plane*, the front is referred to as *anterior* or *ventral*; the back is referred to as *posterior* or *dorsal*. When a *transverse* or *horizontal* plane is used, the area above the plane is referred to as *superior*, or *cranial* or *cephalic*, and the area below the plane is termed *inferior* or *caudal*. Areas farther from the *medial* or *midsagittal* plane are *lateral*; those closer to the plane are *medial*. When referring to points relative to where the arms and legs attach to the body, those farther away are *distal*; those closer are *proximal*. Figure 4-4 illustrates the body planes. Table 4-9 summarizes the directional terms.

Body Cavities

The body's vital organs are contained in cavities. The cranial cavity houses the brain. The spinal cord is located within the spinal cavity. The chest, or thoracic, cavity holds the lungs and heart. Below the diaphragm, the abdominopelvic cavity holds other vital organs, including the intestines, stomach, reproductive organs, bladder, and liver. See Figure 4-5 to view the body cavities.

Body Positions

Body positions refer to the physical orientation of the patient, as when preparing for an examination of procedure. *Prone* describes the body lying face-down, whereas *supine* describes lying face-up. *Lateral* refer to lying on one's side.

Abdominal Regions and Quadrants

Special terms that identify location on or within the abdomen include nine regions and four quadrants.

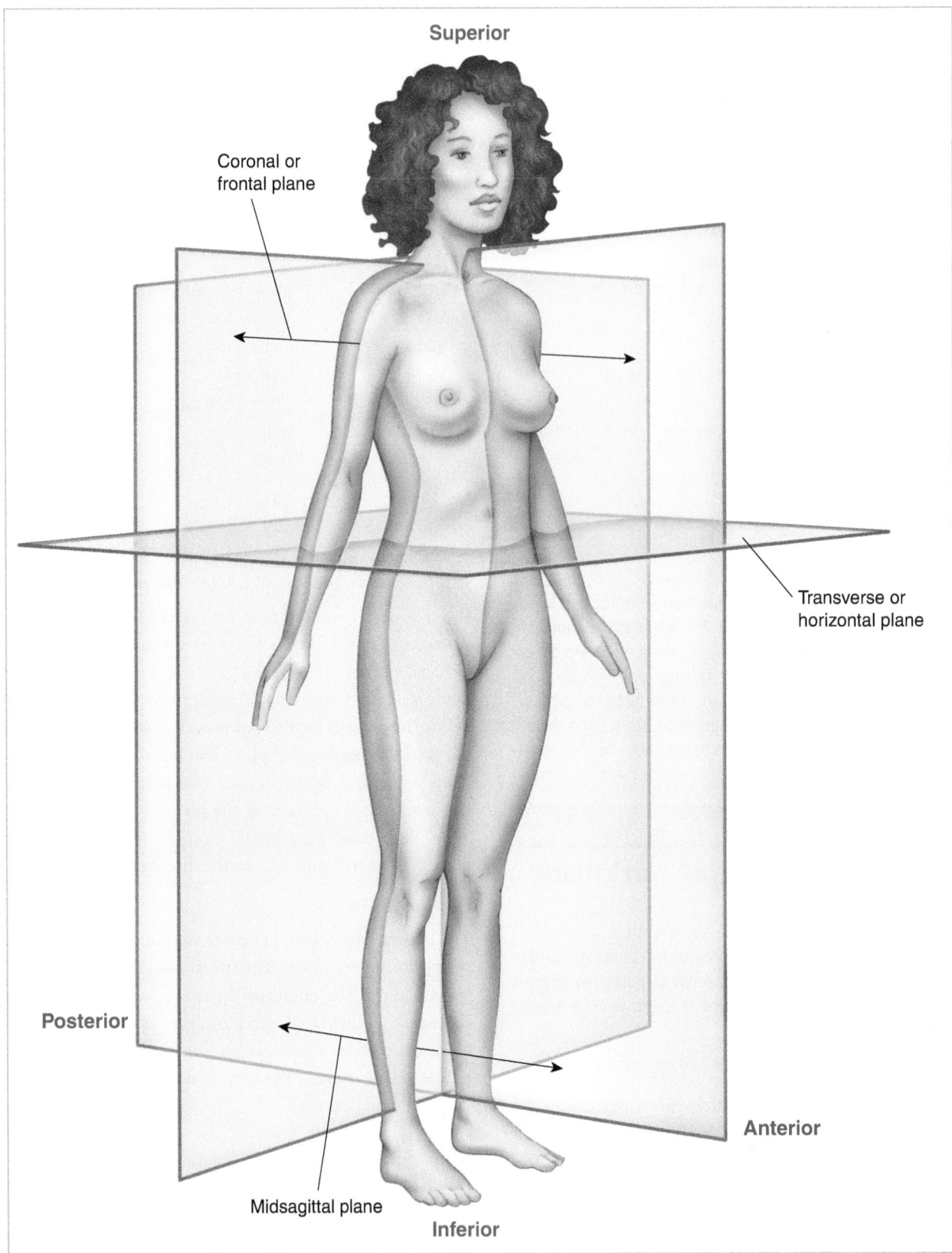

Superior

Coronal or
frontal plane

Transverse or
horizontal plane

Posterior

Anterior

Midsagittal plane

Inferior

FIGURE 4-4 Planes of the body and directional terms.

TABLE 4-9 | Directional and Positional Terms

Term	Description	Example
Superior	Above, in an upward direction, toward the head	The head is *superior* to the neck of the body.
Anterior (ventral)	In front of or before, the front side of the body	The breasts are located on the *anterior* side of the body.
Posterior (dorsal)	Toward the back, the back side of the body	The nape is the back of the neck and is located on the *posterior* side of the body.
Cephalic	Pertaining to the head	A *cephalic* presentation is one in which any part of the head of the fetus is presented during childbirth.
Medial	Nearest the midline or middle	The umbilicus is a depressed point in the *medial* area of the abdomen.
Lateral	To the side, away from the middle	In the anatomical position, the arm is located on the *lateral* side of the body.
Proximal	Nearest the point of attachment or near the beginning of a structure	The *proximal* end of the humerus (upper bone of the arm) forms part of the shoulder joint.
Distal	Away from the point of attachment or far from the beginning of a structure	The *distal* end of the humerus joins with part of the elbow.
Prone	Lying face-down	The patient lies face-down in a *prone* position so the physician can examine the back side of the body.
Supine	Lying face-up	The patient lies on her back on the exam table in a *supine* position.

The nine regions of the abdominopelvic cavity are illustrated in Figure 4-6A. These terms might be used to indicate where the medical assistant must prepare the patient's skin for a surgical procedure. Keep in mind that, in anatomy, "right" and "left" refer to the person's right and left, not right and left as you look at the person. The nine abdominopelvic regions and the organs located in these regions are as follows:

- The *umbilical region* is where the umbilicus, or navel, is found and contains the umbilicus, jejunum, ileum, and duodenum.
- The *epigastric region* is above the umbilical region (several centimeters above the navel) and contains the stomach, liver, pancreas, duodenum, spleen, and adrenal glands.
- The *hypogastric region* is below the umbilical region and contains the urinary bladder, sigmoid colon, and male and female reproductive organs.
- The *left hypochondriac region* is to the left of the epigastric region and contains the spleen, colon, left kidney, and pancreas.

- The *left lumbar region* is to the left of the umbilical region and containsthe descending colon, left kidney, and left adrenal gland.
- The *left inguinal* or *iliac region* is to the left of the hypogastric region and contains the descending colon and sigmoid colon.
- The *right hypochondriac region* is to the right of the epigastric region and contains the liver, gallbladder, right kidney, right adrenal gland, and small intestine.
- The *right lumbar region* is to the right of the umbilical region and contains the gallbladder, liver, and right colon.
- The *right inguinal* or *iliac region* is to the right of the hypogastric region and contains the appendix and cecum.

The abdomen can also be divided into four quadrants, illustrated in Figure 4-6B. Quadrants are more generalized in location than the nine regions. They are used when it is more difficult to identify a specific anatomic site. A patient might complain of pain coming from an organ that the patient feels may be injured; however, the pain may actually

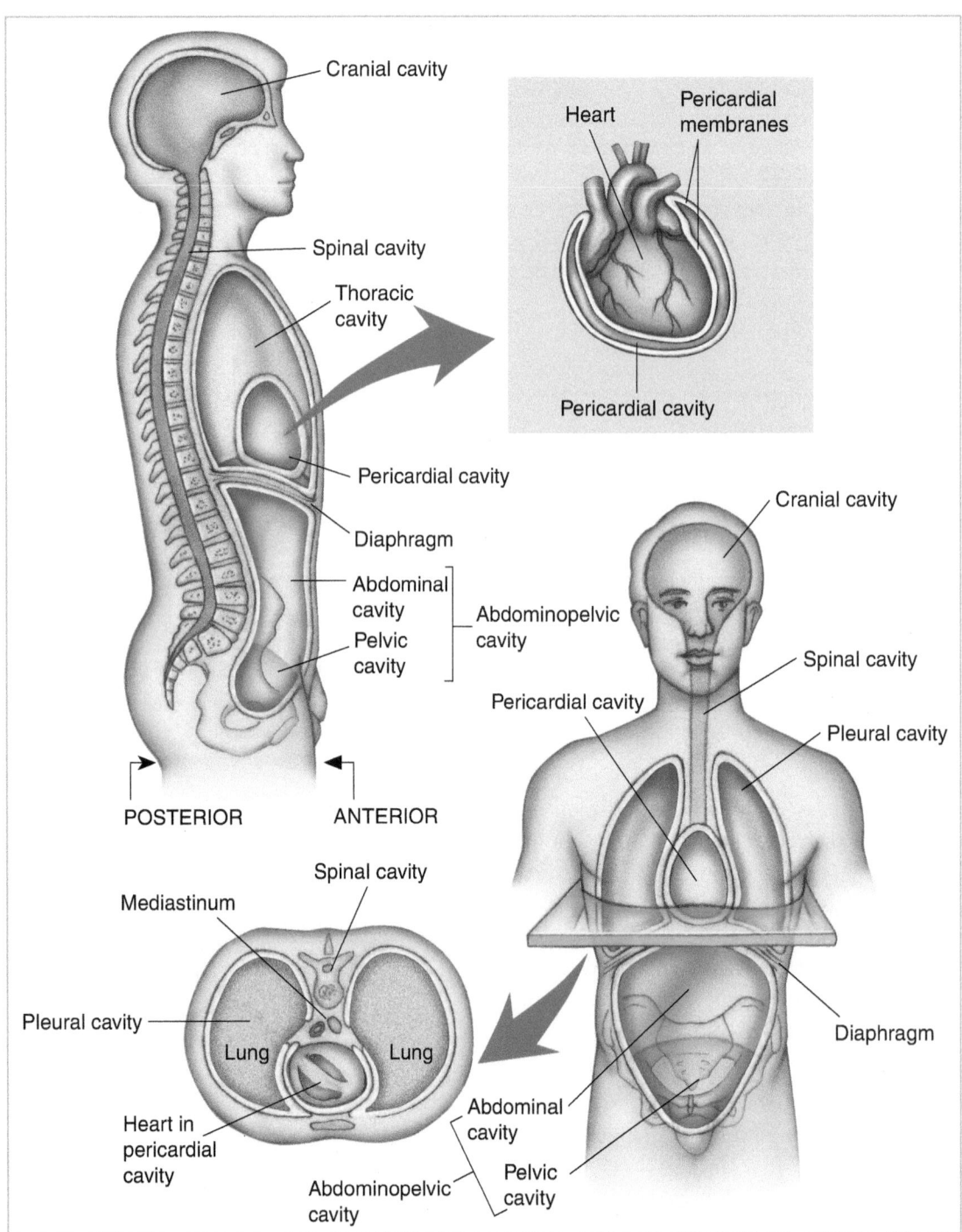

FIGURE 4-5 Body cavities.

be coming from an entirely separate organ. For example, the patient might say, "My stomach hurts." However, the pain felt in that general area might be from the spleen or pancreas, rather than the stomach. Therefore, rather than naming the specific organ or site, the medical assistant identifies the general area, or quadrant. The medical assistant should document the pain as, for example, "left upper quadrant" pain. The four quadrants and the organs they contain are:

- The *right upper quadrant (RUQ)* contains the liver, gallbladder, duodenum, upper portion of the pancreas, and hepatic flexure of the colon.
- The *right lower quadrant (RLQ)* contains the appendix, upper portion of the colon, right ovary, and right fallopian tube in women.
- The *left upper quadrant (LUQ)* contains the stomach, spleen, left portion of the liver, main portion of the

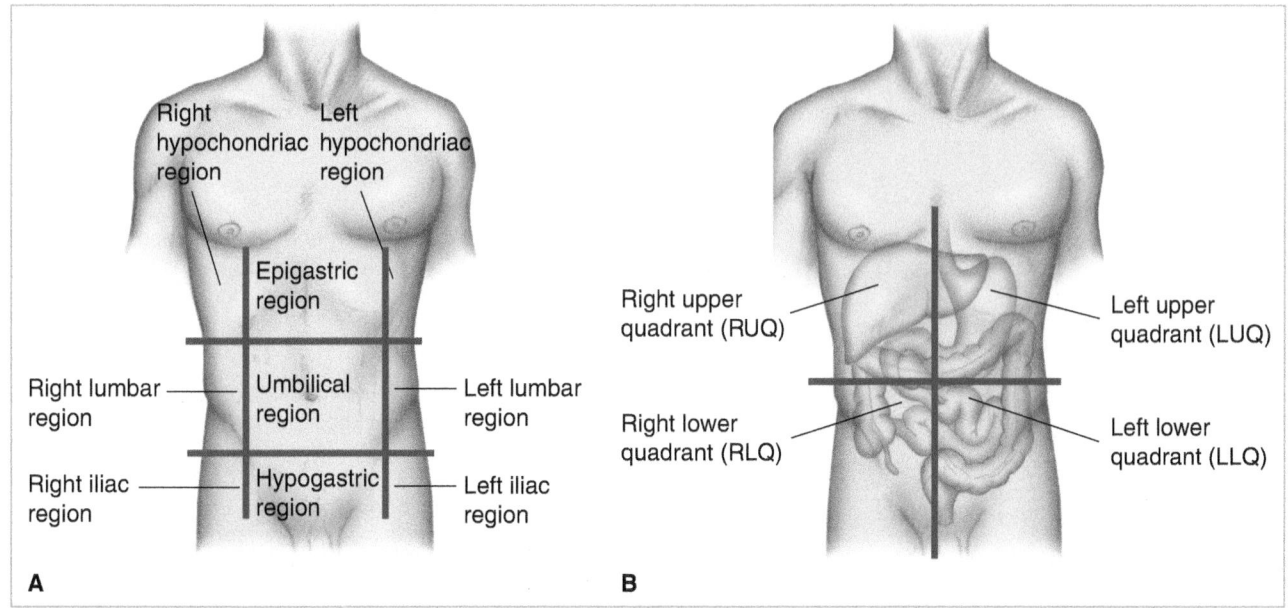

FIGURE 4-6 **(A)** Abdominopelvic regions; **(B)** Abdominal quadrants.

pancreas, left kidney, left adrenal gland, and splenic flexure and lower portion of the colon.

- The *left lower quadrant (LLQ)* contains the sigmoid colon and lower portion of the colon, left ovary, and left fallopian tube.

BODY SYSTEMS AND MEDICAL SPECIALTIES

When studying **anatomy**, which describes the structure of the body, and **physiology**, which describes the functions and processes of the body, it is important to understand that the body contains a number of body systems, also known as organ systems. Each body system has a specific role in body function but may interact with other systems to carry out the role. Physicians can specialize in the diagnosis and treatment of a specific organ system. Their area of study is known as a medical specialty. The following information highlights the role of each system, identifies the name of the physician and specialty, and gives examples of how terminology is used. See Figure 4-7 for an illustration of the systems of the body and their functions. Tables 4-10 through 4-21 list terminology related to each of the body systems.

Integumentary System

The integumentary system includes the largest organ of the body: the skin. The integument also includes hair, oil, nails, sweat glands, fat cells, and other tissues that aid in protection, exchange of heat and fluids, and absorption. The

Professionalism The Life Span

The words a medical assistant uses depend greatly on the age of the patient. If the patient is well educated and understands medical terminology, it is appropriate to use medical terminology when speaking with that patient. However, the vast majority of patients have little knowledge of Latin- and Greek-based terms. Small children may not even understand English very well. The medical assistant should use age-appropriate communication to meet the needs of the patient and ensure that there is clear understanding.

physician who specializes in treating the skin is a *dermatologist*. The specialty of this physician is called *dermatology*.

Placing medication into the layers of the skin is known as intradermal administration (within the dermis or true skin), and placing medication under the skin is referred to as subcutaneous administration (beneath or below the layers of the skin). Inflammation of the skin is known as dermatitis. See Table 4-10 for medical word parts related to the integumentary system.

Skeletal System

The skeletal system consists of bones and joints. Bones, which store minerals, give the body height and movement, and protect and support the body organs. Joints are the places where two or more bones meet. The title of a

Body System		Major Functions
Integumentary system		Protective membrane, temperature regulator, and sensory receptor.
Skeletal system		*Framework and Movement:* Shape, support, protection, and storage place for minerals. Movement is made possible through joints.
Muscular system		*Framework and Movement:* Muscles produce movement, maintain posture, and produce heat.
Nervous system		*Communication and Control:* The nervous system transmits impulses, responds to change, is responsible for communication, and exercises control over all parts of the body.
Endocrine system		*Communication and Control:* The glands of the endocrine system produce hormones, chemical messengers, that provide for communication and control over various parts of the body.
Cardiovascular system		*Transportation and Immunity:* Transports oxygen and carbon dioxide, delivers nutrients and hormones, and removes waste products.
Blood and the lymphatic system		*Transportation and Immunity:* Transports oxygen and carbon dioxide, chemical substances, and cells that act to protect the body from foreign substances. The lymphatic system stimulates immune response, protects the body, and transports proteins and fluids.
Respiratory system		*Distribution and Elimination:* Furnishes oxygen for use by individual tissue cells and removes their gaseous waste product, carbon dioxide.
Digestive system		*Distribution and Elimination:* Digestion, absorption, and elimination.
Urinary system		*Distribution and Elimination:* Produces urine, transports urine, and eliminates urine. The kidneys help maintain electrolyte, water, and acid-base balance of the body.
Reproductive system		*Cycle of Life:* Responsible for sexual characteristics of the male and/or female. Proper functioning ensures survival of the human race.

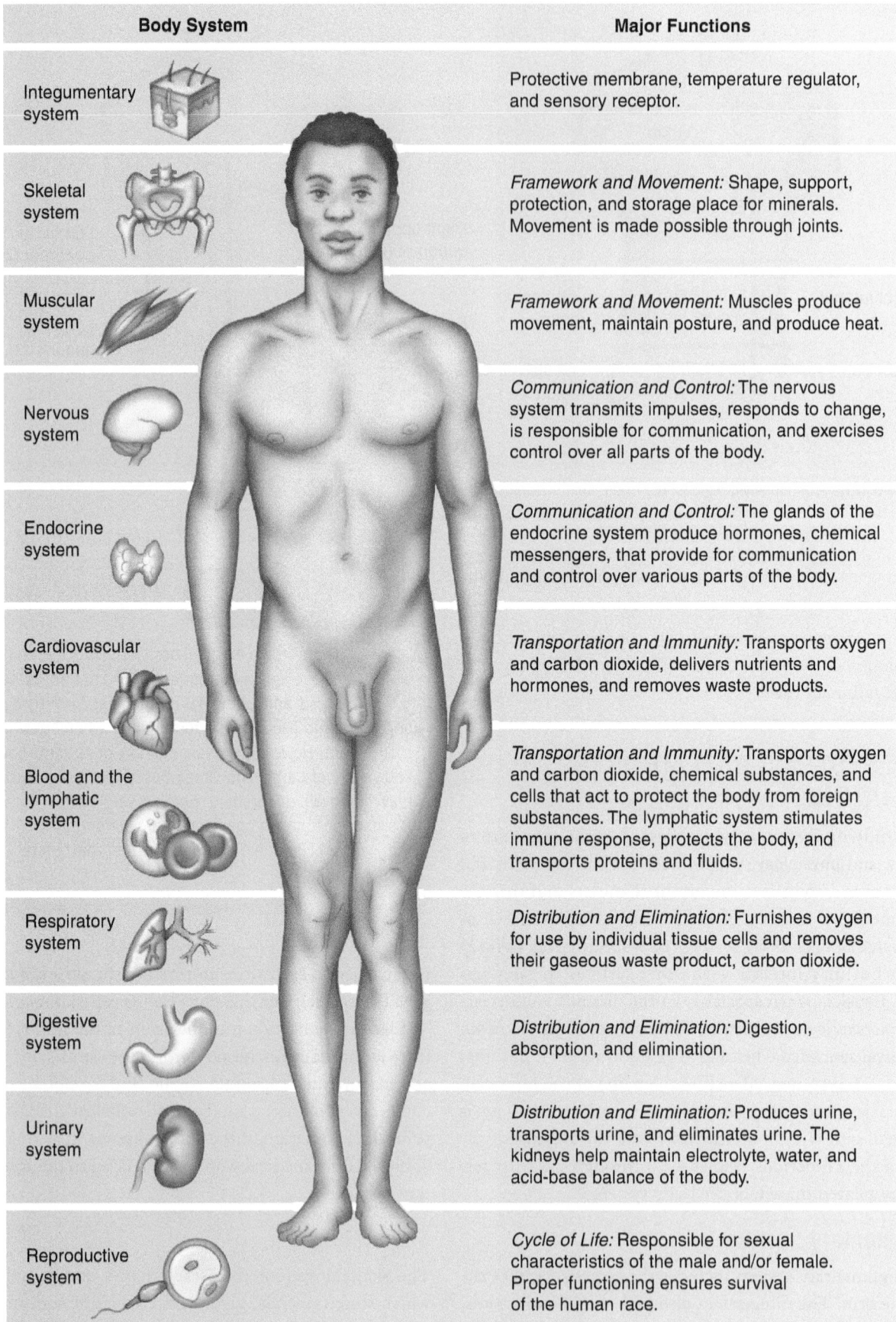

FIGURE 4-7 Body systems and their major functions.

TABLE 4-10	Integumentary System Word Parts
adip/o	fatty deposits
-cyst	fluid-filled sac
dermat/o, derm/o, cutane/o	skin
epi-	upon, above
ex-, ec-	out of
kerat/o	hard or horny
melan/o	black, extremely dark
onycho/o	nail
seb/o	oily
trich/o	hair

TABLE 4-11	Skeletal System Word Parts
ab-	away from
ad-	toward
arthr/o	joint
-blast	immature stage of cell development
circum-	around
-clast	breaking
cost/o	ribs
-malacia	softening
oste/o	bone
por/o	porous

TABLE 4-12	Muscular System Word Parts
bi-	two
delt/o	triangular
dys-	bad, painful
maxim/o	large
my/o	muscle
quad-	four
tax/o	coordination
tri-	three
-trophy	growth
vast/o	large

physician who specializes in treating the bones is an *orthopedist*. (The combining form *orth/o* means "straight," and *ped/o* is the combining form for "foot.") The specialty is *orthopedics*. The combining forms *oste/o* (bone) and *arthr/o* (joint) join with the suffix *-itis* to form the term *osteoarthritis*, which means inflammation of the bones and joints. A specialist in treating arthritis (inflammation of the joints), including rheumatoid arthritis, is called a *rheumatologist*. The specialty of this physician is called *rheumatology*.

Table 4-11 lists medical word parts related to the skeletal system.

Muscular System

The muscular system, which includes muscles, tendons, ligaments, and fascia, consists of soft tissues that help support and move the skeletal system. Muscles assist bones in movement. Tendons connect muscles to bones. Ligaments connect bones to bones. Fascia is the tissue that surrounds muscles. Orthopedists treat conditions of the muscular system, as well as those of the skeletal system.

Two combining forms for muscles are *muscul/o* and *my/o*. Thus, injecting medication into a muscle is known as an intramuscular injection. The heart is also a muscle; thus, inflammation of the heart muscle is termed *myocarditis*. Inflammation of a tendon is *tendonitis*, and inflammation of the fascia is *fasciitis*.

See Table 4-12 for medical word parts related to the muscular system.

Nervous System

The nervous system enables the body to sense changes in the external and internal environments and to experience pain. A physician who specializes in the treatment of the nervous system is a *neurologist*. The specialty is called *neurology*.

Pain is referred to with the suffixes *-algia* and *-dynia*. For example, arthralgia is pain in the joint. A frequently used medication that reduces pain is referred to as an *analgesic*. This word is a combination of *an* (meaning "without") + *algia* (meaning "pain") + *ic* (meaning "relating to"). The brain is an organ of the nervous system. The combining form *cephal/o* means the "head," and *encephal/o* is "in the head." Inflammation of the brain is referred to as *encephalitis*.

Table 4-13 lists medical word parts related to the nervous system.

Special Senses

The special senses include vision, hearing, taste, touch, and smell. A physician who specializes in the treatment of the eye is an *ophthalmologist*. The specialty is *ophthalmology*. An *optometrist* is a nonphysician health care provider who specializes in the care of the eye. The specialty is called *optometry*. An *audiologist* is a physician who specializes in the treatment of hearing disorders. The specialty is *audiology*. *Gustatory* refers to taste, and *olfactory* refers to smell.

TABLE 4-13 | Nervous System Word Parts

-algia, -dynia	pain
arachn/o	spider
-ase, -lysis	to break down
astr/o	star
dur/o	hard
-ethesia	feeling
micr/o	small
mot/o	movement
neur/o	nerve
olig/o	scant

TABLE 4-15 | Cardiovascular System Word Parts

arteri/o	artery
ather/o	fatty plaque
cardi/o	heart
congest/o	filled with fluid
necr/o	death
phleb/o	vein
rhythm/o	heartbeat
-stenosis	narrowing
vas/o	vessel
ven/o	vein

TABLE 4-14 | Special Senses Word Parts

aqu/o	water
gloss/o	tongue
gust/o	taste
lingu/o	tongue
medi/o	middle
ocul/o	eye
olfact/o	smell
ophthalm/o	eye
opt/o	eye
ot/o	ear

TABLE 4-16 | Immune System Word Parts

bacteri/o	bacteria
bas/o	blue
-cyte	cell
eosin/o	rosy pink
leuk/o	white
macro-	large
micro-	small
myc/o	fungus
neutr/o	neutral, absorbs no color when stained
-phage	destroyer, eater

See Table 4-14 for medical word parts related to the special senses.

Circulatory System

The circulatory system consists of the heart, the blood vessels, the blood, and the structures that make up the lymphatic system. A physician who specializes in treatment of the cardiovascular system is a *cardiologist*. The specialty is *cardiology*. An *immunologist* specializes in treatment of the immune system, including the lymphatic system. The specialty is *immunology*.

The cardiovascular system and lymphatic systems are subsystems of the circulatory system. The cardiovascular system comprises the heart and its vessels (arteries, veins, and capillaries). The lymphatic system acts to help ensure the body's fluid balance by gathering fluids that have leaked out of the blood vessels and transporting them back into the blood circulation. The lymphatic system is also related to the immune system, helping to defend the body against disease-causing agents called pathogens.

A narrowing of an artery is *arteriostenosis*. Fatty plaque is referred to by the combining form *ather/o*, so the clogging of an artery by fatty plaques is *atherosclerosis*. The drawing of blood from the vein is phlebotomy. Entering a vein to place a catheter or medication is referred to as an intravenous procedure.

Table 4-15 provides examples of medical word parts related to the cardiovascular system.

Immune System

The immune system protects the body from disease. As stated previously, an immunologist's specialty is immunology, treatment of the immune system.

Cells in the immune system are sometimes named for their color or the color they become when stained, as listed in Table 4-16. White blood cells (leukocytes) defend the body. The suffix *-phil* means "to love." Eosinophils "love" or turn pink when stained, whereas basophils "love" or turn blue. Neutrophils do not change color when stained; they might be said to be neutral in their "love" of colors.

TABLE 4-17	Respiratory System Word Parts
capn/o	carbon dioxide
orth/o	straight
oxyg/o, ox/o, ox/I	oxygen
pharyng/o	throat
-pnea	breath
pneum/o, pneumon/o	air, lungs
pulmon/o	lungs
py/o pus,	infected material
spir/o	to breathe
-thorax	chest

TABLE 4-18	Digestive System Word Parts
aliment/o	digestion
appendic/o, append/o	appendix
cholecyst/o	gallbladder
col/o	colon
dent/o	teeth
enter/o	intestines
gastr/o	stomach
retro-	behind
sigm/o	s-shaped
stomat/o, stom/o, or/o	mouth

TABLE 4-19	Urinary System Word Parts
cyst/o	bladder
-dipsia	thirst
hemat/o	blood
nephr/o	kidney
oligo-	scanty amounts
poly-	many, much
protein-	protein
ren/o	kidney
ur/o, urin/o	urinary
ureter/o	ureter
urethr/o	urethra

Macrophages (*macro* means "large" and *phag/o* means "to eat") are large cells that eat invader cells.

Respiratory System

The respiratory system exchanges oxygen (O_2) in the environment for carbon dioxide (CO_2) in the body. The main organs of respiration are the lungs (*pulmon/o*). A specialist in the respiratory system is a *pulmonologist*. The specialty is *pulmonology*.

The term *pneumon/o* combined with the suffix "itis" makes the term *pneumonitis*, which means inflammation of the lung.

Table 4-17 lists medical word parts related to the respiratory system.

Digestive System

The digestive system either absorbs or rejects food and drugs for the body. The physician with specialized training in the digestive system is a *gastroenterologist*, and that physician's specialty is *gastroenterology*.

The digestive tract begins in the mouth (*stom/o* or *stomat/o* or *or/o*), to the stomach (*gastr/o*), through the intestines (*enter/o*), continuing to the rectum (*rect/o*). Medication given through the mouth is stated as *per os* (po).

See Table 4-18 for medical word parts related to the digestive system.

Urinary System

The urinary system rids the body of excessive fluid and the toxic by-products of metabolism. A *urologist* is a physician with specialized training not only in the urinary system but also in the male reproductive system. The specialty is *urology*. The combined urinary and male reproductive system also is referred to as the *genitourinary* system.

The combining form for the kidney is *nephr/o*, so a physician with specialized training related to the kidney is a *nephrologist*. Urine, formed in the kidneys, flows to the ureters, to the bladder, and out through the urethra. Careful attention must be paid to the spelling of two of the organs of this system. The two ureters (*ureter/o*) drain the urinary bladder (*cyst/o*) into the urethra (*urethr/o*), which leads to the outside of the body. A test used to analyze the content of urine to assess urinary function is urinalysis (U/A).

Table 4-19 lists medical word parts related to the urinary system.

Endocrine System

The endocrine system is the ductless glandular system that controls other body systems by secreting hormones into the bloodstream, which carries them to the various organs. A physician who specializes in treatment of the endocrine system is an *endocrinologist*. The specialty is *endocrinology*.

Endo- means "within" and *–crine* means "to secrete." Endocrine hormones are used within the body. For example, follicle-stimulating hormone (FSH) stimulates ovaries to

TABLE 4-20	Endocrine System Word Parts
andr/o	man
-crine	to secrete
endo-	within
estr/o	woman
exo-	without
gest/o	pregnancy
gonad/o	sexual organs
lact/o	milk
somat/o	body
-stasis	stable

TABLE 4-21	Reproductive System Word Parts
balan/o	penis
cervic/o	neck
crypt-	hidden
gynec/o	female, woman
hyster/o	uterus
labi/o	lip
mamm/o	breast
mast/o	breast
metr/o	uterus
oophor/o	ovary
orchid/o	testis
test/o	testis
testic/o	testis

develop and release an ovum and the testes to develop sperm. Testosterone works in the testes of the male to create secondary sexual characteristics. The pituitary is the master gland of this system, and it gives its name to a synthetic form of oxytocin (pitocin), which is used to stimulate labor in women.

Exocrine glands (*exo-* means "external) secrete hormones into a system of ducts that lead to the outside of the body. Examples of exocrine glands are sweat glands, mammary glands, mucous glands, and tear glands.

See Table 4-20 for medical word parts related to the endocrine system.

Reproductive System

The reproductive system aids in producing offspring. A physician with specialized training in women's health is a *gynecologist*. The specialty is *gynecology*.

Female reproductive organs include the uterus and ovaries. Male reproductive organs include the testes and prostate gland. A urologist is specialized in the diseases and disorders of the male reproductive system as well as both male and female urinary systems. See Table 4-21 for some medical word parts relating to the reproductive system.

Professionalism

The medical assistant must be familiar with medical terminology to promote a professional image. If the patient observes that a medical assistant is unfamiliar with key terms, the patient will lose respect for the medical assistant. Learning medical terminology is a lifelong process, but the professional will look up unknown words and commit them to memory.

BUILDING DIAGNOSTIC AND PROCEDURAL TERMS

Medical terms may describe diagnoses (the patient's condition, injury, or disease) as well as procedures (treatments provided to the patient).

Diagnostic terms and procedural terms are both usually built around a root that identifies the anatomic site involved with a suffix that describes the type of condition or procedure. Diagnostic terms often have a prefix as well. For example, *appendicitis* means inflammation of the appendix (*append* or *appendic* is the word root for appendix, and *-itis* is the suffix for inflammation). *Appendectomy* means surgical excision of the appendix (*-ectomy* is the suffix for excision or surgical removal). An appendectomy might be performed for a patient who has appendicitis. By breaking down a medical term into its parts and looking at the suffix, you can immediately determine whether a diagnosis or procedure is identified. Most procedural terms end with the letter *y*, which denotes a process.

It is common to use the same word root with multiple suffixes to identify slightly different things. For example, if a trachea is removed, it is a trach*ectomy*. If, instead, an opening (or mouth) is placed temporarily into the trachea, it is a trache*ostomy*. *Cis/o* is the combining form for "to cut." Thus, scissors cut. *Excision* means "to cut out or remove." *Incision* means to "cut into."

As noted earlier, an electrocardio*gram* is the written record of the electrical activity of the heart. The electrocardio*graph* is the instrument used to obtain the study. (The electrocardiograph measures the heart's electrical activity

TABLE 4-22 | Examples of Diagnostic Suffixes

Suffix	Meaning
-algia	pain
-cele	hernia, protrusion
-emia	blood in
-itis	inflammation of
-osis	condition of
-pathy	disease
-penia	abnormal reduction in number, lack of
-ptosis	drooping, sagging, prolapse
-ptysis	spitting
-trophy	growth

TABLE 4-23 | Examples of Procedural Suffixes

Suffix	Meaning
-analysis	to assess various parts
-ectomy	to remove
-graphy	to make a written record
-scope	instrument to view
-scopy	to observe
-scopy	process of viewing
-stomy	to create an opening
-tome	instrument to cut
-tomy	to cut into temporarily

and produces the electrocardiogram.) The process of analyzing and producing the written record of the heart's electrical activity is electrocardiography.

See Tables 4-22 and 4-23 for examples of medical word parts relating to diagnostic and procedural terms. Table 4-24 provides examples of word building by body system.

TABLE 4-24 | Examples of Word Building by Body Systems

Body System—Word Parts	Medical Term	Definition
Integumentary System		
cutane/o (skin) + ous (pertaining to)	cutaneous	Pertaining to the skin
melan/o (black) + oma (tumor)	melanoma	Malignant (cancerous) growth composed of melanocytes (black cells that produce melanin)
trich (hair) + oid (resembling)	trichoid	Resembling hair
Skeletal System		
oste/o (bone) + arthr/o (joint) + itis (inflammation)	osteoarthritis	Inflammation of the bone and joint
oste/o (bone) + malacia (softening)	osteomalacia	Softening of the bone
cost/o (rib) + ectomy (excision of)	costectomy	Removal (surgical) of a rib
Muscular System		
quad (four) + plegia (paralysis)	quadriplegia	Paralysis of all four limbs of the body
myo (muscle) + pathy (disease or condition of)	myopathy	Any condition or disease of the muscles
dys (bad or painful) + plasia (formation)	dysplasia	Abnormal development
Nervous System		
an (without) + ethesia (feeling)	anesthesia	To have no feeling, as in surgery when medication causes numbness
arachn/o (spider) + oid (resembling)	arachnoid	Resembling a spider web; one of the meninges (covering of the spinal cord)
neur/o + algia (pain)	neuralgia	Generalized nerve pain

(continued)

TABLE 4-24 | Examples of Word Building by Body Systems (*continued*)

Body System—Word Parts	Medical Term	Definition
Special Senses		
ophthalm/o (eye) + scope (instrument to view)	ophthalmoscope	Instrument to examine the eye
oto (ear) + pyo (pus) + rrhea (flow or discharge)	otopyorrhea	Flow or discharge of pus from the ear
gloss/o (tongue) + rrhaphy (suture)	glossorrhaphy	Suturing of the tongue
Cardiovascular System		
arteri/o (artery) + ectasis (stretching out, dilating)	arteriectasis	Dilation of an artery
cardi/o (heart) + mega (large)	cardiomegaly	Abnormal enlargement of the heart
phleb/o (vein) + stasis (control, stop)	phlebostasis	To stop or control the flow in a vein
Immune System		
leuk/o (white) + penia (abnormal reduction in number or lack of)	leucopenia	Decrease in number of leukocytes in the blood
bacteri/o (bacteria) + lysis (destruction)	bacteriolysis	Destruction of bacteria
myc/o (fungus) + logy (study of)	mycology	Study of fungus
Respiratory System		
pharyng/o (throat, pharynx) + itis (inflammation)	pharyngitis	Inflammation of the throat, sore throat
pneumon/o (lung) + ectomy (excision of)	pneumonectomy	Removal of lung tissue
pneum/o (air) + thorax (chest)	pneumothorax	Accumulation of air in the chest or thoracic cavity typically causing the lung to collapse
Digestive System		
cholecyst/o (gallbladder) + graphy (making a written record)	cholecystography	Process of making a written record of the function of the gallbladder—X-ray study
gastr/o (stomach) + stomy (to create a new opening)	gastrostomy	Making a new opening into the stomach
gastr/o (stomach) + enter/o (intestines) + itis (inflammation)	gastroenteritis	Inflammation of the stomach and small intestine
Urinary System		
nephr/o (kidney) + lith (stone)	nephrolithiasis	Condition of having kidney stones
cyst/o (bladder) + cele (herniation, protrusion)	cystocele	Hernia or protrusion of the urinary bladder
Poly (excessive) + dipsia (thirst)	polydipsia	Excessive thirst, abnormal thirst
Reproductive System		
mamm/o (breast) + gram (recording)	mammogram	X-ray record of the breasts
crypt (hidden) + orchid/o (testis)	cryptorchidism	Condition of having an undescended testicle, hidden
oophor/o (ovary) + hyster/o (uterus) + ectomy (excision of)	oophorohysterectomy	Surgical excision of the uterus and ovaries

SUMMARY

Medical terminology is the foundation of communication in health care. You have been introduced to basic medical terms and how they relate to the anatomy and physiology of the body—the study of the body's structures and functions. To be proficient in the use of medical terminology, you must know how the organs of the body are organized into body systems, each with its own functions and role in working together within the body.

Medical terms are made up of two or more word elements: word root, suffix, prefix, and combining vowel. The word root contains the main meaning and often refers to a body part. A suffix can identify the condition, procedure, or instrument. A prefix further modifies the meaning, for example, indicating quantity or direction. A combining vowel after a prefix or before a suffix completes the word, making it easier to pronounce.

Correct spelling is important in the practice of medical assisting because poor spelling reflects lack of professionalism and can lead to medical errors, for example, when the wrong spelling indicates a word other than the one intended. Plurals are formed according to Latin and Greek, not English, rules of grammar. An understanding of body planes, directions, cavities, positions, and regions is also important in developing a medical vocabulary.

Although medical terminology is often a challenge for the medical assistant, learning the language of medicine is essential in this profession.

4 CHAPTER REVIEW

COMPETENCY REVIEW

1. Define and spell the terms for this chapter.
2. Explain how medical words are formed.
3. Break down the following medical terms into word parts using slashes (/), and then write the meaning of the word.

Example:

gastroenteritis: gastr/o/enter/itis, inflammation of the stomach and intestines

a. urinalysis _____
b. pneumectomy _____
c. mammogram _____
d. hysteroscope _____
e. neurology _____
f. macrophage _____
g. osteoarthritis _____
h. proctoscopy _____
i. blepharoptosis _____
j. atherosclerosis _____
k. cardiopulmonary _____
l. cholecystectomy _____
m. myalgia _____
n. hypertrophy _____
o. dyspnea _____
p. gynecology _____
q. hemostasis _____
r. polydipsia _____
s. sigmoidoscopy _____
t. pyothorax _____
u. dermatome _____
v. leukopenia _____
w. aortostenosis _____
x. hematuria _____
y. orchiopexy _____

PREPARING FOR THE CERTIFICATION EXAM

1. Which of the following is a combining form?
   a. hyper-
   b. –emia
   c. glyc
   d. glyc/o
   e. lip

2. Which of the following is the combining form for the mouth?
   a. gastr/o
   b. enter/o
   c. stomat/o
   d. audi/o
   e. ot/o

3. Which of the following physicians specializes in male reproductive functions?
   a. gynecologist
   b. gastroenterologist
   c. dermatologist
   d. endocrinologist
   e. urologist

4. Which of the following is a combining form for bone?
   a. ophthalm/o
   b. ot/o
   c. oste/o
   d. arthr/o
   e. ather/o

5. Which of the following is the combining form for fatty plaque in blood vessels?
   a. phleb/o
   b. vas/o
   c. arthr/o
   d. arteri/o
   e. ather/o

6. Which of the following is the term for kidney?
   a. cyst/o
   b. nephr/o
   c. ren/o
   d. a and b
   e. b and c

7. Which body system is responsible for using hormones for internal communication?
   a. reproductive
   b. cardiovascular
   c. gastrointestinal
   d. integumentary
   e. endocrine

8. Which word means "under the skin"?
   a. intravenous
   b. intradermal
   c. intramuscular
   d. subcutaneous
   e. oral

9. Which word means "in front of" or "before"?
   a. cephalic
   b. distal
   c. medial
   d. lateral
   e. anterior

10. The word part *-algia* means
    a. enzyme.
    b. bacteria.
    c. hormone.
    d. pain.
    e. medication.

CRITICAL THINKING

Refer to the case study at the beginning of the chapter and use the information you have learned to answer the following questions.

1. In Dr. McWalter's office, Mr. Schultz described pain in the epigastric region. Where is the epigastic region?

2. If Dr. McWalter ordered a test that required Mr. Schultz to be supine, how would you position the patient?

3. Visualize the imaginary lines dividing the abdomen into nine regions. In which region would Mr. Schultz's pain be localized?

ON THE JOB

George Tomlin, RMA, has been working for several years in a specialty practice. He applies for a position closer to his home with better hours and more pay. This office, however, sees patients with a variety of illnesses. For the first time since he graduated from college, he is encountering words and procedures with which he is not familiar.

1. What is the best way for George to review his basic medical terminology?

2. What should George do when he encounters a new word?

3. What are some good ways for him to learn the new vocabulary for his new position?

INTERNET ACTIVITY

Conduct a search of medical terminology sites. Decide which ones you would go to if you needed to define words. Here are a couple of sites to start your search:

- www.medilexicon.com/medicaldictionary.php
- www.quizlet.com/subject (Type "medical terminology" into the search box.)
- www.nlm.nih.gov/medlineplus/mplusdictionary.html (A service of the U.S. National Library of Medicine, National Institutes of Health. Look up medical terms, listen to the pronunciation, and switch to Spanish, if you choose.)
- www.jointcommission.org/facts_about_do_not_use_list (The Joint Commission's "Do Not Use" list of error-prone, often misused, or misunderstood abbreviations to avoid.)

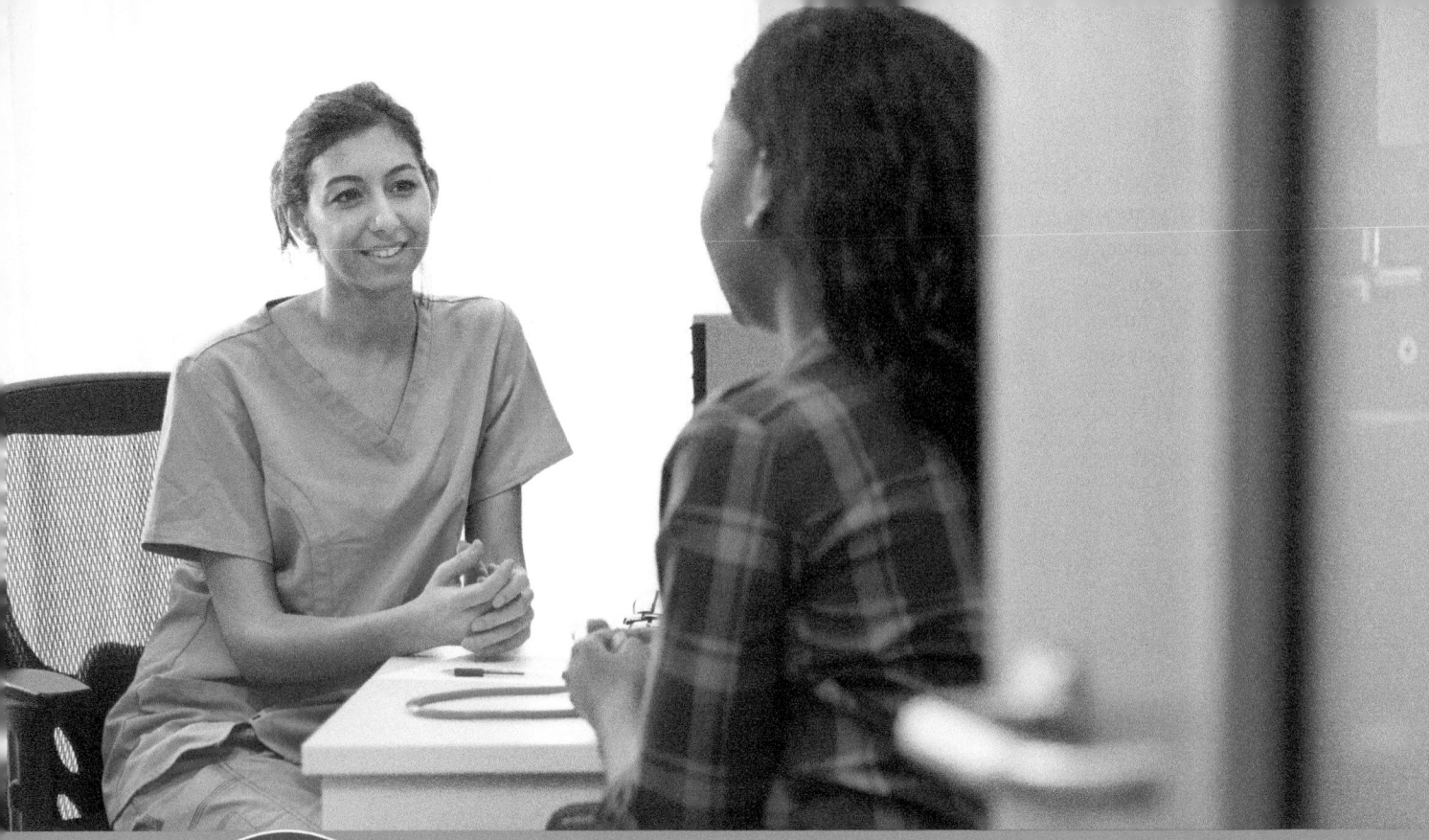

Communication:
Verbal and Nonverbal

Learning Objectives

After completing this chapter, you should be able to:

5.1   Define and spell the terms for this chapter.

5.2   List key components related to interpersonal dynamics.

5.3   Explain the process of communication via the sender–receiver process.

5.4   Identify characteristics of verbal and nonverbal communication.

5.5   List guidelines involved with active listening.

5.6   Compare and contrast assertive, aggressive, and passive communication.

5.7   Identify techniques to overcome communication barriers with patients.

5.8   Explain the difference between adaptive and nonadaptive coping mechanisms.

5.9   List examples of diversity regarding communication in health care.

5.10   Explain the components of intraoffice communication.

5.11   Describe communication as it relates to patient rights.

Yun-qi Yeung, 65 years old, is returning to the medical office to receive the results of a biopsy for prostate cancer screening. Mr. Yeung speaks very little English and is usually accompanied by his son, Lou, for interpretation assistance. Today Lou informs the front desk receptionist that his father is very apprehensive about receiving the results of the biopsy. Later, while in the physician's office, Mr. Yeung and his son find out that the biopsy was positive for the early stages of prostate cancer.

Terms to Learn

active listening	culture	personality
aggressive	empathy	pity
assertive	ethnicity	prejudice
attitudes	ethnocentric	protected health information (PHI)
auditory	exploratory questions	race
authorization	feedback	rapport
behavior	holistic	self-boundaries
bias	integrity	stereotyping
character	kinesthetic	stress
closed-ended questions	leading questions	stressor
compassion	nonverbal communication	sympathy
condescending	open-ended questions	values
consent	passive	verbal communication
coping mechanisms	passive listening	visual

Professional communication skills are a requirement in any environment but are particularly essential in the health care field. As a medical assistant, you will relate to a variety of people, including sick and worried patients, patients of all ages, your physician-employer, fellow staff members, vendors, and even some personal acquaintances of the physician. Some individuals you will interact with will be angry, frustrated, or simply ill and tired. Many patients who come into the physician's office or clinic will have physical or emotional problems that are not the main reason for their appointment. In addition, given the widely diverse population in the United States, you will encounter people from a variety of countries and cultures as well as those from different socioeconomic and education backgrounds. The medical assistant must be able to care for the patient in a holistic fashion and treat everyone with respect, dignity, and courtesy. **Holistic** medicine focuses on the whole patient and addresses the patient's social, emotional, and spiritual needs, as well as the person's physical needs.

It is not enough for the medical assistant to have excellent technical skills. Good interpersonal skills as well as good oral and written communication skills are needed to relate well to patients and fellow staff. In this chapter, you will learn about self-awareness and interpersonal dynamics. You will study the communication process, including directive techniques to improve effective communication, barriers to good communication, and defensive behaviors. Examining diversity issues, communicating in special circumstances, and communicating with special needs patients will help you prepare for various situations you may encounter. Communication in the workplace, working as a member of a team, and understanding some conflict resolution strategies will help in your day-to-day work environment.

INTERPERSONAL DYNAMICS

To communicate effectively in the delivery of health care, you must have a basic understanding of self. Why do you have the personality you exhibit? How do you communicate in everyday situations? Where do the impressions you hold of others originate? In other words, how did you get to be the person you are today? We will examine some concepts related to individuality and relationships with others.

Self-Awareness

Understanding yourself and understanding the differences among others will help you communicate more effectively.

Personality is a sum of the traits, characteristics, and behaviors that make us individuals. We all recognize that there are different personalities, even among close family members and friends.

Character is the sum of the values, attitudes, and behaviors a person exhibits. Psychologists tell us that **values** are a set of standards a person uses to measure the worth or importance of someone or something. **Attitudes** are opinions that develop from our value system. Values are acquired at home, in our family unit, and in the culture we live in, and often they are difficult to change. **Prejudice** is a preformed unfavorable belief or attitude toward members of a certain culture or group often based on little or no experience with or information about the culture or group. Prejudice may be learned from negative experiences but is most often picked up from the prejudices of those around us. Prejudice impacts our actions toward and responses to others. An example of prejudice is viewing individuals with different skin colors as inferior. **Behavior**, the actions others see, is based on our attitudes.

To summarize, values form attitudes, which may include prejudices, and attitudes are reflected in behavior or actions that can be seen by others.

To be an effective communicator in all areas of our lives, it is important to look at our attitudes and our prejudices. How do we see ourselves? How do others see us? Examining ourselves leads to greater self-awareness and can lead to better communication skills. Patients and coworkers expect certain attitudes and professional behaviors to be displayed in the health care setting.

Learning Styles

Examining styles of learning can increase your self-awareness. The three generally recognized learning styles are auditory, visual, and kinesthetic.

Most of us learn by using a combination of these styles, with one style tending to be more dominant. The **auditory** (by hearing) learner is one who retains information better listening to an explanation from a boss or coworker or by hearing a lecture or listening to a CD. People who are auditory learners have difficulty retaining information presented in written format. The **visual** (by seeing) learner, as you would expect, learns better by seeing the information, by reading or looking at drawings, diagrams, or films. Visual learners find it difficult to follow lectures unless visual aids are used with the presentation. The **kinesthetic** (involving movement) learner assimilates knowledge better through hands-on activities, such as experiments, games, lab exercises, and movement—in other words, learning by doing. Such people have difficulty grasping a procedure until they have performed it themselves.

Understanding these learning styles will help prepare you for your role as a patient educator and advocate. You know that most people have one or two preferred styles of learning. If a patient does not seem to easily understand the information you share in one format, for example, by talking to them, try presenting the information in another format such as with visuals or a set of written instructions, or providing a learning-by-doing experience such as having them practice a procedure under your supervision.

THE COMMUNICATION PROCESS

The basic units of the communication process are the sender, message, channel, and receiver. Use the acronym "SMCR" as a memory aid.

S stands for the *sender* of the communication. Who is sending the message?

M represents the *message*. The message can be conveyed by written or spoken words or by behavior.

C indicates the *channel* or method by which the message moves from the sender to the receiver. Channels include the senses: sight, smell, taste, hearing, and touch. Another set of channels are pathways such as the telephone or interoffice mail.

R stands for the *receiver* of the message.

For example, a physician (S) writes a prescription (M) that the medical assistant then reads over the telephone (C) to the pharmacist (R). If any link in this chain is broken, an incorrect message is relayed. What could go wrong? The physician might write the prescription incorrectly, or the medical assistant might relay it incorrectly, or the phone system might break down, or the pharmacist might record the prescription incorrectly. A breakdown at any point in the process would result in miscommunication of the message.

The same holds true if you relay a message to a patient. If the medical assistant (S) explains a procedure (M) verbally to a patient who has a hearing loss (C), then the patient (R) may not hear the message as it was intended.

The communication process, then, is a chain that links a sender (S) and a receiver (R). The sender (S) acts on a stimulus to transmit (encode) a message (M) in a particular form such as verbally or in writing. The message can be transmitted in a variety of ways (C), including face to face, over the telephone, or in a memorandum or an email. The way the receiver (R) translates (decodes) the message may be influenced by the person's age, emotional state, perceptions, education, socioeconomic background, culture, and many other factors.

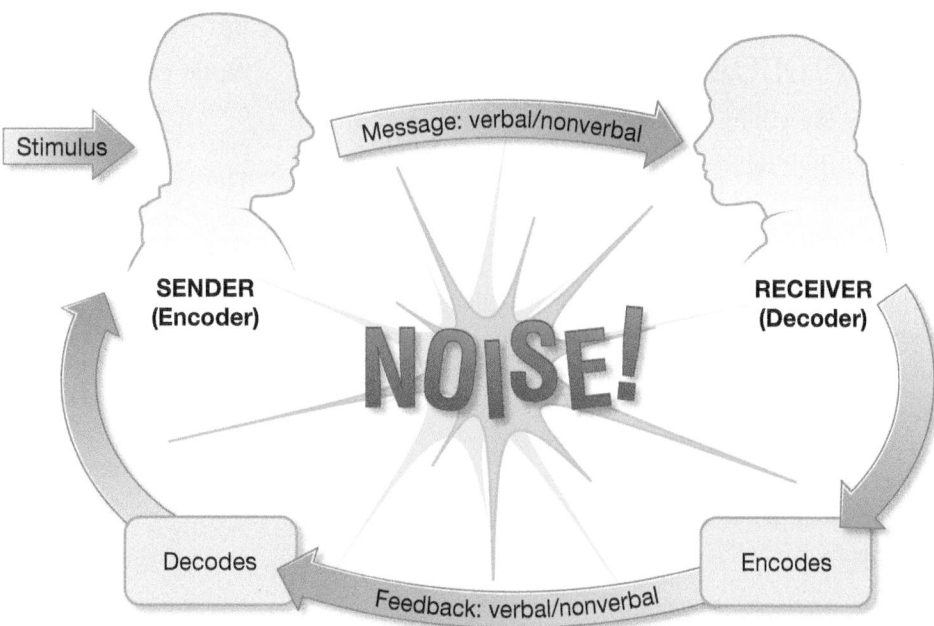

FIGURE 5-1 Face-to-face communication is the richest channel to relay a message from the sender to a receiver.

Channels of Communication

Channels of communication include the various means by which the spoken or written word is communicated from one person to another. Information is said to be "rich" if it accurately conveys to the listener or reader the intent of the speaker. The "richest" information is gained from face-to-face discussion (Figure 5-1). The least rich information is generally obtained from documents that contain a lot of numbers, columns, and tables, such as budget reports. When you want to convey an important message to someone, it is better to do it face-to-face than to put the information into writing.

The face-to-face "rule" of communication is important to remember when you are deciding how to adequately educate patients about their medications. If you put all the important facts into a pamphlet or brochure, the patient may never read it or might look at it but not understand what it means. Face-to-face communication allows you to sense how well the patient understands what you are saying, to ask the patient questions to help confirm understanding, and to give the patient a chance to ask you about anything he doesn't understand.

The three learning styles we discussed earlier—auditory, visual, and kinesthetic—are another important concept to remember when you consider how to communicate information to a patient. Keep in mind that using a variety of styles is a good way to reinforce the message. For example, when providing a written document to the patient (visual), verbally review the information and ask if the patient has any questions about that information (auditory) and, as appropriate, help the patient to practice any actions that will have to be done at home, such as walking with crutches (kinesthetic).

Table 5-1 illustrates the varying degrees of "richness" of various information channels.

TABLE 5-1 | Information Richness Channels

Information Channel (Method of Delivery)	Level of Richness
Face-to-face discussion	Highest
Telephone conversations	High
Written letter/memo (individually addressed)	Moderate
Formal written document (general bulletins or reports)	Low
Fax (facsimile)	Low
E-mail	Low
Internet	Low
Formal numeric document (printouts, budget reports)	Lowest

VERBAL AND NONVERBAL COMMUNICATION

Virtually everything a person does from birth to death is a form of communication. Smiling is a form of nonverbal communication, whereas talking "with a smile in your voice" is verbal communication. Verbal communication is the use of words to convey a message. Nonverbal communication is the language of gestures and actions, which includes body language. In many cases, people are not aware of the image they are projecting with their bodies. The way you hold your arms, make eye contact, gesture, frown, or turn toward or away from the patient frequently conveys much more than mere words could (Figure 5-2).

Box 5-1 offers some examples of messages that convey impatience.

Verbal Communication

Verbal communication involves spoken words, sounds, and tone of voice. Good verbal communication includes appropriate word selection, a positive attitude, and self-boundaries. The sounds a person makes when speaking cover a wide range and can convey vastly different meanings. The tone in which you speak to a patient is vitally important in making a positive impression on the patient and the patient's family. Generally, people will raise their tone at the end of a statement when asking a question and drop their tone when completing a sentence. When the speaker's tone drops, it is appropriate to begin your part of the conversation. Interrupting speakers is a negative behavior that creates a barrier to good communication.

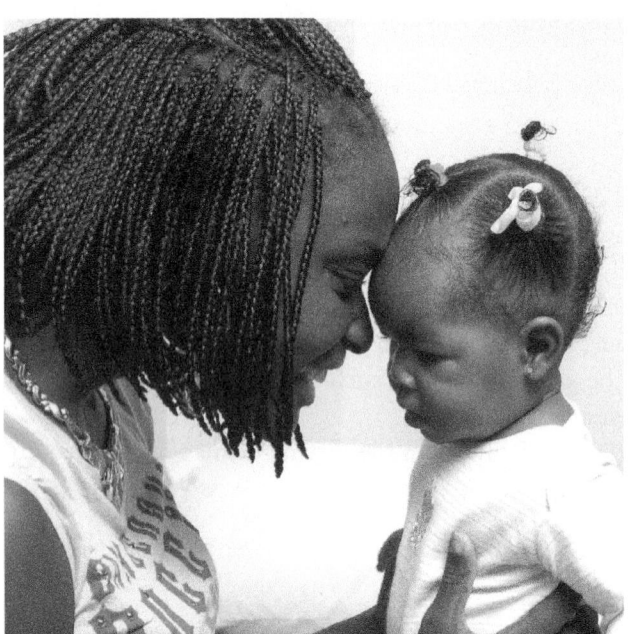

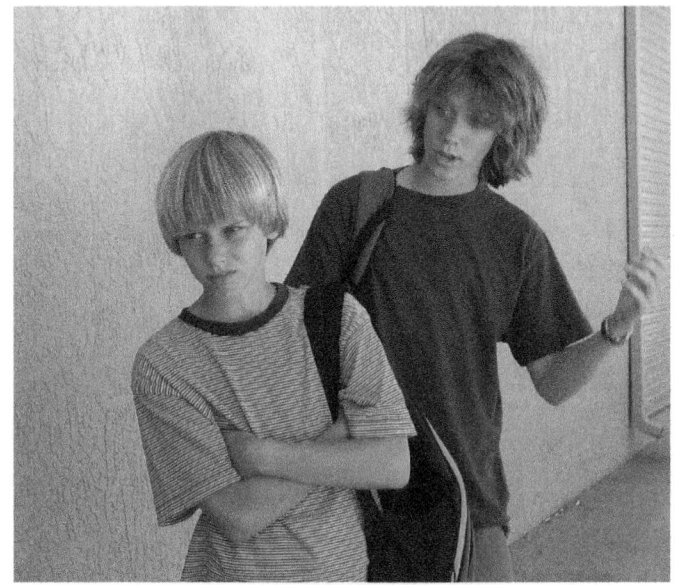

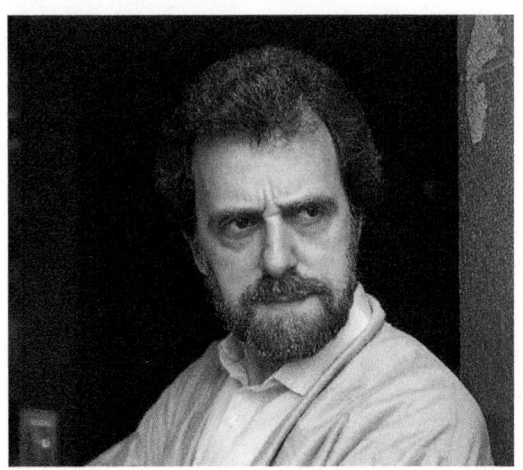

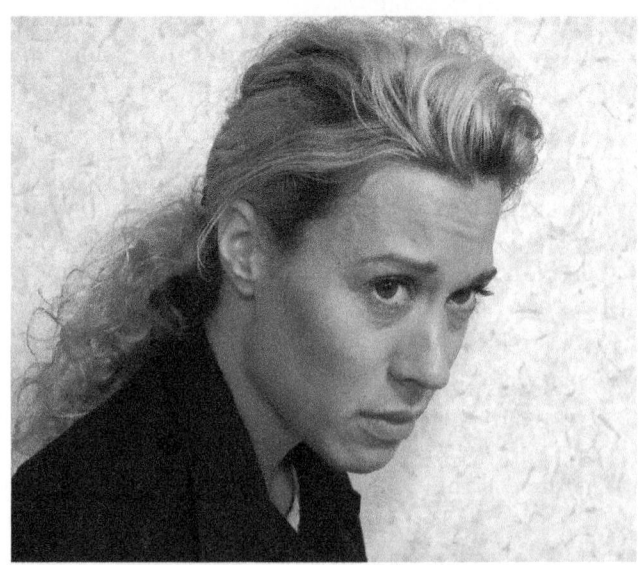

FIGURE 5-2 Nonverbal communications convey strong, powerful messages that may be positive or negative.

BOX 5-1 | **Communication Messages Conveying Impatience**

- Interrupting people when they are speaking
- Answering telephone calls curtly
- Finishing another person's sentence
- Rushing the patient
- Looking at your watch or the clock
- Doing two things at once
- Not looking up from your work when someone approaches
- Rushing around the office

The medical assistant should speak loudly enough to be heard but not so loudly that a patient's confidentiality is compromised. When communicating with patients, you should always be in a private area if the message includes the patient's protected health information (PHI). Speaking clearly and pronouncing your words properly are very important.

Word Selection

Choosing the right words is critical. We can all think of instances when we called a medical facility only to have been spoken to as though we were an annoyance to the person at the front desk. Other times, telephoning the medical assistant was a pleasant experience, and when the conversation was completed, we had a positive feeling. Sarcasm and ridicule have no place in the professional setting. The goal of the medical assistant is to promote an open, comfortable environment for the patient while keeping in mind that the patient is the customer. Choose your words carefully, and take care not to be rude or impatient.

Also be careful not to use technical words or medical language that the patient might not understand. Be aware of the patient's education level and age. For example, when talking with an adult, using the words *stomach* or *abdomen* is appropriate; however, if the patient is a three-year-old child, you might consider using the word *tummy*.

Positive Attitude

The ability to convey a positive attitude is very important. When a patient is present, always involve the patient in your conversation. Excluding the patient—for example, talking about the patient to the patient's parent or spouse but not to the patient himself—is rude. Talking in a manner that is incomprehensible to the patient—"over the patient's head"— is disrespectful. It is important to talk face to face with a patient who is ill or upset, listening carefully and showing concern for the patient's welfare (Figure 5-3). You should be able to demonstrate empathy and sympathy, but be cautious about conveying an attitude of pity for your patients.

Self-boundaries

Word selection and positive attitudes are important aspects of verbal communication. An equally important component

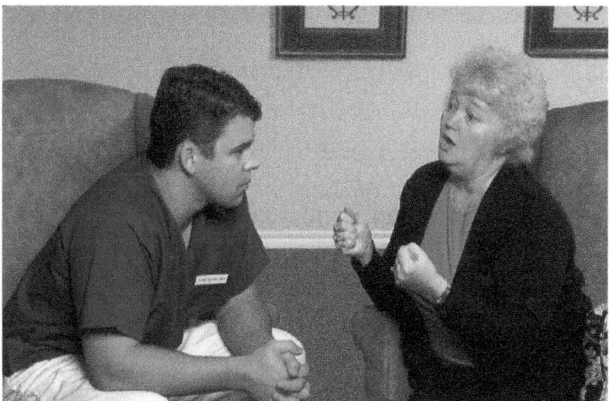

FIGURE 5-3 It is important to act concerned when a patient is upset.

of verbal communication is the concept of **self-boundaries**. This concept will help you to be aware of topics you should *not* discuss with patients. A medical assistant may think that sharing personal information is a way to build rapport with a patient, but this is not professional. In fact, sharing personal information can make patients uncomfortable and may be viewed as a violation of respect and trust from too much intimacy being introduced to the relationship. Recognizing and adhering to self-boundaries will help you, as a medical assistant, to protect your privacy and keep your work and personal lives separate. Also, patients will feel that their health care needs are being met in a secure and therapeutic environment when self-boundaries are maintained.

JUDGMENT CALL

When you are working with others in the office, you should also be aware of their interactions with patients. Let's say you observe another medical assistant talking with a patient, and you hear the patient talking about the recent loss of her husband. The medical assistant responds to the patient, stating, "You poor thing." The medical assistant also starts to cry with the patient. What would you do, if anything, to intervene in this situation? Think about the differences between empathy, sympathy, and pity—and how these attitudes may affect the patient—to help you decide on your action.

Nonverbal Communication

Nonverbal communication is unspoken mannerisms that convey thoughts and feelings. Nonverbal communication generally is unconscious and not easily "faked." For this reason, nonverbal communication often is considered to be a more genuine indicator of a person's feelings than spoken words. It is important that verbal and nonverbal communication send the same message. Nonverbal communication includes the eight behaviors summarized in Table 5-2.

Body language is learned through imitation, by being taught, and by instinct. Patients expect certain types of behaviors, attitudes, and appearance in the health care setting. Medical assistants must be aware of the body language they are using and modify any behavior that could be perceived by patients as inappropriate or negative. For example, appearance is a nonverbal form of communication. Unprofessional attire, visible tattoos, and overpowering perfume can send a negative message.

The gesture of touch is a form of nonverbal communication and a form of body language. Some gestures can be interpreted differently than what the medical assistant might intend. Gently touching a distraught patient's arm can provide reassurance and comfort. However, you must be cautious that the receiver does not misinterpret a touch. In some cultures, for instance, it is considered rude to touch a child's head without permission. At times, abused children can be fearful of even innocent touching. Use caution when touching a patient unless you know that patient well.

TABLE 5-2 | Nonverbal Communication

Behavior	Examples
Posture	Standing or sitting upright, slumping, slouching
Position	Crossed arms or legs, facing a person or turning away
Facial expression	Smiling, frowning, rolling eyes
Territoriality/physical boundaries	Standing too close or too far from someone
Gestures	Waving, pointing, using fingers to indicate numeric amounts
Touch	Physically touching or not touching another person, firm or weak handshake
Mannerisms	Clothing, hairstyle, tattoos; tone of voice; tapping of fingers
Eye contact	Looking toward or away from someone, especially while they are talking

Professionalism The Life Span

Medical assistants devote a significant amount of time interacting with and caring for older adult patients. As the baby boomer generation reaches retirement age and more than likely will have an increased need for medical care, the medical assistant will encounter more older adult patients. Older adults should be treated with respect, as should all patients. It is important not to generalize and treat all older adult patients as frail, confused, and "over the hill." Quite a few people over age 65 are employed full-time, are physically and sexually active, and are raising young families.

Many patients in this age bracket live alone and are eager for conversation and a kind word. Taking a few extra minutes can mean a great deal to the lonely patient.

It is demeaning to call the patient "dear" or "honey." The terms "Mr.," "Ms.," or "Mrs." should be used when addressing patients unless they instruct you to use their first name.

ACTIVE LISTENING

The ability to encourage a patient to communicate effectively is critical when you wish to determine the patient's problems. For example, how can you redirect a patient who is talking about seemingly irrelevant issues? Or how can you get uncommunicative patients to tell you exactly how they are feeling and what they are especially concerned about during today's visit? Each communication experience has unique qualities and must be considered carefully. Before we discuss specific techniques, we need to consider several questions about the overall communication process:

- What is the goal of your communication?
- What message do you want to send?
- What channel or method will be used to deliver the message (written, verbal, face to face, etc.)?
- How will you listen to the response (listening and observational skills)?
- How will you get clarification and feedback?
- Did you meet your goal, or do you need to revise the message (assess or evaluate)?

Listening Skills

Listening involves understanding verbal and nonverbal cues from the patient. You must pay attention to both.

Listening is either active or passive. **Active listening** involves paying complete attention to the speaker, concentrating on the verbal message, watching for nonverbal cues, and offering a response. At times, it is difficult in a medical

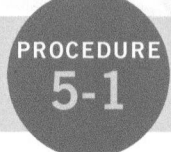

PROCEDURE 5-1

Using Active Listening Skills

Objective ◆ *Use active listening skills to obtain the chief complaint from a patient.*

EQUIPMENT AND SUPPLIES

Patient History Form

METHOD

1. Identify the patient.
2. Smile, and establish eye contact.
3. Seat the patient in an appropriate area.
4. Focus full attention on the patient.
5. Ask the patient the reason for the current appointment.
6. Ask open-ended questions.
7. Do not interrupt the patient.
8. Provide feedback by paraphrasing what the patient says.
9. Observe the patient for signs of needing to give more information.
10. Restate the chief complaint before leaving the patient.
11. Conclude the patient interview in an appropriate manner.
12. Document the chief complaint.

CHARTING EXAMPLE

6/22/YY 4:30 P.M. *cc: gastrointestinal discomfort. Patient states,* "My belly hurts real bad." Nancy Beaumont, CMA (AAMA)

---

office to actively listen when so much activity is happening at once. One skill you will gain with experience is the ability to prioritize simultaneous events. **Passive listening** is listening to someone without having to reply or respond in any way, such as when you are listening as a member of an audience.

How you hear a message is often colored by the message that is being delivered. If it is criticism of your work and you disagree, you hear it one way. If it is praise for your work, you hear it another way. Sometimes you begin formulating a response before the speaker is finished. In any circumstance, if the listener's mind or thoughts wander, the message is received ineffectively, or it may be missed completely by the listener (receiver). Part of effective listening is allowing enough time for the message to be completed and knowing when it is your turn to speak.

With practice we can all become good listeners. Procedure 5-1 provides steps to practice active listening skills to employ with patients as well as with those you will encounter in the workplace. The following are some additional guidelines for good listening:

- Avoid distractions.
- Face the speaker.
- Give the person your full attention.
- Maintain the type of eye contact that is suitable for the culture of the patient.
- Do not be judgmental about what is said.

- Be aware of nonverbal cues.
- Note anything that seems unclear.
- Do not interrupt.
- Maintain personal space.
- Ask questions if you do not understand.

Directive Communication Techniques

The medical assistant can often assist the communication process by directing the patient's comments, using specific communication techniques so that the sharing between the patient and the medical assistant is productive.

Types of Questions

Asking questions is a directive technique. The medical assistant will ask many questions of each patient. It is helpful to

Professionalism

As a health care representative, the medical assistant should set a good example. The medical assistant sets the first impression of the office and in many ways is the marketing representative of the practice. The medical assistant must always present a professional appearance. Good personal hygiene and grooming are a must. Office policy regarding fingernails, jewelry, and general appearance must be followed.

keep in mind the goal of your question before you choose the type of question to ask. Four types of questions are discussed here: close-ended, open-ended, exploratory, and leading.

Closed-ended questions can be answered with a yes or a no. Often these types of questions are appropriate to obtain background information, such as "Is your mother still living?" However, at times you may ask a patient, "Do you understand what I mean?" and the patient will answer, "Yes" even if the patient does not comprehend what you are saying. Usually this happens because the patient does not want to be bothersome or appear unintelligent. You need to consider the situation carefully when you use close-ended questions.

Open-ended questions are those that require more than a yes or no response. Such questions can be useful in gaining feedback or drawing out patient information. An example of an open-ended question is "What were you doing when you got dizzy?" By applying the directive method of using open-ended questions, you will be able to obtain information that the physician will require to treat the patient.

Exploratory questions are used to ask the patient for further information to more fully discuss the subject. For example, if a patient says, "My head hurts," an exploratory question would ask, "Where does it hurt?" or "How long have you had this pain?" In this example, other exploratory questions would seek information about type of pain, when it started, and when it occurs. The medical assistant is often the person the patient feels more comfortable speaking to and questioning. It is important to be empathetic and endeavor to put the patient at ease.

Leading questions are those questions in which part of the answer is in the question. For example, when asked, "Do you have to urinate two, three, or four times a night?" the patient then has to select one answer from your choices. This may be helpful in dealing with patients who do not understand English. However, the medical assistant must be careful not to ask a particular leading question in order to get the desired answer instead of a true answer that wasn't included in the question.

Feedback

Feedback, any response to a communication, is critically important when working with patients because you must determine if they truly understand what was said. Feedback can be either verbal or nonverbal. Sometimes the verbal message and the nonverbal message that patients send do not agree. For instance, as a medical assistant you may ask, "How are you feeling?" and the patient might state, "Fine." Because the patient is walking with a painful limp, you doubt the verbal statement. Always try to ask specific questions (e.g.,

"Do you have pain?" "Tell me about your medication," or "Tell me why you came in to see the doctor."). When you document the information the patient provides, write the patient's exact words in quotation marks.

Reflecting

Reflecting is a directive technique in which you mirror the patient's message back to the individual to ensure that you have understood the message correctly. For example, you may say in response to a patient who says he needs an appointment but not on a Wednesday, "You say you can't come in on Wednesdays?" The reflecting technique is also helpful in resolving conflicts and clearing up confusing statements, and it requires more detail from the other person.

Restating

Restating or paraphrasing is repeating the patient's message in your own words. For example, if the patient says, "I won't have any money till next month," you might reply, "I understand you're saying that you won't be able to pay your bill this month. Is that correct?" This technique helps to confirm that both parties understand the message clearly.

Clarification

The ultimate goal in effective communication is to deliver the message so that it is understood clearly. Clarification is a directive technique in which the medical assistant requests more information to better understand what the patient has stated. Many times patients use words such as *a lot* or *much worse* in explaining their symptoms. It is important to ask them to be more specific in order for the physician to accurately diagnose and treat the patient. For example, the patient says, "My right arm hurts a lot." The medical assistant should employ the directive techniques mentioned to clarify this information. The following questions are examples of follow-up questions and statements useful in this situation:

- "You say that your right arm hurts. Is that correct? Show me on your arm where you feel the pain."
- "What kind of pain is it? When did it start? Does it hurt all the time?"
- "Does the pain interrupt your sleep?"
- "Are you taking any medications, including over-the-counter drugs, for the pain?"

Another form of clarification is asking the patient to repeat back to you the instructions you have just given. This will reveal if the patient has clearly understood what you said and gives you the opportunity to repeat anything the patient didn't grasp.

TABLE 5-3 | Directive Communication Techniques

Technique	Description	Example
Open-Ended Question	Encourage the patient to discuss freely.	"Please describe your pain for me."
Closed-Ended Question	Direct the patient to make a yes/no or simple response.	"Are you having pain?"
Exploratory Question	Ask the patient for further information.	"When did the pain start?"
Reflecting	Direct the conversation back to the patient by repeating the patient's words.	Patient: "I'm afraid of what the doctor will find." MA: "You're afraid of what the doctor will find?"
Acknowledgment	Indicate understanding.	"I understand what you are saying."
Restating	State what the patient has said but in different terms.	Patient: "I can't sleep." MA: "You say you're having trouble getting to sleep at night?"
Add to an Implied Statement	Verbalize implied information.	Patient: "I'm usually relaxed." MA: "And today you're not relaxed?"
Seek Clarification	Request more information to better understand.	Patient: "I don't feel good." MA: "Tell me what kind of symptoms you are having."
Silence	Remain silent, or make no gesture in response to a statement.	Patient: "I don't know what's wrong, but something is."

See Table 5-3 for a list of other directive communication techniques, including a description and an example of each technique.

Empathetic Listening

Empathy is the ability to understand what the patient is feeling because you have experienced the same feelings. ("I know how hard it is to lose weight. It's a constant problem for me, but I keep trying because it's important for my health.") Or you can truly imagine yourself in the patient's shoes (thinking, "I don't have that problem, but I can imagine how tough it must be"). **Compassion** is taking positive action based on the empathy you feel (offering a patient in pain to wait in a quiet private area, if available). **Sympathy** is acknowledging the patient's feelings and difficulties even though you have not had the same experience or can't really imagine yourself being in that person's position (thinking, "Wow, it must be really hard to have that kind of weight problem"). **Pity** is feeling sorry for a person, usually in a **condescending** way (thinking "What a poor soul this person is; I'm glad I never let myself go like that"). Patients react much better to an empathetic or sympathetic listener, who really seems to understand their problems, than to a pitying listener, who may seem to be looking down on them.

You can acquire the skill of empathetic or sympathetic listening by using some simple nonverbal techniques: nodding, leaning toward the patient, positioning yourself so you are at the patient's eye level, and indicating by your facial expression that you understand what the patient is saying (Figure 5-4).

Because we all share human emotions, at times you will become distressed over a patient's situation. It is not possible to be a concerned health care provider and remain totally unemotional at all times. If you become upset, you can excuse yourself for a few moments. Realize that your emotions and concerns are another indication why you are the

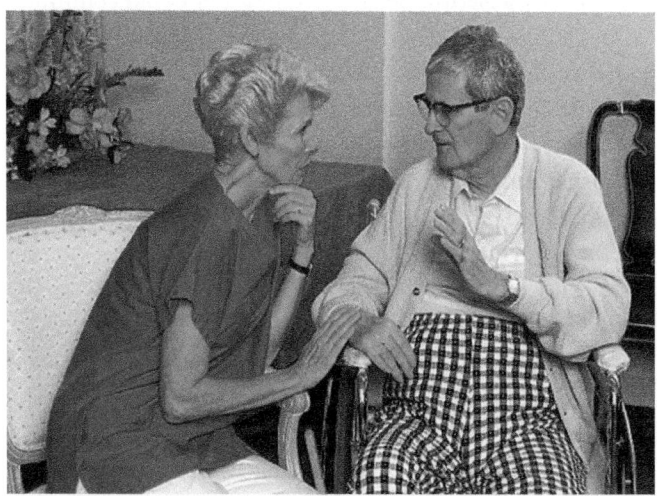

FIGURE 5-4 Empathy draws a more positive response from the patient because it is based on the willingness of the medical assistant to understand what the patient is experiencing.

right kind of person to have chosen the field of health care, a person who is truly concerned for others. Your genuine caring will come across to and be appreciated by the patient.

Discussing Sensitive Issues

Frequently, sensitive issues arise during contact with patients. Discussing issues involving money, such as the patient's bill and personal financial responsibility, can be very sensitive. Before the first office visit, patients should be advised of the physician's charges for specific services or treatment. Inquiries regarding the patient's medical insurance and procedures for payment of fees should also be reviewed before the first visit. Compliance with federal regulations regarding the patient's right to privacy for all health-related information should be addressed at the first visit. This includes reviewing the Health Insurance Portability and Accountability Act (HIPAA) and how the office follows the HIPAA guidelines. When you need to discuss sensitive topics such as these with a patient, the abilities you develop to be assertive without being aggressive will stand you in good stead.

DEVELOPING ASSERTIVE BEHAVIOR TECHNIQUES

Most instances of communication within the work setting involve getting someone else to cooperate with you. Whether you are interacting with a patient or a staff member, communication is your goal, and the methods to achieve cooperation are the same. As a medical assistant, at times you will have to persuade others to listen to you. You can use various behavior styles to communicate with people, and some are more helpful than others. Medical assistants should strive to use **assertive** behavior techniques to aid communication, and avoid **aggressive** and **passive** behavior styles.

Being assertive means making a point in a positive manner by standing firm, making decisions based on your principles or values, and trusting your own ideas or instincts in the situation. It is possible to be assertive without being unpleasant.

By contrast, being aggressive is trying to impose your point of view on others or trying to manipulate them. Aggressiveness is considered a negative behavior, a type of pushiness. In fact, aggressiveness has been compared with bullying or making a verbal attack on someone. Many people resort to aggressive behavior to "win" an argument, to make sure their ideas prevail no matter the negative side effects this may cause, or when they are angry or fearful. Aggressive people tend to be bossy and inconsiderate of the feelings of others.

Passive behavior is compliant or submissive behavior in which people do not let their needs and feelings be known and allow other people to do whatever they choose. Passive behavior by a medical assistant allows patients to run the office and does not show the professionalism needed. It also can be dangerous because it might allow patients to do things or think things that could harm them.

Acquiring the ability to be assertive means that you will learn to offer new ideas, or even unwanted ideas, to people in such a manner that they will not feel threatened. Assertive behaviors include being direct, straightforward, and honest, using positive body language, and using "I" statements such as "I feel."

For instance, suppose you are calling a patient regarding nonpayment of a bill. You will want to gain the patient's acceptance and cooperation. If you start the conversation with an aggressive comment such as "Are you aware that your bill is now two months overdue? When are you going to pay it?" the patient is likely to get angry. The patient could become defensive and hang up on you. Most patients know when they have not paid a bill, and it is not helpful to use threatening language. A better approach would be to identify yourself and indicate that you are helping Dr. Thompson with the monthly billing. In a calm but assertive manner, you ask questions that you hope will prompt a positive response from the patient. These questions might include "How can I help you to clear up these payments? Perhaps we can discuss how you can make a small payment on your account twice a month. What is an amount that you could afford?"

Table 5-4 lists comparative examples of assertive and aggressive questions, comments, and behavior.

Assertiveness is a learned skill that can help you to maintain your self-confidence under stressful conditions. The basis for assertiveness is that everyone has the right to express opinions or beliefs in an appropriate, respectful manner without fear of being humiliated or made to feel guilty. Aggressiveness results in violation of a person's rights during communication. The results of aggressive behavior are resentment and loss of respect. To practice assertive behavior, use the following steps:

- Take a few deep breaths to calm yourself.
- In unemotional tones, describe the behavior that you would like the other person to change.
- Describe how you feel when the behavior occurs.
- State the positive behavior you would like to see.
- Describe the appropriate, reasonable, and enforceable consequences that will result if the person's behavior does not change.

TABLE 5-4 | Comparison of Assertive and Aggressive Behavior

Assertive Behavior	Aggressive Behavior
"This medication works best when it is taken on a regular daily basis."	"You know you can't expect this medication to work when you're not taking it every day."
"Let me find someone who can answer that question for you."	"That's not my job."
"Your behavior is inappropriate."	"Why did you do that? It was stupid."
Knocking on door and then coming into an exam to say, "Excuse me, Dr. Thompson. You are needed on the telephone."	Rushing into an exam room to say, "Doctor, you've got a telephone call."

- Follow through with consequences if the behavior does not change.
- Commend the individual for the behavioral change.
- Evaluate your confrontation.

Communicating with Other Practices and Facilities

Medical assistants spend a good deal of time communicating with other physicians, hospitals, and clinics. These organizations might refer new patients to the medical practice and also are a vital link in the patient care process. In this way, they are vitally important to the economic stability of practices and facilities. Using your skills of courteous assertiveness will be important when you are dealing with professionals outside your practice. Your instructions need to be firm and clear but also polite. You also need to be receptive and understanding of information others share about patient care.

Creating a Customer-Friendly Environment

Medical assistants are the first to encounter the patient in many instances. Therefore, they are responsible for the initial impression the patient has of the practice or facility. The concept of "The customer comes first" should be a primary goal for all health care providers and must be maintained in order to sustain a satisfied client base.

Medical assistants should view the patient as a consumer of health care. Today, patients and family members are more knowledgeable about health care options because of the Internet and other media and sources of information. They no longer place the physician on a pedestal as patients may have done in the days when physicians made house calls. In fact, many patients can experience a certain amount of alienation from their health care providers, because most physicians today are specialists. Specialization can lead to viewing the patient and the patient's injury or procedure as one and the same—"a broken leg" or "an appendectomy"—a viewpoint that is both too narrow and degrading. Instead, the patient should be considered holistically and treated with dignity and respect.

Using good interpersonal skills to establish a positive environment in the health care setting generates a customer-friendly atmosphere and a comfortable workplace. A warm, friendly greeting, showing respect to the patient, being sincere and sensitive, and demonstrating a caring attitude can help set a positive tone.

Greeting Patients

A patient should be greeted within one minute of entering the office. If you are speaking on the telephone when the patient comes in, be sure to acknowledge the patient's presence with a smile and nod. Give your full attention to the patient as soon as you complete the telephone conversation.

Know Your Patient

It is important to understand the patients who come to your office. Become familiar with their background, culture, education level, and socioeconomic status. Knowing and appreciating this information about your patients will help you to build a climate of respect and trust.

It is said that patients don't care how much you know until they know how much you care about them.

COMMUNICATION BARRIERS

As a medical assistant, you can overcome communication barriers by exercising both observation and patience. Communication barriers are factors that prevent a message from being received or that distort its meaning. Identifying and overcoming these barriers is essential for effective communication (Figure 5-5).

Distractions of various types can become communication barriers. External or environmental distractions include factors such as temperature and noise. The medical assistant can usually eliminate these distractions by taking the patient to a quieter location, offering a seat away from an outside door, finding a cooler spot if the patient is too

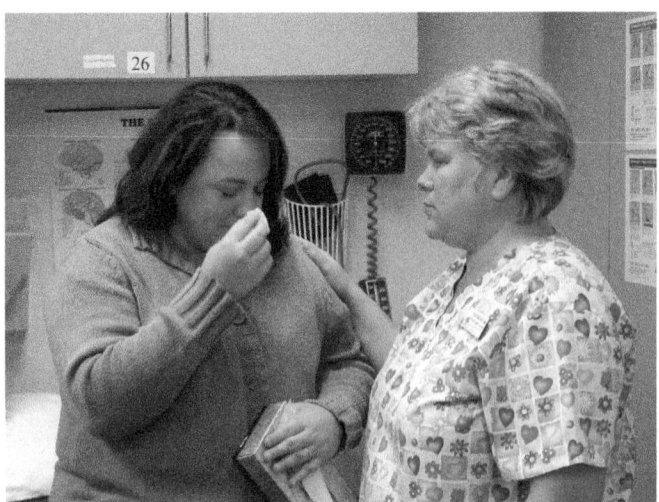

FIGURE 5-5 Effective listening skills demonstrate empathy to the patient and break down barriers to communication.

warm, or providing a blanket if the patient feels cold. Internal distractions, such as pain, hunger, or anger, might not be so obvious, but your skills of observation and empathetic listening may help you to establish communication. Table 5-5 gives examples of internal and external barriers to communication.

An incorrect approach is giving the patient false reassurance. Saying something like "Everything will be all right" can result in the patient's reluctance to talk to you if you give the impression that you don't understand or are dismissing the seriousness of their personal or health-related situation. Such comments can also lead to liability issues for the physician if the patient believes that a promise for recovery has been made.

The medical assistant also may unintentionally put up barriers to communication. Such obstacles include not looking at the patient who is speaking, interrupting the patient, abruptly changing the subject, and—as in the "everything will be all right" example—using meaningless statements to soothe the patient.

Medical assistants must remember that patients come to see the physician because they have a problem. Patients should never be treated in a condescending manner.

Emotions

As a medical assistant, you will experience and witness all types of emotions and feelings. Emotions can vary from person to person because of the person's general emotional makeup or because of that person's past experience.

Medical assistants encounter patients who are frightened, depressed, or angry. How do you know a patient is experiencing such emotions? How can you help that patient? Take time to think through the following scenarios.

- Holly Sutter, CMA, was given a medication order by Dr. Baldwin for Christine Liu. After preparing the medication, she entered the examination room to give Ms. Liu the injection as ordered. Ms. Liu asked, "Am I getting a shot?" Her eyes widened, she began to sweat, and her heart started to beat faster (Figure 5-6). Holly responded by saying, "Yes, I have your injection right here." Ms. Liu stated, "I'm not getting a shot," and walked out of the examination room.

Holly did not recognize that Ms. Liu was displaying fear. Holly was focused only on completing the task of giving the injection. Before Holly entered the examination room with the injection, she should have explained to Ms. Liu that she would be receiving the medication Dr. Baldwin ordered by injection. This would have given Ms. Liu the opportunity to express her negative feelings

TABLE 5-5	Internal and External Barriers to Communication	
Internal Communication Barriers	**External Communication Barriers**
Fatigue	Noise
Disinterest	Temperature
Past experiences with the medical care	Body language
	Odors/scents
Home or work problems	Children (your own or someone else's)
Pain	
Hunger	Language
Anger	Malfunctioning equipment

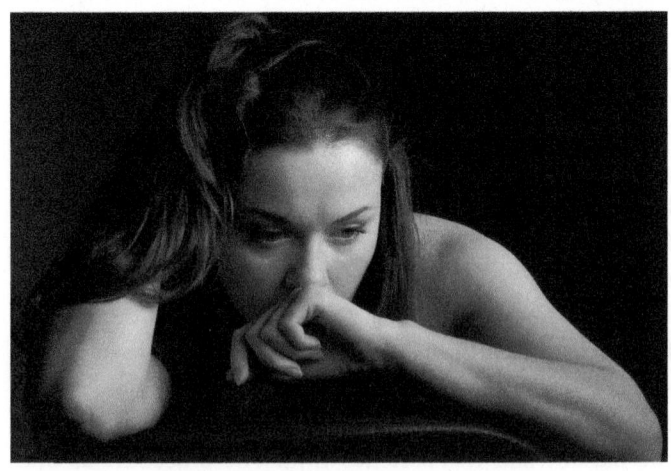

FIGURE 5-6 Emotion: fear.

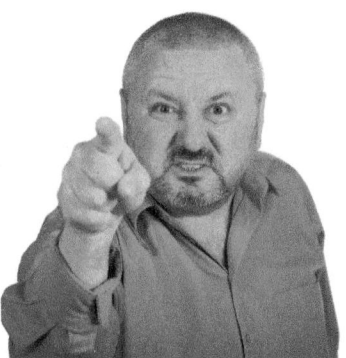

FIGURE 5-7 Emotion: anger.

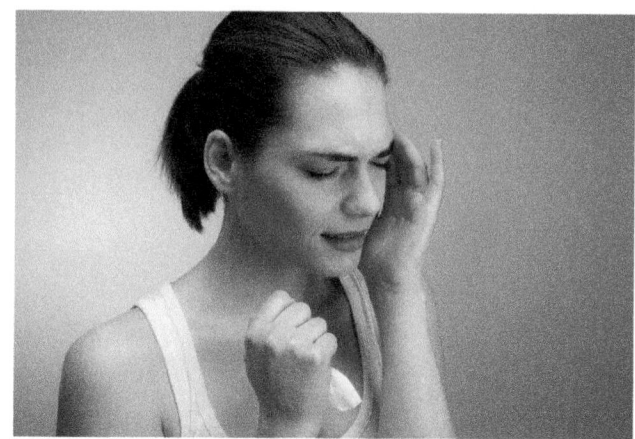

FIGURE 5-8 Emotion: anxiety.

about receiving an injection, and it would have given Holly the opportunity to maintain control over the situation. If unable to help Ms. Liu accept the injection, Holly could have offered to convey Ms. Liu's response to Dr. Baldwin, who might have been able to provide appropriate medication in a different form.

- You are working in the front office when a patient comes to the front reception window and starts screaming, yelling, and cursing at you. Even a patient who doesn't attack you verbally may show signs of anger that you can recognize. How can you recognize and deal with an angry patient?

If a person is angry, a reddish color may appear on the face and ears, eyes may be slightly squinted, lips may be pursed or tightened, and fists may be clenched (Figure 5-7). These are just some of the signs that a person is angry. Once you recognize that a person is angry, remain calm. As long as the patient is not being aggressive, allow him or her to communicate the anger. First, make it clear that you understand the patient is angry. Next, so you can resolve the issue, inquire about what is making the patient angry. During the conversation make sure you are empathic so the patient knows you are concerned about the issue.

- Holly Sutter, CMA, is taking a patient's vital signs when the patient tells her, "I failed all my courses last quarter, and if I fail any more courses I'm going to be kicked out of school." During the conversation, the patient starts crying and tells Holly, "I'm having trouble sleeping, and I am tired of trying so hard in my courses and not succeeding" (Figure 5-8).

During the conversation with the patient, Holly should be empathic and caring. After Holly allows the patient to express his feelings, she should immediately tell the doctor about the conversation and the statements the patient made. It is also important for Holly to document the situation in the patient's medical record.

Professionalism The Law

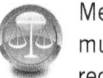 Medical assistants must use caution when communicating with patients. Providing false hopes for recovery or implying that the physician may be able to cure a patient is not only unethical but also can result in liability for the physician and the medical assistant.

Documenting incidents in writing involves careful thought and caution. It is important to chart exactly what occurred and what the patient stated rather than your feelings about the situation. Recording the patient's comment exactly; "I have an overwhelming feeling of hopelessness" is a better indication of the patient's emotional state than the comment "I think the patient is depressed." The latter comment reflects the medical assistant's judgment of the patient's appearance or statement, not what the patient said. As with everything that transpires in the medical environment, the HIPAA regulations regarding confidentiality must be kept in mind.

Stress

Stress is the body's reaction to the world around it. Stress can be emotional, intellectual, or physical. It can also be spiritual, economical, or social. Everyone experiences stress at one time or another (Figure 5-9).

Depending on the level of stress, it can be energizing, motivating, or exhausting. Medical research has shown that a certain amount of stress is not a bad thing. The body's reaction to stress determines if it is good stress (eustress) or bad stress (distress). Stress has also been implicated in various illnesses.

A **stressor** is a real or even an imaginary event that causes stress. Certain major life events such as the death of a loved one, divorce, an unexpected move away from family and friends, unemployment, illness, getting married, delivering a baby, studying for an examination, or purchasing a new car

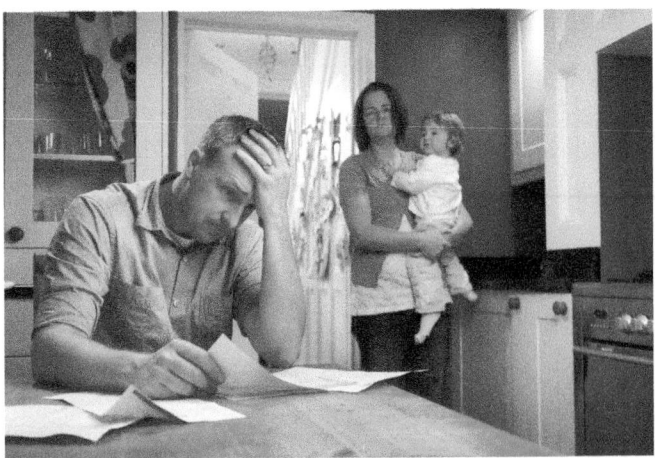

FIGURE 5-9 Signs of stress.

can be stressors. Each of these life events or others may be positive or negative. For a life event to be stressful, it does not always have to be a negative event.

Certain predisposing factors create a tendency or susceptibility to become stressed. These include attitudes and feelings (e.g., emotions such as optimism or pessimism), health habits (e.g., smoking, exercise, drug use, diet), the individual patient's methods for coping, economic and social resources (e.g., income, kind of job, security), and the state of the patient's immune system.

Many patients with a major illness go through a period of depression. The disease may cause emotional changes. In turn, worry about the disease may cause unhealthy habits such as an increase in smoking or drinking alcohol. Patients who have a physical illness such as heart disease, diabetes, or AIDS may become additionally stressed when confronted with the loss of income or a job.

Before you or a patient can cope with stress, you must be able to recognize it and know how you are being affected by it. You will also need to know what event or events are causing the stress. Recommendations for coping with stress include the following:

- Develop a strong support system, including family and friends.
- Find a balance between perfection and fear of failure.
- Eat nutritious meals.
- Avoid harmful habits such as smoking and drinking.
- Participate in physical exercise such as walking, jogging, dancing, biking, and swimming.
- Look outward to develop a social interest by understanding other people's problems and needs.
- Try to see the humor in situations.
- Limit the number of activities to a manageable few.

When you are working as a medical assistant, it will be important for you not to let personal stress affect your job performance. You also will experience stress that is related to work. This type of stress must be left at work when you go home for the night. Personal stress and work stress need to be kept separate and should never interfere with one another.

As part of your job, every day you will be taking care of patients who are sick. This can be emotionally, mentally, and physically draining. Anytime your stress level is too high and you have trouble coping, you must seek support from a close friend or family member. If a close friend or family member is not able to help you, seek help from a professional.

Encountering a patient who is experiencing stress provides an opportunity for patient teaching. After allowing the patient to discuss the stress and stressors, assess the patient's knowledge of the topic of stress. Doing so will establish a starting point for educating the patient. Next, determine the appropriate reading, language, and education level of the patient so that you can select and prepare materials to use to teach the patient about stress. Some of the educational materials that are used in a medical office include videos and patient teaching handouts. When you have completed the patient teaching, you must document it in the patient's medical record.

Symptoms of stress vary from person to person. It is important for you to know what is normal for you and your body. Box 5-2 lists symptoms of stress.

Use of Medical Language

As a medical assistant, you will become adept at understanding and using the language of medicine. Medical abbreviations are often used in communications among people working in the health care field. Most of your patients, however, have little understanding of medical terminology. You may wish to teach patients a few simple terms so they can better understand the physician's instructions about prescriptions, preparation for tests, or follow-up care at home. Otherwise, you must make an effort to avoid using medical terminology or abbreviations when speaking with patients. For example, abbreviations such as *NPO*, meaning "nothing by mouth," are not readily recognized or understood by patients. Always write out or state clear instructions regarding preparations for tests and taking medications. Patients may be reluctant to admit they do not understand, in which case you might assume that they have been properly instructed when they have not. Failure to inform patients in terms they are able to understand could be construed as negligence on the

BOX 5-2 | Symptoms of Stress

Fatigue
Exhaustion
Difficulty falling asleep
Difficulty staying asleep
Restlessness
Tension
Boredom
Lack of interest
Inability to concentrate
Depression

Cramps
Constipation
Diarrhea
Flatulence
Sore muscles
Increased blood pressure
Increased heart rate
Change in eating habits
Increased use of alcohol

part of the health care provider and increase the risk of a lawsuit.

Coping Mechanisms/Defensive Behaviors

A **coping mechanism** is a conscious or unconscious behavior used to respond to a challenging situation. Coping mechanisms can be *adaptive* (positive and helpful) or *nonadaptive* (negative, defensive, and unhelpful). For example, when trying to meet a short deadline, a nonadaptive coping mechanism could be becoming cross with others because of the added stress. An adaptive coping mechanism could be to plan out tasks in advance and ask for assistance when needed. Nonadaptive coping mechanisms, also known as defensive behaviors, can create barriers to communication, whereas adaptive coping mechanisms can enhance communication.

Defense mechanisms operate at a subconscious level to manage stress and anxiety by denying, misinterpreting, or distorting reality. They often hinder self-awareness by preventing people from being sensitive to anxiety. Defense mechanisms can be helpful in dealing with anxiety; however, consistent use of certain defenses leads to the development of either good or self-destructive behavior patterns. For example, the basic human need to be loved and cared for by another person can result in a variety of behaviors when the fear of losing love produces anxiety. One person may be driven to constantly look for love and affirmation by engaging in frequent one-night sexual encounters. Another person may seek and develop a warm, intimate relationship. A third person may be so frightened of not finding love and so fearful of rejection that the person avoids relationships to decrease the anxiety. The management of defense mechanisms may become so time consuming that little energy remains for other aspects of living.

Medical assistants need to be aware of their own and others' coping mechanisms. Patients, when stressed by illness or uncertainty, might exhibit a variety of nonadaptive coping mechanisms. Medical assistants should anticipate this and be prepared to respond in a positive, supportive, compassionate manner. As a member of the health care team, you must beware of using defensive behaviors as coping mechanisms in the professional setting as well as at home. Some examples of negative coping mechanisms are discussed in Table 5-6.

Responding to an Angry Patient

One of the most challenging communication problems is the angry patient. It can be a difficult task for a medical assistant to refrain from taking the patient's comments personally. People have different styles and coping mechanism when they are frightened (Figure 5-10). Many patients who enter the physician's office are fearful of the diagnosis they may hear. Some patients become frightened of the equipment in the office or have a high fear of pain. In addition to fear, another cause of anger is loss of control. If you have been hospitalized, you may be able to relate to this feeling. All these sources of fear or anxiety may make the patient short-tempered about issues such as being misunderstood over the phone, being asked to fill out paperwork when they arrive for an appointment, having to wait too long to see the physician, not understanding instructions from the medical assistant or physician, or not getting the appointment time they want for their next visit.

The responsibility of the medical assistant is to remain calm and use positive communication and professional techniques to direct the patient's anger into a positive channel. Try to defuse the patient's anger. For instance, many patients will gain control over their anger when the medical assistant offers a comment such as "I'm really sorry you feel this way. Let's see if we can solve the problem." You may have to take the patient into a private office if you cannot calm him or her immediately. Disruptive patients can upset

TABLE 5-6 | Nonadaptive Coping Mechanisms

Behavior	Description	Example
Compensation	Substitution of an attitude, feeling, or behavior with its opposite	Mrs. Matthews believes the lump in her breast is cancer. However, she smiles and laughs whenever you talk to her about it.
Denial	Unconsciously avoiding an unwanted feeling or situation	Mr. Morgan cancels an appointment to have a PSA blood test for prostate cancer in spite of having symptoms associated with prostate trouble.
Displaced Anger	Expressing angry feelings toward persons or objects that are unrelated to the problem	Mrs. Matthews is angry at being diagnosed with cancer. She takes this anger out on her family members.
Dissociation	Not connecting one event with another	Mary Sims is a nurse who works with alcoholic patients. In her free time, she drinks to excess.
Introjection	Adopting the feeling of someone else	Mr. Morgan's friends have said that the PSA test is reliable and could relieve his anxiety about having prostate cancer. He believes them and has the test.
Projection	Placing your own feelings on another person	Mr. Morgan becomes irritated when the medical assistant calls to remind him of his appointment. He wrongly decides that she is irritated with him or dislikes him. In reality, he is upset with himself.
Rationalization	Justifying thoughts or behavior to avoid the truth	Mary Sims believes that the appetite-suppressant benefit of smoking offsets the risk of developing cancer.
Regression	Turning back to former behavior patterns in times of stress	Jimmy, who is toilet trained, reverts to bed-wetting during hospitalization.
Repression	Keeping unpleasant thoughts or feelings out of one's mind	Mr. Morgan denies any urinary frequency when questioned by the physician.
Sublimation	Directing or changing unacceptable drives for security, affection, or power into socially or culturally acceptable channels	Mrs. Matthews is worried about having cancer and uses up energy cleaning her house.

others who are waiting to see the physician. Although it is not necessary to give in to a patient's unreasonable demands, it is important to realize that an upset patient is often expressing the need for you to listen carefully, without

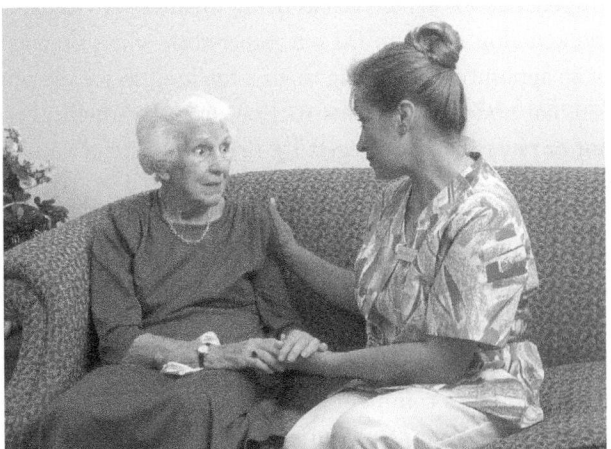

FIGURE 5-10 The medical assistant often has to reassure and comfort the patient before effective communication can take place.

judging, and to assist in solving the problem. Whenever possible, try to direct the patient's comments about a problem to a solution.

In the case of an angry caller, you must remember that no matter how angry or rude a patient becomes, you cannot respond in anger. The role of the medical assistant is to assess or evaluate the situation. Remain calm and speak to the patient in a quiet, calm tone of voice, projecting your concern for the patient in the present situation. Often this will be enough to calm the patient. If that does not work, however, ask your supervisor or office manager for assistance. Alternatively, ask the patient if you may return the call after you have been able to gather more information that will enable you to be of help.

In the case of a patient who becomes abusive or violent, it is necessary to consider the safety of yourself, other staff members, and patients. In such a case, follow office protocols to call for whatever assistance you need. Once the incident has been resolved, be sure to document it appropriately, according to office policies.

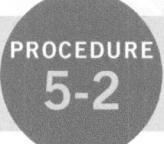

PROCEDURE 5-2

Assisting an Angry or Anxious Patient

Objective ◆ *Interact with a patient who is frightened, angry, or depressed.*

EQUIPMENT AND SUPPLIES

Pen; medical record

METHOD

1. Choose a classmate.
2. Select a quiet part of the classroom to conduct the procedure.
3. Determine who will be the medical assistant and who will be the patient.
4. Have the student who is pretending to be the patient express the emotions of being frightened, angry, and anxious.
5. Once you recognize one of these emotions, remain calm.
6. If the patient is not displaying destructive behaviors, allow the patient to express his feelings without being interrupted (Figure A).
7. Let the patient know that you understand.
8. Inquire about the issue so you can solve it.
9. During the conversation make sure you are empathic so the patient knows you are concerned about the issues.
10. Notify the physician of the conversation.
11. Document the conversation in the medical record.

CHARTING EXAMPLE

3/4/YY 4:00 P.M. Patient expressed concern about not seeing doctor immediately on arrival. Explained physician was delivering baby at hospital and offered patient another appointment later in the day. Patient refused later appointment and agreed to wait in the reception area until physician returned. M. Tyler, CMA (AAMA)

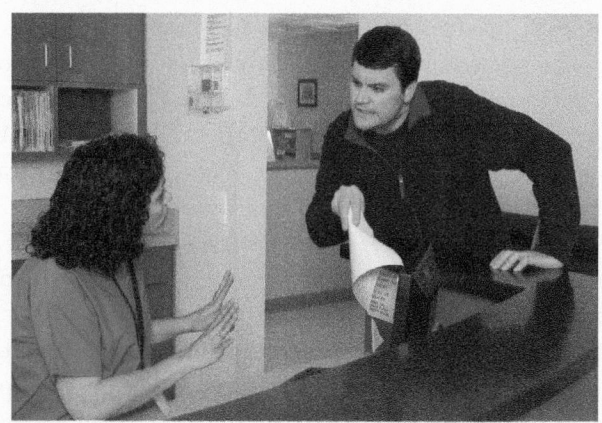

FIGURE A Medical assistants must calm angry patients.

See Procedure 5-2 for a role-play situation in which a patient is feeling fright, anger, and anxiety.

Responding to an Anxious Patient

Many patients exhibit what is known as *white coat syndrome.* This term was derived from the anxiety a patient feels when encountering medical staff, who would generally wear a white coat; however, attire is often more varied in today's medical atmosphere. Some signs of anxiety are trembling, flushing, perspiring, fidgeting, talking excessively, and remaining unusually quiet. Hypertensive patients who suffer from white coat syndrome should have their blood pressure measured at the beginning and the end of the visit to get a more representative value when the patient has had the opportunity to calm down and feel at ease. To deal with anxious patients, use the communication skills you have learned in this chapter: Speak calmly,

reassure patients, smile, touch them respectfully on the hand, and be empathetic.

COMMUNICATION AND DIVERSITY

As a medical assistant, you will encounter special circumstances when dealing with patients. It is likely that at some time you will encounter a patient who is terminally ill, is visually or hearing-impaired, is mentally or emotionally impaired, or is physically challenged in some other way. Regardless of the circumstances, all these patients must be treated with respect, understanding, and professionalism.

Medical assistants act as a coach, of sorts, to their patients. Although this concept is further described in the "Patient Education" chapter, it is essential to understand that the medical assistant must help coach their patients in regards to providing encouragement and support and adapting to their specific needs. Making adaptations in communication techniques to help a patient in a challenging situation is a necessary component of the medical assistant's skill set.

Patients with Sensory Impairment

Patient with special needs may require extra sensitivity, patience, and empathy on the part of the medical assistant. Here we consider several types of individual patients, along with some procedural guidelines.

The Hearing-Impaired Patient

Hearing loss can vary from a slight loss to total deafness. Total hearing impairment is considered by many to be the most difficult of all handicaps, because it can keep people isolated from communication and social interaction. A child who cannot hear will have difficulty speaking, because learning speech involves imitating the speech of others. Many hearing-impaired individuals communicate by means of sign language. Figure 5-11 shows the alphabet in sign language. Basic sign language is not difficult to learn. Simple phrases in sign language should be a part of every medical professional's knowledge base. Hearing-impaired patients often bring an interpreter to the medical office. Figure 5-12 shows a medical assistant using an interpreter with a patient who has hearing loss.

The manner in which you try to communicate will differ depending on whether the patient has a hearing aid, can lip-read, or has a family member or interpreter along for the appointment. Loss of hearing is a frequent but frustrating result of aging. The following are some guidelines to help someone with hearing impairment:

- Select a quiet environment to communicate with the patient.
- Reduce outside noise as much as possible.
- Never shout. Speak slowly and clearly.
- If the patient does not understand you the first time, rephrase the statement.
- Explain everything carefully before performing a procedure.
- Face the patient when speaking.
- Make sure light is on your mouth and not behind you. Light behind you may put shadows over the mouth and inhibit the patient's ability to lip-read.
- Have a paper and pen available so that the patient can communicate in writing.
- Always provide written instructions or pamphlets for patient education purposes.

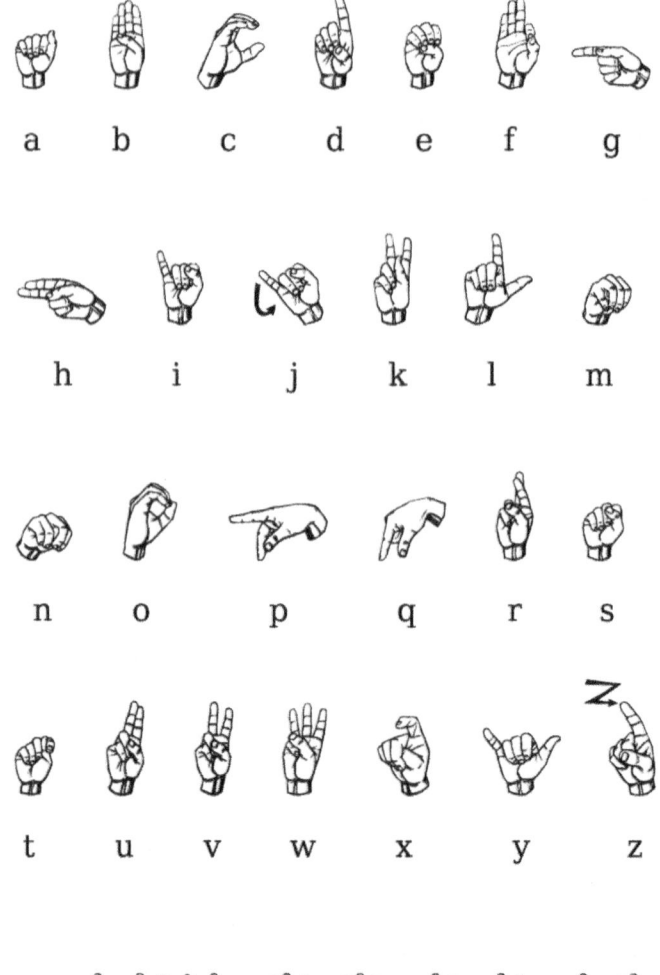
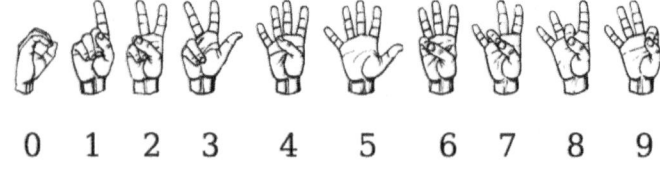

FIGURE 5-11 The American Sign Language alphabet.

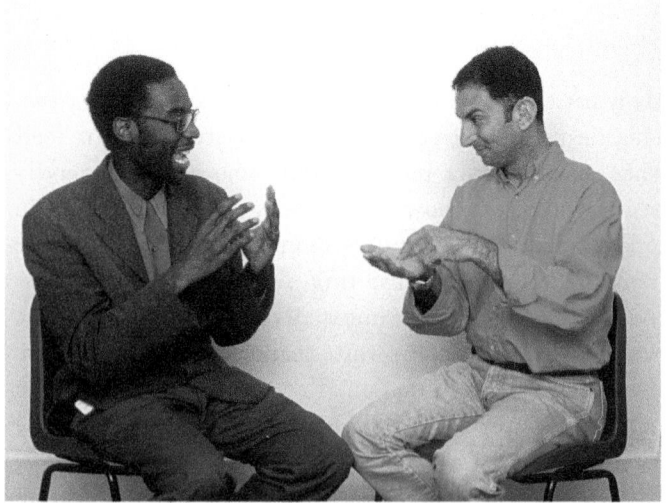

FIGURE 5-12 A hearing-impaired patient using an interpreter.

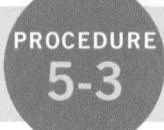

Assisting the Hearing-Impaired Patient

Objective ◆ *Use effective communication skills to assist a hearing-impaired patient to prepare for a physical examination.*

EQUIPMENT AND SUPPLIES

Paper and pencil

METHOD

1. Identify the patient.
2. Reduce external noise as much as possible.
3. Smile, establish eye contact, and face the patient.
4. Speak slowly, and do not shout.
5. Provide a careful explanation of the procedure.
6. Provide paper and pencil for the patient to use if desired.
7. Use written information to reinforce the message for the patient.
8. If possible, have the patient repeat your response to ensure that the message was received accurately.
9. Give directions using actions as well as words.
10. Be sensitive to the patient's needs.
11. Employ an empathetic, professional attitude.
12. Notify the physician of any patient concerns.

CHARTING EXAMPLE

6/24/XX 3:00 P.M. Patient is hearing impaired, so gave patient copy of attached handout on preparation for barium enema diagnostic testing. Patient was able to restate preparation steps. Eric Williams, RMA (AMT)

Basic hearing tests or screening tests are often performed by the medical assistant in the physician's office. An audiogram may be ordered by the physician when there is a suspicion of moderate to severe hearing loss. This test will determine the faintest sounds a patient can hear during audiometric testing. Audiometric testing, conducted by an audiologist, tests hearing ability by determining the lowest and highest intensities and frequencies that a person can distinguish. The patient may sit in a soundproof booth and receive sounds through earphones as the technician decreases the sounds or tones. Procedure 5-3 provides the steps to assist a hearing-impaired patient.

The Visually Impaired Patient

Blindness can be present at birth or may develop as a result of a disease, such as diabetes mellitus. Patients who are blind or are partially sighted can remain independent. Specially trained service animals can help the visually impaired patient to be more independent. Figure 5-13 shows a patient with a service dog. The visually impaired patient cannot rely on nonverbal cues that make up much of the communication process for those with sight. The medical assistant can communicate and help the visually impaired patient by remembering to follow the following suggested guidelines:

- Always speak to announce your presence when you are near a blind person.
- Offer to guide the patient into the examination room by offering your arm. Do not grab the patient without offering your arm first.
- Face the patient, and speak clearly.
- Describe the patient's surroundings.

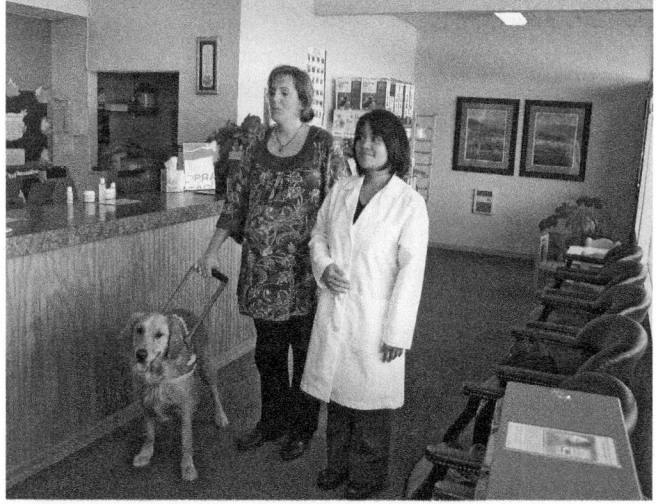

FIGURE 5-13 A visually impaired patient is assisted by a service dog.

- Explain all procedures in detail before beginning.
- Try not to leave the patient alone for any length of time.
- Have available large-print educational materials for patients who might benefit from them.
- Do not be condescending toward the patient.

The Mentally or Emotionally Impaired Patient

Psychology is the science of behavior and the human thought process. This behavioral science is primarily concerned with human beings acting alone or in groups. Normal behavior and abnormal behavior are distinguished from each other in psychology. All social interactions, such as those that occur during the communication process, may pose a problem for some people. As a medical assistant, you will encounter patients, family members, staff, and caregivers who exhibit a wide scope of behavior patterns. Abnormal behavior patterns may be caused by diseases, mental disorders, anxiety, drug abuse, trauma, the aging process, cultural customs, or a combination of several of these causes. Although it is difficult to deal with abnormal behavior, you must be tolerant and respectful of others in all circumstances.

When dealing with an emotionally or mentally impaired patient, it is important to determine, if possible, what level of communication the patient can understand. If a patient has a caregiver, that person may be able to give you tips regarding how to communicate with the patient. In most cases, you should speak slowly and clearly, stay calm, and keep your messages short. If you have to touch the patient for a procedure, be sure first to explain what you are going to do. A caregiver may be able to give you assistance in calming the patient, if needed.

The Physically Challenged Patient

Patients may have a permanent or temporary disability that pose a challenge in mobility. The patient may be using an assistive device, such as a cane or walker, or the patient may be in a wheelchair. Always allow the patient to ambulate and move on their own, offering assistance only when it appears necessary. When communicating and interacting with the patient, treat the patient with respect and dignity. Allow extra time with this patient, and do not appear to be impatient or rushed.

The Illiterate Patient

Illiteracy is the inability to read and write. Just as you cannot assume that everyone speaks English, you cannot assume that everyone knows how to read and write. This can be a challenge when filling out the many forms required in a medical office. If you notice that a patient is not filling out paper work or is taking a long time to do so, you should discreetly ask how they are coming along with the task and if they need any assistance. Perhaps there is a word or question they do not understand and a simple, polite explanation will clarify the meaning and enable them to move ahead. In other cases, it might be appropriate to move the patient to a private area and assist them to read the questions and write down the answers. In all situations, treat patients with respect and never do anything that might make them feel ashamed or inadequate.

The Seriously Ill or Terminally Ill Patient

As a medical assistant, you will come into contact with patients who have a terminal illness. A terminal illness is one that is expected to end in death. This includes many conditions and diseases, including cancer and progressive heart disease.

In cases in which the dying process is slow for the patient, you may have the opportunity to be with the patient on several occasions during office visits. Although there is always hope of recovery or finding a cure through research, it is wise to listen to the patient express her fears and concerns rather than to offer false hope for recovery. When there is no hope of recovery and death is expected within a year, you may be instructed by the physician to refer the patient to the services of Hospice. Hospice can provide the patient with comprehensive physical, palliative, psychologic, and spiritual care until death. After the death, Hospice will support the family, caregivers, and loved ones.

Death is a natural process that everyone must face. People have various ways of coping with their own death based on a variety of influences, including culture, religion, personal experience, and age.

Influence of Culture

People learn what their own culture expects of them at a very early age by observing family and friends as they handle life events such as births and deaths. In some cultures, death is considered a normal end to the life process and is therefore accepted with peace. In other cultures, death may be feared.

The terminally ill patient and family may have already established a very personal approach or method for handling death and dying. You may also have a strong cultural attitude toward death.

Influence of Religion

Religious beliefs play an important role in how patients handle death and dying. Some patients have a strong belief in an afterlife. Other patients follow no particular religious belief. In both cases, the patients' dying process and death can be meaningful and peaceful.

It is considered unacceptable for the medical assistant to attempt to convert the patient to the medical assistant's religious faith. Professionalism mandates that the medical assistant and other staff members recognize and support the patient's right to embrace different religious beliefs.

Influence of Personal Experience

The past experiences of the patient and the medical assistant mold how they approach the topic of death. If the patient has been closely involved with the care of someone who died a painful death, the patient may fear the same kind of death for himself or herself. These patients must be able to discuss their fears. In the same manner, if the medical assistant has had past experiences with the deaths of friends or relatives, it may be easier to assist the patient. On the other hand, patients who have had little exposure to death may have a more difficult time understanding their feelings or expressing their experience.

Influence of Age

Older adults usually have less fear of death than younger people. In some cases, an older adult may not feel well. Also, the patient may have failing eyesight, hearing, and memory and may look at death with relief. If the patient wishes to discuss his approaching death, you should be ready to listen.

Stages of Grief

Dr. Elisabeth Kübler-Ross devoted much of her life to the study of the dying process and working with dying patients. She divided the grief process into five stages that she believes all persons go through (Table 5-7). It is helpful to understand these stages when attempting to help the dying patient. Although these stages relate to death, they can also relate to other losses, such as loss of body organs, health, marriage, or family members. People move between these phases, but not necessarily in a linear fashion.

As the time of death approaches, some of the earlier stages may be repeated. For example, patients who cannot care for themselves may become angry. The critical point to remember when assisting a dying patient is that the grieving period is a normal part of the dying process. The goal is for the patient to eventually accept the loss.

It is also important to understand that family and friends of the patient may be going through the stages of grief at a different pace than the patient. Although the patient may have reached the stage of acceptance, others who love that person may still be in denial, angry, bargaining to gain time, or depressed. You can be most helpful by being as sensitive as possible to the states of emotion of all those who are dealing with that person's death.

Diverse Patient Populations

As a medical assistant, you will come in contact with people from many different cultures. A **culture** consists of the values, beliefs, attitudes, and customs shared by a group of people and passed on through the generations. Behaviors exhibited by the members of a culture are based on their beliefs and values. Health care beliefs may differ widely from those you are accustomed to. As you come in contact with people from cultures other than your own, be aware that diversity can create its own barriers to effective communication. To break through these barriers, you must be tolerant in attitude and treat each patient with respect, dignity, and understanding.

It will also be important for you to be aware of your nonverbal communication and that of the patient. As you research the different cultures in your area, you must learn how nonverbal communication varies across the cultures.

TABLE 5-7	Dr. Elisabeth Kübler-Ross's Five Stages of Grief	
Denial	A refusal to believe that dying is taking place. In this stage, the patient (or family member) may need time to adjust to the reality of approaching death. This stage cannot be hurried.
Anger	At this stage, the patient may be angry at everyone and may express this intense anger at God, family, and even health care professionals. The patient may take this anger out on the closest person. Usually this is a family member. In reality, the patient is angry about dying.
Bargaining	The third stage of grief involves attempting to gain time by making promises in return. The patient may bargain with God. The patient may also indicate a need to talk at this stage.
Depression	This stage is marked with a deep sadness over the loss of health, independence, and eventually life. There is an additional sadness of leaving loved ones behind. The grieving patient may become withdrawn.
Acceptance	The acceptance stage is characterized by a sense of peace and calm. The patient may make comments such as "I have no regrets. I'm ready to die." It is better to let the patient talk and not make denial statements such as "Don't talk like that. You're not going to die."

You must determine if eye contact should be direct or indirect. Not having proper eye placement can interfere with the communication process.

Facial expressions can show a variety of emotions, such as sadness, anger, confusion, and happiness. Facial expressions can also differ from culture to culture. A smile does not always mean kindliness or friendliness; it may also be a sign of fear. It will be important to determine what different facial expressions mean.

Hand gestures also vary across cultures. Some gestures that are accepted in U.S. culture are considered inappropriate in others. It is very important for you to understand the appropriate gestures to use for a particular culture.

Each culture has unique aspects related to medical care. You should be familiar with cultural practices and risk factors for the cultures that are served by the physician practice. Patients from some cultures, such the Haitian culture, believe in magic, so it may take time to build rapport and trust with them. People from other cultures, such as the Amish, may not carry insurance, and thus may prefer to pay cash toward medical bills. In cultures that value large families, such as many Appalachian communities, infertility may carry a stigma. Arabs have been shown to have difficulty metabolizing antiarrhythmics, antidepressants, betablockers, neuroleptics, and opioid agents, so they may experience elevated blood levels and adverse effects when customary dosages are prescribed. Chinese immigrants have an increased incidence of hepatitis B and tuberculosis. Cuban Americans have a high rate of coronary heart disease, hypertension, obesity, type 2 diabetes, and depression. Jewish patients have a higher rate of the genetic disorders called Gaucher's disease and Tay-Sachs disease.

Bias, Prejudice, and Stereotyping

Bias, prejudice, and stereotyping are barriers to effective communication that directly relate to cultural diversity. As discussed previously, culture is defined as the values, attitudes, and behaviors particular to a group of people. **Bias** is an unfair preference for or dislike of something. A bias prevents forming an impartial opinion of someone or something. **Prejudice** is a preformed and unfavorable belief or attitude toward a certain culture or group with little or no information about the culture or group. **Stereotyping** is an idea people hold about the characteristics of a group. These ideas may be true of some members of the group but are unfairly applied to everyone in the group, or they may simply be untrue. Stereotypes are usually negative.

Ethnicity is a classification of people based on a group they are part of. They may be people of the same national origin or the same race or the same religion. People from the same ethnic background are likely to share similar traditions, beliefs, and language.

Race is a classification of people based on their physical or biological characteristics, such as skin color, shape of eyes, hair type, bone structure, or facial features. Race is often used to classify people unfairly and unjustly in a negative way.

People who are **ethnocentric** believe that their cultural background is better than any other. This leads to prejudice, prejudging, and stereotyping, which can negatively impact communication and the acceptance of others.

As a medical assistant, to avoid these negative behaviors, you should adhere to the following behaviors:

- Be aware of your own beliefs.
- Learn as much as possible about other cultures, races, and nationalities.
- Be sensitive to the feelings of others.
- Evaluate information before accepting it as a belief.
- Avoid ethnic jokes.
- Be open to differences.
- When unsure of a patient's cultural beliefs, ask the patient to help you understand.

Language

A patient who speaks a language other than English is at a disadvantage when trying to obtain health care in the United States. Imagine, for a minute, how you would feel if you were traveling in a foreign country and had an accident that required you to go to the hospital. If you did not speak the language in that country, you might not understand anyone in the hospital, and the health care practices also might be very different from what you are accustomed to at home. Your feelings of fear, frustration, and confusion would be increased if you had no one to act as an interpreter. It will help you to be more tolerant if you imagine yourself in the position of the patient who does not speak English or does not speak it well.

You will encounter patients and other health care workers who speak a wide variety of languages. Speakers of Spanish are the second-largest language group, after English speakers, in the United States today. It would be helpful for you to learn a few phrases and some simple words in Spanish to help communicate with Spanish-speaking patients and coworkers. The same is true for patients who speak other languages. If at all possible, when a patient is not completely comfortable with English, you should get someone to interpret for the patient. Perhaps a fellow worker or family member could help. For patients with a limited ability to understand English, speak slowly and clearly (not louder),

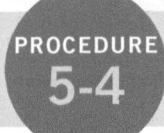

PROCEDURE 5-4

Communicating with a Patient When There Is a Language Barrier

Objective ◆ *Communicate with patients from other cultures.*

EQUIPMENT AND SUPPLIES

Pen or pencil; paper

METHOD

1. Choose a classmate.
2. Select a quiet part of the classroom to conduct the procedure.
3. Determine who will be the medical assistant and who will be the patient.
4. Have the student acting the part of the patient pretend to speak very little English.
5. Be calm, respectful, and considerate (Figure A).
6. Use simple and common words.
7. Avoid using medical terms.
8. Never use slang.
9. Pay attention to your eye contact, facial expressions, and hand gestures.
10. Make the patient feel as comfortable as possible. *Note:* In a real-life situation, if a staff member who speaks the patient's language is available, offer to have that staff member translate the conversation if that would make the patient feel more comfortable.
11. Document the interaction in the patient chart.

CHARTING EXAMPLE

9/30/YY 8:05 A.M. Patient states that he speaks little English. Gave patient handout in Spanish after demonstrating procedure to the patient in the office. C. Glidewell, CMA (AAMA)

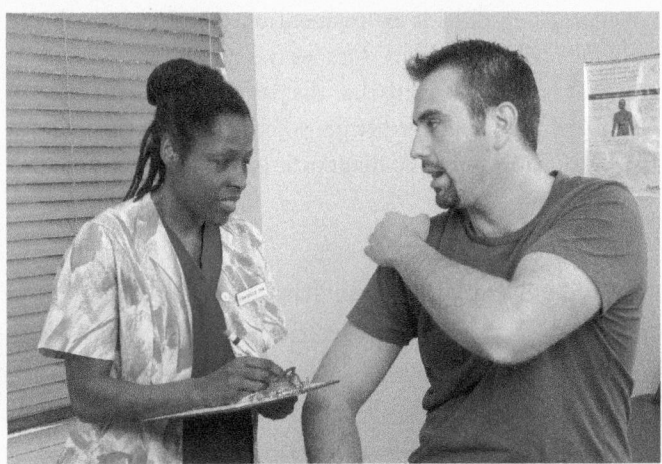

FIGURE A A medical assistant must be prepared to work with a patient who does not speak English.

using simple words or phrases. Smiling and other positive nonverbal cues are helpful. You might try to demonstrate or act out what you want the patient to do. Use pictures, if they are available, to help relay messages, or make a clear drawing to get your point across.

When you are talking to a patient for whom English is not the primary language, use simple and common words. Avoid using medical terms if possible. You should never use slang. It is important for you to determine if the patient understands you. Sometimes patients who do not understand English pretend to understand so as not to seem impolite.

Procedure 5-4 will help you role-play interacting with a patient who does not speak English well.

Professionalism | Cultural Considerations

Medical assistants must work with and provide care for individuals from a wide variety of racial, ethnic, cultural, religious, and socioeconomic backgrounds. In every instance, it is important to respect the individuality of everyone. Patients from other cultures may be completely unfamiliar or unaccepting of the Western model of communication. For example, in Asian cultures it is considered rude to make direct eye contact during a greeting; thus, bowing is often performed, and handshaking is performed with a light grip and diverted eyes. Follow the lead of your patients as best you can by observing how they seem to want to communicate.

Diverse Viewpoints

People from other cultures have different views and customs relating to health care delivery. Your views and customs may not be better than theirs, just different. Patients may have different views about the causes of illness, the treatments, and the behavior expected of the health care provider. In some cultures, illness is thought to be caused by winds or other forces, blood being too thick or thin, or the ill will of others. The best way to learn about the views of someone from another culture is to ask them.

You may not always be successful in encouraging patients from a different culture to relate their symptoms and signs to you. Patients may feel that talking about physical pain is a sign of weakness, or they may be forbidden to mention psychologic problems or to mention certain parts of the body or bodily functions. One of the duties of the medical assistant is to help ensure that the patient complies with the treatment physicians prescribe, whether it is in the form of medication or therapy or diagnostic examinations. It may be necessary to ask for assistance from a family member who understands the issues and can communicate more easily. Table 5-8 lists some diverse cultural traditions.

Religious Diversity

There are many religious beliefs and practices that may affect the interaction and communication between the health care provider and the patient. The medical assistant must become familiar with the various beliefs and practices associated with the religions adhered to by patients. Many religious communities exist in the United States, including Jehovah's Witnesses, Christian Scientists, Orthodox Jews, Mormons (Church of Jesus Christ of Latter-Day Saints), and Amish. These religious groups may have varying beliefs about immunizations, blood transfusion and organ donation, childbirth and fertility, dietary restrictions, and the overall approach to health care delivery. There are also religious holidays that must be observed, so in scheduling appointments, be careful to respect the patient who is unable

TABLE 5-8 | Cultural Traditions in Health Care

Country/Cultural Group	Sick Care Practices	Health Care Beliefs	Family Role in Care
China	Holistic and traditional; includes acupuncture, herbal medicine	Upset in body energy causes disease. Stigma is attached to mental illness. Health promotion is important.	Family takes care of the sick, even in hospital.
Former Soviet Union	Holistic, folk, and Western medical practices	Health promotion is important. Acute sick care is practiced; rehabilitation is not stressed.	Family members provide care in hospital: bathing, feeding, changing linens.
Philippines	Health promotion is important. Mental illness is a disgrace. Evil cast from the eyes of another can cause illness.	Family may give hospital care.	Children feel obligated to care for elderly.
Vietnam	Health care practices contain magical and religious components. Eastern and herbal medicine are important. Self-care and self-medication are used to treat illness.	Only acute sick care is permitted. Health is believed to come from the restoration of yin and yang and hot and cold balance.	Patient care is a family responsibility.
Hispanic/Latino	Health care involves belief in God and fate. Good health may be luck. Believe transgressions or sins may contribute to illness.	Natural and supernatural worlds exist, and body and soul are inseparable. Holistic practices are well accepted.	Family is integral part of the health care process. They are involved in the decision making as to care and treatment of the patient.
Native American	Health care involves belief in religious and spiritual traditions.	Rely on Mother Earth for remedies and healing powers. There must be harmony between the body, mind, and spirit.	Family members, especially elders, are critical to the care of patient. Tribal leader may be consulted for advice in treatment.

to accept an appointment on the date of a religious holiday or special observance.

Gender and Sexual Orientation

Sexual orientation describes what gender someone is sexually and romantically attracted to. A straight person is attracted to people of the opposite sex. Lesbians are women attracted to other women. Gays are men attracted to other men. Bisexual people are attracted to both males and females. Transgender people are those who identify with the opposite gender from what they were born with—from male to female or from female to male. Some transgender people undergo sex change surgery to physically change their sex organs.

You cannot determine a person's sexual orientation by the way they look, or their job, or hobbies. The only way to know is if they tell you. Homophobia is fear and hatred of lesbian and gay people; biphobia is fear and hatred of bisexual people. Regardless of a medical assistant's personal opinions or personal sexual orientation, patients of all sexual orientations should be treated the same.

Socioeconomic Status

A person's socioeconomic status refers to individual and family social status based on income, education, and occupation. Researchers generally classify socioeconomic status as low, middle, or high. Medical assistants work with patients of every socioeconomic status and must be careful not to make assumptions about a person's status or health based on appearance, speech, or other factors. Statistics show that low income and education are strong predictors of many physical and mental health problems, including respiratory viruses, arthritis, coronary disease, and schizophrenia. These might be because of environmental conditions, such as the workplace or housing situation, or they might be a causal factor. For example, mental illnesses can be the root cause of many socioeconomic problems. Medical problems and disabilities can prevent someone from working, thus causing them to lose health insurance coverage; then, high medical bills can use up a person's financial resources, including their home that they once thought was secure.

Likewise, medical assistants should not assume that a person is well-off financially or treat those who are any differently. Do not treat a wealthy person rudely simply because they are wealthy; neither should you give them preferential treatment compared with other patients.

Lifestyle Choices

The phrase *lifestyle choices* refers to the decisions people make about how they live and behave. It can include choices such as where they live, who they live with, what they eat, how they exercise, moral and ethical standards, use of illegal

 Professionalism Cultural Considerations

Many cultures, particularly some ethnic and some religious groups, have strong opinions regarding mental health disorders. In fact, some Asian cultures view the idea of mental illness as a flaw or weakness in a person's character. Those who follow Scientology often strongly oppose psychology, psychiatry, and medications as a means for treating mental illness or depression. Some religious sects believe that mental illness is a form of demon possession or spiritual attack.

These varying views regarding psychology and mental health have an impact on the way a patient receives treatment. Above all else, it is your responsibility to be the advocate for the patient and to place the patient's wishes and beliefs above your own.

substances, and political preferences. Never treat patients differently because of their choices, even if you do not personally agree with them. When choices affect a person's health, provide patient education as directed by the physician. For example, a medical assistant who is an exercise enthusiast should not just randomly start telling an overweight person that they are living an unhealthy lifestyle and should eat differently or exercise more. When the patient is seen for a weight-related condition, such as cardiovascular disease or diabetes, and the physician has asked you to provide education, give the patient the appropriate brochures and instructions according to office policy, and document the education in the patient's chart.

INTRAOFFICE COMMUNICATION

The goal in the medical office should be to establish a sense of **rapport**—an environment of cooperation—with patients, coworkers, supervisors, and vendors. To create this cooperative environment, all the communication skills we have examined in this chapter must be put to use.

Establishing Trust

To communicate effectively in the health care environment and in everyday life, you must establish trust in your relationships and use **integrity** when relating to others. Integrity means being honest and demonstrating moral principles—doing the right thing even when no one is watching. Being open, honest, and firm in your convictions, presenting a professional image, and using positive body language help create a positive environment.

Some of the most difficult communication problems occur with other staff members (Figure 5-14). Good staff

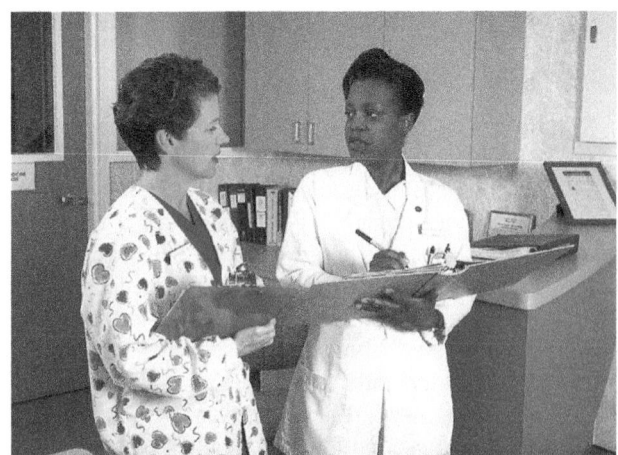

FIGURE 5-14 Staff members often find it difficult to communicate with other coworkers.

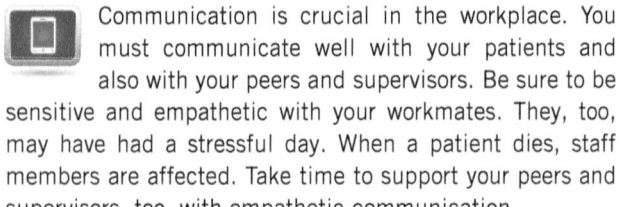
communication depends on positive and respectful interactions. A thoughtless or condescending comment can cause permanent damage to a relationship. To be condescending is to adopt a superior attitude and act as though you are better or smarter than someone else. Withdrawing from the group, feeling angry and hurt, and discussing other staff members behind their backs cause office morale to suffer. Using assertive (positive) behavior with fellow staff means that you assert your own needs without threatening theirs. For instance, if it is your turn to have a holiday off and you have been scheduled to work, it is better to state, "I'm sorry, but I can't work that day. Because I worked overtime on the last holiday, I have made plans for this one." An aggressive (negative) statement, such as "It's not fair; I always have to work on holidays and the others don't," would imply that favoritism or special treatment has been shown to some staff members and might cause the supervisor to become defensive.

Rapport and Team Building

A positive attitude can make the difference between keeping and losing a job. A positive attitude is easier to project if you are happy in your work. The work group you are part of is an important factor in your attitude. Work groups must become a cohesive team. To do this, some degree of socializing is beneficial. Discussions with other staff members about hobbies, travel, sports, family, and friends help to establish trust and understanding. Of course, such discussions need to take place at times and in ways that do not interfere with work.

Gossip is unnecessary, unprofessional, and often results in a negative conversation, usually about someone who is not present. The medical assistant must learn to recognize gossip and not participate in it. Gossip can be extremely hurtful and is destructive to the cooperation needed in the medical facility.

Staffing arrangements are as varied as the types of medical practices. The solo practice with its staff of one; the multiphysician practice with a variety of staff, including an office manager; and the clinic with many registered nurses (RNs) and other types of allied health care workers are only a few of the types of practices in which the medical assistant may work. Whatever the staffing arrangements, the physician or office manager must be clear about the chain of command and convey to the employees the process for following the chain of command. In the solo office with one medical assistant, problems rarely arise. However, in larger practices, the health care professional with most seniority is often the unofficial office manager. This person may not be the most qualified staff member, the most multiskilled, or the most accomplished manager. Friction among coworkers is often a problem in many of these larger practices. To avoid this problem, clearly defined areas of responsibility and authority should be established. An office policies and procedures manual can help resolve conflict about authority and responsibility.

Conflict Resolution

Inevitably, from time to time, coworkers experience strife and conflict. Conflict interferes with establishing rapport and cooperation, which are essential in the workplace. However, at times, conflict can be a positive experience if it resolves issues of disagreement in an appropriate manner.

The policies and procedures manual is a valuable tool when beginning to resolve issues. The manual should state clearly what standards are acceptable in all areas and with all employees of the facility.

Conflicts happen when miscommunication or misunderstanding of the message occurs. If someone offers a feedback or criticism, do not argue with the person or become defensive. Simply say, "Thank you for your thoughts," and continue with what you were doing.

Conflict also can stem from prejudices or preconceived ideas. Medical assistants should be aware of their own tendencies in this area and be careful not to act on them or let them affect their relationships with others.

- Recognize that a problem exists. Recognition may result from a feeling, observation, or conversation with others.
- Describe the problem, and clarify what the basic issue or question is and the factors that affect it.
- Identify alternative methods of resolving the problem. Any alternative method should be considered, even if is not immediately seen as practical.
- Consider how the method or solution will affect those involved.
- Choose the best method for resolving the problem, and implement it.
- As the plan is being put into effect, evaluate the results and adjust the method if necessary.

Problem Solving and Critical Thinking

Regardless of the type of practice, communication is vitally important to keep conflict to a minimum, establish a positive environment, and provide quality health care. Problem solving and critical thinking are necessary skills for health care workers. Problem solving is a way of looking at a problem and ultimately arriving at a decision. Box 5-3 offers helpful steps for problem solving. Most problems have more than one solution. Weighing all the factors involved and evaluating the results will help later with other problems.

Critical thinking (Box 5-4) includes the ability to think imaginatively, solve problems, visualize situations, learn new information, and think logically. Both problem solving and critical-thinking skills are important concepts to employ before trying to resolve any conflict. Box 5-5 illustrates the steps in conflict resolution.

Communicating with Superiors

In dealing with your superiors, as with your coworkers, communication should be kept positive. If conflicts do arise and you need to speak with your superior, choose an appropriate time or ask for an appointment to discuss the matter. Be direct and to the point, and do not promote any gossip you may have heard. If you have been given an order to do something and need clarification on how to complete it, ask for help. Most supervisors would rather be asked a question than have you perform a function about which you are not clear. Show initiative in your daily work. If a task needs to be done, volunteer to do it without being asked, as long as it falls within your job description. Too often, staff members are busy keeping score of which employees do more or less work as compared with others.

Loyalty to Your Employer

You represent your employer or physician every time you speak to a patient or caller. You must support the physician and the physician's reputation in every instance. In your position, you may become privileged to personal information about your employer. Under no circumstances, whether inside or outside the office, should you discuss that personal information. It is perfectly acceptable to state, "I really can't answer that," or "I'm sorry, but I don't know," in response to a patient's or other staff member's questions.

A loyal employee protects and defends an employer when other employees engage in negative conversation. See

- Ask questions.
- Define a problem.
- Examine evidence.
- Avoid emotional reasoning.
- Analyze assumptions and bias.
- Avoid oversimplification.
- Consider other interpretations.
- Tolerate ambiguity.
- Think about your own thinking.

- Communicate your needs in simple terms.
- Know when to express your feelings.
- Do not assume you know the other person's feelings.
- Look at the issue from the other person's perspective.

TABLE 5-9 | Responses That Communicate Loyalty

Question/Comment	Sample Response
"I guess Dr. Thompson can't see me on Wednesday because he's playing golf."	"Dr. Thompson's day off is Wednesday, but he could see you on Saturday."
"I hear Dr. Thompson and his wife are divorcing."	"I really have no information about Dr. Thompson's personal life."
"I've been waiting one hour to see Dr. Thompson. Why is he so slow?"	"I'm sorry you've had a long wait. Dr. Thompson has had many very ill patients today. May I reschedule your appointment?"

Table 5-9 for examples of loyal responses to questions or comments about your employer's personal life.

COMMUNICATION AND PATIENT RIGHTS

Every patient has the right to privacy and confidentiality. Any information about a patient is considered privileged information.

Privacy

Privacy is the health care industry's term for what is commonly known as confidentiality. All patients have the right to have their personal privacy respected and their medical records handled with confidentiality. Your treatment and concern for the patient reflect the physician's high standards of care. The human dignity of each patient must be preserved regardless of the patient's socioeconomic background, race, age, nationality, sexual orientation, or gender. HIPAA, as previously mentioned, was passed in 1996 by Congress. The Privacy Rule, which is part of HIPAA, provides for the federal protection of health information. This rule, although protecting patients' privacy, also allows for patients to have better access to their medical records and to have more control about how and to whom the information can be released. HIPAA designates as **protected health information (PHI)** any facts that, if revealed, potentially could be used to identify the individual. PHI includes the following data elements:

- Name
- Address
- Phone numbers
- Fax numbers
- Dates (birth, death, admission, discharge, etc.)

- Social Security number
- E-mail address
- Medical record numbers
- Health plan beneficiary numbers
- Account numbers
- Certificate or license numbers
- Vehicle identifiers, serial numbers, and license plate numbers
- Device identifiers and serial numbers
- Web Universal Resource Locators (URLs)
- Internet Protocol (IP) address numbers

This means that none of this information can be given out by any means (electronic, paper, or orally) for any reason without the consent of the patient. The patient gives **consent** by signing a copy of the medical office's notice of privacy practices (NPP). The NPP is provided before all new-patient visits and is generally updated once a year with established patients. Although the office must make a good faith effort to obtain the patient's signature, it is not mandatory. The NPP consent covers any information necessary for treatment, payment, and operations (TPO). For any other purposes, the patient must provide a written **authorization** that identifies the type of information to be released, the name of the recipient, and the length of time it for which it is valid. If you are in doubt about whether to release personal patient information, do not do it. Always make sure that you have obtained the appropriate authorization.

Family members can pose special confidentiality problems. If a patient brings a family member into the examination room with them, you might presume that they are giving informed consent to share information with that family member. However, it is prudent to have the patient sign a form specifying with which family members or friends the office personnel may discuss the patient's case. Domestic violence victims may be intimidated into allowing their violent perpetrators to come to the office with them. A wise medical assistant may ask the significant other to leave the room for a few minutes so the assistant can assess whether the patient is safe at home. It is important to let patients know that they can exclude family members from the discussion of their health if they wish.

Advising Patients

As a medical assistant, you are the physician's representative. Because you are part of the staff, wear a uniform, and assist with treatments, patients may view you as an authority figure. The physician advises the patient on a course of treatment or procedure based on the examination and diagnostic test results. You are not permitted to offer your opinion about the physician's diagnosis, discuss the course of action the physician has set forth, or tell the patient what you would do in her position. Those opinions are beyond your scope of practice and could put you and the physician at risk of being sued. If asked by a patient, "What would you do if you were me?" you must not offer advice. Explain to the patient that the physician will be pleased to review the course of action and answer any questions and that you will be happy to arrange for that meeting. A medical assistant giving advice to a patient could be construed as practicing medicine without a license and is a punishable offense in most states.

Patient Decision Making

Patients who have received bad news from the physician or are faced with difficult choices do need help to come to a decision. Your role is to listen empathetically to the patient, ask reflecting or clarifying questions, and make clear the information the physician has related to help the patient come to a decision on a course of treatment. For example, Mrs. Santos has been told by the physician that her breast biopsy was positive and a mastectomy is recommended as soon as possible. When the physician leaves the room, she asks you what she should do. Your response should be, "Mrs. Santos, you seem upset about having to have a mastectomy. What concerns you about the procedure?" If she asks what you would do in her circumstances, you can explain again in simple terms what the doctor has said. You may also obtain approval from the physician to suggest to the patient that she seek a second opinion. Sometimes patients are so nervous in the presence of a physician that they do not hear

information correctly. It would be permissible to give Mrs. Santos written information about the procedure, offer to bring her concerns to the physician, and encourage her to call back once she is home if she has more questions.

SUMMARY

Communication is a necessary requirement for everyday living. In the health care field, the ability to communicate effectively is essential for success, such as when calling and requesting a prescription be renewed, documenting the patient's symptoms and helping the patient be diagnosed properly, providing patient education, arranging travel plans for the physician, and so on. The concern you have for patients will show in your words, actions, gestures, and tone of voice. The values of the office personnel reflect in their attitudes and behaviors. Effective listening is patient centered and requires practice to ensure that you understand the obvious and less obvious needs of the patients. The special needs of some patients may not be the presenting problems when they arrive in the physician's office; however, these special needs must be dealt with to accommodate the patients as much as possible. Special care must be taken with patients who are hearing impaired, do not speak English, cannot see, are angry or anxious, are terminally ill, or are mentally or emotionally impaired. The medical assistant must remain flexible and be able to handle all unusual situations professionally. Although medical assistants should advocate assertively for the patient, they should never become aggressive. They should understand that patients are vulnerable and may engage in defensive behaviors. Therefore, getting honest feedback from patients is vital.

5 CHAPTER REVIEW

COMPETENCY REVIEW

1. Define and spell the terms for this chapter.
2. What would you say to a patient who says that the medication Dr. Thompson gave her last week made her sick?
3. What would you say to the patient who is angry at the delay in the waiting room?
4. What would you say to the patient who complains to you about Dr. Thompson?
5. What should you do if you are unfamiliar with a patient's religious or cultural beliefs?
6. Describe how to communicate to a profoundly deaf patient that she must remove all clothing and put on a gown.
7. Describe some cultural problems that can arise when treating patients from other cultures.

8. Discuss several negative coping mechanisms that you feel you sometimes exhibit. How do they impact negatively on your relationships with others?

9. Gladys Pierce's neighbor calls to see if she kept her appointment because she says Gladys is sometimes forgetful. What would you say?

PREPARING FOR THE CERTIFICATION EXAM

1. Which of the following is an open-ended question?
   a. Do you smoke?
   b. Have you ever had surgery?
   c. Do you take herbal supplements?
   d. Why are you here today?
   e. Are your parents still living?

2. If a patient is hearing impaired, which of the following would you do?
   a. Cover your mouth with your hand when talking.
   b. Stand with your back to the window.
   c. Give written instructions for surgical preparation.
   d. Speak more quickly than usual.
   e. Forego getting informed consent.

3. Which of the following should you say to an angry patient?
   a. "Sit down and be quiet."
   b. "You need to calm down."
   c. "How may I help you resolve this problem?"
   d. "You should have been here on time."
   e. "I need to get the doctor first."

4. A 49-year-old patient has a developmental delay and is highly emotional. What is the best course when approaching the patient in the reception area?
   a. Insist that he sit quietly in the reception area.
   b. Give him a toy truck to keep him occupied.
   c. Find a coloring book for him.
   d. Privately ask the caregiver how best to approach him.
   e. Offer him a cup of coffee.

5. Which of the following comprises the sum of all our values?
   a. behavior
   b. character
   c. beliefs
   d. attitudes
   e. prejudice

6. Which ethnic group makes up the largest number of non–English speakers in the United States?
   a. Hmong
   b. Hispanic
   c. Slavic
   d. Caucasian
   e. Persian

7. Which of the following is *not* a sign of impatience?
   a. tapping your finger
   b. interrupting conversation
   c. walking around the room
   d. sitting down
   e. checking your watch

8. Which of the following is assertive, not aggressive, behavior?
   a. demanding your way
   b. interrupting others
   c. telling others they are wrong
   d. advocating for patients
   e. shouting loudly

9. Which form acknowledges the release of patient information for treatment, payment, and operations (TPO)?
   a. Authorization for Treatment
   b. Notice of Privacy Practices
   c. New Patient Registration Consent
   d. Protected Health Information Authorization
   e. Patient Privacy Notice

10. Mrs. Hamsi has breast cancer. She does not want to offend her doctor, so she yells at her daughter as she leaves the office. What negative coping mechanism is she exhibiting?
    a. denial
    b. depersonalization
    c. depression
    d. displacement
    e. dissociation

CRITICAL THINKING

Refer to the case study at the beginning of the chapter and use what you have learned to answer the following questions.

1. The front desk receptionist informs the medical assistant that Mr. Yeung is very apprehensive. What are some things that the MA should or shouldn't do in this instance?

2. When working with a patient who has an interpreter, is it best to direct questions and comments to the interpreter or toward the patient? Explain your answer.

ON THE JOB

Amy Freeman is a new medical assistant who recently passed the CMA examination. She has carefully studied the HIPAA. When she is locking up the office at night, she notices that a patient's X-ray, bill, and driver's license photocopy have been left on a desk. Which documents, if any, must she put away under HIPAA regulations before leaving for the evening?

INTERNET ACTIVITY

Search using the term *deaf culture* for a chat room for the deaf. Communicate with people with hearing impairment about their culture.

Additional Internet resources for information on hearing, vision, and physical impairment:

- ▶ www.jointcommission.org
- ▶ www.ada.gov
- ▶ www.dol.gov
- ▶ www.ncbi.nlm.nih.gov

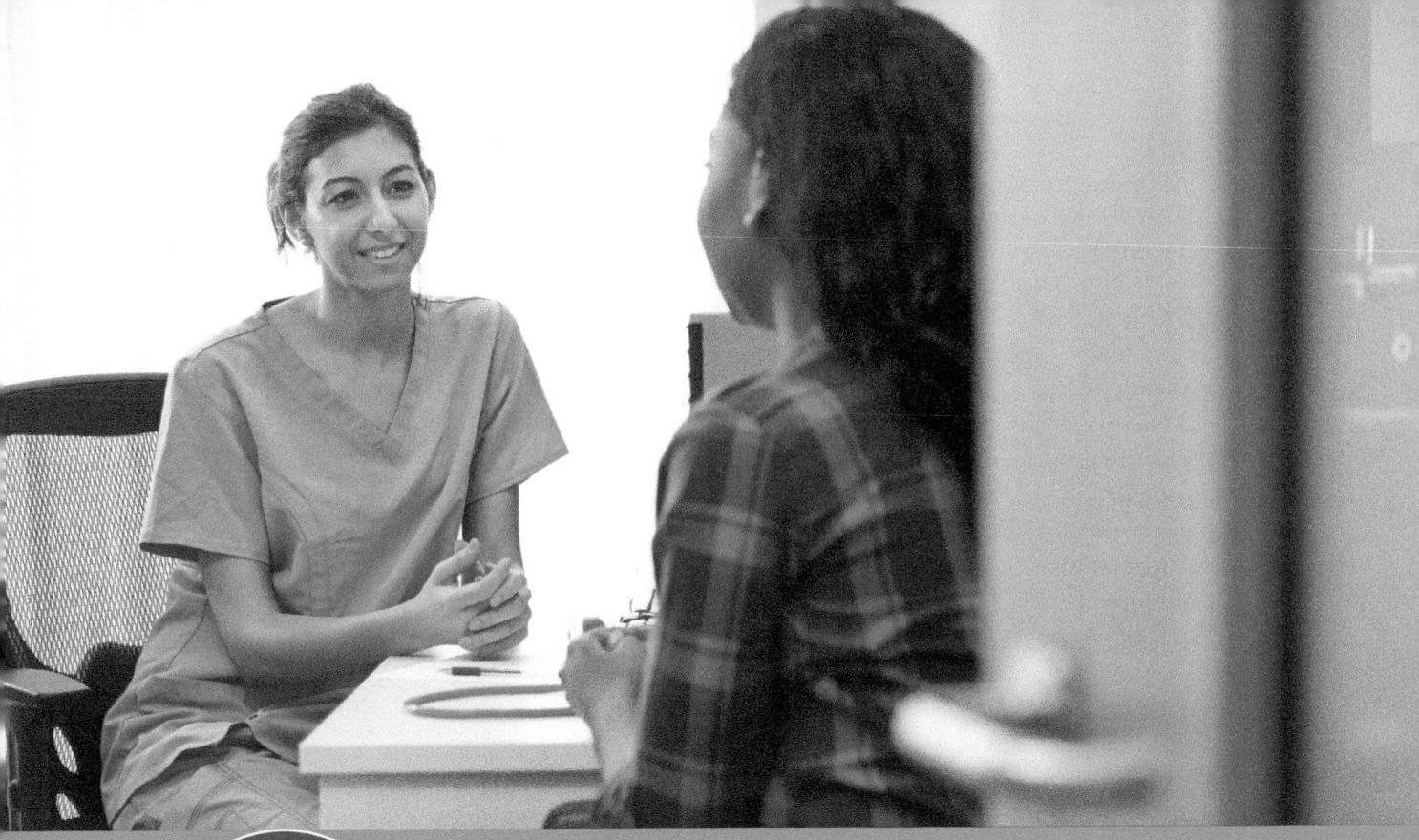

CHAPTER

6

The Office Environment

Learning Objectives

After completing this chapter, you should be able to:

6.1   Define and spell the terms for this chapter.

6.2   Describe Occupational Safety and Health Administration's (OSHA) role in office safety.

6.3   List steps for fire prevention and safety in the ambulatory health care setting.

6.4   Outline the principles for evacuation of an ambulatory health care setting.

6.5   Explain the importance of electrical safety in the ambulatory health care setting.

6.6   Explain the purpose of a safety data sheet (SDS).

6.7   List the steps for the disposal of biological and chemical materials.

6.8   Identify the importance of various safety signs, symbols, and labels.

6.9   Describe the four types of medical waste.

6.10 List safety measures used when responding to an accidental exposure.

6.11 Explain the principles of standard precautions.

6.12 Identify how to select the proper personal protective equipment (PPE) based on expected exposure.

6.13 Differentiate between ergonomics and proper body mechanics.

6.14 Explain the medical assistant's role in a quality assurance program.

Susan Schultz, a medical assistant, prepares a medication for Mrs. Yeung that is to be given by an intramuscular injection technique. She has both safety needles and nonsafety needles at hand for use in this procedure. She has not been told to use only the safety needles and feels more comfortable with the nonsafety style because that is what she was taught in school, so she chooses to use a nonsafety needle. After giving the injection, Susan proceeds to dispose of the needle and syringe in the sharps container. As she places the nonsafety needle on the flip-lid, it begins to slide off. Susan catches it, receiving a needlestick in the process. She continues to put the needle and syringe into the sharps container and finishes attending to the patient.

After dismissing the patient, Susan reports the needlestick to her supervisor, Linda. Linda immediately asks Susan why she chose not to use a safety needle. Susan explains that she did not think she needed to and was not really trained to use them. Linda also asks if the patient is still in the office and how much time has elapsed since the needlestick occurred. Susan tells Linda the patient is no longer in the office and that the needlestick incident occurred approximately 10 minutes ago. Linda immediately asks Cindy, the phlebotomist, to draw several tubes of blood from Susan. Once Cindy is finished drawing Susan's lab specimens, Linda asks Susan to complete an incident report, describing the situation in full. Linda proceeds to call the patient and arrange for Mrs. Yeung to come into the office for lab draws.

Terms to Learn

biohazards

body mechanics

ergonomics

ground fault circuit interrupter (GFCI)

incident report

National Committee for Quality Assurance (NCQA)

Occupational Safety and Health Administration (OSHA)

personal protective equipment (PPE)

quality assurance (QA)

safety data sheet (SDS)

Just as in any workplace, general safety measures, employee safety, housekeeping, proper body mechanics, office security, and measures to ensure a clean, pleasant environment are critical to maintaining the safety and comfort of the medical assistant, the patient, and all employees in the medical office. Additional safety issues may arise in a medical workplace, including biological hazards, blood-borne pathogens, and the handling of drug samples.

GENERAL SAFETY MEASURES

A workplace hazard can be defined as any condition that could affect the health or safety of an employee—either immediately or through long-term exposure. Various federal, state, and local agencies are responsible to enact laws and regulations to protect workers and the public. The **Occupational Safety and Health Administration (OSHA)** is a federal government agency responsible for the safety of all employees of companies operating in the United States. OSHA is concerned with any workplace hazard that may impact the safety of an employee. Other governmental agencies may have standards regarding these factors as well, such as the local fire marshal or local law enforcement agencies. In addition, insurance companies with which the office may contract may have rules and regulations above and beyond these other agencies.

OSHA ensures the safety and health of America's workers by setting and enforcing standards; providing training, outreach, and education; establishing partnerships; and encouraging continual improvement in workplace safety and health. The agency has the authority to inspect a workplace without notification and to levy fines on any deficiencies relating to the health and safety of employees. In addition to the federal agency, each state also has a safety agency that can enact additional safety legislation. State laws can be more strict than federal laws, but if they are more lenient, the federal law still applies.

Many medical offices make the mistake of believing the only OSHA issues they need to be concerned with are the bloodborne pathogens standards. Whereas these regulations are important and will be covered later, many other safety factors fall under the regulations of OSHA.

Matters surrounding workplace hazards are discussed in the material that follows. See Guidelines 6-1 for some general safety measures to adhere to in the office.

Planning for Office Safety

A disaster is any event that can cause injury or damage to a group of people. Disasters that could happen in a medical office or have an effect on the operation of the medical office include fire, flood, tornado, earthquake, hurricane, and explosion. It is important for all employees to be aware of specific plans that have been put in place to protect the safety of the patients as well as the medical office staff. The safety measures discussed in this chapter will provide information on how to evacuate the medical office in the event of a disaster, how to manage fires, as well as dealing with situations that may arise from electrical, mechanical, and chemical accidents. All newly hired employees should be trained in all emergency steps within the first day of employment. This training should be documented in writing to ensure compliance with OSHA regulations. If a particular medical facility has radiation equipment or radioactive materials on site, implementation of further regulations and training regarding safe use and disposal of these items may be required.

Evacuation Plans

A disorganized evacuation can result in confusion, injury, and property damage. Every medical office must have a written evacuation plan that outlines how to safely remove patients and employees from the building during an

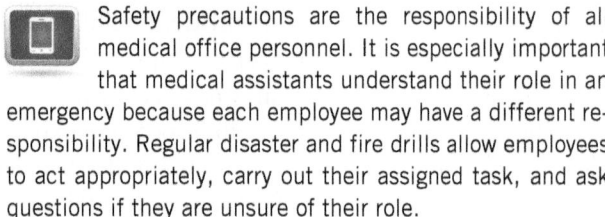

Professionalism   The Workplace

Safety precautions are the responsibility of all medical office personnel. It is especially important that medical assistants understand their role in an emergency because each employee may have a different responsibility. Regular disaster and fire drills allow employees to act appropriately, carry out their assigned task, and ask questions if they are unsure of their role.

Guidelines 6-1

General Safety Measures

- Walk—never run—in a medical office. Even in an emergency situation, move quickly without running.
- Always walk on the right-hand side of the hallway. Wheelchairs and carts bearing patients use the same hallways as do employees and visitors. Some medical facilities position a mirror, on the wall or ceiling, at hallway junctions to prevent collisions.
- Use handrails when on stairways.
- Never carry uncapped syringes with needles or sharp instruments in hallways or between examination rooms.
- Keep floors clear. Immediately wipe up spills or call housekeeping to assist. Never pick up broken glass with bare hands. Follow OSHA standards when cleaning up glass, spilled specimens, and liquids.
- Open doors carefully to avoid injuring anyone on the other side.
- Replace burned-out lightbulbs immediately, especially over exit signs.
- Report all unsafe conditions immediately.
- Wear long hair pulled back and tied to prevent it from coming into contact with hazardous materials or becoming tangled in equipment.
- Wear shoes that cover the entire foot. Open-toe, open-heel, or high-heel shoes are not recommended in the medical office because of the possibility of slipping and injuries.
- Never place food in a refrigerator containing laboratory specimens or refrigerated drugs.
- Do not eat, drink, or smoke in the medical office, except in designated areas.
- Mount file cabinets against a wall to avoid accidental tipping when a heavy top drawer is open.
- Keep floors clean but not so highly polished that they cause slipping. All spills must be cleaned immediately. A hazard sign should always be placed near a wet floor.
- Store all controlled substances (narcotics) in a locked cabinet. A record of all narcotic administration must be maintained according to the Drug Enforcement Administration (DEA) regulations. Any loss of drugs must be reported to the regional office of the DEA immediately. The local police should also be notified.

emergency. During development and implementation of your evacuation plan, think about all possible emergency situations. In some areas of the country these could include hurricanes, whereas in others they could include volcanic eruption. Be sure the plan complies with OSHA's emergency standards. Guidelines 6-2 outlines OSHA's guidelines for developing an evacuation plan.

Evacuation plans must include a floor plan diagram that shows all exits, fire extinguishers, and stairwells, as well as the most direct route out of the building from each area. The floor plan diagrams should be placed in conspicuous areas all around the facility. Figure 6-1 shows an example of a floor plan diagram for evacuation.

Safety Hazards

Medical offices must be prepared for many types of safety hazards. Not only is the safety of employees at stake, as in any business, but the well-being of patients also is of paramount consideration. Common types of hazards include fire, electrical, mechanical, and chemical.

Fire Safety

Fire is one of the most common hazards in any office, including medical offices. Evacuation floor plans, as discussed earlier, should be placed in conspicuous areas all around the facility. They should be large enough to be easily read in dim

light and from a reasonable distance. Before fire drills, it should be determined who will be designated for each area and responsible for ensuring that all patients and staff are able to get out safely.

Portable fire extinguishers should be attached to walls in areas that are no more than 75 feet away from any employee area. Appropriate extinguishers for medical offices are the ABC types, which are capable of putting out many types of fires (Figure 6-2). Each employee should be instructed on the proper use of fire equipment.

Fire extinguishers should be inspected on a regular schedule to ensure effectiveness for use during a fire. A class ABC fire extinguisher is a multiuse device, an all-purpose dry chemical extinguisher that is safe for most fires. Fire extinguishers are classified according to the type of fire they are designed to extinguish:

- Class A—For use on cloth, wood, rubber, paper, and plastic
- Class B—For use on grease, gasoline, or oil-based fires
- Class C—For use on electrical fires caused by appliances, tools, and other equipment that is plugged into an electrical source

When using a fire extinguisher, remember the acronym PASS, which explains how to use a fire extinguisher properly:

- *Pull* the safety pin from the handle of the fire extinguisher.
- *Aim* the extinguisher nozzle at the base of the fire.

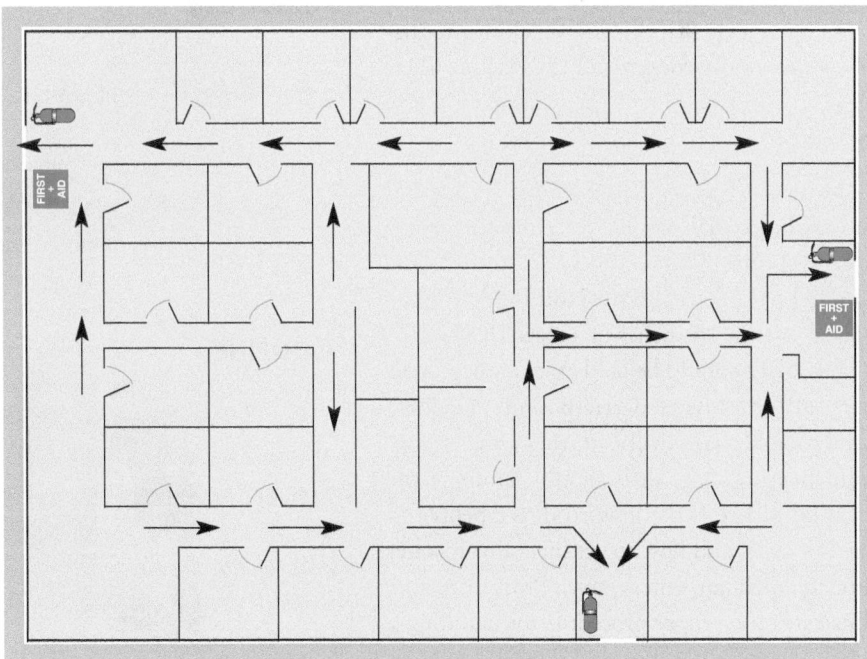

FIGURE 6-1 Example of an evacuation floor plan.

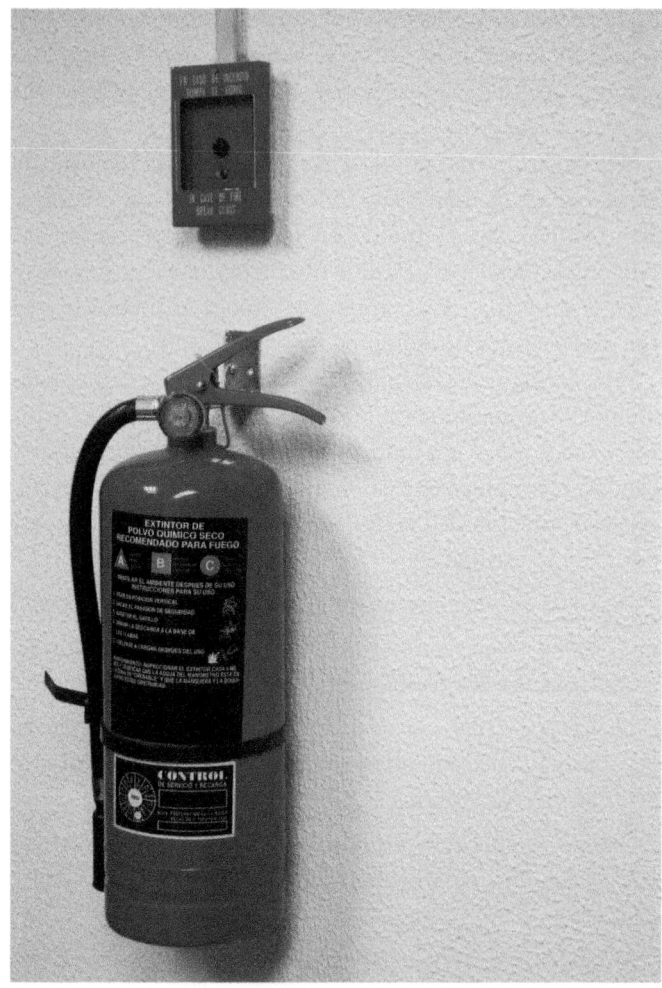

FIGURE 6-2 An ABC fire extinguisher is safe for most fires.

Many offices have adopted the acronym RACE to help employees remember what to do in the case of a fire. RACE stands for:

- *Rescue*
- *Alert*
- *Confine*
- *Extinguish*

Employees should *rescue* other employees and patients from the fire area, *alert* by calling 911, *confine* by closing doors and windows, and *extinguish* the fire. However, do not linger to fight a fire that is not quickly and easily extinguished.

Because of the widespread "No Smoking" policies now in place in medical facilities, cigarettes are not as much of a fire hazard inside the building as they used to be. However, safe disposal systems should be placed outside in designated areas to prevent people from throwing cigarettes into wastebaskets or other trash receptacles.

The following precautions should be in place in the event of a fire:

- Telephone numbers of fire and police departments should be attached to all telephones, including extensions.
- Fire extinguishers should be properly maintained through monthly maintenance checks; the date and initials of the person responsible for testing the equipment should be legible.

- *Squeeze* the handle or lever slowly to discharge the contents of the extinguisher.
- *Sweep* from side to side approximately 6 inches over the fire until it is out.

Most of today's medical offices are located in buildings with smoke detectors and sprinkler systems. Smoke detectors and alarms should be tested regularly. Nothing should be placed within 18 inches of a sprinkler head.

Fire drills should be held at least once a year with all employees participating. An ideal time to hold a fire drill is during a mandatory staff meeting. The drill should reinforce the location of fire exits, how to direct people to the fire exits, and how to act in a calm manner during such an emergency. Procedure 6-1 illustrates the proper procedure for handling a fire in the medical office, and Figure 6-3 shows a basic plan for fire safety.

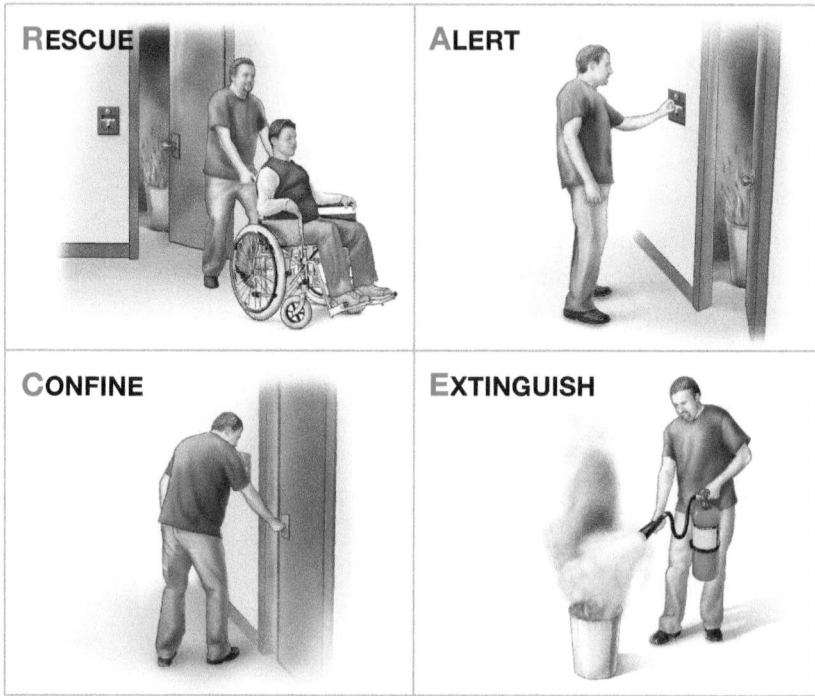

FIGURE 6-3 A fire safety plan like RACE saves lives.

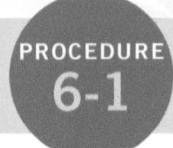

Managing a Fire in the Medical Office

Objective ◆ *Respond to a fire in the medical office.*

EQUIPMENT AND SUPPLIES

Policies and procedures manual; evacuation maps of the office

Note: Planned fire drills should be executed at least annually and preferably more frequently so that all employees know their role and expectations in the event of an actual disaster.

1. As soon as a fire is discovered, **RESCUE** anyone who is in immediate danger from the area of the fire.
2. **ALERT** the staff by activating the established mechanism for signaling fire within the office. This may require pulling the alarm lever or calling a code over the intercom. Call 911 or the local fire department following the same procedure as practiced during fire drills.
3. All staff should calmly and quickly assist in getting all patients out of the office in an orderly manner, following the exit routes on the posted evacuation maps, and using the stairs, if applicable. After each room is evacuated, make sure all doors are closed to **CONFINE** the fire, keeping it from spreading.

4. If the fire is contained, an attempt should be made to **EXTINGUISH** it using the fire extinguisher. However, if the fire is not contained, valuable time should not be spent in attempting to extinguish it. Instead, evacuation should be promptly begun.
5. Use the PASS procedure if it is possible to extinguish the fire:
   - **PULL** the safety pin from the handle of the fire extinguisher.
   - **AIM** the extinguisher nozzle at the base of the fire.
   - **SQUEEZE** the handle or lever slowly to discharge the contents of the extinguisher.
   - **SWEEP** from side to side approximately 6 inches over the fire until it is out.
6. The individual charged with ensuring that all rooms are cleared should quickly go through the office to ensure that no one is left behind.
7. Staff and patients should gather away from the building at the predetermined area.

- Exits and stairways should be clearly marked and free of debris, and a diagram of all exits should be posted near the fire extinguishers.
- File cabinets should be fireproof to protect vital records.

Electrical Safety

Electrical shock is a hazard in the medical office. All equipment should be grounded according to the manufacturer's instructions. Avoid using extension cords, which are both an electrical and a trip-and-fall hazard. No circuit should be overloaded, and surge protectors should be used for all electronic equipment. If surge protectors are not used, a power surge can short-circuit or "fry" the sensitive components of electronic equipment, including computers. You should never plug a surge protector into another surge protector to double the number of outlets.

All electrical cords attached to equipment should be checked regularly for any cracks, loss of insulation, or other problems. Do not use any equipment that has a frayed electrical cord. Always unplug equipment before performing any

maintenance on the device. In wet areas, such as near sinks, a **ground fault circuit interrupter (GFCI)** outlet must be used. GFCIs are designed to protect people from severe or fatal electric shocks. Because a GFCI detects ground faults, it can also prevent some electrical fires and reduce the severity of others by interrupting the flow of electric current. These outlets will break the circuit, or trip, if they become wet, protecting both the user and any plugged-in equipment.

Mechanical Safety

Many pieces of equipment in the medical office can cause harm if they are not used properly. Equipment that could cause harm includes the centrifuge, the autoclave, sterilizers, and oxygen equipment. Always read the entire instruction manual before installing or using any type of equipment. If you have any questions, ask your supervisor for clarification before continuing.

Chemical Hazards

Medical offices may contain chemicals that are hazardous to the human body. Materials may be considered harmful in several ways. **Biohazards** are biological substances, such as medical waste and virus or bacteria samples, that pose a threat to human beings and are potentially infectious. Corrosive materials cause burns, and flammable materials can burst into flames. Toxic materials can cause serious illness or death when there is exposure through skin contact, ingestion, or inhalation.

OSHA has established a Hazard Communication Standard (HCS) that requires employers to disclose toxic and hazardous substances in the workplace. The standard specifies the kind of information the employer must disclose and the manner in which the employer must disclose it. As needed, OSHA issues updated guidelines to reflect current information about toxic and hazardous substances. This information is available under the heading Hazard Communication on the OSHA website: www.osha.gov. The regulations on chemical hazards are available from the U.S. Department of Labor in Washington, DC.

Safety Data Sheets

Under OSHA's HCS, any workplace in which employees may handle a potentially harmful substance must make available to its employees a **safety data sheet (SDS)** for each potentially harmful substance at the workplace containing printed information about that substance. Each SDS—which may also be referred to as a PDS, product data sheet—offers basic information needed to ensure the safety and health of

the user at all stages of manufacture, storage, use, and disposal of a hazardous product. An SDS (or PDS) provides information regarding the hazards of using the product, how to protect yourself from injury by using the appropriate **personal protective equipment (PPE)**—such as gloves, fluid-resistant lab coats, safety glasses, and a surgical mask, face shield, or respirator—and what actions to take if an accidental splash or exposure occurs. SDS's are provided by the chemical manufacturer, distributor, or importer. The information is required to be presented in a consistent, user-friendly, 16-section format (Box 6-1). SDS's must be available to employees and can be kept in a notebook, on a computer, or on a web-based retrieval system. All employees must know where the SDS's are kept and how to access them.

Each office should have an employee who is the designated OSHA compliance officer and is trained and aware of all the required controls for the use and storage of such materials. All employees must have documented annual training regarding OSHA Hazard Communication (HAZCOM).

SAFETY SIGNS, SYMBOLS, AND LABELS

Signs, symbols, and labels are important communication vehicles in the workplace. They notify employees, patients, and the public of potential safety hazards. Warnings should

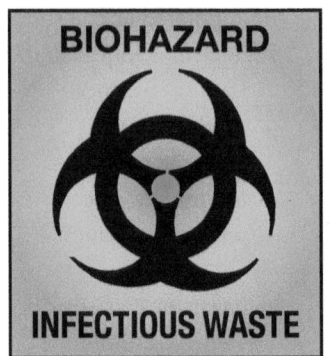

A. Biohazard label

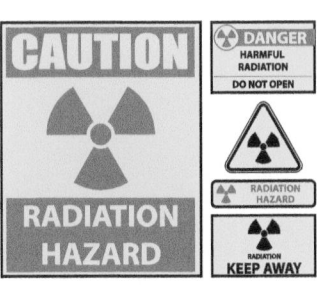

B. Radiation hazard label

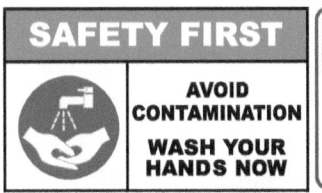
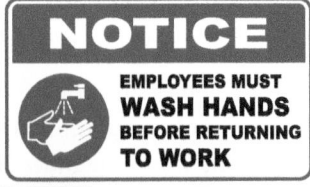

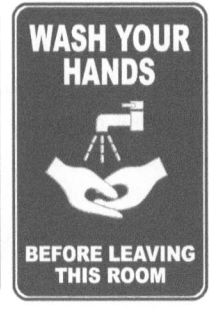
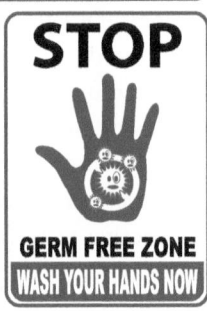

C. Handwashing signs

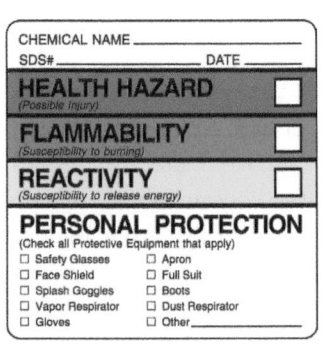

D. Chemical hazard label

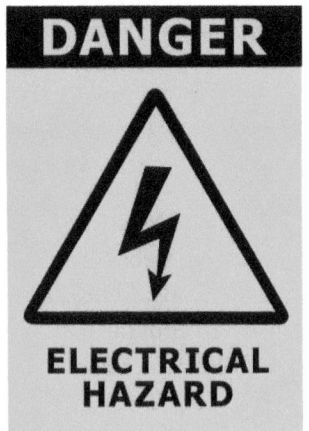

E. Electrical hazard label

F. Fire hazard label

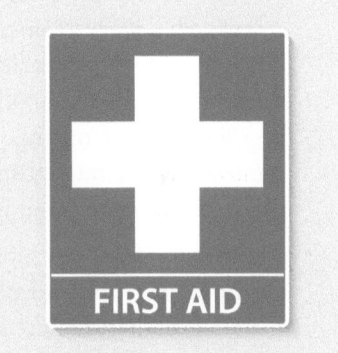

G. First aid sign

FIGURE 6-4 Common warning labels and signs in the medical office.

be placed anywhere a hazard might occur. Informational signs are placed to explain the precautions necessary to avoid a hazard. Warning signs are a reminder of safety precautions and unexpected hazards but are not a substitute for employee training.

Signs are large enough to be recognized from a distance and are usually placed on walls, posts, or equipment. *Labels* are adhesive-backed paper that are intended to be read closer-up and can be affixed to bottles, boxes, or other containers. *Symbols* are graphic images that make it easier to identify the message—a quick glance communicates faster than words and can be understood by those who cannot read English. Commonly used safety warnings appear in Figure 6-4.

Specific color schemes help indicate the type of information the sign or label contains:

- Red signs are prohibitions that warn of an immediate danger, an action that must taken, or an activity to be avoided, for example, a fire hazard.
- Yellow or amber signs warn of precautionary steps that should be taken, for example a biohazard warning.

- Blue signs are mandatory instructions, for example hand washing.
- Green signs promote safety in a positive manner but do not indicate danger, for example, a first aid kit.

Shapes can also be used to communicate the type of information. Discs (circles) provide prohibitions and instructions; triangles are warnings; squares and rectangles are for emergency and informational signs.

Medical assistants should familiarize themselves with these and other safety signs in their workplace. If you see a new or unfamiliar sign, symbol, or label, ask your supervisor to clarify its meaning.

EMPLOYEE SAFETY

Safety is the responsibility of every member of the staff. Whereas it is imperative for the medical office to provide a safe working environment, the staff must also be constantly aware of their surroundings and any possible hazards. Employees must be willing to implement all safeguards to keep themselves and patients safe.

Medical Waste

Hospitals, dental practices, veterinary clinics, laboratories, nursing homes, medical offices, and other health care facilities generate several million tons of hazardous medical waste each year, which includes biological and chemical waste. Biological waste is potentially infectious and includes blood, blood products, body fluids and tissues, cultures, vaccines, sharps, gloves, inoculation loops, and paper contaminated with body fluids. Hazardous chemical waste contains harmful substances, such as germicides, cleaning solvents, and pharmaceuticals. Other types of waste are solid waste and radioactive waste. Medical waste is categorized into four major types:

- **Biological**—Any waste material that has the potential to carry disease. This includes laboratory cultures, blood and blood products from blood banks, operating rooms, emergency rooms, medical and dental offices, autopsy suites, and patient rooms. Infectious waste must be separated from other solid and chemical waste at the point of origin. A licensed medical waste removal agency must dispose of these materials. This is covered in more detail in the following section.

- **Chemical**—Includes substances such as germicides, cleaning solvents, and pharmaceuticals. This waste material can be a causative factor in a fire or an explosion. The safe manner with which to handle and dispose of chemicals is included in the MSDS.

- **Radioactive**—Any waste that contains or is contaminated with liquid or solid radioactive material, such as Iodine 123, Iodine 131, and Thallium 201. Radioactive waste must be clearly labeled as radioactive and must be removed by a licensed disposal agency.

- **Solid**—Waste that does not fall into the previous categories. Solid waste not contaminated with bodily fluid, such as paper gowns, table covers, paper towels, and food, can be generated in many areas of medicine, including patient rooms and surgery suites. Solid waste is not always hazardous but can cause pollution of the environment. Mandatory recycling can reduce the amount of solid waste produced.

Disposal of Medical Waste

OSHA standards require that waste containing contaminated sharps be disposed of in proper containers and identified with biohazard labels, and sharps must be placed in puncture-proof, leak-proof containers. These provisions help protect of employees in medical facilities as well as those who handle the waste downstream.

Medical waste disposal is primarily regulated at the state level, so medical offices must be aware of and follow state and local laws. Most states have regulations covering packaging, storage, and transportation of medical waste. Some states require health care facilities to register and/or obtain a permit. State rules also cover the development of contingency plans, on-site treatment, training, waste tracking, recordkeeping, and reporting.

Written records must be kept of hazardous waste disposed of and should contain the following information:

- Date of treatment
- Amount of waste treated
- Method/conditions of treatment
- Name (printed) and initials of person performing the treatment

OSHA Bloodborne Pathogen Standards and Standard Precautions

Medical offices must follow the OSHA regulations (available from the U.S. Department of Labor in Washington, DC, and on the OSHA website: www.osha.gov) for handling contaminated materials. Offices may opt to contract with a private company to provide assistance in meeting OSHA regulations. OSHA rules and regulations govern all freestanding health care providers and ensure protection from contracting a contagious disease from any body fluids that may be handled by health care workers.

Occupational exposure is defined as a reasonable anticipation that the employee's duties may result in skin, mucous membrane, eye, or parenteral (for example, assisting with procedures involving blood) contact with infectious material. Every employee who has the possibility of occupational exposure to potentially infectious materials must adhere to the OSHA standards. Examples of employees at risk are physicians, nurses, laboratory workers, medical assistants, dental assistants, and, in some cases, housekeeping personnel. The OSHA standards mandate that each at-risk employee must be offered the hepatitis B (HBV) vaccine series within the first 10 days of employment and at the expense of the employer. An employee who refuses the vaccine must sign a waiver declining the vaccine at that time. If an employee later wishes to become vaccinated, the employer must provide the vaccine at that time. OSHA defines the following as body fluids:

- Blood
- Semen
- Amniotic fluid
- Cerebrospinal fluid

- Synovial fluid
- Vaginal secretions
- Pleural fluid
- Pericardial fluid

The best ways to prevent exposure to bloodborne pathogens are wearing PPE, when applicable, and complying strictly with hand hygiene protocol. All PPE must be provided by the employer and readily available for use by the employee. OSHA requires that each medical office have a written Exposure Control Plan to assist in minimizing employee exposure to infectious materials. This plan must be reviewed by all office staff and updated annually. An Exposure Control Plan must include the following:

- **Exposure Determination**—Listing of job classifications within the office to determine at-risk employees (those with potential exposure to infectious materials)
- **Method of Compliance**—Specific measures to reduce the risk of exposure

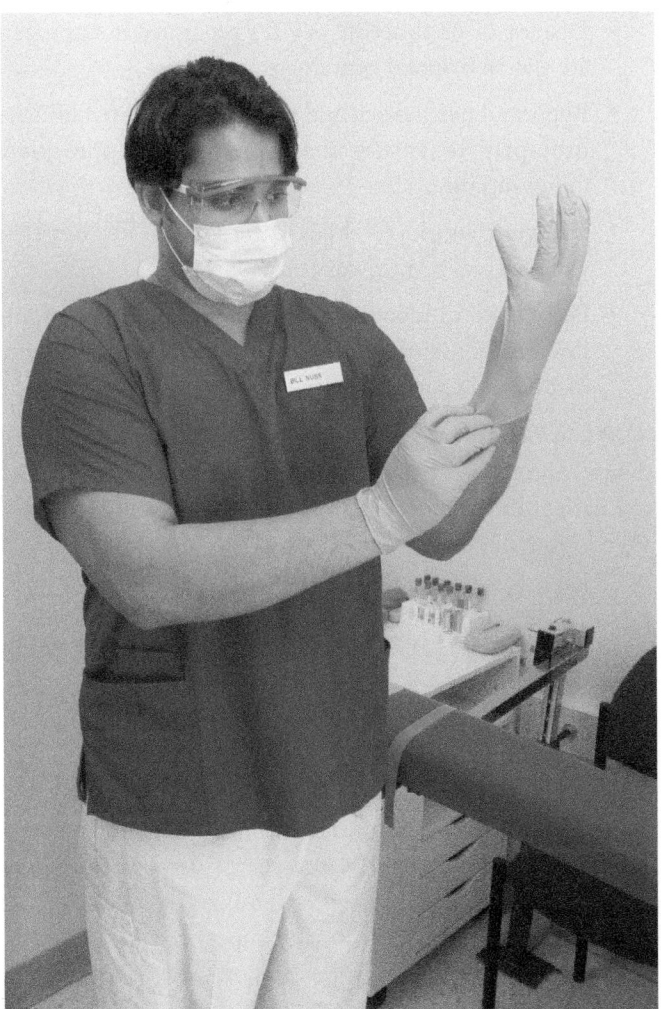

FIGURE 6-5 PPE used to prevent exposure to bloodborne pathogens.

- **Post-Exposure**—Evaluation and follow-up, which specify the steps to follow when an exposure incident occurs

A record for each employee must be kept on file for 30 years after the termination of employment. The record includes documentation of the employee's annual review of the Exposure Control Plan for the facility. In addition, the record must contain information regarding the administration of hepatitis B vaccine series or a waiver signed by the employee within 10 days of initial employment, as well as a copy of any exposure incident reports. These records must be confidential and kept securely under lock and key.

Standard Precautions

The Centers for Disease Control and Prevention (CDC) issued recommendations for protection of health care workers. These became known as the standard precautions. According to standard precautions, all blood and body fluids should be treated as if they are contaminated with any bloodborne pathogen. The most commonly noted diseases related to bloodborne exposure are HIV and HBV. The PPE needed to fulfill the recommendations includes gloves, protective eyewear, masks, and fluid-resistant lab coats. Figure 6-5 shows a medical assistant applying PPE. Table 6-1 describes what

TABLE 6-1	Personal Protective Equipment (PPE) and Clothing	
Clothing and Equipment	**When Used**
Gloves	Anticipate contact with blood, infectious material, open wounds, or broken skin on hands.
	Examples: venipuncture, capillary stick, wound care, injections, minor surgery, cleaning contaminated equipment, such as contaminated surfaces of thermometers
Mask	Anticipate spray with blood or infectious materials. Often used with eye shields.
Eye/Face Shield	Anticipate spray with infectious materials, droplets of blood, or other infectious matter.
	Example: performing blood smear
Gowns, Lab Coats	Anticipate gross contamination of clothing during a procedure.
	Examples: minor surgery, laboratory procedures

protective clothing is appropriate, and Guidelines 6-3 lists details in the use of PPE and clothing.

When selecting the appropriate PPE, keep in mind that some people—medical personnel as well as patients—are highly sensitive to latex used in some disposable gloves. The medical office should keep nonlatex products available for these individuals or simply use nonlatex products exclusively. In addition, the SDS for any given substance will contain information regarding PPE that is necessary for that substance.

Information about standard precautions can be found on the CDC website: www.cdc.gov.

Preventing and Responding to Needlestick Injuries

OSHA estimates 5.6 million workers in the U.S. health care industry are at risk of occupational exposure to bloodborne pathogens via needlestick injuries and other sharps-related injuries. Health care workers who use or may be exposed to needles are at increased risk of needlestick injury. Such injuries can lead to serious or fatal infections with bloodborne pathogens such as hepatitis B virus, hepatitis C virus, or human immunodeficiency virus (HIV). Needlestick injuries can occur before, during, or after performing a procedure involving a needle. The CDC recommends that health care workers can protect themselves from needlestick injuries by following these practices:

- Avoid the use of needles where safe and effective alternatives are available.
- Help your employer select and evaluate devices with safety features.
- Use devices with safety features provided by your employer.
- Avoid recapping needles.
- Plan safe handling and disposal before beginning any procedure using needles.
- Dispose of used needle devices promptly in appropriate sharps disposal containers.
- Report all needlestick and other sharps-related injuries promptly to ensure that you receive appropriate follow-up care.
- Tell your employer about hazards from needles that you observe in your work environment.
- Participate in bloodborne pathogen training, and follow recommended infection prevention practices, including hepatitis B vaccination.

When health care workers experience a needlestick or sharps injury or are exposed to the blood or other body fluid of a patient during the course of work, they should immediately follow these steps:

- Wash needlesticks and cuts with soap and water.
- Flush splashes to the nose, mouth, or skin with water.
- Irrigate eyes with clean water, saline, or sterile irrigants.
- Report the incident to the supervisor.
- Immediately seek medical treatment.

It is especially important that the medical assistant always dispose of needles properly in a sharps disposal container that is puncture-proof, leak-proof, and clearly labelled. If an injury does occur, report it to your supervisor and complete an incident report form. Incident reports are discussed later in this chapter.

Guidelines 6-3

OSHA Guidelines for Using Personal Protective Equipment and Clothing

- The employer must supply the protective clothing and provide cleaning or disposal of it.
- The clothing or other equipment must be strong enough to act as a barrier to infectious materials that might reach the employee's street clothing, work clothing, eyes, mouth, or skin.
- Disposable gloves may not be reused.
- Protective eye equipment must have solid sides to prevent infectious material from entering the eye area from the side.
- All equipment and clothing must be removed and placed in a designated container before leaving the medical office.

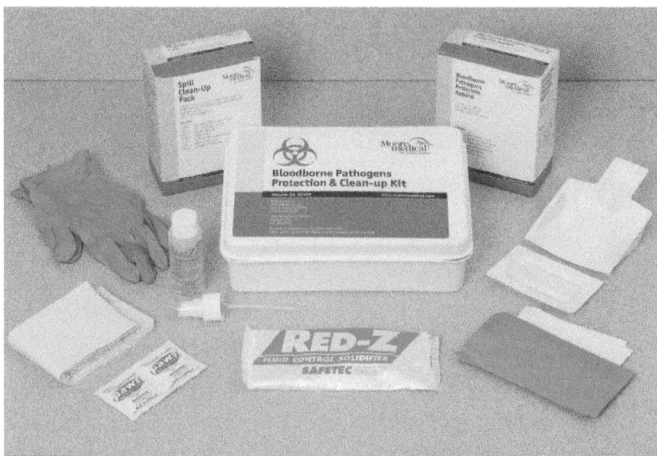

FIGURE 6-6 An example of a commercial spill kit.

Responding to Spills

If infectious material has been spilled, proper procedures must be followed in the cleanup. A spill kit should be used. See Figure 6-6 for an example of a commercial spill kit. Commercial kits are available, but a simple kit can be assembled with the following equipment:

- Plain clay cat litter
- A small dust pan
- A biohazard bag

The cat litter is used as a drying agent to allow sweep-up of the material without spreading it. The material should then be placed in a biohazard bag and disposed of properly with other biohazardous waste.

Most offices contract with outside vendors to pick up, transport, and dispose of biohazardous waste. Typically, the amount paid to the vendor is based on the total weight. From a cost perspective, this is one of the reasons why it is important for waste that is not considered biohazardous to be disposed of in regular trash receptacles. Placing items that have been used but are not soiled, such as used paper gowns or dry exam table paper, in the biohazardous waste container is frowned on.

Responding to Eye Contamination

Eyes can be contaminated as the result of splashes of chemical biological substances. An eyewash station should be available to use in the event that harmful materials enter the eyes, to prevent infection, burns, or damage (Figure 6-7). Most eyewash stations are located close to the laboratory area of the facility or where chemicals are used and may cause contamination of the skin or eyes. The eyewash station should be checked monthly to ensure that it is working

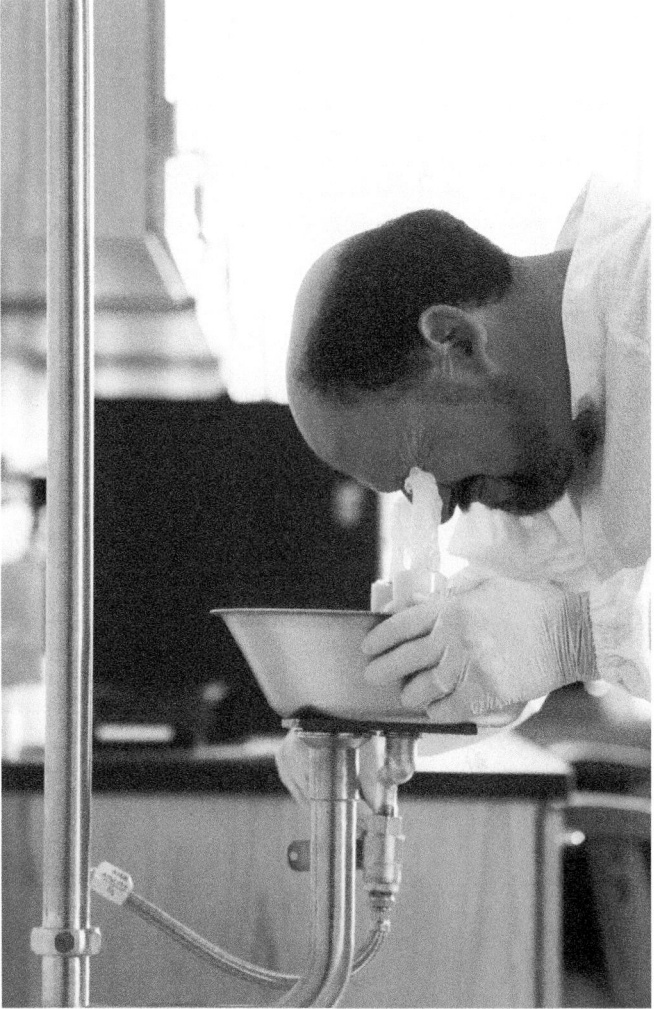

FIGURE 6-7 A commercial eyewash station. In a medical office, the eyewash station is likely to be attached to a sink.

properly. Each eyewash station is accompanied with a set of instructions. Follow the manufacturer's requirements for proper use and maintenance of the device. Procedure 6-2 explains the proper use of an eyewash station.

Housekeeping Safety

All members of the housekeeping department must receive careful instruction regarding OSHA standards. Housekeeping personnel should not empty biohazardous waste and sharps containers; they empty office trash containers only. However, because housekeeping personnel are around potentially infectious materials, they must receive training. If the office contracts with an outside agency for housekeeping duties, the contract should state that all of the agency's employees should be trained in bloodborne pathogen standards and standard precautions. The medical office is then not required to train the personnel.

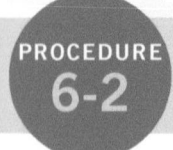

PROCEDURE 6-2

Ensuring Proper Use of an Eyewash Device

Objective ◆ *Use an eyewash station to remove hazardous materials from the eyes.*

EQUIPMENT AND SUPPLIES

Eyewash station attached to a sink faucet; drying towel

1. When an irritant has entered the eye(s), immediately notify a coworker and go to the eyewash station.
2. Remove glasses or contact lenses. *Do not rub the eyes.*
3. Remove the caps or covers from the eyewash device, and start the flow of water.
4. Place head over the stream of water, holding both eyes open. Even if only one eye is affected, both eyes should be washed.

5. For a mild irritation, five minutes of flushing with water should be sufficient. However, if the irritant is a corrosive material, it is recommended to flush for up to 60 minutes to ensure the chemical is thoroughly rinsed from the eyes.
6. Seek medical attention to have the eyes examined.
7. Complete an incident report.

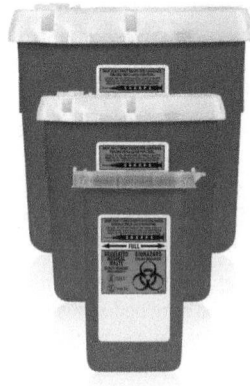

FIGURE 6-8 Examples of waste and hazard containers.

Proper storage of all chemical products is essential for the safety of employees and patients. Figure 6-8 shows examples of waste and hazard containers that may be used, and Procedure 6-3 provides information regarding housekeeping using OSHA guidelines.

PROPER BODY MECHANICS

Medical assistants move, lift, and carry many things, including equipment, supplies, and sometimes even patients. Correct methods of standing and lifting objects help prevent pain and injury. **Body mechanics** is coordination of body

PROCEDURE 6-3

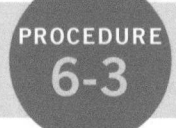

Housekeeping Using OSHA Guidelines

Objective ◆ *Clean and disinfect contaminated surfaces.*

EQUIPMENT AND SUPPLIES

Prepared spill kit; gloves; 1:10 bleach/water solution; dustpan; broom; sharps container; biohazard bag or container

1. Before performing any housekeeping procedures, the employee should ensure the appropriate PPE has been applied (Figure A).

2. For any wet spills, use the prepared spill kit according to package directions.
3. Immediately after exposure to infectious materials, clean and disinfect contaminated surfaces with a 1:10 bleach/water solution. All surfaces must be decontaminated on a regular schedule. This schedule must be posted, signed by

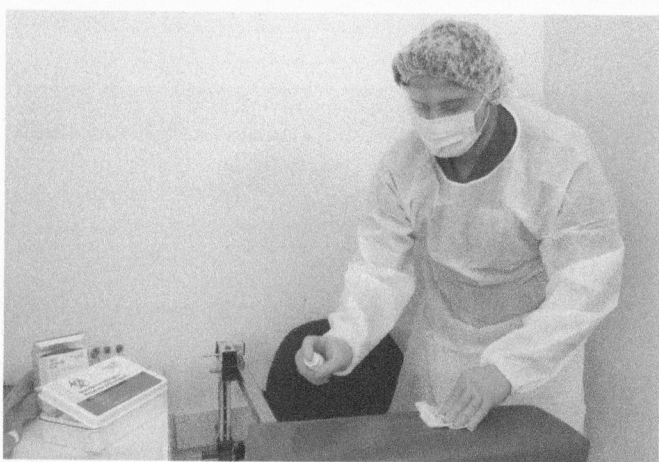

FIGURE A PPE used during spill clean-up.

the person who performs the decontamination, and kept with OSHA records.

4. Properly bag contaminated clothing and laundry in leak-proof, labeled biohazard bags. Contaminated laundry should not be handled or washed at the medical office or with any uncontaminated clothing.

5. Replace a damaged biohazard bag by placing a second bag around the first. Do not remove infectious material from the damaged bag.

6. Biohazardous waste must be removed by a licensed waste disposal service and incinerated or autoclaved before it is placed in a designated landfill area.

7. Use puncture-proof, sealable, biohazard sharps containers for all needles and sharps, such as razors and glass pipettes.

8. Place each sharps container close to the work area, and ensure that each container remains upright.

9. Replace a sharps container when it is two-thirds full.

10. Seal and label each sharps container before placing it with the biohazardous waste for removal by the disposal service.

11. In the event of broken glass, use a dustpan or other mechanical device, such as a hemostat or another type of forceps, to pick it up. Never pick up broken glass with hands.

12. Properly dispose of any PPE used during housekeeping. Failure to do so may result in an OSHA citation.

13. Perform hand hygiene both before and after using gloves.

alignment, balance, and movement. Table 6-2 describes the principles of proper body mechanics and provides a demonstration of proper lifting techniques.

Ergonomics

Ergonomics applies scientific information and data regarding human body mechanics to the design of objects and overall environments for human use. OSHA no longer provides regulations for ergonomics, but it still is an important factor for medical assistants to be aware of. In the medical setting, ergonomics applies to all aspects of the facility. The most common area for problems is the computer workstation. The keyboard should be at elbow height, the monitor at eye level, and the chair adjustable, with a lumbar support. The operator's feet should rest on the floor comfortably, with no strain. A wrist rest and mouse wrist support should be used.

Lighting should be appropriate for the task. Overhead fluorescent lights should not reflect on the computer monitor screens, causing a glare. This can be prevented by adding an antiglare shield to the monitor or tilting the screen so that the light does not hit it directly. Clinical areas should be well lit. Repetitive motions should be limited, and the proper tools should be available for any procedure.

OFFICE SECURITY

Security issues in a physician's office are unique. Medical offices make an attractive target for a thief or addict looking for drugs. Doors and windows must be outfitted with secure locks. Depending on the opening and closing procedures of the office, every employee or designated personnel will have keys to the office. No matter how many keys have been authorized, when a key is reported missing, all locks must be changed.

Many offices have electronic security systems that are activated by the last person who leaves the office and deactivated by the first person who arrives at the office. To activate and deactivate the security system, a predetermined code must be entered into the system. When the first employee enters the building in the morning, an alarm will be activated at the security system company's office if the code is not properly entered within a specified number of seconds. The company will, in turn, alert the appropriate agency, such as fire or police. Depending on the system, an alarm may or may not sound within the building as well.

Security procedures should be implemented during the workday, too, taking into account the need to secure patients and staff, patient medical records, computer stations, medical supplies, and prescription pads from intruders and disorderly persons. The Health Insurance Portability and Accountability Act (HIPAA) has raised awareness of many security issues regarding the privacy of each patient's personal medical history. It is every employee's responsibility to be vigilant when it comes to office security.

If someone is acting suspiciously or demanding money or drugs, it is important to make mental note of such

TABLE 6-2 | Principles of Proper Body Mechanics

Movement	Description
Stoop	• Do not bend from your back. • Stand close to the object you are moving. • Keep your feet 6 to 8 inches apart to create a base of support. • Place one foot slightly ahead of the other. • Bend at the hips and knees, keeping the back straight, and lower the body and hands down to the object (Figure 6-9). • Use the large leg muscles to assist in returning to a standing position (Figure 6-10).
Lift firmly and smoothly	• If you think you cannot move a heavy or awkward load, get help. • Grasp the load by using the large leg muscles. • Keep the load close to the body.
Use the center of gravity for carrying a load	• Keep your back as straight as possible. (Hint: You should not be able to feel your clothing touch your back if you are standing straight.) • Keep the weight of the load close to your body and centered over the hips. • Put the load down by bending at the hips and knees. • When two or more people carry the load, have one person give the commands to lift or move the object.
Pull or push (rather than lift or load)	• Remain close to the object you are moving. • Keep feet apart with one slightly forward. • Have a firm grasp on the object. • If the object is on the floor, crouch down with feet apart. • Bend your elbows, and place hands on the load at chest level. • Keep your back straight. • Push up with your legs in order to stand up with the load.
Avoid reaching	• Evaluate the distance before reaching too far for an object. • Stand close to the object. • Do not reach to the point of straining. • To change direction, point your feet in the direction you wish to go. • Keep the object close to your body as you lower it.
Avoid twisting	• Do not twist your body.

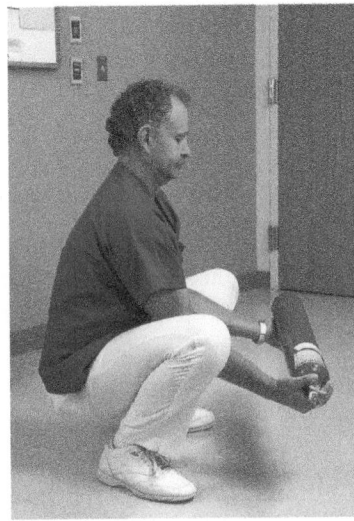

FIGURE 6-9 Correct position when lifting a heavy object off the floor.

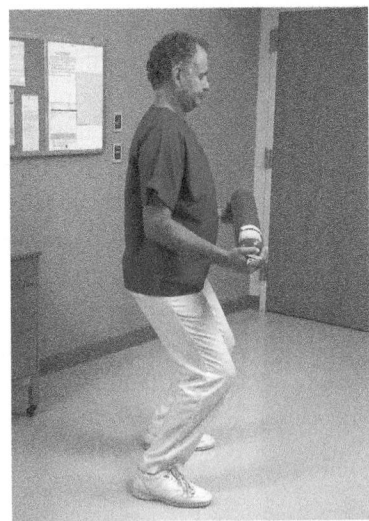

FIGURE 6-10 Use strong leg muscles, keeping back straight, when lifting.

identifying characteristics as the individual's height, weight, facial hair, race, accent, tattoos, and scars. If possible, record this information so you will not be relying solely on memory if you are asked to describe the individual. Immediately report any suspicious concerns to the physician or office manager.

INCIDENT REPORTS

Any unusual occurrence, medical error, or accident is referred to as an incident in the medical setting. A medical error is a preventable negative effect of care, even if it is evident or harmful to the patient. Medical errors include an inaccurate or incomplete diagnosis or improper treatment of a disease, injury, or condition. Following are some examples of accidents, medical errors, and unusual occurrences:

Accidents

- A patient falls on a wet floor.
- A medical assistant receives a needlestick from a contaminated needle.
- A chemical substance is spilled on the floor.

Medical errors

- A housekeeping employee is stuck by a needle (improperly disposed of) while emptying the trash.
- A patient is given the wrong medication.
- Surgery is performed on the wrong site.

Unusual occurrences

- A patient misplaces or loses personal property, such as a hearing aid or eyeglasses, while in the office.
- A prescription pad is missing.
- Syringes or needles are found to be missing from the supply cabinet.
- An employee's purse or wallet is missing.
- A patient is abusive and uses vulgar language.

Whenever any accident, injury, medical error, or unusual occurrence takes place, the employee should immediately notify the supervisor. This is especially important if a needlestick accident or medical error is involved. Time is of the essence to prevent further harm to the patient or, in the case of needlesticks, when drawing blood specimens for baseline testing. The supervisor also will require the employee to immediately complete a written report. This is called the **incident report** and should be completed in black ink or using a computer-based form. An incident report establishes the facts of the event as soon as possible after occurrence and can protect both the employer and the medical assistant against possible lawsuits. Some incidents should also be reported to either the police or to the liability insurance carrier. For example, stolen property should be reported to the police, and a slip and fall should be reported to the insurance carrier. The incident should be described as simply as possible, stating only facts and not opinions. Keep in mind that the incident report may be used as a legal document; thus, only objective information should be included, such as "Patient fell while getting onto exam table." Do not include subjective comments, such as "Patient was not paying attention to what she was doing."

Medical offices should have their own customized forms including incident reports, which should include the following information:

- Names of all persons involved
- Date and time of the incident
- Exact location of the incident (including the address of the medical facility and the location of the incident within the facility)
- Name of the person to whom the incident is reported
- Time of the report
- Brief description of what happened
- Names of all witnesses
- Name and description of any equipment involved in the incident
- Action taken at the time of the incident
- Action taken to prevent a recurrence
- Signature and title of the person completing the report

The incident report, like all other information relating to the patient, is subject to subpoena in litigation (lawsuits). A copy of the incident report should be placed in a master incident report file, the patient's file (if the incident involved a patient), and the employee's file. Figure 6-11 is an example of a paper-based incident report form. In many offices, incident reports can also be completed on the computer (Figure 6-12). Procedure 6-4 explains how to complete an incident report.

Professionalism

Maintaining a professional demeanor in the medical office can prevent many incidents from occurring. Wearing the appropriate apparel and shoes, avoiding excessive jewelry, and pulling back long hair can eliminate hazards that might result in injuries.

INCIDENT REPORT

Name of injured party _____ Date _____

Address _____ Telephone _____

_____

The injured party was: ☐ Employee ☐ Patient ☐ Other _____

Date of accident/incident _____ Time of incident _____

Where did incident occur? _____

Names of witnesses (include titles):

_____ _____

_____ _____

What first aid/treatment was given at the time of the incident?

_____

_____

Who administered first aid? _____

Briefly describe the incident. _____

_____

_____

_____

_____

Names of employees present at time of incident/injury:

_____

What, in your opinion, caused the accident? _____

Follow-up: What steps have been taken to prevent a similar accident? _____

_____

_____

Date _____   Employee's signature _____

Date _____   Supervisor's signature _____

FIGURE 6-11 An example of a typical incident report.

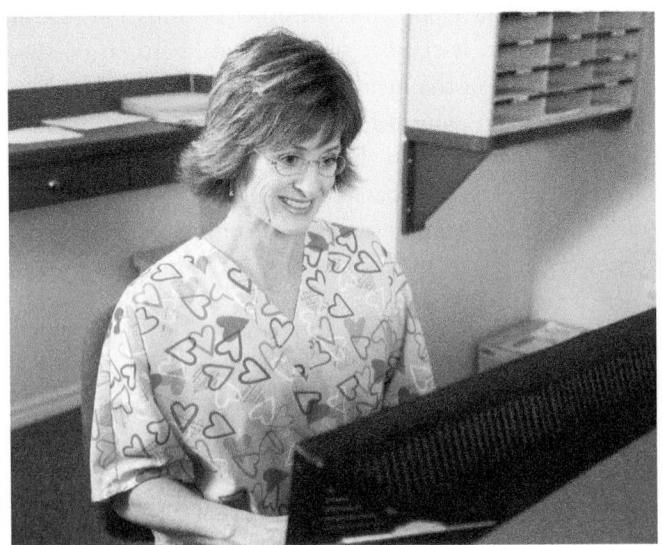

FIGURE 6-12 Incident reports can be completed using the computer in some medical offices.

QUALITY MEDICAL CARE

Quality medical care is an expectation of all patients and requires that the health care team use procedures and techniques that result in the best possible outcome for the patient. In addition, patients must be satisfied with the care and treatment they receive from everyone in the office. Keep in mind that satisfaction does not promise a cure.

The major parameters or attributes of health care that are regularly examined include treatment, outcome, cost/benefit, accessibility, and delivery location. The outcome factor actually requires a measurable change in the health status of the patient that is a direct result of the care received. Cost/benefit refers to the expenditure or cost in terms of time, money, and effort, along with the relationship of this cost to the actual benefit the patient receives. Accessibility to health care refers to the effort a patient must make to receive health care. The American Medical Association (AMA) has defined eight essential elements of quality care (Box 6-2).

QUALITY ASSURANCE

In the early 1960s, the health care industry began to feel an increasing demand from the public for accountability regarding quality care. From that initial swell of public pressure developed a continuing effort on the part of health care providers to deliver satisfactory, achievable excellence in care. **Quality assurance (QA)** is the process of gathering and evaluating information about the services provided (as well as the results achieved) and comparing this information with an accepted standard typically referred to as a benchmark. Benchmarks may apply at a local, state, or national standard level.

Quality assessment measures consist of formal, systematic evaluations of overall patterns of care. The goal of the actual programs and activities of quality assurance have a desired degree of care in a health care setting. The results of the evaluations are then compared with standard results. As deficiencies are identified, recommendations for improvement in care are made. Quality improvement programs (QIPs) use the data gathered by quality assurance and assessment to make quality improvements in health care.

Formal Quality Assurance Programs

A quality assurance program (QAP) in a hospital, ambulatory health care setting, long-term-care facility, or health

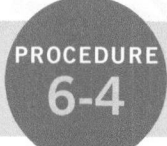

Completing an Incident Report

Objective ◆ *Complete an incident report related to an error in patient care.*

EQUIPMENT AND SUPPLIES

Pen; patient's medical record; computer; incident report, either paper or electronic version

METHOD

1. Upon learning of an error in patient care, immediately inform the physician.
2. Remain calm and professional while explaining the circumstances surrounding the incident.
3. Ask the physician what steps must be taken to rectify or reverse any potential adverse reactions because of the error in patient care. Complete the steps as directed by the physician.
4. Document the error in the patient's medical record. Include information regarding the conversation with the physician and steps taken to rectify the situation, as well as other supporting information.
5. Complete the preliminary information on the incident report. Fill out the following information, which can be found in the patient's medical record: patient's full name, address, and telephone number. Document the date and time that the incident occurred, and indicate where the incident took place.
6. Complete the essential information on the incident report. Carefully document any witnesses to the event, any first aid or treatment that was given to combat reverse

reactions, and who provided the first aid or treatment. Briefly but succinctly describe the incident that occurred, and identify any witnesses. Identify why you think the incident happened. Include follow-up care that may be required, as indicated by the physician.
7. Sign and date the incident report.
8. Have your supervisor sign and date the incident report.
9. In the patient's medical record, document that an incident report was completed.
10. File the incident report in the correct area, as designated by the medical office.

CHARTING EXAMPLE

9/15/20xx. At 8:15 A.M., the patient was accidentally given a pneumonia vaccine rather than the influenza vaccine that was ordered by the physician. I immediately informed Dr. Babcock of the error. Dr. Babcock reviewed the patient's chart and found the patient hadn't had a pneumonia vaccine in three years and that the accidental administration would not be harmful to her health. Both Dr. Babcock and I explained the situation to the patient, who was still in the office. She was irritated but was not extremely upset. She was late for meeting at work so she chose to return to the office next week for her influenza vaccine. An incident report was completed and filed according to office policy. K. Taylor, RMA (AMT)

BOX 6-2 | The AMA's Eight Essentials of Quality Care

- Bring about the optimal improvement in the patient's condition within the earliest time frame possible based on the patient's comfort and physical condition.
- Have an emphasis on early detection and treatment as well as health promotion and disease prevention.
- Receive treatment in a timely fashion without unnecessary delay, termination, interruption, or prolongation.
- Encourage the patient's participation in the decision process regarding treatment.

- Base the treatment on skillful use of technology and the health professional's use of accepted principles of medical science.
- Demonstrate concern for the patient and the patient's family, with sensitivity to the stress caused by illness.
- Achieve the treatment goal through the wise use of technology and other resources.
- Provide adequate documentation in the patient's medical record to facilitate peer evaluation and continuity of care.

maintenance organization (HMO) consists of a system for reviewing records maintained by staff. These records may consist of medical or nursing records, data regarding days of hospitalization or treatment, progress reports, and other statistics that provide a firm indication of the care received by patients. A quality assurance program must include evaluation and educational components to identify and correct problems. Quality assurance programs such as these are required in order for the facility to receive funding by the Public Health Service Act (which defines the requirements) as well as to achieve and maintain accreditation. The basic components of a quality assurance program include the following:

- Establish a QA committee. Representatives from the entire patient care team (such as physician, nurse, and medical assistant) should be part of a QA committee (Figure 6-13).
- Review all clinical and administrative services and procedures. Committee members or an assigned individual can conduct the review. All team members should have a role in the QA process, from designing the QA forms to selecting issues for review. Policies and procedures manuals are also subject to review during this process.
- Set up a structure for identifying items to review. Pay particular attention to problem issues.
- Quantify all issues, for example:
  - Average length of waiting time in minutes to see the physician
  - Number of errors in writing items on patient records
  - Number of insurance claims disallowed per 100 filed
  - Number of failed venipunctures per 50 attempts

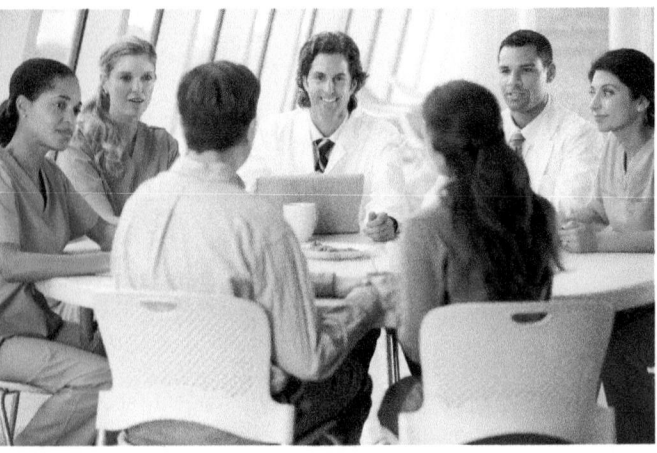

FIGURE 6-13 A quality assurance (QA) committee meeting.

- Limit the number of issues. Set a limit to the number of issues or problems reviewed at any one session. Place emphasis on taking corrective measures.
- Maintain careful records. Review all records, such as incident reports and committee records, and progress or improvement with the entire medical team.

Box 6-3 lists examples of issues that a QA committee might review in a physician's office.

Implementing a Quality Assurance Program

The ultimate goal of a formal QAP is to improve the quality of care so that there is no difference between what should be done and what is being done. Professionals in the field who are experts in a particular health care area develop these norms or standards.

Implementing a QAP requires the development of patient-centered criteria based on acceptable standards of care. Criteria are standards used to compare something in order to make a decision. For example, years ago some

---

BOX 6-3 | Issues Reviewed by a Quality Assurance Committee in a Physician's Office

- Disallowed insurance claims
- Errors in dispensing medications (use incident reports)
- Errors in labeling of laboratory specimens
- Incorrect coding of diagnosis for insurance claims
- Long waiting time for patients
- Adverse reactions to treatments and/or medications (use incident reports)
- Inability to obtain venous blood on the first attempt
- Patient satisfaction (from survey or questionnaire results)
- Patients who leave the office without seeing the physician
- Patient complaints relating to confidentiality (maintain HIPAA compliance)
- Appearance of the office

- Handicapped accommodations including parking availability
- Safety
- Provider availability
- Emergency preparations
- Treatment areas
- Safety and monitoring practices for radiology and laboratory
- Medications
- Infection control
- Patient education/rights
- Medical records
- Collection procedures
- Telephone and reception behaviors

Remember when dealing with older adult patients that they may have balance problems or gait disabilities that make them more prone to falls. Consider this when preparing the waiting room and the examination rooms. Avoid throw rugs, extension cords, or anything that may be a trip-and-fall hazard.

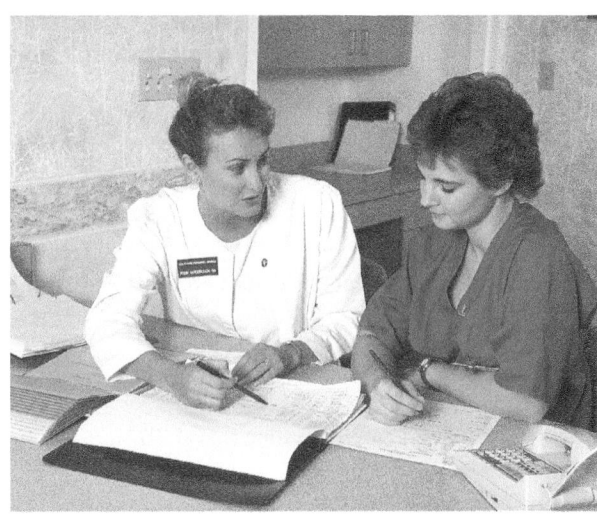

FIGURE 6-14 A medical assistant at a quality assurance (QA) meeting.

patients were discharged from a hospital without being given any formal information or education about what to do when they returned home. Now all hospitalized patients should receive instructions at discharge regarding medications, diet, activity, and follow-up appointments with the physician. This discharge plan is explained to the patient, who then signs the plan and keeps a copy. A copy of the signed plan is also put in the patient's chart, indicating that this instruction took place. A QAP would monitor the discharge planning process. If, for some reason, the discharge plan was overlooked and not provided for the patient, that particular patient would "fall out" in that performance measure and be counted against the facility in the overall percentage.

Medical Assistant's Role in a QAP

The medical assistant is trained in clinical and administrative skills with the expectation for the highest level of performance. To assist the physician-employer, the medical assistant should pay rigorous attention to the quality of care given to patients. Patient satisfaction is a key element in quality of care. The medical assistant may be the first and last person to respond to a patient's complaint or discomfort. Medical assistants have the opportunity to present patients' concerns or complaints at a team QA meeting so that corrective measures can be taken (Figure 6-14). Some of the areas in which the medical assistant may assist the physician with quality assurance are noted in Box 6-4.

Health Plan Employer Data and Information Set

Under Health Plan Employer Data and Information Set (HEDIS), managed care plans that serve Medicare patients must collect data relating to eight categories of performance:

- Effectiveness of care
- Access to and availability of care
- Member satisfaction
- Informed health care choices
- Health plan descriptive information
- Cost of care
- Health plan stability
- Use of service

Medicare, HMOs, and other plans seeking accreditation from the **National Committee for Quality Assurance (NCQA)** must also report data. The NCQA evaluates the quality of health plans in order to help consumers and employers make more informed decisions about their health care. Eventually, most of the health plans (HMOs and preferred provider organizations {PPOs}) with which

---

BOX 6-4 | The Medical Assistant's Role in Quality Assurance

- Resolve patient complaints about items such as billing questions and long waiting times in the reception room.
- Perform patient education regarding diet, laboratory and procedure instructions, and personal care.
- Perform telephone follow-up regarding a patient's condition and progress.

- Double-check laboratory tests performed in the office.
- Verify the results of laboratory tests given over the telephone. Always ask the laboratory to repeat any results that are abnormal or unclear. Request to have a written report sent by mail or fax.
- Bring patient complaints to the attention of the physician.

TABLE 6-3 | Clinical Laboratory Improvement Amendment (CLIA)

Category	Explanation
Waived—Simple Testing (Level I)	Incorrect test results pose little risk for the patient.
	Laboratory is subject to random inspectors only.
	Some physicians' laboratories fall in this category.
Moderately Complex—Intermediate-Level Testing (Level II)	Poses risk to patient if there is an incorrect test result.
	Must be certified by approved accrediting agency.
	Must be staffed by credentialed personnel.
	Must meet quality assurance standards.
Highly Complex—Complex Testing (Level III)	Poses high risk to patient if there is an incorrect test result.
	Must be certified by approved accrediting agency.
	Must be staffed by credentialed personnel.
	Must meet quality assurance standards.

a physician contracts with will be collecting data for the medical practice.

Clinical Laboratory Improvement Amendment

The federal government requires that all clinical laboratories that test human specimens must be controlled. The Clinical Laboratories Improvement Amendment of 1988 (CLIA 1988) divides laboratories into three categories. Laboratory tests are categorized using criteria based on:

- Knowledge necessary to run the test
- Training and experience necessary to perform the test
- Reagents used and preparation of the materials for testing
- Operational steps required to perform the test
- Calibration of equipment, quality control, and proficiency testing requirements

The laboratory categories and criteria are described in Table 6-3.

The Joint Commission

The Joint Commission (TJC), formerly known as the Joint Commission on Accreditation of Health Organizations, headquartered in Chicago, Illinois, is a private, nongovernmental agency that establishes guidelines for hospitals and health care agencies to follow regarding quality of care. It is supported by representatives of the American Hospital Association (AHA), American College of Surgeons, American College of Physicians, and American Dental Association. In addition to forming guidelines for the operation of health care institutions, such as hospitals, ambulatory care facilities, and long-term care institutions,

The Joint Commission conducts surveys and accreditation programs.

The Joint Commission inspectors visit health care facilities and review patient medical records, medical staff organizations, and the general operations of the facility. Some survey and accreditation process indicators are mortality rate (the number of deaths in a given population), frequency of medical complications, nosocomial (hospital acquired) infection rate, and autopsy rate. Based on their assessment, the inspectors issue either a full or a provisional accreditation report. The Joint Commission works with facilities to correct any deficiencies within a specified time frame.

The Joint Commission does not actually have authority or power to take punitive action against a physician or facility for poor treatment. However, the survey results of The Joint Commission are used by other agencies that do have the authority to impose a sanction or penalty, such as the U.S. Department of Health and Human Services.

SUMMARY

Safety measures are an important aspect of the medical office for keeping patients and employees safe. These safety measures include general safety, employee safety, emergency plans (such as for fire, tornado, hurricane, etc.), and the handling of biological hazards and bloodborne pathogens. Proper housekeeping procedures using OSHA guidelines, proper body mechanics, and office security are essential to maintaining a safe and pleasant workplace. The efforts of a medical assistant can be critical in ensuring that all these components are carefully regarded.

6 CHAPTER REVIEW

COMPETENCY REVIEW

1. Define and spell the terms for this chapter.
2. List six safety rules to follow in medical offices.
3. You have been asked to draft the OSHA Exposure Control Plan for your office. What three points must you include in this plan?

PREPARING FOR THE CERTIFICATION EXAM

1. What acronym is frequently used in the event of a fire in the office?
   a. CLIA
   b. RACE
   c. PPE
   d. GFCI
   e. HAZCOM

2. All of the following are safety measures *except*
   a. always walk on the left side of the hallway.
   b. never carry uncapped syringes between exam rooms.
   c. open-toe and open-heel shoes are not recommended in the medical office.
   d. no eating or drinking in the medical office except in designated areas.
   e. floors should be clean but not highly polished.

3. Which of the following is typically used in wet areas such as near sinks?
   a. PASS
   b. RACE
   c. PPE
   d. GFCI
   e. HAZCOM

4. All of the following should be in place in the event of a fire *except*
   a. fireproof file cabinets.
   b. exits clearly marked.
   c. diagram of all exits posted near fire extinguishers.
   d. fire extinguishers that have been maintained with annual maintenance checks.
   e. telephone numbers of fire and police departments.

5. All of the following are examples of PPE *except*
   a. goggles.
   b. respirator.
   c. protective gloves.
   d. absorbent lab coat.
   e. surgical mask.

6. All of the following are major types of medical waste *except*
   a. solid.
   b. infectious.
   c. chemical.
   d. radioactive.
   e. biohazardous.

7. Fire extinguishers should be attached to the wall no more than
   a. 70 feet from an employee area.
   b. 75 feet from an employee area.
   c. 70 feet from an examination room.
   d. 75 feet from an examination room.
   e. 75 feet from the reception area.

8. The governmental agency responsible for the safety of all employees operating in the United States is
   a. PASS.
   b. CLIA.
   c. OSHA.
   d. HIPAA.
   e. OIG.

9. All of the following are considered sources of potential infectious material *except*
   a. sweat.
   b. semen.
   c. cerebrospinal fluid.
   d. amniotic fluid.
   e. pericardial fluid.

10. To help prevent an accidental needlestick, the sharps container should be replaced when it is
    a. half full.
    b. two-thirds full.
    c. three-quarters full.
    d. three-fifths full.
    e. completely full.

CRITICAL THINKING

Refer to the case study at the beginning of the chapter and use what you have learned to answer the following questions.

1. What errors did Susan make in preparing the injection?
2. What tests must be performed as a result of this needlestick?
3. Is Linda responsible for anything in this situation?
4. How would this pertain to OSHA's Bloodborne Pathogens Standards?

ON THE JOB

Bonnie feels that the office is always too cold, so she keeps a heater under her desk. To use the heater, she must run an extension cord across to another electrical outlet. Several times, the safety officer in the practice asks her to discontinue using the heater. Bonnie puts the heater away for a couple of days, then brings it back out when she feels it will not be noticed. The safety officer comes by one day and confiscates the heater and extension cord. Bonnie feels that this is unfair because she is cold during the day. She thinks she should be allowed to use the heater, which allows her to perform her duties in comfort and more efficiently.

1. What OSHA violations are of concern in this situation?
2. Did the safety officer handle the situation correctly the first few times?
3. Did the safety officer have the right to confiscate the heater and extension cord?
4. How might the situation be rectified to make Bonnie comfortable?

INTERNET ACTIVITY

Search the Internet to find private companies that are in business to provide services to help prepare an office to meet OSHA requirements.

Search the Internet to locate medical laboratory exams that are classified under the waived tests according to CLIA standards.

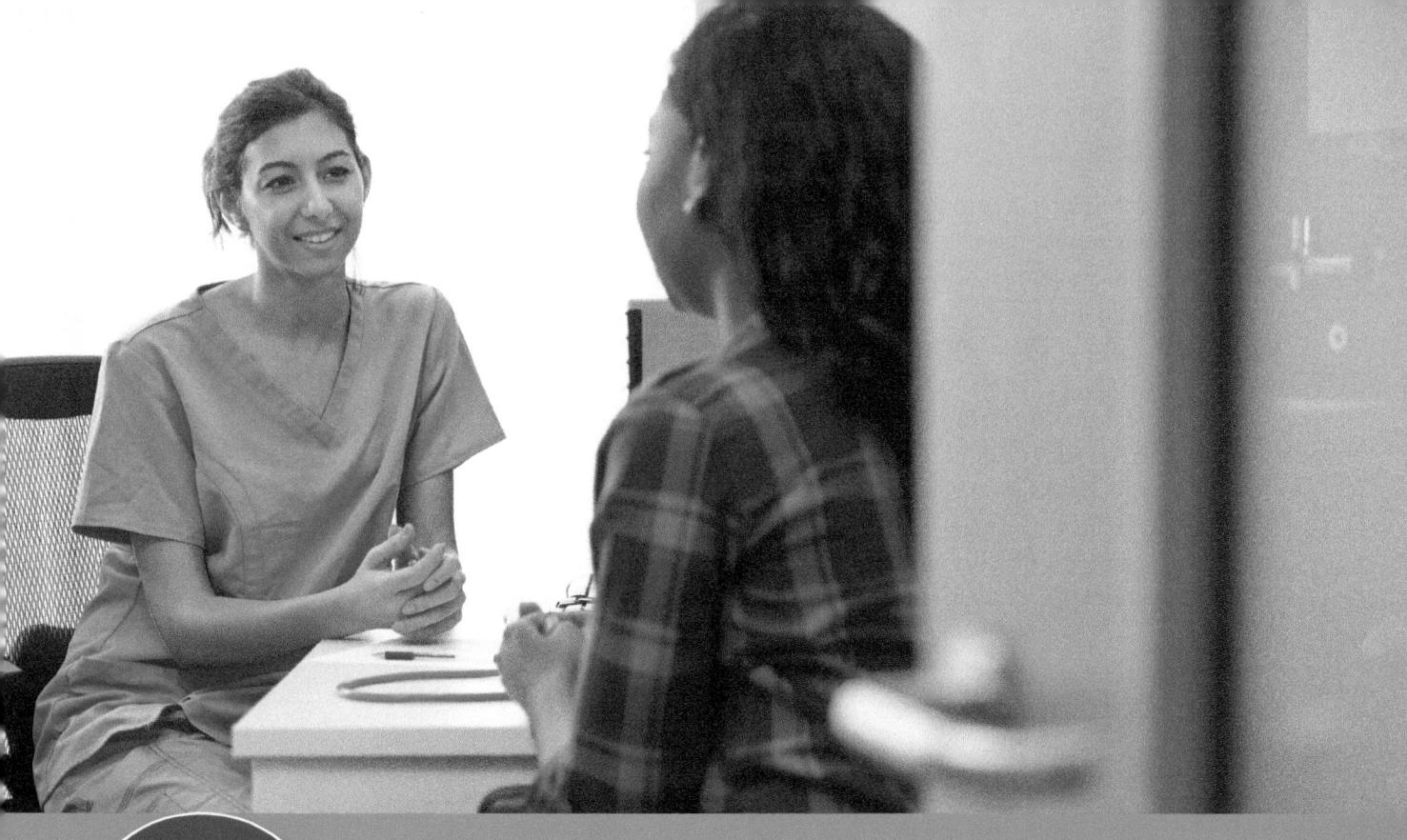

Learning Objectives

After completing this chapter, you should be able to:

7.1   Define and spell the terms for this chapter.

7.2   List proper telephone techniques when answering the telephone in the health care setting.

7.3   Identify guidelines to follow when placing callers on hold.

7.4   List the steps of taking a detailed telephone message.

7.5   Outline HIPAA guidelines regarding patient privacy when making phone calls.

7.6   Explain how to handle various types of telephone calls that are common in a health care setting.

7.7   Identify information needed when handling phone calls related to patient prescriptions.

7.8   Describe the medical assistant's role in telephone triage.

7.9   Explain how to deal with a difficult caller.

7.10 Describe special considerations when placing conference calls.

Carmine DiStefano has been looking for a new physician. He decides to try Pearson Physicians Group because the practice is near his office. When Carmine calls the office to set up an appointment, he is first greeted by an answering system. After he has been given many options, he decides to press "2" to schedule an appointment. Carmine then waits as the system transfers him to the appropriate person. When the transfer is done, he is greeted by Tonya Michaels, a new medical assistant with the practice. Tonya greets Carmine by saying, "Good afternoon. Pearson Physicians Group. This is Tonya. How may I help you?" Although Carmine is left with a cold feeling because he detects an insincere tone in Tonya's voice, he decides to go ahead and schedule an appointment. Tonya then tells Carmine to hold. When she finally returns after more than two minutes, Tonya does not give Carmine a reason for the wait—nor does she offer an apology. Carmine feels annoyed and frustrated and informs Tonya that he will seek services from another physician.

Terms to Learn

answering service	conference call	queue
automated assistance program	enunciation	referral
caller ID	inflection	telephone triage
clarity	pitch	voice messaging system

The telephone is one of the most vital tools used within the medical office. In addition, both the person answering the telephone and the communication used can "make or break" the practice. We have all been at the receiving end of poor telephone etiquette at one point or another. The key within the medical office is to ensure that every telephone encounter is not only courteous but also efficient, accurate, and professional. Many times the patient's first impression of the office is based on the initial interaction with the individual who answers the telephone. Attention to detail is required when answering the telephone, especially when taking important messages or requests for prescription refills.

TELEPHONE TECHNIQUES

If you work in the front office area, much of your day will be spent on the telephone. A fundamental rule to remember when answering your medical office's telephone is that you are in a professional setting and not simply answering the telephone as you would at home. When talking on the phone at home, the conversation is generally more informal and chatty than the style of conversation that is expected in a medical office. It is inappropriate to answer the office line with personal greetings, such as "Hi" or even "Hello." Most offices will provide a script for you to follow when answering the telephone. A pleasant but professional persona and voice must always be presented to your callers.

Telephone use in the medical office should be in an area where other patients and visitors are unable to hear the conversation, determine the nature of the call, or discern who the person is on the other end of the call. Most reception areas are located a short distance from the waiting area so that conversations and phone calls cannot be overheard or, if it is a small office, there may be a window surrounding the reception area to provide privacy for conversations and calls.

Answering the Telephone

Your manner of answering the telephone frequently determines how the conversation will flow. It is also the first impression that callers, including potential new patients, receive of your office. The following are some important techniques that will assist you in answering your medical office's telephone in the most pleasant and professional manner.

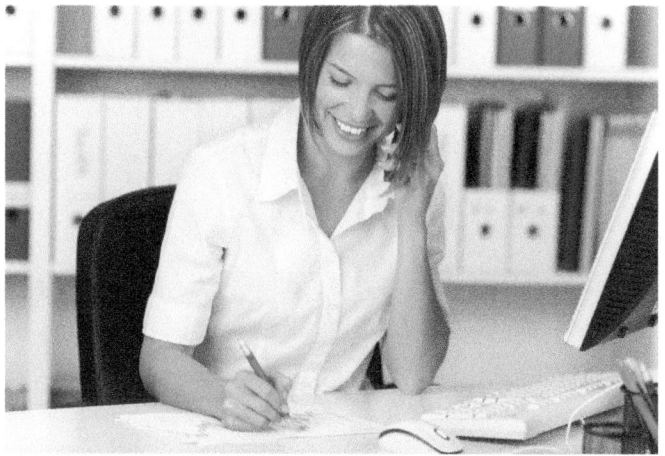
FIGURE 7-1 A pleasant smile can go a long way, even through telephone lines.

Smiling

Always answer the telephone with a smile. A human voice has so many nuances that most callers will be able to sense warmth or indifference in your voice. Until you can become comfortable with smiling when answering the telephone, you may want to look in a mirror as you answer so you can observe yourself and your facial expressions as you speak (Figure 7-1).

Greetings

When the telephone rings in the medical office, it is important that it be answered quickly, generally by the third ring. The medical office supervisor will teach you the office's preferred method of answering the telephone. An appropriate greeting includes the following:

- The name of the office or the physician
- Your name
- Asking the caller how you can be of assistance

An example of a typical office greeting might be "Good morning. Pearson Physicians Group. This is Jessica. How may I help you?" A greeting such as this will help make the patient feel comfortable about contacting your office.

Speech

Many times people overlook the importance of speaking clearly on the telephone. However, speaking clearly is a key element in communicating effectively with patients—on the phone as well as in person. Four elements of speech are commonly considered: clarity, enunciation, inflection, and pitch.

Clarity refers to the quality or state of being understandable. How clear is your voice to the caller? Are you holding the telephone receiver 1 to 2 inches from your mouth so that the best sound gets through to the caller? Many people tend

TABLE 7-1 | Some Words Commonly Misunderstood Because of Poor Enunciation

Word	May be Misunderstood As
Prostate	Prostrate
Ear	Air
Galactorrhea	Galacturia
Homeostasis	Hemostasis
Heart attack	Artifact
Palpation	Palpitation

to drop the receiver so that it sits just below the chin. This does not produce clear sound for the person on the other end of the telephone. The telephone handset should be held in the middle, with the receiver to your ear and the mouthpiece 1 to 2 inches from your mouth. You also must have nothing in your mouth—no gum, candy, food, or liquid—that could garble your words.

Enunciation refers to the clear articulation and pronunciation of words. Being careful not to speak too rapidly helps with word enunciation. Because you may use the same greeting and phrase repeatedly to answer the telephone, it is easy to fall into the habit of speaking too quickly. Slow down and pronounce your words slowly and properly, imagining the person on the other end of the line hearing them for the first time. Correct pronunciation helps minimize confusion for the caller. See Table 7-1 for examples of words that are commonly misunderstood because of poor enunciation. Avoid using regional pronunciations in the office setting. Remember that your patients come from many different cultures and may not understand your particular pronunciation.

Your voice ranges from high to low, depending on how you commonly speak and, often, on the context of your phrase. Have you ever noticed that when you ask a question your voice tends to rise at the end of the phrase? This is an example of the **pitch** of your voice. Be aware of using appropriate pitch when speaking with patients.

Professionalism

 An important aspect of your personal success as a medical assistant—and the success of the medical practice—is your communication skills. Improper grammar conveys an uneducated and unprofessional image. It is important to use proper grammar whenever you communicate, either verbally or in writing, with patients, physicians, or coworkers.

Inflection refers to the changes in pitch and tone of your voice as you utter words and phrases. Remember that speaking on the telephone is an opportunity to display excellent customer service. Try to avoid speaking in a monotone (one single tone). The caller may feel you are bored and not interested in helping.

Identify the Caller

Protection of a patient's information is vital in every medical office and health care facility. It is important to remember that some individuals may seek confidential information by unauthorized means, such as claiming to be the patient or even a specialist treating the patient. Therefore, steps must be taken to protect the patient's medical record. For example, each time a person phones and claims to be a patient, ask for identifying information, including both first and last names, the patient's date of birth, and the last four digits of the patient's social security number. You can check this information against the patient's electronic or paper medical record.

Listening

Listening is a critical part of managing telephone calls. Callers do not like to be asked to repeat information or to be interrupted when they call the office. The average rate of speaking is 125–150 words per minute and the average rate of listening is 400–500 words per minute. This means that you are capable of listening to a flow of words that is faster than the way most people speak. This should be an advantage for the caller, because if you are truly listening to the conversation, you will not have to ask the caller to repeat anything. In addition, you are much less likely to interrupt the caller in the midst of something they are trying to tell you. Listening requires focus and undivided attention. When you are talking with a caller on the phone, do not be engaged in other duties that require your attention. A phone call is not a time for multitasking.

The Business Telephone System

Many types of business telephone systems are in use today (Figure 7-2). Most medical offices use some form of multiline telephone. Some of these multiline phones may have all separate lines, where you must press a particular line's button to answer it; others may have a system that will feed calls to you from a **queue**, or waiting line. More and more offices have systems that answer the initial call with a recording and then direct the call to the appropriate person after the caller chooses an option to meet their needs. Procedure 7-1 details answering the telephone and using the hold function in a professional manner.

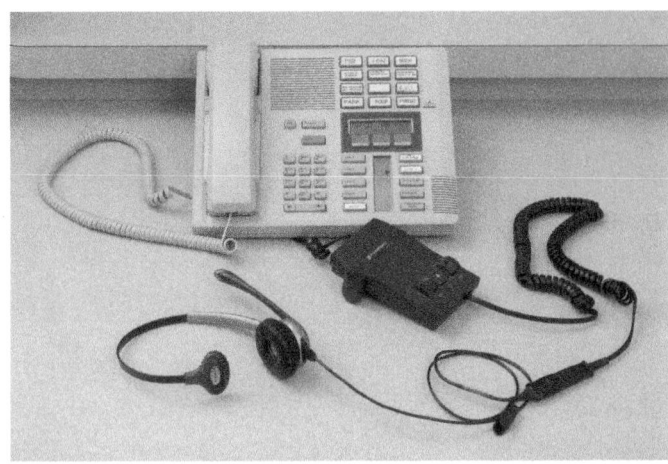

FIGURE 7-2 Choose the telephone unit that offers the features needed in your office.

Whether you answer initially (without an automated system) or an automated system answers (calls are queued), follow the rules for greeting callers stated in Procedure 7-1.

Making Calls

You will have to make calls as often as you answer them. On most business telephones, you will be required to dial 9 to get an outside line, but some systems have an outside line button that you push in order to dial an outside number. Depending on the office's location, you also may need to dial the area code with all calls. Large cities have begun to make this a common practice because of the existence of multiple area codes within a local calling zone.

The telephone calls that you make in the office should be limited to business calls. All offices have different policies regarding the use of the office telephone for personal calls. Some may prohibit them entirely, whereas others may allow them in limited number, or may ask that any personal calls be made on a private line, which may also be referred to as the back line. It is important to keep in mind that the office telephone is for patients and emergencies, so you must keep the lines open and available for business calls only.

Using the Hold Function

One of the most sensitive issues relating to telephone courtesy is the use of the hold function, which permits keeping more than one call on the line at a time. Holding a call is permissible when you are speaking with a caller on one line and another call comes in as long as the situation is handled courteously for both callers. You should never put a call on hold before you have given the caller a chance to say it is an emergency.

Be very mindful of how the hold function is used. Callers should never be left on hold for indefinite periods of time. If

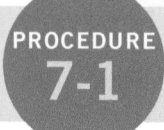

PROCEDURE 7-1

Answering the Telephone and Placing Calls on Hold

Objective ◆ *Ensure that the telephone is answered in a professional manner and that, if necessary, callers are placed on hold appropriately.*

EQUIPMENT AND SUPPLIES

Telephone; message pad; pen; notepad

1. Answer the telephone by at least the third ring, with the mouthpiece 1 to 2 inches from your mouth.
2. Smile and speak clearly, using inflection, a pleasant tone, and a moderate rate of speech.
3. Answer using the greeting your office prefers (e.g., "Thank you for calling Pearson Physicians Group. This is Carlos. How may I help you?").
4. At this point, callers will typically identify themselves. If not, ask callers to identify themselves by their first and last names. Then, if it is an established patient, verify the patient's birthdate or other identifying information against the patient's medical record.
5. Listen to the caller closely to verify the reason for the call, which may include, but is not limited to, the following:
   - A patient calling to schedule an appointment
   - A patient calling to request a prescription refill
   - Another physician's office calling about a mutual patient
   - An insurance company calling regarding a patient's claim
   - A relative or friend of an office employee or physician
6. Once you have determined the reason for the call, act accordingly while providing excellent customer service. In busy offices, you may need to answer more than one incoming telephone line. When this occurs, you will combine the procedure just described with the following steps:

- When you are speaking with one caller and another incoming line rings, you must notify the current caller that another line is ringing and ask if the current caller can hold. Wait for the caller's response, then place the first call on hold.
- Answer the second call following the procedures described above, ask if the second caller can hold, wait for a response, and then place the second call on hold. *Note:* If the second call is an emergency, you would not ask the person to hold but would assist the caller immediately.
- Return to the first call, thank the caller for holding, and continue assisting the person.
  Note: When you return to that caller, do not ask "Who are you waiting for?" because it conveys the impression that you have forgotten about that person.
- Once the first call is completed, return to the second call, thank the person for holding, and continue assisting that caller.
- If the caller asks to speak with another employee who is not readily available and it is necessary to place the call on hold, be sure to check back with the caller about every 30 seconds. This lets the caller know you are actively working to be of help, and it also provides an opportunity for the caller to leave a message instead of continuing to hold.

you anticipate that the call may need to be placed on hold for a long time, offer the patient the option of either continuing to hold or having their call returned.

If you are already speaking with a caller when a second call comes in, it is proper to ask the first caller if you may place her on hold for a moment in order to answer the second call (review Procedure 7.1). Once you have asked this question, be sure to listen for the caller's response before automatically placing the call on hold. It is possible the first caller has a billing question, in which case you may transfer the call instead of placing the caller on hold. It is discourteous to handle the second caller before returning to

the first call. An example of a typical hold-conversation follows:

To First Caller:	"Mrs. Miller, may I place you on hold for a moment? I have another call."
Mrs. Miller:	"Yes, I can hold."
To Second Caller:	"Good afternoon. Pearson Physicians Group. This is Tonya. How may I help you?"
Mr. Thompson:	"This is Bobby Thompson, and I need to make an appointment to see the doctor."

TONYA: "Mr. Thompson, can you please hold?"

MR. THOMPSON: "Yes, I can."

TONYA: "Mrs. Miller, thank you for holding." (Tonya continues with this first call as efficiently and expediently as possible without hurrying the caller.)

When you answer a second call and discover it is an emergency, you must take care of it before returning to the first call. If it is not an emergency, finish the first call before moving to the second. With all calls that you place on hold, try to keep the wait time to a minimum. Nobody likes to be on hold.

Other situations also may require you to place a caller on hold. For example, you may need to access information from the patient's medical record so you can answer a patient's question. When this happens, explain what you need to do and then ask if you may place the patient on hold while you do it. Always wait for a response, then retrieve the information in the timeliest manner possible. If you have trouble getting the information and need more time, let the caller know and offer the option of calling back once you have found the needed information. If the patient agrees it would be best for you to call back, be sure you do just that.

Never leave callers on hold without checking back with them. Communication is key, and it is important that patients understand you are working to help them. To avoid forgetting about a caller on hold, be wary of distractions and do not complete any tasks that are unrelated to helping that caller.

Another situation that requires you to put a caller on hold is when a patient must speak with the doctor or another staff member who is not readily available. In this situation, follow the protocol used in the office where you work. Many physicians only accept calls from other physicians or family members while they are busy seeing patients. Physicians may choose to return patient phone calls during a specified time of day. If this is the policy in the office where you work, let the patient know the physician is seeing patients and when he generally returns calls. If the physician answers patient's calls while seeing patients, make sure the caller is aware that there will be a wait and offer to take a message and relay it to the physician. As much as possible, it is best to keep the telephone lines open. If the caller chooses to wait, you must check on the caller approximately every 30 seconds. Let the caller know that the physician is still unavailable. Then ask if the caller would like to leave a name and phone number so the call can be returned.

Transferring Calls

As you field calls in the medical office, you will find that it is often necessary to transfer or send them from one office telephone extension to another extension in the same office. Most business telephones have a transfer feature. You should follow certain steps to make this a smooth transition for the caller:

1. Once you have identified the person to whom you will be transferring the call, tell the caller the name of this person. This lets the caller know who to expect on the other end of the line as well as who to call back in case the call is disconnected during the transfer process. If you have an extension number available, it is also helpful to provide that number to the caller before transferring the call.

2. When you start the transfer, make sure the caller is aware of your actions. Do not transfer the call without the patient's prior knowledge and consent.

3. Most telephone systems allow you to announce a call that you are transferring. Let the person to whom you are transferring the call know the caller's name and the reason for the call. That person may tell you that she is unavailable to take the call.

4. Do not hang up before you know if the person was available to help the caller.

5. If you get a busy signal when you transfer the call, let the caller know that the line is busy and offer to take a message or let the caller leave a recorded message.

Taking a Message

Medical offices are busy places. Medical assistants often take messages from patients, other physicians, health care facilities, and businesses. Electronic medical records allow telephone messages to be entered directly into the patient's medical record. Many medical offices that don't use electronic records have preprinted telephone messages or notepads used for recording telephone messages. Most calls can be documented in the space provided on the pad. It is important to use the form as a guide for gathering all pertinent information. Occasionally, patients provide much more information than necessary, and you may not know what is pertinent until you near the end of, or have completed, the call. To provide all the necessary information, yet be brief, write down all information provided by the patient and transfer it (in bullet points) to the message screen or preprinted form or, if it is too lengthy, attach it to the message form. Make sure that the intended recipient receives the message.

All messages should include the following information:

- First and last names of the caller (with spelling verified)
- A telephone number including area code at which the caller can be reached for a callback
- The reason for the call
- The name of the person the caller is trying to reach
- The date and time of the call

If at any time you do not understand what a caller has stated, you must clarify the message with the caller. Repeat the message to the patient to ensure accuracy, and always emphasize repetition of the callback number. Inform the patient of a time frame within which they can expect a return call. Double-check that the patient will be able to be reached at the phone number provided during this time frame. If not, obtain an alternative telephone number. If a callback does not occur because the phone number was recorded incorrectly, the caller may interpret it as disrespect or a lack of concern.

All telephone messages regarding a patient should be documented in the patient's medical record as an interaction that occurred between the office and the patient. This may be important should the patient's record be subpoenaed for any legal reason.

It is very important not to throw away but to shred anything that contains patient information. Even the written notes you use to take messages must be shredded if they contain any patient information. It is a violation of the Health Insurance Portability and Accountability Act (HIPAA) privacy rule to place any patient information directly into the trash.

See Procedure 7-2 for instructions on how to take telephone messages.

The Voice Messaging System

In the medical office, you will usually work with a **voice messaging system** for both incoming and outgoing calls. A voice messaging system allows messages (voice mail) to be left or recorded when the medical assistant is unavailable to answer the telephone. If your office uses such a system, inform callers in the initial greeting to hang up and dial 911 if they are calling because of a medical emergency.

You may have to record a message for incoming calls that will be forwarded to voice mail. If you are using such a system, include your full name and request that the caller leave a detailed message including a phone number for a return call. It is also helpful to let patients know, in the voice mail messsage, the time when calls are usually answered. Your voice messaging system should also allow for the caller to dial 0 for immediate assistance.

Professionalism   The Law

Medical assistants must use a level of caution when speaking with patients over the telephone. Never diagnose a patient or give medical advice—only the physician can diagnose and treat patients. When handling calls, always follow your office's protocol manual. Document every call that you have with a patient. Document all details—even seemingly insignificant ones. Never discard any patient information in a trash can. When disposing of patient information, shred it.

When calling patients, you will find that most of them have some form of voice messaging system. This does present a possible problem in the context of patient privacy, because someone other than the patient may pick up the message. Know both your office's policy regarding what kind of message should be left on a patient's voice messaging system and how to adhere to HIPAA guidelines when doing so. This is also discussed later in the chapter.

Call Forwarding

The call forwarding feature allows for incoming calls to be forwarded to another telephone. For example, a physician may wish to forward cell phone calls to a home telephone. You will often use this feature if your office uses an answering service. (Answering services are discussed later in this chapter.)

Caller ID

Caller ID is a popular telephone option. This function allows telephone owners to know who is calling each time the telephone rings. In the office, it is unlikely that you will have caller ID, but many of your patients may have this telephone feature. It is important to understand that a medical office may need to block the office number from showing up on the patient's caller ID. This is because most offices often have multiple telephone lines, some designated for incoming calls and others for outgoing calls. Each of these lines may have a different telephone number. Back lines—those meant only for incoming calls from patients—should be left open at all times. A patient who has caller ID may get the number to one of your back lines. This can become very confusing to both the patient and the staff. Maintaining patient privacy is another reason commonly used to block the medical office's telephone number.

Privacy Manager

Privacy manager is an addition to the variety of telephone options. It allows patients to block access to their home

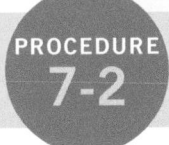

PROCEDURE 7-2 — Taking a Telephone Message

Objective ◆ *Ensure that correct and relevant information is retrieved when taking a telephone message.*

EQUIPMENT AND SUPPLIES

Message form or pad with carbon or carbonless for duplicates; pen; electronic health record, if available

1. Smile before answering the telephone and, in a warm voice, properly answer the telephone.
2. Use a message form to keep a record of the message, or document it directly into the electronic health record.
3. Record the date and time of the call.
4. Record the caller's full name and a callback number with area code for use during office hours. (Always ask the caller to spell his or her name and provide another identifier, such as date of birth or the last four digits of a social security number.) If recording the message in an electronic health record, verify that you have the correct patient record.

5. Document for whom the message is intended.
6. Document the complete message (Figure A). Avoid using abbreviations other than accepted medical abbreviations. Include symptoms (e.g., temperature, rash, vomiting, and duration of symptoms).
7. Repeat the message to the patient to ensure clarity, and emphasize that the correct callback number has been obtained.
8. Thank the patient for calling, inform the patient when to expect a return call, and, before hanging up the telephone, ask if there are any other questions.
9. To indicate that you are the one who took a handwritten message, either write out your first and last name or record the initial of your first name and your last name spelled out. If using an electronic health record, save the message and forward it to the intended recipient.

CHARTING EXAMPLE

Patient Name: Carl Toper   Date of Birth: 9/12/46
Date: 10/29/20XX   Time: 9:15 A.M.   Physician: Dr. Verde
Patient's Telephone Number (Home): 213-555-3424
(Other): 213-555-5946
Medical Record Number: 99574   Allergies: Penicillin
Pharmacy Name: Dispense for You
Pharmacy Telephone Number: 213-555-2359
Prescription Number: N/A
Message Taken By: . . . . Tonya Blue, RMA (AMT)

MESSAGE

Patient called stating he has had nausea and diarrhea since he returned from seeing his grandkids in Seattle last week. On questioning, the patient stated his granddaughter had a fever the day he left to return home. Mr. Toper is wondering if the nausea and diarrhea will cause any problems with his insulin dosing. Per the patient, he will be home all day.

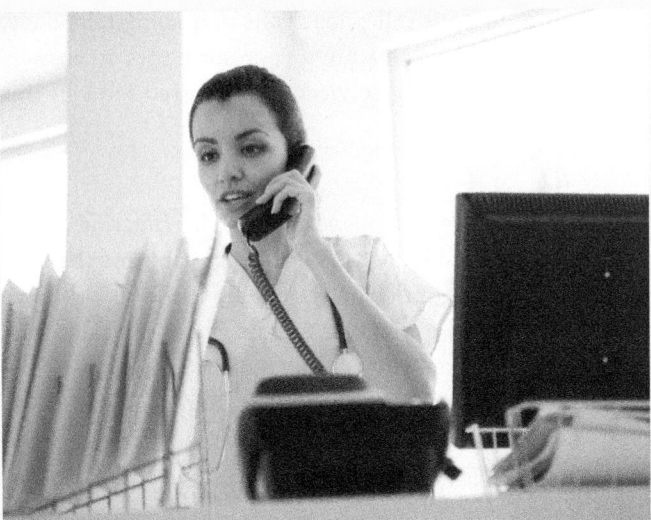

FIGURE A All messages must be documented and placed in the patient's record.

telephones. When you call a telephone number that has privacy manager attached, you will be asked to state from where you are calling, by simply saying the name of the medical practice. Once you have given this information, unless you are cleared, you will be directed to a voice mail system, where you will leave a message.

Headsets

At times you will need to free your hands for administrative duties while still being available to answer the telephone. In such instances, you can use a headset.

Headsets free your hands so you can document calls (Figure 7-3). They are ergonomically correct, as they do not

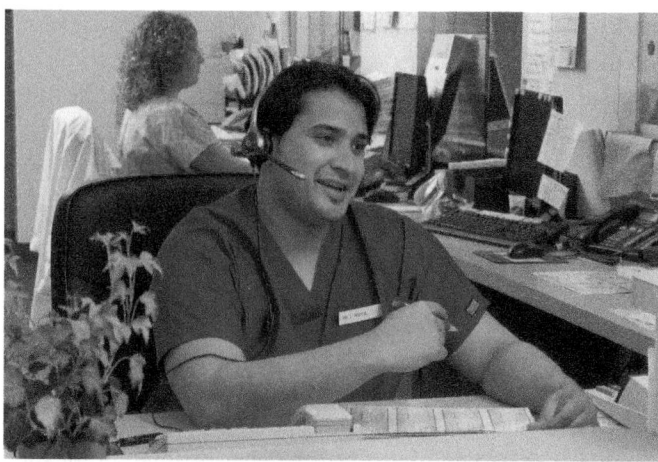

FIGURE 7-3 Headsets are ergonomically correct and allow the medical assistant or receptionist to use both hands for administrative duties, while still being available to answer the telephone.

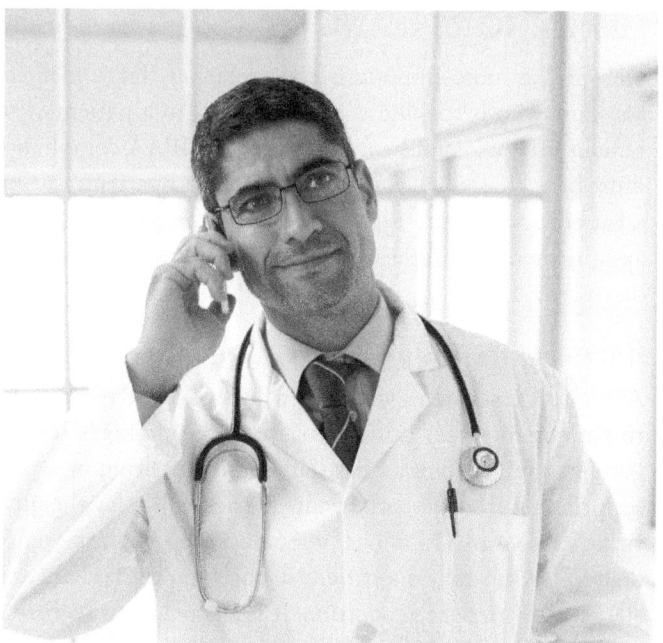

FIGURE 7-4 Many physicians use cell phones to stay in touch with their offices.

cause the neck and shoulder injuries that can result from cradling the receiver on the shoulder. Keep the headset microphone close to your mouth so the caller does not have difficulty hearing or understanding you.

Most telephones have a built-in speakerphone or microphone and speaker. The speakerphone allows you to hear and speak without having to pick up the handset of the telephone. The speakerphone has a few drawbacks, however: Others nearby may overhear your conversation, or the caller on the other end will be able to hear background noise. Patient confidentiality should be a foremost concern when using the speakerphone. It is never appropriate to answer incoming patient calls using a speakerphone unless you are in a private office with the door closed.

Pagers and Cell Phones

Although pagers may not be as commonly used as cell phones, you must know if any physician in your office carries a pager. Most pager systems are easy to use. You simply call the pager number and, when instructed, enter in the callback telephone number. Some offices may use a coded message system. For example, certain numbers may be designated for different types of emergencies or situations. Using a specific number will give the physician a heads-up about the nature of the call. You must learn how your office uses its pager system if it has one; additional information would be found in the office policies and procedures or protocol manual.

Cell phones have become fundamental to business and social life. Most physicians and office managers now use cell phones to conduct day-to-day business (Figure 7-4). Most have replaced their pagers with cell phones, because most cell phones also have a pager function.

Different types of cell phones are available, offering a wide variety of functions. All cell phones provide incoming and outgoing call capability as well as texting. Texting replaces voice mail by allowing the sender to type a message instead of speaking it. This is a preferred practice when the person receiving the call is in a location that does not allow vocal conversation. Smartphones combine the features of a cell phone and a minicomputer and have access to Internet applications and e-mail. Medical offices may use patients' e-mail or texting applications to send appointment reminders to patients.

Cell phones do have a significant disadvantage in that they can interfere with electronic monitors, and for that reason they are not allowed in parts of certain hospitals or procedure rooms of medical offices. Most medical offices prohibit the use of cell phones in the waiting room, not only because of the interference they may cause but because it is not proper etiquette to use a cell phone around other persons. Usually, signage clearly designates where cell phones are and are not allowed. In most cell phone–free zones, pagers are allowed. To understand and keep up to date with rules regarding cell phone and pager use, check frequently with hospitals with which your office regularly communicates.

Proper cell phone etiquette is important everywhere. When receiving or placing a cell phone call, it is recommended that you be at least 10 feet from others and use a low voice when talking.

HIPAA COMPLIANCE

One of the most important considerations for a medical assistant who is making a telephone call to a patient is to remain HIPAA compliant at all times. HIPAA compliance must be exercised when returning a call to a patient, calling a patient with test results, and even calling a patient for an appointment reminder. Each of these scenarios will be discussed.

Return Calls and Callbacks

As a medical assistant, you often will be asked to return calls to patients or other callers. For instance, messages left by patients may contain a question for the physician or a prescription refill request, and your callback will relay the physician's response. Occasionally the physician will ask you to do a follow-up call to a patient to check on the welfare and status of the patient's condition. It is a good measure, before phoning a patient, to review that person's medical record to establish who has been given permission to receive information about the patient. Most medical offices have patients update their privacy notices each year. During the time of this update, the patient can identify who is allowed to receive messages on their behalf regarding their confidential health information.

The first thing to do when phoning any patient is to make sure that it is the patient with whom you are speaking. Start every patient callback by identifying yourself, then asking to speak to the patient. You should not indicate why you are calling until you have the patient on the phone. If the person who answers asks you why you are calling, explain that confidentiality laws prevent you from revealing that information to anyone other than the person you have asked to speak to, unless they have specifically been identified by the patient as someone who may receive confidential information on the patient's behalf.

Leaving a Message

If the patient is unavailable, ask to leave a message to have the patient call you back. You may also have to leave a message on a patient's home telephone or cell phone. Even though cell phones are considered more private, the message must still remain confidential. You must consider the patient's privacy, and if you were to leave a self-identifying message such as "This is Cathy from Carsonville OB/GYN," you may have disclosed confidential patient information. To leave a message, yet maintain patient privacy, consider this appropriate example:

"This is Cathy from Dr. Smith's office, and this message is for Charlene. Please return my call at your earliest convenience. You may reach me at 555-987-6543."

Guidelines to follow when leaving a message for a patient with another person, or when leaving a message on the patient's answering machine or voice mail, remain the same:

- State your name.
- State the name of the patient's doctor for whom you work, *not* the name of the practice.
- State the phone number where you can be reached.
- Do not leave any additional information as it could be a breach of confidentiality laws.

The only time it is acceptable to leave a detailed message with someone other than the patient is if the patient has explicitly stated and has given written permission for messages to be left with specific individuals, as stated in a patient privacy notice. A patient may also state that a phone number, such as a cell phone, is a secure line and it is acceptable to leave a detailed message.

Test Results

A patient may have testing done to confirm a diagnosis or to determine if a treatment is successful. Often patients are eager to receive the results of any tests, whether it is blood work, diagnostic imaging, or other tests ordered by the physician. A medical assistant may be permitted to call a patient with the results of tests that have been performed. However, it is important to note that results may not be divulged to a patient until the physician has reviewed the results and has given verbal or written permission for the medical assistant to share the information with the patient.

Test results are highly confidential information, and patient privacy should remain the utmost concern. When calling a patient with test results, the same protocol should be followed as when leaving a message for the patient. Always make sure that you are speaking with the patient before divulging where you are calling from and why you are calling. Never leave a message that includes the actual test results, even if the patient has given permission stating detailed messages are allowed to be left either with specific individuals or on voice mail. When the patient is unavailable, but a more detailed message is allowed, consider the following example:

"This is Tavia calling from Dr. Smith's office. Shannon, please give me a call at your earliest convenience to discuss your test results. My number is 555-123-1234."

Appointment Reminders

Most offices call patients to remind them of upcoming appointments. Patients should be contacted at least the day before their appointment; however, some offices call patients a week in advance. Calling to confirm appointments is one way to ensure proper management of the physician's schedule. Some offices send e-mail or text message appointment reminders. In order to use text or e-mail appointment reminder systems, the patient must sign an authorization form allowing this method of contact. These methods help reduce breaches of confidentiality because the information is sent directly to the patient.

When a medical office uses telephone-call appointment reminders, the same guidelines should be followed. Although it seems repetitive to mention, the importance of understanding HIPAA compliance and patient confidentially can never be overstated. Again, HIPAA compliance requires the following:

- Never divulge any information to anyone other than the patient.

- When someone answers the phone, ask for the patient by name. "May I please speak with Mary Anderson?"

- If asked for additional information by the person answering the phone, state your first name and the name of the doctor, not the practice. "This is Lydia calling from Dr. Wellington's office."

- Do not leave additional information, unless specific permission has been given by the patient. If allowed, you may state, "This is Lydia calling from Dr. Wellington's office. I'm calling to remind Mary of her appointment. Please have her call the office if she needs to reschedule." By not stating the appointment date and time in the message, you are providing additional patient information. The patient will either remember the time of the appointment or will call the office to confirm the appointment time.

Documentation

All telephone interactions must be documented in the patient's medical record. This is especially important when leaving a message for the patient. It is important to always make a note in the patient's medical record indicating the date and time the message was left. Also include the name of the person with whom a message was left. A patient may call the office angry because they expected a call and never received one. If a call was made to the patient, and a message was left, the documentation in the medical record will help the medical assistant provide the patient with the exact time and date the message was left.

TYPICAL INCOMING CALLS

You will receive many types of calls in the medical office. The following are some types you will handle on a daily basis.

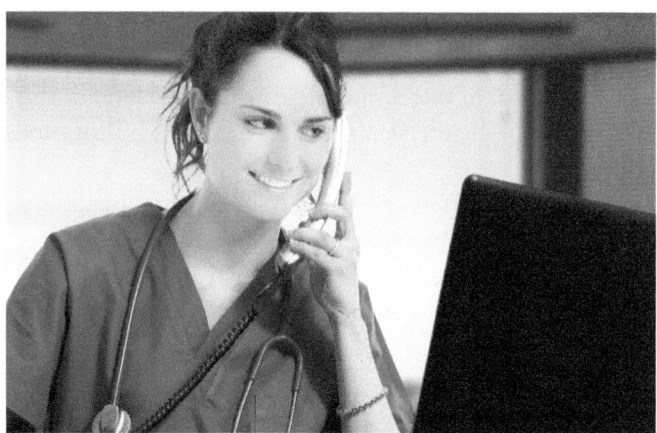

FIGURE 7-5 The medical assistant spends many hours on the telephone assisting patients.

Patient Calls

Most calls coming into the medical office will be from patients (Figure 7-5). They may be calling for an appointment or about insurance, billing, fees, office hours and directions, laboratory results, or prescription refill requests.

Appointment Requests

Appointment requests are among the most common types of calls you will receive in the medical office. These calls often come from patients with health problems of varying degrees of severity or urgency, so you need to follow telephone triage procedures (discussed later in this chapter) to schedule them appropriately. The caller may be a current patient or a new patient. For patients who need routine appointments, offer an appointment time that is convenient for both the patient and the medical office.

Insurance and Billing Questions

Medical offices get many calls from patients with questions about what procedures are covered under their insurance plan, concerns about their billing statement, and many other questions regarding financial aspects of their health care. You may be able to answer some of these questions, but you will direct most callers who have this type of question to the billing department for assistance.

One of the most frequently asked questions is "Why did I get a bill?" Many patients have the misconception that their insurance company will pay the entire bill. You may need to explain to the patient the details of what was billed. In your explanation, you will need to include what steps the insurance company has taken in regard to covering the charges. This could include discussing deductibles, copayments, and coinsurance.

You also may need to explain reasons for denial of certain charges. If you are unable to help with questions concerning insurance coverage, you may refer the patient to the insurance company or employer's human resources department. All of these concepts are discussed later in this textbook in the chapters on medical insurance, billing, and coding issues.

New patients often call before scheduling an appointment to inquire about whether the provider participates with their insurance plan. The medical assistant should have a list of the most common insurance plans with which the practice is affiliated. Specific patient questions regarding provider participation should be directed to the insurance company.

Fees

Specific questions about fees should always be referred to the billing department. Keep in mind that you will usually be unable to give any exact figures until the patient has been seen by the physician.

Office Hours and Directions

Most offices now include the office hours and directions in the office's automated assistance system. However, you may have to handle some of the calls yourself. You should have your office address and hours posted near your telephone for quick reference. It is also a good practice to have directions posted near the telephone. The directions should include routes to the office from all directions—north, south, east, and west.

Follow-Up Calls from Patients

It is common for a physician to have a patient call the office as a follow-up to certain procedures and to relate the status of certain problems. When these calls come into the office, the medical assistant must take a message and convey this information to the physician. Always obtain as much detail as possible from the patient regarding his or her condition when taking messages of this nature.

Referral Requests

Many insurance companies require a **referral** (which documents authorization) from their primary care physician by telephone or fax before patients see a specialist. Referrals are always required for patients in health management organizations (HMOs). Thus, patients may phone to request that a referral be arranged. You must get all the information necessary to place the referral, including the name, address, and telephone number of the specialist's office. This information may be found in the local telephone book, on the

Internet, or in the insurance company's provider book. You also will need to find out the reason the patient is seeing the specialist. You may obtain some of this information from the patient, and you also may need to check the patient's medical record for the diagnosis that the referral references. All referrals need to be approved by the physician before being completed and released to the patient or, as is sometimes required, sent directly from your office to the specialist's office.

Patients Who Refuse to Identify Themselves

Occasionally, you will encounter patients who refuse to identify themselves to you. You must let the caller know that you will not be of assistance without having that person's name and reason for calling. Inform the caller that the physician will not return calls to patients who refuse to identify themselves. If the caller continues to refuse to state his or her name, some offices will ask that the caller write a letter addressed to the physician.

The Persistent Talker

Every medical office has patients who call and draw the staff into long conversations. Because your time is limited, you must end such conversations kindly but promptly. You may simply state to the patient that you are busy helping another patient and apologize for the inconvenience.

TDD Calls

The TDD, telecommunications device for the deaf, is a teleprinter or electronic device for text communication over a telephone line. The caller can type in a message, and the person who receives the call can do the same. This is a very efficient way to communicate with deaf or hearing-impaired patients and clients. Some cell phone companies offer a data-only plan for those who do not need or require verbal communication. Text messaging by cell phone or smartphone can fill the same need.

Nonpatient Calls

Not all telephone calls to the office are from patients. You will find that a large number of calls come from salespeople, hospitals, other physicians, and other health care facilities.

Sales Calls

Answering calls from sales representatives is part of the medical assistant's telephone responsibilities. You may have to become the wall between the salesperson and your physician and office manager. Most physicians will not take any type of sales calls while seeing patients. They may ask you to take messages or ask the sales representative to fax or e-mail the information to them. The same will probably hold true with office managers. They will ask you to take messages for most sales calls so they can return the calls at a more convenient time.

Reports from Hospitals and Other Patient Care Facilities

If your physician has patients in a hospital or nursing facility, you will likely receive calls from those facilities. The facilities often call with reports on the patients' status or changes in their conditions. In many cases, you will interrupt the physician for such calls. To do so, you should knock on the examination room door and let the physician know an important call is on hold. Sometimes you will need only to take a message for the physician. The message may contain information to relay to the physician or may be a request that the physician return the call. In either case, you always should immediately notify the physician so she can determine whether the call should be returned sooner rather than later.

General Office Matters

Some calls received in the office deal with general office business, including telephone calls from accountants or calls regarding suppliers or rented office equipment. These calls should be handled on a case-by-case basis. It is important to carefully screen calls from the office's suppliers. Make sure to obtain the supplier's name and the business's name, address, and telephone number. It is best that the office manager or person responsible handle calls regarding office equipment or supplies.

Physician's Personal Calls

The physician also will receive personal calls in the office. Physicians work long hours and often encourage family members to call them at the office. Most physicians will instruct you how they wish their personal calls to be

Professionalism   The Law

It is always best to err on the side of caution when discussing a patient with someone other than the patient. Be familiar with HIPAA as it applies to the patients seen in your office. For instance, when a patient under the age of 18 seeks medical advice regarding psychiatric evaluation, the patient's information is protected even from the parent or guardian. If any question arises regarding whether you should release the information to the parent or guardian, it is best not to release it and seek guidance from the physician.

handled. In some cases, they will want you to knock on the examination room door and simply state, "Doctor, you are wanted on the telephone." In other cases, physicians may ask you to give them telephone messages as soon as they come out of the examination room. Generally, family members do not wish to interrupt the physician during a patient examination.

Calls from Other Physicians

The physician will let the office staff know how to handle calls from other physicians. The physician may wish to take such calls right away or immediately when finished with an exam. Such calls may relate to a patient consultation and require an immediate answer. In certain circumstances, such as a consult on a patient, the physician receiving the call may want to have the patient's medical record available.

Obscene or Prank Calls

It is not uncommon for offices to occasionally receive an obscene or prank phone call. Hang up immediately if you receive such calls. Inform the office manager of the incident so the manager is aware, especially if it may happen to others in the medical office who answer the telephone. You also may report the call to the telephone company, especially if it is an ongoing problem that seems to involve the same caller. Usually, the telephone company can trace the call.

PRESCRIPTION REFILL REQUESTS

Phone requests for prescription refills are commonly received in medical offices. Because of the high volume of such calls, many offices have a voice mail system to answer most of these calls. The medical assistant is often responsible for taking messages off the voice mail system and responding to them at least twice each day, sometimes more frequently.

The physician must sign off on all prescription refill requests. The physician needs to review the patient's medical record when determining their response to prescription refill requests.

When taking messages of this nature, specific information is required in order for the message to be handled in an efficient manner. See Procedure 7-3 for important information about taking a prescription refill message.

Calling the Pharmacy with a Refill Request

The medical assistant is often responsible for calling the pharmacy with a prescription refill request. However, increasing use of electronic medical records and computerized order entries have decreased the number of times the MA has to call the pharmacy. Rather, the physician reviews the request for a prescription refill and automatically submits the prescription refill request to the pharmacy electronically, eliminating the phone call.

Some offices still use paper records, and sometimes wireless connections and Internet services are interrupted. In these instances, the medical assistant needs to call the pharmacy to submit a refill request. Procedure 7-4 outlines the steps to follow when calling a pharmacy with a refill request.

PROCEDURE 7-3 | Taking a Prescription Refill Message

Objective ◆ *Ensure that correct information is obtained when refilling a patient's prescription.*

EQUIPMENT AND SUPPLIES

Message pad or paper; pen

1. Document the name of the patient. (This name may be different from the name of the caller.) Always ensure the proper spelling of the name because many names are similar.
2. Document the patient's telephone number or callback number.
3. Document the name and dosage of the medication being requested. Ask the caller to spell the medication name if you do not understand what the caller is saying.
4. Document how long the patient has been on the medication.
5. Document the patient's symptoms and why the prescription is still needed.
6. Document the patient's age and (if a child) weight.
7. Ask for the name and telephone number (including area code) of the pharmacy and the prescription number if available.
8. Let the caller know you will forward the message to the physician.
9. Let the caller know you will call back if the prescription cannot be refilled or if the physician has any questions.
10. The refill request must be reviewed by the physician. If the office uses an electronic health records system, the refill request may be documented in the patient's electronic record and the physician would be notified to review the message in the EHR. If the office uses paper records, attach the telephone message to the patient's medical record and give both to the physician to review.

CHARTING EXAMPLE

Patient Name: Lucy Coles   Date of Birth: 4/20/67
Date: 10/24/YY   Time: 10:05 A.M.   Physician: Dr. Rudy
Patient's Telephone Number (Home): 213-555-1234
                              (Cell): 213-555-3496
Medical Record Number: 89564   Allergies: NKDA
Pharmacy Name: Dispense for You
Pharmacy Telephone Number: 213-555-2359
Prescription Number: CC5679
Message Taken By: . . . . Tonya Blue, RMA

MESSAGE

Patient called requesting refill on Celexa 20 mg. Patient stated she is doing well on the medication with no side effects. Patient scheduled for follow-up visit on 12/10/YY. Patient will be at home telephone number until 4:45 P.M.; after that, please call cell phone number above.

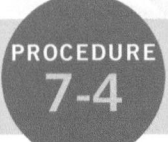

Calling the Pharmacy for a Prescription Refill

Objective ◆ *Use the correct procedure to call a pharmacy to refill a patient's prescription.*

EQUIPMENT AND SUPPLIES

Patient medical record, either electronic health record or paper chart; physician-authorized prescription refill request; telephone

METHOD

1. Review the order for the prescription refill. This is either in the patient's electronic medical record or on the message sheet that was used to take the patient's request for a refill. Make sure that the request includes the following information:
   - Patient's first and last names
   - Patient's date of birth
   - The pharmacy name and phone number
   - The name of the medication, dosage, and instructions—for example, Glucophage XR, 1000 mg, once daily
   - The number to be dispensed and the number of refills allowed—for example, dispense #30, with two refills
   - The prescription number that was previously assigned to the patient's prescription
2. Review the prescription refill request to be certain it was signed and authorized by the physician.
3. Call the patient's pharmacy. When indicated, press the option that will allow you to speak with a pharmacist.
4. State your name and the name of the doctor's office. Inform the pharmacist you are calling to refill a patient prescription. For example, you might say, "This is George calling Dr. Robinson's office with a prescription refill for Brenda Atkinson."
   Note: For clarity, it is often helpful to spell the patient's last name to avoid any confusion.
5. When prompted, provide the pharmacist with the patient's date of birth.
6. Provide all of the prescription information to the pharmacist. A succinct way to state the information is as follows: "Dr. Robinson is ordering Glucophage XR, 1000 mg to be taken once daily. Dispense 30 pills with two refills."
7. The pharmacist will repeat the prescription information to you. Listen closely to make sure there are no errors.
8. If necessary, provide the pharmacist with the prescription number of the patient's original prescription.
9. Thank the pharmacist, and restate your name and the office telephone number in case there are any questions after the phone call is completed
10. Document the phone call in the patient's medical record.

CHARTING EXAMPLE

11/25/20xx ,11:45 A.M.: Prescription refill phoned into Rightway Pharmacy. Rx was authorized by Dr. Robinson; Glucophage XR, 1000 mg, taken once daily, #30 x 2 refills.—George Beachly, CMA (AAMA)

TELEPHONE TRIAGE

Triage is a process used to determine the order or sequence in which patients should be seen for treatment. The severity of the patient's illness or injury determines the order of treatment. **Telephone triage**—determining the order in which to take patient calls—is an issue for the telephone screening process. By asking specific questions, the medical assistant can determine how to handle a patient's problem. Each office should have a policies and procedures manual that provides information regarding the office's preferred method of screening telephone calls.

Most patients call because they feel they need to see the physician. It will be one of your responsibilities to see that the patient is helped in the most appropriate manner. You will need to gather information from the patient. As with all telephone calls, the first thing you'll need to find out is the patient's name and telephone number, in case you become disconnected. Have the patient spell out his or her name to avoid mistakes. During the course of your conversation, ask for some basic demographic information in addition to medical information. Box 7-1 lists information that you should request from the patient. When scheduling the patient, enter the information you received from the patient in the appointment screen and save it in the patient's medical record.

As a medical assistant, you must be careful when screening patients on the telephone. You will be assessing a patient's symptoms. This, however, is very close to exceeding the medical assistant's scope of practice. Make sure that you are closely following the established telephone protocols that were agreed on by the physician. If ever a situation arises that is not covered in the policies and procedures manual, the medical assistant must ask the physician how to handle that particular problem. Follow only the protocols that the physician has approved.

Handling an Emergency Call

Every office should have a written protocol for handling emergency calls. Because you cannot see the telephone

caller, it can be difficult to determine a true emergency when talking to someone over the telephone. It is critical to get the caller's name and telephone number immediately in case you are disconnected. You will then proceed by asking the patient specific questions. Examples of questions you may ask, depending on your office's procedure, are listed in Box 7-2. If an emergency is taking place during the telephone call, alert the physician immediately.

In some cases, the patient may be hysterical or crying. Your job, in a situation such as this, is to calm the patient. If your voice remains calm and reassuring, you may be able to soothe the patient. If the caller is extremely upset, ask if someone else can come to the telephone. Your role is to gain as much information from the caller as possible so that the emergency can be handled quickly. Following are some types of emergencies you may face:

- Allergic reactions (anaphylactic shock)
- Asthma
- Broken bone
- Drug overdose
- Eye injury or foreign body in the eye
- Gunshot or stabbing wound
- Heart attack
- Inability to breathe, or difficulty breathing
- Loss of consciousness
- Accidental poisoning
- Premature labor
- Profuse bleeding
- Severe pain, including chest pain
- Severe vomiting or diarrhea
- Suicide attempt or suicide threats
- High temperature

- What is your name?
- What is your telephone number?
- Where are you?
- What is your relationship to the patient? (If a parent, spouse, friend, or passerby is calling)
- What is the emergency?
- When did the emergency occur?
- How severe is the emergency?
- What are the patient's symptoms? (Problems breathing? Bleeding? Extreme pain? Other symptoms?)
- What has been done for the patient?
- Has anyone called emergency medical services (EMS)?
- Who is the patient's primary physician?

Note: Some specialists, such as obstetricians and cardiologists, may have additional questions they wish to have you ask the caller. These will be specifically stated in a triage notebook or office policies and procedures manual.

The office should have a policy in place for how to handle emergency calls when no physician is present. Many times, medical office policies and procedures direct office staff to send the patient to a nearby emergency department. In this situation, *never* hang up the phone with the patient. Instead, while the patient is on the phone, signal a coworker for help and have your coworker call 911 on behalf of the patient. It is important to remain on the line with the caller until emergency medical services arrive. The office should also have the phone number of the local poison control organization in case the emergency is one that needs this service.

Never take an emergency call lightly. Emergencies can be life threatening. Even if you have questions about whether the call is actually an emergency, you must always assume it is and alert the physician. Malpractice suits have been brought against medical assistants who failed to correctly handle an emergency.

HANDLING DIFFICULT CALLS

You are likely to receive many types of problematic calls in a medical office, and the most important thing to remember when dealing with a difficult patient is not to lose your temper. Difficult patients can vary from those who are angry and yelling to those attempting to obtain confidential information. With any difficult caller, you must keep the situation as calm as possible. It is helpful to remember that the patient, more often than not, is displacing anger and is probably frustrated with some other situation, such as worry over an illness, having had a bad day, or suffering from pain.

When you have a difficult patient on the phone, the best approach is to be empathetic while remaining in control of the situation. Take the time to listen and find out the exact problem. Once you determine the problem, you can begin to help. When patients use inappropriate language, you may choose to tell them that you will not continue to speak with them if they continue to use foul language—if the physician or policies of the office permit you to take such a stand. Everyone, including you, is entitled to a certain level of respect and courtesy. In this case it is appropriate to hang up the call if the caller continues to use abusive language on the phone. Warn the caller that you will take this action before hanging up. Usually the caller will settle down and talk appropriately.

Alternatively, you may choose to ignore the foul language and reply as if the caller has used the most polite and courteous language, maintaining your standards of behavior and ignoring the caller's while attempting to find out if the caller has a real problem you can help with—and with the option to hang up if you determine that person does not have a legitimate problem.

USING A TELEPHONE DIRECTORY

When calling most insurance companies and hospitals, you encounter an automated *telephone directory* or **automated assistance program**—a telephone system that directs callers to the appropriate person through a series of questions.

After the call is answered automatically, the caller is presented with options so that the telephone system can direct the call to the proper person or department. Many large business systems provide additional options. When using one of these systems, it is important to pay close attention to the options that are offered because it can be easy to miss your cue. When you hear an option, the system will instruct you either to press the appropriate button or to state the option verbally. In most systems, if you cannot find an option to fit your needs, you can dial 0 to speak with an operator and direct the call. Document the date, time, and name of the individual you speak with in case you need to follow up in the future. It is also advisable to document a telephone number or extension where you may contact the individual directly.

The term *telephone directory* can also pertain to the telephone book provided to you by your local telephone company. These directories have two main sections: white pages and yellow pages. Usually, the white pages list the names, addresses, and telephone numbers of telephone service customers; the yellow pages list the names, addresses, and telephone numbers of local businesses. Sometimes a directory also contains a white-page business section. In addition, you will find emergency numbers, local government numbers, national area codes, local ZIP codes, and directions on making long distance calls, including international calls. Telephone directories are also available on the Internet and are becoming less used in the office, being replaced by Internet searches for specific information.

Long Distance Calls and Conference Calls

Occasionally, you will be asked to make long distance telephone calls for office business. In the past, a long distance call would be any call outside your area code. This is no longer true. Many larger cities have added area codes within local calling regions. Thus, you must know what is considered long distance in your area. Long distance calls can be very costly, so your office may limit how many are made. You may also be asked, at times, to set up a conference call, which may involve participants in long distance areas. Some offices assign long distance codes to each employee and, before a call being placed, that employee's long distance code must be keyed in. This measure can be used to track potential abuse of long distance calls.

Telephone Logs

Many offices maintain a telephone log to keep track of the long distance calls being made. When the telephone bill arrives, the log and the bill can be compared. This can help to identify any abuses of the business telephone with personal calls. Many logs have you list the name of the person, the facility or company being called, the number being called, the name of the person placing the call, the date and time of the call, the city and state to which the call is placed, the duration of the call, and the reason for it.

Making a Conference Call

A **conference call** is made when several people from different locations wish to have a joint discussion by phone. This means, for example, two physicians at a distance from each other may speak with a patient at a third location at the same time. These calls are more efficient and can save money in the long run because the participants do not have to make several separate long distance calls to relay the same information.

Most business telephone systems allow you to make conference calls without using a telephone operator. You will

need to determine if your telephone system allows you to do so. If your system is not set up for making conference calls, you may ask an operator to place the calls. See Procedure 7-5 for placing a conference call.

Time Zones

Time zones within the United States and foreign countries must be considered when placing long distance telephone calls or arranging conference calls. The continental United States and parts of Canada are divided into four time zones based on their location in the country: Eastern, Central, Mountain, and Pacific. As you move from east to west across the United States, there is a one-hour difference (earlier) in each time zone. For example, if it is 9:00 A.M. in Ohio (Eastern Time Zone), then it is 8:00 A.M. in Illinois (Central Time Zone).

Keep a time zone map posted near your office telephone (Figure 7-6) so you can plan long distance calls based on office hours in each time zone. A call placed at 3:00 P.M. in California will be received in New York at 6:00 P.M., which is usually after offices close. Also keep in mind that most states observe daylight saving time, when the clocks are set either one hour earlier or later. In the spring, clocks are set one hour ahead and in the fall one hour back. Some areas of the country do not observe the time change.

USING AN ANSWERING SERVICE

Many offices use an **answering service** when no one is available in the office. This service can be in effect 24 hours a day or just at designated times such as during the night, during lunch, or during peak hours of the day to relieve office staff.

The system works by forwarding office calls to the service, which is typically located at an off-site location. Answering service personnel answer the calls and inform the patients that the office is closed. They also take some non-emergency messages, which are delivered to the office when you return phone service to your care. When emergency calls come in, the answering service contacts the physician by pager or telephone. If a patient speaks with the answering service, it must be documented just as it would be if the call were answered by office staff. Most answering services fax the calls received, and physicians in turn document their responses and actions related to the call. Once the physician has completed the documentation, the information should be placed in the patient's record.

A fee is attached to answering services, but many offices consider this a necessary service. Offices have the option of using an answering machine or voice messaging system while the office is closed. This option is less expensive, but

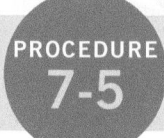

PROCEDURE 7-5

Placing a Conference Call

Objective ◆ *Allow for a discussion via the telephone between three or more parties from various locations.*

EQUIPMENT AND SUPPLIES

Telephone numbers of participating parties

1. Gather the telephone numbers of all participants before beginning the call.
2. Determine the time that everyone will be available for the conference call. You may have to call or e-mail people in advance to determine a convenient time. Be aware of time zone differences when arranging conference calls.
3. Dial 0 for the operator, and provide the name and telephone number (area code first) for each person to be called.
4. The operator will then place a call to each party. When all the participants are on the line, the operator will come back to the original caller (you) and the conversation can begin. If you are placing this call for your physician, he will pick up on your line (Figure A).
5. If you are setting up the conference call ahead of time, tell the operator when you wish the conference call to begin.

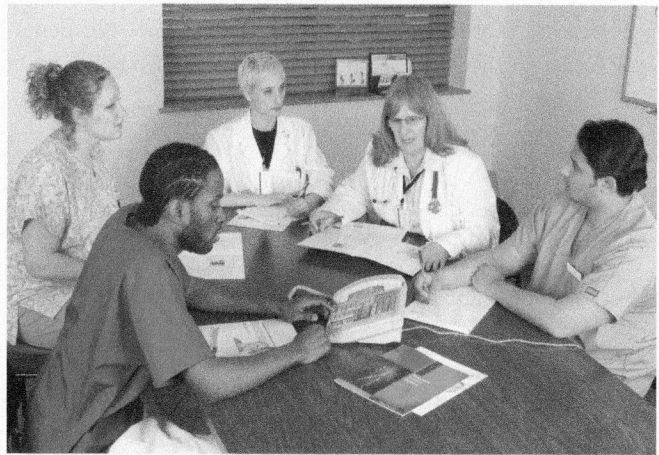

FIGURE A Conference calling by telephone allows three or more persons in different locations to speak with each other at the same time.

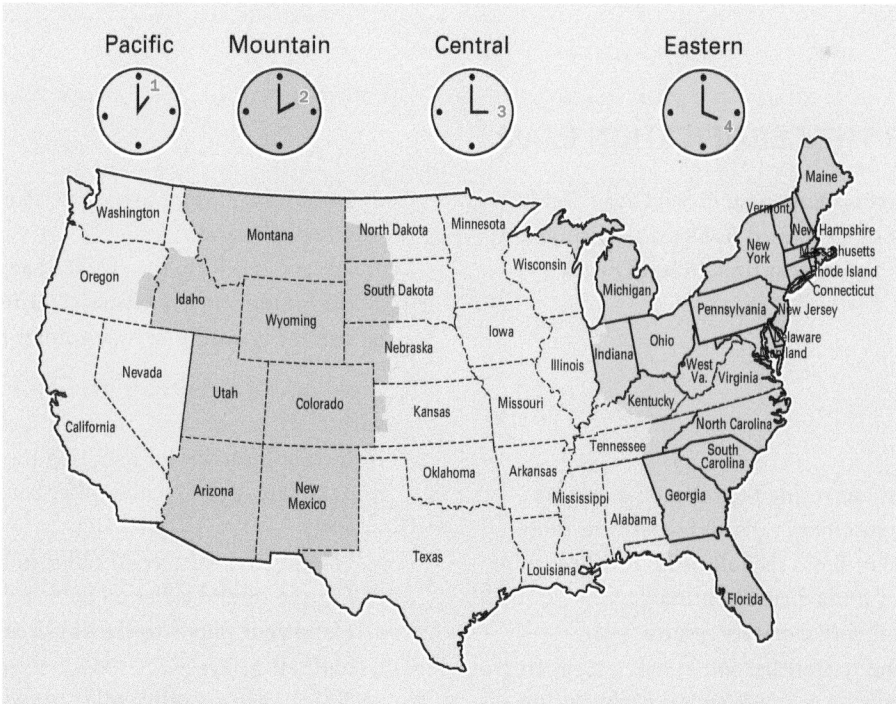

FIGURE 7-6 Having a time zone map located near the telephone will assist you when making long distance calls outside your time zone.

the patients' problems may not be addressed as quickly. If the office uses an answering machine or voice messaging system, you must ensure that the messages are retrieved in a timely manner and that the recorded office greeting provides a number to call in case of emergency.

SUMMARY

Medical assistants devote a good amount of their work day to telephone communication involving incoming and outgoing calls. Most first impressions of the office are generated based on the interaction on the telephone. Always greet the caller warmly and professionally. On a typical day, the medical assistant fields many different types of calls from patients, insurance companies, pharmacies, and others. Keep in mind that your ability to communicate and your telephone skills greatly affect the way others perceive the office where you work. Attention to detail is required while taking telephone messages. You must understand what information is required in order to complete the message. You are representing your office every time you speak. Take each call one at a time, and use the techniques and procedures presented in this chapter to work more efficiently while maintaining patient confidentiality.

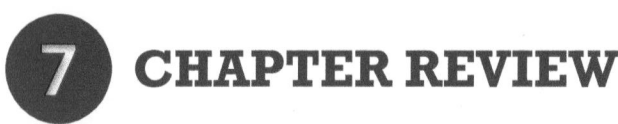

7 CHAPTER REVIEW

COMPETENCY REVIEW

1. Define and spell the terms for this chapter.
2. When it is 9:00 A.M. in New York, what time is it in (a) Pittsburgh, PA; (b) St. Paul, MN; (c) Los Angeles, CA; and (d) Denver, CO?
3. Write a telephone message for a patient who calls for a refill of Estrace 1 mg daily.

4. How might you handle receiving a prank telephone call?
5. Why should you smile when answering the telephone?
6. What do you do when you are helping a patient on one line and another line begins to ring?

PREPARING FOR THE CERTIFICATION EXAM

1. One of your patients is vacationing in San Diego, California, and calls your office located in Detroit, Michigan, at 5:15 P.M. What is the current time in San Diego?
   a. 5:15 P.M.
   b. 4:15 P.M.
   c. 3:15 P.M.
   d. 2:15 P.M.
   e. 1:15 P.M.

2. As the receptionist answering the telephone, you are required to triage incoming calls and determine those that are most urgent. From the following list, determine which call requires immediate attention:
   a. Patient is calling for laboratory results.
   b. Patient is calling to state her son is very groggy this morning and that he was tackled last night during a football game.

   c. Patient is calling to schedule an appointment for a school physical.
   d. Patient is calling to state she has developed hives since beginning a new medication last night.
   e. Patient is calling with a splinter in his knee.

3. A second call comes in while you are already on the phone with a patient. If the second call is an emergency, which is the best behavior for handling the first call?
   a. Take care of the second caller before returning to the first.
   b. Hang up on the second caller and call 911.
   c. Put the second caller on hold and go back to the first.
   d. Hand your phone to the physician to handle the second call.
   e. Tell the second caller to go immediately to the hospital.

4. Which of the following phone calls would necessitate the need to interrupt a physician while they are in an examination room with a patient?
   a. A prescription refill request
   b. A call from a patient regarding their progress while using a new medication
   c. A call from the physician's stockbroker
   d. A call regarding lunch with a pharmaceutical representative
   e. A call from a consulting physician regarding a mutual patient

5. When documenting a telephone message regarding an update on a patient's condition, all of the following must be recorded *except* the
   a. name of the person taking the message.
   b. patient's telephone number.
   c. patient's medical insurance copayment.
   d. time of the call.
   e. date of the call.

6. When answering the telephone, the medical assistant or receptionist should always pay close attention to the following regarding his or her speaking voice *except* for
   a. disinterest.
   b. enunciation.
   c. clarity.
   d. pitch.
   e. inflection.

7. Which of the following is an appropriate greeting for an incoming call?
   a. Thank you for calling. Dr. Smith's office. Please hold.
   b. Good morning. Dr. Smith's office.
   c. Good morning. Dr. Smith's office. This is Jenny. How may I help you?
   d. Good morning. Dr. Smith's office. This is Jenny. Hold, please.
   e. Dr. Smiths's office. This is Jenny.

8. When transferring a call, the receptionist should do several things, *except*
   a. notify the caller you are initiating a transfer.
   b. provide the name of the person to whom the caller is being transferred.
   c. stay on the line until the call has been transferred.
   d. transfer directly to voice mail.
   e. provide the extension number of the person to whom the caller is being transferred.

9. When taking a telephone message for a prescription refill, the following information must be obtained *except* for the
   a. name of the patient.
   b. prescription number.
   c. pharmacy website address.
   d. pharmacy telephone number.
   e. name of the medication.

10. When working in a busy office, it is inevitable that you will need to place callers on hold. Once the caller is on hold, how often should you check back with them?
    a. every three minutes
    b. every two minutes
    c. every one minute
    d. every 30 seconds
    e. every 90 seconds

CRITICAL THINKING

Refer to the case study at the beginning of the chapter and use what you have learned to answer the following questions.

1. How could Tonya have improved Carmine's experience when she went to place him on hold?

2. What should Tonya have done while Carmine was on hold for two minutes?

3. From the start of the conversation with Tonya, Carmine was displeased. What could Tonya have done to improve her communication with the patient?

ON THE JOB

For more than two years, medical assistant Linda Lewis has been employed by Drs. Norek and Klein, who are gerontologists. Also on staff are two registered nurses, a medical laboratory technician, and a medical social worker. The daughter of one of the doctor's patients has just called the office. She is very distraught at the seemingly diminished capacity of her mother and insists on speaking to the doctor.

Linda explains that both physicians only take emergency calls during patient appointment hours but that she will take a detailed message. The caller, however, suggests that not only should her call be considered an emergency but that she will sue the doctor if the call is not handled accordingly.

1. What should Linda do immediately to diffuse the situation?
2. Is this a case when the call should be passed on to one of the registered nurses or the medical social worker?
3. Is this a case when the physician should be interrupted to take the telephone call because of the threat of an impending lawsuit?
4. How could Linda ascertain whether this is indeed an emergency? Is it up to her, as a medical assistant, to make such a determination?

INTERNET ACTIVITY

Use the Internet and research the ways HIPAA has affected the use of the telephone in the medical office.

Administrative Medical Assisting

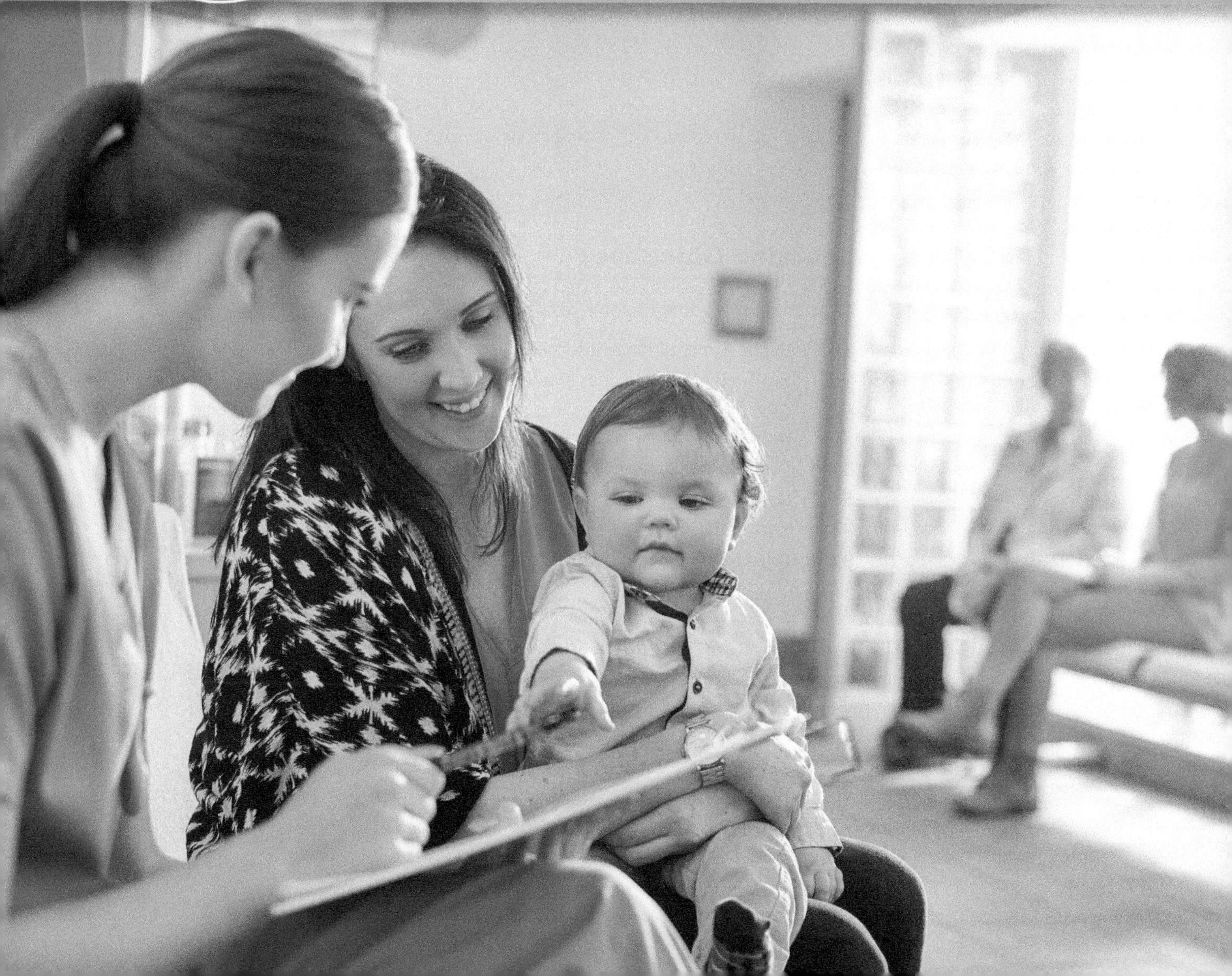

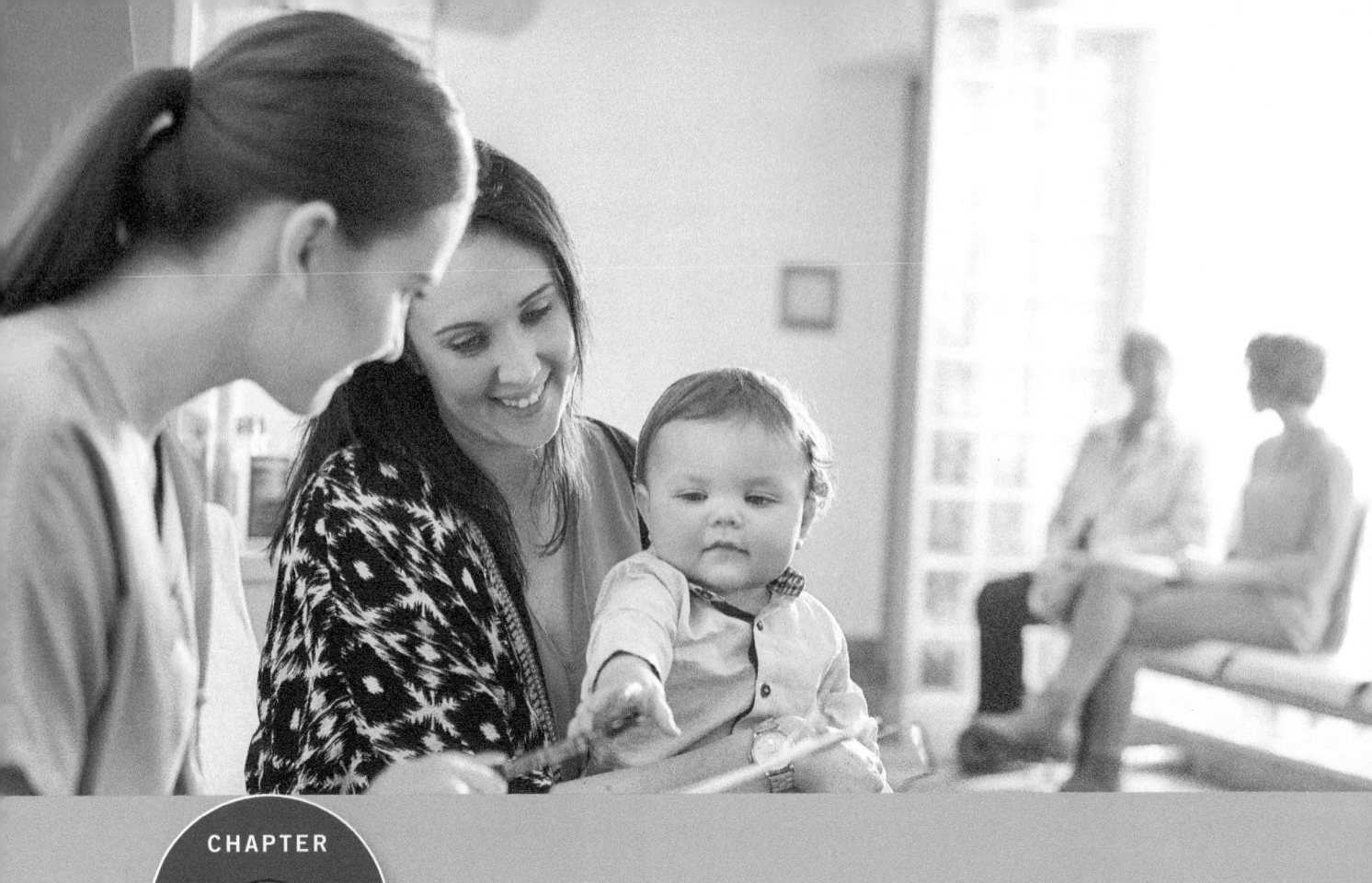

CHAPTER 8

Patient Reception

Learning Objectives

After completing this chapter, you should be able to:

8.1 Define and spell the terms for this chapter.

8.2 Explain the general duties of a receptionist.

8.3 Describe personal qualities that are important to displaying a professional image when working in patient reception.

8.4 Describe the characteristics of a well-maintained reception area.

8.5 Describe the process of opening the medical office for the day.

8.6 Explain the process of checking in a patient from start to finish.

8.7 Describe the process of closing the medical office for the day.

Tania Washington is responsible for opening Pearson Physicians Group on Tuesday and Thursday mornings. She arrives early and is the first employee at the office. There is a patient waiting at the front door to be let inside for his appointment that is scheduled for 45 minutes later, which is when the office is scheduled to open. When Tania opens the door to the office, she sees that the reception room has magazines strewn about, the children's books are not neatly piled, and the trash can has not been emptied.

Terms to Learn

assignment of benefits	demographic	pulling (charts)
collating	encounter form	queuing up
copayment	no-show	receptionist

atient reception requires a multiskilled individual who is able to multitask and whose manner, physical appearance, and tone of voice project a professional, confident, and caring person. A small office has fewer employees than one with several physicians; therefore, the medical assistant who acts as receptionist in a small office may perform many of the other tasks described separately in this chapter.

In the role of **receptionist**, the medical assistant greets and assists incoming patients and performs many important duties that make the office run smoothly and efficiently. Some of these duties are quiet and behind the scenes; others require constant interaction with patients. The medical assistant who functions as a receptionist must do everything possible to ensure patient safety and confidentiality at all times during the office visit.

This chapter has three main sections. First, you learn about the overall duties and responsibilities of a medical office receptionist with special emphasis on personal characteristics and physical presentation. Next you learn about the important responsibilities related to maintaining the reception area. Finally, you walk through the daily workflow in a typical office with a focus on your interactions with patients.

DUTIES OF A RECEPTIONIST

The number of patients as well as the nature of the medical practice—for example, a solo practice or a corporation of several physicians—determine the duties or tasks the

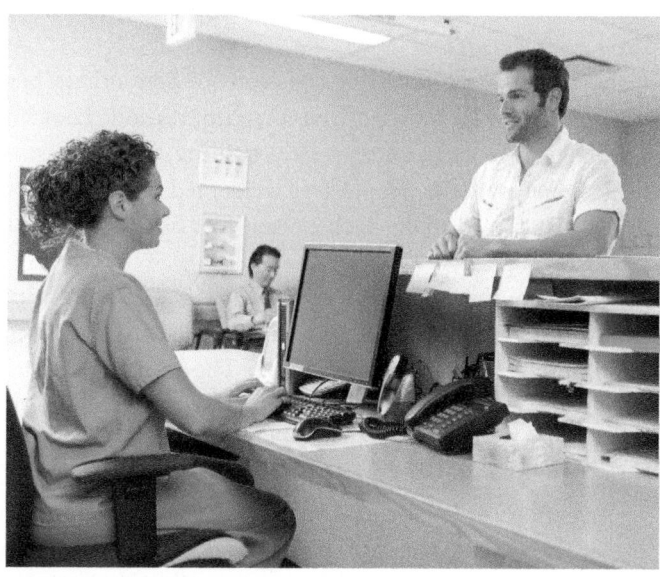

FIGURE 8-1 The medical assistant as receptionist in a medical office.

medical assistant performs in the role of receptionist (Figure 8-1).

The duties of a receptionist can include opening the office, greeting patients on arrival, assisting new patients with completion of the proper forms, collecting copayments, maintaining a clean and safe environment in the reception area, and managing any disturbance or medical emergency in the reception area. In addition, the receptionist may handle incoming telephone calls for the office, schedule returning appointments, and make reminder calls for upcoming appointments. See Box 8-1 for a list of receptionist duties.

BOX 8-1 | Duties of a Medical Receptionist

- Open the office.
- Queue up or pull charts for the next day's appointments.
- Collate patient records.
- Check in patients.
- Greet patients as they arrive and sign in.
- Update patient demographics.
- Help new patients fill out paperwork.
- Collect copayments and balances due from patients.
- Keep the reception area clean and safe.
- Keep office equipment in good working order.

- Manage reception area disturbances.
- Handle reception area emergencies.
- Handle incoming calls.
- Schedule appointments.
- Escort patients to exam rooms.
- Respect patients' time.
- Document patient no-shows.
- Prepare bank deposits.
- Close the office.

Personal Characteristics

As a receptionist, you are probably the first person patients see on entering the office. Your demeanor reflects on the entire office. Patients may choose to stay with a physician or not return based solely on how they feel they have been treated by the receptionist, regardless of how they feel about their medical care.

Receptionists need to be conscious of how others perceive them and give a positive first impression. Looking people in the eye, speaking clearly, smiling, and exercising basic courtesy help people feel welcomed and cared for. You must try to make each person feel he has your full attention.

The receptionist works at the hub of office activity. Many tasks and processes are taking place at the same time, so interruptions are common. The ability to switch between tasks quickly and cheerfully, without becoming irritated or losing track of what you were doing, is important.

Attention to detail and accuracy are also paramount. In the medical field, accurate spelling and numeric skills are vital and can impact a patient's care as well as the financial well-being of the office.

Physical Appearance

Careful grooming, good hygiene, and appropriate dress must be observed, because the medical receptionist's physical appearance also reflects on the entire office. A poorly groomed receptionist could send the unwanted message that the office is poorly maintained and not clean.

Office policy specifies the preferred clothing. In most offices, the clinical staff members all wear uniforms of the same type or color, which may consist of scrubs-type pants and top with a lab coat. The advantages of this type of uniform are that it can be worn by both male and female staff and is relatively inexpensive. Colors and patterns of uniforms are usually determined by the managers of the practice. Shoes must be closed-toe for safety reasons, and some offices ban wearing any shoes without a back, such as clogs. Shoes must be clean and skid resistant. Receptionists and other administrative personnel frequently wear the same style uniform as the clinical staff but without a lab coat, or they may be allowed to wear business-casual dress.

Hygiene, at a minimum, consists of daily bathing, use of a deodorant without a strong scent, good oral care, and clean, well-pressed clothing. Hairstyles and jewelry worn by male and female medical assistants should reflect professionalism, as should makeup. Accessories should be conservative and minimal—generally limited to one finger ring, a watch with a second hand, a name tag, and a professional association pin. Most offices do not tolerate any type of facial or tongue piercings, and tattoos may need to be covered. Long hair should be worn tied back and off the shoulders. Nails should be well trimmed, and only clear polish should be used. No perfumes should be worn, because patients can be allergic to certain scents.

Name pins or tags should be visible at all times. Many offices require a picture ID for security reasons. The photo should be visible to patients; this not a time for vanity or self-consciousness about your picture. ID with a magnetic strip can allow entrance into a secure area and also can be used to clock in and out for hours worked.

Communication Skills

Because medical receptionists spend a lot of time speaking with patients, on the telephone and in person, good communication skills are essential. Good communication requires listening to what others are saying, understanding their needs, and responding in a helpful and nondefensive manner. Refer to the chapter titled "Telephone Techniques" for more information on telephone skills.

MAINTAINING THE RECEPTION AREA

Just as the personal appearance of the receptionist makes a first impression on patients, so does the appearance of the reception area. (The term *reception area* is more positive than the outdated term *waiting room*.) An important but sometimes overlooked role of the medical assistant is taking care of the reception area. This area must be kept clean and free from any hazards that may injure a patient. A soiled or unkempt reception area may cause patients to be concerned about the overall cleanliness and sanitation of the office, including treatment areas.

Neatness

The reception area must be kept clean and organized (Figure 8-2). If patients see a messy, disorganized area, they may wonder about how their information is being handled. Regular cleaning keeps the reception room sparkling, pleasant, and smelling good. The receptionist must monitor the cleanliness and neatness of the room. If the room begins to get messy throughout the day, the receptionist may need to take a few moments to straighten it up. The receptionist may find it most convenient to check the reception room when returning from breaks and lunch. Planning a designated time for waiting area maintenance as part of the regular schedule helps make it easy to remember without interrupting your ongoing work flow. Magazines, brochures, patient education documents, and toys should be arranged neatly. Any papers lying around must be thrown away or destroyed, depending on the information they contain. Spills should be wiped up as soon as they occur.

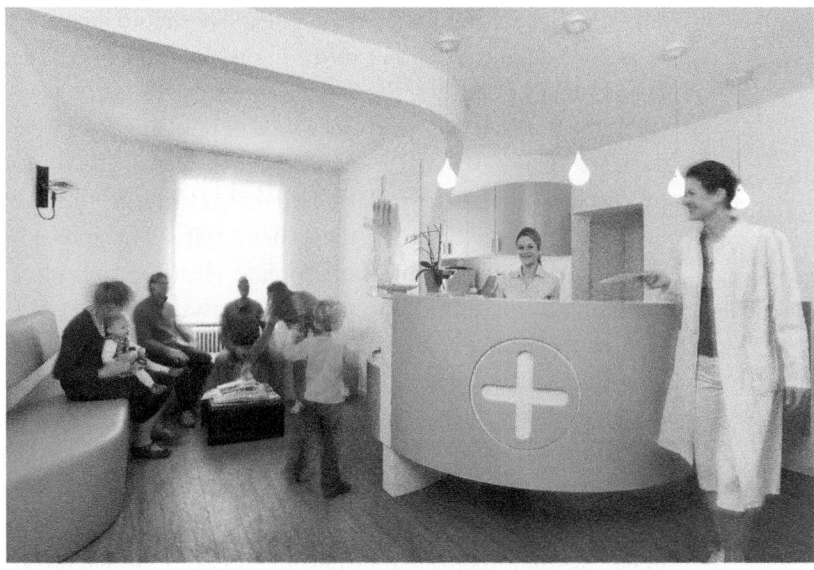

FIGURE 8-2 The medical reception area must be clean, organized, and pleasant.

Cleaning

Routine cleaning should be a high priority in any office and may be done by a professional cleaning service, a designated staff member, or some combination of these. The reception room should be dusted, vacuumed, and mopped every day. Trash containers should be emptied and any glass on the doors or table tops polished and kept free of fingerprints and smudges. It is best not to use commercial air fresheners or fragrances because some patients may be allergic to them.

Periodic deep cleaning is also necessary to keep the reception area healthful and looking its best. Carpets should be shampooed on a quarterly basis by a professional carpet cleaner. Traffic lanes may need cleaning more frequently. Upholstered furniture should be shampooed at least once a year. More frequent deep cleanings may be needed in a particularly busy office or one that sees a lot of children. Windows should be washed inside and out twice a year.

The receptionist is often the contact person for daily interactions with the professional cleaning service. A notebook may be kept at the reception desk in which the office can write any requests to the cleaning service and where the cleaning service can leave notes regarding any issues they may have noticed. Checking this notebook each morning and writing requests in it at the end of each day is a good way to keep communication flowing with outside cleaning contractors.

Furniture Placement

In addition to keeping the reception room clean and organized, the receptionist may also be responsible for placement of furniture. Most offices prefer arranging furniture in conversational groups rather than around the perimeter of the reception area. The path from the entrance to the receptionist's desk should be direct, with nothing in the way to hinder or trip the patient. Offices should have a designated area where patients can pause before approaching the reception desk. A sign may state, "Please wait here until the receptionist calls you." The sign should be placed 6 to 10 feet from the reception desk but out of traffic lanes.

Furniture should be placed to allow access and movement of wheelchairs. This means allowing a relatively straight traffic path approximately 36 to 44 inches wide and providing open space for wheelchairs to park near the seating area. It is also helpful to provide a desk or writing area no more than 36 inches high. At least one portion of the reception counter should be no more than 36 inches high so it is accessible to those in wheelchairs.

The type of furniture found in the office should be appropriate for the patient population. In offices that treat many older adults or frail patients, such as internal medicine and oncology practices, it is best to provide sturdy chairs and couches with seats approximately 20 inches above the floor. It is difficult for older adults and weak patients to rise from low furniture. In a pediatric office, it is helpful to provide plenty of smaller chairs and couches for children. Check for any damaged, soiled, or worn furnishings on a regular basis. Anything that poses a safety hazard should be removed until it is repaired.

Children's Area

Many offices maintain a designated area for children that is supplied with toys, books, and appropriately sized tables and chairs. This helps occupy children while waiting to see the doctor. Parents are responsible for supervising their children while they are in the play area. When straightening up the reception room throughout the day, staff should also straighten up the children's area. Toys should be cleaned and sanitized daily.

Television

Many offices have a television patients can watch while they wait. Typically, educational health information is shown. Whatever the topic, it should always be appropriate for patients. Keep the volume relatively low to minimize the overall noise level in the waiting area.

Lost and Found

It also may be the responsibility of the receptionist to take care of items patients mistakenly leave in the office. The

office may have a lost-and-found box for these items. Many offices try to contact a patient if it is known who the item belongs to. The office may have a policy as to how long unclaimed items are kept before they are thrown away or donated to a local charity.

DAILY WORK FLOW OF THE OFFICE

Although each day is a little different from the day before in the medical office, certain routines and processes are consistent and certain tasks must always be accomplished. The receptionist's day can be divided into opening the office and preparing for the day; working with patients before and after they are seen by medical staff; and closing the office and preparing for the next day.

Opening the Office

The medical assistant who opens the office should arrive 30 minutes before the start of office hours. In addition to the receptionist's friendly smile and welcoming greeting, a well-lighted, clean, and inviting environment does much to cheer patients. The receptionist should begin opening the office by checking the security alarm and disengaging it, turning on all lights, and checking the general status of the reception room, which should be tidy and clean. If the office maintains a communication notebook with the cleaning service, check for any new messages that may alert you to safety or maintenance issues in the office. Any area used for children's toys should be neat and safe. Magazines and books should be stacked or placed in wall racks.

If the office uses electronic health records (EHR), the medical assistant should make sure that computer stations in all the exam rooms and physician offices are turned on. It is also helpful to access each physician's schedule so it is displayed on the appropriate computer monitor or other electronic device.

If the office uses paper charts, the medical assistant should check to make sure all charts are pulled and prepared for that day's patients; this task may often be performed the previous afternoon. Charge slips should be printed in advance for the day with any balances due highlighted.

The cash box should be counted before any patients are seen; it is counted again and balanced at the end of the day. The balance at the beginning of the day should be exactly the same as it was at the end of the previous day. Counting cash should always be performed by two staff members, in each other's presence, to ensure accuracy and security.

A master list of patient appointments should be printed out, and copies of the master list should be placed on the desks of the clinical medical assistants and each of the doctors—but not in areas where patients may be able to see them.

The final task before opening the office is to check the answering service or voice mail. If messages have come in, the receptionist should document all calls, place messages on charts, and distribute them to the appropriate individuals. Occasionally, messages might require immediate action. The receptionist should bring those messages to the attention of the appropriate individual. If additional appointments were made, the receptionist should pull the charts and print encounter forms for these added patients. It may be the responsibility of the opening medical assistant to make sure that all examination rooms are prepared for use. Each office can have other duties for the receptionist based on its particular needs.

Using a spreadsheet or word processing program, create a checklist that lists the opening and closing procedures of the day, with a place for the person(s) performing the duties to sign off or initial as each is completed. A formal checklist helps ensure that nothing is missed. If the person who normally performs the opening or closing is absent, a checklist will help the person filling in to be more confident that everything is properly completed. See Procedure 8-1 for more about opening the office. Table 8-1 shows a sample format for a checklist.

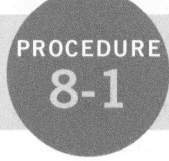

PROCEDURE 8-1 Opening the Office

Objective ◆ *Prepare and set up the office to receive patients and operate efficiently.*

EQUIPMENT AND SUPPLIES

Checklist of opening office procedures; office keys for rooms and files; message forms or pads; master lists of scheduled patients

1. Arrive at least 30 minutes before the first scheduled appointment.
2. Turn on the lights in the patient reception area before the first patient arrives.
3. Check that the heating or air conditioning and computers are working properly.
4. Turn on office equipment such as computers, copiers, printers, and fax machines. Fill all machines with paper.
5. Check the reception room for safety hazards such as frayed electrical cords, a slippery floor, or torn carpeting. Place a warning sign near any safety hazard, and report it immediately to the office manager.
6. Check magazines, and recycle any that are torn, damaged, or outdated.
7. Check for cleanliness, and report inadequate housekeeping services.
8. Unlock file rooms or cabinets where records are kept.

9. Take calls from the answering machine or faxes that may have come in from the answering service. Handle any that need immediate attention.
10. Unlock any money that may be used for the day. Count and balance the money to make sure that the amount is the same as it was when closing the office the day before.
11. Unlock the outer office door.
12. Queue up each physician's appointment schedule on the appropriate computer device, and verify that electronic charts for scheduled patients are accessible. Verify that all paper charts have been pulled and collated, together with a printout of each physician's master appointment list, if using paper records. If a patient has been added to the schedule after the records were pulled, pull, review, and add this patient's record to the other records.
13. Make phone calls to gather any laboratory test information that is missing from any patient's record. Provide the physician(s) and nurse(s) with a copy of the list of any laboratory test information that you have called for but have not yet received.
14. Print the day's patient schedule, and place it on the physician's desk or other designated area.

TABLE 8-1 | Sample Checklist of Opening and Closing Duties

Opening	M 1/2/YY	T 1/3/YY	W 1/4/YY	Th 1/5/YY	F 1/6/YY	Sa 1/7/YY
Turn on the lights.	DM	AP	CR			
Check heating or air conditioning.	DM	AP	CR			
Turn on computers, copiers, and printers.	DM	AP	CR			
Pick up phone messages.	DM	AP	CR			
Closing						
Check for missed orders.	AP	DM				
Document no-shows.	AP	DM				
Prepare medical records for tomorrow.	AP	DM				
Balance cash box.	AP	DM				

Preparing Office Equipment

For an efficient beginning to the day, all office machines such as copiers, computers, printers, and fax machines should be turned on and made ready for use. Many copiers take several minutes to warm up. Paper bins should be filled at the beginning of each day to avoid the frustration of running out of paper while performing an urgent task.

Managing Patient Records

Medical receptionists play an important role in helping physicians be prepared for their day by organizing and preparing patient charts. Much of this work may be done the day before the patient's appointment, in preparation for the next day, but the person opening the office each day is responsible for ensuring that all charts and paperwork are ready. That person may need to retrieve charts for patients scheduled at the last minute or may need to reorganize charts based on schedule changes and telephone messages.

A medical record or chart, which may be either electronic or paper-based, contains physician documentation for each patient visit as well as ancillary information for the patient, such as laboratory reports, radiology reports, operative reports, and reports from consulting physicians. The medical record contains only clinical information. The patient's financial information is stored in the patient file, which is maintained in the financial office, on paper, or on a computer system.

Queuing up (activating or displaying a computerized list) electronic charts or **pulling** paper-based charts is the process of preparing the medical charts of scheduled patients for the physician so that all pertinent information is readily available. The exact steps involved vary by office and depend on how much of the process has been automated. Many offices have automated part or all of the medical records

management process, which greatly simplifies preparation for the next day, because all the computer records for a patient are linked and can be accessed by selecting the appropriate menu item. Some offices can access the patient's record simply by clicking the patient's name where it appears on the appointment schedule. An office that is technologically advanced might not work with any hard copies. Some offices still use paper charts or are in the changeover period from paper to electronic.

Automated systems display a list of appointments for the day. This is accessible to each physician and each person in the back office, including medical assistants who are rooming patients. As each patient checks in, the receptionist checks him off in the computer. The back office is notified that the patient has arrived. After the patient is roomed, the electronic health record can be accessed in the examination room and updated throughout the appointment. The computer reconciles all visits at the end of the day and produces a list of patients who did not appear or for whom certain information, such as charges, is missing. It also generates a list of services provided and charges incurred so that the billing department can finalize all the information and submit it for insurance billing.

When working with physical records, the charts are collated. **Collating** is filing all information and test results for a patient into that patient's medical record, then sorting and organizing the charts in the order in which the patients will be seen. An **encounter form** may be placed with each chart, or it may be added at the conclusion of the visit. An encounter form, also called a charge slip or superbill, is a record of service for billing and for insurance processing. A printed appointment list is placed on top of the collated records. This serves as a checklist to keep track of patient arrivals and completed physician visits. As patients arrive, you verify their names on the schedule, and as they complete their visit and check out, you mark their names off the list or in the EHR. This system helps ensure that patients have checked in and checked out and that all encounter forms are accounted for. A copy of this same list is placed on the physician's desk on the morning of the patient's visit. A list may also be given to the person who is rooming patients that day.

Checking In Patients

In the medical office, greeting the patient is the first interaction in a check-in process that ensures that all the patient information is up to date and prepares the physician for the encounter. The check-in process includes signing patients in, registering new patients and explaining payment policies, updating information for established patients, and preparing encounter forms for the current visit. In all of this, medical receptionists should show courtesy and respect for patients and consideration of their time.

As a staff member, the medical receptionist is required by the Health Insurance Portability and Accountability Act (HIPAA) to always respect patient confidentiality and actively protect their privacy. Be knowledgeable about HIPAA regulations (discussed in detail in the chapter titled "Medical Law and Ethics") and act on them in everything you do. Confidentiality and privacy actions should become second nature to medical assistants.

Be aware of what you are saying and whether you can be overheard by other people. Do not speak with patients about their care around other patients. Speak only in a private area where you cannot be overheard.

The reception area should not function as a social gathering place for staff. Speak with other staff members about patients only when necessary for patient care. Talk with other staff where you cannot be overheard easily, not in a hallway, reception area, or other public area. Never discuss patients by name just to gossip, pass the time, or let off steam. It is disrespectful, and you never know who might hear.

In some offices, the receptionist sits behind a glass partition that slides open easily to personally greet each patient entering the office (Figure 8-3). If the receptionist is on the telephone when a patient enters, looking up and smiling is a good way to acknowledge the patient's presence. The reason for the glass partition is to protect the confidentiality of patients. Always close the partition when you are speaking on the telephone or to medical

office staff members. A violation of confidentiality can be grounds for a lawsuit.

Greeting Patients

If several patients arrive at the same time, they should form a short line next to or behind the sign that states, "Please wait here until the receptionist calls you." This is a privacy and safety measure. It allows any patient currently at the reception desk to speak privately, without other patients close by. It also allows the receptionist to finish phone conversations, money handling, or other sensitive matters out of hearing and viewing distance of patients. However, patients should not be kept waiting more than a few moments. When the receptionist is ready for the next patient, she should make eye contact, smile, and invite the patient forward with a friendly tone of voice and a standardized greeting, such as, "Welcome to City Clinic. I can help you."

Emergency patients or those with a contagious disease should enter the office through a private office entrance (if there is one) and be escorted directly into an examination room. This is done to limit exposure to contagious germs and not to alarm the other patients.

Patients must always take precedence over other visitors to the office, such as a medical supplier or pharmaceutical representative. Schedule such meetings when few or no patients are in the office whenever possible. Nonemergency conversations with other staff persons should always be interrupted to respond to a patient.

Signing In

An electronic or paper sign-in sheet is maintained at the reception desk. The sign-in sheet, which differs from office to office, usually contains space for the patient's name, the time

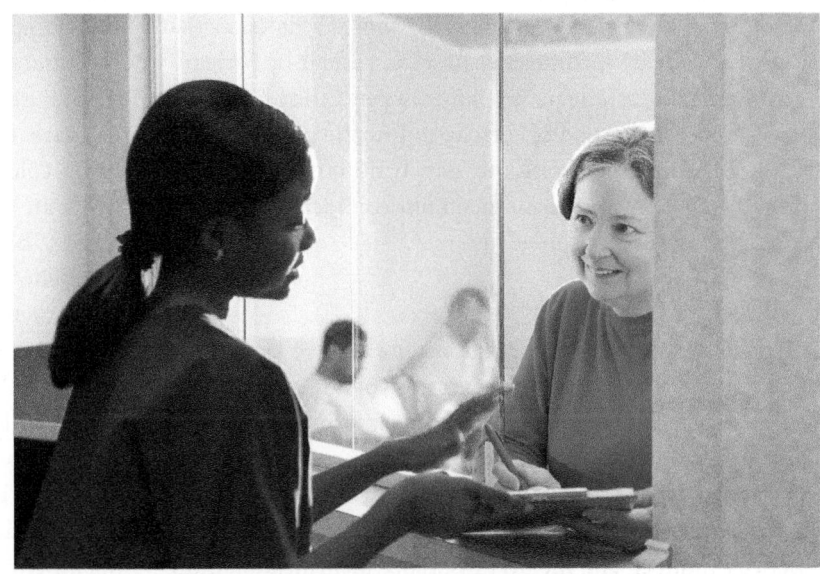

FIGURE 8-3 Each patient is greeted by the receptionist.

of arrival, and the name of the physician the patient will see. The sign-in sheet allows the receptionist to maintain a continuous record of all patients who come into the office.

Be sure the sign-in sheet used in your office is HIPAA compliant.

Electronic sign-in pads are small electronic screens with a stylus that the patient uses to sign in. The signature is stored electronically and is linked to the patient's appointment. Electronic sign-in pads provide complete confidentiality, away from the sight of other patients and they provide a permanent, easily accessible record.

Several types of HIPAA-compliant, paper-based sign-in sheets are available. They should contain only the patient's name, time of arrival, and the physician's name. The reason for the visit should not be listed. When patients arrive and sign in, they should not have access to the names of patients who signed in earlier. Some offices have patients sign in with first names only. It is also a good idea to set out an empty sign-in sheet frequently throughout the day.

Some paper formats use a sticker with carbonless paper underneath. This type of system requires patients to record their information on the sticker, peel off the sticker, and hand it to the receptionist. The information hidden under the carbonless paper is the information for office records, such as patient name, time of arrival, and reason for visit.

A similar sign-in sheet uses shingled tickets with numbered stubs. The patient hands the ticket to the receptionist and keeps the numbered stub. This method allows the office the option of calling patients back by either name or number. However, calling patients back by number has received mixed reviews. Some patients want to be called by name, as going to the doctor is a very personal experience and using numbers is impersonal. Others prefer not to have their name made known in the reception area. This is a decision that must be made by each practice, or even patient by patient.

In some offices, the paper sign-in sheet is filed in a designated folder at the end of the day to provide another record of the patients seen during that day. If the office policy is to destroy the sign-in sheet to maintain confidentiality, make sure these papers are shredded.

Preventing Identity Theft

Medical assistants have an important role in preventing identity theft. Identity theft is illegally obtaining and using another person's personal identifying information, usually for financial gain. Medical identity theft is using this information to obtain medical goods and services. Information sought or obtained includes name, address, birthdate, social security number, and medical insurance identification number. To help prevent identity theft, medical assistants should

verify **demographic** information such as address and birthdate when patients check in. Specifically, ask the patient to state, "What is your address?" or "What is your birthdate?" Do not ask questions that can easily be answered "yes" by anyone, such as "Is your address the same?" or "Is your birthday January 1?" It is advisable to make a copy or electronic scan of a patient's driver's license or state-issued identification at the first visit, then verify it on each subsequent visit by asking patients to show their card. Some offices take a photograph of each patient at the first visit and place it in the electronic health record, so the patient can be visually confirmed at each visit.

Tracking Appointment Status

As patients sign in or call to reschedule throughout the day, the status of the appointment should be marked on the electronic or printed schedule. Not only does this help keep the office organized, it assists in patient follow-up and provides documentation of patients who repeatedly miss appointments.

When using a computerized schedule, the user can make a menu selection to mark each patient as "arrived." Any patients who call to reschedule are automatically marked as "rescheduled" when the new appointment time is entered into the computer. Patients who do not keep their appointment and do not call to reschedule are marked as **no-show**. When the receptionist becomes aware of a no-show, she should note this on the schedule immediately. An electronic scheduling program generates reports to help the office identify no-shows and cancellations and it attempts to reschedule them. When the appointment schedule is linked to the EHR, the computer can make an automatic entry in the medical record regarding the missed appointment.

Offices using a paper-based scheduling system find it helpful to adopt a series of notations or colored highlighting to mark the status of each appointment. For example, if using colored highlighters, the medical assistant can highlight an appointment in green at the time each patient arrives. Blue can be used to indicate patients who reschedule, yellow for those who cancel and do not reschedule, and pink for no-shows. At the end of the day, the receptionist should review the schedule and make a list of all no-shows and cancellations who did not reschedule.

Regardless of whether the patient was rescheduled, place a notation on the patient's record about the failed appointment, the date, any action taken and the result, and the initials of the person performing the documentation. This documentation is important in protecting the physician should there ever be a lawsuit.

No-Shows. At the end of each day, one of the responsibilities of the receptionist is to account for no-shows and verify that the no-show is documented in the patient's chart. The reception-ist must learn and use the procedure for no-shows as stated in the office's policies and procedures manual. Some offices have a standard practice to phone the patient to determine why the appointment was not kept and to reschedule the appointment. A policy to charge for no-show appointments may be in place. However, the patient is responsible to pay the charge personally, because it cannot be billed to insurance. Placing reminder calls to patients the day before their scheduled visit may lower the number of no-shows. A designated staff member, usually the office manager, is responsible for informing the physician of the patient no-shows.

Registering New Patients

After patients sign in, the next step depends on whether the patient is new or established. New patients must fill out a patient registration form, the HIPAA Notice of Privacy Practices (NPP), a medical history form, and a payment agreement. Some offices mail these forms to patients to com-plete at home and submit at the first office visit. Others ask

---

JUDGMENT CALL

Denise and Amy share the receptionist duties in the office of Dr. Johns. Denise has been on maternity leave for the past two weeks and expects to be gone for another six weeks. Dur-ing this time, the office has chosen to use a temporary service to fill Denise's position until she returns. The temp's name is Shalonda. Amy and Shalonda are both responsible for check-ing in patients. When one of the older established patients, Ms. Yun, approaches the desk, Shalonda asks her to complete the information update form. Ms. Yun nods and heads over to one of the chairs in the reception room. After about 30 minutes, Dr. Johns approaches Shalonda and asks where his 11:30 patient is. He has a lunch meeting and doesn't want to be late. Shalonda asks across the reception area, "Ms. Yun, are you about done with that paperwork? The doctor has a lunch meeting and doesn't want to be late." Amy has heard what Shalonda said and asks Ms. Yun to step up to the desk.

Critical Thinking Questions

1. Even though the doctor needs to leave for a lunch meet-ing and is now running 30 minutes behind because Ms. Yun did not complete her paperwork on time, what ac-tions could have been taken to prevent this interaction?
2. What should Amy do?
3. Should Amy tell the office manager about Shalonda's in-teraction with Ms. Yun?

---

new patients to arrive 15 to 30 minutes early to complete the necessary forms.

The patient registration form requests demographic information, such as address, contact information, age, gen-der, education, and insurance information (Figure 8-4). The NPP informs patients of their rights regarding HIPAA. The medical history form records patients' current health issues, as well as past illnesses, family medical history, and lifestyle habits, such as alcohol consumption, smoking, and recre-ational drug use. The payment agreement explains the office's financial and payment policies.

Offices using EHRs may have patients supply the regis-tration information online, or the office may have a com-puter in the reception area that allows the patient to complete registration electronically at the office (Figure 8-5).

When using a paper-based system, place the registration form on a clipboard with a pen attached and ask the patient to complete it while waiting to be seen by the physician.

No matter which registration method is used, provide the patient with clear instructions. Briefly explain the pur-pose of each form. Be sure that patients are able to access all the electronic forms required, and explain how to navi-gate between fields. On paper forms, highlight or circle the sections the patient must complete. Point out if two sides are to be completed. Highlight or draw an arrow where the patient's signature is required. Assist patients who are unable to read and write because of illiteracy or a disability. Realize that many patients who cannot read or write may be embarrassed by this and do not readily admit they are unable to complete the forms. If you believe they may need assistance or it is taking longer than usual for

PATIENT REGISTRATION FORM
(Please Print)

Date: _____

Patient's
Name: _____
     First   Middle   Last

DOB: _____ / _____ / _____
     Month Day Year

Address: _____
     Street   City   State   Zip

Phone: _____ / _____ - _____
     (Area code)

Patient's SS#: _____ - _____ - _____   Driver's License #: _____   Occupation: _____

Method of payment (circle):   cash   check   credit card   insurance co-payment

Primary Insurance Co.: _____   Policy/Group #: _____

Medicare #: _____   Medicaid #: _____

Person
Responsible
For Payment: _____
     First   Middle   Last   Relationship

Address: _____
     Street   City   State   Zip

Phone: _____ / _____ - _____
     (Area code)

Employer Name: _____
     First   Middle   Last

Dept: _____

Address: _____
     Street   City   State   Zip

Phone: _____ / _____ - _____
     (Area code)

Spouse or
Nearest Relative: _____
     First   Middle   Last   Relationship

Address: _____
     Street   City   State   Zip

Phone: _____ / _____ - _____
     (Area code)

How were you referred to this office? _____

_____

Statement of Financial Responsibility: I, _____
do hereby agree to pay all medical charges incurred by the above listed patient. I further understand
that these charges are my responsibility, regardless of insurance coverage.

Responsible Person's Signature: _____

FIGURE 8-4 Patient registration form.

FIGURE 8-5 A computerized patient registration form used by offices with electronic health records.

them to complete the forms, you may quietly ask, "Do you have any questions about the forms? They may be confusing and I'm glad to assist you." You may want to help them in a private area of the office.

Updating Established Patients

Established patients may or may not need to complete paperwork, depending on how long it has been since their last visit. Some offices ask patients to update their medical history, sign new HIPAA forms, and sign new insurance authorizations once a year. At every visit, it is important that the medical assistant ask patients to verbally confirm their current address and telephone number as well as insurance information. This should be done at every visit, even if the patient has been in the office recently. Contact and insurance information can change over the course of even a few weeks. Remember to always speak in a manner to minimize other patients overhearing. HIPAA requires that every attempt be made to protect patient privacy. For example, in a quiet voice, the receptionist should ask the patient, "Mr. Jones, will you please verify your address?"

Explaining Payment Policies

Another important task when greeting both new and established patients is to review or explain your office's policies regarding billing and payment. Along with verbally explaining these policies, it is advisable to give each new patient informational brochures. The patient must also sign an **assignment of benefits** form,

Professionalism   The Law

Medical receptionists should be familiar with the office policy regarding cancellations and no-shows. Scheduling software is useful in tracking and flagging patients with repeated no-shows or cancellations so they can be contacted according to office policy. If the patient fails to keep two or more appointments, the physician should be informed. Lack of patient follow-up can have a negative impact on the patient's health status, and the physician could be held liable. In extreme cases, the physician may choose to terminate the patient from the practice. This requires the physician to send a letter to the patient stating that treatment will be terminated as of a certain date, usually with at least 30 days' notice. The letter should be sent as both certified with return receipt requested and as regular mail.

which authorizes the insurance company to send payments directly to the physician.

Request to see the patient's insurance card(s), and ask the patient politely if any insurance information has changed since they received the card. Also ask returning patients if their insurance has changed since their last visit, and make a copy of the insurance card at least once a year. This can decrease the chances of lapsed coverage. Scan or photocopy both sides of the insurance card(s), and be sure that the copy is legible. This may require using a darker than normal setting on the copy machine. Important information for insurance billing appears on the back of the card. Insurance billing cannot be processed without complete and legible information.

Check the insurance card to determine if a patient copayment is required. Indicate the copayment in the appropriate place on the patient's file. **Copayments** are designated amounts that some medical insurance plans require patients to pay for medical services. Most medical offices expect to receive copayments at the time of service, and some insurance plans require that copayments be collected at each visit rather than billing the patient after the fact. The copayment may be collected before or after the visit, depending on office procedure. The receptionist is often the person in charge of accepting office payments. She may also be responsible for collecting balances on accounts and copayments. It is important to keep excellent records of all incoming money so that balancing at the end of the day is easier.

Depending on the type of insurance the patient has, the receptionist may need to call the insurance company to verify the patient's coverage and the participation status of the physician with whom the visit is scheduled. See Procedure 8-2 for more information on how to register a new patient.

Collecting Copayments

Depending on the type of insurance patients have, they may be required to make a copayment at each visit. Copayments help establish patient financial responsibility and must be paid if the insurance plan requires it. Furthermore, the physician's contract with the insurance company or managed care plan holds the office responsible to collect the copayment at each visit. Generally, it is not allowable to bill the patient for copayment after the visit; it must be physically paid at the time of service. If patients have several visits within a short time, they cannot "save up" and pay all the copayments at one time; they must be paid at each individual visit. Many offices post a sign near the reception desk that states, "Copayments are due at the time of the visit." Although usually it does not matter whether the funds are

collected before or after the patient sees the physician, in most cases it is best to collect the money when the patient signs in. By doing this, you minimize the risk of the patient leaving at the end of the visit without paying. However, some offices prefer to wait and collect the copayment at the conclusion of the visit.

In most offices, patients may pay by cash, personal check, or credit card. Each patient should receive a printed receipt for the payment. The patient may need it for insurance purposes and to document tax deductions, and the medical office's accounting department needs a receipt in order to account for all monies received. A receipt is also a safeguard against financial mishandling or embezzlement. Even if the patient says she does not need a receipt, one should be produced. If the patient does not want to take it with her, you may shred it or place it for confidential destruction. See Procedure 8-3 for more information on how to collect copayments.

Initiating Encounter Forms

The **encounter form** (also referred to as the charge slip or superbill) is used in most medical offices to collect service information for the billing process. The encounter form contains a list of the most common procedure codes, called Current Procedural Terminology (CPT®) codes, and diagnosis codes, called International Classification of Disease (ICD-10-CM) codes, which are reported to insurance companies for reimbursement.

The appropriate encounter form is attached to the medical record of each patient who is to be seen by the physician on that day. Automated offices may print out an encounter form from the computer. Some offices handle the process entirely electronically, so that no paper form is required. In such cases, the codes are determined after the visit, based on the documentation provided by the physician. Some offices use a charge plate system or computer program that

Professionalism

Patients may be confused about the requirements of their insurance policy. As the medical receptionist, you provide a valuable customer service by clearly and politely explaining the patient's financial obligations and the office's payment policies. Most patients are glad to comply with the policies when they understand them and know the expectations. Do not apologize to the patient for requesting payment or explaining financial obligations. Just be matter-of-fact about it. Without proper payments, the medical office would not be able to remain open.

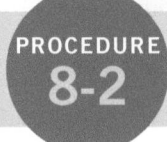

Registering a New Patient

Objective ◆ *Complete a registration form for a new patient.*

EQUIPMENT AND SUPPLIES

For paper-based charts: registration form, pen, clipboard, private area; for electronic health records: computer and possibly online access

Note: If the patient has not completed a registration form before the appointment, the receptionist may need to assist the patient.

1. Gather the supplies.
2. Verify that the patient has not been seen in the office before.
3. Obtain and record the following information from the patient:
   - Full name spelled correctly
   - Date of birth
   - Home address, including zip code
   - Telephone number, including area code
   - Cell phone number, including area code
   - Marital status
   - Employer
   - Employer address
   - Employer telephone number
   - Social security number
   - Insurance information, including group number
   - Insurance subscriber's name
   - Insurance copayment amount (photocopy or scan both sides of the insurance card)
   - Name of the guardian, if applicable
   - Name of the person responsible for payment
   - Address of the person responsible for payment
   - Telephone number of the person responsible for payment
   - Photocopy of the patient's photo ID, such as a driver's license or military ID
4. After the preceding information has been documented, review everything with the patient to ensure accuracy. Double check that each required piece of information has been completed.
5. For patients who are unable to complete the form themselves, document within the record that the patient verbally provided the documented demographic information, verify everything for accuracy, and have the patient sign in the appropriate area. The receptionist completing the form should also sign and date it.
6. Ask the patient to read and sign the HIPAA Notice of Privacy Practices. If the patient declines to sign the form, write a note on the form indicating that the patient refused to sign and, if possible, the reason. The receptionist writing the note should sign and date it. Remember that HIPAA requires that patients be notified of the privacy practices and *asked* to sign the form, but does not *require* a signature. This form is a consent, not an authorization. Patients who do not sign the form can be seen by the physician, and their information can be processed and used in a manner consistent with the privacy notification.

CHARTING EXAMPLE

6/7/YY, 2:00 P.M. Information provided verbally by patient, Rena Jones. On completion of documentation, reviewed information with patient for accuracy. Patient confirmed information correct as noted. L. Ritchie, RMA

imprints the patient's name and identification number on all forms used in the medical office, including the encounter form.

Completing the Check-in Process

When you are done checking in the patient or attending to other needs, it is very helpful to tell the patient exactly what to do next. This may be something like, "You may sit down in any chair to fill out these forms, then bring them back to me when you are done." Do not assume that patients know what you need them to do next.

When patients have completed all the forms, review them to ensure that all are completed correctly in their entirety and that all signatures are in place. If something is missing, politely ask the patient to supply the missing information. When everything is completed, say thank you and ask the patient to have a seat until the doctor is available.

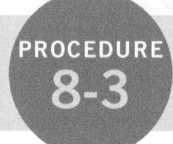

PROCEDURE
8-3

Collecting Copayments

Objective ◆ *Collect a copayment from a patient.*

EQUIPMENT AND SUPPLIES

Computer or ledger card; cash box; credit card terminal

1. Gather the supplies.
2. Access the patient's computerized or paper-based financial account.
3. Verify the patient's identity.
4. Verify that the insurance information on file is current, or obtain updated insurance card and policy information.
5. Look up the amount of the copay for the type of visit the patient has scheduled. Some insurance plans have different copays for different types of visits. The copay for a preventive care visit may be $0, and the copay for a problem-oriented visit may be $10 or $20.
6. Say to the patient, "Your copay today is $_____. How would you like to make payment? We accept cash, check, credit, or debit card."
7. Accept the payment.
    a. If the patient pays in cash, count the money to be certain it is the correct amount. If the patient requires change, lay the patient's payment next to the cash box, remove the amount of change, and count it out to the patient. After the patient accepts the change, place the original money in the cash box. Enter the payment amount and form of payment (cash) on the patient's financial record.
    b. If the patient pays by check, verify that the name and address on the check are correct. Verify that the payment amount is correct and that the check has been signed. Some offices allow the patient to leave the *Pay To* field blank, then use a rubber stamp to apply the

office's name in the appropriate place. This should be done in the presence of the patient. Enter the payment amount, form of payment (check), and check number on the patient's financial record. Place the check in the cash box or other designated place.
    c. If the patient pays by credit or debit card, verify that the name on the card is correct. Ask the patient if debit or credit will be used. Swipe the card in the credit card terminal, select debit or credit, and enter the payment amount. Follow instructions for your specific terminal to complete the transaction. Patients paying by debit need to enter their PIN number. Ask the patient to sign the electronic signature pad or paper slip. If required by your system, verify the last four digits of the card number and the three-digit security code on the back of the card. Enter the payment amount, form of payment (credit or debit card), and credit card transaction number on the patient's financial record. Place the charge card receipt in the cash box or other designated place.
8. Generate a receipt for the patient showing today's visit and the amount paid. Patients paying with a credit card should receive two receipts, one from the credit card terminal that documents the charge to their card and one from the patient's financial account showing the amount posted to the account.
9. Thank the patient for the payment, and give instructions on what to do next, such as, "Thank you. You may have a seat and someone will call you back in a few minutes, when the doctor is ready to see you."

Remember that you should not leave computer screens or paperwork visible where others might see them.

Consideration for the Patient's Time

One of the most common complaints expressed by patients is the excessive amount of time they have to spend in the reception room before being seen by a physician. Patients generally are understanding when they are told the physician has an emergency that has resulted in a schedule delay. However, offices need to ensure that the physician is not

running behind schedule because of errors with the scheduling process.

Patients typically respond well to a quiet explanation from the receptionist regarding how long the wait is expected to be. Be aware of waiting times so that patients are not "forgotten" by the receptionist. Periodically check on your waiting patients. Know the office policy regarding which type of complaint is seen immediately by the physician.

A 20-minute wait is accepted by most patients. If the wait is going to be longer, then you should approach each patient and ask if the patient prefers to wait or wishes to reschedule the appointment. If the expected wait time exceeds 20 minutes, the receptionist should inform the patient as soon as possible. This may mean notifying the patient of the delay either before or after he has checked in. For instance, if the physician is running two hours behind, the receptionist should attempt to contact the patient before arriving at the office and let patient know of the delay. Patients appreciate this because it gives them the opportunity to adjust their schedule to accommodate the later appointment or to reschedule the appointment, if necessary.

Escorting the Patient into the Examination Room

All patients should be personally escorted into the examination room (Figure 8-6). In most instances, this is done by a medical assistant who is assigned to patient care, rather than by the receptionist. If, however, you are asked to help "room" patients, make sure you select the correct record and clearly call the patient by name (or number). To ensure that you have the correct patient and chart, ask the patient to state his or her name and date of birth and check it against the information on the chart. Never use a patient's first name unless the patient has asked you to do so. Walk at the patient's speed, and offer assistance to patients using a wheelchair, crutches, a walker, or a cane. You may wish to make pleasant conversation to make the patient feel at ease. If the patient is a small child or in a wheelchair, make sure you are at eye level when you speak with them.

After the patient arrives in the exam room, clearly explain exactly what articles of clothing the patient should remove. It is important to be specific, because it can extend a patient's appointment time if the physician is unable to perform an examination because the patient has not been correctly prepared. The patient may feel embarrassed if more clothing has been removed than was required. Point out the gown or sheet for the patient to use after undressing, and make sure the patient knows whether the gown is to open in the front or the back. If you suspect a patient needs assistance removing clothing, ask if you may help. If the patient is of the opposite gender from the medical assistant, offer assistance from someone of the same gender, when possible. Always protect the patient's modesty; the patient will appreciate it.

When the patient is situated, state approximately when the doctor will be in to see him. If the doctor is delayed, assure patients waiting in examination rooms that the doctor hasn't forgotten about them. If the patient has to wait in the exam room to see the doctor, make sure that appropriate reading material is available.

If EHRs are used, be certain that no data is visible on the computer screen. This requires that the user log out of the system. When not in use, the computer system may be set up to display a blank screen, generic photographs or graphic images, or health education information. If a paper chart is being used, it is often placed in a slot or box just outside the examination room. The patient's record should be placed in the proper location so that patient information is not visible to anyone walking by. This may require placing the chart in the box so the patient information faces the wall.

Never leave patients alone with their chart. They may read something they do not understand and become upset. There is also the potential that a patient might remove a page or pages, resulting in an incomplete chart. In the worst case, if the patient were someday to bring legal charges against the physician, the incomplete chart might not support the physician's case because of missing documentation. The "golden rule" of documentation is the following: *If it is*

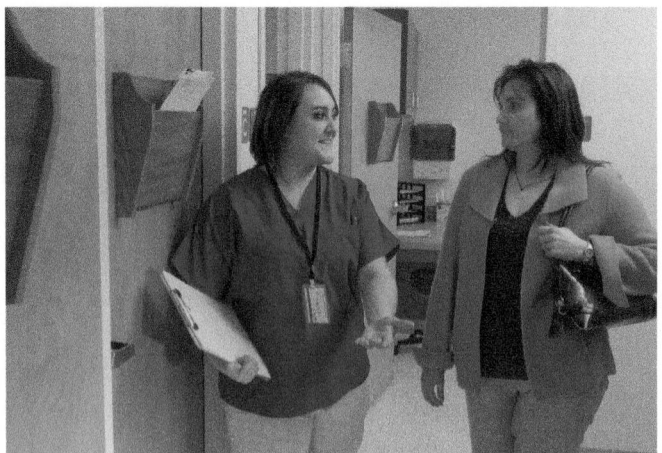

FIGURE 8-6 The medical assistant escorts the patient into the examination room.

not documented, it didn't happen, so it is critical to ensure that information is not removed from the chart or lost.

Completing the Patient Visit

After the physician has completed the exam, return to the examination room and knock before entering. Give the patient instructions about what to do next. For example, you might say to the patient, "You may dress now. The doctor will come back to talk to you shortly," or "Please stop at the reception desk (or other designated area) after you have dressed, and I'll explain the test the doctor has ordered." Offices with EHRs may provide patients with a computer printout that summarizes the visit, treatment prescribed, follow-up instructions, and educational information regarding the patient's condition.

At the end of the visit, the physician indicates on the encounter form what treatment was given, the supporting diagnosis, and the charge. The encounter form is then given to the receptionist or the cashier. Payment or arrangements for payment are made before the patient leaves the office.

All patients are entitled to and should receive a copy of the encounter form before they leave the office. When there is no charge for the visit, as in a follow-up visit after surgery, the physician should write "no charge" or "N/C" on the slip. For accounting purposes, an encounter form number is assigned to each patient, including those with no charge. This makes it possible to track and reconcile all charges and patient visits.

Some offices provide patients with paperwork that summarizes their visit. Double check that each patient receives all their intended material and does not receive someone else's papers.

Make it a point to speak with patients before they leave. Always ask patients if they have any additional questions. In some cases, a patient may need to make a payment, talk to the cashier, make another appointment, or have a specific test or procedure explained. If discussion is needed, it should be done in a private area out of the hearing range and view of other patients. Remember that HIPAA regulations prohibit discussions involving protected health information (PHI) with patients taking place in any area where another patient may overhear.

When a patient is checking out, make it clear when everything is complete by saying, "That takes care of everything today. Please call us if you have any questions. The exit door is to your left. Have a great day."

Patient Education

Although most patient education is provided by the clinical staff, it begins when the patient calls for an appointment. Patient education also occurs at the reception desk and in the reception area. For example, education regarding office hours, policies, insurance form submissions, and after-hours emergency telephone numbers can be handled at the reception desk. The receptionist may be responsible for providing and explaining instructions regarding tests and procedures, such as fasting before a particular blood test. In smaller offices where the receptionist handles insurance processing, education can take place regarding the patient's responsibility in the insurance reimbursement process.

Level of understanding. Always ensure that patient communication is provided at a level the patient understands. It is best to ask the patient to restate what you have said. This offers an opportunity to assess the patient's level of understanding. If it is apparent the patient didn't quite understand the first attempt, reword the information to an appropriate level and ask the patient to restate it again. If the educational information seems to confuse the patient or is extensive, it is best to provide written information for the patient. No matter the level of patient understanding, always stress the importance of calling the office if more instructions or clarification is needed.

Many times patients feel more comfortable asking for clarification from the receptionist or medical assistant than from the physician. If the patient asks a question you cannot answer or are unsure how to answer, do not hesitate to ask the physician or another individual in the office who might be able to help.

Professionalism

Although medical assistants may be concerned that saying, "I don't know the answer to your question" may make them appear unprofessional, the opposite is true. Medical assistants demonstrate a high level of professionalism by knowing their limits and scope of practice, then indicating that they will find someone who can answer the question. It is important for medical assistants to present this in a positive manner and not appear annoyed or frustrated by the patient's question. A positive and polite response would be, "That's a very good question. I don't know the answer myself, so may I find someone who can discuss this with you? It should only take a few minutes." This reassures patients that they have been heard and that the medical assistant is concerned about providing them with an accurate response. It is never appropriate to guess at an answer or give advice about something beyond your scope of training.

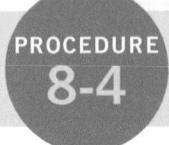

Closing the Office

Objective ◆ *Secure the office properly during nonoperating hours.*

EQUIPMENT AND SUPPLIES

Checklist of office closing procedures; bank deposit forms and envelope/pouch; office keys for rooms and files

1. Allow at least 15 to 30 minutes at the end of the day to close the office.
2. Check all records used during the day for any orders that may have been missed.
3. Check the appointment schedule, and verify that there is an encounter form or posted visit for every patient who came in. Make a list of no-shows and cancellations who did not reschedule.
4. Balance the cash box in the presence of another staff member. Ensure that the total amount of cash and checks matches the amounts recorded by the computer system. Prepare a deposit of the day's receipts. Place the deposit in the office safe unless you will make the bank deposit on your way home. It is wise to have the person designated to make the daily bank deposit vary the time of deposit. Many offices use a courier for this task. For purposes of accounting controls, the person preparing the bank deposit and the person actually making the deposit should be different. Both people should be bonded.
5. Queue up or pull records for patients who will be seen the next day. Place the collated records with the encounter forms attached and the master list of the next day's scheduled patients together in the appropriate place. Also, make a copy of this master list of patients for each physician.
6. Follow office policy regarding computer data backup. This might require verifying that the system is set to automatically back up data, executing a command to start a backup, or replacing back-up media. (See the chapter titled "Computers in the Medical Office" for more information on computer data backup.)
7. Lock all files and file rooms, physician offices, and other individual offices within the medical practice.
8. Turn off electrical equipment and appliances. *Note:* Some equipment, such as incubators, fax machines, and computers, may require 24-hour operation. Check with your supervisor regarding the special requirements of your office.
9. Check all examination rooms to make sure they are clean and supplied for the next day.
   Note: This step may be done by the medical assistant who was in charge of rooming patients that day.
10. Straighten the reception room. Put away all magazines and pick up any toys.
11. Leave any instructions for nighttime cleaning personnel in a designated place.
12. Activate the answering service before leaving. Know the name of the physician who is accepting emergency calls or is on call until morning. Remind the physician who is on call.
13. Lock all doors except the one you will use to exit.
14. Activate the security system if there is one. Turn off the lights per office policy.
15. Lock the door after you exit. Take two steps away, then step forward again to double check that the door is locked.

Closing the Office

Closing the office at the end of the day is a major function of the medical assistant. This function is critical to operating a well-run office. The purposes of closing procedures are to ensure the security of the premises and to prepare in advance for the next day. A list of no-shows and cancellations that did not reschedule should be printed from the computer or manually compiled from a paper-based schedule. The cash box should be counted and balanced in the presence of another staff member and a deposit consisting of the day's cash receipts and checks prepared. Next is queuing up EHRs or pulling paper charts for patients scheduled for the next day. Finally, equipment and lights should be turned off and all doors secured. A procedure for closing the office at the end of the day is presented in Procedure 8-4.

SUMMARY

The receptionist's role can be one of the most demanding and most interesting positions in the medical office.

While attending to the general running of the office, the medical assistant serving as receptionist must greet all patients, assist new patients in registering while obtaining updated health and insurance information, answer calls, schedule patients, open and close the office, contact and document no-shows, and more. All this requires a calm, caring, and organized individual who can keep patient information confidential and protect the safety of the patient during the office visit. The patient is most important.

8 CHAPTER REVIEW

COMPETENCY REVIEW

1. Define and spell the terms for this chapter.
2. Explain the steps to take if you are the first person to arrive and must open the medical office.
3. Describe how a professionally groomed receptionist should appear.
4. Explain what you would do if a patient suddenly collapsed in the reception room.
5. Explain the steps a medical assistant should take to collect a copayment from a patient.
6. Describe the important characteristics of a typical waiting area.

PREPARING FOR THE CERTIFICATION EXAM

1. What are the designated amounts that some medical insurance plans require patients to pay for medical services or medication, usually at the time of service?
   a. insurance premiums
   b. deductibles
   c. copayments
   d. coinsurance
   e. benefits

2. What is the act of collecting all records, test results, and information pertaining to the patient?
   a. filing
   b. collating
   c. tracking
   d. sorting
   e. indexing

3. How often should patients' insurance information be confirmed?
   a. once a year
   b. whenever the medical assistant has time
   c. at every visit
   d. after an insurance claim is denied
   e. when the patient tells you it has changed

4. What form authorizes the insurance company to send payments directly to the physician?
   a. assignment of benefits form
   b. copayment form
   c. patient registration form
   d. encounter form
   e. HIPAA Notice of Privacy Practices

5. When should the receptionist document the fact that a patient doesn't show for an appointment?
   a. on the same day
   b. only if the patient doesn't call to reschedule
   c. immediately
   d. when completing the daily journal
   e. when the office manager tells the receptionist to do so

6. How long are patients typically willing to wait in the office for their appointment before they become agitated?
   a. 50 minutes
   b. 40 minutes
   c. 30 minutes
   d. 20 minutes
   e. 1 hour

7. What is queuing up medical charts?
   a. filing all information and test results for a patient into their medical record
   b. having patients sign in with their name, time of arrival, and the name of the physician to be seen
   c. activating or displaying a computerized list
   d. listing no-show patients at the end of the day
   e. listing the procedure and diagnosis codes reported to the insurance company

8. How should you address a patient when calling her from the reception room to the exam room?
   a. Mrs. Smith
   b. Suzanne Smith
   c. Honey
   d. Suzy
   e. Mrs. Robert Smith

9. What action may the physician take if a patient is a repeated no-show for appointments?
   a. Refer the patient to a physician partner.
   b. Release the patient from the physician's care.
   c. Cancel the patient's insurance.
   d. Write off the patient's balance.
   e. Notify the patient's insurance company.

10. What must *not* be included on a patient sign-in sheet?
    a. name
    b. time of arrival
    c. reason for visit
    d. physician's name
    e. date

CRITICAL THINKING

Refer to the case study at the beginning of the chapter and use what you have learned to answer the following questions.

1. How should Tania handle the patient who is early for his appointment?
2. Tania checks the prior day's schedule and sees that Meghan closed the office on Monday night. How should Tania handle the disheveled reception room?
3. After other staff members have arrived for the day, Tania unlocks the office door. She sees the man from earlier in the morning exit his car and make his way to the door. When he arrives in the office, Tania notices that he has a bloody nose. What should she do with this patient?

ON THE JOB

Dr. Morrison, a child psychiatrist who is in solo practice, employs one medical assistant in her office. This medical assistant is multiskilled, like all medical assistants, and handles essentially all the administrative and clinical tasks in the office.

It is 3:00 P.M. and a parent has just arrived for a 3:30 P.M. appointment with her 10-year old daughter. The child is a new patient of Dr. Morrison and was referred by her attending physician. She has a relatively long history of combative and destructive behavior, and the referring pediatrician is seeking a psychologic evaluation from Dr. Morrison. Psychotropic medication of some sort may be a viable treatment option. The medical assistant has politely asked the mother and daughter to be seated and to fill out some registration forms. The child is acting out—pulling cushions off the reception room couch, wildly ripping the pages of the magazines, whining, and kicking her mother. The behavior seems to be escalating as the mother tries to frantically control her child while, at the same time, follow the instructions of the medical assistant and fill out the registration forms.

1. What, if anything, should the medical assistant do?
2. Would it be appropriate, for example, for the medical assistant to interrupt Dr. Morrison's current session?
3. Might this be considered a medical emergency?

INTERNET ACTIVITY

1. Find out how HIPAA has changed the way the medical office handles patient reception.
2. Look for companies that produce forms that can be used by a medical receptionist.

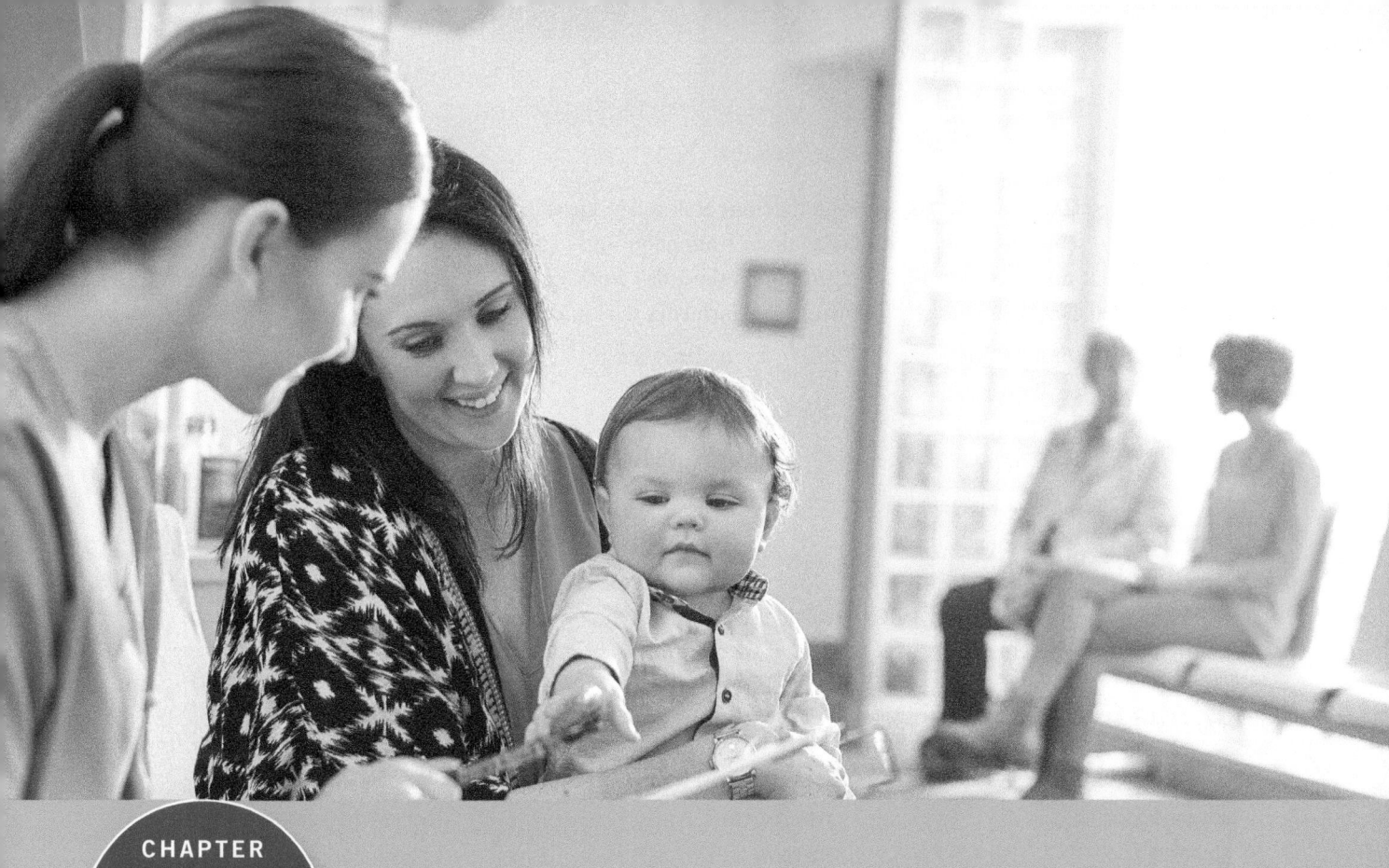

9

Appointment Scheduling

Learning Objectives

After completing this chapter, you should be able to:

9.1   Define and spell the terms for this chapter.

9.2   Describe six types of appointment scheduling methods.

9.3   Identify both advantages and disadvantages to manual and electronic appointment scheduling systems.

9.4   Explain the importance of establishing an appointment matrix.

9.5   List specific communication skills necessary during appointment scheduling.

9.6   Explain the medical assistant's role when dealing with urgent and emergency situations related to appointment scheduling.

9.7   Describe how to maintain the appointment schedule when unplanned adjustments occur.

9.8   Explain the importance of proper documentation when a patient misses a scheduled appointment.

9.9   List critical information that is required when scheduling a patient for a procedure outside the medical office.

Marc Rodgers, CMA (AAMA), is working the front desk today. He is looking ahead to tomorrow's (Friday) schedule. The office usually closes from noon until 1:00 P.M. for lunch. Marc takes note that tomorrow Dr. Miller is working a short day from 11:00 A.M. until 3:00 P.M. Marc sees that Dr. Miller has the following appointments scheduled:

11:00	Laura White	2:00	Rinna Brown
	Joe Tanner		Monica Floyd
	Lucy Smith		Peter Conner
1:00	Justin Ivy		
	Ramona Pierce		
	Lucas Abrams		

At 3:30 P.M., Rinna Brown calls to cancel her appointment for Friday. Shannon Reece wants to know if she can schedule a new patient appointment for tomorrow. Kevin Fowler, a familiar drug representative, wants to know if he can drop in briefly tomorrow.

Terms to Learn

acute conditions	modified wave scheduling	rescheduled
advance booking	new patient	scheduling system
archived	no-show	specified time scheduling
catch-up time	office hours	subpoena
cycle time	open-ended questions	surgery scheduler
double booking	outpatient	tickler file
established patient	overbooking	time patterns
inpatient	patient cancellation	triage
matrix	patient status	wave scheduling

A well-run appointment scheduling function can contribute to positive patient satisfaction and help a medical practice run efficiently. By contrast, poor scheduling practices can create a variety of delays. Offices use a variety of appointment scheduling methods, so medical assistants should be familiar with all of them. Each office chooses the methods that best suit its needs and physician preferences. Medical assistants also need to understand the advantages and disadvantages of both manual and electronic scheduling systems and how to use them.

There are several steps to performing the patient scheduling process for medical assistants to become familiar with. After appointments are made, the schedule needs to be maintained with rescheduling, cancellations, missed appointments, future appointments, and follow-up. Changes to the appointment schedule made by either the patient or the office—including rescheduling, cancellations, and missed appointments—*must be documented* on the schedule and in the individual patient's medical record. Accuracy and attention to detail with patient appointment scheduling is very important because without it, the medical office cannot operate.

APPOINTMENT SCHEDULING METHODS

Office hours are the time span each day that a medical office is open for business. Offices may be open the same hours each day, or they may open earlier or stay open later on selected days to accommodate patients' work schedules. Some offices offer limited weekend hours. Unlike retail establishments, medical offices usually require that patients call the office in advance to schedule an appointment.

The scheduling method used in each office depends on a variety of factors, including physician preference, type and size of practice, equipment availability, staff availability, amount of flexibility required by the physician(s), insurance coverage issues, and patient needs (Figure 9-1). Appointments may be scheduled by telephone, e-mail, or in person (Figure 9-2). Offices use any of several methods to schedule appointments. The following six methods, along with their benefits and limitations, are discussed in this chapter:

- Specified time
- Wave
- Modified wave
- Procedure grouping
- Double booking
- Open hours

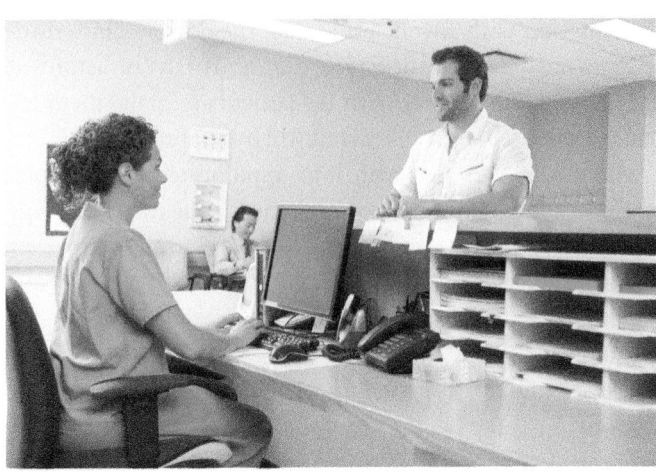

FIGURE 9-2 Scheduling appointments in a physician's office.

Specified Time Scheduling

Specified time scheduling is a format in which each patient is given a specific time slot. The time allocated to each patient depends on the reason for the office visit or the type of examination or testing that is to be done. For example, in some but not all offices, a complete physical examination may require one and one-half hours. In an office based on 15-minute increments, or time slots, this patient would be given six time slots in a row to equal the one and one-half hours needed. No other patients would be scheduled for arrival during this time. The goal of specified time scheduling is to prevent a long **cycletime**—the length of time the average patient spends in the medical office. Scheduling each patient for a specific time based on appointment type, rather than having multiple patients arrive at the same time as might happen with other scheduling methods, helps shorten the cycle time and prevent a large backlog of waiting patients.

The drawback to specified time scheduling is that some patients may not provide enough information about their medical problems at the time the appointment is scheduled even if the receptionist who made the appointment questioned the patient carefully. For instance, consider a patient who is given a 15-minute appointment when the patient actually requires 45 minutes for a thorough physical examination. Because not enough time has been allocated for the visit, the schedule will back up because the next patient is scheduled for 15 minutes later but will have to wait 45 minutes. It is the receptionist's responsibility to get as much information as possible from the patient before scheduling an appointment so the proper amount of time can be reserved for the patient.

Occasionally, patients do not share all the information related to their condition, or they refuse to share any

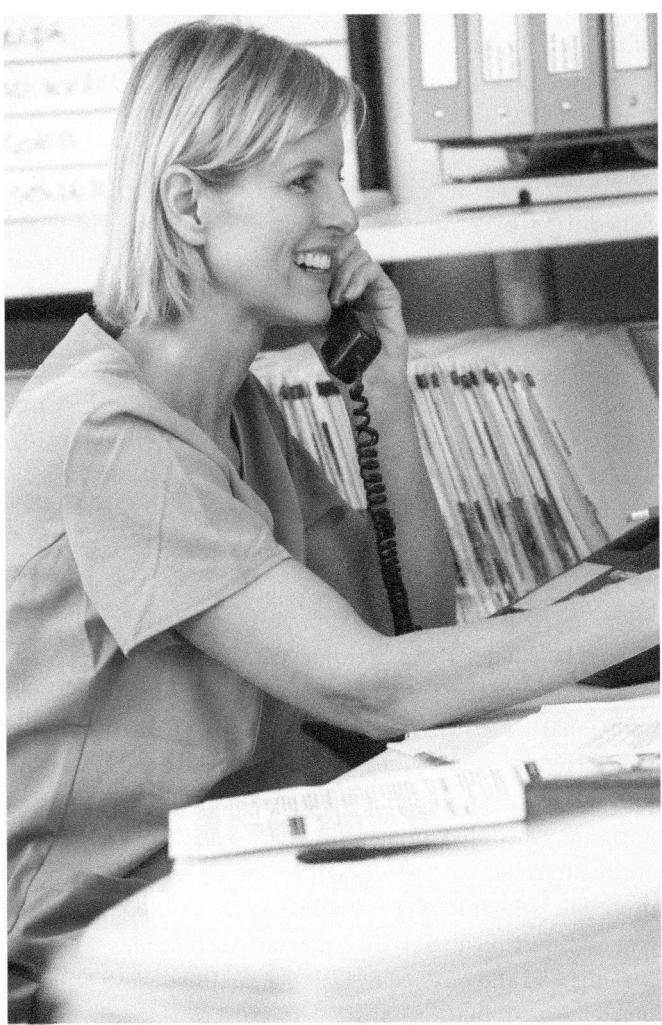

FIGURE 9-1 Scheduling patient appointments by telephone.

information with anyone other than the doctor. This creates special challenges for the receptionist. It is very helpful to try to establish rapport with the patients to make them feel comfortable enough discussing their symptoms, which at times can be very personal. If an appointment is scheduled and the patient ends up requiring more time than was originally scheduled, the physician might have to ask the patient to make another appointment.

Wave Scheduling

Wave scheduling is a system in which all the patients are told to come in at the beginning of the hour in which they are to be seen. Patients are then seen in the order in which they arrive. Because some of the patients require more time, and others may be late, or some may not come in at all, wave scheduling allows for the actual time used by patient appointments to average out over the hour. The goal of wave scheduling is to begin and end each hour on time.

Each hour is divided into equal segments of time, depending on how many patients can be seen within an hour. For appointments averaging 20 minutes, three 20-minute appointments would be scheduled within each hour period, and for appointments averaging 15 minutes, four appointments would be scheduled during the entire hour.

Wave scheduling tends to work well in an office whose patients are often late. The disadvantage is that all patients may arrive at nearly the same time, but the last one signed in will have a longer cycle time. They will have to wait the longest and may not be seen until 45 minutes after arrival. Most patients consider 20 minutes as an acceptable wait time to be seen, so when wave scheduling is used, it is appropriate to advise patients that they should be seen within the hour.

Modified Wave Scheduling

Modified wave scheduling helps avoid the possibility that any patient would have to wait 45 minutes to be seen by the physician. This method also is built on the hour as the base block of time.

There are many variations of modified wave scheduling. For example, assuming an average appointment time with three patients per hour, patients are scheduled to arrive at 10- or 15-minute intervals during the first half hour with no new arrivals during the second one-half hour. All three patients would be seen within the hour period. Patients have a shorter cycle time, and the physician is not delayed while waiting for a late-arriving patient. With this system the physician can still spend 20 minutes with each patient without having to wait for any patients to arrive.

Modified wave scheduling works best for busy offices that tend to have many appointments of approximately the same

length. The disadvantage is that patients with complicated conditions requiring a longer time may need to be scheduled during separate time periods so they don't back up the other patients. Some offices may choose to use specified time scheduling in the morning and wave or modified wave scheduling in the afternoon to accommodate different types of appointments.

Table 9-1 is a comparison chart providing examples of specified time, wave, and modified wave scheduling.

Scheduling by Grouping Procedures

Scheduling by grouping procedures is a system in which patients requiring the same type of examination or procedure are scheduled during a particular block of time. For example, an obstetrician may prefer to have all new patients scheduled together on two mornings a week, because each requires a longer physical examination. An allergist may group all patients requiring skin testing together on three afternoons a week. A pediatrician may do well-baby checkups during particular hours each day. See Figure 9-3 for an example of scheduling by grouping procedures.

Double Booking Scheduling

Double booking is the practice of scheduling two patients to be seen during the same time slot without allowing for any additional time in the schedule. It is considered to be an ineffective but sometimes unavoidable method. For example, if each patient needs a 20-minute appointment, and both are scheduled from 1:00 P.M. to 1:20 P.M., then the entire afternoon's schedule will be late by at least 20 minutes. The schedule is overbooked to accommodate patient requests, but ultimately it can create inconvenience for the patients and the physician. Using a modified wave scheduling helps eliminate this problem because enough time is allowed in the schedule for all the patients.

TABLE 9-1 | Comparison of Scheduling Methods

Specified Time		Wave		Modified Wave	
1.00	Ed Trombley—ear irrigation	1.00	Ed Trombley Jerry Richard Janet Orlando	1.00	Ed Trombley
1.20	Jerry Richard—well-baby checkup with vaccines			1.10	Jerry Richard
1.40	Janet Orlando—PAP smear			1.20	Janet Orlando
2.00	Lena Mezza—well-baby checkup with vaccines	2.00	Lena Mezza David Ingiolo Christina Soave	1.30	
2.20	David Ingiolo—BP check			1.40	
2.40	Christina Soave—skin rash (poss. contagious)			2.00	Lena Mezza
3.00		3.00		2.10	David Ingiolo
3.20				2.20	Christina Soave
3.40				2.30	
4.00		4.00		2.40	

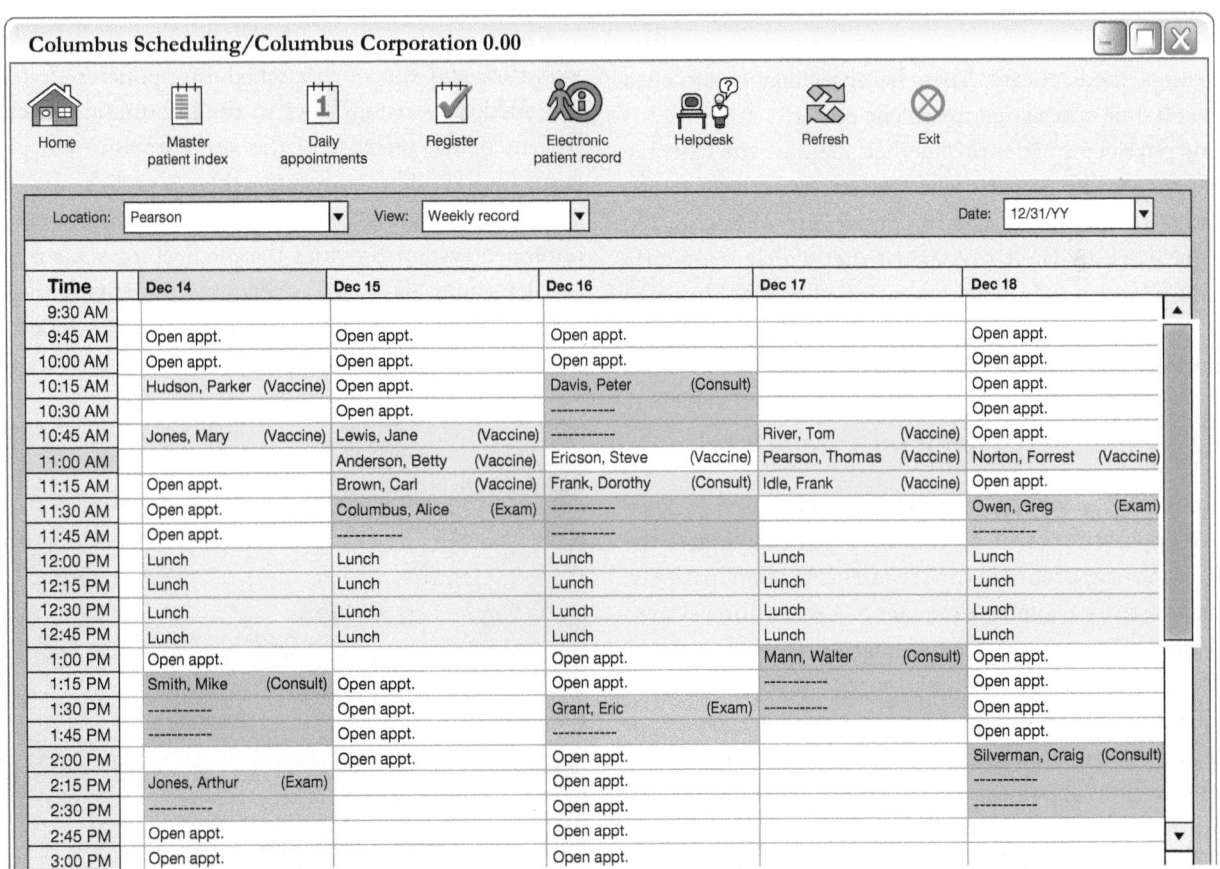

FIGURE 9-3 An example of scheduling by grouping. All immunizations are scheduled for morning appointments.

Open Hours Scheduling

An open office hours system is the least structured of all the systems. The hours in which the office is open are posted, and patients may arrive at any time during those hours. The patients are generally seen in the order of their arrival, unless a patient with an emergent condition arrives, who would then be seen right away. The open hours method is commonly used in urgent care clinics, which are prepared to handle situations requiring immediate, but not life-threatening, medical care. These facilities may be attached to a hospital or other large treatment center.

Some physicians prefer this method, because the schedule is not disrupted by patients who miss appointments. A disadvantage to this method is the possibility of having too many patients arrive at the same time, which frequently results in a longer cycle time than is desirable. The physician and staff can be overworked during peak times of the day but not have any patients during other times.

TYPES OF SCHEDULING SYSTEMS

Each office has a **scheduling system**, or tool, used to keep track of appointments. A scheduling system facilitates the coordination of appropriate time segments for staff, patients, and the practice's available equipment. A scheduling system can be applied to any practice, no matter its size, specialty, or patient load.

Scheduling systems range from a simple notebook with timed slots to a sophisticated electronic health record (EHR) system that links appointments to patients' medical records. Scheduling systems establish the appropriate office process flow and coordination of time with the ability for flexibility as necessary. Table 9-2 summarizes the advantages and

disadvantages of computerized and manual scheduling systems. Highlights are discussed in the following sections.

Computerized Systems

Medical practices of all sizes and specialties can use computers to schedule appointments (Figure 9-4). Computerized systems may be purchased based on the medical practice's specific needs. Some practices purchase a commercial software product, and others contract with a commercial appointment scheduling service. The responsibility of the medical assistant is to understand and follow the computerized appointment system while adhering to Health Insurance Portability and Accountability Act (HIPAA) guidelines. No official government body or standards agency is established to certify a commercial computerized product or service as specifically HIPAA-compliant. However, various public agencies, including the Centers for Medicare and Medicaid, certify or approve computer programs in order for a physician to qualify for participation in research projects or incentive programs. Generally, such programs are HIPAA-compliant. Ultimately, individual health care providers must ensure that any computerized product purchased for the medical practice addresses the specific needs of the practice and its own HIPAA compliance issues, such as patient safety, confidentiality, and security.

Computerized appointment systems help to facilitate workflow and ensure that scheduling policies are followed. The medical assistant keys in the information, such as the patient name, purpose of the appointment, and preferred time frames. The computer then searches for available appointments and provides a list of available times. A computerized system provides the medical assistant the ability to view times, dates, and open appointments with ease and consideration for the appointment criteria. It allows the office manager to allocate the time allowed for various types

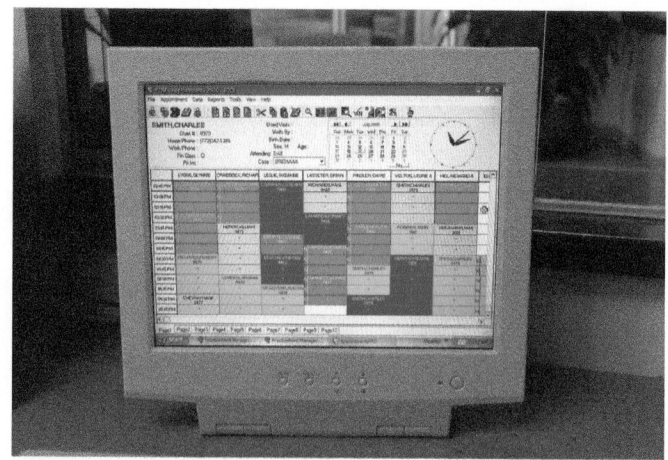

FIGURE 9-4 An example of a computerized scheduling screen.

TABLE 9-2 | Comparison of Computerized and Manual Scheduling Systems

Computerized Scheduling Systems	
Advantages	**Disadvantages**
Quick access to information	Cost of equipment
Ability to track appointment statistics	Time and cost of staff training
Auditing of records and changes	Unavailability during power outage
Linkage of schedule to patient charts	Potential computer failures and data loss
Automated patient reminders	Electronic security breeches
Potential for patients to self-schedule	Need to update software periodically
Ability to search for open appointments	
Legible and easy to read	
Accessible to all staff with security authorization and in multiple rooms or locations	

Manual Scheduling Systems	
Advantages	**Disadvantages**
Always available	Can become messy and illegible due to changes
Minimal staff training required	Physical security; easy to lose or misplace
Inexpensive	Difficulty of tracking statistics
Quick to use	Must double document changes in patient chart
	Reminders must be generated manually
	Cumbersome to search for open appointments
	Difficult to audit changes
	Available only to one person in one place at a time

of appointments, to allow or not allow double-booking, to group appointment types according to the physician's preference, and to set other criteria necessary for smooth scheduling.

An advantage to computerized appointments is the ability to access and view patient appointments with a click or touch of a button. Whether a patient has a future appointment or a series of appointments, the computerized system can produce the information without the need of flipping through the multiple pages of a manual schedule book.

Another advantage of computerized appointment scheduling is the ability to track regular patterns within the medical practice. For example, the office could track the number of no-shows or how many patients were scheduled for the same type of appointment (e.g., flu), and create a report that can be viewed on the computer screen or printed out. This computerized tracking feature provides an excellent analytical tool for audit and identification of the best and most efficient methods within the office. Time management could be modified as needed based on the reports.

Some offices allow patients to schedule their own appointments online. This can be convenient for both the patients

and the medical office. Usually a specific block of appointment times is slotted for self-scheduling by patients. This may be limited to certain types of routine visits, such as annual examinations or routine follow-up. Other types of appointments, such as those to address new or serious problems, might be scheduled only by calling the office.

Even if a practice does not permit self-scheduling by patients, it may provide the option for patients to request an appointment via a secure e-mail or inquiry system linked to the EHR patient portal (a website that allows patient access to limited EHR information and communication with the medical office). Using an online form, patients can indicate the reason for the appointment and the preferred dates or time frames. The message is sent to the scheduler, who reviews the request, assigns an appointment time, and sends a confirmation back to the patient. Technology is rapidly changing in this area, so medical assistants should be prepared to adapt to new systems as they become available.

Disadvantages of computerized scheduling include the cost of equipment and staff training, the potential for electronic security breaches, the cost of power, and the potential for failure because of power outage or computer system breakdown.

Manual Systems

Some medical practices have not converted to computerized systems and instead use manual appointment systems. Manual systems use a hard-copy schedule book and a pen. Appointment books are purchased from various commercial office supply companies and come in a variety of styles, sizes, and features. Each office determines the type of book needed based on the practice's needs and preferences. Refer to Figure 9-5 for a sample of an appointment book. In accordance with HIPAA compliance, patient privacy must be protected at all times when using an appointment book. The book should never be left in an area that is visible to visitors at the reception desk. The appointment schedule for the day should be placed in a secure and private location for approved staff members to reference as needed.

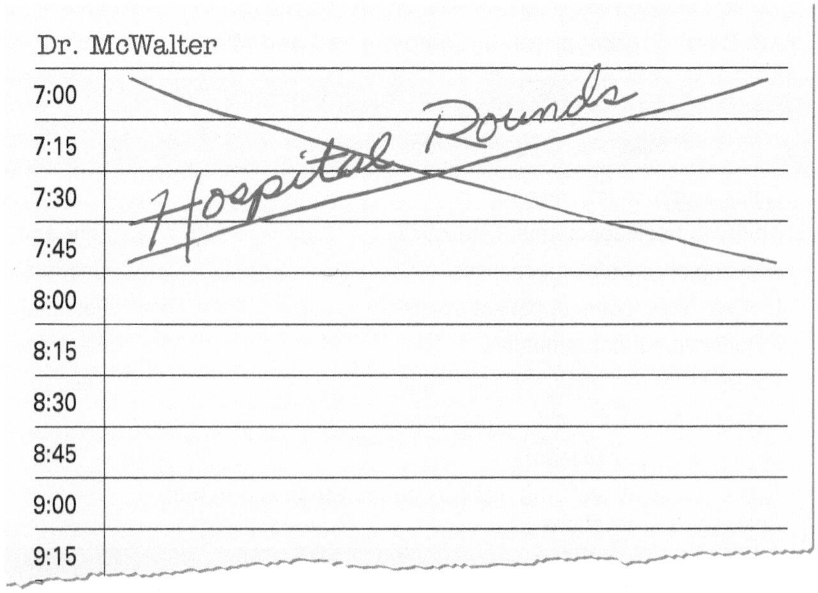

Manual scheduling systems are inexpensive and easy to use, but can become illegible due to frequent changes and do not provide easy access to data and statistics. By their nature, manual systems can be used by only one person in one location.

PATIENT SCHEDULING PROCESS

Every office selects its preferred method for appointment scheduling, in accordance with the needs of the practice. The scheduling process is similar whether it is done electronically or manually. Steps of the process are described in the next sections. Delays may be caused by **overbooking**, when more than one patient is scheduled in the same time slot. Delays are also caused by not allowing enough time on the schedule for patient visits. This usually occurs because inaccurate information is obtained about the reason a patient wishes to see the doctor. Therefore, it is important that the office have clear policies and procedures regarding when overbooking is appropriate and how to assess patient needs over the phone so that adequate time is allotted for them in the schedule.

Form an Appointment Matrix

The first step in the patient scheduling process is known as forming a **matrix**—a grid that shows the availability of each physician, as well as periods of time that are not available for appointments (Figure 9-6). A matrix can be developed in

Dr. McWalter

7:00	
7:15	
7:30	Hospital Rounds
7:45	
8:00	
8:15	
8:30	
8:45	
9:00	
9:15	

FIGURE 9-5 An example of a manual appointment book.

both electronic and manual scheduling systems. Areas of the matrix are crossed out or blocked out to indicate times that are unavailable for appointments—for example, when the physician is making hospital rounds or is in surgery, out to lunch, on a break, returning telephone calls, in meetings, or out of town.

Ideally, a matrix is formed in advance for a period of 3 to 6 months. It is not good practice to prepare a schedule for an entire year, because there may be unexpected changes in the physician's personal or professional schedule. When you create an appointment matrix for a manual system, use a pencil so that changes to the matrix can be easily made in the future. (Use pen to write in individual patient appointments.) Cross out the blocks of time when the physician is unavailable, and write the reason across the blocked-out space.

Identify the Patient and the Need

When a patient calls for an appointment, begin by asking for the patient's name (verifying the spelling if needed), birth date, telephone number including area code, and purpose of the visit. After the patient has described the purpose of the visit, the receptionist should use the office criteria to help determine the type of appointment and the time needed. Occasionally, the receptionist needs to ask open-ended questions to gather enough information to determine what type of appointment the patient needs. **Open-ended questions** require more than a yes or no answer and are used to gather pertinent information. Next, the receptionist needs to determine the availability of facility, equipment, and staff to meet the patient's needs. Based on this

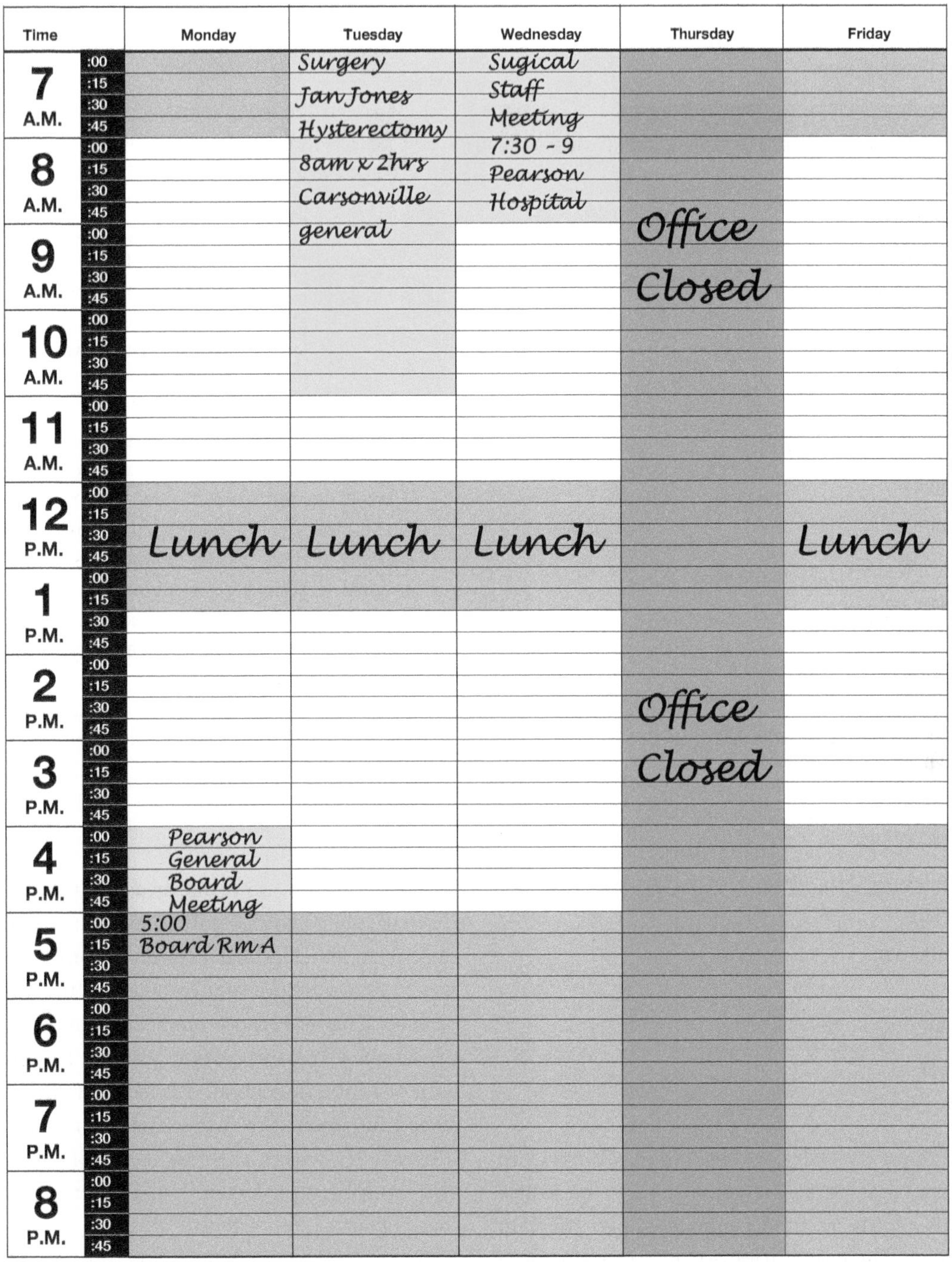

FIGURE 9-6 An appointment schedule with a completed matrix.

Time	Monday	Tuesday	Wednesday	Thursday	Friday
7 A.M.		Surgery Jan Jones Hysterectomy	Surgical Staff Meeting 7:30 – 9 Pearson Hospital		
8 A.M.		8am x 2hrs Carsonville			
9 A.M.		general		Office Closed	
10 A.M.					
11 A.M.					
12 P.M.	Lunch	Lunch	Lunch		Lunch
1 P.M.					
2 P.M.				Office	
3 P.M.				Closed	
4 P.M.	Pearson General Board Meeting				
5 P.M.	5:00 Board Rm A				
6 P.M.					
7 P.M.					
8 P.M.					

information, the receptionist can then discuss available dates and times with the patient. Refer to Table 9-3 for estimates of the amount of time to be allotted for specific office procedures.

Determine Patient Status

Patient status refers to whether a patient is a new or an established patient for your office. This is important to determine because it affects the length of time that should be scheduled for the appointment and what information must be gathered from the patient.

Established Patient Appointments

Any patient who has been seen by the physician within the past three years is considered an **established patient**. In multi-specialty offices, the patient must have been seen by a physician of the same specialty and subspecialty to be considered an established patient. When a patient sees a

TABLE 9-3 | Time Estimates for Specific Office Procedures

Procedure	Time in Minutes
Allergy testing	30–60
Cast check	10
Cast change	30
Complete physical with EKG	60
Blood pressure check	15
Dressing change	15
Minor surgery procedure	30–45
Office visit: Established patient	
Low complexity	5–10
Medium complexity	15–20
High complexity	20–30
Office visit: New patient	
Low complexity	10–15
Medium complexity	15–30
Complete physical	30–45
Pelvic examination with PAP test	30
Patient education	30–45
Postoperative checkup	15–20
Prenatal examination (first visit)	30–60
Prenatal checkup	15
Prostate examination	30
School physical	15–30
Suture removal	10
Well-baby checkup	15

Professionalism

As the receptionist, you need to be able to quickly switch focus from one task to another and not become easily frustrated. You may be answering the phone to schedule appointments at the same time as checking in patients, answering questions, and monitoring the reception area. An important part of customer service is giving your full attention to each task and each patient. Remember to use effective communication skills when scheduling patient appointments. Always project a professional, caring, and willing demeanor to the patient. Use effective listening and speaking skills so you can understand the patient's needs and concerns and so that the patient can understand what you say to them in return.

Listening carefully to the patient's information and requests helps you determine the type of appointment that is actually needed. Try not to make the caller repeat information because you were distracted. If this does occur, do not just ask the same question, such as "What is your phone number?" as though you never asked it before. Instead say, "I'm sorry Mr. Smith, would you mind telling me your phone number again?" A courteous approach helps minimize the patient's frustration about needing to repeat information.

physician of a different specialty or subspecialty, even within the same practice, that person is considered to be a **new patient** to that physician, because a more thorough workup must be performed. These definitions of an established and new patient are suggested by the American Medical Association and are consistent with those required by Current Procedural Terminology (CPT®) codes used for billing.

Established patients have an existing medical record that is accessed each time the patient contacts the physician for an appointment. When established patients call for an appointment, verify their telephone number, address, and insurance information before scheduling the appointment. Maintaining good customer service with established patients includes appointment reminders and observing patient cycle time. Procedure 9-1 provides information on how to schedule established patients.

New Patient Appointments

Before scheduling someone as a new patient, be sure to verify that this person is truly a new patient to the practice or the physician. Medical insurance companies have requirements that must be met to consider the patient as a "new" patient. This is because medical insurance companies compensate new-patient visits at a higher level than established-patient visits. In general, if it has been more than three years since the patient saw a physician of the same specialty and subspecialty within the practice, or if the patient has never been seen by a physician in the practice, you may consider that person a new patient.

Offer the Appointment Time

Avoid asking the patient, "When would you like to come in?" because some patients can become demanding. However, it is acceptable to ask the patient if certain days or times are preferred, given their work schedule and other obligations. To expedite the scheduling process, the receptionist should initially offer only one or two choices of dates, days, and times that meet the patient's schedule preferences. If the patient is unable to accept the offered choice, the receptionist may suggest one or two alternatives. Always state the date, day, and time clearly, and confirm that the patient has correctly understood when the appointment is scheduled.

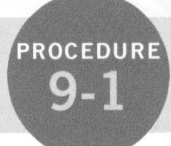

PROCEDURE
9-1

Scheduling Established Patients

Objective ◆ *Use an appointment scheduling system to schedule patients with efficiency.*

EQUIPMENT AND SUPPLIES

Pencil or pen (if preferred by office management); computerized scheduling system or appointment book

METHOD

1. Understand the scheduling system used in your office.
2. If using computerized scheduling, log in to the scheduling system with your user name and password that have been previously established. When scheduling manually, use black or blue ink, so entries cannot be erased. All changes should be crossed out with a single line and a notation such as *R/S* to indicate *rescheduled* or *CX* to indicate *cancelled*.
3. Before scheduling patients, set up a matrix by blocking out all time periods when the physician is not available (hospital rounds, vacation, etc.) for appointments.
4. Schedule appointments by beginning with the first empty appointment in the morning or early in the afternoon, and then fill in the day. Do not schedule appointments at the end of the day with large open gaps in between.
5. For computerized scheduling, access the menu that enables you to search for the correct patient. Some systems allow searching by the patient's birthdate or medical record number. This decreases the chances of pulling up the wrong patient if you have more than one patient with the same name. For manual scheduling, print the patient's full first and last names next to the appropriate time on the schedule. Add Jr. for *Junior* and Sr. for *Senior* if two patients in a family have the same name.

6. For computerized scheduling, verify that the telephone numbers in the system are correct. If they are incorrect, take the time right then to update them. Correct contact information is necessary if the office needs to get in touch with the patient before the appointment. For manual scheduling, ask the patient for current work and home telephone numbers, including the area code. Include a cell phone number if the patient has one. Write these numbers next to the patient's name.
7. Record the reason for the visit on the schedule, using accepted medical abbreviations only.
8. Allow the correct amount of time for the appointment. If an appointment will take more than the minimum time allotted on the schedule, be sure to adjust the length of time as needed. For computerized scheduling, you may specify the length of the appointment by entering the number of minutes, such as 15, 30, or 60 minutes. Some systems may allow you to highlight the time blocks on the screen. For manual scheduling, draw an arrow to indicate that the patient requires two or three blocks of time. In some offices, a line is drawn across the time blocks.
9. After the appointment is recorded, repeat to the patient the date, time, and any special instructions.
10. If the patient is in the office while you are scheduling the appointment, record the appointment on a reminder card and hand it to the patient.

Note: In offices where scheduling is done by computer, follow any on-screen prompts in addition to the steps suggested above.

Some offices schedule patients for an arrival time that is 10 to 15 minutes before the actual "appointment time" of when they expect to see the patient, so patients have time to complete the check-in process. If scheduling for the "appointment time," also inform the patient of the time they should arrive, which is usually earlier. Be clear whether you are giving the patient an "arrival time" or an "appointment time" that requires them to arrive early to complete the check-in process.

After the patient and the receptionist have mutually agreed on the time, either key the information into the computer or write the patient name and telephone number into

the scheduled time slot in the schedule book. If using a computerized scheduling system, remember to click the "save" button as soon as the appointment has been entered.

Confirm the Appointment Details

When you have recorded the patient's name on the schedule, repeat the date and time of the appointment for the patient. This verifies that you have recorded the appointment correctly, and it offers the patient the opportunity to make any corrections. If the patient is making the appointment in person, write the date, day, and time on an appointment card for the patient.

Scheduling a new patient's appointment requires additional time, patience, and effective organizational skills. Always project a professional and positive image with the patient. Using effective communication skills while scheduling the appointment sets the stage for the patient's actual in-office visit and ongoing relationship with the practice. Procedure 9-2 provides instruction on how to schedule new patients.

When scheduling pediatric and older adult patients, it is important to note that they may need specific times and may have other special needs.

Communication Skills for Scheduling

The medical assistant must apply professional, legal, and effective communication skills when scheduling patients for appointments. Following are some professional considerations to follow when communicating with the patient:

- Determine whether you are speaking directly with the patient or to a third party (parent, spouse, adult child) calling on behalf of the patient.

- Use the patient's name on the telephone and in e-mail.
- On the telephone, confirm the appointment by asking the patient to repeat the day, date, time, and location of the appointment.
- E-mailed appointment requests should be initiated by the patient, not the office. It is best for patients to use a secure e-mail system, such as one linked to the office's website or EHR system. When responding to an e-mail, be sure to use proper grammar and correct spelling. Request that the patient provide a return communication for verification of received information. Some e-mail systems allow the sender to request an automatic receipt when the message has been read by the recipient.
- Communicate your desire to meet the patient's requested appointment time. If necessary, provide a brief explanation when offering an alternative time. If it is necessary to provide an explanation, be sure not to use any other patients' names.

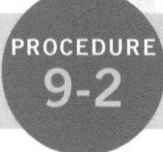

PROCEDURE
9-2

Scheduling a New Patient Appointment

Objective ◆ *Schedule the first visit for a new patient.*

EQUIPMENT AND SUPPLIES

Pencil or pen (if preferred by office management); computerized scheduling system or appointment book

1. Assemble necessary appointment scheduling equipment.
2. Obtain the patient's full legal name and correct spelling, birth date, full address, telephone contacts (home, office, cell), and e-mail address.
3. Record the patient's chief complaint and symptoms.
4. Request the name of the patient's insurance carrier and policy number.
5. Ask how the patient was referred to the medical office (physician referral, friend, colleague, insurance company, etc.).
6. Ask if the patient has a preference for morning or afternoon appointments.
7. Attempt to accommodate the new patient's request for a preferred appointment time.
8. Confirm the day, date, and time of the appointment, and have the new patient repeat the information for verification and mutual understanding.

9. Advise the patient of any need to arrive early, before the official appointment time, to complete paperwork, such as the patient history form and HIPAA consent.
10. Provide the new patient with directions to the office.
11. Inform the new patient of all materials to bring for the first visit, such as insurance card, photo identification, list of current medications, past medical records, current lab, X-ray, and other medical reports, as available.
12. Welcome and thank the new patient by name for selecting your medical office.
13. Forward all information as discussed with the new patient via e-mail or, if time allows, regular mail.
14. Document new patient information in a new medical record.

CHARTING EXAMPLE

1/05/YY 10:25 A.M. New patient appointment scheduled for patient John Samuel on 1/20/YY at 3:30 P.M. Patient requested new patient registration form and patient history form be forwarded to his home address at 1234 Carpenter Road, Smith Station, Chicago. Patient aware he needs to arrive 30 minutes before his appointment. Driving directions provided. L. Battista, RMA

- Be specific and inform the patient of the office policies for cancellations and missed appointments.

- Be sure to gather all pertinent information from the patient, such as name, telephone contacts, e-mail address, reason for visit, insurance carrier, and whether the patient needs directions to the office.

- As with any interaction with a patient, whether on the telephone, via e-mail, or in person, the medical assistant must always be aware of HIPAA regulations and take every measure possible to protect the patient's identity and verify that the individual the caller claims to be is indeed the patient. In addition to the common identifiers such as date of birth or address, many offices require a personal identification number (PIN) or password to ensure security. These provide additional measures to prevent any information from being provided to someone other than the patient.

Responding to Urgent and Emergency Situations

On occasion, unscheduled patients contact the office with a need for an immediate appointment. These include patient emergencies and patients with acute conditions. **Acute conditions** are illnesses or injuries that patients suddenly experience and that require treatment but may not be life threatening.

The medical assistant must listen carefully to all the patient's complaints and assess the seriousness of the patient's condition. If pain is involved, it is important to ask the patient where the pain is located, when it first appeared, the duration of strength or measure of the pain, and if the patient has experienced the same pain before. Ask about any other symptoms the patient feels are important

or distressing. Also ask for the telephone number the patient is calling from and determine if the patient is alone. Always follow office policies and procedures regarding handling emergency situations. The physician should always be informed immediately regarding a potential emergency.

The medical assistant needs to know how to apply triage skills. **Triage** is the process of sorting or grouping patients according to the seriousness of their condition. Triage becomes necessary when more than one seriously ill patient is waiting to see the physician. In general, sudden onset of pain must be considered an emergency until otherwise determined by the physician.

If an emergency exists, as in the case of severe chest pain, then the physician must be informed of the call immediately. If a physician is not available, then the medical assistant should follow office protocol, which may require referring the patient to the nearest emergency department. If the patient is not able to call EMS, then the medical assistant should arrange for an ambulance and emergency medical personnel to transport the patient. Table 9-4 lists acute illnesses that require the patient to be seen by a physician as soon as possible. Table 9-5 lists emergency (life-threatening)

TABLE 9-4 | Examples of Acute Conditions

Earache	Infection that is visible to patient (e.g., a red, swollen area after an injury)
Fever lasting more than 24 hours	
Pain or burning on urination	Pain in abdomen that is not severe
Skin rash	Unusually heavy uterine or vaginal bleeding
Unusual discharge (e.g., blood in urine)	
Eye infection	Sore throat and/or swollen glands

TABLE 9-5 | Examples of Emergency Conditions

Acute allergic reaction	Laceration
Allergic reaction with respiratory distress	Loss of consciousness
Chest pain	Pain or numbness after the application of a cast for fracture
Coma	Poisoning
Convulsions	Severe bleeding
Diabetic reaction	Severe dizziness
Difficulty breathing	Severe nausea, vomiting, or diarrhea lasting more than 24 hours
Drowning/near-drowning	
Drug overdose	
Foreign object in the eye	Severe pain
	Sudden acute illness
Fracture	Sudden paralysis of part or all of the body
Gunshot wounds	
Head injury	Temperature over 104°F

Appointments are cancelled or rescheduled for any number of reasons. Sometimes the patient experiences an unforeseen emergency, is too ill or too fatigued to get to the office, or forgets the appointment. A **rescheduled** appointment is one for which the patient calls before the scheduled time and changes it to, usually, another day and time. A **patient cancellation** is an appointment for which the patient calls the office to say she cannot make the appointment time and does not schedule another appointment. A **no-show** is an appointment for which the patient does not attend the appointment and does not call to reschedule or cancel.

At times, the physician may be delayed or needs to cancel appointments because of an emergency at the hospital or in the office. Delays can also occur if a piece of needed equipment has malfunctioned or building issues arise, such as a power outage. In all such cases, the medical assistant should provide patients with an explanation and reschedule the delayed appointments.

conditions that require immediate physician assistance. Document any phone calls involving emergent medical situations in the patient's medical record. Record the date and time of call, patient's complaint, action taken, information from the physician, and instructions provided to the patient.

MAINTAINING THE SCHEDULE

Unforeseen circumstances arise, so it is unlikely that a single day in a medical office will go by without some type of adjustment needing to be made to the schedule. Changes such as missed appointments, delays, or cancellations occur daily. Remember to remain positive when such situations happen. It is also important to keep the physician's schedule flowing smoothly, without gaps, and to accommodate the patient's scheduling request with a pleasant demeanor.

Rescheduled Appointments

A patient whose personal schedule changes may call the office to reschedule a medical appointment. Ideally, the patient will call at least 24 to 48 hours in advance. First, say, "Thank you for calling to let us know. I can assist you with that." After verifying the patient's identity, confirm the date, time, and purpose of the original appointment to be certain you are rescheduling the correct appointment. The purpose of the appointment provides direction regarding how soon it must be rescheduled. If the appointment is for short-term follow-up on an illness or injury, it should be rescheduled as soon as possible, usually within a few days. If the appointment is for an annual preventive care examination, then rescheduling one or two weeks later may not be a problem. The office scheduling policies should define acceptable rescheduling time frames for various types of appointments. If medical assistants are uncertain regarding the urgency of rescheduling, they should check with their supervisor.

After you determine how soon the appointment must be rescheduled, follow the normal procedures for scheduling an appointment. At the end of the conversation, confirm both the date that was cancelled and the new, rescheduled date and time. In an electronic scheduling system, you can retrieve the original appointment entry and enter the new date and time. The system clears the original time slot so it is available for another patient and reserves the new time slot for the patient calling. The system adds a notation to the appointment, indicating that it was rescheduled. This is helpful to track patients who habitually reschedule in a manner that could harm their health.

In a manual system, use a single line to cross out the patient information in the original time slot and enter it in the new time slot. Add a note next to the original entry that it was rescheduled and the date to document that it is a rescheduled appointment (for example, *R/S 1/10/YY*). Also document the rescheduled appointment in the patient's chart. Erasures should never occur with paper records and appointment books.

Patient Cancellations

Sometimes a patient calls to cancel an appointment but does not schedule a new time. Ideally, the patient will call at least 24 to 48 hours in advance. First, thank them for calling, then verify the patient's identity and the date, time, and purpose of the original appointment to be certain you are rescheduling the correct appointment. Always ask if the

patient wants to reschedule, and politely stress the importance of staying healthy by keeping medical appointments. The purpose of the appointment provides direction regarding how necessary it is for the patient to schedule a different time. If the appointment involves follow-up on an acute injury or illness, then work with the patient to find a suitable time. If the patient refuses or is unable to state an alternative time, conclude the conversation by asking the patient to call back and reschedule as soon as possible. The cancellation should be documented in the patient chart, including the information that you offered the patient alternative times and requested a call back. The physician should be notified of any cancellations that could endanger the patient's health.

In a computerized system, select the appropriate menu item or check-off box to indicate the cancellation. In a manual system, write cancellation (CX) on the appointment schedule sheet. Enter a reminder to follow up with patients who do not call back to reschedule within an appropriate time frame.

Make every attempt to fill a void in the schedule caused by a changed or cancelled appointment. The approach depends on how far in advance the patient calls. If there are several days or weeks until the newly open appointment time, you may be able to offer it to one of the next several patients who call to schedule. Another approach, especially on short notice, is to call the patient who has the last appointment for the day and ask the patient if it is possible to come in earlier. In the event that a long appointment, such as a 90-minute appointment for a complete physical, has been cancelled, you will have to attempt to move up an entire group of patients. Many offices maintain a list of patients who wish to be called if an appointment becomes available at the last minute. This approach is beneficial in maintaining good customer service and is an effective way to help manage the office schedule.

No-Shows

No-shows, also called failed or missed appointments, occur when a patient does not show up to keep an appointment. Missed appointments happen with no warning, so the medical assistant has less opportunity to make satisfactory adjustments. No matter what the reason for a missed appointment, the medical assistant must contact the patient, offer to reschedule the appointment, mention the extra fee if there is one, and document it as a missed and rescheduled appointment in the patient medical record.

Careful, legible documentation of missed appointments is necessary to legally protect the physician from a claim of patient abandonment. For example, if a patient with serious condition accidentally misses an appointment, and the medical practice does not follow-up to reschedule, then the patient's condition worsens, the medical practice could be sued for neglect. Even if a lawsuit is not filed, harm could be done to the patient's well-being. Because of the serious liability associated with missed appointments, all missed appointments must be documented in the appointment schedule *and* in the patient's chart.

Documenting in a Computerized System

In a computerized appointment schedule, select the correct menu item or check-off box associated with the appointment to indicate the no-show or cancellation. Most EHR systems link the appointment schedule to the patient's chart and make an automated entry in the patient's chart that an appointment was missed. It is a good idea to double-check the patient chart to ensure the entry was, in fact, made. Add any information needed to fully explain the missed appointment, including that a follow-up phone call was made to the patient to reschedule.

Documenting in a Manual System

In a manual schedule, write no-show (NS) or cancellation (CX) both on the appointment schedule sheet and in the patient chart. As is done in an electronic system, also add any information needed to fully explain the missed appointment, including that a follow-up phone call was made to the patient to reschedule.

Charges for Missed Appointments

Some medical practices charge patients for no-show appointments. They also might charge for cancelling or rescheduling an appointment on very short notice, perhaps within 24 hours of the original appointment time. If the medical practice has a cancellation or rescheduling charge, patients must be made aware of the policy before they actually cancel or reschedule. Many offices place the cancellation/rescheduling policy in an office brochure that is given to all new patients. State the charge or fee for no-shows or short-notice cancellation/rescheduling and how far in advance an appointment must be changed in avoid the charge. In addition, this information is often posted in the reception area near the front desk.

Patients must pay any cancellation fees personally, because such fees cannot be billed to insurance. It is important to make patients aware of the cancellation policy out of consideration for themselves, other patients, and the physician. Some offices, although they state a cancellation policy, charge patients only if they repeatedly cancel at the last minute or are frequent no-shows.

Future Appointments

Ideally, before leaving the office, the patient will schedule the next appointment. This is known as **advance booking**. Scheduling while the patient is in the office also reduces the number of incoming calls requesting appointments.

Advance booking allows patients to book their next appointment ahead of time. Advance booking is done for regularly scheduled checkups or required follow-up appointments, such as after blood pressure checks or completion of physical therapy treatments. The date and time of the next appointment can be written on an appointment card that also contains the name, address, and telephone number of the physician's practice. Such cards should be given to each patient at the time the next appointment is made (Figure 9-7). In some cases, it may not be possible to schedule the next appointment if the office's appointment matrix is not yet available. For example, if the office maintains a matrix for the next three months, appointments cannot be schedule further out. When this occurs, instruct the patient when to call back, send them a reminder card, or maintain a call-back list of patients who need to be scheduled when the next segment of the matrix becomes available.

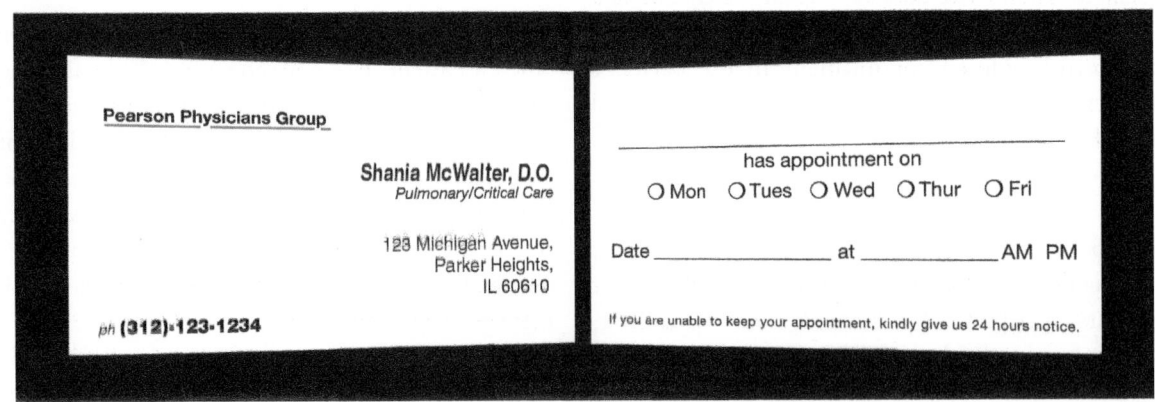

Pearson Physicians Group

Shania McWalter, D.O.
Pulmonary/Critical Care

123 Michigan Avenue,
Parker Heights,
IL 60610

ph **(312) 123-1234**

_____
has appointment on
O Mon   O Tues   O Wed   O Thur   O Fri

Date _____ at _____ AM PM

If you are unable to keep your appointment, kindly give us 24 hours notice.

FIGURE 9-7 The reminder card should be completed and handed to the patient after the appointment is scheduled.

Scheduling appointments is routine work for the scheduler or medical assistant, but for patients it can be very stressful. Frequently, they are not feeling well or are concerned about a problem they are experiencing. They are also worried about being able to obtain a convenient appointment time, because most patients have very busy schedules with work, family responsibilities, travel time, and other obligations.

Remember to treat every patient with courtesy and respect. Give your full attention to each phone call. Be careful to listen to exactly what the patient tells you, and repeat it to be sure you understood correctly. When you need to look up information in the computer system or scheduling book, tell the patient, "I can help you with that. Can you wait a moment while I look up this information?" Do not just respond with silence while you are performing the task, as this may make the patient feel ignored or worry that they have been cut off. If you cannot fulfill the patient's exact request, do not say, "I cannot do that" or "That time is not available." Instead, offer the patient a couple of options, saying, "Unfortunately, that specific (day) or (time) is not available, but I can schedule you for (alternate time) or (alternate day). Would one of these work for you?" This approach helps the patient feel that you are trying to help them.

Follow-Up

Follow-up reminders are considered a good approach for maintaining customer service as well as smart office management to decrease the no-show rate. Follow-up reminders can be provided in writing, by secure e-mail, or by telephone, as selected by the patient. When a patients completes the new patient registration form, they are asked how they wish to be contacted, including their phone number and e-mail address, if desired. They are asked if voice messages can be left at the phone number provided. Medical offices must identify and follow patient preferences for contact. Patients might be in a living or family situation in which they do not want others to know their medical information or appointment schedule. All follow-up methods should include the day, date, and time of the next appointment and instructions on what to do if the patient needs to reschedule.

Tickler file

A **tickler file** is an automated or manual system that notifies the office of certain tasks to be performed. A common application is to generate appointment reminders. A manual tickler file is a small file box with dividers for months of the year and days of the month. Offices usually ask patients to write their name and address on an appointment reminder postcard, then they place it in the tickler file under the month of the appointment. When that month arrives, cards are resorted by day or week of the month. The week before the appointment, the medical assistant mails the reminder card to the patient. Reminders can also be used for patients who are due for a service, such as an annual PAP test or mammogram, but are not currently scheduled.

A computerized scheduling system already stores the dates and times of upcoming appointments. The medical assistant can make a menu selection to print labels, postcards, or letters to all patients with appointments the following week.

Electronic Reminders

Electronic reminders can be sent using secure e-mail or text messages, if approved in advance by the patient. Secure e-mail is a messaging system that is part of the office's EHR system and cannot be accessed without authorization. EHRs often offer a patient portal (a web-based access page) that allows patients to view appointment information and test results. Patients voluntarily sign up for the system and select a user name and password that prevents others from viewing protected health information (PHI). An appointment reminder is scheduled to automatically appear in the patient portal message box a specific number of days before an appointment and contains details about the appointment. A notice is then sent to the patient using a regular e-mail address or text messaging service. This message states that they have a message in the patient portal but does not provide details, because regular e-mail and text messages do not comply with HIPAA privacy rules. The patient must log into the patient portal to access the details. This two-step process keeps the appointment details private, while proactively notifying the patient.

Telephone Reminders

Some offices make reminder calls one to two days before the appointment. Patients might have more than one phone number, so be sure to get approval of the phone numbers that are acceptable for contacting the patient and leaving messages. For example, a patient might approve receiving a phone call at work, but does not want any messages left at that number.

Reminder calls can be performed personally by an individual or using an automated system that announces the appointment details. Individual phone calls made by staff are more personal and provide the opportunity for patients to ask questions or reschedule, but they are time consuming for staff, particularly in large medical offices. An automated system requires less staff time and might be perceived as impersonal by some patients, but they are reliable and can be programmed to call in the evening when it might be easier to reach patients. Regardless of the method used, leave detailed voice mail messages only for patients who have given approval.

It is essential to comply with HIPAA privacy standards when sending reminder postcards or leaving appointment reminder messages on an answering machine or voice mail.

Buffer Time

To eliminate the need to "squeeze in" an emergency or unscheduled appointment, the medical assistant should integrate **time patterns** into the office schedule, if office policy allows. Time patterns are similar to matrixing off time within the schedule to allow for **catch-up time** or unscheduled appointments.

Small blocks of open time can be built into the schedule to help compensate for the extra time that may be needed for unscheduled patients with unforeseen emergencies as well as time during the day when the physician can return telephone calls, catch up on charting, read mail and journals, or rest. Open time is often scheduled at the end of the morning and again at the end of the day. This allows a catch-up period when the morning or afternoon schedule has become delayed. Each physician has an individual preference about when to return phone calls. Some physicians prefer to return all morning telephone calls when they return from lunch, whereas others may work through lunch and return all calls at the end of the day. It is important to inform patients when to expect the physician to return calls. This helps to reduce additional calls from patient(s) wondering when the physician will be calling.

Building this free-time block into the daily office schedule at the same time each day is very important. Every effort should be made not to schedule last-minute, nonurgent appointments during this time.

ARRANGING OUTSIDE APPOINTMENTS

In addition to scheduling patients to be seen in the office, medical assistants also help facilitate patient appointments at other facilities. The most common of these include referral for testing or treatment, **inpatient** admissions, such as when a patient is admitted to the hospital overnight, and **outpatient** procedures, in which the patient comes in only for the procedure, then returns home. Table 9-6 summarizes the patient information the medical assistant needs to provide when scheduling outside appointments.

TABLE 9-6 | Arranging Outside Appointments

Data Needed	Explanation
Patient's full name	Verify spelling of first and last names.
Address	Ask patient to state current address.
Age/date of birth	Verify birth date in patient record.
Telephone number	Ask patient for current number and area code.
Requirement	Type of room or special requirement.
Admitting diagnosis	List the physician's statement from the patient record.
Recent prior admission	Ask the patient for last admission date in any hospital.
Physician's name	List physician's name.
Insurance information	May fax copy of insurance card.
Name of person at insurance company who gave preapproval	Forms are also available from insurance company that gave preapproval.

Scheduling Patient Referrals

Physicians often refer patients to another facility or physician when further treatment or testing is necessary. Ideally, the referral appointment is scheduled as soon as possible. Whether referring a patient to another location or receiving a referral from another physician, the receptionist or referral coordinator must exchange pertinent information regarding the patient's name, contact number, insurance, and referral needs, as well as the referral physician's name, address, and contact number. In some cases, depending on the insurance, precertification (approval) is necessary before scheduling the appointment. Procedure 9-3 reviews the steps to be taken when arranging for a referral appointment. HIPAA allows physicians to share necessary patient information to make a referral. This is disclosed in the HIPAA consent that patients sign when they join the practice. However, shared information should be limited to only what is necessary for the referral. Information unrelated to the reason for the referral should not be shared.

Scheduling Inpatient Admissions

The medical assistant may be responsible for scheduling all patient admissions (admits) to the hospital, because hospital admissions must be initiated by the physician, not the patient. In a large medical practice, a scheduler may take care of all admissions. When scheduling a direct admit to

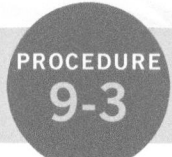

Arranging a Referral Appointment

Objective ◆ *Schedule a referral appointment for the patient.*

EQUIPMENT AND SUPPLIES

Patient chart; telephone; paper; pen; either Rolodex or physician directory; physician request for referral information

METHOD

1. Gather supplies.
2. Open the patient chart, and review the insurance information and physician request for referral.
3. Place a call to the physician's office to whom the patient is being referred.
4. Identify yourself and the physician on whose behalf you are calling. Let the office know you are calling to schedule a referral appointment.
5. First, verify that the practice accepts the patient's medical insurance. If so, continue with the call and provide necessary patient information. If the office does not accept the patient's insurance, thank the practice for its time and notify the physician. The physician will then recommend another physician for the patient referral.
6. If the office accepts the patient's insurance, provide the following information: patient's name, address, telephone number, and reason for referral.
7. The office may ask how soon the patient needs to be seen and will then schedule the patient.
8. Record the referral appointment information in the patient's chart as well as on an appointment reminder card for the patient.
9. Be sure also to record the name of the individual with whom you spoke and the creation of the reminder card.
10. Notify the patient of the date and time of the appointment, and provide the reminder card.
11. Verify that the patient knows the office location. If not, provide clearly written directions.

12. Forward any pertinent information such as laboratory tests or X-rays to the physician's office, and record them in the patient's chart. If faxing information, be sure to place the fax confirmation in the patient's chart.
13. If precertification is required, contact the patient's insurance company and request authorization. Depending on the insurance carrier, this may be done by computer, telephone, or fax. The insurance company will require the following information: specialist's name, telephone number, and reason for the visit or request.
14. If completing the precertification by telephone, document the precertification number and the name and telephone number of the individual who provides the number.
15. Provide the precertification number and pertinent information to the physician's office to which the patient is being referred.

CHARTING EXAMPLE

10/9/YY, 2:15 P.M. Referral appointment scheduled for Patsy Smith. Patient scheduled to see Dr. Kendall on Friday, 10/16/YY, at 10:00 A.M. Verified Dr. Kendall's office participates with patient's insurance. Ms. Smith aware she is to arrive 30 minutes before appointment time to complete paperwork. Patient provided with written information regarding appointment, including driving directions to Dr. Kendall's office. 10/2/YY labs and ultrasound report faxed to Dr. Kendall's office. Confirmation received. D. Joyner, RMA 10/9/YY, 3:00 P.M. Contacted Humana, requested precertification for Ms. Smith's appointment with Dr. Kendall. Spoke with Jim Linday. Precertification authorized #JS123567 valid through 11/16/YY. J. Linday will fax confirmation.D. Joyner, RMA

the hospital (an admission to the hospital directly from a medical appointment), be sure to contact the patient's insurance company for preadmission approval. Procedure 9-4 provides instructions on scheduling inpatient surgical procedures.

Provide the patient with a detailed explanation of the day, date, time, and preparation needed for the admission.

It is always better to place details in writing. Many offices distribute preprinted information to patients. Such information should, however, be personalized with the patient's name. Even when preprinted materials are used, the medical assistant should provide complete, concise, verbal explanations of important points pertaining to the admission/surgical procedure.

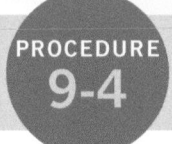

Scheduling an Inpatient Surgical Procedure

Objective ◆ *Schedule an inpatient surgical procedure.*

EQUIPMENT AND SUPPLIES

Patient's chart; patient's insurance card; notepad and pen; written instructions for patient (if required)

METHOD

1. Review the patient's chart for the most current information. Make sure the chart contains the physician's notes and orders regarding the surgical procedure.
2. Verify with the physician the type of procedure for which you are to schedule the patient, and gather the following information from the physician:
   - Category the surgical procedure falls under (routine, elective, urgent)
   - Name of the surgeon to perform the procedure
   - The surgeon's scheduling preference for this type of procedure
   - Estimated length of time for the procedure
   - Estimated length of stay
3. Gather the following information from the patient and patient's chart:
   - Patient's full name, age, sex, and any other pertinent identification or information
   - Physician's current diagnosis
   - Any allergies
   - Special preoperative orders and patient instructions
   - Patient's insurance information
4. Obtain preauthorization from the patient's insurance company, if required.
5. Contact the **surgery scheduler** at the facility and relay the requested surgery information. The surgery scheduler is the person in the hospital or surgery center who schedules the procedure, including the necessary preoperative appointments (e.g., blood work, chest X-ray, etc.), the actual surgery, and postoperative appointments, if necessary.
6. The surgery scheduler will confirm the date and time of surgery and any special instructions to be relayed to the patient.
7. Record the surgery scheduling information in the patient's chart.
8. Record the surgery information on the appropriate physician's schedule.
9. Follow office procedure and the surgeon's request for contacting other members of the surgical team.
10. Instruct the patient on special preparation and admission procedures. Provide written instructions, if available.

CHARTING EXAMPLE

6/5/YY, 9:15 A.M. Spoke with Jenny, surgery scheduler at Pearson General Hospital (PGH). Charles Wolf scheduled for total knee replacement surgery on 6/28/YY at PGH, Dr. Patel, surgeon. Patient aware he is to report to PGH on 6/15/YY at 8:00 A.M. for preoperative assessment and testing. Patient provided with written instructions and verbalized understanding he is not to eat or drink anything after midnight on 6/27/YY. He will call if he has any questions. John Carter, RMA

Scheduling Outpatient Surgery and Outpatient Procedures

Scheduling an outpatient surgery or other procedure is based on the patient's need and diagnosis, type of procedure, insurance carrier, physician, anesthesia requirements (local or general), and facility availability. The medical assistant contacts the surgery scheduling department and makes arrangements with the surgery scheduler. The surgery scheduler may request all patient information, including legal name, telephone contacts, insurance information (for example, prior authorization for some elective surgeries), advance directives, or other preadmittance information. Procedure 9-5 provides instructions on how to schedule an outpatient surgery.

SCHEDULING NONPATIENT APPOINTMENTS

Medical practices may need to schedule appointments for persons other than patients. These appointments may be for sales representatives from various companies—including office equipment, pharmaceuticals, and insurance—or community service leaders. Each visitor needs an appointment to update the staff and physician on the newest product, drug(s),

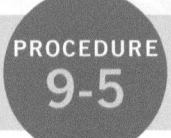

Scheduling an Outpatient Surgical Procedure

Objective ◆ *Schedule an outpatient surgical procedure.*

EQUIPMENT AND SUPPLIES

Telephone; patient's insurance card; notepad; pen; written instructions for patient

METHOD

1. Review the patient's chart for the most current information. Make sure the chart contains the physician's notes and orders regarding the surgical procedure.
2. Verify with the physician the type of procedure for which you are to schedule the patient, and gather the following information from the physician:
   - Category under which the surgical procedure falls (i.e., routine, elective, urgent)
   - Name of the surgeon who will perform the procedure
   - The surgeon's scheduling preference for this type of procedure
   - Estimated length of time for the procedure
3. Gather the following information from the patient and the patient's chart:
   - Patient's full name, age, sex, and any other pertinent identification or information
   - Physician's current diagnosis for the patient
   - Any existing allergies
   - Special preoperative orders and patient instructions
   - Patient's insurance information
   - Days/times patient available for surgery
4. Obtain preauthorization from the patient's insurance company, if required.

5. According to the facility policy, contact the outpatient scheduler at the local hospital or clinic and identify yourself and your office.
6. Instruct the facility about the type of procedure and the amount of time the physician expects to need the operating room.
7. Determine available days at the facility.
8. If possible, offer options to the patient and have the patient choose the best option.
9. Notify the facility of the date and time chosen.
10. Create a patient instruction sheet to include date and time of procedure and necessary preoperative information.
11. Document the conversation in the patient's chart.
12. Document the scheduled surgery on appropriate physician's schedule.

CHARTING EXAMPLE

10/20/YY, 10:30 A.M. Robin Jones scheduled for cervical conization at 12:30 P.M. on 11/9/YY. Patient instructed to arrive at hospital at 10:00 A.M. on day of surgery. Patient was given instruction sheet and stated she understood that she would have to go to the hospital for preoperative testing on 11/3 at 8:00 A.M. Ms. Jones is aware she is not to eat after midnight on the night before surgery—may take morning medications with small amount of water. Patient urged to call with any questions. Celia Ruiz, CMAS (AMT)

equipment, or community issue(s). Most offices have a policy for working with nonpatient visitors and vendor representatives. These appointments should never take priority over patient appointments and may need to be rescheduled if the physician is running late when that particular day comes.

SUMMARY

An efficiently managed medical office requires attention to the scheduling function. The receptionist is responsible for assessing the patient's need for an appointment. Providing the correct amount of time on the schedule for the patient visit works to ensure that the needs of patient and physician

are met. However, the receptionist must remain flexible in scheduling, because patients with emergencies and acute illnesses must be seen immediately. Keep in mind that flexibility is one key to being successful as a health care employee.

A professional and ethical manner is the best approach to handling a schedule that has fallen behind. Quick thinking and planning by rescheduling patients can alleviate stress for the physician who falls behind. Careful documentation and HIPAA compliance regarding all patients who fail to keep appointments, either through cancellation or no-show, can assist the physician in avoiding a lawsuit for abandonment of the patient.

9 CHAPTER REVIEW

COMPETENCY REVIEW

1. Define and spell the terms for this chapter.
2. Write an office policy for scheduling emergency appointments.
3. Role-play instructing a patient on admission to the hospital for a surgical procedure. Use another student as the patient.
4. Correctly document a patient appointment cancellation.
5. Use a computerized scheduling system to integrate patient information and appointment scheduling.

PREPARING FOR THE CERTIFICATION EXAM

1. What is the method of appointment scheduling where no appointments are made and the first patient to sign in is the first patient seen?
   a. wave
   b. streaming
   c. open hours
   d. modified wave
   e. double booking

2. What is the method of appointment scheduling where patients are told to come in at the beginning of the hour in which they will be seen?
   a. wave
   b. streaming
   c. open hours
   d. modified wave
   e. double booking

3. What is a grid that shows available appointment times and periods of nonavailability for each provider?
   a. a cluster
   b. a schedule
   c. a matrix
   d. a calendar
   e. an appointment

4. Which of the following constitutes an emergency appointment?
   a. an 18-year-old college student leaving for school tomorrow needs a physical
   b. 58-year-old woman complaining of heavy vaginal bleeding
   c. 10-year-old child with a 104° fever
   d. 34-year-old woman with sprained ankle
   e. 6-year-old with a 96°F fever

5. Which of the following types of office procedures generally requires the longest amount of time to be scheduled?
   a. Pelvic examination with PAP test
   b. New patient office visit with complete physical
   c. Dressing change
   d. Allergy testing
   e. Prenatal checkup

6. Before calling the surgery scheduler for an inpatient surgery, the medical assistant should gather all of the following *except*
   a. patient's medical insurance information.
   b. physician diagnosis.
   c. dietary preferences.
   d. known patient allergies.
   e. procedure to be performed.

7. If a patient is a no-show for an appointment, the receptionist should do all of the following *except*
   a. record the no-show on the schedule.
   b. record the no-show in the patient's chart.
   c. refer the patient to a specialist.
   d. show the chart to the physician.
   e. if applicable, apply no-show fee to patient's balance.

8. Appointment reminder cards should show all the following *except*
   a. date of next appointment.
   b. time of next appointment.
   c. patient's name.
   d. patient's insurance information.
   e. name of physician patient is seeing.

9. Travis has an appointment at 10:00 A.M., and his room-mate has an appointment the same day with the same physician at 10:20 A.M. What type of appointment scheduling system is Travis's physician using?
   a. double booking
   b. specified time scheduling
   c. wave scheduling
   d. open office hours
   e. modified wave

10. Which condition is *not* an example of an acute condition?
   a. pain with urination
   b. earache
   c. abdominal pain
   d. laceration
   e. eye infection

CRITICAL THINKING

Refer to the case study at the beginning of the chapter and use what you have learned to answer the following questions.

1. Based on Dr. Miller's schedule, what scheduling variation is being used?
2. The office is usually closed from 12:00 to 1:00 P.M. for lunch. New patient visits usually last about one hour. Can Shannon Reece see Dr. Miller tomorrow?
3. How should Marc handle scheduling Kevin Fowler?
4. What needs to be done now that Ms. Brown has cancelled her appointment?

ON THE JOB

A pharmaceutical representative has just arrived at the office of Dr. Joseph Henderson, a board-certified orthopedic surgeon. The waiting room is swarming with patients waiting to see Dr. Henderson, because he was delayed with an unexpectedly complicated lumbar spinal fusion and laminectomy.

The representative is very insistent, almost belligerent, about seeing the physician immediately, even though she did not have an appointment to see him. In fact, the visit was totally unexpected, as the representative had just been in two weeks ago. Last time the representative was in, she gave Dr. Henderson a variety of readily usable and dispensable medications. She has more of the same today—injectable cortisone with Novocain, muscle relaxants, NSAIDs, and even some Tylenol with codeine. Usually, Dr. Henderson is quite receptive to receiving these samples as they help ease the financial burden on his patients for whom he uses or to whom he dispenses the samples. The office is, in fact, running quite low on these particular medications because of Dr. Henderson's heavy patient load.

1. What is your response to the sales representative?
2. Should a representative ever take precedence over scheduled appointments?
3. Does the fact that Dr. Henderson is usually quite anxious to receive any and all samples for his patients enter in as a factor?
4. Does the diminished supply of these samples alter the situation?
5. Can the medical assistant ever accept delivery of any or all of these samples?

INTERNET ACTIVITY

Locate three medical appointment-scheduling software programs on the Internet. Compare and contrast the products, services, features, and costs to fit the needs of a general practitioner's medical practice. Then locate the HIPAA compliance guidelines for appointment scheduling, and develop a useful list for future reference.

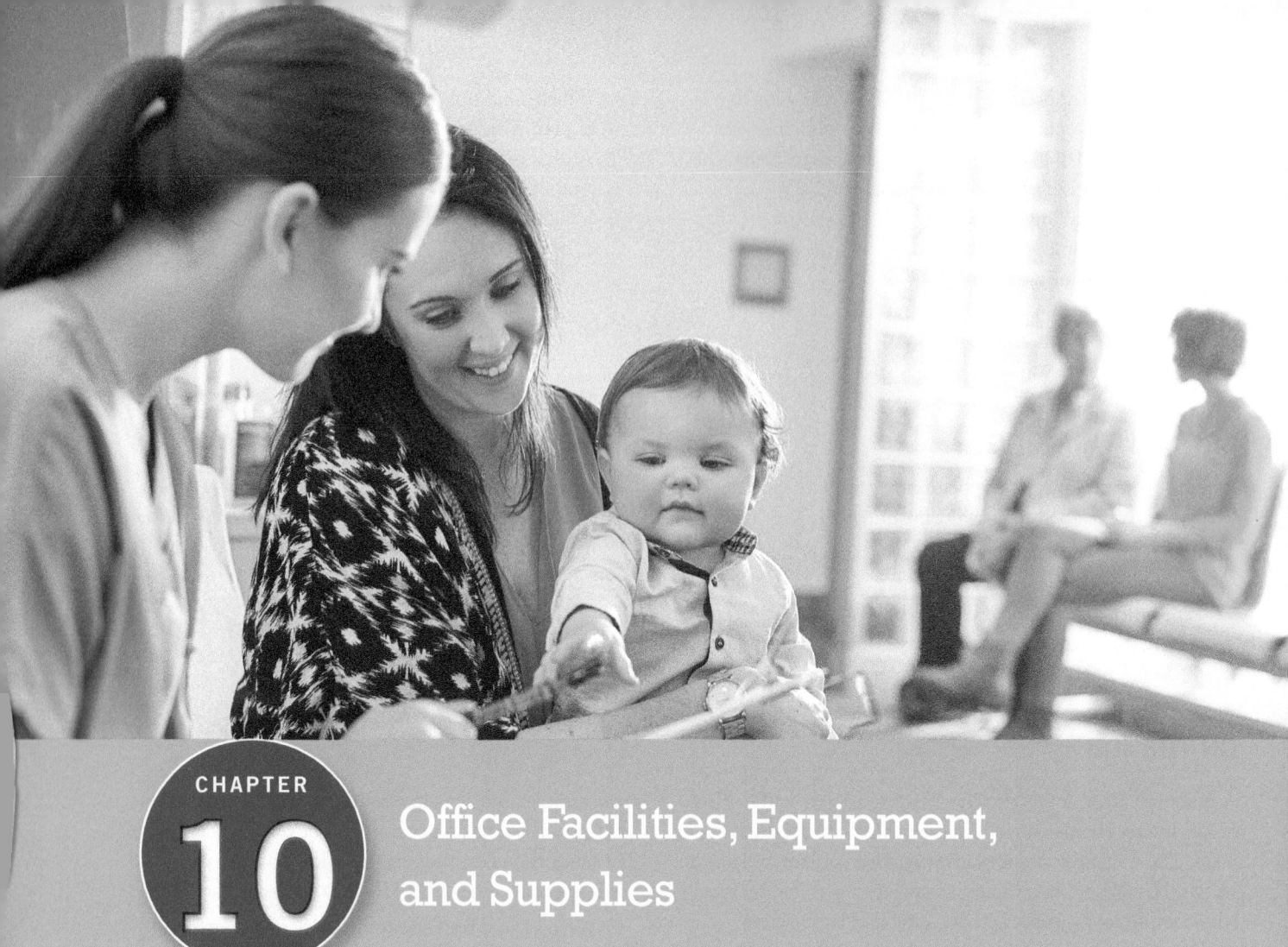

10

Office Facilities, Equipment, and Supplies

Learning Objectives

After completing this chapter, you should be able to:

10.1   Define and spell the terms for this chapter.

10.2   Explain why it is important to consider the Americans with Disabilities Act (ADA) when planning the layout of a medical office.

10.3   Describe elements of effective office flow.

10.4   List considerations that must be taken regarding the purchase and maintenance of capital equipment.

10.5   Describe the functions of various types of medical office equipment.

10.6   Explain why routine maintenance of both administrative and clinical equipment is important in the medical office.

10.7   Describe the differences between capital equipment and expendable supplies.

10.8   List the steps involved in inventory management.

Tania Washington, a medical office manager, arrives at work to find the carpets have just been cleaned and all the patient waiting room furniture is stacked in the hallway. Several patients are starting to walk in the front door. The cleaning crew cleaned the office administration area, and most of the office equipment—including computers and the fax machine—have been moved or unplugged. Tania finds an entire shelf of patient records on the floor and in her work area, and she also notices a few boxes in the hallway that contain patient supplies.

Terms to Learn

Americans with Disabilities Act (ADA)	extended warranty	purchase order (PO)
biomedical equipment	financial life	reorder point
capital equipment	inventory	vendor
clinical equipment	life expectancy	warranty
depreciation	morale	
expendable supplies	office flow	

Every medical workplace should be clean to ensure employee and patient safety and health, the traffic should flow smoothly, and the office should adhere to federal, state, and local safety and health regulations. The physical facility of the medical office plays an important role in staff morale and patient safety. Medical assistants must be aware of the office layout; how to order, use, and maintain office and clinical equipment; and how to manage supplies. As communication processes and technology become more sophisticated, office personnel must stay informed and adhere to the rules that make the medical office safe and protect everyone's right to privacy.

FACILITIES PLANNING

The medical assistant must view the medical office through the eyes of the patient. What does the patient see upon entering the doors and beyond? The pleasant physical atmosphere created by a cheerful, clean office makes an immediate impression on patients. It also enhances the morale of the employees. **Morale** refers to the positive or negative state of mind of employees regarding their work or work environment.

One of the first considerations in planning a medical office facility is the **Americans with Disabilities Act (ADA)**. This legislation protects the rights of the disabled regarding access to employment, public buildings, transportation, housing, schools, and health care facilities. The law requires private facilities used by the public to be easily accessible to disabled individuals, including unrestricted hallways, elevators or ramps, and handicapped-restroom facilities. Furnishings should be arranged to create an easy traffic pattern for patients to follow as they enter and leave the office. The waiting room should have adequate space for wheelchairs to be easily maneuvered.

Patients should walk into a medical office environment that is comfortable and bright. Some medical offices have a reception room with a window that allows patients to look outside during their wait time. External light makes the room well-lit and comfortable. Reception rooms generally should be painted with light colors and have pleasing and tasteful art on the walls (Figure 10-1). Fish tanks are common in medical offices because they are inviting for children and adults to watch. If your office has a fish tank, it is important to regularly maintain the tank for patient safety and cleanliness (and, of course, the well-being of the fish). Be certain to position the tank high enough so children cannot disturb the fish or push over the tank.

OFFICE LAYOUT

Factors to be considered in setting up and maintaining a medical office include the office layout and design, which set the tone, attitude, climate, and culture of the office. Elements of the layout—some of which are mentioned in this chapter and the "Patient Reception" chapter—include the

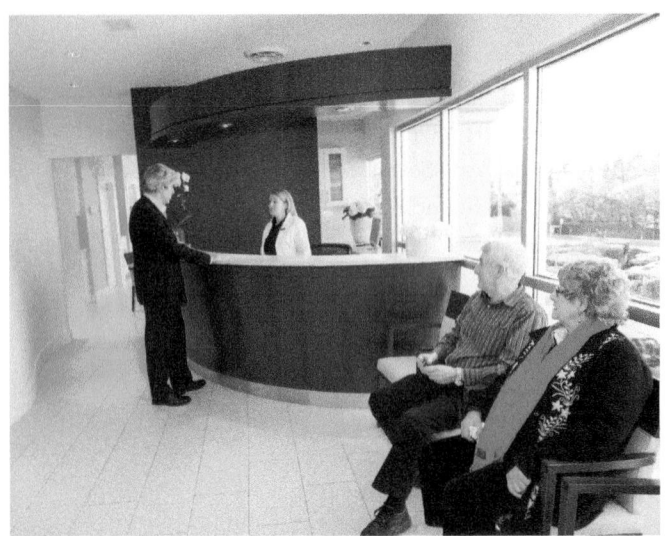

FIGURE 10-1 A reception area should be comfortable and bright.

design of traffic flow, the color of the walls, lighting, room temperature, ventilation, furniture and placement of the furniture, equipment, supplies, and overall organization.

Medical offices are generally divided into two areas: administrative and clinical. The administrative area contains the reception area, where patient processing and scheduling, file storage, payment collections, insurance, billing, and mail processing are performed. Office equipment such as computers, printers, scanners, fax machines, postage meters, calculators, telephone system, paper shredder, dictation and transcribing equipment, and office supplies are also usually located in the administrative area. The reception area often includes a children's play area.

The clinical area contains the examination rooms; physician's office and consultation room; treatment room for office surgical procedures; supply room; clean and contaminated utility areas; restrooms; a laboratory that can house blood drawing, specimen analyzing, and electrocardiogram (ECG) equipment; and, in some offices, a radiology room. Some medical facilities also have a small recovery room with a bed or cot for patients recovering from minor surgical procedures. Specialty practices may have other departments and equipment specific to the types of procedures performed.

Office Flow

The medical facility generally is organized in a way that lends itself easily to teamwork, time management, organized and efficient office equipment usage, and patient movement. This is known as **office flow**. A well-organized office area lends itself

to smooth office flow and reduced cycle time—the length of time the average patient spends in the medical office (Figure 10-2).

The first element of office flow is the patient entrance. The office entranceways should include handrails, elevators, ramps, wheelchair-accessible door frames, patient lifts if necessary, and well-lit walkways. High steps should be marked with reflector tape and should include slip-protection sheets. Doors and door handles should be marked with a push or pull indicator. Keeping doors clean and clear is vital to office aesthetics and patient safety.

Reception Area

The reception area consists of the sitting area for patients and the reception desk. The desk might be enclosed with a

---

Professionalism | The Life Span

Care must be taken to keep the office childproof and kid-friendly. Cover outlets with safety caps. Evaluate the placement of lamps and cords that can be pulled on or tripped over. Also eliminate potential fall hazards that could cause an injury for older adults or disabled individuals, such as loose rugs, toys or other objects on the floor, or freestanding signs that obstruct the traffic flow.

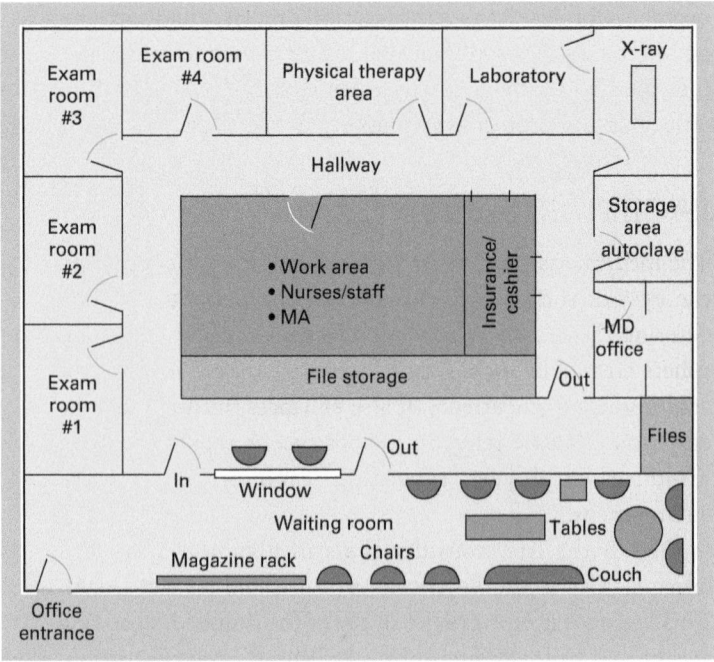

FIGURE 10-2 A typical office layout.

glass partition that can be closed for privacy so that personal medical information cannot be overheard by others in the sitting area. The desk surface should be neat and not contain confidential patient information such as records, an open appointment book, or billing information.

The medical records area should be close to the receptionist's area for quick accessibility to charts needed during telephone calls. The Health Insurance Portability and Accountability Act (HIPAA) states that the medical records area should not be accessible to patients and that patients should not be able to read the labels of the charts. Figure 10-3 shows a typical office file room. Paper medical records are becoming obsolete as they are replaced by electronic records, but most offices still have a certain number of paper records.

Seating that provides good support and can be easily cleaned is most suitable for the patient reception area. Overstuffed chairs and couches should be avoided. Housekeeping staff cannot move such furniture easily. In addition, older adults and the infirm find it difficult to get in and out of deep chairs.

Almost every office provides magazines for patients to read. Materials placed for patient reading must be screened to make sure they meet the standards of your office and would not upset any patients, such as those with strong political or religious viewpoints. Some offices opt to use the patient reception room to provide general patient education on topics such as healthy eating, exercise, and the adverse effects of smoking. Several types of media, such as DVDs, printed literature, and magazines, may be used to present this form of patient education. Typically, the receptionist or another staff member is assigned to keep the reception room, especially magazines and brochures, neatly organized.

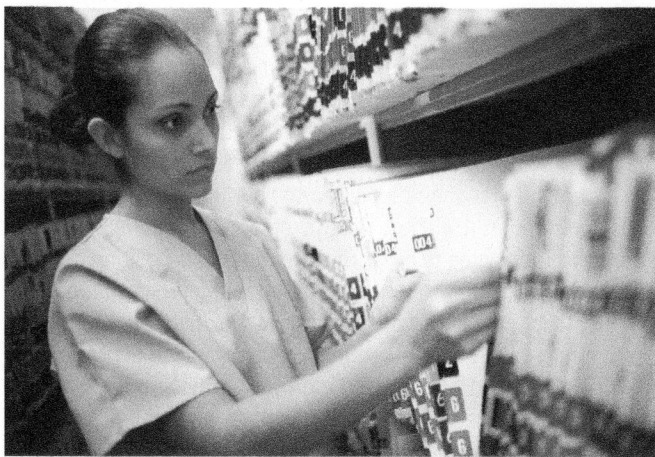

FIGURE 10-3 A typical office file room. (Paper medical records are rapidly being replaced by electronic records.)

Professionalism

Professional medical assistants must strive to keep their immediate work area neat, clean, and organized. This is especially important in the reception area because a patient's first impression of the office, or you personally, may be formed based on the appearance of your work area. Be sure not to allow charts to stack up on the desk or have papers scattered. This may cause the patient to be concerned with how you may take care of their personal information, and this in turn may affect their confidence in the office.

Smoking is not allowed in medical facilities. "No smoking" signs should be placed at the entrance of the building, and a container should be available for the disposal of cigarettes before entering the building. Many states have laws that prohibit smoking immediately outside an entrance, usually within 25 or 30 feet. When this is the case, appropriate signs should be placed outside the door. Some offices place a sign for a designated smoking area at the appropriate distance from the entrance to guide people to the appropriate spot and discourage them from smoking too close to the doors. It is good to monitor the area periodically to ensure that patients do not have to walk through secondhand smoke to enter the office.

A person with a communicable disease who visits the office should be placed in a designated area to minimize spreading the disease. After the visit, the area used should be disinfected immediately.

Patient orientation begins when the patient arrives in the reception area. Clear markings and signs should indicate the location of the registration and check-in desk, office entrance and exits, where patients should sit if more than one doctor is in the office, and restroom locations. Hallways and walkways should be clear of obstructions. In some offices, color-coded indicators on the floor or wall help to facilitate patient flow.

Proper signage helps patients get around the medical office, because it is easy to become disoriented in an area with multiple hallways and doors that look similar. Clearly marked signs assist patients as they exit. When a patient is ready to leave, it is important to confirm the route a patient needs to take to exit the office. For example, if a patient has just been seen by a physician and you are showing the patient out, it is best to lead the way. This helps prevent patients from accidentally walking into another examination room or into private areas of the office. Patients should have a direct, clearly marked route to the check-out desk.

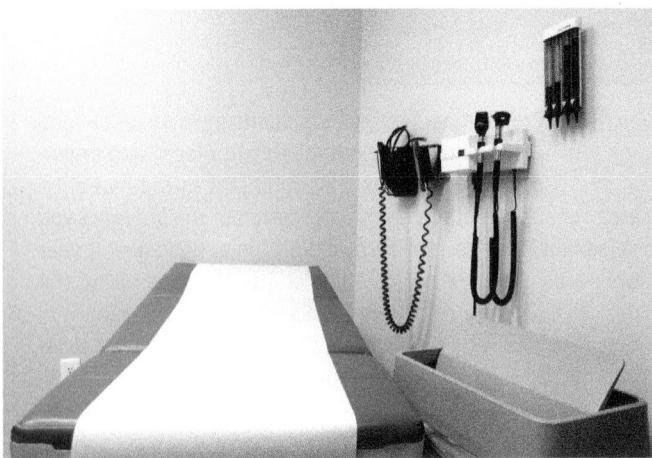

FIGURE 10-4 A patient examination room should be simple and efficiently designed.

Examination Rooms

Examination rooms should contain only furnishings and equipment needed to examine a patient. Most examination rooms have only enough space for the necessities and little else. Figure 10-4 illustrates a typical patient examination room. A sufficient number of instruments and supplies, such as disposable gowns, towels, tissues, and sheets, are kept in examination room supply cabinets. Most examination tables have drawers for the convenient storage of these items. A small sink for hand hygiene, an adjustable gooseneck lamp, chair, small writing desk, examination table, clothes hook, and physician's stool are the only furnishings necessary. Examination rooms should be painted in pleasant and comforting colors. Paintings or pictures can enhance the serenity of the room. Be sure unpleasant odors are not present in the examination rooms. If they are, you might need to close that room until the odor dissipates or the room is sanitized.

The temperature throughout the reception area and examination rooms should be maintained around 72°F. Patients in the examination rooms must frequently disrobe and may be chilled in just a disposable gown. If the examination room is too warm, patients will become drowsy. Controlling the room temperature so that all are comfortable is often one of the most difficult tasks to accomplish in the office because patients have varying sensitivities to heat and cold.

At least one examination room should be configured for a wheelchair-bound patient. It should be larger than a normal-sized examination room to allow both the patient and physician to maneuver comfortably.

Examination rooms should be soundproof so that conversations cannot be heard from one room to another. The examination table should be arranged so that the patient is not exposed when the door is opened. "White noise," such as pleasant, soothing background music, can also filter sounds.

Bathrooms

Bathrooms should be kept clean and odor free. Every bathroom should have hot and cold water, soap, paper towels or another drying system, a trash can, and toilet tissue. Bathrooms also should be large enough to accommodate a wheelchair, and at least one of the bathrooms should meet ADA guidelines for a handicapped restroom facility, such as handrails around the toilet. Although some offices have separate bathrooms for staff members, the same bathroom often is used by both staff and patients. Patient bathrooms should have a shelf or designated area to place urine specimens while patients wash their hands after collecting the sample. This helps minimize the chance of specimens being spilled.

Housekeeping

Housekeeping or medical office cleaning services can be contracted to clean the front office area, clinical areas, and examination rooms every night. Regular housekeeping services are usually not responsible for handling hazardous waste containers. Medical office staff is responsible for disposing hazardous waste (including sharps) in designated containers. Staff members are also responsible for removing the containers from the office or facility (they should follow office procedures). If contracting with an outside cleaning service, the service must operate in compliance with HIPAA standards, particularly if the cleaning personnel accidentally encounter any protected health information (PHI). This requires the cleaning service to sign a HIPAA Business Associate agreement stating members of the service will adhere to HIPAA patient privacy laws and the service will provide the necessary training for its employees.

> ### Professionalism   The Workplace
>
> Flexibility is the key to being a successful health care employee. You may typically work as a clinical medical assistant; however, you may be asked to cover for someone in an administrative position. When asked to cover, you first should check with your immediate supervisor to verify that it will not cause problems within the clinical area and then agree to cover the administrative position. Several benefits come with covering for a fellow employee. Doing so demonstrates that you are truly a flexible team player, which may then be reflected in your performance appraisals. It also is an opportunity to sharpen your skills and work with equipment you may not use all the time in the clinical setting. Take every available opportunity to learn as much as you can about the practice where you work.

OFFICE EQUIPMENT

Office machines and equipment improve efficiency and help maintain effective office flow. Essential office equipment includes a copier, computers, printers, scanners, postage meters, calculators, telephone systems, a facsimile system, and paper shredder (Table 10-1).

New technologies tend to take over the functions of older ones. Some equipment is multi-functional, meaning that one piece of physical equipment serves more than one purpose, such as printing, copying, scanning, and faxing. Offices may have replaced a dedicated fax machine (Figure 10-5) with a scanner and Internet fax services or e-mail. Tasks that once required specialized equipment now can be performed electronically. The functions of a calculator may be performed on a desktop or mobile computer device. A postage meter might be replaced with an electronic postage application supplied by the United States Postal Service. Smartphones and other mobile devices may handle some functions formerly confined to a landline phone system and large desktop computers. If using mobile devices rather than desktop computers or landline phone systems, extra care must be taken not to use such devices in areas where patient information can be seen or overheard, in violation of HIPAA requirements.

The receptionist is often responsible for monitoring certain equipment and learning the many functions of these machines. Knowledge of how to repair small problems, such as clearing paper jams and replacing toner or ink cartridges, is also helpful. It is important that the receptionist attempt to troubleshoot the equipment before calling for service, because solving issues yourself may prevent expensive service calls. Keep a list of phone numbers to call for service for each piece of equipment, if needed. Some service companies place a sticker with their phone number on the piece(s) of equipment they service.

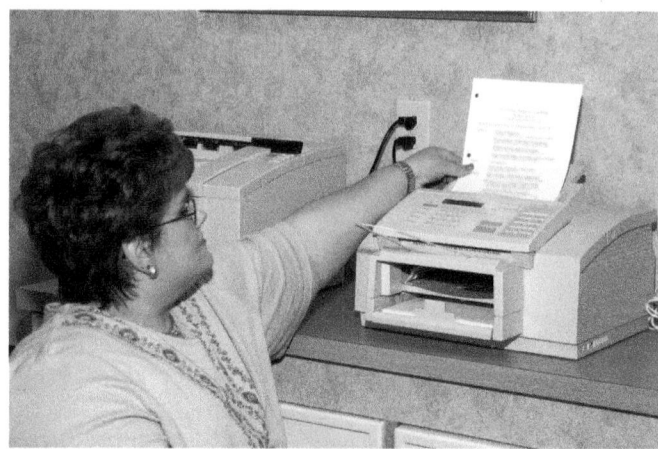

FIGURE 10-5 Fax machines are used in many medical offices, although newer technologies, including scanners, Internet fax machines, and e-mail services, are often used instead to transmit documents.

Capital Equipment

Capital equipment refers to items that require a large dollar amount to purchase (generally over $500) and have a relatively long life. The factor that distinguishes capital equipment from general office supplies is the **life expectancy** (functional life period) of the product. In addition to office equipment, capital equipment also includes examination tables, refrigerators, X-ray and ECG machines, and office furnishings. Capital equipment has longer life than consumable supplies, and its cost is recorded following specific accounting rules.

Capital equipment also has a **financial life**, which is referred to as the depreciation period. **Depreciation** is a loss in value of the product resulting from normal aging, use, or deterioration. An accounting allowance is made for this type of loss of value for tax purposes. This allows the practice to set aside a small amount of money each year toward the eventual replacement of the equipment. Therefore, the office accountant credits capital items differently than general office supplies. A master **inventory**, or list, should be maintained of all the physical assets, or capital equipment, in an office. The inventory list should include the type of equipment, manufacturer, purchase date, serial number, and location. Many offices attach a numbered tag or metal plate with an identification number to each piece of equipment. This helps track where the equipment is located at the current time.

The needs of the office determine the equipment required. Obtaining the equipment requires research to gather equipment information, the actual purchase, delivery, setup, proper training, safe use, and general maintenance. Most medical offices have the following administrative capital equipment:

- **Computers**—Laptops and desktops.
- **Color laser printer**—Used in conjunction with a computer for letter-quality printing. Creates images with a

TABLE 10-1 | Types of Equipment in a Medical Office	
Office Equipment	**Clinical Equipment**
Copier	X-ray machine
Computer	Electrocardiograph (ECG)
Printer	Ultrasonic washer
Scanner	Centrifuge
Postage meter	Endoscope
Telephone system	Pulse oximeter
Facsimile system	Specimen refrigerator
Paper shredder	Urine analyzer

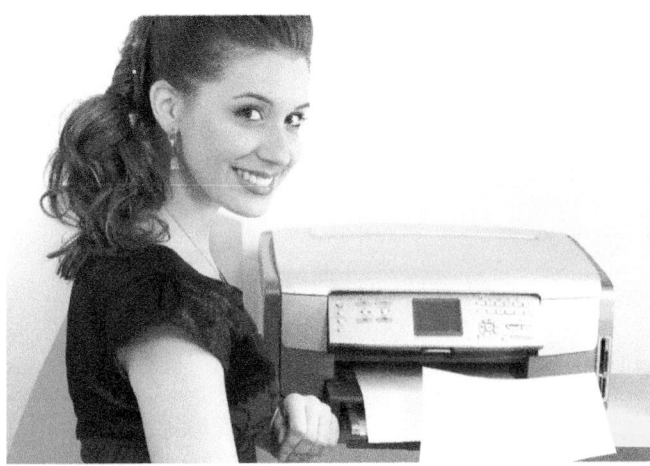

FIGURE 10-6 Copiers should meet the particular needs of the medical office.

laser beam and then transfers the color image to paper with pressure and heat.

- **Telephone system.**
- **Scanners**—Used to "read" and copy text and graphic files, which can be printed out or stored as computer files.
- **Copy machine**—Used to copy, reduce, enlarge, and collate documents in the medical office (Figure 10-6).
- **Postage meter**—Used by offices with large mailings to stamp envelopes and packages (if they have not replaced the meter with electronic postage software).

Purchasing Equipment

When a business determines the need for specific equipment, the purchase process begins. The medical assistant may be asked to research and compare equipment based on the manufacturer, quality, size, service, price, and other determining factors. The medical assistant can search the Internet and can contact local vendors and other offices as part of the fact-gathering quest. Whenever possible, it is wise to identify three to five potential vendors to research. Collecting information, printed materials, and resources helps the physician to make the right choice when actually purchasing the equipment.

Warranties

A **warranty** is a manufacturer's guarantee in writing that its product will perform correctly under normal conditions of use. The warranty provides for a replacement of defective parts at no charge within a certain period of time. An **extended warranty** can be purchased to cover some period of time after the warranty has expired. For example, a copier may have a one-year warranty, but an extended warranty

can be purchased to cover parts replacement after that year has expired.

Be sure to determine exactly what problems are covered by a manufacturer's warranty compared with an extended warranty. In many warranties, only certain kinds of repairs or part replacements are included and others are specifically excluded. Decide if the coverage offered is worth the additional cost of an extended warranty.

Some office equipment that is heavily used, such as a copy machine, has a service contract for preventive maintenance. To avoid a breakdown, a service contract provides maintenance and cleaning of equipment even when it is working properly. A service contract states in detail what problems and service are covered. The dates and frequency of service should be noted carefully.

Literature relating to warranties and preventive maintenance contracts should be kept in a designated location. Because office equipment is expensive, these contracts are important.

Equipment Life and Safety

All equipment purchased comes with a manufacturer's user manual, or instruction manual, that provides instructions about how to maintain the life of the machine and the safety of the user. The medical assistant should read all manuals before using any piece of equipment and have the vendor provide training for the office staff. User manuals provide cleaning, maintenance, and operation directions as well as other important information. The instructions usually place safety of the user first, longevity of the equipment second, and reordering or service information third. User manuals identify default settings for the equipment, how to alter them when needed, and when equipment should be left on and when it should be turned completely off. If a manual for a particular piece of equipment cannot be located, or multiple copies are needed, it is often possible to download the manual from the manufacturer's website.

Procedure 10-1 details procedures for maintaining equipment.

Equipment Records

Records relating to office equipment must be maintained. Receipts for major purchases, operating manuals, instructions, warranties, and repair and maintenance instructions must be kept and filed appropriately. Lists of service people with contact information should be maintained. Many offices maintain a current file of business cards representing the companies from which equipment has been purchased.

An equipment inventory log provides a comprehensive master list of all equipment owned by the office. Typically,

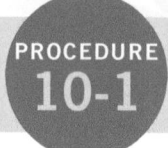

Maintaining Equipment

Objective ◆ *Perform routine maintenance of office and clinical equipment with documentation.*

EQUIPMENT AND SUPPLIES

Equipment maintenance log; access to desired piece of equipment; user manual; pen or pencil

METHOD

1. Plan a time to perform equipment inspection and maintenance when it will not interfere with patient reception and care, such as before or after office hours.
2. Refer to the equipment maintenance log to determine which pieces of equipment are scheduled for inspection and maintenance. Access the user manual or service instructions for each piece of equipment.
3. Note that for certain aspects of inspection and maintenance, the equipment may need to be turned off and unplugged. For other tasks, such as calibration, the equipment may need to be turned on.
4. Visually inspect the equipment, paying special attention to items identified in the user manual. Also check for frayed electrical cords, loose connections, missing screws or fasteners, and loose parts.
5. Perform performance and calibration tests recommended by the manufacturer. Adjust equipment, as needed, according to manufacturer instructions.
6. Clean equipment, and replace lightbulbs, batteries, ink/toner, paper, and other supplies as needed. Always follow manufacturer instructions.
7. In the maintenance log, enter the date of the inspection and your name or initials. Note any problems that require further attention.
8. If the equipment is not operating properly, unplug it and place a sign on it that states, "NOT IN SERVICE. DO NOT USE." Inform the office manager. Telephone the service company to schedule a service call.

it is maintained in the computer and updated by the office manager or other responsible individual. In addition, the office's policies and procedures manual contains a list of equipment used for specific procedures. This is especially helpful for training new employees so they know what is required for specific activities. Table 10-2 provides an example of an office equipment inventory log.

Each piece of equipment should have a maintenance log that documents when regular maintenance is required, when the maintenance occurred, and which individual or company provided the service (Figure 10-7). The maintenance log can

be created and stored on the computer using a spreadsheet or word processing program. In addition to routine maintenance, also document unusual occurrences of equipment on the maintenance log. Memory of what actually happened may fail over time. A written record of exactly what happened and the corrective action that was taken can assist in determining cause as an accident or negligence. An up-to-date maintenance log helps prove that equipment has been properly maintained. The maintenance log may be required by the insurance company and may be subpoenaed if a patient was injured because of equipment failure.

TABLE 10-2	Equipment Inventory Record			
Item	**Serial #**	**Purchase Date**	**Location**
Laptop	XX 12345	2/14/YY	Reception
IBM Workstation	4-190-L1001	9/19/YY	Reception
Hewlett-Packard Color LaserJet Printer	JPHAC15531	9/19/YY	Reception
Ricoh Copier	RC39C452	6/2/YY	Billing

EQUIPMENT MAINTENANCE LOG

Equipment: _Copy Machine_   Location: _Billing Department_
Manufacturer: _Ricoh_   Model: _RC39C452_   Serial # _0987654_
Date purchased _6/2/YY_
Warranty _1 year_   Service Contract _expires 5/31/YY_
Service Phone Number _1-800-555-9999_

Date	Types of Service Performed	Results/Problems	Performed by
1/2/YY	Inspection and cleaning	OK	S. Allen
1/9/YY	Inspection and cleaning	Automatic sheet feeder not working. Called ABC Service.	S. Allen
1/10/YY	Repair auto-sheet feeder	Working	ABC Service
1/15/YY	Changed toner	OK	S. Allen

FIGURE 10-7 Sample equipment maintenance log.

CLINICAL EQUIPMENT

Clinical equipment, also known as **biomedical equipment**, such as an X-ray machine, ECG, ultrasonic washer, centrifuge, endoscope, pulse oximeter, specimen refrigerator, and urine analyzer, is used in patient care. It is especially critical that clinical equipment be maintained in excellent condition so that it does not harm the patient or staff and produces accurate and reliable results. Many pieces of equipment require daily or weekly inspection and simple maintenance. The Clinical Laboratory Improvement Amendments (CLIA), which regulate laboratory testing and equipment, require that testing and calibration be performed according to manufacturer specifications.

The instruction manual for each piece of equipment should list regularly scheduled maintenance, such as visual inspection, performance tests, calibration, cleaning, changing filters, lubrication, replacement of parts expected to wear such as bearings and tubing, and other protocols. Only authorized and trained staff members should perform calibration and maintenance. Some tasks require an outside contractor or biomechanical technician.

A maintenance log should be kept for each piece of clinical equipment that identifies what service is to be performed and at what frequency. The individual who performs the maintenance should sign and date when each task is completed. If a staff member is performing routine inspection and notices a problem, it must be addressed immediately. Do not ignore or delay minor problems, because they could be a sign of a more serious problem or could develop into a more serious problem if not corrected. In the event that clinical equipment is not functioning properly, it should be tagged out by placing a sign on the equipment that clearly states "NOT IN SERVICE. DO NOT USE." Some equipment may have a lockout mechanism that physically locks the equipment or electrical cord to prevent it from being used until it is properly repaired.

Maintaining clinical equipment properly, documenting any problems, and getting it repaired promptly help keep the equipment accurate and reliable, ensure the safety of patients and staff, and protect the physician should there ever be a lawsuit related to a piece of equipment.

SUPPLIES

Office and clinical supplies are vital to the smooth operation of an office and to the ability to provide patient care. Medical assistants may have responsibilities to ensure that an adequate volume of supplies is always on hand, to reorder supplies, to select supply vendors, and to stock supplies. This process is referred to as inventory management. **Expendable supplies**, also called consumable supplies, are items that are used up quickly and have a relatively inexpensive unit cost. Examples of expendable office supplies are found in Table 10-3.

Business Vendors

The medical office uses a variety of **vendors**, or suppliers, to provide all supplies used. Vendors are selected based on several factors, including product price, quality, delivery, and

TABLE 10-3 | Expendable Supplies

Paper Supplies	**Clinical** examination table paper, disposable gowns, drapes, paper towels, sterilization bags and tapes, stationery, ECG paper
	Office photocopy/printer/fax paper, insurance forms, medical chart forms, laboratory order forms, appointment book, receipt book, appointment cards
Clinical Supplies	Disposable speculums, ear and nose speculum covers, catheters, tongue blades, thermometers, cotton-tipped applicators, lubricant, needles, syringes, suture material, dressings, tape, elastic bandages, gloves, goggles, biohazard (red) bags
Office Supplies	Pens, pencils, highlighters, staplers, staple removers, copier/printer/fax ink/toner, CD/DVDs, trash bags

customer service. A reliable supplier is a valuable resource to the practice and can assist in problem solving of supply-related issues, researching products for unique needs, and placing special orders when needed. Types of suppliers include the following:

- Local medical supply houses
- National chains
- Catalogs
- Online
- Group purchasing co-operative (an organization that makes bulk purchases on behalf of several medical facilities and passes the volume discounts on to members)

Suppliers have sales representatives to assist medical offices with the company's products. Representatives usually are assigned to a specific geographic region and, sometimes, to a specific type of health care provider, such as a medical office or hospital. In this way, the sales representative can be knowledgeable about users' needs and serve as an overall point of contact between the vendor and the customer. Sales representatives can help medical offices evaluate the most appropriate product(s) for a specific application. They often can provide or arrange for training for office staff regarding use of the product. Therefore, it is helpful for medical assistants to get to know their vendor representatives. If you have a positive relationship with a sales representative and a problem arises with a product, or you need something on short notice, the sales representative can help troubleshoot the problem, arrange for a replacement, or assist in expediting an order.

Offices should have a policy for how to deal with pharmaceutical representatives, who provide prescription drug samples to physicians. For example, they might request direct access to a physician to discuss the latest drug, but they cannot come in unannounced and expect immediate attention from a physician. There should be a specific time in the schedule for meeting with pharmaceutical representatives that does not interfere with patient care. Each representative should be informed of the time of the appointment and the amount of time allowed. The medical assistant must ensure that such guidelines are followed closely, which might mean announcing when a representative's time has concluded.

It is common for pharmaceutical representatives to schedule a lunch with the office to present their latest products because it is thought that this is a convenient time for physicians. The representative often orders a catered lunch to be delivered to the office or might even host staff at a local restaurant. Offices should establish policy whether this practice is acceptable, the maximum acceptable dollar value of a lunch, how often each company can do this, and the scheduling procedure.

There should also be a maximum dollar value of any gifts that can be accepted by medical office staff from vendors. The purpose is to avoid any improper influence or appearance of bribery. The process of accepting favors or gifts establishes an obligation by the recipient that could result in preferring one company's business, rather than selecting the best products for the office. Even when an individual recipient makes every effort not to show favoritism, others might perceive or interpret that favoritism occurs. Any appearance of an improper relationship must be avoided.

HIPAA Business Associates

Under HIPAA, a business associate is a person or entity who performs activities on behalf of, or provides certain services to, the medical office that involve access by the business associate to PHI. A business associate also can be a subcontractor who creates, receives, maintains, or transmits PHI on behalf of another business associate. Examples of business associates include medical billing services, laboratories, computer vendors who assist with patient records, and answering services. HIPAA rules generally require that medical offices enter into contracts with their business associates to ensure that the business associates will appropriately safeguard PHI. Most vendors and suppliers do not access PHI, so a business associate agreement is not necessary.

Inventory Management

Inventory management requires constant supervision, because a medical office cannot afford to run out of supplies. It can be costly to run out of supplies and have to suddenly make a purchase at full price with additional shipping costs for faster service. The office should maintain a master list of all supplies used, the preferred vendor(s), the quantity normally ordered, the reorder point (explained later), and where in the office they are stored. It is best to track this on the computer using a spreadsheet or word processing software.

Offices maintain an ongoing inventory system that helps to determine when to reorder supplies. There are several ways this can be accomplished:

- **Inventory sheets**—Place an inventory sheet inside the door of each supply cabinet that lists all the supplies stored in that location. Provide space next to each item for staff members to record when they use or remove a supply item.
- **Reminder cards**—Insert color-coded reorder reminder cards into the stack of inventory items. When the card comes to the top of the stack, it is time to reorder.

- **Barcodes**—Use a barcode scanning system with which users scan each item removed from the supply area. This connects to a computer program that monitors supply usage and alerts the user when it is time to reorder.
- **Sticker system**—Removable stickers with an item number or barcode are placed on each item. When the item is taken, the user places the sticker on a sheet, which is monitored by the inventory manager.
- **Supplier initiated**—Some suppliers maintain their own records and notify the medical office when it is time to reorder.
- **Just-in-Time**—Some offices take advantage of a just-in-time (JIT) inventory method. Offices arrange a delivery schedule with suppliers, based on past usage, that delivers the most used supplies on a regular basis, such as twice a week or even daily. This eliminates the need for the office to maintain large stockpiles, eliminates frequent ordering, ensures that the office always has needed supplies, and improves the office's cash flow.

Each of these methods requires that the office establish a **reorder point** for each item. The reorder point is the lowest amount of a supply item the office should have before reordering. It is determined by the frequency with which supplies are used and the amount of time necessary to have the order processed and delivered. The office should also establish specific dates when orders will be placed, so that orders for multiple items can be processed at the same time. For example, an office may order clinical supplies on the 10th of the month and office supplies on the 20th of the month. It is inefficient to place orders multiple times per week or month, because it takes nearly as much time to order one item as it does several. It may also be more costly, because vendors may provide a discount or free shipping when an order exceeds a certain dollar amount. When establishing reorder points for various items, always factor in adequate lead time before the reorder date.

For example, assume that one printer toner cartridge lasts approximately one month and office supplies are ordered on the 20th of each month. It would be advisable to reorder printer cartridges when two remain in inventory. By doing this, if a printer cartridge is replaced on the 25th of the month, there will be an adequate supply to last until the next reorder date and allow time for the order placed on the 20th to be delivered. Having the extra cartridge also provides a buffer in case more than the usual amount of printing is done because of heavy patient flow or billing requirements.

It takes experience to be able to calculate how long inventory items last. However, records can be reviewed to determine when half the supply has been used. Then, by calculating the amount of time it takes to receive a new order, an estimate can be made of when and how much to reorder. Procedure 10-2 details the steps involved in performing an inventory.

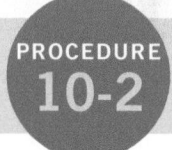

PROCEDURE 10-2 Performing Office Inventory

Objective ◆ *Perform an inventory of office and clinical supplies.*

EQUIPMENT AND SUPPLIES
Inventory sheets; pen or pencil; computer

METHOD

1. Plan a time to review inventory when it does not interfere with patient reception and care, such as before or after office hours. Schedule inventory review to occur immediately before placing an order, so that information is current.
2. Collect and review inventory data from all supply storage locations, depending on the method used to track inventory, such as inventory supply sheets, reminder cards, stickers, or barcode information.
3. Highlight items that have reached or are very near the reorder point.
4. Physically check the remaining supply of any items for which the inventory data are unclear or not available. To do this, locate the supplies in the storage area and physically count how many remain. Discard any clinical supplies that are past the expiration date marked on the package, following office policies and procedures.
5. Enter the date and inventory counts for each item into a computer spreadsheet for future reference when ordering.
6. Plan to place the order within one or two days so the inventory data does not become outdated.

Ordering Systems

When comparing prices, evaluate not only the price of the product itself, but also the availability of volume discounts and added charges such as delivery or shipping costs. Be aware that some companies that offer a low list price may not have the product readily available to ship, resulting in a time delay, or they may charge high shipping costs. Therefore, compare the total cost of the delivered product, which includes the product price, shipping and handling costs, rush delivery costs, and sales tax.

Unit Pricing

The price of the product should be compared on a per unit basis across suppliers, because the price listed by various suppliers may be different for differing quantities. Use basic math skills to compare unit pricing, which requires that all prices refer to the same unit. For example, if ordering cartons of exam table paper rolls, compare the number of feet per roll and the number of rolls per carton. When all these factors are not the same, you may need to do some simple math to create an accurate comparison. Table 10-4 shows an example of a unit pricing comparison for exam table paper from various suppliers. Rolls are of differing lengths, differing quality, and sold in different quantities. To compute the cost per foot, do the following, using Company A as an example:

1. Locate the price per carton. *Example*: $42.69

2. Divide by the number of rolls per carton. *Example*: $42.69/12 = $3.557 per roll

3. Divide again by the number of feet per roll. *Example*: $3.557/125 = $0.028 per foot

4. If desired, divide by 100 to convert dollars to cents. *Example*: $0.028/100 = 2.8¢ per foot

By calculating the price per foot, the medical assistant can easily see prices that range from 1.4¢ per foot to 7.3¢. Reasons for variation include:

- The length of rolls varies from 120 feet to 225 feet.

- The width of the paper varies from 18 inches to 21 inches, so the medical assistant must select the correct width needed.

- The product from Company D is labeled "deluxe" paper and is the most costly.

- Companies A and B sell a carton for the same price, but Company B sells rolls that are 120 feet long, compared with 125 foot rolls from Company A.

- Company B and Company E both sell paper for 3.0¢ per foot, but the paper from company E is 2 inches wider.

- Paper sold in rolls of 225 feet tends to be less expensive per foot than paper sold in shorter rolls.

Company F sells paper for only 1.4¢ per foot. This is half as costly as the other products, so the medical assistant may choose to order a single roll to compare the quality before placing a large order. Sales representatives of various companies might be able to provide samples for the office to test. If the office has been experiencing problems with the quality of exam table paper, the medical assistant may want to contact Company D and request a sample roll of the "deluxe" paper to evaluate if it is worth the additional cost.

Small savings add up for items used in large quantities, such as exam table paper or gloves. For example, even a small medical office can use 100,000 feet of exam table paper per year. Saving a one-half-cent per foot on paper could result in a savings of $500 or more over the course of a year. One staff

TABLE 10-4 | Unit Pricing Comparison

Company	Product	Price per Carton	Rolls per Carton	Feet per Roll	Price per Foot	¢ per Foot
A	Standard exam table paper 18" × 125'	$42.69	12	125	$0.028	2.8¢
B	Standard exam table paper 18" × 120'	$42.69	12	120	$0.030	3.0¢
C	Standard exam table paper 21" × 225'	$69.19	12	225	$0.026	2.6¢
D	Deluxe exam table paper 21" × 1500'	$54.49	6	125	$0.073	7.3¢
E	Standard exam table paper 20" × 125'	$59.95	9	125	$0.053	5.3¢
F	Standard exam table paper 18" × 225'	$3.15	1	225	$0.014	1.4¢

member may use 20,000 gloves per year. Saving one cent per glove could result in a savings of $200 per staff member. However, gloves that are less costly but of poor quality may actually be more expensive in the long run. When gloves tear easily, staff may tend to double-glove (wear two gloves at the same time) or change to new gloves more frequently than otherwise necessary. The lower price may be more than offset by the increased number of gloves used. Staff may become frustrated with the unsatisfactory product, they could be exposed to a greater risk of contamination, and it could look bad to patients.

Discounts

Many vendors provide a discount on supplies when they are ordered in large quantities. This results in a unit cost savings. The drawback to this method is that many offices do not have enough storage space to handle a large inventory of supplies. Some suppliers store excess inventory for the office, delivering it when requested. This allows the office to save money on quantity purchases without needing a lot of extra storage space.

Vendors may provide additional discounts if the medical office signs a contract agreeing to purchase a certain amount of supplies during the year. Contracts or purchase agreements may include payment schedules, shipment times, product discounts, extended warranty, training sessions, and other incentives. In preparation for negotiating contracts, develop a good working relationship with vendors, either in person, on the telephone, in writing, or online.

Other opportunities for obtaining discounts are group purchasing agreements and local buying clubs such as Costco or Sam's Club.

Placing the Order

The process for placing the order is determined by the vendor. Vendors used repeatedly may provide an option to use a manual or online order form that contains previously ordered items, quantities, and item numbers. You may change quantities, delete unwanted items, and add new ones for the new order. This is a tremendous time saver. When ordering from a new or infrequently used supplier, a blank order form must be completed. See Figure 10-8 for a sample supplies order form.

Frequently used vendors usually allow medical offices to open an account and establish credit. This requires the office to supply financial information and references of other suppliers used. When the account is approved, the supplier bills the office via an invoice. If no account has been established, the office must send a check with the order or provide credit card information. Regardless of whether the office has established an account with a supplier or pays with check or credit card, office policy may require that you prepare a formal

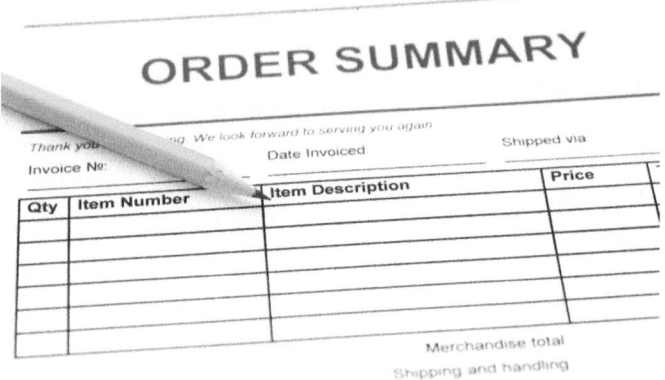

FIGURE 10-8 Sample inventory order form.

purchase order (PO). A PO is a form prepared by the purchaser (the medical office) (Figure 10-9). The PO must be signed by an authorized person in the medical office, such as the office manager or accounting manager. When the vendor bills the office for the order, they place the PO number on the invoice. This enables the office to track the approval and helps protect against unauthorized purchases. Procedure 10-3 explains how to place a supply order.

Receiving an Order

When an order is received, it is important to confirm that it was filled correctly before dispensing supplies to designated areas of the clinic. Open the order when you have time to thoroughly check it. The shipment contains a packing slip that lists every item in the order. Physically locate each item, and compare it to the packing slip to verify that the correct item and correct quantity was shipped. Look for possible notations on the packing slip that indicate a particular product was backordered or shipped separately. Compare the packing slip to the purchase order or order form to verify that the items shipped match the items ordered and that the prices are correct. If there are any variances between the shipment and the order as placed, contact customer service immediately. Do not dispense any items that are incorrect. When everything checks out, staple the packing slip to the purchase order and file them until the invoice is received. At that time, attach the packing slip and purchase order to the invoice to verify that the amount is authorized.

When stocking supply cabinets with newly received supplies, place the newer supplies on the back of the shelf so that older supplies are used first. This is especially important for clinical supplies that have expiration dates. If there are any items that a particular staff member has been waiting for, notify that person that the product has arrived.

Pearson Medical Clinic

PURCHASE ORDER

Pearson Medical Clinic
111 First Avenue
Anytown, NY 11111

The following number must appear on all invoices, bills
of lading, and acknowledgements relating to this PO:
P.O. NUMBER PMC03030303
P.O. DATE 3/3/20YY
TERMS Net 30
F.O.B.
SHIP VIA
ADDRESS CORRESPONDENCE TO:
Name   Mary Manager

TO:
ABC Supply Company
999 Main Street
Anytown, NY 11111

E-mail   Manager@xyz.com
Phone   555-555-5555
FAX#

Sales Tax Rate: 7.50%

QTY	UNIT	DESCRIPTION	UNIT PRICE	AMOUNT
2	Dozen	Product	12.50	25.00
43	Case	Product	0.45	19.35
17	Tube	Product	4.50	76.50
			subtotal	120.85

PLEASE NOTIFY US IMMEDIATELY IF THIS ORDER CANNOT BE SHIPPED COMPLETE ON OR BEFORE: 4/1/20YY	SHIPPING	16.00
	TAX	9.06
	OTHER	
	TOTAL	**$145.91**

FIGURE 10-9 Sample purchase order form.

Drug Samples

The pharmaceutical representatives of drug companies often supply medical offices with samples of medications. A drug sample is a small package of a medication for use by the physician or physician distribution to patients. An inventory list of all sample drugs must be maintained to adhere to Drug Enforcement Administration (DEA) and, in some cases, state regulations (check your local state requirements).

Even though these drug samples are small and "free," the medical office must secure and organize the samples in a locked supply cabinet or drawer. It is advisable to organize drugs by class, storing similar drugs together, such as sedatives, antibiotics, and hypertensive drugs. The expiration dates on drug samples must be carefully monitored. Samples should be rotated like other supplies, with newer samples placed in the back behind samples of the same medication and strength with earlier expiration dates. Expired samples should be discarded following office policies and procedures and in accordance with federal, state, and DEA regulations.

Postage

Because medical offices mail out a large amount of material, using traditional postage stamps can be cumbersome and

PROCEDURE 10-3 Placing a Supply Order

Objective ◆ *Place an order for supplies.*

EQUIPMENT AND SUPPLIES

Inventory sheets; pen or pencil; computer; supply catalogs or website addresses; order form

METHOD

1. Plan a time to place a supply order when it does not interfere with patient reception and care, such as before or after office hours.
2. Review the most recent inventory data. If inventory was counted more than two days previously, it is best to update the information before placing an order.
3. Refer to the catalog, website, or previous order form of each vendor with whom an order needs to be placed.
4. Enter the item number, quantity, and price of each item. Double-check all numbers for accuracy.
5. Prepare a purchase order, if required, and wait for approval before placing the order. Enter the purchase order on the supply order form or attach it to the order (manually or electronically).
6. Submit the order to the vendor using an order form, website, or telephone order line. Verify when delivery can be expected.

---

inefficient. Instead, the office may use a postage meter or electronic postage.

A postage meter is a machine that imprints the postage amount on the envelope or on a strip of adhesive-backed paper that is applied to a package. The postage meter can automatically stamp large mailings. A postage meter with a scale provides the option of weighing letters and packages, then calculates the exact postage required and either prints it directly onto the letter or prints out a strip to be affixed to the package. This method can save significant amounts of money. Metered mail does not have to be stamped with a postmark when it arrives at the post office. Postage is purchased for use with the machine, and as the machine applies postage to letters and packages, the monetary amount in the postage account decreases. When the amount of postage available begins to run low, the medical assistant may either take the meter to the post office or increase the available postage via the Internet if the office has established an account. The meter is occasionally taken into the post office for calibrating (Figure 10-10).

Electronic postage is another option. This method requires the user to apply with and receive approval from the United States Postal Service (USPS) before use. The user also is required to determine the amount of postage required for letters and packages, and then a computer interfaces with the postal system to print the appropriate amount of

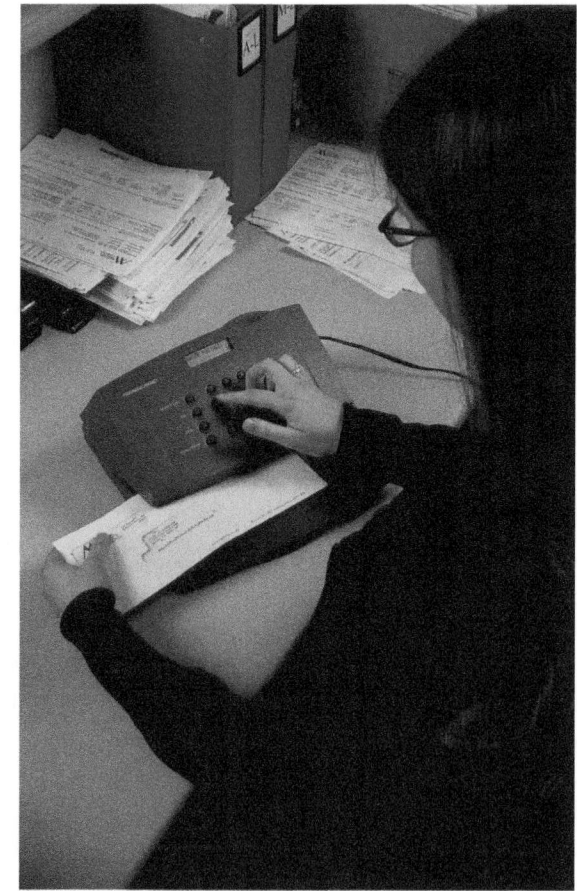

FIGURE 10-10 Postage meters are used for large mailings.

postage. Address labels can be printed at the same time. This method may be used in offices with a lot of bulk mailings.

JUDGMENT CALL

You have noticed that the clinical coordinator has been bringing personal mail in from home and using the office postage meter. The office policy states that the postage meter is to be used strictly for office purposes.

Critical Thinking Question

1. You know the clinical coordinator is not following policy and essentially is stealing from the office. What should you do?

SUMMARY

The office layout contributes to the physical atmosphere, organization, and impression that patients and employees encounter. An organized office layout can affect the office flow, decrease patient cycle time, and positively impact employee morale and patients' attitudes.

The medical assistant must maintain an inventory list for all office equipment purchased, supplies, and drug samples. All staff members should be trained on the use and operational functions of the equipment.

Medical assistants are often responsible for managing and monitoring the office's administrative and clinical supplies and relationships with vendors. This includes maintaining inventory, ordering supplies, and receiving orders.

10 CHAPTER REVIEW

COMPETENCY REVIEW

1. Define and spell the terms for this chapter.
2. Discuss how following the manufacturer's suggestions enhances equipment longevity.
3. Discuss the importance of patient flow.
4. Discuss how inventory control methods contribute to efficient office management.
5. Discuss the handling of pharmaceutical samples in the medical office.

PREPARING FOR THE CERTIFICATION EXAM

1. When asked to seek out a new vendor, the medical assistant should do all the following *except*
   a. gather information about available discounts.
   b. verify delivery procedures.
   c. speak with one vendor.
   d. verify payment policies.
   e. determine ease of availability.

2. When drug samples are left by the pharmaceutical representative, the samples should be kept in a locked cabinet and organized by
   a. class.
   b. shipment date.
   c. alphabetical order.
   d. expiration date.
   e. cost.

3. What is an example of capital equipment found in the medical office?
   a. a computer
   b. computer paper
   c. syringes
   d. a typewriter
   e. computer ink cartridges

4. What room temperature is most comfortable for the majority of patients?
   a. 70°F
   b. 71°F
   c. 72°F
   d. 73°F
   e. 74°F

5. What two distinct areas are typically found in a medical office?
   a. traffic flow and office areas
   b. administrative and clinical areas
   c. reception and staff areas
   d. staff and administrative areas
   e. reception and administrative areas

6. After a vendor is chosen, the medical assistant should expect all of the following *except*
   a. quality assurance.
   b. fast delivery.
   c. unit pricing.
   d. inventory count.
   e. service.

7. Which of the following is classified as clinical equipment?
   a. centrifuge
   b. appointment scheduling system
   c. drug samples
   d. disposable gowns
   e. needles

8. Equipment purchase agreements may include the following *except*
   a. training.
   b. service.
   c. warranty.
   d. office flow.
   e. extended warranty.

9. Which supplies are *not* expendable clinical supplies?
   a. disposable examination gowns
   b. medical chart forms
   c. syringes
   d. goggles
   e. disposable speculums

10. What term describes the physical organization of the office that lends itself to efficient work and patient movement?
   a. optimization
   b. office flow
   c. traffic patterns
   d. ADA guidelines
   e. room management

CRITICAL THINKING

Refer to the case study at the beginning of the chapter and use what you have learned to answer the following questions.

1. What is the first thing you would do to fix the situation after the office carpets were cleaned?
2. What steps should Tania take to get the office organized and ready for patients?
3. What physical precautions should Tania take when handling the boxes?
4. How can office staff work together to expedite patient flow after this disruption?

ON THE JOB

Develop an inventory using an electronic spreadsheet. Create separate headings for the clinical and administrative areas. Under each heading, make a separate list for equipment/machines and expendable supplies. Include purchase date, vendor, and purchase price. For equipment, list the maintenance schedule. For supplies, enter the quantity purchased.

Research prices for a clinical supply item such as gloves, disposable gowns, or tongue blades. Identify at least three vendors, and create a unit pricing comparison to determine which company has the lowest price per item.

INTERNET ACTIVITY

Go to the Americans with Disabilities Act (ADA) website (www.ada.gov) and research the standards for bathrooms in public places that accommodate wheelchairs.

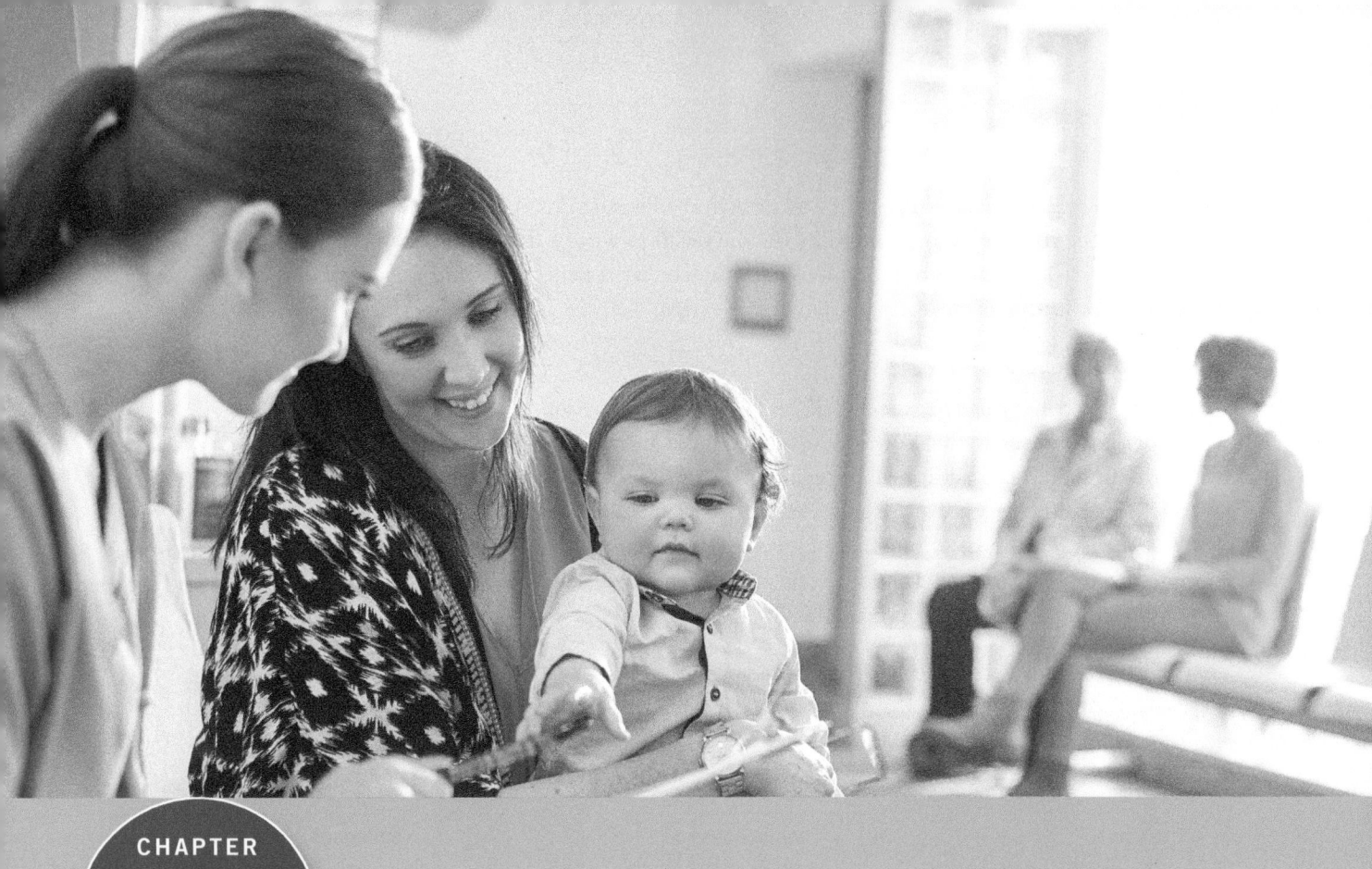

CHAPTER 11

Written Communication

Learning Objectives

After completing this chapter, you should be able to:

11.1 Define and spell the terms for this chapter.

11.2 Explain considerations that should be taken regarding grammar and word choice in written communication.

11.3 List examples for each of the eight parts of speech.

11.4 Describe the standard components of a business letter.

11.5 Describe the difference between block and modified block styles of business letters.

11.6 Explain the importance of both editing and proofreading written documents.

11.7 List the steps for preparing outgoing mail.

11.8 Describe the main classes of mail.

11.9 Explain how incoming mail should be processed in the medical office.

11.10 Describe how electronic technology is applied in professional communication.

Lewis Jordan, RMA, is working with a student in the Pearson Physicians Group externship program. The student has been asked by the physician to write a letter to refer a patient to another physician for a second opinion. The student writes the letter and asks Lewis to review it. Following is the letter written by the extern:

Dear Dr. Johnson

I am referring a patient to your office for further evaluation. I have been seeing this patient for several years now for right metatarsal injury. It is in my opinion that this patient should seek additional information on having the right metatarsal removed. This patient has been in my office on several occasions unable to walk with much swelling.

I trust your medical opinion and would appreciate you advising the proper action to take for this patient. For your review I have enclosed past X-rays. Please feel free to contact my office as soon as possible.

Sincerely,
Dr. J. Ancella

Terms to Learn

active voice	homophones	redundant
ancillary service endorsements	letterhead	reference initials
block style	memos	salutation
complimentary close	modified block style	signature line
constant information	optical character recognition (OCR)	thesaurus
enclosure	passive voice	variables
gender bias	proofread	

Medical assistants draft many types of correspondence to be signed by the physician-employer. These letters must reflect the professionalism of the medical practice. Every piece of correspondence represents the medical office, and impressions of the office can be formed based on the quality of correspondence. The physical appearance of letters depends on the quality of paper, letterhead design, and choice of formats used. However, even the most professional-looking correspondence is quickly and harshly judged when the letter is written in a negative or condescending tone or is filled with grammatical and spelling errors. Correspondence should be positive in tone and well written.

Handling incoming mail requires efficiency in sorting, dating, and reading all correspondence. Correct handling of the mail can save money and time for the medical practice. Handling mail quickly and accurately is paramount.

TONE IN LETTER WRITING

Letters from a medical office must be professional, courteous, businesslike, positive in tone, and protective of the confidentiality of the physician and the patient. This requires some diplomacy. For example, when drafting a sensitive letter requesting payment for a long overdue bill or to advise a patient to seek the services of another physician, the writing should be clear and to the point. The situation should be explained and the expected outcome presented—"Please send a check for (amount due)" or "Please call to make payment arrangements." Threats or derogatory comments are never acceptable in professional correspondence and may have legal consequences for the sender. The following letters are examples of positive and negative tones in writing.

Negative Example:

Dear Mrs. Murray:

You have repeatedly failed to take medications as prescribed and follow my recommended treatment. Because you have again failed to keep an appointment, I am forced to withdraw as your physician, and I request that you find another physician immediately.

Positive Example:

Dear Mrs. Murray:

During your last visit, we discussed the necessity of continuing medical treatment for you to recover fully from your recent medical problems. Therefore, I am concerned that you failed to keep your appointment this week and have not called the office to schedule a new appointment. Your health continues to be important to me, so I am requesting that you call me as soon as possible to discuss future treatment.

If we are unable to reach a mutual understanding about your medical treatment and appointment schedule, I regret that I will not be able to continue as your physician. In that event, you will receive a letter indicating that you have a month's notice in which to secure the services of another physician.

GRAMMAR AND WORD CHOICE

Correct grammar and appropriate word choice in correspondence reflect positively on the overall quality of a medical office. Appropriate word choice includes avoiding the following errors:

- Technical terms
- **Gender bias** (inappropriately indicating either male or female in the language used when referring to people in general)
- Overly long sentences and paragraphs
- Excessive use of the personal pronoun *I*
- Incorrectly used abbreviations
- Passive voice

Each office should have a small library of reference materials that can be used to help with writing tasks. These writing tips are discussed next.

Technical Terminology

When composing a document, consider the recipient, because you normally use different terminology and style when writing for medical professionals than when writing for patients.

When writing to medical professionals or institutions that employ medically trained staff, use of medical terminology is

TABLE 11-1	Medical Terms and Corresponding Synonyms	
Medical Term	Synonym
Carcinoma	Cancer
Cardiac	Heart
Dermatitis	Skin irritation
Diabetes mellitus	Diabetes
Gastric	Stomach
Gynecology	Study of female diseases
Hepatic disease	Liver disease
Hyperglycemic	Excessive blood sugar
Hypertension	High blood pressure
Larynx	Voice box
Leukocytes	White blood cells
Myocardial infarction	Heart attack
Nephrosis	Kidney disease
NPO	Nothing by mouth
Otolaryngology	Study of ear, nose, and throat
Para I	First delivery
Pc	After meals
Thrombus	Blood clot

appropriate, and it is essential that spelling and usage of medical terms are accurate. However, when writing to patients, medical terminology should not be used because they may not be familiar with it and may feel intimidated by it. Table 11-1 lists selected medical terms with corresponding synonyms. The medical terms in the left column are appropriate for correspondence with medically trained personnel (physician to physician, physician to medical record, medical assistant to hospital); the terms in the right column are more easily understood by most patients.

Avoiding Gender Bias

Unfortunately, it is quite common in the medical field to use language that assumes nurses are female and physicians are male. Because this is not an accurate perception, gender-neutral terms are preferred. This means that any reference to a particular gender (male or female) should be eliminated. For example, a male orderly should be referred to as a medical attendant, and "cleaning ladies" should be called housekeepers or cleaning personnel.

Written correspondence must reflect this same neutral bias toward the genders. When writing, do not refer to physicians as males or to nurses and medical assistants as females.

For example, "The patient was referred to a hospital dietitian for diabetic diet instruction. The patient was told to ask her about a food exchange list." This wording assumes the dietitian is a female. A better statement would be "The patient was referred to a hospital dietitian for diabetic diet instruction. The patient was told to ask about a food exchange list." To write in a gender-neutral style, you may have to rewrite the sentence and choose alternative words or phrases.

Sentence and Paragraph Length

Short, concise sentences and paragraphs are preferred in medical writing. Sentence length should never exceed 20 words. Eliminate unnecessary words. Each paragraph should cover only one point. A good paragraph contains two to six sentences. Your reader may stop reading if the paragraph is too long.

Personal Pronoun I

Whenever possible, avoid the use of the personal pronoun *I* in professional writing, which can sound egotistical or threatening. It is better to use *you* and *we*, terms that give the more gracious impression of including the reader in a mutual effort to clear up a misunderstanding. For example, a message such as "I am asking that your overdue balance be cleared up immediately. I will have to take steps to send this account to a collection agency if it is not paid immediately" is negative and unpleasantly personal in tone. When

requesting a patient to pay an overdue bill, it is better to write "We know that you will want to clear up the overdue account. This overdue balance may have been an oversight on your part. If that is the case, kindly remit your payment in the enclosed envelope."

Repetition, Redundancy, and Inflated Phrases

Readers of your correspondence want to know in concise terms what you are telling them. Avoid being **redundant**—repeating the same idea in similar words, expressions, or statements. Examples of expressions that include redundant words are *each and every*, *first and foremost*, and *physician's patient*. These examples can be simplified by writing just *each*, *first*, or *the patient*.

Inflated phrases can usually be eliminated without loss of meaning. Common examples are introductory word groups such as *in my opinion*, *I think that*, *it seems that*, *one must*, and so on. Table 11-2 compares some inflated patterns of writing with concise alternatives.

Active Versus Passive Voice

Active verbs generally make writing more interesting. In the **active voice**, the subject of the sentence performs the

Professionalism The Law

The medical assistant must carefully monitor all dated material to ensure that replies are made on a timely basis. Confidential mail and correspondence, including checks and payments, are handled on a regular basis. This is an important responsibility that may be carried out by a medical assistant. Because the U.S. Postal Service is regulated by the federal government, any tampering or deliberate mishandling of mail is a federal offense.

A nonthreatening tone in correspondence can promote the medical profession to the reader. Any attempts to threaten a patient in writing can lead to charges of harassment. Courteous language, presented in a diplomatic manner, can result in compliance and prevent a lawsuit. The medical assistant must carefully proofread all correspondence before it leaves the office to protect the physician from legal problems. An error in correspondence may not be caught by the physician before signing the document. If you are unsure about proper grammar or spelling, ask someone else to read the document.

TABLE 11-2	Inflated Phrases Compared with Concise Terms	
Inflated	**Concise**
along the lines of	like
as a matter of fact	in fact
at all times	always
at the present time	now, currently
at this point in time	now, currently
because of the fact that	because
by means of	by
by virtue of the fact that	because
due to the fact that	because
for the purpose of	for
for the reason that	because
have the ability to	can
in light of the fact that	because
in the nature of	like
in order to	to
in spite of the fact that	although, though
in the event that	if
in the final analysis	finally
in the neighborhood of	approximately
until such time as	until

TABLE 11-3 | Active Compared with Passive Voice

Active	Passive
The medical assistant took the patient's blood pressure measurement.	The patient's blood pressure measurement was taken by the medical assistant.
The surgeon performed an appendectomy on the patient.	An appendectomy was performed on the patient by the surgeon.
The medical committee reached a decision.	A decision was reached by the medical committee.

action; in the **passive voice**, the subject receives the action. Although both voices are grammatically correct, the active voice is considered more effective because it is simpler, more direct, and less wordy.

To transform a sentence from passive to active voice, make the actor the subject of the sentence. Table 11-3 contains examples of statements in both active and passive voice.

Spelling

Several words in the English language have the same or similar pronunciations but very different meanings and spellings. These words are **homophones** (meaning "same sounds"). They pose problems unless the writer is careful about their usage. Table 11-4 contains some of the most common homophones.

Computer software programs cannot be depended on to correct all word usage errors because they do not "understand" the data input or content of the correspondence. For example, use of the word *effect* or *affect* depends on the context and cannot be determined by the software program. Both spellings are correct, and the context determines which word is correct.

Medical terms are not generally recognized by spell-check software. You may want to research electronic medical dictionaries that are compatible with your word processing program so that medical terms can be recognized by spell-check. In addition, it is always important to have a hard copy medical dictionary available when you are composing documents. See Table 11-5 for examples of the most commonly misspelled medical terms. General rules for capitalization are in Box 11-1.

Plurals

Following are some basic rules for forming plurals of words:

- Abbreviations are formed into plurals by adding an *s* (ECGs, DRGs).
- Plurals of nouns are formed by adding an *s* or an *es* (physicians, suffixes).

Basic rules for forming plurals of medical terms with specific endings are listed in Table 11-6 along with examples for each. More information relating to spelling and grammatical rules of medical terminology can be found in Chapter 4.

Numbers

In general, the numbers 1 to 10 are spelled out—one to ten—in correspondence. For numbers greater than ten, it is acceptable to use the number designation, as in 32, 128, and 1,020. The only exception to this rule is when the number is at the beginning of a sentence. It should then be spelled out. See Table 11-7 for a further description of the use of numbers in correspondence.

Parts of Speech

English grammar recognizes eight parts of speech: noun, pronoun, verb, adjective, adverb, preposition, conjunction, and interjection. Many words function as more than one part of speech. For example, depending on its use in a sentence, the word *cut* can be a noun, as in "The *cut* is fresh," or a verb, as in "The surgeon *cut* into the organ." Table 11-8 provides a quick reference to parts of speech.

Abbreviations

In general, abbreviations are spelled out the first time they appear in a document, with the abbreviation provided in parentheses. On subsequent uses, the abbreviation can be used alone. For example, spell out Health Insurance Portability and Accountability Act (HIPAA) the first time it appears, then use HIPAA in remaining occurrences.

It is best to spell out medical abbreviations in correspondence for clarity, with the possible exceptions of reports sent

---

BOX 11-1 | Rules for Capitalization

First word of:

- Sentences
- Expressions used as sentences
- Each item in a list or outline
- Salutation and closing of a letter

Proper name of person, place, or thing:

- John F. Kennedy
- New York City
- Willis Tower

Noun that is part of a proper name:

- Professor Mary King
- Dr. Shania McWalter
- Michigan Avenue

TABLE 11-4 | Common Homophones

Word	Meaning	Word	Meaning
accept	to receive	lesson	something learned
except	to take or leave out	loose	free; not secured
advice	opinion about what to do for a problem	lose	to be deprived of
advise	to offer advice	pair	set of two
affect	to exert an influence	pare	to trim
effect	result; accomplishment	pear	fruit
all ready	prepared	patience	calm endurance
already	by this time	patients	a doctor's clients
altar	a structure on which religious ceremonies are held	personal	private; intimate
alter	to change	personnel	a group of employees
always	every time; forever	precede	to come before
all ways	every way	proceed	to go forward
bare	naked	quiet	silent; calm
bear	to carry; to put up with	quite	very
brake	something used to stop movement, to stop	right	proper or just; correct
break	to split or smash	rite	a ritual
buy	to purchase	write	to put words on paper
by	near	stationary	standing still
choose	to select	stationery	writing paper
chose	past tense of choose	taught	past tense of teach
cite	to quote	taut	tight
sight	vision	than	besides
site	position, place	then	at that time; next
complement	what makes a thing complete; to complete	their	belonging to them
compliment	an expression of admiration; to praise	they're	contraction of they are
conscience	sense of right and wrong	there	that place or position
conscious	awake; aware	through	by means of; finished
elicit	to draw or bring out	threw	past tense of throw
illicit	illegal	thorough	careful; complete
fair	lovely; light-colored	to	toward
fare	money for transportation, food, or drink	too	also
hear	to sense by the ear	two	one more than one in number
here	this place	waist	midsection
hole	hollow place	waste	to squander
whole	entire; unhurt	weak	feeble
its	of or belonging to it	week	seven days
it's	contraction for it is	weather	state of the atmosphere
know	to be aware of	whether	indicating a choice between alternatives
no	opposite of yes	who's	contraction of who is
lessen	to make less	whose	possessive of who
		your	possessive of you
		you're	contraction of you are

TABLE 11-5 | Commonly Misspelled Medical Terms

abscess	epistaxis	neuron	polyp
additive	eustachian	occlusion	prophylaxis
aerosol	fissure	oscilloscope	prostate
agglutination	glaucoma	osseous	prosthesis
albumin	gonorrhea	palliative	pruritus
anastomosis	hemorrhage	parasite	psoriasis
aneurysm	hemorrhoid	parenteral	pyrexia
anteflexion	homeostasis	parietal	respiratory
arrhythmia	humerus	paroxysmal	roentgenology
bilirubin	idiosyncrasy	pemphigus	sagittal
bronchial	ileum	percussion	sciatica
calcaneus	ilium	perforation	serous
capillary	infarction	pericardium	sphincter
cervical	intussusception	perineum	sphygmomanometer
chromosome	ischemia	peristalsis	squamous
cirrhosis	ischium	peritoneum	staphylococcus
clavicle	larynx	petit mal	suppuration
curettage	leukemia	pharynx	trochanter
cyanosis	malaise	pituitary	venous
defibrillator	malleus	plantar	wheal
ecchymosis	mellitus	pleura	xiphoid
effusion	menstruation	pleurisy	polyp
epididymis	metastasis	pneumonia	prophylaxis

TABLE 11-6 | Rules for Forming Plurals of Medical Terms (Nouns)

Ending	Rule	Example
a	ae	vertebra to vertebrae
ax	aces	thorax to thoraces
ex, ix	ices	apex to apices
is	es	metastasis to metastases
on	a	ganglion to ganglia
um	a	ovum to ova
us	i	nucleus to nuclei
y	ies	biopsy to biopsies
nx	ges	phalanx to phalanges

directly from one physician to another regarding patient care. Only accepted medical abbreviations can be used in medical documentation. The Joint Commission has released a list of unapproved abbreviations, and it is important that the abbreviations on that list are not used anywhere, including medical charts, reports, and insurance documents. A list of accepted medical abbreviations is included in Appendix 1. You can also consult a hard-copy or online medical dictionary or medical abbreviations list.

Error Correction

All correspondence should be error-free because errors reflect negatively on the professionalism of the entire medical office. Word processing has made identifying and correcting errors much easier than it once was. However, a spellchecker does not catch improper word usage or improper use of homophones, so the medical assistant must be attentive to such details.

Word processing allows the writer to display the document on the computer screen, enter the information, and make the necessary changes. This new, corrected document is then saved and printed or e-mailed. Sometimes errors may not be seen until after the document is printed. When that happens, go back into the word processor, make the correction, and reprint the document.

TABLE 11-7 | Use of Numbers in Correspondence

Type	Explanation of When to Use
Decimals	Write using figure without commas (23.04).
Figures	Only numbers (including 1–10) are used in tables, statistical data, dates, money, percentages, and time.
Measurements	Write out in figures (23 inches).
Percentages	Write out in figures and spell out percent (20 percent).
Tables	When typing numbers or placing them in columns, align as follows: • Arabic numerals (1, 2, 3) are aligned on the right. • Decimals (1.33) are aligned on the decimal. • Roman numerals (I, II, III) are aligned on the left.
Time	Do not use zeros when writing on-the-hour time. Use A.M. and P.M. with the time designation (10 A.M., not 10:00 A.M.).

TABLE 11-8 | Eight Parts of Speech

Part of Speech	Definition
Noun	Names a person, place, or thing. *Examples*: medical assistant, office
Pronoun	Substitutes for a noun. *Examples*: I, me, you, he, him, she, her, it, we, us, they, them
Verb	Helping verb: comes before main verb. Main verb: asserts action, being, or state of being. *Examples*: operate, write, speak, obtain, is, are, am
Adjective	Modifies a noun or pronoun, usually answering the questions "Which one?" "What kind?" "How many?" *Example*: responsible medical assistant
Adverb	Modifies a verb, adjective, or adverb usually answering the questions "When?" "Where?" "Why?" "How?" "Under what conditions?" "To what degree?" *Examples*: gently, extremely, nicely, quietly
Preposition	Indicates the relationship between the noun and pronoun that follows it and another word in the sentence. *Examples*: about, above, after, for, in, on, over, through
Conjunction	Connects words or word groups. *Examples*: and, but, nor, or
Interjection	Word used to express strong feeling. *Examples*: oh, hooray, hurrah, ouch

Reference Materials

Every physician's office contains general reference books and medical dictionaries as well as textbooks related to the physician's specialization. A complete office library should include the following:

- A desk dictionary and access to an online dictionary

- A medical dictionary, as well as access to an online medical dictionary, to assist with the correct spelling, pronunciation, acronyms, abbreviations, and meaning of medical terms and diagnoses

- A *Physician's Desk Reference (PDR)* to verify the correct spelling and use of drugs

- Current coding books, including CPT® (Current Procedural Terminology) and ICD-10-CM (International Classification of Diseases)

- A **thesaurus** (which provides synonyms or similar meanings for words), such as *Roget's International Thesaurus*, and access to an online thesaurus

FORMATTING CORRESPONDENCE

Composing letters can be simple when you use an organized approach. Before you begin the letter, think about the point(s) you are trying to make. If it is a long letter, you may want to jot a bulleted list of the points to ensure that you don't overlook anything important. Use the guidelines presented in this chapter. The most important element in writing an organized letter is to make your point quickly.

Business correspondence can use a variety of formats and styles, but most letters include the same standard components. The basic components of a business letter are discussed next, followed by a discussion of various layouts and styles.

Standard Components of the Business Letter

Medical assistants need to learn and use the standard components of a business letter so they project the proper professionalism to those outside the medical practice. Standard components include the heading, date, inside address, salutation, body, closing, and reference initials. In some specialized cases, such as in insurance correspondence, special

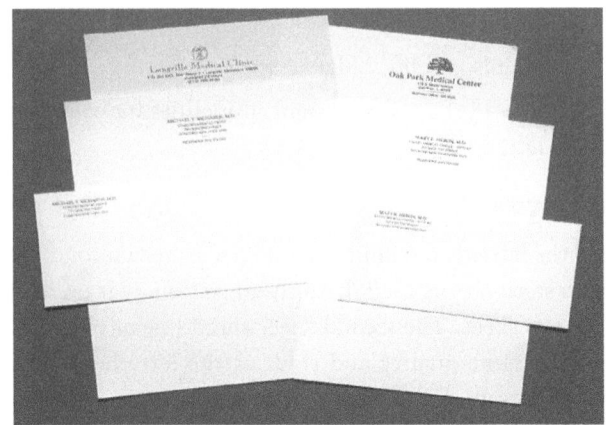

FIGURE 11-1 Various letterhead stationery and envelopes.

components may be added for clarification, such as the insurer's identification number.

Heading

Medical office letters are usually typed on **letterhead**, which is stationery bearing the name of the physician (Shania McWalter, DO) or practice (Pearson Physicians Group), address, telephone number, and fax number, if any. See Figure 11-1 for an illustration of letterhead. If the physician does not use letterhead, the letter should be printed on good-quality bond paper with the return address typed above the date on the upper left side of the paper. Most word processing programs provide templates for letterhead that can be printed at the same time as the letter.

Date

Every correspondence must have the current date. The month must not be abbreviated and must be followed by the numerical day and year (January 1, 2014). The date is usually placed three lines below the letterhead or on line 15 if there is no letterhead. Four to six lines are left after the date before the inside address.

Inside Address

The inside address contains the name, title, company name (if applicable), and address of the recipient of the correspondence. This is typed at the left margin and is single-spaced. If a company name is present (for example, Pearson Physicians Group, Pearson Clinic, or Pearson General Hospital), it must be typed exactly as shown on the company's own letterhead.

All words in the inside address (such as the street name) are spelled out fully. The name of the city is followed by a comma; the two-letter state abbreviation is followed by two spaces (tapping the space bar twice); then the ZIP code is added. If the inside address contains a long line, it may be divided into two lines so that the inside address is in

balance. The second of these two lines would be indented two spaces. See the following example:

Marvin Hammer, MD
123 Bonneymeadow
  Plaza in the Park
Chicago, IL 60610

Business courtesy recommends always including a title with the receiver's name on the inside address.

Salutation

The **salutation**, a courteous greeting, is typed at the left margin and placed two lines below the inside address. The name in the salutation must agree with the name in the inside address. If the letter is going to a physician named McWalter, the salutation would read "Dear Dr. McWalter:" with a colon placed after the salutation. If the person is well known to the writer, the first name is often used, followed by a comma (e.g., "Dear Shania,"). Guidelines 11-1 provides information on using courtesy titles in correspondence.

Body

The body is the main text of the letter and conveys the purpose of the letter. The body begins two lines below the salutation and is single spaced, with double spaces between paragraphs. The paragraphs of the body are either blocked

Guidelines 11-1

Using Courtesy Titles

- *Mr.* is an appropriate courtesy title for men.
- A professional title, such as *MD* or *PhD*, is used instead of the courtesy title.
- *Ms.* is used when the marital status of a woman is unknown or if she is known to prefer the title *Ms.*
- *Mrs.* is appropriate for a married woman if she prefers that title. However, it is always safe to use *Ms.*
- *Miss* is appropriate for unmarried women who prefer that title. It is also used for young girls.
- Two people at the same address with different last names should be addressed individually (e.g., Dr. Shania McWalter and Mr. Allan Radde).
- A capitalized professional title, such as *Owner, President, Manager,* may be placed next to the name or below it, depending on which is a better balance.

  Allan Radde, President   Radde and Associates
  Dinesh Shey, PhD   Department Chair

- If there is no record of the correct spelling of a receiver's name, then call the company or office and ask for the correct spelling.

(with no indentation) or indented (with the first line set in about five spaces from the left margin). A letter may be any length; however, most letters bearing a single message are two to three paragraphs in length and limited to a single page.

Be clear and to the point. The reader should be able to understand exactly what you are writing about within the first two sentences.

Closing

The closing consists of a **complimentary close** containing a courtesy word(s), such as "Sincerely," "Sincerely yours," or "Yours truly." This appears two lines below the end of the body of the letter.

The **signature line** is typed four lines below the complimentary close (to leave room for the signature that is written between the complimentary close and the signature line). The signature line contains the name and title of the writer. If the name and title are on the same line, they are divided with a comma. The personal title of the writer (such as Mr. and Ms.) is not included in the signature line. The exception to this is when the writer may wish to indicate gender to prevent the reader from being confused (for example, Ms. Leslie Lapointe or Mr. Pat Timmons).

The handwritten signature of the writer must be entered directly above the printed signature line before the letter is sent.

Reference Initials

The medical professional uses **reference initials** to indicate who keyed or typed the letter. Reference initials, when used, are placed at the lower left margin in lowercase. For example, if Brandy F. Forthing keyed a letter, she would include the reference initials *bff*.

Enclosure Notation

When other documents are included along with the letter, a notation is made on the letter indicating the **enclosure**. Examples of enclosures are X-ray films, medical records, and brochures. The abbreviation *ENC.* is used, or the word *Enclosure* can be spelled out.

For example:

Enclosures (2)
X-ray lumbar spine
surgical report 12/10/20YY

Copy Notation

In addition to the copy of correspondence kept for office records, a copy of the letter may be sent to someone other than the addressee. This is noted at the bottom left of the letter by typing the letter(s) "c:" or "cc:" before the recipient's name. The title of the recipient is often added.

For example:

c: Jane Paulson, Office Manager

Procedure 11-1 lists important guidelines for composing business letters.

Two-Page Letter

When the letter is too long to fit on one page, a second sheet of plain stationery is used. Letterhead stationery is used only for the top sheet. The second sheet should be of plain bond paper, the same quality and color as the letterhead stationery. A margin of 1 inch is left at the bottom of the first page. The second page and any pages following must begin with the date and subject line of the letter.

Form Letters

When the same letter is sent once or repeatedly to multiple recipients, a form letter can save time for the medical assistant. A form letter contains standard content that is used repeatedly, then personalized with the patient's name, appropriate details such as dates, and the signature of the physician. Figure 11-2 contains an example of a form letter that can be used as a base when constructing a letter of withdrawal.

A computer can individualize the form letter. The body of the letter, the **constant information**, is retained on a computer disk or storage device. The areas of the letter that require personalization, such as the date, inside address, and

FIGURE 11-2 A form letter is used when the same letter is sent to multiple recipients.

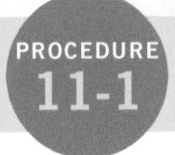

Composing a Business Letter

Objective ◆ *Compose a business letter using proper guidelines.*

EQUIPMENT AND SUPPLIES
Computer or typewriter; office stationery

METHOD

1. Gather necessary information and supplies.
2. Determine the reason for the correspondence. Write down the main purpose of the letter.
3. Make a list of the points you need to cover in the letter. Prepare a rough draft.
4. Arrange the ideas in a logical manner. Make sure the letter has a beginning, middle, and end:
   - The beginning or introduction should be appropriate for the intended reader. Use appropriate greetings and titles.
   - The middle should contain the supporting facts and details. Make sure the content relates to the purpose of the letter.
   - The end should be brief and pleasant and indicate any action that is to be taken by the reader or writer.
5. Use a natural style of writing. Avoid showy language, and avoid medical terms when writing to the layperson. Also avoid inflated phrases (refer to Table 11-2). Use professional language, not slang.
6. Use a positive tone. Negative writing should always be avoided.
7. Pay particular attention to spelling, punctuation, and grammar.
8. Proofread for mistakes—including misspelled, misused words, and missing words—logic, and completeness.
9. Obtain the necessary signatures. Include any enclosures as indicated.

CHARTING EXAMPLE

12/4/YY. Letter written and mailed to patient, Mrs. Ford, requesting that she contact the office to arrange payment for her outstanding balance. Return receipt requested. Copy of letter placed in chart................................B. Castle, CMAS

---

salutation, are called the **variables**. The variables can be stored on a separate CD or database and then merged into the disk or main drive of the computer, which stores the constant information. In this manner, a set of data, such as names and addresses of patients for billing purposes, can be used with a form letter enclosed with the monthly bill.

Letter Styles

Letter style refers to the physical appearance of the letter. Styles vary depending on the purpose. The four letter styles generally used are block, modified block (standard), modified block with indented paragraphs, and simplified, as described below. Block and modified block are used most often in the medical office. Figure 11-3 shows sample letter formats: block, modified block (standard), modified block with indented paragraphs, and simplified.

- **Block style**—The **block style** is formatted with all lines, from the date through the signature line, flush with the left margin. A blank line separates paragraphs as well as the inside address, salutation, body, and close.

- **Modified block style**—In the **modified block** (standard) **style**, the date, complimentary closing, and signature line begin at the center and continue toward the right margin. All other lines are flush with the left margin. This style is often preferred because it has a professional, neat appearance.

- **Modified block style with indented paragraphs**—The modified block style with indented paragraphs is identical to the modified block style just described except that the paragraphs are consistently indented by a designated amount.

- **Simplified style**—In a simplified letter style, all lines are flush with the left margin. The salutation line is omitted. In its place is a subject line, which appears on the third line below the inside address. This subject line is in capital letters and draws the reader's attention to the purpose of the letter. A complimentary closing is also omitted. The signature is also typed in all capital letters on the fifth line below the body. This format is an abbreviated style of writing letters

PEARSON PHYSICIANS GROUP
Shania McWalter, D.O.
123 Michigan Avenue, Parker Heights, IL 60610
(312) 123-1234

August 1, 20YY

Thomas Moore
123 Lee Street
Louisville, KY 40223

Dear Mr. Moore:

With the season for colds and flu fast approaching, it is time once again for flu shots. Supplies have arrived and flu shots will be administered starting October 3. Please call the office to schedule a visit for your flu shot at your earliest convenience.

If you wish to wait to get your flu shot at the time of your next appointment, it is not necessary to call the office. An appointment card with the date and time of your next appointment is enclosed.

Sincerely,

Shania McWalter, D.O.

ENC: Appointment card
c: B. Reed, Office Manager

(A)

PEARSON PHYSICIANS GROUP
Shania McWalter, D.O.
123 Michigan Avenue, Parker Heights, IL 60610
(312) 123-1234

August 1, 20YY

Thomas Moore
123 Lee Street
Louisville, KY 40223

Dear Mr. Moore:

With the season for colds and flu fast approaching, it is time once again for flu shots. Supplies have arrived and flu shots will be administered starting October 3. Please call the office to schedule a visit for your flu shot at your earliest convenience.

If you wish to wait to get your flu shot at the time of your next appointment, it is not necessary to call the office. An appointment card with the date and time of your next appointment is enclosed.

Sincerely,

Shania McWalter, D.O.

ENC: Appointment card
c: B. Reed, Office Manager

(B)

PEARSON PHYSICIANS GROUP
Shania McWalter, D.O.
123 Michigan Avenue, Parker Heights, IL 60610
(312) 123-1234

August 1, 20YY

Thomas Moore
123 Lee Street
Louisville, KY 40223

Dear Mr. Moore:

    With the season for colds and flu fast approaching, it is time once again for flu shots. Supplies have arrived and flu shots will be administered starting October 3. Please call the office to schedule a visit for your flu shot at your earliest convenience.

    If you wish to wait to get your flu shot at the time of your next appointment, it is not necessary to call the office. An appointment card with the date and time of your next appointment is enclosed.

Sincerely,

Shania McWalter, D.O.

ENC: Appointment card
c: B. Reed, Office Manager

(C)

PEARSON PHYSICIANS GROUP
Shania McWalter, D.O.
123 Michigan Avenue, Parker Heights, IL 60610
(312) 123-1234

August 1, 20YY

Thomas Moore
123 Lee Street
Louisville, KY 40223

RE: FLU SHOT

With the season for colds and flu fast approaching, it is time once again for flu shots. Supplies have arrived and flu shots will be administered starting October 3. Please call the office to schedule a visit for your flu shot at your earliest convenience.

If you wish to wait to get your flu shot at the time of your next appointment, it is not necessary to call the office. An appointment card with the date and time of your next appointment is enclosed.

SHANIA MCWALTER, D.O.

ENC: Appointment card
c: B. Reed, Office Manager

(D)

FIGURE 11-3 Examples of four letter formats: **(A)** block style; **(B)** modified block style; **(C)** modified block style with indented paragraphs; and **(D)** simplified letter style.

PEARSON GENERAL HOSPITAL
MEMORANDUM

DATE:

TO:

FROM:

SUBJECT:

c:

FIGURE 11-4 An example of a memo form.

relating to patients. (A variation on the simplified letter style, called semi-simplified, is formatted with all lines flush with the left margin except for the first line of each paragraph. The first line of each paragraph is indented. All other aspects of the simplified letter style apply to this format.)

Interoffice Memoranda

Interoffice memoranda, also called **memos**, are written communications sent to people within the office or organization. They are used to inform personnel about meetings, general changes that affect employees, special projects, or news items. Memos do not require postage and are delivered through interoffice mail.

Memos generally are written using a shortened format developed for that purpose. They may contain a heading much like letterhead stationery to indicate the office where they originated. They contain the word *Memorandum* at the top of the form. Also included are the typed words *DATE*:, *TO*:, *FROM*:, and *RE*: or *SUBJECT*:. The memo form is meant to be used within the office setting and should never be used to send information outside the office. Figure 11-4 illustrates an example of a memo format.

Reports

The medical office often needs to prepare medical or administrative reports to share information needed by other people or organizations. Medical reports provide patient-specific health information whereas administrative reports do not. Examples of a medical report include a referral request of a patient for outside services, a summary of medical findings or status on a patient needed by an outside provider or company (such as an insurance company or an attorney), and a consultation report sent back to a referring physician (Figure 11-5).

March 1, 20YY

PATIENT Rebecca Smith DATE OF BIRTH 07/01/19YY

SUBJECT Follow-up evaluation, neck and back pain

FINDINGS

Patient was seen for follow-up after referral from Dr. Weist on 1/15/20YY. Patient continues to suffer from neck and lower back pain radiating into both arms and both legs with numbness, paraesthesia, and tingling in both arms. She reports moderate relief after trigger point injections on 1/20/20YY and 2/15/YY.

Evaluation today continues to reveal restriction of range of motion of the cervical and lumbar region with tenderness and spasm in the paraspinal musculature. The exam otherwise was unchanged. Palpable trigger points were noted bilaterally in the lumbar paraspinal region.

TREATMENT PLAN

She continues to suffer from ongoing myofascitis, and the doctor's treatment plan will consist of a series of trigger point injections, which were performed again today. She tolerated the procedure well. Instructed patient to ice the region for 15 minutes off and on x 3. She is to continue with treatment program under care of Dr. Weist.

RECOMMENDATIONS

Repeat trigger point injections in two weeks.

PREPARED BY Shawna Curry, MD

(555) 555-5555

FIGURE 11-5 An example of a medical report.

The format of a medical report is dictated by the type of report and the information needed by the recipient and, in general, should include the following items:

- Date on which the report is prepared
- Patient name and date of birth
- Purpose or subject of the report
- Case history including the presenting problem, physical examination and test findings, diagnosis, and treatment provided
- Current medical status of patient
- Treatment plan
- Recommendations
- Name, credentials, and contact information of person preparing the document

Check to be sure that proper patient consent or authorization has been obtained for medical reports. The HIPAA Notice of Privacy Practices (NPP) provides patient consent for any information needed for treatment, payment, and operations (TPO), such as a referral request or treatment report, so specific permission is not required for these. Specific authorization should be obtained for anything that is not routine, such as information requested by an attorney in a lawsuit.

Administrative reports can be intended either for internal use or sent to an outside party. Examples of administrative reports include details of an equipment problem sent to a manufacturer, description of an employee performance issue, or medical practice financial information for a bank. Some reports might use a predetermined form, such as those for personnel matters and financial reporting. The form might come from an outside source, such as a manufacturer or bank. When a predetermined form does not exist, the medical assistant must write the report using narrative description and tables or figures to present details, as needed. All reports should include the date, purpose, and name of the person preparing the report.

EDITING AND PROOFREADING

After the letter has been written, it needs to be edited and proofread. Nearly all letters contain errors after the first draft, because your initial focus is on communicating the content.

Editing

Editing involves reading the final material to check for accuracy and clarity. Read the letter from the point of view of the recipient to be sure you have explained yourself clearly and courteously. When editing medical reports, you cannot change the content of the report or alter the meaning in any way. If you believe the meaning is unclear, you must check with the writer of the report before making content (editorial) changes.

If you are writing a general letter on behalf of another staff person, always give that person the opportunity to review any editing changes you recommend.

When editing material you have composed, such as an informational form letter to be sent to all patients, you can make changes to increase clarity. It is often helpful to set the letter aside for several hours, or until the next day, then reread it to be sure it is clear and complete.

Proofreading

Proofread your document by rereading it to check for errors in content and keying. Proofreading is a critical step in the correspondence process to help ensure accuracy. As already mentioned, the professionalism of the office is judged, in part, by the appearance of correspondence and documents that come from that office. Proofreading cannot be overemphasized. Even small errors, such as omitting commas, are noticed by readers.

Most computer programs provide spellcheck and grammar-check features. Use these tools before printing the document. You may be able to add frequently used medical terms to the spellcheck program so the program does not repeatedly mark these terms as spelling errors.

After printing out a document, read it carefully to catch any content or keying errors. Pay close attention to the spellings of names and procedures. When typing figures, always double-check to make sure all decimal points are placed in the correct position. Look for sound-alike words or word parts, such as *right* and *write* or *anti-* and *ante-*.

Important points to remember when proofreading letters and other documents are listed in Procedure 11-2.

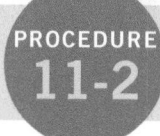

PROCEDURE 11-2

Proofreading Written Documents

Objective ◆ *Draft grammatically correct correspondence with no spelling errors.*

EQUIPMENT AND SUPPLIES

Ruler; pencil; piece of paper; computer; rough draft of a document

1. Access the rough draft of a document that you are working on.
2. Read the document to ensure all points are covered and that thoughts flow logically.
3. Run the computer program spelling and grammar checks, and consider the suggestions made.
4. Save the document, and then print it.
5. Use a ruler, pencil, or edge of a piece of paper to follow each line as you proofread.
6. Check for missing and repeated words.
7. Verify the spelling of proper names and titles.
8. Check where the word breaks occur.
9. Verify numbers in dates, figures, dollar amounts, and time (hours of the day).
10. Read the opening and closing carefully.
11. Proofread at least twice. If still unsure, ask a coworker to review the document.
12. Check the general appearance of the letter for spacing and format.
13. Make the needed corrections, save, and print the document.

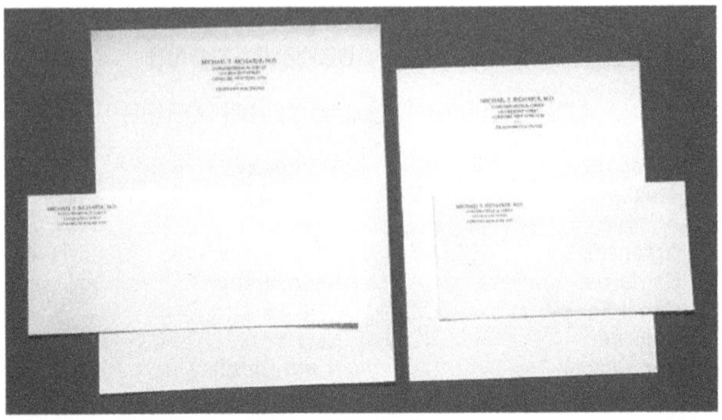

FIGURE 11-6 Letterhead stationery sizes are varied to suit the needs of the sender. Envelopes are sized to match the letter size.

PREPARING OUTGOING MAIL

Letterhead stationery, which contains the name and address of the sender, comes in three commonly used sizes. These sizes are standard, monarch or executive, and baronial. The more common letter sizes with their matching envelope sizes are shown in Table 11-9.

Standard letterhead is used for most office correspondence. Monarch or executive style—a slightly smaller version of standard letterhead—is used by some physicians for their social correspondence. Baronial letterhead is half the size of a standard sheet and is used for brief letters and memoranda. Envelopes are sized to match the letter sizes. See Figure 11-6 for an illustration of letter sizes.

Folding Letters and Inserting into Envelopes

Following are recommended methods for folding and inserting letters into envelopes so the contents can remain confidential and be easily removed. See Figure 11-7 for an illustration of folding a letter.

Number 10 (Standard Business Size) Envelope

1. Bring up the bottom one-third of the letter and fold with a crease.
2. Fold the top of the letter down to ⅜ inch from the first creased edge.
3. Make a second crease at the fold, and place this edge into the envelope first.

Number 6¾ Envelope

1. Bring the bottom edge up to ⅜ inch from the top edge.
2. Make a crease at the fold.
3. Fold the right edge one-third of the width of the paper, and press a crease at this fold.
4. Fold the left edge to ⅜ inch from the previous crease, and insert this edge into the envelope first.

Addressing Envelopes

The U.S. Postal Service (USPS) recommends certain guidelines for addressing envelopes to improve the handling and delivery of the mail. **Optical character recognition (OCR)** equipment used by the USPS scans, reads, and sorts envelopes. For optimal efficiency of OCR scanning, addresses must be typed, using single spacing and all capital letters with no punctuation. A more traditional style of typing envelopes, with the initial letter of each word capitalized and remaining letters in each word lowercased, is still accepted by the USPS.

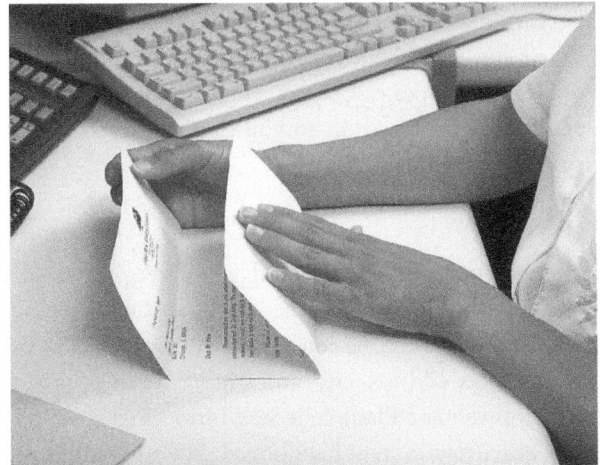

FIGURE 11-7 A well-folded letter fits easily into the envelope and is easily removed by the person who receives it.

TABLE 11-9 | Stationery and Envelopes

Stationery	Dimensions	Envelope	Dimensions
Standard	8½" × 11"	No. 10	9½" × 4⅛"
Monarch or Executive	7¼" × 10½"	No. 7	7½" × 3⅞"
Baronial	5½" × 8½"	No. 6¾	6½" × 3⅝"

TWO-LETTER ABBREVIATIONS

UNITED STATES and TERRITORIES

Alabama	AL	Montana	MT
Alaska	AK	Nebraska	NE
Arizona	AZ	Nevada	NV
Arkansas	AR	New Hampshire	NH
California	CA	New Jersey	NJ
Canal Zone	CZ	New Mexico	NM
Colorado	CO	New York	NY
Connecticut	CT	North Carolina	NC
Delaware	DE	North Dakota	ND
District of Columbia	DC	Ohio	OH
Florida	FL	Oklahoma	OK
Georgia	GA	Oregon	OR
Guam	GU	Pennsylvania	PA
Hawaii	HI	Puerto Rico	PR
Idaho	ID	Rhode Island	RI
Illinois	IL	South Carolina	SC
Indiana	IN	South Dakota	SD
Iowa	IA	Tennessee	TN
Kansas	KS	Texas	TX
Kentucky	KY	Utah	UT
Louisiana	LA	Vermont	VT
Maine	ME	Virgin Islands	VI
Maryland	MD	Virginia	VA
Massachusetts	MA	Washington	WA
Michigan	MI	West Virginia	WV
Minnesota	MN	Wisconsin	WI
Mississippi	MS	Wyoming	WY
Missouri	MO		

FIGURE 11-8 Every state has a two-letter abbreviation.

The last line in the address is the city, two-letter state abbreviation, and ZIP code. It cannot exceed 27 characters in length. See Figure 11-8 for a list of the two-letter state abbreviations.

The bottom margin of the No. 10 envelope (standard business size) should be ⅝ inch with 1-inch margins on the left and right sides. The No. 6¾ envelope should have a 2-inch margin on the left side with the address 12 lines from the top of the envelope.

A return address for the sender should be placed in the upper left corner in the event the letter must be returned to the sender. Envelopes can be preprinted with the address of the sender in this position so you don't have to type the return address each time.

ZIP Codes

Addresses on outgoing mail should have a five- or nine-digit ZIP code. If you do not have the ZIP code for the recipient in your records, it can be looked up on the USPS website using the street address, city, and state. The five-digit ZIP (Zone Improvement Plan) code was introduced in 1963 to increase efficiency in mail handling. USPS added four more digits to the ZIP code 1983. These four digits follow a hyphen placed after the first five digits and identify the

block of the street where the address is located. The nine-digit ZIP code has eliminated many handling steps at USPS collection and distribution centers and has improved service.

CLASSES OF MAIL

The classes of mail as designated by the USPS vary according to weight, type, and destination. Mail is weighed in ounces and pounds. The most common classes of mail include first class, priority, priority express, and package services. Table 11-10 describes these classes of mail. The USPS revises mail classes and specifications from time to time, so it is a good idea to check current rules before planning a large mailing or shipment.

USPS Extra Services

Extra services offered by the USPS and often used by medical offices include certified mail, certificate of mailing, registered mail, insurance, mail recall, tracing lost mail, and returned mail.

TABLE 11-10 | Classes of Mail

Type	Description
First Class	Letters, postcards, business reply cards; letters weighing less than 13 ounces; sealed and unsealed, handwritten or typed material
Priority	First-class mail weighing more than 13 ounces; maximum weight of 70 pounds; postage calculated based on weight and destination. Delivery is expected within one, two, or three days.
Periodicals	Newspapers and periodicals that have received second-class mail authorization; not allowed for newspapers and periodicals mailed by the general public
Standard Mail	Advertisements, circulars, newsletters, small parcels, merchandise
Package Services/ Standard Post	Merchandise, catalogs, printed material, computer media
Priority Express Mail	Available seven days a week; up to 70 pounds in weight and 108 inches around; expected delivery; shipping containers are supplied; pickup service in some areas. Offers overnight delivery to most addressed in the United States.

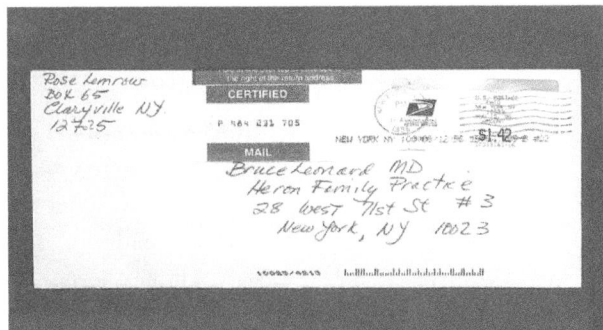

FIGURE 11-9 Items that would be difficult to replace bearing legal significance are sent by certified mail.

Certified Mail and Return Receipt

Mail that includes contracts, mortgages, birth certificates, deeds, and checks, which are not valuable themselves but would be difficult to replace if lost, can be mailed as certified mail (Figure 11-9). Such items are mailed at the first-class rate with an additional fee for the certified mail status. Certified mail requires the signature of the recipient.

If it is necessary to dismiss a patient from the practice, the patient must receive the notification in writing. Certified mail with a Return Receipt requested is used when documentation is needed that the patient did indeed receive the letter. As already noted, certified mail by itself requires the signature of the recipient when it is delivered. Return Receipt allows the sender to receive and actually see the signature of the recipient, which can then be kept on file. This protects the physician and the practice if the patient who received the letter later claims not to have received it.

Certificate of Mailing

For a small fee, a Certificate of Mailing can be obtained at the post office. This document serves as proof that mail was posted. This is useful for mailing items that need to be postmarked by a certain date, such as tax returns and reports to insurance companies.

Registered Mail

Registered mail is the safest way to send first-class or priority mail because it is tracked at each stage as it moves throughout the mail system. Registered mail is insured for the value declared at the time of registration. A fee is paid for this service, and a signed record is kept for each piece of registered mail.

The USPS includes a tracking number on the receipt you get when you mail something from the post office by priority, priority express, or registered mail. The tracking number can be entered on the USPS website to confirm the progress of the item through the postal system and its delivery.

Insurance

Insurance can be purchased for packages and priority mail. The sender is then reimbursed for the content if this mail is lost or damaged. The sender receives a receipt at the time of purchasing the insurance. This receipt, along with the damaged goods, must be presented when reimbursement is necessary.

Mail Recall

If mail has been placed in a mailbox or given to a postal carrier by mistake, it can be recalled by the sender. The sender can call the post office and request that the item be held for pickup. When the sender goes to the post office to reclaim the mail, that person is asked to complete a "Sender's Application for Recall of Mail." This should be done as soon as possible after mailing, because if the mail has already been delivered, it cannot be recalled.

Tracing Lost Mail

All receipts for mailed goods should be retained until receipt of the mail has been acknowledged. If the mail has not arrived after a reasonable period of time, the post office will attempt to trace it upon request. However, first-class mail is not easy to trace because no receipt exists. A special form must be completed to request this service.

Returned Mail

When mail has been returned and marked "Undeliverable," new postage must be applied before remailing to a new address. It is advisable to place the contents into a new envelope with the correct address and new postage.

Special Address Services

Special address services can assist the medical office to identify the current address for patients who have moved, ensuring that they receive correspondence and bills. These services, called **ancillary service endorsements**, enable you to give the USPS specific instructions for how to handle mail that is undeliverable. First-class mail is forwarded to the new address for one year, free of charge, and, if undeliverable, returned to the sender for free. When mail is forwarded, the sender is not normally notified. You must use an ancillary service endorsement to be informed of the recipient's new address.

Undeliverable mail is handled differently depending on the class of mail, the endorsement you use, and how recently the customer moved. Ancillary service endorsements commonly used by medical offices include the following:

- **Address service requested**—The mail piece is forwarded, and the sender receives a notice of the new address.

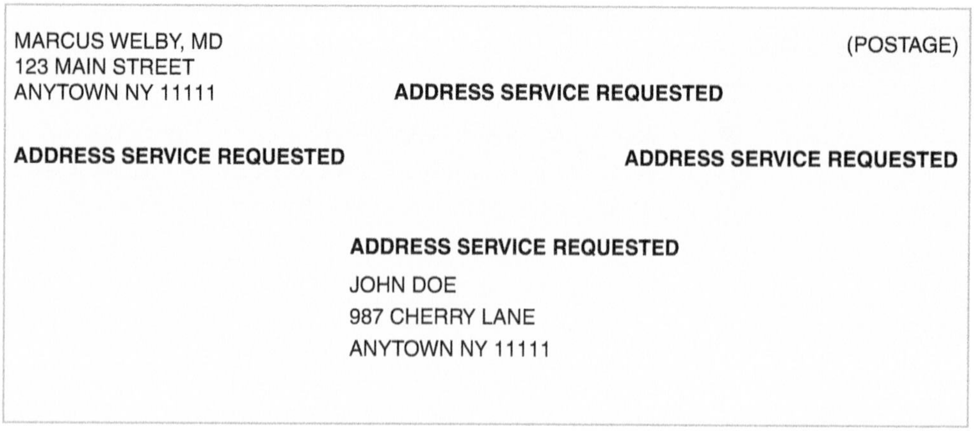

```
MARCUS WELBY, MD                                    (POSTAGE)
123 MAIN STREET
ANYTOWN NY 11111          ADDRESS SERVICE REQUESTED


ADDRESS SERVICE REQUESTED        ADDRESS SERVICE REQUESTED


              ADDRESS SERVICE REQUESTED
              JOHN DOE
              987 CHERRY LANE
              ANYTOWN NY 11111
```

FIGURE 11-10 Envelope showing four options for placement of ancillary service endorsements.

- **Return service requested**—The mail piece is returned to the sender with the new address attached.

- **Change service requested**—The sender receives a notice of the new address, but the mail piece is neither forwarded nor returned.

- **Forwarding service requested**—The mail piece is forwarded for 12 months; in months 13 through 18, the mail piece is returned to the sender with the new address attached.

Some of these actions have fees associated with them when the mail piece is returned or a new address is provided. The endorsement must be placed in one of four positions (Figure 11-10):

- Directly below the return address

- Directly above the delivery address area

- Directly to the left of the postage area and below or to the left of any price marking

- Directly below the postage area and below any price marking

SIZE REQUIREMENTS FOR MAIL

The USPS standardizes envelope sizes for machine-sort mail. Minimum mail sizes have been established. Domestic mail must be at least 0.009-inch thick. A further restriction on size requires that mail ¼ inch or less in thickness must be 3½ inches in height and at least 5 inches long. Mail not meeting this requirement is considered nonstandard and is subject to additional fees.

Although postage for packages is generally based on the package's weight, items that are bulky and lightweight are charged a surcharge. Following are some general guidelines for preparing mail to be metered:

- Separate domestic mail from international mail. Separate mail to Canada or Mexico from other international mail.

- Face all letter-size envelopes in the same direction. Make sure none are upside down. When mailing letter-size envelopes, flaps must be sealed or tucked in.

- Try not to overstuff letter-size envelopes. If this is not possible, seal the envelopes with tape.

- All envelopes larger than a No. 10 must be sealed before being sent.

- Keep the top right corner of each mailing piece clear of markings. This is where the postmark appears.

The medical assistant should always consult the USPS for specific mailing, size, weight, and pricing requirements to ensure the outgoing mail is properly prepared. This may include either a visit to the nearest post office or browsing the USPS website. If mail is sent with inadequate postage, it is returned to you, the sender, which delays the mailing process. The USPS has customer service specialists for business services. If planning a large mailing, it is helpful to meet with a business service representative at your main post office.

 Professionalism **The Workplace**

Approximately 12 percent of the population moves each year, so the medical office must be diligent about maintaining current addresses for patients. It is important to verify patients' addresses every time they come in or telephone the office. USPS ancillary service endorsements have fees associated with them, which are worthwhile, but can become costly if relied on as the main way to update addresses. One approach is to place the endorsement on all outgoing patient mail, because you are charged only for the ones for which the patient has moved and the address correction is sent to you. Used in this way, ancillary service endorsements are a safety net to catch address changes that may be missed for patients who do not come into the office frequently.

TABLE 11-11 | Correspondence Handling Guidelines

Type of Correspondence	Typical Recipient
Checks (insurance or patient payments)	Check is routed to finance and a copy of the check is routed to patient accounting/billing
Insurance explanation of benefits (EOB)/remittance advice (RA)	Patient accounting/billing
Consultation reports	Physician
Utility bills	Office manager/finance
Periodicals and magazines	Recipient named on label
Confidential mail	Recipient named on envelope
Advertising circulars	Department named on the mail piece/office manager. (Note: Some advertising circulars are of interest to the recipient/department because they contain valuable offers or product updates, whereas others are "junk mail" and can be discarded.)
Legal correspondence	Office manager
Medical reports/test results	Physician
Equipment notices	Office manager

INCOMING CORRESPONDENCE

Medical offices receive a wide variety of correspondence in the mail, so medical assistants must sort the incoming mail, identify what each piece is, and route it to the appropriate person. They need to become efficient at recognizing different types of correspondence and know how to handle them. Reports, test results, and other correspondence received from outside health providers should be stamped with the date received, scanned into the patient's EMR (if office protocol), and routed to the appropriate physician for review without delay.

Table 11-11 summarizes types of correspondence and the person in the office who typically receives it. This is a general guide; the procedures of individual offices must be followed.

To facilitate time management within the medical office, each piece of mail should be handled only once. For ease and efficiency in handling large amounts of mail, follow the steps in Procedure 11-3.

ELECTRONIC TECHNOLOGY

Electronic technology can be used to send correspondence without using paper and takes several forms, including e-mail, instant messages, text messages, and fax. You may be accustomed to abbreviating words when sending messages using electronic technology with friends; however, this is not acceptable for electronic communications sent from an office. The tone of the message should remain as professional as if you were keying in a letter to be sent through the USPS. Box 11-2 highlights

BOX 11-2 | Precautions When Using Electronic Technology

- Verify that you have the complete e-mail address of the recipient and have entered it correctly.
- Always be specific on the subject line, such as "4th Quarter Financial Statements" rather than "Reports."
- Include a salutation with the recipient's name, such as "Hi, John" or "Dear Dr. Smythe."
- Sign the message with a full signature block that includes your name, position, employer name, address, telephone number, and e-mail address.
- Reply only to those who need to read your message. Do not use the Reply All feature unless everyone who received the original e-mail needs to read your response.
- Respond to e-mails within 24 hours, even if you do not have a complete answer to give the sender.
- Remember to "attach" any files that must be sent with the e-mail message.
- Do not use capital letters in an e-mail because it looks like yelling.
- Use punctuation correctly.
- Spell correctly and use standard abbreviations only, such as using *you*, not *u*.
- Never send an e-mail if you are upset or angry.
- Avoid using your work e-mail for personal purposes, including sending jokes to others.
- Do not send or receive personal e-mails while you are at work.
- Do not use your personal e-mail account to send work-related messages.

Opening and Sorting the Daily Mail

Objective ◆ *Sort and distribute the medical office's daily mail.*

EQUIPMENT AND SUPPLIES

Date stamp; stamp with the name of the medical office; ink pad; paper clips; pencil

METHOD

1. Gather the supplies needed to process the mail. Process the mail as soon as possible after it arrives, because it often contains time-sensitive documents and information that physician and staff members are waiting for.
2. Sort the unopened mail into piles for first-class, personal or confidential, advertising circulars, and magazines.
3. Discard and recycle unwanted advertising mail.
4. Stamp the current date and time of arrival on each piece of mail. Purchase a rubber stamp and pad from an office supply store so that the date can be changed each day.
5. Stamp the name of the medical office across all periodicals and newspapers.
6. Set aside and do not open mail marked "Personal" or "Confidential." Place it unopened in the physician's inbox unless otherwise instructed.
7. Lay all the envelopes with flaps down to reduce the motions involved in opening a large amount of mail. Use a letter opener to cut open the top edge of each envelope.
8. Remove enclosures from the envelope and attach them to the envelope with a paper clip. Place the envelope on top of the enclosures. Do not staple anything because staples might have to be removed later and could damage sensitive materials, such as X-rays. If an enclosure is noted in the correspondence but is not in the envelope, next to

mention of the enclosure write "No" with your initials to indicate it was not included. Clip the opened envelope to the mail until the mail is completely processed. In some cases, a return address is only on the envelope and not on the inside correspondence.

9. Annotate the mail. An annotation consists of writing a short comment in pencil to indicate the purpose of the letter and underlining the critical portions of the letter. If another document is referred to in the letter, then take initiative by pulling it from the file and attaching it to this correspondence.
10. The office should have a separate policy for opening mail that contains checks in payment of bills, such as those from insurance companies and patients. Usually this requires the following steps:
    - Stamp the back of the check in the designated area with the endorsement stamp for the medical office's bank account.
    - Make a photo copy of each check.
    - Attach the copy of the check to the paperwork that was included with the check, such as an explanation of insurance benefits or patient statement.
    - Enter the amount of the check and the payer in the daily cash log, which may be maintained either as a computer document or as a physical logbook.
    - Place the original check in the daily cash box.
    - Route the copy of the check and attachments to the appropriate person in the patient accounting department.
11. Route the mail immediately after opening it. Another department or physician may be waiting for the document.

---

precautions to use when sending messages using electronic technology.

E-Mail

E-mail is the shortened form of *electronic mail*. E-mail may include letters, memos, reports, and pictures. E-mail messages may be sent over telephone lines, cables, computers, and satellites. E-mail allows the medical assistant to edit, correct, and transmit documents very quickly to another location. E-mail cannot be used if an original signature is

required on the document. When creating e-mail, remember that it is considered part of the patient's record and part of office management; therefore, all standard proofreading and confidentiality guidelines apply.

Some offices use e-mail to confirm office visits. Every office has a particular format to use for this purpose.

If e-mail is offered to patients as a mode of communication, it is imperative to check your e-mail inbox frequently to avoid liability. E-mail is not efficient for use in emergencies because you do not know when someone will

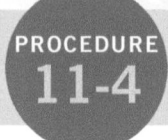

Creating and Sending a Business Letter Using E-mail

Objective ◆ *Compose and send a business letter using e-mail.*

EQUIPMENT AND SUPPLIES

Computer with e-mail application; names and e-mail addresses of all recipients; location of computer files that should accompany the e-mail

METHOD

1. Gather necessary information and supplies.
2. Open the e-mail computer application.
3. Enter the e-mail address of the recipient in the "To" field. Be sure it is spelled correctly and contains the organizational domain after the @ sign, such as maryjo@clinic.com.
4. Determine whether additional people need to receive a copy of the letter. If so, enter their e-mail addresses in the "To" field if they are primary recipients, or in the "CC" field if they are receiving it for informational purposes only.
5. Enter the topic of the letter in the "Subject" or "RE" field. The subject should be as specific as possible, such as "Order 12345." Avoid nondescript subject lines such as "Question" or "Update."
6. Enter a personal salutation in the box for the main message, such as, "Dear Dr. Jones" or "Hi Susan."
7. Write the content of the letter following the steps in Procedure 11-1.
8. Pay particular attention to spelling, punctuation, and grammar. Run the spellchecker on the letter. Proofread for mistakes not caught by the spellchecker, such as missing words and words that are spelled correctly but potentially misused, such as *they're* vs. *their*.
9. Sign the letter with your name, position, company name, address, telephone number, and e-mail address.
10. Attach any needed files.
11. Re-check the recipient, content, and attachments, and then click Send.

check or respond to an e-mail. As always, it is imperative to adhere to HIPAA privacy and security laws when using e-mail.

Attachments are computer files that can be sent with an e-mail message. Sometimes offices e-mail new patients the forms that need to be completed for the first visit. A specific set of menu commands must be executed to attach the message, so remember to complete this step. It is easy to forget to send the attachment in the rush of responding to a message. It is best to use only file formats that most people's computers can read, such as PDF, DOC or DOCX. Formats such as spreadsheets (XLS) or PowerPoint (PPT) might be used when sending files to coworkers or other businesses.

When you receive an attachment from someone, use a virus detection program to check the file for computer viruses before saving it. Then be sure to save the file to your computer so you have it for future reference.

Procedure 11-4 explains how to prepare a business letter using e-mail.

Instant Messages

Instant messages (IMs) are a way to communicate via computer with another person in real time. The content of an instant message appears on the recipient's computer screen immediately after it is sent. Some offices allow users to instant message each other both internally (within the office) or externally. The internal instant message format is usually connected to the office computer server and allows messages to be sent quickly from person to person. External instant messages are generally linked to an account that is purchased from an Internet service provider. In such accounts, you establish your own screen name and password so you can access and communicate with external users with instant messages. External instant messages are not secure and should not be used to communicate protected health information.

It is important to remember that instant messages are not permanent documents and cannot be attached to a person's medical records or used in a court of law.

Text Messages

Text messages are written messages sent and received via a cell phone number. The recipient can read the message on the phone screen and reply, if necessary. Text messaging should be used with caution to communicate with patients because the information is not secure, meaning that anyone with access to the phone potentially can read the message. Some offices use text messaging for appointment reminders, *with the patient's prior authorization.*

Facsimile (Fax)

The fax machine is another way to send a written communication electronically. The fax is an exact duplication of a document that is transmitted to another location via the

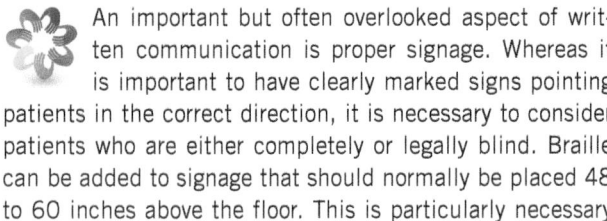

facsimile (fax) machine. Telephone lines are used to transmit fax documents; thus, fax numbers look identical to telephone numbers. To fax a document, insert the original document into the fax machine, dial the receiver's fax phone number, and when the connection is made the document is transmitted over the telephone lines, resulting in a printed document at the receiver's fax machine. The first page of the transmission should be a cover sheet, which identifies the sender (company, name, and telephone and fax numbers), telephone number of the receiver, date, and number of pages. It should contain a message that requests the recipient to notify the sender if the fax has been received in error and also asks the recipient to destroy the document after notification. Fax cover letters must be HIPAA compliant.

Many offices use Internet fax services. Or they may have a scanner and send the scanned image attached to an e-mail. If these newer technologies are used for sending images of documents, the office may no longer have a fax machine.

Professionalism | The Workplace

E-mail has become one of the most commonly used forms of written communication within the office. Most likely, you will find yourself receiving as well as composing e-mails to and from coworkers, patients, and other business associates. It is common courtesy to respond to any incoming e-mails as soon as possible. Set aside time each day to respond to your incoming e-mail. If it appears that you may not be able to respond within the same day, let the sender know you have received the e-mail and will respond either on a given day or when the information requested is available. If you are out of the office for a day or longer, you can set up an auto-response, which is a message automatically sent to each person who e-mails you to inform them when you will be back in the office and who to contact in your absence.

REFLECTION ON THE MEDICAL PRACTICE

Medical assistants often are responsible for preparing interoffice memos and letters to patients. The letter you send is a direct reflection on the physician and the medical office as a whole. If the letter is filled with errors, contains an incorrect diagnosis, or is sent to the wrong patient, it reflects poorly on the medical office and can harm the physician's business. If your responsibilities as a medical assistant include letter writing, it is always a good idea to have someone in the office review your correspondence. To facilitate time management within the medical office, you can use a form letter that you or the physician has created. Proofread each document and check for inappropriate content, misspellings, grammatical or punctuation errors, and margin restrictions.

Professionalism | The Law

HIPAA privacy laws apply to e-mail equally with any other form of communication. E-mail messages that contain protected health information (PHI) must be transmitted securely. Electronic encryption technology should be installed so that the message cannot be intercepted and read by an unauthorized party. Many offices provide a secure messaging system that patients can use to contact the office. The system usually resides on the office's server, or the secure server of a service company, and you must issue patients a password to use it. This method is much safer than using publicly available e-mail services that are not secure.

SUMMARY

The responsibilities of the medical assistant relating to office correspondence are multifaceted. These include being able to draft correspondence using correct grammar and style and efficiently handling mail. Effective mail handling includes using the most efficient and cost-saving form of mail service. These responsibilities must be handled in a professional, courteous, and diplomatic manner. You can demonstrate competence as a medical assistant by handling written communication correctly.

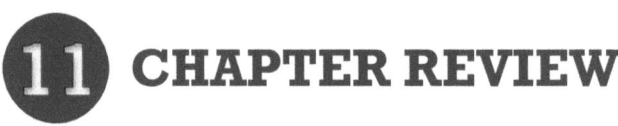

11 CHAPTER REVIEW

COMPETENCY REVIEW

1. Define and spell the terms for this chapter.
2. How would you track a missing piece of mail?
3. Address an envelope using the method recommended by the USPS for use with optical character recognition (OCR) equipment.
4. Describe what types of material you would send by certified mail.
5. Type a short letter using both block and modified block with indented paragraph styles.
6. Why do you think companies (and medical offices) use letterhead stationery?

PREPARING FOR THE CERTIFICATION EXAM

1. What type of mail service should be used when mailing a document that bears legal significance and would be difficult to replace?
   a. insured mail
   b. registered mail
   c. special delivery
   d. certified mail
   e. special handling

2. Which ancillary service endorsement should be used when you want the mail piece forwarded and a notice of the new address sent to the sender?
   a. Address Service Requested
   b. Return Service Requested
   c. Change Service Requested
   d. Forwarding Service Requested
   e. Correction Service Requested

3. Which of the following designates a standard business envelope?
   a. No. 6¾
   b. No. 7
   c. No. 9
   d. No. 10
   e. No. 11

4. How many lines (spaces) below the letterhead should the date be placed when composing a business letter?
   a. three
   b. four
   c. five
   d. six
   e. two

5. Which classification of mail should be used to mail merchandise, catalogs, printed material, and computer media?
   a. first-class
   b. priority
   c. package services/standard post
   d. standard mail
   e. periodicals

6. What is the name of a courteous greeting at the beginning of a business letter?
   a. heading
   b. salutation
   c. body
   d. closure
   e. enclosure

7. What is the two-letter abbreviation for Alabama?
   a. AB
   b. AK
   c. AL
   d. AM
   e. AA

8. What is the maximum length of the last line of the address on an envelope that contains the city, two-letter state code, and the ZIP code?
   a. 25
   b. 26
   c. 27
   d. 28
   e. 24

9. What is the letter format in which all lines begin at the left margin, a salutation is used, and paragraphs are not indented?
   a. simplified letter
   b. block letter
   c. modified block letter
   d. semi-simplified letter
   e. semi-block letter

10. What information should be stamped on all incoming mail?
    a. name of the medical office
    b. date received
    c. name of the recipient
    d. name of the person opening the mail
    e. date sent

CRITICAL THINKING

Refer to the case study at the beginning of the chapter and use what you have learned to answer the following questions.

1. According to the standard practices of written communication, is this letter okay? If not, explain why.
2. In what voice is this letter written?
3. If you were Lewis and you needed to rewrite the letter, what would you change about the letter? Why?

ON THE JOB

Diane Webb, a medical assistant at Pearson Physicians Group, has been asked to proofread the following letter, which was prepared by a temporary assistant. Follow the rules for proofreading, grammar, capitalization, and spelling found in this chapter to correct the errors in this letter. Type this letter using the modified block style, and prepare it for Dr. Shania McWalter's signature.

Dear Docter Stacey:

I right this letter to inform you that I am pleased that you would chose me to present at your conference. Its a great complement.

Their are several cases which I can site. I would like you're recommendation because I no you will be frank with me. We must all ways be discrete and conscience of patience's rights when presenting cases relating to there conditions. We must remain mindful that patients have there legal rites.

I have the following X-ray studies which I can include: xyphoid process, greater trocanter, peretoneal abcess, left calcanus, fracture of right clavical, and a fractured ileum and ischeum. Let me know which of these rentgeneology studies you would prefer.

Please advise me on how to procede.

Sincerely yours,

Dr. Shania McWalter

INTERNET ACTIVITY

Access the Internet, and locate information on how to write professional medical letters. Research other information you may need, such as your extended ZIP code, an online dictionary, a medical dictionary, a thesaurus, and e-mail etiquette guidelines.

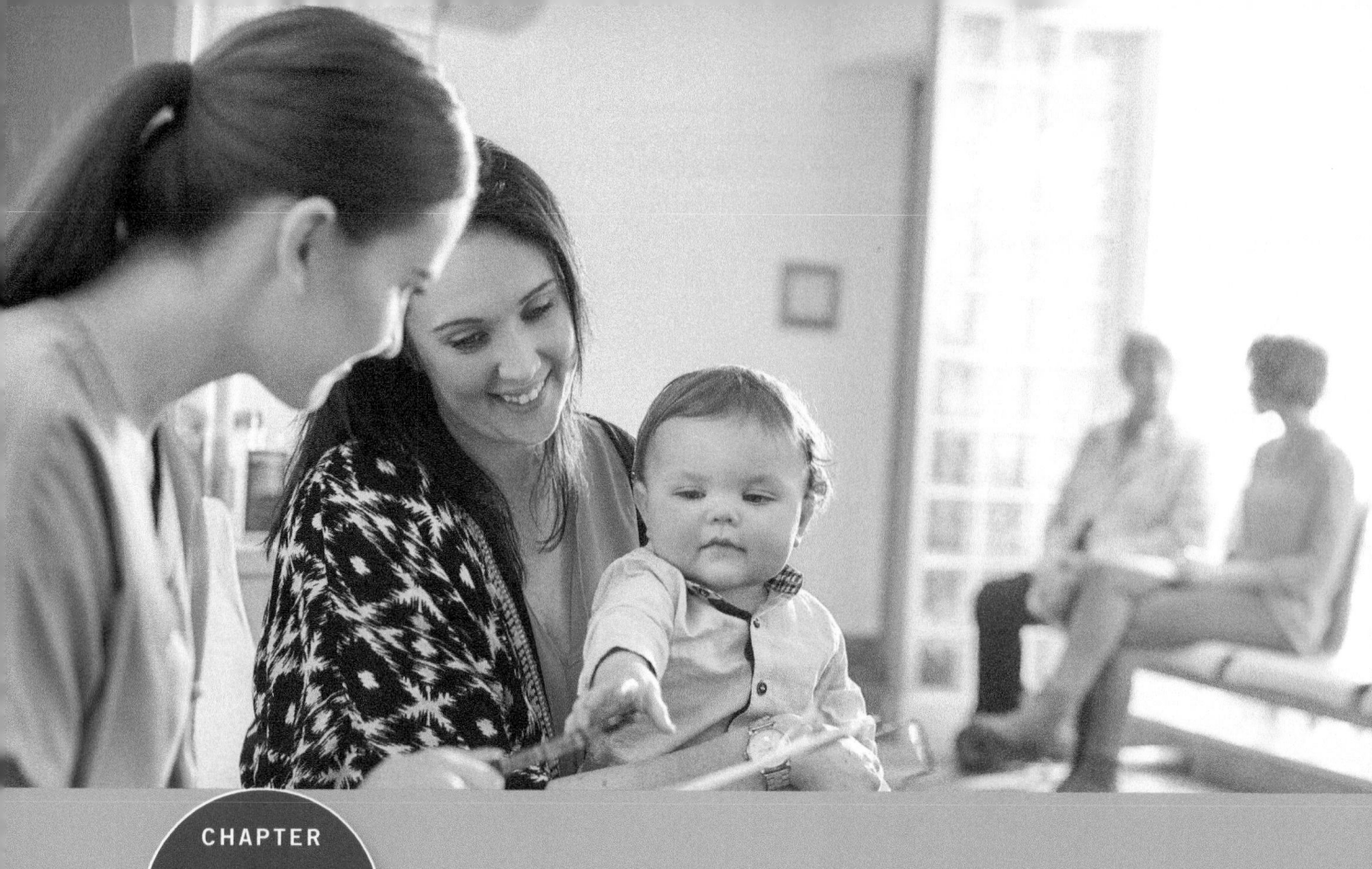

Computers in the Medical Office

Learning Objectives

After completing this chapter, you should be able to:

12.1   Define and spell the terms for this chapter.

12.2   Explain examples of how computers are used in medicine.

12.3   List the differences among the types of computers that are used in the medical office.

12.4   Describe the functions of the various types of computer hardware.

12.5   Explain the difference between input and output devices.

12.6   Describe the HIPAA Security Rule as it applies to computer system security.

12.7   Explain why it is important for a medical office to back up data.

12.8   Explain how the computer is used for electronic communications.

12.9   List the benefits and drawbacks that pertain to the use of social media in the medical office.

12.10 Identify issues to consider in selecting a new computer system.

12.11 List four methods used for implementing ergonomics at your workstation.

Case Study

Samra Belkovich is a medical assistant who works for Pearson Physicians Group. She has been asked to develop some continuing education materials for a community service project that the office will conduct at the local shopping mall. She is assigned to locate the most current information, design and develop the materials for distribution, and include marketing materials for the event and for the office.

Terms to Learn

administrative safeguards	firewall	physical safeguards
application	gigabyte (G or Gb)	practice management software (PMS)
backup	hardware	printer
bandwidth	input devices	random-access memory (RAM)
central processing unit (CPU)	Internet	read-only memory (ROM)
clock speed	Internet service provider (ISP)	Security Rule
cloud computing	kilobyte (K or Kb)	social media
computer	megabyte (M or Mb)	software
database	megahertz (MHz)	spreadsheet
electronic health record (EHR)	memory	storage devices
electronic protected health information (e-PHI)	microprocessor	technical safeguards
	monitor	touchscreen
e-mail	mouse	universal serial bus (USB)
encrypt	operating system	virus protection
ergonomics	output devices	word processor
file cleanup	password	World Wide Web (WWW)

Computers play an important role in the efficient operation of a medical office. Depending on the size of the medical practice, some or all of the functions normally performed in the front office may be done with computers and specialized software programs. To be successful in both the administrative and clinical areas of a medical facility, the medical assistant must be familiar with computers and how they are used. After reviewing the general uses of computers in medicine and the types of computers used, this chapter discusses computer hardware components; types of software; computer system security, including the HIPAA Security Rule; electronic communication via the Internet and World Wide Web; tips for selecting a computer system; and maintaining your own health and well-being through proper computer ergonomics.

USE OF COMPUTERS IN MEDICINE

Advances in technology have enabled medical offices to function with increased efficiency using computers. Computers are

a fundamental piece of operating equipment that can enhance the quality of patient care through data collection, eliminating duplication of work, and decreasing errors. Figure 12-1

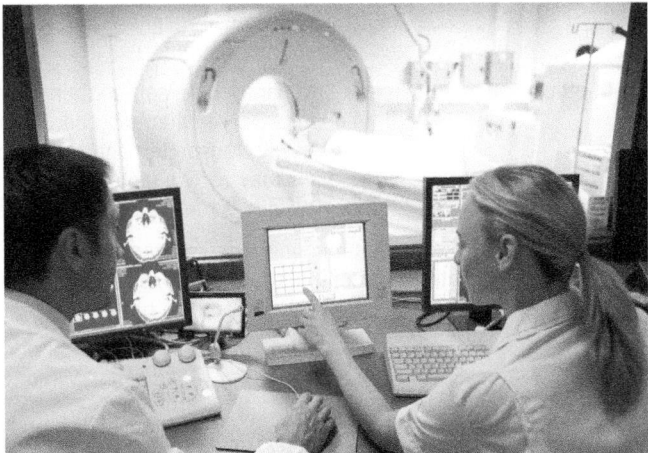

FIGURE 12-1 Computerized tomography (CT) is used to perform a brain scan.

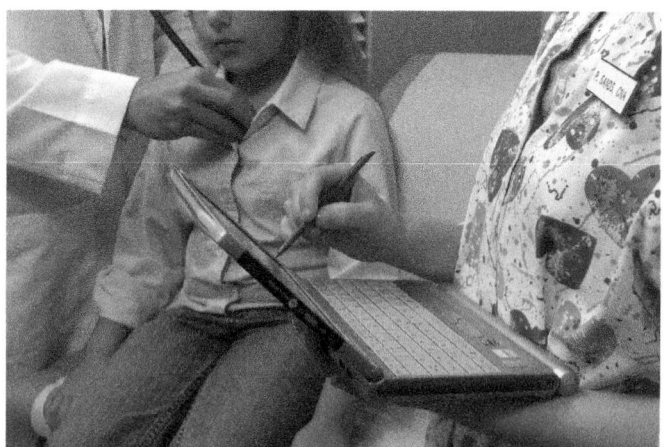

FIGURE 12-2 Medical assistant uses a laptop computer for bedside charting.

illustrates one of many ways computers have become invaluable in diagnosing, monitoring, and reporting the patient's progress. Medical assistants may be responsible to make entries in software programs for electronic health records, electronic bookkeeping, billing, insurance processing, appointment scheduling, inventory data, and many other functions (Figure 12-2). These responsibilities mean that medical assistants must be computer literate. Not only must medical assistants have adequate computer skills, they must also stay current as technology continues to advance.

TYPES OF COMPUTERS

The first modern electronic computer, the ENIAC, was commissioned by the U.S. Army in 1943 and unveiled to the public in 1946. It contained approximately 17,500 vacuum tubes, 6,000 manual switches, and 5 million soldered joints. The machine covered 1,800 square feet of floor space, weighed 30 tons, and consumed 160 kilowatts of electrical power. State-of-the-art for its time, it could perform over 5,000 calculations per second but had less memory and less functionality than one of today's handheld calculators.

In 1971, the development of the microchip, also called a microprocessor, revolutionized computers. A microchip is a silicon wafer less than 1/8 square inch in size. Each microchip contains multiple layers of electronic circuitry that controls computer operations. The first microchip could process 60,000 instructions per second, 12 times as many as the ENIAC. Microchips progressed rapidly to the point where today's chips process billions of instructions per second.

As computers have evolved, many of their characteristics have changed: size, processing speed, processing capacity, storage, and ease of use. Most medical offices use computers for at least a few tasks, and some offices are highly automated. Computers come in various sizes and capacities designed for different types of tasks. Table 12-1 defines the

TABLE 12-1 | Types, Sizes, and Uses of Computers in the Medical Office

Type/Size	Uses in the Medical Office
Server	The central computer is a network that provides resources and directs traffic of other computers in the network. May be attached to multiple screens of any size. CPU case weighs 20 to 60 pounds. Monitors and other peripherals contribute additional weight. Powered by electrical current.
Desktop	Remains in one place with one or multiple monitors. May be used for scheduling, accounting, medical records, and patient registration. Monitor, keyboard, mouse, and CPU case with drives are separate components. Screen size unlimited. CPU case weighs 10 to 30 pounds. Monitors and other peripherals contribute additional weight. Powered by electrical current.
Laptop	Screen and keyboard form a self-contained case. May have a standard- or substandard-size keyboard, with or without a separate 10-key numeric pad. May have a slot for an internal disk drive. Integrated touchpad can replace mouse. Easily transported and can be connected to the network for access to information and applications. Physicians may carry a laptop from room to room for access to electronic health records. Screen size 13 to 17 inches. Weighs 3 to 10 pounds. Powered by a battery or electrical current.
Notebook	Self-contained unit with substandard-size screen and keyboard. This is the smallest size computer that runs standard computer applications such as word processing and spreadsheets. Weighs 2 to 3 pounds. Screen size 9 to 12 inches. Powered by a battery or electrical current.
Tablet	Touchscreen, used primarily for viewing information with limited input. May have a soft keyboard (visible on screen). Screen size 7 to 10 inches. Weighs about 1 pound. Powered by batteries.
Handheld	Multifunction device that may contain a phone, e-mail reader, and Internet browser, such as smartphones and personal digital assistants (PDA). Can be carried in the pocket or on the belt. Handy for viewing information such as medical reference guides. Requires special miniaturized versions of software called apps. Does not run standard computer applications. Limited use for input. Powered by batteries.

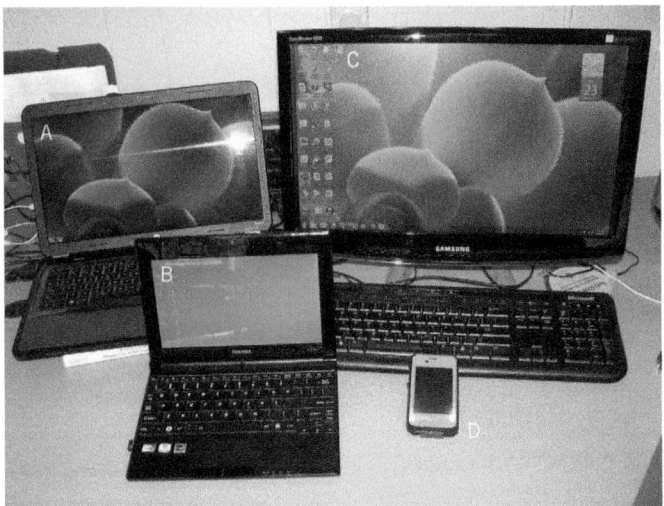

FIGURE 12-3 Types of computers: **(A)** laptop; **(B)** notebook; **(C)** desktop; **(D)** smartphone.

types, sizes, and uses of computers in the medical office. Figure 12-3 shows various types of computers.

Computers may be standalone or part of a network. A standalone computer is self-contained and does not connect with any other computer. A network is a group of computers linked together with cables or wireless (Wi-Fi) connections so that they can share resources, such as software, printers, and data. Individual computers connected to a network are called workstations. Workstations consist of, at a minimum, a monitor and keyboard. In some systems, they may also have their own hard-disk drive and central processing unit (CPU) (described later). Most medium and large medical offices, and many small ones, use computer networks.

Table 12-2 lists different types of hardware, software, and storage components. Table 12-3 lists commonly used computer terms.

TABLE 12-2 | Hardware, Software, and Storage Components

Hardware	Software	Storage
Central processing unit (CPU)	Operating system	Memory • ROM • RAM
Peripherals • Monitor • Keyboard • Mouse • Printer • Modem • Scanner • Speakers	Applications • General purpose • Medical administration • Clinical	Hard disks • Optical drives (internal and external) • Memory cards • USB drives

COMPUTER HARDWARE

A **computer** is a programmable machine, or system of **hardware** (Figure 12-4) that responds to a specific set of instructions and performs a list of instructions in programmed language called **software** and makes use of storage devices to retain the data in the computer when the computer is turned off. Generally, computers require the following hardware components to function:

- **Central processing unit (CPU)** is the brain of the computer that executes the specific set of instructions.
- **Memory** is a computer's capacity to store data and programs on a temporary or permanent basis. Memory is provided by various physical storage devices.
- **Storage devices** make it possible for a computer to permanently retain large amounts of data even when the computer is turned off. Common storage devices include internal and external hard disk drives, optical devices such as CDs or DVDs, USB drives, and memory cards.
- **Input devices**, such as keyboards and scanners, feed data and instructions into a computer.
- **Output devices**, such as display screens, printers, and other devices, allow the user to see what the computer has accomplished.

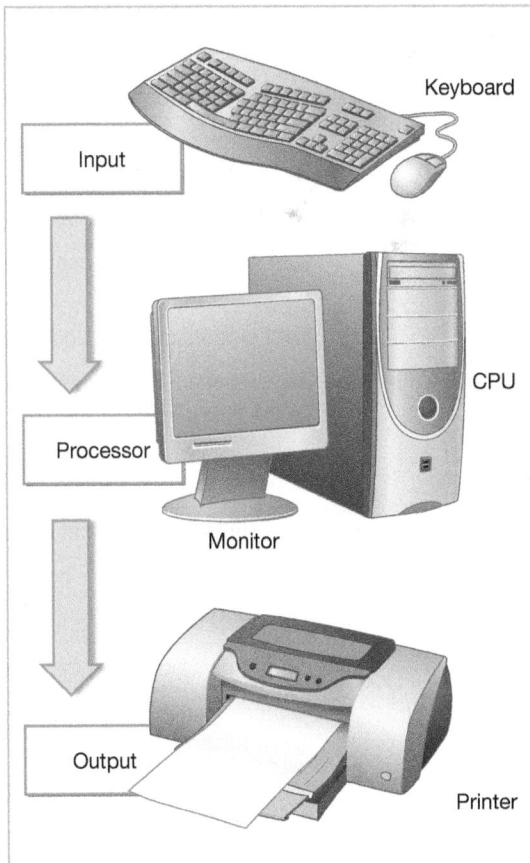

FIGURE 12-4 Components of a computer system.

TABLE 12-3 | Frequently Used Computer Terms

Term	Definition
Backup	A copy of data or software created at periodic intervals to help protect against data loss.
Batch	Data stored for processing at periodic intervals.
Boot	To start up the computer.
Debug	Process of eliminating errors from input data. Also used to refer to the process of identifying a problem in malfunctioning hardware or software.
Disk drive	A device that reads disks using a magnetic or optical read/write head.
Download	The act of receiving data from another computer or storage device.
Downtime	Time a computer cannot be used because of maintenance or mechanical failure.
E-mail	Use of appropriate hardware and software (modem, computer, telephone, etc.) to allow transmission of electronic messages between users on separate computers.
Encrypt	To code or scramble computer data so that it is unreadable by anyone who does not have the decoding key.
File	A collection of data stored in one unit, identified by a filename.
File folder	An electronic tool that stores related files together. Also known as a directory.
Hard copy	A printed copy of data in a file.
Hardware	The physical equipment that is used by a computer to process data.
Input	To enter data into the computer system; data entered into the system.
Network	A system of two or more computers linked together for the purpose of sharing information.
Keyboard	An input device, similar to a typewriter keyboard.
Log in (2 words)	The act of entering a username and password to gain access to a software application.
Login (1 word)	The combination of a username and password that authorizes an individual to open a software application or access certain features.
Menu	A list of options available to the software user.
Modem	Hardware device that converts digital signals to analog signals for transfer over communication lines or links.
Output	Data produced by the computer system.
Password/Security code	A secret sequence of characters that allows an authorized computer operator access to certain programs or features.
Peripheral	Device required for the input, output, processing, and storage of data; includes mouse, disk drives, keyboards, monitors, and printers.
Software	A computer program that allows users to perform a specific task.
Transfer	The act of uploading or downloading data.
Upload	The act of sending data from one computer or storage device to another.
Username	A short name that uniquely identifies an individual to a computer system or software application.
Wireless/Wi-Fi	Technology that uses radio waves, rather than wires or cables, for communication between peripherals and a CPU, or between computers and a network or the Internet.
Write-protect	Feature of storage devices that allows the data to be seen but not changed.

The Central Processing Unit (CPU)

The CPU acts as a traffic controller, directing the computer's activities and sending electronic signals to the right place at the right time. The time it takes for the electronic signals to come and go is measured in **megahertz (MHz)**. One megahertz equals 1 million cycles per second. The higher the MHz, the faster the computer. At the heart of the CPU is the **microprocessor**. Microprocessors have three characteristics: instruction set, **bandwidth** (the amount of data that can be transmitted in a fixed amount of time), and **clock speed** (the speed at which the CPU can process instructions). The higher the numbers, the greater the power of the CPU.

Memory

A computer's memory is measured and stored in kilobytes, megabytes, or gigabytes. A byte is one character of information. Each **kilobyte (K or Kb)** is 1,024 bytes of information. A **megabyte (M or Mb)** is 1,024 kilobytes, or a little over 1 million bytes of information. A **gigabyte (G or Gb)** is 1,024 megabytes, or a little over 1 trillion bytes of information. The higher the number of bytes, the more information a particular storage media can hold.

Computer memory is divided into **read-only memory (ROM)** and **random-access memory (RAM)**.

- ROM is internal permanent storage that contains the hard-coded, permanent programming instructions that make the computer operate. Users cannot access or change the data in ROM.

- RAM is the active memory of the computer while it is turned on. This is the memory needed to run software and store any data that have not been saved. RAM is active only as long as the computer is on. When the computer is turned off, or powered down, information stored in RAM is lost.

Storage Devices

To save data after the computer is turned off or after a program is closed, users must have one or more storage media. Types of storage media have evolved over the years. At one time, magnetic tape and 8-inch soft plastic disks were used. Today, the most common storage media are hard disks, CD/DVDs, and USB drives. An internal hard disk is located inside the computer case with no direct access by the user. An external hard disk is located in a sealed case that connects to the

Professionalism | **The Workplace**

Professionalism includes understanding the differences between terms that appear to be similar, but have specialized meanings in certain contexts. Two easily confused terms in the world of computers are *disk* and *disc*. Although both of these words describe computer storage devices, they identify different technology. *Disk* refers to magnetic media such as hard disks and 3 ½-inch storage disks. *Disc* refers to optical media, such as CDs and DVDs. However, you may encounter situations in which people overlook the differences and use *disk* for both types of media. (*Disc* is also the spelling preferred for most medical terms, such as *spinal disc*.)

computer with a cable. Other disk drives, such as those for CDs and DVDs, may be internal or external. An internal drive is mounted inside the computer case, with an access slot facing out. External drives are encased in metal or plastic and connect to the CPU with a cable. Although storage devices are highly portable, any devices that contain protected health information (PHI) must be safeguarded and transported in a secure manner. Figure 12-5 shows a variety of storage devices.

Hard Disks

A hard disk is a rigid metal disc (a flat, round object) that uses a magnetic head to record data for permanent storage.

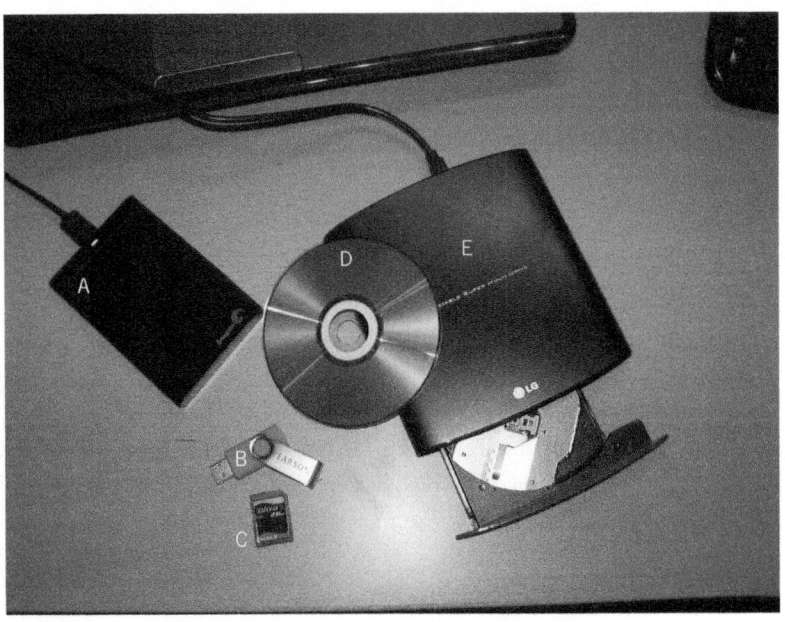

FIGURE 12-5 Storage devices: **(A)** external hard-disk drive; **(B)** USB drive; **(C)** memory card; **(D)** optical disc (DVD); **(E)** optical disc drive.

The terms *hard disk* and *hard disk drive* and *hard drive* often are used interchangeably. Nearly all computers have at least one internal hard disk drive used to store application software and large quantities of user-generated data. External drives may be used for data backup. The CPU controls access to the hard disk. Accessing data on an internal hard-disk drive is usually faster than accessing data on any other media. Although application software stored on the hard disk cannot and should not be modified, user-generated data on a hard drive can be saved (written), retrieved at a later time by a software program, modified, and saved again.

Optical Discs

Optical discs, commonly known as CDs and DVDs, are rigid polycarbonate discs that store data long term. A laser burns data onto the disc with a light, rather than magnetically, as is the case with most hard disks. *CD* stands for "compact disc." *DVD* stands for "digital video disc" or "digital versatile disc." CDs and DVDs range in size from 3 to 7 inches, the most common size being 4.75 inches. A DVD can hold much more information than a CD of the same size, because DVDs record data in layers and can be recorded on both sides.

Application software and reference books are often distributed to users on a CD or DVD. Empty discs can be purchased and used for data that you save to that disc for storage. DVDs are ideal to record presentations that combine sound and graphics.

CD/DVDs are identified by their storage capacity (MB or GB) and one of the following formats (abilities to accept data):

- Read only (ROM) refers to a disc that comes with data already on it, such as a software application or reference data. After the original data are saved to the disc, it cannot be changed.

- Write-once (R) refers to a blank disc on which users can save data one time, but cannot later change or erase the data.

- Read/write (RW) means that the data stored on the disc can be rewritten multiple times. There are several variations of RW discs, labeled +R, –/+R, RW+, and RW–, each with slightly different specifications. When purchasing CD/DVDs, be certain to specify the exact format needed.

USB Drives

A portable **universal serial bus (USB)** drive, also known as a jump drive, thumb drive, or flash drive, is a portable storage device, smaller than a finger, that can store many gigabytes of data. USB devices can be purchased in a variety of sizes, styles, and shapes depending on the need. As a courtesy to their patients, some medical facilities place the patient's medical record on a password-protected flash drive that allows the patient to carry the record from office to office. This is especially helpful for patients with several physicians who are not all linked to the same electronic health records system.

Memory Cards

Memory cards, also called flash cards or smart cards, are small wafers, less than 1 inch by ½ inch in size, encased in plastic, used to store data. They are inserted into a designated slot in the computer or a card reader device to access the data. Memory cards are used to store a wide range of data files, such as audio and video clips, images, and text documents, and are frequently used in digital cameras and smartphones.

Input Devices

Input devices enable the user to generate information that will be used or stored by the computer. Common input devices are a keyboard, mouse, microphone, and scanners. Graphic tablets and barcode scanners are other types of input devices.

Keyboard

The keyboard is a set of keys used to input data that consist of words and numbers. Although the exact layout may vary slightly among manufacturers, a keyboard is designed with alphanumeric keys, navigation keys, function keys, and conjunction keys (Figure 12-6):

- Alphanumeric keys are the letters of the alphabet and numbers from 0 to 9, used to type text and enter numbers.

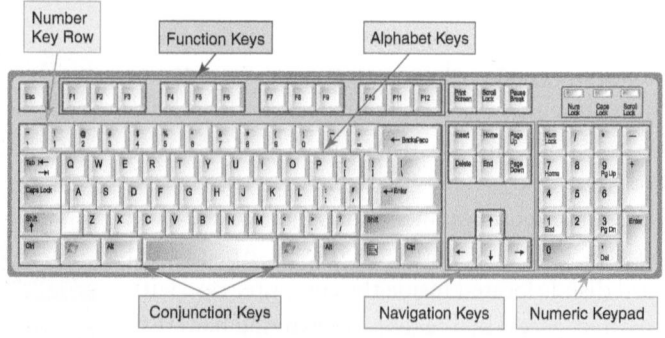

FIGURE 12-6 Typical keyboard layout.

- Navigation keys assist the user in moving through a document or menu, such as Tab, Backspace, Page Up, Page Down, and Home.
- Function keys are used by application software programs to provide shortcuts to executing specific commands. These are usually numbered F1 through F12 and have different functions in different and programs. F1 usually brings up a Help window.
- Conjunction keys, such as Ctrl (Control), Alt (Alternative), and Shift, are held down at the same time as other keys to execute specific commands that vary with different programs.

The commands performed by function keys and conjunction keys are different for each software program, so you must refer to the users' manual and onscreen tips to make the best use of these features.

Mouse

A **mouse** is a small oblong device that the operator rolls over a hard, flat surface to control the movement of the cursor on the monitor. The mouse contains at least one button, and up to three, each performing different functions, depending on the program in use.

Touchscreen

A **touchscreen** is a display that includes sensors that detect the touch of a finger or stylus. In this way, the computer monitor functions as an input device as well as an output device. Because the touchscreen accepts inputs directly through the screen, the computer does not require another input device, such as a mouse or keyboard. Touchscreens often provide a soft keyboard that appears on the screen when alphanumeric input is needed. Touchscreens are commonly used for portable devices, such as tablets and smartphones, electronic sign-in pads, and computer kiosks, such as a patient education or facility navigation booth.

Microphone

A microphone allows the user to speak to a computer and issue commands or record a message. Voice recognition technology (VRT) is software that allows the user to speak into a microphone and translates the spoken words into commands or text. VRT may require the user to provide several samples by reading the names of certain commands or words to "train" the software to understand speech patterns. VRT is a useful hands-free method to execute commands on the computer rather than using a keyboard or mouse. Some physicians use it to dictate progress notes and reports; some hospital medical records departments also use VRT.

Page Scanner

A page scanner creates a digital image of printed paper records and converts them into a format the computer can read, using optical character recognition (OCR). After the document has been converted into an appropriate format, it can be saved, imported into another program, printed, or used for any other purpose as a file. Scanners are used for a variety of office tasks, but most often they are used to convert the patient's paper record or reports into a digital form that can be attached to the patient's electronic health record.

Card Scanner

A card scanner, also called a card reader, functions similarly to a page scanner, but is sized to accept insurance cards, driver's licenses, and government-issued identification cards. The user inserts the card into a slot, and the machine scans both sides of the card directly into the patient's electronic health record. Card scanners save time, improve the accuracy of information, and save paper because the card does not need to be photocopied before scanning.

Digital Camera

A digital camera records pictures. Instead of the image being stored on film, it is stored digitally and can be downloaded to a computer system. Many offices with electronic health records use digital cameras to take pictures of their patients and then download the pictures into the patient's record. The camera sometimes can be attached to the computer and downloads the picture automatically. Having photographs stored in the medical record helps the staff ensure they match the patient with the right record.

Output Devices

Output devices enable the user to obtain data from the computer in a usable format. Common output devices are monitors, printers, and speakers.

Monitor

The **monitor** is the display screen that allows the user to see information on the computer. Most monitors are able to display anywhere from 16 to over 1 million different colors (Figure 12-7). Monitors are available in a variety of sizes and styles similar to television screens. The screen size is measured in inches diagonally, from one corner to the opposite diagonal corner.

Printer

A **printer** is used to transfer information from the computer monitor onto paper, also known as hard copy. The most

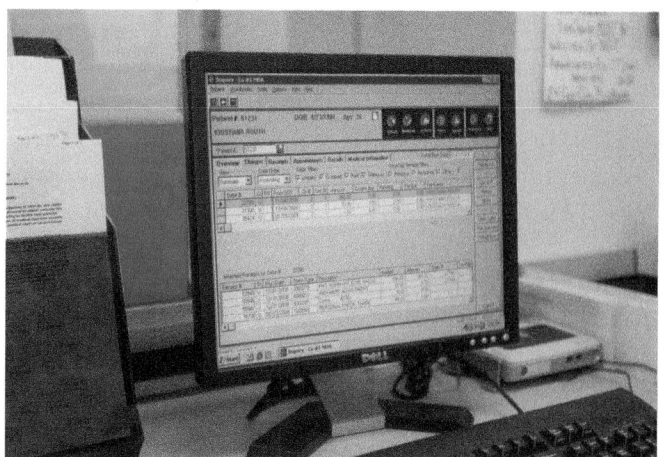

FIGURE 12-7 Color monitor for a computer system.

popular printer options are inkjet and laser. An inkjet printer works by forming dots when the ink is blown onto the paper. Inkjet printers can print graphics and in color if the proper ink cartridges and software have been installed.

Laser printers use light to burn toner onto the paper, similarly to a copy machine. Laser printers are faster and quieter than inkjet printers and can produce typewritten-quality work. Laser printers are available in black-and-white and color.

Some offices use dot-matrix printers for multipage forms, such as carbonless NCR forms, which inkjet and laser printers are not able to print. (Unlike inkjet and laser printers, dot-matrix printers use a striking head, which releases the dye contained in an NCR form.) Although they are useful in printing NCR forms, dot-matrix printers are noisier, have poorer print quality, and are not as fast as inkjet and laser printers.

Medical assistants must know how to load paper into the printer, replace toner or ink cartridges when empty, release paper jams, and perform other minor printer maintenance.

Installing Computer Hardware

Medical assistants may occasionally need to install a new piece of hardware, such as a printer or scanner. Each piece of hardware comes with installation instructions. Hardware installation may require you to also install software that controls the operation of the component, called a device driver. The device driver software is usually packaged with the hardware. Updates may be available on the Internet. Procedure 12-1 explains the steps for installing computer hardware.

COMPUTER SOFTWARE

Software, also called a program, contains the instructions that allow the computer to perform its functions. **Operating system** software is the basic software that allows the computer to run,

manages computer hardware resources, and enables application software to function. The operating system runs whenever the computer is on. Examples of operating systems are Windows, iOS, Mac OS, and Unix.

For a computer to perform most practical tasks, **application** software is also required. A medical office uses several application software programs. Some are general purpose applications, common to most computer users, whereas others are specialized with limited use for a medical office or business. Specific types of applications are discussed in the following sections.

The office should maintain a software inventory log that records each software program purchased and the computer it was installed on. This can be set up in a spreadsheet or word processing program. Also, keep a copy of the purchase receipt and cross reference it to the software inventory log. A copy of a paper receipt can be kept in a notebook designated for this purpose or scanned into the computer. This provides necessary proof of purchase should the office ever be audited to verify legitimate versus illegally pirated software. Figure 12-8 provides an example of a software inventory log.

General Purpose Applications

General purpose applications commonly found on computers include a word processor, spreadsheet, database management, presentation software, and desktop publishing. Internet browsers and e-mail clients, discussed later in this chapter, are also general purpose applications. A suite, such as Microsoft (MS) Office, is a coordinated collection of several applications, including a word processor (MS Word), a spreadsheet (MS Excel), a database management program (MS Access), presentation software (MS PowerPoint), and a desktop publishing program (MS Publisher).

Word Processor

Word processor applications make it possible to create, edit, store, and print written documents such as letters, manuscripts, transmittals, and many other professional documents. Word processing programs can visually enhance a document's appearance with formatting features, such as boldface, italics, font choice, and color. The word processor also allows the user to create a document, save it, retrieve it

Software Inventory					
Computer Location/ID	Software Name and Version	Date Installed	Purchase Date	Place of Purchase	Receipt Number
Reception #1	MS Word 2010	6/2/YY	6/1/YY	ABC Computer	12345

FIGURE 12-8 A software inventory log.

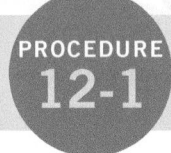
Installing Computer Hardware

Objective ◆ *Follow a general process for installing computer hardware components.*

EQUIPMENT

Computer on which hardware is to be installed; new hardware and all packaging; office equipment inventory log

METHOD

1. Plan a time to install hardware when it does not interfere with patient reception and care and when you are not likely to be interrupted, such as before or after office hours.
2. Check the make, model, and compatibility to ensure it meets your expectations of what was to be purchased.
3. Open the box that contains the hardware, being careful to not cut anything inside the package. Do not throw anything away.
4. Locate the installation manual and parts list.
5. Unpack the box, and check off each item on the parts list as you locate it. Thoroughly check all packing materials. Look for small items that may have dropped to the bottom of the box or that may be packaged in a small envelope or plastic bag. When you think you are done, review the parts list one more time, and again check off every item to be certain you have it. Set the packing materials to one side, but do not throw anything away. If any parts are missing, call the manufacturer at the phone number usually located on the parts list.
6. Read through the installation instructions one time, without performing any of the tasks. This helps you become familiar with the overall installation process, because the details for installing each piece of hardware are unique to that component.
7. Collect any additional materials or information the installation instructions refer to, including tools, such as a screwdriver, or any special information, such as existing passwords, equipment codes, or similar items of information.

8. If installing an internal component, such as new internal drive or memory chips, turn the computer off, unplug it, and open the case. If installing an external component, note if the computer is to be turned off or left on. Anytime instructions state to turn off the computer, also unplug it from the wall. This protects both you and the hardware.
9. Follow the manufacturer's installation instructions, checking off each step as you complete it. Do not skip or change the order of any steps. Reread each step to be sure you follow it correctly.
10. If required, install any software that may accompany the hardware. Some components require you to install a device driver (software instructions needed for the component to communicate with the CPU). You may need to access the manufacturer's website to download the most recent version of the driver.
11. Follow the manufacturer's instructions to test the operation of the newly installed component. This may require starting or restarting the computer.
12. If the component does not function properly, read the troubleshooting instructions or FAQ (Frequently Asked Questions) information usually included in the installation guide.
13. Complete the required registration and warranty forms. These may be included in the package, or you may be able to do this online.
14. Record the addition of the equipment on the office's equipment inventory log.
15. Locate the component's user manual or operating manual, and file it in the appropriate location, per office policy. Sometimes the manual must be downloaded from the manufacturer's website.
16. Retain all packing materials for at least 30 days in the event that the product needs to be returned or exchanged.

at a later time, and work on it again. Documents can be shared so that multiple people can read or contribute to the document, and changes or suggestions from different readers can be shown (tracked) in color. Corrections can easily be made. Using a printer, multiple copies of a document can be created. In the medical office, a word processor typically is used to create correspondence with patients, physicians, and

insurance companies. A word processor program also may be used to create patient education materials, such as office brochures or handouts.

Spreadsheet

Spreadsheet applications allow users to manipulate data by rows and by columns. Users input values into specific spreadsheet cells and use electronic formulas to calculate new numbers. Data from other programs, such as an accounting program or medical billing program, can be imported into a spreadsheet for further analysis. In the medical office, a spreadsheet is typically used to analyze data and statistics, including income, expenses, insurance claims, and patient-specific data. It can also be used to track information, such as inventory, and create checklists.

Database Management

Database management applications are electronic filing systems. The database software application is used to create collections of information that can be sorted and retrieved quickly. Any application that stores large quantities of similar information uses a database, including accounting systems, name and address lists, and medical coding software. A general-purpose database program allows the user to define the type of information to be tracked and to create a customized application.

Presentation Software

Presentation software is used to create slide presentations. Information can be imported from a word processor, if desired, to reduce the need to retype information that may already exist. Presentation software may be used to develop slide presentations for patient education and run as a continuous loop on the waiting room monitor and for presentations the office manager or physician will deliver to outside groups.

Desktop Publishing

Desktop publishing software combines features of a word processor with graphic design capability to produce a sophisticated document more easily than a word processor can accomplish. One option is to create the text in a word processor where it is easier to edit and then import it into a desktop publishing program to add the graphic component. Depending on the software used, it might be possible to provide the document electronically to a professional printing service for production. In a medical office, desktop publishing software typically is used to create patient education brochures, newsletters, signs, and announcements.

Specialized Medical Office Applications

Specialized software helps streamline tasks unique to a medical office or business more efficiently than can be accomplished with general purpose applications. Such programs often incorporate features of a word processor, spreadsheet, or database management program tailored to the unique needs of the medical field. Many companies that market specialized software provide the option of customizing portions of it to the needs of your office. The most

common types of specialized software used in medical offices are a practice management system, electronic health records, and accounting.

Practice Management Software

Practice management software (PMS) is a comprehensive software program that manages many of the administrative and business functions of a medical practice. Functionality may include the following:

- Appointment scheduling
- Patient registration
- Coding and charge entry
- Billing and claims processing
- Electronic claims submission
- Patient and insurance payment posting
- Patient statements and collections
- Patient reminders and correspondence
- Reimbursement management
- Reports and analysis

Medical practice management programs offer many benefits. After entering patient information into the program only once, the practice can schedule an appointment, record charges and payments, generate an insurance form, print a statement (including notices of delinquency accounts or aged accounts), track the number of days required to receive payment from the insurance company, identify unpaid accounts, and write a reminder letter or postcard to the patient about an upcoming appointment.

Several practice management programs are available. All of them provide similar functions. However, each program operates differently, including slightly different screens, menu, and commands, so it is important that new employees understand the specific operation of the management program used in their office. Most offices provide a one- or two-day training session for new users.

Electronic Health Records

An **electronic health record (EHR)**, sometimes referred to as an electronic medical record (EMR), is a computerized version of a patient's medical history. At their simplest, EHRs are computerized versions of patients' charts but, when fully implemented, they are networked, real-time, patient-centered records, designed to collect and share information from all providers involved in a patient's care. Networked EHRs may be found in medical offices associated with a hospital network of providers. Data can be created, managed, and viewed by authorized providers and staff from across all entities within the network.

Accounting

The accounting department uses specialized software to enter, maintain, and generate reports on information related to a medical office's financial operations. Typical accounting software functions include general ledger (GL), accounts payable (AP), accounts receivable (AR), payroll, and budgeting. Insurance and patient billing tasks are performed using the patient accounts module of practice management software. Payments are entered into the patient accounting module to track each patient's account status and into the accounting department's AR module to track the overall financial status of the practice.

Installing Computer Software

To use software, it must be installed, or loaded, onto the computer and configured. The installation files are usually accessed on a CD, DVD, or file downloaded from the Internet. The specific steps vary for each application, so it is important to read the instructions that accompany the software and read all on-screen prompts. Procedure 12-2 explains the general steps for installing computer software.

Troubleshooting Common Computer Problems

Because of the complexity of computer systems, users will experience difficulties with hardware or software at some point. Medical assistants should be familiar with common issues and how to troubleshoot them. General troubleshooting procedures include the following:

- Close all open applications and windows.
- Check for obvious hardware issues:
  - Verify that that all cords are securely connected at both ends.
  - Check or change batteries on devices that use them, such as a mouse.
  - Be sure that required components, such as printers, are powered on and filled with paper.
- Reopen the application in which the issue occurred. Try to recreate the problem by repeating the same keystrokes as when it first occurred. Write down each keystroke and menu selection performed.
- Press the F1 key to access the Help window, if one is available. Search for a solution to the problem in the Help window.
- If an error message appears, write down exactly what it says.
- Restart the computer. (In Windows, select the *Start* button, and then select *Restart*.)

- Reopen the application in which the issue occurred. Try again to recreate the problem.
- If the problem persists, shut down the computer, turn off the power, wait for a few minutes, and then restart it. (In Windows, select the *Start* button, and then select *Shut Down*.)
- Restart the computer, and reopen the application.
- If possible, conduct an Internet search to see if others have experienced the problem and suggest solutions. Access the software manufacturer's website for more specific help.
- Verify that the most current version of the software is installed by checking the manufacturer's website and identifying the current version number. The installed version number of most applications can be found on the *About* tab or *File, Information* tab.
- If the problem persists, contact your system administrator or technical support.

Remember to remain patient and calm throughout the troubleshooting process. If necessary, step away from the computer for a few minutes and come back with a clear mind. Do not let patients see your frustration, and do not discuss computer issues with patients. Doing so could undermine patients' confidence in the medical office or make them feel like their problems are unimportant.

COMPUTER SYSTEM SECURITY

Legal standards of confidentiality and compliance required by the Health Insurance Portability and Accountability Act (HIPAA) apply to all patient records, both paper-based and electronic. It is important to reassure patients that their information is managed appropriately within the medical office. It is absolutely essential for the medical assistant to understand that other patients should not be able to see computerized records any more easily than paper records. This may require some thought and planning when a computer system is used for record keeping in the front office.

HIPAA Security Rule

HIPAA regulations include the **Security Rule**, which provides national standards for protecting **electronic protected health information (e-PHI)**. Covered entities are required to implement three types of safeguards: administrative, physical, and technical.

Administrative Safeguards

Administrative safeguards are the policies and procedures that a medical office develops to ensure the security of e-PHI.

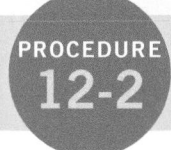
Installing Computer Software

Objective ◆ *Follow a general process for installing computer software.*

EQUIPMENT

Computer on which hardware is to be installed; new hardware and all packaging; office equipment inventory log

METHOD

1. Plan a time to install software when it does not interfere with patient reception and care and when you are not likely to be interrupted, such as before or after office hours.
2. Check the name, version, and compatibility printed on the software package to ensure it meets your expectations of what was to be purchased.
3. Open the box that contains the software, being careful to not cut anything inside the package. Do not throw anything away.
4. Locate the installation manual and parts list.
5. Unpack the package, and check off each item on the parts list as you locate it. Thoroughly check all packing materials. Recheck the parts list to be certain you have everything. Set the packing materials to one side, but do not throw anything away. If any items are missing, call the manufacturer at the phone number usually located on the parts list.
6. Read through the installation instructions one time, without performing any of the tasks. This helps you become familiar with the overall installation process.
7. Collect any additional materials or information the installation instructions refer to, including any existing passwords, equipment codes, or similar items of information.
8. Unless otherwise instructed by the manufacturer's instructions, turn on or reboot the computer to clear its memory. Verify that all software programs and Internet browsers are closed.
9. In most cases, you will be instructed to insert a disk or CD into the DVD drive. The setup program or Installation Wizard usually starts automatically. If it does not start, refer to the installation instructions regarding how to start it.

10. In some cases, you may be installing a program that was downloaded from the Internet. If this is the case, you will probably need to unzip a compressed file and click on the installation program (usually setup.exe) to begin the installation process. Note: Download software only if approved by office policy and only if authorized for office use. Do not download software for personal use under any circumstances.
11. Respond to the prompts that appear on the screen. The first prompt usually asks you to accept the software licensing agreement. Then you usually need to enter the name of the user and the company. Accept the program's default suggestions for installation location (folder) and file locations unless your office computer policy provides other guidelines.
12. When installation is complete, you usually will be asked to restart the computer. Verify that the software functions as expected, following manufacturer's instructions. If there are none, start the program and test its major functions by performing sample tasks.
13. If the software does not function properly, read the troubleshooting instructions or FAQ (Frequently Asked Questions) included in the installation guide. Some companies provide a technical support phone number to call should there be problems.
14. Complete the required registration and warranty forms. These may be included in the package, or you may be able to do this online.
15. Record the addition of the equipment on the office's software inventory log.
16. Locate the software user manual, and file it in the appropriate location, per office policy. Sometimes the manual must be downloaded from the manufacturer's website.
17. Retain all packing materials for at least 30 days, in the event that the product needs to be returned or exchanged.

Examples are designation of a privacy officer, conducting training programs about protecting PHI, and writing contingency plans for backup and recovery of data in emergencies.

Physical Safeguards

Physical safeguards are the controls a medical office has in place to prevent unauthorized persons from physically accessing patient data. Examples are proper positioning of workstations, visitor sign-in and escort, and procedures for protecting e-PHI when hardware is added or removed.

Computer systems must be placed in a secured and private space, such as an area of the office where there is limited public walk-through traffic. Computer screens should be positioned so they cannot be easily seen by patients. Both a screen saver and a privacy screen block others from viewing the computer screen. A screen saver projects an image or texture that covers up the screen at the touch of a key without removing any data. A privacy screen is a physical barrier that prevents passersby from viewing the monitor. Access to the computer or workstation should be locked with a password when no one is at the desk.

Technical Safeguards

Technical safeguards are electronic protections to prevent unauthorized access over networks and to **encrypt** (scramble or encode) all e-PHI. Examples are data validation, password systems, firewalls to prevent unauthorized intrusion, and data encryption.

It is imperative that patient records are accessible only to those who are authorized to use them. Keeping electronic patient records safe requires each user to have a unique password. Medical practice management programs often have several tiers of security, allowing the system administrator (the person in charge of the computer program) to limit access for patient records to those who need to see them. For example, the person who does appointment scheduling in a particular practice may not need to see a patient's financial records. The system administrator can lock the appointment scheduler out of financial records or can assign limited access to the data.

Security Practices

Although there are many details involved when implementing the HIPAA Security Rule, three of the most important practices that medical assistants encounter are the use of passwords, regular data backup, and system maintenance.

Passwords

Passwords prevent unauthorized users from accessing software and information. Each user must enter a username and **password**, followed by an acceptance key (ENTER or RETURN), to access a program. Passwords not only help protect against strangers accessing the medical office software, they also limit staff access to the specific area(s) of a program to which they are authorized. Examples of access limitations include the following:

- Clinical staff may not be authorized to view a patient's financial information.
- Financial staff may not be authorized to view a patient's medical information.
- Billing staff may be able to view, but not change, a patient's diagnoses.

When a medical office uses multiple secure software applications, such as practice management, EHR, and accounting, staff members have separate passwords for each application, as well as for the system as a whole. It is important to guard passwords carefully. They should not be shared with coworkers or written where someone else can see them. You should never allow coworkers to borrow your password or use your computer while you are logged in. If you need to let someone use your workstation, log out and allow the other person to sign in with their own password. When you have completed your task at the computer or need to step away for even a minute, log off or sign off your password before walking away. This prevents others from using your password inappropriately.

Many systems require a specific formula for a password. For example, it may need to be eight characters long and include letters, numbers, and special characters (such as !, @, #, $). When choosing a password, avoid using the names of family members or birthdates that could be easy for someone else to guess. If you must write down your password, keep it in a secure place and do not identify it as a system password. Many medical offices require you to change your password every 30 to 90 days.

Access Logs. Health care organizations are required to maintain logs that track individuals who have accessed patients' health records. This is used as a safeguard to ensure that unauthorized personnel are not accessing information they shouldn't be. The Health Information Technology for Economic and Clinical Health (HITECH) Act requires that the access of e-PHI be tracked. The log should identify the date and time of access, the name of the person accessing the record, the information accessed, and the action taken by the user, such as viewing, changing, deleting information, and so on. HIPAA requires that disclosure of any PHI, paper or electronic, be tracked, including the date of disclosure, name of the entity or person (and their address, if known) receiving the disclosed PHI, description of the PHI disclosed, and the purpose for the disclosure. Patients are entitled to receive the access and disclosure information, upon request.

Data Backup

Data **backup** involves copying all files from the computer to an external medium, such as an external hard drive or optical disc. Backup provides a safeguard in the event of a system failure, fire, or equipment theft because the original files can be retrieved from the backup media and restored to the computer for users to access. The noun or adjective *backup* refers to the process of saving data or the actual saved data. The verb *back up* refers to the action of copying the data to an external source.

Any computer medium that stores data can be used for backup, including online and remote backup services. Online and remote backup services must comply with HIPAA requirements for business associates and sign a

HIPAA Business Associate's agreement because they are handling PHI. Such services should be investigated thoroughly to ensure they will guard PHI. Any violation or misuse of PHI by an outside service comprises patient privacy, reflects poorly on the medical office, and brings liability because the medical office ultimately is responsible.

A backup routine should be performed once per day, outside normal business hours when no one is using the system. Ideally, the system administrator should schedule backups to execute automatically, but in a smaller office, office personnel might be responsible to oversee and implement the backup routine.

Four types of backups can be performed, each with its own advantages and disadvantages:

- In *system imaging*, a mirror image is created of all of software, configuration files, and user data that is organized from a technical perspective exactly the same as the source system. This enables restoration of the system exactly as it existed on the original computer(s). It requires a great deal of time and storage space to accomplish, so generally is done periodically but not every day.

- In a *full backup*, all data on the computer is copied to backup media, but software applications and configuration files are not copied. This enables restoration of the most current user data, but does not protect against loss or damage to software. The time and storage required can be considerable.

- In an *incremental backup*, all files that have changed since a specific date are backed up. This enables restoration of most user data without the time and space requirements of a full backup. Files that were changed before the date of the incremental backup must be restored from an earlier backup. For example, an office might do a full backup once a month, then incremental backups daily.

- In a *differential backup*, all files that have changed since the last full backup are copied. This method usually requires the least time and storage space. However, it can be difficult to identify the last time a file was changed, so you might need to look through several dates of backup media to locate the desired file.

Backups are created using software designed for this purpose that compresses, encrypts, and indexes the data. The specialized software saves space and makes it easier to find files. The software can be configured to automatically execute at a specific day and time, designate the type of backup to be performed, and identify which files should be backed up. Procedure 12-3 outlines how to perform data backup.

Depth of backup data is necessary for maximum protection, meaning that several days or weeks of data should be kept on hand at any given time. Therefore, different media should be used for each day or each backup; do not simply reuse the same media and save over previous backups. Just as computer disks fail, backup media also can fail, so you need to be able to access the "next oldest" backup should the most recent one fail. Office policy should specify how often backups are to be made and how long they should be kept. Table 12-4 shows a sample backup and retention schedule.

TABLE 12-4 | Sample Data Backup and Retention Schedule

Day	Type of Backup	Retention
1	SYSTEM IMAGE	1 year
2	Full	1 month
3	Incremental	1 week
4	Incremental	1 week
5	Incremental	1 week
6	Incremental	1 week
7	Incremental	1 week
8	Full	1 month
9	Incremental	1 week
10	Incremental	1 week
11	Incremental	1 week
12	Incremental	1 week
13	Incremental	1 week
14	Incremental	1 week
15	Full	1 month
16	Incremental	1 week
17	Incremental	1 week
18	Incremental	1 week
19	Incremental	1 week
20	Incremental	1 week
21	Incremental	1 week
22	Full	1 month
23	Incremental	1 week
24	Incremental	1 week
25	Incremental	1 week
26	Incremental	1 week
27	Incremental	1 week
28	Full	1 month
29	Incremental	1 week
30	Incremental	1 week

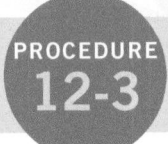

PROCEDURE 12-3   Performing Data Backup

Objective ◆ *Follow a general process for backing up computer data.*

EQUIPMENT

Network server computer; backup software; login name and password; software user instruction manual; backup media

METHOD

1. Gather the equipment and supplies.
2. Select a time to perform the backup that does not interfere with patient-related responsibilities. Identify a time when other computer users are not using the system.
3. Refer to the office's policy on computer backups to determine the type of backup to be performed on this day: system imaging, full, incremental, or differential.
4. Log in to the data backup software with the username and password assigned to you.
5. Respond to the prompts on the screen or make appropriate menu selections to perform the backup tasks: (Note: The specific menu selections and order in which steps are performed varies for each brand of software.)
   a. Select the type of backup to be performed.
   b. Select the computers, drives, folders, and files to be backed up.
   c. Enter a name for the backup, such as *2017_01_01_Full*.
   d. Insert the backup media in the designated drive or slot.
   e. Click *Start*.
6. You usually do not need to watch the computer monitor during the entire backup process, but you should watch it for the first few minutes to make sure the backup has started as intended. Check back periodically to confirm it is progressing as expected. If necessary, insert additional media when prompted (because the original disc is full).
7. Remove the media at the conclusion of the backup when prompted.
8. Label the media with the date and type of backup.
9. Verify that the backup name appears in list of available backups in the software.
10. Close the software application.
11. Make arrangements for the backup media to be transported to a designated off-site storage location. Ensure that all media are stored securely before, during, and after transport.
12. Return the computer to its normal operating screen.

Backup media should be stored in a secure location outside the office. All HIPAA safeguards for protecting PHI must be followed. Confidentiality is mandatory, and access to backup files should be carefully guarded.

System Maintenance

System maintenance involves a variety of tasks that help keep the system operating smoothly and protect it against outside abuse. Outside invaders include hackers, crackers, viruses, and cyberbullies that access confidential information and commit identity theft. Three forms of maintenance are virus protection, firewalls, and file cleanup.

A **virus protection** program is software that scans the computer data to detect and disable malicious virus programs that can harm your data. Ideally, the system administrator installs virus protection software and schedules it to run on a regular basis. In addition, such software can scan all files and e-mail downloaded to the system.

A **firewall** is a hardware- or software-based barrier that prevents outsiders from detecting the existence of your computer on an electronic network and, if detected, prevents them from entering the system.

File cleanup procedures include hard-disk defragmentation and deletion of temporary Internet files, cookies, and Internet history. Ideally these are scheduled by the system administrator to run automatically.

Professionalism

Most patients accept computer technology as a part of conducting any business. Some patients, however, are fearful that unauthorized persons may have access to their records. By using discretion in the handling of all medical records, the successful medical assistant conveys to the patient that confidentiality is of the utmost importance to the practice, thus reassuring the patient.

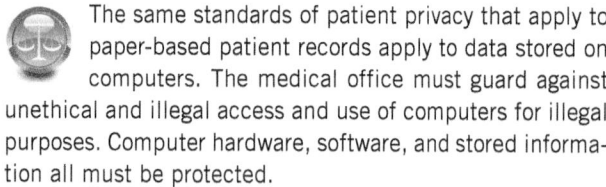

The same standards of patient privacy that apply to paper-based patient records apply to data stored on computers. The medical office must guard against unethical and illegal access and use of computers for illegal purposes. Computer hardware, software, and stored information all must be protected.

Employees must be educated and trained to understand the importance of security methods to prevent loss or damage to valuable equipment and programs. Informed employees can follow the proper procedures to report suspicious occurrences within the workplace. Medical assistants must have an understanding of their own liability and the physician's liability in the processing of medical records.

Every medical office has policies about the use of company computers for personal purposes. It is important that you understand the policies of your office and follow them. You never should use your computer for personal activities, access personal e-mail, or browse the Internet for personal reasons during your paid working hours. If personal use of the computer is allowed in your office, you should use that privilege only during break times or when off-duty. Do not save personal files on company media. If allowed, you may save files on your personal media, such as a portable flash drive. However, office policy may prohibit use of personal media as a precaution against viruses or malware. Remember that the medical practice owns the equipment and is entitled to view any and all information stored on it. For security reasons, the medical practice must be able to track what activities people have performed and what websites they have viewed. This applies to both work-related and personal activities. Do not use the computers in your workplace to access or store information that you do not want your employer to see.

ELECTRONIC COMMUNICATION

Electronic communication is central to most medical offices, so medical assistants must be familiar and comfortable with various ways to communicate. This includes Internet applications such as the World Wide Web, social media, and cloud computing. Medical assistants also should become skilled at using the Internet to access work-related information. Use of e-mail and electronic signatures is also reviewed.

The Internet

The **Internet** is a computer network of thousands of interfacing networks and millions of computers worldwide. Various organizations develop technical aspects of this network and set standards for creating Internet-based applications, but no governing body is in control of the Internet. Access is obtained through a commercial **Internet service provider (ISP)**. While using the ISP and a modem connection, you can browse the Internet for a wide variety of services: electronic mail, file transfer, reference information, interest group membership, interactive collaboration, multimedia displays, real-time broadcasting, shopping opportunities, breaking news, and much more.

Internet technology has allowed many medical insurance companies to offer electronic claims services or electronic media claims (EMC). EMC service speeds up the insurance claim process and puts the payment for services rendered into the practice's bank account in as few as three working days. Such access can be obtained through a clearinghouse or remote computer with transfer to multiple insurance carriers.

Private companies use Internet technology to offer patients a way to store their medical records in one place on the Internet. When patients use this technology, called a personal health record (PHR), they decide if they want to share their medical information, and if so, who may have access to it and what, specifically, can be shared.

JUDGMENT CALL

In the past, several medical office staff abused their Internet privilege, and as a result the medical office where Janis, a medical assistant, works has developed a strict policy on using the Internet for personal business, especially any shopping sites. Prohibited sites are blocked, and when an employee accesses one of these sites, the computer screen immediately turns red, and a report is filed with the information services (I/S) department at the main office.

Dr. Black has asked Janis to gather information about new computers for the office. While she is searching the Internet for information, her computer screen turns red, and the message is as follows: "A report on Internet activity has been forwarded to the I/S supervisor." Janis is immediately concerned because she knows several people have been reprimanded as a result of such messages, and one person was recently fired for visiting prohibited Internet sites. What should Janis do?

World Wide Web

The **World Wide Web (WWW)**, or the Web, created in 1989 by Tim Berners-Lee, is the user part of the Internet. The Web uses servers to provide a graphical user interface and hypertext links to navigate, find information, and link to new resources. Many companies, including medical practices, own a website, which is a collection of web pages (screen views) that provide information about their services. Most medical office websites provide information about the physicians, the services, hours of service, and scheduling information. Some provide the ability for patients to schedule their own appointments or send a secure message to the office requesting an appointment. Websites may also include information about the office's financial policies and provide registration forms for new patients to download and fill out. When the office changes its hours, adds or changes services, or updates its forms, it is important to update the website immediately so that patients receive the most current information.

The World Wide Web provides access to a great deal of information. Its convenient and user-friendly environment makes it easy for patients to research information about a new medication or for medical office staff to use as a tool to further educate members of the health care team.

Social Media

Social media are websites where users interact with each other in a community-like atmosphere. They may include discussion forums, user-generated content websites, and social networking websites, such as Facebook, Twitter,

TABLE 12-5	Websites That Provide Reliable Health Information	
Organization	**Website Address**
American Academy of Family Physicians	http://www.aafp.org http://familydoctor.org
American Academy of Pediatrics	http://www.aap.org
American Cancer Society	http://www.cancer.org
Centers for Disease Control and Prevention	http://www.cdc.gov/ diseasesconditions
Mayo Clinic	http://www.mayoclinic.com/ health-information
National Institutes of Health (MedlinePlus)	http://www.nlm.nih.gov/ medlineplus
Nemours Children's Health System	http://kidshealth.org
U.S. Department of Health and Human Services (Healthfinder)	http://healthfinder.gov
WebMD	http://www.webmd.com

LinkedIn, Instagram, and Pinterest, where people post brief messages, photos, and videos about their life and interests (Figure 12-9). Some sites are more business oriented, such as LinkedIn, and are used as an employment networking tool. Businesses, including medical offices, may post a page about their services on a social networking website as a convenience for patients. The medical office can post short news updates on their social networking page, and patients may

Professionalism

It is important to use and direct patients to health-related websites that contain reliable information created by experts in the medical field. Websites created by government agencies, such as Medicare, the National Institutes of Health (NIH), and Centers for Disease Control and Prevention (CDC), provide reliable and useful information. Websites created by hospitals and recognized medical organizations, such as the American Cancer Society, WebMD, and the American Academy of Pediatrics, are also reliable. Do not use or direct patients to user-developed or collaborative websites such as Wikipedia, eHow, and About.com. Anyone, regardless of their credentials, can write information for these websites. Therefore, you cannot and should not rely on the information to be accurate, up-to-date, and appropriate. Table 12-5 provides website addresses for several organizations that provide reliable health information.

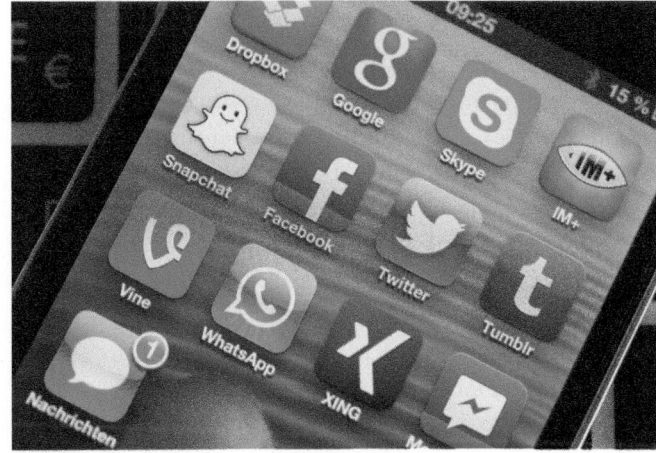

FIGURE 12-9 Patients can access social media sites to read and post information about medical offices using their computers or smartphones.

post comments in response. Users can "friend" or "follow" other users, which identifies people they want to keep in touch with, so that they can view all the comments another person posts.

Some sites allow patients to rate medical offices and share their impressions and experiences. Facebook provides this option on a business's profile page. Sites such as Healthgrades and RateMDs are specifically geared to the medical field and allow patients to rate individual physicians. A rating is a numeric "grade" on a scale of 1 to 5 or 1 to 10 that reflects the patient's experience. A review is a verbal comment in which patients describe their encounter in greater detail. Patients can check the ratings and reviews of a medical office or physician before deciding whether to make an appointment. A customer service "rule of thumb" is that a satisfied customer will tell three people, whereas a dissatisfied customer will tell 10 people. However, a dissatisfied customer whose complaint is resolved quickly is likely to become a loyal customer. Therefore, it is important that medical offices monitor patient satisfaction and act quickly to address any complaints.

Because social media is an increasingly common way for people to communicate and to vent their frustration with negative experiences, medical offices should designate an employee to monitor all social media sites used by the office. Many sites allow the business to post a response or comment as well. Although social media should never be used as the primary method of addressing a patient's complaint, and confidential information should never be discussed, it can be helpful to let everyone know that you are taking appropriate action. For example, you could post a general response such as "Thank you for letting us know your concern. I have contacted you by telephone to assist you. Meredith Mason, RMA."

Although social media can be quite enjoyable as a personal activity, medical assistants must use care in the information they post. If you identify your place of employment in your personal online profile, remember that anything you post could reflect on the medical office, positively or negatively. If you are friends with anyone who is also a patient at your office, do not discuss information about the office or information about the person's medical condition on a social networking site, or anywhere online.

Also keep in mind that many employers search social media to learn more about job applicants. Some even request that you provide links to your social networking pages. Anything you post, even as a joke or in a moment of indiscretion, can become public knowledge and reflect on the type of person you are. Social networking sites provide privacy setting

BOX 12-1 | Social Guidelines for Medical Offices

- Establish separate accounts for personal and professional use.
- Do not post identifiable patient information online.
- Safeguard patient privacy and confidentiality at all times.
- Use privacy settings that are a part of each online application, but realize they are not foolproof.
- Monitor the Internet to see what information others see about you.
- Correct any incorrect information immediately.
- Maintain appropriate professional boundaries with patients online.
- Monitor patients' ratings and reviews of your medical office on social media sites.
- When you see incorrect or inappropriate information posted by or about another medical practice, let them know in a considerate and professional manner.
- Recognize that online actions and content can reflect negatively on you and on the medical practice, and can have consequences for a long time.

options to limit who can see your information, but these may not completely protect your privacy or may not work as you expect.

Several medical associations have published guidelines for maintaining the medical office's social media presence, which are summarized in Box 12-1.

Cloud Computing

Cloud computing refers to applications and services offered over the Internet among a shared group of users. Cloud computing provides constant availability of data and applications, wherever Internet access is available. Using cloud services may be less expensive than purchasing a dedicated application program or service, because the cost is spread across many users. One popular service is online backup.

Professionalism   The Life Span

Older patients may not be very familiar with computers and computer terminology. It may be necessary to spend more time explaining how computers are used to assist in patient care. Some may have basic knowledge of Internet use. If they wish to research a health-related topic, help them by providing a list of reputable websites dedicated to patient education.

If this type of service is used, the medical office must be absolutely certain that HIPAA privacy and security regulations are adhered to by the site owner.

Using the Internet to Access Information

Medical assistants may need to use the Internet to access information related to patient care, patient education, regulations, and insurance companies. By learning to search for and locate reliable information, medical assistants can provide valuable resources for the medical practice. Procedure 12-4 explains the steps for using the Internet to access information related to the medical office.

E-Mail

E-mail, short for electronic mail, is a method of sending messages to others using the Internet. Users must establish an e-mail account with their ISP or a web-based e-mail service such as Gmail, Yahoo, Hotmail, or Microsoft Network (MSN). Users select a short name to identify them that becomes part of their e-mail address. Other people use this address to identify where messages should be sent. Using a special application program, called an e-mail client, users can write and receive messages and maintain an address book. Computer files such as word processing documents, spreadsheets, and photographs can be attached, or linked, to an e-mail, which the receiver can download and view.

It is quite likely that your medical office has an established e-mail account and that each staff member is assigned an e-mail address for work-related correspondence. It is important to use this address only for messages related to your job. You should maintain a separate e-mail address for personal use. E-mail sent on behalf of your medical office should follow business standards for use of proper English, grammar, spelling, and professionalism.

Electronic Signatures

An electronic signature is a set of encrypted characters that identifies, or authenticates, that the sender of a document, or a party to an agreement, is who he claims to be. Electronic signatures are legally recognized and are becoming increasingly accepted in the business world. EHR uses electronic signatures to identify who enters each piece of information into the patient's chart. Electronic signatures may also be used to sign contracts and other legal documents. However, some organizations still prefer that documents be physically signed with the paper document to be returned via the U.S. Postal Service or, possibly, scanned and returned via e-mail.

SELECTING A COMPUTER SYSTEM

Medical assistants may become involved in selecting a new computer system for the office. In a small office, they may be responsible for many of the selection activities. In a larger office, they may be asked for input, feedback, or to be a member of a team that works on certain aspects of system selection.

The first phase of selection of a computer system should focus on the software to be used. Important questions to answer include:

- How will the computer system be used?
- How many people will be using the computer system?
- Is current software meeting the needs of the practice? What new features are needed?
- Does everyone who uses it understand how to use it?
- Will the current programs transfer to a new system? Will the new system have the ability to interface with the hospitals in the area?
- If there are satellite offices, how do those offices exchange information with the main office?
- What new functionality and applications are needed?

After establishing how the computer(s) are to be used and what applications are required, hardware requirements can be established:

- How much storage space is needed now and for several years into the future?
- How many devices of each type (server, desktop, laptop, etc.) are needed?
- Do some areas, such as accounting and medical records, require more than one monitor per user?
- How will the system be backed up?
- What peripherals are needed?

Storage space requirements are determined by the number and type of software applications to be used and the amount of data to be stored. Software applications are constantly increasing in size, so be liberal in estimating storage and memory requirements. A good rule of thumb is to generously estimate the amount of storage needed, then at least double that amount. Storage space is becoming increasingly less expensive each year, so it is best to not skimp in this area.

After the hardware and software analysis has been completed, it is time to look at the products on the market:

- Do some manufacturers have a better service record than others?
- What happens if the computer system malfunctions?

Using the Internet to Access Health Information

Objective ◆ *Use the World Wide Web to locate reliable health information related to the medical office.*

EQUIPMENT

Computer (powered on) with Internet browser

METHOD

1. Open the Internet browser (a software program designed to access the Internet and World Wide Web) on the computer. Examples of Internet browsers are Internet Explorer, Chrome, and Firefox.
2. If you have a preferred website, such as one of those listed in Table 12-5, you may navigate directly to the site by keying the website address into the address bar. Press ENTER to navigate to the website. Skip to step 8 below.
3. Navigate to a search engine (an Internet-based application that searches websites for information) using one of the following methods:
   - Many Internet browsers use a particular search engine by default and open the search page when you open the browser.
   - If you have a preferred search engine, type its address in the address bar at the top of the browser (such as www.google.com or www.bing.com).
   - Type the words "search engine" in the address bar. The screen will display a list of popular search engines from which you can select.
4. Locate the search window on the search engine screen. The search bar is usually a white box with button displaying the word "Search" or "Go," with the image of a small magnifying glass next to it.
5. In the search bar, key in a few specific keywords or phrases to describe your topic. Press ENTER or click the button next to the search bar to activate the search. Examples are *influenza* to locate general information about the flu, *children flu* to locate information about how the flu affects children, or *flu* 2014 to locate information about flu strains in the year 2014.
6. Review the search results on the screen. The screen will display a list of topics, each with a brief excerpt. The website address usually appears immediately under the topic title. Read the topic titles, website names, and contents to locate the most relevant results. Try to determine the sponsoring organization such as a medical organization or government website. Many of these will contain the extension *.org* or *.edu* or *.gov*. Search results are usually several pages long. To navigate to additional pages to see more results, left-click on the page number of the desired page (located at the top or bottom of the search results screen).
7. Left-click on the topic title to navigate to the desired website.
8. Upon arriving at the website, identify the organization or sponsor of the website to ensure the information is reliable. The name may appear at the top of the screen. You can also look for a menu bar that contains the link "About Us." If the website address ends in .com and does not identify the sponsor, it is most likely a commercial site established to attract users who generate advertising revenue. Avoid such sites.
9. Determine if the page has the information you need. Read the title of the screen you have arrived at. Also read the menu choices, which may appear near the top of the page or on the left-hand side of the screen. Often, search engine results are very specific and the link takes you directly to the information you need. Other times, you may need to navigate through the menus to find the desired information or to conduct a second search within the site itself.
10. If necessary, search for more information on the website using one of the following methods:
    - Explore the menu options by moving the mouse over each item and clicking on it, if necessary.
    - If a menu bar containing letters of the alphabet is present, click on the letter of the term you wish to search for.
    - Locate an internal search box near the top or left-hand side of the screen that enables you to search within the site. Enter keywords or a phrase related to the topic you are searching for.
11. Decide how to save the information using one of the following methods:
    - To print the page, click a printer icon that appears on the page, if available. Or you may be able to right-click your mouse to bring up a menu that provides a print option.
    - Bookmark, or save the link, to the bookmark manager or favorites list in your browser. This stores the link so that you can return at a later time. The steps to do this vary slightly for each browser.
    - To e-mail a copy or link for the page, click an envelope icon that appears on the page, if available. You may e-mail it to yourself or to the person who requested the information.

12. Repeat the steps as necessary. When done, close the browser.
    Tips for conducting an Internet search:
    - Conduct multiple searches using slightly different keywords or synonyms such as *flu* and *influenza*, or *bird flu* and *avian flu*.
    - Use a different search engine, which may produce different results.
    - Use the Advanced Search options available on most search engines.
    - Enter the keywords as a question, such as "When should I get a flu shot?"

- Place a minus sign (–) before each word to "omit a word," such as *flu – children* to eliminate any results about how the flu affects children. Place a space before the minus sign, but not after it.
- Place a plus sign (+) before a word to view results with the exact word and no variation; for example, *+ fractures* would give results for "fractures" but not "fracture" or "fractured."
- Use quotation marks to view results that contain the exact wording of a phrase.

- Who pays to have the computer system fixed? Is a warranty provided?
- How will users be trained and supported?

This information will help establish the capital budget, the funds used to acquire the system, and the ongoing operating costs, such as training, supplies, and maintenance. Identify a support system of computer professionals who can provide ongoing technical assistance and quick on-site service for computer software and hardware problems. The office may wish to purchase a service contract to take effect when the warranty covering parts, repair, and service expires. Training contracts are available with firms that provide employee training on new software and hardware.

Computer system selection is a large responsibility. Although the final decision usually rests with a financial manager, it is a good idea to gather input from everyone who uses the system. The system's users can make or break the success of an installation because those who are unhappy with the selection are not as apt to use the system to its fullest capability, and this ultimately costs the practice money. Therefore, to make sure that the money invested in a system is well spent, it is imperative that as many users as possible be involved in the selection process.

COMPUTER ERGONOMICS

Computer **ergonomics** is the process of designing a computer workstation that is well-suited to a user's physical needs. Extended use of a computer with improper ergonomics can lead to physical problems. If you are a longtime computer user, you might have noticed the occasional discomforts that accompany spending lengthy periods of time in front of the computer. As use and hours on the computer continue over the years, the discomfort could become part of the daily routine when you sit down to use a computer. To safely incorporate computer use in your daily routine and to work effectively, you should be aware of some ergonomic tips, such as how to appropriately position computer equipment (Figure 12-10).

Your Chair

When sitting in your chair, make sure that you set your hips as far back as they can go in the chair. Adjust the seat height so your feet are flat on the floor and your knees are at the same level as, or slightly lower than, your hips. Adjust the back of the chair to a 100-degree to 110-degree reclined angle. Make sure your upper and lower back are supported. It may be necessary to use inflatable cushions or small pillows. If you have an active back mechanism on your chair, use it to make frequent position changes. For chairs with armrests, adjust them so that your shoulders are relaxed; remove the armrests if they are in the way.

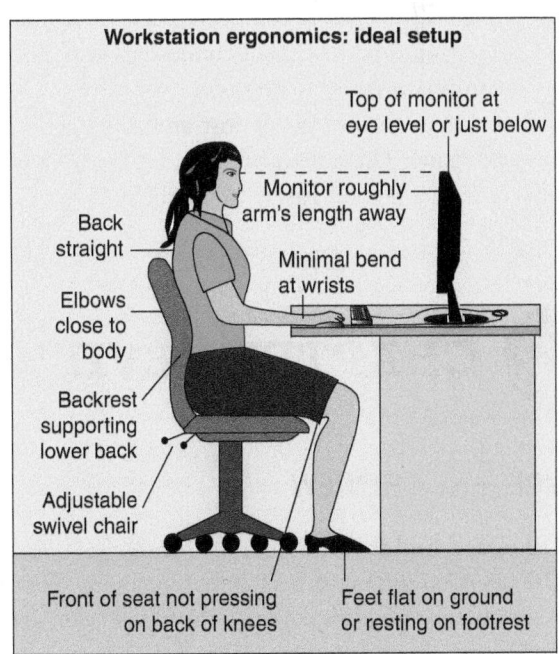

FIGURE 12-10 Ergonomically correct desk, chair, and keyboard.

Your Keyboard

An articulating keyboard tray allows you to adjust the angle and height of the keyboard and can provide optimal positioning of input devices. However, it should accommodate the mouse, provide leg clearance, and have an adjustable height and tilt mechanism. The tray should not push you too far away from other work materials, such as your telephone. It is helpful if you pull up close to your keyboard and position it directly in front of your body. If possible, adjust the keyboard height so that your shoulders are relaxed, your elbows are in a slightly open position, and your wrists and hands are straight. Wrist rests can help to maintain neutral postures and pad hard surfaces. However, the wrist rest should only be used to rest the palms of the hands between keystrokes.

The keyboard, mouse, mouse pad, and other input devices should be cleaned regularly with an appropriate cleaner to keep them functional and reduce the spread of germs.

Your Monitor

Incorrect positioning of the monitor screen and source documents can result in awkward posture and muscle tension. Adjust the monitor and source documents so that your neck is in a neutral, relaxed position. Your monitor should be centered directly in front of you, above your keyboard. Position the top of the monitor approximately 2 to 3 inches above seated eye level. To reduce glare, it may be helpful to place the screen at right angles to windows and adjust curtains or blinds. Optical glass glare filters, light filters, or secondary task lights can also help reduce glare.

If you have difficulties reading the print on a monitor, talk with your optometrist about computer eyeglasses that provide appropriate vision correction.

A computer monitor attracts dust and fingerprints that can obscure vision. Use a designated monitor wipe to clean your monitor on a regular basis to keep the surface clean.

Your Body

Once you have correctly set up your computer workstation, use good work habits. No matter how perfect the environment, prolonged, static postures inhibit blood circulation and take a toll on your body. Take short 1- to 2-minute stretch breaks every 20 to 30 minutes. After each hour of work, change to a noncomputer task for at least 5 to 10 minutes. Always try to get away from your computer during lunch breaks. Avoid eye fatigue by resting and refocusing your eyes periodically. Look away from the monitor, and focus on something in the distance. Rest your eyes by covering them with your palms for 10 to 15 seconds. Use correct posture when working. Shift your position as much as possible.

If you are susceptible to chronic back or neck problems, talk with your physician and physical therapist about the best way to set up your workstation to minimize stress. They can also provide you with appropriate exercises and stretches to do throughout the day.

SUMMARY

The use of computers is essential for medical offices to meet the process flow of business today. Computers enhance quality patient care through data collection, eliminate duplication of work, and decrease errors. Computers enable input, processing, output, and storage of medical data. In medical offices, computer use is especially valuable in eliminating some of the more time-consuming tasks associated with appointment scheduling, charting, billing, and insurance processing. Computers are composed of many parts, including the microprocessor, CPU, monitor, keyboard, and printer. Safety on the computer includes regular maintenance, passwords, antivirus protection, and HIPAA compliance. The successful medical assistant is a computer-literate professional who deals easily with the challenge of finding new and efficient ways to use available technology.

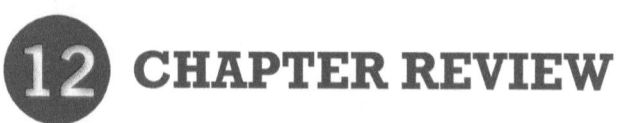

12 CHAPTER REVIEW

COMPETENCY REVIEW

1. Define and spell the terms for this chapter.
2. Using a microcomputer, boot up the computer. Notice what information is displayed on the screen before the computer is "ready" to work. What disk operating system is being used? What software applications are available?

Are any security codes required to use the programs listed? If so, what are they?

3. Discuss the HIPAA Security Rule, including the three types of safeguards and three security practices.

4. Explain three types of websites that provide reliable health information and why it is important to use only reliable sites.
5. Select a word processing program, and type a simple letter reminding a patient that a blood pressure check is due. Use the spell-check feature before printing the letter.
6. Enter a patient's information into a practice management software database. Use yourself and your own information as the data.

PREPARING FOR THE CERTIFICATION EXAM

1. What type of printer is fastest and most quiet?
   a. inkjet
   b. dot-matrix
   c. laser
   d. word processor
   e. scanner

2. Which is considered a hardware element of computers?
   a. systems
   b. scanner
   c. diskettes
   d. central processing unit
   e. magnetic tapes

3. Which is *not* an advantage of a medical database management program?
   a. have to enter patient information only once
   b. can measure storage capacity
   c. can track days before payment is received from insurer
   d. can print delinquency notices
   e. can schedule appointments

4. Which is *not* recommended to establish computer security and protect patient information?
   a. screen saver to cover up the screen
   b. tiers of security that limit access to patient information to authorized employees
   c. a standard password used by everyone in the office
   d. screen positioned away from patients
   e. use of firewalls

5. What is computer downtime?
   a. data entry operations including additions, deletions, and modifications
   b. a copy of work or software batch data stored for processing at periodic intervals
   c. garbage in, garbage out
   d. time of maintenance
   e. processing of information in a very small amount of space

6. What is the name for a list of options available to the computer user?
   a. password
   b. menu
   c. DOS
   d. boot
   e. prompt

7. The ergonomic concerns related to computing may be all of the following *except*
   a. document.
   b. keyboard.
   c. body.
   d. chair.
   e. monitor.

8. Which office function *cannot* be performed by word processing?
   a. User can correct errors on the screen before printing takes place.
   b. User can print X-ray films.
   c. User can input information using a typewriter-like keyboard.
   d. User can generate form letters.
   e. User can see the copy that will be printed before it is printed.

9. Which of the following is considered a software element of computers?
   a. peripherals
   b. mouse
   c. floppy disks
   d. medical billing programs
   e. monitor

10. Which of the following websites would be considered a reliable source of cancer prevention information?
    a. the website of a major hospital that has a cancer specialty center
    b. the blog of an individual nurse who has worked with cancer patients
    c. a discussion board for patients with cancer
    d. Wikipedia
    e. a personal blog from a patient who is a cancer survivor

CRITICAL THINKING

Refer to the case study at the beginning of the chapter and use what you have learned to answer the following questions.

1. Where should Samra begin?
2. Which software programs should she use to design and develop the educational materials and the marketing materials?
3. What should she do to become more familiar with the software features to design the materials?

ON THE JOB

Elizabeth Maxwell, a medical assistant for Dr. Casey, often works at the front desk. One of Dr. Casey's patients, Stephanie Cross, has arrived for a scheduled appointment. On her way in, Stephanie saw a neighbor leaving the office. She asks Elizabeth to look on the office system and tell her why her neighbor was in to see Dr. Casey.

Later the same day, Diana Mulderr, who sits at the desk next to Elizabeth, has forgotten her computer password. She asks to use Elizabeth's password "just for today."

1. What should Elizabeth tell Stephanie Cross?
2. Is it ever permissible to use the computer to look up information on patients for personal reasons?
3. What should Elizabeth tell Diana Mulderr?

INTERNET ACTIVITY

When researching information on the Internet, it is important that the websites used are reputable and provide accurate information. Perform a search using any of the search engines (a website that allows you to search the entire Web for related websites) available to you. Search for health-related websites. Make a list of 10 websites, and comment on each: ease of use, relevant information, clarity, and so on.

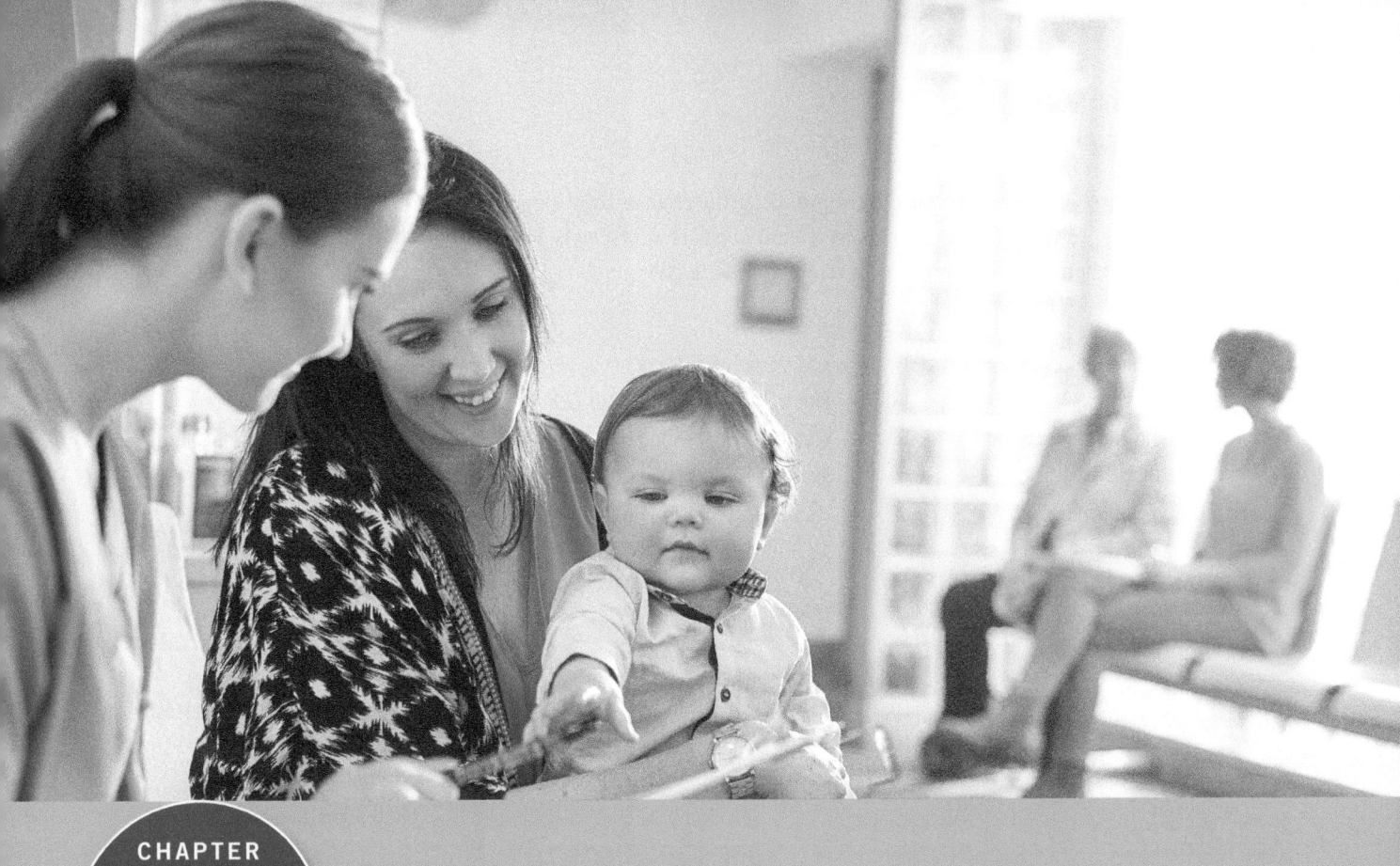

The Medical Record

Learning Objectives

After completing this chapter, you should be able to:

13.1 Define and spell the terms for this chapter.

13.2 Compare and contrast electronic and paper-based records.

13.3 Outline the history of electronic health records.

13.4 Explain the purpose of meaningful use as it applies to electronic health records.

13.5 Describe the HITECH Act as it relates to adopting electronic health records.

13.6 Describe the differences between electronic health records and practice management systems.

13.7 List the benefits of utilizing electronic health records.

13.8 Explain the ownership of medical records.

13.9 Explain special considerations when releasing medical records.

13.10 Describe the differences in organizing a medical record according to problem-oriented and source-oriented methods.

13.11 Describe the components of SOAP charting.

13.12 List the types of information contained in a patient's medical record.

13.13 Identify equipment and supplies needed to create, maintain, and store paper medical records.

13.14 Describe indexing rules related to filing paper medical records.

13.15 Identify long-term storage options for paper medical records.

13.16 Differentiate between how electronic and paper-based records are used in the office.

13.17 Explain the medical assistant's role in computerized physician order entry.

Pearson Physicians Group is considering making the change from paper to electronic health records. The physicians have assembled a team consisting of Lewis Jordan and Tania Washington to gather information relating to this possible change.

Terms to Learn

active records

alphabetic filling

certified EHR technology

chronological medical record

closed records

collating

computerized physician order entry (CPOE)

covered entities

digital signature

digitized signature

electronic health record (EHR)

electronic medical record (EMR)

electronic signature

exception report

Health Information Technology for Economic and Clinical Health Act (HITECH)

inactive records

login

meaningful use

medical record

microfiche

microfilm

numeric filing

Office of the National Coordinator for Health Information Technology (ONC)

personal health record (PHR)

problem-oriented medical record (POMR)

source-oriented medical record (SOMR)

subjective, objective, assessment, and plan (SOAP)

terminal digit filing

token signature

An **electronic health record (EHR)**, sometimes called an **electronic medical record (EMR)**, is a computerized version of a patient's medical history. At their simplest, EHRs are digitized images of paper records but, when fully implemented, they are networked, real-time, patient-centered databases that collect and share information from all providers involved in a patient's care. In general, EMR refers to a digital version of a patient chart kept in a single provider's office, whereas an EHR includes information beyond the provider's office that originally collected the data. The intent of an EHR is to share information across all organizations and providers involved in a patient's medical care, such as the primary care provider, specialists, laboratory, and so on.

Few medical offices are entirely paper-based, and few offices have a completely paperless environment that can result from a fully implemented EHR network. Most medical practices have some components of an EHR and operate somewhere along the continuum from an entirely paper-based medical record to an entirely automated environment. The trend is rapidly moving toward an increased level of automation because of the evolution of technology and legislation that pays providers financial incentives for implementing EHRs. To simplify terminology in this text, no distinction between EMR and EHR is made; EHR is used exclusively.

Most medical assistants work with EHRs at some point during their career. If you work in an office that currently has very little automation, you will most likely be involved in adding components of an EHR sooner or later. Offices that already have well-developed EHRs need to upgrade and expand the system from time to time.

This chapter discusses the purpose and history of EHRs, differences between EHRs and paper-based documentation, and benefits of EHRs. You will also learn about privacy and security concerns, various documentation formats, and components of a medical record. Finally, you will learn about implementing an EHR system.

PURPOSE AND HISTORY OF ELECTRONIC HEALTH RECORDS

An EHR provides a computerized means of gathering, documenting, and storing information about the patient and the care that the patient received in the medical setting. The same information found in a patient's paper chart is found in an electronic chart; however, electronic records are stored and accessed using a computer. EHRs allow access to patient information by multiple physicians and hospitals through the use of electronic networking and communications. Networked EHRs are often found in medical offices associated with a hospital network of providers. Data can be created, managed, and consulted by authorized providers and staff from across all entities within the network. Authorized providers can immediately access medical information from remote locations.

Appropriate Use of Terminology

As a medical assistant, you may encounter a variety of terms for what is now referred to as the electronic health record. When computers first came into use, the term *computer-based medical records* referred to paper-based records that had been scanned, then stored on the computer rather than in file cabinets. As computers gained in popularity and software was developed, the term *electronic medical record (EMR)* became popular. The term *electronic health record (EHR)* was adopted to describe the ability to share computerized patient information among providers. In 2003, the Institute of Medicine of the National Academies (IOM), which was a driving force behind EHRs, adopted EHR as the preferred and exclusive term to describe all types of computerized medical records, whether based in a single office or shared among a network of providers. Legislation, including the 2009 HITECH Act that provides incentive payments for implementing EHRs, uses the term electronic *health* record only. Therefore, it is recommended that medical professionals use only the term electronic *health* record, or EHR.

Personal Health Records

A **personal health record (PHR)** is health information that the patient stores electronically on a computer or on a secure Internet site. This allows patients to maintain electronic records of their own health information such as immunizations, medications, and surgeries. A PHR is maintained by an individual patient, whereas an EHR is maintained by health care providers.

PHRs have several benefits for patients. Patients may choose to share their PHR information with their usual providers. PHRs also give patients a means of sharing health information with new providers, should they move or need medical care while travelling. PHRs can increase patient participation in their own care. Viewing a trend of lab results or blood pressure readings can motivate patients to take medications and keep up with lifestyle changes that have improved their health. PHRs can also help families become more engaged in the health care of family members.

PHRs are provided by third-party vendors and consist of either a software application patients can install on their personal computer or an Internet-based portal that allows patients to store information on a website. Patients fill in the information from their own records and memories, and the information is stored on patients' computers or the Internet. The advantage is that patients are in control of their health information and can access it or share it with any provider. The disadvantage is that providers cannot directly update or verify the accuracy or completeness of the information. Patients must be careful to select a PHR provider that follows stringent privacy practices, so the privacy of their medical information is not compromised.

A tethered PHR is a function of provider-based EHRs that allows patients to access their EHR online. This is discussed later in the chapter. Eventually, patients may be able to link their standalone PHRs with their doctors' EHRs, creating their own health care "hubs."

History and Legislation

Although EHRs have been around since the Mayo Clinic began using them in the 1960s, ambulatory care has been slower than inpatient facilities to adopt the technology. Since President Bill Clinton (1993–2001) took office, the federal government has searched for ways to reduce medical errors and health care costs. President Clinton established the Agency for Healthcare Research and Quality (AHRQ) to research techniques to accomplish this. President George W. Bush (2001–2009) established the **Office of the National Coordinator for Health Information Technology (ONC)** and pushed for the adoption of technology that would reduce medical errors, improve health care quality, and reduce expenditures. President Barack Obama (2009–2017) identified EHR as a priority for his administration and approved legislation to promote the widespread adoption of EHR. Future presidents undoubtedly will continue these efforts.

HITECH Act Funding Incentives

In 2009, Congress passed legislation that made funding available for EHR implementation for the first time. The **Health Information Technology for Economic and Clinical Health (HITECH) Act**, which is part of the American Recovery and Reinvestment Act of 2009 (ARRA), includes financial incentives for providers who adopt EHR and demonstrate its use in ways that can improve quality, safety, and effectiveness of care. The goal of the funding is to encourage providers to adopt EHR sooner than they otherwise would, because Congress believes EHR can help improve quality of care and reduce costs. The ONC, Centers for Medicare and Medicaid Services (CMS), and other agencies within the Department of Health and Human Services (HHS) are working together to establish the criteria for the funding of EHRs. Under the incentive program, eligible Medicare providers can receive as much as $44,000 over a five-year period; eligible Medicaid providers can receive as much as $63,750 over six years.

Meaningful Use

Meaningful use refers to a set of criteria for how EHRs are used that providers must meet to receive incentive payments. The criteria are being phased in over three stages, from 2011 onward. Medicaid providers receive the first year of incentive payment when they adopt, implement, or upgrade **certified EHR technology**. Stage I (2011–2012) focused on data capture and sharing. Stage II (2014) focused on advanced clinical processes. Stage III (2016) focused on improved outcomes. To qualify for payments, providers must demonstrate meaningful use of certified EHR in ways that can be measured. Meaningful use criteria are grouped into five patient-centered areas that relate to health care priorities.

- Improve quality, safety, and efficiency
- Engage patients and families
- Improve care coordination
- Improve public and population health
- Ensure privacy and security for personal health information

Examples of meaningful use criteria include:

- E-prescribing
- Electronic exchange of health information to improve quality of health care
- Submission of information on clinical quality measures

Certified EHR Technology

Certified EHR technology gives assurance to purchasers that a specific EHR system provides the features necessary to meet the meaningful use criteria. Certification also helps providers and patients be confident that the electronic health information technology (IT) products and systems they use are secure, can maintain data confidentially, and can work with other systems to share information. A certified EHR meets the following criteria:

- Includes patient demographic and clinical health information, such as medical history and problem list
- Provides clinical decision support
- Supports physician order entry
- Captures and queries information relevant to health care quality
- Exchanges electronic health information with, and integrates such information from, other sources

Projected Savings

The purpose of the incentive payments is to accelerate adoption of EHRs. The Congressional Budget Office (CBO) anticipates that approximately 90 percent of doctors and 70 percent of hospitals will be using comprehensive electronic health records by 2019. It estimates that the accelerated adoption will eliminate redundant services and tests, thus saving Medicare $4.4 billion from 2011 to 2019. CBO estimates that, during the same time period, the HITECH Act will save the government approximately $12 billon on direct spending in the Medicare, Medicaid, and Federal Employee Health Benefits programs.

Differences Between Electronic and Paper-Based Records

Although EHRs contain the same information as paper-based medical records, they do not look like paper records or function in the same way. Medical assistants should be aware of differences in documentation formats, medical record components, and retention and storage requirements. Medical assistants need to be flexible and willing to learn new procedures and processes, because technology is always improving and EHR systems must be updated or replaced periodically.

Different Documentation Formats

EHRs provide a more flexible documentation format than paper-based records. Paper-based medical records are organized according to a chosen documentation format that is generally used consistently for all records and all encounters. Examples of documentation formats are the chronological format, SOAP (Subjective, Objective, Assessment, Plan), POMR (problem-oriented medical record), and source-oriented medical record. In contrast, documentation formats in the EHR can often use different documentation formats, making use of the best system for the particular task. Depending on the system, users may have a choice of documentation formats. The most common method for documenting progress notes is SOAP charting, but data can easily be sorted or retrieved based on problems or chronology (date order). This flexibility makes the documentation process relatively easy and adds functionality, because information can be accessed in a number of ways. Such flexibility is possible because of the underlying database that identifies and indexes data elements.

Different Medical Record Organization

EHRs store various types of information, just as paper-based records do, such as physical examination notes, lab results, operative reports, and consultation reports. In a paper-based record, the file folder is divided into sections that are labeled for each type of report. In an EHR, each type of report is accessed with a unique menu selection. The advantage of EHRs is that information is linked and cross-referenced. For example, when a progress note documents that the physician ordered a laboratory test, an EHR can provide a link that allows the user to view the results of the lab test without needing to exit the screen and navigate to a different part of the program.

Collating EHRs

The time-consuming task of **collating** paper-based medical records is eliminated when using an EHR. Test results and reports are delivered to the office electronically. A queue provides a computerized list of all new reports, which the physician must review and approve. When this is accomplished, the reports are electronically filed in the patient's EHR. Depending on the system, this may be accomplished automatically or a staff member may need to designate which patient record each report belongs to.

It is not necessary to pull and organize medical records for patients scheduled for the next day, because all the information is already in the EHR. Each staff member who works with the patient can click on the appointment screen or select the patient from a list and instantly access a patient's record.

Difference Between EHR and Practice Management Software

An EHR is different than a practice management system (PMS), which was discussed in the chapter titled "Computers in the Medical Office". An EHR system manages medical records of individual patients and, when fully implemented, networks with offices of other health care providers to share information regarding specific patients. A PMS manages administrative and business functions of a medical practice, including appointment scheduling, patient registration, and insurance billing. A PMS also can generate a variety of business reports related to these areas. A PMS does not store clinical information, aside from that used for billing, such as diagnostic and procedure codes.

BENEFITS OF EHR SYSTEMS

One of the key features of an EHR is that it can be created, managed, and consulted by authorized providers and staff across multiple health care organizations. A single EHR can bring together information from current and past doctors, emergency facilities, school and workplace clinics, pharmacies, laboratories, and medical imaging facilities. This interactivity offered by EHR provides benefits not possible from paper-based records. For example, EHRs enable providers to do the following:

- Review medications prescribed by other providers to avoid duplication or medication interactions.

- Access a patient's medical history to more quickly identify a problem or risk factor.

- View imaging studies electronically to better understand the progression of a patient's condition.

Physicians and their staffs must retrieve paper files from separate and often large rooms, in contrast to electronic records that are easily accessible on a computer. In large offices where patients might see multiple providers, EHRs allow physicians to easily locate patients' laboratory results, consultations, X-rays, and examination findings from other providers. Benefits of EHRs include improved diagnostics and patient outcomes, improved patient participation, and improved efficiencies, resulting in cost savings.

Most electronic health records systems can be configured to work according to an office's specific needs. Some offices implement more features than others. With the incentives for EHR implementation under the HITECH Act, an increasing number of offices have added EHR functionality. Box 13-1 lists the functions many of these systems provide.

BOX 13-1 | Functions of an EHR

The following can be documented in an EHR:
- Progress notes
- Timestamps on documentation entries
- Prescriptions electronically transmitted to the pharmacy
- Patient education information given to the patient
- Digital photos of the patient and the patient's condition
- Automatic recording of vital signs and diagnostic tests
- Electronically reported lab results, imaging studies, and other medical tests, as well as graphs of such data

- Graphs of height, weight, and blood pressure data
- Letters to or about patients
- Consultation reports
- Electronic data transmission to other health care providers
- Telephone calls with patients
- Capability to search electronically for patients with a certain condition or of a certain age or geographic location

---

Improved Diagnostics and Patient Outcomes

EHRs can improve the ability to diagnose diseases and reduce—even prevent—medical errors, improving patient outcomes. Because providers have reliable access to a patient's complete health information, they see a comprehensive picture of the patient's status, which helps diagnose patients' problems sooner.

The medical office can perform many tests in the office and have the results appear immediately in the EHR. This can be done with a number of laboratory tests on blood and urine samples, digital X-rays, Holter monitors, and spirometers. In some cases, thermometers and blood pressure cuffs can be linked to the EHR to allow automatic recording of vital signs (Figure 13-1).

Improved Documentation

EHRs help providers to complete documentation more quickly, more consistently, and in more detail than occurs with paper-based documentation. Most EHR programs have drop-down menus or selection lists that allow the user to choose information or symptoms from a preprogrammed list (Figure 13-2). For example, when the user inserts a diagnosis of "diabetes," the software may display a list of symptoms common to the condition, such as excessive thirst or frequent urination. The physician selects the symptoms reported by each specific patient. Many EHR programs also

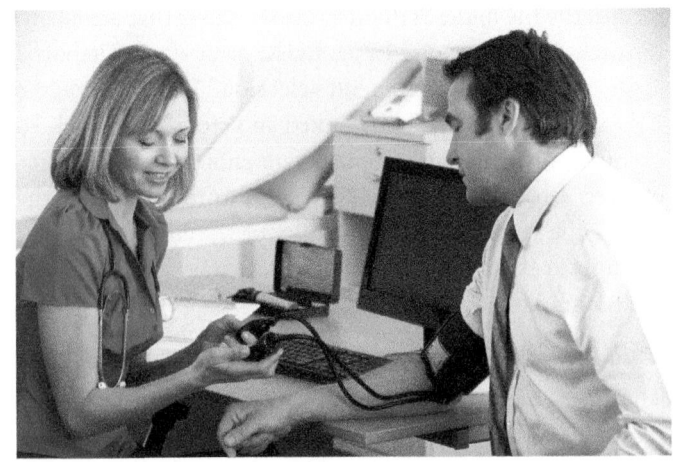

FIGURE 13-1 A blood pressure cuff can be linked to the electronic health record software to allow automatic recording of pressure readings.

include lists of possible diagnoses for the physician to choose from based on the symptoms the patient lists. For example, if the patient complains of excessive thirst and frequent urination, the program might offer "diabetes" as a possible diagnosis for the physician to consider.

Improved Care Coordination

EHR systems can decrease the fragmentation of care by improving care coordination. Better care coordination can lead to better quality of care and improved patient outcomes.

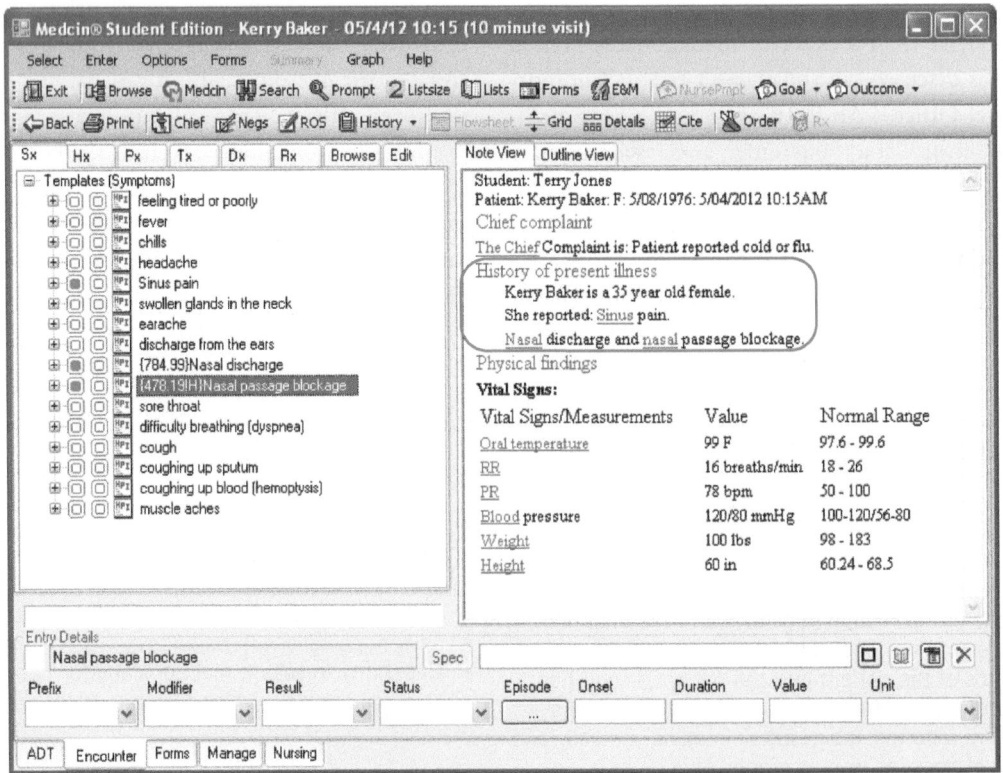

FIGURE 13-2 An example of a selection list used to identify symptoms.

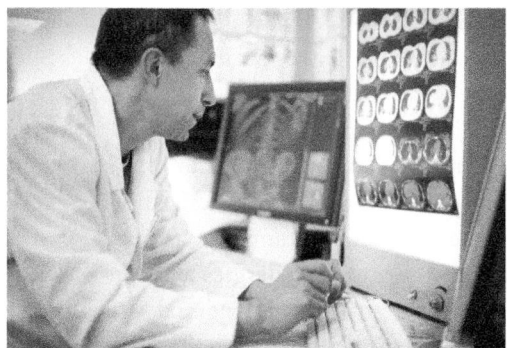

FIGURE 13-3 EHR systems enable providers to view patient records across organizations.

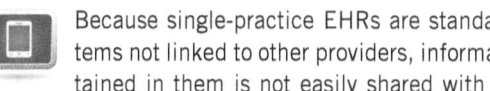
When patients interact with a variety of providers, such as primary care physicians, specialists, nurses, technicians, and other clinicians, it is easy for care and communication to become fragmented. Each member of the health care team has a unique perspective of the patient, based on the area of specialty. Because the EHR enables all providers to see who else is caring for the patient, they can access information they might not see in a paper-based system. This enables providers to consolidate fragmented facts and clusters of symptoms into a cohesive understanding.

Better availability of information can also reduce the chance that one specialist will not know about an unrelated (but relevant) condition being managed by another specialist (Figure 13-3). This is especially important with patients who see multiple specialists, transition between care settings, and receive treatment in emergency settings.

Because EHRs contain all of a patient's health information in one place, it is less likely that providers will have to spend time ordering—and reviewing the results of—duplicate tests and medical procedures.

Avoiding Medical Errors

Better availability of patient information can reduce medical errors and unnecessary tests. EHRs can be used to alert health care providers to possible medication reactions. This is especially helpful when treating patients who are being co-treated by several specialists. The software typically has a built-in safeguard mechanism that alerts the prescribing physician to any contraindicated medications that a patient might be taking.

One of the most convincing arguments for converting paper medical records to an electronic format is patient safety. In 1999, the Institute of Medicine published a report called "To Err Is Human: Building a Safer Health System." This report stated, "At least 44,000 people, and perhaps as many as 98,000 people, die in hospitals every year as a result of medical errors that could have been prevented." One of

the institute's recommendations was to move to EHRs. Their conclusions suggested that some medical errors are caused by indecipherable (unreadable) handwriting, a problem that would be eliminated if health care providers made their entries electronically rather than in handwritten form.

Some states have enacted legislation to address the issue of bad handwriting and medical errors in relation to prescriptions. Such laws may require that all prescriptions written by physicians be electronically submitted to pharmacists or be printed rather than written in cursive handwriting.

Improved Patient Participation

Providers and patients who share access to electronic health information can collaborate in informed decision making. Patient participation is especially important in managing and treating chronic conditions such as asthma, diabetes, and obesity. Providers can give patients full and accurate information about all their medical evaluations. They can also provide information after an office visit or a hospital stay, such as self-care instructions, reminders for other follow-up care, and links to web resources.

Providers can manage appointment schedules electronically and exchange e-mail with their patients. Quick and easy communication between patients and providers may help providers identify symptoms earlier. It also can help providers to be more proactive by reaching out to patients.

Online Patient Access

Online patient access allows patients to look up portions of their EHR via the Internet. This is sometimes called a *tethered PHR*, because the personal health information is maintained by the provider, not by the patient. Using a secure, password-protected system, patients can access their laboratory results, dates of immunizations, or medication history. For example, they can view the trend of their lab results over the last year. Having such information available is especially helpful for patients when they travel or need to seek emergency care with someone other than their primary care providers. The advantage of accessing EHR information online, compared with the PHR, is that the information in the EHR is directly based on official test results and information that providers enter. The disadvantage, compared with PHRs, is that patients usually have limited ability to change or add information. If the patient moves or changes to a different network of providers, she may not be able to include updates to the EHR in the same system.

Health Maintenance

EHRs provide information that can be managed to promote health maintenance among patients. Medical offices send reminder cards or letters to patients regarding the need for upcoming services. These are typically used to remind patients of the need for a colonoscopy, a mammogram, a yearly physical, immunizations, or well-child checkups. The administrative medical assistant can use the software program to print these reminders.

Some medical clinics send informational flyers to patients on a regular basis. An example is a flyer that is sent during flu season that describes the signs and symptoms of the flu along with prevention tips. The prevention tips are intended, in part, to encourage readers to come into the physician's office for a flu vaccine.

The medical assistant can create a list of patients according to specific parameters. For example, if the office has recently welcomed to the staff a physician who specializes in allergies, the medical assistant can create a list of patients who have been treated for allergies and can use that list to send a letter or an e-mail to patients to let them know of the availability of the new physician.

Improved Efficiency and Cost Savings

Health care providers have found that EHRs help improve medical practice management by increasing practice efficiencies and cost savings. Less time spent charting, as a result of more efficient documentation with EHRs, means that more time can be devoted to patient care. Box 13-2 summarizes cost savings made possible by EHRs.

EHRs allow medical staff to easily transmit patient information to patients' health insurance companies when requested rather than having to photocopy the paper records and send them via the postal service. However, keep in mind that it is just as important to follow Health Insurance Portability and Accountability Act (HIPAA) guidelines for releasing medical records electronically as it is for releasing photocopies of the patient's paper medical record.

Multi-User Accessibility

Unlike a paper-based medical record, a patient's EHR can be accessed and used by more than one staff member at a time. For example, the billing office might have the patient's medical record open on a computer screen while accessing information needed for coding a specific procedure. At the same time, the physician might have the same patient's file

---

BOX 13-2 | Cost Savings with an EHR System

EHRs can contribute to cost savings in many areas:

- Reduced transcription costs
- Reduced chart pull, storage, and re-filing costs
- Improved and more accurate reimbursement coding with improved documentation for highly compensated codes
- Reduced medical errors through better access to patient data and error prevention alerts
- Improved patient health/quality of care through better disease management and patient education
- Improved medical practice management through integrated scheduling systems that link appointments directly to progress notes, automate coding, and manage claims

- Time savings with easier centralized chart management, condition-specific queries, and other shortcuts
- Enhanced communication with other clinicians, labs, and health plans through:
  - Easy access to patient information from anywhere
  - Tracking electronic messages to staff, other clinicians, hospitals, labs, etc.
  - Automated formulary checks by health plans
  - Order and receipt of lab tests and diagnostic images
  - Links to public health systems such as registries and communicable disease databases

open on a separate computer screen to input treatment notes. This increases efficiency because staff members do not need to locate the patient's record, nor do they have to wait until one person is finished with it before another can use it.

Electronic Signatures

Most EHRs provide an **electronic signature** component that is based on the individual's **login** (user name and password). An electronic signature, or e-signature, is an electronic indication of intent to agree to or approve the contents of a document. The United States E-SIGN Act defines an electronic signature as an "electronic sound, symbol, or process, attached to or logically associated with a contract or other record and executed or adopted by a person with the intent to sign the record." E-signatures are legal in business and are accepted in health care and EHRs.

Three types of e-signatures are commonly used in EHRs:

- A **digitized signature** is an electronic image of a hand-written signature. The signature may be obtained in real-time, such as when a patient signs a consent form, or may be a previously saved image file, such as when a physician's written signature is scanned into the computer for use on letters. Such a file must be kept secure with limited access. Digitized signatures are the least secure type of e-signature.

- A **token signature** is a type of e-signature in which the user must click a button, enter a personal identification number (PIN), or complete a biometric scan, such as a fingerprint, to record the electronic signature. This type of signature is more secure than a digitized signature because it requires an action by the signer to implement the signature.

- A **digital signature** is the most secure type because it is an encrypted (scrambled) signature with multiple layers of security that prevent it from being used by unauthorized persons.

After an entry is made in the patient's chart, the staff member or physician clicks "Signature" and the entry is electronically signed. Because the electronic signature is based on the computer login information, it is imperative that user names and passwords are not shared and are changed often.

Staff Communication

EHRs can aid in communication among staff members regarding specific patients. An example is a patient who has an outstanding account balance. The billing staff member may need to see the patient during the next visit with the physician. The billing staff member can post a message alert in the patient's chart that is seen by the receptionist when the patient checks in. The alert allows the billing staff

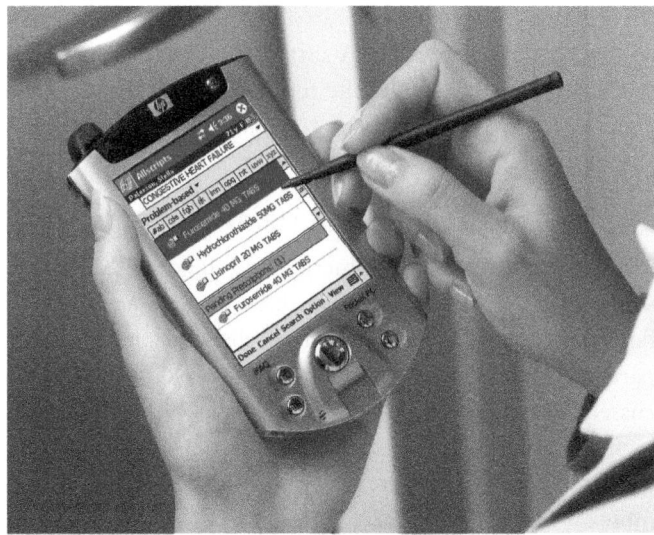

FIGURE 13-4 Medical assistants can quickly pull up a patient record when a phone call is received.

Professionalism   The Workplace

When it is necessary to communicate with another staff member regarding a patient and to send an alert, keep your communication professional. This means to use proper medical terms and correct grammar, and not to make personal comments about patients or staff members. Unlike a sticky note that may be thrown away after the appropriate staff member reads it and responds, the alert you send in the EHR may become part of the patient's permanent, legal record.

member to have the receptionist direct the patient to the billing office before the visit.

Charting patient information, such as telephone calls, is easily done within the EHR (Figure 13-4). Typically the software contains a section for adding information, such as telephone calls or conversations with the patient and the patient's family that occur in the office and are related to the patient's medical care. When the receptionist documents a telephone call in the EHR, the message can be flagged and sent electronically to the appropriate medical assistant or physician without having to get up, pull the patient's chart, and carry the chart and message to the person.

OWNERSHIP OF THE MEDICAL RECORD

The **medical record** is a legal document, a permanent record, and a tool used by staff members to communicate within their office and with other offices regarding the services delivered to the patient. It can also be subpoenaed by the courts as evidence. HIPAA established that the patient owns the information in the medical record and has the right to control under what circumstances, and with whom, it is shared.

The Medical Record as a Legal Document

Medical staff must follow meticulous standards regarding what information to document, how to document it, and how to correct errors. Everything that is done during a patient's medical visit, ordered over the telephone, or discussed with a patient by telephone or e-mail must be documented in the medical record. Any activities not documented are considered not to have occurred. This leads to the common saying in health care, "If it wasn't documented, it wasn't done."

Documentation should be factual, based on statements of the patient and the physician's assessment. The patient's statement of the problems, symptoms, reason for the encounter, and questions should be written in quotation marks using the exact words of the patient when possible. Patient statements are recorded under the subjective (S) portion of the progress notes. The physician's findings of the physical examination and test results are recorded under the objective (O) portion of the progress notes. The physician's diagnostic opinion is recorded under the assessment (A) or impression portion of the progress notes. The physician's recommendations and plan for further testing and treatment are recorded under the plan (P) portion of the progress notes.

Entries in paper medical records should be written in black ink. Handwriting should be clear and easy to read by anyone. Sign and date all entries.

Ownership of the Medical Record

Patients own the information in their medical records, but the facility that created the information owns the physical or electronic record. Patients have the right to view their medical records, so medical offices must have a procedure in place to facilitate this. Usually this involves the patient making a request in advance and setting a time when a staff member can review the records with the patient. Before allowing a patient to view the record, make sure either the physician or the office manager has given approval. If the physician determines it could be detrimental for the patient to read the record, as may be the case in a mental health facility or with files related to the treatment of mental health disorders, access to this portion of the record can be denied. These situations are discussed later in this chapter.

A staff member should always be present when a patient reviews the record. This provides someone who can help

Professionalism   The Workplace

Remember that information in the medical record should be factual. The patient's chart is not the place to document your opinion or internal office problems. Statements such as "Injection was not administered because of lack of staffing," or "Patient very angry with physician" are subjective opinions of staff and do not belong in the medical record. Instead, state the facts, such as "Patient stated, 'I am very upset that the physician did not call me sooner.'"

orient the patient and answer questions about the content. It also serves as a security measure so that a patient does not write in the record, tear pages out, or alter it in any way. Patients may request that changes be made to the medical record. The physician is not obligated to make the change(s), but the nature of the patient's request must be clearly documented within the medical record.

Ownership of Radiology Images

Radiology images can be stored digitally or on film. Regardless of which method is used, the original image is almost always the property of the medical facility that performed the X-ray. Written reports prepared by the radiologist are sent to other physicians at the request of the patient, but the image generally remains in the original office so that it can always be located and accessed for future examination and comparison.

With the increase in digital imaging and electronic health records, many physician offices are electronically linked to large radiology centers or those affiliated with hospitals. This enables physicians to access an image and report electronically, without having to request a physical copy. Radiology facilities are often able to provide patients with a CD or DVD containing the image. Patients may share the image with other physicians or keep it for their own reference.

Professionalism   The Workplace

HIPAA established that patients own the information in their medical record because it is a history of their medical care. As a medical assistant, you must be able to explain to patients that the physician owns all the physical files or electronic media that contain this information, although patients have a right to see and have a copy of their medical records.

When physical films are used, physicians can loan their films to referring physicians for further examination. When the review is complete, the film must be returned to the original facility. Because films are a permanent record of the patient at a particular moment, they must be preserved carefully. It is possible, in some locations, for the patient to obtain a copy of a physical film. The patient might have to pay for the copy to be made.

HIPAA and Confidentiality of Records

The HIPAA Privacy Rule applies to health information created or maintained by **covered entities**, which are health care providers, health plans, and electronic claims clearinghouses that engage in certain electronic transactions. The Office for Civil Rights (OCR) is responsible for implementing and enforcing the privacy regulation.

HIPAA requires that covered entities follow privacy and security rules for protected health information (PHI), regardless of whether it is stored on paper or electronically. These include:

- Provide reasonable and appropriate safeguards to protect the integrity and confidentiality of health care information.
- Train personnel to protect confidentiality of health care information.
- Provide policies and procedures on security and confidentiality protective measures within the medical office.

Medical information can be shared by a wide range of people, both inside and outside the health care industry. Generally, access to medical records is obtained when the patient agrees to let others see them. Occasionally, patient medical information is used for health research and (in accordance with HIPAA) may be disclosed to public health agencies such as the Centers for Disease Control and Prevention (CDC). Specific names or other identifying information are not given to researchers.

Transporting Medical Records

Medical records should never be removed from the office or taken home to complete work. The risk of loss of confidential irreplaceable information is too great. In the rare circumstance that information is needed outside the office for a legitimate reason, obtain clearance from the office manager or physician. This can occur when records must be transferred between office locations or have been subpoenaed for legal purposes.

If providing information from a medical record has been approved, select only the information that is absolutely essential and, preferably, make a photocopy for the approved

recipient, leaving the intact original in the office. Medical records, whether originals or copies, must be transported in a locked briefcase or box with no data visible from the outside. The container should be clearly labeled with the recipient's name, address, and phone number. Ideally, a warning label is also attached, stating something similar to:

THIS PACKAGE CONTAINS CONFIDENTIAL INFORMATION THAT IS PROTECTED BY FEDERAL LAW. DO NOT OPEN. IF FOUND, PLEASE CALL 555-555-5555 IMMEDIATELY.

The person who is responsible for transporting the files must keep the files in her personal, physical control at all times. Upon delivering the package, the person who delivers it must have the recipient sign a receipt.

In the unthinkable situation that medical records are lost outside the office, the event must be reported as a HIPAA breach. Loss of medical records is a serious problem, and staff involved must take the required legal and ethical action of reporting it, regardless of any repercussions that may follow. The patient involved and the United States Department of Health and Human Services (HHS) must be notified regarding the nature and extent of the breach. In the event that more than 500 patients are affected, prominent media outlets in the area and certain other authorities also must be notified with the same information. Each medical office has a privacy officer who is responsible for reporting and managing HIPAA breaches.

Releasing Medical Records

Because patients own the information in their medical records, they have the legal right of "privileged communication" and access to their records. All new patients receive the medical office's Notice of Privacy Practices (NPP) on their first encounter and annually thereafter. In so doing, they consent to the use and disclosure of PHI for treatment, payment, and operations as defined by HIPAA. For all other uses, patients must explicitly authorize release of their records in writing. Authorization can be obtained

Professionalism The Law

In 2013, updated regulations about HIPAA breaches went into effect. The definition of a breach was broadened, and enforcement standards were strengthened. HHS contends that no data breach is too small to be reported, and must be reported any time the security or privacy of PHI is compromised. Recent fines for noncompliance and resolution have ranged from $50,000 to $2.25 million.

Samantha is the file clerk at Dr. Frasier's clinic. Her older adult neighbor, Mr. Wheeler, has requested a copy of his medical records. The office policy states that all patients are entitled to a copy of their records once per calendar year at no charge. Mr. Wheeler has already received his one set of copies for this year. Samantha knows he was recently diagnosed with lung cancer and referred to a specialist at the local teaching hospital. Mr. Wheeler asks Samantha if she will please not charge him for this set of records because his disability check is all that he has and he knows that his upcoming medical treatments will cost him several thousand dollars out of pocket. What should Samantha do?

using a paper or electronic form. An example of a release form appears in Figure 13-5. Procedure 13-1 outlines how to obtain a patient's authorization to release medical records.

Patients also can request a copy of their medical records. Because some records are large and require excessive duplicating time and expense, the physician may charge a reasonable fee to provide this service. Some states specify the allowable fee that may be charged.

Health care providers have specific procedures for handling and releasing medical records because of the confidential information contained in the records, as well as the

FIGURE 13-5 A release form for medical records.

federal and state laws concerning HIV, mental health, and substance abuse information.

Persons Authorized to Release Records

Generally, a patient's medical record can be released only if that patient authorizes it. However, there are some exceptions to the rule. The following persons, in addition to the patient, usually can sign a release:

- Parents of minor children
- Legal guardian
- Agent (someone the patient selects to act on his or her behalf through a health care power of attorney)

Under some circumstances a minor, rather than the parent, must sign the release. Emancipated, married, and mature minors are allowed to sign a consent to release medical information. If you have questions about who can authorize release of patient records, check with your office manager.

Specially Protected Medical Information

Federal law provides special protection for substance abuse treatment records. There is one exception to the HIPAA standard that allows sharing of PHI for treatment purposes. Psychotherapy notes may only be disclosed with *explicit* patient authorization except when they are used by the originator of the notes or for a covered entity's supervised mental health education and training purposes.

Some state laws also provide special protection for HIV/AIDS information and mental health records. Such protections preempt the HIPAA privacy rule because they are more stringent than HIPAA regulations regarding PHI.

The Doctrine of Professional Discretion allows physicians to restrict the release of mental health records to their patients if the doctor believes the patient is not able to handle the information that is presented. These laws are meant to encourage people with these problems to obtain the medical treatment they need without fear. To obtain a copy of the records or have them sent somewhere else, the patient may need to sign a form that identifies the specific information being released.

Disclosure Without Authorization

Although medical records are confidential, at times they can be released without a patient's explicit authorization. In special cases, records may be released to the following:

- Health care workers who have a need for the records to care for a patient
- Qualified people or organizations that perform services, such as data processing, medical record transcription, microfilming, administrative functions, or other related services

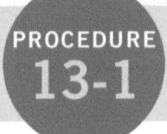

PROCEDURE
13-1

Completing a Request to Release Medical Records

Objective ◆ *Obtain a signed patient authorization to release medical records to another person or organization.*

EQUIPMENT AND SUPPLIES

Electronic medical records release form and electronic signature pad, or paper medical records release form and black pen; information about the specific records to be released; name and address of the recipient; patient's mailing address, if patient is not physically present

METHOD

1. Gather all supplies and information. Log in to the EHR, and access the medical records request screen.
2. Verify the identity of the patient if you have not already done so.
3. Confirm with the patient the information requested, the intended recipient, and the recipient's address.
4. Fill in the corresponding fields on the form or screen for the patient's name, the information requested, and the name and address of the intended recipient.
5. Ask the patient to sign and date the form in the designated place.
6. Visually verify the signature and date to ensure the form was completed correctly.
7. Inform the patient approximately when the information will be released, according to office policy.
8. If the patient is not present, print out the form and highlight the spaces to be completed. Place the form and return instructions in an envelope, apply postage, and mail.
9. Save the screen in the EHR, and confirm that the request is to be sent to the medical records department. If using a paper form, route the completed form to the medical records department.
10. Thank the patient, and ask if there is anything else you can assist with.
11. Close the patient's electronic health record.
12. Log off the system.

- Qualified people or organizations for approved research and education functions
- Certain government authorities, as permitted or required by law, to investigate or regulate health-related issues such as child abuse, communicable diseases, and prescription drug abuse
- Certain lawyers and parties in a lawsuit if a patient's medical condition is an issue in the suit

Generally, strict rules apply to those who receive medical information. For example, they often are required to maintain procedures to protect the patient's confidentiality and prevent release of medical information and patient identity.

The Role of the Medical Assistant Regarding Medical Records

The medical assistant plays an important role in the management and maintenance of medical records to help ensure an efficiently run medical office. Four standards in the use of medical records must be followed:

- **Accuracy**—Because medical records are legal documents and can be used in a court of law, the physician

must be able to trust the accuracy of the data. Remember never to guess about information and double-check your work to help ensure accuracy.

- **Timeliness**—Do not wait to update records; make it an office habit to update records at the time of service or daily. This includes documenting telephone calls, filing lab reports, and documenting office visits.
- **Accessibility**—Make sure that the files are properly filed and easily accessible. If there is a patient emergency, for example, the medical history will be needed immediately.
- **Legibility**—Pay particular attention to numbers and spelling in both paper and electronic records. Spell out words rather than abbreviate. Handwritten medical records must be easily read by anyone.

Making Corrections in the Medical Record

Medical staff occasionally can make errors when documenting. When this happens, the errors must be corrected as soon as possible. The correction should be made by the individual who made the original entry.

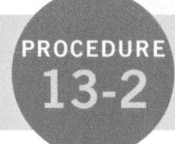

PROCEDURE 13-2 Correcting an Entry in the Electronic Health Record

Objective ◆ *Correct an entry in the electronic health record in an accurate manner following legal protocol.*

EQUIPMENT AND SUPPLIES
Computer with electronic health record software

METHOD

1. Log in with your assigned user identification name and the password you previously created.
2. Identify the correct patient EHR in which the error was made.
3. Locate the error within the record.
4. Review the rules associated with the software you are using for correcting or making an addendum to a patient's record.
5. Make the appropriate correction within the medical record, according to the steps required within the software program.
6. Complete the signature process, according to the steps required within the software program.
7. Verify that the change made is correct and reflects the change you intended.
8. Save the changes.
9. Close the patient's electronic health record.
10. Log off the system.

If you notice a possible error by someone else, bring it to that person's attention in a tactful and professional way. Do not simply hand the person the medical record and say, "You need to fix this" or "You made a mistake in this record." Instead, approach the person in a nonjudgmental manner, such as "I have a question for you. When I was reviewing this record, I noticed that you entered the date January 15. That day was Sunday, so I wonder if you would take a look at this and determine if it is what you intended to write."

Specific procedures must be followed for correcting entries in both paper and electronic records. See Procedure 13-2 for making changes to a medical record.

Correcting Electronic Records

When documenting in an EHR, errors may be corrected before saving the entry by deleting as you would with any other type of computer program. The entry is automatically dated and signed electronically when saved.

When the correction is identified after the record is saved, the steps to make the correction depend on the software. Generally, the user marks the erroneous information for deletion and enters the correct information. The original entry is not truly deleted because, just as with paper records, the original entry must still be viewable. The correction may be viewed on a separate screen or may appear with a line drawn through the entry (Figure 13-6).

> *Patient complains of ~~right~~ left leg pain.*

FIGURE 13-6 Errors in the electronic health record must be corrected as soon as possible. Most often, the user crosses out the error and enters the correct information, as shown in this example.

Correcting Paper Records

In a paper medical record, do not erase or totally obliterate the original error with products such as correcting fluid. Draw a single line through the error so the original entry can still be seen, and enter your initials and the date above the single line with the word "Error." Then write in the correction (Figure 13-7). If an error is made while using a typewriter, it should be corrected as any other typewritten errors are corrected. However, if the error is noted later, then you must draw a line through the error, enter your initials and

---

Progress Notes

5-20-xx 2³⁰pm Patient presents for staple removal
S/P hysterectomy on 5-10-xx. Patient states " I'm
improving, yet still tire easily." Explained to patient
she may feel this way for the next 2 ~~years~~   error 5-20-09 RG
months. Rita Gill, RMA

FIGURE 13-7 An example of a corrected chart notation.

Progress Notes
3-13-XX 10 $\frac{15}{am}$ wt. 135, BP 130/78 Temp 98.2°F
Patient presents for follow-up visit Re: B.P medication
Patient states he feels much better. Sam Smithick, CMA (AAMA)
3-14-XX Late entry, to be added to 3-13-XX entry. Fasting
lipid profide drawn and sent to HBC lab. Sam Smith CMA (AAMA)

FIGURE 13-8 An example of a late entry to the medical record.

the date, and write in the correction. Obliterating information is considered to be tampering with a legal document.

When an entry is made to the medical record later than the date on which it should have been made, list the date of entry and also describe the original date of service (Figure 13-8).

PRIVACY AND SECURITY OF EHRs

EHRs must comply with HIPAA requirements for privacy and security. Many people believe that EHRs are more secure than paper medical records because access is more easily controlled. However, if EHRs are accessed by unauthorized or malicious parties, severe damage can result.

Logins

EHRs provide the ability to identify who has entered and accessed patient information, which is not always possible with a paper-based record. Each computer user has a unique login to access the computer system. The login is the combination of a username and password to access the computer network. Additional logins may be required for different applications. Because each person has private login information, the software can track the activity of each user and identify who made the entry, change, or deletion. With paper records, it is not always obvious who last had a record and who made the latest changes. Box 13-3 provides guidelines for creating and using usernames and passwords.

> **Professionalism** The Life Span
>
> It is important for the medical staff to be respectful of the various levels of comfort patients may have with storing their medical information on a computer. Staff members must take every opportunity to educate those who are not comfortable with the idea. Most individuals in their 40s and younger have grown up with computers and use a computer in their daily lives. However, patients in their 60s and older might not be as comfortable with the idea of using a computer to store their most personal medical information and prefer a paper chart because it is something they can touch and hold.

> **Professionalism** The Workplace
>
> Be aware of the policies in your office regarding access to your own or a family member's medical records. An employee who is also a patient of the practice cannot access their own or a family member's records. If an employee attempts to access either, that employee may be terminated. If you inadvertently access a family member's record, close the record immediately and notify your supervisor you have mistakenly accessed the record. Offices must have the capability to run audits and see which patient's charts have been accessed and by whom.

Each station must be logged off when the user is away from the desk, and computer screens must not be viewable by other patients while private patient information is displayed on the screen.

Laptops and Mobile Devices

Special security requirements are necessary when PHI is accessed with, or stored on, portable or mobile devices. Wi-Fi (wireless networking) allows users on mobile devices such as laptops, notebook computers, touchscreens, tablets, personal digital assistants (PDA), or even smartphones to access data.

Three levels of security must be observed: hardware, data transfers, and data storage. Hardware security refers to the physical device. Users must safeguard their mobile devices so they do not fall into the wrong hands. The device itself should be protected by a password so that it cannot be activated without an access code. All software or "apps" on the device must also provide one or more layers of password authorization to be used, just as they do on a desktop computer or workstation.

Data transfer security refers to the transmission of data. When mobile devices are used to access a central EHR database, the data being transferred is at risk of being intercepted during the transmission process. To protect against this occurring, data transfers must be encrypted, meaning that the data are scrambled in such a way that they cannot be intercepted by an unauthorized user. The process to encrypt and decode data is integrated into the application software used to access the EHR.

Data storage security refers to access to PHI. There may be times when users need to download and store PHI on the mobile device itself. Only PHI that is absolutely necessary should be stored on mobile devices. PHI should be

BOX 13-3 | Password Guidelines

Medical assistants need to create or update their passwords frequently for various computer systems. Each application has its own requirements for the formatting or construction of the username and password. It is important to know how to create a secure password that cannot be guessed by unauthorized parties.

1. When accessing a system for the first time, the system administrator usually provides a temporary login. This is a username and temporary password that you change the first time you access the computer system.
2. The username is often assigned by the system administrator to provide consistency among all staff members and ensure that no username is repeated. Example: The username for Mary R. Jones could be **mary.jones**, **jones.mary**, **mjones**, **mrjones**, or a similar combination of the first and last names.
3. Enter the username in the box provided on the screen when prompted by the software. Pay special attention to capitalization and punctuation, such as a period that may divide the first and last names. Some systems are case-sensitive, meaning that you must use capital letters and lowercase letters as provided by the system administrator. Press the Tab or Enter key as instructed.
4. Enter the temporary password in the box provided on the screen. Pay special attention to key the letters and numbers accurately. For security reasons, you are not able to see the actual characters you type on the screen. Instead you see a dot (.) or star (*) for each character entered.
5. You will be prompted to enter a new, permanent password. You are usually given instructions regarding how many characters in length the password should be, and

the type of characters required. An example would be 8 characters long, including at least one letter, one number, and one special character such as ! @ # $ % ^ & *. Sometimes, you may be required to use at least one uppercase and one lowercase letter. Do not create passwords that would be easy for someone else to guess, such as your name, the name of your child or pet, your birth date, or your phone number.

6. An example of a good password is **brWd84*%** because it contains a capital letter, three lowercase letters, two numbers, and two special characters. To make it easier to remember, you could enter only the consonants or only the vowels from a word you can remember, such as a favorite place.
7. The system prompts you to enter the new password a second time. This ensures that you typed what you intended to type. If you do not enter the exact same characters both times, the system presents an error message stating that the passwords do not match. Reenter the original password, and then enter the duplicate again.
8. Systems with highly sensitive information, such as EHRs, may require you to change your password periodically, such as every 90 days. Systems can keep track of passwords you have used in the past and may prohibit you from reusing a previous password or creating a password that is too similar to your current one. Frequently changing passwords can be a challenge. One way to meet these requirements without forgetting the password is to keep part of the password, such as the letters, the same, and then change the numbers and special characters.

---

deleted as soon as possible after the need has been fulfilled. The stored data must be encrypted to prevent unauthorized access. If the data were not encrypted and the device fell into the wrong hands, the data could potentially be stolen. Confidential medical details could be revealed, and identity theft could also occur. Either of these incidents would be a HIPAA violation that must be reported to authorities.

Backing Up Electronic Health Records

Medical offices must use data backup systems to safeguard the information contained on office computer systems, including patient medical records. This is typically done on a daily basis and, in most offices, the computer backup system is programmed to execute automatically. By having daily backup files, the medical office is not as likely to lose computer data, even if the entire computer system goes down. Data backup is discussed in the chapter titled "Computers in a Medical Office."

DOCUMENTATION FORMATS

To create an organized medical record that multiple providers can access and use, each office must establish an organizational scheme or documentation format. The documentation format specifies where in the medical record various types of information are stored and provides an outline that providers should follow when documenting an encounter. Each practice uses a format specific to its needs, so everyone in an office should follow the same charting system.

The most common documentation formats are

- Chronological medical record
- Problem-oriented medical record
- SOAP charting
- Source-oriented medical record

See Box 13-4 for a summary list of standard categories and reports that are covered in more detail in this chapter.

Chronological Medical Record

The **chronological medical record** follows the patient over a period of time, with each visit consisting of a new entry by date, rather than by symptom or diagnosis. Although this is one of the most common types of medical records, it does make some diagnoses, such as hypertension, more difficult to track through multiple visits. For such diagnoses, a problem-oriented medical record might be more appropriate.

Problem-Oriented Medical Record

The **problem-oriented medical record (POMR)**, developed by Dr. Lawrence Weed in 1970, identifies patient problems and organizes the chart by those problems.

The functional aspect of this type of charting is the patient problem list found at the front of the chart (Figure 13-9). As new problems and diagnoses are identified, they are noted on the problem list, helping the health care provider to identify trends in the patient's medical history or emerging diagnoses. POMR also provides health care providers and physicians who do not already know a specific patient an overview of previous visits and problems at a glance. A POMR has four parts:

- **Database**—Consists of the physical examination, the patient history, and the results of baseline laboratory or diagnostic procedures.
- **Problem list**—List of patient problems that is kept in the front of the chart much like a table of contents would be. The problem list assigns each problem a number with the date. The problem can be further explained by information in the database. Each problem the patient has experienced is titled and numbered in the problem list. Because each patient problem is numbered, that number can be referenced throughout the medical record when needed. Throughout the rest of the history, problems are referred to numerically. If one is resolved, the date of resolution is placed next to the problem listed. If a new problem arises, it is assigned a number and listed with the date.
- **Plan**—Indicates a written plan for each numbered problem identified on the problem list. The plan may include tests to be ordered, treatment plans, or plans for patient education about specific problems. The treatment plan is a very important part of the medical record because it tells what is intended for the patient. Each treatment plan should have a title and should reference the problem number with which it is associated.
- **Progress notes**—Made up of several sections that follow a specific format; the first letter of each section title (Subjective, Objective, Assessment, and Plan) spells out the word SOAP. Thus, this portion of the POMR is known as SOAP notes. Sometimes E is added to create SOAPE if evaluation is completed. All progress notes should be maintained in chronological order. Each progress note also references the patient problem number.

SOAP Charting

The **subjective, objective, assessment, and plan (SOAP)** charting method, as just discussed, organizes the progress notes within documentation of an encounter into four distinct parts: subjective, objective, assessment, and plan. The subjective information gathered from the patient—the things that the patient believes he is seeing a physician for—is usually the same as a chief complaint (CC). This usually includes statements the patient makes about symptoms the patient has experienced, such as pain or dizziness or anxiety. The objective information is composed of the data gathered during the visit—such as vital signs, weight change, fevers, blood work, physical examination results, and any other observable and measurable data. The assessment is the physician's preliminary diagnosis. The plan section of the chart discusses the strategy for care of this patient (Figure 13-10). The SOAP method of documenting a medical record is described in Table 13-1.

NAME _____ AGE _____
OCCUPATION _____ SOC. SEC.# _____

	BLOOD PRESSURE	VISION Without Glasses	Diagnostic Tests	Results
Height _____	**Sitting**	Far R20/ L20/		
Weight _____	R / :L /	Near R / L /		
Build _____		**With Glasses**		
(Sm.Med.Lg.Obese.)	**Standing**	Far R20/ L20/		
Pulse _____	R / :L /	Near R / L /		
Resp. _____		Tonometry R ___ L ___		
Temp. _____	**Lying**	Colorvision _____ (Ishihara plates missed)		
	R / :L /	Peripheral Fields R ___ L ___		

AUDIOMETRIC TESTING		250	500	1000	2000	4000	8000		
	R	___	___	___	___	___	___		
	L	___	___	___	___	___	___		
	Gross Hearing _____								

PULMONARY FUNCTION

Initial Problem List

_____
_____
_____
_____
_____
_____
_____
_____
_____
_____
_____
_____
_____
_____
_____
_____
_____
_____
_____
_____
_____
_____
_____

Employment status _____ Physician's signature _____
DATE _____

FIGURE 13-9 An example of a medical history sheet to list patient problems.

The POMR and SOAP methods can be combined in one chart, making for a very concise, clear set of information on any patient. A problem list for the patient in the example given in Table 13-1 might appear as follows:

- **Problem List**
  2/14/20YY
  Problem No. 1: Diabetes
  Problem No. 2: Hypertension, essential
- **Plan**
  2/14/20YY
  Problem No. 1: Diabetic exchange diet

Regular insulin, 20 units subQ daily each morning
Monitor blood sugar levels during day
Problem No. 2: Norvasc 2.5 mg. daily
Monitor blood pressure weekly

- **Progress Note**
  2/14/20YY
  Problem No. 1: Diabetes
  S—Patient states thirst has diminished and hunger lessened
  O—Urine +2, FBS positive, gained 4 pounds in past 3 weeks, skin turgor good

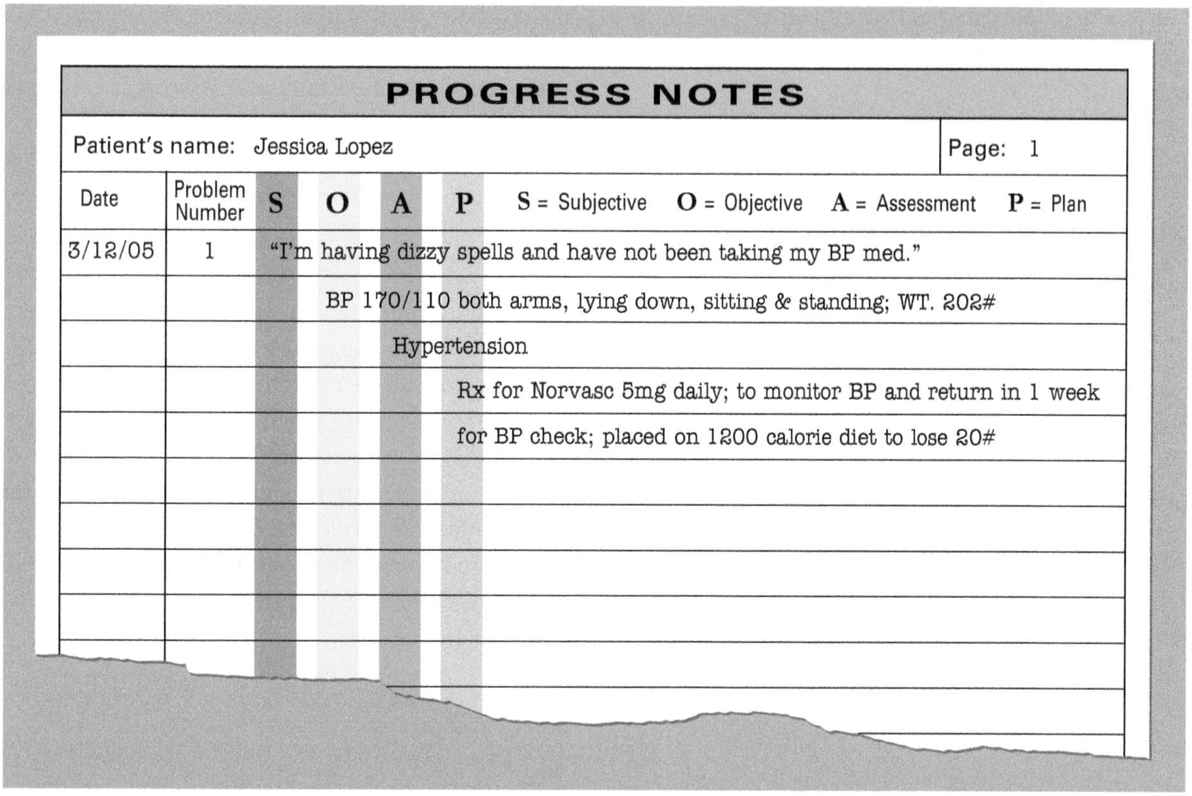

PROGRESS NOTES

Patient's name: Jessica Lopez		Page: 1
Date	Problem Number	S O A P — S = Subjective O = Objective A = Assessment P = Plan
3/12/05	1	"I'm having dizzy spells and have not been taking my BP med."
		BP 170/110 both arms, lying down, sitting & standing; WT. 202#
		Hypertension
		Rx for Norvasc 5mg daily; to monitor BP and return in 1 week
		for BP check; placed on 1200 calorie diet to lose 20#

FIGURE 13-10 An example of SOAP charting.

TABLE 13-1 | SOAP Charting Description and Examples

S	Subjective symptoms provided by the patient or family. The actual patient's words are recorded.	Example: "I'm thirsty and eating all the time, but I'm not gaining any weight. I feel tired all the time."
O	Objective findings from vital signs, physical examination, and laboratory and diagnostic tests.	Example: B/P: 158/96; T: 98°F; P: 76; R: 16 Skin turgor (resiliency) poor. Wt. 10# less than 6 weeks ago Urine 4 + sugar, FBS positive
A	Assessment, including the physician's diagnosis.	Example: Uncontrolled diabetes
P	Plan including recommended treatments, further tests, medications, consultation, surgery, and physical therapy.	Example: Dx: Lab tests for diabetes Tx: Begin diabetic diet and insulin. Instruct on diet and exercise follow-up.

A—Diet and medication effective

P—Continue medication, monitor blood sugar level daily, adjust insulin levels per instruction, return visit in 2 weeks

Problem No. 2: Hypertension

S—Patient states no complaints related to high blood pressure

O—BP 138/86, down 10 points in past 3 weeks

A—Medication effective

P—Continue with medication and patient monitor of BP weekly; come in for check in 2 weeks

Source-Oriented Medical Record

The **source-oriented medical record (SOMR)** is commonly used in medical clinics. Patient information is organized in sections for various purposes, such as history and physical, insurance, progress notes, medications, laboratory, and consultations. Information in each section is maintained in reverse chronological order with the most recent information seen first. Progress notes are included with each patient encounter, whether it is an office visit, telephone call, or written communication. Each office determines which sections to be used and in what order they are to appear in the medical chart. With this method, it can be more complicated to identify and locate past medical problems, treatments, and results.

COMPONENTS OF THE MEDICAL RECORD

A standard medical record is one of the most important items in an office setting. It is imperative that you be familiar with all components of it, such as medical forms and reports, to maintain the integrity and accuracy of patient records. Each patient's medical record contains the same categories of material, but information is unique to each patient. For example, all patient charts contain a patient registration form and family medical history, but not every patient has a consultation report from another physician or a surgical report. Medical reports are filed in the medical record with tabs that label the source, such as lab, X-ray,

consultations, and special studies. If information is not properly organized in the patient's medical record, errors can occur. It is very important that you organize the patient's medical record according to facility policy. Procedure 13-3 outlines how to create a patient's medical record. Procedure 13-4 explains how to organize a patient's medical record.

Patient Registration

The patient registration form usually includes demographic information, such as the patient's full name, address, contact information (including home phone, work phone, cell phone, and e-mail address if applicable), date of visit, age, date of birth (DOB), Social Security number, driver's license number (if applicable), medical insurance information, and person responsible for payment. The form should also request the patient's occupation, marital status, number of children (if applicable), and emergency contact information.

PROCEDURE
13-3

Creating a Patient's Medical Record

Objective ◆ *Establish a new medical record file for a patient.*

EQUIPMENT AND SUPPLIES

EHR software; patient registration form; file folder and forms (for paper records)

METHOD

Electronic Records:

1. Log in to the EHR software using the username and password previously created.
2. Select the menu item to create a new patient or a new chart.
3. Refer to the patient registration form to complete the patient information requested on the screen, such as name, address, birthdate, and so on.
4. Save the information.
5. Visually confirm that the record has been created by the EHR system.
6. Identify the medical record number. Write it on the patient registration form.
7. Scan in or link any existing information, paperwork, documentation, etc. according to procedures for the EHR software.

8. Save the medical record, and sign out of the system.

Paper Records:

1. For paper medical records, identify the medical record number following office procedures and write it on the patient registration form.
2. Insert the patient registration form in the designated location in the front of the file.
3. Create a file folder label with the patient's medical record number or name, following office procedures.
4. If using a preassembled chart, visually check that all the required forms appear in the chart, in their proper locations, according to office policy.
5. If necessary, collect the necessary or missing forms and insert in the designated location in the chart, according to office policy.
6. Insert any existing completed paperwork for the patient in the designated location.
7. File the chart, following the filing protocol outlined in office policy.

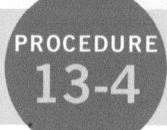

PROCEDURE 13-4

Organizing a Patient's Medical Record

Objective ◆ *Update the patient's medical record by filing new information in the correct place and correct record.*

EQUIPMENT AND SUPPLIES

Patient medical record; assorted documents (paper or electronic) for filing in record

METHOD

Electronic Records:

1. Log in to the EHR with your username and password.
2. Access the record of the desired patient. Confirm the medical record number, patient name, address, and date of birth.
3. Access the menu for importing or linking external documents.
4. Follow the onscreen prompts or menu selections to scan in paper documents or link to existing electronic files. Ensure that each file is associated with the correct purpose, such as laboratory results or consultation reports.
5. When prompted for a date for the record, enter the date the report was issued, not today's current date. The EHR will automatically sort the records in chronological or reverse chronological order, as designated by the user.
6. Verify that all documents have been scanned or imported. Exit the patient's record.

Paper Records:

1. Verify that you have the correct patient record for the patient documents you have been given. Confirm medical record number, patient name, address, and date of birth.
2. File documents in reverse chronological order with the most recent record at the beginning of the section, in the correct areas of the file, according to your facility policy. For example, file laboratory reports with other laboratory reports within the lab section, and with the most recent report on top.
3. Return the medical record to the correct place in alphabetic or numeric order with other patient files.

Family and Medical History

The patient's family and medical history is listed on a form separate from the registration form. This information should include the patient's current medical problem with details of present illness (CC), as well as family medical history, patient's past medical history, past surgeries, allergies, and current prescription and over-the-counter medications. The family and medical history form should request a list of herbal medications and recreational drugs used by the patient. It also should contain the patient's social and occupational history, including the amount of exercise done by the patient, whether the patient uses tobacco and the type of tobacco product, and alcohol use.

Managed care insurance plans often require that the patient's current chief complaint be entered into the medical record using the patient's own words. When recording the patient's own words, be sure to use quotation marks. Relevant past family and social history is also vital, as well as the patient's medication history. Inventory of body systems also is usually included as part of the patient's history (Figure 13-11).

Physical Examination Results

The comprehensive physical examination screen in an EHR, or form in a paper chart, provides the content and results of the examination, such as the patient's general appearance,

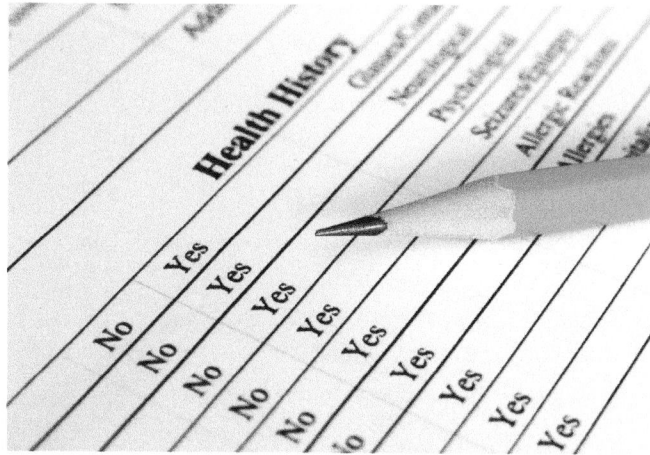

FIGURE 13-11 The patient describes the current problem and medical history form on a separate form.

nutrition, and blood pressure (BP), as well as the examination of the head—eyes, ears, nose, and throat (EENT)—mouth, and scalp. Results of examination of the neck and thyroid; thorax; breast; heart and lungs; abdominal, pelvic, genital, and rectal areas; and skin examinations are recorded. Lymphadenopathy (abnormal enlargement of the lymph nodes), as well as overall impression and treatment plan, are also documented. Not all patients receive general physical examinations.

Diagnostic Test Results

All results from diagnostic tests performed on patients in the office, a laboratory, or a hospital must be tracked for easy accessibility, should the physician need to consult them (Figure 13-12). In an EHR, they should be scanned in if they are not already linked. In a paper chart, test results must be filed in the appropriate section of the chart. Reports from various organizations will have a slightly different appearance; for example, laboratory results issued by different labs will be formatted slightly differently. Distinct types of reports also appear differently; for example, a laboratory report looks different than a hospital report. To identify the

type of report, medical assistants must read the name of the report and the organization that issued it.

Informed Consent Forms

A signed informed consent form documents that a patient understands and consents to a treatment offered and has knowledge of the potential outcome and side effects of that treatment, including the expected outcome if the treatment is not performed. The form must contain the patient's signature, the physician's signature, a witness's signature, and the date. Moreover, it is important to note that the patient may withdraw consent if that patient so wishes. Should a patient choose to withdraw consent or refuse a procedure, it must be clearly noted in the patient's chart. Some medical offices require a patient to sign a "Refusal of Treatment" form.

Diagnosis and Treatment Plan

The diagnosis and treatment plan should include the physician's diagnosis (statement of what is wrong with the patient), the plan to care for the problem, and all options and instructions presented to the patient.

Patient Correspondence and Follow-Up Care

Any patient correspondence sent by the medical office, including procedures, follow-up visits, medical office care, and notations involving the patient, should be included in the patient's medical record. The date each piece of correspondence was mailed should be noted in the chart, along with the initials of the individual who completed the action. Documentation of telephone calls—often a separate log—as well as correspondence with or about the patient from all sources, such as laboratories, health care agencies, and referred consultations, are also added to patient records. Any correspondence received from the patient should be scanned in or filed.

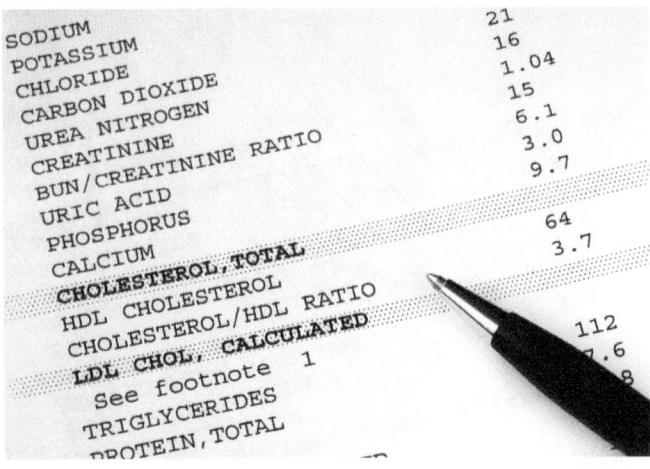

FIGURE 13-12 Laboratory test results.

Clinical Progress Note

A clinical progress note is the physician's narrative description of updated findings and treatments, such as the SOAP note discussed earlier in this chapter. Progress notes supplement documentation of the comprehensive history and physical. They are commonly used for inpatient stays in which the physician sees the patient each day and does not need to perform a full examination each time, or an outpatient seen frequently for a chronic condition.

Flow Sheet

Flow sheets document findings and treatments through the use of check marks and short notes rather than a longer text-based narrative. They help consolidate a large amount of details, such as vital signs, onto a single page for quick reference.

Consultation Report

In many situations, a physician asks another physician to provide an opinion on a patient's case. Typically, the physician requesting the consultation, also called the attending physician, sends a letter of introduction to the physician who will provide the opinion, also called the consulting physician. The letter of introduction includes a brief synopsis of the tests and results already performed. The consulting physician generally examines the patient and then dictates a report. The report is then sent to the attending physician (the requesting physician). The consultation report typically includes the following:

- Patient's name and medical record number
- Date of consultation
- Medical transcriptionist's initials
- Referring physician
- Reason for the consultation
- Physical and laboratory evaluations
- Consulting physician's impression and recommendations

It is appropriate to close this report, which is supplied in letter format, with a complimentary close, such as "Thank you for allowing me to participate in the care of this patient."

Operative Report

The operative report describes a surgical procedure. The surgeon is expected to dictate this report as soon as possible, preferably immediately after the procedure is completed. The heading of the report lists the surgeon's name, date of procedure, name of the procedure, preoperative diagnosis, and postoperative diagnosis. The body of the report is a narrative that describes the actual procedure in detail, including the following information:

- Type and amount of anesthetic agent used
- Location and length of incisions
- Layers of skin and tissue that were incised
- Types of instruments used
- Tissues and organs (if any) removed
- Structures visualized
- Gross (naked eye) observations and findings
- Materials that were used in closing the wound
- Estimated amount of blood loss
- Sponge and needle count

The report concludes by stating the condition of the patient at the end of the procedure, such as "Patient tolerated procedure well," "Patient awake and responding," or "Patient taken to recovery room." Any specimens sent to pathology are also identified.

Pathology Report

The pathology report is generated by the pathologist as the result of examining tissue and organs removed during a surgical procedure (such as a biopsy) or an autopsy. A pathology report focuses on microscopic (histology and cytology) findings, as well as gross (naked eye) description of tissues or organs. This report is related to disease findings and not laboratory findings, which are conducted on body fluids. An autopsy report is a pathology report generated after a patient's death to determine the cause of death.

Radiology Report

A radiology report, completed by a radiologist, documents results of diagnostic procedures, such as X-rays, CT (computerized tomography) scans, MRI (magnetic resonance imaging) scans, nuclear medicine procedures (scans of bone, thyroid, and other body parts), and other fluoroscopic examinations.

Discharge Summary

The discharge summary is completed by the attending physician for every hospitalized patient and summarizes the hospitalization. It explains why the patient was admitted, a summary of the patient's history, and a review of what occurred during the hospitalization. A discharge diagnosis is included in this report, and the patient's condition on leaving the hospital is noted.

Charts, Tables, and Graphs

Some medical reports are accompanied with charts, tables, or graphs that summarize trends in the patient's condition

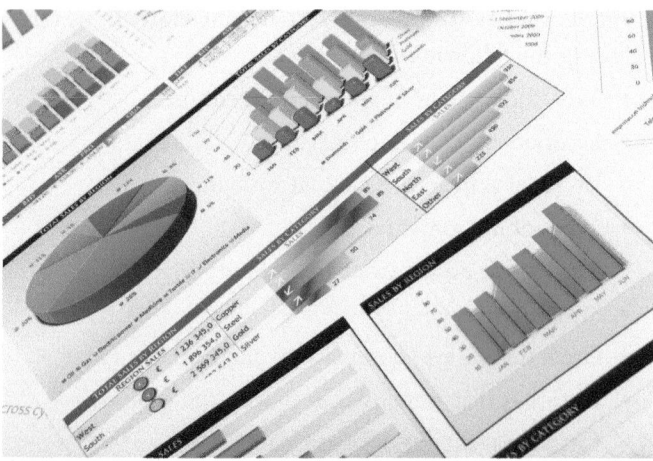

FIGURE 13-13 Charts, graphs, and tables can show trends in a patient's medical condition.

and compare them to averages. For example, laboratory results might show a trend line of a patient's glucose or cholesterol over a period of time with a comparison to the normal values (Figure 13-13).

Additional Reports

Other reports may be required concerning a patient, such as an emergency room report, a psychiatric note, and results of special procedures, such as a cardiac catheterization or an autopsy.

Medical Transcription

Offices using paper charts might use dictation and medical transcription to create the medical record. The physician verbally dictates information regarding a patient encounter, such as a physical examination or operative procedure, which is stored in an electronic audio format, such as a recording tape, CD, electronic chip, or other device. The transcriptionist listens to the audio file and types the exact information into a word processor or dictation program. The resulting document is printed and stored in the patient's medical chart, if physical charts are maintained, or transferred electronically to the EHR, if electronic health records are used.

Medical transcriptionists are medical professionals who have excellent keyboarding and grammar skills, knowledge of medical terminology, and a desire for accuracy and efficiency. The medical transcriptionist must understand words, know where and how to apply them, and use correct English grammar. This includes an understanding of etymology, phonetics, synonyms, acronyms, antonyms, homonyms, and eponyms.

Medical records must be professionally prepared, following appropriate formats. They should be free of errors and correctly filed. Medical records are always subject to possible subpoena by a court of law. The same professional standard

relating to confidentiality is necessary when handling transcription, because patient health information is involved, even though the transcriptionist may never see the patient.

IMPLEMENTING AN EHR SYSTEM

When medical offices decide to implement an EHR system, it is important to have a plan. Although you are not responsible for selecting and implementing an EHR system, you are an important stakeholder who will be affected by changes to it. Other stakeholders are physicians, business office staff, patients, and even suppliers and payers. Medical assistants can provide valuable input into what functions are needed for a smooth patient care process, office efficiency, and security of PHI regulated by HIPAA. They also can advocate for features that make it easy for patients to access their own health information.

The conversion from paper to EHR format typically is done over a period of time. Some clinics are able to use a scanner to scan documents from the patient's paper medical record to the electronic record. Other clinics might need to enter information from the paper chart to the electronic record manually. The process depends on the type of EHR software being used and the preferences of the medical staff.

The United States Department of Health and Human Services recommends six steps to implement an EHR system, as described next.

Step 1. Assess the Practice Readiness

The first step in EHR implementation is to evaluate the goals, needs, and financial and technical readiness of the medical practice. Consider the following areas:

- Are administrative processes organized, efficient, and well documented?

- Are clinical workflows efficient, clearly mapped out, and understood by all staff?

- Are data collection and reporting processes well established and documented?

- Are staff members computer literate and comfortable with information technology?

- Does the practice have access to high-speed Internet connectivity?

- Does the practice have access to the financial capital required to purchase new or additional hardware?

- Are there clinical priorities or needs that should be addressed?

- Does the practice have specialty-specific requirements?

The assessment step helps provide a good understanding of the current strengths of the practice and areas that should be improved before implementing an EHR. Often, these goals relate to patient quality, patient satisfaction, practice productivity and efficiency, improved quality of work environment, and, most important, the overall goal: improved health care.

Step 2. Create a Plan

Planning draws on the information gathered during the assessment phase to outline the practice's EHR implementation plan. Some of the issues that must be considered are the following:

- Which processes and functions will be implemented first, second, third, and so on?
- Will historical patient records be scanned into the EHR, or will existing records continue to be accessed on paper with only new encounters to be stored in the EHR?
- Will a dual system be used during the transition, meaning that records will be maintained both on paper and in the EHR until staff are sure the EHR system functions as expected?
- Who will provide the training?
- How long will implementation require?
- How much of staff members' time will be required to make the transition?

Step 3. Select or Upgrade to a Certified EHR

There are a number of steps involved in choosing the right EHR system for your practice. Eligible health care professionals and eligible hospitals must use certified EHR technology to achieve meaningful use and qualify for incentive payments. Medical offices may select an EHR system based on the system(s) used by major hospitals in the community. This strategy enables physicians to access patient data from the office or the hospital. They can review patients' medical histories with other providers who also use the same hospital.

Step 4. Conduct Training and Implement an EHR System

EHR implementation involves the installation of the EHR system and associated activities such as training, mock "go-live," and pilot testing. The EHR implementation plan and schedule (developed during the planning phase) should be followed and executed during this phase. Software companies that sell EHR software should provide the medical office with training for the staff to learn to use the system. This training should be attended by everyone within the office who uses the software, including the physicians. Often, one member of the medical office staff is designated as a mentor or in-house resource person for using the EHR system. This person may receive additional training. In addition, training materials, such as manuals and DVDs, should be supplied for use in training future staff members. Software companies should supply the office with contact information to reach a technical support person in the event a question or concern with the new software arises.

Step 5. Achieve Meaningful Use

To be eligible for financial incentive payments, providers must demonstrate meaningful use of EHRs as defined by the HITECH Act. This is accomplished over a period of several years and involves meeting criteria established by ONC.

Step 6. Continue Quality Improvement

This final phase involves reassessing what you have learned from training and everyday use of the system. It emphasizes continuous evaluation of your practice's goals and needs after the formal EHR implementation period has concluded. The goal is to continue improving workflows that achieve the individual practice's goals and needs while leveraging the functionality of EHRs. Often, what happens during the implementation phase is very different from what was planned. The practice needs to continuously evaluate its processes to ensure that the practice is functioning efficiently to achieve staff and patient satisfaction.

Professionalism   The Law

It is possible that the medical office where you work may be the only practice in the area that has converted to an EHR system. Other physicians in the area may have plans to convert to an EHR system but may still be using paper. When another physician forwards information such as a consult notice or laboratory results on a mutual patient, it arrives as a paper document. To convert the information on paper into an electronic format to be used in your office, the paper must be scanned and entered into the EHR and flagged for the physician to review. After the information has been entered into the EHR, the original document may either be stored securely or shredded, according to the office policy. If the policy states that paper documents are to be destroyed, the document should be shredded, either on-site or by the company hired to accomplish this task.

FILING, STORAGE, AND RETENTION OF PAPER MEDICAL RECORDS

Choosing the type of file system for paper-based medical forms and reports, in accord with the file folder coding system used in the office, is an important decision, because all files must be maintained within that system. The three categories of files or records in a medical office are active, inactive, and closed:

- **Active records** are those of patients who have been seen within the past three years and are currently being treated. Each medical practice has its own policy regarding what constitutes an active file, but the range is usually three to five years.

- **Inactive records** are those of patients who have not been seen within the past three years or another time period determined by office policy. These files are still maintained by the office but are generally kept in a separate storage file cabinet, which may be located off-site. These patients have not received a formal notification that the physician has terminated caring for them. They may return when a medical problem develops.

- **Closed records** are those of patients who have actively terminated their contact with the physician. This occurs when they move away or ask to have their records sent to another physician, or death occurs. These files can be placed in storage boxes or converted and saved on a computer disk, CD, microfilm, or other media. These files are referred to as archives because they are no longer needed but must be kept for legal reasons.

Fireproof cabinets are used to file documents such as patient records, tax records, insurance policies, and cancelled checks.

File Storage

Three types of file storage commonly used in a physician's office are vertical, lateral, and movable:

- **Vertical files**—Set up with two to four stacked pull-out drawers holding up to a hundred files per drawer. This type of file storage system is heavy and space consuming.

- **Lateral files**—Set up with shelves that allow files to be easily pulled off them. A color-coded system for visual recognition of files is often used.

- **Movable files**—Set up with electrically powered or manually controlled file units that move on stationary tracks in the floor. This type of open filing system saves space, because the file units can be moved close together when they are not needed. This system is also useful for books and journals, because the floor can be reinforced when the track is installed.

File Folders and Guides

File folders are designed to meet special needs. The top or side edge contains tabs at spaced intervals. An identification label is attached to the top tab in a vertical file cabinet or to the side edge of the file in a lateral file cabinet. Sometimes these are color-coded for each physician or type of insurance.

Divider guides, made of heavy pressboard, separate files in drawers or on shelves into subsections using a letter (e.g., A, B, C, A–B, Invoices, etc.) or by patient number.

An out-guide is a placard that indicates a file has been removed. It is placed in the file drawer when a folder is removed to indicate where the folder should be returned. You can write on the out-guide who removed the file and when it was removed. This is especially helpful in a large office when trying to locate charts. The out-guide is usually a distinctive color, such as red, to indicate a file is missing (Figure 13-14).

Labels

The main purpose of the label on the file is to identify what is in the file, such as the patient's name or medical record number. However, the label also can include a color-coded stripe that can be used for other purposes, such as identifying the primary care physician.

Offices also use special alert labels on charts to bring attention to patient allergies, required copayments, and year of last visit. These alert labels help the staff find pertinent information at a glance (Figure 13-15). For instance, a patient's allergy to penicillin is quickly identified if a bright sticker that indicates the allergy is visible on the

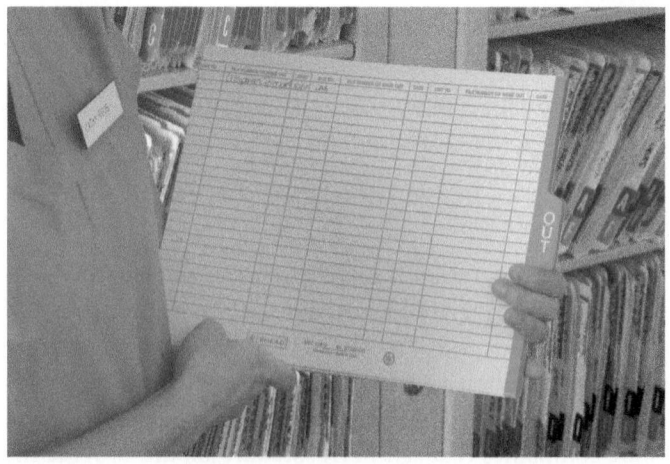

FIGURE 13-14 An example of an out-guide.

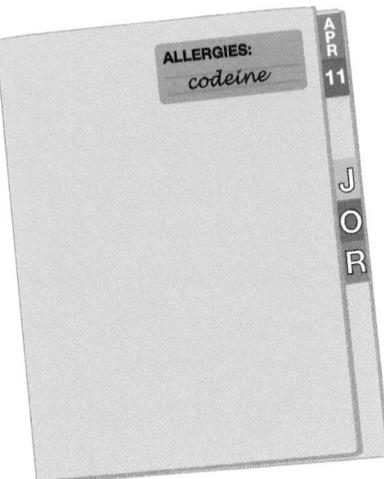

FIGURE 13-15 Using alert labels enables the medical staff to quickly identify important information such as allergies.

outside of the chart. It is important to update the information at every visit.

Color-Coded Label Systems. To decrease the number of misfiled charts and aid in file retrieval, many medical record departments use a system of color-coded file labels (Figure 13-16). This system assigns a unique color for each number from 0 to 9 and for each letter A to Z. Labels are placed on the edge of each file folder that correspond to the first several characters of the medical record number or other identifier. Colored bands on each label are visible when the files are shelved. When files are correctly placed, the colored bands all have the same pattern. In this manner, any misfiles are easily seen. Filing records is simplified because the correct color band can be located on the file shelf. Two popular color-coding methods using a numeric system are the Ames Color File System and the Smead Manufacturing Company's method. Other color-coded methods use an alphabetic system.

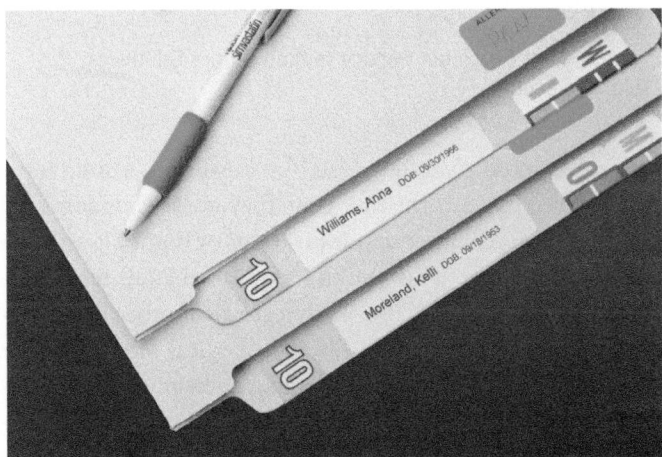

FIGURE 13-16 A color-coded record.

Rules for Filing

Three commonly used systems for filing or indexing paper medical records are alphabetic, numeric, and subject filing. Because the numeric system provides the most privacy, it is most commonly used for medical records; however, alphabetizing is a component of all the methods and is explained in detail here. Color coding is used in all three systems to assist in locating files, refiling, and preventing misfiling.

Alphabetic System

Alphabetic filing sequences names in the order of the alphabet. In this system, the name Abbott would be filed before Bacon because A comes before B in the alphabet. If the first letter is the same, then move to the second letter in the name: Abbott is filed before Acker. This requires that medical assistants know the alphabet well and are quickly able to determine which random letter comes before another. There can be confusion when filing Jacob James Jergens Jr. and Jacob James Jergens III, or determining how correspondence from 23rd Avenue Clinic should be filed.

The key to alphabetic filing is to divide the names and titles into units (first, second, and third). The unit is the portion of the name that is used for filing or indexing purposes. For example:

- Unit 1: Last name (Jergens)
- Unit 2: First name (Jacob)
- Unit 3: Middle name (James)

The first letter of each unit is then used to determine where the file is to be placed. When filing a large number of files, use the first letter of the first unit and place all the files from A to Z in order. Then take each group of A files and use the second letter and consecutive letters to place them in order. If the entire first unit is the same, as in Smith, then move on to the second unit and third unit. For example, Smith, Loren comes before Smith, Michael, which comes before Smith, Michelle. Table 13-2 describes basic rules for

TABLE 13-2 | Rules for Alphabetic Filing

Rules	Example
Names are filed: last name, first name, middle name (or middle initial). Each letter in the name is a separate unit.	Krause, Marvin K. is placed before Krause, Marvin L.
Initials come before a full name.	Brown, H. is placed before Brown, Henry.
Hyphenated names are treated as one unit. This applies to the names of individuals and businesses.	Amy Freeman-Smith is indexed under F for Freeman. It is considered Freemansmith for indexing purposes.
Titles (and initials) are disregarded for filing but placed in parentheses after the name.	Dr. Beth Ann Williams is indexed as Williams, Beth Ann (Dr.).
Married women are indexed using their legal name. The husband's name can be used for cross-referencing.	Mrs. Mary Jane Smith is indexed as Smith, Mary Jane (Mrs. John).
Seniority units, such as Jr. and Sr., are filed in alphabetic order.	Jacob James Jurgens, Jr. comes before Jacob James Jurgens, Sr.
Roman numeral designations are filed alphabetically under the letter "I."	Jurgens, Jacob James III is indexed before Jurgens, Jacob James, Jr.
Mac and Mc can be filed either alphabetically as they occur or grouped together depending on the preference of the office. Be sure that everyone follows the same rule.	Option 1: File each alphabetically as it occurs: Mabrey, MacBride, Martin, McAuliffe, McBride, McMartin; Option 2: File Mc as though it begins with "Mac": Mabrey, McAuliffe, MacBride, McBride, McMartin, Martin
Foreign language names are indexed as one unit.	Mary St. Claire is indexed as Stclaire, Mary. Carol van Dammis indexed as Vandamm, Carol.
If company names are identical, the address—by state, then city, then street—may be used in the index. The ZIP code is not used to index files.	ABC Drugs, 123 Michigan Blvd., Chicago, IL is indexed before ABC Drugs, 1450 N. Ash, Kalispell, MT.
If individuals' names are identical, use the birthdate or mother's maiden name. Avoid using an address, because that can change.	Mark Richard Jones is indexed as Jones, Mark Richard (05/12/65) and Jones, Mark Richard (02/12/89).
Disregard apostrophes.	Megan O'Connor is indexed as OConnor, Megan.
Business organizations are indexed as they are written.	Lincoln Memorial Hospital is correct.
Disregard short terms, such as *a, and, the,* and *of.*	The Whitefish Drug Store is indexed as Whitefish Drug Store (The).
Numeric characters are indexed before alpha characters.	23rd Avenue Clinic is indexed before the Nineteenth Street Medical Center. A separate file is set up for all numeric files.
Names with religious titles, such as Sister Mary Murphy, are to be filed with the last name first, and then with the religious title.	Murphy, Sister Mary.
Compound words are filed as they are written.	South West Physician Service is filed before Southwest Physician Service.

alphabetic filing. Procedure 13-5 lists steps to follow when using the alphabetic filing system.

Numeric Systems

A **numeric filing** system sequences folders in numerical order. A patient identification number is assigned to each patient's medical record. This generally is a six-digit number divided into three sections of two digits each (e.g., 05-72-21).

Identification numbers are assigned using either unit-number or serial number filing. A unit-number filing system is most commonly used by hospitals. A number is assigned to patients the first time they are seen or admitted to a hospital. All other hospitalizations or hospital visits use the same number. This method requires that all records be kept at the same location. With a serial-number filing system, the patient receives a different medical record number for each hospital visit. The patient acquires multiple records that are stored at different locations. For example, a hospitalization, laboratory work, and a mammogram all receive different numbers and are filed within their own systems.

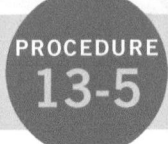

Filing a Record Alphabetically

Objective ◆ *File a patient record in the correct order, using the alphabetic method for filing.*

EQUIPMENT AND SUPPLIES

Patient record; alphabetic files

METHOD

1. Locate medical record files or medical record room.
2. Observe the name on the record to be filed.
3. Records are filed in alphabetic order by last name first, then first name, then middle name or initial. Each letter in the name is a separate unit. Locate the set of records containing the same last name as the record to be filed.
4. Within the set of records containing the same last name as the record to be filed, locate the records with the same letter of the first name as the record to be filed.
5. Using the alphabet as a guide, place the record to be filed after the record that comes before it in the alphabet but before the record that comes after it in the alphabet.
6. A name with only an initial first name is filed before a full name. (Brown, H. is filed before Brown, Henry.) The filing rule "Nothing before something" is a useful tool here.

7. Hyphenated names are treated as one unit. (Mary Freeman-Smith is indexed as Freemansmith, Mary.)
8. Disregard apostrophes. (Megan O'Connor is indexed as Oconnor, Megan.)
9. Titles and initials are disregarded for filing, but placed in parentheses after the name. (Dr. Beth Ann Williams is indexed as Williams, Beth Ann, [Dr.].)
10. Married women are indexed using their legal name. The husband's name can be used for cross-referencing.
11. Seniority units, such as Jr. and Sr., are filed in numeric order from first to last.
12. Numeric seniority terms are filed before alphabetic terms.
13. After placing the file between the two records before and after it in the alphabet, check once more to be sure the file is properly placed.
14. If there is a marker or out-guide in place of the removed record, then take out the marker when replacing the file.

The assigned numbers are kept in an accession record in which numbers in sequential order (1, 2, 3, 4, 5, 6 ...) have a name placed next to them as each new name is entered. This record can also be maintained on the computer.

There are several types of numeric filing that use identification numbers, including straight numeric filing, terminal-digit filing, middle digit filing.

Straight Numeric Filing. The simplest numeric method is the straight numeric filing system in which each record is filed sequentially based on its assigned number from 0 to 9. The numbers used in this system begin at 01 and continue upward.

Example:	01	101	886
	02	102	887
	03	103	888
	04	104	889

In this type of system, the file space is depleted rapidly as new files are added to one section. This requires constant reshifting of files to make room for new files.

Terminal-Digit Filing. **Terminal-digit filing** sequences folders based on the last two digits of the ID number, from 00 to 99, and evenly distributes the files within the entire filing system. This eliminates the need for frequent reshifting of files, providing enough space was designated when the filing system was set up. Filing using terminal digits requires dividing the files into 100 primary sections, starting with 00 and ending with 99. The three sections of numbers assigned to each file are designated as tertiary, secondary, and primary sections, respectively. To file a record with the number 05-72-21 using this system, find the file section matching the patient's primary digits (21). Within that section, match up the secondary digits (72) and file the record according to the tertiary digits (05).

Example:	05	72	21
	Tertiary	Secondary	Primary

Middle-Digit Filing. Using the same six-digit numbering system as for the terminal-digit system, the middle-digit filing system places the middle digits as the primary numbers. In this example, find the section marked 72, within that section find the 05 area, and then file the record according to the tertiary digit, 21.

Example:	05	72	21
	Secondary	Primary	Tertiary

Subject Matter

Filing by subject matter is used for general files, such as invoices, correspondence, résumés, and personnel records. This method is adequate as long as the files are relatively small. If these files become large, then another method, alphabetic or numeric, must be devised.

Cross-Referencing

Because of the large number of files processed in a busy office and the confusion over surnames—(e.g., how stepchildren's names are filed for easy access), cross-referencing of files is recommended. Cross-referencing places an informational message in the file to alert the health worker that a file can be found under another name. For example, if Mrs. Henry Watts also uses her maiden name, Farideh Rahman, then a file insert into Henry Watts's file could state, "See Rahman, Farideh for Mrs. Henry Watts." Cross-referencing can be a simple but useful tool for finding and avoiding misplaced records.

Locating Missing Files

One of the most time-consuming and frustrating activities relating to medical records is locating a misplaced file, also referred to as a missing file. Ideally, everyone who takes a file from a cabinet should add that file name or number to a master file sheet. In addition, an out-guide should be placed in the file indicating a record was removed.

When a file cannot be easily located, it is important to conduct a thorough search of the office. It is absolutely essential that the missing file be located as soon as possible and returned to its proper location. Not only is the information needed by a staff member, you must ensure that the file is not in a location where it can be viewed by unauthorized persons. To locate missing files, consider these tips:

- Look at the file folders near the location where the missing file "should" appear in the file cabinet. It is possible for one folder to be mistakenly placed inside another folder.

- If the patient was recently in the office, or is scheduled for the current day or next day, look in the normal locations where such files are placed.

- Scan the file racks for folders that may be out of sequence. Use of color-coded file labels greatly simplifies this task.

- Check common areas, such as the copy machine, scanner, and fax machines.

- Check with the receptionist, transcriptionist, coding, and billing departments.

- Ask each staff member, including physicians, to conduct a thorough search of the desktops, inbox, and personal file drawers. Remind people to check inside other recently used files in case one folder was nested inside another.

The ability to locate files quickly is an indicator of quality assurance. When internal or external auditors review medical records for completeness and accuracy, they randomly identify which records to review from a master list of patients. Upon concluding the review of records, they also report to management the number of records that could not be located. A record that cannot be located for an audit represents a record that would not be found if needed to respond to a patient emergency or other request.

If a systematic search takes place, the file can usually be located quickly. However, sometimes a single piece of paper, such as a laboratory report, cannot be found because it has been mistakenly filed in the wrong folder. These are nearly impossible to locate. If it cannot be found, you must get another copy of the paper from the original source (e.g., a laboratory or radiology report).

The best way to avoid losing a file is to handle all records methodically and carefully.

Tickler Files

A tickler file is used to remind medical assistants of an event or action that will take place at a future date. The tickler file contains patients' names and telephone numbers, dates when action or activities should occur, and actions to take. The tickler files should be reviewed daily so that actions are taken on time (e.g., tickler files can be used as reminders to call patients to set appointments, to pay certain invoices, or to send fees for the physician's license renewals).

Collating Paper Records

Collating is the process of gathering and organizing information. All the outside reports must be available in the medical record before the patient's scheduled visit. Medical assistants need to collect all information pertaining to a patient who is scheduled to be seen by the physician—including all records, test results, and other information and reports—and organize it into appropriate sections of the patient's chart.

Pulling charts is usually done the day before the scheduled appointment. Verify that test results or reports have been filed into the appropriate sections of the chart. It is important that this information be available when the physician sees the patient, especially because sometimes the sole purpose of the patient's visit is to follow up on those results. Automated offices may be able to generate an **exception report**, a computerized report that lists all procedures ordered but with no results on record. This facilitates the follow-up.

If information such as tests or lab results ordered at the last visit has not been received, you need to follow up. Call the appropriate facilities to retrieve the results. In the patient's chart, document the date, time, name of person with whom you spoke, and expected action regarding the requested information. You may take oral results and record them as a verbal report, but request that the hard copy results be faxed to the office as soon as possible. When you are provided with an oral report, document the information on a message pad and flag it for the physician's review, because the physician may request further reports depending on the findings. However, when the original physical copy of the report is received, place that in the patient's record as well. This is done quite often by the clinical medical assistant. In some offices and laboratories, a fax machine can be used to send reports between facilities.

Normally, reports should be organized, reviewed, and filed as they come in, to avoid a backlog or misplaced reports. This way, everything is ready for the patient's next visit and for any consultations that may be needed between visits. Each office should have policies and procedures for handling outside reports.

Long-Term Storage

Medical offices need to provide for long-term storage of medical records. Files must be kept safe from fire, flood, or other damage. This is often a challenge because of the amount of space required. Records may be maintained in their original hard-copy form or transferred to other media such as electronic (scanned images), **microfilm** (miniaturized photographs of records), or **microfiche** (sheets of microfilm). If the office does not have enough space to store the files internally, space can be rented in another office or building. Medical record storage also may be outsourced to a business that specializes in managing and housing medical documents. Investigate the business to ensure that it is reputable and HIPAA-compliant, and that the files will be safe and accessible.

Retention of Electronic Records

Requirements for long-term retention of patient data are the same for both paper-based and computerized records. The advantage of EHRs is that data are more convenient and less costly to store, and the EHR can be located and accessed more easily.

Because computer data require a small amount of space compared with paper-based records, EHRs do not need to be converted to another format for long-term storage. Usually, a large amount of historical data can be maintained in the main EHR system. Data for patients who have left the practice can be archived so that they do not unnecessarily occupy disk space. Most software has a built-in function that removes unneeded data from the program and saves them in a compressed format that requires less space. In this way, the data can be accessed if needed but do not encumber the software.

Ideally, all medical records should be retained forever. However, this is impractical in many circumstances. Although there are no universal answers, the following can provide you with general guidelines:

- The medical record is critical in a medical liability action and its loss may considerably harm the physician in the defense of a claim. At a minimum, retain records until the statute of limitations expires.

- Each state varies somewhat on the legal time limits (statute of limitations) to keep records and documents. In many cases, the statute of limitations is two years, but the timing does not begin until the point of discovery of damage and the connection between that damage and the treatment. In some circumstances, this could be many years later. Special rules apply when treating a child or an incompetent patient, in which case the time period is longer.

- Most states require that all patient records be retained for two to seven years after the last treatment or seven years after the patient reaches the age of majority (age 18 or 21 in most states), whichever comes last.

- The American Medical Association recommends keeping medical records for ten years.

- In selected circumstances, you might consider saving the more complex records or those records with known serious patient problems for a longer period of time.

- Keep immunization records as long as practical, because patients may need to access them at a future date.

Destruction of Medical Records

If a physician cannot retain patient records indefinitely, consideration must be given to the method of destruction. As with any office policy, a medical record destruction policy should follow a written procedure. The procedure should achieve the following:

- Outline the length of time records will be kept.

- Define which records will be kept on-site and which off-site.

- Designate a person to be responsible for deciding what to keep and what to purge.

- Produce a log that details which patient records have been destroyed and why, when, and how they have been destroyed.

- Provide a method of disposal (e.g., shred, pulp, or incinerate) that destroys all information in the record. Deleting information from an EHR simply removes it from the software application, but the data remains on the storage device and can be retrieved. If possible, physically destroy the storage medium, such as a disk or tape. Otherwise, you can use a HIPAA-compliant utility program that permanently removes any trace of the data from the storage media. It is best to hire an IT professional familiar with HIPAA standards to ensure the data is completely removed and irretrievable.

Patient confidentiality must not be jeopardized because of an inadequate method of destruction. Many medical offices hire the services of a business that handles the destruction of paper or electronic medical records. That service must agree to abide by HIPAA guidelines.

OFFICE FLOW WITH ELECTRONIC AND PAPER MEDICAL RECORDS

Although the functions of the medical office are the same regardless of whether electronic or paper medical records are used, the work flow is different. Table 13-3 compares the differences in patient flow when using electronic and

Professionalism The Life Span

Medical staff should respect the various levels of comfort patients may have with storing their medical information on a computer. Staff members must take every opportunity to educate those who are not comfortable with the idea. Most individuals in their 30s and younger have grown up with computers and use a computer in their daily lives. However, patients in their 60s and older may not be as comfortable with the idea of using a computer to store their most personal medical information and may prefer a paper chart because it is something they can touch and hold.

paper-based records. Two important differences in work flow are point of care documentation and computerized physician order entry.

Point of Care Documentation

Point of care documentation is the ability of providers to document the patient encounter in the examination room and enter information into the computer while the patient is present. This improves the quality of documentation, because physicians no longer have to remember what occurred during the visit when they document at the end of the day. In addition, the EHR screen prompts physicians to enter all required information and alerts them when an important item is missing. Lastly, the physician can ask the patient about any details necessary to complete the description of symptoms or the course of the illness (Figure 13-17).

Many medical offices have computer terminals in each examination room, which allow medical personnel to add information to the patient's EHR, download test results, or research past medication records while the patient is in the room. In some offices, the physician or medical assistant uses a laptop or portable electronic tablet to enter patient data into the computer system. In some cases it is possible to automatically enter vital signs and diagnostic test results from the equipment directly into the EHR.

Medical assistants also need to become familiar with how to document at the point of care, computerized physician order entry, how to make corrections in the medical record, and file retention and storage.

Computerized Physician Order Entry

Computerized physician order entry (CPOE) is the ability of providers to order tests, prescriptions, lab work, and referrals using the computer, rather than writing them on paper, mailing or faxing them, or placing a telephone call (Figure 13-18). Patients do not need to remember to take the order with them to their encounter because the office transmits it electronically. Not only is the order generated and sent electronically, it also is saved in the patient's EHR. Results are returned to the ordering physician and recorded in the patient's EHR.

Meaningful use criteria require a CPOE for a medical office to receive incentive payments. Only licensed health care professionals, including credentialed medical assistants, are allowed to enter orders into the CPOE system for it to count toward meaningful use. "Credentialed" means to obtain a certification or registration from a national credentialing organization, other than the educational institution and employer.

Process	Paper-Based Method	EHR Method
Schedule appointment	• Determine whether the patient is new or established. • Write down information such as patient name, address, telephone numbers, insurance information, and current complaint. • Page through a paper scheduling book to find available appointments.	• Access established patient information on the computer. Create the beginning of an electronic chart for new patients. • Confirm and update patient name, telephone numbers, insurance information, and symptoms in the software program. • Electronically search for available appointment times.
Verify insurance benefits	• Call the insurance company to verify patient coverage. • Write down information on a benefits verification form.	• Electronically confirm the patient's health insurance coverage using secure Internet site or direct portal. • Update coverage information in computer.
Send appointment reminder	• Create and mail appointment reminder notice. • Personally call patient to remind of appointment.	• Software generates printed reminder notice to be mailed. • Software calls the patient and leaves a brief message to remind the patient of an appointment. • Software may set a reminder for office personnel to make the phone call.
Prepare new patient chart	• Gather paper file folder, color-coded labels, patient registration form, forms needed by medical staff. • Create medical record number. • File chart in appropriate location until day of patient visit. • Maintain separate physical charts for each family member. • Create a new separate chart when a patient has workers' compensation or auto insurance claims.	• Enter patient data into the computer, following prompts for required information. • Software generates a new medical record for new patients. • Medical record is immediately accessible whenever needed. • Electronically link records for family members. • Electronically link separate records for the same patient, such as medical and workers' compensation.
Prepare established patient chart for visit	• Locate the patient's paper chart. The chart may be in use by another staff member or physician, or it may be misfiled. • Add appropriate forms so it is ready for use the following day. • File chart in appropriate location until day of patient visit.	• Medical record is immediately accessible whenever needed. Multiple staff members may access the chart at the same time.
Complete patient paperwork	• Ask patient to come in early to complete paperwork, or mail forms to patient in advance of visit. • Review forms to ensure that all information is complete. • File in patient chart.	• Patient accesses the practice's secure website to enter needed patient information. • Software alerts alert staff of any missing information. • Complete patient information forms at kiosk in the medical office reception area. • When the patient arrives in the office, escort patient to an examination room, where a medical assistant fills out the patient information form on the computer while the patient is present to answer any questions.
Room patient/ Take vital signs	• Clinical medical assistant takes vital signs, such as blood pressure, pulse, and temperature. • Write the information in the patient's paper medical chart.	• Take the patient's vital signs, and enter the information into the electronic health record. • Software records vital signs from measurement equipment connected to the computer system.

(continued)

Process	Paper-Based Method	EHR Method
Perform physical examination	• Physician reviews the forms the patient and medical assistant have completed. • Physician documents encounter during and after the appointment. • Physician may dictate findings, which are transcribed by a medical assistant or a transcription service, then added to the patient's paper chart.	• Physician accesses the patient's EHR in the examination room. • Physician documents findings and recommendations while interviewing and examining the patient. • Documentation is complete at the end of the encounter.
Order tests or prescriptions	• Write a prescription by hand and give to patient to take to pharmacy. Call pharmacy with the prescription request. • Write an order for lab test or X-rays by hand, and give to patient to take to the laboratory or radiology facility of choice. • Patient must remember to bring the written order to the appointment.	• Enter prescription request into the EHR, electronically sending it to the patient's pharmacy and recording it in the patient's chart at the same time. • Generate the order for lab tests or X-rays electronically, often with the ability to send the order to the radiology facility or laboratory of the patient's choice. • When patient arrives for the lab test or X-ray, the facility accesses the order in the EHR and performs the procedure.
Provide health education literature to patient	• Locate the appropriate brochures to give to patient.	• Software prints a visit summary with appropriate health education information, based on diagnoses and tests selected by the physician.
Make referral	• Phone the consulting physician to schedule appointment. • Copy and send any needed medical records before the appointment. Consulting physician writes a summary report of the visit and mails to the referring physician.	• Possibly schedule the appointment electronically. • Consulting physician accesses EHR to review pertinent medical history. • Consulting physician enters findings and summary report into EHR.
Receive test results	• Test results are mailed to the office. • File all reports in patient's chart. • Pull the patient's paper chart and provide to physician to review the results along with the patient's chart. • Monitor any test results not received. Follow up with patient by phone or letter to ensure test was obtained. Follow up with facility by phone or letter to request results.	• Receive tests results electronically. • Results are automatically linked to the patient's EHR. • The physician is alerted by the system that results are available, which can be viewed on the computer. • Software generates a report of tests ordered but no results received. Contact the facility electronically to request results. Software generates a telephone list or printed reminders to follow up with patient.
Contact patient for follow-up	• Facility that provides the test mails a copy of the results to the patient. • Call or write to the patient when follow-up is needed.	• Send a secure e-mail to the patient regarding test results. • Generate a telephone list for patients who need to be called about the results. • Patient views the results, and physician comments online through a secure patient access portal.
Assign diagnostic and procedure codes	• Staff pulls the patient's chart and assigns appropriate codes. May need to look in several sections of the chart to obtain all needed information.	• Staff accesses the patient's EHR and views needed information. • Software may generate preliminary codes for staff to verify, update, or change.
Bill insurance company	• Complete paper billing forms or rekey all patient information into a standalone billing program.	• Link EHR data to billing module, and submit claims electronically to insurance companies.

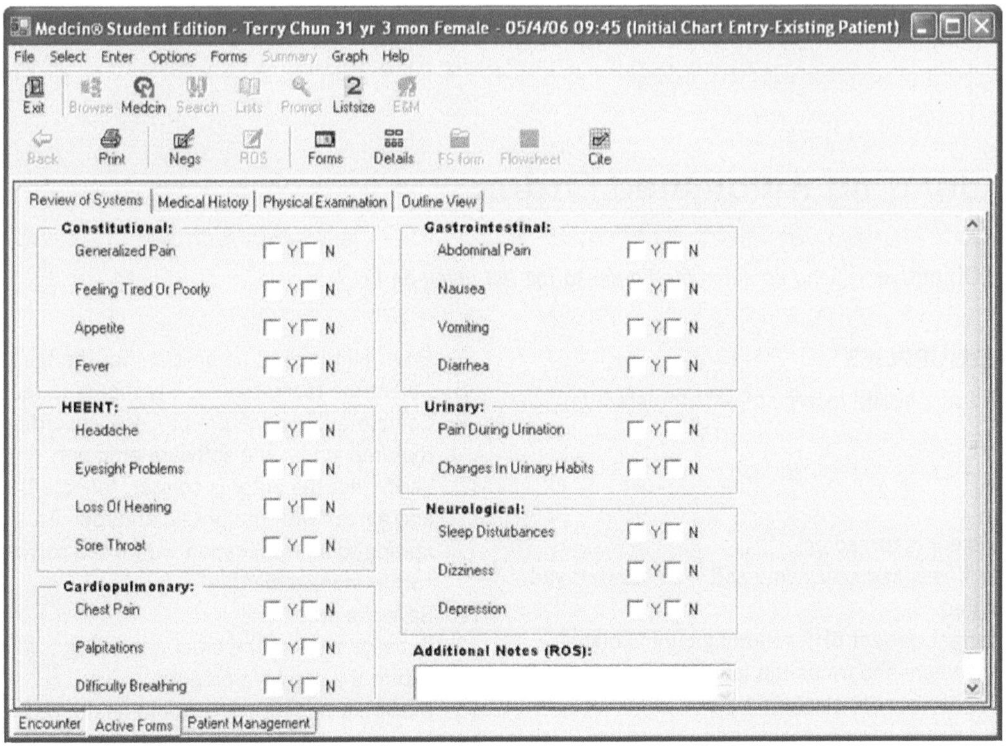

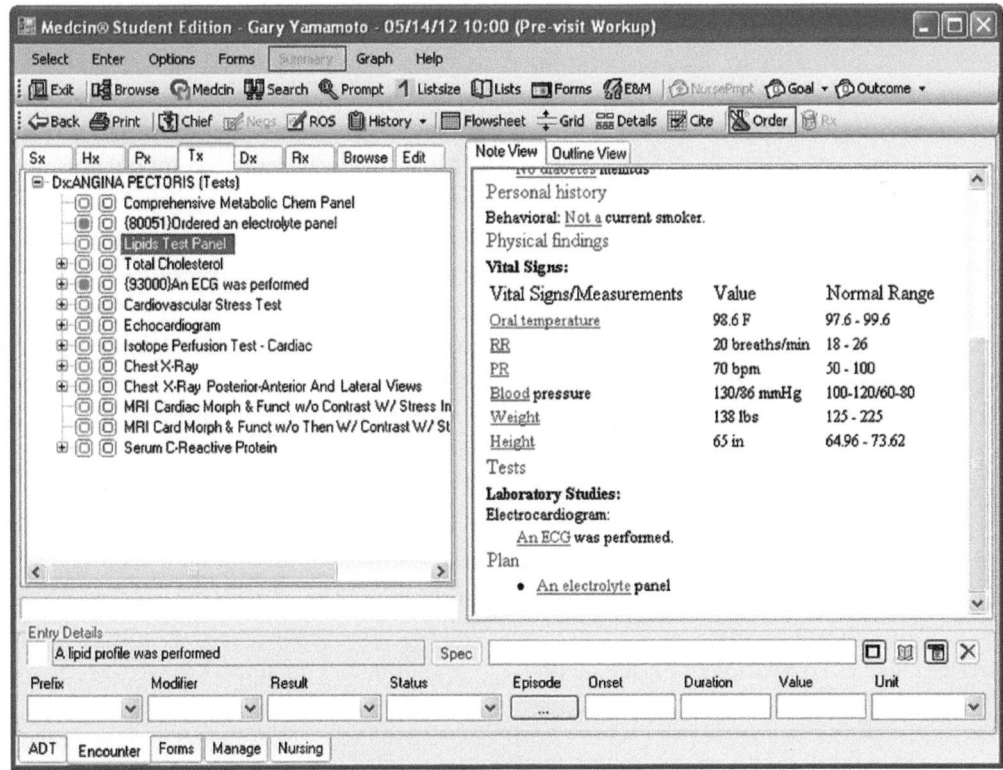

FIGURE 13-17 An example of an intake screen in an electronic health record.

FIGURE 13-18 An example of an EHR screen used to order a laboratory test.

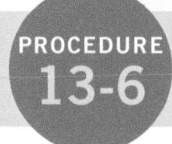

Sending Automated Orders

Objective ◆ *Send an automated order to the lab using an EHR.*

EQUIPMENT AND SUPPLIES

Computer with electronic health record software; orders from the physician

METHOD

1. Be sure the system is turned on.
2. Log in with your assigned user name and the password you previously created.
3. Identify the correct patient EHR following clinic policies.
4. Ask the patient where she wants the lab order sent. Verify that the facility can accept electronic orders.
5. Locate the order entry screen, according to the steps required within the software program.
6. Select laboratory procedures, type of procedure, and specific type of test based on software.
7. Enter all required parameters for the test selected.
8. Select the laboratory facility that is to receive the order.
9. Complete the signature process, according to the steps required within the software program.
10. Verify that the entry is correct, reflects the test intended, and agrees with the physician order. This may require navigating to a new location within the software such as "order management."
11. Save the order.
12. Activate or send the order according to the steps required within the software program.
13. Close the patient's electronic health record.
14. Log off the system.

Refer to Procedure 13-6 to learn general procedures for sending automated orders.

SUMMARY

An electronic health record (EHR) provides a computerized means of gathering, documenting, and storing information about the patient and the care received in the medical setting. The same information found in a patient's paper chart is found in an electronic chart; however, electronic records are stored and accessed using a computer. A personal health record (PHR) is health information that the patient stores electronically on a computer or on a secure, central Internet site. Benefits of EHRs include improved diagnostics and patient outcomes, improved patient participation, and improved efficiencies, resulting in cost savings.

As medical practices make the transition to EHRs, medical assistants need to know how to transfer their knowledge of traditional records to a computerized system. In particular, they should be aware of differences in documentation formats, medical record components, and retention and storage requirements. They also need to become familiar with how to make corrections in the medical record, document at the point of care, and follow HIPAA privacy and security requirements. Both electronic and paper medical records must comply with HIPAA legislation for privacy and security.

Medical assistants can provide valuable input into what functions are needed for a smooth patient care process, office efficiency, and security of protected health information (PHI) regulated by HIPAA. They can also advocate for features that make it easy for patients to access their own health information. The conversion from paper to EHR format is typically done over a period of time and requires a great deal of planning and organization.

COMPETENCY REVIEW

1. Define and spell the terms for this chapter.
2. Explain how the use of EHRs can help to avoid medication prescription errors.
3. Why would it be important for all staff members, even those with extensive computer experience, to attend a training session for new electronic health records software?
4. Explain how a medical office might enter a letter from an outside medical facility into a patient's electronic health record.
5. Explain the types of electronic signatures.
6. Discuss the steps in implementing an EHR system.
7. How would using electronic health records save time over using paper medical records?
8. Why should a medical office shred papers that contain patient information once those records have been entered?
9. Describe where you would find Emma Holmes's file. She has not been seen by Dr. Williams for two years, and there has been no communication with her. Is this an active, inactive, or closed file?
10. You are missing a file for Sean Roy. Discuss what process you would use to find it.
11. Mr. Crosby is angry and demanding that you give him his medical chart so that he can take it to another physician. How do you handle Mr. Crosby's anger and his request for his medical file?

PREPARING FOR THE CERTIFICATION EXAM

1. Which of the following can the medical staff typically do using an electronic health record system?
   a. locate possible contraindications with prescribed medications
   b. allow two or more staff members to access the same patient file at the same time
   c. save time looking for charts
   d. fax medical records to other medical offices
   e. all of the above

2. Which of the following is a reason patients may want to access their own medical records online?
   a. view their current medications
   b. view the date of their vaccination
   c. read their current lab report
   d. see when they are due for their annual exam
   e. all of the above

3. What is point of care documentation?
   a. the ability of patients to access their medical records online
   b. the ability to take patients' vital signs using an instrument connected to the computer and have results automatically entered
   c. the ability of providers to access patient information from remote locations
   d. the ability of providers to document the patient encounter in the examination room

   e. the ability of patients to complete their medical histories online, before they arrive for the appointment

4. All of the following are functions of an EHR *except*
   a. electronic data transmission to other health care providers.
   b. search for certain types of conditions for a group of patients.
   c. ease of access by others.
   d. prescriptions printed.
   e. electronic graphs of lab results.

5. All of the following are benefits of using an EHR *except*
   a. communicating between staff members.
   b. health maintenance.
   c. advertising purposes.
   d. putting records online.
   e. avoiding medical errors.

6. What is the most convincing argument for converting paper medical records to an electronic format?
   a. easier for staff to use
   b. patient safety
   c. saves time
   d. communication with staff
   e. health maintenance

7. How frequently should computers containing EHR information be backed up?
   a. every hour
   b. every four hours
   c. every day
   d. every two days
   e. every week

8. What is the name of the legislative act that provides financial incentives to providers who implement EHRs and meet meaningful use criteria?
   a. HIPAA
   b. CBO
   c. ONC
   d. HITECH
   e. CPOE

9. Which of the following would be last if filed alphabetically?
   a. Jacob James Jurgens III
   b. Jacob James Jurgens Jr.
   c. Jacob James Jurgens Sr.
   d. Jacob James Jurgens
   e. Jacob James Jurgens II

10. Travis Williams has been assigned the patient ID number 386492. To search for his file, you look under 64, then 38, then 92. What system are you using?
    a. unit numbering
    b. straight numbering
    c. terminal-digit filing
    d. middle-digit filing
    e. service numbering

CRITICAL THINKING

Refer to the case study at the beginning of the chapter and use what you have learned to answer the following questions.

1. While gathering information, Lewis and Tania developed a list of pros and cons for converting to electronic health records. What might have been included on their list?

2. The office has decided to make the conversion to EHRs. Once all records have been converted, what should be done with the original paper charts?

3. The office has recently received in the mail a typed consultation report from a local oncologist regarding a mutual patient, Yun-qi Yeung. What should be done with this report now that the office has converted to EHRs?

ON THE JOB

Dr. Jonas runs a private practice. He admits patients and makes rounds in two local hospitals. He uses one type of EHR software in his private office and two other packages in the two hospitals. Not only must Dr. Jonas learn three software systems, but he also may at times be unable to move patient information between those systems because of incompatibility. What might Dr. Jonas do to address these issues?

INTERNET ACTIVITY

Search the Internet for the newest legislation in your home state regarding the handling of medical records. Write a summary of the article, and discuss with your class whether the legislation adds to efficiency when dealing with medical records or creates unnecessary obstacles.

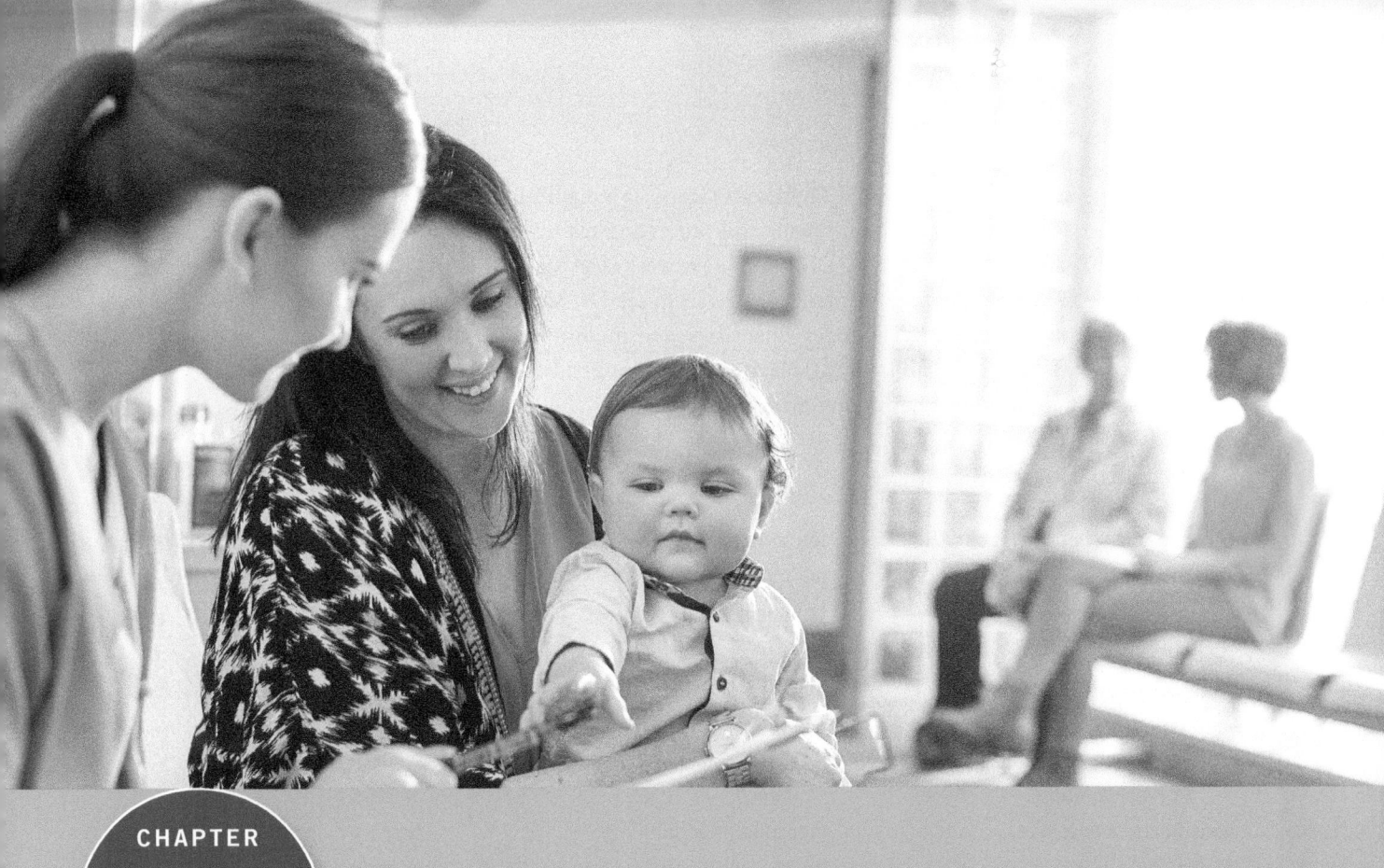

Learning Objectives

After completing this chapter, you should be able to:

14.1 Define and spell the terms for this chapter.

14.2 List key concepts regarding the Patient Protection and Affordable Care Act (PPACA).

14.3 Explain the medical assistant's role related to health insurance claims.

14.4 Identify terminology specifically related to health insurance policy and provisions.

14.5 Explain the purpose of the Genetic Information Nondiscrimination Act of 2008.

14.6 Describe different managed care plans.

14.7 Compare and contrast private and government health insurance plans.

14.8 Differentiate between third-party liability insurance and disability income insurance.

14.9 Outline the steps for a patient referral based on managed care guidelines.

14.10 Describe how to verify eligibility of services.

14.11 Describe how to obtain precertification of services.

14.12 Explain how to gather information needed for filing third-party claims.

14.13 List the steps for filing a third-party claim.

14.14 Describe HIPAA regulations regarding electronic transactions.

Case Study

Lewis Jordan, RMA, works at Pearson Physicians Group as a medical billing and insurance clerk. His duties include verifying insurance and processing claims. Sylvia Baker is a new patient and has an appointment to see Dr. Miller next week. She has Blue Cross/Blue Shield insurance. Mark Flannery is also a patient. He was in to see Dr. Miller last month, and the claim for his care was rejected. The codes, quantities, and modifiers were all correct on the CMS-1500. Lewis receives a call from Mr. Flannery, who is angry, because he has been billed for his last visit and has already paid his copayment.

Terms to Learn

Advance Beneficiary Notice (ABN)

allowed amount

assignment of benefits

beneficiary

birthday rule

capitation

Centers for Medicare & Medicaid Services (CMS)

certificate of coverage

CHAMPVA

claim

clean claim

clearinghouse

CMS-1500

coinsurance

Consolidated Omnibus Reconciliation Act (COBRA)

coordination of benefits (COB)

copayment

covered

Current Procedural Terminology (CPT®) code

deductible

denied claim

dependent

elective procedure

eligibility

exclusion

fee schedule

fee-for-service (FFS)

formulary

gatekeeper

group health insurance (GHI)

health insurance exchange (HIE)

health maintenance organization (HMO)

individual mandate

Item

locum tenens

managed care

managed care organization (MCO)

Medicaid

medical necessity

Medicare

Medicare Severity Diagnosis Related Groups (MS-DRG)

Medigap (MG)

member

national provider identifier (NPI)

noncovered

nonparticipating provider

participating provider

Patient Protection and Affordable Care Act (PPACA)

personal injury protection (PIP)

point-of-service (POS)

preauthorization

preexisting condition

preferred provider organization (PPO)

premium

prepaid plan

primary care provider (PCP)

primary payer

primary policy

private health insurance

referral

relative value unit (RVU)

resource-based relative value scale (RBRVS)

secondary payer

secondary policy

third-party payer

TRICARE

UB-04

unbundling

usual, customary, and reasonable (UCR)

verification of benefits (VOB)

waiting period

workers' compensation

The purpose of medical offices is to provide needed health care services to patients. Medical offices bill insurance companies and patients to receive payment for their services. They must receive accurate payment in a timely manner to hire staff, pay bills, and continue serving patients. Insurance **claims** are bills that the medical office sends to insurance companies, on behalf of patients, for medical services. Preparing insurance claims accurately is vital to the success of any medical practice. To continue serving patients, medical offices must operate as a business, including collecting payment for services.

This chapter is presented in three sections:

- *Health Insurance Policies* describes the past, present, and future development of health insurance in our country, provides an overview of policy provisions and terminology, and introduces the types of health insurance plans and types of insurance coverage.

- *Health Insurance Payers* introduces the various types of government and private payers as well as disability policies. The role of state insurance commissioners is also discussed.

- *Health Insurance Claims* walks medical assistants through the details of gathering accurate patient information and preparing the CMS-1500 claim form, both on paper and electronically.

HEALTH INSURANCE POLICIES

Medical assistants are best able to assist their patients to understand their health insurance when they have a good understanding of this complicated field. Insurance provides protection against or compensation for specific types of risk, loss, or ruin. It is a contract in which an insurance company agrees to pay a sum of money to the insured in the event of a defined contingency, such as death, accident, or illness, in return for the payment of a premium by the insured. Health insurance was not designed to cover all costs associated with health care but rather to assist the patient with expenses incurred for medical treatment. This section reviews the changing role of health insurance, introduces common health insurance terminology, describes the types of insurance plans, and summarizes the type of services covered under insurance.

The History and Purpose of Health Insurance

Because health insurance began over 150 years ago, in its original form, it bears little resemblance to the modern array of plans and services. Health insurance in the United States began in the mid-1800s as disability income insurance, when insurance was used to replace the income of people injured in accidents or ill from certain diseases. The first group policy giving comprehensive benefits was offered by Massachusetts Health Insurance of Boston in 1847. Insurance companies issued the first individual disability and illness policies around 1890.

As medical care advanced in the early 1900s, there was a greater need for insurance that covered hospital expenses. Hospital insurance coverage began in 1929 when a group of schoolteachers in Texas formed a contract with a local hospital to guarantee up to 21 days of hospital care for a premium of $6 per year. This plan became popular, and other groups of employers joined the plan, which eventually became known as the Blue Cross Plan.

Employee benefit plans became popular in the 1940s and 1950s. The unions that represented large groups of workers bargained for better benefit packages, including tax-free, employer-sponsored health insurance.

During the 1950s and 1960s, government programs began to cover health care costs. In 1965, the federal government enacted two programs for health care reimbursement: Medicare, designed for the elderly, and Medicaid, targeted to low income families. These two programs marked a substantial infusion of funding to the health care system, which became a major force in the expansion of health care services in the decades that followed.

The 1970s and 1980s saw a rapid rise in the cost of health care as a result of advancing technology and funding from Medicare and Medicaid. Congress passed the federal HMO Act of 1973, which allowed the use of federal funds and policy to promote health maintenance organizations (HMOs), which provide managed care to participants. **Managed care** is intended to reduce inefficiencies in medical care and thus provide better care at a lower cost. Soon, the majority of employer-sponsored group insurance plans moved from the traditional insurance plans they had previously provided to the less expensive managed care plans. In the 1980s, a new hospital payment program called Diagnosis Related Groups (DRG) was implemented by Medicare to help control spending.

By the mid 1990s, most Americans who had health insurance were enrolled in managed care plans. Many insurance companies had adopted hospital payment programs based on DRGs. By the end of 1995, individuals and companies paid for about half the health care received in the United States with the government paying for the other half through Medicare, Medicaid, and other programs.

In contrast to other industrialized countries in which governments finance health care and oversee the delivery system, Americans must find their own source of health insurance or apply for government programs if they qualify.

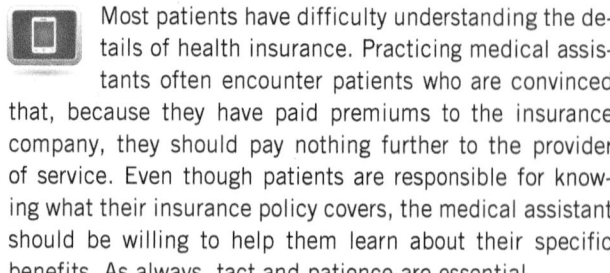

About 60 percent of Americans have health insurance through an employer-sponsored plan.

Despite the many options available for health insurance, it is estimated that 45 to 50 million Americans have no health insurance coverage. Often this is because individuals do not have or do not qualify for employer-based coverage, do not qualify for federal programs, and cannot afford individual policies. For these patients, many offices establish a sliding fee scale that charges fees based on a patient's financial ability to pay. Some cities also have free or low-cost clinics established and run by volunteers or not-for-profit agencies.

The Patient Protection and Affordable Care Act

In 2010, Congress passed the **Patient Protection and Affordable Care Act (PPACA),** also referred to as the Affordable Care Act (ACA) and Obamacare, because it was passed under the administration of President Barack Obama. PPACA represents the most significant reform of the health care system since Medicare and Medicaid were established. The goal of PPACA is to help decrease the number of uninsured Americans and reduce the overall costs of health care.

PPACA established the **health insurance exchange (HIE)** to create a more organized and competitive market for buying health insurance. HIEs are organizations that offer a choice of health insurance plans, certify the plans that participate, and provide consumer information regarding options. They primarily serve individuals buying insurance on their own and small businesses with up to 100 employees. Each state may establish its own HIE or may opt, instead, to allow the federal government to establish and operate it for the residents of that state. Each state's department of insurance provides information about HIEs available on the Internet and identifies whether the state sponsors its own HIE or whether residents should use the federal site (www.HealthCare.gov).

As of 2014, PPACA requires most people to have health insurance and requires them to pay a tax penalty if they do not. This is commonly known as the **individual mandate**

because it requires individuals, rather than organizations, to acquire the insurance. PPACA also expanded the income criteria for who is eligible for Medicaid, the government program for low-income families. If all states implement the expansion, an additional 21.3 million individuals could gain Medicaid coverage by 2022, a 41 percent increase. As PPACA got underway, some states had implemented the expansion of Medicaid although others had not.

With the cost of health care and health insurance coverage rising far beyond the rate of inflation in America, most experts agree that the U.S. health care system will have to change dramatically in the future. PPACA is expected to have a significant impact on health care delivery and health insurance in the years to come. It should decrease the number of uninsured people, improve health outcomes, streamline health care delivery, and increase overall expenditures on health care. However, the exact impact of PPACA is unknown and will be experienced over the course of many years. Also, further changes to the health care system are likely to occur in the future.

The Role of Medical Assistants in Health Insurance Claims

Medical assistants play a vital role in the health insurance claims process in the medical office. Not only do they help gather information from patients, they must be able to answer patients' questions regarding how health insurance works and how amounts owed are determined for any given procedure. Medical assistants must also be able to verify patients' insurance coverage and explain that coverage to the patients. In addition, medical assistants must know how to prepare health insurance claims accurately, follow up on past-due claims, and pursue unpaid amounts.

Developing skills in this area enables the medical assistant to be an advocate for patients, helping them obtain the benefits they are eligible for and helping them understand the reasons why a cost is not covered.

Just as in other areas of medical assisting, the medical assistant's involvement in the insurance billing area depends on the type of practice. In a large physician's office, a separate department often handles most of the insurance matters. In a smaller office, the medical assistant may have more responsibilities in this area. Regardless of the type or size of office, in every situation, the medical assistant is a vital team player who helps patients access their insurance benefits.

Policy Provisions and Terminology

Just as medical assistants need to understand medical terminology to work in a medical office, a knowledge of insurance terminology is critical to helping patients use their health insurance policies. In many situations, there are multiple terms that essentially have the same meanings. In other situations, terms that seem similar to the layperson have different and specific meanings in the world of health insurance. It is important to become familiar with the variations most common in your geographic area. Patients often are unfamiliar with their insurance benefits and may not understand the terms they hear. Medical assistants who understand insurance terms can advocate for patients and communicate in ways that patients understand.

Members and Their Families

Health insurance, also called medical insurance, is a contract between an insurance carrier and the person who owns the insurance policy, known as the **member**, subscriber, insured, or policyholder. For those who receive insurance through their employers, the member is the employee. For those who buy individual policies, the member is the person who purchased the plan. For those covered by government policies, the term **beneficiary** often is used and refers to the individual who qualifies for the program. **Verification of benefits (VOB)** is the process to determine the patient's **eligibility**—that is, to determine if a patient is qualified to receive coverage/paid benefits according to the insurance policy guidelines.

Many commercial policies allow members to include family members on the plan. Family members are called **dependents** and may include a spouse or unmarried domestic partner, children, and stepchildren. Inclusion of family members is not automatic, and it is possible for members to elect to include some, but not all, family members to be covered by a policy. The member must obtain, fill out, and submit forms from the employer or the insurance company to elect, or specifically designate, dependents' coverage. The medical assistant needs to ask the patient, and possibly call the insurance company, to determine who is eligible for benefits under a given policy. It is also important to know exactly how each dependent is legally related to the member.

Members have an opportunity to update dependent coverage each year when the policy renews and under certain circumstances can make changes during the year. Therefore, it is important to verify eligibility at each visit.

Premiums

To purchase a commercial health insurance policy, the policyholder pays a **premium** to the insurance carrier. The premium is usually paid in monthly installments for the next month's coverage. In group coverage, the employer often pays the majority of the premium and employees authorize the remainder to be deducted from paychecks. If dependent coverage is selected, the premium is higher. Some government plans require a premium as well.

Fee Schedules

Health care providers establish a **fee schedule**, which lists the charge for each service they provide, such as a physical exam or a flu shot. A fee schedule is normally organized by type of service and **Current Procedural Terminology (CPT®) code**. CPT codes are codes established by the American Medical Association to identify specific medical, surgical, and diagnostic services. Providers can set their charges in any manner they desire; however, in most states they are required to charge the same fee to every patient and every insurance company. They cannot legally discuss their fees with other providers and use that information to set prices, a practice known as price fixing.

The charge on the fee schedule is known as the provider's usual charge. Insurance companies are not required to pay providers' usual charges. Insurers can use any method they desire to establish a payment level. The amount that insurance companies consider to be an appropriate fee is called the **allowed amount**. Physician and insurance company fees are discussed in detail later in this chapter.

Out-of-Pocket Expenses

Few health insurance plans cover 100 percent of the cost of the care patients receive, so patients are responsible for several different kinds of out-of-pocket expenses. These are medical expenses that patients are personally responsible for paying.

Deductibles. Before the insurance plan pays any benefits, patients often have a **deductible** to meet. The deductible is a monetary amount patients must pay to the provider for health care services before health insurance benefits begin to pay. There are no universal rules or laws regarding deductibles. Deductible amounts might be as low as $100 or as high as $20,000. Plans with low deductibles tend to have higher premiums than plans with high deductibles. Some government plans also have deductibles. When calculating benefits and amounts owed, subtract the deductible from the allowed charge, then apply the percentage or dollar amount covered by insurance.

In some policies the deductible may not be required for all services. A sick visit may require a deductible, but under PPACA a preventive care visit does not. This is to encourage patients to seek preventive care. When patients include family members on the policy, there is usually an individual deductible and a family deductible. The individual deductible is the maximum deductible that any given family member must pay. The family deductible is the maximum deductible for all family members combined.

Copayments and Coinsurance. After the deductible is met, most patients still have out-of-pocket expenses they must pay. **Copayments** are fixed dollar amounts that patients pay at the time of service, such as $5 or $10 per visit. **Coinsurance** is a fixed percentage of charges that patients pay. An 80/20 coinsurance plan means that the insurance company pays 80 percent of approved charges (after the deductible is met), and the patient pays 20 percent. A 70/30 plan means that the insurance company pays 70 percent of approved charges, and the patient pays 30 percent. Different types of visits or different types of providers may have different copayment or coinsurance amounts. For example, under PPACA, preventive care has no copayment or coinsurance, whereas sick care does. A specialist visit may require a higher copayment or coinsurance than a primary care visit. The specific rules are set by the insurance company and clearly spelled out in the patient's policy. Most government programs require a copayment or coinsurance.

When calculating benefits and amounts owed, first subtract the deductible owed from the allowed amount. Then, calculate the coinsurance amount by multiplying the remaining balance times the coinsurance percentage. Finally, subtract the copayment or coinsurance amount from the remaining balance. Procedure 14-1 demonstrates how to calculate the patient responsibility portion of the bill.

When medical offices bill patients' insurance, patients sign an **assignment of benefits**, which authorizes the insurance company to pay benefits directly to the provider. This helps ensure that the provider is paid in a timely manner and simplifies the billing process. If a patient refuses to sign the assignment of benefits, the insurance company should send payment to the patient. Then the patient pays the provider's bill. In this case, the medical office should consider requiring the patient to pay in full at the time of service or establish a regular payment plan. The concern is that the patient may forget about the provider's bill and spend the insurance payment on other expenses rather than paying the provider.

In managed care plans and government programs, assignment of benefits is usually part of the provider's contract and, as a result, is automatic.

Preexisting Conditions

Historically, health insurance plans had **exclusions**, rules that limited when and how much the insurance plan is required to pay in benefits. Many of these restrictions are being eliminated as a result of PPACA. Starting in 2014, all group insurance policies must offer coverage to everyone who applies, regardless of **preexisting conditions**. A preexisting condition is any condition a patient was diagnosed with or treated for, including receiving prescription medications, before beginning coverage with a new insurance plan. Health insurance companies are not allowed to charge more to people with preexisting conditions, and they also cannot exclude coverage of the condition from the insurance policy. This rule applies to group coverage, such as that offered by an employer, but not to individual policies that people purchase on their own.

HIPAA compliance. Under HIPAA, a preexisting condition is covered without a **waiting period** when the patient has been continuously insured for the 24 months before joining the new plan. This allows patients to change jobs and retain preexisting condition coverage without added waiting periods, even when they have chronic illnesses. Patients should save the HIPAA **certificate of coverage** that the previous insurance plan mails out after coverage has terminated. This letter documents the nature and length of coverage with the plan. Patients submit it to the new plan to establish proof of continuous coverage. If patients have had more than one insurance plan during the previous 24 months, they should submit certificates of coverage from each plan. Even when patients have not been insured the 24 months before joining new insurance plans, HIPAA legislation restricts insurance companies from requiring patients to wait any longer than 12 months from the dates their new insurance coverage began to begin coverage for preexisting conditions. PPACA also places restrictions on exclusions for preexisting conditions.

In 2008, the United States Congress passed the Genetic Information Nondiscrimination Act (GINA). Similar to exclusions due to preexisting conditions, this act makes it illegal for health plans to deny an individual health care coverage because that person may have a genetic predisposition to developing a disease in the future. This act also makes it illegal for health insurance companies to charge individuals higher premiums solely based on genetic predisposition. It is also important to note that this act of Congress also prohibits employers from denying hiring or promotion considerations, in addition to firing current

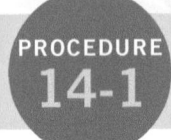

PROCEDURE 14-1

Calculating Patient Financial Responsibility

Objective ◆ *Calculate the patient's financial responsibility using the charges, deductible, coinsurance, and allowed amounts.*

EQUIPMENT AND SUPPLIES

Pen; paper; insurance verification of benefits form; patient's insurance identification card; Remittance Advice form; calculator

METHOD

1. After the patient's insurance coverage has been verified, locate the information on the verification form regarding the deductible and coinsurance amount.

   Example of Patient Benefits

Annual deductible: $100
Coinsurance: 20%.

2. Inform the patient of the deductible amount that needs to be paid after the beginning of the calendar or fiscal year, before insurance payments become effective.
3. Explain to the patient that the amount charged for any particular procedure in the medical office will likely be reduced to a lower amount, called the allowed amount, when processed by the insurance carrier.
4. After the insurance payment is received, use the remittance advice (RA) form to identify the amount the insurance carrier allowed on the claim.

   Example of Charges and Allowed Amounts Shown on RA

Service	Charges	Allowed Amount
Examination	$95.00	$72.00
X-ray	$75.00	$51.00
Laboratory work	$102.00	$80.00
Total	**$272.00**	**$203.00**

5. Calculate the total allowed amount by adding together the allowed amount for each service.
6. Subtract the deductible from the total of the allowed charges.
7. Multiply the remaining allowed amount by the coinsurance percentage to determine the patient's coinsurance amount.
8. Add the deductible to the coinsurance amount to determine the amount the patient needs to pay out of pocket for the visit.
9. Explain the figures to the patient, and collect the fees.

Example Calculation of Patient Responsibility

	Total Allowed	$203.00
	Deductible	−$100.00
(Step 6)		$103.00
(Step 7)	Coinsurance amount	$103.00 × 20% = $20.60
	Patient Responsibility	
	Deductible	$100.00
	Coinsurance	+$20.60
(Step 8)	Total Owed	$120.60

---

employees, based on their genetic predisposition for developing diseases in the future.

Medical Necessity

The fact that a physician determines that a patient needs a particular service or supply item does not mean that the insurance company or payer will agree. **Medical necessity** is the process of establishing the medical need for services or procedures provided. When billing, every procedure code billed must be associated with one or more diagnostic codes that support the need for the procedure. Coding is discussed in the chapters titled "Diagnosis Coding" and "Procedure Coding."

Medical necessity is one of several criteria payers use to determine if, and how much, they will pay for a particular service. One of the reasons that payers establish medical

TABLE 14-1 | Examples of Medical Necessity Criteria

Criterion	Appropriate Example	Inappropriate Example
Improve a patient's condition	Physical therapy to treat an acute back injury	Ongoing physical therapy to maintain general back comfort
Evidence-based practice	Medications proven to benefit patients based on scientific studies	Experimental drugs or treatments
Rendered by appropriate provider	Patient going to internal medicine or family practice physician to diagnose an initial symptom of stomach pain	Patient going directly to gastroenterologist and having many expensive tests performed to diagnose an initial symptom of stomach pain
Least restrictive setting	Suture removal in physician's office; outpatient cataract surgery	Suture removal in the emergency department; inpatient cataract surgery without a medical reason
Not for patient or physician convenience	Liposuction for medical reasons	Liposuction for cosmetic reasons

necessity rules is to avoid paying unscrupulous providers who might provide a service just so they can receive payments rather than because the patient actually needs the service or would benefit from it. It also helps prevent patients from demanding services they do not need, such as expensive tests or cosmetic surgery.

Each payer establishes its own definition of medical necessity and writes it into each insurance policy. Table 14-1 lists common criteria for medical necessity and examples of each. By law, Medicare can pay only for services that are medically necessary, which is defined as services and supplies that:

- Are needed to diagnose or treat a medical condition or improve the functioning of a malformed body member
- Meet the standards of good medical practice in the local area
- Are not mainly for the convenience of the patient or physician

In addition to a general definition of medical necessity, payers may also establish criteria for specific conditions, such as limiting the number of physical therapy visits for back pain; requiring an X-ray before ordering a more expensive MRI; or restricting the age and frequency of preventive screening, such as a screening mammogram every two years for women over a certain age. When providers recommend a treatment that varies from the insurance company's standard list, they may need to obtain preauthorization and provide special reports to justify the service. For some conditions, specific medical necessity criteria are not public information, and patients may learn of them only after a claim is denied. A **denied claim** is a claim that was processed and found to be ineligible for payment.

Insurance plans may limit coverage or require preapproval for **elective procedures**, those that are nonemergent but may benefit the patient. Emergency procedures are those that must be performed immediately to save the patient's life, limb, or vision. Elective procedures can be scheduled at a later time and include a broad range of procedures, such as back surgery, joint replacement surgery, lesion removal, vision-correction, gastric-reduction procedures, and even cosmetic surgery. Some elective procedures may be considered medically necessary, based on the patient's health condition, and others may not.

Medical assistants should not manipulate codes in a way that distorts or alters the diagnoses and procedures as documented in the medical record. This is unethical and fraudulent. Medical assistants do need to be certain they accurately describe everything that was done for the patient and the reasons for which the services were provided.

Types of Insurance Plans

Health insurance plans are classified either as indemnity plans or managed care plans. Indemnity plans impose few restrictions on patients, whereas managed care plans seek to control costs by limiting patients' choices.

Indemnity Plans

Before the 1980s, indemnity plans were common. Indemnity means to pay for the loss experienced by another person. In health insurance, indemnity plans cover a patient's health care expenses with few restrictions. Also called fee-for-service (FFS) plans, they allowed patients to seek care with any covered health care providers for any covered services. Neither the list of physicians that patients could see nor the fee schedules were prearranged. Insurance companies reimbursed health care providers the actual fee charged for each service. This practice is believed to have contributed to the rapid rise of health care costs. Indemnity plans are rare today and, if available, are among the most expensive because they do not contain managed care or cost-control measures.

Managed Care Plans

Managed care plans, also called **managed care organizations (MCOs)**, are companies that attempt to control the cost of health care while providing better outcomes. Managed care plans contract with physicians, hospitals, and other providers to offer services for a lower fee. Then they contract with government programs, private health insurance companies, and self-insured plans to promote an exclusive network of **participating providers** or preferred providers. When patients use participating providers, they are responsible for lower out-of-pocket costs for deductibles, coinsurance, and copayments than if they select a **nonparticipating provider**, one not

on the preferred list. Box 14-1 highlights advantages and disadvantages of managed care plans.

Medical assistants should inform patients whether providers participate with the patients' health plans. A provider may be participating with some patients' MCOs and nonparticipating with others. Most offices ask about health insurance coverage the first time patients call. When in doubt, ask patients for their insurance information and then call the company or research the information online.

Managed care plans are not a separate type of insurance but rather are a way of offering services to patients who are enrolled in a group health plan, self-insured plan, or individual health plan. Managed care plans also offer services to Medicare Advantage programs, Medicaid, and workers' compensation. Managed care companies are regulated primarily by federal laws. Well-known managed care plans include Kaiser Permanente, Group Health Cooperative, Anthem, and Humana.

The most common types of managed care plans are health maintenance organizations (HMOs), preferred provider organizations (PPOs), and point-of-service (POS) plans, which are described next.

Health Maintenance Organizations. **Health maintenance organizations (HMOs)** are managed care plans that cover members only when those members seek care from a list of health care providers and suppliers who have contracted with the HMO (Table 14-2). The list of approved providers is usually somewhat limited and may be restricted to a specific clinic. An open-panel HMO is one in which providers treat both HMO patients and non-HMO patients. A closed-panel HMO is one in which physicians see only the patients of a specific HMO.

Most HMOs require each patient to choose a **primary care provider (PCP)** who belongs to the network of covered providers. The primary care provider is the caretaker or **gatekeeper** and arranges for specialist services or hospitalizations. The

---

BOX 14-1 | Advantages and Disadvantages of Managed Care

Advantages

- Smaller out-of-pocket expenses for the patient
- Nominal copayment
- No deductible for some plans
- Contains health care costs
- Pays for authorized services
- Fee schedules established
- Preventive medical treatment usually covered

Disadvantages

- Increased amount of paperwork
- Preauthorization requirements
- Lower reimbursement rates
- Limited provider choices
- Renewal of coverage not guaranteed
- Specialized care limited at times
- Referrals limited at times
- Limited flexibility
- Unapproved or unauthorized treatments not covered

TABLE 14-2 | Types of Health Maintenance Organizations

Type of HMO	Description
Exclusive provider organization (EPO)	A managed care contract with a smaller network of providers under which the employer agrees to not use any other networks in return for favorable pricing.
Group model HMO	HMO in which the managed care company contracts with multispecialty groups.
Independent provider association (IPA)	An association formed by physicians with separately owned practices that contracts with managed care plans.
Network model HMO	HMO that contracts with two or more group practices, or a group practice plus a combination of staff physicians and independent physicians.
Staff model HMO	HMO in which the managed care company hires the physicians, and owns the clinic sites and possibly the hospital.

specific payment rules vary among plans, but usually, copayments and coinsurance amounts are very low, often with no deductible. When members seek care from providers not on the list, they must pay for the costs out-of-pocket.

To help make health care more cost efficient, HMOs encourage patients to take advantage of preventive health care services such as annual physicals, colonoscopies, and mammography. Under PPACA, preventive services do not have cost-sharing requirements.

HMOs are the most restrictive type of health plan because of the limited number of approved providers. However, they typically provide members with a greater range of health benefits for the lowest out-of-pocket expenses.

Preferred Provider Organizations. The **preferred provider organization (PPO)** contracts with physicians and facilities to perform services for PPO members at a lower rate than for nonmembers. The PPO gives subscribers a list of network providers whom they may see for a lower cost. They usually do not have to obtain a referral or preauthorization to see a specialist within the network. However, major medical procedures usually do require preauthorization. If a patient chooses to receive treatment from an out-of-network or nonpreferred provider, she is responsible for higher out-of-pocket expenses and, often, higher deductibles.

A PPO differs from an HMO in two ways:

- The PPO is a **fee-for-service (FFS)** program and is not based on a prepayment (also known as prospective payment) or capitation program, as is the case for the HMO. Thus, the providers and hospitals, designated as PPOs, are reimbursed for each medical service they provide.

- The PPO members or enrollees are not restricted to certain designated providers or hospitals. The PPO member may receive care from a non-PPO provider;

however, they will generally have to pay more out-of-pocket expenses when they do this.

PPOs manage cost containment in the following ways:

- They negotiate fees with providers that are less than the current market fees.

- They offer financial incentives for PPO members to use a PPO provider.

- They carefully monitor the quality and type of services offered by PPO providers.

Physicians can belong to multiple PPOs. It is also possible that not all the physicians in a medical practice belong to the same PPOs. When this occurs, medical assistants should assist patients by scheduling them with physicians who are part of their approved network.

Point of Service Plans. A **point of service (POS)** plan offers a primary HMO provider network and a secondary PPO provider network, allowing patients to choose which plan to use at the time they seek care. Out-of-pocket expenses are lowest when using HMO providers, somewhat higher when using preferred providers in the PPO, and most costly when using out-of-network providers. A POS plan provides patients with the maximum flexibility and choice when seeking services and also provides cost-effective options for those willing to use the HMO network for their care.

Types of Service Coverage

Type of coverage refers to the specific services covered under the plan. Each insurance policy is tailored to include the benefits most desired and most affordable for each group or individual. Understanding some of the most common alternatives for coverage types enables medical assistants to clarify for patients what can be expected from their policies (Table 14-3). In addition to determining the source of

TABLE 14-3 | Types of Health Insurance Service Coverage

Coverage	Description
Hospital services	Inpatient hospital care such as room and board, and facility fees for special services including operating room, radiology, and laboratory.
Physician services	Physicians' fees for hospital visits, office visits, and nonsurgical procedures.
Surgical services	Surgeon and anesthesiologist fees for surgery performed in a hospital, doctor's office, or outpatient surgical center.
Preventive care	Annual preventive care examinations, immunizations, and screening tests.
Ancillary services	Supplemental riders for prescription drugs, vision, dental, and alternative care.
Disease-specific	Supplemental insurance for specific chronic or terminal illnesses, such as cancer, heart disease, stroke, Alzheimer's disease, Parkinson's disease, multiple sclerosis, and kidney failure.
Catastrophic care	Emergency safety net to protect against unexpected, high-cost medical services only. All routine and sick care is paid out-of-pocket.

patients' insurance, medical assistants need to determine what type of coverage they have.

Medical assistants need to identify how a patient's insurance relates to the specific services being provided in a specific situation. Research, attention to detail, careful communication, and patient advocacy are skills that successful medical assistants use in the insurance arena.

Many patients have prescription drug coverage that helps pay for the cost of prescription drugs. Prescription drug coverage is an add-on plan to the main insurance policy and often has a separate deductible and different copayment or coinsurance provisions. The dispensing pharmacy, not the prescribing physician, bills the prescription drug plan. Plans typically have a **formulary**, a list of drugs approved for coverage. Usually the formulary is subdivided into two or more tiers with each tier having a different level of coverage (Figure 14-1). There may be some drugs that are not on the formulary at all. Patients need to present evidence of

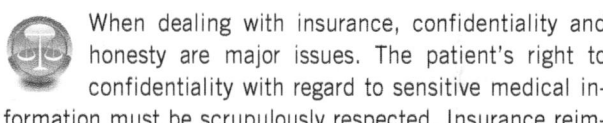

Professionalism   The Law

When dealing with insurance, confidentiality and honesty are major issues. The patient's right to confidentiality with regard to sensitive medical information must be scrupulously respected. Insurance reimbursement, as it is currently structured, provides a constant temptation to do what is necessary to recover the full amount of charges. As a successful medical assistant, be careful to release only information authorized by the patient and avoid becoming involved with insurance fraud in any manner.

medical necessity to receive coverage for nonformulary drugs. Medical assistants can advocate for patients if their plan does not cover a specific drug the provider prescribed. They can help identify potentially similar medications from the formulary or from a lower tier of the formulary that the provider could evaluate and consider prescribing for the patient. This could create a financial savings to the patient while maintaining safe and high-quality care.

HEALTH INSURANCE PAYERS

In addition to the type of managed care and the type of service coverage, a patient's insurance benefits are also determined by the type of payer. **Third-party payers** are organizations that pay for health care services on behalf of the patient. In legal terms, the physician is the first party, the patient is the second party, and the payer is the third party. Third-party payers include several government programs, over 1,300 private insurance companies, workers' compensation, and automobile "med pay" or personal injury protection (PIP) insurance.

Tier 1: Generic $10 copayment
Penicillin G Sodium
Penicillin V Sodium
Trimox

Tier 2: Preferred name brand $15 copayment
Avelox (tablet)
Timentin

Tier 3: Non-preferred name brand $30 copayment
Avelox (solution)
Penicillin G Procaine
Piperacillin Sodium
Zosyn

FIGURE 14-1 Sample tiered drug formulary for antibiotics.

Medical assistants need to understand the various types of third-party payers, because each has separate, and sometimes conflicting, rules about coding and billing.

Private Health Insurance

Private health insurance, also called commercial health insurance, is coverage for health care services offered by private corporations, such as Aetna, Cigna, or United Health Care, and not-for-profit organizations, such as Blue Cross and Blue Shield. The three major sources of private health insurance are group health plans, self-insured plans, and individual insurance. Each insurance company and each plan offered by a company may have different requirements for coding and billing. Typically, the provider's coding and billing departments maintain files on the requirements of each plan. Most laws regarding private health insurance companies are determined by each state's legislature and implemented by the state Department of Insurance. Coverage amounts and premiums vary according to policy type.

Group Insurance

Group health insurance (GHI) is a policy offered to groups of people in which the risk or cost of insurance is spread across everyone equally. Employers and unions contract with a private insurance company to provide a specific list of benefits to its employees. Group insurance is usually the least expensive type of insurance, because statistics show that a few people in a group use a large amount of services but many people in the group use few if any services. Everyone pays the same rate for protection, so the high costs of a few members are shared equally by everyone in the group. The most common groups are the employees of a company and the members of a union.

It is common for an employer to allow employees to select among a variety of benefit packages from the chosen insurance company, so two patients with the same employer and the same insurance company can have different benefits. It is important for medical assistants to determine the specific benefits available to each patient so they give patients incorrect information about benefits. Often this information is available online through the insurer's secured website or by calling the insurance company.

Ask to see the patient's insurance card at every office visit (Figure 14-2). Just because a patient had a particular type of insurance one month does not mean they have the same insurance or the same policy the next month. Scan or make a photocopy of both sides of the card and return it immediately to the patient. In addition to placing a copy of the card in the patient's chart or linking it to the electronic health record (EHR), you also may wish to write the insurance plan

FIGURE 14-2 Sample of an insurance card.

number on the patient's chart or create an electronic note in the EHR. Verify the patient's name with a form of photo identification. Compare the name on the insurance card with the name on the photo ID.

It is important to determine when coverage begins for a patient who has recently changed jobs. Employer-based coverage typically begins with the next calendar month following 30, 60, or 90 days of employment, but this time frame can vary. It is also important to determine when coverage ends for a patient leaving a job. Coverage may end the last day of employment, the end of the month, or the end of the following month. Procedure 14-2 describes how to interpret information on a patient's insurance card.

Blue Cross/Blue Shield Plans

Patients may have Blue Cross (BC) and Blue Shield (BS) plans through group health coverage or individual insurance. Historically, BC plans provided hospital service benefits and BS plans provided physician service benefits. Patients may have a BC plan, a BS plan, or a combination BCBS plan, depending on the geographic area. It is important to remember that each BCBS plan is separate and unique in terms of benefits, cost sharing, and other requirements, just as private commercial insurance companies are unique from each other.

BCBS coverage includes fee-for-service (FFS) traditional coverage, managed care plans, a federal employee program (FEP), Medicare supplemental plans, and health care anywhere plans. The type of coverage is indicated on the member ID card. Most BCBS member ID numbers begin with three letters that are a code indicating the member's home plan. It is essential to include these letters when reporting the member ID number on a claim. Because there are many types of BCBS plans, there are many types of insurance cards.

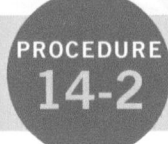

Interpreting Information on an Insurance Card

Objective ◆ *Identify information on an insurance card needed for billing.*

EQUIPMENT AND SUPPLIES

Patient insurance card; photocopy machine or card scanner

METHOD

1. Ask to see the patient's insurance card. If he has more than one insurance plan, ask for each plan's card.
2. Confirm that the card displays the patient's or policyholder's name. If the patient's spouse, or in the case of a child, parent, is the policyholder, then that person's name might be on the card instead of the patient's.
3. Scan or make a photocopy of both the front and back of the card, according to office procedures.
4. Return the card(s) to the patient and thank him.

5. On the front of the card, locate the following information:
   - Name of the insurance company and plan name
   - Member or policyholder identification number
   - Member or policyholder's name
   - Group number, if applicable
   - Primary care physician's name, if applicable
   - Copayment or coinsurance amount
6. On the back of the card, locate the following information:
   - Physician services telephone number
   - Preauthorization telephone number and instructions
   - Insurance plan website
   - Electronic claims submission number
   - Mailing address for claims

Each BCBS processes its own claims, so medical assistants need to verify the correct filing address. When the provider is contracted with a local BC or BS plan, they are usually able to submit the claim to their contracted plan, which will either process it or forward it to the sponsoring plan.

Self-Insured Plan

Self-insured health plans, also called self-funded, are offered by large employers or unions that, rather than purchasing group health insurance, set aside money in a reserve fund and pay for employees' medical expenses from the fund. States regulate how much money employers must set aside to ensure that they will have enough money to pay catastrophic (high-cost) medical expenses. An employer or labor union that self-insures does not purchase a policy through a commercial insurance company. Instead, they set aside a large pool of money, or reserve, and use that fund to reimburse employees for their health care expenses. Sometimes they contract with a third-party administrator (TPA), an outside company that processes the paperwork for claims, but any payments come from the employer's or labor union's funds, not an insurance company.

Other Sources of Coverage

Although employers are the primary source of private insurance coverage, patients have other options for

obtaining health insurance. A patient who leaves a job with group coverage may continue the insurance under COBRA (see below). Unemployed or self-employed individuals may also purchase individual coverage on their own or through an HIE.

COBRA Coverage. When employees have been covered under group insurance and leave employment, they may have the opportunity to continue the group coverage at their own expense. The premium is the same as that for the group, but because often the employer has been paying a large portion of the employees' premium, patients may be surprised at the cost of the premium. Nonetheless, the premium is usually less, and the benefits better, than an individual policy. This option allows employees to keep insurance in force until they obtain new insurance coverage. The federal **Consolidated Omnibus Reconciliation Act (COBRA)** requires employers to extend health insurance coverage at group rates, usually for up to 18 months, to any employee who is laid off, quits, or is fired, except under certain circumstances. COBRA coverage is available to employees who work for employers with 20 or more employees.

Individual Health Insurance Policies. Another type of insurance plan is the individual plan or policy, which individuals buy directly through insurance carriers. These plans are often the most expensive because group rates are unavailable.

The benefits are often not as generous as group policies, resulting in higher deductibles and other out-of-pocket expenses. The minimum level of benefit package for individual insurance policies is regulated by each state and, in some states, only a few companies offer individual policies because of restrictive requirements. Employees who have been on a COBRA plan may be able to convert to an individual policy with the same insurance company when the COBRA benefits expire, but the group rates and benefits will no longer apply.

Health Insurance Exchanges. Since 2014, private health insurance can be purchased through an HIE. The purpose of HIEs is to create an organized and competitive market for buying health insurance. They are aimed primarily at consumers purchasing insurance on their own and small businesses of up to 100 employees. HIEs offer consumers a choice of health insurance plans and certifies the plans that participate. They also provide information to help consumers better understand their options. Policies offered through HIEs must meet a minimum set of criteria and are rated as platinum, gold, silver, or bronze, each with a specific set of benefits. Each level has different premiums. Some states run their own HIEs whereas others opt to participate in the federal government-sponsored exchange. The federal government also offers technical assistance to help states with their own exchanges.

The Office of the Insurance Commissioner

Each state has an Office of the Insurance Commissioner, which is a valuable resource for both the medical office and the patient. When medical assistants or patients believe claims were incorrectly processed and appeal attempts have been fruitless, they can file formal written complaints with the state's insurance commissioner. It is important to involve patients in this process, because they are the consumers the insurance commissioner is charged with

protecting. Patients may be reluctant to appeal to the commissioner on their own initiative, because they are unfamiliar with the process. One good approach is for medical assistants to write a letter on behalf of the patient and ask the patient to sign it. Sometimes informing the insurance company that the patient intends to file a complaint with the insurance commissioner can inspire insurance carriers to review previously denied claims.

Government Insurance

The federal and state governments provide health insurance for designated groups of people, such as older adults, the disabled, military personnel and retirees, and injured workers. Each of these programs has its own eligibility requirements and benefit structure. These are entitlement programs for which beneficiaries qualify based on specific criteria. An overview of these programs follows.

Many Americans who do not have private insurance receive health insurance benefits from the state or federal government. Government programs include **Medicare**, a federal program for persons over age 65, the disabled, and end-stage renal disease (ESRD) patients; **Medicaid**, a federal/state program primarily for low income people; **TRICARE**, for active duty and retired service personnel and their families; and **CHAMPVA**, for veterans with service-related disabilities. Third-party liability plans provide coverage for injuries. These include **workers' compensation**, which provides coverage for employees for job-related injuries or illnesses, and automobile **personal injury protection (PIP)**, which pays for injuries sustained because of an automobile accident. PIP insurance is required in most states and is offered by private insurance companies.

Medicare

Medicare (MCR), established in 1965, is a federal program that provides health insurance for approximately 43 million Americans, including people aged 65 and older, patients who have been disabled for more than 24 months, and patients with end-stage renal disease (ESRD). Medicare is the single largest payer of health care services in the United States.

The program is administered by the **Centers for Medicare & Medicaid Services (CMS)**, formerly known as the Health Care Financing Administration (HCFA). CMS contracts with private companies called Medicare Administrative Contractors (MACs) to educate and work with providers, process claims, and perform other functions.

All members receive Medicare identification cards that list their names, identification numbers, plans (Part A, Part B, or both), and effective dates (Figure 14-3).

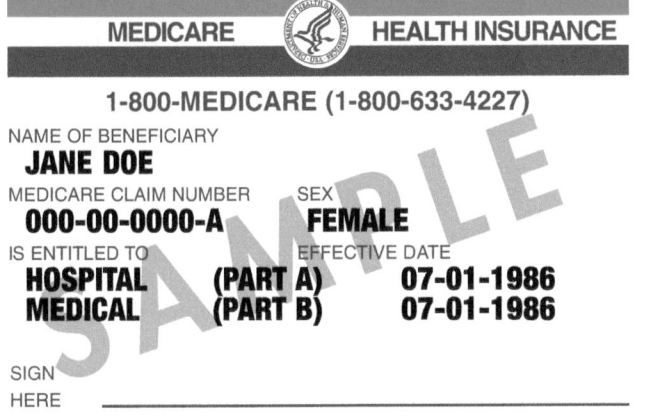

FIGURE 14-3 Sample Medicare identification card.

Medicare claims should be submitted within 365 days of date of service. Claims submitted later than that are denied with no appeal rights. Therefore, it is very important to be certain that all service information is entered into the billing system immediately so that claims can be prepared. If there is any missing information, the medical office needs a procedure, such as a tickler file or exception report, to flag these claims and ensure that the needed information is obtained and entered into the billing system and that the claim is submitted as soon as possible. Although 365 days seems like a long time to file a claim, when information is missing, it is easy to set the claim aside and forget about. If the filing deadline is missed, the claim will not be paid and the medical office will lose the reimbursement. Patients cannot be personally billed if a claim is denied because it was not submitted on time.

There are a few exceptions to the 365-day filing rule. When Medicare is the secondary payer and the primary payer issues payment directly to the beneficiary, but the beneficiary has not provided the primary payment information necessary to file the secondary claim, an extension might be granted. When a third payer is involved, additional time might be allowed. Certain other unusual services that are reviewed by the MAC might qualify for an extension as well. Be sure to identify these claims and clarify the billing procedure and timeframes with the MAC well before the 365-day deadline.

The Medicare program has major component parts called Part A (hospital insurance), Part B (provider coverage), Part C (Medicare Advantage), and Part D (prescription drug).

Participating Providers. Medicare must accredit any health care providers who wish to participate in its program in a process very similar to the application process of a managed care plan. Because most health insurance plans follow Medicare's lead when it comes to accreditation and fee schedules,

it is crucial for medical assistants or office managers to stay up-to-date by consulting Medicare's published guidelines or website. As of July 2005, Medicare requires most medical offices to file medical claims electronically. Clinics with 10 or fewer full-time employees may be allowed to continue to bill claims on paper.

Medicare Part A. Medicare Part A coverage is hospital insurance that covers most care for patients in the following settings or who receive certain specialized services:

- Inpatient hospital (for up to 90 days in a given period of time)
- Skilled nursing facility (SNF) (facility for long-term care where patients must be monitored by nursing staff regularly) for given periods
- Home (medical care)
- Hospice care at home or in a hospice facility (comfort care provided to patients who have six or fewer months to live)
- Inpatient psychiatric treatment
- Respite care (care provided in a skilled nursing facility on a short-term basis for patients normally treated at home).

Citizens who receive Social Security benefits are automatically enrolled in Medicare Part A benefits with no premiums. Those who do not qualify for Social Security may purchase Medicare Part A by paying a premium. Patients owe deductibles and coinsurance for most services in Part A.

Medicare Part B. Medicare Part B covers such services as physician care, therapy, and laboratory testing on a fee-for-service basis. Because Part B is voluntary, members must pay income-based premiums to enroll. In 2016, the standard monthly premium was $104.90 for those with individual incomes of $85,000 or less and couples with income of $170,000 or less. Patients also have out-of-pocket expenses under Part B. There is an annual deductible ($166 in 2016) that increases each year and 20 percent coinsurance on most services.

EXAMPLE: *Medicare Fee Schedule (MFS)*

A participating physician sees a Medicare patient for an office visit.

Normal charge: $118.00

MFS rate: $100.00

Reimbursement is calculated as follows:

Medicare payment: $100 × 80% = $80

Patient coinsurance: $100 × 20% = $20

Contractual allowance: $118.00 − $100.00 = $18.00

The Medicare payment is sent to the physician.

One very important aspect to billing Medicare is a form called the **Advance Beneficiary Notice (ABN)** or waiver (Figure 14-4). The ABN must be signed by patients before receiving covered services that may be denied payment by Medicare. If, during the encounter, physicians recommend services that may be denied, patients need to be informed and given the opportunity to accept or decline the service, knowing they are obligated to pay if Medicare does deny it. If patients do not understand that Medicare could deny the service, they are not obligated to pay for it and cannot be billed for it. Medical assistants are vital to facilitating this, because they are the link between the medical care and the billing rules. Medical assistants need to review the ABN with the patient and obtain a signature before the service is provided. The ABN notifies patients that the service may not be paid by Medicare, and patients agree to be responsible for payment. Medicare does not allow the ABN to be completed after the service is provided.

To understand when the ABN is needed, it is important to understand how Medicare classifies its services. **Noncovered** services are those that are not eligible for reimbursement under any circumstance and do not require an ABN to be completed. **Covered** services are those potentially eligible for reimbursement; however, they are not automatically paid. Covered services must meet medical necessity and other criteria, such as frequency, to be paid. If services do not meet these criteria, Medicare payment may be denied. It is the providers' responsibility to become familiar with what covered services may be denied under what circumstances, based on their specialty. The ABN must be specifically written to identify each patient's particular circumstance and service.

EXAMPLE: *ABN*

Medicare limits how often B-12 injections are given, depending on the diagnosis. In a particular situation, the physician may recommend more than the stipulated number of injections, believing the patient will receive the most benefit. The medical assistant asks the patient to sign the ABN and agree to pay for the additional injection if Medicare denies payment.

Medicare has very specific rules about what services can be billed together. For example, Medicare will not pay for an office visit and an injection on the same day unless the office visit was clearly a distinct service, such as a physical examination. Many surgical procedures are bundled, meaning that multiple procedures are covered with one charge. For example, a surgeon who performs an abdominal hysterectomy (removal of the uterus) with oophorectomy (removal of the ovaries) and salpingectomy (removal of the fallopian tubes)

must bill one charge only, which includes all three procedures. To bill this as three separate services is called **unbundling**, which is considered fraud.

Medicare Part C: Advantage Plan. Medicare Part C is managed care, known as Medicare Advantage plans. Formerly known as Medicare + Choice, these plans are offered by private insurance companies and encompass Parts A, B, and, usually, D. The benefit to the patient is potentially more comprehensive care at the same or lower cost than Medicare. The disadvantage, as with any managed care plan, is that the choice of providers is limited. Patients keep their Medicare identification card and receive an additional card from the Advantage plan. Because patients might not understand the difference between the two cards, it is a good practice for medical assistants to ask patients if they belong to an Advantage plan or have another identification card. When billing, the claim is sent to the Medicare Advantage plan, not the MAC.

Medicare Part D. Medicare Part D coverage, also called prescription drug coverage, is offered by private insurance companies through contracts with Medicare and provides limited benefits for prescription drugs. Patients choose from a variety of private plans, each of which may cover different medications, and select the one that covers the majority of their most costly prescriptions. Patients pay premiums, deductibles, and coinsurance. Members covered by Medicare may opt to purchase Part D coverage, which covers both name-brand and generic prescription drugs at participating pharmacies. Not all drugs are covered under every plan, so patients need to determine which plans cover their most common or most expensive medications.

Medical assistants can assist patients by providing them with complete medication lists. The Medicare website for patients, www.medicare.gov, has a prescription drug plan finder tool to assist patients to evaluate their options. Medicare Part D has an annual deductible, copayments or coinsurance, a maximum benefit level, and a stop loss for patients who have out-of-pocket costs over a certain level. The deductible and stop loss levels are updated annually.

Medigap Plans. **Medigap (MG)** is a private insurance policy that supplements Medicare coverage, to fill "gaps" in Part A and Part B coverage. In most states, patients choose from 10 standardized plans labeled Plan A through Plan N (some letters are no longer used). Medigap policies are used only with Original Medicare, but not with Medicare Advantage plans. All Medigap plans cover the patient's coinsurance. Each type of Medigap plan (A–N) covers different expenses, such as coverage of deductibles for Parts A

A. Notifier:

B. Patient Name: **C. Identification Number:**

Advance Beneficiary Notice of Noncoverage (ABN)

NOTE: If Medicare doesn't pay for **D.** _____ below, you may have to pay.
Medicare does not pay for everything, even some care that you or your health care provider have good reason to think you need. We expect Medicare may not pay for the **D.** _____ below.

D.	E. Reason Medicare May Not Pay:	F. Estimated Cost

WHAT YOU NEED TO DO NOW:
- Read this notice, so you can make an informed decision about your care.
- Ask us any questions that you may have after you finish reading.
- Choose an option below about whether to receive the **D.** _____ listed above.
  Note: If you choose Option 1 or 2, we may help you to use any other insurance that you might have, but Medicare cannot require us to do this.

G. OPTIONS: Check only one box. We cannot choose a box for you.
☐ **OPTION 1.** I want the **D.** _____ listed above. You may ask to be paid now, but I also want Medicare billed for an official decision on payment, which is sent to me on a Medicare Summary Notice (MSN). I understand that if Medicare doesn't pay, I am responsible for payment, but **I can appeal to Medicare** by following the directions on the MSN. If Medicare does pay, you will refund any payments I made to you, less co-pays or deductibles.
☐ **OPTION 2.** I want the **D.** _____ listed above, but do not bill Medicare. You may ask to be paid now as I am responsible for payment. **I cannot appeal if Medicare is not billed**.
☐ **OPTION 3.** I don't want the **D.** _____ listed above. I understand with this choice I am **not** responsible for payment, and **I cannot appeal to see if Medicare would pay.**

H. Additional Information:

This notice gives our opinion, not an official Medicare decision. If you have other questions on this notice or Medicare billing, call **1-800-MEDICARE** (1-800-633-4227/**TTY:** 1-877-486-2048).
Signing below means that you have received and understand this notice. You also receive a copy.

I. Signature:	J. Date:

Form CMS-R-131 (03/11)   Form Approved OMB No. 0938-0566

FIGURE 14-4 Advance Beneficiary Notice Form (ABN).

and B, skilled nursing facility coinsurance, foreign travel, and other specific expenses. Patients need to select the policy that best meets their personal needs. Medigap is billed after Medicare has determined its portion of the payment. Medical assistants should ask patients if they have a Medigap policy so that information can be included on the billing to Medicare.

Medicare and Other Health Insurance (OHI). Patients may have other health insurance (OHI) in addition to Medicare. CMS requires providers to be vigilant in determining when Medicare is obligated to pay first and when they are the **secondary payer**. These are known as Medicare Secondary Payer (MSP) rules. When Medicare is the secondary payer, they pay a lower portion of the bill than when they are the **primary payer**. Medicare provides a detailed questionnaire on the CMS website that medical assistants should review with patients to determine MSP. In general, Medicare is primary to Medicaid and secondary to most other insurance, including workers' compensation, liability, and TRICARE, or when covered by a spouse's group health policy.

Medicare and Locum Tenens

A *locum tenens* (a Latin term meaning "place holder") physician is one who substitutes for a patient's regular physician during that physician's absence, such as illness or vacation. This substitute physician is not part of the regular physician's medical practice and generally has no practice of his or her own but, rather, moves from one practice to another to fill in for absent physicians. There are medical staffing agencies that specialize in providing *locum tenens* physicians for a medical practice's short-term needs. Medicare provides specific criteria that must be met to allow the medical practice to bill and receive payment for services provided by the *locum tenens* physician as though the regular physician performed the services. (When the criteria are met, append modifier -Q6 to the procedure code on the CMS-1500 form for the

service(s) provided by the *locum tenens* physician.) (Modifiers are discussed further in the chapter titled "Procedure Coding.") The regular physician pays the substitute physician directly for services provided. This process streamlines the billing for both physicians.

Medicaid

Medicaid (MCD) coverage is a health benefit program for low-income patients. CMS establishes the general plan requirements, but states have considerable latitude in determining eligibility and coverage rules. The federal government provides funds to every state, and every state adds its own funds to cover qualified enrollees.

Medicaid programs offer coverage on a month-to-month basis in most states, which means that just because Medicaid covered the patient in a previous month, it doesn't mean that the patient is covered this month. *Medical assistants must verify Medicaid eligibility each month the patient comes in.* Many states provide patients with identification cards that medical offices can swipe through a card reader to verify a patient's current eligibility. Some states provide electronic or online verification. If the patient is new to Medicaid or the state does not provide for electronic verification, a paper coupon is presented at the time of service. Because every state runs its own Medicaid program, identification cards or coupons differ.

JUDGMENT CALL

It is the second day of the month, and Johanna Sparks has arrived for a follow-up appointment regarding her blood pressure. When Miriam, the receptionist, asks for a copy of Johanna's insurance card, the patient states she does not have it with her. The patient was seen last week for her six-week postpartum visit and presented her Medicaid card at that time. Ms. Sparks asks why Miriam cannot just use the copy of the card from last week. What should Miriam do?

Low-income older adult or disabled patients often have both Medicare and Medicaid coverage. Medicare is always primary in these cases, and Medicaid is secondary. Often, Medicare's reimbursement rate is higher than what Medicaid allows, resulting in no Medicaid payment. When physicians accept assignment of benefits from both Medicare and Medicaid, or participate in both programs, those physicians must accept what the two agencies together pay as payment in full for covered services. They cannot balance bill, which is charging patients for amounts not covered by insurance. In these cases, balance billing is illegal. To do so can result in fines and removal from the Medicare and Medicaid programs as a participating provider.

If you are working for a Medicaid provider, you should become familiar with your state's Medicaid identification card and eligibility verification system, because these tools provide critical information about patients' coverage, eligibility, and financial responsibility.

TRICARE

TRICARE, formerly called CHAMPUS, is a federal program that provides health care benefits to families of current and retired military personnel. The active duty service member is called a sponsor. Eligible family members are called beneficiaries. To be eligible for TRICARE, sponsors and beneficiaries must be enrolled in the Defense Enrollment Eligibility Reporting System (DEERS).

TRICARE offers three plans, each with different types of benefits:

- TRICARE Standard, a fee-for-service plan
- TRICARE Extra, a PPO
- TRICARE Prime, an HMO

All TRICARE enrollees are automatically enrolled in TRICARE Standard and TRICARE Extra. Most patients with TRICARE Standard and TRICARE Extra owe copayments and deductibles. TRICARE Prime is an optional plan that enrollees must specifically enroll in and requires no copayments or deductibles. Medical assistants should be alert to the fact that TRICARE's deductible year begins October 1.

TRICARE requires participating providers to submit claims within 60 days of the date care was provided. Nonnetwork providers have up to one year from the date the care was provided to submit claims.

CHAMPVA. The Civilian Health and Medical Program of the Veterans Administration (CHAMPVA) is a federal program that covers the health care expenses of the families of veterans with total, permanent, service-related, covered disabilities and the spouses and dependent children of veterans who died in the line of duty. Patients with CHAMPVA coverage may use any civilian health care provider, without preauthorization.

If a patient has other coverage besides CHAMPVA, the other coverage should be billed first. By law, CHAMPVA is always the secondary payer, with the following exceptions: Medicaid, State Victims of Crime Compensation, and supplemental CHAMPVA policies.

Third-Party Liability Insurance

Third-party liability insurance is insurance in which someone other than the patient is ultimately responsible for the medical bills, usually because of injury or negligence. The most common of these are workers' compensation insurance and property and casualty insurance.

Workers' Compensation Insurance

Workers' compensation (WC) insurance covers employees injured in the workplace or suffering from a workplace-related illness. Occupational injuries are those that occur during the course of employment, but do not have to occur on company property or while work duties are being performed. WC covers accidents that occur off-site, such as while driving on company business or at a remote work site, and those that occur during a paid break. Occupational illnesses are conditions that arise from short- or long-term exposure to a workplace hazard or condition, such as dust, chemical allergens, radiation, repetitive motion, and loud noises.

All employers must offer WC, except in Texas. Each state establishes its own requirements for WC insurance but must comply with federal minimums. Insurance can be obtained from a state-managed fund, private insurers, or self-insured by the employer. Some states do not allow private insurers to offer workers' compensation policies, so coverage must be obtained from the state or through self-funding. Federal laws cover workers in Washington, DC, coal miners, federal employees, and maritime workers.

A workers' compensation claim is initiated by filing the First Report of Illness or Injury. The First Report describes the circumstances of the illness or injury, the expected plan of care, and expected prognosis. Most states have a specific form that must be used for the First Report. Medical assistants need to be familiar with how the filing process works in their state.

Benefits to the injured worker include coverage of the cost of medical care related to the illness or injury, wages for time lost from work because of illness or injury, death benefits for survivors when the accident is the cause of the worker's death, and rehabilitation or retraining benefits that enable the worker to return to work or learn a different line of work if necessary.

WC has three types of claims:

- Nondisability (ND) claim—One in which the worker was injured and treated by a physician, but no time was lost from work

- Temporary disability (TD) claim—One in which the worker is able to return to previous or modified work at a later time

- Permanent disability (PD) claim—One in which no further improvement is expected and the worker is unable to return to work

To ensure the program runs properly, health care providers must keep good records on workers' compensation cases. This includes verifying patients' injuries with employers and contacting insurance companies to obtain claim numbers and verify the date of injury on file. Medical assistants must become familiar with their state requirements for preauthorization. They should also create new medical records

and financial records for patients with work-related injuries, to maintain confidentiality and keep reporting and claim filing accurate. The labor department of most states provides free physician reporting forms and claim information for injured workers.

Property and Casualty Insurance

Property and casualty insurance is insurance on homes, cars, and businesses. The "property" portion protects the policyholder (person or business) against the loss of or damage to physical property they own. The "casualty" portion protects the policyholder against legal liability for losses caused by injury to others, including medical expenses of those injured. When patients are injured in an accident involving automobiles, watercraft, and private or public property, they may file a claim with a property and casualty (P/C) insurance company.

The most common form of P/C insurance that medical assistants encounter is automobile insurance. Automobile insurance policies often include medical payments ("med pay") coverage or personal injury protection (PIP), which pays for medical expenses incurred as the result of an automobile accident. However, they may also encounter P/C insurance for boating and personal watercraft accidents and any type of injury caused by the negligence of another person or entity.

P/C insurance is regulated by each state's Department of Insurance, not by federal or HIPAA laws that govern health insurance companies. P/C companies tend to have specialized requirements and their own forms for submitting claims. They often contract with external bill review companies to review medical claims and recommend payment amounts. Medical assistants should keep a file of these requirements for each P/C company they deal with.

Professionalism   The Law

Workers' compensation programs and automobile injury policies are not HIPAA-defined health plans. Separate rules established by each state govern these types of claims. By filing a WC claim, the patient automatically authorizes the release of medical information related to the injury to be released to process the claim. However, be careful to not release information about any other illnesses or injuries. It is a good idea to establish a separate medical record (electronic- or paper-based) and a separate financial record for injury claims of an established patient, to make it easier to keep the information separate.

Short- and Long-Term Disability Income Insurance

Disability income (DI) insurance reimburses a patient for lost wages because of a nonwork-related disability that prevents the individual from working. Disability income insurance is offered by federal, state, and private sources. Benefits are based on a percentage of employees' wages, often 66 percent, because benefits are not subject to income tax. Lost wages because of a work-related disability are covered by workers' compensation insurance; lost wages because of a disability related to an automobile or other liability accident are covered by liability insurance.

Short-term disability provides coverage for a brief period of lost wages immediately following the inability to work. Policies might have a short waiting period—for example, five to ten days—before benefits begin. Benefits typically are paid for anywhere from 60 days to one year, although the exact time frames are determined by each state and each insurance plan. It is intended as temporary income replacement until long-term disability begins.

Long-term disability provides coverage for a longer period of lost wages. Typically there is a waiting period—or elimination period—lasting from 60 days to two years before benefits are paid. Policies vary regarding how long benefits are paid, ranging anywhere from one year to life.

With only a few exceptions, disability insurance does not pay for medical treatment; therefore, medical assistants do not often bill a disability plan for medical services. However, medical assistants may need to assist patients who are applying for disability coverage or benefits by providing information from the medical record regarding a patient's past health history or current disability. Even though patients have disability insurance, they may not have medical coverage because they are not employed and cannot afford or are not eligible for individual health insurance policies.

Family Medical Leave Act

The Family Medical Leave Act (FMLA) is federal legislation that entitles eligible employees of covered employers to take unpaid leave for specified family and medical reasons. Group health insurance coverage must be continued under the same terms and conditions as if the employee had not taken leave. In addition, the employee's job is protected during leave. As a result, some patients might be on a qualified FMLA leave from employment and still have group health insurance coverage during this time. Eligible employees are entitled to 12 or 26 work weeks of leave in a 12-month period, depending on the specific circumstances. To qualify for FMLA, patients must submit evidence of the medical need to their employer.

Patients applying for FMLA will provide the medical office with a form to be completed and signed documenting the patient's need.

Working with Fee Schedules

As a result of the growth of managed care and ongoing concerns about controlling health care costs, insurance companies use a variety of methods to determine how much to pay providers. Medical assistants need to understand how the payment method impacts the medical practice.

Physician Fee Schedules

Providers may use a variety of methods in determining their fee structure (the amount charged for each procedure performed). Physicians are free to set their fees at any level they believe fairly reflects the cost of providing a service and the value of their professional judgment and skill. The most common methods used to establish fees are charge-based fees and resource-based fees.

Charge-Based Fee Schedules. A charge-based fee schedule is determined by comparing the fees that other providers charge for similar services. To determine how their fees for specific services compare with other providers of the same specialty, they may purchase information from a nationwide fee database. For each procedure code, the database reports the average fee amounts, as well as the highest and lowest amount, charged by similar providers within a ZIP code region. It shows the percentage of providers with charges above or below that amount. Based on this research, providers can decide if their fees should be on the high, low, or midpoint of the range.

Resource-Based Fee Structures. Resource-based fee structures, also called relative value systems (RVS), are determined objectively, based on the factors that contribute to a provider's costs. Three types of costs are considered:

- Work—The difficulty level for the provider to perform the procedure
- Practice expense—The amount of office overhead involved in the procedure
- Malpractice—The relative risk that the procedure presents to the patient and the provider

These cost elements, also referred to as the **relative value unit (RVU)**, are added together to determine the fee for a particular procedure.

Medicare's Resource-Based Relative Value Scale. The Medicare physician fee schedule (MPFS) is a list of approved Medicare fees for each procedure. The **resource-based relative value scale (RBRVS)** is Medicare's relative value system formula. Medical offices receive a comprehensive MPFS from Medicare each year that is usually programmed into the computer system, so medical assistants do not normally need to calculate individual fees. However, it can be helpful to have a basic understanding of how Medicare determines its fees.

The RBRVS formula has three components:

- National relative value unit (RVU)
- Geographic adjustment factor (GAF)
- National uniform conversion factor (CF)

The RVU reflects the type of work a physician does, office overhead expense, and the cost of the provider's medical malpractice insurance. An RVU of 1.0 represents the average procedure. A more complicated procedure has a higher RVU, and a less complicated service has a lower RVU. The second component of RBRVS, the GAF, considers the area of the country in which a physician practices, adjusting higher or lower based on that area's cost of living. The third component of RBRVS, the CF, is a dollar amount used to convert the RVU and GAF for each service into the price that Medicare allows. Each year, Medicare adjusts the CF according to the cost-of-living index.

The RBRVS formula helps ensure that Medicare providers are reimbursed equally for the same service, with appropriate adjustments for costs in various parts of the country.

Insurance Plan Fee Schedules

Insurance companies are not obligated to pay the amount the physician charges and usually establish their own reimbursement schedules. Before agreeing to participate with any insurance plan, health care providers should review the reimbursement schedules the managed care companies provide in detail. After contracts are in place, physicians have little leverage to adjust payment amounts and may find that some, or all, fees are lower than they can afford to accept. Insurance companies may adopt a reimbursement schedule based on provider fees, or they may use a risk-based approach.

Fee-Based Reimbursement. Fee-based reimbursement determines the payment amount in relation to the provider's published fee schedule. Most commonly, this is determined based on the usual, customary, and reasonable (UCR) fee or based on a negotiated discount. The most traditional reimbursement method is a UCR schedule maintained by each insurance company. The insurer is not required to publicize its UCR, so the practice learns by experience the amount each company approves.

An insurance company calculates what it determines to be an average or customary price among providers of the same specialty and in the same geographic area. This is the approved or allowed amount. When a provider's actual charge is less than the allowed amount, the insurer calculates payment based on the actual charge. Providers cannot increase their charge for a given service to selected insurance companies to receive higher payment. When providers' charges are more than the insurance allowed amount, the insurance calculates payment based on the allowed amount. This method of determining insurance payments is **usual, customary, and reasonable (UCR)**.

- The *usual fee* is what a physician usually charges for a procedure or service.
- *Customary* refers to the fee charged for the same procedure by the majority of physicians with the same or similar training. This fee is also based on the socioeconomic and geographical area.
- A *reasonable* fee is what a physician charges for a modified procedure or service that is more difficult and requires more time and effort than a standard procedure.

Insurance companies that use the UCR method allow the lowest of the usual, customary, or reasonable fee. When calculating benefits and amounts owed, the first step is to identify the allowed charge.

A common reimbursement method of PPOs is a negotiated fee schedule. The managed care plan develops a list of fees for providers that they agree to accept. Fees may be determined based on a percentage of the provider's usual fee (for example, 80 percent) or may be arrived at through negotiation.

Risk-Based Reimbursement. Risk-based reimbursement methods are those in which the provider shares responsibility for minimizing the cost of care. Insurance companies believe this type of reimbursement discourages physicians from ordering unnecessary or costly procedures. The disadvantage is that it may also discourage physicians from providing medically necessary services because of potential financial penalties.

Capitation. The most common risk-based reimbursement for physicians is **capitation**. Capitation, which literally means "per head," pays providers a flat amount per member per month, regardless of the services the patient uses. If a patient comes in many times, or not at all, the provider receives the same payment. This method is most often used by HMOs. The objective of capitation is to put the responsibility and risk on the provider to manage the patient's care in a cost effective, yet medically appropriate, manner. These are also referred to as **prepaid plans**.

Per Diem. For inpatient care, a *per diem* or per day payment method might be used. The insurance company pays the facility a flat amount per day the patient is in the hospital, regardless of the services provided. This method places much cost management on the facility to provide the services that are medically appropriate because they will not be paid more if they provide unnecessary services. The risk is partially shared with the insurer, who pays more for a longer stay than a shorter one. However, there may be a maximum number of days that the insurance company pays for any given condition.

Per Case. Per case payment is also used for hospitals. Under this method, the insurance company pays the hospital a preestablished amount per patient for the entire stay, based on the patient's diagnosis, regardless of how long the patient is in or what services are provided. Medicare uses a form of per case reimbursement, called **Medicare Severity Diagnosis Related Groups (MS-DRG)**, because patients with similar conditions and care requirements are classified or grouped together and all are eligible for the same amount of reimbursement.

The details of each MCO contract are different; there are no general rules. The medical assistant needs to become familiar with the details of each contract the provider has to be sure the billing and payment are appropriate.

Most *per-diem*, per-case reimbursement methods have provisions for outliers, patients who incur costs significantly greater or less than the average amount because of complications or other medically related factors the provider cannot control. Payment for outlier cases is increased or decreased by the insurance company, based on the provider's contract.

HEALTH INSURANCE CLAIMS

There are many steps involved in converting a patient encounter into a paid insurance claim. Each step needs to be completed in a timely and accurate manner for providers to receive correct payment for their services. The exact procedures are not the same in every office, but the general process is similar. The process begins with the medical assistant gathering accurate patient information. Next, the claims must be prepared and submitted, either electronically or on paper. Finally, payments must be posted and medical assistants must follow up on unpaid claims to be sure that all monies due are received.

Gathering Patient Information

The first step in receiving proper reimbursement for insurance claims is obtaining accurate patient information or demographics. The life cycle of an insurance claim begins when the patient calls the physician to make an appointment, a patient arrives at the emergency department, or a

physician admits a patient to the hospital. Although providers do not code or bill for scheduling an appointment, the insurance process begins when providers begin collecting insurance information. When time allows, patients preregister by completing paperwork regarding their health condition and insurance before the appointment. The provider verifies eligibility with the insurance company through a telephone call or secure website to determine if the patient is covered by insurance and what services are covered or require preauthorization.

Each new patient in the medical office should complete a registration form (Figure 14-5) that is verified at each visit and updated annually. The provider verifies eligibility with the insurance company through a telephone call or secure website to determine if the patient is covered by insurance, the services covered, and preauthorization requirements.

After obtaining pertinent patient demographics, medical assistants must identify the name and birthdate of the insured. When the patient is the spouse or child of the insured, the medical assistant must ask the patient for the additional information. The assistant needs to know if the patient is covered by more than one plan. If so, the assistant then must determine which plan is primary and which is secondary.

Medical assistants must photocopy both sides of patients' insurance identification cards when patients arrive for their first visits. The front of an insurance card typically contains the name and identification number of the insured or member. Each patient is uniquely identified by a member identification number assigned by the insurance company. Patients have a different number with each separate insurance plan they may have.

The back of the card typically has the mailing address for claims and a payer number that is used when filing electronic claims. Insurance telephone numbers appear on the front or

Professionalism The Law

Patient registration forms include a place for patients to authorize the release of their medical information to process insurance claims. This is required by the CMS-1500 billing form. HIPAA allows medical offices to share patient information with insurance companies that is necessary to process the claim because such information is part of the treatment, payment, and operations provision. Patients consent to this when they receive the medical office's notice of privacy practices. Insurance claim forms give patients' names, addresses, birthdates, diagnoses, and types of treatment.

Patient Account #: V611

Allied Medical Clinic
NEW PATIENT REGISTRATION FORM
(Please Print)

Today's Date: _____   PCP: Marcus Wellman, MD

PATIENT INFORMATION

Patient's Last Name: ANDREWS	First: THERESA	Middle: L	☐ Mr. ☒ Mrs.	☐ Miss ☐ Miss/Ms.	Marital status (circle one) Single / (Mar) / Div / Sep / Wid

Is this your legal name? ☒ Yes ☐ No	If not, what is your legal name?	(Former name):	Birth Date: 06/08/1967	Age:	Sex: ☐ M ☒ F

Street Address: 4569 Avenue K, APT. 120	Social Security #: 332-49-0432	Home Phone: (972) 555-4448

P.O. Box:	City: PLANO	State: TX	ZIP Code: 12345

Occupation: CLERK	Employer: TOWN DRUG STORE	Employer Phone: (972) 555-5593

Chose clinic because/Referred to clinic by (please choose one): ☐ Dr.   ☒ Insurance Plan   ☐ Hospital

☐ Family   ☐ Friend   ☐ Close to home/work   ☐ Yellow Pages   ☐ Other

Other family members seen here: **REASON FOR THIS VISIT:** Chest Pain

INSURANCE INFORMATION
(Please give your insurance card to the receptionist.)

Person Responsible for Bill: THERESA ANDREWS	Birth Date: / /	Address (if different): SAME	Home Phone: ( )

Is this person a patient here?   ☒ Yes   ☐ No

Occupation:	Employer:	Employer Address:	Employer Phone: ( )

Is this patient covered by insurance?   ☒ Yes   ☐ No

Please indicate primary insurance: TRUSTMARK PPO	Claims Mailing Address:	P.O. Box 12345	Green Bay, WI	12345
	Phone: 800-555-9863			

Subscriber's Name: SAME AS PATIENT	Subscriber's S.S. #: 332-49-0432	Birth Date: / /	☐ M ☐ F	Group #: 2038831	Policy #: 332490432	Co-payment: $20.00

Patient's Relationship to Subscriber: ☒ Self ☐ Spouse ☐ Child ☐ Other

Name of Secondary Insurance (if applicable):	Subscriber's Name and DOB:	☐ M ☐ F	Group #:	Policy #:

Patient's Relationship to Subscriber: ☐ Self ☐ Spouse ☐ Child ☐ Other   Claims Address:

IN CASE OF EMERGENCY

Name of Local Friend or Relative (not living at same address): LUCILLE MCGOWEN	Relationship to Patient: FRIEND	Home Phone: (469) 555-2001	Work Phone: (972) 555-9648

The above information is true to the best of my knowledge. I authorize my insurance benefits to be paid directly to the physician. I understand that I am financially responsible for any balance. I also authorize ALLIED MEDICAL CENTER or the insurance company to release any information required to process my claims.

Theresa Andrews

_____   _____
Patient/Guardian Signature   Date

FIGURE 14-5 Sample new patient registration form.

back of cards. Typically, one number is for "customer or member service" and another is for "providers." Medical assistants call the latter for information on patients' coverage or claims.

Verification of Benefits

After obtaining insurance information from patients, medical assistants should verify coverage with the insurance company. To verify coverage, medical assistants contact the insurance company to determine which services are covered. They should confirm the following information and record the answers on a verification of benefits (VOB) worksheet (Figure 14-6). A similar form might be integrated into the EHR or practice management system (PMS).

Patient's Name: _____ Chart #: _____ Appt. Date: _____
D.O.B._____ Policy ID # _____ Gr# _____
Policyholder: _____ DOB: _____
Insurance Co. Name: _____ Referral# Required: ❏ No ❏ Yes
Telephone #_____ Referral #: _____
Mailing Address: _____
Employer's Name: _____
Employer's Phone #: _____
Effective Date: _____ Lifetime maximum: _____
Pre-Cert Required: ❏ Yes ❏ No

Deductible Met:
Copay _____ Deductible_____ ❏ No ❏ Yes
Pays @_____%
Exclusion/Preexisting: _____
Chief Complaint/Diagnosis: _____
Insurance Rep's Name: _____ Ext# _____
Voice Tracking #: _____ Date: _____ Time: _____
Verified by _____ Date: _____

FIGURE 14-6 Verification of benefits worksheet.

- What is the effective date of the policy?

- Who is the insured?

- Is the type of service the patient is seeking (office visit, laboratory test, X-ray, etc.) covered?

- What are the deductible, copayment, and coinsurance amounts for this service?

- Is a referral or preauthorization required for this service?

- Where should a paper claim be submitted? For electronic claims, what is the payer number?

- What is the full name and phone number of the person you spoke to?

Insurance companies might have a separate phone number for verification. The process may be completely automated or may include personally speaking with a representative. It is becoming more common for insurance companies to offer the option of verifying benefits online through a secure website, especially if the physician is a preferred provider. It is worthwhile to make arrangements to perform verification online, because it is usually faster and more convenient for medical assistants.

Verifying benefits with the insurance company is not a 100 percent guarantee of payment, because there may have been recent changes in the patient's status that have not been input into the insurance company's computer system at the time of verification, such as adding or dropping coverage. Procedure 14-3 demonstrates how to verify eligibility.

Determining Coordination of Benefits

Patients can be covered by more than one insurance plan. Most often this is because spouses each have a group health plan and each has purchased coverage for the other or that both spouses elect to cover their children under both policies. Insurance companies, in cooperation with state insurance commissioners, have established specific rules that determine which is the **primary policy**, the one billed first, and which is the **secondary policy**, the one billed second. This process of determining which company is primary and which is secondary is **coordination of benefits (COB)**. Patients do not have the option of specifying which insurance should be primary or secondary. Table 14-4 summarizes commonly used rules for determining the order of benefits.

The **birthday rule**, explained in Table 14-4, relies only on the month and day of the parent's birthday. The year is not used. The insurance commissioners of most states have agreed to use the birthday rule. If a state does not use the birthday rule, the COB rules of the plan apply. Medical assistants need to ask about this when verifying benefits.

Obtaining Authorizations and Referrals

Authorizations and **referrals** are approvals patients must receive before receiving certain services or procedures to

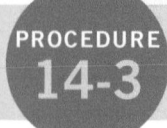

PROCEDURE 14-3   Verifying Eligibility

Objective ◆ *Verify a patient's insurance eligibility in order to determine the covered services and patient's financial responsibility.*

EQUIPMENT AND SUPPLIES

Insurance identification card; patient's registration form; insurance verification of benefits worksheet; telephone or computer; paper; pen

METHOD

1. Look at the patient's registration form to locate the patient's birthdate and the patient's relationship to the insured.
2. Look at the patient's insurance identification card to locate the name of the insured (policyholder), the insured's member identification number, and the telephone number of the insurance company.
3. Call the insurance company at the provider customer service telephone number listed on the insurance identification card or access the insurance company's secure website, if available.
4. When the customer service representative answers the call, write down the name of the customer service representative and the date and time of the call.
5. Verify the spelling of the policyholder's name and birthdate.
6. Verify the patient's name and birthdate.
7. Verify coverage for the type of service to be rendered, including frequency or number of visits.
8. Verify when preauthorization is needed.
9. Verify the patient's financial responsibility for the deductible, copayment, or coinsurance amounts.
10. Verify the coordination of benefits rules if more than one policy covers the patient.
11. Verify the provider's participating or nonparticipating status.
12. Verify the address to which insurance claims are to be mailed or the payer number needed for electronic billing.

TABLE 14-4 | Summary of Coordination of Benefits Rules

Situation	Primary Policy	Secondary Policy
Spouses or partners are covered by each other's policy	Patient's policy	Spouse's or partner's policy
Children covered by policies of both parents, married	Policy of the parent whose birthday (month and day) comes first in the calendar year (birthday rule)	Policy of the parent whose birthday comes second in the calendar year
Children covered by policies of both parents, married, who share the same birthday (month and day)	Policy that has been in force the longer length of time	Policy that has been in force the lesser length of time
Children covered by policies of two biological parents and one stepparent	Custodial parent's policy or as determined by court decree	2nd: Stepparent's policy 3rd: Noncustodial parent's policy

comply with insurance company rules. Before scheduling any nonemergency procedures or costly tests, medical assistants should call insurance carriers both to verify patients' eligibility for those services and to complete any needed **preauthorizations**. Preauthorization, called precertification by some third-party payers, is the process of contacting the patient's insurance carrier to obtain permission for patients to receive prescribed procedures. This generally involves submitting a form to the insurance company that explains the service, the reasons the patient needs it, and the anticipated cost. The insurance company reviews the request and, if approved, provides a preauthorization number that should be reported when the service is billed. Procedure 14-4 explains how to obtain authorization for a procedure.

Obtaining Insurance Company Authorizations

Objective ◆ *Obtain authorization from an insurance company for a procedure.*

EQUIPMENT AND SUPPLIES

Patient insurance information (i.e., ID number, birthdate of the insured, name and telephone number for customer service provider at the insurance company); paper and pen; description of the procedure the doctor has prescribed, including Current Procedural Terminology (CPT) code; patient's diagnosis pertaining to the needed procedure; location where procedure is to be performed (e.g., office, outpatient surgery, inpatient hospitalization); date by which the procedure must be performed

METHOD

1. Write down the date and time of the call, the name of the insurance company, and the name of the insurance company representative on the phone.
2. Give the insurance company representative your name and your office's/physician's name.
3. Give the insurance company representative the name of the patient, the name of the insured, and the insured's ID number.
4. Let the representative know what the procedure is your doctor has prescribed for the patient and the date by which the procedure must be performed.
5. Provide the representative any other requested information (e.g., procedure code, diagnosis code, place where the procedure is to be performed).
6. Write down the authorization number the representative provides.
7. Ask the representative if any supporting documentation (e.g., chart notes, operative report, laboratory report, pathology report) is needed with the CMS-1500 billing form. If so, write down the required documentation.
8. Keep all preceding information in the patient's file for reference in case the claim is not paid by the insurance carrier.

Insurance companies are required by law to have an appeals process for patients to use when a preauthorization request is denied. The medical office and patient need to communicate and work together to file an appeal and work through the progressive steps of the appeal process. Preauthorizations may be valid for a limited period of time, such as 60 or 90 days. Medical assistants should make the physician and patient aware of any such time limit, so the procedure can be scheduled in a timely manner. If patients do not receive the procedure within that time frame, a new request must be submitted.

When patients require specialist care, managed care plans may require referrals from patients' PCPs. Medical assistants who work for PCPs may be asked to arrange those specialist referrals, which entails verifying which specialists are covered under patients' managed care plans. To accomplish this task, assistants can phone insurance carriers' customer service departments or look online, understanding that online information may not be completely up-to-date. When a specialist is selected, it is a good idea to verify current participation with the specialist's office. Medical assistants in specialist offices must ensure that patients' PCPs have arranged referrals before those patients visit the specialists'

offices. Procedure 14-5 explains how to obtain a managed care referral.

HMOs may penalize physicians who fail to obtain an authorization or referral before rendering service. Many insurance carriers deny claims that are not properly

JUDGMENT CALL

Lisa Moss brings her 10-year-old son, Larry, to the clinic for an ear infection. She explains to the medical assistant, Marilou, that Larry is covered by both her and her husband's group health insurance policies. She states that her husband's policy covers preventive care at 100 percent, whereas her policy does not, because the physician is not in the plan's network. Ms. Moss asks Marilou to bill her husband's insurance policy for the visit. Marilou makes copies of both insurance cards. When she checks the birthdates, she finds that Lisa's birthdate is 2/10/1980 and her husband's birthdate is 7/25/1981.

Critical Thinking Question

1. Should Marilou accommodate Ms. Moss's billing request? How should Marilou explain the birthday rule to Ms. Moss?

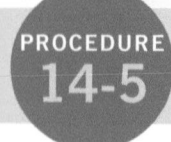

Obtaining Managed Care Referrals

Objective ◆ *Obtain a referral authorization from a managed care company.*

EQUIPMENT AND SUPPLIES

Telephone; patient's medical chart; name and telephone number of patient's primary care provider

METHOD

1. Call the patient's primary care provider's office, and ask for the person in charge of referrals.
2. Give the referral assistant the patient's information, including name and birthdate.
3. Inform the referral assistant of the need for a referral to the physician, including the reason for the patient's visit in the medical office.
4. Ask the referral assistant if any information from the patient's file is needed to process the referral.
5. Ask the referral assistant when to expect the referral. If needed, provide the office fax number for information transmittal.
6. Document the content of the telephone call in the patient's file.
7. Notify the physician and the patient of the content of the telephone call.

preauthorized. In managed care, physicians are prohibited from billing patients for services denied because of lack of authorization. In effect, the physicians perform the procedures for free. With penalties this severe, it is imperative that health care providers verify the need for referrals and authorizations before providing service.

Documenting Insurance Company Calls

Although achieving comprehensive, in-depth knowledge of all insurance plans is unrealistic, administrative medical assistants should know where to find answers and information. Many insurance companies provide coverage information online. Insurance companies' website addresses typically appear on patients' identification cards. These resources are recommended for general information, not procedure authorization. When assistants have questions about patients' insurance coverage, the best place to call is the provider customer service departments of the patients' insurance carrier.

Medical assistants should document any calls made to an insurance carrier in the patient's financial record, including date and time, telephone number used, person on the phone, reference number, and information obtained. The reference number is created by the insurance carrier's electronic system when information about the phone call is entered. If the medical assistant has to call back regarding an issue discussed during the phone call, the reference number enables the insurance carrier to quickly locate the precise record. All data

becomes part of a patient's permanent financial record and can be referenced should there ever be a discrepancy between what the medical assistant was told by the insurance carrier and how the insurance carrier processed the claim.

Preparing Health Insurance Claims

After the proper patient information has been gathered and the service has been provided, medical assistants prepare the claim to submit to the insurance company. Whether submitting claims electronically or on paper, specific guidelines must be followed.

National Provider Identifier

The **national provider identifier (NPI)** is a unique, 10-digit number assigned to health care providers by the CMS. NPI use was mandated as part of HIPAA administrative simplifications language, as of May 2007. Before that date, each health insurance company issued its own identification number. The Medicare number was the unique provider identification number (UPIN).

NPI numbers must be used by all HIPAA-covered entities when submitting health insurance claims. A covered entity is any provider who submits electronic claims to Medicare. Specialists who receive referrals from other physicians must report their own NPI number on the CMS-1500 claim form, as well as the NPI of the referring physician. Not only does each individual provider have an NPI, but the facility or medical group that bills for individual providers also has a facility or group NPI. Both the rendering provider NPI and group NPI are reported on the CMS-1500 in designated locations.

CMS-1500 Claim Form

Although most physicians submit insurance claims electronically, some smaller offices still use paper forms. Regardless of which submission method is used, the same information is required. Medical assistants must submit all paper claims using the **CMS-1500** form, a uniform billing format used for medical claims (Figure 14-7). Dental claims are prepared using the American Dental Association (ADA) standard form. The ADA form and the CMS-1500 are the only two insurance claim forms medical assistants use to submit paper claims. Effective April 2014, a new version of the CMS-1500 was required, to make the data required on paper forms consistent with the data required for electronic claims. This version of the form is officially referred to as the CMS-1500 (02/12).

The boxes to be completed on the CMS-1500 form are referred to as **Items**, blocks, or form locators. The form is divided into two major sections: Patient and Insured Information (Items 1–13) and Physician or Supplier Information (Items 14–33). The top right margin is the Carrier's Area and is used to print the insurance company's address on the form.

The National Uniform Claim Committee (NUCC), chaired by the American Medical Association (AMA), maintains and updates the CMS-1500 form. NUCC also provides specific guidelines for completing a CMS-1500 claim form that are consistent with those for preparing electronic claims. NUCC guidelines are published in the *1500 Health Insurance Claim Form Reference Instruction Manual*, which is updated each year in July and can be accessed on the World Wide Web at www.nucc.org.

TRICARE, CHAMPVA, Medicare, Medicaid, and workers' compensation carriers each have their own rules for completing the CMS-1500 form. Private insurance companies also have their own variations. Because guidelines for completing the CMS-1500 vary at the state and local levels, the medical assistant should check with the local intermediaries and private carriers. For Blue Cross Blue Shield claims, the medical assistant should refer to the provider manual for her state's Blue Cross Blue Shield plans for guidelines.

When completing the form, medical assistants abstract data, meaning they use several source documents to find the required information. It is the medical assistant's responsibility to locate all needed data on established documents and accurately transfer it to the CMS-1500 form. Medical assistants obtain most information for completing the CMS-1500

from the patient registration form, the insurance card, the encounter form (Figure 14-8), and the medical record:

- The patient registration form provides information about the patient's and insured's name, address, birthdate, and related data.

- The insurance card provides information on the insurance policy, identification number, group number, mailing address for claims, basic coverage, and copayment.

- The encounter form provides the date of service, services rendered, and treating provider. The encounter form may contain fees; if it does not, the medical assistant may need to refer to the clinic's fee schedule for charges. The encounter form or patient registration form may contain the clinic's address, tax identification number, and NPI numbers, or the medical assistant may need to refer to other office records for this information. Many names are used for the encounter form, including charge slip, routing slip, superbill, or multipurpose billing form.

- The medical record provides additional details that may not appear on the encounter form, such as the date the illness, injury, or hospitalization began, supporting documentation for the diagnosis, and procedure reports.

Medical assistants may also need to refer to the RA of a denied claim, referral forms, or other documents to complete some claims.

Table 14-5 provides general guidelines for completing the form and identifies the most common source documents needed for each item. Accuracy in identifying and transferring the data is essential. A single transposition in a critical field such as name, identification number, birthdate, or CPT code could cause the claim to be rejected. A few extra minutes spent proofreading data helps prevent the need to rework claims later. An example of a completed CMS-1500 form appears in Figure 14-9. Procedure 14-6 guides you through the process of how to complete a CMS-1500 form.

Professionalism | The Workplace

Before working with insurance claims, it may be helpful to practice filling out paper CMS-1500 forms. Become familiar with each section, and find out what information is required by the various insurance companies to complete the forms and avoid the claim being rejected. If possible, also become familiar with the software used to submit electronic claims. Most software companies provide a tutorial for you to work with before working with actual claims.

HEALTH INSURANCE CLAIM FORM

APPROVED BY NATIONAL UNIFORM CLAIM COMMITTEE (NUCC) 02/12

PICA ▢▢

1. MEDICARE	MEDICAID	TRICARE	CHAMPVA	GROUP HEALTH PLAN	FECA BLK LUNG	OTHER	1a. INSURED'S I.D. NUMBER	(For Program in Item 1)
▢ (Medicare#)	▢ (Medicaid#)	▢ (ID#/DoD#)	▢ (Member ID#)	▢ (ID#)	▢ (ID#)	▢ (ID#)		

2. PATIENT'S NAME (Last Name, First Name, Middle Initial)

3. PATIENT'S BIRTH DATE MM DD YY   SEX M ▢ F ▢

4. INSURED'S NAME (Last Name, First Name, Middle Initial)

5. PATIENT'S ADDRESS (No., Street)

6. PATIENT RELATIONSHIP TO INSURED   Self ▢ Spouse ▢ Child ▢ Other ▢

7. INSURED'S ADDRESS (No., Street)

CITY ____ STATE

8. RESERVED FOR NUCC USE

CITY ____ STATE

ZIP CODE ____ TELEPHONE (Include Area Code) ( )

ZIP CODE ____ TELEPHONE (Include Area Code) ( )

9. OTHER INSURED'S NAME (Last Name, First Name, Middle Initial)

10. IS PATIENT'S CONDITION RELATED TO:

11. INSURED'S POLICY GROUP OR FECA NUMBER

a. OTHER INSURED'S POLICY OR GROUP NUMBER

a. EMPLOYMENT? (Current or Previous) ▢ YES ▢ NO

a. INSURED'S DATE OF BIRTH MM DD YY   SEX M ▢ F ▢

b. RESERVED FOR NUCC USE

b. AUTO ACCIDENT? ▢ YES ▢ NO   PLACE (State) ____

b. OTHER CLAIM ID (Designated by NUCC)

c. RESERVED FOR NUCC USE

c. OTHER ACCIDENT? ▢ YES ▢ NO

c. INSURANCE PLAN NAME OR PROGRAM NAME

d. INSURANCE PLAN NAME OR PROGRAM NAME

10d. CLAIM CODES (Designated by NUCC)

d. IS THERE ANOTHER HEALTH BENEFIT PLAN? ▢ YES ▢ NO If yes, complete items 9, 9a, and 9d.

READ BACK OF FORM BEFORE COMPLETING & SIGNING THIS FORM.
12. PATIENT'S OR AUTHORIZED PERSON'S SIGNATURE I authorize the release of any medical or other information necessary to process this claim. I also request payment of government benefits either to myself or to the party who accepts assignment below.

SIGNED ____ DATE ____

13. INSURED'S OR AUTHORIZED PERSON'S SIGNATURE I authorize payment of medical benefits to the undersigned physician or supplier for services described below.

SIGNED ____

14. DATE OF CURRENT ILLNESS, INJURY, or PREGNANCY (LMP) MM DD YY QUAL. ____

15. OTHER DATE QUAL. ____ MM DD YY

16. DATES PATIENT UNABLE TO WORK IN CURRENT OCCUPATION MM DD YY FROM ____ TO MM DD YY

17. NAME OF REFERRING PROVIDER OR OTHER SOURCE

17a. ____
17b. NPI ____

18. HOSPITALIZATION DATES RELATED TO CURRENT SERVICES MM DD YY FROM ____ TO MM DD YY

19. ADDITIONAL CLAIM INFORMATION (Designated by NUCC)

20. OUTSIDE LAB? ▢ YES ▢ NO $ CHARGES

21. DIAGNOSIS OR NATURE OF ILLNESS OR INJURY Relate A-L to service line below (24E)   ICD Ind. ____

22. RESUBMISSION CODE ____ ORIGINAL REF. NO. ____

A. ____ B. ____ C. ____ D. ____
E. ____ F. ____ G. ____ H. ____
I. ____ J. ____ K. ____ L. ____

23. PRIOR AUTHORIZATION NUMBER

24. A. DATE(S) OF SERVICE						B. PLACE OF SERVICE	C. EMG	D. PROCEDURES, SERVICES, OR SUPPLIES (Explain Unusual Circumstances)		E. DIAGNOSIS POINTER	F. $ CHARGES	G. DAYS OR UNITS	H. EPSDT Family Plan	I. ID. QUAL.	J. RENDERING PROVIDER ID. #
From			To					CPT/HCPCS	MODIFIER						
MM	DD	YY	MM	DD	YY										
1														NPI	
2														NPI	
3														NPI	
4														NPI	
5														NPI	
6														NPI	

25. FEDERAL TAX I.D. NUMBER   SSN ▢ EIN ▢

26. PATIENT'S ACCOUNT NO.

27. ACCEPT ASSIGNMENT? (For govt. claims, see back) ▢ YES ▢ NO

28. TOTAL CHARGE $

29. AMOUNT PAID $

30. Rsvd for NUCC Use

31. SIGNATURE OF PHYSICIAN OR SUPPLIER INCLUDING DEGREES OR CREDENTIALS (I certify that the statements on the reverse apply to this bill and are made a part thereof.)

SIGNED ____ DATE ____

32. SERVICE FACILITY LOCATION INFORMATION

a. NPI ____ b. ____

33. BILLING PROVIDER INFO & PH # ( )

a. NPI ____ b. ____

FIGURE 14-7 CMS-1500 (02/12) claim form.

CARRIER → PATIENT AND INSURED INFORMATION → PHYSICIAN OR SUPPLIER INFORMATION →

ENCOUNTER FORM

Patient Information		Payment Method		Visit Information	
Patient I.D. #		**Primary**	TRUSTMARK PPO	Visit Date	
Patient Name	Theresa Andrews	Primary I.D. #	332490432	Visit #	3/15/20YY
Address	4569 Ave. K #120	Primary Group #	2038831	Rendering Physician	
City/State	Plano, TX 12345	**Secondary**		Referring Physician	
Phone	972-555-4448	Secondary I.D. #		Reason for Visit	Chest Pain
Date of Birth	06/08/1967	Secondary Group #			
Age		Cash/Credit Card			
		Other Billing			

E/M Modifiers	Procedure Modifiers	DIAGNOSIS:
53 – Discountinued Procedure	22 – Unusual, excessive procedure	BRONCHOPNEUMONIA WITH FLU J11.08
24 – Unrelated E/M service during postop.	50 – Bilateral procedure	J18.0
25 – Significant, separately identifiable E/M	51 – Multiple surgical procedures in same day	
32 – Mandated service	52 – Reduced/incomplete procedure	
57 – Decision for surgery	55 – Postop. management only	
	59 – Distinct multiple procedures	

CATEGORY	CODE	MOD	FEE	CATEGORY	CODE	MOD	FEE
Office Visit – New Patient				**Wound Care**			
Minimal office visit	99201			Debride partial thickness burn, small <5% total body surface	16020		
20 minutes	99202			Debride partial thickness burn, medium (e.g., whole face or whole extremity, or 5% to 10% total body surface area)	16025		
				Debride partial thickness burn, large (e.g., more than 1 extremity, or greater than 10% total body surface area)	16030		
30 minutes	99203			Debride wound, not a burn	11000		
45 minutes	99204			Unna boot application	29580		
60 minutes	99205			Unna boot removal	29700		
Other				Other			
Office Visit – Established				**Supplies**			
Minimal office visit	99211			Lt compress band <3"/yd	A6448		
10 minutes	99212	X	35.00	Lt compress band >=3"<5"/yd	A6449		
15 minutes	99213			Lt compress band >=5"/yd	A6450		
25 minutes	99214			Cast, fiberglass	A4590		
40 minutes	99215			Self-adher band w>=3" <5"/yd	A6454		
Other				Foley catheter	A4338		
General Procedures				CTLSO Infant Immobilizer	L1000		
Anoscopy	46600			Kerlix roll	A6220		
Audiometry	92551			Oxygen mask/cannula	A4620		
Breast aspiration	19000			Sleeve, elbow or heel	E0191		
Cerumen removal	69210			Sling	A4565		
Circumcision	54150			Splint, ready-made	A4570		
DDST	96110			Splint, wrist or ankle	S8451		
Flex sigmoidoscopy	45330			Sterile packing	A6407		
Flex sigmoidoscopy w/ biopsy	45331			Surgical tray	A4550		
Foreign body removal–foot	28190			Other			
Nail removal	11730			**OB Care**			
Nail removal/phenol	11750			Routine OB care	59400		
Trigger point injection	20552			Postpartum care only (separate procedure)	59430		
Tympanometry	92567			Antepartum 4-6 visits	59425		
Visual acuity	99173			Antepartum 7 or more visits	59426		
Other Chest X-ray	71020	X	53.00	Other			
Other				Other			

Other Visit Information: _____

Lab Work to Order: _____

Referral to: _____

Provider Signature: <u>Marcus Wellman, MD NPI # 9998887776</u>

Next Appointment: _____

Fees:

Total Charges: $88.00

Copay Received: $20.00

Other Payment: $_____

Total Due: $68.00

Allied Medical Clinic 1933 E. Frankford Rd. Carrollton, TX 12345 972-555-5482

FIGURE 14-8 A sample encounter form.

TABLE 14-5 | Instructions for Completing the CMS-1500 (02/12) Claim Form

Item Number, Name, and Use	Source Document
Carrier Area (top, right-hand margin) The carrier block is located in the upper center and right margin of the form. To distinguish this version of the form from previous versions, the Quick Response (QR) code symbol and the date approved by the NUCC have been added to the top, left-hand margin. Enter the insurance plan's mailing address for claims from this policy. Up to four lines are allowed in the address. If an address contains only three lines, use the first two lines, leave the third line blank, and enter the city, state, and zip code on the fourth line. Be sure to verify the address. Some insurance companies have different addresses and different PO boxes for different types of plans, such as group, individual, or government. When printing page numbers on multiple page claims, print the page numbers in the Carrier Block on Line 8 beginning at column 32. Page numbers are to be printed as: Page XX of YY. This is generally done by clearinghouses when printing an electronic submission on the paper CMS-1500 claim form.	Insurance ID card
Items 1–13: PATIENT AND INSURED INFORMATION	
Item 1: Type of Insurance Item 1 identifies the type of insurance the patient carries. The form lists five government plans: Medicare, Medicaid, TRICARE/CHAMPUS, CHAMPVA, and FECA/Black Lung. There are two other options: Group Health Plan and Other. Other indicates health insurance including HMOs, commercial insurance, automobile accident, liability, workers' compensation, and, usually, BCBS. Mark an X in only one box.	Insurance ID card
Item 1a: Insured's ID Number In Item 1a, enter the insured's insurance ID number as reflected on the insurance card. The insured could be the patient, or it could be someone else such as spouse, mother, or father. If the patient can be identified by a unique member identification number, the patient is considered to be the "insured." Report the patient as the insured in the insured data fields (Items 1a, 4, 5, and 7) and not in the patient fields (Items 2 and 5). For workers' compensation claims: Enter employee ID. For other property and casualty claims: Enter the federal tax ID or SSN of the insured person or entity.	Insurance ID card
Item 2: Patient's Name In Item 2, enter the name of the patient who received services. This information is input as last name, first name, and middle name or initial. The spelling should match the insurance card exactly. If the name on the card is misspelled, then the name on the claims form should be spelled the same way until the patient provides a new card with the correct spelling. *When the patient is the insured, then it is not necessary to report the patient's name in Item 2.*	Patient registration form Encounter form
Item 3: Patient's Date of Birth/Sex In Item 3, enter the patient's date of birth and sex/gender. Enter the date of birth using the eight-digit format: MMDDCCYY. Enter an X in the correct box for male or female. If gender is unknown, leave blank. Do not try to guess the gender based on the patient's name.	Patient registration form Encounter form
Item 4: Insured's Name Item 4 is the name of the person who is the insured. This may or may not be the patient. The insured's name should be entered as last name, first name, middle name or initial. A hyphen can be used for hyphenated names. If the patient can be identified by a unique Member Identification Number, the patient is considered to be the "insured." Report the patient as the insured in the insured data fields (Items 1a, 4, 5, and 7) and not in the patient fields (Items 2 and 5). For workers' compensation claims: Enter the name of the employer. For other property and casualty claims: Enter the name of the insured person or entity.	Insurance ID card

TABLE 14-5 | Instructions for Completing the CMS-1500 (02/12) Claim Form (*continued*)

Item Number, Name, and Use	Source Document
Item 5: Patient's Address Enter the patient's home address and telephone number in Item 5, *if different from the insured's* address and telephone number. This information is taken from the patient information form when the patient registers in the office. The address includes the street name and number, city, state (two-letter abbreviation), and zip code. Do not use commas, periods, or other punctuation in the address. Do not use the # sign for apartment numbers. When entering a nine-digit zip code, include the hyphen. "Patient's Telephone" does not exist in the electronic claims standard, so NUCC recommends that the phone number *not* be reported. For workers' compensation and other property and casualty claims: If required by a payer to report a telephone number, do not use a hyphen or space as a separator within the telephone number.	Patient registration form
Item 6: Patient's Relationship to the Insured After Item 5 has been completed, in Item 6 enter an X in the correct box to indicate the patient's relationship to the insured. Options include Self, Spouse, Child, or Other. If the patient is the insured person, the "Self" entry is marked here. Only one box can be marked. *If the patient is a dependent, but has a unique member identification number* and the payer requires the identification number be reported on the claim, then report "Self," because the patient is reported as the insured.	Patient registration form
Item 7: Insured's Address In Item 7, enter the insured's address. This information should include the street name and number, city, state (two-letter abbreviation), and zip code. "Insured's Telephone" does not exist in the electronic claims standard, so NUCC recommends that the phone number not be reported. For workers' compensation claims: Enter the address of the employer.	Patient registration form
Item 8: Reserved for NUCC Use This field was previously used to report "Patient Status." "Patient Status" does not exist in the electronic claims standard, so this field has been eliminated. This field is reserved for NUCC use. The NUCC will provide instructions for any future use of this field.	Patient registration form
Item 9: Other Insured's Name If Item 11d is marked YES to indicate that other group health coverage exists, also complete Items 9 and 9a–d; otherwise, leave them blank. Item 9 indicates that there is another policy that may cover the patient. When there is additional group health coverage, enter the other insured's full last name, first name, and middle initial of the enrollee in another health plan if it is different from that shown in Item 2. If there is no secondary policy, leave this field blank.	Insurance ID card
Item 9a: Other Insured's Policy or Group Number Enter the policy number or group number of the secondary insurance policy in Item 9a. Enter the number exactly as it appears on the insurance card.	Insurance ID card
Item 9b: Reserved for NUCC Use Item 9b was previously used to report date of birth of the insured of the secondary policy. This data does not exist in the electronic claims standard, so this field has been eliminated. This field is reserved for NUCC use. The NUCC will provide instructions for any future use of this field.	
Item 9c: Reserved for NUCC Use Item 9c was previously used to report insured's employer or school. This data does not exist in the electronic claims standard, so this field has been eliminated. This field is reserved for NUCC use. The NUCC will provide instructions for any future use of this field.	
Item 9d: Insurance Plan Name or Program Name In Item 9d, enter the name of the secondary insurance plan, if any. This information is taken directly from the secondary insurance card. Enter the name exactly as it appears on the card.	Insurance ID card

(continued)

Item Number, Name, and Use	Source Document
Item 10a–c: Is Patient's Condition Related To? Item 10 identifies whether the patient's visit was related to an employment accident, auto accident, or other accident. Enter an X in the correct box. Mark YES when filing workers' compensation claims, auto accident claims, or claims for other types of injuries. Any item marked "YES" indicates there may be other applicable insurance coverage that would be primary, such as automobile liability insurance. Primary insurance information must then be shown in Item 11. Mark NO when the patient's visit does not pertain to an accident. If this box is not marked, or marked incorrectly, the claim could be delayed.	Encounter form Medical record
Item 10d: CLAIM CODES Claim codes or condition codes, originally used on institutional claims, identify additional information about the patient's condition or the claim. A limited number of these codes are reported on the CMS-1500. The condition codes approved for use on the CMS-1500 Claim Form are available at www.nucc.org under Code Sets. For Medicaid claims: Condition codes are required to report the reason for an abortion. For workers' compensation claims: Condition codes are required when submitting a bill that is a duplicate or an appeal. (Original Reference Number must be entered in Box 22 for these conditions.) Do not use condition codes when submitting a revised or corrected bill.	
Item 11: Insured's Policy Group or FECA Number If Item 4 is completed, then also complete Item 11. Item 11 identifies the insured's policy group number listed on the insurance card. This number should be entered exactly as it appears on the insurance card. For workers' compensation claims for federal employees: Enter the FECA number (nine-digit alphanumeric identifier).	Insurance ID card
Item 11a: Insured's Date of Birth/Sex In Item 11a, list the date of birth of the insured that appears in Item 1a. Use the eight-digit format MMDDCCYY. Mark an X in either male or female accordingly. If gender is unknown, leave blank.	Insurance ID card Patient registration form
Item 11b: Other Claim ID Item 11b is used only for workers' compensation or property and casualty claims. Enter the qualifier Y4 (Property Casualty Claim Number) to the left of the vertical, dotted line. Enter the identifier number to the right of the vertical, dotted line.	Insurance ID card Patient registration form
Item 11c: Insurance Plan Name or Program Name Item 11c identifies the insurance plan name. The information should be taken directly from the insurance card and spelled exactly as it appears on the card. Some payers require an identification number of the primary insurer rather than the name in this field.	Insurance ID card
Item 11d: Is There Another Health Benefit Plan? In Item 11d, indicate whether there is another health benefit plan, in addition to the one shown in Item 1a. If there is another plan, mark YES with an X and enter the information into Item 9a–d. If there is no additional insurance plan, mark NO.	Patient registration form
Item 12: Patient's or Authorized Person's Signature Item 12 is where the patient or guarantor signs, allowing the release of any medical information to the insurance company for billing purposes. This release is only valid for billing information. Any other request for records requires a formal release of information form to be signed by the patient or guarantor. This signature is good for one year from the date it is signed and should be updated annually. The words "Signature on File" or "SOF" may be printed here in place of a signature if a current signature is on file in the patient's chart. In this case, do not enter a date. If the patient signs the form, enter the date in the six-digit format (MM/DD/YY) or eight-digit format (MM/DD/CCYY). If there is no signature on file, leave blank or enter "No Signature on File."	Patient registration form

Item Number, Name, and Use	Source Document
Item 13: Insured's or Authorized Person's Signature Item 13 is where the patient or insured signs, authorizing the insurance company to reimburse the physician or supplier directly. The words "Signature on File" or "SOF" may be printed here in place of a signature if a current signature is on file in the patient's chart. In this case, do not enter a date. If the patient signs the form, enter the date in the six-digit format (MM/DD/YY) or eight-digit format (MM/DD/CCYY). If there is no signature on file, leave blank or enter "No Signature on File." Not required for government claims such as Medicare, Medicaid, or workers' compensation because those programs automatically send payment directly to participating providers.	Patient registration form
Items 14–33: PHYSICIAN OR SUPPLIER INFORMATION	
Item 14: Date of Current Illness, Injury, Pregnancy Report the first date of the current illness, injury, or pregnancy in Item 14. Use the six-digit (MMDDYY) or eight-digit format (MMDDCCYY). For a pregnancy, report the first day of the woman's last menstrual period (LMP). Enter one of the following qualifiers to the right of the vertical dotted line to identify which date is being reported. 431 Onset of Current Symptoms or Illness 484 Last Menstrual Period If this information is not known, leave blank.	Encounter form Medical record
Item 15: Other Date Item 15 reports other dates related to the patient's condition or treatment. Use the six-digit (MMDDYY) or eight-digit (MMDDCCYY) format. Enter the applicable qualifier between the vertical, dotted lines after the word "Qualifier" to identify which date is being reported. 454 Initial Treatment 304 Latest Visit or Consultation 453 Acute Manifestation of a Chronic Condition 439 Accident 455 Last X-ray 471 Prescription 090 Report Start (Assumed Care Date) 091 Report End (Relinquished Care Date) 444 First Visit or Consultation Previous pregnancies are not a similar illness. Leave this field blank if unknown.	Encounter form Medical record
Item 16: Dates Patient Unable to Work in Current Occupation In Item 16, list the dates the patient is unable to work because of his illness or injury. These dates are required when filing workers' compensation or disability claims. Use the six-digit (MMDDYY) or eight-digit format (MMDDCCYY). If the information is not required, leave blank.	Encounter form Medical record
Item 17: Name of Referring Physician or Other Source Item 17 requests the name of the provider who referred, ordered, or supervised the services on the claim. Some insurance companies, such as health maintenance organizations (HMOs) or exclusive provider organizations (EPOs), require the referring provider to be reported here. Enter the provider's last name, first name, and credentials. Enter the applicable qualifier code to the left of the vertical, dotted line. If multiple providers are involved, enter one provider using the following priority order and qualifier: 1. DN Referring provider 2. DK Ordering provider 3. DQ Supervising provider	Encounter form Referral form

(*continued*)

Item Number, Name, and Use	Source Document
Item 17a: Other ID # Enter the non-NPI identification number of the referring, ordering, or supervising provider in Item 17a, if required by the plan. In the Qualifier field, enter the two-character designation of what type of ID number is being reported: 0B State License Number 1G Provider UPIN Number G2 Provider Commercial Number LU Location Number (This qualifier is used for Supervising Provider only.)	Referral form
Item 17b: NPI Number Enter the NPI number of the referring, ordering, or supervising provider in Item 17b.	Referral form
Item 18: Hospitalization Dates Related to Current Services Enter the hospital admission and discharge dates the patient was hospitalized as an inpatient. If not discharged, leave discharge date blank. Use the six-digit (MMDDYY) or eight-digit format (MMDDCCYY).	Encounter form Medical record
Item 19: Additional Claim Information Item 19 is required by some payers to report certain identifiers such as alternate provider numbers and provider taxonomy codes. Each identifier requires a two-character qualifier. Refer to the most current instructions from the applicable public or private payer regarding the use of this field. NUCC provides a list of qualifiers to be used. For workers' compensation: Enter the type of attachment or supplemental claim information if required. Enter PWK followed by the NUCC approved code(s) for report type and transmission type.	
Item 20: Outside Lab Item 20 is used only if lab tests appear in Section 24. If the physician's office is billing on behalf of an outside lab, mark YES. This indicates that an entity other than the entity billing for the service performed the purchased services. Enter the purchase price under Charges, and complete Item 32. If the lab tests were performed by the provider's office, mark NO. If no lab tests were ordered, leave this Item blank.	Encounter form Medical record
Item 21: Diagnosis or Nature of Illness or Injury In Item 21, enter the patient's ICD diagnosis code(s) for this claim. In the upper-right corner, enter the number to identify which version of codes is being reported: **9** ICD-9-CM **0** ICD-10-CM Enter between one and 12 codes, in order of priority. Line 1 is the primary diagnosis. Do not enter the decimal point as part of the code number because it is implied. Do not enter narrative descriptions. Ensure that the diagnosis codes support the medical necessity of the services (CPT codes) listed in Item 24D. Relate each diagnosis (A-I) to the lines of service in 24E by letter (A, B, C, etc.).	Encounter form Medical record
Item 22: Resubmission Code and/or Original Reference Number If required, use Item 22 on resubmitted claims to report the payer's reference number for the original claim. Enter the appropriate bill frequency code left justified in the left-hand side of the field. 7 Replacement of prior claim 8 Void/cancel of prior claim Consult with the payer for specific instructions on the use of this Item.	RA Phone call to insurance company
Item 23: Prior Authorization Number Some insurance plans, such as those of HMOs and PPOs, require a prior authorization number. If required, when preauthorization is obtained from an insurance company for services, enter the number assigned in Item 23. HMOs may require that referral numbers be entered here. If this field is left blank when the payer requires prior authorization or referral, the claim will be denied. If no prior authorization is required, leave blank.	Referral form

Item Number, Name, and Use	Source Document
SECTION 24	
The six service lines in Section 24 are divided horizontally to accommodate submission of supplemental information. Enter the service information in the *white* portion of each line. Each CPT code must be entered on a separate line.	
When the same CPT code is provided on nonsequential dates, use a separate line for each date and repeat the CPT code. When the same CPT code is provided multiple times on a single date, enter the date once in Item 24A and enter the number of procedures in Item 24G. When the same CPT code is repeated on sequential dates, enter the beginning and ending dates Item 24A (From and To) and enter the number of procedures in Item 24G. Enter the appropriate NUCC qualifier and code for supplemental information in the *shaded* portion.	
(*Note:* Refer to the current NUCC *1500 Health Insurance Claim Form Reference Instruction Manual* for the list of qualifiers and examples of how to enter supplemental information.)	
Providers must verify requirements for supplemental information with the payer. Supplemental information that may be entered includes: • Narrative description of unspecified codes • National Drug Codes (NDC) for drugs • Vendor Product Number–Health Industry Business Communications Council (HIBCC) • Product Number Health Care Uniform Code Council–Global Trade Item Number (GTIN), formerly Universal Product Code (UPC) for products • Contract rate • Tooth numbers and areas of the oral cavity	
Item 24A: Dates of Service	Encounter form Medical record
In Item 24A, enter the dates of service for the service provided as listed in the CPT code. Use the six-digit format (MM/DD/YY). Use a separate line for each CPT code. When the same CPT code is provided on multiple, sequential dates, enter both the From date and the To date.	
When there is only one date of service for a CPT code, as is frequently the case in physician offices, payers require varying formats for this Item. Some payers require both the To and From dates to be entered. Some require that only the From date be listed.	
Item 24B: Place of Service	Encounter form Medical record
Place of service in Item 24B is a mandatory field because it describes the place where the procedure or service was performed. The most common places of service are the physician's office, hospital, emergency department, or skilled nursing facility. Enter the Place of Service Code (see following list) in the white portion of this field. Note that the CMS has stated that if the place of service is other than the provider's normal location in FL32, the place of service must be fully written out in Item 32. Consider this example: The patient was an inpatient (hospital), and the physician saw the patient in the hospital for an evaluation and management service. Therefore, code 21 (see following list) would be entered in Item 24B and the name and address of the hospital entered in Item 32.	

Common place of service codes include the following:
  11 Physician's office
  20 Urgent care facility
  21 Inpatient hospital
  22 Outpatient hospital
  23 Hospital emergency department
  31 Skilled nursing facility	

(*Note:* A complete list of POS codes can be found at www.cms.gov and also in the front of the CPT manual.)	
Item 24C: EMG (Emergency)	Encounter form Medical record
Item 24C is used only with Medicaid to indicate whether the service was provided on an emergency basis. Enter Y for YES. Leave blank for NO or not applicable. The definition of an emergency is defined differently by each payer.	

(continued)

TABLE 14-5 | Instructions for Completing the CMS-1500 (02/12) Claim Form (*continued*)

Item Number, Name, and Use	Source Document
Item 24D: Procedures, Services, or Supplies In Item 24D, enter the CPT or HCPCS code to identify the procedures, services, or supplies provided. Also enter up to four modifiers in Item 24D. Do not enter the narrative description of the code. Enter each unique CPT or HCPCS code on a separate line. Use only the white portion of the line for CPT and HCPCS codes. If more than six codes are required, continue the claim to a second page. Do not use the gray portion of the line to accommodate more than six codes.	Encounter form Medical record
Item 24E: Diagnosis Pointer Item 24E indicates the reference letter (A–L) of the diagnosis code in Item 21 as it relates to each service or procedure. If more than one diagnosis is attached to a single procedure or service, enter the primary diagnosis first, followed by the additional diagnoses. Up to four letters may be entered, with no spaces or commas between them. Do not enter the actual code number, only the reference letter. Be certain that each CPT code has a corresponding diagnosis code to justify the need. Some payers, such as Medicare, require only one diagnosis reference number per service.	Encounter form Medical record
Item 24F: Charges Enter the charge for each CPT or HCPCS code listed. The amount should be entered without a decimal point or dollar sign. Enter 00 in the cents area if the charge is an even dollar amount. If multiple units are entered in Item 24G, the charges should reflect the total charges for amount of the procedure *times* the number of units. It is not a per unit charge. The charge entered should be the provider's established fee schedule, not the discounted or contracted rate. Medicare claims should contain the Medicare fee schedule charge.	Encounter form Physician fee schedule
Item 24G: Days or Units Enter the number of units per procedure or service provided to a patient in Item 24G. If multiple units are entered in 24G, the charges should reflect the amount of the procedure multiplied by the number of units. This field is most commonly used for multiple visits, units of supplies, anesthesia units or minutes, or oxygen volume. If only one service is performed, enter "1." For anesthesia, report the number of *minutes*. Report units for anesthesia services only when the code description includes a time period (such as "daily management"). When required by payers to provide supplemental information such as the National Drug Code (NDC) units in addition to the HCPCS units, enter the applicable NDC units' qualifier and related units in the shaded line. The following qualifiers are to be used when reporting NDC units: F2 International Unit, ML Milliliter, GR Gram, UN Unit.	Encounter form Medical record
Item 24H: EPSDT Family Plan Use on Medicaid claims only, to identify whether the patient is receiving her services through Medicaid's Early and Periodic Screening, Diagnosis, and Treatment (EPSDT) program. Enter "Y" for yes or "N" for no or follow state-specific guidelines.	Insurance (Medicaid) ID card
Item 24I: ID Qualifier If the insurance plan requires use of a plan-specific provider ID number for the provider who delivered the service, enter the code for type of plan in the shaded portion of 24I. Otherwise, leave blank.	Office records
Item 24J: Rendering Provider Report the provider rendering the service. Enter the NPI number in the unshaded area of the field. When a substitute provider (*locum tenens*) was used, enter that provider's information here. If the insurance plan also requires use of a plan-specific provider ID number for the provider who delivered the service, or the provider does not have an NPI, enter Qualifier in 24I and enter the other ID number in the shaded portion of 24J. Otherwise, leave the shaded portion blank.	Encounter form Medical record
Item 25: Federal Tax I.D. Number In Item 25, enter the provider's federal tax ID number or the employer identification number (EIN) of the billing entity. This number should be consistent with the billing provider listed in Item 33. Do not enter hyphens with numbers. The appropriate box (SSN or EIN) should be marked with an X.	Encounter form Office records

Item Number, Name, and Use	Source Document
Item 26: Patient's Account Number In Item 26, enter the patient's account number assigned by the medical office. The computer system used in the office generates the number, and it should be entered on the claim. This in turn will allow for the account number to appear on the remittance (RA) form, which makes it easier to locate the correct patient to post insurance payments.	Encounter form Medical record
Item 27: Accept Assignment? This field indicates that the provider agrees to accept assignment under the terms of the payer's program.	Encounter form Office records
Item 28: Total Charge Enter the total charges, added together from those listed in Item 24F. The charges should be checked for accuracy to ensure proper reimbursement. Do not use decimal points or dollar signs in this entry. Enter 00 in the cents field if the amount is a whole number.	Calculator
Item 29: Amount Paid Enter the amount paid by the patient or other insurance policies. When submitting secondary claims, enter this amount after the primary RA is received and payment is posted. A secondary claim is printed to be sent to the secondary insurance carrier along with a copy of the primary insurance carrier's RA. Do not use decimal points or dollar signs in this entry.	Encounter form
Item 30: Reserved for NUCC Use Item 30 was previously used to report "Balance Due." This data does not exist in the electronic claims standard, so the field has been eliminated. This field is reserved for NUCC use. The NUCC will provide instructions for any use of this field.	
Item 31: Signature of Physician or Supplier Including Degrees or Credentials In Item 31, enter the legal signature of the physician or supplier who has provided the services to the patient along with professional credentials (M.D., PA-C, or NP). "Signature on File" or "SOF" is also acceptable in this Item. Enter a six-digit date (MM/DD/YY), eight-digit date (MM/DD/CCYY), or alphanumeric date (Month 30, 20YY). A signature stamp may be used instead of a written signature. The stamp must leave a clear, nonsmeared image on the claim.	Typed Signature stamp
Item 32: Name and Address of Facility Where Services Were Rendered Item 32 identifies the name of the facility where services were provided, if other than the billing provider. Enter the name, address, ZIP code, and NPI number. When more than one supplier is used, use a separate CMS-1500 form for each supplier.	Encounter form Medical record
Item 32a: NPI Number Enter the NPI number of the service facility location in Item 32a. Only report a Service Facility Location NPI when the NPI is different from the Billing Provider NPI.	Encounter form Office records
Item 32b: Other ID Number If required by the insurance plan, enter the qualifier and plan-specific ID number in the shaded portion.	Encounter form Office records

Item 33: Billing Provider Information and Phone Number
 	
Enter the provider's or supplier's billing name, address, zip code, and phone number in Item 33. This should be the same entity as the Tax ID in Item 25. Enter the phone number in the area to the right of the field title. Electronic claims require a physical location, not a PO Box, and NUCC recommends that the physical address be entered on the CMS-1500 form as well. Enter the name and address information in the following format:
 	
    First line: Name
    Second line: Address
    Third line: City, state, and zip code
	Encounter form
	Office records

Item 33a: NPI Number Enter the NPI number of the billing provider in Item 33a.	Encounter form Office records
Item 33b: Other ID Number If required by the insurance plan, enter the Qualifier and plan-specific ID number in the shaded portion.	Encounter form Office records

HEALTH INSURANCE CLAIM FORM

APPROVED BY NATIONAL UNIFORM CLAIM COMMITTEE (NUCC) 02/12

CARRIER

☐☐ PICA   PICA ☐☐

| 1. MEDICARE ☐ (Medicare#) | MEDICAID ☐ (Medicaid#) | TRICARE ☐ (ID#/DoD#) | CHAMPVA ☐ (Member ID#) | GROUP HEALTH PLAN ☐ (ID#) | FECA BLK LUNG ☐ (ID#) | OTHER ☒ (ID#) | 1a. INSURED'S I.D. NUMBER (For Program in Item 1) 9999999 |

| 2. PATIENT'S NAME (Last Name, First Name, Middle Initial) BROWN MELISSA J | 3. PATIENT'S BIRTH DATE MM 05 DD 21 YY 1962 SEX M☐ F☒ | 4. INSURED'S NAME (Last Name, First Name, Middle Initial) BROWN JOHN |

| 5. PATIENT'S ADDRESS (No., Street) | 6. PATIENT RELATIONSHIP TO INSURED Self☐ Spouse☒ Child☐ Other☐ | 7. INSURED'S ADDRESS (No., Street) 897 FIRST STREET |

| CITY | STATE | 8. RESERVED FOR NUCC USE | CITY PARKER HEIGHTS | STATE IL |

| ZIP CODE | TELEPHONE (Include Area Code) ( ) | | ZIP CODE 60600 | TELEPHONE (Include Area Code) (555) 1239999 |

| 9. OTHER INSURED'S NAME (Last Name, First Name, Middle Initial) | 10. IS PATIENT'S CONDITION RELATED TO: | 11. INSURED'S POLICY GROUP OR FECA NUMBER DC000 |

| a. OTHER INSURED'S POLICY OR GROUP NUMBER | a. EMPLOYMENT? (Current or Previous) ☐ YES ☒ NO | a. INSURED'S DATE OF BIRTH MM 01 DD 11 YY 1961 SEX M☒ F☐ |

| b. RESERVED FOR NUCC USE | b. AUTO ACCIDENT? ☐ YES ☒ NO PLACE (State) | b. OTHER CLAIM ID (Designated by NUCC) |

| c. RESERVED FOR NUCC USE | c. OTHER ACCIDENT? ☐ YES ☒ NO | c. INSURANCE PLAN NAME OR PROGRAM NAME HEALTHY WAY INSURANCE CO |

| d. INSURANCE PLAN NAME OR PROGRAM NAME | 10d. CLAIM CODES (Designated by NUCC) | d. IS THERE ANOTHER HEALTH BENEFIT PLAN? ☐ YES ☒ NO If yes, complete items 9, 9a, and 9d. |

READ BACK OF FORM BEFORE COMPLETING & SIGNING THIS FORM.

| 12. PATIENT'S OR AUTHORIZED PERSON'S SIGNATURE I authorize the release of any medical or other information necessary to process this claim. I also request payment of government benefits either to myself or to the party who accepts assignment below. SIGNED SOF DATE | 13. INSURED'S OR AUTHORIZED PERSON'S SIGNATURE I authorize payment of medical benefits to the undersigned physician or supplier for services described below. SIGNED SOF |

| 14. DATE OF CURRENT ILLNESS, INJURY, or PREGNANCY (LMP) MM DD YY QUAL. | 15. OTHER DATE QUAL. MM DD YY | 16. DATES PATIENT UNABLE TO WORK IN CURRENT OCCUPATION FROM MM DD YY TO MM DD YY |

| 17. NAME OF REFERRING PROVIDER OR OTHER SOURCE 17a. 17b. NPI | 18. HOSPITALIZATION DATES RELATED TO CURRENT SERVICES FROM MM DD YY TO MM DD YY |

| 19. ADDITIONAL CLAIM INFORMATION (Designated by NUCC) | 20. OUTSIDE LAB? ☐ YES ☒ NO $ CHARGES |

| 21. DIAGNOSIS OR NATURE OF ILLNESS OR INJURY Relate A-L to service line below (24E) ICD Ind. 0 A. F410 B. F17210 C. Z8249 D. Z825 E. F. G. H. I. J. K. L. | 22. RESUBMISSION CODE ORIGINAL REF. NO. 23. PRIOR AUTHORIZATION NUMBER |

24. A. DATE(S) OF SERVICE From MM DD YY	To MM DD YY	B. PLACE OF SERVICE	C. EMG	D. PROCEDURES, SERVICES, OR SUPPLIES (Explain Unusual Circumstances) CPT/HCPCS	MODIFIER	E. DIAGNOSIS POINTER	F. $ CHARGES	G. DAYS OR UNITS	H. EPSDT Family Plan	I. ID. QUAL.	J. RENDERING PROVIDER ID. #
1	12 01 20YY	12 01 20YY	11		99203		ABCD	85 00	1		NPI	1234567890
2	12 01 20YY	12 01 20YY	11		85025		ABC	95 00	1		NPI	1234567890
3	12 01 20YY	12 01 20YY	11		93000		ABC	75 00	1		NPI	1234567890
4	12 01 20YY	12 01 20YY	11		80053		ABC	75 00	1		NPI	1234567890
5	12 01 20YY	12 01 20YY	11		36415		ABC	75 00	1		NPI	1234567890
6											NPI	

| 25. FEDERAL TAX I.D. NUMBER 750246810 SSN☐ EIN☒ | 26. PATIENT'S ACCOUNT NO. B2 | 27. ACCEPT ASSIGNMENT? (For govt. claims, see back) ☒ YES ☐ NO | 28. TOTAL CHARGE $ 345 00 | 29. AMOUNT PAID $ | 30. Rsvd for NUCC Use |

| 31. SIGNATURE OF PHYSICIAN OR SUPPLIER INCLUDING DEGREES OR CREDENTIALS (I certify that the statements on the reverse apply to this bill and are made a part thereof.) PHIL WELLS MD 12/01/20YY SIGNED DATE | 32. SERVICE FACILITY LOCATION INFORMATION a. NPI b. | 33. BILLING PROVIDER INFO & PH # (555)5551234 PEARSON MEDICAL CLINIC 123 UNKNOWN BLVD PARKER HEIGHTS IL 66666-6789 a. 151317216 b. |

PHYSICIAN OR SUPPLIER INFORMATION

NUCC Instruction Manual available at: www.nucc.org   **PLEASE PRINT OR TYPE**   APPROVED OMB-0938-1197 FORM 1500 (02-12)

FIGURE 14-9 A completed CMS-1500 (02/12) claim form.

PROCEDURE 14-6

Completing a CMS-1500 Claim Form

Objective ◆ *Identify required data and accurately complete a paper-based CMS-1500 claim form.*

EQUIPMENT AND SUPPLIES

New Patient Registration Form for Theresa Andrews (Figure 14-5); Encounter Form for Theresa Andrews (Figure 14-8) (Table 14-5): instructions on completing the CMS-1500 Claim Form; blank CMS-1500 form (photocopy Figure 14-7 or obtain from instructor); black pen; calculator

METHOD

Refer to Table 14-5 to identify how each field is to be completed and where to find the information. Print all information neatly, in capital letters, with a pen. Erasing, crossouts, write-overs, and white-out may not be used. You may wish to fill in a draft form in pencil, and then recopy it in ink when finished.

1. Enter the insurance company name and mailing address in the Carrier Area. You will find all insurance information on the New Patient Registration Form.
2. Check the correct box in Item 1.
3. Enter the insured's ID number in Item 1a.
4. Enter the patient's name in Item 2, if it is different from the insured's number.
5. Complete Item 3, using MMDDCCYY date format.
6. Complete Item 4.
7. Leave Item 5 blank because it is the same as Item 7.
8. Complete Item 6.
9. Complete Item 7. Note there are three lines of information to complete.
10. Leave Item 8 blank.
11. Leave Item 9a to 9d blank because there is no secondary insurance.
12. Complete Items 10a, 10b, and 10c.
13. Leave Item 10d blank.
14. Enter the group number in Item 11.
15. Complete Item 11a, using MMDDCCYY date format.
16. Leave Item 11b blank.
17. Enter the insurance plan name in Item 11c.
18. Mark NO in Item 11d.
19. Enter "SOF" in Item 12.
20. Enter "SOF" in Item 13.
21. Leave Item 14 to Item 19 blank.
22. Enter the first diagnosis code in Item 21, line A. You will find all information related to the visit on the Encounter Form.
23. Enter the second diagnosis code in Item 21, line B.
24. Enter the 1 to identify the ICD-10-CM code set in the top right corner of Item 21, next to the label "ICD Ind." You will find this information in Table 14-5 under the instructions for Item 21.
25. Leave Item 22 and Item 23 blank.
26. In Item 24A, line 1, enter the date of service in both the FROM and TO fields.
27. Enter the place of service code in Item 24B. You will find this in Table 14-5 under the instructions for Item 24B.
28. Leave Item 24C blank.
29. Enter the CPT for the office visit code in Item 24D.
30. In Item 24E, enter "A B" to designate that both diagnoses on lines 21A and 21B relate to this service.
31. Enter the fee for the office visit in Item 24F.
32. Enter 1 for units in Item 24G.
33. Leave blank Item 24H and Item 24I.
34. Enter the physician's NPI number on the unshaded portion of 24J. You will find this on the Encounter Form next to the physician's signature.
35. Repeat these steps for Item 24A, line 2 for the chest X-ray.
36. Enter the EIN in Item 25, and mark X in the appropriate box. You will find this at the bottom of the Encounter Form.
37. Enter the patient's account number in Item 26. You will find this on the New Patient Registration Form.
38. Mark YES in Item 27.
39. Add up the total charges in column 24F. Write the total in Item 28.
40. Leave Item 29 and Item 30 blank.
41. Enter the physician's signature, credentials, and the date in Item 31. Be certain to stay within the lines of the box.
42. Enter the name and address of the clinic in Item 32. You will find the clinic information at the bottom of the Encounter Form.
43. Enter the clinic's group NPI number in 32a.
44. Leave Item 32b blank.
45. In Item 33, enter the clinic's phone number in the top right corner.
46. Enter the clinic's name and address in Item 33.
47. Enter the clinic's NPI number in Item 33a.
48. Leave Item 33b blank.
49. Proofread your work. Check spelling and numbers against your source documents.
50. Check your claim against the sample CMS-1500 form in Figure A.

HEALTH INSURANCE CLAIM FORM

APPROVED BY NATIONAL UNIFORM CLAIM COMMITTEE (NUCC) 02/12

TRUSTMARK PPO
PO BOX 12345

GREEN BAY WI 12345

[ ][ ] PICA

PICA [ ][ ]

| 1. MEDICARE (Medicare#) ☐ MEDICAID (Medicaid#) ☐ TRICARE (ID#/DoD#) ☐ CHAMPVA (Member ID#) ☐ GROUP HEALTH PLAN (ID#) ☐ FECA BLK LUNG (ID#) ☐ OTHER ☒ (ID#) | 1a. INSURED'S I.D. NUMBER (For Program in Item 1) 332460432 |

2. PATIENT'S NAME (Last Name, First Name, Middle Initial)

3. PATIENT'S BIRTH DATE — MM 06 | DD 08 | YY 1967   SEX M ☐ F ☒

4. INSURED'S NAME (Last Name, First Name, Middle Initial)
ANDREWS THERESA

5. PATIENT'S ADDRESS (No., Street)

6. PATIENT RELATIONSHIP TO INSURED
Self ☒ Spouse ☐ Child ☐ Other ☐

7. INSURED'S ADDRESS (No., Street)
4569 AVENUE K APT 120

CITY   STATE

8. RESERVED FOR NUCC USE

CITY
PLANO   STATE TX

ZIP CODE   TELEPHONE (Include Area Code) ( )

ZIP CODE
12345   TELEPHONE (Include Area Code) (972) 5554448

9. OTHER INSURED'S NAME (Last Name, First Name, Middle Initial)

10. IS PATIENT'S CONDITION RELATED TO:

11. INSURED'S POLICY GROUP OR FECA NUMBER
2038831

a. OTHER INSURED'S POLICY OR GROUP NUMBER

a. EMPLOYMENT? (Current or Previous) ☐ YES ☒ NO

a. INSURED'S DATE OF BIRTH MM 06 | DD 08 | YY 1967   SEX M ☐ F ☒

b. RESERVED FOR NUCC USE

b. AUTO ACCIDENT? ☐ YES ☒ NO   PLACE (State)

b. OTHER CLAIM ID (Designated by NUCC)

c. RESERVED FOR NUCC USE

c. OTHER ACCIDENT? ☐ YES ☒ NO

c. INSURANCE PLAN NAME OR PROGRAM NAME
TRUSTMARK PPO

d. INSURANCE PLAN NAME OR PROGRAM NAME

10d. CLAIM CODES (Designated by NUCC)

d. IS THERE ANOTHER HEALTH BENEFIT PLAN? ☐ YES ☒ NO   If yes, complete items 9, 9a, and 9d.

READ BACK OF FORM BEFORE COMPLETING & SIGNING THIS FORM.
12. PATIENT'S OR AUTHORIZED PERSON'S SIGNATURE I authorize the release of any medical or other information necessary to process this claim. I also request payment of government benefits either to myself or to the party who accepts assignment below.

SIGNED   SOF   DATE

13. INSURED'S OR AUTHORIZED PERSON'S SIGNATURE I authorize payment of medical benefits to the undersigned physician or supplier for services described below.

SIGNED   SOF

14. DATE OF CURRENT ILLNESS, INJURY, or PREGNANCY (LMP) MM | DD | YY   QUAL.

15. OTHER DATE QUAL.   MM | DD | YY

16. DATES PATIENT UNABLE TO WORK IN CURRENT OCCUPATION FROM MM | DD | YY   TO MM | DD | YY

17. NAME OF REFERRING PROVIDER OR OTHER SOURCE

17a.
17b. NPI

18. HOSPITALIZATION DATES RELATED TO CURRENT SERVICES FROM MM | DD | YY   TO MM | DD | YY

19. ADDITIONAL CLAIM INFORMATION (Designated by NUCC)

20. OUTSIDE LAB? ☐ YES ☐ NO $ CHARGES

21. DIAGNOSIS OR NATURE OF ILLNESS OR INJURY Relate A-L to service line below (24E)   ICD Ind. 0
A. J1108   B. J180   C.   D.
E.   F.   G.   H.
I.   J.   K.   L.

22. RESUBMISSION CODE   ORIGINAL REF. NO.

23. PRIOR AUTHORIZATION NUMBER

24. A. DATE(S) OF SERVICE From MM DD YY — To MM DD YY	B. PLACE OF SERVICE	C. EMG	D. PROCEDURES, SERVICES, OR SUPPLIES (Explain Unusual Circumstances) CPT/HCPCS	MODIFIER	E. DIAGNOSIS POINTER	F. $ CHARGES	G. DAYS OR UNITS	H. EPSDT Family Plan	I. ID. QUAL.	J. RENDERING PROVIDER ID. #
1	03 15 20YY 03 15 20YY	11		99212		AB	35 00	1		NPI	9998887776
2	03 15 20YY 03 15 20YY	11		71020		AB	53 00	1		NPI	9998887776
3										NPI	
4										NPI	
5										NPI	
6										NPI	

25. FEDERAL TAX I.D. NUMBER   SSN EIN ☐ ☒
444555666

26. PATIENT'S ACCOUNT NO.
V611

27. ACCEPT ASSIGNMENT? (For govt. claims, see back) ☒ YES ☐ NO

28. TOTAL CHARGE
$ 88 | 00

29. AMOUNT PAID
$

30. Rsvd for NUCC Use

31. SIGNATURE OF PHYSICIAN OR SUPPLIER INCLUDING DEGREES OR CREDENTIALS (I certify that the statements on the reverse apply to this bill and are made a part thereof.)
MARCUS WELLMAN MD
SIGNED   3/15/YY   DATE

32. SERVICE FACILITY LOCATION INFORMATION

a.   b.

33. BILLING PROVIDER INFO & PH # (972) 5555482
ALLIED MEDICAL CENTER
1933 E FRANKFORT RD
CARROLLTON TX 12345-6789
a. 1112223334   b.

NUCC Instruction Manual available at: www.nucc.org   **PLEASE PRINT OR TYPE**   APPROVED OMB-0938-1197 FORM 1500 (02-12)

FIGURE A A completed CMS-1500 (02/12) claim for Procedure 14-6 (Theresa Andrews).

Secondary Policies

When patients have a secondary insurance policy, it is billed after the primary policy has paid. This is because the secondary payer needs to know how much the primary policy paid to determine benefits. In some cases the secondary policy may pay 100 percent of the balance remaining, and in other cases it may not. The calculations depend on the provisions of each policy.

To bill secondary insurance, medical assistants create a CMS-1500 form, attach a copy of RA from the primary payer, and send the entire package to the secondary payer.

The secondary CMS-1500 is identical to the one sent to the primary with two changes:

- Enter the name and address of the secondary payer in the Carrier Area.

- Enter the amount paid by the primary policy company in Item 29.

When an office uses computer software to create CMS-1500 forms, the software normally generates a form for the secondary company with the required changes. When submitting electronic claims, some insurance companies automatically forward the RA information to the secondary

company, eliminating the need for a second billing by the medical office.

Electronic Transactions

One of the purposes of HIPAA is to standardize how electronic transmissions are handled. Electronic transactions, also called electronic data interchange (EDI), are exchanges involving the computerized transfer of health care information between two parties for specific purposes, such as a health care provider submitting medical claims to a health plan for payment. Version 5010 is the set of standards used for all health care transactions.

Each process that was once handled on paper has a corresponding electronic format. Just as the CMS-1500 form is the standard for paper claims, the 837P is the standard format for electronic claims. Each data element in the 837P corresponds to a field on the CMS-1500. In addition to submitting claims, medical assistants may use electronic transactions for tracking claim status, receiving RAs, coordination of benefits, eligibility inquiries, referrals, and authorization requests.

Electronic claims, also called electronic media claims (EMC), are the leading method of claims submission by providers. Electronic claims are never printed on paper and can be submitted to the insurance carrier via direct data entry, direct wire, telephone line via modem, or disc. When claims are sent electronically to the insurance carriers for processing, an electronic signature is used to verify that the information received is true and correct. Medicare requires electronic transmission of claims for providers with 10 or more employees or facilities with 25 or more employees. Paper claims are not processed for these submitters.

Electronic claims have a number of advantages:

- Administrative costs are lower because fewer personnel hours are needed to prepare forms, and supply and postage costs are lower.

- Fewer claims are rejected because technical errors are detected and corrected before the claim arrives at the payer.

- Processing is faster with fewer errors. An electronic claim is received by the payer in minutes. The payer does not have to perform data entry, so there is less opportunity for errors to be introduced. In addition, most claims can be automatically adjudicated by the computer, rather than being processed by a claims analyst.

- Errors can be corrected faster. If errors are found on claims by carriers or the claim is denied, the office is notified immediately and medical assistants can begin work on resolving the issue.

- Payment is faster. Payment can be transferred electronically to the provider's bank, eliminating delays in cash flow. These payments are referred to as electronic remittances. Medicare is required by law to process electronic claims in 14 days, and is prohibited from processing paper claims for at least 28 days after receipt.

Electronic claims also have disadvantages:

- Claims transmission can be disrupted occasionally because of power failures or computer hardware or software problems that might require claims to be resubmitted.
- Many patient billing programs cannot create an electronic attachment, so when a claim attachment is required, the electronic claim must be sent separately from mailed attachments, which sometimes causes problems for the payer in matching up the two. In some cases, the claim must instead be submitted on paper when it must be accompanied by a claim attachment.

Medical assistants enter patient, insurance, and service information into practice management software, which then converts the data into the standard format required by HIPAA. Claims may be submitted daily, weekly, or on any schedule the office determines is best.

Electronic claims are submitted through a **clearinghouse**, a billing service, or directly to the carrier. A physician who plans to use electronic billing must contact all major insurers and carriers for a list of the vendors approved to handle electronic claims, and must have a signed agreement with each. Each carrier has special electronic billing requirements and is knowledgeable in which systems meet their criteria and which are compatible in format. Insurance carriers also provide information about how to submit an electronic bill for patients who have secondary coverage.

Medicare, Medicaid, TRICARE, and many private insurance carriers allow providers to submit insurance claims directly to them with no "middle man." In this type of system, the medical practice must have special software or the physician must lease a terminal from the carrier to key in claims data. The data are transmitted via modem (dedicated telephone line) directly to the carrier's computer for processing. Medicare provides software and training for electronic submissions of Medicare claims. Procedure 14-7 describes how to prepare an electronic insurance claim.

If the physician is not sending the data directly to the carrier, they may use a clearinghouse. A clearinghouse is a company that receives claims from providers, processes them through a series of audits to check for errors, and then forwards them to the appropriate insurance carrier in the required data format. Clearinghouses may charge a flat fee per claim or charge a percentage of the claim's dollar value. It is very important for physicians' practices to negotiate the best possible fee for using a clearinghouse's services.

The clearinghouse conducts an audit to determine if any data on the claim is incorrect or missing. A claim with incorrect or missing information is a dirty claim, and is not transmitted to the carrier. The results of the audit are sent back to the provider from the clearinghouse in the form of an audit/edit report. The medical assistant needs to correct any claims with incorrect data (as indicated on the audit/edit report) and resubmit them to the clearinghouse. When the claims are corrected and resubmitted to the clearinghouse, they are **clean claims**, which are then formatted and forwarded to the carrier. Each time the claim is returned, there is an additional charge, so the medical assistant should ensure that clean claims are transmitted initially.

Paper Claims

The CMS-1500 form must be used when submitting claims on paper. The form was developed so it could be used with optical character recognition (OCR). OCR scanners read printed or typed text and convert it to data that a computer can process, rather than having the data rekeyed. The CMS-1500 form is printed in a specific color of red ink so that it is recognizable by OCR scanners. The red portion drops out, or becomes invisible to the scanner, so the scanner can read only the data entered. The office should not attempt to reprint or copy the form on a color device because the dropout red does not reproduce accurately. Original approved forms must be used.

Filing Timelines

Most insurance carriers accept claims up to one year from the date of service, although some have much shorter timelines, such as 90 days. After filing timelines pass, claims are considered past timely filing limits and will likely be rejected. With most managed care plans, claims rejected because of timely filing limits cannot be billed to the patient. To avoid rejection, it is best to submit claims soon after service is rendered.

Supporting Documentation

Many insurance plans require supporting documentation, such as chart notes, surgical/operative reports, laboratory reports, and pathology reports, before they agree to pay for certain, usually high-cost, services such as surgeries. When calling insurance carriers to obtain preauthorization for services, medical assistants should ask customer service representatives if they need supporting documentation with the

Completing Electronic Insurance Claims

Objective ◆ *Identify required data and accurately complete computer screens needed to create and submit an electronic insurance claim.*

EQUIPMENT AND SUPPLIES

Computer with medical billing software; patient medical chart; fee slip for patient's visit

METHOD

1. Log in to the patient accounting software with the username and password previously created.
2. Choose the patient's account ledger in the computer billing software.
3. Verify that the fee slip is for the patient with the account opened on the computer.
4. Enter the charges and coding as appropriate.
5. Complete the patient insurance information field.
6. Enter the patient's information, including address, telephone number, and birthdate.
7. Enter the insured's information, including address, telephone number, and birthdate.
8. Enter the patient's relationship to the insured.
9. Enter the insured's identification and group number.
10. Check the appropriate box to indicate the patient has authorized the release of information to the insurance company.
11. Check the appropriate box to indicate the patient has assigned the benefits (payment) to the provider.
12. Check the appropriate boxes to indicate if the visit was related to an accident.
13. If the visit was a result of an accident, enter the accident's date.

14. Enter information regarding a referring physician, if applicable.
15. Enter information regarding the dates of hospitalization for these charges, if applicable.
16. Enter the treating provider's name, address, telephone number, national provider identification (NPI) number, and Internal Revenue Service (IRS) tax identification number.
17. Enter information regarding the facility where the services were performed if not performed in the provider's office.
18. Check the appropriate box to indicate the provider accepts assignment.
19. Review all information on the screen for accuracy and completeness.
20. Following the instructions for the software application, select the menu item to transmit electronic claims. Usually, all claims entered into the computer during the day (or week) can be sent at the same time.
21. Following the instructions for the software application, select the menu item to download a transmission report that lists all claims sent in the current batch. Review the report to verify that all claims were received.
22. Identify the reason for any claims that did not transmit. These claims are flagged as "failed" or "did not transmit" or similar wording. A code or abbreviation for the failure is provided. Look up the meaning of the code or abbreviation in the manual provided by the claims clearinghouse or software vendor. Correct the error(s) and resubmit.

insurance claim forms. Sending proper documentation with the initial billing, when required, helps avoid delayed payment. Most claims that require attachments must be prepared on paper, although there is an increasing ability for insurance companies to accept electronic attachments.

The insurance company may ask for additional documentation while reviewing the claim. The request usually comes in the form of a letter. When replying to such requests, medical assistants should be certain to identify exactly what information is being requested and respond specifically. It is not necessary to send a voluminous amount of records when only one or two specific items are requested. Box 14-2 lists steps to take to help avoid claim form rejection.

UB-04 Claim Form

The **UB-04**, also known as the CMS-1450, is the claim form used by inpatient hospitals (Figure 14-10). The electronic format for claims submission of inpatient services is the 837I. The National Uniform Billing Committee (NUBC), chaired by the American Hospital Association (AHA), maintains and updates the UB-04 form. NUBC also provides specific guidelines for completing a UB-04 claim form that are consistent with those for preparing electronic claims. The form contains 81 form locators, or boxes, that must be completed:

- 1-41 Patient information
- 42-49 Billing information

INPATIENT

1 Any Hospital		2 Any Hospital			3a PAT CNTL # 1234		4 TYPE OF BILL
123 Any Street		456 Any Street			b MED REC # 98765		0111
Philadelphia	PA 19103	Philadelphia	PA 19103	5 FED. TAX. NO. 221234567	6 STATEMENT COVERS PERIOD FROM 11 03 06 THROUGH 11 04 06	7 RESERVED	

8 PATIENT NAME	a Patient ID if different from Sub	9 PATIENT ADDRESS	a 1234 Main Street				
b Doe, John		b Philadelphia			c PA	d 19111	Country code if other than USA

10 BIRTHDATE	11 SEX	12 DATE	ADMISSION 13 HR	14 TYPE	15 SRC	16 DHR	17 STAT	18	19	20	21	CONDITION CODES 22 23 24 25 26 27 28	29 ACDT STATE	30
03 20 1971	M	11 03 06	08	3	3	12	01	Condition Codes Required identifying Events					PA	RESERVED

31 OCCURRENCE CODE DATE	32 OCCURRENCE CODE DATE	33 OCCURRENCE CODE DATE	34 OCCURRENCE CODE DATE	35 OCCURRENCE SPAN CODE FROM THROUGH	36 OCCURRENCE SPAN CODE FROM THROUGH	37
a						FUTURE USE
b Occurrence and Occurrence Span Codes may be used to define a significant event that may affect payer processing						

38		39 CODE VALUE CODES AMOUNT	40 CODE VALUE CODES AMOUNT	41 CODE VALUE CODES AMOUNT
John Doe 1234 Main Street Philadelphia, PA 19111		a A1 952:00		
		b Value Codes and amounts required when necessary to process claim		
		c		
		d		

	42 REV.CD.	43 DESCRIPTION	44 HCPCS/RATE/HPPS CODE	45 SERV. DATE	46 SERV. UNIT	47 TOTAL CHARGES	48 NON-COVERED CHARGES	49	
1	0129	Semi-Private	200.00		2	400:00	0:00	Future Use	1
2	0250	Pharmacy			1	50:00	0:00		2
3	0360	OR Services				100:00	0:00		3
4									4
5									5
6									6
7									7
8									8
9									9
10									10
11									11
12									12
13									13
14									14
15									15
16									16
17									17
18									18
19									19
20									20
21									21
22									22
23	PAGE 1 OF 1	CREATION DATE	TOTALS ►			550:00	0:00		23

	50 PAYER NAME	51 HEALTH PLAN ID	52 REL INFO	53 ASG BEN.	54 PRIOR PAYMENTS	55 EST. AMOUNT DUE	56 NPI 2222222222		
A	Independence Blue Cross	Report HIPAA National	Y	Y	Required when indicated payer has paid amount to Provider	Amount estimated to be due	57 1234567890		A
B	Secondary Payer	Health Plan Identifier					OTHER Secondary		B
C	Tertiary Payer	when mendatory					PRV. ID Tertiary		C

	58 INSURED'S NAME	59	60 INSURED'S UNIQUE ID	61 GROUP NAME	62 INSURANCE GROUP NO.	
A	Doe, John	18	ABC12345678900	Watch Repair, Inc.	1234	A
B	Secondary					B
C	Tertiary					C

	63 TREATMENT AUTHORIZATION CODES	64 DOCUMENT CONTROL NUMBER	65 EMPLOYER NAME	
A	02468	491234	Watch Repair, Inc.	A
B	Secondary			B
C	Tertiary			C

66 K50115	A Use A through Q to report "Other Diagnosis" if applicable	E	F	G	H	68 Reserved
0	J	K	L	M	N	O	P	Q	

69 ADMIT DX K50115	70 PATIENT REASON DX May be used to report reason for visit	71 PPS CODE DRS	72 ECI May be used to report external cause of injury	73 Reserved

74 PRINCIPAL PROCEDURE CODE DATE	a OTHER PROCEDURE CODE DATE	b OTHER PROCEDURE CODE DATE	75 Reserved	76 ATTENDING NPI 2222222222 QUAL 16 1234569822
0D1B0Z4 08 26 YY				LAST Smith FIRST David
c OTHER PROCEDURE CODE DATE	d OTHER PROCEDURE CODE DATE	e OTHER PROCEDURE CODE DATE		77 OPERATING NPI QUAL
				LAST FIRST

80 REMARKS	81CC a B3 292N00000X	78 OTHER NPI QUAL
May be used to report additional	b Secondary	LAST FIRST
information.	c Tertiary	79 OTHER NPI QUAL
	d	LAST FIRST

UB-04 CMS-1450   APPROVED OMB NO.   NUBC™ National Uniform Billing Committee   THE CERTIFICATIONS ON THE REVERSE APPLY TO THIS BILL AND ARE MADE A PART HEREOF.

Red = Required
Black = Situational/Required, if applicable/Reserved

FIGURE 14-10 Inpatient hospitals bill using the UB-04 form or its electronic equivalent.

- 50-65 Payer information
- 66-81 Diagnosis and procedure information.

NUBC guidelines are published in the *Official UB-04 Data Specifications Manual*, which is updated each year in July and can be accessed on the World Wide Web at www.nubc.org.

SUMMARY

Most patients coming into the medical office have some form of health care insurance. Health insurance was not designed to cover all costs associated with health care but rather to assist the patient with expenses incurred for medical treatment. The 1980s and 1990s saw a rapid rise in the cost of health care, because of advancing technology and funding from Medicare and Medicaid. Congress passed the federal HMO Act of 1973, which allowed use of federal funds and policy to promote health maintenance organizations (HMOs). As a result, the majority of employer-sponsored group insurance plans moved to less expensive managed care plans. In 2009, Congress passed the Patient Protection and Affordable Care Act (PPACA), which established the health insurance exchange (HIE) to create a more organized and competitive market for buying health insurance.

Health insurance plans are classified either as indemnity plans or managed care plans. Indemnity plans impose few restrictions on patients, whereas managed care plans seek to control costs by limiting patients' choices. Managed care plans contract with physicians, hospitals, and other providers to offer services for a lower fee. Then, they contract with government programs, private health insurance companies, and self-insured plans to promote an exclusive network of participating providers or preferred providers.

Third-party payers are organizations that pay for health care services on behalf of the patient and include private health insurance as well as government plans such as Medicare, Medicaid, workers' compensation, and military insurance (TRICARE and CHAMPVA). The medical assistant should have a working knowledge of each type of insurance to be able to quickly and accurately process insurance forms.

Insurance companies are not obligated to pay the amount the physician charges and usually establish their own reimbursement schedules. An insurance company calculates what it determines to be an average or customary price among providers of the same specialty and in the same geographic area. This is the approved or allowed amount. When a provider's actual charge is less than the allowed amount, the insurer pays the actual charge. When providers' charges are more than the insurance-allowed amount, the insurance pays the allowed amount. This method of determining insurance payments is usual, customary, and reasonable (UCR).

The first step in receiving proper reimbursement for insurance claims is obtaining accurate patient information. Each new patient in the medical office should complete a registration form (review Figure 14-5) that is verified at each visit and updated annually. After the proper patient information has been gathered and the service has been provided, medical assistants prepare the claim to submit to the insurance company. Whether submitting claims electronically or on paper, the same information is required and specific guidelines must be followed for each format. Medical assistants must submit all paper claims using the CMS-1500 form, a uniform billing format used for medical claims. The 837P is the standard format for electronic claims. Each data element in the 837P corresponds to a field on the CMS-1500. In addition to submitting claims, medical assistants may use electronic transactions for tracking claim status, receiving RAs, coordination of benefits, eligibility inquiries, referrals, and authorization requests.

COMPETENCY REVIEW

1. Define and spell the terms for this chapter.
2. Explain the birthday rule and when it is used.
3. What are the two important components of an HMO?
4. How does a PPO differ from an HMO?
5. Explain the purpose of verifying benefits.
6. How much does the following patient owe? Total charges: $125.00, allowed amount: $110.00, amount paid by insurance: $88.00, coinsurance: 20%

7. What is the name of the standardized form used to submit insurance claims? What information must be included on this form?
8. List five ways to avoid rejection of insurance claims.

PREPARING FOR THE CERTIFICATION EXAM

1. What provision of PPACA helps people who need to purchase health insurance to do so?
   a. Medicare
   b. Medicaid
   c. HIE
   d. TEFRA
   e. GHI

2. How many days from the date of service is considered to be timely filing by most insurance carriers?
   a. 20
   b. 30
   c. 45
   d. 120
   e. 365

3. What is the monetary amount patients must pay to the provider for health care services before health insurance benefits begin to pay?
   a. premium
   b. copayment
   c. deductible
   d. coinsurance
   e. allowable

4. What is Medicare's per-case reimbursement method?
   a. RVS
   b. RBRVS
   c. UCR
   d. MS-DRG
   e. FFS

5. Where on the CMS-1500 form should the name be entered when the patient is also the insured?
   a. Item 2 Patient's Name
   b. Item 4 Insured's Name
   c. Both Item 2 and Item 4
   d. Item 6 Patient's Relationship to Insured
   e. Item 9c Insurance Plan or Program Name

6. What is the process of determining which company is primary and which is secondary?
   a. assignment of benefits
   b. verification of benefits
   c. preauthorization
   d. point-of-service plan
   e. coordination of benefits

7. Using the birthday rule, the parent who is usually primary when billing for a child's services is the parent who
   a. has a birthday earlier in the year.
   b. has a birthday later in the year.
   c. is older.
   d. is younger.
   e. is randomly selected by the insurance company.

8. Which type of service may require an authorization from the insurance company?
   a. emergency room visit
   b. elective joint replacement surgery
   c. removal of foreign body from the eye to save an injured worker's vision
   d. annual preventive care visit
   e. treatment for strep throat

9. Which type of insurance is *not* covered under HIPAA?
   a. HMOs
   b. Medicare
   c. TRICARE
   d. workers' compensation
   e. all of the above are subject to HIPAA

10. Which Medicare program covers physician care, therapy, and laboratory testing on a fee-for-service basis?
    a. Part A
    b. Part B
    c. Part C
    d. Part D
    e. Medigap

CRITICAL THINKING

Refer to the case study at the beginning of the chapter and use what you have learned to answer the following questions.

1. What steps should Lewis take to verify Sylvia Baker's insurance?

2. List some reasons the claim for Mr. Flannery care could have been rejected.

3. How should Lewis handle Mr. Flannery's angry call?

ON THE JOB

Patient Kenya Hilbert arrives for an appointment and gives the medical assistant, Portia Milstine, MA, her insurance card. Portia notices that the insurance company is Healthy Way Insurance and that Ms. Hilbert works for the Exact Accounting Company, a large company near the medical clinic. She recalls that this morning Josiah Campbell came in and that he also had Healthy Way Insurance and also works for the Exact Accounting Company. When she verified his benefits, she learned that preventive care is covered at 100 percent, and for other services, patients must pay a $20.00 copayment. The office is busy this afternoon, so Portia wonders if she really needs to take the time to verify the benefits for Ms. Hilbert. After all, it looks like she has the exact same insurance that Mr. Campbell had, and she already verified his benefits.

1. Is it necessary to verify the benefits for Ms. Hilbert because she has the same insurance company as Mr. Campbell and they work for the same company? Why or why not?

2. What would happen if Portia told Ms. Hilbert that her visit today will be covered 100 percent by her insurance company, based on what she learned about Mr. Campbell's insurance with the same company?

3. What methods could Portia use to verify benefits?

INTERNET ACTIVITY

Most third-party payers maintain websites to provide the public with information about services and benefits. Conduct an Internet search to find the government's website for Medicare beneficiaries, Medicaid in your state, and Blue Cross or Blue Shield in your state or region. What information on the sites would be useful for patients? What sections of each site would be useful for medical assistants?

Some states have set up their own health insurance exchange (HIE), and others use the federal HIE at www.healthcare.gov. Find out how your state handles HIEs, and locate the appropriate website so that you can refer patients to it when needed.

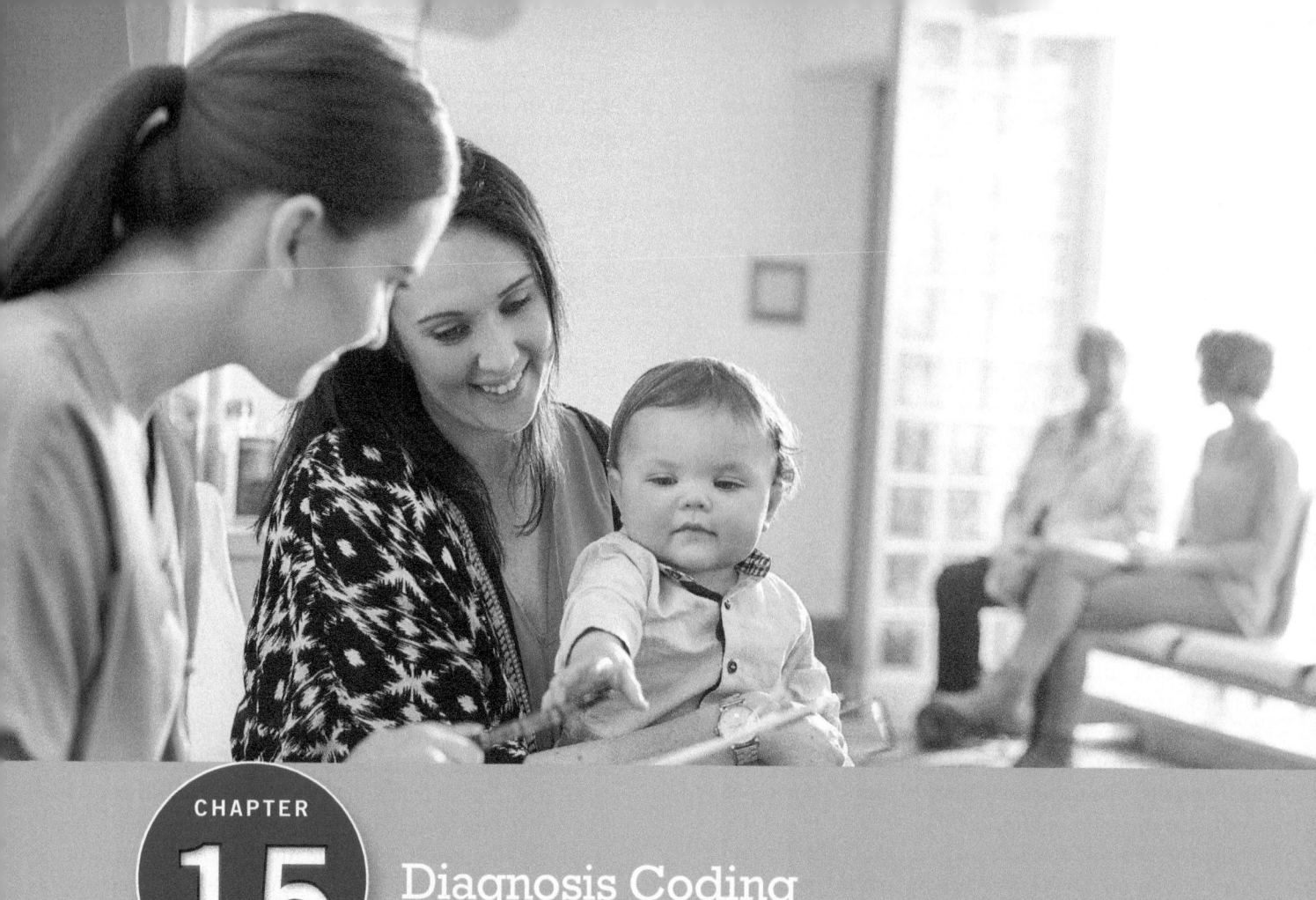

Learning Objectives

After completing this chapter, you should be able to:

15.1 Define and spell the terms for this chapter.

15.2 Explain the medical assistant's role in diagnostic coding.

15.3 Describe the history of diagnostic coding.

15.4 List the expected benefits of the conversion to ICD-10.

15.5 Explain the organization of the ICD-10-CM manual.

15.6 Describe the purpose of each section of the ICD-10-CM manual.

15.7 Describe how to use the ICD-10-CM coding system to assign a diagnostic code.

15.8 Identify situations that require special diagnostic coding considerations.

Sophia DiStefano, a 5-year-old female, is seen by Dr. Salpega. He diagnoses Sophia with bilateral chronic serous otitis media because this visit is the third bout of otitis media she has had within the past seven months. Dr. Salpega asks that David Dolan, a Registered Medical Assistant, conduct an audiometry screening on Sophia. He also suggests that Edvige, Sophia's mother, consider having Sophia undergo a bilateral tympanostomy and tube placement for a more permanent treatment of the chronic otitis media.

Terms to Learn

abuse	ICD-10-CM	procedure coding
category	Index to Diseases and Injuries	qualified diagnosis
chapter	Index to External Causes	section
code	Main Term	subcategory
combination code	medical coding	subterm
compliance	multiple coding	Table of Drugs and Chemicals
conventions	Office of the Inspector General (OIG)	Table of Neoplasms
diagnosis coding	Official Guidelines for Coding and Reporting (OGCR)	Tabular List
etiology		uncertain diagnosis
first-listed diagnosis	Patient Protection and Affordable Care Act (PPACA)	verify
fraud		

Medical coding is the process of assigning alphanumeric characters that represent the diagnoses doctors give their patients (**diagnosis coding**) and the services they provide (**procedure coding**). Diagnosis codes are listed in **ICD-10-CM** (International Classification of Diseases, Clinical Modification) manual. These codes are used by all health care providers, including physicians. Procedure codes used by physicians and outpatient hospitals are listed in the CPT (Current Procedural Terminology) manual. Procedure codes used by inpatient hospitals are listed in the ICD-10-PCS (International Classification of Diseases, Procedure Coding System) manual.

MEDICAL CODING

In medical coding, the combination of diagnosis codes and related procedure codes provides the basis for health care reimbursement. The Health Insurance Portability and Accountability Act (HIPAA) mandates the approved code sets for all covered entities, such as medical offices, that handle claims related to health care services. On a broader scale,

medical codes are used to compile and report statistics—within the United States and worldwide—regarding health status and health trends.

Physicians are responsible to code and bill for all the services they personally provide in medical offices, outpatient settings such as ambulatory surgery centers, and inpatient settings such as hospitals. This chapter, "Diagnosis Coding," focuses on how to assign ICD-10-CM diagnosis codes for patients seen in medical offices. The chapter titled "Procedure Coding" focuses on how to assign the CPT procedure codes.

The Role of Medical Assistants in Coding

Medical assistants usually do not perform medical coding as a regular part of their job because most offices hire or contract with professional certified coders who are trained in the details of assigning medical codes. However, the need may arise occasionally for medical assistants to research a code. In addition, medical assistants are among the few employees of medical offices who are trained in both the administrative and the clinical aspects of health care.

Therefore, medical assistants can fill an important role in the communication and understanding of medical codes in the following ways:

- Assist in communication between coders and physicians when a question arises.

- Provide appropriate diagnosis codes when an insurance preauthorization is required for a procedure or when a patient is referred to another provider for a procedure or consultation.

- Facilitate communication with attorneys who may need information about medical codes related to injured patients they represent. (Specific written authorization by patients is required for the release of protected health information {PHI} to attorneys.)

- Answer patient questions about the meanings of codes on their insurance claims or other paperwork.

- Review or facilitate medical documentation to help ensure it provides adequate specificity (detail) for coding.

Medical coding requires knowledge of anatomy and physiology; clinical procedures; local, state, and federal regulations; and attention to detail. Medical assistants should understand the scope and limitations of their training in medical coding, should provide assistance whenever possible, and should consult with a certified coder whenever they are not completely confident regarding the coding information requested.

History of Diagnosis Coding

Diagnosis coding began in 1893 with French physician Jacques Bertillon. Dr. Bertillon created the Bertillon Classification of Causes of Death, which the American Public Health Association (APHA) adopted in 1898. Historically, diagnosis coding was used to track the study of disease and causes of death. As the medical field became more sophisticated, so did the coding system. The system that began as a short list of diseases has now become a highly detailed classification of over 70,000 codes, each consisting of three to seven characters. Table 15-1 provides highlights of the history of diagnosis coding.

Overview of ICD-10-CM

ICD-10-CM is an update and major revision to the ICD-9-CM, which was used in the United States from 1979 to 2015 for diagnosis reporting.

TABLE 15-1 | The History of Diagnosis Coding

Date	Event
1893	French physician Jacques Bertillon creates the Bertillon Classification of Causes of Death.
1898	American Public Health Association (APHA) adopts the Bertillon Classification.
1901	APHA publishes the first coding manual, called the International Classification of Diseases (ICD), Volume I.
1910	APHA begins publishing updates to ICD approximately every 10 years.
1948	The World Health Organization (WHO), an arm of the United Nations (UN), takes responsibility for maintaining and publishing updates to what has become ICD-6.
1965	United States passes legislation authorizing government-funded health care programs for older adults (Medicare) and low-income families (Medicaid). United States publishes an adaptation of ICD-8 tailored to the needs of clinicians in this country, called International Classification of Diseases, Adapted (ICDA-8).
1979	WHO publishes ICD-9, and the United States publishes an adapted version, called International Classification of Diseases, 9th revision, Clinical Modification (ICD-9-CM). The United States begins publishing annual updates to ICD-9-CM to refine the code set and keep pace with changes in medicine. The United States requires clinicians to report ICD-9-CM codes to receive reimbursement from Medicare and Medicaid.
1994	WHO publishes ICD-10 for worldwide reporting of morbidity and mortality data. The United States develops a clinical modification but does not implement it.
1999	The United States begins using ICD-10-CM for coding and classification of mortality data from death certificates.
2009	The United States passes legislation requiring the use of ICD-10-CM on October 1, 2013.
2012	The United States postpones the implementation of ICD-10-CM by clinicians one year, to October 1, 2014.
2014	The United States postpones implementation of ICD-10-CM until after October 1, 2015.
2015	The United States implements ICD-10-CM/PCS on October 1, 2015.

TABLE 15-2 | Comparison of Codes in ICD-9-CM and ICD-10-CM

Feature	ICD-9-CM	ICD-10-CM
Number of codes	16,000	70,000+
Code length	3 to 5 digits	3 to 7 characters
Code structure	3 digit category 4th and 5th digits for etiology, anatomic site, manifestation	3 character category 4th, 5th, 6th characters for etiology, anatomic site, severity 7th character used for additional information
First character	always numeric, except E-codes and V-codes	1st character is always alphabetic
Subsequent characters	all numeric	2nd character is always numeric; all other characters may be alphabetic or numeric
Decimal point	mandatory after 3rd character, except E codes where decimal point is after 4th character	mandatory after 3rd character on all codes
Placeholders	none	character "X" is used as a placeholder in certain 6- and 7-character codes

Because of numerous differences between ICD-9-CM and ICD-10-CM, the transition to the new coding system was one of health care's top priorities. Planning for ICD-10-CM began many years in advance, to analyze systems, update administrative processes, coordinate activities with vendors, train staff, and establish budgets for these activities. The overall process to plan for, implement, and monitor the ICD-10-CM transition required approximately five years.

Everyone who is part of the health care system or uses its data is impacted by the change to ICD-10-CM, including providers, payers, regulators, vendors, claims clearinghouses, medical billing services, researchers, educational institutions, and support staff in each of these settings. All computer systems that collect, transmit, receive, or store diagnostic data needed updating to accommodate the expanded length, format, and structure of codes. These changes further impacted the budgets of organizations and the productivity of workers.

Industry leaders expect that ICD-10-CM will bring many benefits to the health care field over the next several years, including more accurate, detailed data about health trends, fewer coding and billing errors, and an overall savings of time and money.

Table 15-2 compares ICD-9-CM with ICD-10-CM. Table 15-3 lists expected benefits of ICD-10-CM.

Compliance

Compliance simply means following the rules. Health care providers must follow rules established by multiple federal, state, and county government agencies. Some rules are specific to health care, and others pertain to any type of business. Companies and organizations establish compliance programs to actively keep informed about regulations, educate employees, and make sure that everyone in the company is cooperating.

Violating coding and billing rules can be classified as fraud or abuse. Knowingly billing for services that were never given or billing for a service that has a higher reimbursement than the service actually provided is **fraud**. Mistakenly accepting payment for items or services that should

TABLE 15-3 | Expected Benefits of ICD-10-CM

- Detailed diagnosis codes reduce the need for attachments to claims.
- Provides more detailed and higher quality data for tracking quality, safety, and effectiveness of health services.
- Expected to save time and money in the long run.
- Consistency across codes and more specific code descriptions help reduce coding errors.
- Combined with the increased use of electronic health records, the new code set provides more consistent and more detailed data for physician use.
- Advancements in technology and medical practice are reflected in the organization and description of codes.
- The coding system in the United States becomes more consistent with that used in other countries.
- Public officials can better track and respond to domestic and international public health threats.
- The structure of the new code set provides the flexibility to add codes, as needed, in the future.

not be paid as a result of improper coding and billing practices is **abuse**. Examples of fraud or abuse (depending on whether they are done knowingly or by mistake) are billing for a noncovered service, assigning a more costly code to a lesser service, or coding in a way that does not follow national or local coding guidelines. Investigation of Medicare fraud and abuse is primarily the responsibility of the Department of Health and Human Services (HHS) **Office of the Inspector General (OIG)**. The purpose of the OIG is to fight waste, fraud, and abuse in Medicare, Medicaid, and more than 300 other HHS programs.

The OIG provided guidance to assist health care entities to develop effective internal controls to help them be aware of and follow the requirements of federal, state, and private health plans. The OIG believes that health care institutions that adopt and implement compliance programs significantly reduce fraud, abuse, and waste. Compliance programs identify internal controls to help providers be aware of and follow the requirements of federal, state, and private health plans. The OIG has issued sample compliance programs that include seven major characteristics (Table 15-4).

The **Patient Protection and Affordable Care Act (PPACA)**, passed in 2010, mandates compliance programs for providers who contract with Medicare and Medicaid. The timeline for defining and implementing compliance programs has not yet been established.

TABLE 15-4 | Characteristics of a Compliance Program

1. Develop and distribute written standards of conduct, policies, and procedures that address specific areas of potential fraud.
2. Designate a high level manager to be the chief compliance officer who oversees compliance activities.
3. Develop and implement education and training for employees.
4. Establish a process for reporting exceptions.
5. Develop an internal system to respond to accusations or reports of improper activities, and implement disciplinary measures when appropriate.
6. Develop an auditing and monitoring system.
7. Investigate and correct system-wide problems and develop policies regarding employment or retention of sanctioned individuals.

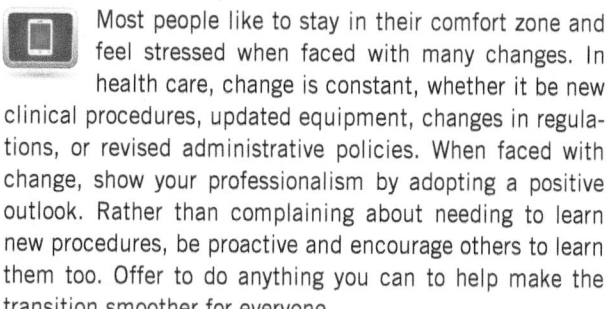

Professionalism   The Workplace

Most people like to stay in their comfort zone and feel stressed when faced with many changes. In health care, change is constant, whether it be new clinical procedures, updated equipment, changes in regulations, or revised administrative policies. When faced with change, show your professionalism by adopting a positive outlook. Rather than complaining about needing to learn new procedures, be proactive and encourage others to learn them too. Offer to do anything you can to help make the transition smoother for everyone.

Professionalism   The Law

All providers and their staff members have a responsibility to be aware of the billing and coding rules established by the federal government and to follow them. Just as telling a police officer, "I didn't see the speed limit sign" does not mean you won't get a speeding ticket, you cannot plead "ignorance" about health care laws.

ORGANIZATION OF THE ICD-10-CM MANUAL

ICD-10-CM provides the codes that identify the diagnoses physicians give patients. ICD-10-CM lists over 70,000 diagnostic codes in one volume. ICD-10-CM codes are updated annually and take effect October 1 of each year. Code changes are published by the National Center for Health Statistics (NCHS) and the Centers for Medicare and Medicaid Services (CMS), in conjunction with the World Health Organization (WHO). Medical assistants should use the edition of the ICD-10-CM that was in effect on the date of service.

Several companies publish the ICD-10-CM manual, so the exact order of information may vary, based on which publisher's book is used. A table of contents page near the front of the manual outlines the contents, organization, and page numbers of the ICD-10-CM (Table 15-5). CMS provides electronic files for ICD-10-CM, which can be downloaded (www.cms.gov).

Introductory Material

The introductory material in the beginning of the ICD-10-CM provides important information for medical assistants. Not only does it provide instructions on how to use ICD-10-CM, it also includes the Official Guidelines for Coding and Reporting (OGCR), universal conventions, and publisher-specific conventions.

Conventions

Conventions are specialized rules, abbreviations, formatting, and symbols that alert users to important information. These

TABLE 15-5 | Organization of the ICD-10-CM Manual

Type of Information	Name of Section	Purpose
Introductory material	Preface Introduction How to Use the ICD-10-CM ICD-10-CM Conventions ICD-10-CM Official Guidelines for Coding and Reporting	Information and rules on how to use the manual.
Index	ICD-10-CM Index to Diseases and Injuries (Index) ICD-10-CM Table of Neoplasms ICD-10-CM Table of Drugs and Chemicals ICD-10-CM Index to External Causes	Alphabetical list of diseases and injuries, reasons for encounters, and external causes. Two tables provide quick lookups, one for neoplasms and one for drugs and chemicals causing injury. Coders must always reference one of these indices or tables when searching for a code.
Tabular list	ICD-10-CM Tabular List of Diseases and Injuries	Numerical list of diseases and injuries, reasons for encounters, and external causes. Provides additional instruction on how to use, assign, and sequence codes. Coders must always reference the Tabular List to verify a code, after consulting the Index, and before assigning the final code.

are described at the beginning of the manual. A key to selected symbols usually appears at the bottom of each page. Certain conventions are universal to all ICD-10-CM manuals, and others are specific to each publisher. Conventions that are an official part of the ICD-10-CM code set are explained in the OGCR and appear in Table 15-6. The most important of these for medical assistants are *Excludes1* and *Excludes2*. These notations explain which codes cannot be used together, as explained next.

ICD-10-CM codes are alphanumeric, meaning they consist of both letters and numbers. The letters are usually written as uppercase but are not case sensitive. Either uppercase or lowercase letters may be used with no change in meaning.

Excludes1. Excludes1 notes appear immediately under a code in the **Tabular List**. The note is followed by a list of other conditions and codes. Excludes1 means that the condition represented by the code and the condition listed as excluded are mutually exclusive and should not be coded together. When an Excludes1 note appears under a code, none of the codes that appear after it should be used with the code where the note appears. This occurs frequently with conditions that may be either congenital or acquired.

EXAMPLE: *Excludes1*

K55 Vascular disorder of intestine

Excludes1: necrotizing enterocolitis of newborn (P77.-)

The second condition, necrotizing enterocolitis of newborn, is not included in codes that begin with K55 Vascular disorder of intestine, and the codes are mutually exclusive. A patient cannot have both conditions. When coding for necrotizing enterocolitis of newborn, the correct code begins with P77, not K55.

Excludes2. Excludes2 notes also appear immediately under a code in the Tabular List. The note is followed by a list of other conditions and codes. Excludes2 means that the condition excluded is not part of the condition represented by the code, but the patient may have both conditions at the same time. These conditions are not mutually exclusive. When an Excludes2 note appears under a code, it is acceptable to use the main code and the excluded code if the patient is documented to have both conditions.

EXAMPLE: *Excludes2*

K86.0 Alcohol induced chronic pancreatitis

Excludes2: alcohol induced acute pancreatitis (K85.2)

The second condition, alcohol induced acute pancreatitis, is not included in code K86.0, but may be reported together with it, if the documentation states that the patient has both the acute and chronic forms of the condition.

Seventh Character. The seventh character of an ICD-10-CM code is reserved for special use, most commonly the episode of care for injuries. The seventh character must be assigned

TABLE 15-6 | ICD-10-CM Conventions

Convention	Meaning/Use
– Short dash	**Index and Tabular:** Additional characters should be assigned in place of the –. The additional characters may be numbers or letters.
( ) Parentheses	**Index and Tabular:** Nonessential modifiers that describe the default variations of a term. These words are not required to appear in the documentation to use the code.
: Colon	**Tabular:** Appears after an incomplete term that requires one or more modifiers following the colon to be classified to that code or category.
[ ] Square brackets	**Tabular:** Synonyms, alternative wording, explanatory phrases **Index:** Indicates sequencing on etiology/manifestation codes or other paired codes. The code in square brackets [ ] should be sequenced second.
And	**Tabular:** Means "and/or"
Boldface (Heavy type)	**Index:** Main terms **Tabular:** Code titles
Code Also	**Tabular:** More than one code may be required to fully describe the condition.
Code First/Use Additional Code	**Tabular:** Provides sequencing instructions for conditions that have both an underlying etiology and multiple body system manifestations and certain other codes that have sequencing requirements.
Excludes1	**Tabular:** Mutually exclusive codes. None of the codes that appear after this term should be used with the original code itself.
Excludes2	**Tabular:** The code(s) listed after this term are not part of the condition represented by the code but may be reported together if documented.
Includes notes	**Tabular:** Begin with the word "Includes" and further define, clarify, or give examples.
Inclusion terms	**Tabular:** A list of synonyms or conditions included within a classification.
Italics (Slanted type)	**Tabular:** Exclusion notes, manifestation codes.
NEC	**Index and Tabular:** Not Elsewhere Classifiable. The medical record contains additional details about the condition, but there is not a more specific code available to use.
NOS	**Tabular:** Not Otherwise Specified. Information to assign a more specific code is not available in the medical record.
See	**Index:** It is necessary to reference another Main Term or condition to locate the correct code.
See Also	**Index:** Coder may refer to an alternative or additional Main Term if the desired entry is not found under the original Main Term.
With	**Tabular:** In a code title, means "both" or "together."
With/Without	**Tabular:** Within a set of alternative codes, describe options for final character.
X	**Tabular:** A placeholder in codes with less than six characters that require a 7th character extension. The X itself has no meaning and is not replaced with an actual number or letter. In some codes, the X is used to reserve room for future expansion.

from the Tabular List. When a seventh character is required on a code of five or fewer characters, add the placeholder X to fill out the empty characters in the code.

Placeholders. The character X appears in certain codes that are four, five, or six characters long. It is used in two ways:

- Some codes that are five or six characters long use the X to reserve a position for future use. In the examples that follow, X is used to hold the fourth position of the

code open for future use and has no meaning. The fifth and sixth characters are part of the core code.

- J09.X1 Influenza due to identified novel influenza A virus with pneumonia

- M01.X21 Direct infection of right elbow in infectious and parasitic diseases classified elsewhere

- When codes that are four or five characters long require a seventh character for special purposes, the placeholder X is used to fill in any empty positions. In the example that follows, the core code is S69.80. The seventh characters A and D identify the initial and subsequent encounter for the injury and must appear in the seventh position, so X is used to expand the length of the code.

- S69.80XA Other specified injuries to the wrist, initial encounter
- S69.80XD Other specified injuries to the wrist, subsequent encounter

Official Guidelines for Coding and Reporting

The ICD-10-CM **Official Guidelines for Coding and Reporting (OGCR)** are rules that provide directions for how to code selected conditions and establish the rules for how to identify which diagnoses should be reported on a claim for any given patient (Figure 15-1). HIPAA requires that coders adhere to OGCR when assigning ICD-10-CM diagnosis codes. The OGCR also explain the conventions that are universal within the ICD-10-CM code set.

Index to Diseases and Injuries

The **Index to Diseases and Injuries** (Index) lists conditions, diseases, and reasons for seeking medical care. Index entries are organized alphabetically by **Main Term** and **subterms** that aid in locating the most appropriate code. After identifying preliminary codes in the Index, verify them in the Tabular List. Final code selection should never be based only on the Index.

Although most conditions and reasons for the encounter are located in the Index to Diseases and Injuries, ICD-10-CM has three additional references for specialized purposes.

- **Table of Neoplasms**—Neoplasms are indexed on the Table of Neoplasms, located under "N" in the alphabetic Index. Some publishers may place this table at the end of the Index (Figure 15-2).
- **Table of Drugs and Chemicals**—Poisonings, adverse effects, and underdosing are indexed on the ICD-10-CM Table of Drugs and Chemicals, which is located at the end of the Index in most manuals (Figure 15-3).
- **Index to External Causes**—External causes of illness and injury are located in a separate index, the ICD-10-CM Index to External Causes, which follows the Table of Drugs and Chemicals in most manuals (Figure 15-4).

Tabular List

The Tabular List is an alphanumerically sequenced list of all diagnosis codes, divided into 21 chapters based on cause, or **etiology**, and body system. After locating the diagnosis in the Index, medical assistants need to **verify** the code by referencing the Tabular List. To verify a code means to consult the Tabular List to read detailed code descriptions, conventions, and instructional notes, and to assign additional specificity. Medical assistants need to know where to find the beginning of each chapter, because the beginning of the chapter provides global instructions that apply to all codes within the chapter. Table 15-7 shows the organization of the Tabular List and the code ranges for each chapter. Most chapters begin with a unique letter of the alphabet.

---

4. Chapter 4: Endocrine, Nutritional, and Metabolic Diseases (E00-E89)

a. Diabetes mellitus

The diabetes mellitus codes are combination codes that include the type of diabetes mellitus, the body system affected, and the complications affecting that body system. As many codes within a particular category as are necessary to describe all of the complications of the disease may be used. They should be sequenced based on the reason for a particular encounter. Assign as many codes from categories E08 – E13 as needed to identify all of the associated conditions that the patient has.

1. **Type of diabetes**
   The age of a patient is not the sole determining factor, though most type 1 diabetics develop the condition before reaching puberty. For this reason type 1 diabetes mellitus is also referred to as juvenile diabetes.

2. **Type of diabetes mellitus not documented**
   If the type of diabetes mellitus is not documented in the medical record the default is E11.-, Type 2 diabetes mellitus.

3. **Diabetes mellitus and the use of insulin**
   If the documentation in a medical record does not indicate the type of diabetes but does indicate that the patient uses insulin, code E11, Type 2 diabetes mellitus, should be assigned. Code Z79.4, Long-term (current) use of insulin, should also be assigned to indicate that the patient uses insulin. Code Z79.4 should not be assigned if insulin is given temporarily to bring a type 2 patient's blood sugar under control during an encounter.

FIGURE 15-1 Example of the Official Guidelines for Coding and Reporting.

HOW TO CODE DIAGNOSES

Coding begins and ends with the patient's medical record. Medical assistants abstract, or summarize, information from the medical record to code for services and the reasons they were provided.

	Malignant Primary	Malignant Secondary	Ca in situ	Benign	Uncertain Behavior	Unspecified Behavior
-shoulder NEC	C76.4-	C79.89	D04.6-	D36.7	D48.7	D49.89
-sigmoid flexure (lower) (upper)	C18.7	C78.5	D01.0	D12.5	D37.4	D49.0
-sinus (accessory)	C31.9	C78.39	D02.3	D14.0	D38.5	D49.1
--bone (any)	C41.0	C79.51	–	D16.4-	D48.0	D49.2
--ethmoidal	C31.1	C78.39	D02.3	D14.0	D38.5	D49.1
--frontal	C31.2	C78.39	D02.3	D14.0	D38.5	D49.1
--maxillary	C31.0	C78.39	D02.3	D14.0	D38.5	D49.1
--nasal, paranasal NEC	C31.9	C78.39	D02.3	D14.0	D38.5	D49.1
--overlapping lesion	C31.8	–	–	–	–	–
--pyriform	C12	C79.89	D00.08	D10.7	D37.05	D49.0
--sphenoid	C31.3	C78.39	D02.3	D14.0	D38.5	D49.1
-skeleton, skeletal NEC	C41.9	C79.51	–	D16.9-	D48.0	D49.2
-Skene's gland	C68.1	C79.19	D09.19	D30.8	D41.8	D49.5
-skin NOS	C44.90	C79.2	D04.9	D23.9	D48.5	D49.2
--abdominal wall	C44.509	C79.2	D04.5	D23.5	D48.5	D49.2
---basal cell carcinoma	C44.519	–	–	–	–	–

FIGURE 15-2 Example of the Table of Neoplasms.

Substance	Poisoning, Accidental (unintentional)	Poisoning, Intentional Self-harm	Poisoning, Assault	Poisoning, Undetermined	Adverse Effect	Underdosing
Aconitum ferox	T46.991	T46.992	T46.993	T46.994	T46.995	T46.996
Acridine	T65.6X1	T65.6X2	T65.6X3	T65.6X4	–	–
-vapor	T59.891	T59.892	T59.893	T59.894	–	–
Acriflavine	T37.91	T37.92	T37.93	T37.94	T37.95	T37.96
Acriflavinium chloride	T49.0X1	T49.0X2	T49.0X3	T49.0X4	T49.0X5	T49.0X6
Acrinol	T49.0X1	T49.0X2	T49.0X3	T49.0X4	T49.0X5	T49.0X6
Acrisorcin	T49.0X1	T49.0X2	T49.0X3	T49.0X4	T49.0X5	T49.0X6
Acrivastine	T45.0X1	T45.0X2	T45.0X3	T45.0X4	T45.0X5	T45.0X6
Acrolein(gas)	T59.891	T59.892	T59.893	T59.894	–	–
-liquid	T54.1X1	T54.1X2	T54.1X3	T54.1X4	–	–
Acrylamide	T65.891	T65.892	T65.893	T65.894	–	–
Acrylic resin	T49.3X1	T49.3X2	T49.3X3	T49.3X4	T49.3X5	T49.3X6
Acrylonitrile	T65.891	T65.892	T65.893	T65.894	–	–
Actaea spicata	T62.2X1	T62.2X2	T62.2X3	T62.2X4	–	–
-berry	T62.1X1	T62.1X2	T62.1X3	T62.1X4	–	–

FIGURE 15-3 Example of the Table of Drugs and Chemicals.

Coding is to be performed to the highest level of certainty. Only conditions, diseases, and symptoms documented in the medical record can be coded and billed. If the medical record is incomplete or inaccurate, it should be corrected or amended before attempting to code.

Diagnosis coding involves three basic steps:

1. Identify the first-listed diagnosis.

2. Research the diagnosis in the Index.

3. Verify the code(s) in the Tabular List.

**Abandonment (causing exposure to weather conditions)
(with intent to injure or kill) NEC** X58
Abuse (adult) (child) (mental) (physical) (sexual) X58
Accident (to) X58
-aircraft (in transit) (powered)—*see also* Accident, transport, aircraft
--due to, caused by cataclysm—*see* Forces of nature, by type
-animal-rider—*see* Accident, transport, animal-rider
-animal-drawn vehicle—*see* Accident, transport, animal-drawn vehicle occupant
-automobile—*see* Accident, transport, car occupant
-bare foot water skiier V94.4
-boat, boating—*see also* Accident, watercraft
--striking swimmer
---powered V94.11
---unpowered V94.12
-bus—*see* Accident, transport, bus occupant
-cable car, not on rails V98.0
--on rails—*see* Accident, transport, streetcar occupant
-car—*see* Accident, transport, car occupant
-caused by, due to
--animal NEC W64
--chain hoist W24.0
--cold (excessive)—*see* Exposure, cold
--corrosive liquid, substance—*see* Table of Drugs and Chemicals
--cutting or piercing instrument—*see* Contact, with, by type of instrument
--drive belt W24.0
--electric
---current—*see* Exposure, electric current
---motor (*see also* Contact, with, by type of machine) W31.3
----current (of) W86.8
--environmental factor NEC X58

FIGURE 15-4 Example of the Index to External Causes.

It is important to keep in mind that the diagnosis must describe (1) the reasons that the specific service was provided, and (2) related medical conditions that may affect the specific service. Diagnosis codes should not repeat a patient's entire problem list. The problem list is a comprehensive list of all active conditions that often appears in the front of the medical record, but it does not document the reason(s) for a specific encounter.

A patient's condition can require one or several codes, depending on the complexity of the patient's condition, the number of complications and comorbidities, and the organization of the coding manual. For many diagnoses, such as diabetes, a **combination code** identifies the condition and various manifestations or two conditions that commonly occur together. Other situations require **multiple coding**—reporting several codes to fully describe the condition.

EXAMPLE: *Code actively managed conditions*

The physician sees a patient for a sinus infection, who also has chronic gastric reflux. The physician prescribes an

TABLE 15-7 | ICD-10-CM Tabular List

Chapter	Title	Code Range
Chapter 1	Certain infectious and parasitic diseases	A00-B99
Chapter 2	Neoplasms	C00-D49
Chapter 3	Diseases of the blood and blood-forming organs and certain disorders involving the immune mechanism	D50-D89
Chapter 4	Endocrine, nutritional, and metabolic diseases	E00-E89
Chapter 5	Mental, behavioral, and neurodevelopmental disorders	F01-F99
Chapter 6	Diseases of the nervous system	G00-G99
Chapter 7	Diseases of the eye and adnexa	H00-H59
Chapter 8	Diseases of the ear and mastoid process	H60-H95
Chapter 9	Diseases of the circulatory system	I00-I99
Chapter 10	Diseases of the respiratory system	J00-J99
Chapter 11	Diseases of the digestive system	K00-K95
Chapter 12	Diseases of the skin and subcutaneous tissue	L00-L99
Chapter 13	Diseases of the musculoskeletal system and connective tissue	M00-M99
Chapter 14	Diseases of the genitourinary system	N00-N99
Chapter 15	Pregnancy, childbirth, and the puerperium	O00-O9A
Chapter 16	Certain conditions originating in the perinatal period	P00-P96
Chapter 17	Congenital malformations, deformations, and chromosomal abnormalities	Q00-Q99
Chapter 18	Symptoms, signs, and abnormal clinical and laboratory findings, not elsewhere classified	R00-R99
Chapter 19	Injury, poisoning, and certain other consequences of external causes	S00-T88
Chapter 20	External causes of morbidity	V01-Y99
Chapter 21	Factors influencing health status and contact with health services	Z00-Z99

antibiotic for the acute sinus infection and inquires how the gastric reflux is doing, but does not further evaluate, treat, or manage it. The medical assistant codes only the sinus infection.

ICD-10-CM code: J01.90 Acute sinusitis, unspecified

EXAMPLE: *Code all relevant medical conditions*

A diabetic patient comes into the office for a second-degree burn on the right hand. The physician treats the burn and indicates that the diabetes may slow the healing process and requires more frequent follow-up visits as a result. The medical assistant codes both the burn and the diabetes. The first-listed diagnosis is the burn. The secondary diagnosis is diabetes.

ICD-10-CM codes: T23.201A Burn of second degree of right hand, unspecified site, initial encounter

E11.9 Type 2 diabetes mellitus without complications

EXAMPLE: *Use a combination code when one is available*

A patient with type 1 diabetes sees an ophthalmologist because of changes in vision. The physician examines the patient and diagnoses moderate nonproliferative retinopathy due to diabetes. The medical assistant assigns a combination code that describes both conditions.

ICD-10-CM code: E10.339 Type 1 diabetes mellitus with moderate nonproliferative diabetic retinopathy without macular edema

EXAMPLE: *Use multiple codes when required*

A patient presents with a skin abscess on the abdomen. The physician prescribes antibiotics. A culture and sensitivity test is positive for the organism *Staphylococcus aureus* that is responsive to methicillin. The medical assistant codes for skin abscess and notes that the coding manual instructs to also code for the causal organism.

ICD-10-CM codes: L02.211 Cutaneous abscess of abdominal wall

B95.61 Methicillin susceptible Staphylococcus aureus infection as the cause of diseases classified elsewhere

The following coding steps provide the practical details needed to patiently and accurately execute the process. This discussion is oriented toward office-based coding.

Abstract Diagnostic Information

Medical assistants abstract information from the medical record to identify the information necessary to code for services and the reasons they were provided. When coding for office-based or other outpatient services, medical assistants refer to the patient registration form, the encounter form,

visit notes, lab and radiology reports, and operative reports for outpatient procedures. Often the physician indicates a diagnosis code on the encounter form, but medical assistants may need to verify it against the medical record. Look for a definitive diagnostic statement by the physician regarding the reason for the visit. The diagnosis might be indicated with the word *Impression* or, in SOAP notes (Subjective, Objective, Assessment, Plan), under A (*Assessment*). This is the **first-listed diagnosis**, formerly known as the primary diagnosis, the reason chiefly responsible for the services provided.

Uncertain diagnosis or **qualified diagnosis** is a diagnosis accompanied by a term such as *possible, probable, suspected, rule out (R/O),* or *working diagnosis,* indicating the physician has not determined the root cause. For outpatient coding, do not use uncertain diagnoses. Instead, look for the patient's signs or symptoms that are part of the patient's chief complaint. The chief complaint is a statement in the patient's own words of the reason for the visit. Signs are indications of a condition that the physician can observe or measure, such as a rash. Symptoms are indications reported by the patient that the physician cannot observe or measure, such as a headache.

CRITICAL THINKING

Refer to the Case Study at the beginning of the chapter.

1. With what type of otitis media was Sophia diagnosed?
2. Does the condition occur in the right ear, left ear, or bilaterally?

Research Codes in the Index

After determining the diagnosis in the patient's medical record, use the ICD-10-CM coding manual to assign the actual code number. The first step in using the coding manual is to identify the diagnosis in the Index. Using the Index involves three steps:

1. Locate the Main Term.
2. Read the subterms and modifiers.
3. Identify the preliminary code(s).

Identify the word(s) from the first-listed diagnosis to be looked up as the Main Term in the Index (Figure 15-5). The Main Term is always boldfaced with an initial capital letter in the Index. The Main Term may be any of the following:

- A condition, such as *Fracture*
- A disease, such as *Pneumonia*
- Reason for a visit, such as *Screening*
- Eponym (a disease or condition named after an individual), such as *Colles' fracture*

- Abbreviation or acronym, such as *AIDS*

- Nontechnical synonym (a word similar in meaning), such as *Broken* instead of fracture

- An adjective, such as *Twisted*

Some Main Terms, such as *Disease*, are rather generic with pages of subterms, but others, such as *Duroziez disease*, are quite specific and list only one code.

Main Terms usually do not include anatomic sites. To locate a condition that affects a specific site, look up the condition itself as the Main Term. Then read the subterms to locate the anatomic site (Figure 15-6).

EXAMPLE: *Anatomic sites are not Main Terms*

A medical assistant needs to code for an ankle sprain. She looks in the Index under A for the Main Term *Ankle*,

---

Gastrinoma
-malignant
--pancreas C25.4
--specified site NEC—*see* Neoplasm, malignant, by site
--unspecified site C25.4
-specified site—*see* Neoplasm, uncertain behavior
-unspecified site D37.9
Gastritis (simple) K29.70
-with bleeding K29.71
-acute (erosive) K29.00
--with bleeding K29.01
-alcoholic K29.20
--with bleeding K29.21
-allergic K29.60
--with bleeding K29.61
-atrophic (chronic) K29.40
--with bleeding K29.41
-chronic (antral) (fundal) K29.50
--with bleeding K29.51
--atrophic K29.40
---with bleeding K29.41
--superficial K29.30
---with bleeding K29.31
-dietary counseling and surveillance Z71.3
-due to diet deficiency E63.9
-eosinophilic K52.81
-giant hypertrophic K29.60
--with bleeding K29.61
-granulomatous K29.60
--with bleeding K29.61
-hypertrophic (mucosa) K29.60
--with bleeding K29.61
-nervous F54
-spastic K29.60
--with bleeding K29.61
-specified NEC K29.60
--with bleeding K29.61
-superficial chronic K29.30

FIGURE 15-5 Example of the Index to Diseases and Injuries.

Anisocytosis R71.8

Anisometropia (congenital) H52.31

Ankle—*see* condition

Ankyloblepharon (eyelid) (acquired)—*see also* Blepharophimosis

filiforme (adnatum) (congential) Q10.3

total Q10.3

FIGURE 15-6 Example of Index entry for an anatomic site with a cross-reference.

and finds an entry with the cross-reference *Ankle—see condition*. The condition is a *sprain*. She looks under *S* for the Main Term *Sprain* in the Index. Under *Sprain*, she locates the subterm *ankle*. The subterm entry *ankle* provides additional subterms for the exact site and type of sprain.

Subterms are words indented two spaces under the boldfaced Main Term that further describe variations of the condition. Examples of types of subterms are:

- Etiology: Pneumonia, *allergic*

- Coexisting condition: Pneumonia, *with influenza*

- Anatomic site: Pneumonia, *interstitial*

- Episode: Pneumonia, *chronic*, or similar descriptors

Subterms often have second-, third-, and additional-level subterms, each level being indented another two spaces under the preceding level. The meaning of each indented level includes the subterm at the previous level. It is important to carefully follow the sequence of subterms and subsequent levels of subterms to locate the most specific code. Figure 15-7 shows an example of an Index entry with multiple levels of subterms.

When the Main Term or subterm is too long to fit on one line, a carryover line is used. Carryover lines are indented more than two spaces from the level of the preceding line. It is important to read carefully to distinguish between carryover lines and subterms.

Main Terms or subterms may contain instructional notes, such as *see* or *see also*, which direct the user to other entries. For example, *Pleurobronchopneumonia—see Pneumonia, broncho-*. This directs the user to the appropriate entry for the code needed. In this example, the user should look under the Main Term *Pneumonia* and the subterm *broncho-* to locate the code for *Pleurobronchopneumonia*.

Entries under the Main Term may contain special formatting, such as slanted brackets, indicating that multiple coding may be required. The second code in slanted brackets is

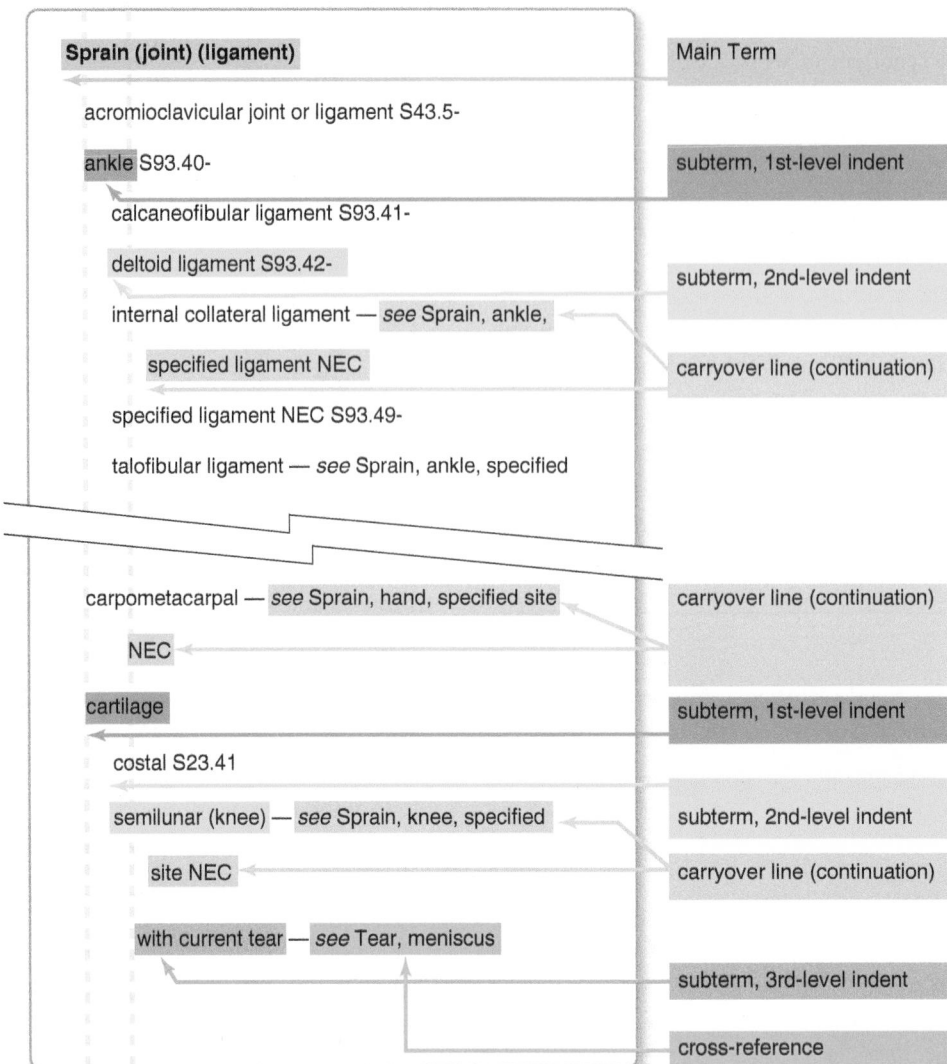

FIGURE 15-7 Example of Index entry with Main Term and indented subterms.

required in addition to the first code to completely describe the condition.

When the appropriate subterms are located, the preliminary code(s) appears immediately to the right. It is helpful to jot down the appropriate preliminary codes before verifying in the Tabular List. Never use the Index to make the final code selection.

CRITICAL THINKING

Refer to the Case Study at the beginning of the chapter.

1. What is the Main Term to be looked up in the Index?
2. What subterms should be located?
3. What cross-referencing instruction appears next to the fourth-level subterm *serous*?
4. What code is suggested in the Index?

Verify Codes in the Tabular List

Preliminary codes found in the Index must be verified in the Tabular List to confirm the code description and assign additional characters that specify details of the condition, such as laterality (the side of the body) and episode of care. Look for the preliminary code number in the Tabular List, which lists codes in alphanumeric order. The Tabular List contains 21 **chapters** based on etiology or the body system. The chapter numbers do not correlate directly with the code numbers. Review Table 15-7. Chapters are divided into **sections** with boldfaced or highlighted headings. Within the sections, the actual code numbers are tabulated in three levels: **category** (three-character entries), **subcategory** (four- and five-character entries), and **code** (the most specific entry that requires no additional characters) (Figure 15-8). It is helpful to learn the specific meanings of

Level	Example
Chapter	Chapter 10 Diseases of the respiratory system (J00-J99)
Block	Influenza and pneumonia (J09-J18)
Category	J15 Bacterial pneumonia, not elsewhere classified
Subcategory	J15.2 Pneumonia due to staphylococcus
	J15.21 Pneumonia due to staphylococcus
Code	J15.211 Pneumonia due to staphylococcus

FIGURE 15-8 Organizational structure of ICD-10-CM chapters.

these designations, because the terms are used frequently in coding instructions.

Before verifying and finalizing the code, medical assistants must interpret the conventions that appear with the code and its category. Tabular List conventions include punctuation, instructional notes, and symbols. Conventions may appear on the same line with the code, above it, below it, or at the beginning of a subcategory, category, section, or chapter. Look carefully for any information that may be relevant to the code selection. Additional information may direct you when to use a different code or an additional code, depending on your original diagnostic statement. Figure 15-9 shows an example of conventions in the Tabular List.

ICD-10-CM codes can be between three and seven characters in length (Table 15-8). There is no general rule regarding how many characters any given code must have. The number of characters is determined after reading the instructional notes and conventions available in the category. Use the most specific code available for each condition. Most coding manuals display a symbol or color-coding with entries that provide a more specific code.

Within a preliminary code or category, the Tabular List often provides options for anatomic site, laterality, with or without manifestations, and other details. When provided, these details must be coded with additional characters to assign a code with the highest level of specificity.

The seventh character of an ICD-10-CM code is reserved for special use, most commonly the episode of care. Episode of care characters do not appear sequentially within the Tabular List. They appear at the beginning of a subcategory or category and apply to all codes within that division. Be certain to review the subcategory and category headings thoroughly to locate the correct seventh characters when required. It sometimes requires a little detective work and reviewing several pages of codes to locate the appropriate listing (Figure 15-10).

As a final check, with coding manual instructions fresh in your mind, refer back to the original documentation and verify that all conditions of the code agree with the medical record. If a discrepancy arises, work through the process again from the beginning. Procedure 15-1 summarizes how to assign ICD-10-CM diagnosis codes.

K29 Gastritis and duodenitis

Excludes1: eosinophilic gastritis or gastroenteritis (K52.81)
Zollinger-Ellison syndrome (E16.4)

K29.0 Acute gastritis
Use additional code to identify:
alcohol abuse and dependence (F10.-)
Excludes1: erosion (acute) of stomach (K25.-)
K29.00 Acute gastritis without bleeding
K29.01 Acute gastritis with bleeding

K29.2 Alcoholic gastritis
Use additional code to identify:
alcohol abuse and dependence (F10.-)
K29.20 Alcoholic gastritis without bleeding
K29.21 Alcoholic gastritis with bleeding

K29.3 Chronic superficial gastritis
K29.30 Chronic superficial gastritis without bleeding
K29.31 Chronic superficial gastritis with bleeding

K29.4 Chronic atrophic gastritis
Gastric atrophy
K29.40 Chronic atrophic gastritis without bleeding
K29.41 Chronic atrophic gastritis with bleeding

FIGURE 15-9 Example of the Tabular List and instructional notes (conventions).

TABLE 15-8 | Examples of ICD-10-CM Codes with Varying Number of Characters

Code Length	Code	Description
3-characters	I10	Essential (primary) hypertension
4-characters	F52.8	Other sexual dysfunction not due to a substance or known physiological condition
5-characters	K70.30	Alcoholic cirrhosis of liver without ascites
6-characters	L89.511	Pressure ulcer of right ankle, stage 1
7-characters	T22.761A	Corrosion of third degree of right scapular region, initial encounter
7-characters with placeholder X	O33.4XX0	Maternal care for disproportion of mixed maternal and fetal origin, fetus 1

S94 Injury of nerves at ankle and foot level

The appropriate 7th character is to be added to each code from category S94
A - initial encounter
D - subsequent encounter
S - sequela

    S94.0 Injury of lateral plantar nerve
        S94.02 Injury of lateral plantar nerve, right leg

Final codes with placeholder X and episode of care characters:

S94.02XA Injury of lateral plantar nerve, right leg, initial encounter
S94.02XD Injury of lateral plantar nerve, right leg, subsequent encounter
S94.02XS Injury of lateral plantar nerve, right leg, sequela

FIGURE 15-10 Example use of a placeholder (X) and episode of care characters.

Professionalism

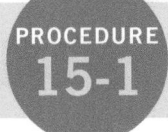

Patients may not understand the diagnosis stated on the encounter form or insurance statement. This may be especially true of patients with multiple chronic conditions. The medical assistant can help patients with any questions they may have concerning the encounter form by patiently explaining the information in terms that are easily understood.

CRITICAL THINKING

Refer to the Case Study at the beginning of the chapter.

1. When verifying the code in the Tabular List, what information is needed to assign the correct code?
2. What is the final diagnostic code and description for Sophia's encounter?

Performing ICD-10-CM Diagnostic Coding

Objective ◆ *Assign ICD-10-CM codes based on documentation.*

EQUIPMENT AND SUPPLIES

Patient's medical chart; current ICD-10-CM coding manual; superbill with doctor's written diagnosis

METHOD

1. Locate the patient's diagnostic code(s) or description on the encounter form or in the chart notes.
2. Verify that the diagnostic code(s) or description on the encounter form also appears in the patient's chart in the form of a patient complaint (subjective finding) or a test finding (objective finding).
3. Look in the Index of the ICD-10-CM coding manual to find the Main Term. Search the subterms for the most specific description, and identify the preliminary diagnosis code.
4. Look up the preliminary code(s) in the Tabular List. Confirm that the written description matches the chart notes. If in doubt, check with the physician.
5. Read and apply the conventions in the Tabular List. Assign any additional characters required.
6. Assign the code for each diagnosis, beginning with the appropriate first-listed diagnosis.

Coding for Special Situations

Many diagnoses require advanced coding skills to accurately capture the details of a specific patient's situation. Table 15-9 summarizes how to code for diagnoses that may present special challenges. Because some of these may exceed some medical assistants' experience, they should show their professionalism by recognizing when additional expertise is required. Medical assistants may work in offices that hire certified coders to assign and audit diagnosis codes.

Reporting incorrect diagnosis codes on an insurance claim can create problems such as improper reimbursement, inaccurate patient medical history, and fraud. Whenever medical assistants are unsure of how to select a code, they should reach out to their supervisor or a certified coder.

TABLE 15-9 | Coding for Special Situations

Condition	Coding Steps
Burns	**Index (Main Term):** Use *Burn* for burns caused by heat. Use *Corrosion* for chemical burns. **Subterms:** Anatomic site and degree (first, second, third). **Tabular List:** Assign code for the highest degree of burn at each site. Assign additional code for percentage of body surface affected by third-degree burns. Assign external cause codes where applicable.
Diabetes	**Index (Main Term):** *Diabetes* **Subterms:** Select *type 1, type 2, due to drug or chemical, due to underlying condition.* **Additional subterms:** Type of complication(s), if any. **Tabular List:** Verify the combination code for the type of diabetes and complication.
External causes	**Index (Main Term):** Use the Index of External Causes. Locate the event that caused the injury, such as accident, fall, burn, bite. For the first encounter, assign additional codes indexed under *Activity, Place of occurrence*, and *Status*. **Subterms:** Accidents are classified as *transport* and *nontransport*. Transport accidents are listed by type of vehicle, such as boat, car, or motorcycle. Also identify whether the victim was a *driver* or a *passenger*. **Tabular List:** Verify the description and assign a seventh character for episode of care.
Fractures	**Index (Main Term):** *Fracture, pathological* or *Fracture, traumatic.* **Subterms:** Anatomic site and type **Tabular List:** Verify all details of the fracture, and assign characters for laterality and episode of care.
HIV	**Index:** *Human* + subterm *immunodeficiency virus.* **Subterms:** Subterms include the following: *asymptomatic, contact, counseling, dementia, exposure to, laboratory evidence.* Use default code B20 for symptomatic HIV/AIDS. **Tabular List:** Verify the code. Assign additional codes for any AIDS-related conditions.
Hypertension	**Index (Main Term):** *Hypertension* **Subterms:** Comorbidities **Tabular List:** Verify the code and comorbidities.
Influenza	**Index (Main Term):** *Influenza* **Subterms:** Locate the specific type of virus and manifestations. **Tabular List:** Verify the type and manifestation(s).
Neoplasms	**Index (Main Term):** Look up the clinical name of the tumor, such as melanoma or carcinoma. Carcinoma and many other tumors are coded using the Table of Neoplasms (review Figure 15-2). **Table of Neoplasms:** Locate the row for the anatomic site and the column for the behavior (malignant, benign, cancer in situ). **Tabular List:** Verify the code, noting any additional characters required and other instructional notes.

(continued)

TABLE 15-9 | Coding for Special Situations (*continued*)

Condition	Coding Steps
Obstetrics	**Index (Main Term):** *Pregnancy*
	Subterms: Subterms include the following: *complicated by, management affected by, supervision of.*
	Tabular List: Verify the appropriate trimester. Assign as many codes as necessary to describe all complications. Assign a code for the preexisting medical condition when appropriate. Assign a code from Z3A.- to identify the weeks of gestation.
	Index (Main Term): *Delivery*
	Subterms: Select *cesarean* or *complicated by.*
	Tabular List: Assign as many codes as necessary to describe all complications. Assign a code from Z38.- to identify the outcome of delivery.
Poisonings and adverse effects	**Index (Main Term):** Use the Table of Drugs and Chemicals (review Figure 15-3).
	Table of Drugs and Chemicals: Locate the substance in the left-hand column. Locate column for the intent for the poisoning (injury due to substance that should not be consumed or an overdose of a medication) as: *accidental, self-harm, assault, undetermined; adverse effect* (injury resulting from a medication taken as prescribed), *underdosing* (injury resulting from taking too little of prescribed medication).
	Tabular List: Verify the substance and intent. Assign seventh character for episode of care.
Well Visits, Health Status (Z-codes)	**Index (Main Term):** *Encounter for, Examination, Status (post), History-personal, History-family*
	Subterms: Select the type of encounter or status, as applicable.
	Tabular List: Verify the code; note any sequencing instructions.

SUMMARY

Medical coding is the process of assigning alphanumeric characters that represent the diagnoses patients have and the services they receive. Medical assistants play an important role in communication and understanding of medical codes. The diagnosis coding system that began as a short list of diseases in 1893 has now become a highly detailed classification of over 70,000 codes, each consisting of three to seven characters. ICD-10-CM is the HIPAA-mandated code set for diagnostic coding used for billing and reimbursement. Health care providers must follow billing and coding rules established by multiple federal, state, and country government agencies.

The introductory material to the ICD-10-CM manual provides instructions on how to use ICD-10-CM, outlines the Official Guidelines for Coding and Reporting (OGCR), and lists universal conventions and publisher-specific conventions. Medical assistants abstract information from the medical record to identify the information needed to code for services and the reasons they were provided. After determining the diagnosis in the patient's medical record, they research the code in the Index using a Main Term and subterms to locate preliminary codes that describe the condition(s). The codes found in the Index must be verified in the Tabular List to confirm the code description and assign additional characters that specify details of the condition, such as laterality and episode of care. Many diagnoses require advanced coding skills to accurately capture the details of a specific patient's situation. Whenever medical assistants are unsure of how to select a code, they should reach out to their supervisor or a certified coder.

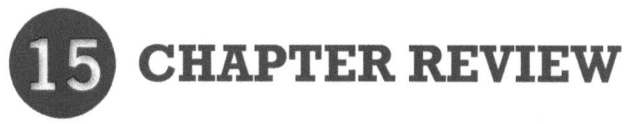

15 CHAPTER REVIEW

COMPETENCY REVIEW

1. Define and spell the terms for this chapter.
2. Discuss the role of medical assistants in diagnostic coding.

3. Name, locate, and explain the purpose of each section of the ICD-10-CM coding manual.

4. Explain how to abstract diagnostic information from the medical record.
5. Identify and locate in the Index the Main Terms and subterms for a diagnostic statement.

6. Explain how to verify codes in the Tabular List.
7. Discuss how to code for special situations.

PREPARING FOR THE CERTIFICATION EXAM

1. What convention identifies two codes that are mutually exclusive and cannot be used together?
   a. Code also
   b. Excludes1
   c. NEC
   d. See also
   e. Excludes2

2. Which of the following is *not* a benefit of ICD-10-CM?
   a. Detailed diagnosis codes reduce the need for attachments to claims.
   b. Provides more consistent and more detailed data for physician use.
   c. Allows anyone in the office to perform diagnosis coding.
   d. Reflects advancements in technology and medical practice.
   e. Provides the flexibility to add codes in the future.

3. What term describes knowingly billing for services that were never given or billing for a service that has a higher reimbursement than the service actually provided?
   a. fraud
   b. maximizing
   c. unbundling
   d. flexible billing
   e. abuse

4. When do annual updates to ICD-10-CM codes take effect each year?
   a. January 1
   b. April 15
   c. July 1
   d. October 1
   e. November 15

5. What character functions as a placeholder in ICD-10-CM?
   a. 0
   b. 9
   c. #
   d. A
   e. X

6. Which section of the ICD-10-CM manual is an alphanumerically sequenced list of all diagnosis codes, divided into 21 chapters based on cause and body system?
   a. Index to Diseases and Injuries
   b. Index to External Causes
   c. Tabular List
   d. Table of Neoplasms
   e. Table of Drugs and Chemicals

7. Which of the following is a combination code?
   a. E10.339 Type 1 diabetes mellitus with moderate nonproliferative diabetic retinopathy without macular edema
   b. L02.211 Cutaneous abscess of abdominal wall
   c. J01.90 Acute sinusitis, unspecified
   d. K55 Vascular disorder of intestine
   e. B95.61 Methicillin susceptible Staphylococcus aureus infection as the cause of diseases classified elsewhere

8. Main Terms in the Index may be any of the following *except*
   a. condition.
   b. eponym.
   c. abbreviation.
   d. adjective.
   e. anatomic site.

9. What is the maximum length of an ICD-10-CM code?
   a. 4
   b. 5
   c. 6
   d. 7
   e. 8

10. What should medical assistants do when they are unsure of how to select a code for a particular situation?
    a. ask the physician
    b. search the Internet
    c. ask a certified coder
    d. assign a generic code
    e. use the placeholder character

CRITICAL THINKING

Refer to the case study at the beginning of the chapter and use what you have learned to answer the following questions.

1. Why is it necessary for David to code for the specific condition *chronic serous otitis media* rather than a nonspecific condition such as *otitis media*?

2. Why must David be sure to code for the *bilateral* nature of the condition?

3. What are the benefits of having over 70,000 diagnosis codes?

ON THE JOB

Lisa Medina, a certified coder, performs medical coding for a large multi-specialty clinic. You have just been hired as Lisa's assistant. She has asked you to review the encounter forms for the day, on which physicians have checked off the diagnoses of each patient. You notice that Dr. Parker, an endocrinologist, has checked off the box for *Diabetes unspecified* for most of his patients without checking off any manifestations or complications. You think this is unusual because many diabetic patients do have complications.

1. What are the options for handling this situation?
2. Which option would you select?
3. Give three reasons for your choice.
4. Who should you consult before acting on your choice?

INTERNET ACTIVITY

Perform an Internet search for "medical coding ethics." What organizations offer a code of ethics for coders? Discuss why a code of ethics is necessary. What guidelines in a code of ethics for coders stand out to you?

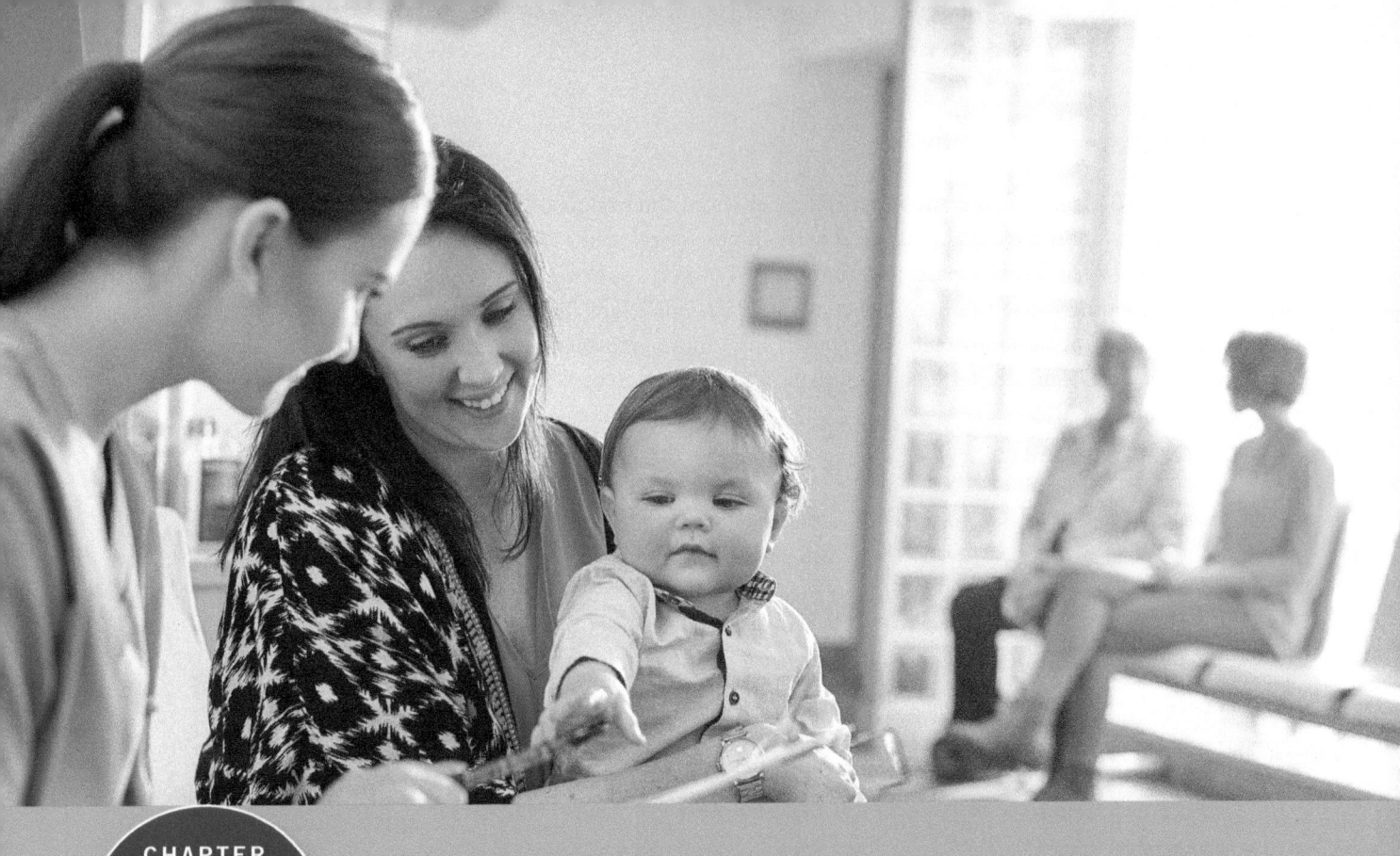

Procedure Coding

Learning Objectives

After completing this chapter, you should be able to:

16.1   Define and spell the terms for this chapter.

16.2   Explain the medical assistant's role in procedure coding.

16.3   Describe the history of procedure coding.

16.4   Explain medical necessity as it applies to coding.

16.5   Explain the difference between fraud and abuse.

16.6   Compare and contrast the effects of upcoding and downcoding.

16.7   Describe the organization of the procedural coding manual.

16.8   Describe how to use the procedural coding system to assign a procedure code.

16.9   Describe the use of the HCPCS coding manual.

Sophia DiStefano, a five-year-old female, experienced three bouts of otitis media within the past seven months and was diagnosed with chronic otitis media. Following an audiometry screen two weeks ago, Dr. Salpega recommended surgery to correct the underlying problem. Sophia's mother signed an informed consent for the procedure. Today, Dr. Salpega performs a bilateral tympanostomy (tube placement) for a more permanent treatment of the condition. David Dolan, a Registered Medical Assistant, needs to code for the procedure.

Terms to Learn

abuse

add-on code

audit

bundling

category

Centers for Medicare and Medicaid Services (CMS)

common descriptor

contributing factors

coordination of care

counseling

Current Procedural Terminology (CPT®)

downcoding

edits

established patient

Evaluation and Management (E&M)

examination (E, Ex)

face-to-face time

fraud

global period

guidelines

Healthcare Common Procedure Coding System (HCPCS)

history (H, Hx)

indented code

Index

instructional notes

key component

Level I codes

Level II codes

Main Term

medical decision making (MDM)

medical necessity

modifiers

modifying term

new patient

outpatient

parent code—see standalone code

patient status

presenting problem

procedure coding

procedures

professional component

relative value unit (RVU)

resequenced code

section

semicolon (;)

special instructions

standalone code

subcategory

subheading

subsection

surgical package

Tabular List

technical component

unbundling

upcoding

Procedure coding is the act of assigning alphanumeric characters to the procedures and services that physicians and health care facilities provide to patients. Providers determine the fee they wish to charge for each procedure code that is used to bill insurance companies. Each procedure code must be reported in conjunction with a diagnosis code that identifies the reason the procedure was performed. Since 1966, procedure codes have been standardized, which has rendered coding both more efficient and more accurate. Accuracy in procedure coding is essential, because incorrect or inadequate coding may lead to denial or delay of insurance claims. Improper reporting of procedure codes could be grounds for allegations of fraud or abuse.

OVERVIEW AND HISTORY OF PROCEDURE CODING

Current Procedural Terminology (CPT®) is a listing of five-character alphanumeric codes and descriptions used to report outpatient medical services and **procedures**. The Health Insurance Portability and Accountability Act (HIPAA) mandates the use of CPT by covered entities that handle electronic claims related to outpatient health care services.

As a result, CPT is the standard for efficient and effective communication among health care providers, regulators, and payers. The CPT manual is a published by the American Medical Association (AMA). The AMA holds all copyrights and privileges to the content of the manual.

The Role of the Medical Assistant in Procedure Coding

Medical assistants most often are involved with assigning procedure codes to basic procedures and services provided in the medical office or healthcare setting. Medical assistants might work in offices that use certified coders to assign and audit procedure codes, so the extent to which a medical assistant is involved in procedure coding varies from one office to the next.

Medical assistants must be sure that all patient care information is properly documented in the patient's medical record. The adage "If it isn't charted, it wasn't done" applies. To perform accurate and complete procedure coding, health care providers must keep adequate, accurate, and complete patient medical and billing records.

In addition to providing services in the medical office, physicians also provide services in other settings such as an ambulatory surgery center, outpatient hospital departments such as radiology or cardiac catheterization lab, and inpatient hospitals. Although the services are provided in a location other than the medical office, physicians are still responsible for coding and billing the services they provide in those settings. These services usually require more complex coding than basic office services and are coded by a certified coder who has advanced training.

Medical assistants primarily are involved with services provided in the office setting, which is the focus of this chapter. Medical assistants should understand the scope of their training and recognize when they need to reach out to a certified coder for assistance.

The History of CPT Coding

Before the mid-1960s, most patients paid for their services out-of-pocket. When they had health insurance, they submitted their own claims to insurance companies and were reimbursed directly. There were no standard medical billing forms or procedure codes. Reimbursement was cost-based, meaning that the insurance companies paid whatever fees providers charged.

With the passage of Medicare and Medicaid in 1965, the health care industry recognized the need to standardize the description of health care services. The Health Care Financing Administration (HCFA), now known as the **Centers for Medicare and Medicaid Services (CMS)**, assigned the task of developing codes to the American Medical Association

(AMA). The AMA developed and published the first edition of CPT in 1966 and has been responsible for CPT codes ever since. The first edition of CPT primarily contained surgical procedures with limited sections on medicine, radiology, and laboratory. Codes were four numbers in length.

In 1970, the second edition of CPT was published, which expanded surgical procedures and identified them as diagnostic or therapeutic. It also added procedures relating to internal medicine and expanded the other sections of the manual. The third edition was published within a few years and, in 1977, the fourth edition, still in use today, was adopted. At this time, a process was established to update the code set on a regular basis.

In 1983, the federal government adopted CPT as part of its Healthcare Common Procedure Coding System (HCPCS). This action mandated the use of HCPCS/CPT to report services billed to Medicare Part B. In October 1986, state Medicaid agencies were required to use HCPCS. In 1987, as part of the Omnibus Budget Reconciliation Act, HCFA mandated that CPT be used to report outpatient hospital surgical procedures.

The passage of the HIPAA in 1996 required that uniform standards be established for electronic transactions. This occurred October 16, 2003, when CPT was designated as a mandated procedure code set for covered entities for physician services and most other types of outpatient claims.

CPT codes must be used on the CMS-1500 claim form and its electronic equivalent, the 837P. To standardize medical fees and increase the accuracy of the coding process, in 1992 the U.S. Congress developed a system that assigned a **relative value unit (RVU)** to every health care procedure or treatment.

Today, the CPT manual covers all procedures approved by the Food and Drug Administration (FDA). The CPT lists over 9,000 procedure codes. CPT is updated every year, with changes taking effect January 1. Code changes are published by the AMA in conjunction with CMS. CPT updates are made to clarify code descriptions and incorporate new technologies and equipment. HIPAA requires that you use the edition of the CPT that was in effect on the date of service.

Professionalism The Law

 Imagine that, on January 3, you are coding services for patients seen during the past week. For patients seen on December 31, you must use the CPT manual for the old year. For patients seen on January 2, you must use the CPT manual for the new year. Also remember that the effective date for CPT manuals is January 1. This differs from the effective date for ICD-10-CM diagnosis coding manuals, which is October 1.

Overview of CPT Coding

Procedure codes identify billable services provided to patients. Medical offices report CPT procedure codes on CMS-1500 forms and electronic claims to identify the services provided and the cost of those services. Physicians are paid for CPT codes, but diagnosis codes are required to explain the reason(s) for the encounter or the reason services were provided, also known as **medical necessity**.

EXAMPLE: *Billable Service*

An established patient presents in the office complaining of a sore throat. The physician performs a problem-focused history, a problem-focused examination, and straightforward medical decision making. The physician then takes a throat culture, which will be processed in the office, to check for strep throat. The medical assistant reports an evaluation and management CPT procedure code that identifies the complexity of the encounter. An additional laboratory CPT procedure code is reported for the strep test. The ICD-10-CM diagnosis code identifies the sore throat, which was the reason for the visit and for the lab test.

On the CMS-1500 form, each CPT code must be cross-referenced, or linked, to one or more diagnosis codes that identify the medical necessity. Diagnosis codes are entered in Item 21. Date(s) of service, CPT codes, charges, and related information are entered on lines 1 through 6 of Item 24. In column 24E, enter the letter from Item 21 (A through L) that corresponds to the diagnosis that supports the medical necessity of each service (Figure 16-1). Each service must be linked to one or more diagnosis codes. A diagnosis code can be linked to as many services as appropriate.

Insurance companies and other payers establish their own medical necessity guidelines. They define clinical criteria that must be met for the service to be covered under the policy. Although a physician considers a service to be medically necessary for a patient, it might not meet the insurance company's criteria and, as result, not be covered. The physician might choose to talk with the patient to discuss alternative options if the medical necessity guidelines of the insurance company are not fully met. The patient can choose to have the service provided anyway, realizing that the insurance policy would not pay for it and the patient would need to personally cover the cost. See Procedure 16-1 for more information on using medical necessity guidelines. Medical necessity also was discussed in the chapter titled "Medical Insurance".

Medical assistants may find it challenging to find the most appropriate and accurate code for each patient encounter. For example, patient encounters for what is commonly referred to as an "office visit" are reported with one of 30-plus codes, depending on a number of circumstances surrounding the visit. However, only one code is correct in any given situation, so medical assistants must become familiar with the nuances among codes that may appear to be similar. Likewise, more than 50 codes exist for a patient who receives sutures for a wound. The correct code is based on the location, length, and depth of the wound. Medical assistants need to be familiar with all the criteria for coding services offered by their office to be certain they select the accurate code.

Federal Compliance

It is improper to code for a more complex service than what was actually provided in the hope of receiving higher reimbursement. Doing so is considered to be fraud and carries severe penalties, including fines and possible imprisonment. This should not scare medical assistants but should make them aware of the importance of their role and the need for accuracy. Medicare places the responsibility for knowing the rules on providers (and by extension their coders). Medicare's stance is that once they publish a rule, providers should know about it and follow it.

Although HIPAA is best known for its privacy rules and health care transaction standards, it also created several programs to further control fraud and abuse in health care. One of these provisions increased the amount of money the Office of the Inspector General (OIG) could spend to

FIGURE 16-1 CMS-1500 form showing linkage of CPT and diagnosis codes.

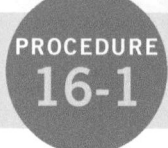

Using Medical Necessity Guidelines

Objective ◆ *Access and apply insurance companies' medical necessity guidelines.*

MATERIALS

Copy of patient's insurance card; patient's electronic health record; telephone; paper and pen

METHOD

1. Refer to the patient's medical record, and identify the service provided or planned. Make sure that the documented diagnosed justifies the procedures being performed. If possible, identify the visit's applicable ICD-10-CM diagnosis and CPT procedure code(s).
2. Refer to the patient's insurance card, and identify the telephone number for physician services.
3. Call the insurance company's physician services phone number. Request to speak to someone regarding medical necessity guidelines.
4. Provide the customer service representative with the name and CPT code of the service provided or planned.
5. Request that the medical necessity guidelines be faxed or e-mailed.
6. Upon receipt, verify that the medical necessity guidelines received are for the service desired.
7. Read the specific criteria that must be met, which might include patient age, gender, diagnosis, previous treatments and results, and treatment plan.
8. Compare the criteria to the medical record and make sure that all of the requirements are met.
9. When done, highlight any requirements not met. Provide this information to the physician, who then will decide whether to order additional tests and treatments, or provide a different service.

---

investigate fraud and abuse. It also increased the penalties for violations. The OIG is a division of the United States Department of Health and Human Services (HHS) that investigates fraud, abuse, and other non-compliance matters in the Medicare and Medicaid programs. The Department of Justice (DOJ) also is responsible to investigate and prosecute medical billing fraud and abuse.

Reporting incorrect codes on an insurance claim can create problems such as improper reimbursement, fraud, and inaccurate patient medical history. When uncertain of the best code, it may be tempting to "guesstimate" and assign an approximate code. This practice may result in **upcoding**, which is coding for a higher level of service than what was actually provided to gain higher reimbursement. Guessing could also result in **downcoding**, which is coding for a lower level of service than what was actually provided, to avoid potential fraud or abuse. Downcoding may seem prudent to avoid fraud, but it deprives the medical office of reimbursement to which it is legally entitled.

Fraud and Abuse

Fraud and abuse are separate types of billing violations. **Fraud** is the act of intentionally billing for services that were never given or billing for a service that has a higher reimbursement than the service actually provided. This includes both upcoding and downcoding. Upcoding is viewed as an attempt to gain higher reimbursement. Downcoding also bills for a service that was not provided. It could also be an attempt to gain partial reimbursement for a more complex procedure that is not covered. Fraud includes making false statements or representations of material facts to obtain a benefit or payment for which no entitlement would otherwise exist. The violator may be a physician or other practitioner, a hospital or other institutional provider, a clinical laboratory or other supplier, an employee of any provider, a billing service, a beneficiary, a Medicare employee, or any person in a position to file a claim for Medicare benefits. Examples of fraud may include knowingly doing any of the following:

- Billing for services not provided
- Billing for services not documented
- Misrepresenting the diagnosis to justify payment
- Billing for appointments that the patient failed to keep
- Altering documentation to receive a higher payment amount

- Soliciting, offering, or receiving a kickback (a financial incentive provided by another physician, laboratory, hospital, or pharmaceutical representative for using their services)
- Unbundling (billing for separate services that are included in a single procedure code)
- Falsifying certificates of medical necessity, plans of treatment, and medical records to justify payment
- Upcoding (billing for a service at a higher level than was actually provided)
- Downcoding (billing for a lesser service to gain partial reimbursement for a more complex procedure that is not covered)

Abuse is improper behavior and billing practices that result in improper financial gain but are not fraudulent. Abuse includes any practice that is not consistent with the goals of providing patients with services that are medically necessary, meet professionally recognized standards, and are fairly priced.

Examples of Medicare abuse may include:

- Charging excessively high fees for services or supplies
- Billing for services that were provided, but not medically necessary
- Routinely filing duplicate claims for the same encounter, even if they do not result in duplicate payments
- Billing for supplies that were given to the patient, but not medically necessary

Fraud and abuse schemes can be carried out by individuals acting alone or with others, to or by institutions.

Perpetrators might even use sophisticated telemarketing and other promotional techniques to lure consumers so they can obtain identity information or to provide unnecessary services that can then be billed. Rather than focusing on a single victim, most fraud schemes attempt to defraud several private and public sector victims at the same time.

The CMS website offers information to consumers and patients to encourage them to identify and report fraud. Figure 16-2 lists potential warning signs of fraud that could be seen in direct communication between a health care provider and a patient or in communication between the provider and a medical assistant, who is asked to relay the information to the patient.

OIG expects providers and their staff to keep themselves informed about legal and illegal behaviors. As in all areas of health care, ignorance is no excuse. The CMS website provides several resources, including newsletters, webpages, conference calls, and online training, to help providers be informed. When medical assistants are unsure regarding a coding or billing issue, they may consult with the physician, a colleague, or a professional organization.

Because this chapter provides an introduction to procedure coding, medical assistants should be aware of coding situations that require the attention of a certified coder. Examples of such situations include those requiring multiple CPT codes, complex operative procedures, and those with many choices in the CPT Tabular List. Whenever medical assistants are unsure of how to select a code, they should reach out to their supervisor or a certified coder.

Perpetrators of fraud may make statements such as the following:

- The test is free; the doctor needs only your Medicare number for his records.
- Medicare wants you to have the item or service.
- The medical office knows how to get Medicare to pay for it.
- The more tests the patient takes, the cheaper they are.
- The equipment or service is free; it will not cost the patient anything.
- Routinely waive copayments without checking on ability to pay.
- Advertise "free" consultations to Medicare beneficiaries.
- Claim they represent Medicare.
- Use pressure or scare tactics to sell high-priced medical services or diagnostic tests.
- Bill Medicare for services the patient does not recall receiving.
- Use telemarketing and door-to-door selling as marketing tools.

FIGURE 16-2 Warning signs of fraud.

ORGANIZATION OF THE CPT MANUAL

The CPT manual consists of an introduction, Tabular List, Index, and several appendices. Medical assistants need to become familiar with the organization of the CPT manual so that they can find needed information quickly. Various

editions or publishers may organize the features differently and may not include some features. The content and labeling of specific topics sometimes changes from year to year when the manual is updated. For this reason, it is important to become familiar with the specific edition of the manual you use and to review the new edition for changes each year.

Introductory Matter

Introductory matter provides valuable reference material for medical assistants. This information appears within the first several pages of the CPT manual, before the code listing begins, and, in some editions, inside the front and back covers.

The introductory matter provides a table of contents by page number, instructions for use of the codebook, and other valuable information, depending on the version of the manual used. Possible inclusions are a review of medical terminology and anatomic plates.

Inside the front cover, or within the first few pages, most CPT manuals include a list of commonly used symbols, **modifiers**, and place-of-service codes. These are provided for quick reference for users who fully understand the correct use of these items. Inside the back cover of most CPT manuals commonly used medical abbreviations are listed.

Index

The **Index** lists procedures and services in the CPT manual alphabetically by **Main Term** and **modifying terms** that aid in locating the most appropriate code or range of codes. The CPT coding process begins with the Index. After identifying potential codes in the Index, users should verify them in the Tabular List. Never make the final code selection based only on the Index, even if only one code appears.

Tabular List

The **Tabular List** is a numerical listing of all CPT codes, divided into Category I, Category II, and Category III. The Tabular List provides the official descriptions of CPT codes and the guidelines for using them. When coding, medical assistants first search for a code in the Index, then verify it in the Tabular List.

Category I

Category I codes, which compose the bulk of the CPT. They describe widely used services and procedures approved by the FDA. The CPT manual does not specifically label codes as Category I. Rather, Category I codes carry the names of the six **sections**. Although most of the codes are in numeric order, the Evaluation and Management (E&M) are first in the section. E&M codes are the most frequently used and are used by all medical specialties, so they are placed first for convenience. Other codes are used more selectively, based on the specific services provided by each office. The majority of this chapter discusses Category I codes.

Category II

Category II codes are optional codes used to collect and track data for performance measurement. They consist of four numbers followed by the letter F. They identify certain services or test results that contribute to quality patient care and are usually included in a routine examination or other service. Examples include documentation of:

- Disease-specific assessments (heart failure, osteoarthritis)
- Certain types of care plans (prenatal flow sheet, pain management)
- Select patient history elements (fall history, tobacco use history)
- Components of physical assessment (blood pressure, weight, mental status)
- Test results (mammogram, oxygen saturation)

By using Category II codes, the medical office reduces the amount of time spent auditing charts to collect this information. The codes themselves are not billable and carry a charge of $0, but Medicare pays physicians a financial incentive for reporting Category II codes for data collection purposes.

Category III

Category III codes are temporary codes for data collection and for tracking the use of emerging technology, services, and procedures. The codes are four numbers followed by the letter T. If a category III code is available, medical assistants should use it in place of a Category I code.

Category III technology and procedures may be in the FDA approval process. Services may be items that the AMA is considering adding to Category I.

Appendices

The CPT manual has appendices that provide reference information. Several appendices summarize codes designated with special symbols throughout the CPT manual. Other appendices provide technical information used in offices that perform specialized procedures, such as nerve conduction studies, cardiac catheterization, or genetic testing. The appendices used most often by medical assistants in the medical office setting include the following:

Appendix A—*Modifiers* presents a complete description of modifiers applicable to the current year codes. Modifiers are two-digit alphanumeric codes appended to CPT or Level II codes to further describe circumstances. An abbreviated list of commonly used modifiers may appear inside the front cover, but medical assistants should develop the habit of referring to Appendix A until they are familiar with the details of how a specific modifier is to be used. Use of modifiers is introduced later in the chapter.

Appendix B—*Summary of Additions, Deletions and Revisions* is useful at the beginning of the year when the new CPT codes are released. Medical assistants can quickly cross-reference the CPT codes on encounter forms to Appendix B to determine the codes commonly used in their office that might be affected by the annual revision.

Appendix C—*Clinical Examples* provides examples of E&M code scenarios for many medical specialties. These should not be used for coding but for learning and understanding how various patient encounters might be coded. The most commonly used E&M codes each have at least one example.

HOW TO ASSIGN CPT PROCEDURE CODES

Proper coding begins with the right tools: a current year CPT coding manual, a HCPCS manual (which will be described in detail later in this chapter), a medical dictionary, and completed documentation in the medical record. Outdated coding tools can provide outdated codes, and outdated codes risk claim delay or denial. HIPAA requires that the current year coding manual be used, determined by the patient's date of service. Every service or procedure must be documented, in electronic or paper form, before coding can begin. When medical assistants are asked to code records with incomplete service or procedure documentation, they should route the records back to the health care providers who performed the services to complete all necessary documentation. Although rerouting may delay insurance claim submission, in the long run it is faster and more effective than submitting inaccurate or incomplete claims.

Procedure coding consists of three basic steps:

1. Abstract procedures from the patient's medical record.
2. Look up the procedure(s) in the Index.
3. Select and verify the code in the Tabular List.

Each of these steps is discussed in the next sections, and the additional sub-steps are demonstrated in detail. Medical assistants need to patiently and accurately execute the process of procedure coding.

Step 1. Abstract Procedures from the Patient's Medical Record

Medical assistants abstract diagnosis and procedural information from the medical record to code for services and the reasons they were provided. Coding must be performed to the highest level of certainty, meaning that all relevant information in the record should be coded, but missing information should not be assumed or coded. If the medical record is incomplete or inaccurate, it should be corrected or amended following proper procedures before attempting to code.

There are a number of documents within the medical record that contain information needed for coding. When coding for office-based or other outpatient services, medical assistants refer to the encounter form, visit notes, in-house lab and radiology reports, and operative reports for outpatient procedures. When coding for services that physicians provide to inpatients, medical assistants refer to the daily rounds sheet, which lists the patients seen in the hospital; daily progress notes; and operative reports for inpatient procedures.

It is important to keep in mind that, when performing procedure coding, medical assistants must code and bill only for the services actually delivered on a specific date by a specific provider. Do not bill for services previously completed, performed by a different provider, or ordered to be completed in the future.

EXAMPLE: *Identifying Services to Code*

A patient, Henry, makes a follow-up visit to Dr. Jessop related to back pain. Dr. Jessop discusses Henry's progress and current condition, performs a physical examination, reviews X-rays taken by the hospital outpatient department, adjusts Henry's medication, provides therapeutic ultrasound, and orders a magnetic resonance imaging (MRI) study. The medical assistant, Heather, codes for the two services that Dr. Jessop performed today:

- E&M visit
- therapeutic ultrasound

Heather does *not* code for the following services, because Dr. Jessop did not perform them today:

- The X-ray was performed previously at another location.
- The E&M medical decision-making component includes Dr. Jessop reviewing the X-ray, adjusting the medication, writing the prescription, and ordering the MRI.
- The patient fills the prescription at the pharmacy.
- The MRI will be performed in the future at another location.

Abstracting procedures from the patient's medical record involves three steps:

1. Identify the primary service or procedure.
2. Identify secondary services or procedures.
3. Identify the quantity of each procedure.

Identify the Primary Service or Procedure

Often the physician indicates procedure codes on the encounter form, but it is wise to verify the codes on the encounter form against the medical record. When abstracting from the medical record, be certain not to write in the record. Make a photocopy of the pertinent pages that you wish to annotate or highlight, or keep a separate paper for notes. Remember to shred copies of medical records when you are done with them.

First, look for the chief complaint or reason for the visit. Then, identify the primary procedure or the main service provided during the encounter. Often, this may be the E&M encounter—the history, examination, and medical decision making (recommendations). It is common for the E&M to be the only service provided.

Identify Secondary Services or Procedures

Medical assistants should identify the secondary procedures, which are additional services documented in the medical record in addition to the primary procedure. Secondary procedures are coded in the same way as primary procedures and prioritized from highest cost to lowest cost on the CMS-1500 form. This is because many insurance companies pay the first procedure in full but discount additional procedures performed at the same time. Generally, the E&M is identified first, with additional procedures to follow.

Identify the Quantity of Each Procedure

For many procedures, such as E&M, the quantity is one. For services such as removal of lesions, identify the type and number of lesions removed. For services based on time, identify the number of minutes spent providing the service, then convert to the unit of time required by the code description. For example, therapeutic ultrasound is reported in 15-minute increments, so when 30 minutes of treatment are provided, report 2 units on the CMS-1500 form.

Step 2. Look Up the Procedure(s) in the Index

For each procedure, use the Index to locate the preliminary code(s). This involves determining the Main Term, modifying terms, and codes or code ranges. Never code directly from the Index. After completing this step, you must verify the code(s) in the Tabular List. Using the Index involves three steps:

1. Identify the Main Term.
2. Review the modifying terms and/or instructional notes.
3. Identify the preliminary code(s).

Identify the Main Term

The Main Term is the word you look up in the Index to find the code(s). The CPT Index classifies Main Terms in four ways. Medical assistants may use any of these methods to locate a code in the Index. If one method does not provide adequate information, then another method can be used (Figure 16-3).

1. Look up the name of the *procedure* or *service*, such as *Endoscopy* or *Splint.*
2. Look up the name of the *organ* or *anatomic* site, such as *Colon* or *Tibia.*

3. Look up the name of a *condition* or *disease*, such as *Fracture* or *Polyp.*
4. Look up the *eponym* (a disease or condition named after an individual), such as *Colles fracture*; an abbreviation or *acronym,* such as *AIDS*; or a nontechnical *synonym* (a word similar in meaning), such as *Removal* instead of *Excision.*

Medical assistants should be aware that in the CPT Index, Main Terms include organs and anatomic sites, whereas in ICD-10-CM, anatomic site is not an option in the Index. Because there are many choices of how to locate a Main Term, a good guideline is to search in this order: eponym or abbreviation; procedure or service; organ or anatomic site; disease or condition; and synonym.

The Main Term is always boldfaced with each word beginning with a capital letter. Some Main Terms are broad, with several pages of modifying terms, such as *Excision*, and others are quite specific with only a single code, such as *Color Vision Examination.*

Review the Modifying Terms and Instructional Notes

Main Terms rarely provide the exact code needed. Frequently, Main Terms function as major headings that have up to three levels of modifying terms. Modifying terms are descriptive words in the Index that appear indented under the Main Term to further describe the service or procedure. When modifying terms appear, it is important to review the entire list of options before selecting the most specific term (Figure 16-4). Medical assistants should be aware that modifying terms are different from two-digit modifiers that are appended to Category I codes.

Search method	Examples		
	Repair of Colles Fracture	Electrocardiogram	Removal of cataract
Eponym	Colles fracture	–	–
Acronym/abbreviation		EKG	–
Procedure name	Repair	Electrocardiogram	Phacoemulsification
Anatomic site	Wrist	Heart	Eye
Condition	Fracture	–	Cataract
Synonym	–	Monitoring	Removal, Excision

FIGURE 16-3 Alternative methods for locating the CPT Main Term.

Type of convention	CPT Alphabetical index entry
Main term	→ **Endoscopy**
Instructional note	→ *See* Arthroscopy; Thoroscopy
First modifying term	→ Anus
Second modifying term	→ Ablation
Third modifying term and code	→ Polyp xxxxx

FIGURE 16-4 Example of CPT conventions in the Index.

The first level of modifying terms is aligned on the same margin as the Main Term, but in smaller, non-boldfaced type. The second and third levels of modifying terms are each indented several spaces beyond the previous level. They further describe the Main Term, in reference to anatomic site, such as *Endoscopy, Anus*; extent, such as *Excision, Clavicle, Partial*; procedure, such as *Electrocardiography, 24-Hour Monitoring*; or similar descriptors.

When the Main Term or modifying term is too long to fit on one line, a carryover line is used. Carryover lines are indented the same number of spaces as the beginning of the line. It is important to read carefully to distinguish between carryover lines and modifying terms.

Main terms and modifying terms contain instructional notes, such as *see* or *see also*, which direct the user to synonyms for the code. For example, the entry *Pneumonotomy— see Incision, Lung* instructs the user to look under the Main Term *Incision* and the modifying term *Lung* to locate the codes for removal of the lung. In Figure 16-4, the instructional note *See Arthroscopy; Thoroscopy* directs the user to other Main Terms that may also be useful.

Codes next to a Main Term might be single codes, a range of codes, or a nonsequential list, as follows:

- A single code is one code that is presented for a specific modifying term, such as *Polyp* (Figure 16-4).
- A range of codes is presented with a hyphen "-", such as the entry for *Bone Graft, Harvesting 2XXXX-2XXXX*.
- Nonsequential codes are presented with a comma ",". Commas indicate that three codes should be reviewed, but the intervening code numbers are probably not applicable.

Identify the Preliminary Code(s)

When the appropriate modifying terms are located, the preliminary code(s) is printed immediately to the right. It is helpful to jot down the potential appropriate codes before verifying in the Tabular List, being careful not to transpose any digits. Never use the Index to make the final code selection. Even if only one code appears, it must be verified in the Tabular List to be certain the code selection is accurate and to read any instructional notes.

Step 3. Verify the Code in the Tabular List

All codes must be verified in the Tabular List to ensure that the description accurately describes the service provided. Medical assistants also need to read the guidelines, special instructions, and instructional notes printed in the Tabular List. Verifying the code in the Tabular List involves seven steps:

1. Locate the preliminary code(s) in the Tabular List.
2. Interpret Tabular List conventions.
3. Select the code with the highest level of specificity.
4. Review the code for bundling, add-on codes, and quantity.
5. Append modifiers, if needed.
6. Compare the final code with the documentation.
7. Assign the code.

Locate the Preliminary Code(s) in the Tabular List

Look for the preliminary code number in the Tabular List, where codes are arranged in numerical order. The Tabular List contains six sections, each of which is divided into **subsections, subheadings, categories**, and **subcategories** based on anatomy, procedure, condition, or descriptor. Medical assistants should be aware that because of the expanding nature of the code set, some codes are not in strict numerical order. These are **resequenced codes** and are highlighted with the symbol # for easy identification.

Interpret Tabular List Conventions

Before medical assistants verify and finalize the code, they first need to interpret the conventions presented with the code. CPT codes are five-digit numbers with no decimal point, and a description to the right. Tabular List conventions include formatting, punctuation, verbal instructions, and symbols. Conventions may appear on the same line with the code, above it, below it, or at the beginning of a subcategory, category, subheading, subsection, or section. Look carefully for any information that may be relevant to the preliminary code selection, because this additional information may direct you to use a different code or an additional code. The Tabular List conventions of the semicolon, verbal instructions, and symbols are discussed next.

Semicolon. In the Tabular List, an important convention is the use of the **semicolon (;)** and indented code descriptions. To conserve space and avoid repeating common terminology, some of the procedure descriptors in the Tabular List are not printed in their entirety, but rather refer back to a common portion of the procedure descriptor listed in a preceding entry. The **standalone code** or **parent code** is the one whose description is left-justified and begins with a capital letter. The shared portion of the code before the semicolon is the common descriptor, which is shared with indented codes. The portion after the semicolon is the unique descriptor that applies to only one code number.

The **indented code** description is indented three spaces and begins with a small letter. This description is the unique descriptor for that code number. The unique descriptor must be combined with the shared descriptor from the standalone code to obtain a full description of the code. Within a series of indented codes, medical assistants *must* refer back to the preceding standalone code to determine the common descriptor of the indented code(s). Indented codes describe variations on the standalone code, such as an alternative anatomic site, alternative procedure, or extent of services.

An indented code should not be billed together with the parent code. They are considered two distinct procedures or services. The common descriptor is simply a space-saving convention in the printed book.

Guidelines and Instructions. The CPT manual provides several types of narrative instructions that guide medical assistants in proper coding:

- **Guidelines** are instructions that appear at the beginning of each of the six sections and apply to all codes in that section. Guidelines also list commonly used modifiers and provide subsection information.

- **Special instructions** are directions within each section describing specific rules and definitions for use of codes within a particular category or subcategory. Read and interpret the special instructions before assigning a code, even if it means going back to the top of the page or a previous page to find them.

- **Instructional notes**, which appear in parentheses, direct the user to alternative codes for closely-related procedures or to codes that must or must not be used together.

Symbols. Symbols in the Tabular List alert the user to certain circumstances that may affect use or interpretation of codes. A key appears at the bottom of each page. Medical assistants should become familiar with these meanings.

Select the Code with the Highest Level of Specificity

There is no universal rule that defines how many codes need to be reviewed to identify the one with the highest specificity. Sometimes, the best code is the first one listed; other times, there may be a dozen or more codes to review and additional ones to cross-reference. There also is no universal rule that describes how precise the correct code will be in its description. For example, many codes on the integumentary system include the size of the area treated, but the size is usually a range, such as 1.1 cm to 2.0 cm. If a treatment covers 1.5 cm, there is not a more specific code or modifier to describe the exact size. The medical record often contains more detail than what is coded. Only by carefully interpreting the conventions associated with each code, category, and section can one be certain. As medical assistants become experienced in a particular office, they become very familiar with the most frequently used codes.

Review the Code for Appropriate Edits

Carefully review code descriptions, instructional notes, and special instructions one more time to be certain that the code selected is accurate. **Edits** are specific coding and billing criteria that are checked for accuracy based on predetermined rules. Payers' computer systems reject claims that violate edit rules. Edits that should be reviewed are bundling, add-on codes, and quantity definitions.

Bundling Edits. Pay special attention to **bundling** edits, frequently triggered by the words *includes* and *not separately reportable*. These words indicate that multiple services are included in a single code. The words *report separately* or *use in conjunction with* indicate that additional codes should be used.

Add-On Codes. **Add-on codes** should be verified. Use of add-on codes may be limited to only a few codes that are listed in instructional notes. For example, when coding for discectomy of multiple disks, the code for each additional interspace is reported in addition to a specific primary procedure code.

Quantity Edits. CPT codes differ regarding how the quantity of procedures is to be reported. This information is provided in the code description or special instructions.

Codes that include a time-based element also vary in how quantity is reported. For example, codes for certain physical therapy treatments describe 15 minutes of treatment with a quantity of *1* on the CMS-1500 form, Item 24G. Thirty minutes of treatment is reported with a quantity of *2* on the CMS-1500 form, Item 24G.

Append Modifiers, If Needed

Modifiers are suffixes consisting of two digits or two characters that are appended to CPT codes to report a service or procedure that has been modified by some specific circumstance without altering or modifying the basic definition or CPT code. Modifiers affect the complete description of a service and frequently have a significant impact on reimbursement and coding compliance. Use of modifiers can be described in the instructional notes, special instructions, or guidelines. The experience of the coder is an important factor when determining if the situation calls for modifiers.

The proper use of modifiers can speed up claims processing and increase reimbursement. Improper use of CPT modifiers may result in claim delays or denials. A complete list of modifiers appears in the CPT manual in Appendix A with their full definitions. Modifiers are used for a variety of reasons:

- To report only the professional component of a procedure or service
- To report a service mandated by a third-party payer
- To indicate that a procedure was performed bilaterally
- To report multiple procedures performed at the same session by the same provider
- To report a portion of a service or procedure that was reduced or eliminated at the physician's discretion
- To report a portion of the surgical package provided by other than the primary surgeon
- To report assistant surgeon services

The modifiers most commonly used in an office-based setting. For more information on modifiers, refer to Appendix A in the CPT manual.

Compare the Final Code with the Documentation

As a final check, with coding manual instructions fresh in your mind, refer back to the original documentation and verify that all conditions of the code agree with the medical record. If a discrepancy arises, work through the process again from the beginning.

Professionalism   The Workplace

Reporting incorrect procedure codes on an insurance claim can create problems such as improper reimbursement, fraud, and inaccurate patient medical history. When uncertain of the best code, it may be tempting to "guesstimate" and assign an approximate code. This practice may result in upcoding, which is coding for a higher level of service than what was actually provided to gain higher reimbursement. Guessing could also result in downcoding, which is coding for a lower level of service than what was actually provided, to avoid potential fraud or abuse. Downcoding may seem prudent to avoid fraud, but it deprives the medical office of reimbursement to which it is legally entitled.

CODING FOR EVALUATION AND MANAGEMENT SERVICES

Evaluation and Management (E&M) codes describe patient encounters with a physician for the evaluation and management of a health problem. They are the most frequently used codes in most medical offices. Although E&M codes begin with the numbers 99, they are located out of numerical sequence in the CPT manual. The E&M section is the first section at the front of the manual. This placement is for convenience, because they are the most commonly used section of CPT codes.

Usually, the physician marks the E&M code on the encounter form. Medical assistants need to ensure that documentation in the medical record is consistent with the codes checked off. Offices should **audit** bills on a regular basis. Auditing is a detailed process that verifies that every detail of the E&M code is clearly documented. An internal audit is one conducted by the office whereas an external audit is one conducted by an outside organization, such as Medicare. To prepare for an internal audit, follow these steps:

- Access the patient's record in the electronic health record (EHR) system. Locate the physician's documentation of the encounter to be audited within the chart.
- Retrieve a copy of the insurance claim to identify the code(s) billed for the date of service being audited. If the audit is done before billing, retrieve the coding worksheet that identifies the code intended to be billed.
- Refer to a copy of the *Documentation Guidelines* for Evaluation and Management services published by the Centers for Medicare and Medicaid Services, or a similar document from the patient's insurer.

The auditing process involves reading the documentation, comparing it to the *Documentation Guidelines* to identify the specific criteria met during the encounter, determining the level of service of documented, then comparing it to the code assigned or billed. If there is a discrepancy, the coder should recode the encounter so it matches the services documented.

E&M coding possesses some differences from the rest of CPT coding. The key steps for E&M coding are summarized next. This provides a general overview of the criteria for E&M coding. Additional details can be found in the E&M section guidelines in the CPT manual and professional reference resources. The general process for coding E&M services includes the following steps:

1. Identify the type of service.
2. Determine the key components, contributing factors, or time spent with the patient.
3. Compare the final code with the documentation.
4. Identify bundled and separately billable services.
5. Append modifiers, if needed.

Step 1. Identify the Type of Service

The first step in coding E&M services is to identify the category and subcategory of service, before trying to determine the specific code. The category and subcategory identify the general location, type of service, and type of patient. These elements must be selected correctly before a code can be assigned. Identifying the type of service involves three steps:

1. Identify the category.
2. Identify the subcategory.
3. Read the reporting instructions.

Identify the Category

E&M codes are selected based on the category of service. A category may describe the location of service, such as office visit or hospital inpatient visit, or the type of service, such as consultation, critical care, or preventive care. This can be confusing because the *Office Visit* category does not list all services provided in the medical office. Office-based services also appear in other categories, such as *Consultation* and *Preventive Care*. It is important to be familiar with CPT definitions of these services, which are described in special instructions at the beginning of each subsection.

Identify the Subcategory

Most E&M categories are further subdivided based on patient status (new vs. established), location (office vs. inpatient), frequency (initial vs. subsequent), or other relevant characteristics. Special instructions in the subsections describe these criteria. Commonly used terms are discussed next.

Medical assistants frequently need to determine **patient status**—that is, to distinguish between **new patients** and **established patients**. This criterion is used for office visits and preventive care. For coding purposes, a new patient is one who has not received any professional services from the physician, or another physician of the same specialty or subspecialty who belongs to the same group practice, within the past three years. An established patient is one who has received professional services from the physician, or another physician of the same specialty or subspecialty who belongs to the same group practice, within the past three years. Upon looking at the Tabular List, you see that all of the codes listed appear under the heading *Evaluation and Management*.

Some codes are determined based on whether the patient is an **outpatient** or an inpatient. An inpatient is someone who has been formally admitted to a facility with written admission orders from a physician. All others are considered outpatients, even though they may occupy a hospital bed. For example, observation status and emergency department patients are outpatients. Observation status is a designated type of care in which a patient is hospitalized for monitoring, but not formally admitted.

Certain codes describe the frequency of the encounter and identify whether this is the first encounter with a particular physician (or substitute from the same specialty and subspecialty) for the current hospital admission. The first, or initial, encounter requires a more extensive history and examination than subsequent visits during the same admission. Be aware that the meanings of initial and subsequent for CPT codes are different from the ICD-10-CM definitions for the initial and subsequent episodes of care.

Read the Reporting Instructions

Each category and subcategory within the E&M section contains definitions and instructions that describe key terms, how the codes are to be reported, and what may be bundled into the code description. Even though the instructions can sometimes be lengthy, take time to read and understand what is being said. For example, when reporting critical care services, special instructions provide examples of what constitutes critical care, where it can be provided, and the age of the patient appropriate for the codes. In addition, the instructions list the CPT codes that are bundled into critical care and cannot be reported separately.

Step 2. Determine the Key Components and Contributing Factors

Within each subcategory, there are three to five levels of codes, in increasing order of complexity. It is necessary to determine the **key components** or other criteria used for code selection within each subcategory of E&M codes.

Many codes are based on the extent of the history (H), the examination (E), and the medical decision making (MDM). Other codes are based on time or age. A summary of the three key components (H, E, MDM) follows. More detailed guidelines can be found in the CPT guidelines and advanced coding texts.

History

History (H, Hx) describes the background, onset, and progression of the patient's current condition. The complexity of the history may be classified as follows:

- **Problem focused**—Patient's problem is small; he has only one chief complaint and gives a brief history of his present illness or problem.

- **Expanded problem focused**—Patient's problem is mild to moderate; he has more than one chief complaint and/or a more extensive history of his present illness or problem.

- **Detailed**—Patient's problem is moderate to severe, and he has pertinent past, family, and/or social history that is directly related to his current problem.

Each of these levels of history has specific definitions in the CPT manual and official documentation guidelines.

Examination

Examination (E, Ex) describes the complexity of the physical assessment of the patient. The complexity of the examination may be classified as follows:

- **Problem focused**—A limited examination of the affected body area is done.

- **Expanded problem focused**—A limited examination of the affected body area is done along with other related organ systems.

- **Detailed**—An extended examination of the affected body area and other related organ systems is performed.

- **Comprehensive**—A general multisystem examination is performed.

Each of these levels of examination has specific definitions in the CPT manual and official documentation guidelines.

Medical Decision Making

Medical decision making (MDM) describes the complexity of establishing a diagnosis or selecting a management option. The four types of medical decision making are:

- **Straightforward**—Minimal diagnoses, minimal complexity, and minimal risk of complications.

- **Low complexity**—Limited diagnoses, limited complexity, and low risk of complications.

- **Moderate complexity**—Multiple diagnoses, moderate complexity, and moderate risk of complications.

- **High complexity**—Extensive diagnoses, extensive complexity, and high risk of complications.

Each of these levels of medical decision making has specific definitions in the CPT manual and official documentation guidelines.

The specific E&M code is assigned based on how it meets the criteria of the key components. The criteria for each component are described in the code definition in the CPT manual. Some categories of E&M codes require that all three key components be at the level specified in the code description or a higher level to assign the code. Other categories require that only two of the key components be at the level specified in the code description or a higher level to assign the code. The number of components required is stated in the code description.

Contributing Factors

Contributing factors are **counseling, coordination of care**, and nature of the **presenting problem**. These factors rarely determine the E&M code, but should be consistent with the code selected.

- **Counseling**—Provider's discussion with the patient and/or a family concerning the patient's diagnosis, test results, impressions, prognosis, risks and benefits of treatment options, and instructions for management of the condition.

- **Coordination of care**—Working with other providers or agencies to provide the patient with needed care, such as referral to home health care.

- **The presenting problem**—The primary reason the patient is seeing the provider.

E&M codes take the following into consideration in determining the nature of the presenting problem:

- **Minimal**—The problem may not require the presence of the physician, but service is provided under the physician's supervision.

- **Self-limited or minor**—The problem runs a definite and prescribed course, is temporary, and is not likely to permanently alter the patient's health status.
- **Low severity**—The problem has a low risk of causing the patient's death without treatment, and full recovery is expected.
- **Moderate severity**—The problem has a risk of death without treatment; there is an uncertain prognosis or an increased likelihood the problem will cause permanent health problems for the patient.
- **High severity**—The problem has a high risk of causing the patient's death without treatment, or there may be a high probability of prolonged functional impairment to the patient as a result of this condition.

Time is also a consideration in E&M coding. Codes with the three key components also include an indication of the amount of **face-to-face time**, which is the time that the physician typically spends with the patient and family. Although E&M codes with the three key components should never be selected based on time, there are situations in which a code level can be increased based on time. When the time spent in counseling and coordination of care is more than 50 percent of total visit time, time may be considered a controlling factor to qualify for a higher level E&M code. Documentation needs to indicate the total amount of time spent with the patient and family, the amount of time spent in counseling and coordination of care, and a description of why the additional time was required.

Step 3. Verify the Final Code with the Documentation

As a final check, with coding manual instructions fresh in your mind, refer back to the original documentation and verify that all conditions of the code agree with the medical record. If a discrepancy arises, work through the process again from the beginning.

After verifying documentation against CPT guidelines, special instructions, and code descriptions, finalize the appropriate code and enter it into the computer system. Be certain to double-check the accuracy of the code number, as transpositions easily occur.

Step 4. Identify Bundled and Separately Billable Services

Medical assistants must determine which services are bundled in the E&M code and which should be billed separately. This ensures that coding is accurate, no fraud is committed, and the office receives reimbursements for all services provided.

The following services are included in an E&M code:
- Discussions with patients and their families about the current problem
- Physical examination
- Reviewing test results, reports from other providers, and records of outside services
- Ordering tests and services
- Writing prescriptions
- Scheduling procedures
- Obtaining preapproval or preauthorization
- Providing instructions and education to patients and their families

Certain E&M codes, such as those for critical care, include a more specific list of bundled services. Surgical codes include postoperative follow-up. When an office or emergency department encounter develops into another E&M service with the same physician on the same date, they may be combined into one code. For example, when a physician sees a patient in the emergency department, and then admits the patient, the emergency department services are bundled into E&M code for the hospital admission.

Identify other services provided in the office that may be billed in addition to the E&M code, such as:
- Venipuncture
- Immunizations
- ECGs
- X-rays
- Lab tests performed in the office

Step 5. Append Modifiers, If Needed

Certain modifiers are used specifically for E&M coding to tell payers that an E&M service should be reimbursed and not bundled into another service. Refer to the CPT manual for more information about modifiers.

CODING FOR SPECIAL SITUATIONS

In addition to coding for office visits, medical assistants sometimes need to code for surgical procedures, radiology (X-rays), and laboratory tests. Each of these services has special rules that must be followed. Often, a certified coder handles coding for these services, but medical assistants need to be aware of the special requirements in the event they need to answer questions or provide information to another staff member. See Procedure 16-2.

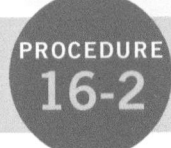

16-2   Performing Procedural Coding

Objective ◆ *Assign CPT codes based on documentation.*

MATERIALS

CPT coding manual; superbill/encounter form; patient's medical record

METHOD

1. On the superbill, locate the procedure code the physician has circled.
2. Identify the primary and secondary services or procedures performed, as stated in the medical record.
3. Locate the Main Term in the Index.
4. Review the modifying terms and instructional notes associated with the Main Term.
5. Identify the preliminary code(s) associated with the most appropriate modifying term(s).
6. Locate the preliminary code(s) in the Tabular List.
7. Interpret the conventions used in the Tabular List.
8. Select the code with the highest level of specificity.
9. Review the code for appropriate bundling, add-on codes, and quantity.
10. Determine if modifiers are required.
11. Verify the final code against the documentation.
12. Assign the code.

JUDGMENT CALL

During the five years Audrey has worked for Dr. Suarez, the physician has often asked her to bill for services he did not perform. Audrey has never objected, in part because she feels patients are unharmed by the practice. She also believes she is blameless, because she receives no additional money from the process.

One day Audrey arrives at work to find that Dr. Suarez has been arrested. Later, the physician is convicted and sentenced to two years in jail. The office closes, and Audrey loses her job. Audrey begins a job search but finds that her association with Dr. Suarez is affecting her negatively. In fact, several potential employers have turned her away as a result. One of those employers said, "I'm sorry, but we just can't trust someone who worked for a doctor involved in insurance fraud." How could Audrey have avoided this situation?

Coding for Surgery

Surgical procedures can be performed in the medical office, at an ambulatory surgery center, or at a hospital. The same codes are used for a given procedure, regardless of where it is performed. The location of the service is indicated on the

CMS-1500 in Item 24B. The surgical section of CPT is the largest section and is divided into 14 subsections by body system. CPT defines the services included in the CPT surgical package. It also provides rules on bundling and unbundling that must be followed.

CPT Surgical Package

All CPT surgery codes include the **surgical package**, also known as the global surgical concept. The surgical package includes specific services, in addition to the operation, that cannot be billed separately. Bundled services, outlined in the CPT Surgery Section guidelines, include:

- One related E&M encounter on the date immediately before or on the date of procedure, subsequent to (following) the decision for surgery

- Preparing the patient for surgery, including local infiltration, topical anesthesia

- Performing the operation, including normal additional procedures, such as debridement

- Evaluating the patient in the postanesthesia recovery area

- Immediate postoperative care, including dictating operative notes, talking with the family and other physicians

CHAPTER 16 Procedure Coding **411**

- Writing orders
- Typical postoperative follow-up visits for normal uncomplicated care

The **global period** refers to the number of days surrounding a surgical procedure during which all services relating to that procedure—preoperative, during the surgery, and postoperative—are considered part of the surgical package. Medicare defines postoperative follow-up periods of 0, 10, or 90 days, based on the type of procedure. At inpatient facilities, preoperative testing performed done within three calendar days of the procedure, also is bundled into the procedure payment.

Third-party payers have varying definitions of what constitutes a surgical package and varying policies about what is in the surgical package, including the number of follow-up days. Therefore, it is important to ask about the surgical package criteria when certifying for surgery with a third-party payer. By doing so, the office knows in advance which services may or may not be billed separately in addition to the surgical procedure.

The surgical package does not include certain services. Code these services separately for reimbursement in addition to the surgical package fee:

- Complications, exacerbations, recurrence requiring additional services
- Ongoing care (other than the surgical procedure) for the condition for which a procedure was performed
- Care for coexisting conditions or injuries

Bundled Codes

In addition to the surgical package, CPT codes may include multiple procedures that are commonly performed together. Many surgical code descriptions include a phrase such as *with or without* or other language to include or exclude incidental services. The CPT subsection notes and guidelines may indicate that a particular code includes certain related or supporting procedures. **Unbundling** occurs when separate procedures are reported that should have been included under a bundled code. This practice is illegal and results in denial of a claim and, possibly, fines.

Coding for Radiology

Medical offices can take certain X-rays in the office, so the physician has the results immediately. This also avoids requiring patients to travel to a different location for the X-ray. The codes in the Radiology section report radiologic services performed by or supervised by a physician. The process of performing a radiology examination includes several steps:

- **Order the examination**—A physician or other qualified health professional writes an order for the test, often as part of an E&M encounter. There is no code for ordering a radiologic examination because it is included in the other services provided by the ordering physician.
- **Perform the actual imaging**—The radiologic examination itself is reported by the provider or facility that actually provides the service. Creating the image, including personnel and equipment, is the **technical component** of a radiology code. When only the technical component is provided, the facility appends the modifier –TC.
- **Analyze and report on the examination results**—A qualified physician reviews the image results and writes a report that details the findings. This is the **professional component** of a radiology code and is bundled into the same code used to report performing the test. When a physician provides only the professional component, the medical assistant appends the modifier –26.

When a physician provides both the technical and professional components of a radiology service, the medical assistant bills the full code with no modifiers.

The Radiology section is divided by modality, or imaging method (Table 16-1). Each modality subsection is further divided by anatomic site.

Some radiologic procedures, such as X-rays, are coded based on the number of views taken of the anatomic site. Each view is an image made from a different direction or angle, such as anterior and posterior (A/P). When reviewing the codes for a particular procedure, be sure that the number of views identified in the code description matches the number of views documented in the chart or report.

To locate codes for radiology procedures, look up the modality or imaging method as the Main Term and the anatomic site as the modifying term.

Coding for Pathology and Laboratory

Medical offices with a certified laboratory can perform certain lab tests in the office. This often gives the physician the results immediately, while the patient is still in the office, and avoids the need for the patient to travel to a different location. The codes in the Pathology/Laboratory section cover services provided by physicians or by technicians under the supervision of a physician. The process of performing a laboratory test includes several steps:

TABLE 16-1 | Radiological Modalities (Methods)

Method	Description
Computerized tomography (CT)	A 3-D image created using X-rays to make a series of cross-sectional images in an area of the body.
Fluoroscopy	A real-time, moving X-ray image, usually viewed on a monitor.
Magnetic resonance imaging (MRI)	An image created using powerful magnets and radio waves.
Mammography	An image of the breasts, or mammary glands, created using low-dose X-rays.
Positron emission tomography (PET)	An image created using a radioactive substance called a tracer to show how organs and tissues are functioning.
Radiation Oncology	A form of cancer treatment that uses high-energy ionizing radiation to shrink or kill tumors. Also called radiation therapy.
Ultrasound (US)	An image created using sound waves, useful to view soft structures within the body.
X-ray	A picture created using radiation particles, used primarily for solid structures within the body.

- **Order the test**—A physician or other qualified health professional writes an order for the test, often as part of an E&M encounter. Do not code for writing orders.

- **Obtain and handle the sample**—The collection method used to obtain the sample is coded separately, such as a biopsy, venipuncture, capillary stick, or arterial puncture.

- **Perform the actual test**—The test itself is reported within a series of codes and it include. Performing the test, including personnel and equipment, is the technical component of a laboratory code.

- **Analyze and report on the test results**—A qualified physician reviews the test results and writes a report that details the findings. This is the professional component of a laboratory code and is bundled into the same series code used to report performing the test.

The Pathology and Laboratory section is divided by type of test (Table 16-2), the type of specimen, and the substance being tested for. To locate a CPT code for a laboratory or pathology procedure, look up the name of the test, the substance tested for, or the type of specimen in the Index. Procedures and services are listed in the Index under the following types of Main Terms:

- Name of the test, such as urinalysis, drug test

- Procedure, such as hormone assay or fine needle aspiration

- Abbreviations, such as CBC, RBS, TLC

- Panel of tests, under Blood Tests

- Type of specimen, such as blood or urine

The Pathology and Laboratory section provides codes for organ or disease-oriented panels 80047–80076 series. A panel is a group of tests ordered together to detect particular diseases or malfunctioning organs. When a panel is reported, all the listed tests must have been performed with no substitution. If not all the tests listed in the panel code were performed, then list the individual CPT code for each test that

TABLE 16-2 | Types of Laboratory Tests

Type of Test	Description
Chemistry	Quantitative tests for the amount of asubstance contained in a specimen
Microbiology	Tests that identify the presence and type of microorganisms in a specimen
Hematology	Blood tests to determine cell counts of various types of blood cells
Immunology	Tests on antigens, allergens, or antibodies
Cytopathology	The microscopic examination of cells from anywhere in the body to detect conditions and determine if neoplasms are benign or malignant
Pathology	The visual examination of body structures or tissue, with or without a microscope

was performed, not the code for the panel. Panels were developed for coding purposes and should not be interpreted as clinical standards for testing.

Some medical practices have laboratory equipment and perform their own testing. In-office labs must be certified by the Clinical Laboratory Improvement Amendment (CLIA) of 1988, which awards three levels of certification. The lowest level allows in-office certified labs to perform dipstick urinalysis and urine pregnancy. If the medical practice does not have a lab but obtains the specimen for the lab, the venipuncture code can be billed for obtaining the blood sample. As in every medical setting, the Occupational and Safety and Health Administration (OSHA) regulates safety.

Although Medicare does not allow physicians to bill for lab work they did not perform, other third-party payers do. When a medical practice has a contract with a lab and pays the lab for the work, the medical practice can bill for the tests reported. The modifier -90 is attached to the code for the lab test. On the CMS-1500, Item 20 must be checked "Yes" and the fee that the medical practice pays the lab must be entered under "Charges" in Item 24F. Finally, Item 32 must report the name, address, and NPI of the laboratory.

When the medical office collects a specimen to be sent to an outside lab for processing, code only the specimen collection and handling.

Coding for Medicine

The Medicine section of the CPT manual contains codes for reporting diagnostic testing, noninvasive or minimally invasive procedures (procedures that do not require a surgical incision), and treatments from all areas of medical practice, as well as some nonphysician providers. Examples include vaccines, psychiatry, ophthalmology, cardiology, allergy, neurology, infusion therapy, audiology, and physical and occupational therapy.

Codes in this section are, in general, divided by medical specialty. To locate codes in the Index, look up the name of the procedure, such as electrocardiogram, or the condition for which it is provided.

Immunizations and Vaccinations

Immunizations and vaccinations are a service commonly provided in medical offices. Immunizations require two codes, one for administering the immunization and the other for the particular vaccine or toxoid that is administered. Codes for administering the vaccines are divided based on the age of the patient and whether counseling was

provided to parents of children. Add-on codes are provided when more than one immunization is administered at the same encounter.

To locate codes for administration of the vaccine, look for the Main Term *Immunization Administration* in the Index. To locate codes for the product administered, look in the Index for the name of the product, such as *DTaP* or *Typhoid*. You may also look up the Main Term *Vaccines*, and then select the appropriate modifying term for the specific product.

THE HEALTHCARE COMMON PROCEDURE CODING SYSTEM (HCPCS)

The **Healthcare Common Procedure Coding System (HCPCS)**, called "Hick Picks" by coders, is a set of codes developed and maintained by CMS for the reporting of professional services, nonphysician services, supplies, durable medical equipment (DME), and injectable drugs. HCPCS has two levels of codes. A third level was discontinued at the end of 2003.

CPT codes are HCPCS **Level I codes** for professional services.

Level II codes are alphanumeric codes that begin with a letter, followed by four numbers. Typically, when professionals refer to "HCPCS codes," they are referring to Level II codes. Level II codes cover supplies, DME, drugs, nonphysician providers, and certain physician services for Medicare and Medicaid. When CPT and HCPCS codes exist for the same service, with the same description, use the CPT code. When procedure descriptions differ, use HCPCS Level II codes, because these codes are required by Medicare and Medicaid. They are mandated by HIPAA as a uniform code set for insurance carriers, but implementation is in progress. Be sure to check with private carriers to verify if they accept HCPCS Level II codes. Reimbursement for supplies and equipment is usually faster when HCPCS codes are used, because they are more specific than using the generic CPT code for supplies. A list of the categories in Level II appears in Table 16-3. Level II codes are updated on a quarterly basis; the manual is published annually in October. Quarterly updates are available on the CMS website at www.cms.gov.

The HCPCS Level II coding manual contains an Index and a Tabular Listing. As with the other coding manuals, first use the Index to locate the item or service, and then refer to the Tabular List to verify. Many DME manufacturers print a suggested HCPCS code on the item packaging. This

TABLE 16-3 | Level II HCPCS Codes

Service	Code Range
Transportation services, medical and surgical supplies, miscellaneous	A0000–A9999
Enteral and parenteral therapy	B0000–B9999
Temporary hospital outpatient PPS	C0000–C9999
Dental procedures	D0000–D9999
Durable medical equipment (DME)	E0000–E9000
Procedures and services, temporary	G0000–G9999
Alcoholic and drug abuse treatment services	H0000–H9999
Drugs administered other than oral method	J0000–J8999
Chemotherapy drugs	J9000–J9999
Temporary codes for DMERCS	K0000–K9999
Orthotic and prosthetic procedures and devices	L0000–L9999
Medical services	M0000–M9999
Pathology and laboratory	P0000–P9999
Temporary codes	Q0000–Q9999
Diagnostic radiology services	R0000–R9999
Private payer codes	S0000–S9999
State Medicaid agency codes	T0000–T9999
Vision	V0000–V2999
Hearing services	V5000–V5999

TABLE 16-4 | HCPCS Modifiers Used for Medical Office Services

Modifier	Description
AH	Clinical psychologist
AJ	Clinical social worker
E1	Upper left eyelid
E2	E2
E3	Upper right eyelid
E4	Lower right eyelid
F1	Left hand, second digit
F2	Left hand, third digit
F3	Left hand, fourth digit
F4	Left hand, fifth digit
F5	Right hand, thumb
F6	Right hand, second digit
F7	Right hand, third digit
F8	Right hand, fourth digit
F9	Right hand, fifth digit
FA	Left hand, thumb
GA	Signed advance beneficiary notice (ABN) form on file (for Medicare patients)
LT	Left side
PC	Professional courtesy
Q6	Service provided by a *locum tenens* physician
RT	Right side
SA	Nurse practitioner with physician
TC	Technical component

Source: www.cms.gov

is a useful aid but always verify the HCPCS code in the manual. Many entries in the manual also contain cross-reference information to Medicare reimbursement rules for the specific item or service.

HCPCS Level II also contains alphanumeric modifiers that can be used with either Level I CPT codes or Level II codes. The most commonly used modifiers are those that designate specific anatomic sites of procedures and non-physician provider types (Table 16-4). Many additional modifiers exist for specific Medicare and Medicaid reimbursement situations. One of the most important of these is the modifier -GA, which indicates that a Medicare Advanced Beneficiary Notice (ABN) form was signed by the patient when a covered service is expected to be denied. Through experience, medical assistants become familiar with the specific requirements for their medical office.

SUMMARY

Procedure codes identify billable services provided to patients. Current Procedural Terminology (CPT) is a listing of five-character alphanumeric codes and descriptions used to report outpatient medical services and procedures. The CPT manual is published and copyrighted by the American Medical Association. The Health Insurance Portability and Accountability Act (HIPAA) mandates the use of CPT by covered entities that handle electronic claims. Medical assistants may work in offices that use certified coders to assign and audit procedure codes, so the extent to which a medical assistant is involved in procedure coding varies from one office to the next.

Medical offices report CPT procedure codes on CMS-1500 forms and electronic claims to identify the services provided and the cost of those services. Physicians are paid for CPT codes, but diagnosis codes are required to explain the reason(s) for the encounter or the reason services were provided. It is improper to code for a more complex service than what was actually provided, in the hope of receiving higher reimbursement. Doing so is considered fraud and carries severe penalties, including fines and possible imprisonment.

The CPT manual consists of an introduction, Tabular List, Index, and several appendices. Symbols in the Tabular List alert the user to certain circumstances that may affect use or interpretation of codes. Procedure coding consists of three basic steps: (1) abstract procedures from the patient's medical record; (2) look up the procedure(s) in the Index; (3) select and verify the code in the Tabular List.

Each section of CPT contains codes for a specific type of procedure. Evaluation and Management (E&M) codes describe patient encounters with a physician for the evaluation and management of a health problem. They are the most frequently used codes in most medical offices. The surgical section of CPT is the largest section and is divided into 14 subsections by body system. CPT defines the services included in the CPT surgical package. It also provides rules on bundling and unbundling that describe when multiple services are included in one code and when they should be reported with separate codes. The codes in the Radiology section report radiologic services performed by or supervised by a physician. Medical offices may take certain X-rays in the office, so that the physician has the results immediately. Laboratory codes are reported for tests performed in the medical office that is certified by the Clinical Laboratory Improvement Amendment (CLIA). The Medicine section contains codes for reporting diagnostic testing, noninvasive or minimally invasive procedures, and treatments for all areas of medical practice, such as vaccines, psychiatry, ophthalmology, cardiology, allergy, neurology, infusion therapy, audiology, and physical and occupational therapy.

HCPCS codes are used to report professional services, nonphysician services, supplies, durable medical equipment, and injectable drugs.

16 CHAPTER REVIEW

COMPETENCY REVIEW

1. Define and spell the terms for this chapter.
2. Assign CPT codes to the following scenarios. Underline the Main Term. Use the CPT manual to look up each procedure in the Index. Read all the modifying terms to help you select the preliminary code. Verify the code in the Tabular List. Write the code on the line provided.
   a. Extracapsular cataract removal with insertion of intra-ocular lens prosthesis (1 stage procedure), using the phacoemulsification technique _____
   b. Tonsillectomy and adenoidectomy for a 13-year-old patient_____
   c. Pulmonary stress test _____
   d. Chest X-ray, 4 views _____
   e. Administration of a measles, mumps, and rubella (MMR) vaccine for a seven-year-old child with parental counseling (2 codes) _____
   _____

PREPARING FOR THE CERTIFICATION EXAM

1. How many digits do CPT codes have?
   a. three
   b. four
   c. five
   d. six
   e. seven

2. Which section of the CPT manual should be consulted first, when assigning a code?
   a. Index
   b. Tabular List
   c. Table of Contents
   d. Appendix A
   e. Appendix B

3. What information is reported in column 24E of the CMS-1500 form?
   a. the procedure or service provided
   b. the charge for the service
   c. the date of service
   d. the CPT code billed
   e. the diagnosis that supports the medical necessity of the service

4. What does "CPT" stand for?
   a. Correct Procedural Terminology
   b. Current Procedural Terminology
   c. Correct Payment Terminology
   d. Current Physician Terminology
   e. Current Professional Terminology

5. What is the portion of a test or procedure in which a qualified physician interprets the results and writes a report?
   a. technical component
   b. professional component
   c. global package
   d. bundling
   e. results reporting

6. Which of the following is an eponym?
   a. Colles fracture
   b. EKG
   c. HIV
   d. wrist
   e. excision

7. What symbol in the Tabular List identifies a resequenced code that does not appear in strict numerical sequence?
   a. ⊘
   b. ✗
   c. #
   d. •
   e. ►◄

8. What is the common descriptor?
   a. a code description that is left-justified and begins with a capital letter
   b. a code description that is indented three spaces and begins with a small letter

c. the portion of a code description in boldface type

d. the portion of a code description that appears before the semicolon

e. the portion of a code description that appears after the semicolon

9. What is a bundling edit?

a. multiple codes required to report a single service

b. multiple services are included in a single code

c. multiple procedures performed at the same session by the same provider

d. billing for a service at a higher level than was actually provided

e. intentionally billing for services that were never given

10. Which coding violation occurs when a provider codes for a more complex service than was actually provided?

a. upcoding

b. downcoding

c. bundling

d. unbundling

e. abuse

CRITICAL THINKING

Refer to the case study at the beginning of the chapter and use what you have learned to answer the following questions.

1. Should David code and bill for the audiometry screening? Why or why not?

2. What is the diagnosis related to Sophia's procedure? How can David ensure that the diagnosis is correct?

3. What procedure code should be assigned for a bilateral tympanostomy with local anesthesia? Is a modifier necessary?

ON THE JOB

Lisa Medina, certified medical coding specialist, processes insurance claims for a large internal medicine practice. You have recently been hired as Lisa's assistant, and she has asked you to verify the accuracy of a group of claim forms. As you review the forms, you notice that one of the doctors regularly checks the superbill used in the office at one E&M code level higher than the actual level of service provided.

1. Name some of the options for handling this situation.

2. Tell which option you would select.

3. Give three reasons for your selection of this particular option.

4. Whose advice might you seek before acting on your choice?

INTERNET ACTIVITY

1. There are many places to purchase ICD-10-CM and CPT coding books. Search the Internet to find the cost of the ICD-10-CM and CPT coding books and coding software. In what months are the new editions of the ICD-10-CM and CPT coding books available?

2. Conduct an Internet search for "Department of Justice medical billing fraud" to learn about recent investigations and actions. Share your findings with your classmates.

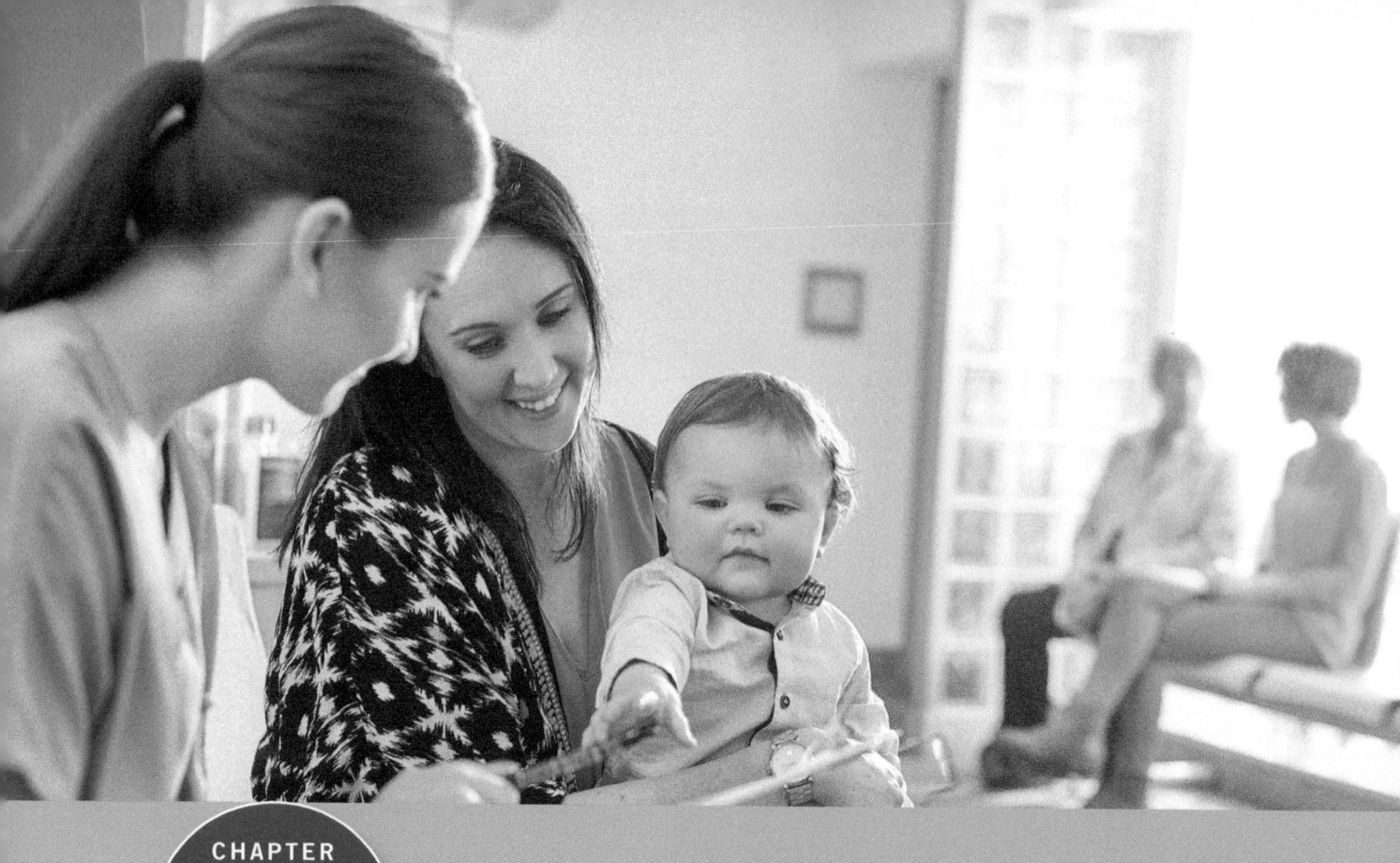

Patient Billing and Collections

Learning Objectives

After completing this chapter, you should be able to:

17.1   Define and spell the terms for this chapter.

17.2   Describe the medical assistant's role in patient accounting.

17.3   Identify types of adjustments made to a patient's account.

17.4   List the types of information that are part of the patient's billing record.

17.5   Describe systems used for maintaining accounts receivable.

17.6   Outline the procedures for aging accounts.

17.7   List information that should be included when discussing a patient's financial obligation for services.

17.8   Identify security precautions that should be taken when accepting various forms of payment.

17.9   Interpret information that is found on a remittance advice (RA)/explanation of benefits (EOB).

17.10 Outline solutions for denied claims.

17.11 Describe the differences between monthly and cycle billing.

17.12 Explain various fee adjustments.

17.13 List reasons a patient's account may be delinquent.

17.14 Identify laws that govern collection.

17.15 Describe considerations that must be taken when working with a collection agency.

Molly McConnley arrives at Pearson Physicians Group without an appointment at 3:45 P.M. She is complaining of radiating pain in her left leg and is visibly walking with a limp. Dr. Miller agrees to see Ms. McConnley because his last patient for the day has just checked out. While Dr. Miller is examining Ms. McConnley, Samra Belkorich, the medical assistant, begins to create a new encounter form for her. Samra realizes that Ms. McConnley owes Pearson Physicians Group $328 for a procedure that was performed. No payment has been made to Ms. McConnley's account for the past two months.

Terms to Learn

account balance	cycle billing	patient statement
account note	day sheet	payment
accounts receivable (AR)	days in AR	pending
adjustment	debit	posted
Allowed Amount	denied claim	practice management system (PMS)
appeal	disallowance	professional courtesy (PC)
AR aging analysis	electronic remittance advice (ERA)	reason codes
bad debt	explanation of benefits (EOB)	received on account (ROA)
balance billing	financial hardship	reconcile
bulk remittance	internal control	rejected claim
cash discount	late fee	remittance advice (RA)
charge	ledger card	skip
collection agency	line item posting	statute of limitations
contractual allowance	monthly billing	trace
copayment	patient account	Truth in Lending form
credit	patient accounting	user log
current	patient ledger	

uality patient care is the primary concern of any medical practice. However, revenue is necessary to maintain a viable business. Active management of the flow of funds into the practice is a vital, but sometimes neglected, responsibility. Medical assistants must understand the components of accounts receivable, collect and reconcile insurance payments, prepare patients' bills, extend credit when necessary, and collect balances from patients. To maintain a sound billing and collection system, the medical assistant actively helps patients understand their financial responsibility to the doctor.

OVERVIEW OF PATIENT ACCOUNTING

Accounting is the system of reporting the financial results of a business. **Patient accounting** refers to the functions of the accounting department related to recording charges and payments for services provided to patients. Each **patient account** is a record of the charges and payments for a specific patient. The total of all patients' accounts combines to create **accounts receivable (AR)**. AR is money owed to a business by customers in exchange for goods or services that have already been provided. In medical offices, AR refers to amounts

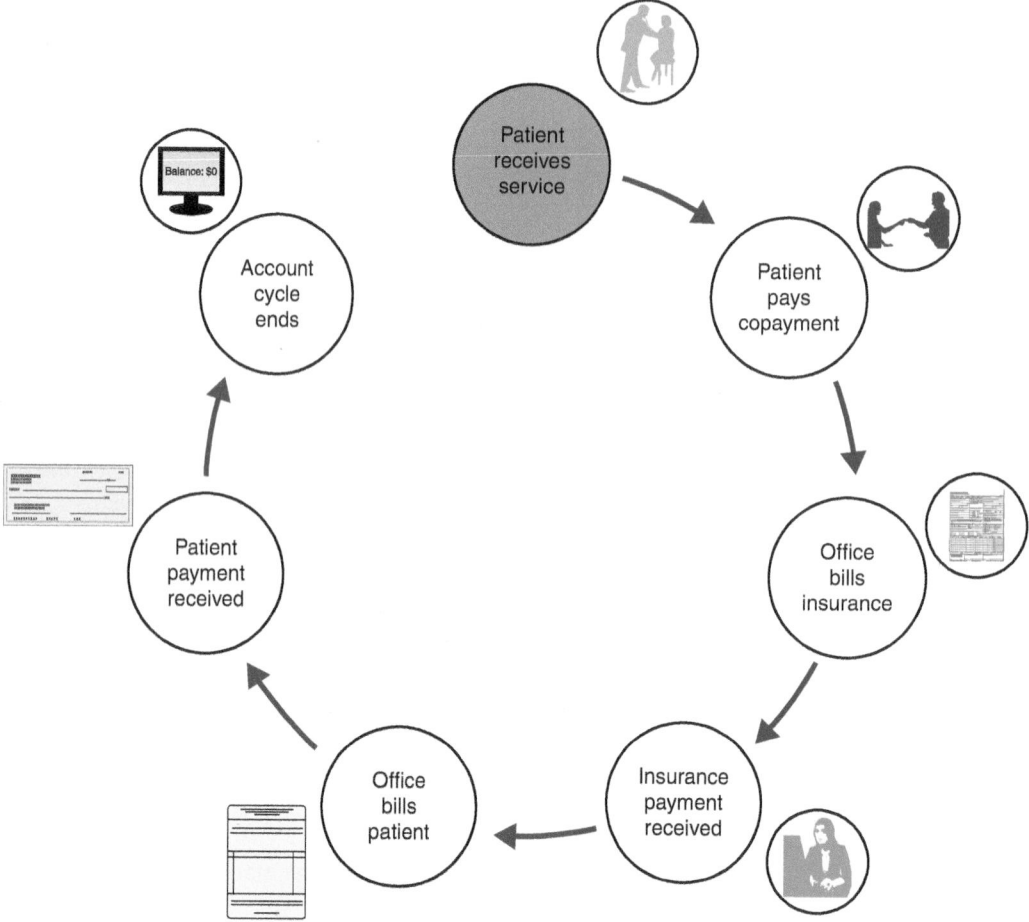

FIGURE 17-1 Accounts receivable cycle.

owed by patients and their third-party payers (such as Medicare and insurance companies) for services provided to patients. AR is expressed as the total dollars owed by all patients on a specific date. Each time a service is provided and a bill is issued, the AR increases. Each time a payment is received, the AR decreases. A lower AR is better than a higher AR. Figure 17-1 illustrates the AR cycle.

The Medical Assistant's Role in Patient Accounting

Medical assistants play a valuable role in patient accounting because they often are the link between the billing office and the patient. They fill one of the few positions that routinely have contact with both the administrative aspects and clinical aspects of a medical office. The type of involvement varies based on the type and size of medical practice as well as the balance between clinical and administrative duties in the job description. In some practices, medical assistants bear the primary responsibility of maintaining patient accounts. In other settings, the patient accounting function might be outsourced to a medical billing service or the office might

hire staff specially trained in patient accounts management. Regardless of the extent of their role, medical assistants must be knowledgeable about the overall process, the terminology, and the special problems that may arise, so they can be a liaison and educator for the patient.

Accounts Receivable Transactions

AR transactions are financial events that either increase or decrease the **account balance**, the amount of money a patient owes. Medical offices work with three types of AR transactions:

- **Charge**—The monetary cost for services or supplies that increases the account balance. In accounting terms, a charge is referred to as a **debit**.

- **Payment**—The receipt of money that decreases the account balance. In accounting terms, a payment is referred to as a **credit**. Payments are sometimes entered with the abbreviation **ROA**, which means "**received on account**."

- **Adjustment**—A positive or negative change to a patient's account balance that does not involve the exchange of money or the addition of a charge for services. Examples of adjustments will be discussed throughout the chapter, such as:

- Nonsufficient funds (NSF) check
- Collection agency transaction
- Credit balance
- Third-party allowance

Most adjustments are credits that are subtracted from the account balance, such as a discount, write-off, or **contractual allowance** (as explained in Box 17-1).

Day Sheets

A **day sheet** is a running total of all patient account transactions each day and is an important tracking and monitoring tool. Transactions recorded include the following:

- Charges for patient services
- Patient copayments made at the time of service
- Insurance payments received in the mail
- Patient payments received in the mail
- Adjustments, such as account write-offs and contractual allowances

When using a computerized system, medical assistants enter each transaction as it occurs, then generate a report at the end of the day. Day sheet reports that cover longer time periods, such as a week or a month, can also be generated. Figure 17-2 shows an example of a day sheet report. The balance at the end of the day identifies the amount by which the

---

BOX 17-1 | Adjustments

Adjustments are changes made that affect the patient's balance but are not a new charge or payment. They can occur when the physician reduces a fee or has signed a participating provider fee schedule. For example, imagine that a physician's usual charge for a surgical procedure is $1,500, but the participating provider contract states that the physician agrees to accept a fee of $1,200 as payment in full. The $1,200 allowed amount is divided between the insurance company and the patient's coinsurance, such as $1,000 due from the insurance company and $200 coinsurance due from the patient. The physician's office must enter an adjustment for $300, known as the contractual allowance ($1,500 − $1,200 = $300).

AR increased (positive number) or decreased (negative number) during that day.

The day sheet should be reconciled daily to the following:

- **Individual encounter forms**—First, compare the encounter forms to the appointment schedule. Every patient visit on the appointment schedule should have an encounter form. Then, compare the individual encounter forms to the charge (debit) entries on the day sheet. There should be an entry on the day sheet for each encounter form produced during the day. When there is no charge for the appointment, as may be the case for a postoperative follow-up visit, a charge of $0 can be entered for tracking purposes.

Pearson Medical Clinic Day Sheet Report 6/1/20YY							
Date	Account	Patient Name	Description	Debit	Payment	Adjustment	Balance
6/1/20YY	14001	Patient 1	Office visit	$ 100.00			$ 100.00
6/1/20YY	14001	Patient 1	Copayment-cash		$ (10.00)		$ 90.00
6/1/20YY	14123	Patient 123	Post-op follow up visit	$0.00			$ 90.00
6/1/20YY	14007	Patient 7	Nurse visit	$ 50.00			$ 140.00
6/1/20YY	14014	Patient 14	Patient payment-mail		$ (75.00)		$ 65.00
6/1/20YY	14053	Patient 53	Annual physical	$ 150.00			$ 215.00
6/1/20YY	14006	Patient 6	Insurance payment		$(123.51)	$ (1.50)	$ 89.99
6/1/20YY	14087	Patient 87	Office visit	$ 100.00			$ 189.99
6/1/20YY	14087	Patient 87	Copayment-credit card		$ (20.00)		$ 169.99
TOTALS				**$ 400.00**	**$ (228.51)**	**$ (1.50)**	**$ 1,149.97**

FIGURE 17-2 Example of a day sheet report.

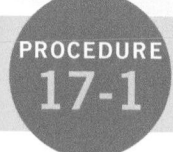

PROCEDURE 17-1

Obtaining Accurate Patient Billing Information

Objective ◆ *Obtain accurate billing information from patients.*

MATERIALS

Practice management system (PMS) software; new patient registration form; patient's health insurance card

METHOD

1. Open the computerized practice management system to the screen to add a new patient or to the patient's existing account screen.
2. Ask the patient for the completed patient registration form, which would have been mailed out before the visit or given to the patient upon arrival to complete.
3. Read the information on the registration form, and ask the patient to clarify any unclear or missing information. Be sure to verify the name, address, and phone number of the person financially responsible for the account. Repeat back to the patient any information they give you.

4. Ask the patient for the medical insurance card, and scan it into the PMS if a card scanner is used by the office. (See the chapter titled "Computers in the Medical Office.") If the office does not use a card scanner, manually enter the insurance company name, policy number, policyholder name, and claims mailing address into the corresponding screen in the PMS.
5. If the patient has an existing account in the PMS and does not need to complete an updated patient registration form, review the existing information. Read the information to the patient and ask them to verify it, such as:
   - Do you still live at 123 Main Street?
   - Is your phone number 555-123-4567?
   - Is your insurance plan XYZ?
   - Do you have any other medical insurance?
6. Refer to the chapter titled "Medical Insurance," Procedure 14-3 Verifying Eligibility to verify the patient's insurance information.

- **Total charges from encounter forms**—Using a calculator, add up the charges from the individual encounter forms to compute total charges. This number should match the total for the charges (debit) column on the day sheet.
- **Bank deposit**—Compare the amount of the bank deposit (cash and checks) for the day to the total for the payment (credit) column on the day sheet. These numbers should be the same unless credit card payments were received. Subtract any credit card payments from the payment column on the day sheet, because these are not part of the bank deposit. Most day sheet reports are able to provide separate totals for cash, check, and credit card payments to aid in this step of the reconciliation.

Patient Billing Record

Patient billing information includes patient demographics and the patient ledger. Patient demographics include the patient's name, address, marital status and children, employer, and health insurance information. Gathering patient information is discussed in the chapter titled "Medical Insurance." Procedure 17-1 discusses obtaining

accurate patient billing information. The **patient ledger** is a chronological record of the charges, adjustments, payments, and current balance for a specific patient (Figure 17-3). The patient ledger may also be referred to as the **ledger card**, which is a carryover from the days of manual billing when patient transactions often were recorded on a 5-by-7-inch card. In a computerized patient accounting system, transactions are added to the patient ledger at the time they are entered into the computer.

Attention to accuracy is essential when entering a patient account number or patient name, to ensure that transactions are **posted** to (entered into) the proper account. Transactions posted to the wrong account can be time consuming to track down because the charge or payment is posted to the overall system, so the daily totals balance. However, when posted to the wrong patient's account, the account balance and billing will be incorrect for two patients—the patient whose account was posted in error and the patient to whose account the transaction should have been posted. Such errors are usually not identified until a patient complains that there is a mistake in the account—seeing either an extra charge or a payment that does not belong to that person or missing a

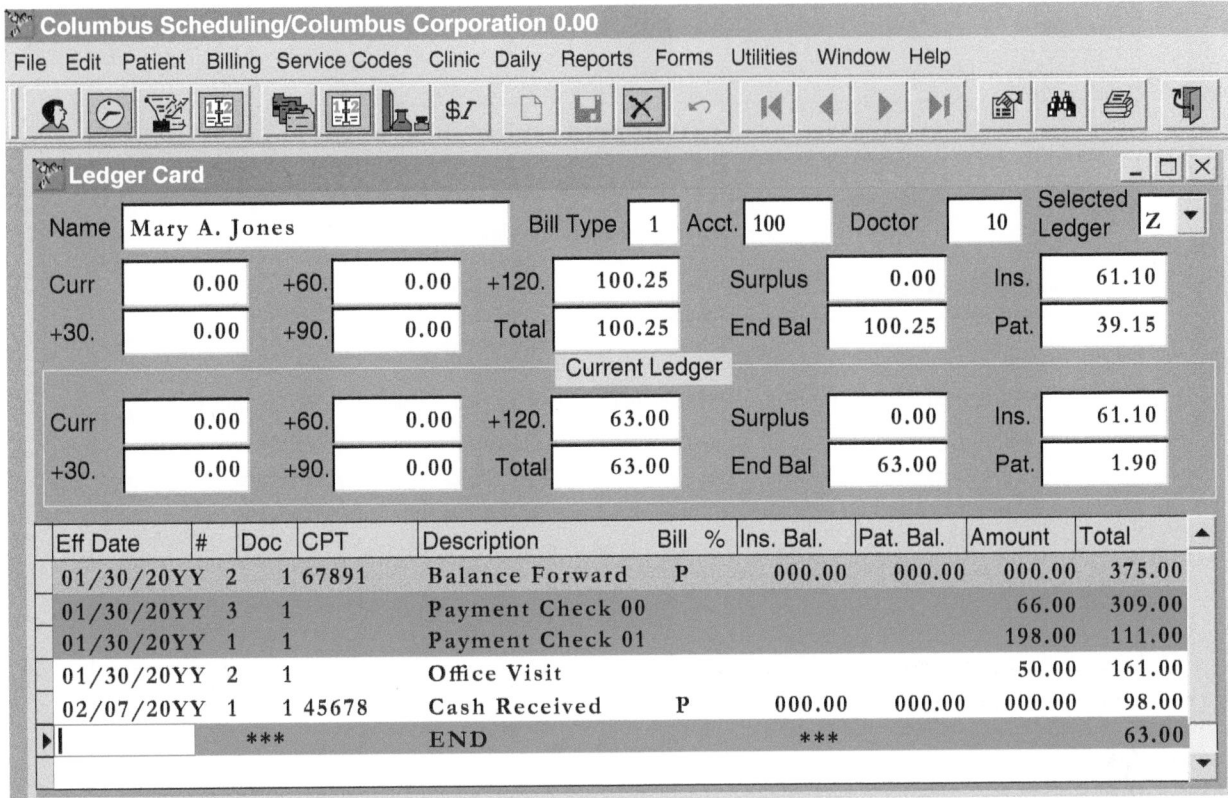

FIGURE 17-3 Example of a patient's ledger in practice management software.

charge or payment that should have been posted. You have to find the original transaction, determine which account it was posted to, remove it from that account, and reassign it to the correct account.

Accounts Receivable Systems

Patients' financial records are maintained separately from their medical records. Some patients have more than one financial account, called a patient account. A separate account should be established for claims that are billed to workers' compensation or third-party liability insurance, such as injuries from automobile accidents. Each new injury or illness related to workers' compensation or third-party liability should have its own patient account. Medical treatment for these conditions should be documented in a separate medical record. Offices use practice management software or a manual system to track patient accounts activity.

Patient Accounting Software

Most offices perform patient accounting using a computer program. Patient accounting software is also referred to as a **practice management system (PMS)**. The PMS may consist of modules, or components, that can be purchased separately and added as a small practice grows (Figure 17-4).

Every PMS provides similar functions. However, each program operates slightly differently, including slightly different screens, menu, and commands, so it is important that new employees understand the specific operation of the PMS used in their office. This is accomplished through training classes, video demonstrations, user manuals, and online help references.

To access the system, every employee must have a unique login, which consists of a username and password. Only those employees with a job-related need to access the information should have logins. Employees must log off the system whenever they are not using it or leave their workstations. They should not let others access the system using their login. The system automatically records the user who enters or changes each piece of information in the program. The system administrator sets permissions for each user that control the features of the PMS each user is allowed to view, enter, or change. The system must be able to maintain a **user log** that identifies who accessed the system, the information accessed, and when (date and time) information was accessed. The office manager or system administrator should review the user logs regularly to ensure there has been no unauthorized access.

Procedures 17-2 and 17-3 show the steps for using a computerized billing system and for correcting account posting errors.

The Pegboard System

The pegboard system, sometimes called the write-it-once method, is a manual bookkeeping system for patient

Component	Description
Appointment scheduling	Schedule patient appointments.
Patient registration	Enter patient demographics and insurance information.
Coding and charge entry	Enter charges for services using ICD–10–CM diagnosis codes and CPT® procedure codes.
Billing and claims processing	Print CMS-1500 insurance claims.
Electronic claims submission	Submit insurance claims electronically.
Patient and insurance payment posting	Post patient payments by form of payment. Post insurance payments to specific patients and specific dates of service.
Patient statements and collections	Print statements with line item details on amounts owed by patients.
Patient reminders and correspondence	Prepare and print letters to patients.
Reports and analysis	Produce reports to identify practice trends and accounts receivable status.

FIGURE 17-4 Typical components of software for a practice management system (PMS).

accounting. It consists of interrelated forms that are placed onto the pegboard and used with a master day sheet. It is an efficient system because the forms have a carbon ribbon attached or are on special paper that permits entering charges, payments, and adjustments onto the master day sheet, the encounter form, and the patient's ledger card at the same time. Box 17-2 discusses how to use a pegboard system, should you be employed in an office that still uses one.

BOX 17-2 | Using a Pegboard System

Some offices still use manual pegboard systems. The following information summarizes how to record various types of transactions using a pegboard system. Refer to the instructions that accompany the specific system for details.

1. Place a new day sheet and a strip of encounter forms on the pegboard, making sure they are fastened securely into the pegs.
2. Complete the information required at the top of the day sheet (date and page number).
3. Carry balances forward from the previous day sheet, and enter them in the designated location. These include all column totals, the previous day's total, and accounts receivable balances.
4. Remove the encounter form from the pegboard, and clip it to the front of the patient's chart. The physician enters the procedure performed that day on the appropriate line of the encounter form, fills in the diagnosis, and signs the form after seeing the patient. The CPT procedure code is included on the encounter form for ease of processing. The encounter form is then given to the receptionist by the medical assistant or the patient.
5. *To post charges:* Place the ledger card under the next receipt (which also functions as a charge slip). Write the amount charged, pressing firmly and evenly to make an impression through multiple pages to the day sheet.
6. *To post patient payments:* With the ledger card aligned as stated in the previous step, enter the amount paid and payment method (cash, check, or credit card) into the appropriate column.
7. *To post adjustments:* With the ledger card properly aligned, enter the amount of the adjustment in the appropriate column. When the adjustment is a discount or write-off that deducts from the account balance, enter the amount in parentheses and be certain to subtract the amount when doing the math. When an adjustment is made (e.g., a discount given to another health professional), subtract it from the balance due from the insurance company. Always follow the facility's policy on adjustments.
8. *To post refunds:* When a credit balance exists or the patient is entitled to a refund, request the approval of the physician or office manager according to office policy. With the ledger card properly aligned, enter a negative adjustment amount, write a description of the reason for the refund, and enter the check number used to issue the refund.

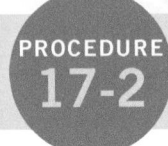

Using a Computerized Billing System

Objective ◆ *Post patient accounting transactions accurately (charges, payments, adjustments) using a computerized practice management system (PMS).*

EQUIPMENT AND SUPPLIES

Computer with a PMS; source document for the transaction, such as the encounter form for charges; check, cash, or credit card for payments; information supporting the need for an adjustment

METHOD

1. Log in with your username and password previously created.
2. Review the rules associated with the PMS for entering transactions.
3. Access the appropriate patient account. Double-check the patient name and birthdate to verify that you have the correct patient.
   - Accounts can easily be confused among patients with the same or similar name and when multiple family members are served.
   - Some patients may have more than one account, such as an account for private insurance and an account for a workers' compensation or personal injury claim. Verify that you have the correct account for the transaction to be entered.
4. The PMS tracks the date, time, and identity of the person making the entry, based on the login information provided. If this is not the case, add your name, date, and time in the description field of each entry made.
5. Complete the transaction according to the steps that follow for the type of transaction.

To post charges:

1. Access the menu item for entering new charges.
2. Enter the date of service and the CPT procedure code(s) marked on the encounter form.
3. The PMS normally fills in the service description and dollar amount based on the CPT code. Verify that these are accurate and match what you expect.
4. Enter or verify the ICD-10-CM diagnosis code. When a patient has a new diagnosis, enter the ICD-10-CM code. When a patient is seen repeatedly for the same condition, the diagnosis code may carry over from one encounter to the next. The PMS normally fills in the diagnosis description. Verify that the description matches the encounter form.
5. Repeat the process for additional procedures.
6. Review the data entered to be sure it is correct.

To post payments:

1. Access the menu item for entering new payments.
2. Enter the date of the payment and the purpose of the payment. Examples are patient copayment, patient coinsurance, payment on account, and insurance payment.
3. Enter the dollar amount. Some systems require you to enter a decimal point and some systems automatically enter the decimal point and assume that the last two digits you enter should be placed to the right of the decimal point. If the system enters the decimal point for you, you must enter the final two zeroes for whole dollar amounts, such as "1000" for $10.00.
4. Select the form of payment (check, cash, credit card) from the menu. Enter the check number in the designated spot.
5. Repeat the process for additional payments on the same account.
6. Review the data entered to be sure it is correct.
7. Save the data, if required.
8. If the patient is making payment in person, print a receipt, following the steps required by the PMS.

To post adjustments:

1. Access the menu item for entering adjustments.
2. Enter the date of the adjustments and the purpose of the adjustments. Examples are insurance disallowance, cash payment discount, and professional courtesy. You can usually access these options in a menu.
3. Enter the dollar amount, being careful to indicate if it is a positive or negative adjustment.
4. Add any necessary comments, notes, or descriptive information to document the reason for the adjustment. You may be able to do this in the description field of the adjustment entry, or you may be able to enter a free-form **account note**. The account note is a feature that allows you to enter more detailed information than is possible in the description field. The account note may appear as an additional line item in the patient ledger, or it may be attached to an existing line item, depending on the software used.
5. Compare the computer screen to the source document to verify that the entry was entered correctly.

After the transaction has been entered:
(Take special note of the following steps, because they should be performed at the conclusion of most PMS procedures.)

1. Save the data, if required, and exit the patient's account.
2. Write or stamp the date posted and your name or initials on the source document, according to office procedures.
3. File the source document in the appropriate location, according to office procedures.
4. Log off the system when you are done posting for all patients.

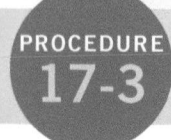

Correcting Account Posting Errors

Objective ◆ *Identify and correct a charge or payment posted to the incorrect patient account using a practice management system (PMS).*

EQUIPMENT AND SUPPLIES

A description of the error identified; computer with PMS software; source document (check, encounter form, or similar) supporting the transaction affected

METHOD

1. Errors in patient accounts may be identified by patients who report noticing a charge or payment that is not theirs, or that a charge or payment that should appear is missing. Errors may also be identified when posting payments that do not match up to the charges on the account.
2. Turn on the computer. Log in to the patient accounting program with the username and password previously established.
3. Access the account of the patient known to have an error.
4. Identify whether the error involved a charge, payment, or adjustment.
5. Identify the date on which the original transaction occurred or was posted.
6. Locate the source document. For an error involving a payment, pull a copy of the patient check or insurance RA/EOB from the paper or electronic files of past payments. For an error involving a charge, pull a copy of the encounter form from the paper or electronic files of past encounter forms.
7. Read the details on the source document, and identify the patient and account to which it should have been posted.

8. Reverse the entry on the account posted in error. Refer to the instructions for the PMS, because functions and steps vary based on the program.

Tips:
- Some programs may allow you to enter a negative charge or a negative payment, and others require you to post the correction as adjustment. Enter the current date, a description of the error, and the amount. A useful description or account note is "Posted in error, transfer to account # 999."
- Do not include the name of the other patient in the description because you do not want this information to print out on the billing statement. You may post details in an account note, if the PMS allows you to activate an option for the *not* to print on patient statements.
- For an error involving a payment, enter a positive adjustment, because you need to increase the account balance.
- For an error involving a charge, enter a negative adjustment, because you need to decrease the account balance.
- Determine if additional steps may be required to repost the CPT procedure codes to generate an insurance claim or to link a payment to the correct date of service and insurance check.
- The PMS tracks the date, time, and identity of the person making the entry, based on the login information provided. If this is not the case, add your name, date, and time at the end of the description.

Account 222 SMITH HARRY J					
Date	Transaction #	Description	Charges/ Debits	Payments/ Credits	Balance
6/1/20YY	12345	Office Visit	$150.00		$ 150.00
7/1/20YY	23654	Transaction # 12345 posted in error. Transfer to account # 999.	($150.00)		$ 0.00

Reversing entry to account #222 for a charge posted in error that should have been posted to account #999.

9. Post a correcting entry to the account that should have been posted originally. Refer to the instructions for the PMS, because functions and steps vary based on the program.
Tip: Follow the suggestions in step 8, with the following changes:
- For an error involving a payment, enter a negative adjustment, because you need to decrease the account balance.
- For an error involving a charge, enter a positive adjustment, because you need to increase the account balance.
- Add a description or account note that explains the reason for the correction.

Account 999 GILBERT MARY A					
Date	Transaction #	Description	Charges/ Debits	Payments/ Credits	Balance
7/1/20YY	23654	Charge for 6/1/20YY posted to wrong account. Transferred from account 222.	$150.00		$150.00

Correcting entry to account #999 for a charge posted in error to account #222.

10. Write a note on the source document describing the correction.

> 7/1/20YY Posted to account 222 in error. Made correcting entries in PMS and posted to account 999. Dave Gao, MA

Example of documentation on the source document that was posted in error.

11. Double-check all entries. Refile the source document.
12. Place a telephone call to both patients. Briefly explain the error, and apologize for any confusion. Remember not to reveal the name of the other patient whose account was involved in the error. Send both patients an updated account statement.
Tips:
- If the patient is not available, do not leave a detailed voice message, because it would violate patient confidentiality if someone else were to listen to the message. In addition, patients may become upset when they receive a message about an error on their account, because they might be unable to call the office immediately.

> "Mr. Smith, this is Dave from Pearson Medical Clinic. I want to let you know that we found an error on your account and have corrected it. A charge intended for another patient was mistakenly posted to your account. We removed the charge, and you will not be billed for it. I apologize for any inconvenience or confusion. I will send you an updated statement of your account."

> "Ms Gilbert, this is Dave from Pearson Medical Clinic. I want to let you know that we found an error on your account and have corrected it. A charge for your visit on June 1 was mistakenly posted to another account. We have posted the visit on your account and will bill your insurance for it today. I apologize for any inconvenience or confusion. I will send you an updated statement of your account."

Example script for phone calls to patients explaining account errors.

- If you cannot reach the patient within two days, write a short letter similar to the phone call examples and send it to the patient with the updated account statement.
13. If the error involves a charge, determine if the charge was billed to the insurance company. Also identify whether the claim was paid. Contact the insurance company that was billed in error, explain what happened, and ask how to proceed.
Tips:
- If you do not notify the insurance company that it was billed in error, you are at risk of fraudulent billing.
- If you accept a payment for the erroneous charge, you must refund it to the insurance company either by writing a check or through a deduction on a future payment. The insurance company will explain how the refund should be handled.
- Do not send a refund or return the check without receiving specific directions from the insurance company; otherwise, the returned funds may not be posted correctly by the insurance company.
- If both patients involved are with the same insurance company, you must still contact the insurance company to correct the error. Do not assume that because the insurance company still owes the same dollar amount the errors will balance each other out.
14. If the error involves a payment that was posted to the wrong account in your system, but the visit was billed correctly to insurance, you do not need to contact the insurance company. Simply enter the necessary corrections in your patient accounting system.
15. Log out of the patient accounting system.

Accounts Receivable Analysis

AR should be constantly monitored to ensure that bills are being paid as expected and to identify accounts that are past due. AR is evaluated in terms of age, or how long the money has been owed. AR analysis is performed using two types of reports: days in AR and aging analysis.

Days in AR

The statistic **days in AR** is the average number of days that money has been owed to the practice. This is calculated by dividing the total AR dollar amount by the average daily revenue of the practice. The lower this number is, the better, because it means that the practice is able to collect payment rapidly. A good number is 45 days. An AR over 90 days, or three months, is a poor number and indicates that the financial health of the practice could be improved. When payments are over 90 days past due, they are very difficult to collect. Figure 17-5 shows how to calculate the days in AR.

Days in AR varies depending on the type of medical practice, the payer mix (the percentage of revenue from different classes of third party payer, such as private insurance, Medicare, Medicaid, workers' compensation, and so on), and level of automation. Examples of how AR can vary include the following:

- Practices that send most insurance claims electronically tend to have a lower AR than those that send a large portion of insurance claims on paper, because electronic claims are received and processed more quickly by insurance companies than paper claims.

- Practices with a high percentage of Medicare patients that submit claims electronically tend to have a lower AR because Medicare is required by law to process electronic claims within 14 days of receipt but does not process paper claims for at least 28 days.

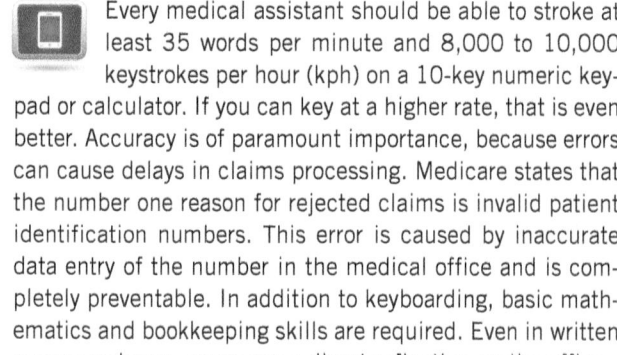

- Practices with a high percentage of patients injured in automobile accidents tend to have a higher AR because auto insurance/personal injury protection (PIP) tends to take longer to process claims than health insurers. In addition, many of these insurers require that claims be submitted on paper.

- Practices with a high percentage of patients who have plans with high deductibles and high coinsurance tend to have a higher AR because it takes longer to collect the patient portion of the bill.

AR Aging Analysis

An **AR aging analysis** is a report that categorizes a company's accounts receivable according to the length of time since it has been billed (Figure 17-6). Typically, time periods used are:

- 0 to 30 days
- 31 to 60 days
- 61 to 90 days
- 91 to 120 days
- over 120 days

Accounts less than 30 days old are considered **current** and of minimal cause for concern. Accounts aged 31 to 60 days should be reviewed to identify those that should have been paid already. For example, if a practice bills Medicare electronically and typically receives payment within 14 to 21 days, any Medicare accounts over 30 days old should be investigated. Nearly all accounts older than 60 days should be reviewed at least once a month so that the reason for nonpayment can be identified and corrected.

AR analysis can be performed by varying the parameters of the aging analysis report.

Description	Amount	Calculation
(A) Total annual revenue	$1,000,000.00	Based on previous year.
(B) Total AR amount	$150,000.00	Based on current financial statement.
Calculation of days in AR		
(C) Average daily revenue	$2,739.73	(A) $1,000,000.00/365 days (To be more precise, you can take the actual revenue for the past 90 days, divided by 90.)
Days in AR	55	(B) $150,000.00/(C) $2,739.73

FIGURE 17-5 Example of calculation of days in accounts receivable (AR).

Pearson Medical Clinic Accounts Receivable Aging Analysis Report As of 6/30/20YY				Days Outstanding				
Account	Patient Name	Amount Owed	Insurance	0–30	31–60	61–90	90–120	120+
14001	Patient 1	$ 150.00	Healthy Way		$ 100.00		$ 50.00	
14002	Patient 2	$ 120.00	Healthy Way	$ 60.00			$ 60.00	
14003	Patient 3	$ 250.00	XYZ HMO			$ 125.00	$ 125.00	
14004	Patient 4	$ 900.00	ABC Auto	$ 225.00	$ 250.00	$ 150.00	$ 75.00	$ 200.00
14005	Patient 5	$ 58.00	Medicare	$ 58.00				
14006	Patient 6	$ 80.00	None			$ 80.00		
14007	Patient 7	$ 175.00	Medicare	$ 175.00				
14008	Patient 8	$ 222.00	Medicaid	$ 165.00	$ 57.00			
14009	Patient 9	$ 450.00	Workers Comp	$ 250.00	$ 150.00	$ 50.00		
14010	Patient 10	$ 75.00	None	$ 75.00				
14011	Patient 11	$ 357.00	XYZ HMO	$ 223.00	$ 81.00	$ 53.00		
14012	Patient 12	$ 100.00	Healthy Way	$ 100.00				
	TOTAL	$ 2,937.00		$1,331.00	$ 638.00	$ 458.00	$ 310.00	$ 200.00
	Percentage			45%	22%	16%	11%	7%

FIGURE 17-6 Example of an accounts receivable aging analysis report.

For example, separate reports can be generated for patients and insurance companies because each has unique payment and follow-up considerations. Separate reports can be generated for each type of payer, such as Medicare, private insurance, HMOs, and even individual insurance companies. Generating custom reports can be helpful for offices with a large number of accounts, so that it is more efficient to drill down and identify the problem areas.

COLLECTING PATIENT PAYMENTS

Patients need to understand office policy about financial matters. They need to know how much they will be charged, how much they are personally responsible to pay, and when they need to pay it. They also need to know their options if they feel they cannot afford to pay all that they owe. Mutual understanding of financial arrangements helps to minimize problems of collection for delinquent accounts.

Patient Financial Obligations

Patients have a financial obligation to pay for their medical services and are entitled to an accurate estimate of them. The initial visit to the office should include information on fees,

payment, and financial arrangements. Patients should be given information such as the following:

- Charges for services
- Participating insurance plans
- Insurance billing practices
- Payment of deductibles, coinsurance, copayments, and balances
- Accepted forms of payment (cash, check, credit card, electronic benefit transaction (EBT) cards)
- Payment plans for those who don't have insurance

Many financial policies and procedures can be addressed in a booklet or office brochure given to the patient. Information about payment policies and fees should be posted near the reception desk where patients can readily see and read it, particularly when copayments are due at the time of service. This helps patients become aware of office procedures and encourages discussion of such matters. The chapter titled "Medical Insurance" discusses medical insurance plans in detail.

Patients who need surgical or other medical procedures should be made aware as early as possible of fees, insurance allowances, and methods of payment, so they can plan for these medical expenses. Such information is especially important because procedures can be expensive and many insurance plans do not cover the full cost. Some offices establish a payment plan so patients can make payment over an extended period of time. Legal requirements for payment plans are discussed later in this chapter. Patients must understand that they have the ultimate responsibility for all charges.

Refer to the chapter titled "Medical Insurance," in which Procedure 14-1 provides details on how to calculate patient financial responsibility.

Professional Fees

The fee is determined by the physician or the practice's partners after considering the time and services involved as well as the prevailing fee in the community. The economic level of the community, including whether the area is considered urban or rural, and the average fee charged by physicians in the same specialty are factors that determine the prevailing fee. The prevailing fee is referred to by insurance companies as the customary fee when establishing a fee schedule known as usual, customary, and reasonable (UCR).

Some medical offices display a sign that explains fee policy. The sign might include actual fees for services. A printed fee schedule should be available for quick reference. The medical assistant, if instructed by the physician, should be able to quote fees or a range of fees from this schedule. This schedule is approved by the physician and is updated as needed. Medical offices should post in a prominent area for patients to view a notification that states, "Payment is due at the time of service."

Collecting Copayments

A **copayment** is a fixed amount that patients' insurance policies may require them to pay for certain types of visits. For routine office visits, the amount is usually between $5 and $30. Some insurance plans require copayments for visits when the patient is sick but not for preventive care. The purpose of the copayment, from the insurance company's point of view, is to establish a financial responsibility for the patient that encourages the patient to use good judgment in seeking care. If patients were to have no financial responsibility, they might feel free to use medical services when they were not really needed. Under the Patient Protection and Affordable Care Act (PPACA), most insurance companies cannot require copayments for preventive care so that patients are encouraged to maintain their health through preventive care services. Insurance companies also benefit when patients use preventive care to detect and avoid more serious health problems. The patient pays the copayment to the physician, not the insurance company. This amount is deducted from the insurance company's allowed amount when calculating benefits.

When a copayment is required by the insurance policy, providers are required to collect it. Providers do not have the option to routinely waive copayment obligations and tell the patient they will simply accept whatever the insurance plan pays. To routinely waive copayments is considered to be the same as if the provider were to misrepresent the actual fee to the insurance company.

Managed care contracts often require that the copayment be paid at the time of the visit and may not allow providers to bill patients at a later time. Managed care organizations want patients to be aware of the cost of service every time they receive service. Even when patients plan to see a provider frequently, as may occur with a chiropractor, the copayment may need to be collected at each visit and not grouped so several copayments are paid at the same time.

Accepting Copayments

Be courteous and professional when asking patients for payment. A good approach is to say, "Your copayment today is $10. Would you like to pay with cash, check, or a credit card?"

After processing the payment, always generate a numbered receipt for each payment received. A numbered receipt

Professionalism

Patients can become easily confused about insurance matters. Although technically patients are responsible for knowing how their health insurance plan works, this is rarely the case. You can provide a great deal of support to patients by helping them understand their insurance. If you cannot answer their questions immediately, offer to research their questions. In particular, you should become familiar with the managed care plans in which the physicians in your practice participate and the Medicare and Medigap programs.

Professionalism | Cultural Considerations

When working with patients, it is important not to make assumptions regarding the relationship between a man and a woman as well as with any children involved. For instance, when identifying the policyholder of an insurance plan, rather than saying, "Is he the patient's father?" it would be more appropriate to ask, "How is he related to the patient?" Being careful about words spoken can help eliminate awkward or embarrassing situations.

is necessary because it is an **internal control**, a procedure that helps ensure all financial matters are handled properly and helps discourage unethical workers from stealing. A PMS can print a receipt after the payment is entered into the patient's account. In a manual system, a receipt book with prenumbered receipts and a carbonless copy of each receipt should be used. Even when patients say they do not want a receipt, you still need to create one for tracking purposes.

When the transaction is complete, thank the patient for the payment and give specific instructions regarding what to do next, such as "Thank you. You may have a seat until we call you." When patients pay after they have seen the provider, say, "Thank you for coming today. You are done now. Please use the exit door at the right."

Lock the payment in the cash drawer or other designated location for checks and credit card receipts. Do not leave the cash drawer unlocked between transactions. Never leave an unlocked cash drawer unattended.

Security Precautions

Most offices allow patients to pay using cash, checks, or credit/debit cards. Although there is a small cost to the medical practice for each credit/debit card transaction processed, most offices find that patients appreciate being able to use this form of payment and are more likely to pay on time. Be familiar with the office policies and procedures for accepting payment from patients.

All forms of payment carry a small risk of being fraudulent. The medical office is not obligated to accept a specific form of payment and always has the right to refuse any currency, check, or credit card that they are not confident is valid. Table 17-1 shows tips for handling and verifying each form of payment.

A check that "bounces" or is returned for nonsufficient funds (NSF) is the same as not getting paid at all and requires immediate action. This can happen because of a minor problem with the patient's bank account, or it could be intentional. It is best to call the patient and ask if they are aware of the returned check. They might let you know what happened and tell you it is all right to redeposit the check. In this case, include the check in the next deposit, and verify that it clears. Many times, this solves the problem.

If the redeposit also is returned or you suspect some other problem, action must be taken. You must reverse the patient's payment in the PMS using an adjustment and send a certified letter to the patient. In most cases, the patient is allowed eight days to present valid funds before you take legal action. Procedure 17-4 explains how to post an NSF check in the PMS.

COLLECTING INSURANCE PAYMENTS

To post insurance payments, medical assistants must read and interpret the remittance advice (RA) or explanation of benefits (EOB), enter data into the PMS, and follow up on unpaid claims. After the payer has processed the claim, the provider receives a check or electronic deposit and a RA/EOB. Depending on the sophistication of the provider's PMS, the payment may be automatically posted to the patient's account or the medical assistant may need to manually enter it into the computer or manual patient accounting system. If the medical assistants are responsible for posting payments, they also **reconcile** the RA/EOB. They compare the RA/EOB to the original bill to verify that each service billed was paid in the amount expected.

Remittance Advice/Explanation of Benefits

After an insurance carrier has processed a claim, a check is sent to the health care provider with a **remittance advice (RA)** statement, also known as an **explanation of benefits (EOB)**. Technically, a RA is a statement sent to the provider and the EOB is a statement sent to the patient and usually has slightly different formatting. In some situations, the terms are used interchangeably. The RA/EOB lists the name of the patient, the name of the insured, the date of service, the amount billed, the amount allowed, the amount paid, and the amount the provider may bill the patient. Medical assistants must check RAs/EOBs to ensure all services that were billed are accurately listed and that the payment matches the amount in the insurance company contract.

Large insurance carriers may send a **bulk remittance** and check or electronic deposit as payment for several patients. A bulk remittance lists multiple claims and multiple patients, and provides the same information for each that a single RA/EOB does. A bulk remittance reduces paperwork and enables the insurance company to issue one check for several claims or several patients. When you post a bulk payment in the PMS, a software feature allows you to enter the check or payment number and total payment amount once, and then distribute the amount among multiple claims or multiple patients.

The format and contents of individual RAs/EOBs vary based on the benefit plan and the services provided, but they always provide policy information, service information, and payment information (Figure 17-7). No universal paper form for explaining benefits is available. Terminology varies on RAs/EOBs from different insurance companies. For example, some RAs/EOBs show the "**Allowed Amount**" and others show "Approved Amount" or similar terminology. As

TABLE 17-1 | Security Tips for Accepting Various Forms of Payment

Cash	Checks	Credit/Debit Cards
• Count the money audibly in the patient's presence. This confirms the amount the patient gives you. Even if she gives you only one bill, restate the face amount, such as "$10." • Check the legality of all currency, using a counterfeit detection pen or scanner available from office supply companies. • If change is needed, lay the money given by the patient on your desk while making change. Do not put it into the cash box until the transaction is complete, so that there is no question about how much the patient gave. • Count the change audibly as you give it to the patient.	• The patient's name (or parent/guardian) is printed on the check. • The patient's current address is printed on the check. • The bank on which the check is drawn is clearly identified. Many practices do not accept checks from out-of-state or out-of-area banks. • The check is prenumbered. • The bank routing number, account number, and check number should appear in MICR print at the bottom of the check. • The current date is written on the check. Do not accept a postdated check, one that bears a date that has not yet occurred. • Do not agree to wait additional time before depositing the check. Both postdating and waiting invalidate the check with the State Attorney, should legal action be required. • The correct name of the practice appears in the payee field. Some practices use an ink stamp to stamp the practice name in the payee field. Stamp the check in the presence of the patient. Do not accept a check with a blank payee field. • Do not accept a check for an amount greater than the patient's charge and make change to the patient in cash. • The dollar amounts written in numbers and in words should be identical. • The check is signed in your presence. The signature matches that on the proof of identity. • Write the proof of identity on the face of the check, such as a driver's license number or government issued identification number. • Write your initials on the check next to the proof of identity. This establishes you as a witness to the transaction, should legal action be required. • Call the issuing bank to verify the validity of the check if you have any concerns. Excuse yourself and place the call where the patient cannot hear you. Because of privacy concerns, some banks may not give out information about the account balance. • Speak with the bank the medical office uses to learn more about security features used to identify valid checks.	• Be familiar with the operating instructions for the electronic card reader. • Take care when entering the dollar amount to verify it is accurate. • Some PMS scan be interfaced with the card reader in such a way that the transaction is automatically entered into the patient's account. When this is the case, always double-check that the entry transferred correctly. • The name printed on the card matches the patient's name exactly. • The expiration date is later than the current date. • The signature on the back of the card reasonably matches the signature on the driver's license, government identification card, or other document. • Write down the three-digit code from the back of the card on the credit card processing slip or enter it in the designated place in the PMS. • Do not process a transaction for an amount greater than the patient's charge and make change to the patient in cash. • Allow patients making debit card transactions to enter a personal identification number (PIN) to complete the process. • Patient's signature on the credit card slip or transaction screen should reasonably match the signature on the back of the card. • Do not accept cards that are past the expiration date, cards that have no signature, or cards that cannot be read by the electronic card reader. • Return the card to the patient and say, "Thank you. Here is your card." This helps ensure that you don't accidentally forget to return the card. • Do not keep the patient's credit card number on file, for security reasons. • Do write down the issuing bank and last four digits of the card number, in the event that you need to refer to the card used for the transaction. • If, in the future, you need to issue a fund for services or supplies paid for with the card, you must credit the amount to the specific card used to make the original payment.

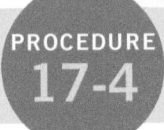

Posting NSF Checks

Objective ◆ *Post entries to a patient account that has experienced a check with non-sufficient funds (NSF).*

EQUIPMENT AND SUPPLIES

Copy or image of the returned check; NSF notification from your bank that identifies a fee charged to your account; computer with practice management system (PMS) software

METHOD

1. Log in with your username and password previously created.
2. Access the appropriate patient account. Double-check the patient name and birthdate to verify that you have the correct patient and account type.
3. Access the appropriate menu item according to the procedures for the PMS. You may be able to reverse the payment using the payments menu, or you may need to enter it as an adjustment.
4. Select the adjustment type for an NSF check.
5. Enter the date the check was returned and dollar amount of the original check.
6. Enter a description such as "Check # 111 returned NSF."
7. Access the menu for adjustments. Select an item type for "bank fees."
8. Enter the date the check was returned and the dollar amount of the processing fee charged by your bank.
9. Enter a description such as "Bank fee for NSF Check # 111."
10. Review the entry to verify that the date and amount were entered correctly.
11. Save the data, if necessary.
12. Access the menu to create a patient statement. Print a statement.
13. Access the menu to create a patient letter. Select or create a letter to the patient that explains: "Your check number 999 for $00.00 was returned to our office because of lack of funds in your account. In addition, the medical office was charged a fee of $00.00 for the processing of the check. You are responsible to reimburse us for this cost, in addition to paying for the original service. A statement is enclosed that shows the current balance on your account. Please remit payment within eight days by MM/DD/YY or call the office to make payment arrangements."
14. Make a photocopy or scanned image of the returned check for your records.
15. Mail the letter, the patient statement, and the returned check via certified mail.
16. Complete the steps in Procedure 17-2 for **After the transaction has been entered**.

---

a medical assistant, you eventually will become familiar with the forms and terminology used by the carriers with whom your practice contracts, but you should review every RA/EOB carefully before you enter data. Most RAs/EOBs provide a key that explains the meaning of various terms used.

Insurance carriers often use **reason codes** or remark codes on the RA/EOB to identify reasons for payment adjustments and denials. These are usually three- or four-character alphanumeric codes for which a key appears on the face or back of the RA/EOB. Reason codes provide important information about how the insurance company processed the claim.

For claims submitted electronically, an electronic RA/EOB is referred to as an **electronic remittance advice (ERA)**. ERAs are required to follow HIPAA electronic transaction standards for content, organization, and formatting. Reason codes are standard on ERAs. ERAs make it possible for payment information to be automatically posted to the patient accounting system. Medicare provides software that allows you to download and view the ERA if your PMS does not perform this function (Figure 17-8).

An RA/EOB is not always accompanied by payment. It can give the status of **pending** claims, those awaiting additional information, and **denied claims**, those that were received but for which no payment was made. A **rejected claim** is one that is never accepted into the payer's computer system because of invalid information, such as an invalid patient identification number or invalid ICD-10-CM or CPT codes. Rejected claims do not usually appear on RAs/EOBs because they were not accepted into the payer's system. A report from the electronic claims

Explanation of Benefits

This is not a bill.

06/08/20YY ③

① **Healthy Way Insurance**

⑤	**Your ID Number:**	W125370058
④	**Subscriber Name:**	CHRIS PATIENT
⑦	**Patient Name:**	CHRIS PATIENT
⑥	**Claim Number:**	K100925-0038
②	**Group Name:**	XYZ Company

If you have questions, contact us:

By Mail:

Healthy Way Insurance
PO Box 0000
Chicago IL 10000

CHRIS PATIENT
999 MAIN STREET
ANYTOWN IL 99999

Provider Information

⑧ **KRISTEN COUGHLIN MD**
   2525 NE 44TH ST
   ANYTOWN IL 99999

By Phone/E-mail:

Local: 425-555-3000
Toll Free: 1-800-555-6004
E-mail: abc@hwins.xxx

Provider Name: ⑨	Date(s) of Service	Service(s) Provided ⑩	Amount Charged ⑪	Allowed ⑫	PPO Savings	Non-Cov'd Amount ⑮	Deductible ⑭	Copay ⑬	Co-Ins. %	Paid ⑯	Patient's Responsibility ⑰	See Notes Section
KRISTEN COUGHLIN MD	05 07 20YY 05 07 20YY	99123 Office Visit	125.00	66.94	58.06				6.69	90	60.25	6.69	PPU
KRISTEN COUGHLIN MD	05 07 20YY 05 07 20YY	94010 Breathing Capacity Test	72.00	28.31	43.69				2.83	90	25.48	2.83	PPU
		TOTALS	197.00	95.25	101.75	0.00	0.00	9.52		85.73	9.52	

Other Insurance Paid Amount — 0.00
(*) See Notes Adjustment — 0.00
Final Paid Amount/Check — 85.73   # 43984431

Total Payment to Provider: *******85.73   **Total Payment to Enrollee:** *******0.00

NOTES:

THANK YOU FOR USING A
PARTICIPATING PROVIDER

PPU   THIS IS YOUR PLANS PARTICIPATING PROVIDERS CONTRACTUAL ALLOWANCE FOR
      THIS SERVICE PROVIDER AGREES TO REDUCE THE FEE TO THE AMOUNT
      ALLOWED

DEDUCTIBLE

YOU HAVE MET 200.00 OF YOUR 200.00 DEDUCTIBLE FOR 01/01/20YY–12/31/20YY

KEY:

Policy Information:
1. Insurance company name
2. Name of employer or group
3. Date the EOB statement was finalized
4. Member's or insured's name and ID number
5. Patient's identification number as it appears on his ID card
6. Control number assigned to the claim

Service Information:
7. Name of the person who received the service (the patient)
8. Provider's name
9. Dates of the services provided (DOS)

10. Procedures performed (CPT codes)
11. Total charge for each procedure

Coverage Determination:
12. The contractual allowed amount
13. Patient's copayment or coinsurance amount
14. Patient's deductible
15. Noncovered procedures or amounts
16. Total payment to the provider
17. The total amount that is the patient's responsibility

FIGURE 17-7 Example of a Remittance Advice/Explanation of Benefits statement.

clearinghouse used to transmit the claim usually identifies those that were rejected.

Box 17-3 explains how to reconcile a RA/EOB.

Posting Insurance Payments

Insurance payments should be posted with great attention to detail and accuracy. One insurance check can include payment for several services (as reported with CPT codes), for several dates of service for the same patient, or for several patients. When posting an insurance check, the money must be properly allocated among all patients included in the check and to each specific charge for each date of service. This is called **line item posting**, because payment is allocated

to each charge line on the claim (such as the CMS-1500 or electronic claim). Procedure 17-5 demonstrates how to enter insurance payments.

After you post the patient's payment to the specific date and procedure, you sometimes need to enter an adjustment. An adjustment is a positive or negative change to a patient's account balance, such as a correction, change, discount, or write-off.

If the provider is participating in the plan, the medical assistant adjusts off (subtracts) the difference between the billed amount and the allowed amount so that the patient is not billed. When providers contract with insurance carriers, they must accept the allowed amount of the claim as

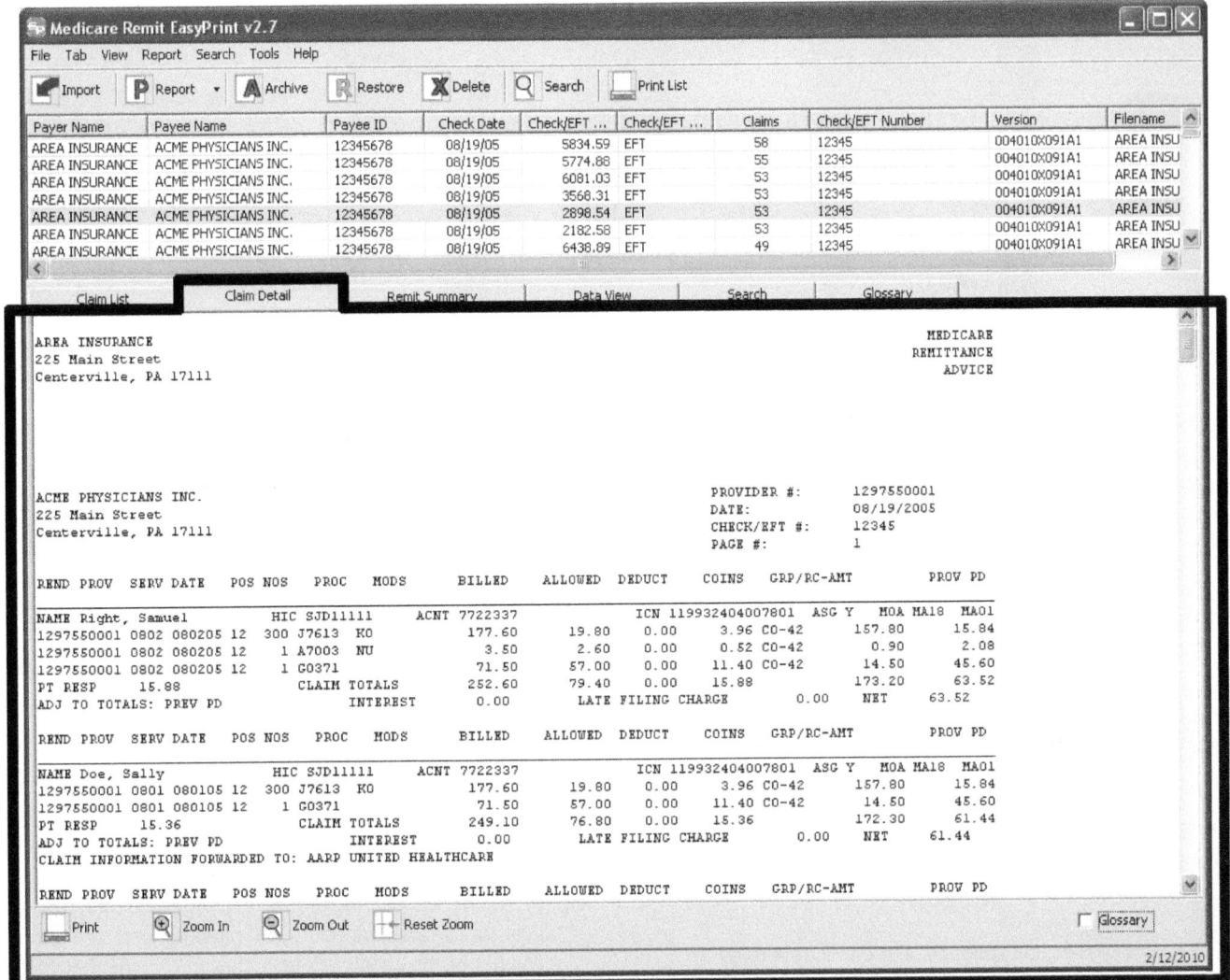

FIGURE 17-8 Example of a Medicare Electronic Remittance Advice (ERA).

BOX 17-3 | How to Reconcile a RA/EOB

Dr. Rippon saw patient Casey Price for an annual checkup. The charge for the service is $150. Kelley Sanders, MA, bills Healthy Way Insurance. Dr. Rippon is a participating provider. Review the portion of the RA/EOB that follows and determine:

How much did the insurance company pay?

How much does Dr. Rippon need to write off as a contractual allowance?

How much should Kelley bill Mr. Price?

Healthy Way Insurance allowed $132.43 for this service.

Healthy Way Insurance paid 90% of the allowed amount or $119.19 ($132.43 × 90%).

Kelley must enter an adjustment to write off the contractual allowance of $17.57 ($150.00 − $132.43).

Mr. Price owes 10% of the allowed amount or $13.24 ($132.43 × 10%).

Charge	Allowed	Deductible	Coinsurance (10%)	Paid (90%)	Contractual Allowance
$150.00	$132.43	$0	$13.24	$119.19	$17.57

Portion of a Remittance Advice (RA) or Explanation of Benefits (EOB).

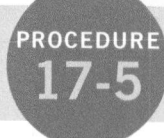

Posting Insurance Payments

Objective ◆ *Post single and bulk insurance payments to patients' accounts using a practice management system (PMS).*

EQUIPMENT AND SUPPLIES

Remittance advice (RA)/explanation of benefits (EOB); copy of check; computer with PMS

METHOD

1. Log in with your username and password previously created.
2. Access the menu item for posting payments.
3. Enter the date the check was received, the payer, the dollar amount, and the check number in the designated fields.
4. Select the account of the patient the payment is for. Verify that you have the correct name, the correct family member, and the correct account type for the payment to be posted.
5. Select the date of service covered by the payment.
6. Select the first line item for the date of service.
7. Enter the dollar amount for the following:
   • Payment amount
   • Copayment, coinsurance, and deductible owed by patient
   • Noncovered items that are patient responsibility

   • Contractual allowance (write-off) for participating provider contracts
   • Disallowance that is to be billed to the patient for nonparticipating provider contracts
8. Post additional line items in the same way.
9. Verify that the total of line item entries, plus any amount already paid by the patient, equals the total charge for each date of service.
10. If more than one date of service is included in the check, repeat the process for any additional dates of service.
11. Verify whether the balance on the claim should be billed to the patient or to a secondary insurance policy.
12. Enter any necessary account notes or descriptive information, according to office policies.
13. Review all numbers to verify that data was entered accurately. Save the data, if necessary.
14. Repeat this process for any additional dates of service for the same patient.
15. If the check includes payments for multiple patients, repeat this process for additional patients, until the entire amount of the check has been posted to patient accounts. Complete the steps in Procedure 17-2 for **After the transaction has been entered.**

---

payment in full. **Balance billing** is billing the patient for the difference between the billed amount and the allowed amount. When providers are participating with a managed care plan, balance billing violates the provider's contract with the insurance carrier. When providers are not contracted with a carrier, they are required to balance bill.

When patients have defined copayment amounts, those copays should be collected at the time of service. When patients owe coinsurance or deductible amounts, medical assistants bill patients for those amounts after receiving the RA/EOB and payment from the insurer.

Claims Follow-Up

Claims follow-up is an important part of the insurance billing process, because medical assistants must ensure that all claims are processed and paid correctly by the insurance company. When a claim is not paid in full, the medical

assistant must determine the reason(s) and continue to follow up until all questions about the payment are appropriately resolved. Some claims might be delayed, meaning it takes longer than usual to receive payment. Other claims may contain specific services that are denied, and some claims may be denied in their entirety.

Most PMS software can print a variety of reports that list past due claims, making it easy to identify those that require further investigation. An AR aging analysis report lists the outstanding insurance claims and identifies how long it has been since each claim was submitted. Most computer systems provide options to identify the accounts to include in an AR aging report. For example, you can generate a report that lists only Medicare claims, or only claims for a specific payer. This is useful when a practice has a large number of patients with the same insurance carrier or HMO, so that claims from the same payer can be managed together.

Each state has its own guidelines that outline the time frame within which an insurance carrier must pay or deny a claim. Any claims that have not been processed within that time frame are subject to interest in the amount allowed by state law. As a general rule, you should call the insurance carrier regarding any claims that have not been paid or denied within 45 days of submission on paper, or within 20 days of submission electronically.

When payment is denied for one service or for the entire claim, the medical assistant needs to **trace** the claim, or investigate the reason. Usually the reason is stated on the RA/EOB, but the medical assistant may need to call the insurance company for clarification. Solutions may involve obtaining additional information from the patient, asking the coding department to review the documentation and the codes assigned, or providing copies of documentation. The provider needs to respond to insurance company inquiries quickly, because any delay by the provider adds to the time it takes to receive payment. Procedure 17-6 discusses how to respond to a denied insurance claim.

In general, unless the explanation given on the RA/EOB is clear and acceptable, you should call the insurance carrier to trace the claim. If the insurance carrier states it does not have the claim on file, request a fax number to send the

PROCEDURE 17-6 Responding to a Denied Insurance Claim

Objective ◆ *Identify the reason for a denied insurance claim, correct the error, and resubmit the claim.*

EQUIPMENT AND SUPPLIES

Patient's account in the practice management system (PMS), including patient insurance information (i.e., ID number, birthdate of the insured, name and provider customer service telephone number of insurance company) and details of the procedure the doctor performed, including CPT code, patient's diagnosis, place of service, and date of service; paper and pen; copy of the remittance advice (RA)/explanation of benefits (EOB); any documentation of the service having been preauthorized by the office

METHOD

1. Organize all materials.
2. Call the insurance company's provider customer service phone number as listed on the patient's insurance identification card.
3. Write down the date and time of the telephone call, the number called, and the name of the customer service representative on the phone.
4. Introduce yourself and your medical office to the customer service representative, and then provide the patient's identification number and date of service.
5. If the service was preauthorized, give the preauthorization number to the customer service representative.
6. Ask the customer service representative why the procedure was not paid as anticipated.
7. If there is an error processing the service for payment, ask if any other information is needed to process the claim correctly. Also ask when the office can expect payment for the procedure.
8. If the customer service representative says the claim was processed correctly, request the reason for the denial.
9. If the reason for the denial was lack of supporting documentation, ask if faxing the information is a solution. If the answer is yes, get the customer service representative's direct fax line and fax the needed documentation.
10. If the reason for the denial requires an appeal be filed, ask the customer service representative to explain the insurance company's process for appeals. Also request a written procedure for appeals.
11. Thank the customer service representative for the assistance. Ask if the representative can give you a direct phone number should you have any further questions. A direct phone number is one that goes to that individual, usually with voice mail, rather than going through the call center.
12. Write down any pertinent information, such as where to mail the appeal and what information the appeal should contain.
13. Call the patient with the findings, and get the patient involved as needed.
14. Create an account note in the PMS that describes the details of the telephone call.

EXAMPLE OF ACCOUNT NOTE

12/18/YY. Contacted Marty Shapiro at United Healthcare. He stated that check in the amount of $169 for services rendered to patient was sent on December 12, 20YY. Call back if not received by next week. R. Young, CMAS

claim directly to the customer service representative for personalized processing. You also might be told that there is an error on the claim. Sometimes, you are able to clarify the error over the phone; other times, the claim must be resubmitted. Always document phone calls made to an insurance carrier, noting the date and time of the call, the name of the person spoken to, and the results of the call, including any commitment by the insurer to reprocess or pay the claim. Also request the reference number or confirmation number that identifies the call in the insurance company's computer system, in case you have to call again. This information can usually be entered using an account note in the PMS.

Rejections, Denials, and Appeals

Claims are sometimes denied or rejected, many times for errors the medical office made. Incorrect identification numbers, incorrect birthdates, missing diagnosis codes, and missing supporting documentation all delay payment of insurance claims (Table 17-2). Attention to detail in the claim submission process saves time and effort in the end.

A rejected claim is one that never entered the carrier's system because of an incorrect identification number or similar technical problem. These are often returned to the provider by the electronic claims clearinghouse. A rejected claim should be corrected and resubmitted as a new claim, because it has not yet been accepted into the payer's claims processing system.

Of claims that do enter the carrier's system, some claims or parts of claims might not be paid. In these cases,

be careful to differentiate between denied claims and disallowances:

- A denied claim is one the carrier received and processed but did not pay because of benefits or coverage issues. The reason for denial is usually listed on the RA/EOB.

- A **disallowance** is the amount of the charge that is above the maximum allowable fee. Benefits are applied by the insurer only to the allowed amount. When a provider is contracted with an insurance company, the amount disallowed by the insurer is the contractual allowance and must be written off. In other words, the amount approved by the insurer is accepted as payment in full, and the patient is not billed for the disallowed amount. However, the patient may be responsible to pay a portion of the allowed amount under the coinsurance or copayment provision. When the provider is not contracted with the insurance company, the amount disallowed by the insurance company must be billed to the patient.

If the reason for payment reduction cannot be determined, or if you (the medical assistant) or patient disagrees with the reason, you should place a telephone call to the insurance company. If a corrected claim needs to be resubmitted, contact the insurance company for specific directions on how to do this so it will not be automatically rejected by the system. Denied claims that are resubmitted

TABLE 17-2 | Reasons for Denied Claims and Solutions

Reason for	Denial Solution
Need supporting documentation	When calling for preauthorization of any procedure, ask the insurance company customer service representative if supporting documentation is required. If so, copy the chart notes, operative report, laboratory report, or other documentation and send it in with the CMS-1500 billing form.
Diagnosis code does not match procedure performed	Before sending the claim, look at the diagnosis codes the physician assigned to the patient in the ICD-10-CM coding manual to verify that the code matches the diagnosis.
Patient is no longer eligible for coverage	Before scheduling a procedure, call to verify coverage with the insurance carrier.
Missing information on the claim	Proofread all data entered into the PMS and all CMS-1500 claim forms before sending to determine any missing information.
Preauthorization was not obtained	Before scheduling a procedure, call to verify coverage with the insurance carrier.
Patient age or gender does not match the procedure	Proofread all data entry to ensure accuracy.
Past timely filing limits	Submit all insurance claim forms in a timely manner, usually within 30 days of the date of the procedure.

as new claims, rather than corrected claims, are usually rejected because of a duplicate date of service.

Submitting a formal **appeal** involves more time and research than submitting an initial claim. Additional information and paperwork must be supplied, and detailed clinical information from the physician also might be requested by the carrier. Be sure to find out exactly what the insurance company requires, because it is not helpful to send more information than what is requested. Because the appeals process is time consuming, it is often not done properly or consistently.

Before submitting an appeal, the first step is to know and follow the appeals policy of the payer. For example, you must submit the appeal in a timely manner because there is often a cutoff date for doing so. Most practices learn about the appeals policies of the major plans they work with by referring to physician administrative manuals, contracts, and newsletters. You may also call the insurance plan to learn about specific policies.

An appeal includes writing a letter or completing a form that clearly states why the provider believes the denial is not justified. It is best to be clear and factual rather than emotional, angry, or threatening when writing appeal letters. Attach the RA/EOB and any supporting documentation to the letter. Some plans provide paperless review procedures, which may allow you to upload the documents on the payer's website or complete online forms with the required information. The PMS may be able to generate a customized letter or appeal form based on the information you enter.

Send a copy of the appeal to the patient. Because health care coverage is an agreement between the patient and the insurance carrier, better results may occur when the patient requests the appeal. For this reason, you should always ask the patient to become involved in the appeal process.

Balance Billing

After all insurance payments are received and follow-up is complete for a claim, the office sends the patient a bill for any deductible, coinsurance, or patient responsibility amounts that have not been paid, which may or may not include balance billing. Balance billing is the practice of billing patients for the difference between the physician's actual charge and the amount allowed by insurance. Balance billing is handled differently for participating and nonparticipating providers.

When providers have a participating or preferred provider contract with the insurance company, they agree to accept the insurance-allowed amount as payment in full and cannot balance bill patients. Balance billing of patients by a participating or preferred provider is a contract violation.

When the provider is nonparticipating or not contracted with an insurance company, the patient is responsible for the entire balance not covered by insurance and must be balance billed. The provider cannot opt to write off the disallowance, except in well-documented cases of patient financial hardship. To charge the insurance company the full fee, but not bill the disallowance to the patient, is viewed as misrepresenting the physician's true fee to the insurance company. If the physician is willing to accept a lesser fee, then that is the fee that must be billed to the insurance company to begin with.

When setting up the patient's account in a PMS, the software provides a check-off box or menu selection to indicate whether a patient should be balance billed. It is important to use this feature appropriately and consistently.

BILLING PATIENTS

Patient billing is the process of sending the patient a statement for the dollar amounts not covered by insurance and includes following up on unpaid bills and extending credit when necessary. Payment at the time of service is preferred, because it significantly reduces the costs of billing, such as to the cost of paper and forms, postage fees, and the use of human resources. Because most patients have a health insurance policy that covers a significant portion of the fees, the office submits a claim to the insurance company before collecting from the patient. Patients without insurance must be billed for any amounts not paid at the time of service.

Patients with health insurance may be required by their insurance policy to pay a copayment at the time of the visit. As noted earlier, copayments may be required only for certain types of visits, such as seeing the physician for a specific complaint or illness, but may not be required for preventive care. A patient's PMS account, electronic health record (EHR), or paper medical record can be flagged with the amount of copayment required so the receptionist can collect copayments before the patient is seen by the physician.

Patients with insurance might owe money after the insurance company has paid, for a variety of reasons:

- Copayment was not collected at time of service.
- The patient must pay a deductible amount before the insurance benefits start.
- Coinsurance is due on a portion of the service.
- The patient received services or supplies not covered under the insurance policy.
- The insurance policy has paid out the maximum benefit allowed by the policy.

- The provider is nonparticipating with the patient's insurance company, and the patient owes the disallowed amounts.

The Billing Cycle

In general, the faster you bill a patient or insurance company, the faster you receive payment. Patients are billed by sending them **patient statements** (Figure 17-9). Billing methods depend on the preferences and policies of the medical office. Billing may be performed internally by the physician's office or prepared externally by a medical billing service.

The medical assistant must have a thorough understanding of office policy with regard to the timing of billing—when during the month patient bills are sent. The timing of issuing patient bills affects the cash flow of the practice. Inform patients of when billing statements will be mailed when they register with the practice. Follow the billing schedule consistently, so that patients can plan their expenses and so that the office has a predictable cash flow. If a change is made to the billing schedule, patients should be notified. This can be done by enclosing a notice of billing policy changes in each statement at least two months before the change.

There are two types of billing cycles: monthly billing and cycle billing.

Monthly Billing

In **monthly billing**, statements for all patients are generated once a month, on the same day each month. The preparation of patient statements is a labor-intensive process that may require several days of full-time work. This is usually followed by several days of heavy incoming call volume from patients who have questions about their bills. Payments tend to arrive in the mail in one large wave, requiring extra time to post payments. When time is required for labor-intensive projects such as patient

billing, time is detracted from other office duties, so arrangements must be made to ensure that all duties are adequately staffed.

Cycle Billing

In **cycle billing**, approximately 25 percent of patient accounts are billed each week (Figure 17-10). The workload of preparing statements and responding to patient questions is distributed evenly throughout the month. Cash flow also is distributed evenly throughout the month, which not only disperses the work of posting payments, but it is usually better for practice finances to have a steady flow of cash. Cycle billing also helps to better disperse incoming calls from patients. When the workload of patient billing is evenly distributed throughout the month, it is easier to fulfill these duties along with other office responsibilities.

FIGURE 17-9 Example of a patient statement.

Details of the statement:

Pearson Medical Clinic

PT STMT OUTSOURCE
PO BOX 52432
PHOENIX AZ 85072–2222

(1)

(2)
For all billing questions
Please call 1-800-555-5555 x9999

SEND TO:
(3) PAUL N. PATIENT
321 MAIN STREET, APT 102
ANYTOWN USA 12345

IF PAYING BY VISA OR MASTERCARD, FILL OUT BELOW (4)

VISA (5) MASTERCARD (6)
CARD NUMBER   AMOUNT
SIGNATURE (7)   EXP DATE (8)

STATEMENT DATE	PAY THIS AMOUNT	ACCOUNT NO
05/03/20YY	$429.40	101576 (9)

CHARGES AND PAYMENTS MADE AFTER STATEMENT DATE WILL APPEAR ON THE NEXT STATEMENT (10) SHOW AMOUNT PAID HERE $

REMIT AND MAKE CHECKS PAYABLE TO:

(11) PT STMT OUTSOURCE
PO BOX 52432
PHOENIX AZ 85072-2222

Please check box if above address is incorrect
☐ or insurance information has changed, and
please indicate change(s) on reverse side

STATEMENT

PLEASE DETACH AND RETURN TOP PORTION
WITH YOUR PAYMENT IN ENCLOSED ENVELOPE

Date of Service	Claim Number	Charges	Medicare Payment	Other Payment	Adjustments	Total Patient Payment	Last Patient Payment Date	Amount Due from Patient	Message (see back)
03/01/YY–03/05/YY	Q403008C	$429.40	$00	$00	$00	$00		$429.40	
(12)	(13)	(14)	(15)	(16)	(17)	(18)	(19)	(20)	(21)

Current	31–60 Days	61–90 Days	91–120 Days	Over 120 Days		AMOUNT DUE	$429.40
$429.40	$00	$00	$00	$00		(23)	

(22)

If payment has been sent, please disregard this notice.
(24)

(25) PT STMT OUTSOURCE
PO BOX 52432
PHOENIX AZ 85072-2222
Tel: 1-800-555-5555 x9999

SEE REVERSE SIDE FOR IMPORTANT BILLING INFORMATION (26)

Legend:

1. Name and remittance address of medical office
2. Phone number of billing office
3. Name and address of person receiving services
4. If paying by charge card, check box indicating which type
5. Card number if paying by charge
6. Amount paying by charge
7. Signature of card holder
8. Expiration date of charge card
9. Patient Account Number
10. Amount paid by patient
11. Remittance Address
12. Service dates of claim
13. Claim Number
14. Total charges on claim
15. Amount paid by Medicare (if applicable)
16. Amount paid by other insurance (if applicable)
17. Adjustments taken (if applicable)
18. Amount owed by patient (if applicable)
19. Date of last patient payment
20. Amount due for claim
21. Message Code See explanations on back of statement
22. Age of unpaid balance
23. Total Amount due from Patient
24. Statement messages
25. Name and remittance address of
26. Phone number of billing office

Billing Date	Patient Names Beginning With
7th	A–F
14th	G–L
21st	M–R
28th	S–Z

FIGURE 17-10 Example of a cycle billing schedule.

Procedure 17-7 describes how to prepare patient statements using a PMS. Box 17-4 discusses how to prepare patient ledgers manually.

Fee Adjustments

Medical offices make adjustments to patient statements and fees when an unusual situation exists. These include late payment fees, cash discounts, professional courtesy, and financial hardship.

Late Fees

Many businesses charge a **late fee** when customers do not pay their bills on time, and many medical offices do the same. A late fee policy encourages patients to pay their bills on time. Late payments hurt the cash flow of the medical practice, which can be costly, because the practice might need to borrow money temporarily to cover the cash shortage until more funds arrive in the mail. The medical office should have a clearly defined late payment policy that specifies at what point a late fee is charged and how the late fee is calculated. Late fees may be a preset dollar amount, such as $3 per month, or a percentage of the balance due, such as 1 percent per month.

PROCEDURE
17-7

Preparing Patient Statements

Objective ◆ *Produce patient bills using a computerized practice management system (PMS).*

EQUIPMENT AND SUPPLIES

Computer with a PMS; printer; window envelopes compatible with statement format; stamps, postage meter, or other method of applying postage

METHOD

1. Fill the printer with patient statement forms, if used, or plain paper.
2. Log in with your username and password previously created.
3. Access the menu for creating patient statements.
4. Select the statement format to be used.
5. Enter the parameters for the patients to be billed, such as:
   - A preset definition for "cycle 1," "cycle 2," and so on
   - The section of the alphabet to be billed, such as "last name beginning with A" through "last name beginning with F"
   - The payer type, such as Medicare patients or HMO patients
   - Names of specific patients
   - Patients with an account balance within a specified range, such as "accounts over $10.00"
   - Patients with account balances over "x" days old (This can be useful if the office policies call for printing special reminder notices, writing personal notes, or affixing a reminder sticker to such statements.)

6. Complete any other information required by the PMS, such as a reminder message or late charge policy to be printed on the statement.
7. Print the statements. The PMS automatically updates the patient accounts to document that a billing statement was sent.
8. Complete the steps in Procedure 17-2 for **After the transaction has been entered**.
9. Collect the statements from the printer, and organize a work area for folding and stuffing. If special patient statement forms are used, remove the forms from the printer so that the next staff member does not unknowingly print on the forms.
10. As you handle each statement, review it to verify that it is readable, complete, properly aligned on the paper, and undamaged. Set aside those statements that may need to be checked or reprinted.
11. Affix any reminder stickers used by the practice. Fold each statement neatly in such a way that the address appears in the window of the envelope.
12. Insert the statement in the envelope, and check the front to verify that the entire address is visible.
13. Seal the envelope, and affix postage. Mail the statements according to office procedures.
14. Reprint those statements that are not usable, following the preceding steps. Shred the unused statements to maintain patient privacy.

Medical offices that do not use a PMS system, or whose PMS system does not print patient statements, may use manual patient ledgers. Manual patient ledgers may consist of cards that are filled in with an ink pen or typewriter, or may be a computer template form that stands on its own and is not related to a larger patient accounting or practice management system (PMS).

1. Write, type, or key into the computer the patient's name in the following format: last name first, first name, middle initial.
2. Enter the patient's mailing address, including zip code, and the residential address, if different.
3. Enter the patient's telephone number, including area code. If applicable, enter the patient's home, work, and cell phone numbers.

4. Enter the patient's insurance information including name, address, and telephone number of the insurance company, subscriber name and ID, group number, and effective date.

If the previous ledger card has been filled to capacity, you must forward the ending balance from the previous card onto the new ledger card. When using pegboard and other manual systems, medical offices often make a photocopy of the ledger card and mail it in place of patient billing statements. When doing this, verify that the patient's mailing address is positioned in such a way that it is visible through the window on the envelope.

Information regarding the late payment policy should be provided in the initial information provided to patients about financial policies and printed on patient statements. A late fee cannot be assessed if the patient is not properly notified in advance.

Cash Discount

When patients do not have health insurance, the medical office can offer a reasonable discount to patients who pay in full at the time of service, known as a **cash discount**. The discount reflects the savings a practice realizes by not having to bill insurance. However, if the patient must be billed or extended credit, there is no basis for a cash discount. Giving extreme cash discounts can be viewed by insurance companies as misrepresenting the physician's true fees, because the physician is charging insurance more than what the physician is actually willing to accept.

Professional Courtesy

Professional courtesy (PC) is a discount or fee reduction a physician opts to give to other physicians, staff, family members, or clergy. Professional courtesy reductions must be clearly documented in the patient's account. Some physician's offices ask the patient to sign a letter stating that the patient was provided a service and was not charged out of professional courtesy. Place a copy of this letter in the patient's financial file or scan it into the PMS.

The amount of professional courtesy must be deducted from any claim sent to insurance. Medical offices cannot waive a portion of the fee for the patient but bill the insurance company the full amount of the fee. Such a practice is viewed as misrepresenting the physician's true fee to the insurance company.

Financial Hardship

Financial hardship refers to the inability of the patient to pay. The physician may choose to provide service at no charge or a very low charge to patients experiencing financial hardship. Each office is free to set its own criteria and policy for financial hardship, but the patient's financial situation must be well-documented. Financial documentation may include copies of a tax return, paycheck stub, or comparison of income to the federal poverty level. Patients should sign a letter stating that they are unable to pay the normal fee and request a financial hardship waiver. Medical practices must be cautious and restrained about how often this is done, because if it happens too often, insurance companies may claim the physician is misrepresenting the true fee.

Overpayments and Refunds

At times, situations arise that result in an overpayment on a patient's account. The most common reasons this may occur are:

- Duplicate entries, such as a charge entered twice, in error
- Miscalculation of the amounts owed
- Double payments by patient or insurance company

The overpayment might result in a credit balance on the account, but does not always do so. For example, if there is an overpayment of one service, but claims for subsequent services are still outstanding, there might not be a credit balance on the account as a whole. One of the advantages of line item posting of insurance payments is that it helps track the services that have been paid, those that have not, and those that may have been paid twice in error.

Whenever it is discovered that an overpayment occurred for a specific service, it must be addressed immediately. You should always review any possible overpayment with your supervisor.

Insurance Company Refunds

The medical office is legally obligated to notify insurance companies of any overpayment that may have been made in error. Physicians cannot consider overpayment of one date of service as a trade-off or "down payment" toward other services for the same patient. Even when the mistake is a result of an error by the payer, the practice is held responsible for correcting the situation. This is especially true in regard to Medicare. Knowingly keeping a Medicare overpayment is fraud, because the practice is keeping federal money that it is not legally entitled to. The practice is expected to keep adequate records that enable it to identify overpayments on any specific claim.

When an insurance company overpayment is suspected, pull copies of all relevant claims and RAs/EOBs from your paper or electronic files. First, review all the calculations to verify that an overpayment was made and the amount in question. Then, place a call to the insurance company and explain your findings. The insurance company will tell you how to handle the refund. If the practice does a large volume of claims with the insurer, the insurance company might process the refund as a deduction from a future check, so that no additional money needs to change hands. Medicare, Blue Cross/Blue Shield, and workers' compensation programs often do this. If you do a limited amount of business with the insurer, you may need to write a check to the insurance company. Be certain to document such transactions, including sending the check via certified mail, so that if there is a future question whether you reimbursed them, you have the documentation needed. The decision of how to handle the refund is up to the insurance company, not the medical office. The medical office should enter the refund as an adjustment on the patient's financial account, even when the refund is deducted from a future payment. It is best to include a special designation in the PMs specifically for this purpose.

Overpayments by insurance companies should never be made to the patient.

Patient Refunds

Patients may be owed a refund if there was a miscalculation regarding the deductible, copayment, or coinsurance amount, or they mistakenly paid the same bill twice. Refunds to patients, after being approved by your supervisor, are made using the same method of payment that the patient used. Payments originally made with cash or check should be refunded with a check. Be certain that the patient's original check has cleared all the way through the banking system before issuing a refund check. Payments made with a credit card must be refunded to the exact same credit card used for the original transaction. This is usually required by the merchant credit card vendor (the company providing the office's credit card processing services) as proof against any future claims by the patient. Procedure 17-8 explains how to post a refund to the patient's account. A refund is entered into the patient's account using a designated adjustment code in the PMS.

Medical offices should have a procedure to request approval for a refund and to request a refund check be issued by the accounting department. Become familiar with the policy and refer to it each time a patient refund is needed. If you issue a refund to a patient in error, it will be extremely difficult to recoup the money.

Credit Policy

Payment at the time of service is the ideal method of collection. Know the office policy regarding patients who are not prepared to pay at the time of service. Depending on the type of practice and the reason for the appointment, the patient may be asked to reschedule. To avoid this situation, it is helpful to remind patients when they schedule an appointment that they will be expected to make their copayment at the time of the visit. Some offices also ask whether the patient will be paying by cash, check, or credit card. If the office policy is to allow patients to be seen without making their required payment, a billing statement should be prepared and mailed to the patient, requesting payment immediately.

When the patient will be responsible for a significant out-of-pocket amount, such as with surgery or similar procedures, credit arrangements often must be made. This is best done during the patient's initial visit before the surgery or

---

JUDGMENT CALL

Keri, the receptionist in Dr. David's office, is training a new employee to help out in the front office. Keri and the new employee will be responsible for making patient appointments and processing the monthly patient statements. Keri is aware that Mr. Wallace has a balance of $2,400, and after several attempts to communicate with him and his failure to respond to payment requests, his account is about to be turned over to collections. As Keri looks at the next day's schedule, she notices the new employee has scheduled Mr. Wallace for an annual physical. What should Keri do?

PROCEDURE 17-8 — Processing Credit Balances and Refunds

Objective ◆ *Post the appropriate entries to a patient account that has a credit balance using a practice management system (PMS).*

EQUIPMENT AND SUPPLIES
Computer with a PMS; source document that identifies the reason for the credit balance and authorizes the refund to be made; refund check, RA/EOB, or credit card slip

METHOD

1. Log in to the PMS using your previously established username and password.
2. Access the patient's account.
3. Locate the charge that was overpaid.
4. Select the menu item to enter an adjustment and the type of adjustment.
5. Enter the dollar amount to be refunded. This will be a positive adjustment (debit) that increases the account balance.

6. Enter a description or account note to explain the reason for the adjustment. Be as detailed as possible.
7. Verify that all entries are correct.
8. If a check is to be sent to the insurance company or the patient, access the correspondence menu and generate a letter that explains the refund.
9. Complete the steps in Procedure 17-2 for **After the transaction has been entered**.
10. Mail the letter and check via certified mail.

EXAMPLE ACCOUNT NOTE
3/1/20YY Refunded $20.00 to patient because patient mistakenly paid the copayment for 2/15/YY twice. Check # 9999...David Gao, MA.

---

procedure is performed. Never wait until after the procedure is completed to discuss payment arrangements. All necessary information should be gathered from the patient with regard to demographics, insurance, deductibles, employment, and signatures.

If the patient cannot pay in full at the time of service and has no insurance, then the office can consider billing the patient for services and extending credit. If credit is extended and it is determined that the patient will make set payments to the physician in more than four installments, the patient must sign a **Truth in Lending form** (Figure 17-11). This form must clearly state the amount financed, the finance charge, and the total amount of the payments. When no finance charges are to be assessed, that fact should be stated on the form. The original form is given to the patient, and a copy is retained by the doctor and must be kept on file for two years. The disclosure must be very specific, and the patient must sign it in the medical assistant's presence. Credit bureaus operate as sources of credit data on individuals. They can supply data verifying a patient's employment, residence, and payment history. The medical office must be sure that it is working with a reputable credit bureau.

COLLECTING PATIENT BALANCES

Every medical office should have a collection policy in place to provide a clear and consistent method of handling sensitive financial situations. The medical assistant must understand the collection policy and must administer it uniformly and fairly according to the physician's directives.

Delinquent Accounts

Accounts that are extremely overdue become very difficult and costly to collect. Patients must be educated about billing and collection procedures so that they have a clear understanding of what is expected of them financially. Encourage patients to openly discuss problems or questions they might have with respect to their bills.

The reasons that a bill becomes delinquent may include:

- The patient believes that insurance will cover the bill.
- The patient is unable to pay.
- The patient has a misunderstanding about the fee.
- The patient does not feel that the bill is important.

Failure to collect delinquent accounts affects the medical practice in many ways. Patients who owe money may stay

ANNUAL PERCENTAGE RATE The cost of your credit as a yearly rate.	FINANCE CHARGE The dollar amount the credit will cost you.	AMOUNT FINANCED The amount of credit provided to you or on your behalf.	TOTAL OF PAYMENTS The amount you will have paid after you have made all payments as scheduled.
%	$	$	$

Your Payment Schedule will be:

Number of Payments	Amount of Payments	When Payments are Due

Security: You will have a security interest in the following described property: (property description) _____

Late Charge: If any part of a payment is unpaid for 10 days after it is due, I may be charged 5% of the amount of payment.
Prepayment: (Scheduled Installment Earnings Method): If I pay off early, I may be entitled to a refund of part of the Finance Charge and I will not have to pay a penalty. (True Daily Earnings Method): If I pay off early, I will not have to pay a penalty.
Additional Information: See the contracts documents for any additional information about nonpayments, default, any required repayment in full before the scheduled date, and prepayment refunds and penalties.

Annual Percentage Rate	Finance Charge	Amount Financed	Total of Payments
The cost of your credit at a yearly rate.	The dollar amount your loan will cost you.	The amount of credit provided to you or on your behalf.	The amount you will have paid after you have made all scheduled payments.
10.16	71,855.17	71,600.00	151,455.017

FIGURE 17-11 Example of Truth in Lending form.

away from the office out of embarrassment because of their financial situation. Failure to collect delinquent accounts may imply guilt on the part of the physician as to the quality of care that the patient received. Ultimately, failure to collect delinquent accounts burdens the entire practice as a result of lost revenue.

Most practices have a collection process in place that includes noting the patient's account status in that patient's record. This is especially helpful if the patient calls the office to schedule an appointment or inquire about medication refills.

The medical assistant must determine, in a timely manner, the reason that payments are overdue and then implement the collection process. The medical office may consider a "write-off" policy for small dollar amounts because the cost of the collection efforts would be greater than the amount to be collected. For example, if the patient's bill is $80 and the cost of collection efforts exceeds $20, the billing office can refer to the office's policies and procedures manual to determine the specific threshold amount for collection services. To implement a write-off, enter an adjustment on the patient's account using a special designation for this purpose.

Collection Techniques

The medical office might employ several methods of collection. The physician decides office policy regarding collection of overdue payments; the medical assistant has the responsibility to carry out the policy consistently and fairly. Reminder notices, telephone calls, collection letters, and finally a collection agency may be used.

A personal interview can be a very effective collection method. The patient who is seen in the office for an appointment and has an outstanding account is readily available for discussion with the office staff. This is the time to tactfully and privately bring attention to the overdue account and to make arrangements with the patient for payment.

Reminder notices in the form of stickers or printed notes can be placed on patient statements asking for their prompt attention to a past due bill, and encouraging the patient to contact the office if there is a question about the past due bill. If no payment or contact is made, then a reminder letter

TABLE 17-3 | Laws Governing Collection

Law	Description
Notice on "Use of Telephone for Debt Collection" from the Federal Communications Commission	Provides guidelines for the specific times that credit collection phone calls can be made. It prohibits using the telephone for harassment and threats. Telephone calls for the purposes of collections must be made between the hours of 8:00 A.M. and 9:00 P.M.
Fair Debt Collection Practices Act of 1978	Provides a guide for determining what are considered the fair collections practices for creditors.
Equal Credit Opportunity Act of 1975	Prohibits discrimination—unfair treatment—in the granting of credit. This law mandates that women and minorities must be issued credit if they qualify for it, based on the premise that if credit is given to one patient it should be given to all patients who meet the same criteria.
Fair Credit Reporting Act of 1971	Provides guidelines for collecting an individual's credit information. Individuals are able to learn what credit information is available about them. Consumers can correct and update this credit information.
Truth in Lending Act of 1969	Requires a full, written disclosure concerning the payment of any fee that will be collected in more than four instalments. Also referred to as Regulation Z of the Consumer Protection Act.

is sent. It should not be a form letter but rather an individual letter that lets the patient know that the account is being reviewed and that there is concern about the unpaid debt. Tactful, professional telephone calls may also become part of the collection process and sometimes can be more effective than the letter.

Regulations

Several laws have been enacted to provide protection against unscrupulous collection practices that harm individuals. The medical assistant is responsible for following the administrative procedures these laws require (Table 17-3), so you must be familiar with these laws, and you also must be familiar with your particular state laws when applying collection techniques. Procedure 17-9 provides basic rules and guidelines to assist in the task of making collection calls. Violation of these rules could be a federal offense.

Telephone Collections

A telephone call at the right time and in the right manner can be more effective than a letter. The medical assistant must be sure to make the call tactful, brief, and to the point. All conversation should be conducted only with the debtor or guarantor, the person legally responsible for payment. This might or might not be the patient. A firm commitment to make payment by a specific date or according to a specific schedule should be obtained before ending the conversation. When you call and find the debtor is unavailable,

leave only a message stating that the individual should contact the office.

Collection Letters

A personalized letter has many advantages over an impersonal form letter. Patients who receive the personalized letter may feel that their account has received individual attention and feel more obligated to respond. Personalized letters based on a standard template are easy to create using word processing software. A PMS also might provide a letter writing feature. The letter can be inserted with the monthly statement. The letter should inquire why the bill has not been paid. There should be an offer to assist the patient with making payment arrangements. The letter must convey the message that action will be taken to resolve the payment obligation. Procedure 17-10 provides basic rules and guidelines to assist in drafting a collection letter. Figure 17-12 shows an example of a reminder collection letter.

Collection Agencies

When none of the other collection methods are successful in obtaining payment for services, the office can consider using an outside collection agency. A **collection agency** is an outside company that specializes in collecting payment for unpaid bills. The physician should approve all accounts being sent to a collection agency or being written off. Once a patient's account is in the hands of a collection agency, most offices terminate the physician–patient relationship,

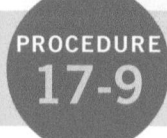

Making Collection Calls

Objective ◆ *Place a call to a patient requesting payment.*

EQUIPMENT AND SUPPLIES

Patient's account in the practice management system (PMS); demographic information; telephone; black ink pen

METHOD

1. Based on the collection policy of the office, determine how many days overdue the bill must be before the first call is made.
2. Access the patient's account in the PMS, and review the account activity before placing the call.
3. Find a quiet area of the office in which to work while placing collection calls. Patients do not want their financial business shared, even unintentionally, with others, and background noise may be distracting.
4. Collection calls should only be made Monday through Saturday from 8:00 A.M. to 9:00 P.M. Do not call on Sundays or holidays.
5. Locate the patient's telephone number, and place the call.
6. When the call is answered, confidently ask to speak with the patient. Do not share information with anyone other than the patient or responsible party.
7. If the patient is unavailable, you may leave a message; however, the message should simply state the caller's name, who the message is for, and the telephone number where the caller may be reached.

8. When speaking with the patient, politely introduce yourself and ask if this is a good time to talk. If the patient tells you it is not a good time, ask what time would be better, and make a note of that in the chart. Call back the patient at the stated time.
9. When speaking with the patient, be polite, project confidence, and state the facts and purpose of the call. Never threaten an action you do not intend to take.
10. Ask the patient if there is a reason for nonpayment. If the patient is able to provide a reason, document the response.
11. Ask the patient when you might expect payment, and document that response as well.
12. Politely thank the patient and repeat the terms agreed on.
13. Document the interaction with a note in the patient's account.

EXAMPLE OF ACCOUNT NOTE

12/18/20YY. Spoke with Mrs. Ross regarding delinquent account. Patient stated she has recently lost her job and has been unable to keep up with her financial obligations. Mrs. Ross has agreed to make two payments of $20 each, due on the 1st of the month. Patient will contact the office if she is unable to make the payment. C. Wood, CMA

---

using the proper notification procedure as determined in the office manual.

Selecting a Collection Agency

Typically, collection agencies are used as a last resort. If a collection agency is used by the office, it should be chosen carefully. Some collection agencies have a dedicated department for medical bills. If possible, interview the collection agency before choosing one. Reputable agencies have references that can be checked and readily discuss their collection methods and HIPAA compliance practices. Further checks can be done with the Better Business Bureau and national credit agencies. Ask other medical offices which agency they use.

Because most practices are reluctant to use a collection agency, they sometimes delay sending accounts to the agency until they have been overdue for a long time. However, the longer the medical office waits to send an account to a collection agency, the less likely the collection agency will be able to collect it. If an office sends only extremely old accounts that are unlikely to be collectable, the agency has no incentive to put effort into collections, because usually the agency is paid only when a patient payment is received.

Working with a Collection Agency

When working with collection agencies, medical assistants must be familiar with how collection agencies charge for

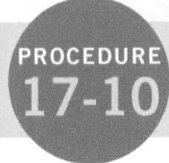

PROCEDURE 17-10

Writing a Collection Letter

Objective ◆ *Compose a collection letter requesting payment.*

EQUIPMENT AND SUPPLIES

Patient's ledger; demographic information; computer; black ink pen

METHOD

1. Based on the collection policy of the office, determine at what point the first letter is sent.
2. Review the account activity in the patient's account in the PMS.
3. Access the correspondence module of the PMS, or open the word processing program. Compose a rough draft of the letter, using proper formatting, grammar, and punctuation.
4. In the first paragraph, summarize the reason for the letter and any payments the patient has made on the account.
5. In the second paragraph, state the desired action of the patient. This may simply be to contact the office, or it may specifically state the expected payment amount and dates of the expected payment. Ensure that the letter is written in a polite tone without any threats for lack of compliance.
6. In the third paragraph, or closing paragraph, thank the patient in advance for prompt attention to the matter and encourage the patient to contact the office.
7. When the rough draft is complete, read through the document again, checking for spelling, grammar, and formatting errors.
8. Correct any errors, then print and sign the document.
9. Make a copy of the letter, and place it in the patient's file or scan it into the computer and attach it to the patient's account.
10. Place the letter in an addressed envelope, and mail it to the patient. In the PMS, enter a note in the patient's account indicating the day the letter was mailed.

EXAMPLE OF ACCOUNT NOTE

3/29/YY. Letter mailed to Mr. Elders requesting payment by4/29/YY. See copy of letter in patient record. J. Levy, RMA

---

services, how patients are notified, and how to manage the patient's account after turning it over.

Be certain to include the only minimum necessary information when turning over an account for collection, such as the balance due, itemized statements showing the dates and amounts of transactions, and contact information. Do not include a diagnosis or other medical information, because this is a violation of the patient's privacy and HIPAA guidelines, and the collection agency does not need this information to collect the balance due.

The patient must be notified that the account will be referred to a collection agency if it is not paid by a certain date. Typically this is accomplished through a series of precollection letters. After the patient has been notified, the account must be turned over to collection as stated. If it is not, the notification could be considered an idle threat and the practice could be subject to a lawsuit. After the account has been turned over, no further collection attempts can be made by the physician's office. If the patient contacts the office after the account has been turned over for collection, the patient should be referred to the collection agency for payment arrangements.

The physician's office must be aware of the costs involved when using a collection agency. A flat fee may be charged for precollection activities or for fairly recent accounts. For older accounts, most companies charge a percentage of the amount collected, called a contingency, which can range from 25 to 50 percent. The contingency percentage is higher for older accounts and lower for newer accounts. For example, the patient may have an outstanding balance of $1,000 that is sent to collection. The agency sends letters and makes telephone calls to the patient requesting payment. The patient makes a payment of $500 to the collection agency, the agency charges approximately half ($250) of the amount collected, and the balance is forwarded to the office. The remaining $500 is written off by the office as **bad debt**, an amount owed and not collectable. An adjustment is entered onto the patient's account for this purpose.

Pearson Physicians Group
Shania McWalter, D.O.
123 Michigan Avenue, Parker Heights, IL 60610
(312) 123-1234

Date

Patient Name
Street Address
City, State and ZIP Code

Dear Patient:

Your balance of $400.00 has been on our books for 18 months. Normally at this time, because your payment is long past due, your account would be handed over to our collection agency. However, we prefer to hear from you regarding your preference in this matter.

Please check one of the following options, and return this letter to our office:

☐ I would prefer to settle this account. Payment in full is enclosed.

☐ I would like to make regular weekly/monthly payments of $_____ until this account is paid in full. My first payment is enclosed.

☐ I don't believe that I owe this amount for the following reasons(s):

_____

_____

_____
patient's signature

Failure to return this letter will result in turning this account over to a collection agency.

Sincerely Yours,

Shania McWalter, D.O.

FIGURE 17-12 Example of a collection letter.

The patient's account balance can be handled in the patient accounting system in one of two ways. The physician's accountant should advise the practice which method to use. One method involves writing off the balance as bad debt in the patient's ledger and transferring the amount due to a separate account designated for collections. Payments received through the collection agency are credited against the collections account, with a notation of the patient account involved. This method clearly separates true receivables that are collectible from patients from those sent to collections. A second method is to leave the balance owed on the patient's account, post the collection payment to the account when received, and then write off the balance as bad debt. This method makes it easier to track the status of specific patient accounts.

In either method, the collection agency fees may be entered as an adjustment against the account or entered as an expense in the general ledger. Procedure 17-11 provides instructions on how to post a payment from a collection agency.

Special Problems

Even with the best billing and collection system, problems may arise, thus making collection a challenge for even the most efficient medical offices. Special situations involve skip tracing, bankruptcy, claims against estates, and the statute of limitations.

Skip Tracing

A **skip** is an individual who has a balance due and has moved without leaving a forwarding address. Skip tracing is the process of locating the individual. Skip tracing is a collection problem that requires immediate action because the greater the amount of time it takes to locate the skip, the less likely it is that you will receive payment. Skips can be traced by checking the registration form to confirm addresses, calling all telephone numbers, and calling all references without divulging the nature of the call. Placing the notice *Address Service Requested* on the outside of the mailing envelope directs the U.S. Postal Service to notify you of the person's new mailing address, if available. The postal service may charge a fee for this service, but it is a sound investment.

Bankruptcy

A patient who files for bankruptcy is protected by the court. When notice is received of a patient's bankruptcy, all collection attempts must cease and the medical office must file a claim for payment with the courts.

Claims Against Estates

When a patient dies, a bill should be sent to the estate of the deceased. Contacting next of kin will provide information regarding who is the administrator of the estate. It is important to follow-up on collection of bills to avoid giving any impression of physician's fault for medical care of the deceased patient.

Statute of Limitations

Statute of limitations refers to the amount of time a legal collection suit may be brought against a debtor. This time varies from state to state and should be verified with state agencies. If you have accounts that are more than two or

PROCEDURE 17-11

Posting a Payment from a Collection Agency

Objective ◆ *Post payments from a collection agency in a practice management system (PMS).*

EQUIPMENT AND SUPPLIES

Calculator; computer with a PMS; collection agency payment

METHOD

1. Log in to the PMS using your previously established username and password.
2. Access the patient's account or the bad debt account, depending on the method used to track accounts sent to collection.
3. Access the menu to post a payment.
4. Enter the date the payment was received.

5. Choose "Collection Agency" to indicate the source of the payment.
6. Enter the dollar amount of the check.
7. Access the menu to post an adjustment.
8. Post an adjustment for the amount of the collection agency fee or enter the fee as an expense in the accounting system.
9. Post an adjustment to write off the remaining balance as bad debt.
10. Verify that all entries are accurate.
11. Complete the steps in Procedure 17-2 for **After the transaction has been entered**.

three years old, you should investigate the statute of limitations in your state before spending time, effort, and money to collect the debt.

SUMMARY

The professional health care facility should have an office policy regarding fee setting, billing, and collection. The goal of such policy is to protect the financial well-being and goodwill of the medical practice. Medical assistants must be knowledgeable of the overall process, the terminology, and the special problems that may arise, so they can be a patient liaison and educator.

Patient accounting refers to the functions of the accounting department related to recording charges and payments for services provided to patients. Patients' financial records are maintained separately from their medical records. Accounts receivable (AR) is the amounts owed by patients and their third-party payers for services provided to patients. AR transactions are financial events that either increase or decrease the account balance, the amount of money a patient owes. AR is evaluated in terms of age, or how long the money has been owed using two types of reports: days in AR and aging analysis.

Providers are required to collect the copayment from the patient. To routinely waive copayments is the same as if the provider were to misrepresent the actual fee to the insurance company. When posting an insurance check, the money must be properly allocated among all patients included in the check and to each specific charge for each date of service. When payment is denied for one service or for the entire claim, the medical assistant needs to trace the claim, or investigate the reason, which is usually stated on the explanation of benefits (EOB).

Patients are billed by sending them patient statements, which can be printed on either a monthly basis or in a cycle in which 25 percent of bills are sent each week. Medical offices make adjustments to patient statements and fees when unusual situations exist, such as late payment fees, cash discounts, professional courtesy, and financial hardship. Every medical office should have a collection policy in place to provide a clear and consistent method of handling sensitive financial situations when patients do not pay on time. When none of the other collection methods are successful in obtaining payment for services, the office can consider using an outside collection agency, which is an outside company that specializes in collecting payment for unpaid bills.

17 CHAPTER REVIEW

COMPETENCY REVIEW

1. Define and spell the terms for this chapter.
2. With a fellow student, role-play a telephone conversation you would have with Samuel Jones, a patient who is unemployed, to collect a $225 bill overdue for 60 days.
3. Write a sample collection letter from Dr. Shania McWalter to Samuel Jones, based on the previous question.
4. What statements can you make to a patient to encourage payment at the time of service?
5. Discuss the legal and ethical considerations involved when making collection calls.
6. Name the three forms of payment and security tips for accepting each.

PREPARING FOR THE CERTIFICATION EXAM

1. What report provides a running total of all patient account transactions each day?
   a. patient ledger
   b. day sheet
   c. AR aging analysis
   d. tracing report
   e. daily schedule

2. What is accounts receivable?
   a. money owed to collection agencies for funds collected
   b. money owed to the practice for services received
   c. money received by the practice from insurance companies
   d. money owed to the insurance companies for overpayment
   e. money received by insurance companies from the patient

3. What should you do when a patient leaves no forwarding address?
   a. close the patient's account
   b. write off the patient's balance
   c. send the account to a collection agency
   d. contact local law enforcement
   e. print "Address Service Requested" on the mailing envelope

4. Who approves which accounts to turn over to collections?
   a. office manager
   b. physician
   c. administrative accounts representative
   d. bookkeeper
   e. billing manager

5. What are the days in AR number for a practice that has $250,000 in AR and average daily revenue of $4,200?
   a. 12
   b. 25
   c. 42
   d. 60
   e. 69

6. How much does the patient owe when she sees a participating provider for the following service? Office visit $110.00. Allowed amount $93.00. Coinsurance 20 percent.
   a. $15.23
   b. $17.00
   c. $18.60
   d. $20.00
   e. $22.00

7. Line item posting of a bulk remittance is posting a payment amount for each
   a. charge line.
   b. date of service.
   c. patient.
   d. physician.
   e. check.

8. What should the office do when notified that a patient has filed for bankruptcy?
   a. attempt to contact the patient
   b. write off the balance
   c. send a reminder letter
   d. contact the patient's attorney
   e. file a claim with the courts

9. What is a chronological record of the charges, adjustments, payments, and current balance for a specific patient?
   a. payment history
   b. patient reconciliation
   c. EOB
   d. patient ledger
   e. aging analysis

10. When is it permissible to place collection calls?
   a. Monday through Saturday from 8:00 A.M. to 9:00 P.M.
   b. Monday through Friday from 8:00 A.M. to 5:00 P.M.
   c. Sunday through Saturday from 10:00 A.M. to 4:00 P.M.
   d. Monday through Saturday from 9:00 A.M. to 5:00 P.M.
   e. Monday through Friday from 10:00 A.M. to 4:00 P.M.

CRITICAL THINKING

Refer to the case study at the beginning of the chapter and use the information you have learned to answer the following questions.

1. How should Samra handle the situation with Ms. McConnley?

2. When Ms. McConnley is ready to check out, she informs Samra that she does not have any cash to pay her $25 copayment. How should Samra respond?

3. Is it necessary for Samra to make any notations in the patient's chart?

ON THE JOB

(A) Collection Letter

Services were rendered to Jeffrey Boylan on October 1. It is now 45 days since Mr. Boylan received care, and he has not yet made a payment on his outstanding balance of $150. At this point, the office's policy requires that a reminder letter be sent. Compose a collection letter to Mr. Boylan in accordance with HIPAA and office guidelines. Address: Mr. Jeffrey Boylan, 14 Meadow Road, Anytown, State 12345

(B) Tracking Claims

Drake Scott, CMA (AAMA), is responsible for processing insurance claims for a large medical clinic. You have just hired Anne Obermark, CMA (AAMA), to work with Drake in processing insurance claims. You determined that Anne will be responsible for tracking claims.

1. Why is it important for Anne to track insurance claims processed through the clinic?

2. What AR report should Anne use to identify the claims that require follow-up? What should she look for on this report?

3. Anne finds five claims that have not been paid in the past three months. What should she do to obtain payment?

INTERNET ACTIVITY

Your office is considering using a collection agency. Conduct an Internet search of collection agencies in your local area. Create a comparison grid that identifies how long each has been in service, who their clients are, which ones specialize in medical bill collections, and how to arrange for service. Identify the top three companies you would recommend that the office contact for more information and references.

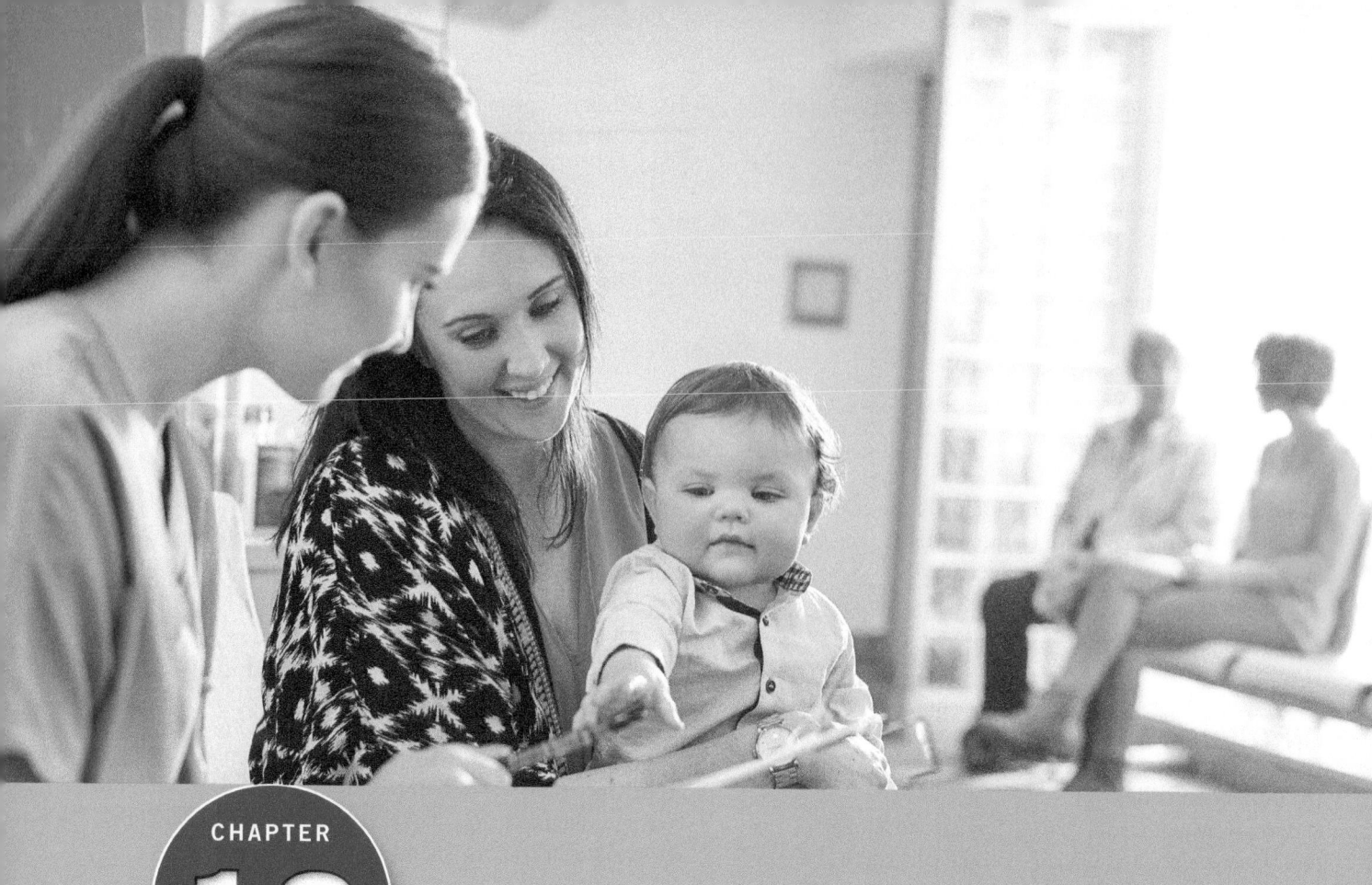

CHAPTER

18

Banking and Practice Finances

Learning Objectives

After completing this chapter, you should be able to:

18.1   Define and spell the terms for this chapter.

18.2   Describe banking procedures that are common to a medical practice.

18.3   Explain the role of a medical assistant related to practice finances.

18.4   List safety precautions that can be implemented to prevent financial fraud.

18.5   Identify information found on checks.

18.6   Describe considerations that must be taken into account when accepting a check as a form of payment.

18.7   Describe different forms of endorsement.

18.8   List the steps related to completing a bank deposit.

18.9   Identify common recurring monthly expenses.

18.10 Describe the steps for reconciling a bank statement.

18.11 Explain how the Fair Labor Standards Act (FLSA) impacts a medical practice.

18.12 List options available for managing payroll.

18.13 Explain different types of payroll withholdings.

Tania Washington is a medical office co-manager for Pearson Physicians Group. She is in charge of managing the financial matters of the group practice. It is the end of the day, and Tania needs to collect the deposit slip, checks, and petty cash drawer from the front office. Susan hands Tania all the materials and leaves work for the day.

Terms to Learn

accounting

accounts payable (AP)

accounts receivable (AR)

American Bankers Association (ABA) number

asset

blank check

bookkeeping

cancelled checks

cash disbursement

credits

debits

deductions

deposits

disbursement account

double-entry bookkeeping

embezzlement

endorsement

exempt

Fair Labor Standards Act (FLSA)

Federal Insurance Contributions Act (FICA)

Federal Unemployment Tax Act (FUTA)

fidelity bond

financial agent

gross wage

hourly

internal controls

invoice

liability

magnetic ink character recognition (MICR)

negotiable instrument

net pay

nonexempt

nonsufficient funds (NSF)

online banking

overtime

packing slip

paid time off (PTO)

payee

payer

petty cash

power-of-attorney (POA)

purchase order

reconciliation

remittance slip

salaried

separation of duties

stale check

State Unemployment Tax Act (SUTA)

stop-payment order

surety bond

third-party check

voucher check

W-2 form

W-4 form

withholding

The financial life cycle of a medical practice begins with providing services and receiving payment. The money received in payments pays the bills of the practice that are necessary to keep the practice running. The amount left over after paying bills is called earnings, profit, or equity. Some or all of this money is paid to the partners or other investors.

The medical assistant's responsibilities for maintaining control of the medical office's banking and bookkeeping procedures are twofold. First, absolute accuracy is necessary when working with bank deposits, reconciliation of funds, and all related bookkeeping activities. The second responsibility relates to the trust that the physician has placed on the employee for handling cash, checks, and accounts. The medical assistant acts as the agent for the physician and must be vigilant to help safeguard the practice against financial fraud.

This chapter provides an introduction to the financial functions and banking procedures of a medical practice. Procedures discussed in this chapter include working with checks to accept payments, make deposits, and pay bills. At the end of the month, the bank statement must be reconciled. Finally, medical assistants need to understand the payroll process.

FINANCIAL FUNCTIONS

Maintaining accurate financial records to be used by the accountant can be one of the medical assistant's responsibilities. Therefore, it is important to be familiar with basic financial functions. These include bookkeeping, accounting, accounts receivable, accounts payable, and prevention of fraud, which are discussed next.

Bookkeeping

Bookkeeping is the recording of financial transactions and is a precise skill that requires attention to detail. Bookkeeping is a continual process and should be done on a daily basis. Most offices use computer software for bookkeeping. However, bookkeeping is still performed manually in some smaller offices. The medical assistant or office manager might perform bookkeeping, or the medical practice can hire a bookkeeper. All receipts and charges should be entered immediately into a computerized accounting system or manual journal. Receipts, in duplicate, must be written for all money received. One copy is given to the patient, and one copy stays in the office file.

Transactions are classified into five types of accounts:

- **Asset** (resources)
- **Liability** (debts)
- Income (revenue)
- Expense (purchases)
- Equity (earnings)

Each of these has many sub-accounts.

The basic accounting equation is:

$$Assets - Liabilities = Equity$$

The financial activity of a business is recorded using a method called **double-entry bookkeeping** because every transaction affects two accounts by increasing one and decreasing the other. Thus, each transaction is entered twice. Accountants refer to these entries as **debits** and **credits**. Any increase in expense (debit) must be offset by a decrease in assets or increase in liability (credit). For example, a purchase of paper increases office supplies (expense) and decreases cash (asset) or increases accounts payable (liability).

The chart of accounts is a listing of the categories used to track the sub-accounts of assets, liabilities, income, expenses, and equity (Figure 18-1). Each account is assigned a number that must be recorded when entering financial data. Some computerized systems show the user the verbal description of the account and enter the corresponding account number automatically.

Accounting

Accounting is the system of reporting the financial results of a business. The purpose of accounting is to make an analysis, a statement, or a summary about financial matters. At the end of each month, business owners, including physicians, review

Account	Name	Type
1100	Operating cash	Asset
1200	Petty cash	Asset
1300	Accounts receivable	Asset
1400	Equipment	Asset
2100	Account payable	Liability
2200	Payroll	Liability
2300	Accrued taxes	Liability
2400	Dept	Liability
3100	Patient services	Revenue
3200	Interest income	Revenue
4100	Utilities	Expense
4200	Rent/lease	Expense
4300	Liability insurance	Expense
4400	Salaries	Expense
5100	Partners' equity	Equity

FIGURE 18-1 Example of a chart of accounts.

financial statements for the month that report the amount of money received and spent, assets owned, liabilities owed, and the profit or earnings of the operation. This information helps physicians evaluate the financial health of the practice and identifies changes that might be desirable. Many physicians hire an accountant or accounting service to prepare tax returns and to prepare financial statements that are used to obtain bank financing. If the physician is in a partnership with other physicians, the accountant's financial statements assist in dividing the earnings among the partners.

Accounts Receivable

Accounts receivable (AR) is money owed to the medical practice for services provided. In most offices, the majority of AR consists of reimbursement from insurance companies and other third-party payers on behalf of patients. A lesser portion of AR is due directly from patients for copayments, coinsurance, deductibles, and noncovered items. Amounts due from patients who do not have insurance are also part of the AR.

Accounts Payable

Accounts payable (AP) is money that the medical office owes to vendors, suppliers, utility companies, and others for services rendered. The following are examples of AP expenditures:

- Office supplies (paper, pens, computer supplies)
- Medical supplies and equipment

- Equipment repair and maintenance
- Housekeeping/janitorial service
- Utilities (telephone, Internet, electric, heat, and water)
- Income taxes
- Payroll
- Occupancy (rent, lease, or mortgage)

Records relating to accounts payable include the following:

- **Purchase order** (a document produced by the medical office that authorizes the buyer to place an order)
- **Packing slip** (a document the shipper sends with the product that lists the item(s) in the package)
- **Invoice** (a bill from the shipper that documents the total amount due)

When paying a bill, the medical assistant, or bookkeeper, should confirm that the purchase order, packing slip, and invoice agree regarding the quantity and cost of items ordered, delivered, and paid. These three documents should be stapled together or scanned, together with the check stub and filed in the appropriate location in the office.

Banking

The basic banking functions are depositing funds, writing checks, transferring funds between bank accounts, withdrawing funds, and reconciling statements. Most of the funds that come into a medical office are from the collection of accounts receivable.

The medical office uses funds (money) in a checking or savings account to pay business-related expenses. A bank account used for paying out, or disbursing, funds is called a **disbursement account**. When funds are moved from one account to another or used as cash, transactions must be managed in a systematic manner and accurately documented. Monthly statements for both checking and savings accounts must be reconciled or balanced to determine what money is available for use.

Bank records are subject to government examination because the federal government regulates banking practices. In addition, the accountant for the medical practice needs accurate records for preparation of federal, and perhaps state, tax returns. Because the medical assistant is not present when the accountant reviews the books, all information the medical assistant has entered must be clear and accurate. The income and expenses reported on the medical office's income tax return must be verifiable against deposits and expenditures from the office's bank accounts.

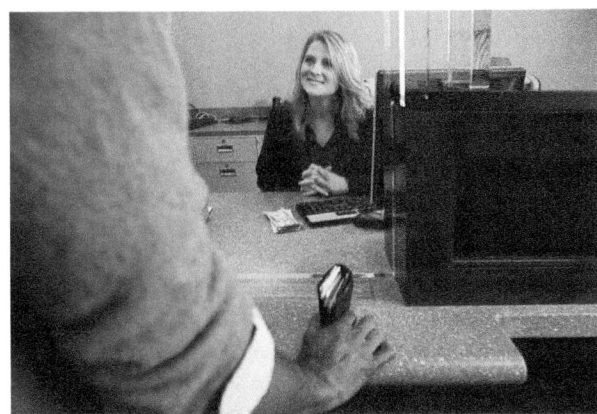

FIGURE 18-2 Bank teller assisting with customer service.

Types of Bank Accounts

Banks offer both checking and savings accounts for their customers (Figure 18-2). A checking account is the most common type of disbursement account because it allows the owner of the account to withdraw money from the account by writing checks, which are used as payment for outstanding debts (bills). Cash can also be withdrawn from a checking account. Checking accounts are not usually interest-bearing accounts. Some accounts earn interest if there is a minimum balance in the account. Generally, the bank charges a fee, or service charge (e.g., $5 per month), to maintain the account.

A savings account is an interest-bearing account in which funds not needed for daily expenses can be placed. Interest is earned monthly or quarterly. This means the bank calculates a certain percentage (such as 2 percent) based on the average balance during a month and pays that amount to the account. Cash can be withdrawn from a savings account or transferred into a checking account. There is usually a limit to the number of monthly withdrawals allowed before a fee is assessed. Savings accounts generally are not disbursement accounts because funds must be transferred to a checking account to use or an electronic transfer must be initiated.

A money market account is an investment tool with check-writing privileges and usually pays a higher interest rate than traditional savings accounts. It typically requires a minimum balance of $500 to $5,000, depending on the institution. Money market accounts can be used as disbursement accounts, but the number of checks that can written each month might be limited.

Computerized Accounting Systems

Many offices use computerized accounting systems to manage their finances. This is a time- and cost-savings and greatly reduces the risk of miscalculations. A computerized accounting system enables you to enter the data in real time,

Professionalism The Workplace

Speed and accuracy with the numeric keypad is essential. The placement of number keys on a computer keyboard numeric keypad and on a manual 10-key calculator are similar. Touch-typing is the skill of being able to accurately key in information without watching the keyboard. This enables you to keep your eyes on the source document, which speeds data entry. Some employers require job applicants to take a keyboarding test before scheduling an interview. A minimum acceptable 10-key rate is 8,000 to 10,000 keystrokes per hour (ksh). For jobs requiring a lot of data entry, a 10-key rate of 15,000 ksh or higher is desirable.

eliminates the need for redundancy, and implements double-entry bookkeeping automatically.

Customized reports can be generated easily for any time period desired, such as daily, weekly, monthly, quarterly, and annually. Year-end reports can be provided to an outside accountant for allocation of earnings among the partners and income tax preparation. Computer entries should always be backed up with source documents such as invoices and purchase orders. Computerized accounting systems may be able to integrate seamlessly with the patient accounting system, so that patient accounts are always in balance with the overall practice income and AR.

Each user of a computerized accounting system should have a unique login, which consists of a username and password. You may be asked to change your password periodically, such as every 30, 60, or 90 days. The system administrator sets permission levels for each user, which provides access only to the functions of the software required to perform job duties. The software creates a user log that identifies when each user was logged in and data that each viewed, entered, or modified. Never share your password with another employee, and do not allow anyone to use your computer while you are logged in.

Online Banking

Most banks provide an **online banking** service to their customers. Online banking provides the customer with bank account access 24 hours a day, 7 days a week, using a secure website established by the bank. Customers can perform most transactions online that previously required the account holder to physically go to the bank.

Online banking functions include all of the following: account reconciliation, bill payments, viewing account activity including deposits and processed checks, checking account balances (the total amount of money in the account),

and transferring money between accounts. Another advantage of online banking is the ability to download data from the bank website directly to the customer's accounting software.

Online banking is a paperless system, so it is important that records be kept in the office. When a bill is paid, it must be noted in the accounts payable (AP) records to ensure that the office's records are up-to-date.

Banks require a highly secure system of usernames, passwords, and other security features to access the account. The medical practice should restrict access to online accounts to only a few individuals and should change the logins frequently.

The Role of Medical Assistants in Practice Finances

The role of medical assistants in practice finances varies by office. Medical assistants frequently are involved in one or more aspects of accounts receivable and, in smaller offices, can have some responsibilities for accounts payable or banking. Medical assistants are multiskilled staff members who need to be flexible and willing to help wherever needed. They must be knowledgeable of financial policies and procedures and able to follow them exactly as written. Accuracy and attention to detail are mandatory, because even minor errors have a far-reaching impact on the practice. Finally, legal and ethical behavior is essential. Awareness of legalities and the ability to practice high ethical standards are mandatory for medical assistants involved in practice finances.

Preventing Financial Fraud

Fraud and **embezzlement** (unauthorized taking of funds) are of great concern for all businesses, and medical practices are no exception. The staff is often close-knit, and physicians place a great deal of trust in their staff, including medical assistants. Often, because of the stress of managing a practice, physicians rely heavily on one or two individuals to handle financial matters. After all, the physician went into medicine to care for patients, not to become a financial manager.

The risk is that when any person is entrusted with too much financial responsibility, the opportunity for fraud and embezzlement exists. Usually it begins in a seemingly innocent way, such as appropriating a small "loan" for oneself to make it through a difficult personal situation, with full intent of repaying the practice before anyone notices. Such situations rarely resolve as intended, and the individuals soon may feel entitled to "borrow" more funds as repayment for all their hard work for the physician. They may rationalize that because there appears to be a large amount of money flowing through the practice, diverting a small amount will not make much difference. The situation can spiral out of control rapidly, and by the time it is discovered, physicians may find they have lost hundreds or thousands of dollars to someone they considered to be "family."

This is a concern to medical assistants for two reasons. First, you never want to put yourself in a situation where you could be tempted to do something you never imagined you were capable of. Second, you want to make sure that you do not get blamed for the potential wrongdoing of another staff member. Fortunately, the accounting field defines a system of checks and balances, called **internal controls**, that helps prevent these things from occurring.

Separation of Duties

Separation of duties is a set of internal controls that reduce the risk of fraud and embezzlement by dividing financial responsibilities into distinct tasks and assigning each task to a different individual. The concept behind separation of duties is that any person who has multiple roles in handling finances has the opportunity to abuse those privileges and powers. No single person should have control over the entire life span of a transaction. This means that the same person should not be able to initiate, record, authorize, and reconcile a transaction, such as accepting money from patients, recording it in the computer, making the deposit, and reconciling the bank statement. Figure 18-3 provides examples of internal controls for a medical office.

Bonding

Medical offices should have business insurance that protects the business against losses of property and assets because of theft and physical damage. One component of business insurance is a **fidelity bond**, or employee dishonesty coverage. Bonding not only helps protect the business against theft, it can discourage employees from trying to steal because they know they will be aggressively investigated by the insurance company. The insurance company is not sympathetic to the dishonest employee's point of view, regardless of the reasons that may be given for stealing.

Employers can choose from three types of fidelity bonds, each with different requirements and different levels of coverage:

- Rotate financial duties among staff members, especially those involving cash and deposits.
- Issue numbered receipts for all patient payments made in the office.
- Assign two people to count the cash at the end of the day.
- The person who accepts copayments should be different from the person who makes the deposit.
- The person who prepares insurance bills and patient statements does not post payments.
- The person who posts payments does not pay bills.
- Write-offs and refunds must be approved in writing by the physician.
- The physician, outside accountant, or other person with little involvement in other financial transactions reconciles the bank statement and reviews all cleared checks.
- Login information for the computerized accounting system is changed frequently and never shared with another staff member.
- Do not allow any other person to access the accounting system while you are logged in.
- Establish electronic permissions for each authorized user of the computer system, so that each person is limited in the information they can enter or change.
- Review system user logs regularly that document who has accessed various aspects of the accounting system.
- Conduct background checks and credit checks before hiring new employees.
- Bond all employees.
- Authorize a limited number of people to sign checks. Require two signatures on checks over a certain dollar amount.
- Require purchase orders for all nonroutine expenses. The person who authorizes purchase orders should not write checks.
- Require written authorization of any payments not associated with an invoice.
- Keep blank checks in locked cabinet with limited access.

FIGURE 18-3 Examples of internal controls.

- **Name schedule fidelity bond**—Each time the medical office hires an employee it wants to bond, it must submit the employee's name to the insurance company to activate coverage. To have a claim accepted, the employer must be able to prove that the specific individual committed the theft.

- **Blanket position fidelity bond**—Everyone who works in a specific position is bonded, and new employees are added automatically. Claims do not require proof of the specific individual who committed the theft.

- **Primary commercial blanket bond**—All employees are covered as a single unit, and individual names are not submitted. Claims are based on the total amount of the loss, not on how many employees may have been involved.

Some businesses require employees who handle cash to personally purchase **surety bond** insurance as a condition of employment. The bonding company evaluates each applicant's background for eligibility. The individual is responsible to pay the application fee and monthly premium.

Professionalism The Law

The United States Department of Labor sponsors the Federal Bonding Program to encourage companies to hire people who are considered high-risk. Bond coverage is provided for *any* person with a risk factor in his personal background that may cause employers to question his honesty. Examples are ex-felons, substance abusers, persons discharged from the military with a dishonorable discharge, and those with poor credit history or bankruptcy. People in these groups have difficulty obtaining jobs that involve handling money because the company's existing fidelity bond excludes such employees from coverage.

The Federal Bonding Program issues bonds to employers, free of charge. The employer is then able to obtain the worker's skills while minimizing the risk of employee dishonesty. Individuals who know that their background may cause an employer concern can obtain federal bonding before applying for a job. This improves their chances of being hired but does not require a company to hire them. Each state administers the Federal Bonding Program through its job office, often called a Workforce/One-Stop office. The toll-free number to locate your state's office is 1-877-US2-JOBS.

Professionalism The Workplace

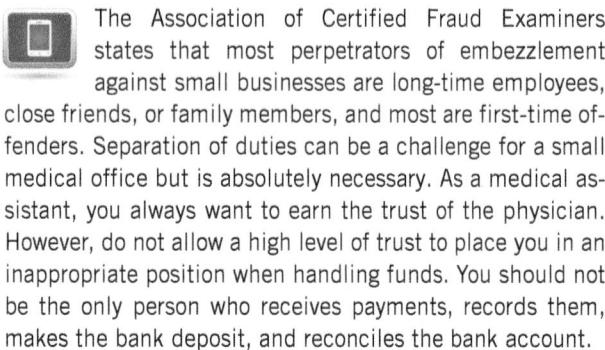

The Association of Certified Fraud Examiners states that most perpetrators of embezzlement against small businesses are long-time employees, close friends, or family members, and most are first-time offenders. Separation of duties can be a challenge for a small medical office but is absolutely necessary. As a medical assistant, you always want to earn the trust of the physician. However, do not allow a high level of trust to place you in an inappropriate position when handling funds. You should not be the only person who receives payments, records them, makes the bank deposit, and reconciles the bank account.

You need to insist on a separation of duties to protect your own integrity, as well as to protect the physician. At the very least, two people should prepare and sign off on the deposit, and the person who reconciles the bank account should not be responsible for making deposits or writing checks. If necessary, suggest that the physician hire an outside accountant to reconcile the bank statements each month. Although this may seem like an inconvenience to the physician at first, ultimately your honesty and concern for the physician's security will be appreciated. You do not want to be in a position where you could be falsely accused of mishandling the finances. You want to ensure that the physician's financial matters are organized in such a way as to protect against fraud or embezzlement, whether you are personally present.

CHECKS

Working with checking accounts is a basic banking function. Checking account activities include accepting checks, depositing checks, writing checks, transferring funds between accounts, and reconciling accounts.

A check is a written order to a bank to pay or transfer money to an individual, business, or other entity. A check, which is payable on demand, is considered a negotiable instrument. A **negotiable instrument** is one that actualizes, or permits, the transfer of money to another person. To have a negotiable instrument, the check must:

- Be written and signed by an authorized payer of the check
- State a sum of money to be paid
- Be payable on demand or at a fixed date in the future
- Be payable to the holder (payee) of the check

Most offices maintain the checkbook as part of an accounting software package. Checks must be purchased that are compatible both with the software program and with the printer used to print checks. If checks are to be written manually, they can be purchased from the bank or a company that specializes in printing checks. Manual checks can be provided as single checks in a pad or in a page format with several checks per page that can be stored in a notebook. Medical offices can also use a duplicate or write-it-once check system in which a carbon strip on the back of the check allows a record of the check to be made when the check is written.

Information on Checks

Standard information is included on all checks regardless of the bank that issues them. See Figure 18-4 for a labeled example of the standard parts of a check. This preprinted information includes the following:

- Name and address of the **payer** (person signing the check to release the money)
- Name of the bank on which the check is drawn
- Preprinted sequential number on each check
- Space to enter the full date
- American Bank Association (ABA) number that identifies the bank on which the check is drawn
- "Pay to the order of" space in which to enter the name of the **payee** (person or company to receive the money)
- Space in which to write the amount of the check in words
- Small box or space in which to enter the amount of the check in numbers

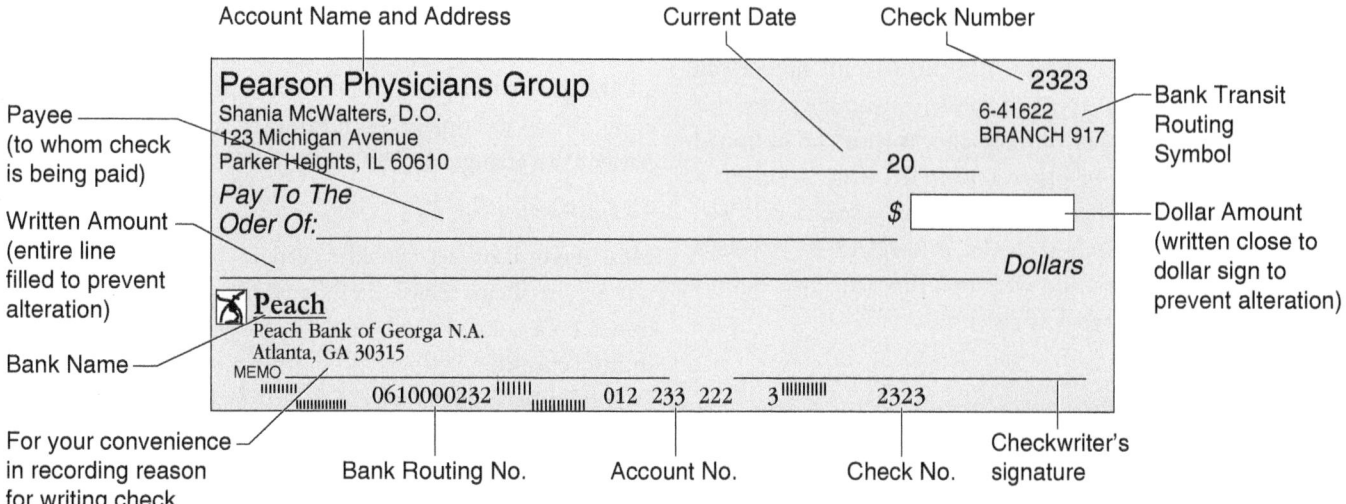

Labels around the check:
- Account Name and Address
- Current Date
- Check Number
- Payee (to whom check is being paid)
- Written Amount (entire line filled to prevent alteration)
- Bank Name
- For your convenience in recording reason for writing check
- Bank Transit Routing Symbol
- Dollar Amount (written close to dollar sign to prevent alteration)
- Bank Routing No.
- Account No.
- Check No.
- Checkwriter's signature

Check text:
Pearson Physicians Group
Shania McWalters, D.O.
123 Michigan Avenue
Parker Heights, IL 60610

2323
6-41622
BRANCH 917

20 ____

Pay To The Oder Of: ____

$ ____

____ Dollars

Peach
Peach Bank of Georga N.A.
Atlanta, GA 30315
MEMO ____

0610000232 012 233 222 3 2323

FIGURE 18-4 Labeled parts of a check.

- Space for the signature of payer
- Preprinted name and address of bank
- Magnetic ink character recognition (MICR) figures used for bank processing of the check

The blank spaces on a check must be completed in order for a bank to honor and cash the check.

ABA Number

The **American Bankers Association (ABA) number** is located in the upper-right corner of a printed check. It is printed as a fraction on a business check or as a straight series of numbers (1–109/210) on a personal check. The ABA originated this number to identify the area where the bank issuing the check is located, as well as to identify the individual bank.

Magnetic Ink Character Recognition

Magnetic ink character recognition (MICR) is a system of combining characters and numbers located at the bottom left side of checks and deposit slips. The MICR is read by high-speed machinery, increasing the speed and accuracy of processing bank statements and check sorting. It also facilitates the bookkeeping process within the bank. Printed on each check, the MICR consists of three series of numbers. The first series of numbers is the bank routing number that identifies the bank and its location. The second series of numbers identifies the individual account. The third series of numbers is the check number, which matches the preprinted number in the upper-right corner of the check. During bank processing, additional numbers are printed across the bottom of the check to indicate the amount of the check.

Check Security

An unused check is referred to as a **blank check** because it contains only the preprinted account information but no payment information. A blank check is as vulnerable as cash in the hands of the wrong person because payment information can be filled in, along with a forged or stamped signature, and cashed. Blank checks must be stored in a securely locked location to which only one or two people have access.

If signature stamps are used, they should be kept in a locked location that can be accessed only by the person whose name is on the signature stamp, such as the physician. Unsecured signature stamps can easily be misused by a dishonest person, because they eliminate the need to forge a signature, so the recipient of the check and the bank cannot tell it was written inappropriately.

Advantages of Checks

Checks are recommended for all business transactions because they provide a level of security and documentation not available through any other means. Advantages of checks include the following:

- Safety of funds
- Convenience
- Ease of maintaining records
- Documentation of money transfers
- Reliability of records for tax purposes
- Summary of deposits from receipts
- Protection while money is in the bank account (banks carry insurance to cover loss)
- Stop-payment orders that can be issued by the payer to protect any lost or stolen checks

Special Purpose Checks

In addition to account checks that the account holder can issue, there are several types of check instruments used for special purposes. Special purpose checks must be obtained directly from a bank or other authorized institution for a specific transaction. These include cashier's checks, certified checks, bank drafts, limited checks, money orders, traveler's checks, voucher checks, and warrants. Box 18-1 lists definitions of the different types of checks.

Accepting Checks

An office policy should be in place to guide staff regarding accepting checks from patients as payment for services. Most of the time, it is acceptable for patients to pay for services with a personal check. When a check is received, it should be inspected for validity and locked in a secure location, such as the cash box.

Financial Agents

Some patients may have a **financial agent**, another individual who is authorized to sign the check on the patient's behalf. This may be implemented through a **power-of-attorney (POA)** document or because the financial agent is a designated cosigner on the bank account. A notation should be made in the patient's computer account or financial file regarding who is permitted to sign checks for the patient. If a POA grants this power, the medical office should request a copy of the document each time it is used, because the patient can change the POA at any time.

Third-Party Checks

Most medical offices consider certain checks risky and may not accept them. These include third-party checks, checks drawn on an out-of-town bank, cash-back checks, and "paid in full" checks.

A **third-party check** is a check written by a party unknown to you. You are considered the first party in this process because the medical office is the one collecting the money. The patient (the second party), the payee, has received a check from another person (the third party) to pay that patient's medical bill. You are at risk in accepting a third-party check, because you do not know the payer who has signed the check and have no contact information on the payer. The check might be invalid, and there might not be funds available in the original account to cover the check. Third-party checks should not be accepted unless they come from a known source, such as an insurance company or guarantor (financially responsible party), for a bill the medical office submitted.

BOX 18-1 | Special Purpose Checks

- *Cashier's checks* are written using the bank's own check or form and are issued by the bank. A cashier's check guarantees the money is available because the bank deducts the money from the purchaser's checking or savings account when the check is issued. The purchaser can also pay cash for the check. There is usually a charge for this service.
- *Certified checks* are written on the payer's own check form, then stamped by a teller to guarantee that funds are available to redeem the check. The bank withdraws the money from the payer's account when it certifies the check.
- *Bank drafts* are checks that are drawn up by a bank against funds (money) that are deposited to its account in another bank.
- *Limited checks* are issued on special check forms that contain a preprinted maximum dollar amount for which the check can be written. There may also be a time limit during which the check is valid or must be cashed. Limited checks are used for payroll checks and insurance payments.
- *Money orders* are prepaid payment orders that can be purchased from banks, the United States Postal Service, and other authorized agents. A money order is purchased with cash, plus a service fee. Money orders are safe to accept as payment, because they are prepaid and there is no chance that the funds will be taken back. Many consider money orders to be safer than personal checks or cashier's checks. Money orders are frequently used by individuals who do not have bank accounts when a check is needed, because it is recommended that cash not be sent through the mail.
- *Traveler's checks* are prepaid checks from an authorized agent that can be used in place of cash. They are preprinted in dollar amounts similar to currency ($10, $20, $50, $100, $500, and $1,000) and are prepaid at the time the user obtains them. Considered a safe means for carrying money when traveling, traveler's checks are also convenient because most places accept a traveler's check and only the original purchaser can cash it. There is a space for two signatures of the payer: one at the time of purchase and another when the check is cashed. The payee is able to compare the two signatures, thus protecting the payer in the event the check is stolen or lost. People purchasing traveler's checks are advised to always sign the checks at the time of purchase before leaving the bank.
- *Warrants* are not actually negotiable checks. They are statements issued to indicate that debts should be paid. For example, an insurance adjuster may issue a warrant indicating that a fire insurance claim should be paid. This warrant then becomes authorization to the insurance company to issue a check as payment.

You might encounter situations in which the insurance company pays the patient instead of the medical office. The patient brings the insurance check to the office, applies a special endorsement in which the patient signs the check over to the office, and then the office adds its endorsement and deposits it. Some automobile insurance companies do not recognize an assignment of benefits in which the patient authorizes the insurance company to pay the physician directly. In such cases, office policy may allow you to accept a third-party check, because you know who issued the check and the face value of the check is the amount the patient owes.

Out-of-Town Banks

Checks from accounts outside the local area are generally not accepted unless the payer is an established patient. It is difficult to collect payment if a check is not good, you might have little contact with a patient from out of town, and it might not be easy to reach an out-of-town bank concerning the validity of a check, before accepting it.

Cash-Back

A cash-back check is a check that a person writes for more than the amount owed so that the payee will refund the difference in cash. This is an easy way for the check writer to obtain cash. For example, a payer who owes $30 would write a check for $50 and request $20 in "change." Some retail establishments, such as grocery stores, accept such checks, but medical offices should never accept checks for more than the amount owed. This practice increases the risks associated with accepting personal checks, such as nonsufficient funds, and places an unnecessary burden on medical offices to manage the cash box.

"Paid in Full"

Checks written with the statement added "Paid in Full" should be avoided. Patients sometimes write this on their check when they believe they no longer owe any money to the physician. If you deposit the check, you acknowledge that this is correct. Therefore, if the patient still owes money on the bill and you deposit the check, you might have difficulty collecting any further payments.

Endorsement of Checks

To transfer money from one person to another, the check must be endorsed. According to federal banking regulations, an **endorsement** is placed on the back of the check within the top 1.5 inches on the left side of the check as it is turned over. The upper-left corner is referred to as the "trailing edge" of a check. If the endorsement is not placed within this designated area or extends beyond the 1.5-inch mark, it can be refused by a bank.

An endorsement can consist of either a payee's written or rubber stamped signature. To discourage theft, checks should be endorsed "For Deposit Only" as soon as they arrive in the mail or are accepted from a patient.

It is common procedure in a medical office to endorse checks as soon as they are received. This often is done with an endorsement stamp that contains the doctor's name, the account number, and the name of the bank. Some checks specify that the check must be cashed within a set period of time, such as 90 or 180 days. If the check has not been presented for payment within the time suggested on the check, it is considered a **stale check**.

Endorsements are regulated by the Uniform Negotiable Instrument Act. A check that has been transferred to more than one person (third-party payer) has more than one endorsement on the back. Types of endorsements are discussed in Table 18-1.

Bank Hold on Accounts

Occasionally, a bank places a *hold* on funds in a checking account. Before allowing anyone to draw on those funds, an Uncollected Funds Hold (UCF or UFH) may be attached to the deposited funds that must "clear" before the bank knows the funds are present. This typically occurs with checks written for large sums. The bank does not actually credit the account in which the money was deposited until the check has been processed and the funds paid to the payer's bank. These funds cannot be used by the depositor until the check or funds have cleared and the hold is removed. The bank notifies the depositor of the length of time for the hold.

Returned Checks

A check may be returned by the bank for a variety of reasons. When this occurs, a notice detailing the reason for the return is also included with the check. Checks are returned, for example, when the payee name, date, or signature of payer is

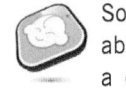

Professionalism The Life Span

Sometimes an older adult who is physically unable to write a check, or who cannot see to write a check, designates an agent to write and sign checks for him or her. Most often it is a family member. This is an arrangement the person has made with the bank, and it is a perfectly legitimate and legal way to handle finances. When money is owed to the doctor's office, it is usually the agent who writes the check for the patient, but it is credited to the patient's account.

TABLE 18-1 | Endorsements

Endorsement	Description	Example
Blank	Signature of the payee. After being endorsed, the check can be cashed by anyone. This is not used in the business office.	*Shania McWalter*
Restrictive	Specifies the money's purpose, such as "For Deposit Only." It is considered the safest endorsement because if the check is misplaced, no one else should be able to cash it.	PAY TO THE ORDER OF FIRST TOWN BANK FOR DEPOSIT ONLY SHANIA MCWALTER, D.O. 123–123456
Special	The payee signs the check over to another person. This type of endorsement should not be accepted by a medical office unless the check is from an insurance company that paid the patient. The medical office should re-endorse the check below the first endorsement.	*Jon Ulrich pay to the order of Shania McWalter, D.O.* PAY TO THE ORDER OF FIRST TOWN BANK FOR DEPOSIT ONLY SHANIA MCWALTER, D.O. 123–123456

missing. If a check is returned with the payee's name or date missing, it is acceptable for the medical assistant to fill in the date and physician's name. If the payer's signature is missing, then the check must be returned to the payer. It is always wise to place a telephone call to a patient with the reasons for returning the check. All checks should be reviewed before adding a written or stamped endorsement for deposit.

Nonsufficient funds (NSF) in the payer's account and the stop-payment order, issued by the payer, are two of the more serious reasons for the return of a check. In the case of NSF, the payer's account does not have enough money to cover the amount of the check, so the bank returns it to the payee. The medical office should contact the writer of the check and ask how he or she wishes to make the payment. The patient (payer) may state that funds are now available in the account and ask that the check be resubmitted. To resubmit a check, write the word *Resubmit* on both the face and the back of the check, make out another deposit slip, and resubmit it. Many banks charge a fee to the depositor if a deposited check is NSF. This charge should be passed on to the patient.

Some medical offices have a policy that if a check is returned for NSF, they do not resubmit the check. They request the payment be made immediately, with cash, money order, or a cashier's check. A cashier's check guarantees payment, because it is written on a check drafted by a bank. Offices may also accept payment in the form of a certified check, which is a check written on the patient's check but is

Professionalism **The Workplace**

As a medical assistant working in the administrative office, you may be the individual responsible for discussing the office financial and check handling practices with the patients. This is an important rule because it safeguards the patient and the physician from loss of money through carelessness. Many offices provide their patients with an informational pamphlet prepared specifically for your office with guidelines and options for payment of services. Patients should also be instructed not to send cash through the mail.

guaranteed by the bank because money has been set aside in the patient's account.

If a **stop-payment order** has been issued by the payer, then the bank does not allow the funds to be disbursed. The bank indicates that you should contact the payer with the terms" Refer to Maker" on the item notice. This procedure is used when a check has been lost or stolen.

DEPOSITS

Making deposits is a basic banking function. **Deposits** are cash, checks, and money orders placed into a bank account after being received. Medical offices can make deposits to checking accounts and savings accounts. Office policies and procedures should outline into which accounts funds should be deposited. Offices vary on specific methods of handling deposits, but the following procedures are usually followed:

- Prepare and make deposits daily.
- Maintain all records of daily receipts (for checks, cash, money orders, and credit card transactions) in a safe location.
- Compare the total on the deposit slip against the total on the day sheet for checks and cash.
- Keep a duplicate copy of deposits on file in the office. Photocopy the deposit slip before submitting it to the bank. Some offices copy checks for later reference.
- Keep bank receipts for deposits on file in the office.
- Immediately record deposits in the checkbook.

The frequency of making deposits may depend on several factors. If there is a significant distance between the office and the bank, deposits might not be made as frequently as if the bank were closer to the office. Most banks provide courier service to businesses, in which the bank sends a bonded person to personally pick up your deposit and deliver it to the bank for processing. Large offices might make several deposits per day to help reduce the possibility of losing money. It is important to remember that the sooner money is deposited, the sooner it is available to pay bills. Until cash and checks can be deposited, they should be stored in a safe or other secure location that is not accessible to patients or unauthorized staff members.

Completing the Deposit Slip

A deposit slip is completed every time a deposit is made into a bank account. The slip indicates the total dollar amounts of cash and checks being deposited. Entries on the slip should be printed in black ink. Currency (coins and bills) is totaled separately from checks. Procedure 18-1 lists steps for preparing deposit slips. See Figure 18-5 for an example of a deposit slip.

Compare the total on the deposit slip against the day sheet totals for cash and checks. If the two figures do not match, look for the error in several ways:

- Recalculate the math on the deposit slip.
- Verify each item on the deposit slip is entered correctly.
- Look for transposed numbers.

- If the error is still not found, subtract the difference between the deposit slip and the day sheet, then search for an item with that number.
- Look for checks that might have been omitted from the listing on the deposit slip.

Credit card payments are not included in the deposit because they are deposited electronically by the merchant credit card company that handles the office's credit card transactions.

Computer-Generated Deposit Slips

The accounting software program usually can generate a deposit slip for you based on payments entered into the computer since the last deposit. This helps ensure the accuracy of the numbers and guarantees that the deposit slip reconciles with the day sheet. Any payments that were missed or not entered into the software for another reason do not appear on a computer-generated deposit slip. You must match the physical checks and cash with the deposit slip to verify that all monies are accounted for. You also should run a total of the physical checks to verify that they match the amount on the deposit slip.

Deposit to Savings Accounts

When the amount in a checking account becomes greater than the amount needed to cover the checks written on the

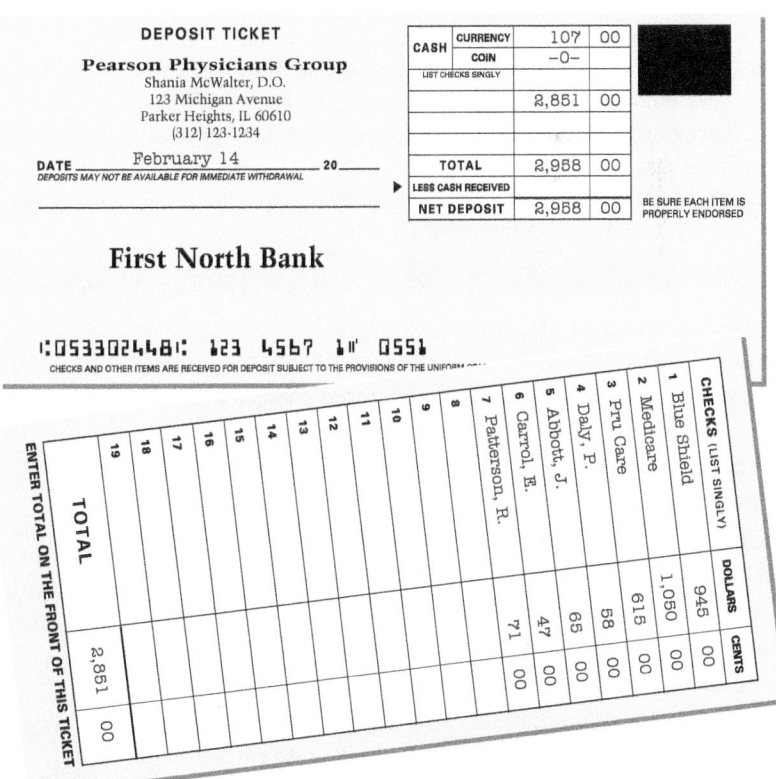

FIGURE 18-5 An example of the front and back sides of a deposit slip.

Preparing a Bank Deposit

Objective ◆ *Complete a bank deposit slip.*

EQUIPMENT AND SUPPLIES

Pen; deposit slip; checks and currency to be deposited; endorsing stamp; calculator

METHOD

1. Verify that each check has been endorsed. If any checks were not previously endorsed, apply the endorsing stamp to the back of the check.
2. Complete the information on the front of the deposit slip:
   - Account name (if not preprinted)
   - Account number (if not preprinted)
   - Date of the deposit
3. If there is cash to be deposited, enter the total amount of the cash in the designated space on the deposit slip beside the CASH indicator. In the CURRENCY box, list the total amount of all cash paper money to be deposited. In the Coin box, list the total of all the cash coin money to be deposited. Organize the currency bills in descending order by face value, with all bills face-up. For instance, group $100 bills together face-up, then all $50 face-up, and so on.
4. List each check to be deposited on a different line. If you have more checks than fit on the front, list each additional check on the reverse side of the deposit slip. List money orders last.
5. On each numbered line, write the name of the person who wrote the check and the dollar amount of the check.
6. List each check in a different numbered box.
7. Use a calculator to add all the checks entered on the reverse side of the deposit slip, and enter the total of the checks in the space at the bottom of the deposit slip that reads TOTAL. This amount is also placed on the front of the deposit slip in the space that reads TOTAL FROM REVERSE SIDE.
8. Use the calculator to add the total amount of the cash and the checks being deposited. List this amount in the space labeled TOTAL and in the space labeled NET DEPOSIT on the front of the deposit slip.
9. Verify your totals.
   - Add all the dollar amounts listed on the deposit slip *in reverse order* from what you did the first time. The total should be the same.
   - Then, go through the stack of checks and add up the amounts as written on the checks. This total should match the one written on the deposit slip.
   - Do the same for currency and coins.
   - If there is any discrepancy, even 1 cent, check for transposition errors when writing the numbers on the deposit slip and for keying errors on the calculator. If you cannot find the error, ask someone else to review the deposit.
10. Place the deposit slip and the cash and checks listed on the slip in an envelope for deposit to the bank.

---

account, cash and checks can also be deposited or transferred into a savings account to earn more interest than in a checking account. Office policy should specify the conditions in which deposits should to be made into a savings account, or it may require that all funds be deposited in the checking account first for tracking purposes, then transferred to the savings account in a separate transaction. Transferring funds from a checking account to a savings account can be done by check or electronically, if the office uses online banking.

A savings account is set up with a register similar to those used with checking accounts. The register is used to maintain a record of deposits, withdrawals, interest earned, and account balance. The bank sends statements on savings accounts monthly or quarterly.

Making the Deposit

Deposits can be made to both the checking and savings accounts in person, by mail, by night depository, or picked up by a bank courier. When a deposit is made in person, a receipt is issued at the time the deposit is made. When a deposit is made by any other method, a receipt is sent back to you by mail. Cash should never be sent in the mail, but can be deposited in a night depository or when using a bank courier. Use a locking money bag that has a locked zipper for cash deposits not delivered in person.

A night depository is a bin or slot on the outside of the bank. You need to obtain a night depository key from the bank and use money bags with security locks. The deposit slip, cash, and checks are placed in the bag and then placed in the bin at the end of the day when the bank may be closed. For security purposes, the office might require that two people take the deposit to the bank together.

Some banks offer a free courier service for businesses. You can schedule a pickup on a regular basis, such as daily or three times per week, or call in advance when a pickup is needed. Use a locking money bag if cash is deposited using a courier.

Online banking might allow you to deposit checks electronically. To accomplish this, you need to scan the front and back (with endorsement) of each check, then follow the bank's procedures for uploading the scanned images. When making an electronic deposit, the physical check is never transmitted to the bank. Such checks must be clearly marked as having been deposited electronically and stored in a secure location so they are not mistakenly redeposited. Currency and coins cannot be deposited electronically.

It is preferable that one designated person be responsible for the deposits and another for the accounts receivable records. This is an internal control that promotes separation of duties.

Accepting and Depositing Cash

Cash can be accepted as a form of payment. However, most patients pay either with check or credit card. Currency should be checked with a counterfeit detection device. Prenumbered receipts must be issued, in duplicate, for all cash payments. The patient receives one copy, and the office retains the second copy. Having large amounts of cash in an office poses a security risk and also offers the potential for the embezzlement of funds. Large cash amounts may necessitate making bank deposits more than once a day to minimize cash on hand.

Saving Documentation

Documents relating to banking procedures should be saved in an organized manner. In addition to banking documents, such as copies of deposit slips and check stubs, your records must include the following proofs of business expenses:

- Receipts
- Vouchers for expenses and salaries
- Invoices
- Statements from suppliers
- Proof of payments

Supporting documents should be saved in a file with check numbers of payments written on the document. After the bank statement has been reconciled each month, it should be stored with the **cancelled checks** as further documentation of business activity. Remember that business expenses are subject to auditing by the Internal Revenue

Service (IRS). Good record keeping is essential when providing documentation to the IRS.

PAYING BILLS

All bills should be paid by check for documentation and control purposes. The only exception to this policy would be very small payments, such as daily newspaper delivery and public transportation costs that can be made from petty cash. However, it is advisable that all payments, even the daily newspaper, be paid from accounts established with appropriate vendors.

Cash disbursement refers to a payment made to creditors from the accounting asset account labeled "Cash." Usually, the disbursement is made by check, not currency. Payment by check provides a permanent document for proof of payment and tax purposes.

An office policy must be established regarding how often checks are written—such as weekly, biweekly, semimonthly, or monthly. The bill-paying schedule must match a schedule of when funds are available for payment of office expenses. For instance, your office policy might be to send patient statements at the end of the month for payments that are due on the first of the next month. In this case, you may not want to write checks against your account to pay office expenses during the last week of the month if the account balance is typically low.

The office banking policy should indicate who is responsible for writing and signing checks. A smart policy is to separate the responsibilities; one person (the medical assistant) should write the checks, and another person should be authorized to sign them (office manager or physician). In some medical offices, two authorized signatures are required to transfer funds from one account to another or to write checks over a certain dollar amount, such as $1,000. These practices are internal controls designed to promote the separation of duties.

Scheduling Bill Payment

Payment of bills is referred to as an accounts payable function. Bills should be scheduled for future payment as they arrive in the office. When using computerized accounting software, enter the invoice information and due date into the computer. When the designated payment date arrives, the software reminds you that a bill needs to be paid.

It is a good idea to schedule reminders for bills at least one week before the actual due date so the checks or payment for them are mailed several days in advance, allowing adequate time for delivery by the due date. Payments that do not arrive at the vendor's site by the due date are subject to late fees. Although a late fee may be a small charge of a few dollars, it is an unnecessary expense that can add up over time.

It is not necessary to pay bills on the day they arrive, because they are generally not due for 30 days. During that 30-day period, the money can remain in an interest-bearing account. Some vendors offer a discount if payment is included with the order or paid within a certain number of days, such as payment within 10 days. Because this discount could be as much as 10 to 20 percent, it is wise to take advantage of it.

A schedule for paying recurring monthly expenses can be established in the accounting software. Examples of recurring monthly expenses may include the following:

- Insurance premium(s)
- Rent or mortgage
- Waste removal
- Utilities, including telephone charges
- Housekeeping and maintenance expenses
- Laundry
- Equipment rental, such as a copy machine
- Taxes
- Maintenance contracts for equipment
- Medical and office supplies
- Postage

Bills that are the same amount and paid at the same time each month can be automatically prescheduled. One example of a recurrent bill is the office rent, which is typically the same amount each month and is due on the same day of each month. For some offices, there may be an annual, bimonthly, or quarterly lease arrangement. In this case, the lease money may be paid up to one year in advance. The bills for the electricity, the water, the telephone, and the gas vary in amount from month to month but are still due on the same day each month.

When possible, try to consolidate bill paying activity to once or twice a month. This is an efficient use of time and allows for a planned transfer of funds from a savings account to a checking account to cover these expenses.

Writing Checks

Writing checks is a basic banking function. The check writing process must be handled carefully to avoid errors. Methods for writing checks vary from office to office, depending on the preferences of the physician and the accountant. Procedures 18-2 and 18-3 provide instruction for the proper procedure to follow when writing checks using accounts payable software and writing manual checks, respectively. Box 18-2 explains how to use a pegboard or write-it-once system to write checks.

Checks must be printed from the computer, typewritten, or legibly handwritten in ink so they cannot be altered. Never use a pencil to write checks. No blank space should be left before the name of the payee, the written dollar amount, and the numbered dollar amount. This is to prevent another person from altering any of these items. The signature cannot be typewritten. See Figure 18-6 for an example of a correctly written check.

In some cases, the amount of the check is imprinted or embossed by a check-writing machine that requires a key, combination, or password to access. This helps protect against forgery and alteration of the check. All the other information is entered by hand. Checks with stubs may need to be detached from the stub for typing. However, the stub must be completed immediately.

Checks can be prepared in a batch at designated times each month and given to the physician to sign. Attach all source documents, such as invoices and statements, to the check for the physician to sign.

Writing a check payable to "Cash" is not advised. Such checks are easily cashed, because they have no payee designated and have been signed by the payer. When you need to

---

BOX 18-2 | Write-It-Once System

The write-it-once system is a manual check writing system that requires that checks be written by hand. A pegboard system, check register sheet, and checks with a carbonized writing strip on the back are used for this method. Checks with the carbonized strip on the back edge are placed on top of the check register, lining up the first line of the check register with the writing line of the first check. All information that is written on the check (e.g., payee or dollar amount) appears on the check register sheet as a permanent record.

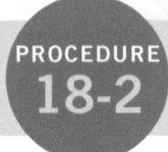

PROCEDURE 18-2

Paying Bills with Accounts Payable Software

Objective ◆ *Pay bills and print checks using computerized accounting software.*

EQUIPMENT AND SUPPLIES

Computer with accounts payable (AP) software; invoices; purchase orders; checks; printer; scanner; software user manual

METHOD

Log in to the accounts payable system with your username and password previously established.

To enter bills:

Note: Some offices create electronic copies of invoices and purchase orders that require that someone scan them into the system, save the file in a specific location, and name the file according to specific rules. Other offices work directly from paper invoices and purchase orders. Some bills may be able to be paid using an online "bill pay" service offered by your bank.

1. Organize the paper documents to be entered or access the location of the electronic images according to the instructions for your system.
2. In the software, access the menu for entering bills or invoices. Select the task to enter a new bill.
3. Select the name of the vendor from a preestablished list of vendors.
   - If the vendor is not in the system, select the menu item to enter a new vendor and key in the following information, according to procedures for your software: vendor name, address to which payment should be mailed, phone number, contact person, e-mail address, your account number, payment terms, and any other information requested.
4. Enter the following information: invoice number, dollar amount due, due date.
5. Select the type of expense, such as shipping or office supplies. This information may be automatically completed by the system for expenses such as rent and utilities. You may need to enter an account number that identifies the type of expense.
6. Enter the date you wish to be reminded to pay the bill.
7. Verify the accuracy of all data and save, if necessary.
8. On the source document, write "Entered by (your name) on (current date)." You may have an ink stamp that provides a format, with space to enter your name and date.

9. Repeat for all bills. Double-check all entries against your source documents to verify that you did not miss any invoices. File source documents in designated location. Log off the system.

To print checks:

1. Load checks into the printer. Follow the procedures for your combination of printer and software regarding how to orient the checks: face up or face down, and top edge first or bottom edge first.
2. Access the menu to pay invoices that were previously entered.
3. Enter the applicable range of due dates for invoices you wish to pay.
4. Review the screen that lists invoices to be paid and manually add or delete any, as needed.
5. Select the menu option to print checks. Enter or confirm any other required information such as check date.
6. Select or verify the printer and check format, if necessary. Select the menu option to begin printing.
7. Collect the checks from the printer. Review them to verify that all documents are legible and properly aligned. Reprint any misprinted or damaged checks.
8. Log off the system.
9. Remove blank checks from the printer tray and put them back in their designated location. Verify that the cabinet or drawer is locked.
10. Collate the checks with supporting documents such as purchase order or invoice. Route to the appropriate person to sign the checks.

After the checks are signed:

1. Review each check to verify that all checks have the required signature(s).
2. Detach check stub and attach to the supporting documents. File source documents in the designated location.
3. Place checks in window envelopes. Verify that the mailing address appears completely within the window. Apply postage and mail.

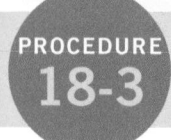

PROCEDURE 18-3

Preparing Manual Checks

Objective ◆ *Prepare a handwritten check.*

EQUIPMENT AND SUPPLIES

Blank checks with stub or record; black ink pen; invoice, purchase order, or other supporting documentation; security envelope; postage

METHOD

1. Identify the lowest-numbered unused check.
2. Fill in the check stub or check record before writing the check.
3. Use a black ink pen to complete check and stub.
4. Write the full date in the designated place. Date the check on the day it is written. Never postdate a check. (Postdating a check means writing a future date on a check.)
5. Write the name of the payee on the "Pay to the order of" line. Use care when spelling the name of the payee. Do not use abbreviations or titles such as MD. Leave no space either before or after the payee's name. If space remains after the name, draw a straight line from the name to the end of the space.
6. Write the amount of the check, using numbers in the designated area. Verify that the amount agrees with the invoice.
7. Write the dollar amount in words on the second line, usually labeled "Pay." Verify that it agrees with the numeric dollar amount.
8. Record your account number with the vendor, invoice number, and/or purpose of the check (example: "Office Supplies") on the memo line at the bottom left of the check.
9. Fill in all blank spaces, and leave no room for anyone to add anything. Always begin writing or figures at the extreme left of the space.

10. It is not advisable to write checks for less than one dollar. In addition to the time spent on bookkeeping for such a small amount, many banks place a service charge for each check written. This can be costly. However, when you must write a check for less than one dollar, use care. Write out the amount with the word "only" indicating to the reader that the amount is less than one dollar. Do not cross out the word *dollars.*
11. Prepare the check to be signed. Remove the check from the register, being careful not to tear it. Attach the invoice and any other supporting documentation behind the check with a paperclip. The individual signing checks should be the owner of the bank account or that person's authorized agent. In some offices, the office manager is authorized to sign checks for the physician.
12. Look over the check carefully to ensure all spaces have been filled in.
13. Subtract the amount of this check from the "Balance Brought Forward" line in the check register. Write this amount as the new balance brought forward. Check the math for accuracy.
14. After the check is signed, place it in an envelope with the remittance slip from the invoice. Address the envelope or, if using a window envelope, verify that the complete address is visible in the window. Seal the envelope, attach postage, and mail.
15. File the invoice and other supporting documentation in the designated location in the office.

write a check for petty cash, write it immediately before departing for the bank or, if possible, prepare a handwritten check after you arrive at the bank. Banks usually require that the person cashing the check endorse it in the teller's presence.

Completing the Check Stub

A check stub provides a permanent record of the date, amount, payee, and purpose of the check. The check stub has

room to place the new balance, which is obtained by subtracting the current check from the previous balance. See Figure 18-7 for an illustration of a correctly completed check stub. When using accounting software, the program prints the check stub at the same time as the check.

Accounting software may issue a **voucher check** instead of a check with a stub. They are frequently used for payroll because more details can be printed on a voucher than on a check stub. Voucher checks comprise a full page and contain

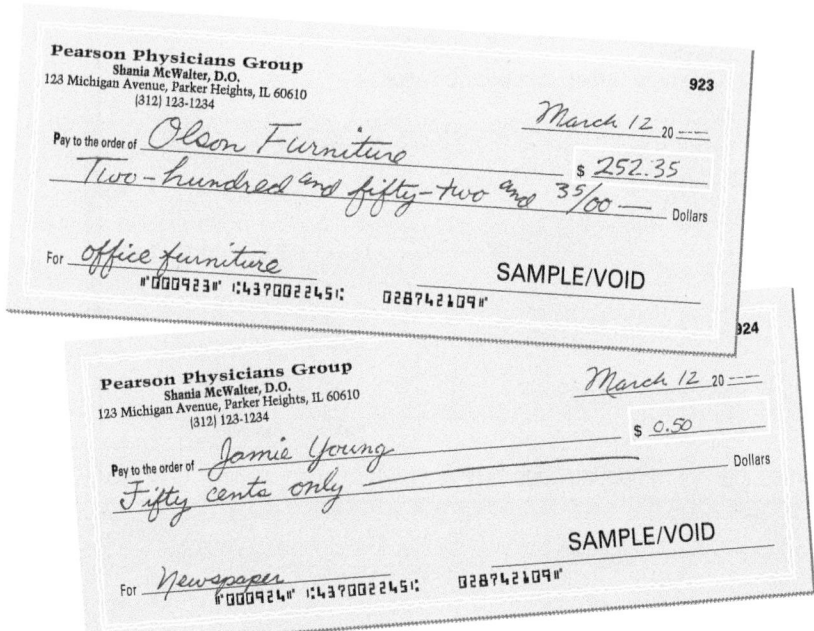

FIGURE 18-6 Correctly written checks.

No. 1028	BALANCE FORWARD	727	18
DATE *March 10* 20 *11*			
TO *Hanneman's*			
Health Supply			
FOR *Bandages*			
	THIS CHECK	32	45
Tax Deductible ☐	BALANCE	694	73

FIGURE 18-7 Correctly completed check stub.

two or three detachable sections for transaction information (Figure 18-8). One-third of the page contains the actual check; a second section provides details about the transaction, such as any payroll deductions, account to which the check is to be credited, or reason for issuing the check; the third section, if any, is an identical copy of the second section that the payer keeps as a record of the transaction. The payer files the third section with the original invoice or other source documents.

Errors in Writing Checks

Banks are very suspicious of alterations on a check. If you make a mistake when you write a check, such as writing out a different dollar amount than appears in the boxed space for the numeric amount, or the payee name is written in the space meant for the handwritten dollar amount, the check is not valid. In this case, draw a line through the check and write VOID, in ink, in large letters on the face of the check. Keep the voided check so that it is not considered missing when the bank statement is reconciled. If the check has already been signed, many people tear off and discard just the signature and keep the remainder of the check for a record.

Mailing Checks

Care should be used when mailing checks so that the check amount is not visible through the envelope. Checks printed from computer software often print the address of the vendor on the check, to be used with a window envelope. Security (opaque) envelopes can be purchased for use with checks. Other methods include placing the check in a piece of folded paper or actually folding the check in half. When mailing a payment to a vendor for an item or a service received, a **remittance slip**, or tear-off stub from the invoice being paid, is usually mailed along with the check. The vendor's address often appears on the remittance slip, which should be positioned so it appears in the window of the envelope provided by the vendor. Do not staple the check to the invoice, because it could cause the check to tear, making it unacceptable for deposit.

Petty Cash

Petty cash is a small amount of cash kept in the office to use for incidental purchases that require cash, such as reimbursements or postage due. For example, petty cash is used for

Professionalism

For many patients, money owed is a touchy and uncomfortable subject. Always address this topic in a calm, nonjudgmental way. If a patient requests to make payment arrangements, provide information on the office policy and offer to assist with the details. Although this requires extra time, patients will appreciate your helpfulness. Also, they are more likely to pay their bills if they feel you are willing to work with them. Always follow the office policy, and never veer from it. In this way, your honesty in dealing with money issues will never be questioned.

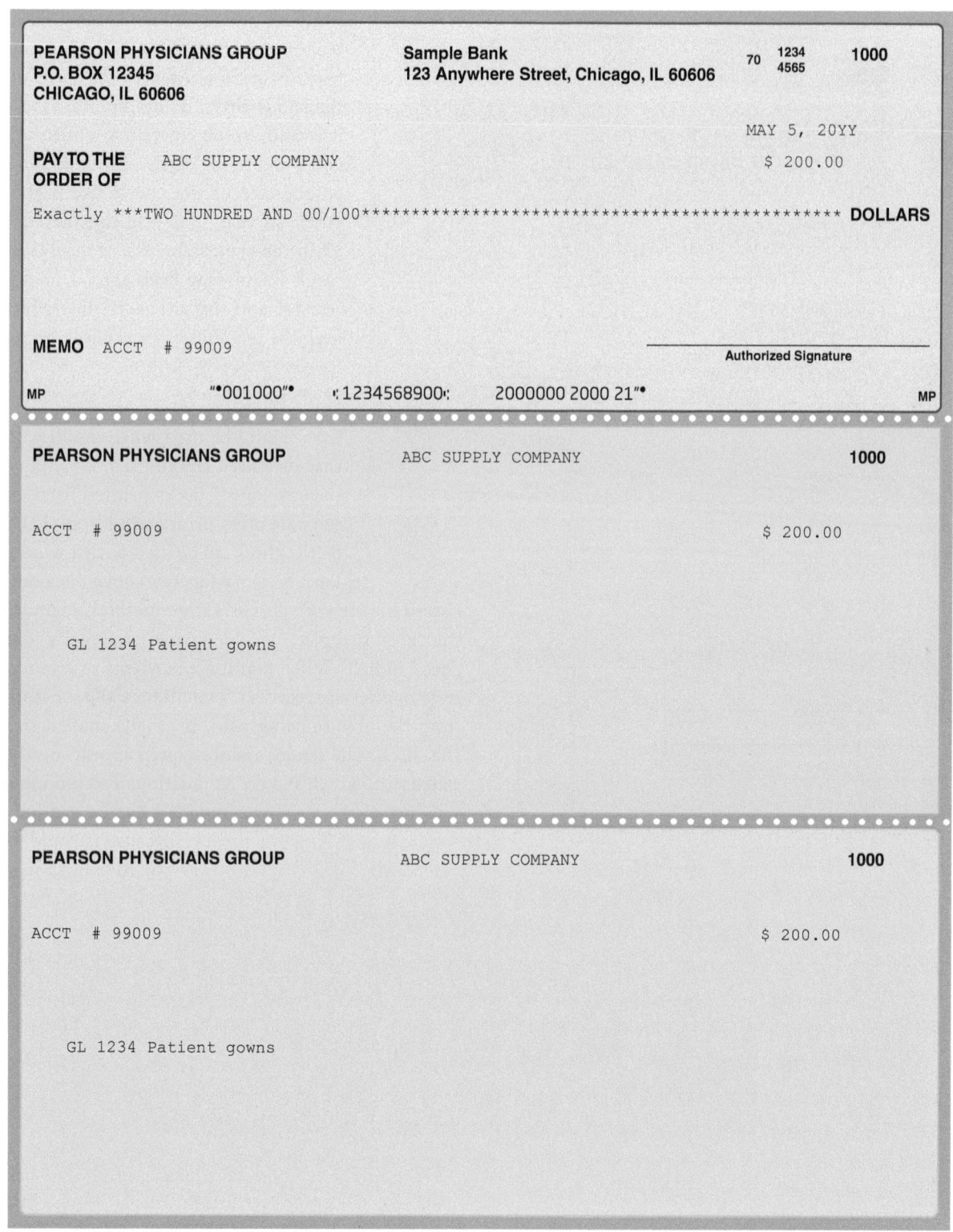

FIGURE 18-8 Example of a voucher check.

postage due on certified mail or other letters received in the office. Petty cash is kept completely separate from any cash received from patients. The two should not be intermixed and, preferably, handled by different staff members.

The amount of petty cash varies from office to office, but usually ranges from $50 to $100. Each expense paid for from petty cash must be recorded in a daily financial log or receipt pad. When the amount of money in petty cash drops to a predetermined level, such as $10, a check is written to replenish the funds.

At the end of a designated period (usually a week or a month), petty cash is reconciled and replenished. Count the money in the petty cash drawer, and total the receipts for money taken out of the petty cash drawer. The total of receipts plus money should equal the amount placed in the drawer at the beginning of the period. The cash used during the period is replaced to make the total cash available in the drawer equal to the beginning amount.

Petty cash is usually handled by one responsible office person and by a substitute in that person's absence. The petty cash drawer should be kept in a secure place within the office and should be locked at all times.

BANK STATEMENTS

The purpose of a statement from the bank is to confirm the amount of funds that are in each account. The bank statement can identify errors that may have been made by the office bookkeeping system or by the bank.

A monthly bank statement includes all transactions that have been processed. On some bank statements, charges against are labeled as debits, and additions to an account are labeled as credits. The statement lists checks that have been processed and paid out to the medical practice's creditors by the bank, deposits, and fees charged by the bank against the account. Figure 18-9 is an example of a typical bank statement.

STATEMENT OF ACCOUNT

FIRST NORTH
BANK OF CHIGAGO
123 East Pearson, Chicago, IL 60611
(312) 321-1000

Pearson Physicians Group
Shania McWalter, D.O.
123 Michigan Avenue,
Parker Heights, IL 60610

144808
PAGE 1 OF 1
STATEMENT PERIOD
FROM 08/01/11
THRU 08/31/11
CUST # 300-30-3000

---------------- ADVANTAGE CHECKING ACCOUNT ----------------

ACCOUNT NBR DD	12345	BEGINNING BALANCE	$2,646.63
AVG COLL BAL	$4,732.52	DEPOSITS/CREDITS	$8,000.00
MINIMUM BAL	$2,502.88	INTEREST PAID	$.00
TAX ID NUMBER	300-30-3000	CHECKS/DEBITS	$7,871.32-
		SERVICE CHARGES	$5.00-
		ENDING BALANCE	$2,770.31
		# DEPOSITS/CREDITS	1
		#CHECKS/DEBITS	11

DATE	DESCRIPTION		AMOUNT	BALANCE
08/01	BEGINNING BALANCE			$2,646.63
08/01	CK#	872	24.95-	2,621.68
08/06	CK#	879	3.00-	2,618.68
08/08	CK#	883	75.00-	2,543.68
08/14	CK#	885	15.80-	2,527.88
08/15	CK#	886	25.00-	2,502.88
08/19	DEPOSIT		8,000.00	10,502.88
08/26	CK#	887	32.00-	10,470.88
08/26	CK#	888	2,500.00-	7,970.88
08/28	CK#	890	70.00-	7,900.88
08/28	CK#	889	125.57-	7,775.31
08/28	CK#	884	5,000.00-	2,775.31
08/31	MONTHLY MAINTENANCE FEE		5.00-	2,770.31
08/31	ENDING BALANCE			$2,770.31

CHECK REGISTER

CHECK#	DATE	AMOUNT	CHECK#	DATE	AMOUNT
872	08/01	24.95	886	08/15	25.00
879*	08/06	3.00	887	08/26	32.00
883*	08/08	75.00	888	08/26	2,500.00
884	08/28	5,000.00	889	08/28	125.57
885	08/14	15.80	890	08/28	70.00

* INDICATES NON-CONSECUTIVE CHECK NUMBER(S)

FIGURE 18-9 A typical bank statement.

Bank statements include the following information:

- Account number
- Average daily balance
- Minimum balance
- Tax ID number
- Beginning balance
- Deposit history, including credit card transaction deposits
- Interest/credits
- Checks and debits
- Service charges
- Ending balance

Many banks also provide an image of the front and back of each check. This is an internal control that makes it possible to verify that no one changed the payee or payment amount after the check was recorded in the books or computer system.

Reconciliation

Account reconciliation is a basic banking function. **Reconciliation** is the process of comparing the data on the bank statements with the records maintained in the medical office. The purpose of reconciliation is to match the account activity and totals against the medical office records (Figure 18-10) to identify and correct errors.

Bank statements should be reconciled as soon as they are received, and errors should be corrected immediately. Office policy may indicate an exact date when reconciliation should take place. For separation of duties, the person who opens and reconciles the bank statement should be someone other than

Bank Reconciliation Form		
Bank Statement Date:		/ /
Ending Balance from Bank Statement		$
Add Deposits in Transit:		
Deposit Date	Amount	
/ /	$	
/ /	$	
/ /	$	
/ /	$	
/ /	$	
Total Deposits in Transit		+ $
Subtotal		= $
Subtract Outstanding Checks:		
Check Number	Amount	
	$	
	$	
	$	
	$	
	$	
	$	
	$	
	$	
	$	
	$	
	$	
	$	
	$	
	$	
	$	
	$	
	$	
	$	
	$	
	$	
	$	
Total Outstanding Checks		- $
Adjusted Statement Balance		= $
Checking Account Balance		$
Difference (should = 0 when balanced)		$

FIGURE 18-10 Bank reconciliation form.

the person who prepares the checks and makes the deposits. This is an internal control that helps prevent embezzlement of funds. In a small office in which there are few staff members to share the duties, this is the one function that must be performed by an independent person, even if it means that the physician does it or an accountant is hired to do it.

Savings account statements should be reconciled like checking accounts, although the process is easier because there are usually fewer transactions.

JUDGMENT CALL

Dr. Lysacek's bookkeeper resigned last week, and the position has not been filled. Because it is a small office, Ashleigh Fletcher, MA, has been counting daily cash receipts and making the deposits each day. Today Dr. Lysacek asks Ashleigh to reconcile the bank statement that just arrived. Ashleigh recalls the information she learned in school about separation of duties. How should she respond to Dr. Lysacek's request?

For interest-bearing accounts, the interest earned is usually based on the average daily balance (the average amount of money in that account during the period covered by the statement). Interest credited or service fees charged to the account, as shown on the bank statement, should be recorded in the checking account register before beginning the reconciliation.

The bank statement lists processed checks in numerical order. Any checks that are listed in nonconsecutive order may be indicated with an asterisk (*). For instance, you may have check numbers 1301 and 1303 showing as processed, with an asterisk beside check number 1303. This should prompt you to look in the check register for check 1302, which may be a voided check or a check that has not yet been cashed.

The reverse side of the bank statement provides a form to assist in reconciling the bank statement and contact information on how to handle errors or questions about the statement. Procedure 18-4 lists step-by-step instructions for reconciling a bank statement. Box 18-3 shows an example of bank statement reconciliation.

Computerized Reconciliation

Computerized statement reconciliation works in a manner similar to manual reconciliation, except that the calculations are performed by the computer.

- Access the menu option for bank statement reconciliation.
- Key in the ending balance shown on the bank statement.
- The computer screen displays a list of deposits, cleared checks, and fees.
- Check off each item on the screen that matches an item on the bank statement.
- The computer highlights any discrepancies on the screen that you need to fix.
- When you are done, the computer displays a message that the account is balanced.

Reconciling a Bank Statement

Objective ◆ *Reconcile a bank statement for a checking account manually.*

EQUIPMENT AND SUPPLIES

Current and previous bank statements; cancelled checks (if returned by the bank); checkbook stubs

METHOD

1. Compare the beginning balance of the current statement with the ending balance of the previous statement. These should be the same.
2. Write the current ending balance in the appropriate space on the reverse side of the bank statement.
3. Compare deposits noted on the statement against your records or receipts by making a check mark next to each correct number.
4. List separately all outstanding deposits. These are deposits made toward the end of the month that have not been included in the current statement. Add these together and place the total on the reverse side of the statement in the space provided.
5. Add the ending balance to the total of deposits not already included and write this amount on the TOTAL line.
6. Compare the value of the checks listed on the statement with the value listed in the checkbook or check stubs, and place a check mark next to each correct number.

7. Note all numbers missing from the sequential list of check numbers; these are checks that have not yet cleared your bank (outstanding checks). List all outstanding checks. Add the total for outstanding checks and place that figure on the line indicated on the back of the statement.
8. Subtract the total figure for checks outstanding from the previous total on the back of the statement to determine the current balance. This amount should agree with the amount in your checkbook or stub balance.

EXAMPLE

1. Ending bank balance shown on this statement: $ _____
   ADD (+)
2. Deposits not credited in this statement, (if any) $ + _____
3. TOTAL $ = _____
   SUBTRACT (−)
4. Checks outstanding $ − _____
5. BALANCE $ = _____

PAYROLL

Payroll is generally the largest category of AP expenses in a medical office. Preparing payroll requires calculating worked hours, wages, and deductions for the entire staff, printing and distributing checks, and sending monies withheld to the appropriate places. Payroll may or may not include the physician, depending on how the office structure is set up for accounting and tax purposes. Payroll checks are generally issued weekly, biweekly, or monthly. These result in the following pay periods for a year:

- Weekly—52 pay periods a year (Employees are paid every week on the same day of the week.)

- Biweekly—26 pay periods a year (Employees are paid every two weeks.)

- Semimonthly—24 pay periods a year (Employees are paid on predetermined dates during the month, for example, on the 15th and 30th of every month.)

- Monthly—12 pay periods a year (Employees are paid on the same date every month.)

The physician determines the type of pay period to be used. All employees are then paid at the same time.

Fair Labor Standards Act

The **Fair Labor Standards Act (FLSA)** is a federal law that regulates work conditions and pay. Most states also have labor regulations that must be followed. FLSA classifies employees as **exempt** or **nonexempt** from earning **overtime** pay for hours worked in excess of 40 hours per week. The classification is determined by pay rate, pay method, and the type of job. Most employees are nonexempt and must be paid for overtime hours. In general, exempt employees must earn a certain amount per week or per year (specified by the United States Department of Labor), be paid by salary, and perform certain types of high-level administrative, executive, or professional job duties.

BOX 18-3 | Example of Reconciling a Bank Statement

Ashleigh Fletcher, MA, needs to reconcile the bank statement for July. First, she compares the July beginning balance to the ending balance of the June statement, which she reconciled last month. Both amounts are $17,907.11, as they should be. The balance in the checkbook is $16,478.35.

Step	Process		Result
1	Ashleigh locates the ending balance on the July statement, which is $15,478.32. She enters this amount on the reconciliation form that appears on the back of the bank statement.		$15,478.32
2	Ashleigh compares each deposit shown in the checkbook to those listed on the bank statement. She places a check mark next to each item as she verifies it, both in the checkbook and on the bank statement. She finds two deposits in the checkbook that were made after the closing date of the statement, so they do not appear on the statement. She writes these numbers in the space provided on the reconciliation form and totals them:		

8/1/20YY $ 456.33
8/2/20YY $ 774.12

                     $1,230.45   + $1,230.45

She identifies the amount of the monthly service charge of $10.00 on the bank statement. She enters this amount into the checkbook and subtracts it from the current checkbook balance ($16,478.35 − 10.00 = $16,468.35).

Step	Process		Result
3	Ashleigh adds the amount of deposits not yet credited to the ending bank balance.	=	$16,708.77
4	Ashleigh compares each check shown in the checkbook to those listed on the bank statement. She places a check mark next to each item as she verifies it, both in the checkbook and on the bank statement. She finds three checks in the checkbook that did not clear before the closing date of the statement, so they do not appear on the statement. She writes these numbers in the space provided on the reconciliation form and totals them:		

#1529 $ 45.16
#1531 $ 67.00
#1533 $ 128.26

           $ 240.42   − $240.42

Step	Process		Result
5	Ashleigh subtracts the amount of outstanding checks from the total of deposits in the previous step. This amount agrees with the balance in the checkbook, so she knows all funds are accounted for and the checking account is in balance.	=	$16,468.35

Summary of RULES

Step 1: Enter the ending statement balance.
Step 2: Enter all deposits made but not yet credited on the bank statement.
Step 3: ADD the numbers in steps 1 and 2.
Step 4: Enter the total dollar amount of checks written but not showing as cleared on the bank statement.

Step 5: SUBTRACT the amount in step 4 from the amount in step 3. This amount should equal the balance shown in your checkbook.

Tip: *If you need to reconcile bank statements manually, consider creating or downloading from the Internet a template that allows you to enter the data into a spreadsheet. Doing so saves time because it eliminates the risk of calculation errors when totaling a long list of numbers.*

The definition of a workweek for the purpose of calculating overtime is determined by the employer and does not have to be Sunday through Saturday. The overtime pay rate is 1.5 times the normal pay rate. An employee whose regular pay rate is $15.00 per hour has an overtime rate of $22.50 for each overtime hour worked.

Hourly employees are paid a specific amount for each hour worked, plus overtime pay. They do not earn wages for any time they are not at work, unless the employer has made provision for **paid time off (PTO)**, such as pay for a specific number of hours of sick time, vacation time, or holidays. PTO is not required by law.

Salaried employees receive a predetermined amount of money every pay period that is not dependent on the number of hours worked within the pay period. Unless the salaried employee is classified as nonexempt, that employee is not entitled to overtime. Regardless of whether the employee works 40 hours or 50 hours in a week, the pay remains the same.

Methods for Managing Payroll

Managing payroll requires meticulous record keeping. Errors can affect the income of employees of the medical office, as well as practice finances, and carry severe financial penalties. Several systems may be used for calculating and issuing payroll checks. They include outsourced payroll, in-house payroll software, and in-house manual payroll.

Outsourced Payroll

Many offices contract with an outside payroll company to relieve the office of time-consuming and detailed record keeping. Basic services offered include calculating payroll and tax obligations, printing and distributing checks, and producing reports. Additional services can include direct deposit, payroll tax filing, issuing W-2 forms, 401(k) deductions, and tracking of employee benefits. Most payroll services guarantee the accuracy of their work and defend the company and pay tax penalties if any discrepancies or errors are found. Figure 18-11 summarizes benefits of contracting with an outside payroll service.

Although contracting with an outside payroll service can save a significant amount of time and expense, the medical office is still responsible for certain activities, such as collecting new employee paperwork, reporting employee hours each pay period, and making funds available for payroll. Procedure 18-5 discusses how to work with a payroll service.

- Frees up staff time for patient-related duties
- Reduces the cost of processing payroll
- Ensure accurate reporting
- Guarantees no tax penalties for filling errors
- Offers employees direct deposit of their checks
- Keeps technology current
- Maintains up-to-date knowledge of payroll tax regulations
- Eliminates dependence on a particular employee
- Minimizes the need for employee training on payroll tasks
- Provides direct source to answer employee payroll questions

FIGURE 18-11 Benefits of outsourced payroll.

Payroll Software

For offices that choose to keep payroll in-house, several software packages are available that are used to calculate payroll and tax withholdings and print payroll checks. Each employee has an account within the software in which wage in-formation and tax exemptions are stored (Figure 18-12). Tax rate schedules must be updated each year. The amounts calculated for withholding can be performed more accurately using a computer than manually. Doing payroll

---

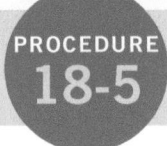

PROCEDURE 18-5

Working with an Outside Payroll Service

Objective ◆ *Prepare the information required by an outside payroll service to process payroll.*

EQUIPMENT AND SUPPLIES

Employee time records; computer or calculator; telephone or computer with Internet connection; new employee paperwork; documents regarding any changes needed to employee information, such as new address, new banking information, new pay rate, etc.; payroll journal or payroll reporting forms; contact information for the payroll service or its secure website for payroll customers

METHOD

The office is responsible to transmit payroll information to the payroll service each pay period. This may be done using the Internet, telephone, or fax. The procedures for each method of transmission are different. Using the procedures for the applicable transmission method, perform the following steps.

1. Review all employee paperwork to verify it is complete and accurate.

2. Enter the total hours worked for each employee, indicating the number of hours to be paid at the regular pay rate and the number of hours to be paid at the overtime rate.
3. Enter the number of hours of paid time off (PTO) for each employee. This may be divided into sick time, holidays, and vacation.
4. Enter information regarding new employees, terminated employees, change in status, change in pay, change in withholding or deductions, etc.
5. Verify all data entered for accuracy and omissions.
6. Save the data if working online, transmit the data via fax, or telephone the payroll company to report the numbers verbally. Write down the confirmation number for the submission.
7. After the payroll service processes the information, you are notified of the amount of funds needed for payroll and withholding. Transfer the designated amount of money to the appropriate bank account used for payroll.

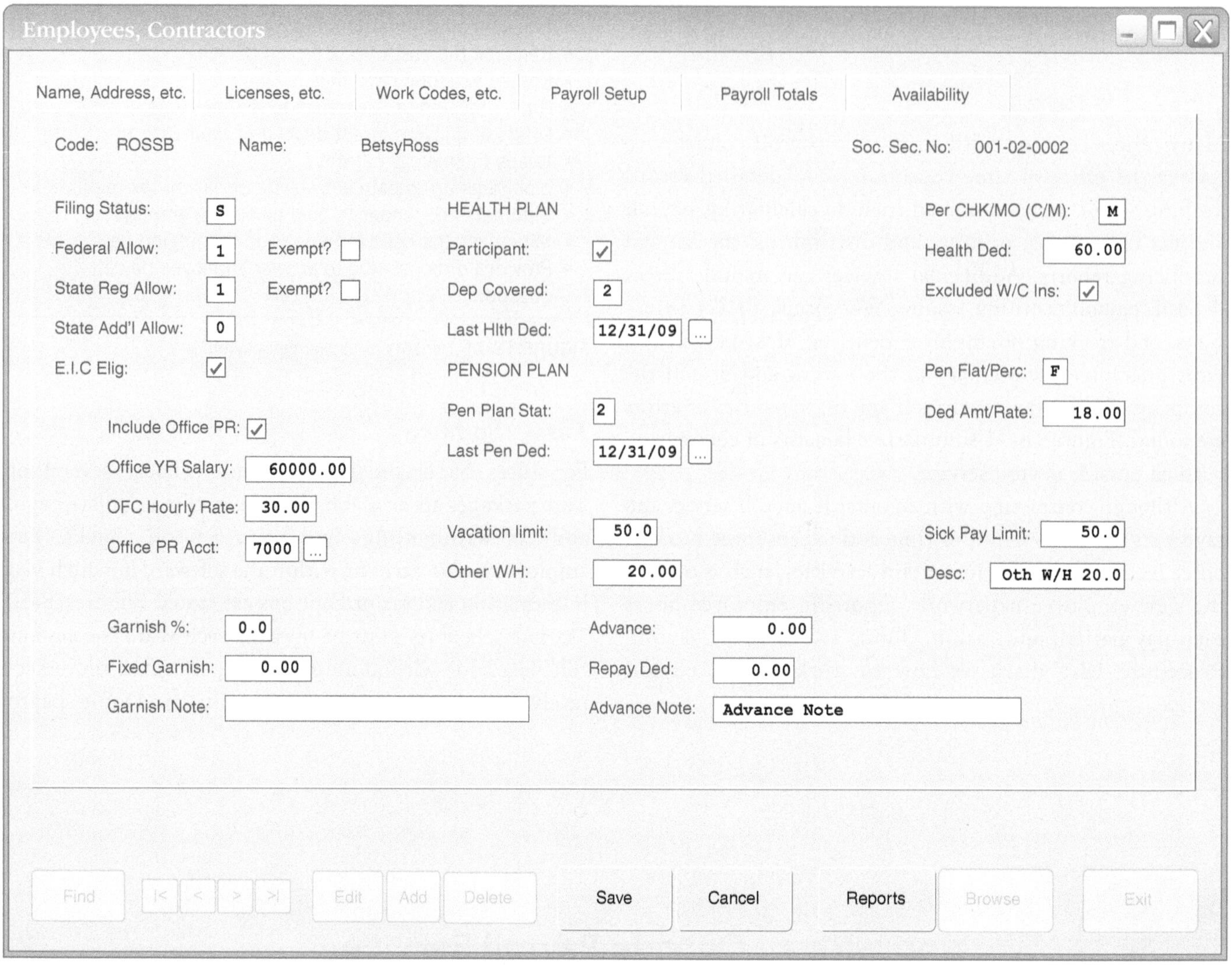

FIGURE 18-12 Example of an employee setup screen in a computerized payroll program.

in-house requires staff members who are knowledgeable in payroll law.

Manual Payroll

Small offices with few staff members may choose to keep payroll manually, performing all calculations with a calculator and handwriting checks. Accurate records are needed for documentation of gross income, tax withholding, and each check issued for all employees. The write-it-once pegboard system is an efficient method of doing manual payroll, because most of the payroll record can be accomplished with a single entry.

Deductions

The employee's payroll check is determined by first calculating the **gross wage**, then subtracting

required and voluntary deductions, which produces the **net pay**, often referred to as take-home pay. Figure 18-13 shows how to calculate gross wages for hourly and salaried employees. **Deductions** are money withheld from the employee's paycheck for taxes, health and life insurance premiums, and other benefits. Figure 18-14 provides an example of computerized payroll processing and the deductions that may be taken.

Hourly Employee
Hourly wage × Number of hours worked = Gross wage
Example:
$15 per hour × 40 hours worked = $600
Salaried Employee
Annual Salary amount/number of pay periods in the year = Gross wage
Example:
$52,000 per year/52 pay periods = $1,000

FIGURE 18-13 Gross pay calculation.

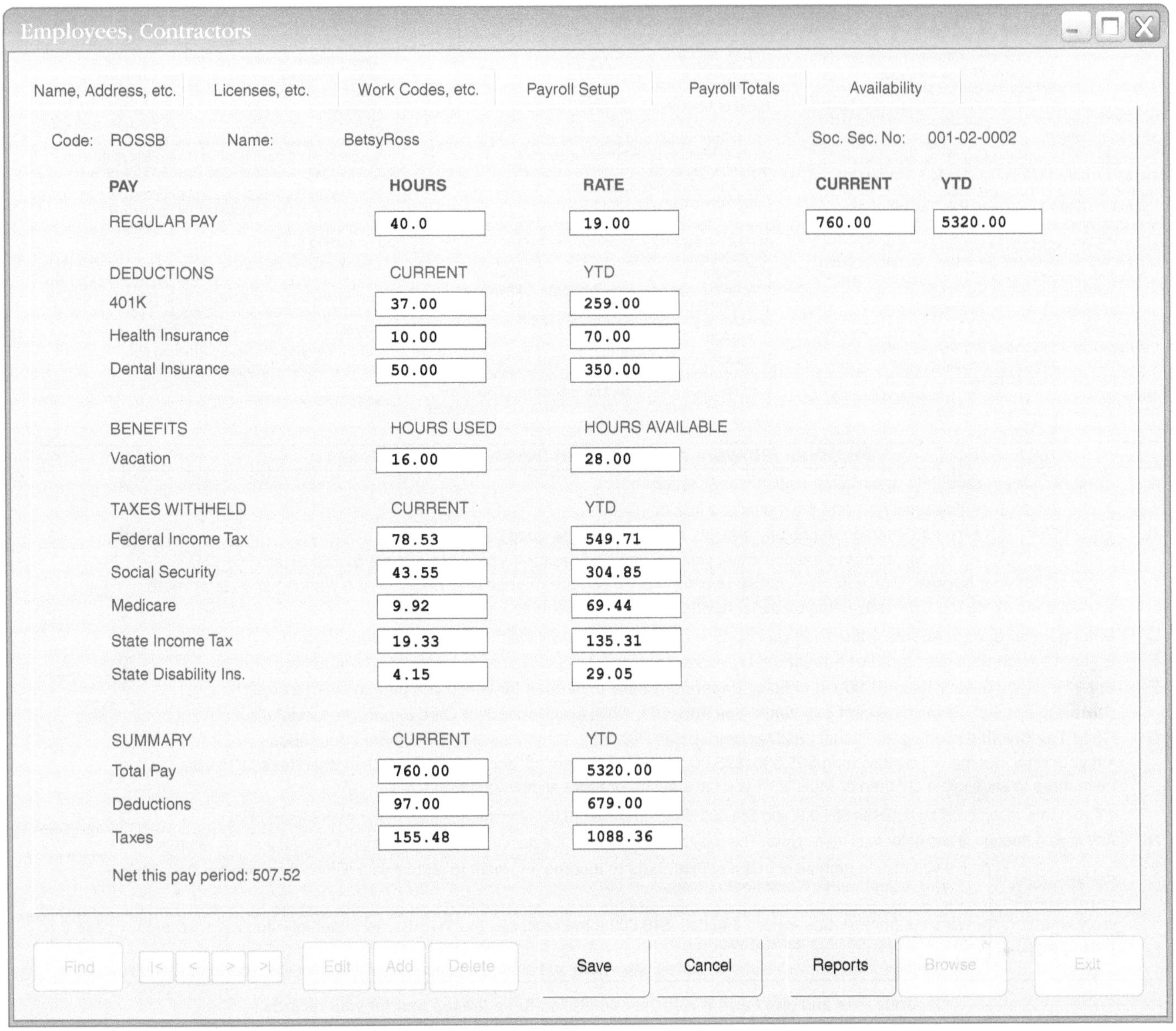

Employees, Contractors

Name, Address, etc. | Licenses, etc. | Work Codes, etc. | Payroll Setup | Payroll Totals | Availability

Code: ROSSB   Name: BetsyRoss   Soc. Sec. No: 001-02-0002

PAY	HOURS	RATE	CURRENT	YTD
REGULAR PAY	40.0	19.00	760.00	5320.00

DEDUCTIONS	CURRENT	YTD
401K	37.00	259.00
Health Insurance	10.00	70.00
Dental Insurance	50.00	350.00

BENEFITS	HOURS USED	HOURS AVAILABLE
Vacation	16.00	28.00

TAXES WITHHELD	CURRENT	YTD
Federal Income Tax	78.53	549.71
Social Security	43.55	304.85
Medicare	9.92	69.44
State Income Tax	19.33	135.31
State Disability Ins.	4.15	29.05

SUMMARY	CURRENT	YTD
Total Pay	760.00	5320.00
Deductions	97.00	679.00
Taxes	155.48	1088.36

Net this pay period: 507.52

Find | |< | < | > | >| | Edit | Add | Delete | Save | Cancel | Reports | Browse | Exit

FIGURE 18-14 Example of a computerized employee payroll record.

Required Deductions

Withholding is the deduction of federal, state, and city taxes from gross wages. The employer pays the tax amount withheld to the government on behalf of the employee. When employees file their annual tax returns, the amount withheld during the year is deducted from the amount owed at tax time.

Government regulations require that records must be maintained for each employee containing the following information:

- Amount of gross pay
- Social Security number of the employee
- Number of exemptions of each employee (taken from W-4 form completed by the employee at the time of hire)
- Deductions for federal, state, and city taxes and Social Security
- State disability insurance and unemployment tax, where applicable
- Any pretax deductions, such as 401(k) contributions

The federal government mandates employers to withhold and report three types of taxes: federal income tax, Social Security—also known as the **Federal Insurance Contributions Act (FICA)**, and Medicare. Federal income taxes are based on a percentage of the employee's total gross income. To determine the amount of money to be withheld from each paycheck, employees must complete a **W-4 form** when hired (Figure 18-15).

Form W-4 (20YY)

Purpose. Complete Form W-4 so that your employer can withhold the correct federal income tax from your pay. Consider completing a new Form W-4 each year and when your personal or financial situation changes.

Exemption from withholding. If you are exempt, complete **only** lines 1, 2, 3, 4, and 7 and sign the form to validate it. Your exemption for 2013 expires February 17, 2014. See Pub. 505, Tax Withholding and Estimated Tax.

Note. If another person can claim you as a dependent on his or her tax return, you cannot claim exemption from withholding if your income exceeds $1,000 and includes more than $350 of unearned income (for example, interest and dividends).

Basic instructions. If you are not exempt, complete the **Personal Allowances Worksheet** below. The worksheets on page 2 further adjust your withholding allowances based on itemized deductions, certain credits, adjustments to income, or two-earners/multiple jobs situations.

Complete all worksheets that apply. However, you may claim fewer (or zero) allowances. For regular wages, withholding must be based on allowances you claimed and may not be a flat amount or percentage of wages.

Head of household. Generally, you can claim head of household filing status on your tax return only if you are unmarried and pay more than 50% of the costs of keeping up a home for yourself and your dependent(s) or other qualifying individuals. See Pub. 501, Exemptions, Standard Deduction, and Filing Information, for information.

Tax credits. You can take projected tax credits into account in figuring your allowable number of withholding allowances. Credits for child or dependent care expenses and the child tax credit may be claimed using the **Personal Allowances Worksheet** below. See Pub. 505 for information on converting your other credits into withholding allowances.

Nonwage income. If you have a large amount of nonwage income, such as interest or dividends, consider making estimated tax payments using Form 1040-ES, Estimated Tax for Individuals. Otherwise, you may owe additional tax. If you have pension or annuity income, see Pub. 505 to find out if you should adjust your withholding on Form W-4 or W-4P.

Two earners or multiple jobs. If you have a working spouse or more than one job, figure the total number of allowances you are entitled to claim on all jobs using worksheets from only one Form W-4. Your withholding usually will be most accurate when all allowances are claimed on the Form W-4 for the highest paying job and zero allowances are claimed on the others. See Pub. 505 for details.

Nonresident alien. If you are a nonresident alien, see Notice 1392, Supplemental Form W-4 Instructions for Nonresident Aliens, before completing this form.

Check your withholding. After your Form W-4 takes effect, use Pub. 505 to see how the amount you are having withheld compares to your projected total tax for 2013. See Pub. 505, especially if your earnings exceed $130,000 (Single) or $180,000 (Married).

Future developments. Information about any future developments affecting Form W-4 (such as legislation enacted after we release it) will be posted at *www.irs.gov/w4*.

Personal Allowances Worksheet (Keep for your records.)

A	Enter "1" for **yourself** if no one else can claim you as a dependent	**A** _____
B	Enter "1" if: { • You are single and have only one job; or • You are married, have only one job, and your spouse does not work; or • Your wages from a second job or your spouse's wages (or the total of both) are $1,500 or less. } . . .	**B** _____
C	Enter "1" for your **spouse**. But, you may choose to enter "-0-" if you are married and have either a working spouse or more than one job. (Entering "-0-" may help you avoid having too little tax withheld.)	**C** _____
D	Enter number of **dependents** (other than your spouse or yourself) you will claim on your tax return	**D** _____
E	Enter "1" if you will file as **head of household** on your tax return (see conditions under **Head of household** above) . .	**E** _____
F	Enter "1" if you have at least $1,900 of **child or dependent care expenses** for which you plan to claim a credit . . .	**F** _____
	(**Note.** Do **not** include child support payments. See Pub. 503, Child and Dependent Care Expenses, for details.)	
G	**Child Tax Credit** (including additional child tax credit). See Pub. 972, Child Tax Credit, for more information.	
	• If your total income will be less than $65,000 ($95,000 if married), enter "2" for each eligible child; then **less** "1" if you have three to six eligible children or **less** "2" if you have seven or more eligible children.	
	• If your total income will be between $65,000 and $84,000 ($95,000 and $119,000 if married), enter "1" for each eligible child . . .	**G** _____
H	Add lines A through G and enter total here. (**Note.** This may be different from the number of exemptions you claim on your tax return.) ▶ **H** _____	

For accuracy, complete all worksheets that apply.
{ • If you plan to **itemize** or **claim adjustments to income** and want to reduce your withholding, see the **Deductions and Adjustments Worksheet** on page 2.
• If you are **single and have more than one job** or are **married and you and your spouse both work** and the combined earnings from all jobs exceed $40,000 ($10,000 if married), see the **Two-Earners/Multiple Jobs Worksheet** on page 2 to avoid having too little tax withheld.
• If **neither** of the above situations applies, **stop here** and enter the number from line H on line 5 of Form W-4 below. }

------------------------------ **Separate here and give Form W-4 to your employer. Keep the top part for your records.** ------------------------------

Form **W-4**
Department of the Treasury
Internal Revenue Service

Employee's Withholding Allowance Certificate

▶ Whether you are entitled to claim a certain number of allowances or exemption from withholding is subject to review by the IRS. Your employer may be required to send a copy of this form to the IRS.

OMB No. 1545-0074

20**YY**

1 Your first name and middle initial	Last name	2 **Your social security number**

Home address (number and street or rural route)	3 ☐ Single ☐ Married ☐ Married, but withhold at higher Single rate.
	Note. If married, but legally separated, or spouse is a nonresident alien, check the "Single" box.
City or town, state, and ZIP code	4 If your last name differs from that shown on your social security card, check here. You must call 1-800-772-1213 for a replacement card. ▶ ☐

5	Total number of allowances you are claiming (from line **H** above **or** from the applicable worksheet on page 2)	**5**	
6	Additional amount, if any, you want withheld from each paycheck	**6**	$
7	I claim exemption from withholding for 2013, and I certify that I meet **both** of the following conditions for exemption.		
	• Last year I had a right to a refund of **all** federal income tax withheld because I had **no** tax liability, **and**		
	• This year I expect a refund of **all** federal income tax withheld because I expect to have **no** tax liability.		
	If you meet both conditions, write "Exempt" here . . . . ▶	**7**	

Under penalties of perjury, I declare that I have examined this certificate and, to the best of my knowledge and belief, it is true, correct, and complete.

Employee's signature
(This form is not valid unless you sign it.) ▶   **Date** ▶

8 Employer's name and address (Employer: Complete lines 8 and 10 only if sending to the IRS.)	9 Office code (optional)	10 Employer identification number (EIN)

For Privacy Act and Paperwork Reduction Act Notice, see page 2.   Cat. No. 10220Q   Form **W-4** (2013)

FIGURE 18-15 W-4 form used by employees to request IRS withholding.

Example of FICA and Medicare Deductions					
Gross Wages:	$1,000.00				
	Employee %	Employee $	Employer %	Employer $	Total $ Paid
FICA	6.2%	$62.00	6.2%	$62.00	$124.00
Medicare	1.5%	$14.50	1.5%	$14.50	$ 29.00
Total		$76.50		$76.50	$153.00

FIGURE 18-16 Example FICA and Medicare deductions.

The Federal Employer's Tax Guide provides tables to determine the amount of withholding that are built into computerized payroll programs. Separate tables are provided based on marital status, the number of exemptions, and the frequency of pay periods.

Federal income tax rates vary from 10 percent to nearly 40 percent of gross wages, based on a person's total income.

The percentages for Social Security and Medicare taxes are the same for everyone, up to a certain income level. Half is deducted from the employee's check and half is paid by the employer. Figure 18-16 shows how this works.

Individual states may also have payroll withholding requirements for income tax, worker's compensation, unemployment tax, and short-term disability insurance for employees.

Voluntary Deductions

Voluntary deductions are those not required by the government but requested by the employee for fringe benefits. Voluntary deductions often include premiums for health, life, and disability insurances, pension plan contributions, and union dues. After processing payroll, the employer forwards the money withheld to the appropriate vendors who provide the various services.

Deposit Requirements

Employers must pay the federal tax money withheld from employee paychecks at the end of each period or month. The Internal Revenue Service (IRS) imposes a severe penalty for failure to deposit this money. In addition to depositing income tax withholding, FICA, and Medicare taxes, employers must also pay federal unemployment taxes and estimated income taxes on the business itself. Employers must file a quarterly report (Form 941: Employer's Quarterly Federal Tax Return) on April 30, July 31, October 31, and January 31. If an employer fails to remit tax payments as required, the responsibility remains with the employer. The government does not hold employees responsible for amounts deducted by the employer but not submitted.

Federal Unemployment Tax. Every employer must contribute to unemployment taxes as mandated under the

Federal Unemployment Tax Act (FUTA). If the employer is making payments into a state unemployment fund, this can generally be applied as credit against the FUTA tax amount. FUTA is the sole responsibility of the employer. It is based on the employee's gross income but must not be deducted from the employee's wage.

FUTA deposits are calculated quarterly, and the amount due must be paid by the last day of the first month after the quarter ends. Therefore, for the first quarter of the year ending on March 31, the payment must be made by April 30. An annual FUTA report must be filed to the federal government using Form 940 each year.

State Unemployment Tax. All states have unemployment compensation laws, generally referred to as the **State Unemployment Tax Act (SUTA).** Most states require only the employer to make payments toward this fund. However, a few states require both the employer and employee to make a payment. In this case, the employer withholds the required amount from the employee's paycheck. Each state's regulation concerning tax requirements should be checked carefully before preparing the payroll.

Year-End Reporting

The **W-2 form** (Figure 18-17) is a federally required tax report that lists the employee's annual gross income; federal (income, Medicare, and Social Security), state, and local taxes withheld; taxable fringe benefits, such as tips; and the employee's net income for the year.

W-2 forms must be delivered by January 31 for the preceding calendar year. For example, W-2 forms indicating wages earned in the year 2017 must be mailed to employees by January 31, 2018. The employer provides three copies of the W-2 form to each employee, one each for federal and state filing

Professionalism The Law

The importance of making federal tax deposits cannot be understated. Businesses experiencing cash flow problems may be tempted to use the money for operating expenses, believing that the situation will soon improve and they will "catch up" on deposit requirements by the end of the year. Unfortunately, this may not happen and the amount owed can escalate quickly. Not only does the business face large tax penalties for not making deposits, it can easily accumulate an unpaid tax debt that is more than it can possibly pay, even if finances improve.

22222	**a** Employee's social security number	OMB No. 1545-0008		

b Employer identification number (EIN)		**1** Wages, tips, other compensation 32094.40	**2** Federal income tax withheld 5559.06
c Employer's name, address, and ZIP code **Pearson Physicians Group** **123 Machigan Avenue** **Parker Heights, IL 60610**		**3** Social security wages 32094.40	**4** Social security tax withheld 1989.85
		5 Medicare wages and tips 32094.40	**6** Medicare tax withheld 465.37
		7 Social security tips	**8** Allocated tips
d Control number B1-049097-0	**9**		**10** Dependent care benefits
e Employee's first name and initial Last name Suff.	**11** Nonqualified plans		**12a** Code
	13 Statutory employee ☐ Retirement plan ☒ Third-party sick pay ☐		**12b** Code
	14 Other		**12c** Code
			12d Code
f Employee's address and ZIP code			

15 State Employer's state ID number	**16** State wages, tips, etc. 32094.40	**17** State income tax 1305.46	**18** Local wages, tips, etc.	**19** Local income tax 412.97	**20** Locality name C A S D I

Form **W-2** Wage and Tax Statement   **20YY**   Department of the Treasury—Internal Revenue Service

Copy 1—For State, City, or Local Tax Department

FIGURE 18-17 W-2 form issued to employees at the end of the year.

and one for the employee's file. W-2 forms are generally prepared by the person or company that prepares payroll checks.

SUMMARY

Banking is a critical office procedure that requires careful handling of money and records. A thorough understanding of banking procedures and terminology is vital to running an efficient medical office. Great trust is placed in the medical assistant to handle the physician's banking needs with accuracy. Medical offices should adopt a system of checks and balances in financial matters called internal controls to ensure separation of duties. Several different people should be involved in the handling and recording of funds, and reconciling bank statements, so that opportunities for fraud and embezzlement are minimized.

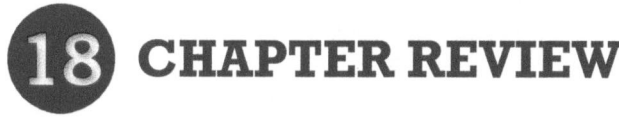

18 CHAPTER REVIEW

COMPETENCY REVIEW

1. Define and spell the terms for the chapter.
2. Using your own bank statement, reconcile it to your checkbook records.
3. Create and complete a check and check stub in the amount of $10.65 drafted to Bill Jay.
4. Call a local bank and request information regarding the various options for checking and savings accounts.
5. Create a bank deposit slip for $23.10 in cash and checks for $54.00, $21.25, $110.00, $29.00, and $9.25.
6. Explain the separation of duties, and list five internal controls that can be implemented to accomplish this.

PREPARING FOR THE CERTIFICATION EXAM

1. What is the name of a check that becomes void because it was not cashed within the time stated on the check?
   a. certified check
   b. limited check
   c. cashier's check
   d. stale check
   e. old check

2. Who is the person the check is made out to?
   a. maker
   b. payee
   c. payer
   d. teller
   e. recipient

3. What is the code number found in the lower-left corner of a printed check?
   a. MICR
   b. withdrawal number
   c. registration number
   d. account number
   e. OCR

4. What is the name of a check written on the payer's own check form but guaranteed by the bank?
   a. cashier's check
   b. voucher check
   c. certified check
   d. limited check
   e. paycheck

5. What is the frequency of payroll when employees are paid on two set dates every month?
   a. bimonthly
   b. semimonthly
   c. biweekly
   d. semiweekly
   e. biannually

6. What is the gross annual wage?
   a. amount of money the employee takes home in a year
   b. amount of money the employee takes home each pay period
   c. amount of money the employee earns in a year before deductions
   d. amount of money the employee earns in a pay period before deductions
   e. amount of money the employee pays into a fund every year

7. What is a prepaid payment order that can be purchased from banks, the United States Postal Service, and other authorized agents?
   a. cashier's check
   b. certified check
   c. voucher check
   d. money order
   e. payroll check

8. Which type of endorsement is the safest to use in the business office?
   a. blank
   b. special
   c. restrictive
   d. limited
   e. exclusive

9. By what date must an employer provide W-2s to employees?
   a. December 31
   b. January 1
   c. January 31
   d. April 1
   e. April 15

10. What procedures reduce the risk of fraud and embezzlement by dividing financial responsibilities into distinct tasks and assigning each task to a different individual?
    a. job descriptions
    b. bonding
    c. separation of duties
    d. background checks
    e. statement reconciliation

CRITICAL THINKING

Refer to the case study at the beginning of the chapter and use the information you have learned to answer the following questions.

1. As Tania reviews the checks for deposit, she realizes that one of the checks collected for a patient's copayment is postdated two days in advance. The office has a clear policy regarding not accepting postdated checks. The deposit slip, which today lists 18 checks, already includes the postdated check. What should Tania do?

2. While reviewing the petty cash drawer, Tania realizes that $5 is missing and unaccounted for. How should Tania handle this situation?

ON THE JOB

Your office has decided to contract with an outside payroll service to handle the preparation of paychecks. Contact three payroll services in your area, and find out what services they provide, how much they charge, and what steps are required to get established with them. Write a short report that summarizes your findings for the physician and office manager.

INTERNET ACTIVITY

Call your bank and get its online address. Then go to the Internet and access the bank's home page. If you do not have a bank account, call several local banks and go to their home pages. List the steps in setting up an online banking account.

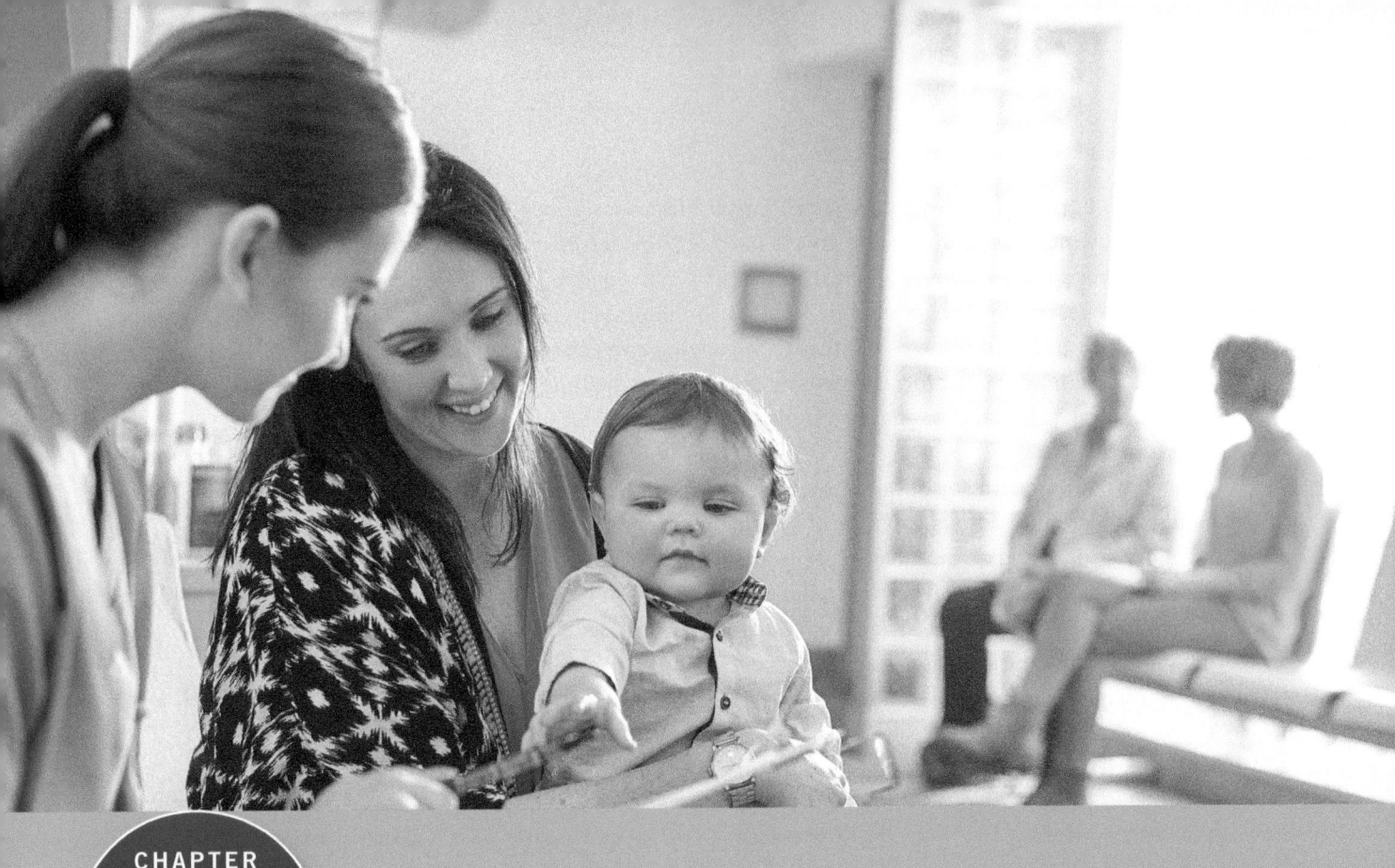

19

Medical Office Management

Learning Objectives

After completing this chapter, you should be able to:

19.1 Define and spell the terms for this chapter.

19.2 Describe how to implement a systems approach to medical office management.

19.3 List at least 10 duties of a medical office manager.

19.4 Identify time management principles.

19.5 Describe characteristics of common leadership styles.

19.6 Identify types of questions that are illegal to ask during an employee interview.

19.7 List topics that should be covered during a new employee's orientation and training period.

19.8 Differentiate between a personnel policy manual and an office policies and procedures manual.

19.9 Describe how to assist the physician with work-related travel arrangements.

19.10 Identify key principles related to marketing a medical practice.

Tania Washington is an office manager at Pearson Physicians Group. The group's business has been growing steadily, and the office is in need of a new certified medical assistant. Tania decided to put an advertisement in the local newspaper and on the newspaper's employment website. She received many résumés in response to the posted position. She took a couple days to sort through the résumés and the accompanying cover letters, removing all that did not meet the minimum qualifications as well as those with spelling and grammatical errors. On Monday, she contacted several individuals who had the best résumés and set up interviews for the week.

Before speaking with any of the candidates, Tania wrote a set of questions she would use for all candidates. She also made notes of specific questions she wanted to ask pertaining to the information found on each applicant's résumé or cover letter.

Tania's first interview went very well, but it was difficult to read the application form that the applicant completed. The second applicant had recently had her tongue pierced, and at times it was very difficult to understand her speech. The third applicant had the least experience but looked very professional, wrote neatly, and spoke well.

Terms to Learn

at-will employment	grievance	sexual harassment
bullying	itinerary	solvent
colleagues	probationary period	
discriminatory	seniority	

To provide quality patient care, the entire office must be well managed. Although medical assistants do not begin their careers as office managers, you may eventually fill such a role. Office management requires special administrative and communication skills as well as effective time management. Planning activities, delegating tasks, and effectively using personnel require careful attention to how time is managed.

This chapter discusses the systems approach to office management and the role of the office manager. Then, specific responsibilities of the office manager are discussed, including creating a team atmosphere, hiring effective staff members, and developing office policies. Several documents are important for a medical office to run smoothly. These include the personnel policy manual, the office policies and procedures manual, and patient information booklets. Finally, physician travel arrangements, speaking engagements, marketing, and customer service are discussed.

SYSTEMS APPROACH TO OFFICE MANAGEMENT

Current management philosophy recommends a systematic approach when managing a medical office. Under this approach, the functions of an office are categorized into systems that must function simultaneously and be integrated into a whole system: the medical office. For example, the administrative component of a medical office can be divided into the following systems:

- Personnel management
- Employee records
- Financial management (including banking, billing, collections, and insurance)
- Scheduling
- Facility and equipment management (including computers)
- Clinical office management

- Communication (written and oral, including patient education)
- Legal concepts

The clinical component of managing an office can be considered a system by itself. Brief descriptions of the various systems that form the medical practice follow.

Personnel Management Responsibilities

Personnel management duties include recruitment and selection, probation, performance and salary review, discipline, and maintenance of employee records.

The recruitment and selection process is used when a medical practice must replace a staff member who has left or when more staff are needed for an expanding practice. For new employees to successfully transition into their positions, an orientation is required. During orientation the new employee will learn about the office and the new position and about the expected duties and responsibilities associated with the new position. Large offices and clinics often have formal orientation training sessions that employees attend before beginning their day-to-day assignments.

Personnel management usually requires an annual performance review of each employee, at which time a merit raise in salary may be granted if the employee's performance has been acceptable. At times it is necessary to discipline an employee. It is advisable not to wait until the annual review to discipline the employee. This should occur as soon as discipline is warranted. These topics are discussed in greater detail in this chapter.

Employee Records

Federal law requires records to be maintained for every employee. These include the following payroll records:

- Social Security number of the employee
- Number of exemptions claimed by the employee (W-4 form)
- Gross wages (pay earned before taxes are withheld)
- Deductions for federal income tax, Social Security, and Medicare; state income tax and other local taxes, as applicable

Financial Management

Financial management includes banking, billing, collections, and insurance collections. This critical area is responsible for tracking the income necessary to keep the practice **solvent**, or capable of paying its bills and salaries.

Scheduling

Scheduling includes both patient scheduling and staff scheduling. Effective and efficient scheduling of staff can contribute significantly to the satisfaction level of the practice at several levels. If the office staff is continuously scheduled inappropriately, it affects employee morale and may cause discontent among the physicians and patients. Yet there must be some flexibility with the staff schedule to allow for unanticipated occurrences, such as sick days and business appointments.

Facility and Equipment Management

Facility and equipment management includes facility layout and planning, inventory, maintaining safety and Occupational Safety and Health Administration (OSHA) standards, and equipment replacement.

Clinical Office Management

The clinical aspects of office management are separate from the administrative aspects. Managing the clinical aspects of a medical office requires training of clinical personnel, keeping track of medical supplies, purchasing supplies when the stock is low, making sure that the physician's requests are met, and ensuring that proper procedures are followed. The office manager may handle safety issues (such as employee hepatitis B injections) and OSHA regulations, or a clinical coordinator or nurse manager may do so.

Communication

An office manager's ability to effectively communicate at all levels is very important and will contribute significantly to the cohesiveness of the staff. This includes written communication; oral communication, including verbal and nonverbal; and patient education.

Legal Concepts

Physicians typically use attorneys to assist with handling legal documents and issues. However, medical assistants must have an understanding of legal terminology and be aware of legal requirements with which the medical office must comply.

ROLE OF THE OFFICE MANAGER

The office manager is the coordinator for business activities conducted in the office. Each office varies, but the general duties include the following:

- Acting as liaison between staff and the physician-employer
- Conducting performance and salary reviews

TABLE 19-1 | Manager's Responsibilities to Employee and Physician-Employer

To Employee	To Physician-Employer
Interview	Increase efficiency of office
Hire/terminate	Meet with physician to discuss problems/plans
Orientate/train	Manage calendar for physician
Arrange work schedules	Assist with meetings
Arrange vacation coverage	Update physician on insurance changes related to Medicare fee schedules
Conduct performance evaluations	Order CPT® and ICD code books and current pharmacology books annually
Consult with physician regarding salary increases	Renew insurance policies and pay premiums

- Delegating responsibilities to staff
- Orienting, developing, and training staff
- Improving office efficiency
- Maintaining the office policies and procedures manual
- Overseeing Health Insurance Portability and Accountability Act (HIPAA) compliance
- Planning and conducting staff meetings
- Preparing patient education materials
- Providing guidelines for patient education
- Recruiting, hiring, and firing
- Supervising cash, banking, and payroll operations
- Supervising employees on a day-to-day basis
- Supervising the purchase and storage of equipment and supplies

Along with the knowledge needed to run an efficient medical office, an office manager needs effective administrative and communication skills. Medical assistants who have demonstrated these skills may seek to be promoted into this position. The following are other qualities or skills observed in good managers:

- Ability to organize
- Ability to communicate effectively at all levels
- Ability to enforce policy, when necessary
- Ability to resolve conflicts
- Creativity
- Diplomacy
- Excellent judgment
- Flexibility
- Leadership and take-charge initiative
- Objectivity

- Sense of fairness
- Willingness to continue to learn and promote the same behavior in staff members

The office manager's time is generally spent on employee and administrative issues. The employees, on the other hand, spend most of their time working with patients. A good office manager strives to establish and implement a team approach to management by including all staff in the decision-making process. Ultimately, the manager must make the final decision in conjunction with the physician-employer, but compliance with decisions is much greater when employees have had the opportunity to participate and contribute to the process. Table 19-1 describes responsibilities the office manager has to the employees and also to the physician-employer.

Many office managers are promoted based on **seniority**—a status gained by being the individual who has worked for the physician the longest. This is not always a wise practice because not everyone is a skilled manager, and even individuals who have experience or have completed management classes are not always the best candidates. When no internal candidate has the necessary skills for the office manager position, the physician-employer seeks an outside candidate. This is usually accomplished by posting an advertisement under the medical heading of the employment section of the

Professionalism

The office manager has an important position and should always set the standard of professionalism. In addition to the physicians and other providers, the office manager should be a role model for the office staff. Office managers must dress appropriately, be prompt and courteous, and take firm charge of the medical office.

local newspaper and relevant websites. In some cases, the physicians' **colleagues** (fellow members of the profession) may recommend a qualified candidate for the position.

Time Management

An effective office manager must be able to successfully manage time. If the manager is organized, the office is usually organized. Time management requires the ability to multitask and prioritize important tasks to complete them on schedule. This is quite different from doing every task as it comes along. The office manager generally has little control over the tasks presented. The control lies in how the tasks are handled and delegated.

One of the main responsibilities of the office manager and medical assistant is to manage routine office functions so the physician is free to concentrate on practicing medicine. When routine tasks, such as opening the daily mail, searching for a drug sample to give to a patient, and dealing with pharmaceutical and other sales representatives, are handled by the office manager, the physician has time to devote to administrative and patient-related tasks that only the physician can do.

Before establishing a time management system, it is important to define the office goals with the physician. Physicians' goals vary from simple to complex and from long term to short term. Examples of goals are collecting all payments at the time services are provided, reorganizing or computerizing billing, adding a partner or new service, writing a textbook, or planning for early retirement.

After goals have been established, priorities can be set using a to-do list. As tasks come to the office manager's attention, each item is assigned a priority designation of 1, 2, or 3, depending on how critical the item is to completion of goals. For example, ordering supplies that are running out is a priority 1, whereas rearranging a linen cupboard or a file drawer might be a priority 3. Priority 1 items must be done first and priority 3 last. It is often tempting to do the easier tasks first because they take less time and show an immediate accomplishment. Good time management would determine that the inventory order should be placed immediately and the priority 3 items should be delegated to someone else or completed later, if necessary. It is a good idea to date a to-do list and to cross off or check items as they are accomplished. This can be done on the computer, as part of a calendar application, or on paper. Box 19-1 shows an example of one type of to-do list.

Make every attempt to perform each task, such as handling mail, only once. Mail should be handled immediately, if possible, and all mail-related duties should be completed at the same time. As mail is opened, it must be quickly

BOX 19-1 | Medical Office To-Do List

Priority	To-Do: _____ Date: _____
2	Order paper supplies.
1	Arrange Dr. Williams's air transportation to medical convention next week.
2	Prepare performance appraisal for J. Jones.
3	Reorganize storeroom.
1	Prepare convention speech.
1	Place ad for new medical assistant.
3	Ask Janet to remove old magazines from reception room.
1	Call for pap test report for Ms. Kohut.
2	Block out schedule matrix for next quarter.
1	Prepare agenda for Thursday's staff meeting.

sorted according to importance, delivered to the appropriate recipients, or organized for follow-up action, as necessary.

When leaving a telephone message, it is advisable to leave detailed voice mail messages, whenever possible, because it can actually save time. Leaving a detailed message during the first call can prevent having to make another telephone call. An exception would be when calling a patient when only your name and phone number should be left, to protect the patient's privacy.

Never trust anything to memory in the medical office, because so much activity occurs that it is easy for something to slip from memory. Always write down complete instructions from the physician and information from the patient, another employee, or a supplier. It is best to maintain one small record book and keep all notations in that book rather than have several separate pieces of paper with information that can be misplaced. Many medical assistants carry a small notepad and pen in their pocket at all times.

Some offices require that the in-basket of the day's mail and incoming laboratory reports be emptied before the end of the day. This is a good time management technique to develop.

Monthly Planning

The office manager may wish to develop a system in which the office schedule for the entire month is laid out on a calendar. All physicians' conferences, staff meetings, vacations, accountant meetings, and other vendor visits should be noted. One of the office manager's tasks is to approve and decline vacation requests from staff members. It is important to list staff vacations on a calendar because it helps to prevent overlapping of vacations, which can leave an office short-staffed. This calendar should be placed in an accessible location. It may be helpful to purchase an erasable-style wall calendar so that corrections and changes can be made easily.

The manager creates and updates the physician's calendar. It is not necessary to include staff vacations on the physician's calendar. However, the office manager's own vacation schedule and days off should be included in both the physician's calendar and the staff calendar. Many physicians use the electronic calendar on a mobile device in which they enter all hospital rounds, meetings, conferences, and time away from the office. It is wise to compare the office calendar with the physician's calendar on a periodic basis and to update the office's master calendar as necessary.

Using a software-based calendar application, the office manager can create separate schedules that all appear on the same calendar. For example, the office manager could define a calendar for staff, one for personal tasks, and one for the physician. The office manager can view and manage all the schedules but send each person only the information that pertains to her.

Staff Meetings

Staff meetings should be held on a regular basis to promote communication and the flow of important information. Many of the best ideas for office improvement are a result of suggestions made at staff meetings (Figure 19-1). Staff members may wish to have direct communication with the physician, but this is often not possible in a large practice. The office manager can help to resolve this problem by asking the physician(s) to attend all or part of regularly scheduled staff meetings. If it is necessary to hold weekly meetings because of the nature of the practice, then the physician(s) should be invited monthly to accommodate busy schedules.

Meetings may need to be scheduled for periods when the staff members' work schedules overlap, either because

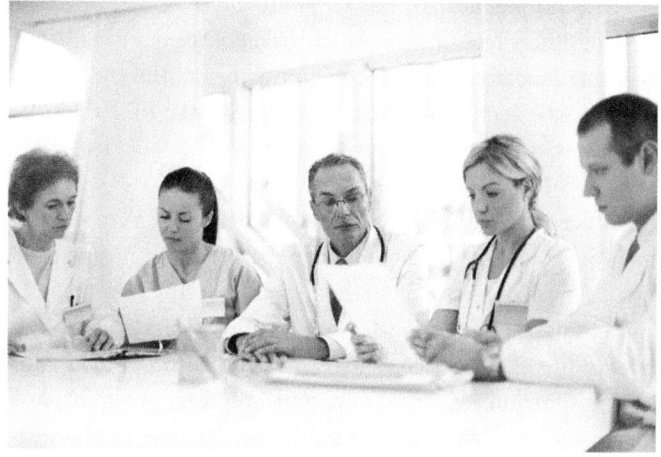

FIGURE 19-1 Regular staff meetings increase the efficiency of the medical office staff.

of shift changes or staggered hours, or before or after regular office hours. For instance, if the practice is open from 9:00 A.M. to 9:00 P.M. on Thursdays, the meetings could be scheduled for 4:30 P.M. or 5:00 P.M. when all the staff would be present. The meeting time needs to be blocked into the scheduling matrix so that it does not overlap with patient appointments. Or the meetings may be scheduled at 8:00 A.M. before the office opening. If attendance at staff meetings is mandatory, then staff members must be compensated for any meeting that is outside their normal work schedule.

The office manager usually conducts staff meetings and facilitates team interaction. The office manager determines the time and date for the meeting and also prepares the agenda, frequently with input from the physician and other staff. The key to a good meeting is a concise agenda that identifies items for discussion, such as staff responsibilities, and limits the time allotted. Focusing staff meetings and discussions in this way limits the amount of time wasted. Generally, the minutes, including names of the individuals attending the meeting, are recorded for future reference and distributed for review before the next meeting. See Box 19-2 for an example of an office staff meeting agenda. Procedure 19-1 shows how to prepare and hold a staff meeting.

Motivating Employees

Motivating employees is vital to maintaining a positive working environment and an efficiently run medical office. Qualities that employees expect from management include respect, ownership of personal space or environment, a sense of affiliation with the practice, fair compensation, acknowledgment, recognition, emotional rewards, communication, honesty, visibility of the management, empathy, trust, and equal treatment of all staff.

Respect from management is a basic need of all employees. The office manager should greet employees in a pleasant manner, always acknowledge their hard work, and never reprimand them in front of their peers. The manager should be accessible and listen to employees when they need to talk and should consider their suggestions seriously. Satisfied employees are one of the best resources that the office manager has in running an efficient medical office.

In the medical office, many people often share one space. If possible, each employee should have some personal space. Preferably this would be a desk, but it may just be a small table or a locker located somewhere in the office. Allowing employees to place pictures in the area in which they work most often makes the employee feel settled and, in turn, tends to produce a greater level of productivity.

Pearson Physicians Group
Staff Meeting Agenda

Date: December 19, 20YY
Time: 4:30–5:30 P.M.
Place: Staff Conference Room

Time	Agenda	Person Responsible
4:30	Introduction of new staff	T. Washington, Office Manager
	Review of last meeting's minutes	
4:35	New policies	
4:45	Problems with insurance	L. Turner/Insurance Coding Clerk
4:55	OSHA protocol for needlesticks	K. Wall/Lab Tech
5:05	Vacation schedules	T. Washington
5:10	New office location	Dr. McWalter
5:20	New business	Tania Washington
5:30	Meeting adjourned	

Creating a sense of affiliation to the medical office is often achieved by making simple considerations. Sharing in the highlights of staff members' lives, such as throwing a small birthday celebration or recognizing a special event (marriage or birth of a child), helps employees feel part of the office community or "family." Bringing the staff together with special events outside the office, such as a company picnic, can also increase the sense of affiliation.

Generally, employees want to feel that they are being fairly compensated for the amount of work they produce. If an employee feels that the quality and quantity of work produced is not reflected in pay, the employee may seek a position elsewhere. One of the office manager's responsibilities is to make sure that all staff are appropriately compensated.

There are other rewards beyond pay. Employees need encouragement, recognition, and acknowledgment of their

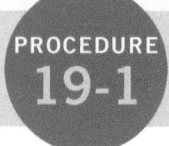

PROCEDURE
19-1

Following Staff Meeting Procedures

Objective ◆ *Explain and present the necessary steps to preparing and running a staff meeting.*

EQUIPMENT AND SUPPLIES

Agenda items received from staff; meeting agenda; means of keeping time (watch, clock, stopwatch, etc.); room for the meeting; any audio or video equipment that may be needed

METHOD

1. One week before the meeting, request agenda items from the staff.
2. Before the meeting, create a meeting agenda with all topics to be discussed. On the agenda include the date, time, and place of the meeting. Identify who will be running (facilitating) the meeting (most often, the office manager). Assign a length of time to each topic and a person who is responsible for that topic.
3. Start the meeting on time.
4. Begin by briefly covering the previous meeting.
5. Try to stay on schedule as much as possible.
6. Allow for time at the end of the meeting to have open discussion of any new business.
7. Adjourn the meeting.
8. After the meeting, have the minutes of the meeting typed and distributed to all involved.

work, such as awards for meeting or exceeding set goals. Praise should be given to employees using a method that does not make them feel awkward. Some employees prefer public recognition, whereas others prefer private recognition. For example, an employee who prefers private recognition appreciates receiving a card from the office manager recognizing the achievement rather than a large poster hung at the entrance to the workplace. Many offices now incorporate a questionnaire at the time of new employee orientation that asks how the employee prefers to be recognized. In general, a combination of personal and public recognition is most effective.

Communication is essential to managing an efficient office and maintaining a cohesive work atmosphere. Employees like honest, straight talk from their employers. It is always best for employees to receive news directly from their manager rather than through rumors. The office manager should always inform staff of both the positive and the negative issues affecting the practice.

It is essential for the office manager to be available to the employees. Being visible to employees creates a positive rapport, and any problems that may arise can often be dealt with swiftly and efficiently. A manager should not hide in an office, staying busy with business affairs. Employees are very aware of their manager's behavior, especially during the time spent in the office. The office manager needs to lead by example. For example, the office manager should be mindful of her own arrival and departure times to the office. It is difficult for the office manager to maintain credibility when counseling an employee regarding tardiness when she is late several times per week.

An office manager often can gain a great deal of loyalty from employees through empathy. Although the office manager is a figure of authority to the employee, honest communication and a sincere regard for the employee's well-being go a long way in creating a comfortable and productive workplace.

Leadership Styles

The ability to make appropriate calls of judgment, the willingness to learn new ideas, staying calm during stressful situations, always maintaining a professional attitude, and good listening skills are all attributes of good leaders. As an office manager, you are the team leader of the medical office. Think back to good managers you have had in the past. What attributes made them good managers? Was it their knowledge, or was it that they were easy to approach, or both? If you think back, you may find traits in former managers that you can incorporate into your own behavior to create your personal style of office management.

Leadership style refers to the predominant way a manager makes decisions and relates to others in the office. The four types of leaders are authoritarian, democratic, permissive, and bureaucratic. Each type of leader is distinct and responds to different motivators. Knowledge of different management styles may help you fine-tune your own management style and give you ideas on how to benefit your employees.

Each leadership style has benefits and downfalls. Most managers find they exercise one particular style the majority of the time; however, they may shift to a different management style if the situation calls for it. For example, an office manager might be a democratic leader the majority of the time, but if a fire breaks out in the office, the manager may switch to an authoritarian style.

Authoritarian

Authoritarian leaders tend to be very direct. They make most decisions on their own without the input of others. They are strong decision makers but may not be viewed as team players. Authoritarian leaders tend to want respect and obedience from their staff members and might even use fear to achieve staff obedience. The need for power and absolute authority often motivates this type of leader. Authoritarian leaders work best in times of great stress and crisis situations.

Democratic

A *democratic leader* concentrates more on the relations among staff members and emphasizes teamwork within the office. This type of leader tends to be motivated from within to provide a comfortable work environment for all. With a leader of this style, you often find very open communication. Democratic leaders are more receptive to new ideas from staff members, which helps to create an atmosphere of cooperation among the staff, instituting greater participation in the decision-making process. This style of leadership often leads to a contented staff.

Permissive

Permissive leaders are very open with the staff. They are not strict with rules and policies. Like the democratic leader, the permissive leader is self-motivated. In many situations, she allows staff members to make their own decisions and does not interfere with staff processes. However, medical offices must keep an ordered environment, and at times permissive leadership can lead to disorganization and even hazardous conditions.

Bureaucratic

Bureaucratic leaders are very strong at enforcing rules. Their motivation comes from external means. They prefer to rely on established management methods for office matters.

Bureaucratic leaders tend to be rigid and set in their ways. The staff often find the bureaucratic leader to be distant and formal.

Types of Authority

For any manager to enact and enforce the rules that are necessary to run an efficient medical office, she must establish a level of authority. A manager may establish several types of authority or power, which are used depending on what the situation calls for. Types of authority and power include the following:

- **Reward-based power**—Incorporates rewards or some type of enticement in exchange for better job performance and teamwork. When managers use rewards to exact greater productivity from their employees, they are exercising a form of power over their employees. The degree to which this works depends on the level of reward that the employee wants and receives.

- **Legitimate authority**—Authority and responsibility are given to people based on their title. The president of a company holds legitimate authority: the power of the title of president.

- **Expert authority**—Given to those who have a great deal of knowledge. This is earned through experience and education.

- **Referent power**—Given out of high regard and respect. It comes with a person's likability and even success in the field.

- **Informative power**—The power wielded by those with information that others want or need.

- **Connective power**—The idea that if you know the right people you can get what you need—is one reason to network at local organizations. As a student, it is never too early to start making connections.

With all authority comes the ability to abuse or overuse it, which can lead to distrust of the manager. The effects of overuse of authority depend on the type of power wielded by the individual. With reward power, one downfall is that the employees can become reliant on rewards. Once this happens, the power becomes coercive, which is a negative power because it uses fear to motivate employees. The employee may be afraid of punishment or that the manager may withhold certain rewards to gain cooperation. Also, there is the possibility of jealousy among employees. They may have the perception that someone is getting more attention or rewards than someone else, and thus the idea of favorites emerges. Misused legitimate power leads to fear of the person with the title or even the title itself. In the misuse of informative

power, you often see avoidance, a sense of unfairness, and a bit of hostility. Expert, referent, and connective powers all tend to lead to the same effects when misused: a perceived level of manipulation and intrusion among those affected.

CREATING A TEAM ATMOSPHERE

For a medical office to run at its most efficient level, the staff must work as a team. This can be difficult for the office manager to manage. Still, the office manager is in charge of strengthening and enhancing the team atmosphere. The following are some factors that must come together to create a successful office team:

- **Size**—A team should have enough members to generate ideas and accomplish work, but not so large it becomes unmanageable.

- **Team personalities**—Use teams composed of a variety of personalities and skill sets so that weaknesses of one person can be offset by strengths of another.

- **Responsible team members**—All members of the team must be held accountable for their actions.

- **Unified team approach**—Team members must agree on the purpose and goals.

Every team must have a leader, and the office manager must realize that he is the team leader. Other team leaders may emerge from the team itself.

Managers should treat all members of a team equally. Showing favoritism, perceived or real, to one or two employees can easily break down any team atmosphere.

Managers also must show that they are an integral part of the team. Employees become more confident and content in their jobs when they know that their manager is willing to help out with employee duties when assistance is needed. Most successful managers adopt the attitude, "I would not ask the employee to do anything I haven't already done or to do anything I wouldn't be willing to do." For instance, if two members of the office team are both out sick, a manager who answers the telephone or files medical records in their place shows team members a vital component to teamwork.

In some medical offices, it also might be necessary to have several levels of leaders among the office team. For example, one team leader might work at the front desk, and another might have clinical duties. To keep the team unified and productive, all team leaders must be highly organized, have a good deal of energy, and support the other team leaders.

Team Size

The size of a group can greatly affect the dynamics of how it functions. Small groups often become very intimate.

Close bonds may form, but because of the small group dynamics, they also tend to be very unstable. As groups grow larger, they tend to become more stable but experience a loss of group intimacy. This information is important to know when assembling a team. A smaller group has a more relaxed atmosphere, whereas a larger group has a more rigid structure. In similar fashion, the smaller the office, the easier going it may be. Larger multiphysician offices tend to be much more formal and systematic as a whole, but employees may be very close within their own small groups, such as a group of receptionists or clinical medical assistants.

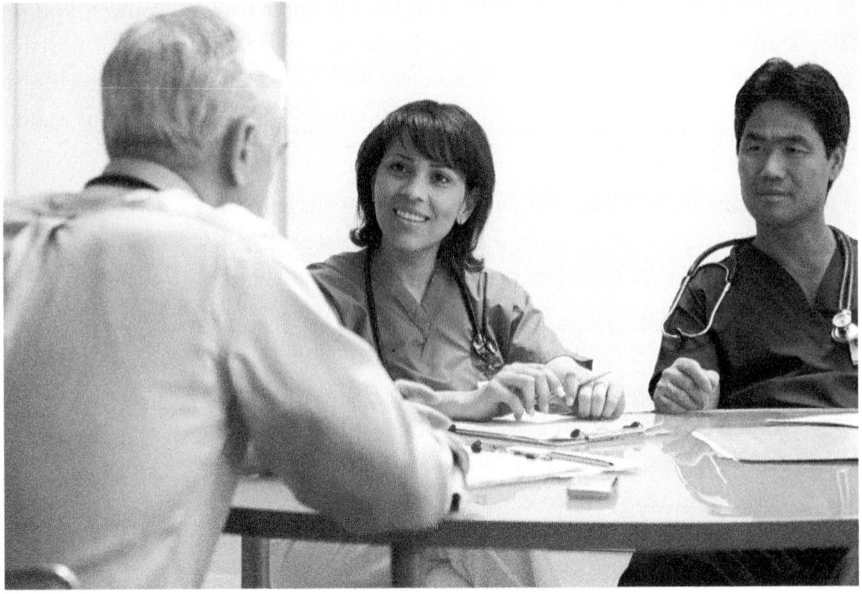

FIGURE 19-2 A medical office requires teamwork.

Team Personality and Skills

Creating a team atmosphere can begin during the hiring process by allowing some staff members to help in the hiring process. Participants must be made aware of legal and illegal interview questions. It is important that the staff understand what the office manager is looking for in potential employees. Staff members may be able to provide some insight into the personality of the job candidate, which would be helpful in maintaining a cohesive team atmosphere. Ultimately, the office manager and physician have the final say in the hiring of the candidate, but this process lets the staff know that their opinions also matter.

It takes the right mix of people to create a strong team. It is never a good idea to fill an office with people who are similar in personality and leadership style. Often, similar weaknesses manifest in the day-to-day business of the office, which defeats the goal of efficiency and teamwork. A manager should look for staff members who complement each other's talents and traits. For example, one member of the staff who is really good with computers but is weak in filing is complemented by a staff member who is weak in computers but an excellent filer. Creating this mix provides the foundation for a strong team (Figure 19-2).

Within any given team, the different team members take on various roles. These roles can be task-oriented or nurturing in nature. Task-oriented roles include the information seeker, the information giver, the coordinator, the energizer, the evaluator or critic, and the recorder. These roles all focus on the goal toward which the team is working. Nurturing roles may include the encourager, the harmonizer, the compromiser, and the follower. A team member may take on one or many roles within the team.

Team Accountability

As a team, members must hold each other accountable for their actions. If something goes wrong, the team must come together to locate and fix the problem. This means that the team should not attack or try to blame a problem on any one member. They must find where, as a team, they lost track and how they can prevent a similar problem from reoccurring.

Team Purpose and Goals

The team must find a way to work together. Ensure that you have the correct personalities and talents. Encourage team members to concentrate on a single goal. Successful teams work with the same purpose in mind and approach a problem or task using similar means. This helps reduce potential conflict among the team members as they work out problems.

Any team has some weaknesses, so it is important for the office manager to monitor the progress of the team. Clinical and administrative employees might tend to divide themselves into separate teams. The employees might feel comfortable with this type of division, but it usually puts strains on running the practice. The office manager must prevent this from happening. When possible, it is good practice to have staff members switch places occasionally or shadow another employee (e.g., have those who are usually front-office employees trade with or accompany those who are more accustomed to back-office duties). This helps team members to experience the duties and responsibilities of the office as a whole. When employees are not working toward the goal of a cohesive team, the manager might wish to use team-building exercises. Many companies offer team building workshops to help office managers strengthen their office teams.

HIRING EFFECTIVE STAFF MEMBERS

The office manager needs to hire new staff from time to time when someone leaves the office or a new position is created. Recruitment can begin in-house, which means that the job vacancy is posted within the medical office so existing employees may apply for the vacant positions before the position is advertised elsewhere. If no internal candidates are interested or qualified, several methods may be used to seek applicants.

Advertising the Position

There are many ways of advertising for open positions. These include placement of job advertisements in newspaper and trade journals, professional organizations, the Internet, formal training programs, and employment agencies, which charge a fee to be paid by the employer to the agency if an agency's candidate is hired. Local training programs in colleges are also excellent resources.

The newspaper or Internet is often the best way to reach your local population. Many online providers offer options for job advertisements. Advertisements should describe the position and the required qualifications accurately. This prevents the office from receiving too many résumés from unqualified applicants. If you are too general in your description, you may receive an excess of applicants. However, being too specific can cause the opposite problem: You might receive a very limited number of individuals applying for the position.

After you have advertised and received résumés, you must begin the task of sorting through each applicant's résumé. One commonly used sorting method includes first removing résumés that do not show the appropriate educational requirements, certifications, licensure, or work experience for the position that has been advertised. Next, it is helpful to remove résumés that have obvious errors, such as poor grammar and spelling. At that point, office managers are usually left with the candidates they believe show the most promise for the position. At this point, the interview process begins.

Conducting Interviews

Interviewing often begins with short telephone interviews in which the office manager speaks with applicants and asks a few pertinent questions regarding their background, experience, and availability. This gives a different perspective on candidates than a résumé can provide and helps the manager eliminate candidates who may not be qualified. It also provides insight into a candidate's telephone skills. Those who pass the telephone interview are invited to submit a job application and schedule an in-person interview.

A job application is a uniform method of gathering information and comparing candidates, as compared with résumés, because the information on résumés received in the mail varies in form and content from one candidate to another. Job applications can be completed either online or on paper form (Figure 19-3). You may choose to send an application by mail and have applicants bring it with them

EMPLOYMENT APPLICATION FORM

Directions: Answer all questions using black ink (print).

PERSONAL NAME			
(LAST)	(FIRST)	(MI)	
ADDRESS-STREET	CITY	STATE	ZIP
PHONE NUMBER:	SOCIAL SECURITY NUMBER:		
POSITION DESIRED:			
EXPECTED SALARY OR HOURLY WAGE:			

EDUCATION			
NAME OF SCHOOL	ADDRESS	DATE(S)	DEGREE/CERTIFICATE
HIGH SCHOOL			
VOCATIONAL/TECHNICAL			
COLLEGE			
OTHER			

WORK EXPERIENCE – Give present position (or last position held first).			
JOB TITLE:	EMPLOYER	ADDRESS	DATES
DUTIES PERFORMED:			
JOB TITLE:	EMPLOYER	ADDRESS	DATES
DUTIES PERFORMED:			
JOB TITLE:	EMPLOYER	ADDRESS	DATES
DUTIES PERFORMED:			

REFERENCES – List three persons (other than relatives) who have known you for at least 2 years		
NAME/TITLE	ADDRESS	TELEPHONE NUMBER

APPLICANT'S SIGNATURE ______________________________ Date

FIGURE 19-3 A standard employment application form may be used.

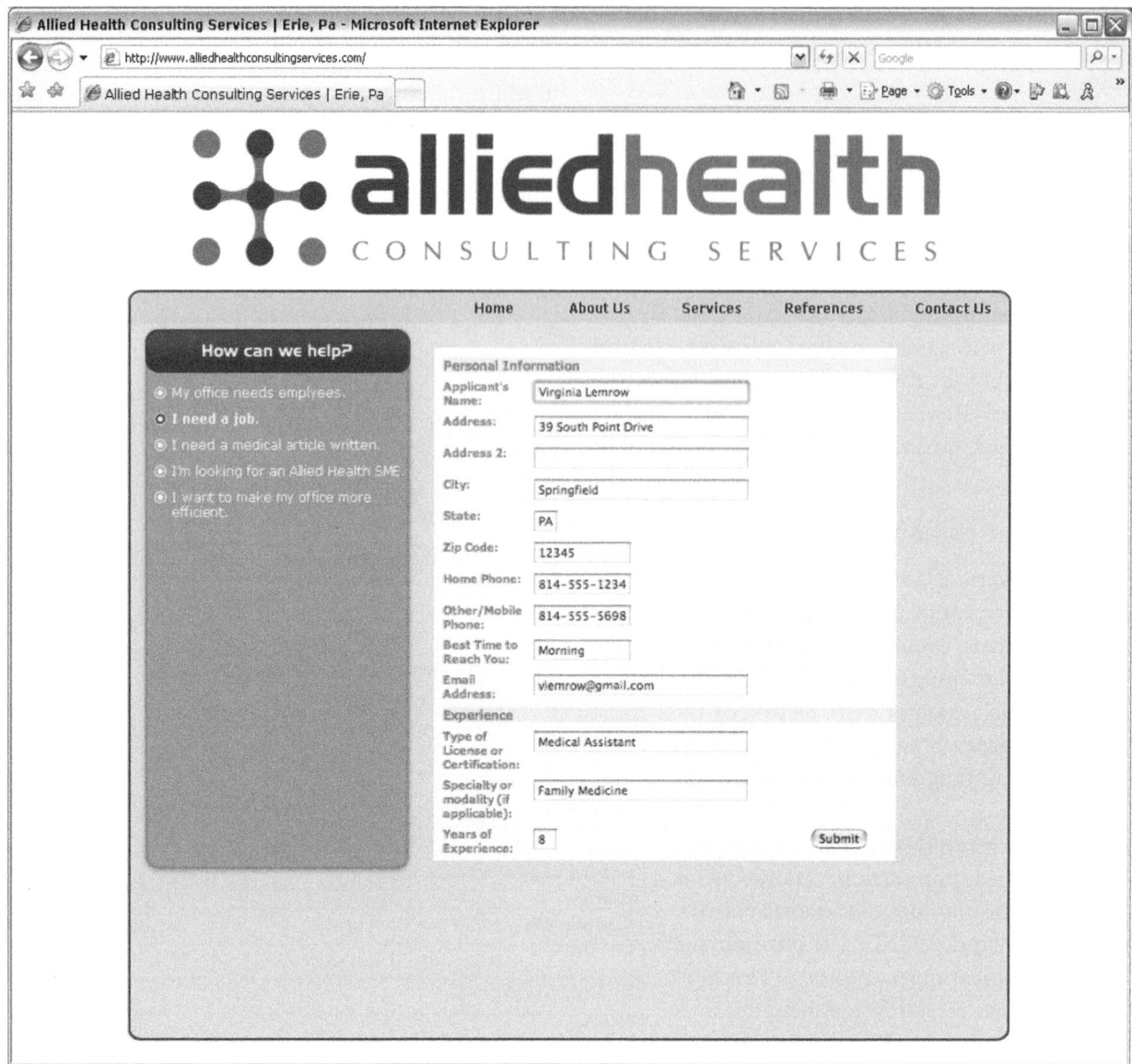

FIGURE 19-4 Example of an online employment application and posting of a résumé.

to the interview. Alternatively, you can provide the link for them to access the online version (Figure 19-4). Online applications give the manager the opportunity to review the application before the interview. However, there also are benefits to having the applicant fill out the form at the time of the interview. You are able to see how the applicant handles filling out forms under a time constraint. You also get to see the applicant's handwriting. Legible handwriting is important to have because employees need to read others' documentation, notes, and instructions. The last thing you learn from this process is how adept the applicants are at completing a requested task. Do they follow directions and complete every line, or do they take shortcuts? Their actions can indicate how they might handle on-the-spot tasks that may need to be resolved quickly and efficiently.

Important aspects of the applicant should be assessed. Is the applicant dressed appropriately? Does the applicant reflect a professional appearance? Is the résumé neatly prepared? The answers to these questions give insight into the type of employee the applicant might make and whether he or she may fit into your current team.

Interview Questions

Many questions can be asked in an interview, but some are not recommended or not allowed by law. You must keep in mind the fair-employment practice (FEP) laws that affect hiring. Title VII of the Civil Rights Act of 1964, later amended as the Equal Employment Opportunity Act (EEOA) of 1972 (and further amended in 1990), prohibits discriminating against applicants based on race, color, religion, sex, or national origin both during the interview and on the application.

State and federal equal opportunity laws do not clearly forbid employers from making preemployment inquiries that relate to, or disproportionately screen out, members based on race, color, sex, national origin, religion, or age. However, such inquiries can be used as evidence of an employer's intent to discriminate, unless the questions asked can be justified by some business purpose. Therefore, inquiries about organizations, clubs, societies, and lodges of which an applicant may be a member, or any other questions that could indicate the applicant's race, sex, national origin, disability status, age, religion, color, or ancestry, generally should be avoided. Similarly, employers should not ask for a photograph of an applicant. If needed for identification purposes, a photograph may be obtained after an offer of employment is made and accepted (www.eeoc.gov/laws/practices).

For example, asking an applicant questions such as "Did you have difficulty finding a babysitter today?" or "Do you plan to have children?" generally is considered **discriminatory**, or prejudicial treatment, and therefore should not be asked. However, you can ask applicants if they are able to come to work as scheduled, if they can arrive on time, and if they foresee anything that would interfere with their job attendance or performance.

Employers are explicitly prohibited from making preoffer inquiries about disability, including alcoholism and drug addiction, which are protected under the Americans with Disabilities Act (ADA). Under the law, employers generally cannot ask disability-related questions or require medical

examinations until after an applicant has been given a conditional job offer. This is because, in the past, this information was frequently used to exclude applicants with disabilities before their ability to perform a job was evaluated.

Employers are permitted to ask limited questions before a job offer is made about reasonable accommodation. This is permitted if the employer reasonably believes that the applicant may need accommodation because of an obvious or voluntarily disclosed disability, or where the applicant has disclosed a need for accommodation. Employers also can ask if the applicant will need an accommodation to perform a specific job duty. If the answer is yes, the employer can ask what the accommodation would be.

The employer cannot ask any questions about the nature or severity of the disability before a job offer is made. However, after making a conditional job offer, an employer can ask any disability-related question or require a medical examination as long as all individuals selected for the same job are asked the same questions or made to take the same examination.

Refer to Table 19-2 for more information on asking interview questions.

Assessing a Good Fit

Learning important information about applicants is key to making sure that they would be a good fit for your practice. You may want to ask them about past office experience and what types of physicians they have worked with before.

Another good idea is to test applicants' ability to think on their feet. It has been an increasing practice to give applicants

TABLE 19-2 | Types of Interview Questions

Recommended/Allowed	Not Recommended
Can you work on Saturday (if the job requires it)?	Do you have a disability? (Illegal to ask)
Can you arrive at work by 8 A.M. every day?	Are you an alcoholic? (Illegal to ask)
Are you able to work on your feet for eight hours?	Have you ever been a drug addict? (Illegal to ask)
What training and education did you receive in the military?	How old are you?
What is your experience performing the duties of this job?	Are you an immigrant?
Will need an accommodation to perform a specific job duty? What would be the accommodation?	Where were you born?
Have you ever been convicted of a crime?	What church do you go to?
Do you currently use illegal drugs?	What religious holidays do you observe?
	Are you married?
	Do you have children?
	Do you have trouble hearing?
	Have you ever been arrested?
	What type of military discharge did you receive?
	Do you have a car? What kind of car do you have?

off-the-cuff questions to see how they respond. You are not looking for a correct answer but wish only to see how they reason through the question. Do they give up and guess, or do they try to make a logical guess by thinking through the possibilities? Many managers also give applicants situational questions. For example, you may wish to ask how they would handle a patient who is upset about a test result.

As discussed in the sections on creating a team atmosphere, it is sometimes a good idea to allow certain staff members to ask questions of the applicant. Again, staff members can give feedback on whether they feel the applicant fits with the other staff.

While interviewing, applicants are also forming opinions regarding whether they want to work for the practice. Present the positive aspects of the work environment and provide a brief tour of the office to give them a sense of the practice. Discuss challenges the applicant may encounter, and ask how she would handle them. Ask applicants what questions they have for you. Often you can learn as much about applicants by the types of questions they ask as you can by how they answer your questions.

It is important to find the right employee for every position. Always look beyond experience and knowledge to the applicant's personality. To maintain a positive team atmosphere, sometimes it is better to hire someone with a little less experience but is a good personality fit for the office.

You may choose to have your top applicants come back for second interviews. You may wish to have the physician or other staff members interview these applicants and to provide another opportunity for the candidate to ask questions of you.

Checking References

The next step in the selection process is to check the references of the applicants. This is done by conducting a brief telephone interview with the person(s) referenced by the applicant. After interviewing all the applicants of interest and checking their references, it is time to decide whom to hire.

Hiring the Applicant

After you have verified the references of your applicants, you can begin the process of selecting your top choices for the position and making an offer. It may happen that you call your top choice and offer the position but the applicant declines your offer. In such a case, you would then offer the position to your next choice.

The new employee should receive a job description and written confirmation of the job offer that includes the salary

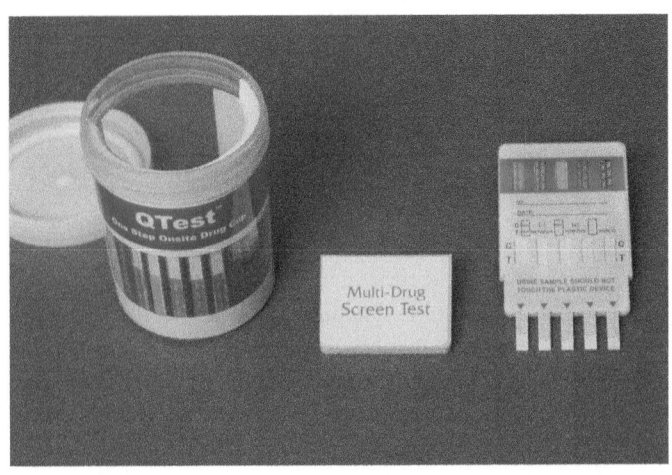

FIGURE 19-5 Example of equipment used for a urine drug screen that a medical office may require before employment.

and benefits offered. The office manager usually signs this letter. After an applicant has accepted the position, all other applicants should be notified, either by telephone or in writing, that the position is filled.

Some medical offices require a post offer drug screen (Figure 19-5), acceptable credit report, acceptable criminal background check, preemployment physical (which may include tuberculosis [TB] testing and hepatitis B immunization), and body mechanics testing and training. The new employee should be provided with information regarding scheduling the appropriate tests and completing the appropriate forms required for the position either before the offer of employment or at the time the offer is made.

Professionalism | Cultural Considerations

Many medical office managers seek to hire applicants who are multilingual, particularly if a medical office is situated in a region that is highly populated with a specific ethnic group. For instance, states in the southern part of the United States may be more populated with Spanish-speaking individuals, because Texas borders Mexico and Florida is in close proximity to Cuba and Puerto Rico. Thus, a medical assistant who is bilingual in Spanish and English would be very desirable in those states. Many areas on the west coast find it beneficial to hire staff who are fluent in one of the many Asian languages or Russian. Being multilingual is often a deciding factor between two candidates who are both equally qualified for a position in a medical office. Skills in communicating with American Sign Language for the deaf are valuable also. Medical assistants should include all fluent languages on their résumés.

The candidate must be made aware that the offer of the position is contingent on satisfactory completion of required screenings and that the offer may be withdrawn if a required screening is failed or not completed.

New Employee Probation

The first three months (90 days) usually constitute a **probationary period**, or trial period, for new employees. This time frame allows the supervisor to observe the new employee at work and to determine if he or she is suited to the position. During this probationary period, an employee can be terminated without cause.

Orientation and Training

An effective manager has an organized, efficient method of orientation and training for all new hires. The time and effort pays off in the long run, because it ensures that all employees receive the same information. Many offices have an orientation checklist, which is used to verify that all topics are covered.

The following is a list of the basic subjects that should be covered during new hire orientation:

- Work hours and schedule, including overtime approval procedures
- Office layout (locations of the restroom, break room, employee parking, employee entrances, etc.)

- Dress code
- Smoking policy
- Lunch and break times and location
- Job description
- All employment records—including I-9s (Figure 19-6), emergency contact information, affidavit of citizenship, insurance enrollment, and so on
- OSHA Bloodborne Pathogens Standards and standard precautions—including request for a waiver form for hepatitis B vaccine
- Health Insurance Portability and Accountability Act (HIPAA) training
- Fire safety—locations of fire extinguishers (Figure 19-7), exit procedures, stairwell locations (Figure 19-8)
- Confidentiality (obtain signature on confidentiality statement)
- Policies and procedures manual (Employee should read and sign a statement that the document has been read and understood.)
- Physician's work preferences—how the physician and the team prefer to work, including examples to help the medical assistant understand the role

Smaller offices with fewer employees may conduct orientation sessions on the job as the new employee begins working. This is not ideal but is often necessary. Orientation materials and a schedule can be developed to assist in this training process.

Although some workplace rules and policies may have been covered during the interview process, they should be repeated after the person is hired. Reiterating these issues during orientation can prevent confusion and errors. A confident employee is an effective employee.

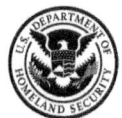

Employment Eligibility Verification

Department of Homeland Security

U.S. Citizenship and Immigration Services

USCIS
Form I-9
OMB No. 1615-0047
Expires 03/31/2016

▶ **START HERE.** Read instructions carefully before completing this form. The instructions must be available during completion of this form.
ANTI-DISCRIMINATION NOTICE: It is illegal to discriminate against work-authorized individuals. Employers **CANNOT** specify which document(s) they will accept from an employee. The refusal to hire an individual because the documentation presented has a future expiration date may also constitute illegal discrimination.

Section 1. Employee Information and Attestation (Employees must complete and sign Section 1 of Form I-9 no later than the **first day of employment**, but not before accepting a job offer.)

Last Name (Family Name)	First Name (Given Name)	Middle Initial	Other Names Used (if any)

Address (Street Number and Name)	Apt. Number	City or Town	State	Zip Code

Date of Birth (mm/dd/yyyy)	U.S. Social Security Number	E-mail Address	Telephone Number
	☐☐☐-☐☐-☐☐☐☐		

I am aware that federal law provides for imprisonment and/or fines for false statements or use of false documents in connection with the completion of this form.

I attest, under penalty of perjury, that I am (check one of the following):

☐ A citizen of the United States

☐ A noncitizen national of the United States (See instructions)

☐ A lawful permanent resident (Alien Registration Number/USCIS Number): _____

☐ An alien authorized to work until (expiration date, if applicable, mm/dd/yyyy) _____ . Some aliens may write "N/A" in this field. (See instructions)

For aliens authorized to work, provide your Alien Registration Number/ USCIS Number **OR** Form I-94 Admission Number:

1. Alien Registration Number/USCIS Number:_____

OR

2. Form I-94 Admission Number: _____

	3-D Barcode Do Not Write in This Space

If you obtained your admission number from CBP in connection with your arrival in the United States, include the following:

Foreign Passport Number: _____

Country of Issuance: _____

Some aliens may write "N/A" on the Foreign Passport Number and Country of Issuance fields. (See instructions)

Signature of Employee:	Date (mm/dd/yyyy):

Preparer and/or Translator Certification (To be completed and signed if Section 1 is prepared by a person other than the employee.)

I attest, under penalty of perjury, that I have assisted in the completion of this form and that to the best of my knowledge the information is true and correct.

Signature of Preparer or Translator:	Date (mm/dd/yyyy):

Last Name (Family Name)	First Name (Given Name)

Address (Street Number and Name)	City or Town	State	Zip Code

🛑 *Employer Completes Next Page* 🛑

Form I-9 03/08/13 N   Page 7 of 9

FIGURE 19-6 The I-9 form.

Section 2. Employer or Authorized Representative Review and Verification

(Employers or their authorized representative must complete and sign Section 2 within 3 business days of the employee's first day of employment. You must physically examine one document from List A OR examine a combination of one document from List B and one document from List C as listed on the "Lists of Acceptable Documents" on the next page of this form. For each document you review, record the following information: document title, issuing authority, document number, and expiration date, if any.)

Employee Last Name, First Name and Middle Initial from Section 1:

List A Identity and Employment Authorization	OR	List B Identity	AND	List C Employment Authorization
Document Title:		Document Title:		Document Title:
Issuing Authority:		Issuing Authority:		Issuing Authority:
Document Number:		Document Number:		Document Number:
Expiration Date *(if any)(mm/dd/yyyy)*:		Expiration Date *(if any)(mm/dd/yyyy)*:		Expiration Date *(if any)(mm/dd/yyyy)*:
Document Title:				
Issuing Authority:				
Document Number:				
Expiration Date *(if any)(mm/dd/yyyy)*:				
Document Title:				3-D Barcode Do Not Write in This Space
Issuing Authority:				
Document Number:				
Expiration Date *(if any)(mm/dd/yyyy)*:				

Certification

I attest, under penalty of perjury, that (1) I have examined the document(s) presented by the above-named employee, (2) the above-listed document(s) appear to be genuine and to relate to the employee named, and (3) to the best of my knowledge the employee is authorized to work in the United States.

The employee's first day of employment *(mm/dd/yyyy)*: _____ **(See instructions for exemptions.)**

Signature of Employer or Authorized Representative	Date *(mm/dd/yyyy)*	Title of Employer or Authorized Representative		
Last Name *(Family Name)*	First Name *(Given Name)*	Employer's Business or Organization Name		
Employer's Business or Organization Address *(Street Number and Name)*	City or Town		State	Zip Code

Section 3. Reverification and Rehires *(To be completed and signed by employer or authorized representative.)*

A. New Name *(if applicable)* Last Name *(Family Name)* First Name *(Given Name)*	Middle Initial	B. Date of Rehire *(if applicable) (mm/dd/yyyy)*:

C. If employee's previous grant of employment authorization has expired, provide the information for the document from List A or List C the employee presented that establishes current employment authorization in the space provided below.

Document Title:	Document Number:	Expiration Date *(if any)(mm/dd/yyyy)*:

I attest, under penalty of perjury, that to the best of my knowledge, this employee is authorized to work in the United States, and if the employee presented document(s), the document(s) I have examined appear to be genuine and to relate to the individual.

Signature of Employer or Authorized Representative:	Date *(mm/dd/yyyy)*:	Print Name of Employer or Authorized Representative:

Form I-9 03/08/13 N

Page 8 of 9

FIGURE 19-6 *(continued)*

LISTS OF ACCEPTABLE DOCUMENTS
All documents must be UNEXPIRED

Employees may present one selection from List A
or a combination of one selection from List B and one selection from List C.

LIST A		LIST B		LIST C
Documents that Establish Both Identity and Employment Authorization	**OR**	**Documents that Establish Identity**	**AND**	**Documents that Establish Employment Authorization**
1. U.S. Passport or U.S. Passport Card		1. Driver's license or ID card issued by a State or outlying possession of the United States provided it contains a photograph or information such as name, date of birth, gender, height, eye color, and address		1. A Social Security Account Number card, unless the card includes one of the following restrictions: (1) NOT VALID FOR EMPLOYMENT (2) VALID FOR WORK ONLY WITH INS AUTHORIZATION (3) VALID FOR WORK ONLY WITH DHS AUTHORIZATION
2. Permanent Resident Card or Alien Registration Receipt Card (Form I-551)				
3. Foreign passport that contains a temporary I-551 stamp or temporary I-551 printed notation on a machine-readable immigrant visa		2. ID card issued by federal, state or local government agencies or entities, provided it contains a photograph or information such as name, date of birth, gender, height, eye color, and address		
4. Employment Authorization Document that contains a photograph (Form I-766)				2. Certification of Birth Abroad issued by the Department of State (Form FS-545)
		3. School ID card with a photograph		
5. For a nonimmigrant alien authorized to work for a specific employer because of his or her status: **a.** Foreign passport; and **b.** Form I-94 or Form I-94A that has the following: (1) The same name as the passport; and (2) An endorsement of the alien's nonimmigrant status as long as that period of endorsement has not yet expired and the proposed employment is not in conflict with any restrictions or limitations identified on the form.		4. Voter's registration card		3. Certification of Report of Birth issued by the Department of State (Form DS-1350)
		5. U.S. Military card or draft record		
		6. Military dependent's ID card		4. Original or certified copy of birth certificate issued by a State, county, municipal authority, or territory of the United States bearing an official seal
		7. U.S. Coast Guard Merchant Mariner Card		
		8. Native American tribal document		5. Native American tribal document
		9. Driver's license issued by a Canadian government authority		6. U.S. Citizen ID Card (Form I-197)
		For persons under age 18 who are unable to present a document listed above:		7. Identification Card for Use of Resident Citizen in the United States (Form I-179)
6. Passport from the Federated States of Micronesia (FSM) or the Republic of the Marshall Islands (RMI) with Form I-94 or Form I-94A indicating nonimmigrant admission under the Compact of Free Association Between the United States and the FSM or RMI		10. School record or report card		8. Employment authorization document issued by the Department of Homeland Security
		11. Clinic, doctor, or hospital record		
		12. Day-care or nursery school record		

Illustrations of many of these documents appear in Part 8 of the Handbook for Employers (M-274).

Refer to Section 2 of the instructions, titled "Employer or Authorized Representative Review and Verification," for more information about acceptable receipts.

FIGURE 19-6 (*continued*)

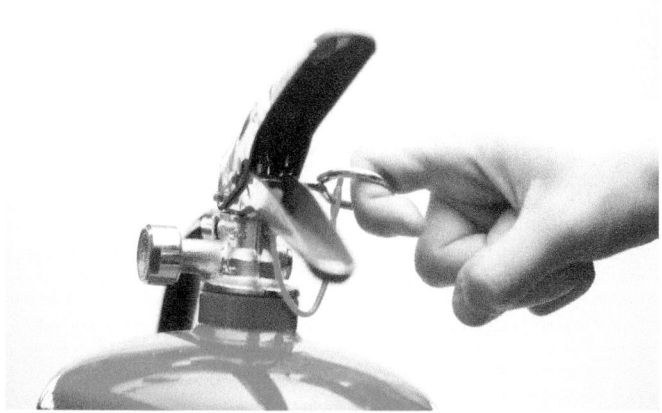

(A) Pull the pin on the upper handle of the fire extinguisher.

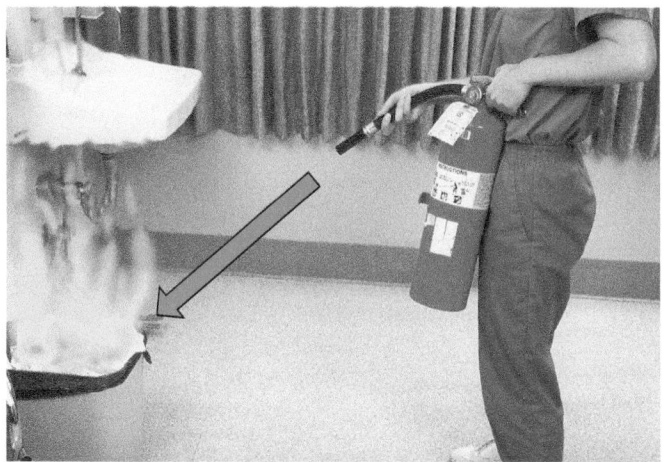

(B) Aim low toward the base of the fire.

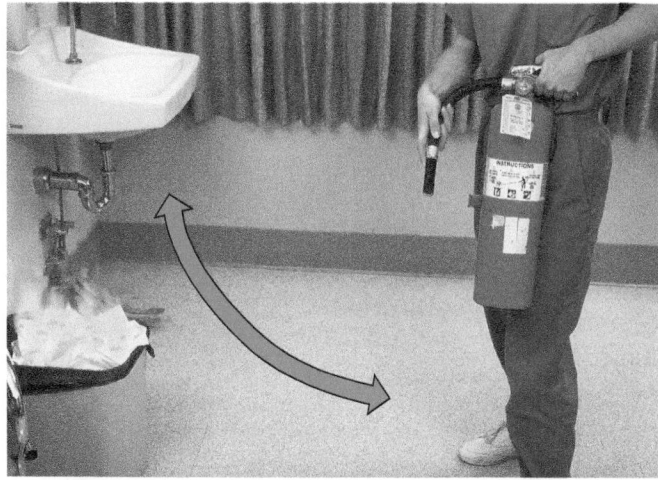

(C) Sweep the area from side to side.

FIGURE 19-7 It is important for new employees to know the location of all fire extinguishers.

At-Will Employment

At-will employment means that there is not an explicit contractual relationship between the employer and employee, and that the company is free to terminate the employment

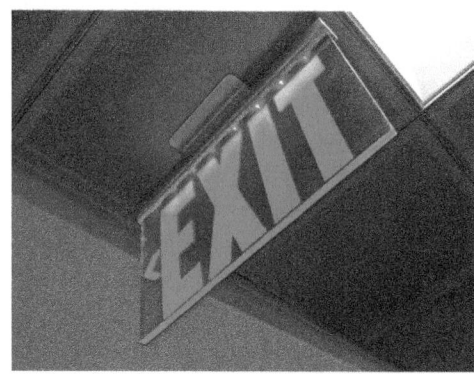

FIGURE 19-8 New employees should be shown all exits in case of an emergency.

relationship without just cause. The nature of the at-will relationship is discussed in most employee handbooks, together with the explicit statement that acknowledging acceptance of the employee handbook does not constitute an employment contract. There are variations from state to state in how this policy is interpreted by the courts. It is best to consult with a qualified labor attorney regarding personnel actions.

At the same time, there are reasons for which an employee *cannot* be terminated. Employers cannot engage in discriminatory practices against protected classes of employees, which means they cannot terminate someone because of gender, race, age, or physical handicaps. When the employer, or labor union if applicable, outlines disciplinary steps that must be taken to terminate an employee, then the company must follow these policies. Employers cannot terminate an employee because of involvement in union activity or, in most states, for retaliation against an employee for doing something that complies with public policy. For example, an employee could not be terminated for filing a complaint to the state department of health regarding unsafe practices in a medical office.

It is best to maintain thorough personnel records regarding disciplinary action, so that the company can back up its claim that a disciplinary action or termination was not discriminatory or for a prohibited reason.

Performance Evaluations

Performance evaluations provide employees feedback on how well they are performing in their assigned positions. They also provide the opportunity for managers to introduce new goals for staff. The employee should be encouraged to voice concerns and make suggestions for increasing the morale and productivity of the staff.

Types of Evaluations

The office personnel manual should clearly delineate the types of performance reviews and the time intervals at which they are to be given. Following is a list of types of reviews.

- **Orientation or training**—Observe the new employee, and every few days ask the employee how the training is going. Make sure the employee has the materials, equipment, and supplies needed to perform the job. Ask the employee if he or she has any questions regarding policy and if supervision is being provided, and continue to reinforce the idea that you are available to address questions or concerns.
- **Routine performance review**—Performance reviews are normally performed at 90-day, 6-month, and yearly intervals. A description of what a performance review will cover and the intervals at which reviews will be conducted should be stated in the policies and procedures manual; a review should not come as a surprise to the employee. Many offices offer the staff member the opportunity to do a self-evaluation before the meeting. This allows the employee the chance to think about his or her performance to date and to formulate any concerns. Approximately one hour should be devoted to this meeting. Figure 19-9 is an example of a form that may be used in a routine evaluation.

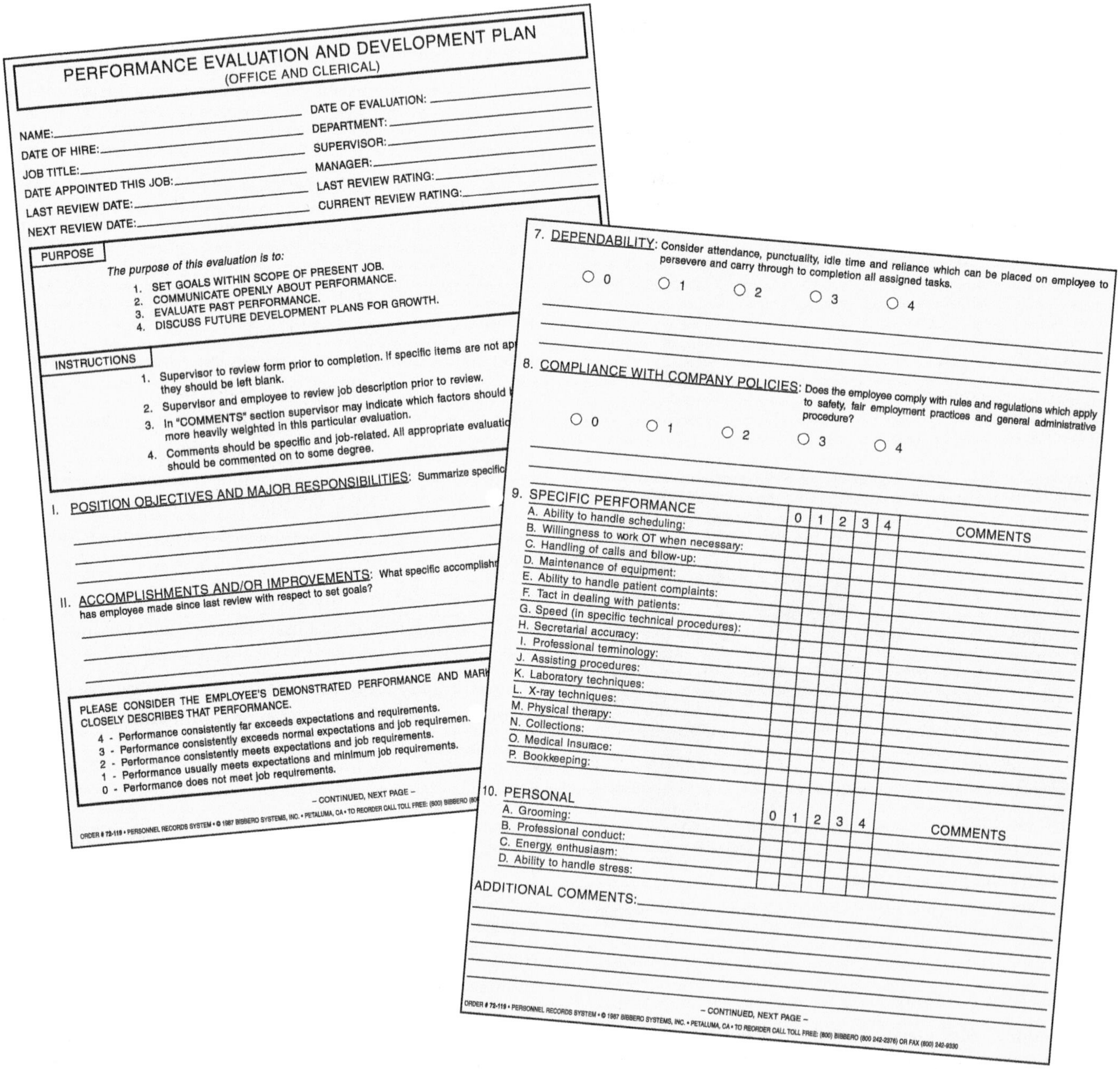

PERFORMANCE EVALUATION AND DEVELOPMENT PLAN
(OFFICE AND CLERICAL)

NAME:
DATE OF HIRE:
JOB TITLE:
DATE APPOINTED THIS JOB:
LAST REVIEW DATE:
NEXT REVIEW DATE:
DATE OF EVALUATION:
DEPARTMENT:
SUPERVISOR:
MANAGER:
LAST REVIEW RATING:
CURRENT REVIEW RATING:

PURPOSE

The purpose of this evaluation is to:
1. SET GOALS WITHIN SCOPE OF PRESENT JOB.
2. COMMUNICATE OPENLY ABOUT PERFORMANCE.
3. EVALUATE PAST PERFORMANCE.
4. DISCUSS FUTURE DEVELOPMENT PLANS FOR GROWTH.

INSTRUCTIONS

1. Supervisor to review form prior to completion. If specific items are not ap they should be left blank.
2. Supervisor and employee to review job description prior to review.
3. In "COMMENTS" section supervisor may indicate which factors should more heavily weighted in this particular evaluation.
4. Comments should be specific and job-related. All appropriate evaluati should be commented on to some degree.

I. POSITION OBJECTIVES AND MAJOR RESPONSIBILITIES: Summarize specific

II. ACCOMPLISHMENTS AND/OR IMPROVEMENTS: What specific accomplish has employee made since last review with respect to set goals?

PLEASE CONSIDER THE EMPLOYEE'S DEMONSTRATED PERFORMANCE AND MAR CLOSELY DESCRIBES THAT PERFORMANCE.
4 - Performance consistently far exceeds expectations and requirements.
3 - Performance consistently exceeds normal expectations and job requiremen.
2 - Performance consistently meets expectations and job requirements.
1 - Performance usually meets expectations and minimum job requirements.
0 - Performance does not meet job requirements.

– CONTINUED, NEXT PAGE –

ORDER # 72-119 • PERSONNEL RECORDS SYSTEM • © 1987 BIBBERO SYSTEMS, INC. • PETALUMA, CA • TO REORDER CALL TOLL FREE: (800) BIBBERO

7. DEPENDABILITY: Consider attendance, punctuality, idle time and reliance which can be placed on employee to persevere and carry through to completion all assigned tasks.
○ 0 ○ 1 ○ 2 ○ 3 ○ 4

8. COMPLIANCE WITH COMPANY POLICIES: Does the employee comply with rules and regulations which apply to safety, fair employment practices and general administrative procedure?
○ 0 ○ 1 ○ 2 ○ 3 ○ 4

9. SPECIFIC PERFORMANCE	0	1	2	3	4	COMMENTS
A. Ability to handle scheduling:						
B. Willingness to work OT when necessary:						
C. Handling of calls and blow-up:						
D. Maintenance of equipment:						
E. Ability to handle patient complaints:						
F. Tact in dealing with patients:						
G. Speed (in specific technical procedures):						
H. Secretarial accuracy:						
I. Professional terminology:						
J. Assisting procedures:						
K. Laboratory techniques:						
L. X-ray techniques:						
M. Physical therapy:						
N. Collections:						
O. Medical Insurace:						
P. Bookkeeping:						

10. PERSONAL	0	1	2	3	4	COMMENTS
A. Grooming:						
B. Professional conduct:						
C. Energy, enthusiasm:						
D. Ability to handle stress:						

ADDITIONAL COMMENTS:

– CONTINUED, NEXT PAGE –

ORDER # 72-119 • PERSONNEL RECORDS SYSTEM • © 1987 BIBBERO SYSTEMS, INC. • PETALUMA, CA • TO REORDER CALL TOLL FREE: (800) BIBBERO (800 242-2376) OR FAX (800) 242-9330

FIGURE 19-9 Example of an employee performance evaluation form.

- **Poor performance review**—This type of review is conducted when there have been obvious deficiencies in the performance of the employee. It should offer the employee an opportunity and help to improve. This kind of review also provides a framework for documenting the poor performance and sets the stage for possible dismissal.
- **Salary reviews**—A review of the employee's salary when a shift in job responsibilities occurs.

Conducting a Performance Evaluation

Preparation is the key for effective performance evaluations. The appraisal should be given in a nonjudgmental manner and should focus on the entire review period, not just recent events. The manager must look at the employee's performance as a whole. The employee's job description should be reexamined and the most important aspects of the position identified. It is important to target specific areas of performance.

Following are some questions the manager should ask her- or himself to help achieve effective management goals when conducting a performance evaluation:

- How can improvement be achieved?
- How can I, as the manager, help the improvement?
- How can I remain fair and even?
- How will I handle the possibility of a negative response from the employee?

During the interview, the discussion of the job description and required duties should provide the employee the opportunity to voice any frustration. The manager should be open to understanding problems the employee may be experiencing. At the same time, the manager should reinforce what is expected of the staff member. Teamwork should be emphasized.

The manager should rate how well the employee has met defined performance expectations. Before assigning a rating, each rating must first be defined: What factors determine outstanding performance? What determines a good versus a poor performance? Objectively rate the employee's performance, and provide the employee work examples that support your ratings.

In addition to evaluating quantifiable job skills, the evaluation should also consider the employee's social interaction skills, many times referred to as their "soft skills." How does the employee get along with the other members of the office team? How does the employee interact with the patients? Depending on the employee's position within the office, it may be more important to excel in one set of skills than another.

In this general evaluation, it is also important to give the employee new goals to strive to meet before the next scheduled

evaluation. The employee should be told about areas in which he might improve work performance and ways to help achieve the suggested goals, such as educational seminars and conferences. If possible, the evaluation meeting should end on a good note. Ideally, the employee should leave the meeting with the feeling that something valuable was gained from the review. Regular evaluations offer the chance for a productive give-and-take beyond day-to-day interactions.

In situations in which employees are not performing up to the standard set for them, they should be counseled at the time the concerns arise. It is best for the formal performance evaluation *not* to be the first time the employee has heard your concerns. At the very least, it is a good idea to inform the employee at the start of the meeting that you have some concerns. This prevents the employee from being surprised when you begin to explain the problems with his or her performance. All conversations regarding performance should be documented, so that if termination is necessary at some future time, you have evidence that you tried to work with the employee to improve the items of concern. Such documentation may satisfy the legal requirements for evidence that a termination is not based on discrimination.

Most employees look at an evaluation as the chance to be given or to ask for a raise in pay. There are several schools of thought regarding whether raises should be tied to performance reviews or done at a separate time. Regardless of the method chosen, the personnel manual should clearly define when and how salary adjustments will be done.

Box 19-3 lists possible topics to cover during the review of front-office personnel. Typically, clinical staff are evaluated either by the clinical coordinator or physician, because they are the persons primarily working with the clinical employee. Finally, as in all aspects of medical office management, everything said during the evaluation should be documented objectively, leaving personal opinions aside.

Disciplinary Process

Occasionally, it is necessary to discipline an employee when employment rules are violated. Discipline may take the form of a probationary period or, for more serious offenses, outright dismissal.

For frequent tardiness or absenteeism, an employee can be placed on probation and told that if the situation occurs again within a set period of time (e.g., 30 days or 3 months), the employee will be discharged. In some facilities, both verbal and written warnings are issued before corrective action is taken. Investigating every employee incident prevents someone from being fired for false reasons. For instance, diabetic employees may appear to be on drugs when they are, in fact, having a diabetic reaction.

Telephone technique
Daily balance of cash box
Accurate filing
Appointment scheduling
Communication and interaction with others
Treating patients with respect
Prioritizing tasks
Managing time effectively
Working neatly
Following directions
Cheerfulness and interest in the patient's comfort
Punctuality and attendance record

Grammar and spelling
Appropriate appearance and hygiene
Performance as a team member

ADDITIONAL TOPICS FOR A CLINICAL MEDICAL ASSISTANT'S REVIEW

Accurate and concise charting
Ability to anticipate the needs of the doctor
Knowledge of procedures
Willingness to help fellow team members
Continuing education

Because of the sensitive nature of medical work, certain situations may result in immediate discharge. These include intoxication, drug use, breach of patient or office confidentiality, and sleeping on the job. The employee must be sent home on suspension while the incident is investigated. If the allegations prove to be true, then the employee is dismissed. It is best to have a witness present when dismissing an employee.

Any employee incident must be carefully documented and include the time, the date, and an objective statement regarding what happened. This statement is placed in the employee's file. Document the incident immediately after it has occurred.

Human Resource Documentation

The office manager is responsible for maintaining human resource documentation related to employees and physicians. This information is needed not only for compliance purposes, but outside organizations such as insurance companies, hospitals, and accrediting organizations also require it. By having documentation well organized, it is easy to retrieve when needed. Information includes the following:

- **Licensure or certification**—Clinical staff in the medical office are either licensed or certified. For example, physicians and registered nurses are licensed, and medical assistants are certified. The office must keep copies of the current license or certificate, as well as information about when it needs to be renewed. If the license or certificate is allowed to expire, the professional cannot provide service.

- **Continuing education units (CEUs)**—Licensure or certification often requires that the professional obtain continuing education each year or each renewal period. When a provider takes an educational course or workshop, the sponsoring organization issues a certificate

that identifies the topic, date, and number of credits. The office should maintain copies of all continuing education taken. Staff other than physicians generally are responsible to maintain their own records, so check the office policy to see how this is handled in your office.

- **Training**—In addition to CEUs, keep records of any training completed, including basic life support (BLS) and advanced cardiovascular life support (ACLS). Also include any specialized classes, certifications, or skills training that qualify a provider to perform specific services or procedures.

- **Fees and dues**—Renewal of a license or certificate requires that the professional pay a renewal fee. Professional organizations also require annual dues. The medical office pays this for physicians. Other staff members often pay fees and dues personally, but the office might have a policy to reimburse staff for certain expenses. The office should keep receipts of all fees paid on behalf of physicians or other staff members.

In addition to the basic information listed above, offices must identify any additional documentation required by the physician's specialty board or other licensing or accrediting organizations. Set up and maintain a set of files, or electronic file folder, to store this information. Whenever a class is taken or a license is renewed, make it a habit to place a copy in the designated folder. This saves time and frustration compared with tracking it down, usually in a rush, at the time it is needed.

POLICIES

Each medical office should have a personnel policy manual as well as a manual of office policies and procedures.

Personnel Policy Manual

The personnel policy manual, also known as the employee handbook, contains information for the employee about the employer–employee relationship, the work environment, and the expectations of the particular medical facility. This manual contains general information about office policies relating to dress and behavior codes, punctuality, office safety, and the role of the employee in an emergency, such as a fire. It usually describes the circumstances or grounds for dismissal, such as sleeping or drinking while on the job, as well as breach of confidentiality on or off the job. OSHA guidelines and standard precautions may be included in the personnel policy manual or may be found in a separate OSHA handbook.

Employees should be provided with specific information about the following issues or benefits:

- Compensation and reimbursement for work-related activities, such as attending conventions and continuing education or degree courses, and parking fees
- Emergency leave
- **Grievance** (complaint) process
- Health benefits
- Holidays
- Jury duty
- Overtime policy
- Pension plan
- Performance review and evaluation
- Probationary period
- Sick leave
- Termination of employment
- Vacation
- Work hours, including flex time

An office manager knows that an updated personnel policy manual can be a useful tool when providing employee counseling. A well-designed personnel policy manual remains flexible enough in its design to allow for revisions, if and when policies change. Manuals for small offices consist of several pages that are copied on site. In large practices, the manual may be bound and copied at a printing service.

The personnel policy manual is often the first piece of office literature that the employee is asked to read. Employees should be asked to sign a statement indicating they have read and understood the information it contains. The signed statement should be placed in the employee's personnel file.

JUDGMENT CALL

Office manager Tania Washington recently hired Lisa, a medical assistant, who is currently in the 90-day probationary period. Today, Lisa arrived at work wearing slip-on shoes. Although the toe was closed, the heel was open, which is against office policy. Tania asked Lisa to come into her office and reminded her of the office dress code that prohibits open-heeled shoes for safety reasons. Lisa said, "I used to work at Main Street Clinic, and they have a lot more employees than this office does. I wore these shoes all the time there and never got in trouble. Why are you on my case?"

Critical Thinking Questions

1. How should Tania respond to help Lisa understand the difference between the policies of the two offices?
2. How do you think Lisa feels, and how should Tania view her feelings?
3. What should Tania do if Lisa wears the same shoes again?

Workplace Sexual Harassment

Workplace **sexual harassment** is unwelcome sexual advances, requests for sexual favors, and other verbal or physical harassment of a sexual nature. It can include offensive remarks about a person's sex. The perpetrator can be the victim's supervisor, another supervisor, a coworker, or even someone who is not an employee.

The employer must maintain a workplace where people are comfortable to work without being the target of unwanted sexual advances. Although employees are free to date each other outside the workplace, professional behavior is expected at all times in the medical office. It is inappropriate for supervisors to date direct subordinates. If two people meet at work and subsequently marry, it is best if one accepts a position that allows their relationship to flourish without needing to be concerned about workplace subordination.

It is against the law to create a hostile work environment in which employees must accept unwanted advances or listen to inappropriate talk. If sexual or romantic advances are made toward the medical assistant and are not appreciated, the medical assistant should make it clear that the advances must stop. If they do not stop, the medical assistant should report the incident(s) to a supervisor. Supervisors are held accountable under the law for maintaining a workplace that is free of sexual harassment. *Quid pro quo* is the Latin term for giving something for something else. It is used in reference to pressure for sexual behaviors forced on someone not wanting them in return for promotions or rewards. Any inference of sexual quid pro quo should be reported to supervisors.

Workplace Bullying

Workplace **bullying** is repeated mistreatment of employees that can involve verbal abuse, humiliation, intimidation, threatening behavior, and interference or sabotage of work duties. Bullying can be carried out by supervisors, peers, or even subordinates. A survey by the Workplace Bullying Institute identified that 9 percent of employees in the United States report currently being bullied, and 26 percent report having been bullied in the past. Managers must be aware that workplace bullying exists and make it clear to staff members that it is unacceptable. It is important also to educate employees about this problem and encourage witnesses and victims to report incidents immediately.

Office Policies and Procedures Manual

Medical offices should have a policies and procedures manual describing how to carry out tasks within a particular medical practice. This manual varies in content from the personnel policy manual. The policy and procedures manual provides detailed descriptions of the standard operating procedure (SOP) and how to perform specific administrative and clinical tasks.

Policy refers to a plan of action, such as "It is office policy that all employees receive hepatitis B (HBV) vaccination." The procedure describes the steps to be performed to carry out the policy. For example, "A series of three injections of HBV will be administered over a seven-month period of time, free of charge, to the employee." The terms *policy* and *procedure* are used interchangeably in many offices.

The primary functions of a policies and procedures manual are to

1. List the tasks to be performed within the office, including equipment needed to complete the procedure

2. Standardize the procedure for each task

3. Describe job responsibilities and titles

The policies and procedures manual, when properly updated, is an excellent reference tool for the new employee, because it provides guidelines for performing specific tasks. Temporary or substitute employees also find it valuable.

Ideally, the policies and procedures manual is contained in a loose-leaf binder that allows the addition of new pages for ease of updating. Each policy is numbered and dated. As the policy is updated, the number remains the same, but the date changes to indicate the revision. The manual should be clearly labeled and available for employees to read.

New policies and procedures are usually distributed or posted for employees in addition to being added to the policies and procedures manual. In some offices, the staff is asked to initial the corner of the policy to indicate they have read it.

Table 19-3 contains a list of information that should be included in a policies and procedures manual. Writing and updating this manual is often a job function of the medical assistant or the office manager. Although one person may have primary responsibility for development of the manual, the best manuals incorporate the input from a variety of personnel. The physician should always provide the final review of all written policies and procedures.

TABLE 19-3 | Contents of an Office Policies and Procedures Manual

Content	Description
Routine Clinical Tasks	Clinical tasks such as venipuncture, taking vital signs, ECGs, assisting with physical examinations, assisting with pap test and other laboratory tests
Special Procedures	Surgical tray setup for individual physicians, assisting with special exams such as proctological exams, using specialized equipment such as ultrasound
Emergency Procedures	Protocol for handling telephone and office emergencies, description of equipment used for emergency care such as mouth shield for CPR, proper sequence for alerting physician, and 911 emergencies
Quality Assurance	Procedures for maintaining quality control over all laboratory testing and procedures
OSHA Compliance	Compliance regarding needles, other sharps, specimens, personal protective equipment, regulated waste control, hepatitis B vaccine, laundry disposal, and contaminated equipment

TRAVEL AND SPEAKING ENGAGEMENTS

The medical assistant might be asked to assist the physician in making travel arrangements for medical meetings or in preparing for medical speaking engagements. Travel arrangements can include making hotel, flight, and car rental reservations, and sometimes preparing a printed travel **itinerary** for the trip.

When making the travel arrangements, the physician might wish to use a local travel agent or one of the many Internet sites available for booking flights and hotels. It is important to find out what the physician's preferences are before making any plans. The physician may prefer a non-smoking hotel room and only business-class flight tickets. Make sure the reservations are in line with the wishes of the physician.

When putting together the travel itinerary, which is the travel plan, obtain all the flight, hotel, car rental, and meeting or engagement information. Flight information includes travel dates, airline name, flight number, confirmation number or e-ticket number, and departure and arrival times. The hotel information includes the hotel name, address, telephone number, reservation dates, and confirmation number. Also, assemble car rental reservations and any information pertinent to the meeting that the physician is attending. Keep a copy of the itinerary at the office, and give a copy to the physician.

When helping a physician to prepare for a speaking engagement, you can help in a variety of capacities. It might include doing research. Be sure to provide all source material with any research that you reference and cite. The physician may ask you to create handouts for the presentation. When doing so, ensure that impeccable spelling and grammar are used. Always obtain the physician's approval on the handout before making numerous copies. The physician may also ask you to create a computer presentation. Various software programs can assist you in creating a presentation.

MEDICAL PRACTICE MARKETING AND CUSTOMER SERVICE

Marketing a medical practice involves various activities to promote the services of a physician or group of physicians to a population of patients. Marketing lets the community know about a new office. It can also help improve the image of an established office to compete with the new offices and to retain patients. Always remember that outstanding customer service can be a valuable marketing tool. Many marketing tools can be developed in-house with the aid of

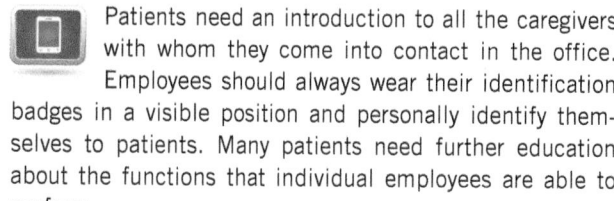

Patients need an introduction to all the caregivers with whom they come into contact in the office. Employees should always wear their identification badges in a visible position and personally identify themselves to patients. Many patients need further education about the functions that individual employees are able to perform.

Patient information booklets are one of the best ways to educate the patient about the functions of the staff and medical office. Whereas verbal instructions are still necessary, the booklets can enhance learning. Medical assistants need to involve the entire staff in the production of patient literature.

computer software. Other times, it is cost-effective to hire an outside company that specializes in marketing for medical practices.

Patient Information Booklet

A patient information booklet and a variety of patient teaching materials can be developed in-house. These materials should provide patient information regarding office hours, payment guidelines, appointment and cancellation policy, the telephone answering service, information about the physician(s), after-hours availability, directions to the facility, and parking information. A good patient information booklet can reduce the number of questions received by telephone from patients, enhance the office's image, and reduce the number of patients who fail to remember instructions.

Instruction booklets can be used for patients with special needs or to teach methods of disease prevention.

Developing and using a format and design is described in Procedure 19-2. A patient information booklet containing vital office information should be handed to each new patient at the time of registration or mailed before the first appointment. Patient information materials never diminish the need to give personal instructions to the patient. They simply augment, or reinforce, patient teaching.

Target Market

When marketing a medical office or facility, one of the first things to look at is the target market of the physician(s). What kinds of services are being offered? This can affect the physician's office location. A new geriatric medical practice has a better chance of doing well if it is located near retirement communities rather than within communities composed mostly of young families.

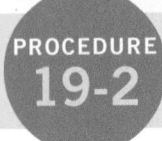

Developing a Patient Information Booklet

Objective ◆ *Develop a booklet to inform patients about services provided by your medical office.*

EQUIPMENT AND SUPPLIES

Computer; design software (if including images); high-quality paper; printer (or an independent printing service)

METHOD

1. Make the booklet as appealing as possible. Leave a white border around all page edges. Use large print for the older adultreader's benefit. The booklet should be small enough that it fits easily into a pocket or purse.
2. Write the booklet with the reader in mind and at a reading level appropriate for the target audience. Avoid the use of technical medical terms. Never use medical abbreviations in patient literature.
3. Avoid long paragraphs of explanation. Keep the sentences short and concise, and use as many bulleted points as possible.
4. Provide a list of the regular office hours.
5. List any special services offered by the practice or clinic, such as patient education classes or blood pressure testing programs.
6. Explain the procedure for having a prescription refilled.
7. Explain the procedure for processing medical insurance forms.
8. Include a general statement about payment of fees, especially if payment is expected at the time of delivery of services. Do not discuss specific fees in patient brochures.
9. Provide information about the physician and the staff. For example, "Dr. McWalter is in general practice specializing in family practice. Our pediatrician is Dr. Conway. Our physicians are on staff at two hospitals: Northwestern Memorial Hospital and Children's Memorial Hospital." Include the name and telephone number of the office manager, the personnel responsible for insurance processing, and the patient educator.
10. State what procedure to follow in case of an emergency. For example, instruct the patients to call 911 if the emergency is life threatening. Also, provide a 24-hour emergency telephone number. Ask the patient to keep this number near the telephone.
11. Include a telephone number at the end of the brochure where additional information may be obtained.
12. End the brochure by thanking the patient for taking the time to read the literature.

After assessing the target market and the needs of the target group, types of services the practice could offer can be determined and tailored to meet the expectations and needs of the target market. Services may include new procedures that could benefit patients' needs.

After you have determined your services, a plan must be developed and put into place. The first step is to look for any problems or opportunities that may come about in the execution of the plan. The plan should describe specific steps that need to be implemented, who is responsible for these steps, and a reasonable time frame. Many ventures have failed because of poor planning. When the plan has been executed, it is a good idea to review the plan to determine if it has or has not met expectations. Make note of any particular problems that may have arisen and the positive lessons that may have been learned in the process.

Marketing the Practice

A medical practice may be promoted in many ways. Some marketing plans may require large expense budgets to implement the plan. However, some marketing tools are available free or at low cost.

Free Marketing and Public Relations

One of the best ways of promoting a practice is by word of mouth, which is completely free. Many patients choose their physician based on friends and family recommending their own physician. Word of mouth is built on a base of good customer service. Another method of promoting a practice is through public relations activities, such as local charities and events. Involvement in the community helps spread the office's name and show that it is a participating member of the community. Goodwill in the community can translate into growing the practice.

Websites

A practice website is commonly used for marketing a medical practice. This can be done using simple website-building software or hiring a website firm. It is important to determine the main objective of the website and then plan the content that supports that goal. Is it simply providing one-way information to the patient regarding the practice? Or does the website provide a patient portal for interactive communication that allows the patient to ask questions, complete forms, and so on and have the physician or medical office staff member respond? Would the patient be able to access various forms and procedure instructions? Will patients be able to request appointments online? It is important to always consider HIPAA laws, confidentiality, and security requirements if interactive communication is the goal of your office's website. Keep the site easy to use. Graphics should be simple, fonts should be easy to read, and colors should be pleasing to the eye. You then have to choose a web server to support your site. Many options are available and need to be researched. Some are free but add advertisements to your site. Others require a fee.

Customer Service

One of your most potent marketing tools depends entirely on the level of customer service delivered to the patient. Just as word of mouth can bring you many customers, it can also drive them away if poor services are provided. A satisfied patient might share an experience with three or four people, but one dissatisfied patient often complains to a dozen people. As a result, negative reviews spread faster than positive ones.

The patient, like a customer, responds positively or negatively to his or her experience at the medical office. What impression does the patient have? Is the staff helpful and empathetic? Is the staff attentive and considerate of the patient's time and condition? It is important that all patients are treated with respect and concern. Box 19-4 includes spoken phrases that might leave the patient with a poor view of a medical office's customer service abilities. The most successful practices provide excellent customer service for their patients, which in turn usually means increased profits as a result of increased patient volume.

BOX 19-4 | Phrases That Decrease Customer Service Level

"It's not my job."	"I can't."
"I don't know."	"You're wrong."
"It's not my fault."	"It's not my problem."
"What do you want?"	

SUMMARY

A smooth-running office requires attention to many factors, including staff training, effective time management skills, up-to-date policies and procedures manuals, and careful attention to detail. Using a systems approach to office management, the functions of an office are categorized into systems that must function simultaneously and be integrated into a whole system, which is the medical office. The office manager is the coordinator for business activities conducted in the office. Along with the knowledge needed to run an efficient medical office, an office manager needs effective administrative and communication skills.

The medical office staff must work as a team, taking into account the team size, a variety of personality and skills, individual accountability, and overall purpose and goals. The office manager is also responsible for hiring effective staff members, by carefully advertising the position, screening applicants, conducting interviews, and providing adequate new employee orientation, training, and performance evaluations.

The personnel policy manual contains information for the employee about the employer–employee relationship, the work environment, and the expectations of the particular medical facility. The policies and procedures manual provides detailed descriptions of the standard operating procedures (SOP) and how to perform specific administrative and clinical tasks.

The medical assistant may be asked to assist the physician in making travel arrangements for medical meetings or in preparing for medical speaking engagements.

Maintaining good customer service is key to keeping a contented patient base while enhancing the possibility of growing the practice.

COMPETENCY REVIEW

1. Define and spell the terms for this chapter.
2. Prepare an office procedure for any one of the following tasks: appointment scheduling, patient reception process, taking vital signs, OSHA guidelines.
3. Prepare a monthly calendar for the month of December, showing staff vacations and office coverage.
4. Develop a patient information booklet for your own physician's practice.
5. Prepare an employee policy for taking vacation days.

PREPARING FOR THE CERTIFICATION EXAM

For the following questions, choose the best answer:

1. For completion of the I-9 form, the employee must present an acceptable document from which of the following?
   a. List A only
   b. List B only
   c. List C only
   d. List A only OR one each from List B and C
   e. Lists A, B, and C

2. All of the following should be found in an office policies and procedures manual *except*
   a. OSHA compliance.
   b. routine office tasks.
   c. special procedures.
   d. termination.
   e. emergency procedures.

3. Which of the following laws affect the hiring of a new employee?
   a. EEOC
   b. AMA
   c. Title IV of the Civil Rights Act
   d. OSHA
   e. EEOA of 1972

4. During new employee orientation, all of the following should be covered *except*
   a. personalities of coworkers.
   b. personnel policy manual.
   c. policies and procedures manual.
   d. HIPAA training.
   e. work hours.

5. All of the following records are required for employee payroll *except*
   a. gross salary.
   b. I-9.
   c. W-4.
   d. 1099.
   e. Social Security number.

6. All of the following are factors that contribute to a successful office team *except*
   a. unified approach.
   b. responsible members.
   c. size.
   d. job duties.
   e. personalities.

7. All of the following are qualities or skills found in good office managers *except*
   a. organization skills.
   b. effective communication skills.
   c. subjectivity.
   d. flexibility.
   e. creativity.

8. Patient instruction booklets should be
   a. used in place of individual instructions.
   b. used to standardize instructions.
   c. used to prevent lawsuits.
   d. used for vision-impaired patients.
   e. used only with hearing-impaired patients.

9. Routine performance reviews are normally performed at all of the following intervals *except*
   a. 30 days.
   b. two months.
   c. three months.
   d. six months.
   e. one year.

10. Which of the following leadership styles is motivated by external means?
   a. bureaucratic
   b. permissive
   c. democratic
   d. authoritarian
   e. none of the above

CRITICAL THINKING

Refer to the case study at the beginning of the chapter and use the information you have learned to answer the following questions.

1. Where else could Tania have advertised the job opening?
2. Why is it important for Tania to have her applicants fill out paperwork by hand?

3. Which applicant do you think Tania should hire? Consider if personal appearance should outweigh professionalism. Explain your answer.

ON THE JOB

Sarah Egan is the office manager in Dr. Williams's practice. Nell Jacobs, who has worked as a CMA (AAMA) in the office for one year, has frequently been absent or tardy on Mondays. Sarah suspects that Nell has a drinking problem. However, Nell has never arrived at the office intoxicated—until today. Sarah has just observed Nell stumbling in the parking lot when getting out of her car. Her speech is slurred, and her breath has a fruity odor that Sarah thinks could be alcohol. Nell does not appear to understand anything that Sarah is saying to her.

1. Given the situation, as the office manager, what should Sarah do immediately regarding Nell?
2. If Sarah decides to send Nell home, should she call Nell's husband to come and get her, or, perhaps, insist that Nell go home in a cab?

3. Does Sarah have an obligation to tell Dr. Williams about her suspicions regarding Nell?
4. Should this incident become part of Nell's employment record?
5. Is this incident grounds for firing an employee?
6. Because Nell is a CMA (AAMA) and works with patients, is it within Sarah's rights to demand a blood and urine screening for alcohol and drugs?
7. Should the police be notified of the incident?
8. If Nell is indeed intoxicated or under the influence of alcohol or drugs, is Sarah obligated to refer Nell to counseling at an alcohol and drug rehabilitation facility?

INTERNET ACTIVITY

Research the different methods that the Internet provides for advertising job opportunities available at your medical office.

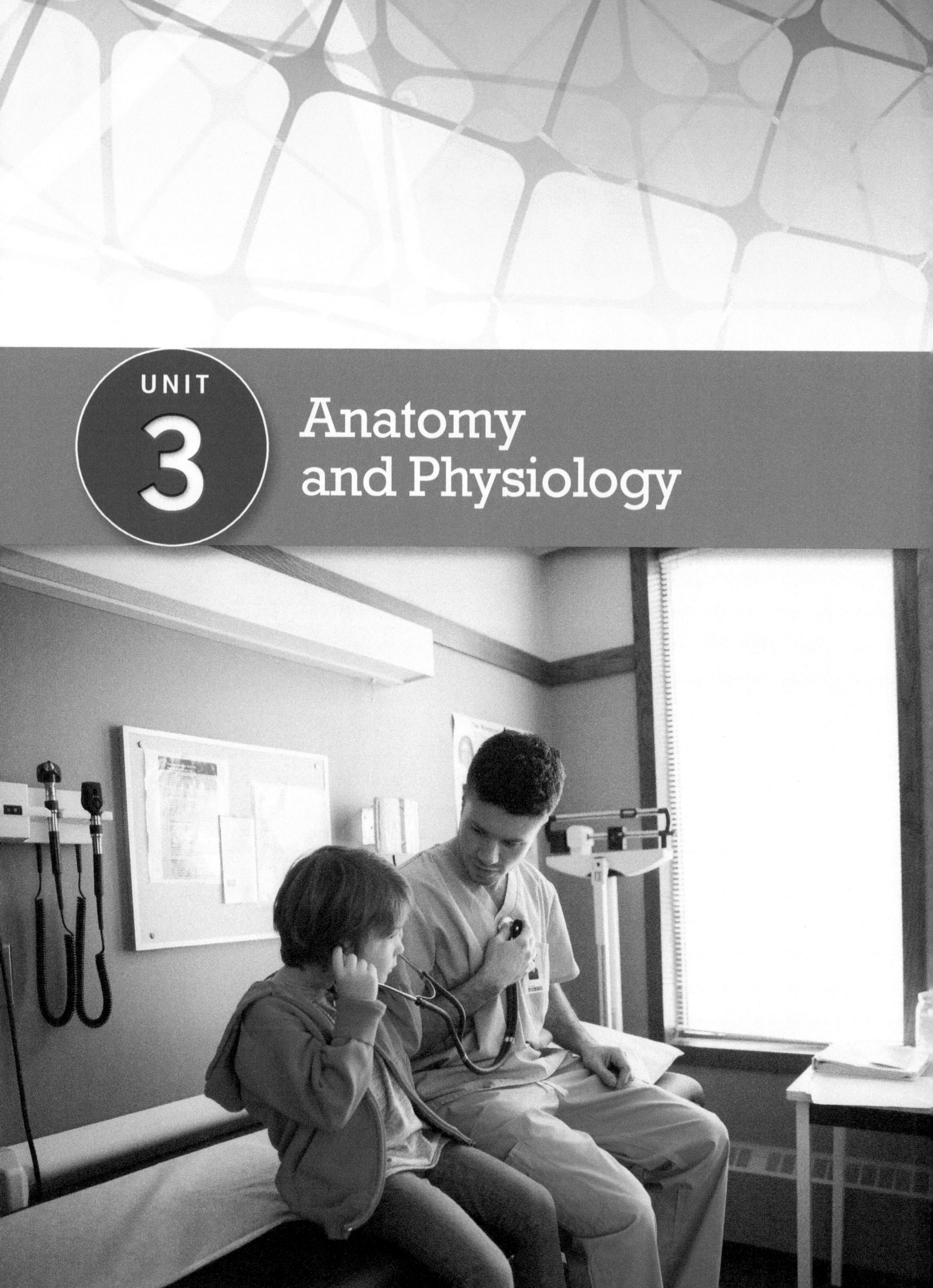

UNIT
3

Anatomy and Physiology

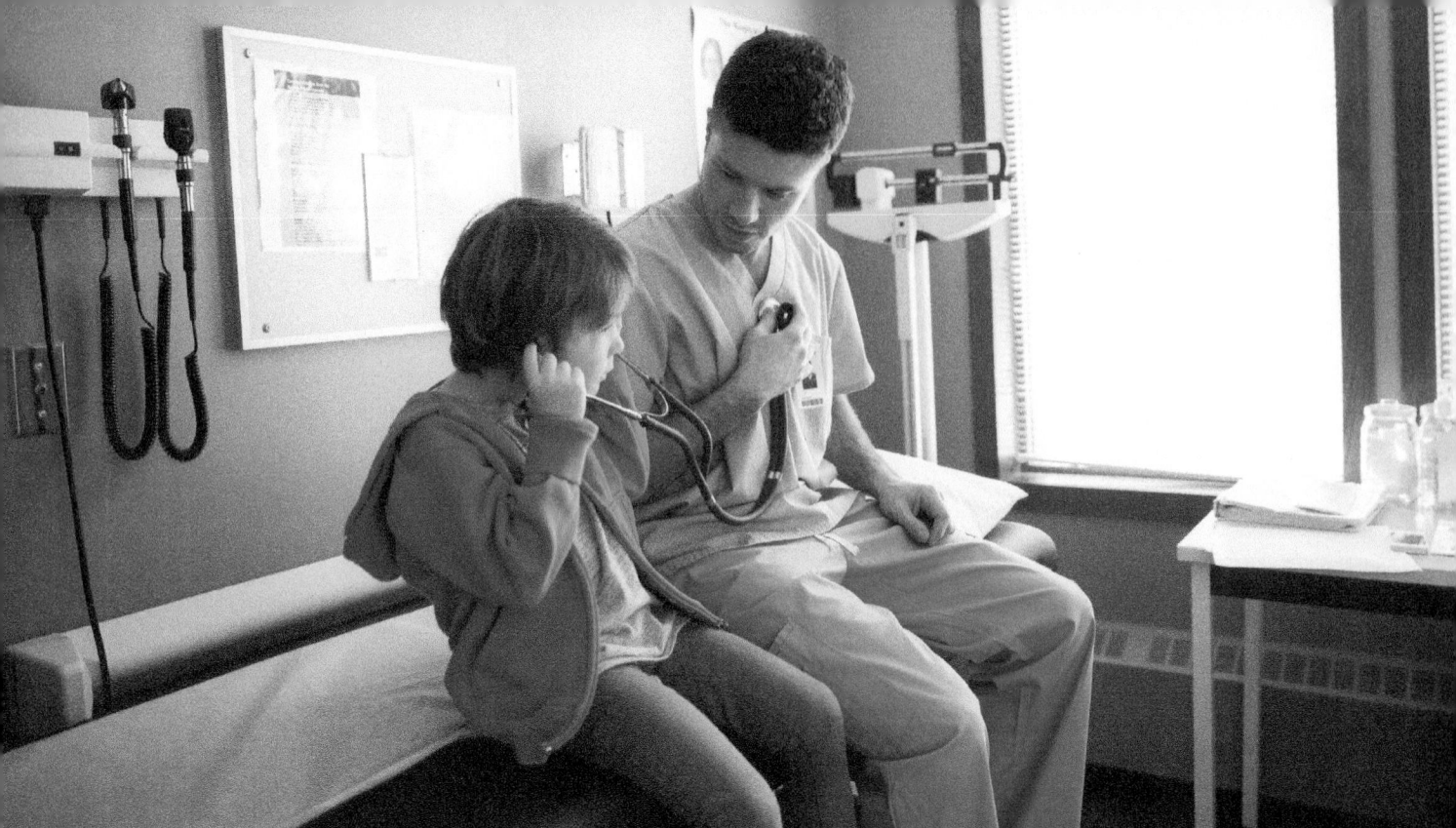

Body Structure and Function

Learning Objectives

After completing this chapter, you should be able to:

20.1   Define and spell the terms for this chapter.

20.2   Explain the structural organization of the human body.

20.3   Describe the functions of cellular structures.

20.4   Explain types of cellular division.

20.5   Describe the types of tissues found in the human body.

20.6   Identify the systems of the human body.

20.7   List the major organs in each body system.

20.8   Describe the normal function of each body system.

20.9   Explain how chemistry is associated with the human body.

20.10   Explain the relationship between genetics and DNA.

20.11   Identify diseases and disorders related to genetic mutations.

Lucy Gutierrez is completing her medical assisting practicum and has the opportunity to shadow a medical assistant who works in a genetics clinic that is a part of Pearson General Hospital. This shadowing opportunity will last for two weeks. Lucy is very excited about this possibility because genetically acquired diseases have always intrigued her.

Terms to Learn

active transport	Down syndrome (trisomy 21)	neurons
albinism	electrolyte	nuclear membrane
anabolism	filtration	nucleus
anatomy	flagella	organelles
atom	fragile X syndrome	organs
attention-deficit/hyperactivity disorder (ADHD)	gametes	osmosis
catabolism	genetics	passive transport
cell	hemochromatosis	pathophysiology
cell membrane	hemophilia	phenylketonuria (PKU)
chromosomes	heredity	physiology
cilia	homeostasis	ribonucleic acid (RNA)
cleft palate	interphase	sickle cell anemia
color deficiency	Klinefelter's syndrome	spina bifida
congenital disorder	meiosis	striated
cystic fibrosis (CF)	metabolism	systems
cytokinesis	mitosis	talipes
cytoplasm	molecule	Tay-Sachs disease (TSD)
deoxyribonucleic acid (DNA)	muscular dystrophy	tissues
diffusion	mutation	Turner's syndrome

The human body is a complicated and intricate organism composed of millions and millions of cells. To understand the workings of the human body, it is important to understand its **anatomy** (the study of the structure of an organism) as well as its **physiology** (the study of the function of an organism). Various factors, including age, genetic predisposition, and environmental influences, can lead to the development of diseases and disorders within the body. The study of these diseases and disorders is termed **pathophysiology**.

From the tiniest cell to a complex organ system, the body is composed of increasing levels of organization, which are discussed later in this chapter. All these parts are intended to function in a normal unified state. By adjusting for constant changes in the environment, the body and its systems work together to maintain a constant state of balance in which all systems of the body work together and function cohesively. This is known as **homeostasis**, which is a fundamental characteristic of all living things. When homeostasis is not maintained and an imbalance occurs, diseases and disorders form within the body.

Body temperature, nutrient and waste concentrations, and salinity and acidity are examples of mechanisms that our bodies use to sustain life. These properties each have chemical reactions that keep us alive as our bodies strive to maintain homeostasis. Homeostasis is relevant to all body systems.

THE HUMAN BODY: LEVELS OF ORGANIZATION

The human body is organized by increasing levels of organization. The units of organization from simplest to most complex include atoms, molecules, organelles, cells, tissues, organs, organ systems, and the complete organism (Figure 20-1). The organ systems within the body depend on each other to maintain a homeostatic balance.

Atoms

Atoms are the most basic level of organization. An **atom** consists of at least one proton, which is a positively (+) charged particle; at least one neutron, which is without an electrical charge; and at least one electron, which is a negatively (−) charged particle. Protons and neutrons constitute the majority of the atomic mass and reside within the nucleus. Electrons revolve around the nucleus of the atom. Protons, neutrons, and electrons form together in different combinations to create elements. There are 118 recognized elements on the Periodic Table of Elements; however, only 13 of these elements are found in the human body in amounts that are considered greater than trace amounts. Trace amounts are found in quantities of less than 0.01 percent. Table 20-1 lists the 13 common elements found in the human body.

Molecules

A **molecule** is a chemical combination of two or more atoms that forms a specific chemical compound. For example, a water molecule (H_2O) has two hydrogen atoms and one oxygen atom that are chemically joined together. A single drop of water is composed of millions of water molecules.

Molecules can move and thus can take the form of solids, liquids, or gases. Molecules are farthest apart in the form of gases and are closest together, moving slowly, in solid formation. Multiple molecules combine to make cells.

TABLE 20-1 | Elements Found in the Human Body

Symbol	Element	Symbol	Element
C	Carbon	N	Nitrogen
Ca	Calcium	O or O_2	Oxygen
Cl	Chlorine	P	Phosphorus
H	Hydrogen	K	Potassium
I	Iodine	Na	Sodium
Fe	Iron	S	Sulfur
Mg	Magnesium		

Cells

A **cell** is the smallest functional unit of life. This microscopic unit is the building block of the human body. There are millions and millions of types of cells and, although some are a part of a larger organism, many are organisms unto themselves. Our bodies have bone cells, nerve cells, fat cells, reproductive cells, skeletal muscle cells, blood cells, and smooth muscle cells, to name just a few. Though each cell has a unique function and feature, many features are recognized among all cells. Every cell has three common components: the cell membrane, cytoplasm, and the nucleus.

Cell Membrane

The outer covering of the cell is the **cell membrane**. Cell membranes have the capability of allowing some substances to pass into and out of the cell while denying passage of other substances. This selective permeability allows individual cells to receive nutrition and dispose of waste, just as the human being eats food and disposes of waste. The cell membrane also helps maintain the cell's shape.

The surface of some cells, such as in the respiratory system, is covered with small hairlike projections called **cilia**. These cilia aid in increasing the overall surface area of a cell. Cilia work by propelling substances along a cell's surface, which increases the cell's ability to absorb water and nutrients. **Flagella** are similar in structure to cilia. These are taillike structures that, for example, enable a sperm cell to move through the reproductive tract.

Cytoplasm

Cytoplasm is a jellylike substance found between the cell membrane and the nuclear membrane. Cytoplasm is 80 percent water and is generally clear in color, resembling the uncooked white of an egg. The rest of the cytoplasm is composed of proteins, ions, and nutrients. Cytoplasm provides storage and work areas for the cell. **Organelles** are structures found within cytoplasm. Each organelle has a specific function and purpose to maintain the vitality of the cell. Organelles include the endoplasmic reticulum, ribosomes, Golgi apparatus, mitochondria, lysosomes, and centrioles (Figure 20-2). The functions of these organelles are found in Table 20-2.

Nucleus

The **nucleus** is responsible for the cell's metabolism, growth, and reproduction. Because of this, it is considered the control center of the cell. The **nuclear membrane** is a double-layered sac that houses the nucleus. It controls what is allowed to enter and exit the nucleus. The chromosomes of the cell are within the nucleus. Genetic information and

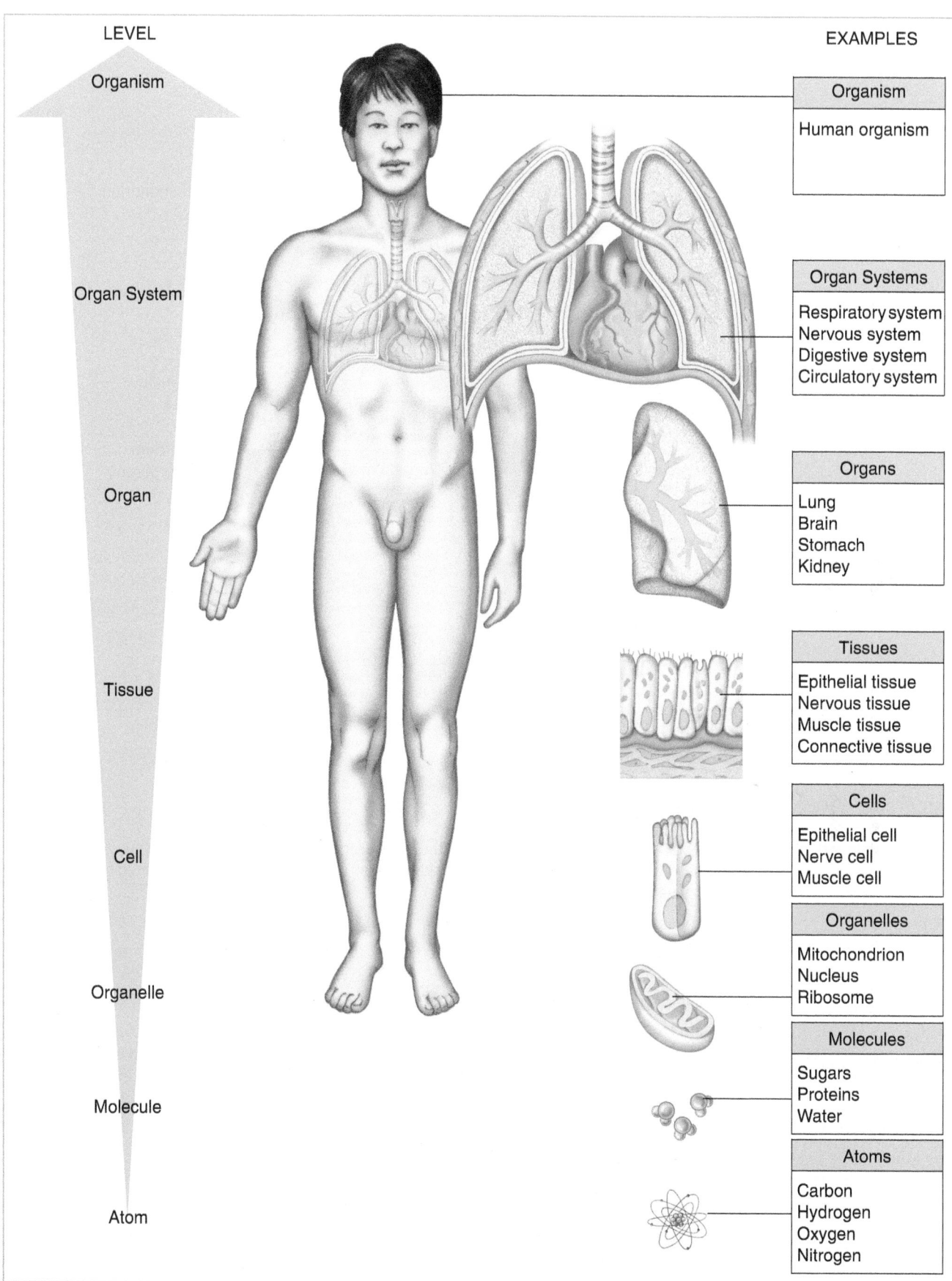

LEVEL

Organism

Organ System

Organ

Tissue

Cell

Organelle

Molecule

Atom

EXAMPLES

Organism

Human organism

Organ Systems

Respiratory system
Nervous system
Digestive system
Circulatory system

Organs

Lung
Brain
Stomach
Kidney

Tissues

Epithelial tissue
Nervous tissue
Muscle tissue
Connective tissue

Cells

Epithelial cell
Nerve cell
Muscle cell

Organelles

Mitochondrion
Nucleus
Ribosome

Molecules

Sugars
Proteins
Water

Atoms

Carbon
Hydrogen
Oxygen
Nitrogen

FIGURE 20-1 Organization of the human body.

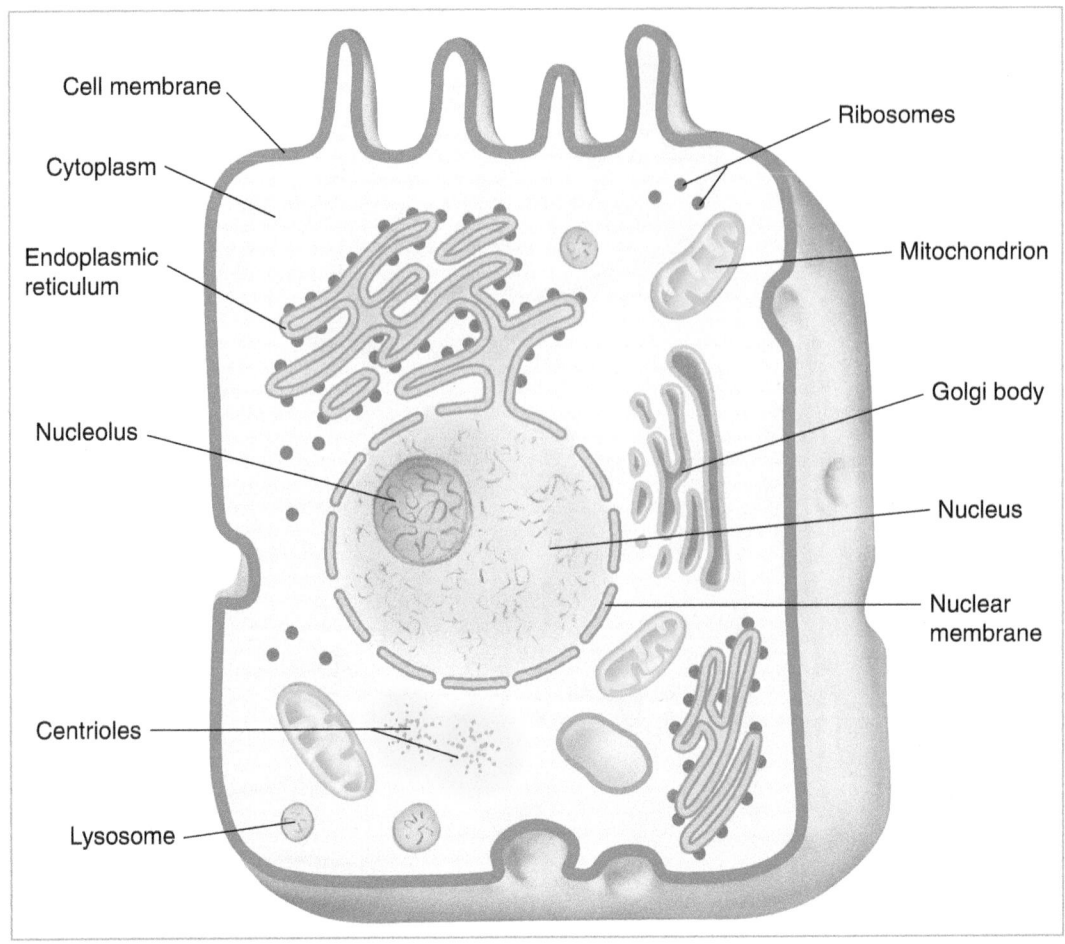

FIGURE 20-2 Major parts of the cell and the structures located inside the cell.

TABLE 20-2	Cellular Organelles and Their Functions	
Endoplasmic reticulum	A tubular network that is attached to the nuclear membrane. Rough endoplasmic reticulum has ribosomes embedded within, giving it a bumpy appearance; smooth endoplasmic reticulum does not have embedded ribosomes.
Ribosomes	Responsible for the production of protein that is essential to the vitality of the cell.
Golgi apparatus	A saclike membranous structure that sorts, modifies, and transports various proteins throughout the cell.
Mitochondria	Considered the powerhouse of the cell, it is responsible for the production of adenosine Triphosphate (ATP), a form of cellular energy.
Lysosomes	Sometimes considered the "stomach" of the cell, the lysosomes are the sites of digestion of proteins, lipids, and carbohydrates. Anything that is not digested by the lysosome is sent to the cellular membrane for removal from the cell.
Centrioles	These paired organelles are found lying at 90-degree angles near the nucleus. Centrioles are involved in cellular division.

familial characteristics are carried within the **chromosomes**. One gene represents one segment of **deoxyribonucleic acid (DNA)**. Each gene also occupies a specific site on the chromosome, as if it has a permanent address. In the human body, each cell contains 23 pairs of chromosomes for a total of 46 chromosomes in each cell.

DNA provides the cell's blueprint, or genetic makeup. DNA is shaped in a double helix: two long chains of nucleic

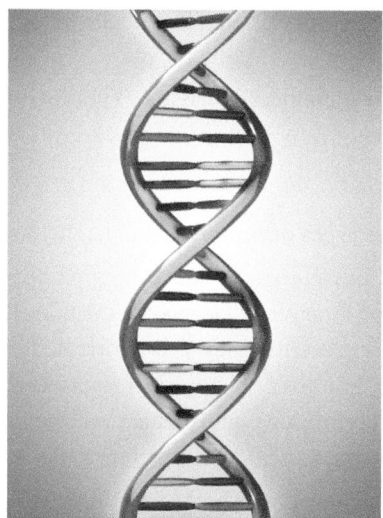

FIGURE 20-3 Two long strands of nucleic acid twist to form DNA.

acid that twist around each other (Figure 20-3). DNA is mandatory for cellular reproduction. **Ribonucleic acid (RNA)** is a single chain of chemical bases. RNA takes the form of messenger RNA (mRNA) and transfer RNA (tRNA), among others.

The nucleic functions include the following:

- Storage and organization of genes and chromosomes
- Transport of genetic products
- Production of messages through RNA (via mRNA and tRNA)
- Production of ribosomes
- Uncoiling of DNA to replicate key genes

Cell Division: Mitosis and Cytokinesis

Cell division must occur to create and replenish cells throughout the tissues and organs of the body. A cell divides into two new cells via the processes of mitosis and

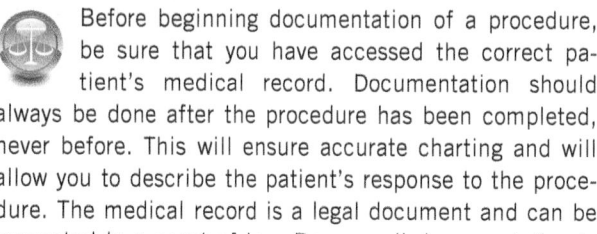
cytokinesis. First, the cell replicates each of its chromosomes. Then, during **mitosis**, the nucleus of the cell divides, with each half of the new nuclei containing an identical set of chromosomes. There are five stages of mitosis: prophase, prometaphase, metaphase, anaphase, and telophase (Figure 20-4). These phases are described in Table 20-3. As you read through the stages in Table 20-3, examine each correlating image in Figure 20-4. At this point, after mitosis, the two new nuclei with their individual sets of chromosomes are still contained within the one original cell.

Mitosis is usually followed immediately by **cytokinesis**, which divides the cytoplasm, organelles, and cell membrane, completing the division of the original cell into two new daughter cells. After cell division, each new cell, just like all cells of the human body, has 23 pairs of chromosomes, for a total of 46 chromosomes.

The period of time that a cell exists when it is not actively dividing but rather is preparing for the division process is called **interphase**. During the interphase period, the cell is busy performing its normal selected function.

Cells tend to have a very short duration, or lifespan. Mitosis and cytokinesis allow them to be renewed on a regular basis.

Meiosis

Meiosis is the cellular division of reproductive cells. Through meiosis, cells reduce their chromosomal number from 46 to 23 to form **gametes**. In a male, each gamete is a sperm cell. In a female, each gamete is an ovum (egg). When two gametes (one from each parent) are combined through sexual reproduction, a zygote is formed. The zygote, a cell that now contains 46 chromosomes, 23 from each parent, is the earliest stage of an embryo.

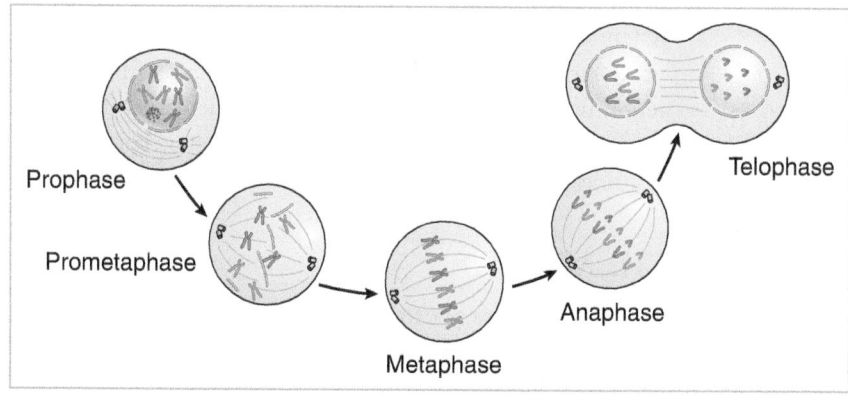

Prophase

Prometaphase

Metaphase

Anaphase

Telophase

FIGURE 20-4 Stages of mitosis.

TABLE 20-3 | Stages of Mitosis

Stage	Description
Prophase	Centrioles, which have previously replicated, move to opposite ends of the cell, creating spindle fibers between them.
Prometaphase	The nuclear membrane begins to dissolve, and the centrioles move to the poles of the cell.
Metaphase	The chromosomes move to the middle and line up along the center of the cell as the spindle. This center is called the equatorial plate.
Anaphase	The new daughter chromosomes, which are termed chromatids, begin to move to the opposite ends of the cell and away from each other.
Telophase	The chromatids are now at two far ends of the cell. Cytoplasm division occurs (cytokinesis), and the mitosis process is completed.

Tissues

The next level of organization is the formation of tissues. Specialized cells that have the same function and purpose group together to form **tissues**. Four types of tissues are found within the human body: epithelial, connective, muscle, and nerve (Figure 20-5).

Epithelial Tissue

Epithelial tissue is arranged in a flat formation and is sheet-like in appearance. It forms the outer layer of skin, lines the walls of body cavities, and covers the surface of organs. It is also the forming tissue that comprises certain glands, ducts, and tubes. Functions of this tissue include absorption, secretion, excretion, and protection.

Connective Tissue

Connective tissue is the most copious form of tissue in the human body. It has a vast assortment of functions, which include forming a support network for organs of the body, covering muscles, and connecting muscles to bones and bones to joints. Connective tissue can be further classified into three distinct categories:

- Connective tissue proper: This tissue is either loose like adipose (fat) or dense like collagen.

- Fluid connective tissue: This includes both blood and lymph.

- Supporting connective tissue: This includes cartilage and bone.

Muscle Tissue

There are three types of muscle tissue in the human body:

- **Striated** muscle tissue has a striped appearance and forms voluntary muscles. Skeletal muscles are called voluntary because they are controlled by conscious thought. You may choose to flex your biceps, which is a voluntary muscle, and this action of purposeful flexing demonstrates control by your will.

- Involuntary or smooth muscle tissue is controlled by the autonomic nervous system. It is also known as visceral muscle tissue, as it lines the walls of hollow organs (viscera) such as the stomach. A person does not consciously control movement of involuntary muscles. An example is the involuntary muscles that are used to digest food, which happens automatically through the digestive process and not by a person's conscious effort.

- Cardiac muscle tissue, which forms the heart muscles, is a specialized form of striated muscle that is under the control of the autonomic nervous system.

Nerve Tissue

Nerve tissue, composed of **neurons** (nerve cells), acts as the functional unit of the nervous system. Nerve tissue has two properties: excitability and conductivity. Nervous cells, and in turn nervous tissue, are active, which demonstrates the excitability property. Because nerve cells transmit impulses and coordinate activities in the body, nerve tissue is said to be conductive.

BODY ORGANS AND SYSTEMS

A group of tissues with a similar function comes together to form **organs**. Organs work within body systems. Body **systems** are groups of organs that work together toward the same purpose: to sustain life within the human body. The major functions of each body system are identified in Figure 20-6. The major organs and associated structures found within each of the systems are discussed in Table 20-4.

CHEMISTRY

For cells to receive nourishment and eliminate wastes, materials must be transported both into and out from the cell. This can be done via passive or active transport.

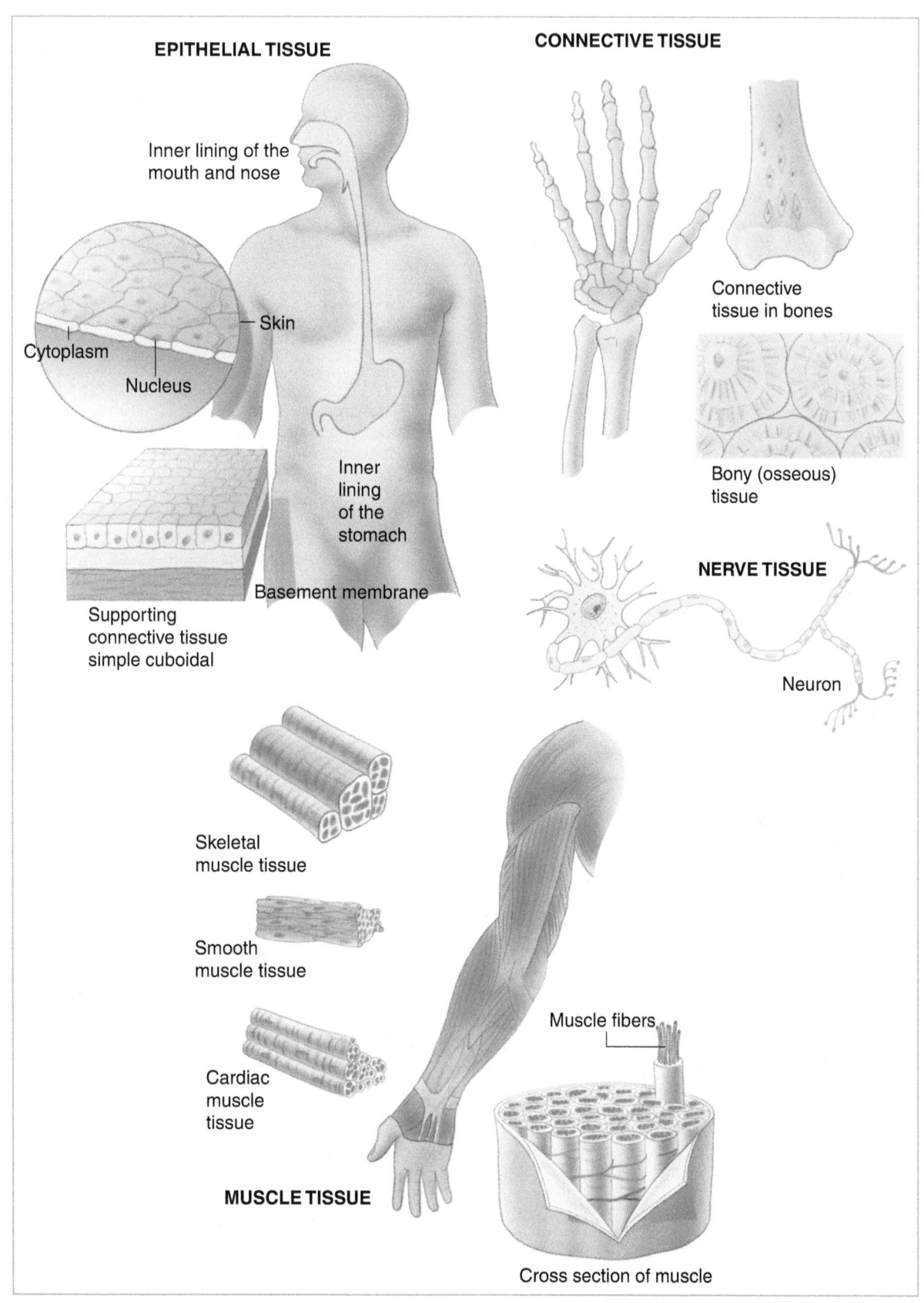

EPITHELIAL TISSUE

Inner lining of the mouth and nose

Skin

Cytoplasm

Nucleus

Inner lining of the stomach

Basement membrane

Supporting connective tissue simple cuboidal

CONNECTIVE TISSUE

Connective tissue in bones

Bony (osseous) tissue

NERVE TISSUE

Neuron

Skeletal muscle tissue

Smooth muscle tissue

Cardiac muscle tissue

Muscle fibers

MUSCLE TISSUE

Cross section of muscle

FIGURE 20-5 Types of tissue in the human body.

Organ System		Major Functions

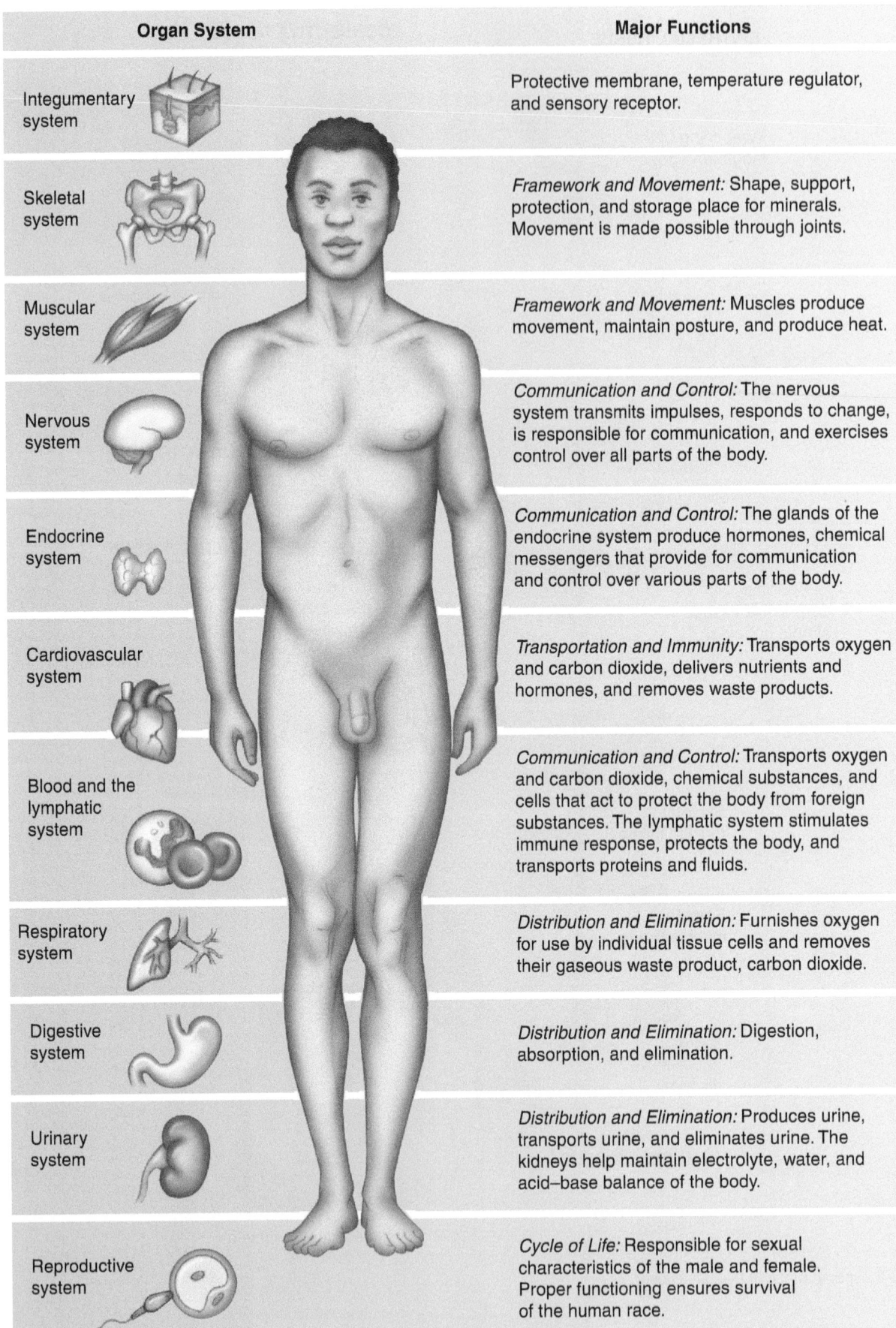

Integumentary system
Protective membrane, temperature regulator, and sensory receptor.

Skeletal system
Framework and Movement: Shape, support, protection, and storage place for minerals. Movement is made possible through joints.

Muscular system
Framework and Movement: Muscles produce movement, maintain posture, and produce heat.

Nervous system
Communication and Control: The nervous system transmits impulses, responds to change, is responsible for communication, and exercises control over all parts of the body.

Endocrine system
Communication and Control: The glands of the endocrine system produce hormones, chemical messengers that provide for communication and control over various parts of the body.

Cardiovascular system
Transportation and Immunity: Transports oxygen and carbon dioxide, delivers nutrients and hormones, and removes waste products.

Blood and the lymphatic system
Communication and Control: Transports oxygen and carbon dioxide, chemical substances, and cells that act to protect the body from foreign substances. The lymphatic system stimulates immune response, protects the body, and transports proteins and fluids.

Respiratory system
Distribution and Elimination: Furnishes oxygen for use by individual tissue cells and removes their gaseous waste product, carbon dioxide.

Digestive system
Distribution and Elimination: Digestion, absorption, and elimination.

Urinary system
Distribution and Elimination: Produces urine, transports urine, and eliminates urine. The kidneys help maintain electrolyte, water, and acid–base balance of the body.

Reproductive system
Cycle of Life: Responsible for sexual characteristics of the male and female. Proper functioning ensures survival of the human race.

FIGURE 20-6 Organ systems of the human body.

TABLE 20-4 | Major Organs and Structures within the Body Systems

Body System	Organs and Structures Within	Body System	Organs and Structures Within
Integumentary system	• Skin is the outermost structure • Underlying structures include sweat (sudoriferous) glands, fat (adipose) glands, hair follicles, and other connective structures	Blood and lymphatic system	• Red blood cells, white blood cells, and platelets • Plasma • Bone marrow • Spleen • Thymus • Lymph (fluid) • Lymph nodes
Skeletal system	• Bones • Joints	Respiratory system	• Nose • Mouth • Pharynx • Larynx • Trachea • Bronchi • Lungs
Muscular system	• Muscles • Ligaments • Tendons	Digestive system	• Mouth • Esophagus • Stomach • Small intestine • Large intestine • Rectum • Anus • Liver • Gallbladder • Pancreas • Appendix
Nervous system	• Brain • Spinal cord • Nerves	Urinary system	• Kidneys • Ureters • Bladder • Urethra
Endocrine system	• Thyroid gland • Parathyroid gland • Adrenal glands • Pituitary gland • Pineal gland • Ovaries • Testes • Stomach and pancreas also are considered a part of the endocrine system because they produce hormones.	Reproductive system	Female: • Vagina • Cervix • Uterus • Fallopian tubes • Ovaries Male: • Penis • Prostate gland • Seminal vesicles • Vas deferens • Testes

Passive transport does not require the cell to use energy; however, it does involve certain processes, including diffusion, osmosis, and filtration. **Diffusion** is the movement of dissolved particles from an area of greater concentration to an area of lesser concentration until they are evenly distributed. **Osmosis** is a form of diffusion whereby water is pulled through a membrane, once again moving from areas of greater to lesser concentration. **Filtration** requires some form of pressure to diffuse dissolved particles through membranes.

Active transport, by contrast, requires cellular energy to carry materials from an area of lesser concentration to an area of greater concentration. The cellular energy used in active transport is adenosine triphosphate (ATP). Through active transport, cells are able to obtain what they need from tissue fluid. This can be done through two methods:

- **Phagocytosis**—In this method, the cell engulfs a solid particle, such as a bacterium.
- **Pinocytosis**—In this method, the cell "drinks" the fluid required.

Electrolytes

An **electrolyte** is a molecule that conducts electricity. When dissolved in water or other bodily fluids, electrolytes break down into ions that are either positively or negatively charged. Ions that are positively charged are called *cations*. Ions that are negatively charged are called *anions*.

Cells use electrolytes to maintain voltage or electrical force across their cell membranes. This is especially important in neurons as well as in heart and muscle cells. Electrolytes are also used to carry electrical impulses to other cells.

The body's fluids—including blood, plasma, and interstitial fluid (the fluid between cells)—contain high concentrations of the electrolyte sodium chloride (NaCl). Other electrolytes found in the human body include sodium (Na^+), potassium (K^+), chloride (Cl), calcium (Ca), magnesium (Mg), bicarbonate (HCO_3), phosphate (PO_4), and sulfate (SO_4).

It is essential for your body to maintain proper electrolyte levels within the blood, even though changes to the body occur quite frequently. The kidneys are responsible for maintaining these levels. Consider the example of heavy exercise: Heavy exercise results in a loss of electrolytes from sweating. The body, by means of the kidneys maintaining electrolyte balance, is able to maintain homeostasis even though changes to the body, such as sweating, are occurring.

Electrolytes that are lost must be replaced to keep their concentrations in body fluids constant. That is why sodium chloride or potassium chloride is added to many sports drinks. Sugar and flavorings are also added, not only to make sports drinks taste better, but also to provide the body with extra energy.

Metabolism

Metabolism consists of all the chemical processes in the body that maintain life, including the production and release of energy. Energy is required as the body replenishes cells, repairs damage, and accommodates to the surrounding environments.

Two processes are involved in metabolism: anabolism and catabolism. **Anabolism** is a process of chemical reactions that work together to build things up, such as creating molecules from smaller components. Anabolism requires

energy to complete its task. **Catabolism** is a chemical process that works to break down larger units into smaller units. Consider food that is being digested. Digestion is a catabolic process because it breaks down the food that we eat into smaller particles that can be used by our body for nourishment. In contrast to anabolism, catabolism releases energy during its process.

GENETICS AND HEREDITY

Genetics is the study of the hereditary makeup of animals or plants. As mentioned earlier in this chapter, a person's genes are made up of DNA. Organized in chromosomes that are located in the nucleus of each cell, DNA controls the structure and function of the entire body. Each person's DNA and genetic makeup are inherited from the person's parents and other ancestors.

Genetic Engineering

Changes that occur to an organism's existing DNA are the result of genetic engineering. Although some genetic changes may happen naturally, genetic engineering is generally considered to be the use of technology by scientists intentionally to make changes to the genetic makeup. This increasingly popular field of science is still relatively new. Because genetic engineering is so new, its effects are not yet fully known, and controversy surrounds whether genetic engineering is safe or ethical.

Genetic Fingerprinting

Everyone's DNA has the same chemical structure. The differences between individuals lie in the order of the base pairs that are the building blocks of the DNA. There are millions of base pairs in each person's DNA, meaning that each person has a different DNA sequence by which he can be identified. The analysis and identification of a person's unique genetic makeup is known as genetic, or DNA, fingerprinting. Identical twins provide the only instance in which two people carry the same genetic fingerprint.

DNA fingerprinting is achieved by obtaining a small amount of a person's DNA—usually from hair, semen, vaginal fluid, blood, or saliva, but any part of a human can be used. This piece of DNA is put through various tests to extract and isolate part of the strand of DNA. This is done by using chemicals, such as enzymes, and electricity to separate the different parts of the DNA. The sample analysis shows the DNA patterns. If two patterns from two DNA samples match, they are very likely to have come from the same person. In the case of proving parentage, DNA from the child is matched to that of the people requesting the test. The tests show the relationship of these people to the particular child by matching both the maternal (mother's) and paternal (father's) DNA fingerprints to the child's. If the DNA fingerprint shows significant similarities, then the people participating in the test are the parents.

Genetics, Heredity, and Disease

As already mentioned, **heredity** is the genetic transmission from parent to child. The genes for certain traits are passed down in families from parents to children, and hereditary traits are determined by specific genes. Individuals carry two genes for each trait: one from the mother's egg and one from the father's sperm.

Genetic Disorders

Genetic disorders are medical conditions that are caused by mutations in a single gene or a set of genes. A **mutation** is a change in the DNA sequence of a gene. The genes are not responsible for genetic disorders and diseases; the mutations that result from improper operations of normal genes are responsible for genetic disorders and diseases.

A genetic mutation may develop at any point during a person's lifetime; genetic mutations do not present only at birth. A genetic disorder that is present and may be diagnosed at birth is described, specifically, as a **congenital disorder**. Common congenital disorders include the following:

- **Albinism** is a congenital but nonpathological disorder. A recessive gene mutation causes hereditary lack of pigment in the skin, hair, and eyes. The patient may complain of photophobia (excessive sensitivity to light) and be prone to sunburn because protective melanin is not present.

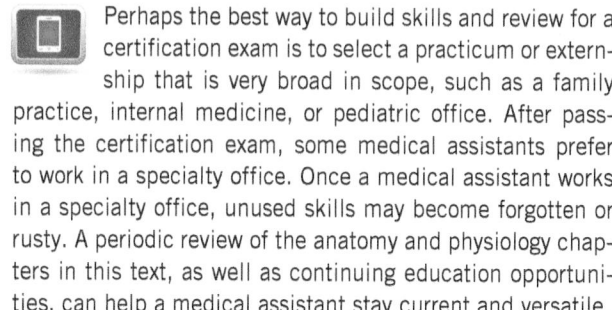

Professionalism The Workplace

Perhaps the best way to build skills and review for a certification exam is to select a practicum or externship that is very broad in scope, such as a family practice, internal medicine, or pediatric office. After passing the certification exam, some medical assistants prefer to work in a specialty office. Once a medical assistant works in a specialty office, unused skills may become forgotten or rusty. A periodic review of the anatomy and physiology chapters in this text, as well as continuing education opportunities, can help a medical assistant stay current and versatile.

- **Attention-deficit/hyperactivity disorder (ADHD)** is a disorder that can affect both children and adults characterized by difficulty focusing attention and organizing and completing a task. The cause may be genetic factors, and the disorder is 10 times more prevalent in boys than in girls. No cure is known, but treatment often includes medications or counseling to help with behavior modifications or developing strategies to deal with the disorder. Dietary modifications, including avoiding certain foods or food additives, may also be recommended if these are determined to be part of the cause of hyperactivity. Symptoms of ADHD may subside or even disappear with time.

- **Cleft palate** (Figure 20-7) is a congenital defect in the roof of the mouth that occurs when the palatine bones of the skull do not close properly. The cleft causes a passageway between the mouth and nasal cavities. It may also be associated with a cleft upper lip, and it affects females more often than males. Initially, the

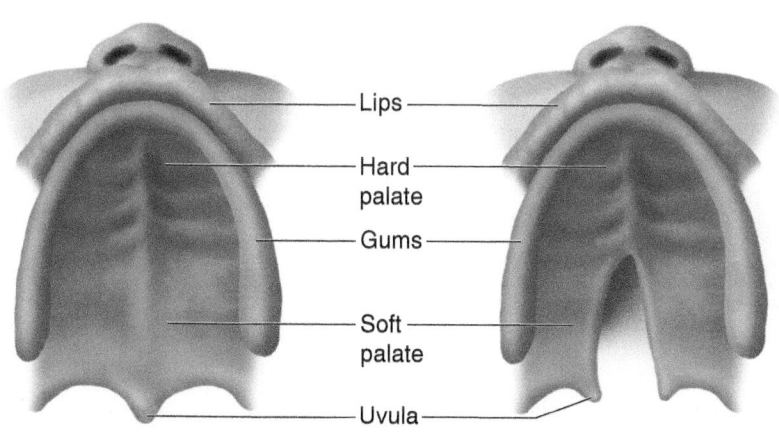
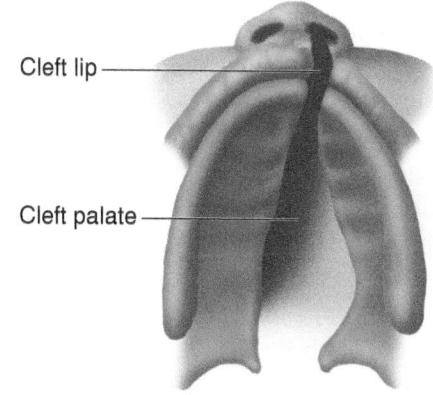

Lips — Hard palate — Gums — Soft palate — Uvula

Normal palate in infant

Partial cleft palate

Cleft lip — Cleft palate

Complete cleft palate and cleft lip

FIGURE 20-7 Cleft palate.

infant has special needs for feeding. Surgical repairs are usually performed within the first year of life and are generally successful in repairing the defect.

- **Color deficiency** is a disorder that was previously called color blindness. It often entails difficulty in distinguishing between reds and greens. It is an inherited, sex-linked disorder, usually passed from mother to son. In total color deficiency, the person is unable to perceive any color at all because of a defect in or absence of cones in the retina.

- **Cystic fibrosis (CF)** is generally diagnosed during childhood. This genetic disease is characterized by mucosal changes that cause the mucus to become sticky, dry, and dense. Passages within the lungs and pancreas are those that most commonly become obstructed by the thick build-up of mucus. The Cystic Fibrosis Foundation explains that recent advances in treatment have advanced the predicted median survival age close to 40 years. This is a vast improvement to the survival rate that prevailed during the 1950s, when many children succumbed to this disease during their elementary school years.

- **Down syndrome (trisomy 21)** is a disorder caused by an extra chromosome present at the 21st chromosomal pair (hence the name). This genetic mutation occurs during meiosis and cellular reproduction. A few of the major features seen include marked sloping of the forehead, a short broad hand with a single palmar crease (known as a simian crease), and a flat nose. A mother who gives birth after the age of 40 has a higher risk of delivering an infant with Down syndrome. Amniocentesis is generally used as a tool for diagnosing this disorder. See Figure 20-8 for a photo of someone with this anomaly.

- **Fragile X syndrome**, also known as Martin-Bell syndrome, Marker X syndrome, and FRAXA syndrome, is the most common form of inherited mental retardation. Individuals with this condition have developmental delays, variable levels of mental retardation, and behavioral and emotional difficulties. They may also have characteristic physical traits that tend to become more evident as the child grows and develops. Some of these traits include elongated and narrow face, large ears, and a protruding forehead and jawline. Other characteristics might include very flexible fingers, flat feet, and, in males, enlarged testicles after puberty. Generally, males with Fragile X are affected with moderate mental retardation and females with

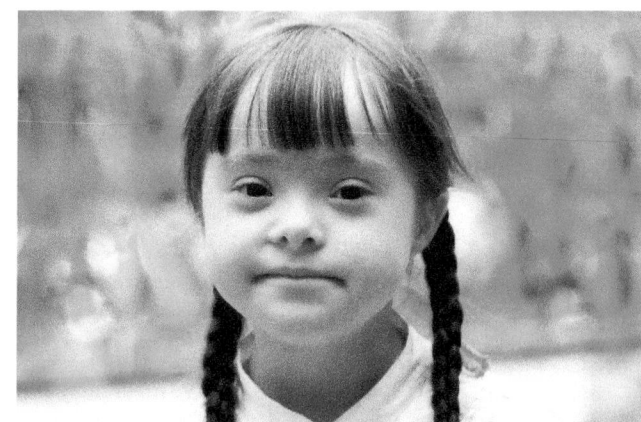

FIGURE 20-8 Girl with Down syndrome.

mild mental retardation. Fragile X is caused by a mutation in the *FMR-1* gene, located on the X chromosome. The role of this gene is unclear, but it is thought to be important to early development.

- **Hemochromatosis** is characterized by an extreme accumulation of iron within the body. Those most commonly afflicted are of European descent, mainly Caucasian, nearly 4 in 100 of whom are born with this genetic disorder. Hemochromatosis patients are believed to absorb excessive amounts of iron from the diet. Because the human body has limited ways of eliminating the absorbed iron, the iron accumulates over time in the liver, bone marrow, pancreas, skin, and testicles. The accumulation of iron in these organs causes them to function poorly. Patients with early hemochromatosis have no symptoms and are unaware of their condition. The disease may be discovered when elevated blood iron levels are noted as a result of routine blood testing. In males, symptoms may not appear until 40 to 50 years of age. Iron deposits in the skin cause darkening of the skin. Because females lose iron through menstrual blood loss, they develop organ damage from excessive iron accumulation on average 15 to 20 years later than men.

- **Hemophilia** is a hereditary, sex-linked disorder in which blood coagulation time is greatly increased. Hemophiliacs bleed more easily and for a longer period of time because it takes so long for their blood to clot. This genetic disorder is caused by a recessive gene mutation in the X chromosome. Females carry the recessive gene and transmit the disorder to their male offspring.

- **Klinefelter's syndrome** is a congenital endocrine disorder affecting males. Many symptoms go unnoticed until puberty. Symptoms include small and firm

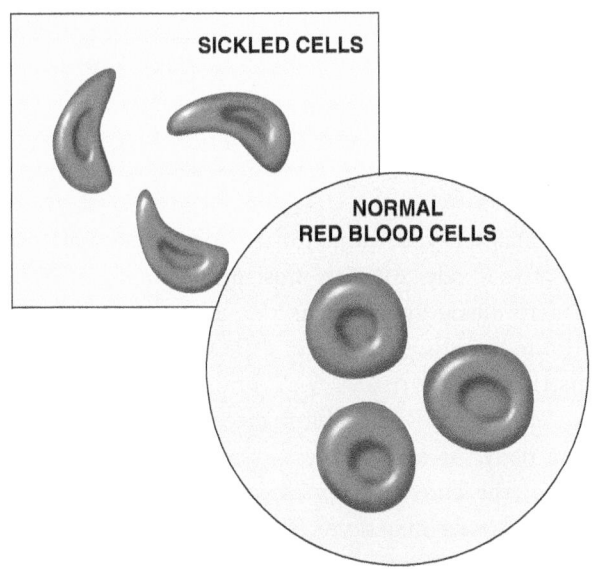

FIGURE 20-9 Sickled and normal red blood cells.

testes, small penis, tall stature, weak bones, low energy levels, and excessive breast tissue, which is termed *gynecomastia*. This disorder also can lead to shyness, learning difficulties, and attention disorders.

- **Muscular dystrophy** is a progressive wasting, or atrophy, and weakening of muscle. More common in males, this genetic disease has various forms. The most common type is Duchenne muscular dystrophy, which accounts for 50 percent of all cases. The onset is at an early age, and the patient is usually confined to a wheelchair by the age of 12. Death often occurs within 10 to 15 years of onset of symptoms. Unfortunately, there is no successful treatment, although physical therapy and exercise are recommended to prevent more atrophy of muscles.

- **Phenylketonuria (PKU)** is caused by a recessive gene mutation. A defective enzyme causes the body to be unable to oxidize the amino acid phenylalanine into tyrosine. If the condition is not treated early, mental retardation occurs as a result of brain damage. Many states require testing at birth to detect PKU.

- **Sickle cell anemia** (Figure 20-9) is a hereditary, chronic form of anemia that is caused by a recessive gene mutation. Also known as Hemoglobin SS disease, it is most common in people of African or Mediterranean descent.

- **Spina bifida** (Figure 20-10) is a congenital neural tube defect. It develops when the vertebrae in the spine do not form correctly around the spinal cord. Symptoms vary greatly and depend on the severity of the disease. In some cases, the spinal cord and its membranes may protrude outside the body and be evident at birth. Most often the abnormality occurs in the lumbar region.

- **Talipes** is an inherited deformity of the foot. It is commonly referred to as clubfoot. Special orthopedic shoes can help with walking, and casting of the foot may also be a treatment option. In some cases surgery is required.

- **Tay-Sachs disease (TSD)** is an inherited disorder characterized by a genetic mutation that targets the nervous system. Specific ethnic groups are more commonly

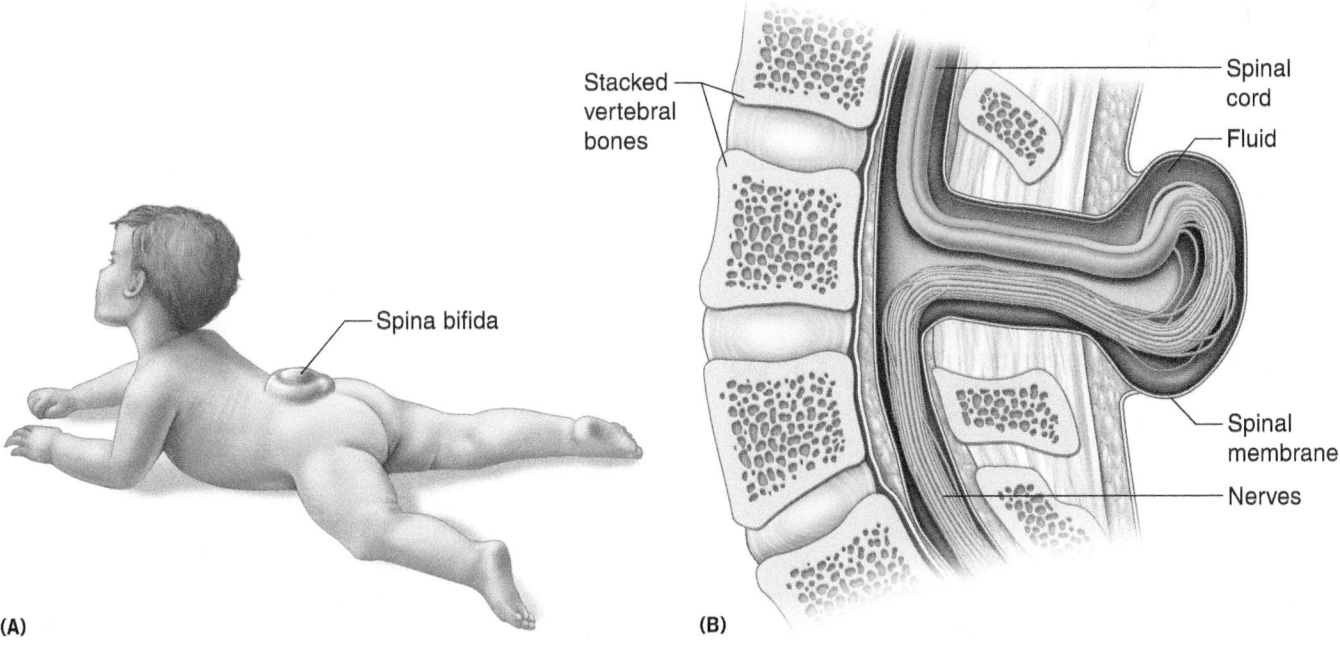

FIGURE 20-10 (A) An infant with spina bifida; **(B)** the spinal cord protrudes from the body.

afflicted with this disease, including those of central and northern European Jewish (Ashkenazi) or French-Canadian ancestry. This terrible disease afflicts babies, most often around the age of 6 months. Progressive symptoms develop quickly, and the baby slowly becomes paralyzed; first there is a lack of smiling and movement, then total paralysis occurs. Unfortunately, most children with TSD die before their fifth birthday. At this time, there is no known cure.

- **Turner's syndrome** is a congenital disorder caused by all or part of one of the X chromosomes becoming lost before or immediately after conception. Intelligence may be impaired, amenorrhea (absence of menstruation) may be present, and the patient is usually short in stature.

SUMMARY

In this chapter, you learned of the organizational components of the body. As with most matter in the world, our bodies are made up of atoms that form molecules. These in turn form cells. A group of cells with similar functions forms tissues, and tissues with similar functions form organs. These organs then form systems that make up the human body. As each of these systems performs a specific function, the body can remain in homeostasis. Although disease processes may occur, the body is remarkable in its ability to fight off infections or, in some cases, as in cellular development, even to regenerate.

The systems of the body include the integumentary, skeletal, muscular, nervous, cardiovascular, immune, respiratory, digestive, urinary, endocrine, and reproductive systems.

The cell, like a city, stores information and uses molecules to perform work, thus creating waste that requires disposal. Parts of the cell include the nucleus, cell membrane, endoplasmic reticulum, cytoplasm, ribosomes, lysosomes, centrioles, mitochondria, ribosomes, and Golgi apparatus.

Body processes can be active or passive. Active transport uses energy, whereas passive transportation happens without energy consumption. Metabolism is comprised of two partnering processes: anabolism and catabolism.

Genetics is a relatively new science with a lot of potential to help patients. Each person, unless a twin, has a unique genetic fingerprint. Understanding familial and inherited characteristics and disease risk can help the medical assistant to gather appropriate data from patients. Knowledge of congenital disorders can help predict the risk that a child may inherit one.

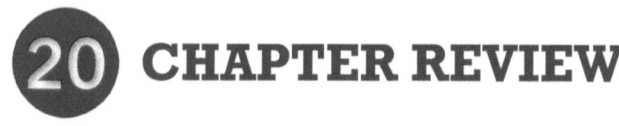 **CHAPTER REVIEW**

COMPETENCY REVIEW

1. Define and spell the terms for this chapter.
2. List the organization of the body from atom to organism.
3. List five parts of the cell and their functions.
4. What are the three types of muscle tissue?
5. What are the four functions of epithelial tissue?
6. What are the two properties of nerve tissue?
7. Which part of the cell is known as the control center, and why?
8. Compare and contrast anabolism and catabolism.
9. Select five genetic disorders and describe their pathology.

PREPARING FOR THE CERTIFICATION EXAM

1. Which part of the cell allows for selective permeability?
   a. cytoplasm
   b. cell membrane
   c. vacuole
   d. Golgi body
   e. endoplasmic reticulum

2. Which of the following systems is responsible for regulating body temperature and acting as a sensory receptor?
   a. reproductive
   b. respiratory
   c. cardiovascular
   d. integumentary
   e. nervous

3. Talipes is also known as
   a. PKU.
   b. anemia.
   c. club foot.
   d. fragile X syndrome.
   e. cleft palate.

4. This organelle is considered the "powerhouse" of the cell:
   a. Golgi apparatus.
   b. nucleus.
   c. lysosome.
   d. mitochondria.
   e. ribosome.

5. This is the term for a positively charged particle:
   a. atom.
   b. proton.
   c. electron.
   d. molecule.
   e. neutron.

6. Which cell structure is responsible for the production of ribosomes?
   a. nucleus
   b. cytoplasm
   c. endoplasmic reticulum
   d. Golgi body
   e. mitochondria

7. Which phase directly follows prophase during mitosis?
   a. prometaphase
   b. cytokinesis
   c. anaphase
   d. metaphase
   e. telophase

8. Which genetic disorder is a hereditary, sex-linked disorder that affects blood coagulation?
   a. Klinefelter's syndrome
   b. muscular dystrophy
   c. hemophilia
   d. fragile X
   e. hemochromatosis

9. The lung is considered a/an
   a. organ system.
   b. organelle.
   c. cell.
   d. tissue.
   e. organ.

10. What is responsible for carrying electrical impulses to other cells?
    a. ions
    b. cations
    c. electrolytes
    d. anions
    e. plasma

CRITICAL THINKING

Refer to the case study at the beginning of the chapter and use the information you have learned to answer the following questions.

1. Lucy finds that many patients have a variety of genetically related diseases and disorders. She is particularly interested in the patient cases that deal with trisomy 21, as her younger cousin was born with it. What is the more common term for trisomy 21, and how is it generally diagnosed before birth?

2. If you were in Lucy's position, what would you like or dislike about having the opportunity to shadow and work in a genetic clinic of a hospital?

3. Lucy is learning that the genetic clinic at Pearson General Hospital has had an unusually high number of cases of children with Tay-Sachs disease (TSD) over the past 15 years. Which cultural groups are most often afflicted with TSD?

ON THE JOB

Kara is a medical assistant for an OB/GYN office. Kara is working with Dr. Miller, who is about to tell his patient Barbara Klemens that the results of her amniocentesis are not favorable. The test reveals a chromosomal anomaly that is present in patients with Down syndrome.

1. What is the alternate term for Down syndrome that is commonly used in the medical field? Why is it given this name?

2. What are some physical characteristics of Down syndrome?

3. Who has a higher risk of delivering an infant with Down syndrome?

INTERNET ACTIVITY

Use the Internet to find information pertaining to an amniocentesis procedure.

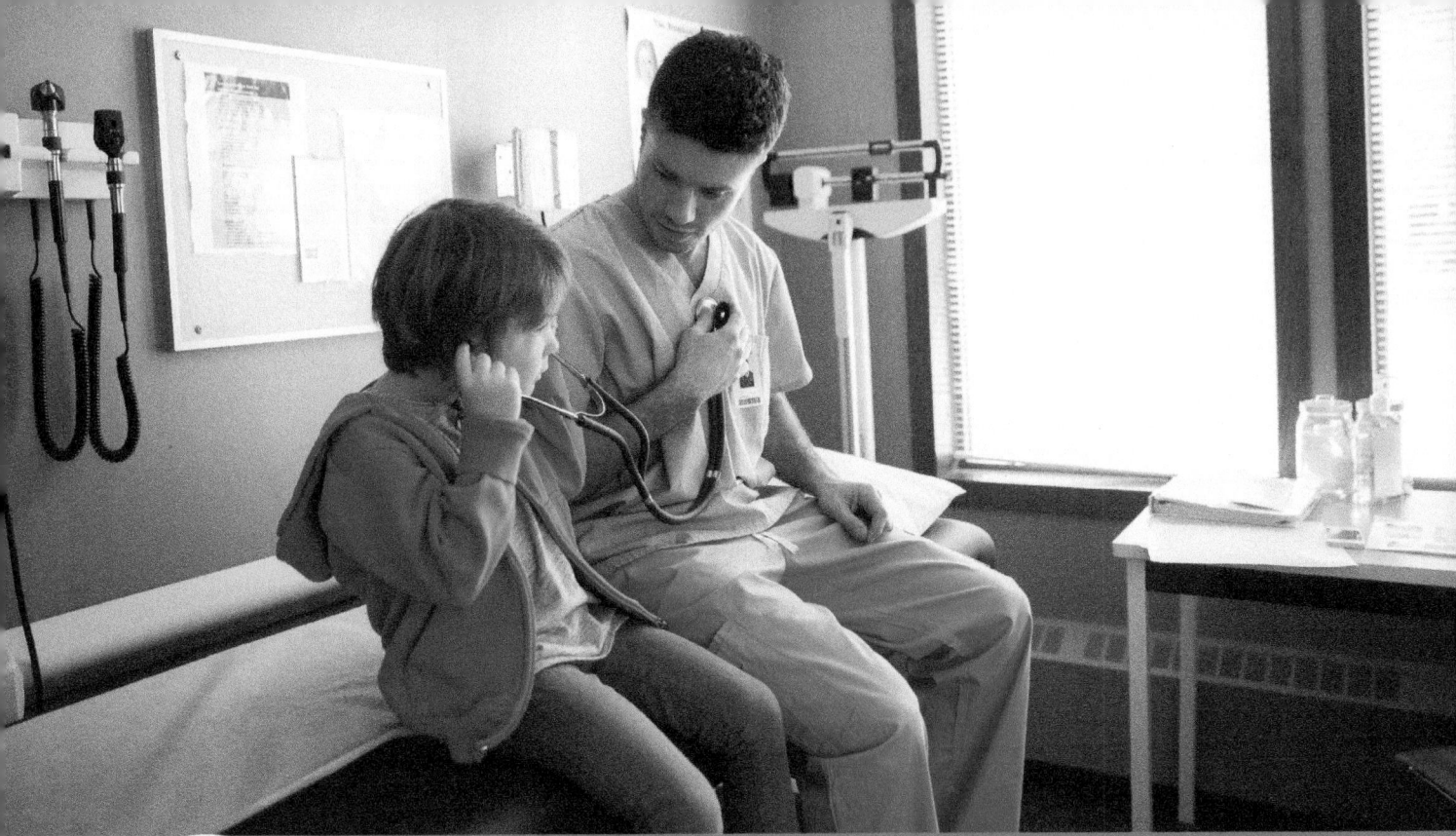

21

The Integumentary System

Learning Objectives

After completing this chapter, you should be able to:

21.1   Define and spell the terms for this chapter.
21.2   List and describe the functions of the skin.
21.3   Identify the location of each layer of skin
21.4   Describe the function of each layer of skin.
21.5   Describe the functions of accessory organs of the skin.
21.6   Differentiate between basal cell carcinoma, squamous cell carcinoma, and malignant melanoma.
21.7   Describe how the integumentary system changes between childhood and older adulthood.
21.8   Identify pathology associated with the integumentary system.
21.9   Describe various forms of skin care treatments that are used to reverse the signs of aging.

Julie Yeung is a 29-year-old patient of Pearson Physicians Group. Julie, of Italian descent, and her husband, Lou, of Chinese descent, have not been successful conceiving a child. She has recently been diagnosed with an ovarian disorder known as polycystic ovarian syndrome. Today, she is seeing Dr. Miller for increased dark-hair growth on her face and chin.

Terms to Learn

acne vulgaris	folliculitis	rosacea
alopecia	furuncle	scabies
bacteremic	herpes simplex	sebaceous glands
basal cell carcinoma	herpes zoster	seborrheic dermatitis
benign	hirsutism	sebum
callus	impetigo	squamous cell carcinoma
carbuncle	keloid	sudoriferous glands
cellulitis	keratin	tinea capitis
contact dermatitis	lunula	tinea corporis
corn	malignant	tinea cruris
decubitus ulcer	malignant melanoma	tinea pedis
dermis	matrix	urticaria
dysplastic nevus	melanin	verrucae
eczema	melanocytes	vesicles
epidermis	pediculosis	vitiligo
erythema	psoriasis	

Weighing more than 6 pounds and covering more than 3,000 square inches, the skin is the largest organ of the human body. Skin and its accessory structures constitute the integumentary system. Accessory structures of the integumentary system include hair, nails, sebaceous (oil) glands, and sudoriferous (sweat) glands.

FUNCTIONS OF THE INTEGUMENTARY SYSTEM

The skin works in multiple ways to provide homeostasis for the body. The five main functions of the integumentary system are protection, regulation, sensation, absorption, and secretion. By providing these functions, the integumentary system, along with the other body systems, can maintain the internal conditions that are essential to the function of the body.

Protection

Intact skin serves as a protective barrier to the internal structures and compartments of the body. The skin prevents harmful agents (such as bacteria, viruses, and pollution) from entering the body. Cuts and abrasions, which open the skin causing it not to be intact, allow harmful microbes to enter the body. The skin guards the body against the sun's ultraviolet rays by producing a protective pigmentation called melanin. Vitamin D, which is essential to the body, is also produced by the skin.

Regulation

The skin also helps regulate body temperature. When body temperature rises and requires cooling, the blood vessels in the skin dilate and bring more blood to the surface of the skin where heat from the blood is more easily released. While this is occurring, the body's sweat glands begin to secrete sweat that evaporates to cool the body.

If the body needs to conserve heat, the blood vessels in the skin will constrict, moving heat-carrying blood away from the skin and circulating it to the muscles and internal vital organs to keep them warm. Both the constriction and the dilation of blood vessels in the skin are reflex actions initiated by the nervous system. The regulation of body temperature is an example of how the integumentary system and the nervous system work together to maintain homeostasis.

Sensory Reception

The skin contains millions of microscopic nerve endings that act as sensory receptors. Again, the integumentary system and the nervous system work together, in this case for the function of sensation. Each nerve ending is specialized to provide a specific type of sensory reaction. Sensory reactions include responses to pressure, traction, heat, cold, pain, and more. The nerve endings and their sensory receptors send information to the cerebral cortex of the brain. When the message reaches the brain, an appropriate response is triggered. For example, if the hand touches a hot pan and senses heat and pain, a message is sent to the brain, which sends back a signal to remove the hand from the hot pan (Figure 21-1).

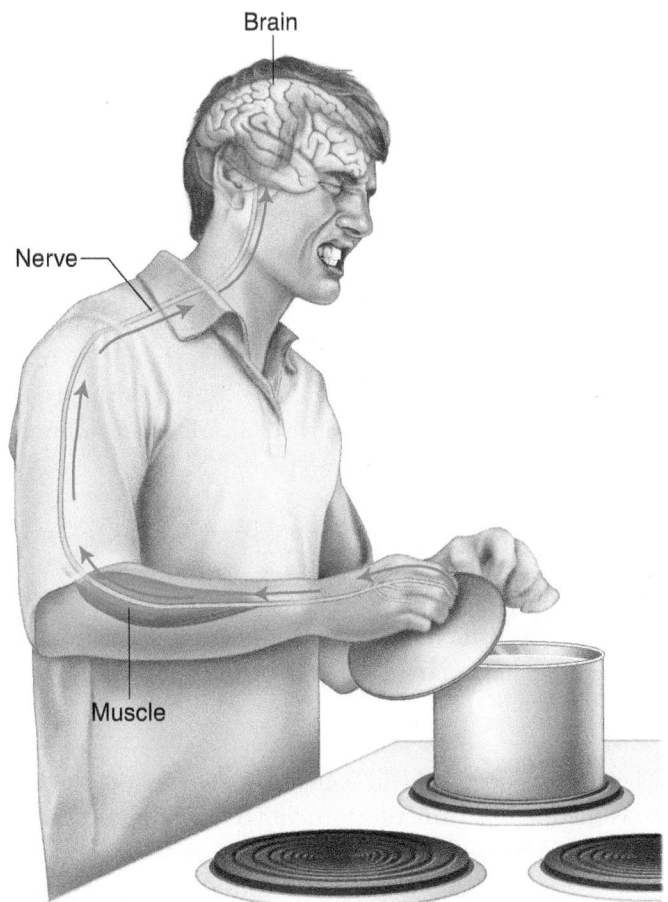

FIGURE 21-1 The integumentary and nervous systems work together to recognize specific sensations, such as heat and pain.

Absorption

Absorption is another function of the skin. Transdermal (through-the-skin) medications take advantage of this capability of the skin to absorb substances. Transdermal drugs are often administered by placing medicated patches on various parts of the body. Placement is chosen based on the most effective location to deliver the specific medication. Examples of transdermal medications are those intended to prevent motion sickness and those that provide hormonal therapy, including birth control patches. Another form of transdermal medication is a medicated paste. For example, nitroglycerin paste is applied to the chest to regulate certain heart conditions.

Both transdermal patches and medicated pastes have time-release properties that allow the medications to be absorbed through the skin and into the bloodstream slowly, at a desired rate, rather than all at once.

It is important to note that the medical assistant who administers or applies a transdermal medication should always wear protective gloves. The gloves act as a protective barrier to prevent the medication intended for the patient from entering the medical assistant's bloodstream.

Secretion

The skin contains millions of sudoriferous glands, which secrete perspiration, or sweat, and sebaceous glands, which secrete oil for lubrication. Perspiration is composed mostly of water with small amounts of salt and other chemical compounds. If the secretions are allowed to accumulate, especially around body hair in the axillary region, bacteria will begin to grow, creating body odor. Sebaceous glands produce sebum, which acts to protect the body from dehydration and the possible absorption of harmful substances. Both sudoriferous and sebaceous glands are discussed as accessory organs of the skin later in this chapter.

STRUCTURES OF THE SKIN

The skin is composed of three layers: the epidermis, the dermis, and the subcutaneous layer (Figure 21-2).

The Epidermis

The **epidermis** is divided into four layers or strata: the stratum corneum, stratum lucidum, stratum granulosum, and stratum germinativum.

Stratum Corneum

The stratum corneum, the outermost layer of skin, consists of dead cells filled with the protein **keratin**. Keratin works to firm and strengthen the skin. The stratum corneum forms a

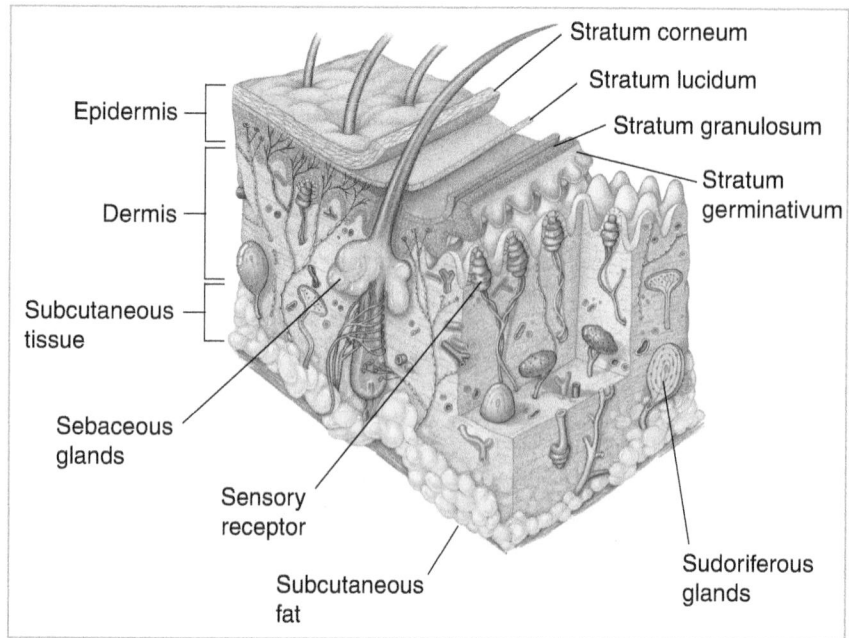

FIGURE 21-2 The integument: the epidermis, the dermis, subcutaneous tissue, and its appendages.

protective covering for the body. The thickness of the layer varies based on the body part that is being covered, some layers being thicker than others. For example, consider the soles of the feet and the palms of the hands. Because of the ongoing pressure on their surfaces, the soles of the feet and the palms of the hands have thicker layers than do the surfaces of areas such as the eyelids or forehead.

Stratum Lucidum

The stratum lucidum is a translucent layer lying directly beneath the stratum corneum. In thinner skin, this layer is often absent. Cells in this layer are either dead or dying.

Stratum Granulosum

The stratum granulosum consists of several layers of living cells that are in the process of becoming part of the stratum lucidum and stratum corneum. These cells are actively becoming keratinized, or hardened, after they lose their nuclei.

Stratum Germinativum

The stratum germinativum contains several layers of living cells that are still capable of mitosis, or cell division. This layer, occasionally referred to as the mucosum, is most responsible for the regeneration of the epidermis. If this layer is damaged, as from a severe burn, the skin is unable to regenerate itself, and skin grafting must be done. This layer also contains the **melanocytes**, the cells that produce **melanin**. Melanin is the pigment that gives the skin its color. The varying amounts of melanin that may be produced allow individuals to have varying shades of skin tones. The absence of melanin in the skin, hair, and eyes is an inherited disorder known as albinism.

The Dermis

The **dermis** is the middle layer of the skin and is often referred to as the "true skin." It is composed of connective tissue containing nerves and nerve endings, blood vessels, sebaceous and sweat glands, hair follicles, and lymph vessels. The dermis is further divided into two layers: the papillary layer and the reticular layer.

- The papillary layer is the thin upper layer of the dermis adjacent to, or attached to, the bottom part of the epidermis. It is made up of loose connective tissue with fingerlike projections (the papillae) that extend into the epidermis. Papillae form the ridges that are fingerprints.

- The reticular layer is the thicker lower layer of the dermis. It consists of dense connective tissue that supports blood vessels and nerves as well as hair roots, sebaceous and sudoriferous glands, and nails.

The Subcutaneous Layer

The subcutaneous layer is the innermost layer of the skin. Subcutaneous tissue is composed of loose connective tissue with small lobes of fat. Subcutaneous tissue helps support, nourish, insulate, and cushion the skin. It contains larger blood vessels and nerves than those found in the dermis. Medical assistants must be familiar with the subcutaneous layer of the skin, because many medications are administered here via subcutaneous injection.

ACCESSORY STRUCTURES OF THE SKIN

The accessory structures of the skin include the hair, nails, sebaceous glands, and sudoriferous or sweat glands.

Hair

The visible portion of hair is the shaft. The root of the hair is embedded within the follicle. A loop of capillaries enclosed in connective tissue is the hair papilla. The papilla is found at the base of each hair follicle. The pilomotor muscle is attached to the side of each follicle. Contraction

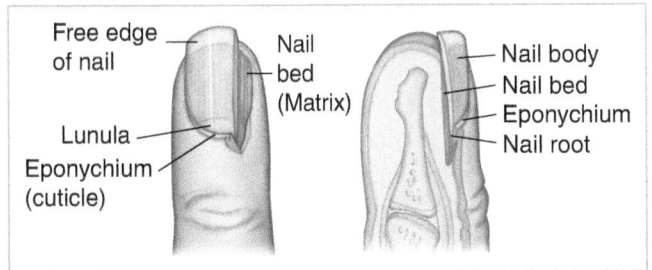

FIGURE 21-3 The fingernail, an appendage of the integument.

of the pilomotor muscle causes goose bumps, or the sensation of the hair standing on end. This may be the result of an emotional reaction or may be the skin's attempt at self-warming. With the exception of the palms of the hands and the soles of the feet, the entire body is covered by a very thin layer of hair.

Hairs that surround the eyes, ears, and nose act as a protective barrier, filtering out foreign particles and preventing their entrance into the sensory organs.

Nails

Fingernails and toenails are horny cell structures of the epidermis and are composed of hard keratin. A nail consists of the body, the root, and the **matrix**, or nail bed (Figure 21-3). The **lunula** is the crescent-shaped white area at the base of the nail. Average nail growth is about 1 mm (0.04 in.) per week. A lost fingernail may take 3½ to 5½ months to regrow, whereas a lost toenail may take as long as 6 to 8 months to regrow. Nail growth may be adversely affected by disease, nutritional deficiencies, and hormonal insufficiencies.

Sebaceous Glands

Located in the dermis, the **sebaceous glands**, or oil glands, secrete **sebum**. Sebum is made of fat and the debris of dead fat-producing cells. The function of sebum is to protect and waterproof hair and skin. The endocrine system regulates the amount of secretion of the sebaceous glands, which also varies with age, pregnancy, and puberty.

Sebaceous glands can usually be found in hair-covered areas where they are contained in hair follicles but can also be found in the hairless areas of the lips, eyelids, penis, labia minora, and nipples. At the hairless areas, sebum rises to the surface through ducts. The sebaceous glands of a fetus in utero secrete vernix caseosa, a "waxy" or "cheesy" white substance found coating the skin of the newborn baby.

Sudoriferous Glands

Predominant in the palms of the hands and the soles of the feet, **sudoriferous glands**, or sweat glands, occur in nearly all regions of the skin. Sweat glands are coiled, ball-shaped structures that are located in the dermis or subcutaneous layers. Sweat glands secrete perspiration, which helps to cool the body by evaporation. It is estimated that the body loses 0.5 L of fluid per day via sweat.

COMMON PATHOLOGY OF THE INTEGUMENTARY SYSTEM

Skin is vulnerable to many disorders because it is the most exposed of all the body systems. Skin disorders have multiple signs. There are common and specific skin lesions that may evidence specific diseases or disorders. A skin lesion is simply any part of the skin that does not resemble the surrounding skin, or a variation in the skin. Many skin lesions are **benign** in origin, meaning they are noncancerous. A variety of common skin lesions are shown and described in Figure 21-4.

Common diagnostic methods and tests used to identify and treat the pathological conditions discussed in this section are described in Table 21-1.

Skin Cancer

The most common of all cancers, skin cancer affects more than one million people each year in the United States. These cancers occur when normal skin cells undergo a change during which they grow and multiply without normal controls. Those with lighter and fairer skin, as well as natural blondes and redheads, are more prone to skin cancer.

As the abnormal cells multiply, they form a mass called a tumor. As a result of their uncontrolled growth, **malignant** (cancerous) tumors encroach on neighboring tissues, especially lymph.

Like many cancers, skin cancers start as precancerous lesions that can develop into cancer because of the quick reproduction of abnormal cells and skin changes. Health care professionals often refer to these changes as dysplasia. One example of this is a **dysplastic nevus**, or an abnormal mole. People with dysplastic nevi often have a lot of them, perhaps one hundred or more. They are usually irregular in shape, with notched or fading borders. Dysplastic nevi may be either flat or raised, and the surface may be smooth or rough ("pebbly").

The three major types of skin cancers are:

- Basal cell carcinoma
- Squamous cell carcinoma
- Malignant melanoma

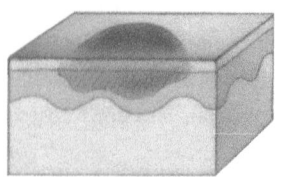

A macule is a discolored spot on the skin; freckle.

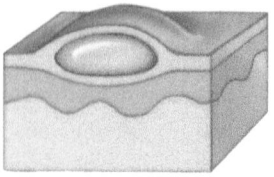

A wheal is a localized, evanescent elevation of the skin that is often accompanied by itching; urticaria.

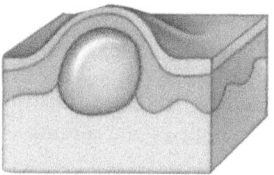

A papule is a solid, circumscribed, elevated area on the skin; pimple.

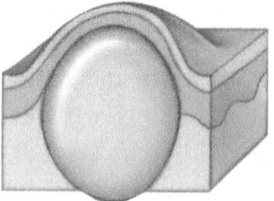

A nodule is a larger papule; acne vulgaris.

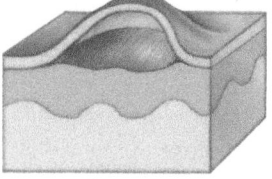

A vesicle is a small fluid filled sac; blister. A bulla is a large vesicle.

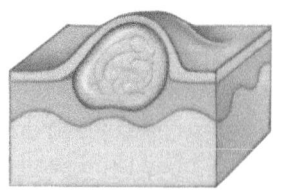

A pustule is a small, elevated, circumscribed lesion of the skin that is filled with pus; varicella (chickenpox).

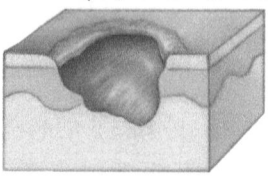

An erosion or ulcer is an eating or gnawing away of tissue; decubitus ulcer.

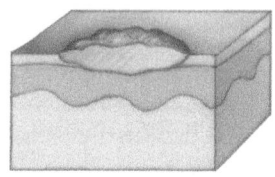

A crust is a dry, serous or seropurulent, brown, yellow, red, or green exudation that is seen in secondary lesions; eczema.

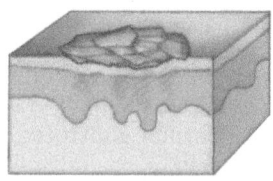

A scale is a thin, dry flake of cornified epithelial cells; psoriasis.

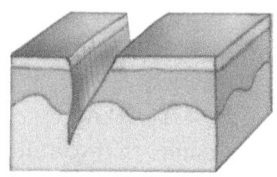

A fissure is a crack-like sore or slit that extends through the epidermis into the dermis; athlete's foot.

FIGURE 21-4 A skin lesion may be harmless and benign or evidence of an illness or disorder.

Basal Cell Carcinoma

Basal cell carcinoma, the most common form of skin cancer, is a malignant tumor most often caused by overexposure to the sun and ultraviolet rays. It may often appear as a change in the skin, such as a growth, irritation, or sore that does not heal or as a change in a wart or mole. Though the nose is the most common site, it also occurs on the head, neck, back, chest, or shoulders.

Signs and Symptoms. Signs of basal cell carcinoma can vary and may include skin changes such as the following:

- Firm, pearly bump with visible and spider-like tiny blood vessels (telangiectasias)
- Red, tender, flat spot that bleeds easily
- Small, fleshy bump with a smooth, pearly appearance, often with a depressed center
- Smooth, shiny bump that may look like a mole or cyst
- Scarlike patch of skin, especially on the face, that is firm to the touch
- Bump that itches, bleeds, crusts over, and then repeats the cycle and has not healed in three weeks
- Change in the size, shape, or color of a wart or mole

Treatment. Because basal cell carcinoma usually grows and progresses slowly, it often can be detected and successfully treated in its early stages of development. The most common treatment is surgery to destroy or remove the entire skin growth, including a margin of cancer-free tissue surrounding the growth. Another treatment option is a type of surgery called Mohs micrographic surgery, originally known as chemosurgery. This microscopically controlled surgery removes the cancerous lesion one layer at a time until the tumor is completely removed. Mohs surgery is highly effective, with cure rates higher than 90 percent. Additionally, cryosurgery and laser surgery are treatment options for basal cell carcinoma. Cryosurgery uses freezing as a mechanism to kill the cancer cells, whereas laser surgery uses a beam of light to destroy the cells that make up the tumor. Overall treatment for skin cancer varies, depending on the size and location of the cancer as well as the age and overall health of the patient.

Squamous Cell Carcinoma

Squamous cell carcinoma is a malignant tumor that affects the middle layer of the skin. Changes to an existing wart, mole, or other skin lesion could indicate this form of skin cancer as may the development of a new growth that ulcerates and does not heal well. Squamous cell carcinoma has a

TABLE 21-1 | Procedures and Diagnostic Tests Related to the Integumentary System

Procedure/Test	Description
Adipectomy	Surgical removal of fat.
Biopsy	Removal of a piece of tissue by syringe and needle, knife, punch, or brush to examine under a microscope as an aid to diagnosis.
Cauterization	Destruction of tissue with a caustic chemical, electrical current, freezing, or hot iron.
Chemobrasion	Abrasion of skin using chemicals; also called chemical peel.
Cryosurgery	Use of extreme cold to freeze and destroy tissue.
Curettage	Removal of superficial skin lesions with a curette or scraper.
Debridement	Removal of foreign material or dead tissue from a wound.
Dermatoplasty	Transplantation of skin or skin grafting. May be used to treat large birthmarks (hemangiomas) and burns.
Electrocautery	Destruction of tissue with an electric current.
Exfoliative Cytology	Scraping cells from tissue and then examining them under a microscope.
Frozen Section	Taking a thin piece of tissue from a frozen specimen for rapid examination under a microscope. Often performed during a surgical procedure to detect cancer.
Fungal Scrapings (FS)	Scrapings taken with a curette from lesions, placed on a growth medium, and examined under the microscope to identify fungal growth.
Incision and Drainage (I&D)	Making an incision to create an opening for the drainage of material, such as pus.
Laser Therapy	Removal of skin lesions and birthmarks using a laser that emits intense heat and power at close range. The laser converts frequencies of light into one small beam.
Lipectomy	Surgical removal of fat.
Marsupialization	Creation of a pouch to promote drainage by surgically opening a closed area, such as a cyst.
Needle Biopsy	Use of a sterile needle to remove tissue for examination under a microscope.
Rhytidectomy	Surgical removal of excess skin to eliminate wrinkles. Commonly referred to as a facelift.
Skin Grafts	Transfer of skin from a normal area to cover another site. Used to treat burn victims and after some surgical procedures.
Sweat Test	Test performed on sweat to determine the level of chloride. Increased skin chloride occurs in some diseases, such as cystic fibrosis.
Tzanck Test	Microscopic examination of a small piece of tissue that has been surgically scraped from a pustule. The specimen is placed on a slide and stained; then the type of viral infection causing the pustule can be identified.

high cure rate if it is detected and treated early, but neglect can allow the cancer to spread, causing great disability or even death. Along with exposure to sunlight and ultraviolet rays (including those from tanning beds), risk factors include genetic predisposition (skin cancers are more common in those who have light-colored skin, blue or green eyes, and blond or red hair), chemical pollution, and overexposure to X-rays or other forms of radiation. Exposure to arsenic, which may be present in some herbicides, presents another risk for development of skin cancers.

Signs and Symptoms. Similar to basal cell carcinoma, signs of squamous cell carcinoma include any skin lesion, growth, or bump that is small, firm, reddened, nodular, coned, or flat in shape. Squamous cell carcinoma also presents as a lesion whose surface is scaly or crusted. Squamous cell carcinoma may be located on the face, ears, neck, hands, or arms. Occasionally, the growth may occur on the lip, mouth, tongue, or genitals.

Treatment. The treatment for squamous cell carcinoma varies with the tumor's size, depth, location, and how much it has spread or metastasized. Surgical removal of the tumor, which includes removal of the skin around the tumor (wide excision), is often recommended. Microscopic shaving (Mohs micrographic surgery) may remove small tumors. Cryosurgery and laser surgery are also used in the treatment of squamous cell carcinoma. Skin grafting may be needed

- In children, skin conditions can be acute or chronic, local or systemic, and some can be congenital (inherited). Age-related skin conditions include milia (the white pimples occurring in newborns) and acne (red pustules occurring in puberty).
- Skin infections in children present as systemic infections with symptoms such as fever and malaise. Because the sebaceous glands do not produce sebum until the child is about 8 to 10 years old, a child's skin is drier and chaps more easily. For that reason, it is important to teach children good hygiene and skin care habits at an early age.

The Older Adult

- As a person ages, the papillae grow less dense, and the skin becomes looser. Less collagen and fewer elastic fibers are present in the upper dermis, and the skin loses its elastic tone, causing wrinkles to occur more easily. The occurrence of premalignant and malignant skin lesions may also increase with aging, especially on the nose, eyelids, and cheeks. Among skin cancers found in older adults, 80 percent are basal cell carcinomas.
- By age 50, approximately half of adults have some gray hair. The scalp hair continues to thin in men and women as aging progresses, and the hair becomes dry and brittle. The nails may flatten and become more discolored, dry, and brittle.

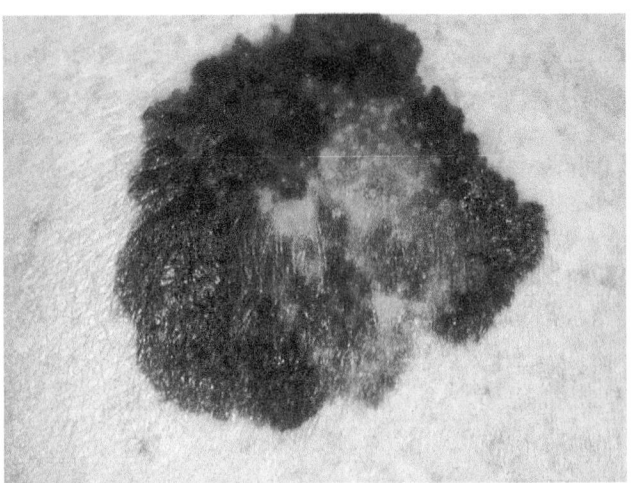

FIGURE 21-5 Melanoma.

The Glasgow 7-point scale also identifies signs and symptoms of melanoma. The symptoms and signs (see the following list) can occur anywhere on the skin, including the palms of the hands, soles of the feet, and nail beds. In this scheme, change is emphasized along with size. Bleeding and sensory changes occur relatively late. The Glasgow 7-point scale includes:

- Change in size
- Change in shape
- Change in color
- Inflammation
- Crusting and bleeding
- Sensory change
- Diameter greater than 7 mm (0.28 in.)

Treatment. The key to successful treatment of melanoma is early diagnosis. Patients identified with localized, thin,

if wide areas of skin are removed. The tumor may also be reduced in size by radiation treatments. Chemotherapy tends to be minimally effective; however, it can be used if surgery and radiation fail.

Malignant Melanoma

Originating in the melanin-producing melanocytes of the skin, **malignant melanoma** develops when the melanocytes do not respond to the normal control mechanisms of cellular growth. This often occurs in the melanocytes of a preexisting mole. The abnormal cell growth within the mole may then invade nearby structures or spread to other organs in the body (metastasis), invading and compromising the function of those structures or organs (Figure 21-5).

Signs and Symptoms. Malignant melanomas are usually diagnosed by using the ABCDE rule (Table 21-2), which is an excellent way of identifying changes of significance in a mole. This ABCDE method means checking the mole for the following: asymmetry, border irregularity, color variegation, diameter greater than 6 mm (0.24 in.), and elevation above surrounding tissue.

TABLE 21-2	The ABCDEs of Melanoma Changes in a Mole	
A—Asymmetry	The mole does not have two halves that match each other.
B—Border	The border is ragged, notched, or blurred together.
C—Color	Color is uneven; shades of black, brown, or tan are present; areas of white, red, or blue may be present.
D—Diameter	There may be a change in size, and the mole is typically greater than 6 mm in diameter.
E—Elevation	The mole sits above the surrounding tissue.

small lesions nearly always survive. For those with advanced lesions, the outlook is poor in spite of progress in systemic therapy.

Acne Vulgaris

Acne vulgaris (acne) is a common skin condition that occurs when oil and dead skin cells clog the skin's pores (Figure 21-6). It most often affects teens, with more than 85 percent of them developing at least a mild form of this condition. This occurs because of hormonal changes and the fact that the skin becomes oilier during the teenage years. Some women of childbearing age also develop acne before their menstrual cycle, again because of the hormonal changes occurring in the body. Whereas mild acne is merely annoying, severe acne can lead to emotional and physical scars.

Signs and Symptoms. The skin blemishes of acne vulgaris are often red and swollen because the blocked follicles that occur with acne provide an environment in which bacteria can multiply rapidly, causing inflammation. With mild cases of acne, only whiteheads and blackheads may be present. At times, these may develop into an infection in the skin pore (pimple). Severe acne can mean hundreds of pimples or sores that can cover the face, neck, chest, and back. Cystic lesions are pimples that are large and deep. These lesions are often painful and can leave scars on the skin.

Treatment. The severity of acne will determine the most useful and beneficial treatment. Treatment could include lotions or gels applied to blemishes or sometimes entire areas of skin, such as the chest or back (topical medications) and oral antibiotics. Sometimes the health care provider will combine treatments to get the best results and to avoid the development of bacteria that are resistant to antibiotics.

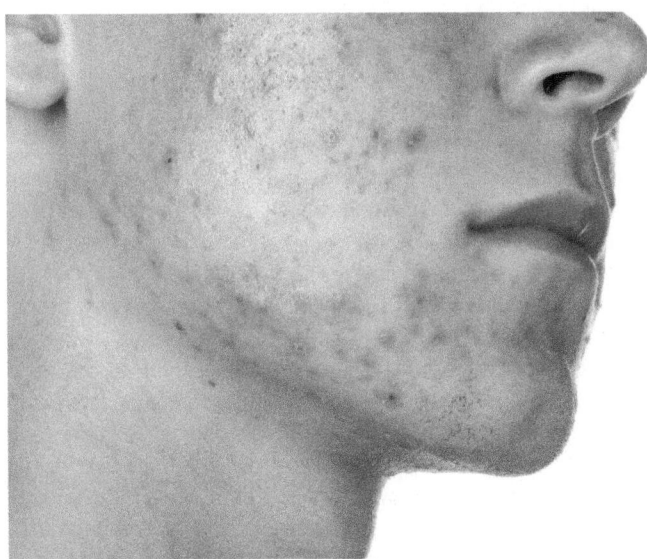

FIGURE 21-6 Acne vulgaris.

Alopecia

Alopecia is baldness or loss of hair. The most common form is male-pattern baldness, also known as androgenic alopecia. Women may also experience alopecia. Alopecia areata is another type of hair loss, involving patches of baldness that may come and go. Alopecia areata affects about 1 in 100 people, mostly teenagers and young adults (Figure 21-7). Alopecia can be an inherited disorder, or it can be caused by hormonal changes, nutritional deficiencies, and stress. Additionally, alopecia is a common side effect of chemotherapy; a treatment for cancer.

Signs and Symptoms. Alopecia areata causes patches of baldness that are about the size of a large coin. They usually appear on the scalp but can occur anywhere on the body, including the beard, eyebrows, and eyelashes. There are usually no other symptoms.

Male-pattern baldness, androgenic alopecia, is hereditary. It is called male-pattern baldness because it tends to follow a set pattern. The first stage is usually a receding hairline, followed by thinning of the hair on the crown and temples. When these two areas meet in the middle, a horseshoe shape of hair remains around the back and sides of the head. Eventually the person may be completely bald. Women's hair gradually thins with age, but women tend to lose hair only from the top of the head. This usually becomes more noticeable after menopause.

Treatment. Drugs and lotions are available that can be rubbed on the scalp to treat male- and female-pattern baldness. However, these do not work for everyone and effects are not long lasting. Shampoos and formulas are available for improving circulation to the scalp, and some people try herbal treatments. Hair transplants are also used to help the appearance of hair loss, although these treatments can be expensive and often are not covered by medical insurance.

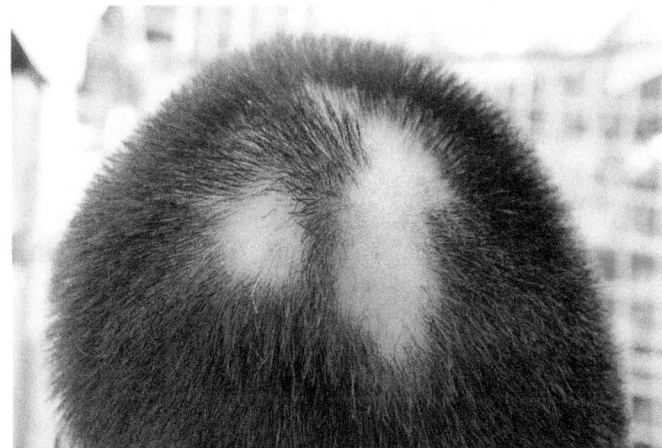

FIGURE 21-7 Alopecia.

Unfortunately, hair loss can lead to problems with confidence and self-esteem.

Cellulitis

Cellulitis is an acute, spreading bacterial infection below the surface of the skin. A cut, an abrasion, or an ulceration may precede cellulitis, because it commonly appears at a break in the skin. It can also be a result of local trauma, such as an animal bite. Very rarely is cellulitis caused by the **bacteremic** spread of infection (i.e., bacteria arriving from a distant source via the bloodstream). Risk factors for cellulitis include diabetes and impairment of the immune system. Cellulitis is not contagious, because it is an infection of the skin's deeper layers: the dermis and subcutaneous tissue. The epidermis provides a cover over the infection.

Signs and Symptoms. Cellulitis is characterized by **erythema** (redness), warmth, swelling, and pain. Fever, chills, and enlarged lymph nodes may also accompany this infection (Figure 21-8).

Treatment. Topical and oral antibiotics are administered for treatment of cellulitis. Commonly, penicillin-based antibiotics are used because they are most effective against staphylococcus (staph) infections that cause cellulitis. If the patient is allergic to penicillin or culture tests indicate staph is not the cause of infection, other antibiotics will be prescribed. In severe cases of cellulitis, IV antibiotics might be required.

Contact Dermatitis

Contact dermatitis is an allergic reaction caused by the skin coming in contact with an irritating substance. Causes of contact dermatitis often include exposure to poison ivy (Figure 21-9), poison oak, lotions, detergents, other chemicals, or nickel, which is a metal commonly used in jewelry or jean snaps.

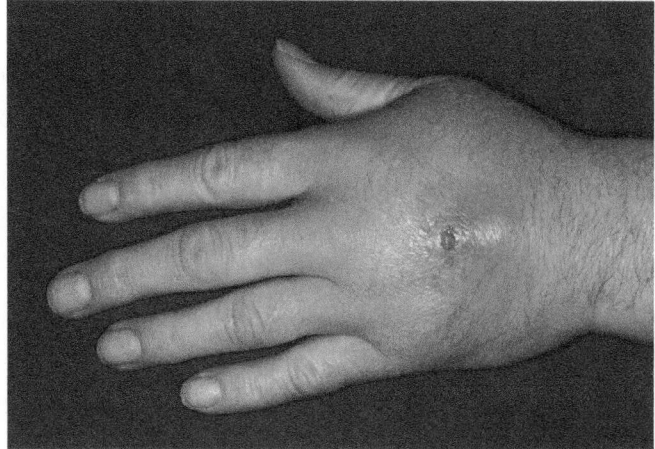

FIGURE 21-8 Cellulitis.

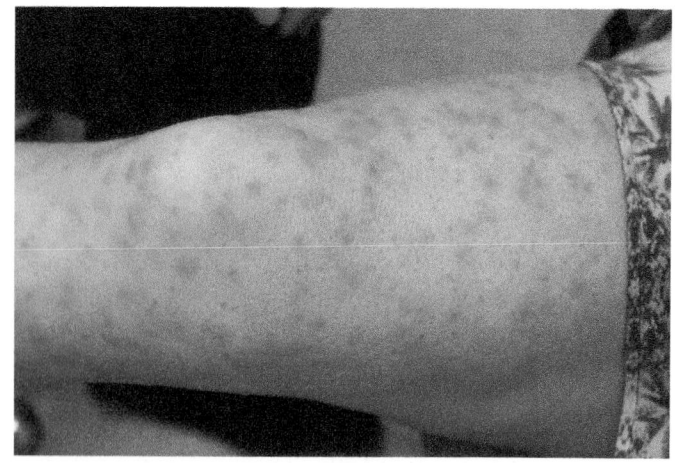

FIGURE 21-9 Contact dermatitis resulting from poison ivy.

Signs and Symptoms. With contact dermatitis, the obvious response is red, irritated skin, but **vesicles** (small blisters) and rash may also result. Oftentimes, itching and pain may be present. Serious allergic reactions may result in urticaria, or hives.

Treatment. This form of an allergic reaction is mostly treated with antihistamines (antiallergy medicines) and topical corticosteroid creams to reduce the inflammation. Widespread or excessively uncomfortable reactions may also be treated with systemic corticosteroids (oral medications) that help to further decrease the inflammation caused by the allergic reaction.

Calluses and Corns

Calluses and corns are excessive growths of the stratum corneum layer of the epidermis. They often occur on the hands

> ### Professionalism — Cultural Considerations
>
> In many cultures, modesty is very important, and being sure that a patient is properly draped is a major consideration. The medical assistant can always ask the patient if the medical team should know anything regarding special draping, and who needs to be present during the examination. Always be very respectful of the patient's rights and need for modesty.
>
> Some cultures may use special tattoos or marks as part of their heritage, and it is important to be respectful of these marks because they may have special meaning to the patient. Being judgmental about such adornments is never acceptable. If a patient has body piercings, they may require special attention because of the potential for infection. Always note any swelling or redness around a piercing site, and report it to the physician in a professional manner without doing or saying anything to embarrass the patient.

and feet. Both calluses and corns can be caused by physical bone deformities; however, they also can be caused by such other factors as ill-fitting shoes and unprotected hands during manual labor.

Signs and Symptoms. A **callus** is an area of thickened skin that does not have an identifiable border. It may appear grayish-yellow, brown, or even red. It may cause no pain, or it may produce tenderness, throbbing, or burning. A **corn**, on the other hand, has a distinct border with various textures. Corns appear most often on the feet. Though corns may be hard or soft, they are generally painful.

Treatment. Treatment becomes necessary when corns or calluses become burdensome or painful. Although patients with diabetes must be treated by a podiatrist to decrease the chance of infection and maximize wound healing, most other patients can treat corns and calluses by themselves. Placing a bandage on the corn or callus to reduce friction is beneficial, as is applying lotions or creams to soften the rough and hardened corns or calluses.

Decubitus Ulcer

A **decubitus ulcer**, also called a pressure sore or bedsore, is an area of skin and tissue that breaks down. Such ulcers typically occur when constant pressure is maintained on a specific area of the skin, such as on the coccyx. The constant pressure on the area decreases the blood supply, causing death to the affected tissue. Patients who have been lying in bed for too long without being repositioned or patients who are in wheelchairs may be susceptible to these skin conditions. In addition to the coccyx, common locations for a decubitus ulcer include hips, sacrum, heels, ankles, shoulders, back, and the back of the head.

Signs and Symptoms. Signs of decubitus ulcers vary with their stages (Figure 21-10). According to the National Pressure Ulcer Advisory Panel, the following are the four stages of decubitus ulcers:

- **Stage I**—A reddened area on the skin that does not blanch (turn white) when pressed. This is an early stage, and if the pressure is kept off the area, healing may occur.
- **Stage II**—The skin has a blister or an open sore. The area around the site may be red and irritated.
- **Stage III**—The skin breakdown looks like a crater with damage to the tissue below the skin.
- **Stage IV**—The wound becomes so deep that damage occurs to the tissues beneath the initial ulcer, including damage to bone and muscle.

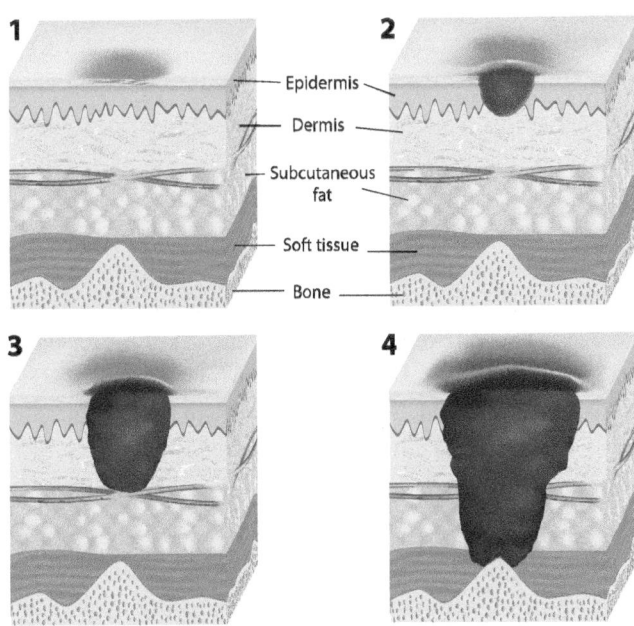

Stages of Pressure Sores

FIGURE 21-10 Pressure sores, or decubitus ulcers, occur from tissue breakdown caused by constant pressure.

Treatment. Treatment of decubitus ulcers begins with relieving pressure through the use of support surfaces and repositioning. Support surfaces may include special pillows or cushions that are water- or air-filled. Foam cushions and sheepskin pads are also used. Repositioning the patient to relieve pressure from the sore spot must be routine. Decubitus ulcers are typically debrided (i.e., cleaned of all toxins and then medicated and covered with special dressings to help in healing). Protecting the wound from any further injury is essential to protect the patient from infections, systemic sepsis, and other serious complications.

Eczema

Eczema, or atopic dermatitis, is a chronic skin condition caused by an allergic-type reaction of the skin. Though there is no known definitive cause, heredity tends to play a role. For those afflicted with eczema, typically a family history of allergies and eczema is present. Eczema is common during infancy and childhood and often disappears in adulthood.

Signs and Symptoms. Common signs include areas of red and swollen skin caused by itching, scaling, and rashes. Adults may also suffer from chronic episodes of eczema.

Treatment. Treatment depends on the stage, or appearance, of the lesions that have formed on the skin. Lesions may be dry, scaly, or have a "weeping" appearance. Weeping lesions are treated with mild soaps and dressings, whereas severe cases and dry scaly lesions may be treated with mild antiitch lotions or low-potency topical corticosteroids. Very severe cases may require treatment with systemic corticosteroids and topical immunomodulators (TIMs). Sometimes short periods of time in a tanning bed are useful to dry up lesions, but this treatment should only be approached while under a physician's supervision.

Furuncles and Carbuncles

A **furuncle**, or boil, is an abscess of a hair follicle and the adjacent subcutaneous tissues. A **carbuncle** is a collection of furuncles. The microbe involved in the disease process is usually *Staphylococcus aureus* (staph), which normally lives harmlessly on the skin. When an opening in the integument invites the microbes into the subcutaneous tissue, painful furuncles grow.

Signs and Symptoms. Furuncles can be red to purple in appearance and are generally painful. The area surrounding the furuncle tends to become tender to the touch. The center is generally white or yellow and is filled with pus. Carbuncles can be anywhere from the size of a pea to the size of a golf ball and are similar in color to furuncles.

Treatment. The customary treatment for these disorders is incision and drainage followed by application of an antibiotic. Patients must be taught not to squeeze furuncles because that will cause the microbes to spread. Handwashing is the best prevention for the spreading of microbes.

Folliculitis

An infection or inflammation of the hair follicles is known as **folliculitis**. Although folliculitis can occur anywhere body hair is present, it most often appears in areas that become irritated by shaving or the rubbing of clothes or where follicles and pores are blocked by oils and dirt. Common sites of folliculitis include the face, scalp, armpits, and legs (Figure 21-11).

Signs and Symptoms. General signs of folliculitis include a reddened rash; raised, red, often pus-filled lesions around hair follicles (pimples); pimples that eventually crust over and occur in areas of a high concentration of hair follicles, such as the face (especially in men's beards and moustaches), armpits, scalp, and groin; and itching at the site of the rash and pimples.

Treatment. Treating folliculitis generally involves minimizing damage to hair follicles by avoiding clothing that will rub against the skin, shaving with an electric razor instead of a blade razor, and keeping the skin clean, using soap and water and skin cleansers. Treatment of folliculitis usually includes application of antibiotic ointments.

Herpes Simplex

Herpes simplex primarily affects the mouth or the genital area. There are two strains of herpes simplex viruses:

- Herpes simplex virus type 1 (HSV-1) usually affects the face, including the lips and mouth (Figure 21-12). Acquired during childhood, it is the most common herpes simplex virus. HSV-1 is characterized by lesions inside the mouth or on the lips, including fever blisters and cold sores.

- Herpes simplex virus type 2 (HSV-2) is sexually transmitted. Oral and genital lesions are common. Some people do not display any signs or symptoms. However, left untreated, the virus can also lead to complications such as meningoencephalitis (infection of the lining of the brain and the brain itself) or an infection of the eye. Cross-infection of type 1 and 2 viruses may occur from oral-genital contact.

The herpes virus can infect a fetus and cause congenital abnormalities. A newborn born vaginally to a mother with an active genital herpes infection is highly susceptible to the virus.

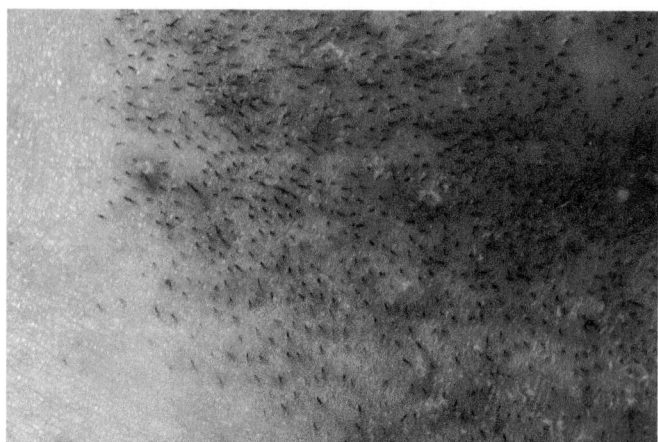

FIGURE 21-11 Folliculitis.

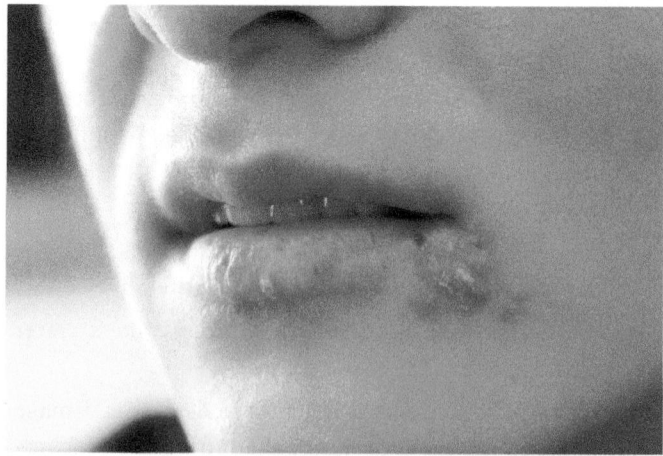

FIGURE 21-12 Blisters caused by HSV-1.

Signs and Symptoms. Outbreaks of herpes simplex seem to coincide with lack of rest, high stress, exposure to the sun, and even menstruation. General signs and symptoms of herpes simplex include the following:

- Mouth sores
- A burning or tingling sensation followed by the development of genital lesions
- Blisters or ulcers on the mouth, lips, gums, or genitalia
- Fever blisters/cold sores
- Fever—may be present especially during the first episode
- Lymph node enlargement in the neck or groin

Treatment. There is no cure for the herpes virus; it will always remain in a person's body. During times of nonactive inflammation, the virus lies dormant. Mild cases of herpes simplex may not require any form of treatment. With HSV-1, the cold sore will generally disappear within two weeks. Over-the-counter medicated lip balms and salves can be helpful to ease the symptoms and speed healing. As treatment for HSV-2, prescription antiviral medications may help expedite healing and lessen the number of outbreaks. Dietary and nutritional supplements may also prove to be helpful, but they should be used only under the direct supervision of a physician.

Herpes Zoster

Herpes zoster, which is also known as shingles, is a viral infection that causes a painful rash. It is caused by the varicella zoster virus, which also causes chickenpox. Once a person has been infected with chickenpox, the virus lies dormant in the nerves. After the virus reactivates, it is diagnosed as shingles or herpes zoster. Herpes zoster is transmitted through direct contact with the fluid inside the red blisters. Before the development of blisters, the person afflicted with the virus is not contagious.

Signs and Symptoms. Herpes zoster can be very painful. Often along with pain, a burning, tingling, and itchy feeling may be experienced. A red rash with fluid-filled blisters begins to develop, and numbness or sensitivity in an affected part of the body may also occur. In serious conditions, the skin can remain painful and sensitive to the touch; this is known as postherpetic neuralgia. Most of these symptoms occur on one side of the body, wrapping around from the back to the sternum, following the path of the nerve where the virus had been dormant. Headache, fever, and chills are also common symptoms.

Early treatment can help shorten a shingles infection and reduce the risk of complications, but prevention by vaccination (Zostavax) is ideal.

Treatment. Oral antiviral medications are generally prescribed, preferably within 48 to 72 hours of the first sign of the rash. Corticosteroids are sometimes prescribed to reduce swelling and pain. If the pain is severe—particularly if the patient develops postherpetic neuralgia—the health care provider may prescribe oral analgesics or a skin patch that contains a pain-relieving medication.

Hirsutism

Hirsutism is a condition of thick abnormal hair growth that affects men and women, though women are more commonly affected by and diagnosed with the disorder. Often with this skin disorder, women have a pattern of hair growth that is typically found on males.

Signs and Symptoms. Women will develop thick and dark hair growth. Common areas for the excessive hair growth include the face and chest. It is common for women of certain cultural descent, such as those from the Mediterranean region, to naturally have darker and more hair growth than lighter, fairer-skinned women. However, hirsutism is often linked to endocrine disorders, such as problems with the ovaries or adrenal glands.

Treatment. Treatment consists of removing the unwanted hair through shaving, plucking, waxing, or using depilatory creams. Electrolysis and laser hair removal are more permanent forms of hair removal; however, they are more costly. Physicians may also prescribe medications that block androgen hormones, helping to decrease the amount of hair growth. These medications may take six to eight months to begin working.

Impetigo

Impetigo is a skin infection caused by bacteria. It is most common in children and is very contagious. Impetigo can originate in intact skin but also can be secondary to a preexisting skin condition or trauma.

Signs and Symptoms. Impetigo is characterized by round, crusted, oozing spots that grow larger day by day (Figure 21-13). It may affect the skin anywhere on the body but commonly occurs in the area around the nose and mouth. A honey-colored crust often develops from blisters that burst and ooze fluid.

Treatment. The treatment for impetigo varies, depending on the severity. Mild cases of impetigo often resolve through the use of mild cleansing, removal of crust formations, and

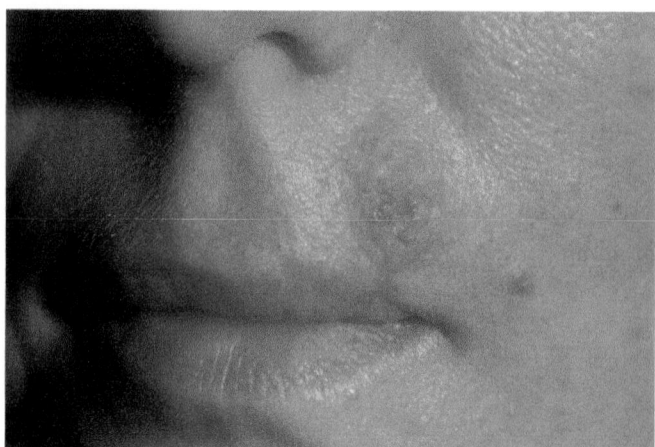
FIGURE 21-13 Impetigo.

topical antibiotic ointment. More severe cases of impetigo may require the use of oral antibiotics.

Keloids

A **keloid** is a type of skin lesion that can appear following a surgery or injury; however, keloids also sometimes appear spontaneously after minor inflammation. Keloids can grow and extend past the original site of injury. This separates them from hypertrophic scars, which are similar to keloids but remain confined to the area of injury. Burns and piercings have also been known to produce keloids.

Signs and Symptoms. These unsightly skin blemishes can appear thickened and raised and red or pink in color (Figure 21-14). These skin lesions also have a dome-like appearance. Keloids tend to be itchy and bothersome, as well as tender to the touch.

Treatment. Various treatments are available for keloids. Some of the most common include cortisone injections, surgery,

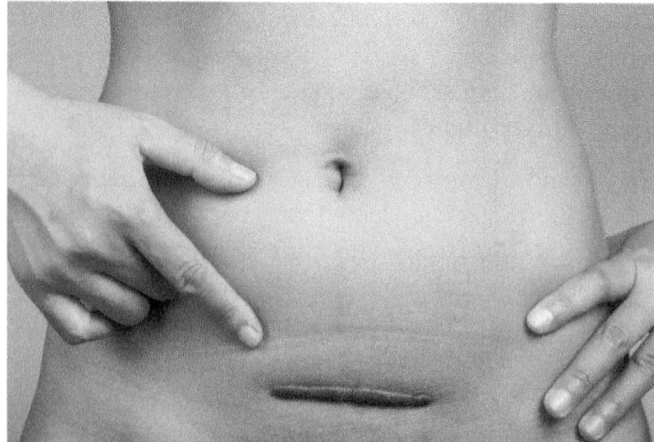
FIGURE 21-14 Keloid.

and laser removal. Additional forms of treatment include cryosurgery, interferon injections, and application of silicone sheets.

Pediculosis

Pediculosis is an infestation of lice in the form of eggs, larvae, or adult lice. Under suitable conditions of exposure, anyone may become louse-infested, as pediculosis is easily transmitted from person to person during direct contact. It is not caused by uncleanliness, which is a common myth. Forms of pediculosis include *Pediculus humanus capitis* (head louse), *Pediculus humanus corporis* (body louse), and *Pthirus pubis* (pubic louse). Head lice are commonly found in school and institutional settings. They are often transmitted with the sharing of hats, combs, or clothing. Body lice generally reside along the seams of clothing. This form of lice is commonly found in places that are both crowded and unsanitary. Pubic lice, also known as crabs, are usually sexually transmitted.

Symptoms. The most common symptom of all forms of lice is itching. Head lice tend to cause itching around the back of the head or around the ears. Itching surrounding the genitals is an indicator of pubic lice. Body lice tend to travel to the body to feed on skin and then return to clothing.

Treatment. Prescription and nonprescription medications are available for the treatment of pediculosis. Pyrethrian-based medicated shampoos and cream rinses do not require a prescription, whereas Lindane-based shampoos do.

Nit combs are also available to help remove nits (lice eggs) from hair. To ensure that nits have not survived, retreatment after seven to ten days is recommended.

Psoriasis

Psoriasis affects an estimated 7.5 million Americans. Though it can develop at any age, psoriasis develops most commonly between ages 30 and 50. This condition has genetic and autoimmune characteristics. Psoriasis is thought

Professionalism | The Workplace

Patients with integumentary problems may have diseases that are contagious to the personnel in the medical office. Although all medical offices must practice standard precautions to prevent disease transmission, it is especially important that the medical assistant wear gloves when touching the skin of patients with contagious illnesses. Increased sanitization practices might also be required for exam tables and other surfaces that might come in contact with highly contagious skin conditions.

to be caused by a buildup of dead skin cells that, rather than shedding off, pile and form scaly patches. Though it can be unsightly, psoriasis is not contagious.

Signs and Symptoms. Psoriasis is characterized by episodes of redness, itching, and thick, dry, silvery scales on the skin. Joint pain may also accompany this condition. Its onset can be gradual or abrupt. Flare-ups have been attributed to infections, obesity, and lack of sunlight, as well as sunburn, stress, poor health, and cold climate. When the case is severe and widespread, large quantities of fluid can be lost, causing dehydration and severe secondary infections that can be serious.

Treatment. The extent and severity of psoriasis determines the course of treatment. Treatment involves analgesics, sedatives, intravenous fluids, retinoids, and antibiotics. Mild cases are treated at home with topical medications such as prescription or nonprescription dandruff shampoos, cortisone or other corticosteroid creams, and antifungal medications. Severe lesions may require hospitalization for proper treatment.

Rosacea

Rosacea is a disorder that primarily affects the facial skin, often characterized by flare-ups and periods of remission. This condition affects an estimated fourteen million Americans—and most of them do not know they have it.

Signs and Symptoms. Signs of rosacea include redness on the cheeks, nose, chin, or forehead. Other signs include small visible blood vessels on the face, bumps on the face, and watery or irritated eyes. Over time, the redness becomes ruddier and more persistent.

Treatment. Therapies and medications are available to treat the symptoms associated with rosacea such as topical antibiotic or cortisone-based creams. Currently, a cure is not available for rosacea. Avoiding extreme temperatures and temperature changes, reducing alcohol intake, and the use of sunscreen can help prevent or mitigate rosacea outbreaks.

Scabies

Scabies is a highly contagious disorder of the skin. It is caused by the human or scabies itch mite. Scabies is spread by direct personal contact, such as by shaking hands, or by indirect contact, like sharing infected articles such as clothing, bedding, or towels. Common among schoolchildren, roommates, and sexual partners, scabies is usually found where people are crowded together.

Signs and Symptoms. As the female lays her eggs, a very small zigzag blister marks her trail. It is fairly difficult to see this; however, symptoms and signs such as intense itching and a red rash around the area are more obvious. The sides of the fingers, backs of the hands, wrists, heels, elbows, armpits, inner thighs, and waistline are common locations for scabies (Figure 21-15).

Treatment. Since Roman times, sulfur has been used as a scabicide. Sulfur is most often used in a cream or ointment with a 6 to 10 percent concentration. Corticosteriods and antihistamines are often used to relieve itching.

Seborrheic Dermatitis

Seborrheic dermatitis is an inflammatory condition of sebaceous or oil glands caused by an increase in sebum. This disorder is most common in infants and children and is frequently known as cradle cap.

Signs and Symptoms. Some of the classic signs and symptoms of seborrheic dermatitis include yellow or white scales that attach to the hair shaft, thick or patchy crusts on the scalp, itching, soreness, and dandruff.

Professionalism The Law

Because examination of the skin often requires that clothes be removed, be very careful to ensure that plenty of sheets are available for draping the patient, so that only the area being examined can be seen and the patient is otherwise covered. This protects the patient's right to privacy and confidentiality during the examination. Be sure that the door to the exam room is completely closed, and never permit anyone else to enter unless the patient is completely covered. To help the patient feel comfortable, follow your facility protocols regarding assisting the physician during a skin examination.

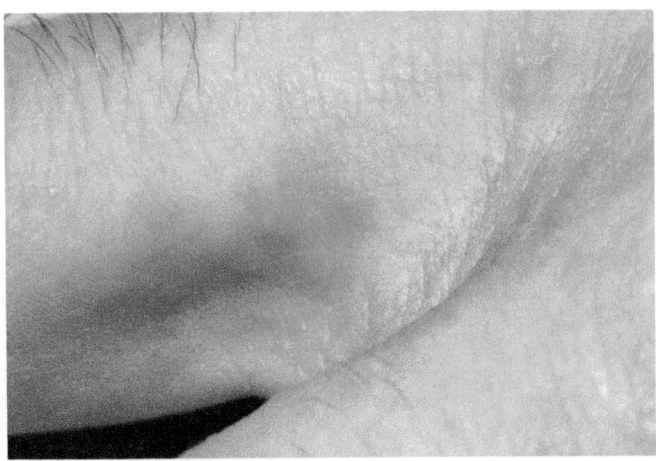

FIGURE 21-15 Scabies.

Treatment. This form of dermatitis is treated with medicated low-strength creams. Although there is no prevention, shampooing the scalp daily with medicated shampoo can alleviate the problem by reducing the amount of oil on the surface of the scalp.

Tinea

Tinea is any of several fungal infections of the skin. **Tinea corporis**, sometimes called ringworm, is not actually a worm but an integumentary disorder. Caused by a fungus, it can appear anywhere on the body. If the fungus is on the head, it is called **tinea capitis**. On the foot, it is known as **tinea pedis**, or athlete's foot. When found in the genital area, it is referred to as **tinea cruris**, more commonly referred to as jock itch. Elsewhere on the body, the fungus is called tinea corporis (Figure 21-16).

Signs and Symptoms. Tinea usually presents in the form of a ring, often with itchy, red, scaly patches.

Treatment. Tinea is treated with antifungal creams or oral antifungal agents. Over-the-counter medication is available, but if the infection is severe, a prescription medication may be required.

Urticaria

Urticaria, also known as hives, is a red, raised, severely itchy rash caused by acute hypersensitivity to medications, food, or environmental stimuli (Figure 21-17). The major concern related to urticaria is that it can obstruct the airway by causing airway constriction, which occurs with a severe allergic reaction termed *anaphylaxis*. Because of the possibility of airway constriction, ask patients about allergies before an injection and observe after an injection or allergy test for wheezing or other indication of breathing problems for the length of time the physician specifies.

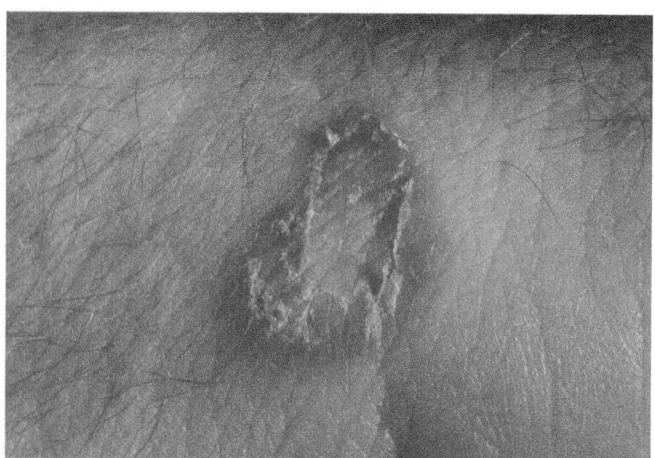

FIGURE 21-16 Tinea corporis.

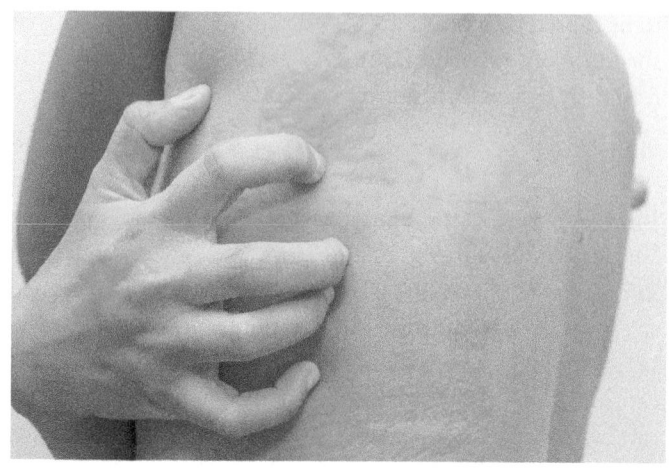

FIGURE 21-17 Urticaria (hives).

Signs and Symptoms. Signs include localized areas of pink, itchy, swollen patches of skin. It is common for burning or stinging sensations also to be felt. Hives may vary in size from the diameter of a pencil eraser to the diameter of a cereal bowl. Many times, the hives may overlap, forming even larger areas of irritation and swelling.

Treatment. Treatment consists of removing the causative allergens and treating with antihistamine and, in severe cases, epinephrine.

Vitiligo

Vitiligo, also known as leukoderma, is a disorder that causes white patches and large areas of decreased pigmentation to form on the skin. These patches form from the destruction of melanocytes, the cells that produce melanin for pigmentation. This disease is often linked to immune system disorders, such as Addison's disease or pernicious anemia. Vitiligo also affects those with thyroid disorders.

Signs and Symptoms. Vitiligo is marked by the early or premature graying or whitening of body hair or by the depigmentation of skin or mucous membranes. When the skin is affected, it generally begins to appear on the neck, armpits, elbows, genitals, hands, or knees.

Treatment. The treatment of vitiligo is aimed at evening skin tone and color. This may be done by cosmetic, medical, or surgical means. Using sunscreen and avoiding tanning help make the depigmentation less noticeable. Makeup and self-tanning lotions may also be used to even out the skin tone. Medical treatments may include the use of topical corticosteroid therapy as well as a form of topical ultraviolet therapy. Skin grafting as well as a form of tattooing called micropigmentation may also be successful.

Verrucae (Warts)

Warts, or **verrucae**, are infections caused by viruses in the human papillomavirus (HPV) family. There are at least 60 types of HPV viruses. Warts can grow on all parts of the body, including the skin, the inside of the mouth, the genitals, and the rectal area. A common wart is the plantar wart, which is always located on the soles of the feet.

Signs and Symptoms. The appearance and texture of a wart varies based on its location. Warts may appear grainy, fleshy, and varied in color from flesh-toned to red, pink, or white. Warts may also appear as raised or flat skin lesions. The size of a wart can vary from 1 mm to 1 cm. At times, plantar warts may cause pain in the heel or soles of the feet.

Treatment. Depending on the size, location, and type of wart, various treatments are available. Over-the-counter medicines containing salicylic acid are available. A physician may perform cryotherapy, which freezes the wart; generally, liquid nitrogen is used in this procedure. Physicians may also prescribe various prescription medications. In severe cases, minor surgery may be an option.

SKIN CARE TREATMENTS

Advancing medical technology and the desire to capture a youthful skin radiance and appearance have led to the surging popularity of medical skin care treatments. Many of the procedures that are discussed next are performed by trained and experienced professionals in a dermatologist's office or in a medical spa setting. Along with researching these procedures, patients should always use discretion when choosing a health care professional who specializes in this area of expertise. Often, after many of these procedures, patients are instructed to reduce sun exposure for specified periods of time, depending on the type of treatment performed.

It is important to note that because many of these procedures are considered cosmetic (to improve appearance) rather than medical (to treat a condition or disease), they might not be covered by a patient's medical insurance and the patient may have to pay for these procedures from their own funds.

Botox

Botox is a popular procedure that is indicated for reducing wrinkle lines. Most often, botox is used for frown lines, forehead lines, and wrinkles around the eyes, which are commonly referred to as crow's feet. A very small, diluted amount of the toxin *Clostridium botulinum* is injected into the wrinkle lines. This toxin causes wrinkles to relax and soften, thereby diminishing their visibility. For maintenance, this procedure is usually repeated every four to six months. Side effects of the treatment include headaches, bruising, and eyelid drooping, all of which are temporary.

Chemical Peel

A chemical peel is a type of chemical surgery that uses various acid concentrations to remove old and damaged layers of skin cells. A chemical peel can be performed at one of three levels.

- **Light chemical peel**—The purpose of this peel is to reduce the size of pores, make the skin appear softer, and produce more coloring in the skin. During a light chemical peel, only the top layer of the skin is stripped. The procedure is completed in about an hour and leaves a mild redness to the skin, which disappears as time progresses.

- **Medium chemical peel**—The purpose of a medium chemical peel is to reduce wrinkles. It results in much smoother skin than the light chemical peel can produce. The medium peel results in the top layer and some underlying cells being stripped, causing collagen and elastin to be stimulated. Recovery from a medium chemical peel can last up to 10 days because of the peeling, swelling, and redness that occur after the treatment.

- **Deep chemical peel**—This is an aggressive treatment that can affect the layers of skin down to the dermal layer. This procedure is aimed at reducing all signs of aging in all but certain areas of the face. With this level of chemical peel, skin conditions such as pigmentation disorders and precancerous lesions can be removed. The healing process involves considerable pain, often felt up to 12 hours post surgery. Analgesic medications are required. It may take weeks for additional peeling, swelling, and redness to subside.

Laser Resurfacing

Laser resurfacing is one of the newer treatments available to reduce the signs of aging. Short, pulsated laser beams vaporize damaged or troublesome areas of the skin. Full-face laser resurfacing takes approximately one to two hours, whereas a partial-face resurfacing takes 30 to 45 minutes. The resurfacing results in the stimulation and production of new collagen and skin cells, which results in younger and tighter-looking skin. Immediately following the procedure, antibiotic ointment and sterile dressings are applied to reduce the incidence of infection. The patient returns to the office one to three days after the procedure to have the sterile dressings removed. Analgesics are prescribed for pain relief. Complete healing following laser resurfacing takes approximately 10 to 21 days.

Microdermabrasion

During microdermabrasion, the top layer of dead skin cells is removed to provide the skin with a rejuvenated look. Tiny crystals work with abrasion and suction devices to produce healthier-looking skin. This noninvasive and non-chemical approach is appealing to many patients who do not wish to pursue more aggressive skin-freshening treatments. Candidates for microdermabrasion include those who wish to erase signs of aging, including fine lines,

wrinkles, and sun-damaged skin. As with other skin care treatments, it is important to find qualified professionals to perform this procedure.

SUMMARY

The integumentary system is composed of the skin and accessory organs. The skin is the largest organ of the body and serves protective, regulatory, sensory reception, absorptive, and secretory functions.

The skin provides many protective functions for the body, including preventing infection and preserving the internal environment. Skin also helps to promote optimum temperature levels. The protective function of the skin is supported by several layers: the epidermis (stratum corneum, stratum lucidum, stratum granulosum, stratum germinativum) and the dermis. Accessory organs that support the skin are the hair, nails, sebaceous glands, and sudoriferous glands.

The large integumentary system is prone to disorders. Several types of skin cancer can develop: basal cell carcinoma, squamous cell carcinoma, and melanoma. Other disorders include acne vulgaris, alopecia, cellulitis, contact dermatitis, corns and calluses, decubitus ulcers, eczema, furuncles and carbuncles, folliculitis, herpes simplex and herpes zoster, impetigo, keloids, pediculosis, psoriasis, rosacea, scabies, seborrheic dermatitis, tinea, urticaria, vitiligo, and verrucae.

New techniques in skin care treatments help reverse the signs of aging, including wrinkles and sun damage. Some of the more common treatments include chemical peels, laser resurfacing, and microdermabrasion.

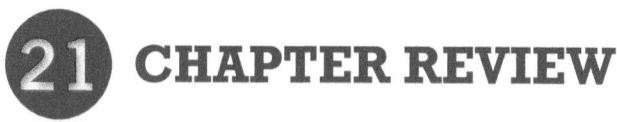 **CHAPTER REVIEW**

COMPETENCY REVIEW

1. Define and spell the terms for this chapter.
2. What is the primary organ of the integumentary system?
3. Name the four accessory structures of the integumentary system.
4. Name the five functions of the skin.
5. Name the three layers of the skin.
6. What is the protein substance in the dead cells of the outer layer of skin that strengthens and firms the skin?
7. Name the four layers of the epidermis.
8. What is the name of the crescent-shaped area of the nail?
9. What is the name of the cell that gives pigment or color to the skin?
10. What are the ABCDEs of skin cancer?

PREPARING FOR THE CERTIFICATION EXAM

1. Which layer is the innermost layer of the epidermis?
   a. stratum corneum
   b. stratum granulosum
   c. stratum germinativum
   d. stratum lucidum
   e. lunula

2. Which skin condition is a form of cancer?
   a. acne vulgaris
   b. psoriasis
   c. urticaria
   d. melanoma
   e. alopecia

3. What is the medical term for baldness?
   a. psoriasis
   b. vitiligo
   c. alopecia
   d. cellulitis
   e. seborrheic dermatitis

4. Which problem may occur if a patient spends too much time in the same position in bed?
   a. eczema
   b. a decubitus ulcer
   c. a furuncle
   d. impetigo
   e. pediculosis

5. What is the lay term for Herpes zoster?
   a. alopecia
   b. impetigo
   c. pediculosis
   d. psoriasis
   e. shingles

6. Which skin care treatment uses various concentrations of acid to remove layers of dead skin?
   a. microdermabrasion
   b. dermabrasion
   c. chemical peel
   d. laser resurfacing
   e. use of medicated lotions and ointments

7. Which skin condition is contagious?
   a. scabies
   b. vitiligo
   c. rosacea
   d. alopecia
   e. keloids

8. Which of the following is a type of skin lesion?
   a. keloids
   b. impetigo
   c. rosacea
   d. tinea
   e. scabies

9. Which of the following is a fungal infection?
   a. furuncles
   b. urticaria
   c. rosacea
   d. tinea
   e. pediculosis

10. Which term is used when a patient is infested with lice?
    a. tinea
    b. pediculosis
    c. furuncles
    d. psoriasis
    e. eczema

CRITICAL THINKING

Refer to the case study at the beginning of the chapter and use the information you have learned to answer the following questions.

1. Dr. Miller diagnoses Mrs. Yeung with hirsutism. What factors listed in the case study support his diagnosis?

2. After discussing treatment options, Mrs. Yeung has decided that she does not want to deal with shaving, waxing, or plucking on a daily basis. What might be a viable treatment option for Mrs. Yeung that addresses her ideals?

INTERNET ACTIVITY

Several organizations have been established to help in the prevention and treatment of diseases affecting the integumentary system. Perform an Internet search to learn more about these organizations and what each provides to people afflicted with specific skin disorders.

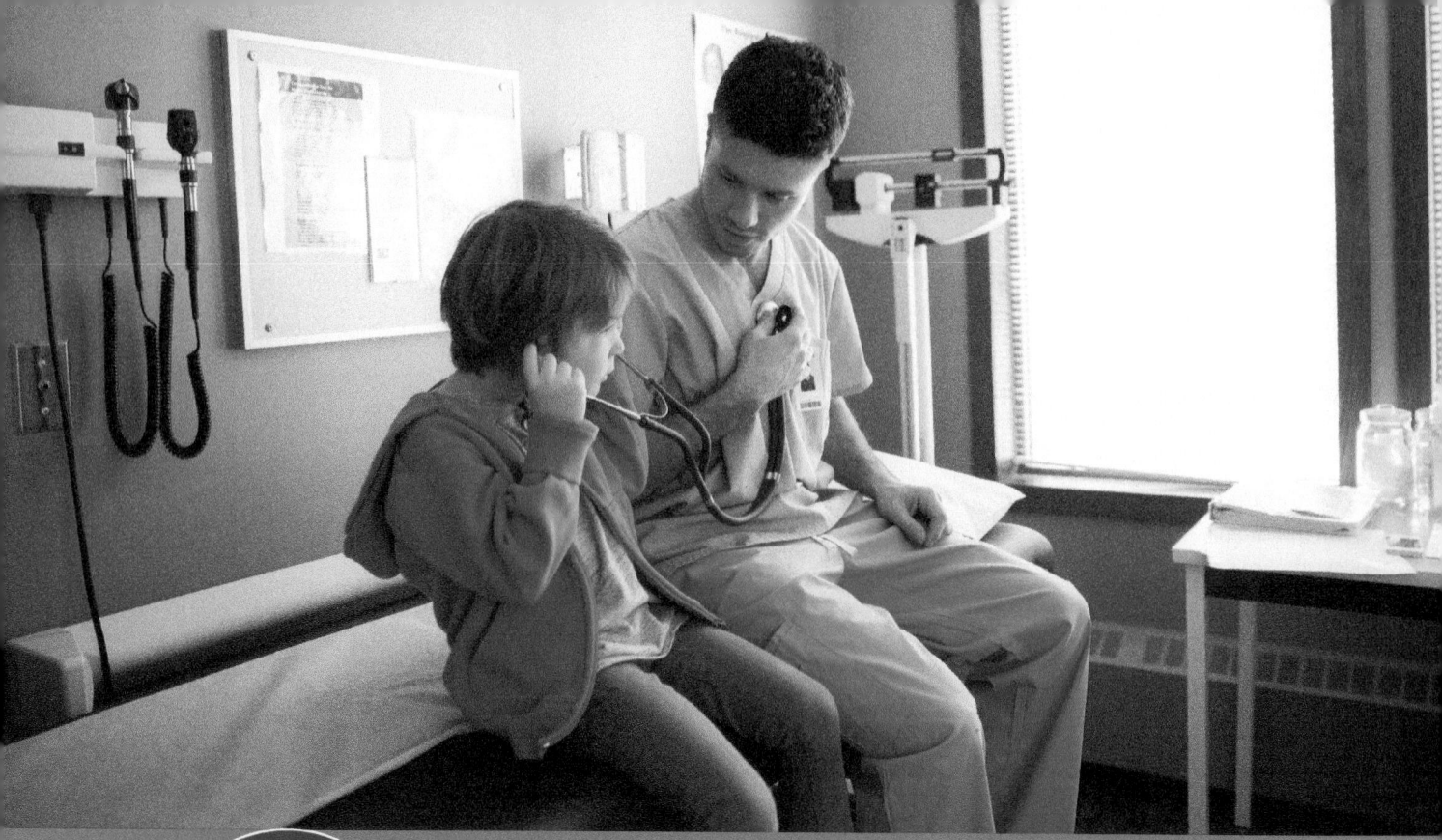

The Skeletal System

Learning Objectives

After completing this chapter, you should be able to:

22.1   Define and spell the terms for this chapter.

22.2   List the six types of bones found in the human body.

22.3   Describe the functions of bones and the skeletal system.

22.4   List structures associated with long bones.

22.5   Compare different types of joints.

22.6   Describe how the skeletal system changes between childhood and older adulthood.

22.7   Identify the location of bones associated with the axial skeleton.

22.8   Identify the location of bones associated with the appendicular skeleton.

22.9   Describe pathology associated with the skeletal system.

Seventeen-year-old Charlie Baker was pitching during a high-school baseball game when he suddenly experienced a sharp pain in his right shoulder after striking out a player of the opposing team. Because of his intense pain, the coach sent him to the emergency department at Pearson General Hospital. Charlie explained to the emergency department physician that the pain occurred immediately after he pitched the ball to the batter. He was trying to throw a fastball.

Terms to Learn

abduction	diarthrotic joint	medullary canal
adduction	dislocation	orthopedic physician
amphiarthrotic joint	dorsiflexion	osteoarthritis
appendicular skeleton	endosteum	osteomalacia
arthritis	epiphysis	osteoporosis
articulation	etiology	periosteum
atlas	eversion	pronation
axial skeleton	extension	protraction
axis	flexion	reduction
bursa	gouty arthritis	retraction
bursitis	hallux valgus	rheumatoid arthritis
cancellous (spongy) bone	hammertoe	rickets
chondrocytes	hemopoiesis	rotation
circumduction	inversion	scoliosis
compact bone	kyphosis	supination
diaphysis	lordosis	synarthrotic joint

The skeletal system (Figure 22-1) makes up the framework of the human body. It is responsible for providing shape and support, protecting internal organs, and serving as a storage place for mineral salts, calcium, and phosphorus. The skeletal system also plays an important role in the formation of blood cells and in providing an area for the attachment of skeletal muscles. Two distinct divisions compose the skeletal system. The 206 bones of the body are divided into the axial skeleton, which is made of 80 bones, and the appendicular skeleton, which consists of the remaining 126 bones. The axial and appendicular skeletons will be discussed later in this chapter.

BONES AND THEIR CLASSIFICATION

It may be surprising to learn that bones are 50 percent water. The remaining 50 percent of bone composition is a rigid, calcified substance known as osseous tissue. Microscopic structures found within the osseous tissue are listed in Table 22-1. Figure 22-2 illustrates the microscopic structures listed in the table.

Bones are classified according to six shapes: long, short, flat, irregular, sesamoid, and sutural (wormian) (Figure 22-3).

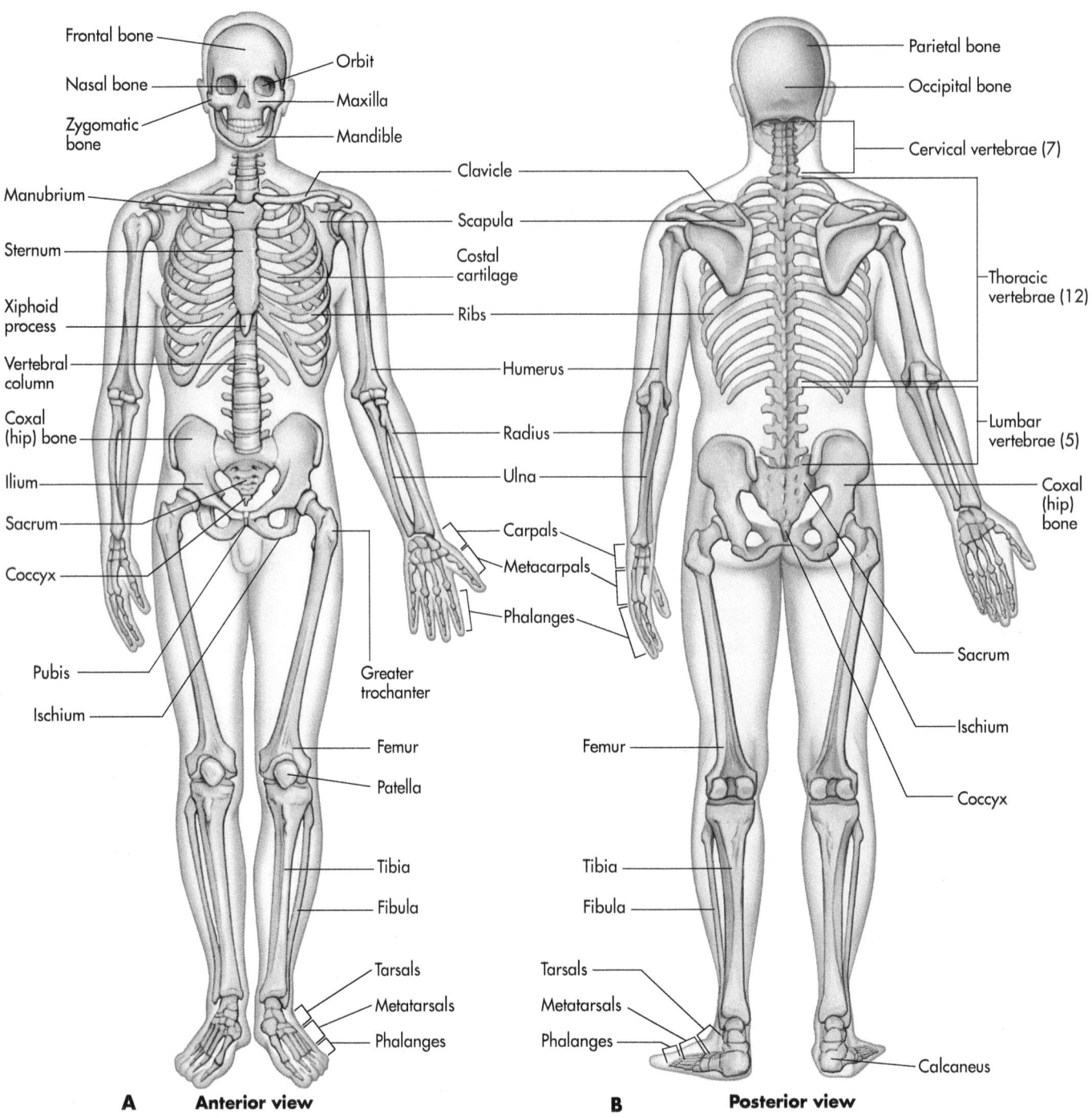

FIGURE 22-1 Anterior and posterior human skeleton.

Functions of Bones

As already noted, the bones of the human skeleton have six main functions:

- Providing shape, support, and the framework of the body
- Providing protection for the body's internal organs
- Serving as a storage place for mineral salts, calcium, and phosphorus

- Playing an important role in the formation of blood cells, as **hemopoiesis**, also called hematopoiesis (formation of blood cells), takes place in the bone marrow
- Providing an area for the attachment of skeletal muscle
- Helping to make movement possible through articulation

TABLE 22-1 | Microscopic Components of Osseous Tissue

Component	Description
Bone Matrix	Intercellular substance of the bone that is made of water, mineral salts, and collagen fibers. Calcium phosphate, the main salt of a bone matrix, makes the matrix very hard.
Osteoblasts	Bone-building cells that create and secrete collagen and other organic compound needed to build the matrix. These cells can later turn into osteocytes.
Osteoclasts	Large cells that digest the old bone matrix and create the holes in the bone.
Osteon	Considered the organizational unit of the bone, composed of the Haversian system.
Haversian System/Central Canal	Runs lengthwise through the bone and is a canal-like system that houses blood vessels and nerves.
Lamellae	Rings of hard matrix surrounding the central canal.
Lacunae	Spaces within the lamella that contain osteocytes.
Canaliculi	Miniature canals that provide a passageway for nutrients and the removal of waste by connecting the lacunae.

Compact Bone and Spongy (Cancellous Bone)

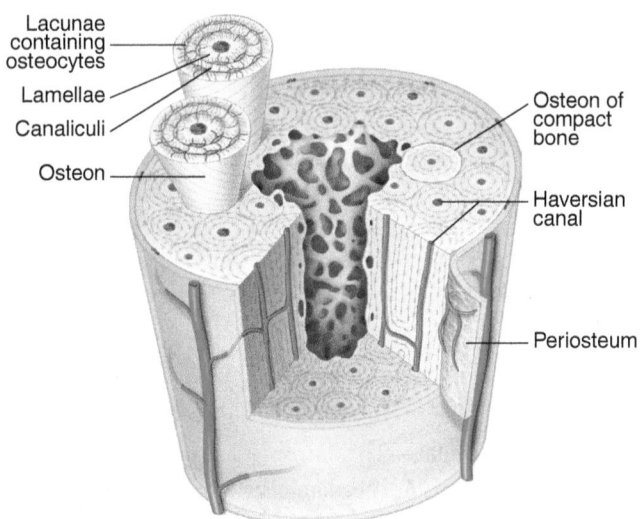

FIGURE 22-2 Microscopic components of osseous tissue.

Structure of a Long Bone

Long bones, such as the tibia, femur, humerus, and radius, have most of the features found in all bones (Figure 22-4). These features include:

- **Epiphysis**—The ends of a developing bone
- **Diaphysis**—The shaft of the long bone
- **Periosteum**—Membrane that forms the covering of bones, except at their articular (of or relating to a joint) surfaces

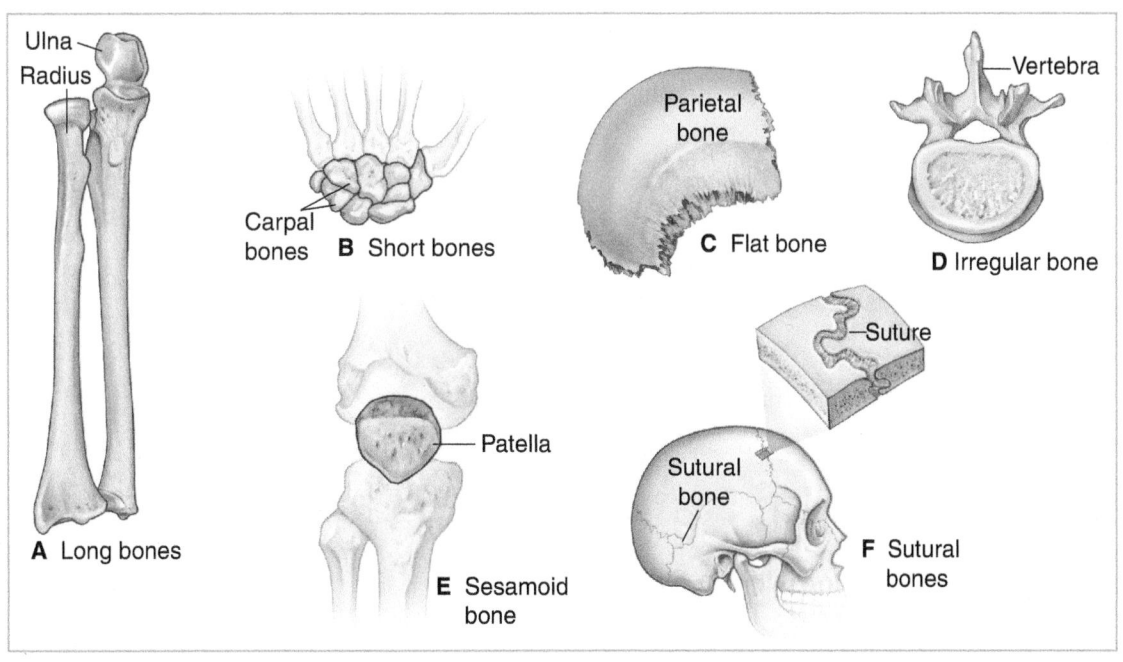

FIGURE 22-3 Classification of bones by shape.

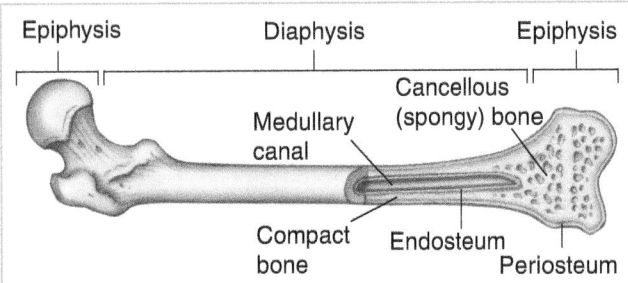

Epiphysis　　　Diaphysis　　　Epiphysis

Cancellous
(spongy) bone

Medullary
canal

Compact
bone

Endosteum

Periosteum

FIGURE 22-4 The features found in a long bone.

- **Compact bone**—The dense, hard layer of bone tissue
- **Medullary canal**—The narrow space or cavity throughout the length of the diaphysis (The medullary canal contains yellow bone marrow, which is made of fat cells.)
- **Endosteum**—The tough, connective tissue membrane lining the medullary canal and containing the bone marrow
- **Cancellous (spongy) bone**—The reticular tissue that makes up most of the volume of bone (The spongy bone contains red bone marrow. Red bone marrow manufactures most of the red blood cells found in the body and is found in the long bone.)

Bone Markings

The positions of various structural features of the bone are indicated by bone markings. These areas on the bone help to mark attachment of tendons and ligaments to muscles,

TABLE 22-2 | Bone Markings

Marking	Description
Condyle	Rounded process of bone that often joins with another bone at a joint.
Crest	Narrow, usually prominent, ridge of bone.
Epicondyle	Raised area on or above a condyle.
Line	Narrow ridge of bone that is less prominent than a crest.
Process	Bony projection.
Trochanter	Very large, blunt, irregularly shaped process.
Tubercle	Small rounded process.
Tuberosity	Large rounded projection that may be roughened.

passageways for blood vessels and nerves, and where bones join (Table 22-2).

JOINTS AND MOVEMENT

A joint, which is also called an **articulation**, is located at the place where two bones connect (Figure 22-5). The positioning of the bones at the joint determines the type of movement that the joint allows. Joints are classified by the three general types of movement they permit. A **synarthrotic joint** does not have a joint cavity where the bones touch, so the joint does not move. An example of a synarthrosis is a cranial suture. where the bones of the cranium meet. An

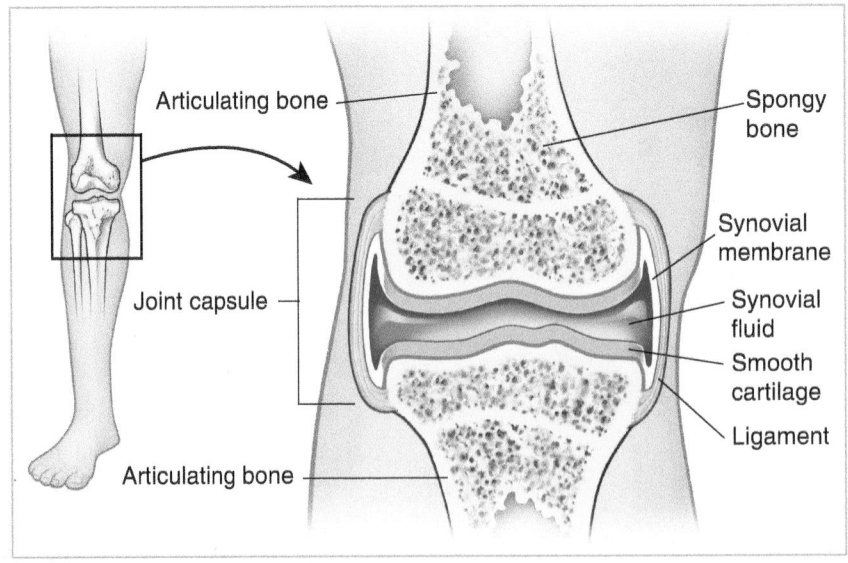

Articulating bone

Joint capsule

Articulating bone

Spongy bone

Synovial membrane

Synovial fluid

Smooth cartilage

Ligament

FIGURE 22-5 A typical joint.

amphiarthrotic joint, such as a vertebra, has limited movement. The most freely moving joint is a diarthrotic joint. Examples of this type of joint are the elbow, wrist, hip, and knee. The diarthrotic joint allows for several types of body movement. These movements are listed in Table 22-3 and illustrated in Figure 22-6.

Professionalism — The Life Span

The Child

- Babies are born with more cartilage and bones than adults. All bones are derived from cartilage. A baby is born with 270 bones. Through bone fusion during infancy, bones of the head and spinal column fuse together.
- During childhood, bones gradually become harder as more minerals are deposited. This hardening process is called ossification.
- Children grow taller as new bone tissue is made in an area between the heads of the long bones and their shafts. This area is known as the epiphyseal growth plate.

The Older Adult

- Women build bone until about age 35 and then begin to lose about 1 percent of their bone mass annually. Men start losing bone mass approximately 10 to 20 years later. During the aging process, most skeletal system changes result from changes in connective tissue. Most bone loss is caused by the loss later in life of bone mineral content, especially calcium salts deposited in the bone matrix. The cartilage becomes hard and brittle.
- Aging results in less joint movement, and, unfortunately, the onset of joint disease is more likely. An example of this is the increased likelihood of developing arthritis with age.

Bone healing also slows in the older adult. It takes much longer for a bone to heal in an adult than a child because the bone cells responsible for bone formation (osteoblasts) begin to have slower and impaired functioning.

Professionalism

The mark of a professional is not being afraid to learn more. Each team member, including the physician and the entire staff, should continue to ask questions, research answers, and learn from the experiences each day provides. Asking questions is the most important method of learning, along with continuing education programs, reading journals, and attending medical conferences. By learning and keeping current with medical information, the medical assistant can assist the medical office in continuing to provide high-quality medical care for all patients.

TABLE 22-3 | Movements of the Body

Movement	Description
Abduction	The process of moving a body part away from the midline.
Adduction	The process of moving a body part toward the midline.
Circumduction	The process of moving a body part in a circular motion.
Dorsiflexion	The process of bending a body part backward.
Eversion	The process of turning outward.
Extension	The process of straightening a flexed limb or the spine.
Flexion	The process of bending (or curving) a flexed limb or the spine.
Inversion	The process of turning inward.
Pronation	The process of lying prone or face down; the process of turning the hand so that the palm points downward.
Protraction	The process of moving a body part forward.
Retraction	The process of moving a body part backward.
Rotation	The process of moving a body part around a central axis.
Supination	The process of lying supine or face upward; the process of turning the palm or foot upward.

THE AXIAL SKELETON

The axial skeleton is the central portion of the skeleton. It is highlighted green in Figure 22-7. As shown in Figure 22-8, the axial skeleton consists of the skull, the sternum, the ribs, the vertebrae, the sacrum, and the coccyx. The head is composed of 22 bones; the skull has 8 bones, and the bones of the face total 14 (Figure 22-9).

The vertebral column, which houses the spinal cord, consists of a series of vertebrae that are connected to form four spinal curves (Figure 22-10). These curves are referred to as cervical, thoracic, lumbar, and sacral. The vertebrae are divided into five regions: the cervical, consisting of the first 7 vertebrae; the thoracic, the next 12 vertebrae; the 5 lumbar vertebrae; the sacral; and the coccyx, or tailbone. The first cervical vertebra, termed the atlas, attaches the spine to the occipital bone at the base of the skull. The axis, the second cervical vertebra, has a pivoting characteristic, allowing the head to turn from side to side.

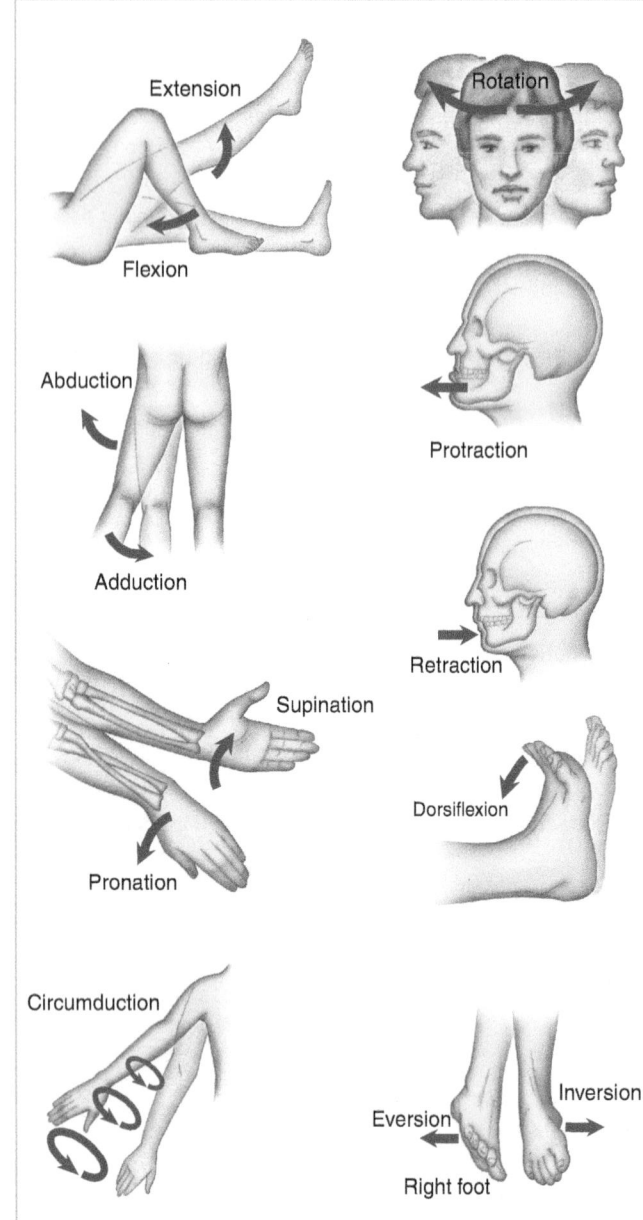

FIGURE 22-6 Types of body movements.

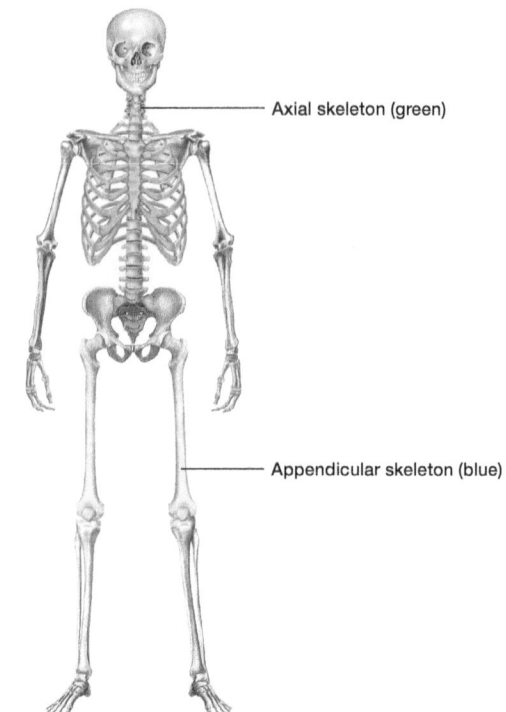

FIGURE 22-7 A contrasting comparison of the axial and appendicular skeleton.

The rib cage is also classified as part of the axial skeleton. The ribs form a protective cage that houses the heart, lungs, and other vital components of the human body. The rib cage consists of 12 pairs of ribs, which are divided into three categories: true ribs, false ribs, and floating ribs (Figure 22-11). There are 7 pairs of true ribs, which connect posteriorly to the spinal column and anteriorly to the sternum via small strips of costal (which means relating to the ribs) cartilage. Three pairs of false ribs follow the true ribs. The false ribs attach to the spine in the back, but rather than attach to the sternum in the front, they attach to costal cartilage of the very last true ribs. Finally, the last two

pairs of ribs are the floating ribs. These ribs are attached only to the spinal column without any point of anterior articulation.

THE APPENDICULAR SKELETON

The **appendicular skeleton**, which is responsible for movement, consists of the upper and lower extremities as well as the clavicles, the scapula, and the pelvic girdle. In Figure 22-7, the appendicular skeleton is shown in blue. Upper extremity bones include the humerus, radius, ulna, carpals, metacarpals, and phalanges. The bones of the lower extremities include the femur, patella, tibia, fibula, tarsals, metatarsals, and phalanges (see Figure 22-12A and B). The pelvic girdle, which is also part of the appendicular skeleton, includes the ilium, ishium, pubis, sacrum, and coccyx (Figure 22-12C).

The male pelvis (Figure 22-13A) is shaped like a funnel, forming a narrower outlet than the female's. It is both stronger and heavier than the female pelvis and therefore is well suited for lifting and running. The female pelvis (Figure 22-13B) is formed to be able to support pregnancy and childbirth. Often described as having a basin-like appearance, the female pelvis is much broader, rounder, and lighter than the male pelvis.

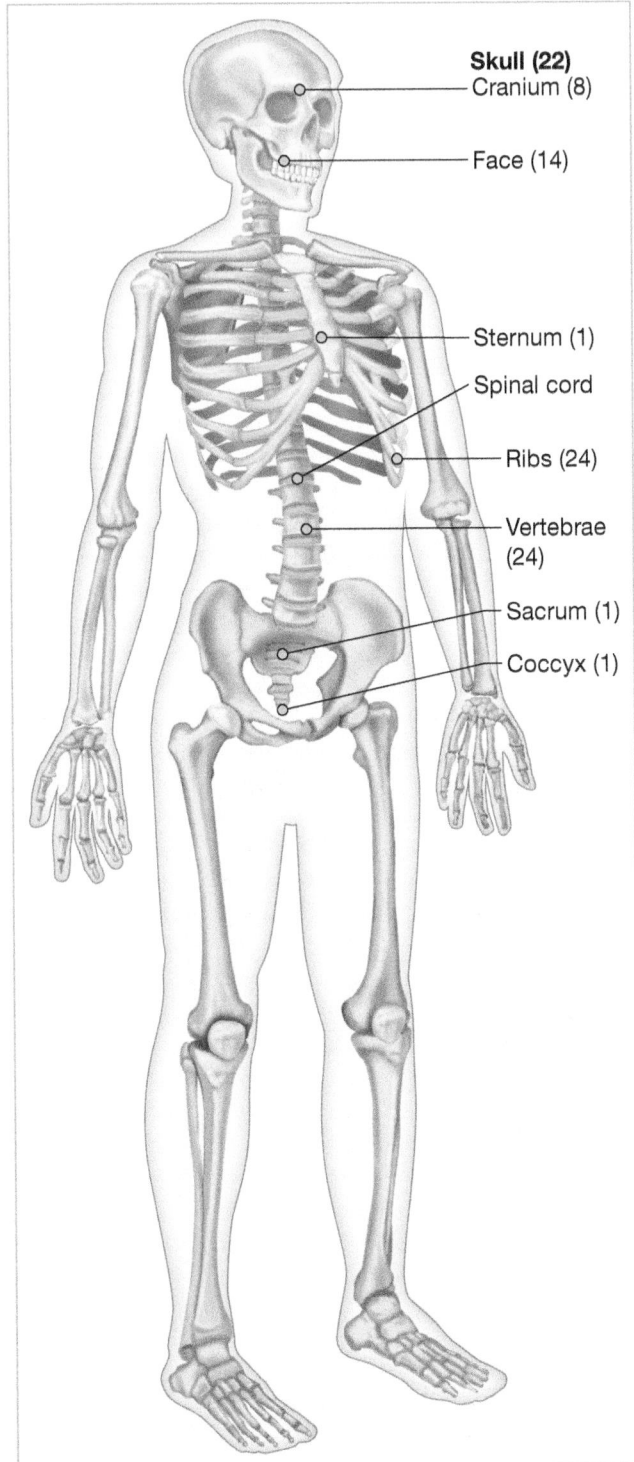

FIGURE 22-8 Bones of the axial skeleton.

COMMON PATHOLOGY ASSOCIATED WITH THE SKELETAL SYSTEM

A number of diseases and disorders associated with the skeletal system are discussed on the following pages. Table 22-4 lists additional disorders associated with the skeletal system.

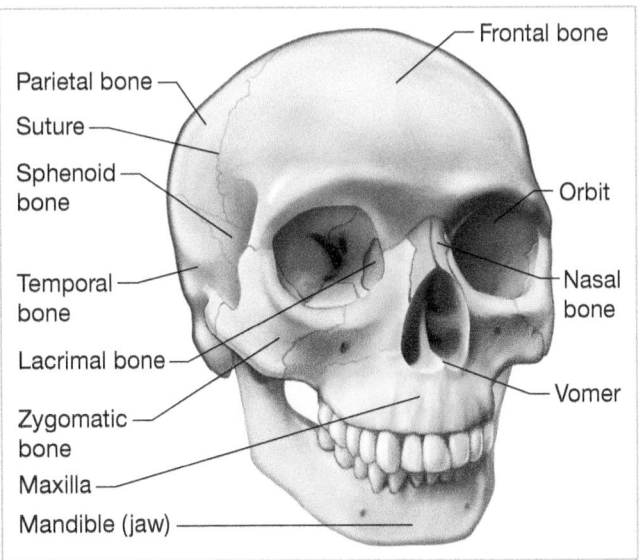

FIGURE 22-9 Cranial and facial bones.

Common diagnostic methods and tests used to identify and treat the pathological conditions related to the skeletal system are described in Table 22-5.

Abnormal Curvature of the Spine

Abnormal curvature of the spine, a portion of the axial skeleton, is often diagnosed as scoliosis, lordosis, or kyphosis (Figure 22-14).

Scoliosis

Scoliosis is an abnormal lateral curvature of the spine. Testing for this type of spinal curvature is often performed during childhood examinations in both physician offices and school settings as part of the child's overall health status review. Because it is tested for frequently at a young age, it is often diagnosed in toddlers, children, and adolescents.

Signs and Symptoms. Many times, a scoliotic spine appears to have an S or C shape. It is generally defined as a curvature of at least 10 degrees to the right or left, measurable on an X-ray. Those afflicted with scoliosis may often appear as if either their shoulders or their legs are uneven.

Treatment. Orthopedic braces often are used to reduce the progression of the abnormal spinal curvature. Physical therapy is also indicated for the treatment of scoliosis with an emphasis on strengthening the muscles of the body's core, including the back and abdomen. In cases of severe curvature or a continual progression of the disease, surgical treatment may be required.

Lordosis

Lordosis, often called swayback, is an exaggerated inward curvature of the lumbar spine.

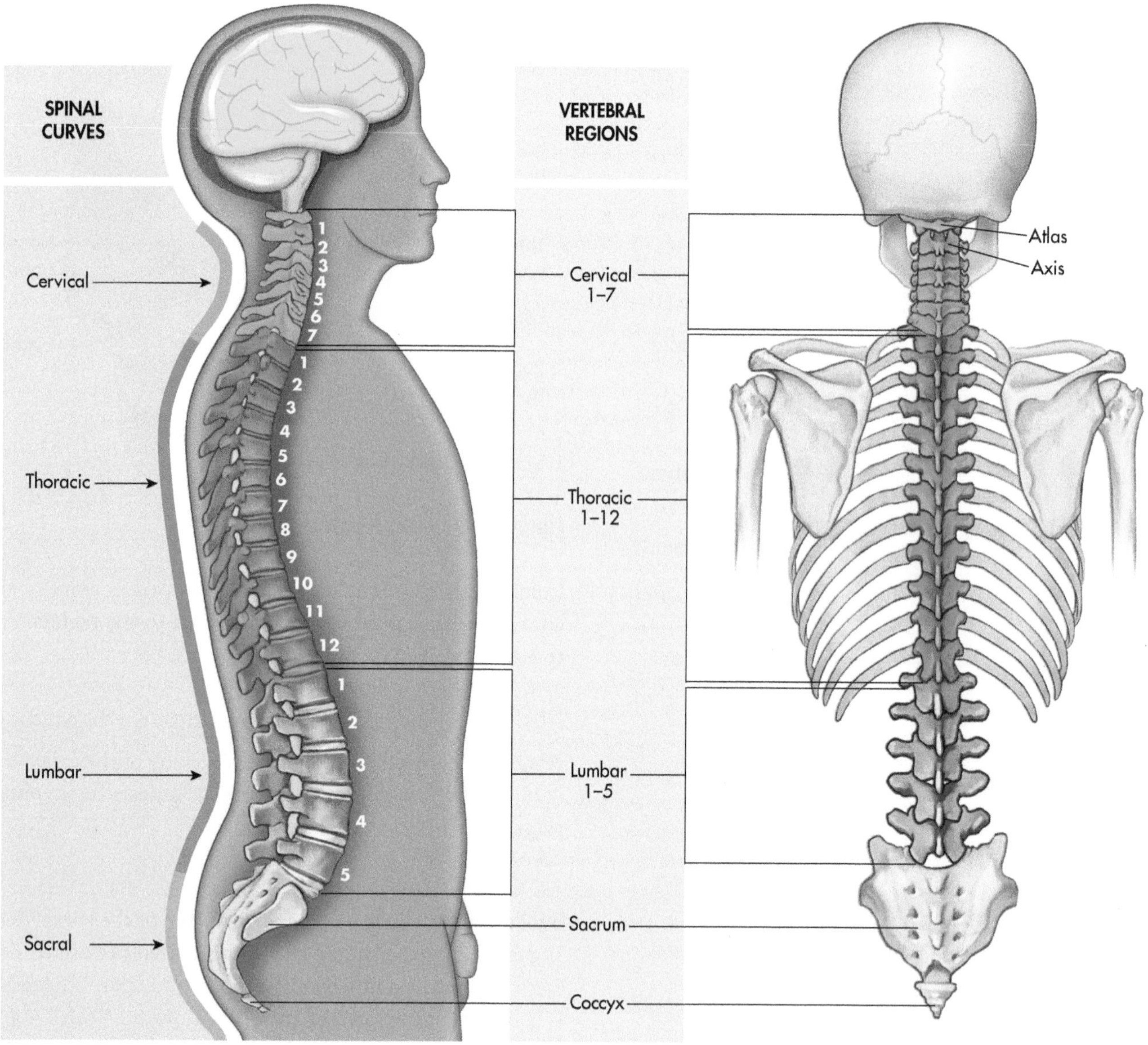

SPINAL CURVES

Cervical

Thoracic

Lumbar

Sacral

1
2
3
4
5
6
7

1
2
3
4
5
6
7
8
9
10
11
12

1
2
3
4
5

VERTEBRAL REGIONS

Cervical 1–7

Thoracic 1–12

Lumbar 1–5

Sacrum

Coccyx

Atlas

Axis

FIGURE 22-10 Vertebral regions showing the four spinal curves.

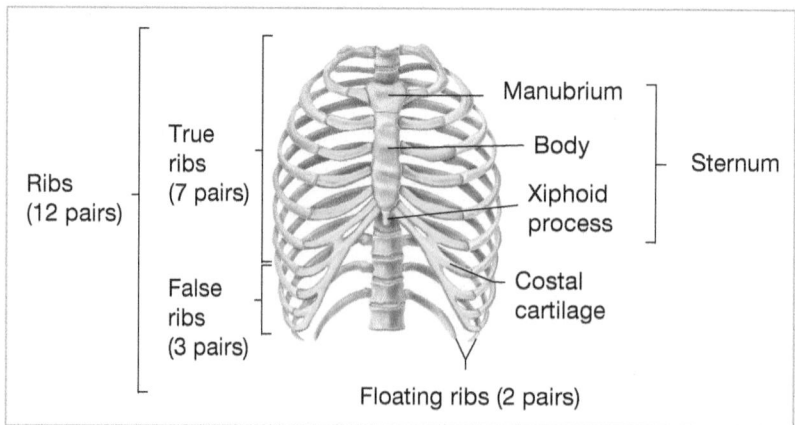

Ribs (12 pairs)

True ribs (7 pairs)

False ribs (3 pairs)

Manubrium

Body

Xiphoid process

Costal cartilage

Floating ribs (2 pairs)

Sternum

FIGURE 22-11 The rib cage.

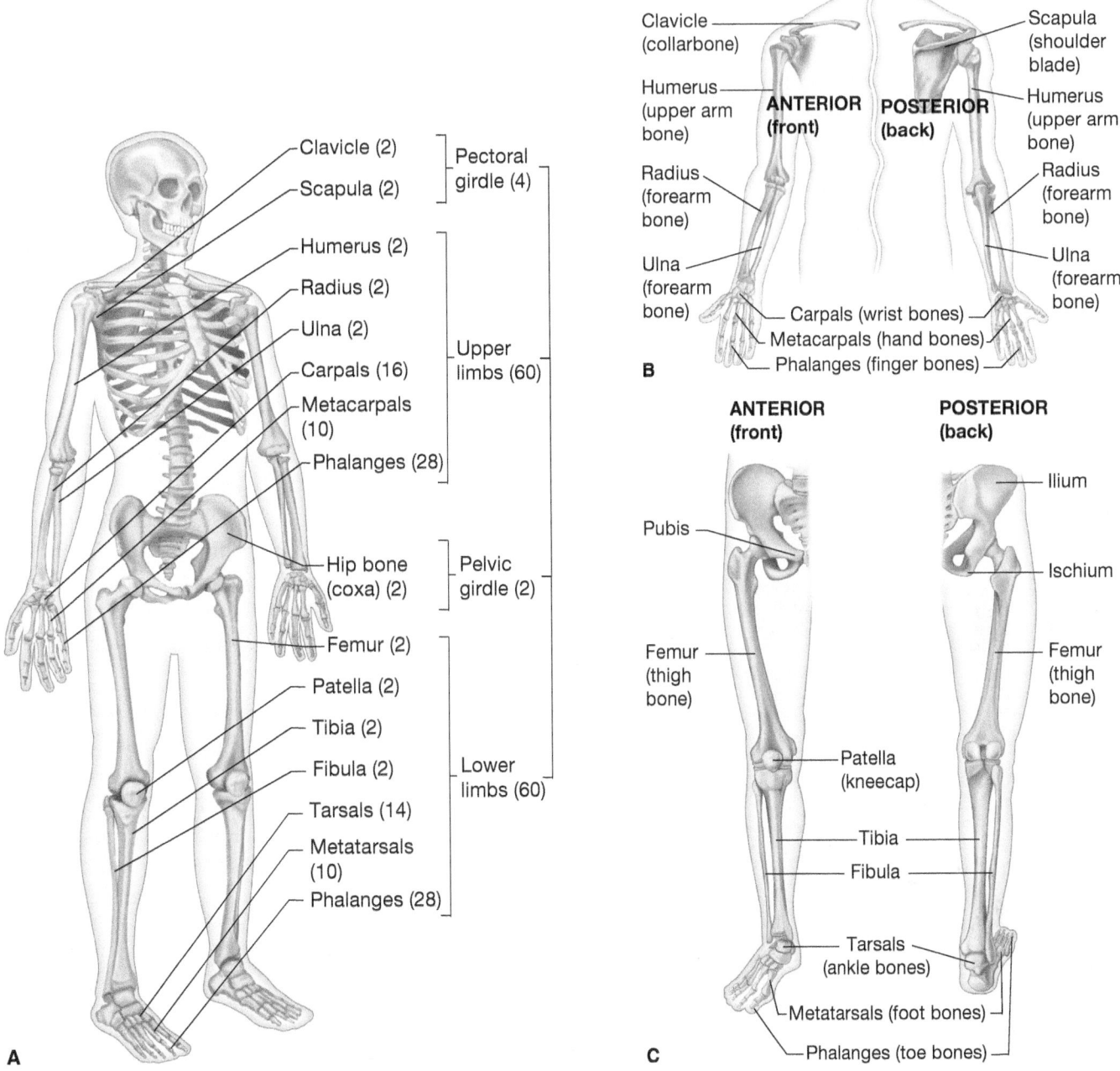

FIGURE 22-12 (A) The appendicular skeleton; **(B)** bones of the upper extremities; **(C)** bones of the lower extremities.

TABLE 22-4 | Additional Disorders of the Skeletal System

Disorder	Description
Epicondylitis	Commonly referred to as tennis elbow; characterized by elbow pain that is a result of repetitive grasping and rotating of the forearm.
Osteomyelitis	Inflammation of the bone and bone marrow caused by infection; can be difficult to treat.
Paget's Disease	A fairly common metabolic disease of the bone with unknown etiology; usually attacks middle-aged and older adult people; characterized by bone destruction and deformity.
Ruptured Intervertebral Disk	Herniation or outpouching of a disk between two vertebrae; also called a slipped or herniated disk.
Spinal Stenosis	Narrowing of the spinal canal causing pressure on the spinal cord and nerves.

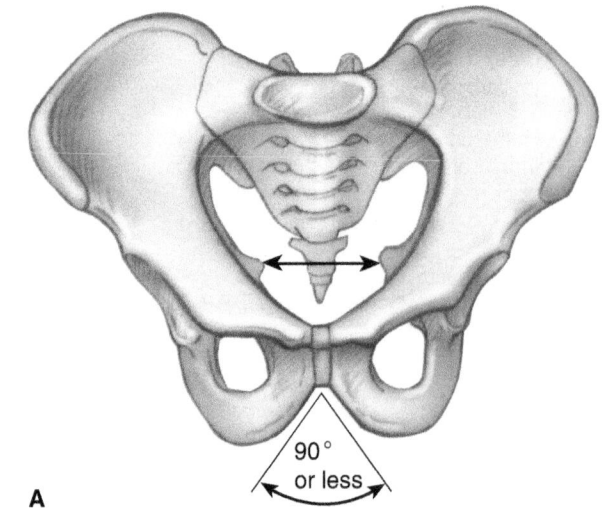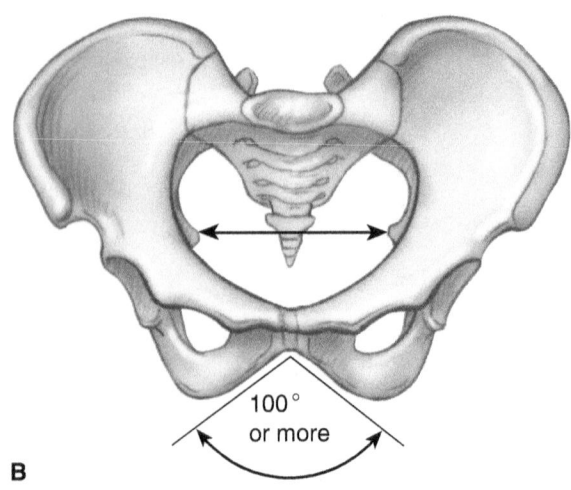

FIGURE 22-13 (A) The male pelvis; **(B)** the female pelvis.

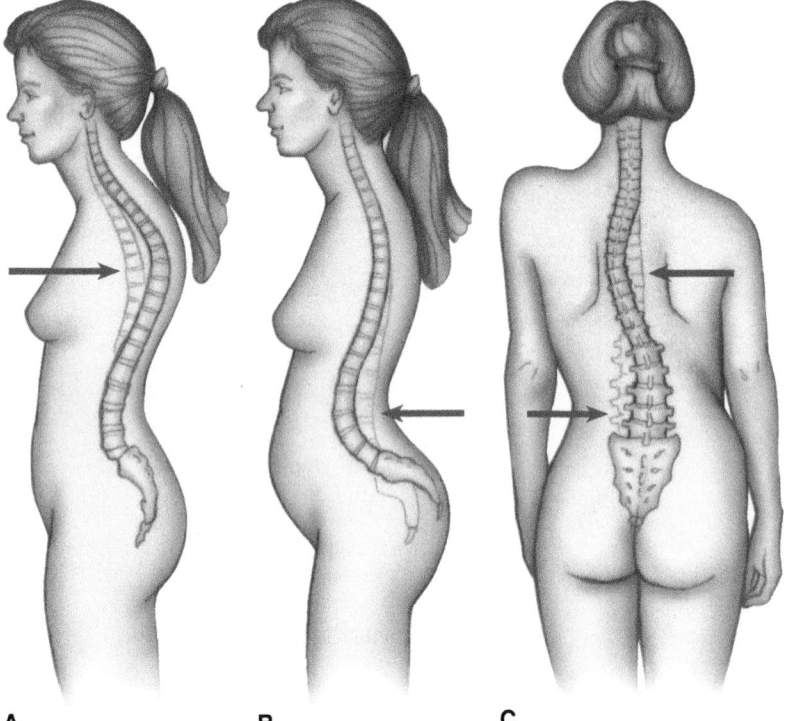

FIGURE 22-14 (A) Kyphosis; **(B)** lordosis; **(C)** scoliosis.

the patient losing excess body weight and by physical therapy to help maintain and strengthen the core of the body. Physical therapy also aims to increase flexibility and range of motion. If diagnosed in children or teens, braces may be implemented to control the curvature.

Kyphosis

Kyphosis, sometimes known as humpback, is an exaggeration of the thoracic curvature of the spine. The exaggeration in curvature may be a result of a congenital defect, a disease process (such as tuberculosis, syphilis, or malignancy), a compression fracture, faulty posture, osteoarthritis, rheumatoid arthritis, rickets, osteoporosis, or other condition.

Signs and Symptoms. The most telling sign of kyphosis is the rounded appearance of the upper back. Symptoms may include fatigue, mild back pain, and either a tender or a stiff feeling within the spine. In severe cases, shortness of breath may occur. In some patients, kyphosis may be the result and an early indicator of osteoporosis. Osteoporosis is discussed later in this section.

Treatment. As with lordosis, the overall health and age of the patient are taken into consideration when developing a treatment plan. Again, physical therapy focusing on the flexibility and strengthening of the spine is common. In addition, the **etiology**, or the cause or source of the patient's disease or disorder, also is considered. For instance, if osteoporosis is a cause of kyphosis, bone-strengthening medications may be prescribed to help lessen the severity of the disease.

Signs and Symptoms. Lordosis is commonly diagnosed in adult men and women who are overweight and carry excess weight in their abdomen, as well as pregnant women. The most glaring sign is a severe inward curvature of the lower back. When diagnosed in children, a prominently protruding abdomen and/or buttocks are the most common signs.

Treatment. Treatment for lordosis depends on the patient's overall health, age, and severity of the condition. The overall goal of treatment is to stop the progression of the curvature and prevent spinal deformity. This may be accomplished by

TABLE 22-5 | Procedures and Diagnostic Tests Related to the Skeletal System

Procedure/Test	Description
Amputation	Partial or complete removal of a limb for a variety of reasons, including tumors, gangrene, intractable pain, crushing injury, or uncontrollable infection.
Anterior Cruciate Ligament (ACL) Reconstruction	Replacing a torn ACL with a graft by means of arthroscopy.
Antinuclear Antibody (ANA)	Blood serum test to measure antibodies present in a variety of immunologic diseases such as rheumatoid arthritis and systemic lupus.
Arthrocentesis	Removal of synovial fluid with a needle from a joint space, such as in the knee, for examination.
Arthrography	Visualization of a joint by a radiographic study after injection of radiopaque contrast.
Arthroplasty	Surgical reconstruction of a joint.
Arthroscopic Surgery	Use of an arthroscope, a lighted instrument with camera/video capabilities, to facilitate performing surgery on a joint.
Arthrotomy	Surgically cutting into a joint.
Bone Densitometry	The use of advanced-technology X-ray equipment that enables the measurement of bone loss in an individual.
Bone Graft	Piece of bone taken from the patient that is (a) used to take the place of a removed bone or a bony defect at another site or (b) wedged between bones for fusion of a joint.
Bone Scan	Use of scanning equipment to visualize bones. It is especially useful in observing progress of treatment for osteomyelitis and cancer metastases to the bone.
Bunionectomy	Removal of the bursa at the joint of the great toe.
Carpal Tunnel Release	Surgical cutting of the ligament in the wrist to relieve nerve pressure caused by the repetitive motion (e.g., typing) that results in carpal tunnel syndrome.
Computerized Axial Tomography	Computer-assisted X-ray used to detect tumors and fractures. Also referred to as CT scan.
C-reactive Protein (CRP)	A blood serum test in which a positive result may indicate rheumatoid arthritis, acute inflammatory change, or widespread metastasis.
Goniometry	Measurement of joint movements and angles via goniometer.
Laminectomy	Removal of the vertebral posterior arch to correct severe back problems caused by compression of the lamina.
Meniscectomy	Removal of all or part of a torn meniscus (knee cartilage).
Myelography	Study of the spinal column after injecting radiopaque contrast.
Phosphorus (P) Blood Test	Testing of the phosphorus level of the blood; level may be increased in osteoporosis and during fracture healing.
Photon Absorptiometry	Measurement of bone density using an instrument for the purpose of detecting osteoporosis.
Reduction	Correcting a fracture by realigning the bone fragment. A closed reduction of the fracture is the manipulation of the bone into alignment and the application of a cast or splint to immobilize the part during the healing process. Open reduction is the surgical incision at the site of the fracture to perform the bone realignment. This is necessary when bone fragments must be removed.
Serum Rheumatoid Factor (RF)	An immunoglobulin present in the serum of 50 to 95 percent of adults with rheumatoid arthritis.
Spinal Fusion	Surgical immobilization of adjacent vertebrae. This may be done for several reasons, including correction of a herniated disk.
Thermograph	Process of recording heat patterns of the body's surface. Used to investigate the pathophysiology of rheumatoid arthritis.
Total Hip Replacement (THR)	Surgical replacement of a hip by implanting a prosthetic or artificial joint.
Uric Acid Blood Test	Measurement of uric acid in the blood; level is increased in gout, arthritis, multiple myeloma, and rheumatism.

Arthritis

Arthritis is the inflammation of one or more joints. Arthritis develops from a breakdown of cartilage in a joint. The breakdown of cartilage can be attributed to a number of factors including joint injury, autoimmune disorders, and normal to excessive wear and tear on the joints. Arthritis can occur at any age; however, it most commonly develops in older adults.

Signs and Symptoms. The symptoms of arthritis vary with every patient depending on the degree of the disease and the joint affected. Universal and classic signs and symptoms of this disease include joint pain and swelling, morning stiffness, warmth and redness around a joint, and decreased ability to move the joint.

Treatment. Treatment for arthritis depends on the age, occupation, and other activities of the patient, the cause and severity of the disease, and the joint that is affected. A modification to daily activities and low-impact aerobic exercise (such as swimming) are helpful. Medications to reduce joint pain and swelling, application of heat or cold, joint protection, and surgery may also be used in treating various levels of arthritis.

Osteoarthritis

Osteoarthritis is the most common type of arthritis and results from joint degeneration caused by years of wear and tear. Joints frequently impacted include the hips, knees, and finger joints of older adult patients. Obesity, a history of trauma, and various genetic and metabolic diseases increase the risk of osteoarthritis. Osteoarthritis is also referred to as degenerative joint disease (DJD).

Signs and Symptoms. Signs associated with osteoarthritis include swelling and fluid accumulation around the joints. In addition to stiffness, an interesting symptom that occurs with osteoarthritis is an aching pain that is associated with changes in the weather. Permanent joint deformity may occur in some cases (Figure 22-15).

Treatment. Treatment of osteoarthritis requires the use of nonsteroidal antiinflammatory drugs (NSAIDs) such as ibuprofen and naproxen, steroid injections to the affected joint, and, in severe cases, joint replacement.

Rheumatoid Arthritis

Rheumatoid arthritis is an autoimmune disorder in which inflammation causes joints to become deformed. In addition to inflammation, increased growth of both cartilage and bone is associated with this autoimmune disorder. Autoimmune disorders are characterized by the body attacking its

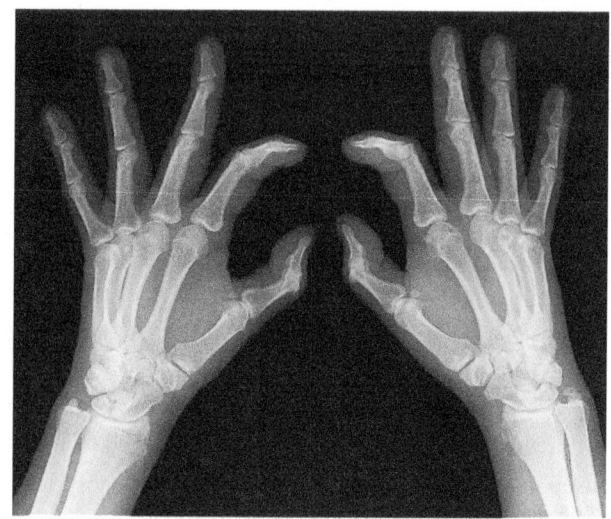

FIGURE 22-15 X-ray showing typical joint changes with osteoarthritis.

own body tissues. This is often caused by abnormal antibodies that circulate throughout the blood system.

Signs and Symptoms. Initial symptoms of rheumatoid arthritis are often difficult to identify as they can be mistaken for other conditions. Some of the early symptoms include fever, fatigue, joint pain, and weakness. Then, as the disease progresses, rheumatoid arthritis is marked by inflammation, joint swelling, and joint deformity (Figure 22-16). Morning joint stiffness is very common, because joints have had limited movement during sleep. Fatigue and loss of appetite are also associated with this disease. In addition to the hands, other parts of the body can be affected. Most commonly, the smaller joints of the body are affected along with the surrounding tissue. The medical assistant must be aware of possible symptoms to obtain relevant information for the physician; this is accomplished by asking patients useful questions and correctly documenting their answers.

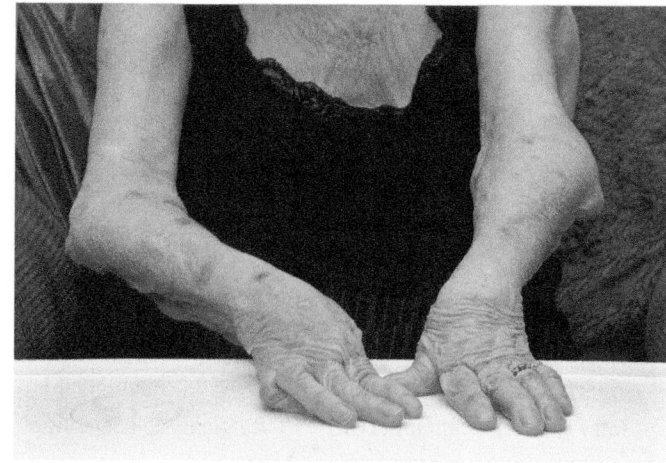

FIGURE 22-16 Typical hand deformities associated with rheumatoid arthritis.

Treatment. There is no cure for rheumatoid arthritis. However, early detection, diagnosis, and treatment may deter pain and joint decay. Medications including antirheumatic drugs, nonsteroidal antiinflammatory drugs, and corticosteroids may be helpful. Nonmedicinal treatments include heat and cold treatments and low-impact exercises. Additionally, eating a balanced diet and getting plenty of rest will help the body with healing.

Gouty Arthritis

Gouty arthritis, also called gout, is a disease caused by the formation and accumulation of uric acid crystals in the joints that result from high levels of uric acid in the bloodstream. The accumulation of these crystals leads to inflammation. The joint most frequently affected is the great toe; however, fingers and hands can also be affected.

Signs and Symptoms. A gouty joint is often very warm and very sore to the touch. After joints have been persistently affected by gout, they may become disfigured. When gouty arthritis affects the joints in the feet, as it commonly afflicts the joint of the big toe, walking can become difficult because of the severe pain associated with the condition.

Treatment. Medications are available to treat gouty arthritis by reducing the levels of uric acid in the bloodstream. A diet rich in colorful fruits and vegetables such as kale, cabbage, leafy green vegetables, red peppers, strawberries, cherries, and blueberries helps to decrease the symptoms of gout. Dietary restrictions include avoiding caffeine, alcohol, liver, and other purine-rich foods.

Bursitis

Bursitis is an inflammation of the **bursa**, which is a small sac of fluid around the joints. This fluid-filled sac cushions and lubricates high friction areas of the joint where tissues rub against each other. Bursitis is generally the result of overuse and trauma to joints, occurring most frequently in the elbow, knee, shoulder, and hip.

Signs and Symptoms. The most common signs and symptoms of bursitis include joint pain and limited mobility, swelling, and tenderness surrounding the joint.

Treatment. Treatment of bursitis usually involves rest, pain medication, steroid injections, aspiration of excess fluid from the bursa, and antibiotics. Physical therapy may also increase, promote, and restore range of motion and movement of the joint.

Carpal Tunnel Syndrome

The carpal tunnel is a narrow passageway in the wrist. The tunnel protects the median nerve to the hand and the nine tendons that bend the fingers (Figure 22-17). Carpal tunnel

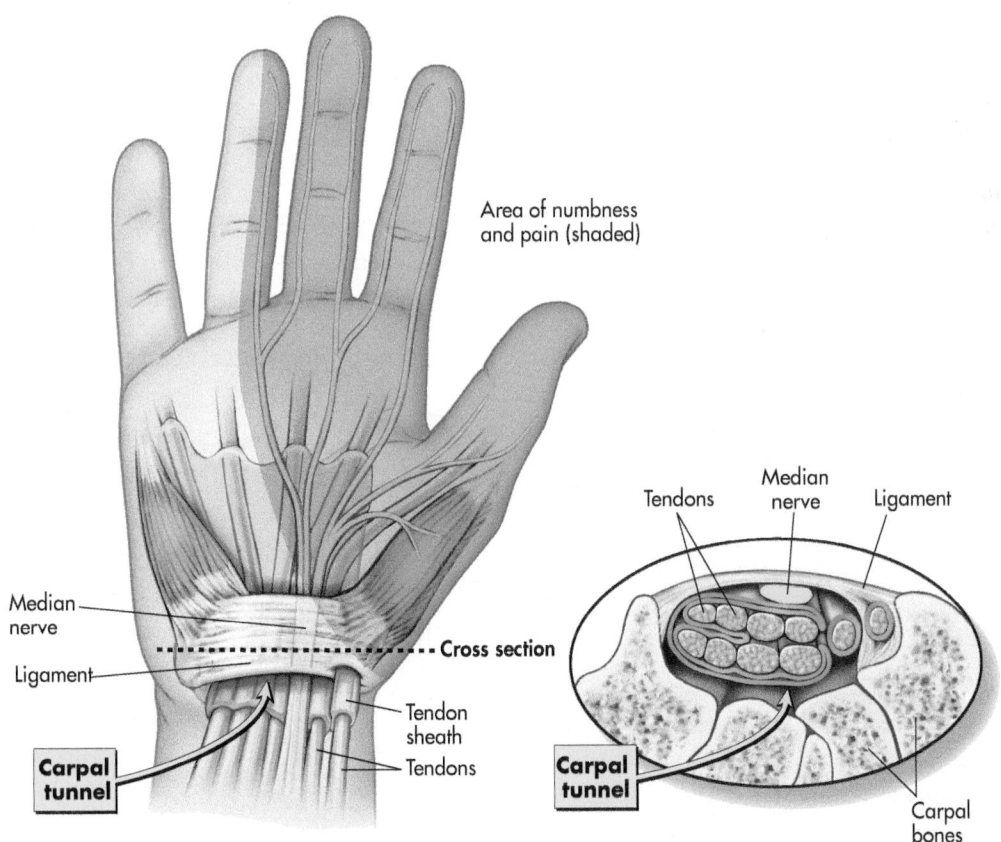

FIGURE 22-17 Cross section of the wrist showing tendons and nerves involved in carpal tunnel syndrome.

syndrome occurs when pressure is placed on the median nerve. Repetitive movements involving the wrist may contribute to the condition, movements as might occur with sports, such as racquetball or tennis, or activities like sewing, driving, assembly-line work, painting, typing, writing, the use of hand tools or vibrating tools, or other similar activities. Certain conditions increase the risk of carpal tunnel syndrome, including obesity, diabetes, and rheumatoid arthritis.

Signs and Symptoms. Pressure placed on the median nerve can produce pain, numbness, and hand weakness. The hands and fingers may feel tingly, itchy, and swollen, even if swelling is not visibly present. It is not uncommon for the pain and numbness to radiate up the arm.

Treatment. Proper treatment of carpal tunnel syndrome can alleviate symptoms of pain and numbness and can restore the normal use of the wrists. Treatment may include the application of wrist splints at night for several weeks. Hot and cold compresses also may be used. Resting the hand and wrist while avoiding the activities that trigger pain is indicated for early treatment. Also, proper ergonomics related to typing and other activities can be useful in preventing this syndrome. Medications used in the treatment of carpal tunnel syndrome include NSAIDs to relieve pain and reduce inflammation. Diuretics (sometimes called "water pills") that remove water from the body by increasing urine production may be prescribed to decrease swelling. Injections of corticosteroids can also help relieve signs and symptoms. If these measures do not provide significant relief, a surgical procedure may be performed to decrease pressure on the median nerve. It is about 85 percent effective in relieving carpal tunnel syndrome.

Fractures

Fractures are bone cracks or breaks of various types and various degrees. Fractures are classified based on the site of the fracture, the nature of the crack or break in the bone, and whether the fracture has caused a break in the skin. Fractures are diagnosed based on an X-ray of the broken bone (Figure 22-18). They may be classified as displaced, which means that the bone has completely separated and is no longer in a straight line (as with its normal anatomical

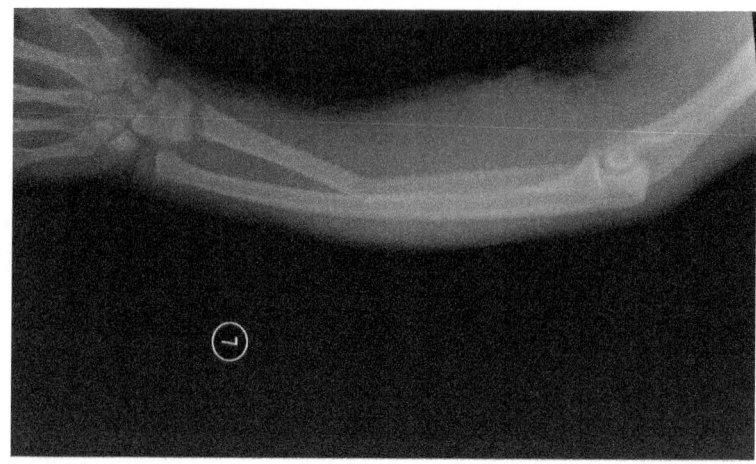

FIGURE 22-18 Fractures are diagnosed based on an X-ray of the broken bone.

position). A nondisplaced fracture still maintains its alignment and structural integrity, even though the bone is broken or cracked.

Signs and Symptoms. The different types of fractures, some of which are illustrated in Figure 22-19, include the following:

- **Closed (simple)**—This type of fracture does not involve a break in the skin. It is completely internal.

- **Open (compound)**—These are more dangerous fractures because the fracture has broken through the skin. Because the integrity of the skin and other tissues is damaged in this type of fracture, the risk of infection or hemorrhage is greater than with a closed fracture.

- **Comminuted**—In this type of fracture, part of the bone is shattered into a multitude of bony fragments.

- **Transverse**—These fractures break the shaft of the bone across its longitudinal axis.

- **Greenstick**—This type of fracture usually occurs in young children, whose bones are still relatively soft.

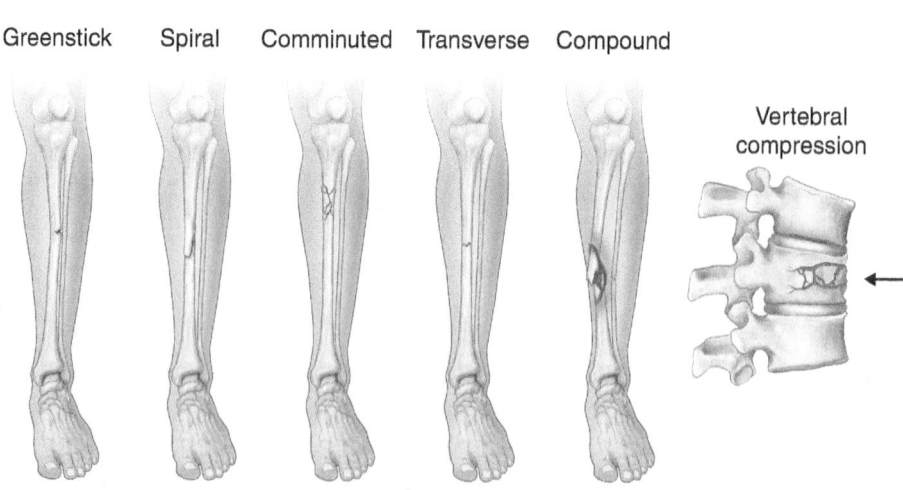

Greenstick   Spiral   Comminuted   Transverse   Compound

Vertebral compression

FIGURE 22-19 Various types of fractures.

Only one side of the shaft is broken; the other side is bent, similar to breaking a green plant stick.

- **Spiral**—Spiral fractures are spread along the length of a bone, and are produced by twisting stresses.
- **Colles'**—Colles' fracture is frequently the result of reaching forward to stop or cushion a fall. This fracture is exemplified by a break in the distal portion of the radius. Colles' fractures are most frequently seen in children and older adults.
- **Pott's**—These fractures occur in the ankle and affect both bones of the lower leg (the tibia and fibula).
- **Compression**—Compression fractures occur in the vertebrae after severe stress, such as when someone falls and lands with a significant amount of force.
- **Epiphyseal**—These fractures are commonly seen in children in areas of bone where the growth plate is undergoing calcification (a hardening process of the calcium in the bones) and the **chondrocytes** (cartilage-forming cells) are dying.

Treatment. Fractures are generally casted by a physician. Today, casts are made using fiberglass (Figure 22-20). An **orthopedic physician** is a physician who treats musculoskeletal conditions. The cast that is applied limits the movement of the affected bone, allowing proper healing to occur. At times, in severe fractures, surgical intervention must be performed. It is common that both pins and metal plating are used to stabilize joints and bones during surgery. Pain and antiinflammatory medications are often prescribed for patient comfort.

Dislocations

A **dislocation** occurs when a bone slips out, or separates from, the joint. Sudden impact on a joint may cause one of the

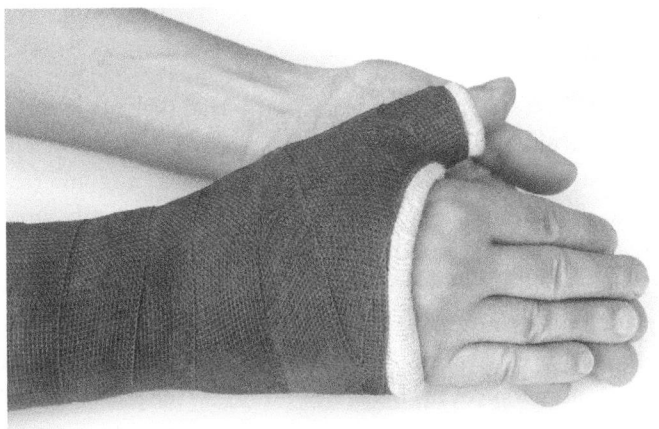

FIGURE 22-20 A fiberglass cast is being used to treat a broken wrist.

Professionalism | **The Workplace**

Patients with injuries to the skeletal system may have trouble walking. It is important to have wheelchairs and hand railings available that are necessary to facilitate movement. The medical assistant may need to walk closely with the patient to ensure safety. If at all possible, place a patient who has trouble walking in an examination room near the reception area to reduce the amount of walking necessary.

bones that meet at that joint to become dislocated. A dislocation usually follows a blow, a fall, or other trauma. Usually the joint capsule and ligaments tear when a dislocation occurs, and often the nerves are injured.

Signs and Symptoms. The visual signs of a dislocation include bones appearing "out of place" or misshapen as well as discolored skin around the joint. The patient will exhibit limited movement, and the joint may appear bruised or swollen. Dislocated joints are intensely painful, and it is generally very difficult to move the affected joint.

Treatment. If a dislocation is suspected, patients generally should seek emergency treatment in a hospital or urgent care setting, as many physicians' offices are not equipped to handle this injury. A procedure known as **reduction** is used to align and reposition the joint, which reduces pain and allows the joint to have proper range of motion. Pain relievers and antiinflammatory medications are often prescribed for patients. At times, general anesthesia is given for reduction procedures that are difficult and must be performed in the operating room.

Osteoporosis

Osteoporosis is characterized by progressive loss of bone density and thinning of bone tissue. Osteoporosis affects more than 25 million Americans, mostly women, and most frequently begins to appear between ages 50 to 70. Individuals who have known decreased bone density or a predisposition to the disease may develop osteoporosis at an earlier age. Individuals with osteoporosis are subject to increased fracture potential, especially in the hips, vertebrae, and wrists. The following individuals have a higher risk factor for the development of osteoporosis:

- Those with a family history of osteoporosis
- Those who do not engage in weight-bearing exercise as part of their lifestyle
- Caucasian women who have never been pregnant and experience early menopause

- Individuals with a history of frequent corticosteroid use
- Individuals who excessively smoke, drink alcohol, and consume diets high in salt, fat, and caffeine
- Individuals who have an insufficient intake of calcium or vitamin D

Signs and Symptoms. Osteoporosis generally has gradual and sometimes hard-to-recognize symptoms. The most common signs of osteoporosis are decreased height and a stooped posture. As mentioned earlier in the chapter, kyphosis can be an early indicator of osteoporosis. Additional signs and symptoms include back pain and frequent fractures throughout the body. Physicians may order bone densitometry screenings to catch the disease in early onset, particularly for those who are considered high risk or who have a family history.

Treatment. Treatment of osteoporosis is aimed at preventing more bone loss; however, the disease itself cannot be cured. Prevention methods include healthy diets that are rich in vitamins and minerals, weight-bearing exercises to strengthen weakened bones, adding calcium and vitamin D supplements to the diet, and medications to help preserve calcium and decrease bone loss.

Hallux Valgus

Hallux valgus is the enlargement of the inner portion of the joint at the base of the big toe. It is most commonly known as a bunion.

Signs and Symptoms. Reddened skin surrounds the inflamed joint of the big toe in hallux valgus. In addition, the joint may be filled with fluid and feel tender to the touch.

Treatment. Properly fitting shoes should be worn. Also, proper padding and cushioning of the joint should be considered. Pain medications and antiinflammatory medications may be used to help deal with the symptoms. Foot surgery may be required for severe cases. The patient may need to be fitted with special adaptive shoes made by an orthopedic shoe specialist.

Hammertoe

Hammertoe is a condition in which the toe bends into a hammer shape or claw shape because of the abnormal flexion of the proximal interphalangeal joint. It is frequently caused by an imbalance between muscle and tendons within the toe. Hammertoe may also be hereditary or result from a traumatic injury to the foot. It can be further aggravated by wearing ill-fitting shoes.

Signs and Symptoms. Pain and visible joint deformation are classic symptoms and signs of this skeletal disorder.

Treatment. Treatment for hammertoe consists of analgesics, splinting, and wearing specially designed footwear. In severe cases, surgical straightening of the toe may be required.

Rickets

Rickets is an early childhood disease caused by a vitamin deficiency in calcium, vitamin D, and phosphate. This disease results in bone deformities, especially bowed legs, from weak bones. Genetics may increase the risk of developing rickets.

Signs and Symptoms. Symptoms include pain and tenderness of the bones, an increased likelihood of bone breakage, impaired growth associated with decreased height, and muscle cramps. Decreased muscle tone and weakness are also present with rickets.

Treatment. Treatment for rickets includes correcting vitamin deficiency by increasing vitamin and mineral intake. Comfort measures, including rest and heat and ice applications, may be taken to relieve the symptoms.

Osteomalacia

Osteomalacia is the adult onset of rickets. As with rickets, deficiencies in calcium and vitamin D are causes for the disease. Additional causes for development of osteomalacia include cancer, liver disease, kidney failure, and side effects associated with antiseizure medications.

Signs and Symptoms. Symptoms and signs of osteomalacia include bone pain, bowing legs, and frequent fractures.

Treatment. The treatment for osteomalacia is very similar to the treatment for rickets, including increasing vitamin and mineral intake and comfort measures to relieve symptoms.

SUMMARY

The skeletal system is divided into the axial skeleton and the appendicular skeleton. The functions of the skeletal system include providing shape and support, protecting internal organs, and production of blood cells. Bones not only store essential minerals but also assist with joints and movement. Therefore, disorders of the skeletal system can seriously impair mobility and the ability to perform activities of daily living. Arthritis is a crippling degeneration of joints. Bursitis is an inflammation of the bursa that lubricates the joints. Carpal tunnel syndrome is caused by excessive repetitive use of the wrists. Fractures can occur from trauma or weakness in the bone. Dislocations occur when a bone slips out of the joint.

Gout is caused by an accumulation of urate crystals. Osteoporosis is damage to the bone caused when the bone becomes porous and weak. Hallux valgus, also known as a bunion, is an overgrowth of the great toe. Hammertoe occurs when the toe bends into a hammer shape. Osteomalacia and rickets are caused when bone softens, sometimes from lack of vitamin D.

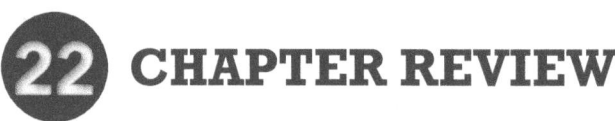

22 CHAPTER REVIEW

COMPETENCY REVIEW

1. Define and spell the terms for this chapter.
2. Name the two main divisions of the skeletal system.
3. Name the six classifications of bone, and give an example of each.
4. Discuss the six main functions of the skeletal system.
5. Name the three general types of joints.
6. Contrast the difference between the three abnormal curvatures of the spine.
7. Describe how the female pelvis differs from the male pelvis.
8. Draw pictures of 3 of the 13 types of body movements found in Figure 22-6.
9. Describe what kind of fracture would commonly occur in a child who falls down the stairs and injures their wrist.
10. What is arthritis?

PREPARING FOR THE CERTIFICATION EXAM

1. Which of the following is also known as a bunion?
   a. hallux valgus
   b. hammertoe
   c. toe dislocation
   d. toe fracture
   e. bursitis

2. Which of the following is caused by the accumulation of uric acid crystals in the joints?
   a. rickets
   b. scoliosis
   c. gouty arthritis
   d. lordosis
   e. osteoporosis

3. Which of the following is an abnormal lateral curvature of the spine?
   a. gout
   b. lordosis
   c. kyphosis
   d. scoliosis
   e. rickets

4. Which of the following is not part of the axial skeleton?
   a. ribs
   b. coccyx
   c. femur
   d. sternum
   e. vertebrae

5. Which of the following is the process of moving a body part around a central axis?
   a. flexion
   b. extension
   c. pronation
   d. rotation
   e. protraction

6. Which of the following is the process of bending the toes upward and backward to relieve a cramp in the calf muscle?
   a. abduction
   b. adduction
   c. dorsiflexion
   d. extension
   e. circumduction

7. What type of fracture does twisting cause?
   a. comminuted
   b. spiral
   c. greenstick
   d. epiphyseal
   e. compound

8. Rickets is caused by a lack of which vitamin?
   a. A
   b. B
   c. C
   d. D
   e. E

9. Which of the following is an inflammation of the bone and bone marrow?
   a. osteomyelitis
   b. osteoarthritis
   c. osteomalacia
   d. osteoporosis
   e. epicondylitis

10. Which bone is not located on the face?
   a. maxilla
   b. mandible
   c. lacrimal
   d. sphenoid
   e. clavicle

CRITICAL THINKING

Refer to the case study at the beginning of the chapter and use the information you have learned to answer the following questions.

1. The emergency department physician suspects that Charlie may have dislocated his shoulder. What are some additional signs and symptoms of a dislocation?
2. The physician informs Charlie he will have to have a reduction to his shoulder; however, it may be painful because of the severity of the injury. Charlie is very apprehensive about the procedure. What is an option that could be considered regarding the reduction?
3. Months after the successful reduction, Charlie developed bursitis in the same shoulder. What are some possible treatment methods for bursitis?

INTERNET ACTIVITY

Find the website of the National Osteoporosis Foundation. Determine what information the organization provides for patients and for health care providers. Use this information to learn how to teach a patient about osteoporosis.

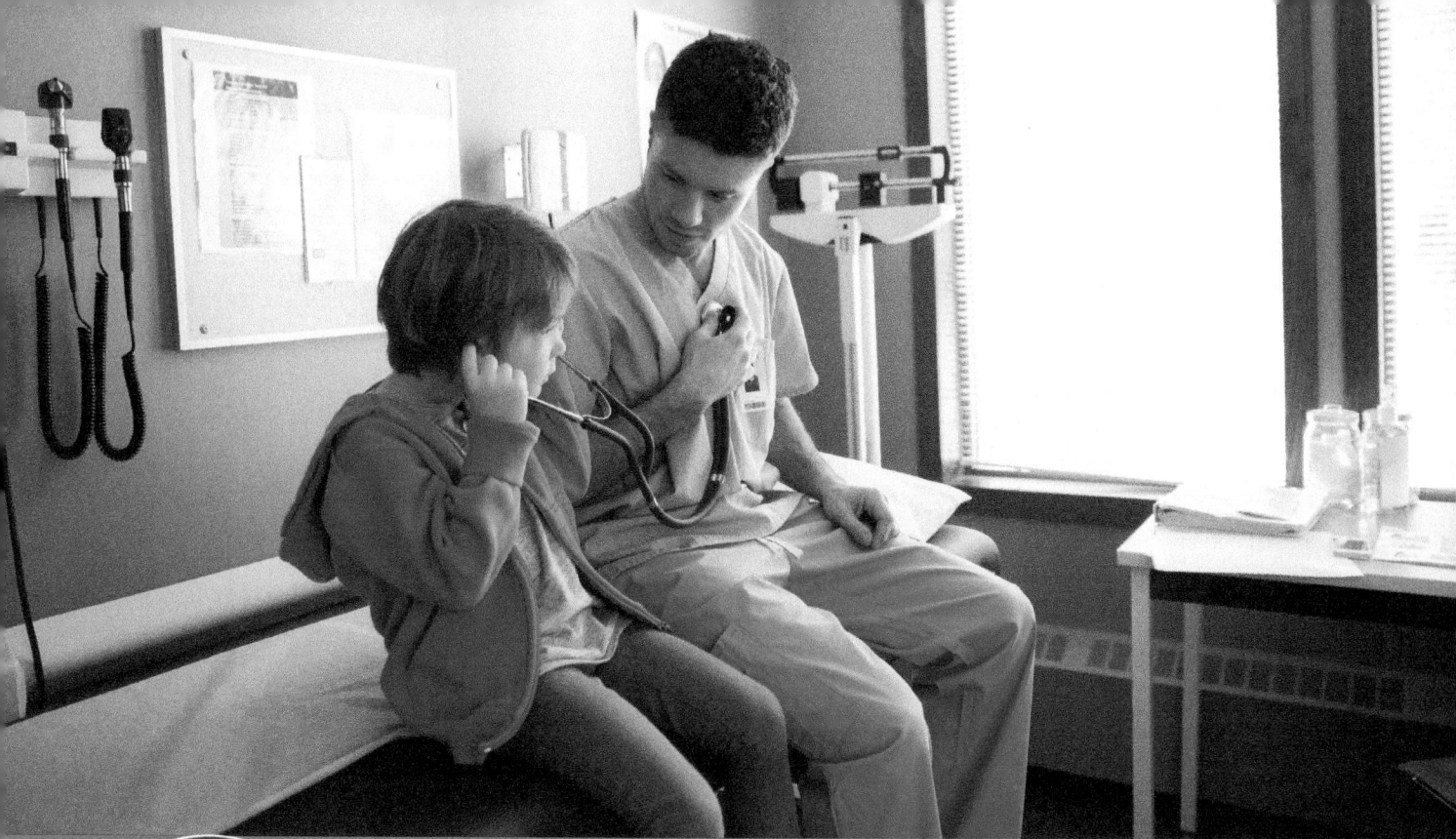

CHAPTER

23

The Muscular System

Learning Objectives

After completing this chapter, you should be able to:

23.1 Define and spell the terms for this chapter.

23.2 Explain the function of muscles.

23.3 Describe the three types of muscle tissue.

23.4 Describe how the muscular system changes between childhood and older adulthood.

23.5 Explain how energy is used by muscles.

23.6 Describe the structure of skeletal muscles.

23.7 List major skeletal muscles found throughout the body.

23.8 Describe pathology associated with the muscular system.

On returning home from a camping trip, 12-year-old Felix Gutierrez noticed a small black bump near his left ankle. He showed his mother, Rosa, who immediately recognized that the black bump was in fact a tick. She immediately attempted to remove the tick but was not sure if she was completely successful.

Terms to Learn

agonist	ligament	sprain
antagonist	Lyme disease	strain
aspiration	muscular dystrophy (MD)	striated
atrophy	myasthenia gravis (MG)	synergist
cardiac muscle	origin	tendon
fascia	oxygen debt	tendonitis
fibromyalgia	prime mover	tetanus
ganglion cyst	skeletal muscle	tonicity
insertion	smooth muscle	

The muscular system is composed of all the muscles within the body. Muscle fibers are made of different lengths and shapes and vary in color from white to deep red. The muscle fibers are held together by connective tissue. The connective tissue is held together by a fibrous sheath called **fascia**. Each fiber within a muscle also has its own nervous system connection with a stored supply of energy in the form of glycogen. Muscle must be supplied with proper nutrition and oxygen to perform properly. The muscular system is well permeated by vessels from both the circulatory and the lymphatic systems.

FUNCTIONS OF MUSCLE

Making up approximately 42 percent of a person's total body weight, muscles serve many functions. The main functions of the muscular system include movement, stability, circulation and respiration, heat production, and aiding in digestion and elimination.

Movement

Nearly all movement in the body can be attributed to a muscle contraction. Therefore, contractibility is considered the main function of the muscular system. Voluntary movement is easy to understand because it is easy to consider muscles required to perform specific, conscious movements such as walking, standing up from a seated position, and even smiling. Involuntary muscle movements do not require conscious thought and therefore aren't thought about very often. More about involuntary muscle movements will be discussed later in this section.

Generally speaking, muscles, where they are attached to bones, internal organs, and blood vessels, are responsible for all types of bodily movement (Figure 23-1).

Stability

Tonicity is the body's ability to maintain posture through a continual partial contraction of skeletal muscles. The muscular system works in conjunction with the skeletal system to provide stability. Without conscious thought, multiple muscles and joints are activated to simply maintain posture, whether standing, sitting, or lying down. Some of the smallest muscles, such as those found in the vertebral column, play an important role in this function.

Circulation and Respiration

The heart is composed of cardiac muscle tissue, which is discussed in the next section of this chapter. The involuntary movement and contraction of the heart muscle (a pumping mechanism) is responsible for circulating blood throughout the body, providing essential nutrients and oxygen to our

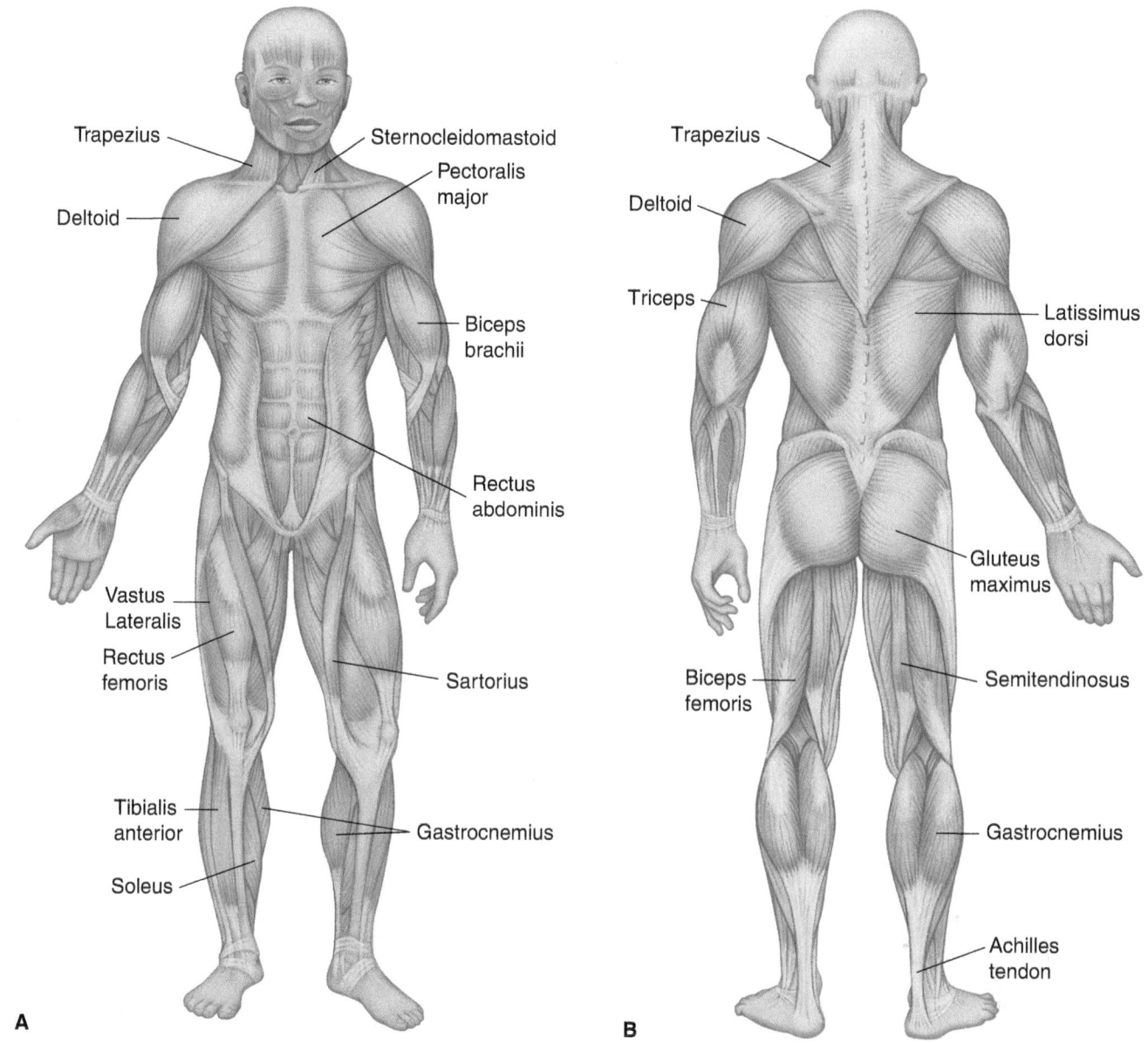

Trapezius
Sternocleidomastoid
Deltoid
Pectoralis major
Biceps brachii
Rectus abdominis
Vastus Lateralis
Rectus femoris
Sartorius
Tibialis anterior
Gastrocnemius
Soleus

A

Trapezius
Deltoid
Triceps
Latissimus dorsi
Gluteus maximus
Biceps femoris
Semitendinosus
Gastrocnemius
Achilles tendon

B

FIGURE 23-1 (A) Selected skeletal muscles (anterior view); **(B)** selected skeletal muscles and the Achilles tendon (posterior view).

systems. Respiration is also controlled by muscle movements. The diaphragm, which is located under the rib cage and separates the thoracic and abdominal cavities, is the major muscle responsible for breathing. Accessory muscles found around the rib cage and in the thoracic cavity also assist in respiration.

Heat Production

Muscles produce heat through the chemical changes involved in muscular contraction. This is what helps the body maintain a normal temperature. As a muscle contracts, it releases heat, making the person feel warmer. As an example, consider a person who is exercising. Exercise requires a lot of muscle contraction, which, in turn, releases a lot of heat. The extra heat causes the person to sweat.

Digestion and Elimination

Muscles that line the digestive tract are made of smooth muscle tissue. The involuntary action of the smooth muscles of the digestive tract transport food through the stomach and intestines. As food is transported throughout the digestive tract, the body is able to absorb vital nutrients and calories necessary for function. At the end of the digestive process, muscles help in eliminating fecal matter from the body.

TYPES OF MUSCLE TISSUE

As already noted, muscle tissue has the ability to contract, or shorten, which produces the movement of internal and external body parts. Breathing, speaking, walking, talking, eating, and almost every other bodily function require the contraction of muscle tissue. The muscles serve as the engines, or powerhouses, of the body and are constructed to provide speed and power. Muscles are composed of about 75 percent water, 20 percent protein, and about 5 percent carbohydrates, lipids, inorganic salts, and nonprotein nitrogenous compounds. The exact composition of various muscles differs.

Three types of muscle cells form three distinct types of muscle tissue. Each type is designed to perform specific functions of the body. The three types of muscle tissue are skeletal, smooth, and cardiac (Figure 23-2).

Skeletal muscle, sometimes called voluntary or **striated** muscle (*striated* means striped in appearance), can perform skeletal movement because it is attached to the bones of the body. Skeletal muscle is responsible for voluntary movements, meaning that it is under conscious control. Skeletal muscle is made up of cylindrical fibers. The nucleus tends to be toward the edge of each striated cell. Because all skeletal cells are striated, the skeletal muscle itself tends to have an overall striped look.

Smooth muscle, or involuntary muscle, is composed of elongated, spindle-shaped cells. Muscles made from these types of cells are also called visceral muscles because they are found in the body's viscera (organs), including organs found in the respiratory tract, urinary system, and digestive system, as well as in the walls of the blood vessels. In contrast to skeletal muscle cells, smooth muscle cells are not striated and their nucleus is centrally located. Smooth muscle is called involuntary muscle because it is not voluntarily controlled, meaning it is not controlled by conscious thought. For example, you do not have to purposely engage the muscles of your digestive system to perform the act of digestion; your body's muscles perform this action voluntarily, or on their own.

Cardiac muscle is found in the heart. The cells of this specific muscle tissue have a single central nucleus and are roughly quadrangular in shape. The cells form a network of branching fibers. Cardiac muscle cells are both striated and involuntary. Cardiac muscle tissues are supplied with nerve fibers that carry messages to and from the central nervous system (brain and spinal cord). Each involuntary contraction and relaxation of cardiac muscle results in a

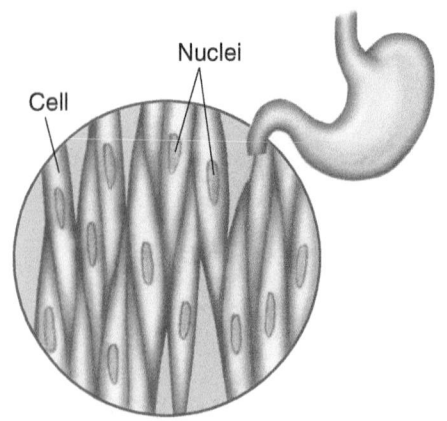
Smooth muscle tissue

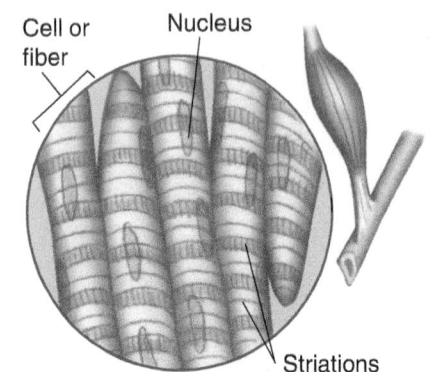
Skeletal muscle tissue

Cardiac muscle tissue

FIGURE 23-2 Types of muscle tissue.

heartbeat, which, as discussed earlier, is responsible for pumping blood throughout the body to deliver oxygen and nutrients. The average resting human heart beats 60 to 80 times a minute.

ENERGY PRODUCTION FOR MUSCLE

Muscles use energy in the form of adenosine triphosphate (ATP), which is a type of chemical energy created within the body's cells. This type of energy is needed for sustained or repeated muscular contractions. ATP can be produced by either aerobic (with oxygen) or anaerobic (without oxygen) means:

- **Aerobic production of ATP**—In the presence of oxygen, the body can use carbohydrates, fats, and proteins to make energy (ATP) that is used by the muscles. When the body uses ATP that is produced aerobically, more energy is available to use. This is the type of energy required for endurance.

- **Anaerobic production of ATP**—The body uses stored glucose, known as glycogen, to make ATP without oxygen. The glycogen, which is the usable form of carbohydrate in the body, breaks down into ATP and lactic acid simultaneously. Generally, this form of energy production is useful for small bursts of energy rather than for endurance.

  Another way of acquiring ATP is breaking down creatine phosphate, which is also done without the use of oxygen. This means of ATP production is limited to skeletal muscles and, as with other anerobic ATP production, provides small bursts of energy.

Oxygen Debt and Muscle Fatigue

When the body uses an excessive amount of oxygen, it must then take in enough oxygen to make up for the shortage and allow the body to recover, or return to a resting state. The amount of oxygen "owed" to the body to enable recovery is called **oxygen debt**.

Oxygen debt may occur when the skeletal muscles are used vigorously for more than one or two minutes, as with exercise. If your body is working hard, it may not be able to take in and absorb enough oxygen to cope with the level of activity. When oxygen is lacking, the body is unable to produce energy through aerobic means and, as a consequence, the anaerobic method of creating energy is activated.

Unfortunately, as already mentioned, anaerobic energy production is only short term, not enough for endurance. The body can only use anaerobic energy for about 60 seconds, depending on the individual. After this, fatigue sets in, making it very difficult to recover. To recover from oxygen debt, the body must increase respiration to bring more oxygen into the bloodstream to reach the muscles. An example is a sprinter running a short distance very fast. At the end of the sprint, the athlete is breathing heavily to compensate for the oxygen debt.

Muscle fatigue usually develops as a result of an accumulation of the lactic acid that is produced along with ATP during anaerobic metabolism. This accumulation of lactic acid decreases the muscle's ability to contract. This causes the muscle to become incredibly fatigued, and muscle cramps may occur. Muscle fatigue may also occur if the blood supply to a muscle is stopped or interrupted or if a motor neuron loses its ability to release a neurotransmitter substance called acetylcholine into the muscle fibers.

STRUCTURE OF SKELETAL MUSCLES

As already mentioned, skeletal muscle attaches to bone and is voluntarily controlled (Figure 23-3). More than 600 different skeletal muscles are responsible for the movement of the body through contractility, extensibility, and elasticity. Various sizes, shapes, and fiber arrangements create a variety of muscles, each of which can perform a specific function, or multiple functions, in the body.

Connective tissue forms several types of coverings for skeletal muscle for the purpose of function and protection. Mentioned earlier in the chapter, fascia is the connective tissue that covers each skeletal muscle and functions to separate the muscles from one another. Information related to additional structures that comprise skeletal muscles is found in Table 23-1.

Attachments to Skeletal Muscles

Actions of skeletal muscles depend greatly on where the skeletal muscles attach to bone. Origin and insertion are the points at which skeletal muscles attach to given structures. The **origin** is a muscle's attachment point to a bone that is primarily fixed or still; the **insertion** is the attachment point of the other end of that muscle to a bone that moves. For example, the biceps muscle has its origin at the shoulder; its insertion point is in the forearm, close to the elbow. The biceps muscle's insertion point near the elbow enables the forearm to flex during muscle contraction, and the other end of the muscle is anchored at the origin point on the unmoving shoulder (Figure 23-4).

Muscles and nerves function together as a motor unit. For skeletal muscles to contract, they must be stimulated by impulses from motor nerves.

Muscles perform in groups that are classified in the following categories:

- **Prime mover** or **agonist**—A muscle that is the primary actor in a given movement. This is the muscle that produces the movement in muscle contraction. For example, when the knee extends, the prime mover is the quadriceps.

- **Antagonist**—A muscle that counteracts, or opposes, the action of another muscle. When the biceps contracts, the triceps relaxes; this is an antagonist pair.

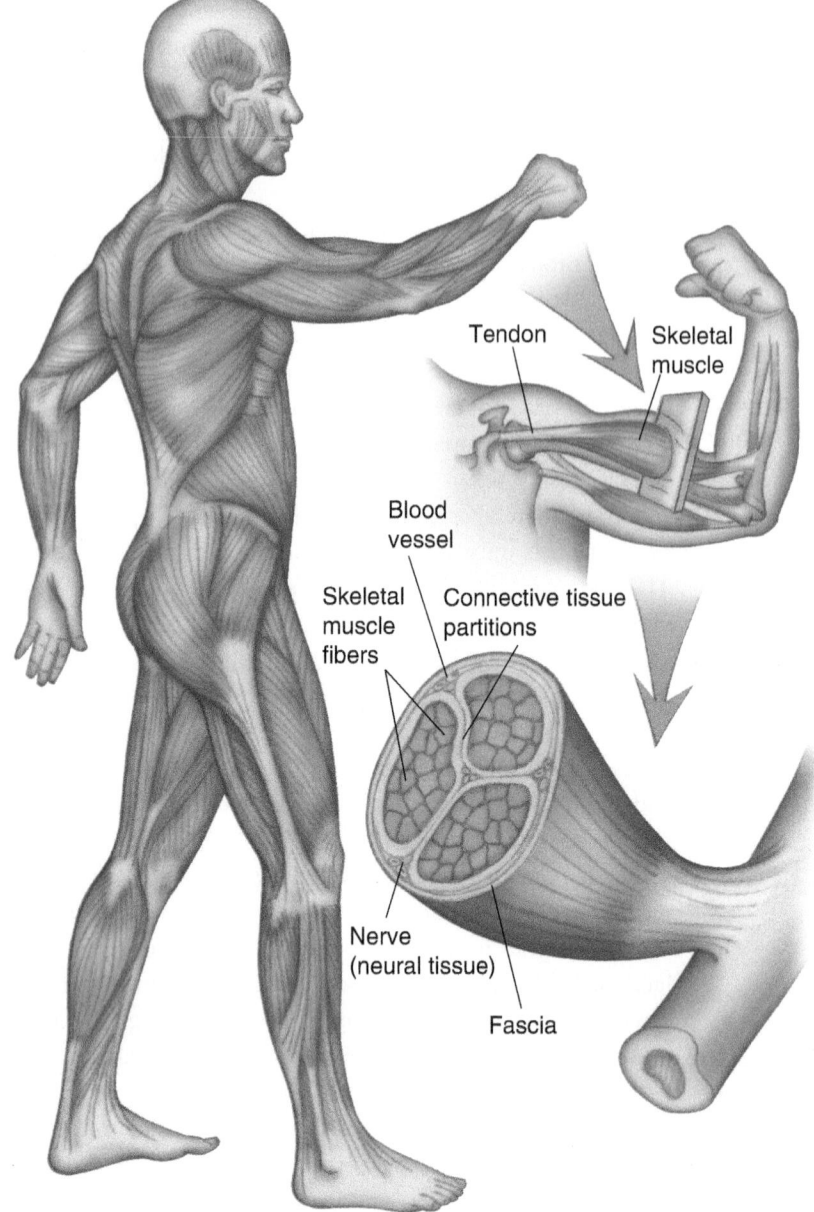

FIGURE 23-3 A skeletal muscle consists of a group of fibers held together by connective tissue. It is enclosed in a fibrous sheath (fascia).

TABLE 23-1 | **Skeletal Muscle Structures**

Structure	Description
Epimysium	A thin fascia that surrounds and covers skeletal muscle. It helps keep skeletal muscles separated from one another.
Perimysium	Made of connective tissue, perimysium divides muscle into smaller sections called fascicles.
Endomysium	A protective covering made of connective tissue that surrounds the individual muscle cell.
Tendon	Thick structure made of fibrous connective tissue. Tendons connect skeletal muscle to bones.
Aponeurosis	A thin, sheet-like tendon that connects muscle to muscle.

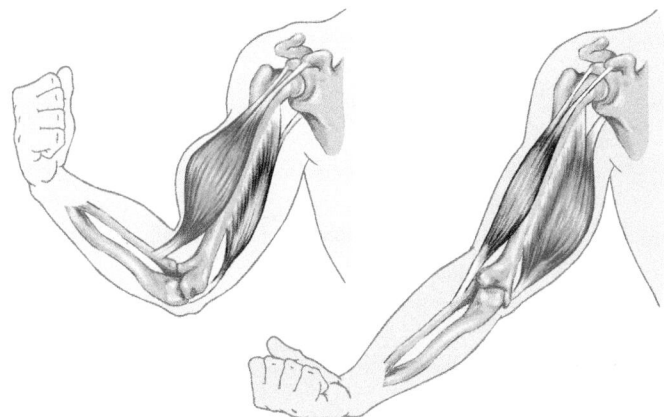

FIGURE 23-4 The origin of the bicep is at the shoulder; the insertion is in the forearm.

- **Synergist**—A muscle that acts with another muscle, most often a prime mover, to produce movement. When performing a squat exercise, the prime mover muscles are the quadriceps and the gluteus maximus, and the synergist muscles are those in the hamstrings group.

MAJOR SKELETAL MUSCLES

When describing the major skeletal muscles, it is important to remember that these muscles are often identified according to their location, size, action, shape, or number of attachments to the muscle. They are usually listed in the following groups:

- Muscles of the head
- Muscles of the arm, wrist, hand, and fingers
- Respiratory muscles
- Abdominal muscles
- Muscles of the pectoral girdle
- Muscles of the leg, ankle, and foot

Muscles of the Head

The muscles of the head include those that move the head, provide facial expressions, and move the jaw (see Figure 23-5). They include the following muscles:

- **Sternocleidomastoid**—Pulls the head from side to side and to the chest
- **Splenius capitis**—Rotates the head and allows it to bend to the side

The muscles that provide for facial expression include the following:

- **Frontalis**—Raises the eyebrows

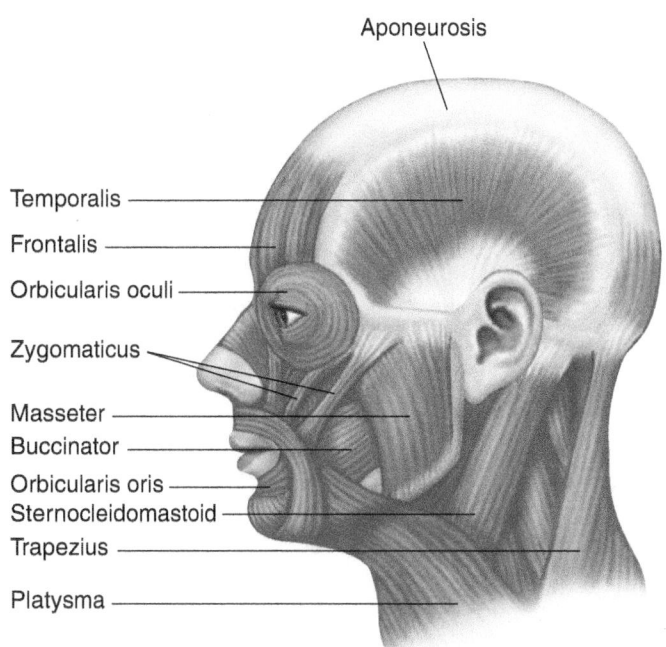

FIGURE 23-5 Muscles of the head, neck, and face.

- **Orbicularis oris**—Allows the lips to pucker
- **Orbicularis oculi**—Allows the eyes to close
- **Zygomaticus**—Pulls up the corners of the mouth
- **Platysma**—Pulls down the corners of the mouth

The muscles of the jaw allow for chewing, or mastication. They include the following:

- **Masseter and temporalis**—Close the jaw

Muscles of the Arm, Wrist, Hand, and Fingers

Figures 23-6 and 23-7 illustrate many of the muscles of the arm, wrist, hand, and fingers.

Muscles that move the upper extremity include those in the arm and forearm:

- **Pectoralis major**—Pulls the arm across the chest and also rotates and adducts the arms
- **Latissimus dorsi**—Provides for extension, adduction, and inward rotation of the arm
- **Deltoid**—Provides for abduction and extension of the arm at the shoulder
- **Serratus anterior**—Also known as the "boxer's muscle," pulls the scapula forward
- **Subscapularis**—Rotates the arm medially
- **Infraspinatus**—Rotates the arm laterally
- **Biceps brachii**—Flexes the arm at the elbow and rotates the hand laterally

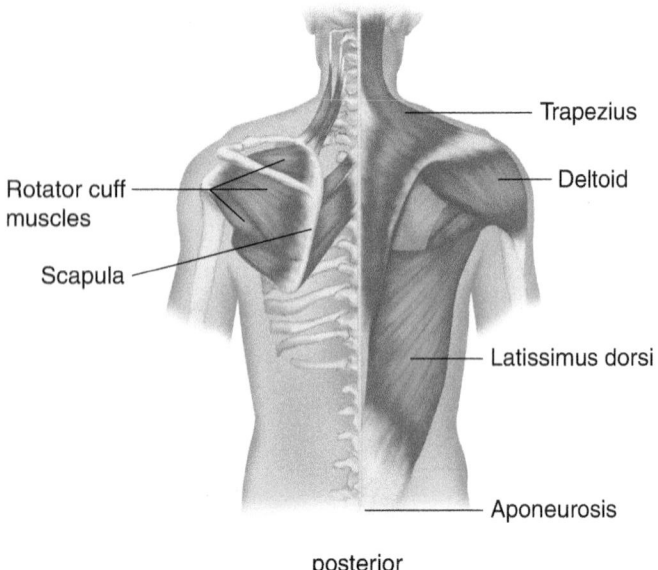

FIGURE 23-6 Muscles of the posterior torso that are responsible for arm movements.

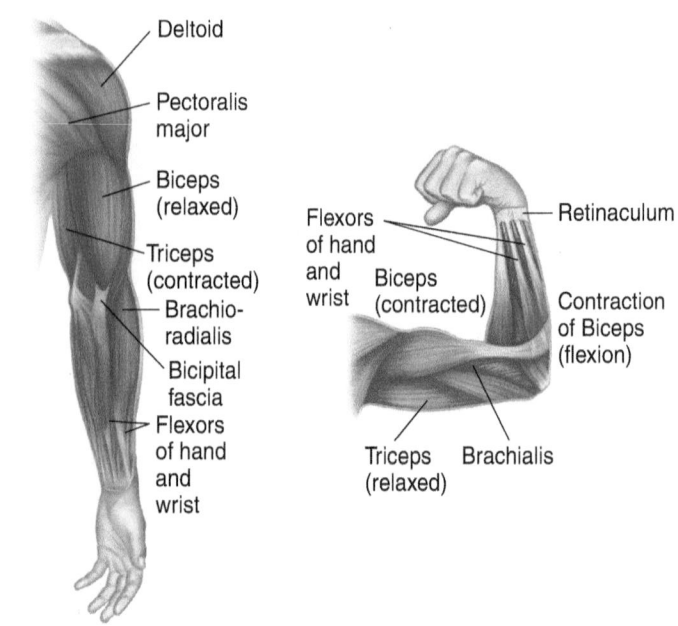

FIGURE 23-7 Muscles of the arm and hand.

- **Brachialis**—Flexes the arm at the elbow
- **Brachioradialis**—Flexes the forearm at the elbow
- **Triceps brachii**—Extends the arm at the elbow
- **Supinator**—Rotates the forearm laterally
- **Pronator teres**—Rotates the forearm medially

Muscles that move the wrist, hand, and fingers include the following:

- **Flexor carpi radialis** and **flexor carpi ulnaris**—Flex and abduct the wrist
- **Palmaris longus**—Flexes the wrist
- **Flexor digitorum profundus**—Flexes the distal joints of the fingers but not the thumb
- **Extensor carpi radialis longus** and **extensor carpi radialis brevis**—Extend the wrist and abduct the hand
- **Extensor carpi ulnaris**—Extends the wrist
- **Extensor digitorum**—Extends the fingers but not the thumb

Respiratory Muscles

The muscles of respiration include the following:

- **Diaphragm**—Separates the thoracic cavity from the abdominal cavity; its contraction causes the process of inspiration
- **External and internal intercostals**—Contraction expands and lowers the ribs during breathing

Abdominal Muscles

The muscles of the abdominal wall include the following (Figure 23-8):

- **External and internal obliques**—Compress the abdominal wall
- **Transversus abdominis**—Also compresses the abdominal wall
- **Rectus abdominis**—Flexes the vertebral column and compresses the abdominal wall

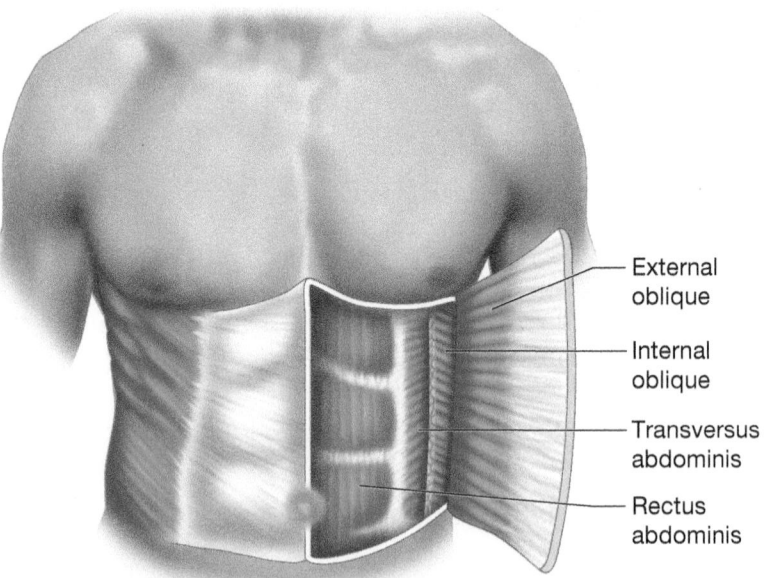

FIGURE 23-8 Abdominal muscles.

Muscles of the Pectoral Girdle

The muscles that move the pectoral girdle, or shoulder, include the following:

- **Trapezius**—Raises the arms and pulls the shoulders downward
- **Pectoralis minor**—Pulls the scapula downward and raises the rib cage

Muscles of the Leg, Ankle, and Foot

The muscles that move the leg include the following (Figure 23-9):

- **Psoas major**—Flexes and externally rotates the hip joint
- **Iliacus**—Flexes the thigh and rotates it medially
- **Gluteus maximus**—Extends the thigh
- **Gluteus medius** and **minimus**—Abduct the thigh and rotate it laterally

- **Hamstring group**—Flexes the leg at the knee and extends the leg at the thigh; muscles in this group include the biceps femoris, semitendinosus, and semimembranosus
- **Quadriceps group**—Extends the leg at the knee; muscles in this group include vastus lateralis, vastus medialis, vastus intermedius, and the rectus femoris
- **Sartorius**—Performs multiple functions including flexing the knee and thigh, abducting the thigh, and enabling the act of being able to sit cross-legged

The muscles that move the ankle and foot include the following:

- **Gastrocnemius**—Flexes the foot and aids in pushing the body forward
- **Tibialis anterior**—Causes dorsiflexion and inversion of the foot

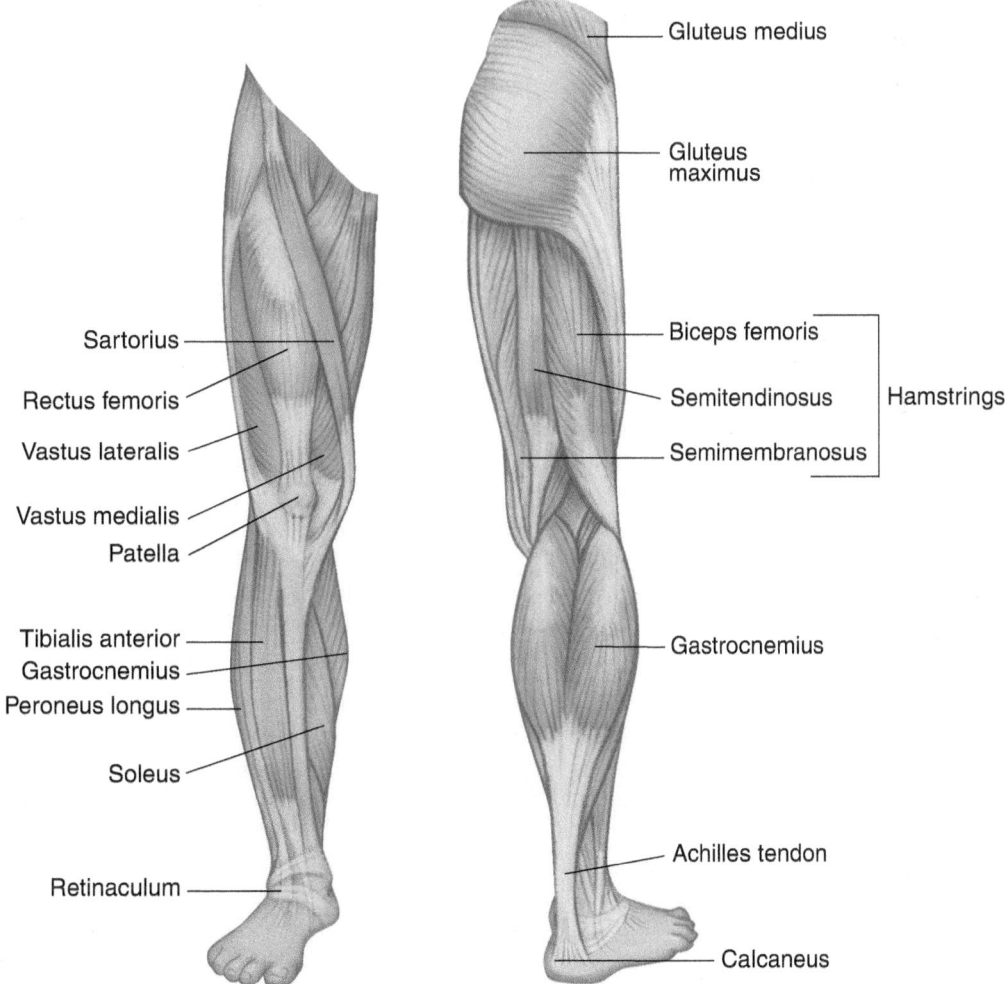

FIGURE 23-9 Muscles of the buttocks, legs, and feet.

- **Peroneus**—Everts the foot and helps bring about plantar flexion
- **Flexor digitorum longus** and **extensor digitorum longus**—Flex and extend the toes, respectively, and assist in other movements of the feet

COMMON PATHOLOGY ASSOCIATED WITH THE MUSCULAR SYSTEM

Because of the sheer number of muscles, the diseases and disorders associated with the muscular system are quite numerous. Muscular disorders are characterized by abnormalities of muscle fibers. In addition, many neurological disorders, such as lesions of the central or peripheral nervous system and abnormalities of neuromuscular transmission, can also produce symptoms that are primarily muscular. Other systemic disorders, including those that are frequently seen in conditions of the cardiovascular, respiratory, and endocrine systems, frequently mimic muscular disorders but do not directly affect muscular function. These systemic disorders account for more than half of all muscular complaints. Table 23-2 identifies diagnostic procedures and tests related to the muscular system.

Atrophy

Atrophy is the loss of muscle mass and strength that occurs when muscles aren't used over a long period of time. Often, atrophy results from bed rest and immobility, but it can also be caused by malnutrition and injury. Atrophy can also be secondary to a primary disease or disorder such as a spinal cord injury, polio, or stroke, to name a few. Lipoatrophy (also known as lipodystrophy) is atrophy of fat tissue. It is common for lipoatrophy to occur at a site of insulin or corticosteroid injections.

Signs and Symptoms. The most common sign of atrophy is the apparent "wasting away" appearance of a muscle group. Frequently, patients have extreme weakness and fatigue associated with atrophic muscle groups.

Treatment. Exercise is the best course of treatment for muscle atrophy. This is done under the care and supervision of a physician and a physical therapist. Isometric exercise of the immobilized muscle can be particularly useful. This form of exercise uses active muscle contractions performed against stable resistance (e.g., tightening the muscles of the thighs or the buttocks). Active exercise of uninjured limbs helps prevent atrophy.

TABLE 23-2 | Procedures and Diagnostic Tests Related to the Muscular System

Procedure/Test	Description
Aldolase	Blood serum test to measure ALD enzyme present in skeletal and heart muscle to diagnose Duchenne muscular dystrophy before symptoms appear.
Calcium	Blood serum test to determine levels of calcium. Calcium is essential for muscular contraction, nerve transmission, and blood clotting.
Creatine Phosphatase (CPK)	Blood serum test to measure the CPK level that increases because of necrosis or atrophy of skeletal muscle, traumatic muscle injury, strenuous exercise, progressive muscular dystrophy, and after heart attack.
Electromyography (EMG)	Study and record of the strength of muscle contractions as a result of electrical stimulation. Used in the diagnosis of muscle disorders and to distinguish nerve disorders from muscle disorders.
Fasciectomy	Surgical removal of the fascia (fibrous membrane) covering and supporting muscles.
Lactic Dehydrogenase (LDH)	Blood serum test to measure the level of the enzyme LDH. It is increased in muscular dystrophy, after damage to skeletal muscles, after pulmonary embolism, and during skeletal muscle malignancy.
Magnetic Resonance Imaging (MRI)	Medical imaging that uses a magnetic field and radio waves as its source of energy. It does not require the injection of contrast medium or exposure to ionizing radiation. The technique is useful for visualizing large blood vessels, the heart, brain, and soft tissues.
Muscle Biopsy	Removal of muscle tissue for pathological examination.
Serum Glutamic Oxaloacetic Transaminase (SGOT)	Blood serum test to measure the level of the enzyme SGOT. It is increased in skeletal muscle damage and muscular dystrophy. This test is also called aspartate aminotransferase (AST).
Serum Glutamic Pyruvic Transaminase (SGPT)	Blood serum test to measure the level of the enzyme SGPT. It is increased in skeletal muscle damage. This test is also called alanine aminotransferase (ALT).

Fibromyalgia

Fibromyalgia is a widespread disorder affecting an estimated three million individuals in the United States. It is characterized by musculoskeletal pain and fatigue. Fibromyalgia occurs more often in women than men. There is no obvious known cause of fibromyalgia, but evidence points to a genetic predisposition that creates a neuromuscular or neuroendocrine abnormality that disturbs usual sensory perception, especially pain signals.

Signs and Symptoms. Symptoms include mild to severe muscle pain and fatigue, sleep disorders, irritable bowel syndrome, depression, and chronic headaches.

The American College of Rheumatology (ACR) has identified specific criteria for the diagnosis of fibromyalgia. The ACR states that a patient must show pain at 11 of 18 trigger or tender points to be considered for a diagnosis of fibromyalgia (Figure 23-10). The patient must also have a history of widespread pain lasting at least three months.

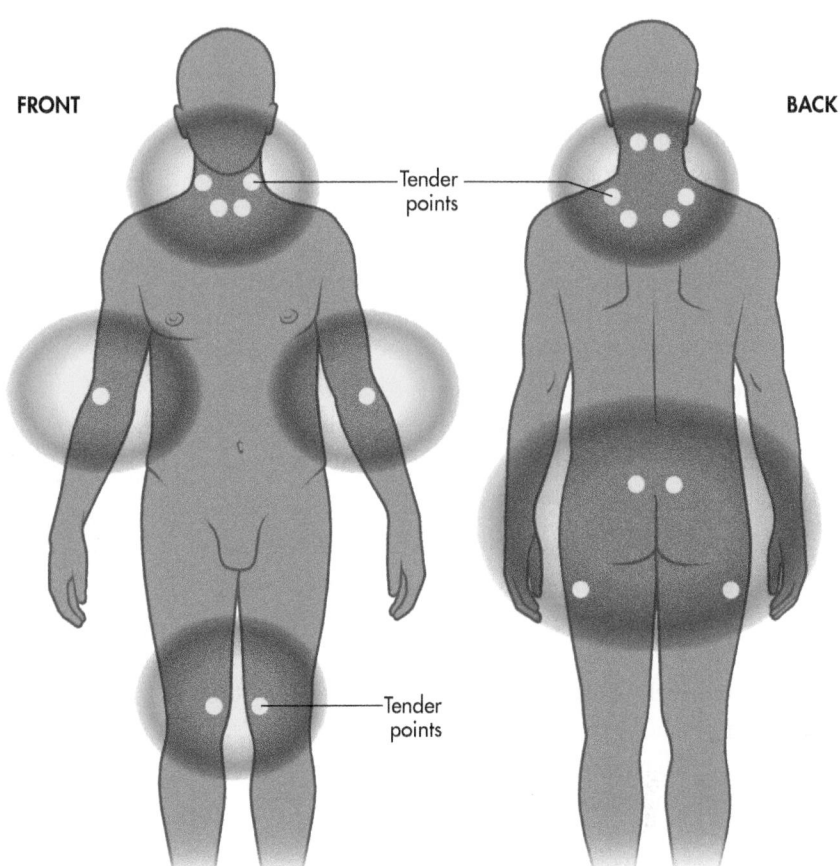

FRONT   BACK

Tender points

Tender points

FIGURE 23-10 The 18 tender points of fibromyalgia.

Treatment. There is no cure for fibromyalgia. Treatment is geared toward improving the quality of life and reducing pain. Sleep is important for many body functions, including tissue repair and antibody production, so the disruption of sleep directly affects the quality of life in a patient with fibromyalgia. Therefore, an emphasis is often placed on improving the patient's sleep as well. Frequently, the medications prescribed for fibromyalgia include muscle relaxants, pain relievers, antiinflammatory drugs, antidepressants, and antianxiety drugs. Other treatments frequently employed include chiropractic, acupuncture, acupressure, relaxation techniques, and massage.

Ganglion Cyst

A **ganglion cyst** is a benign (noncancerous) saclike swelling or fluid-filled cyst. Typically the cysts develop over a joint or tendon. Ganglion cysts occur more frequently in women than in men. It is thought that these cysts are caused by repetitive motions; however, this might not be true in all cases.

Signs and Symptoms. A ganglion cyst is often painless but can be very painful if its location causes it to press on a nerve. Typically, these fluid-filled masses occur on the back of the hand at the wrist, but also on the palm side of the wrist. They may also develop, less frequently, on the top of the foot, on the outside of the knee or ankle, and where the base of the fingers meet the palm of the hand. Swelling may occur, although it is often erratic, developing and disappearing without apparent cause.

Treatment. Treatment is not necessary if the cyst is asymptomatic and painless. Antiinflammatory drugs can be used to reduce swelling and pain. Often **aspiration** (removal by suction of fluid from within the cyst) is performed. This treatment is about 74 percent effective against recurrence of the cyst. If the cyst causes pain or decreased range of motion, surgery may be performed. Even surgical removal of a ganglion cyst is not always 100 percent effective against recurrence.

Lyme Disease

Lyme disease is caused by the *Borrelia burgdorferi* bacterium. It is carried by ticks, frequently found on deer and other wild animals. The bacterium is transmitted through the bite of an infected tick. Prevention of Lyme disease is the best medicine.

Signs and Symptoms. A round bull's-eye rash is typically associated with Lyme disease. This rash is also known as erythema migrans (EM) and generally feels warm to the touch, though it is not generally painful or itchy. Additional symptoms of Lyme disease include headache, fatigue, neck stiffness, and fever. Signs and symptoms of Lyme disease vary from patient to patient, with many of the signs and symptoms also typical of other diseases. Not everyone who contracts Lyme disease develops the hallmark bull's-eye rash. With symptoms mimicking other diseases and lack of the bull's-eye rash, this condition can be difficult to diagnose. Unfortunately, the condition often worsens when left untreated. Prevention measures include wearing long sleeves and long pants while in heavily wooded areas, the proper use of insect repellent, and the prompt removal of any tick that may be lodged in the skin.

Treatment. If Lyme disease is detected early, full recovery is possible. This is accomplished by taking the prescribed round of antibiotic medications. Antibiotics often prescribed include erythromycin, penicillins, or doxycycline. If not detected early, Lyme disease can result in skin, joint, heart, and nervous system disorders. Because Lyme disease is difficult to diagnose with certainty but can have severe consequences, the course of treatment is usually prescribed if Lyme disease is strongly suspected.

Muscular Dystrophy

Muscular dystrophy (MD) is a disease that progressively weakens and causes degeneration of the body's skeletal (voluntary) muscles, thereby reducing the patient's control of movement. It is a genetic disease with more than 30 different forms. Although mostly affecting skeletal muscles, some involuntary muscles including the muscles of the heart may also be affected. Some forms of the MD also impact organ functions. The major forms of MD include the following:

- Duchenne MD
- Becker MD
- limb-girdle MD
- facioscapulohumeral (FSH) MD
- congenital MD
- oculopharyngeal MD
- distal MD
- Emery-Dreifuss MD
- myotonic MD

Signs and Symptoms. Each form of MD has its own set of specific signs and symptoms. However, there are general signs and symptoms that are common in all forms and are specific to muscle groups affected. These include muscle weakness, loss of coordination, and immobility. Signs and

symptoms that are more varied based on the specific form of MD could include difficulty walking and frequent falls, delayed development of motor skills, and mental retardation. Skeletal deformities such as a curved spine, clubfoot, and the formation of a claw hand may occur. Unfortunately, the progression of this disease results in fatality.

Treatment. There is no cure for MD in any form. Treatment is geared toward prolonging and improving the quality of life. Physical therapy is implemented to sustain and build muscle strength and overall flexibility. Some patients may use orthotic devices to provide support, and others undergo corrective orthopedic surgeries. Respiratory therapy is especially important for those whose respiratory muscles and overall respiratory system are affected by the disease. Patients with MD may be prescribed a variety of medications, including corticosteroids that help slow the progression of muscle degeneration and antibiotics to prevent respiratory infections. Anticonvulsants are also commonly used.

Myasthenia Gravis

Myasthenia gravis (MG) is a chronic autoimmune neuromuscular disease. Its name, translated from its Latin origin, means "grave muscle weakness." The hallmark characteristic of this disease is muscle weakness that affects voluntary muscles. MG most commonly occurs in young adult women and older men but can occur at any age. Although MG may affect any voluntary muscle, certain muscles, including those that control eye movements, eyelids, chewing, swallowing, coughing, and facial expressions, are more often affected.

Signs and Symptoms. The primary symptom of MG is muscle weakness. The muscle weakness increases during periods of activity and improves after periods of rest. The muscles involved in MG vary from one individual to the next.

Treatment. Although there is no cure for MG, people living with this disease are not only able to control it but also can lead full and productive lives. Because it is an autoimmune disorder, medications may be given to decrease the production of antibodies that the body perceives as abnormal and a threat. Medications to improve muscle strength as well as neuromuscular transmission are also prescribed. Physicians determine individualized treatment based on the patient's age, symptoms, overall health, and general prognosis of the disease.

Rotator Cuff Tears

The rotator cuff is the area that enables people to reach above their heads and lift with the arms. Rotator cuff tears are

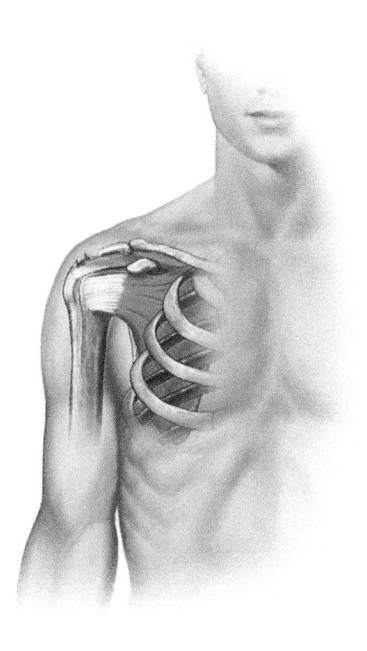

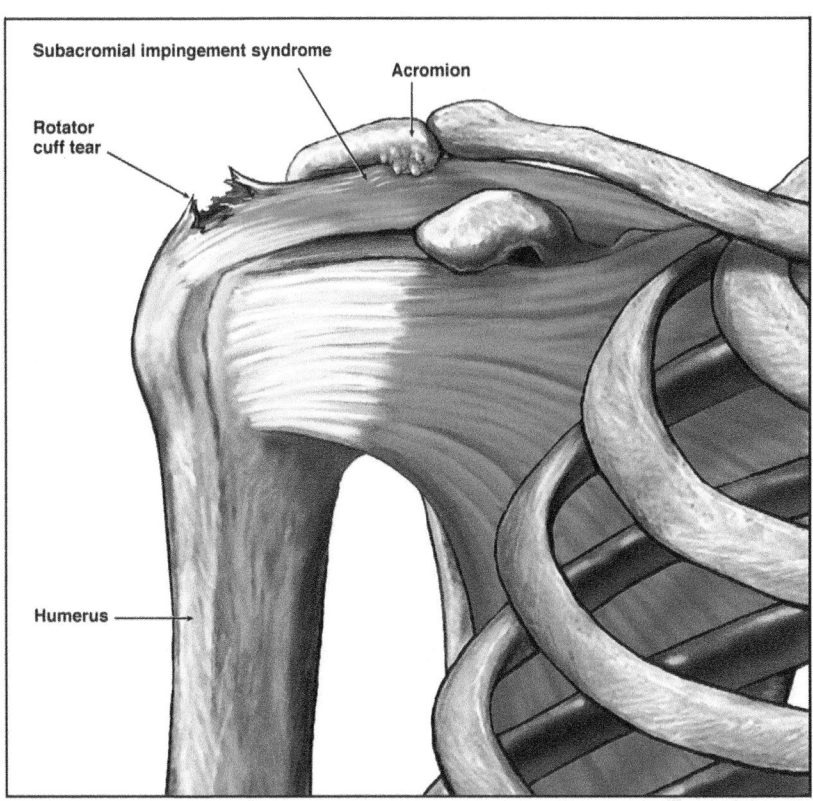

Subacromial impingement syndrome

Acromion

Rotator cuff tear

Humerus

Anterior view of shoulder

FIGURE 23-11 A rotator cuff tear.

increasingly common in the muscles that form the shoulder and their tendons (supraspinatus, infraspinatus, teres minor, and subscapularis) (Figure 23-11). Most rotator cuff tears occur as the result of many years of overuse of the muscles and tendons; however, one single traumatic injury can also cause a rotator cuff tear.

Signs and Symptoms. These tears can cause considerable pain and limit the function and range of motion of the patient. In addition, signs include atrophy of the shoulder muscle and a crackling sensation when moving the shoulder in certain positions.

Treatment. Treatment for a torn rotator cuff includes rest, narcotic and nonsteroidal antiinflammatory drugs (NSAIDs), splinting, physical therapy, and performing range-of-motion exercises. More severe rotator cuff tears may require steroid injections and possibly surgery.

Shin Splints

Shin splints are caused by inflammation of the periosteum of the extensor muscles of the lower leg (particularly the tibia) and surrounding tissues. The condition is usually caused by overuse or improper conditioning of the leg muscles. Shin splints commonly occur with running sports, military

training, and high-impact dancing and in people with flat feet or rigid arches.

Signs and Symptoms. General symptoms and signs of a shin splint include increased pain, tenderness, and possible swelling in the shin area. These effects can cause pain when walking or moving the lower legs.

Treatment. Shin splint treatment includes rest and applying ice or cold compresses to the shin area. Medication such as aspirin and NSAIDs may be used for pain management and to reduce swelling. Treatment also includes the use of proper footwear, which can prevent future episodes.

Sprains and Strains

A **sprain**—a stretching or tearing—is an injury to a **ligament** (connective tissue that connects bones or cartilage, or holds a joint together), whereas a **strain** is an injury to either a muscle or a tendon (which connects muscle to bone). A strain may be the result of a simple overstretching muscle injury, or it could be as severe as a tear to the tendon or muscle.

Sprains

Sprains are very common injuries, especially among athletes. Often a sprain will occur after a ligament has been overstretched or torn, especially in ligaments of major joints such as elbows, knees, wrists, ankles, and feet. Ankle sprains are the most common injury in the United States.

Signs and Symptoms. Typically, the signs and symptoms associated with a sprain include pain, swelling, bruising, and loss of joint mobility and function. Depending on the severity of the sprain, these signs and symptoms vary in intensity. Often the signs and symptoms have a sudden onset as they immediately follow an injury.

Treatment. Sprains are generally treated using the RICE method:

- **Rest**—If the injured joint is a weight-bearing joint, such as the ankle, it is important to use canes, crutches, or other walking devices.

- **Ice**—Ice the sprain with an ice pack or cold compress.

- **Compression**—Compression bandages should be worn around the sprain to encourage proper healing.

- **Elevation**—Elevate the affected sprain as soon as possible after an injury. It is most beneficial to have the strained muscle either above or at the same level as the heart.

Additional treatments may include range-of-motion exercises, physical therapy, and NSAIDs. Surgery, which is a rarity, may be performed when a sprain has been classified as chronic and other forms of treatment are not effective.

Strains

The twisting or pulling of a muscle often results in a strain. Prolonged, repetitive movements generally result in a chronic strain, whereas an acute strain may be caused by improperly lifting a heavy object. In addition, sports including soccer, football, hockey, tennis, gymnastics, and many others tend to place individuals at higher risk for muscle strains.

Signs and Symptoms. Common symptoms associated with a strain include pain, muscle weakness, muscle spasm, and loss of muscle function. Inflammation and cramping, accompanied by swelling, may also be associated with a strain.

Treatment. The treatment for a strain is very similar to that of a sprain. Rest, cold compressions, antiinflammatory medication, and gentle stretching are often helpful. Heat application, as with a heating pad, is also beneficial and should be alternated with applications of cold compresses. At times, a physician may recommend the application of a brace to limit mobility of the injured muscle.

Tendonitis

Mentioned earlier in this chapter, a **tendon** is the band of connective tissue found at each end of a muscle that attaches

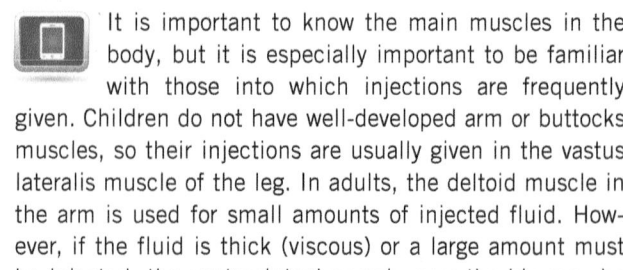

the muscle to a bone. Excessive and repetitive movements are often the cause of **tendonitis** (also spelled *tendinitis*), an inflammation of the tendon, which occurs when the tiny fibers of the tendon begin to tear. The following are the areas commonly associated with tendonitis:

- Elbow and wrist
- Biceps and shoulder
- Hip, leg, and knee
- Achilles tendon

Signs and Symptoms. Pain and stiffness commonly surround the affected area. Also, this condition has been known to cause a burning sensation that surrounds the joint and inflamed tendon. Generally, pain is worse during and immediately after activity, whereas the following day the tendon tends to become stiffer, though it still causes a significant amount of pain.

Treatment. With proper care, tendonitis should lessen with rest over time. However, complete healing may take up to six weeks following the initial injury. The initial approach to treating tendonitis is to support and protect the tendons by bracing any areas of the tendon that are being pulled during use. It is important to loosen up the tendon, reduce the pain, and minimize any inflammation. Physical therapy, including exercises to increase range of motion, has proven to be a very beneficial treatment for tendonitis.

Tetanus

Tetanus can be fatal. It is an infectious disease caused by the bacterium *Clostridium tetani*, which usually enters the body through a puncture, cut, or open wound. *Clostridium tetani* releases a toxin that affects the motor nerves (which stimulate the muscles). This bacterium is commonly found in dust, soil, and manure.

Signs and Symptoms. Tetanus is characterized by profoundly painful muscle spasms all over the body. Most recognized is a locking effect that results in the mouth being unable to open (lockjaw). Difficulty swallowing is experienced because of neck stiffness, along with stiffness of the chest, abdominal, and back muscles. Fevers are also common with tetanus.

Treatment. Preventing tetanus is the best course of treatment. All children should be immunized against tetanus by receiving a full series of five diphtheria, pertussis, and tetanus (DPT, or Tdap) vaccinations, which generally are started at 2 months of age and are completed around 5 years of age. The tetanus and diphtheria (Td) vaccination is now recommended at 11 to 12 years of age if at least five years have elapsed since the last dose of a tetanus and diphtheria toxoid containing vaccine. Follow-up booster vaccination is recommended every 10 years thereafter (i.e., 21 years old, 31 years old, etc.). In adult patients, it is recommended that the patient receive one dose of Tdap as a booster for tetanus, diphtheria, and pertussis during adulthood. It is recommended that the Tdap booster be given at least two years after a Td booster has been administered. Should an unvaccinated person contract tetanus, the likely course of treatment would include the administration of antitoxin, such as tetanus immune globulin, administration of antibiotics, and vaccination.

SUMMARY

The muscular system is composed of specialized cells called muscle fibers. These fibers, when brought together, form muscle, which makes up about 42 percent of a person's total body weight. The purpose of muscles is to create movement, maintain stability, assist in circulation and respiration, assist in heat production, and aid in digestion and elimination. To achieve this, muscles must be supplied with proper nutrition and oxygen.

The three types of muscle are smooth, skeletal, and cardiac. Voluntary muscles, which are striated, move in coordination with decisions from the nervous system, either from the brain or spinal column. Involuntary muscles, which are smooth, are not regulated by the conscious thought of the individual. Cardiac tissue is both smooth and striated. Thus, a person does not voluntarily control whether the heart contracts but can influence its rate or rhythm.

Muscles are named by their purpose, structure, or location. Prime movers (agonists) are the primary actor in a given movement. Antagonists counteract the action of another muscle. Synergists act with another muscle to produce movement.

Muscles receive a lot of wear and tear, and thus many disorders can develop. Among the disorders associated with the muscular system are atrophy, fibromyalgia, ganglion cysts, Lyme disease, muscular dystrophy, myasthenia gravis, rotator cuff tears, shin splints, sprains and strains, tendonitis, and tetanus.

23 CHAPTER REVIEW

COMPETENCY REVIEW

1. Define and spell the terms for this chapter.
2. Name the three types of muscle tissue.
3. What are the two points of attachment for muscles?
4. What are the other names for skeletal muscle?
5. What are other names for smooth muscle?
6. List the six groups of major skeletal muscles.
7. Give examples of internal organs with smooth muscle.
8. What is the name and special property of heart muscle?
9. Why is the rotator cuff especially important to the patient's range of motion?
10. What are the five main functions of muscle?

PREPARING FOR THE CERTIFICATION EXAM

1. Which of the following muscles is located in the arm?
   a. rectus abdominis
   b. gastrocnemius
   c. rectus femoris
   d. triceps
   e. pectoralis major

2. A muscle that is considered a prime mover, may also be termed a/an
   a. synergist.
   b. agonist.
   c. antagonist.
   d. primary muscle.
   e. synergist mover.

3. Which muscle pulls the head from side to side and pulls the head to the chest?
   a. gastrocnemius
   b. biceps femoris
   c. gluteus maximus
   d. deltoid
   e. sternocleidomastoid

4. Which muscle(s) extends the thigh?
   a. tibialis anterior
   b. gastrocnemius
   c. gluteus maximus
   d. extensor carpi ulnaris
   e. external obliques

5. Which of the following diseases is caused by *Borrelia burgdorferi?*
   a. Lyme disease
   b. muscular dystrophy
   c. myasthenia gravis
   d. tetanus
   e. plantar fasciitis

6. Which of the following diseases has a preventative vaccine?
   a. muscular dystrophy
   b. ganglion cyst
   c. fibromyalgia
   d. tetanus
   e. myasthenia gravis

7. Which of the following is a genetic disorder?
   a. muscular dystrophy
   b. Lyme disease
   c. myasthenia gravis
   d. tetanus
   e. ganglion cyst

8. Which of the following separates the thoracic cavity from the abdominal cavity?
   a. peroneus
   b. diaphragm
   c. supinator
   d. pronator teres
   e. trapezius

9. Which of the following is in the pectoral girdle?
   a. gluteus maximus
   b. deltoid
   c. trapezius
   d. internal oblique
   e. frontalis

10. Which of the following is caused by twisting or pulling a muscle or tendon?
    a. sprain
    b. tendonitis
    c. strain
    d. myasthenia gravis
    e. cramping

CRITICAL THINKING

Refer to the case study at the beginning of the chapter and use the information you have learned to answer the following questions.

1. Should Rosa seek medical care for Felix? Explain why or why not.

2. What are some signs and symptoms Rosa should be looking for if she is concerned that her son may have been bitten by a tick infected with the *Borrelia burgdorferi* bacterium?

3. What measures can be taken to prevent being bitten by infected ticks?

INTERNET ACTIVITY

Do an Internet search to learn about resources for families who have members with muscular dystrophy.

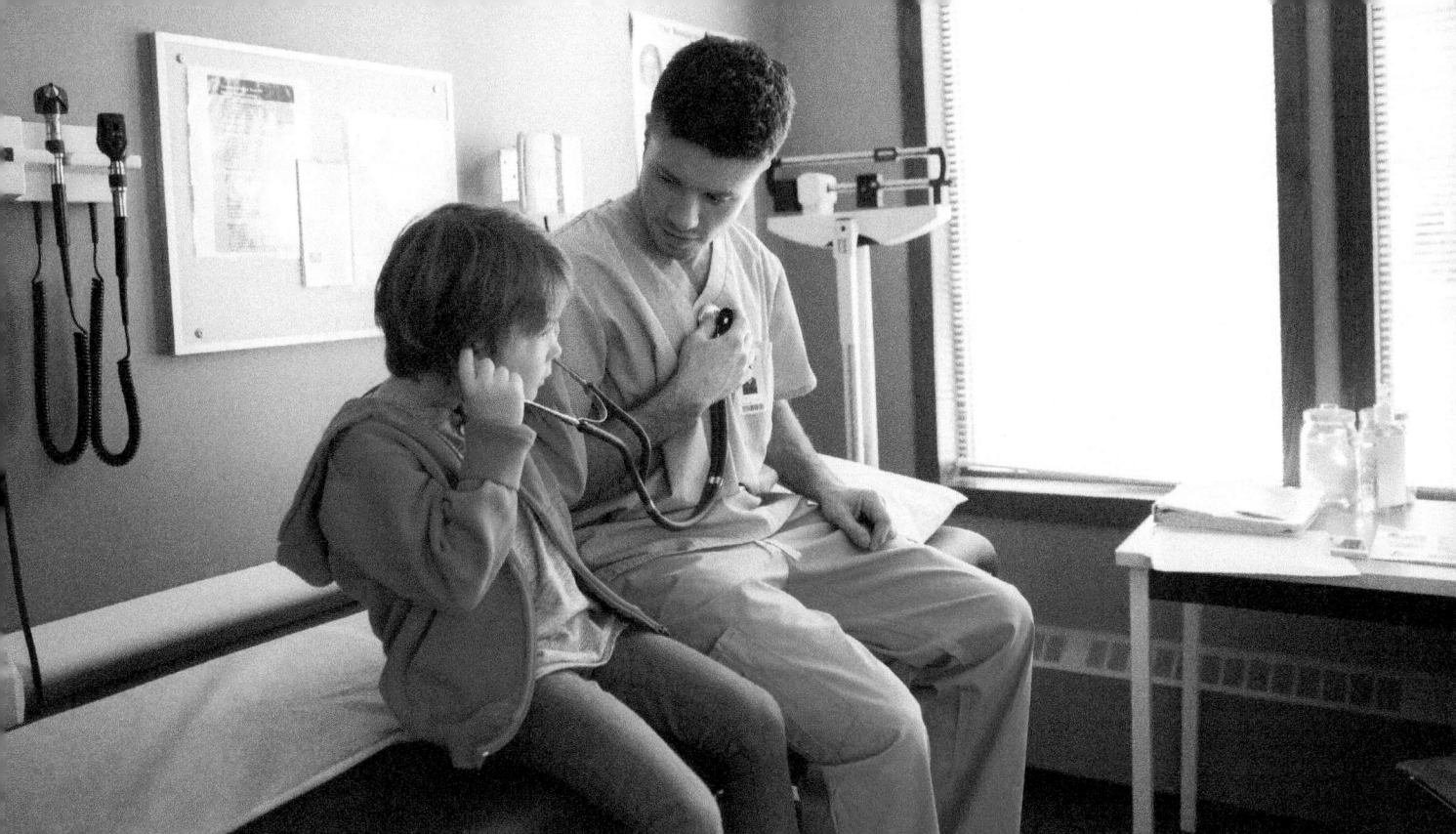

The Nervous System

Learning Objectives

After completing this chapter, you should be able to:

24.1   Define and spell the terms in this chapter.

24.2   Explain the relationship between the different sections of the nervous system.

24.3   List the functions of the nervous system.

24.4   Describe the structural units of the nervous system.

24.5   Describe how the nervous system changes between childhood and older adulthood.

24.6   Explain how nerve impulses are transmitted.

24.7   Detail the functions of the central nervous system based on its various parts.

24.8   Detail the functions of the peripheral nervous system based on its various parts.

24.9   Explain the delicate balance between the sympathetic and parasympathetic nervous systems.

24.10 Identify and explain common pathology associated with the nervous system.

Elena Bramatovich is 67 years old and has been a patient of Pearson Physicians Group for the past seven years. According to her family, Elena's memory and cognitive functions have been decreasing over the past couple of years. Her daughter, Svetlana, has written a letter to Dr. Miller regarding more drastic changes in her mother's behavior. Svetlana informs Dr. Miller that she is concerned that her mother is developing dementia.

Terms to Learn

afferent nerves	epilepsy	Parkinson's disease
Alzheimer's disease	fissure	peripheral nervous system (PNS)
amyotrophic lateral sclerosis (ALS)	gyri	quadriplegia
autonomic nervous system (ANS)	hemiplegia	sciatica
axon	interneurons	seizure
Bell's palsy	meninges	sensory neurons
central nervous system (CNS)	meningitis	sheaths
cerebrospinal fluid (CSF)	motor neurons	somatic nervous system (SNS)
concussion	multiple sclerosis (MS)	stroke
contusion	myelin	sulcus
corpus callosum	neuralgia	synapse
demyelination	neurilemma	synaptic space
dendrites	neuroglia	tract
efferent nerves	neurons	
encephalitis	paraplegia	

The nervous system is an essential and integral component of the human body. It acts to correlate external and internal factors that affect our bodies. For this to occur, the nervous system must gather, store, and decipher both external and internal information. Through careful analysis of this information, the nervous system decides how to respond and react in an appropriate manner to satisfy certain needs. Of these needs, the most important is the need for survival. The nervous system is made up of various subsystems and, although most are interrelated, some are able to function on their own.

SECTIONS AND FUNCTIONS OF THE NERVOUS SYSTEM

The brain and spinal cord make up the **central nervous system (CNS)**. The **peripheral nervous system (PNS)** is made up of nerves that connect the CNS to the other parts of the body (Figure 24-1). Subsections of the peripheral nervous system include the somatic nervous system (SNS) and the autonomic nervous system (ANS). The ANS is further divided into the sympathetic and parasympathetic nervous systems. Each of these divisions of the nervous system is discussed in further detail later in this chapter. Figure 24-2 illustrates the components of the nervous system and how they relate to each other.

The nervous system transfers information via electrical impulses that travel along the length of the nerve cells. The nerve cell processes information from the sensory nerves and initiates an action within milliseconds.

The nervous system is responsible for three separate functions: (1) It detects and interprets sensory information. (2) It then takes that information and makes decisions about how it is being received. (3) Finally, it carries out a motor function based on the decisions made.

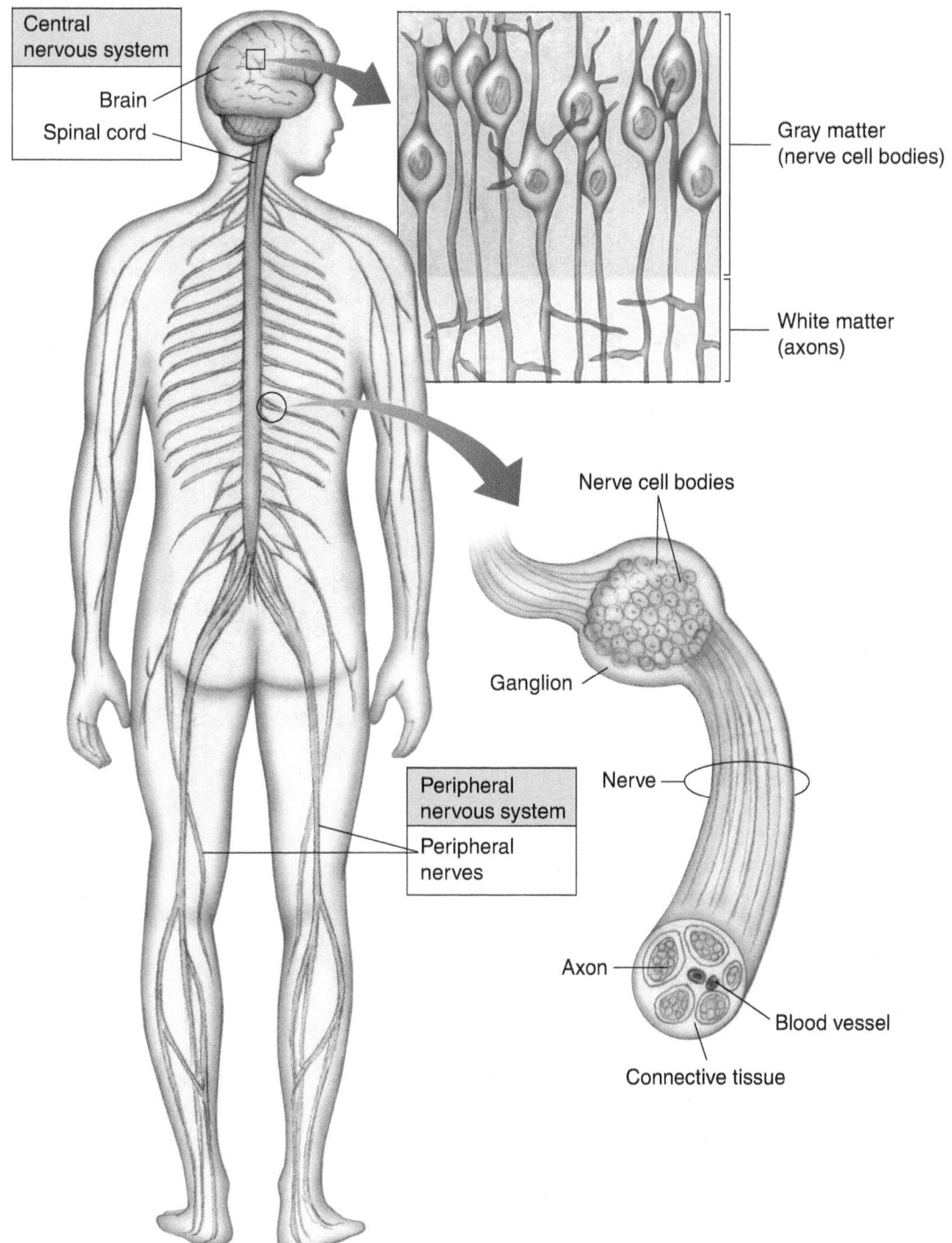

FIGURE 24-1 The nervous system.

STRUCTURAL UNITS OF THE NERVOUS SYSTEM

To understand how the nervous system functions, it is necessary to understand its fundamental structural units. Specialized tissue, nerve cells, fibers, and tracts all work together to execute both simple and complex functions of this intricate system.

Neurons

Nervous system tissue is made up of specialized nerve cells called **neurons** and supporting tissue structures known as **neuroglia**, which are also called *glia*. These supporting structures are further described in Table 24-1. There are three types of neurons: motor neurons, sensory neurons, and

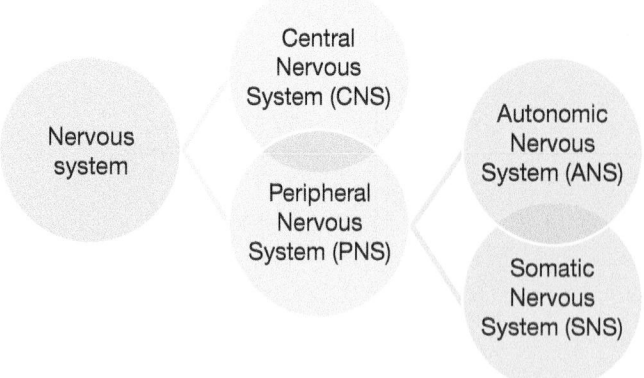

FIGURE 24-2 Components of the nervous system.

TABLE 24-1 | Types of Neuroglia

Structure	Function
Astrocytes	Attach blood vessels to the nerve cells; they are star-shaped in appearance
Microglia	Act to guard the cell and engulf invaders, as in a phagocytic mechanism
Oligodendrocytes	Help to produce the myelin sheath

interneurons. These cells enable the body to interact with its ever-changing internal and external environments.

Motor Neurons

Motor neurons control most of the body's functions, because they cause muscles to contract, glands to secrete, and organs to function properly. Motor neurons are considered **efferent nerves**. *Efferent* means "carrying away." Motor neurons transmit impulses away from neurons in the central nervous system to stimulate a target muscle, organ, or gland.

A motor neuron has processes (projections) known as the axon and dendrites that extend away from it in various directions. (Motor neurons usually have several dendrites and only one axon.) **Dendrites** receive information for the neuron, whereas the **axon** sends information away from the body of the cell. The axon is covered with a fatty insulating substance called the *myelin sheath*. Axons may be several feet long and reach all the way from the cell body to the area that is to be activated. Dendrites resemble tree branches and are unsheathed (Figure 24-3).

Sensory Neurons

Sensory neurons are attached to the sensory receptors of the body and transmit sensory information from these receptors

to the central nervous system through a peripheral process (projection). Sensory neurons lack true dendrites, are sheathed, and more closely resemble axons (Figure 24-4). When information from the sensory neuron is received, the CNS activates motor neurons to respond to the information. As already noted, motor neurons are called efferent nerves, meaning that they carry impulses away from the CNS to other parts of the body. By contrast, sensory neurons are referred to as **afferent nerves** (*afferent* means "carrying toward"), because they carry impulses in the opposite direction, from the body's sensory receptors toward the CNS.

Interneurons

Interneurons are often referred to as associative neurons because they are located entirely within the CNS. These cells

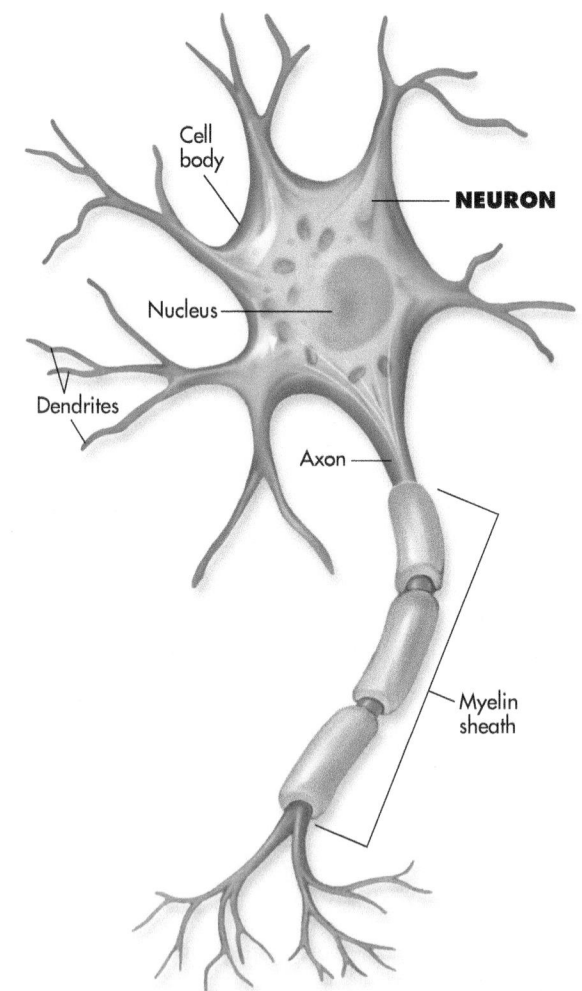

FIGURE 24-3 Motor neuron showing the axon, dendrite, and myelin sheath.

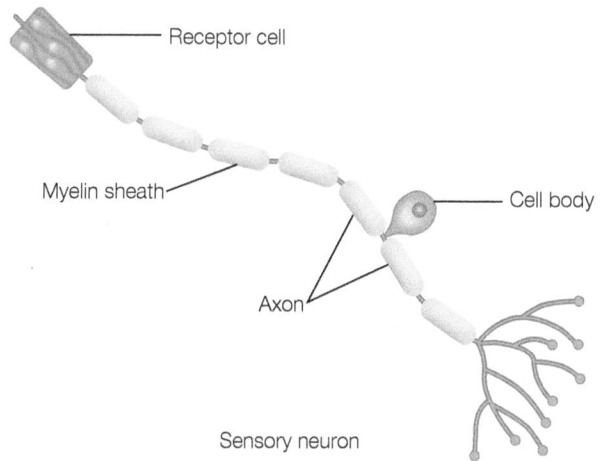

Receptor cell

Myelin sheath

Cell body

Axon

Sensory neuron

FIGURE 24-4 A sensory neuron.

work as a liaison between sensory and motor neurons by mediating their impulses.

Nerve Fibers, Nerves, and Tracts

It is important to understand the correlation between nerve fibers, nerves, and their tracts because these components are all necessary in conducting an impulse.

Nerve Fibers

A nerve fiber is a single elongated process, usually an axon from a motor neuron or a peripheral process from a sensory neuron. The nerve fibers that are found in the PNS are wrapped in protective membranes, mentioned earlier, called **sheaths**. Sheaths are formed by accessory cells and are classified as either myelinated or unmyelinated. Myelin is a thick fatty substance, and myelinated sheaths have both an inner sheath of myelin and an outer sheath, or **neurilemma**, composed of Schwann cells. (Schwann cells are needed for the process of regenerating a damaged nerve fiber.) Unmyelinated sheaths are wrapped only in the neurilemma and, as their name indicates, lack myelin. By contrast, nerve fibers of the CNS do not contain Schwann cells. Thus, damage to nerve fibers of the CNS is permanent, whereas damage to a peripheral nerve can be reversed.

Nerves

A nerve is a bundled unit of nerve fibers found outside the CNS. As noted, nerves are often categorized as afferent (conducting impulses to the CNS) or efferent (conducting impulses from the CNS to muscles, organs, and glands). Some nerves possess the fibers of both afferent and efferent nerves. These special nerves are called mixed nerves.

Tracts

A group of nerve fibers within the CNS is often referred to as a **tract**. All nerve fibers that are housed within the nerve

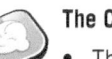

Professionalism   The Life Span

The Child

- The development of the child's nervous system begins when the embryo is about 6 weeks. By the time the child is born, the baby's brain waves can be measured. As the child grows, regular neurological testing can provide the physician with important information that can indicate various neurological disorders. Testing of the child's nervous system includes testing the newborn's reflexes and testing the child as she grows. This includes testing of mental status, motor functions and balance, and the sensory system. Doctors often evaluate these areas during well-child visits that are scheduled to establish growth and development at specific ages.

The Older Adult

- In individuals who do not have neurological disease (such as dementia), intellectual performance tends to be maintained until at least age 80. However, tasks may take longer to perform because of some slowing in central processing. Verbal skills are well maintained until age 70, after which some healthy older adults gradually develop a reduction in vocabulary, a tendency to make semantic errors, and abnormal pronunciation. Other age-related changes are subtle but can be detected as difficulty learning, especially languages, and forgetfulness in noncritical areas. However, this mild forgetfulness is unlike dementia in that it does not impair recall of important memories or affect function.
- With normal aging, the number of nerve cells in the brain decreases. From age 20 or 30 to age 90, brain weight declines by about 10 percent, and the area of the cerebral ventricles (cavities) relative to the entire brain may increase three to four times.

tract must have the same origin, function, and termination. This means that all the nerve cells within the tract have the same starting and ending points and work toward the same purpose. The spinal cord contains sensory tracts that are afferent, which ascend to the brain, and efferent tracts that descend from the brain. The largest nerve tract is the **corpus callosum**, which joins the right and left hemispheres of the brain.

Nerve Impulses and Synapses

A nerve impulse begins with stimulation, which occurs at the receptor. Sensory receptors vary in the complexity of their functions from the simple, such as receptors in the skin that sense pain, to the very complex, such as receptors in the retina of the eye that collect the input necessary for sight. All sensory receptors are specialized to respond to certain stimulations, such as heat, cold, light, pressure, or pain.

When the receptor is stimulated, it reacts by initiating a chemical change or impulse. The transmission of an impulse by a nerve fiber is based on the "all or none" principle, meaning that either there is a response or there is not. The receptor must receive sufficient stimulation to send the impulse, or else the impulse is not transmitted to the brain or other target organ. Each receptor has its own threshold at which it will react to a stimulus, and each will only respond when its threshold is reached.

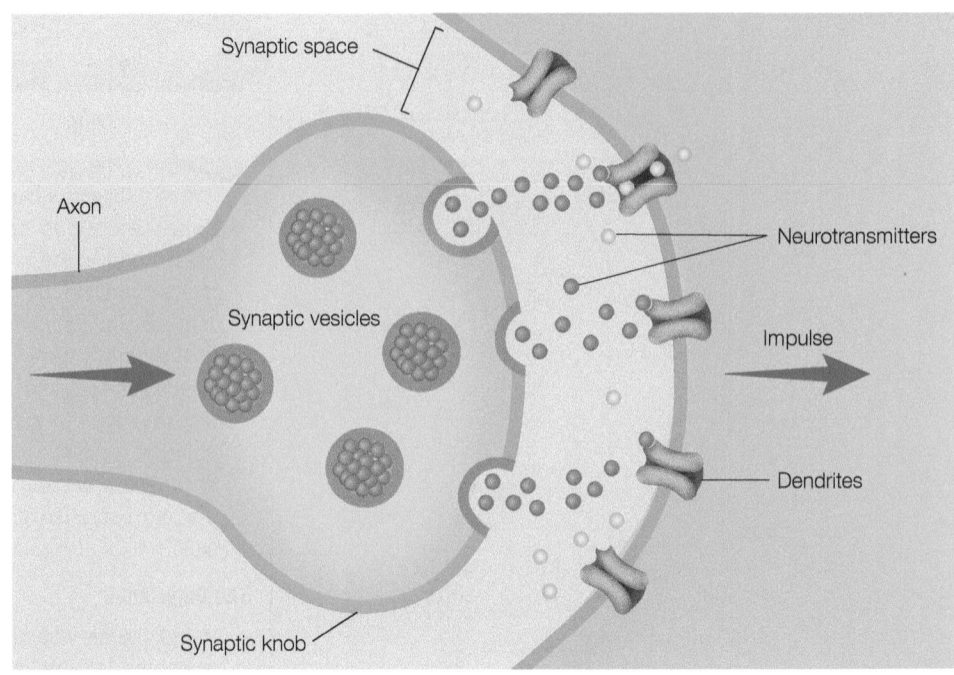

FIGURE 24-5 A synapse.

When a receptor reacts to a stimulus, the resulting impulse is transmitted from the receptor nerve to other nerves. As noted earlier, the axon is the nerve projection that transmits impulses, and the dendrite is the nerve projection that receives impulses. The site at which an impulse is transmitted from the axon of one nerve to the dendrite of another nerve is called a **synapse**. However, the impulse is not transmitted by direct contact. Rather, there is a small gap between axon and dendrite, and the impulse travels across that gap, which is called the **synaptic space**.

To summarize, a transfer of an impulse happens this way:

- The impulse travels down the axon of a nerve all the way to a knob-shaped structure, called the synaptic knob, found at the end of the axon.

- Inside the synaptic knob are vesicles (tiny vessels) that contain chemicals called neurotransmitters. When the impulse reaches them, the vesicles migrate forward to the membrane that covers the end of the synaptic knob.

- Next, the vesicles release the neurotransmitters into the synaptic space.

- The neurotransmitters drift across the space and then bind to receptors on the dendrite of the next neuron on the other side (Figure 24-5).

In this way, the impulse is transmitted from neuron to neuron, in a kind of domino effect, until the impulse reaches its target. The entire impulse transfer from the receptor along all the intervening nerves to the target site takes just a tiny fraction of a second.

CENTRAL NERVOUS SYSTEM

The CNS is composed solely of the brain and the spinal cord. This portion of the nervous system receives impulses from the entire body, processes the information, and responds with appropriate actions. These resulting actions or activities may be conscious or unconscious, depending on the sensory stimuli.

Both the brain and the spinal cord are divided into gray matter and white matter. The gray matter (which is actually gray in color) consists of unsheathed cell bodies and true dendrites, whereas the white matter (which is white in color) consists of the myelinated nerve fibers. In the spinal cord, the arrangement of the gray and white matter in cross section is H-shaped, with the gray matter forming the core of the spinal cord, surrounded by the white matter. In the brain, the reverse arrangement is true. The white matter forms the core of the brain with the gray matter (surface layer) surrounding the cortex.

Brain

The brain is the largest mass of nervous tissue in the body. It is estimated that the male brain weighs about three pounds, the female brain slightly less.

The brain is encompassed by three membranes called **meninges**. These are the:

- **Pia mater**—The pia mater (which means "soft mother") is the innermost, delicate layer of the meninges. Holding blood vessels onto the surface of brain and spinal cord, it lies directly on the top of both.

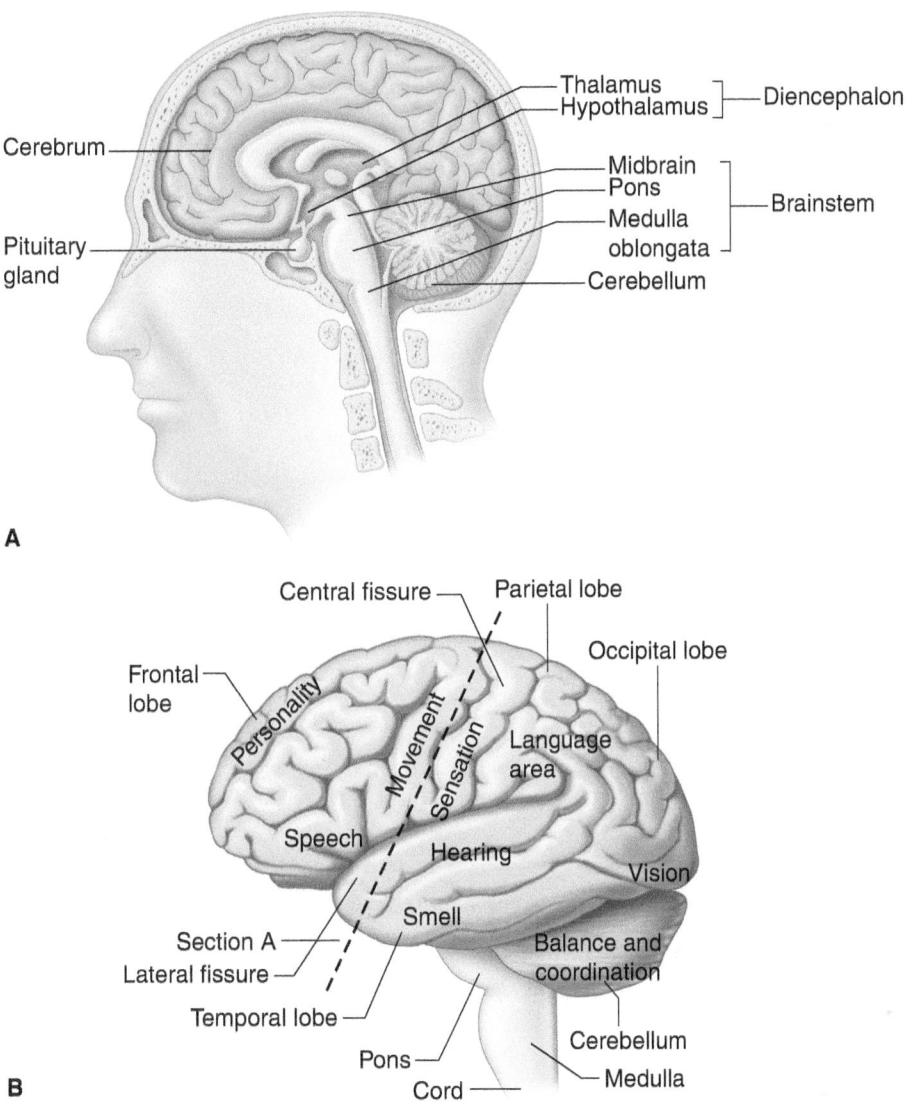

FIGURE 24-6 (A) Sagittal section of the brain; **(B)** lateral view of the brain.

- **Arachnoid mater**—This is the middle layer named for its weblike appearance. (Spiders are arachnids, belonging to the class *Arachnida*.)

- **Dura mater**—The outermost and strongest layer ("tough mother").

The major divisions of the brain, discussed in the next sections, are the cerebrum, the diencephalon, the brainstem, and the cerebellum. The brainstem consists of the midbrain and the hindbrain. The hindbrain is further divided into the pons and the medulla oblongata (Figure 24-6).

Cerebrum

The cerebrum is the largest portion of the mature brain. It is composed of both gray matter and white matter. The cerebrum governs all sensory and motor activity, including sensory perception, emotions, consciousness, memory, and

voluntary movements—which are considered higher brain functions. The cerebrum is divided in one-half, forming two mirror-image portions called cerebral hemispheres. As mentioned earlier, the corpus callosum, the brain's largest nerve tract, connects these two halves of the cerebrum. The surface of the cerebrum is marked by numerous ridges or convolutions, called **gyri**, which are separated by grooves. This surface is known as the cerebral cortex. A deep groove in the brain is called a **fissure**, and a shallow groove is referred to as a **sulcus**. A longitudinal fissure separates the right and left hemispheres of the cerebrum, and a transverse fissure separates the cerebrum from the cerebellum.

Cerebral Cortex. The cerebral cortex is the outer covering of the cerebrum. It houses 75 percent of all the neurons of the entire nervous system. Similar to the cerebrum, the cortex is also composed of gray matter as well as the white matter that lies directly below it. Responsible for interpreting sensory information and initiating body movements, the cerebral cortex also acts to store memories and create emotions.

Lobes of the Cerebral Cortex. Scientists have divided the cerebral cortex into lobes as a means of identifying certain locations in the brain. The lobes, which have been named to correspond to the overlying bones of the skull, are the frontal, parietal, temporal, and occipital lobes. The specific functions of the lobes of the brain are as follows:

- **Frontal lobe**—Deals with reasoning, personality and emotions, problem solving, planning, parts of speech, and movement
- **Parietal lobe**—Perceives stimuli related to touch, pain, temperature, and pressure; recognizes and differentiates size, shape, and color
- **Temporal lobe**—Perceives and recognizes auditory stimuli (hearing) and memory; interprets organizing and sequencing of items and events
- **Occipital lobe**—Is primarily concerned with the aspects of vision; perceives and recognizes printed words

Diencephalon

Literally translated, *diencephalon* means "second portion of the brain." The thalamus and hypothalamus make up the diencephalon. The thalamus is two large masses of gray cell bodies that are connected by a third mass. This portion of the brain serves as a relay center for all sensory impulses with the exception of smell.

As its name implies, the hypothalamus lies beneath the thalamus. It primarily regulates autonomic nervous activity associated with behavior and emotional expression. The hypothalamus also is responsible for regulating thirst and hunger as well as maintaining body temperature. Working with the endocrine system, it helps with a variety of metabolic functions that occur throughout the body, because it produces neurosecretions for the control of water balance, sugar and fat metabolism, and regulation of body temperature.

Brainstem

Structurally resembling a stem, as its name would suggest, the brainstem contains the midbrain, the pons, and the medulla oblongata. Together, these structures relay important information to the cerebrum, including visual, auditory, and other sensory data.

Midbrain. The midbrain is located just below the cerebrum and above the pons. It is associated with visual reflexes and tracking visual movements of the eyes. The two lower segments are associated with the sense of hearing.

Pons. The pons is a broad band of white matter anterior to the cerebellum and between the midbrain and medulla oblongata. The pons contains fiber tracts that link the cerebellum and medulla to higher cortical areas. It plays a vital role in voluntary and involuntary motor control.

Medulla Oblongata. This highly important area of the brain connects the pons and the rest of the brain to the spinal cord. Here, nerve centers vital to the body's survival exert control over the circulation of blood by regulating both the heartbeat and arterial blood pressure. Different areas of the medulla oblongata are also responsible for involuntary bodily functions, including breathing, swallowing, coughing, sneezing, and vomiting.

Cerebellum

The cerebellum is the second largest portion of the brain. It is located in the back of the skull, just above the brainstem and below the cerebrum. The cerebellum plays an important part in the coordination of voluntary movements, muscle tone, and equilibrium It is responsible for adjusting body muscles to automatically maintain posture. Tremors, slower overall movements, and a lack of balance could result from damage to the cerebellum.

Spinal Cord

Measuring approximately 17 to 18 inches (43 to 45 centimeters) long in adults, the spinal cord extends from the base of the medulla oblongata to the junction between the first (L_1) and second (L_2) lumbar vertebrae. The function of the spinal cord is to conduct sensory impulses from the rest of the body to the brain and to send motor impulses from the brain to the rest of the body; this occurs in the white matter. The spinal cord also serves as a reflex center for nerve impulses that do not need to pass through the brain.

Cerebrospinal Fluid

Colorless in appearance, **cerebrospinal fluid (CSF)** is often considered to be the "blood" of the nervous system. Produced by the choroid plexus, which is located in the ventricles (cavities) of the brain, the CSF moves from the ventricles into the connecting canal, and then through the spinal canal and the subarachnoid space that surrounds the brain. CSF has several functions, including serving as a cushion to protect the brain and spinal cord, which float in the fluid, and nourishing the brain and spinal cord with oxygen and glucose. It also acts as a vesicle to carry neurotransmitters, including monoamines, acetylcholine, and neuropeptides.

TABLE 24-2 | Cranial Nerves and Functions

Nerve/Number	Function
Olfactory (I)	Provides sense of smell
Optic (II)	Provides vision
Oculomotor (III)	Conducts motor impulses to four of the six external muscles of the eye and to the muscle that raises the eyelid
Trochlear (IV)	Conducts motor impulses to control the superior oblique muscle of the eyeball
Trigeminal (V)	Provides sensory input from the face, nose, mouth, forehead, and top of the head; motor fibers to the muscles of the jaw (chewing)
Abducens (VI)	Conducts motor impulses to the lateral rectus muscle of the eyeball
Facial (VII)	Controls the muscles of the face and scalp, the lacrimal glands of the eye, and the submandibular and sublingual salivary glands; controls input from the tongue for the sense of taste
Vestibulocochlear (Acoustic) (VIII)	Provides input for hearing and equilibrium
Glossopharyngeal (IX)	Provides general sense of taste, regulates swallowing, controls secretion of saliva
Vagus (X)	Controls muscles of the pharynx, larynx, thoracic, and abdominal organs; controls swallowing, voice production, slowing of heartbeat, acceleration of peristalsis (movement through the digestive system)
Accessory (XI)	Controls the trapezius and sternocleidomastoid muscles, permitting movement of the head and shoulders
Hypoglossal (XII)	Controls tongue movements

Peripheral Nervous System

The PNS is one of the two major divisions of the nervous system—along with the CNS, discussed in the prior section. The PNS is further divided into the SNS and the ANS. The nerves of the PNS connect the CNS to sensory organs (such as the eye and ear) and to other organs of the body, muscles, blood vessels, and glands.

Cranial and Spinal Nerves

Cranial and spinal nerves make up a large component of the PNS. Cranial nerves originate in the brain and are identified by Roman numerals. Symmetrically arranged in 12 pairs to each side of the brain, the nerves are named for the function or area of the body they serve. The 12 pairs of cranial nerves and their functions are listed in Table 24-2. Figure 24-7 shows the relationship of the 12 cranial nerves to specific regions of the brain. The PNS also contains 31 pairs of spinal nerves that are connected to the spinal cord and named for the region of the vertebral column where they exist: 8 pairs of cervical spinal nerves, 12 pairs of thoracic spinal nerves, 5 pairs of lumbar spinal nerves, 5 pairs of sacral spinal nerves, and 1 pair of coccygeal spinal nerves (Figure 24-8).

Professionalism

Many patients come into the medical office under some type of stress, often from either personal or medical issues. It is important that health care professionals try to reduce the patient's anxiety and stress level, whenever possible. Medical assistants can misinterpret a patient's anxiety as anger, which can cause the medical assistant (in turn) to become anxious. The emotions of a health care professional who displays anxiety may be misinterpreted by the patient, adding more anxiety to the mix and creating a viscous circle. Stress can be reduced with a quiet tone, gentle treatment, appropriate information, and relaxed mannerisms from the medical assistant.

Somatic Nervous System

The **somatic nervous system (SNS)**, a division of the PNS, is made up of nerves that connect to the skeletal muscles, the sensory organs, and the skin. It is sometimes referred to as the "voluntary" nervous system because it connects to muscles and other structures that are under voluntary control of the body. In addition to controlling voluntary

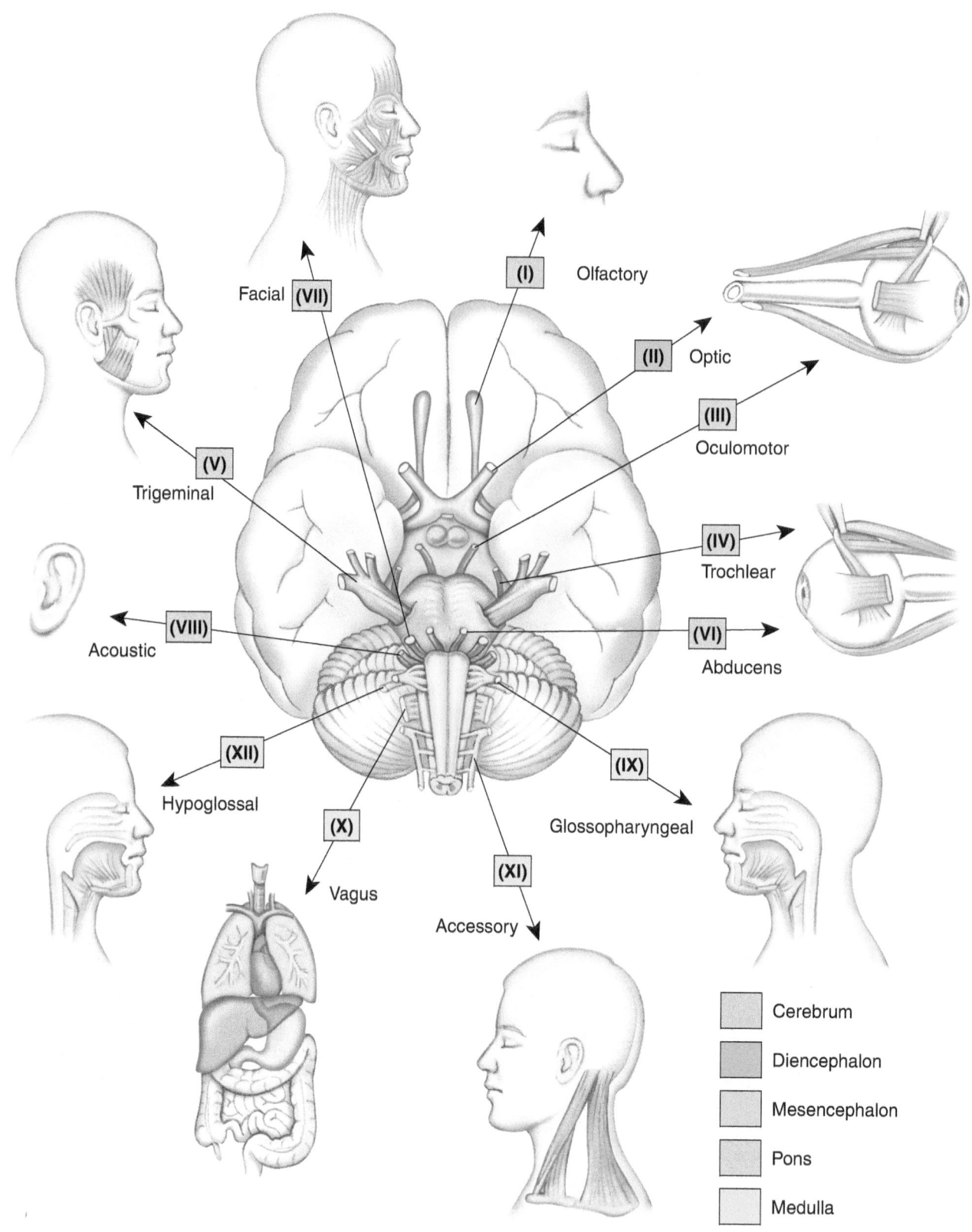

Facial **(VII)**
(I) Olfactory
(II) Optic
(III) Oculomotor
(V)
Trigeminal
(IV) Trochlear
(VIII)
Acoustic
(VI) Abducens
(XII)
Hypoglossal
(X)
Vagus
(XI)
Accessory
(IX)
Glossopharyngeal

Cerebrum
Diencephalon
Mesencephalon
Pons
Medulla

FIGURE 24-7 The relationship of the 12 cranial nerves to specific regions of the brain.

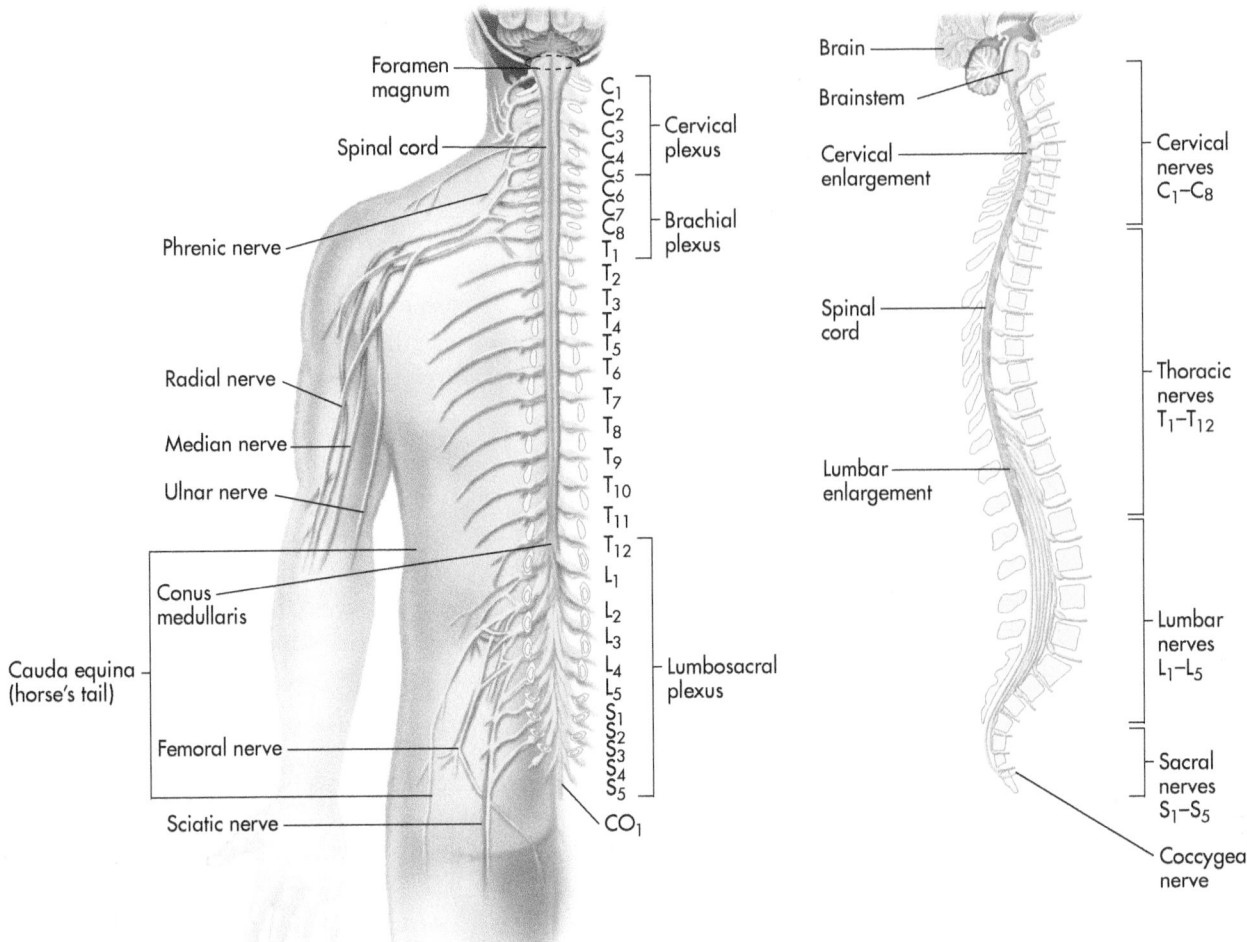

FIGURE 24-8 The 31 pairs of spinal nerves.

muscle movements, the SNS also is responsible for processing sensory information received from the eyes, ears, nose, and touch.

Autonomic Nervous System

The **autonomic nervous system (ANS)**, is another component of the peripheral nervous system. This division controls involuntary bodily functions. Some functions under its control include heart rate, control of smooth muscle tissue, glandular secretion, sweating, and arterial blood pressure. The final division of the CNS occurs with two additional subdivided parts of the ANS: sympathetic and parasympathetic nervous systems. These counteracting systems work together to maintain homeostasis in the body.

Sympathetic Division

The first part of the sympathetic division of the ANS is found in the spinal nerves of the thoracic and lumbar spine. The sympathetic ganglia are masses of nerve cell bodies where the axons of spinal nerve cells enter.

When synapses are activated between the spinal nerves and the sympathetic ganglia, widespread innervation (stimulation) occurs. This activation and stimulation prepare the body for a swift reaction called *fight or flight*. During fight or flight, a person experiences increased alertness with an increase in metabolic rate and other bodily functions. At this point, the SNS stimulates the adrenal gland to release epinephrine (adrenaline). For example, imagine that you are standing in a crowded building when the fire alarm sounds. Smoke is visible at the end of a hallway. At the sound of the alarm and the sight of the smoke, the sympathetic division of your ANS will trigger a response that causes your heart rate and respiration to increase, your blood pressure to rise, and the aforementioned adrenaline rush that rouses you to get out of the building to a safe location.

Parasympathetic Division

The first stages of parasympathetic nervous system response are formed by cranial nerves (III, VII, IX, and X) and sacral nerves (II, III, and IV). The cranial nerve fibers involved serve internal organs of the thoracic, abdominal, and pelvic regions, and the fibers of the sacral spinal nerves serve the lower colon as well as the rectum, bladder, and reproductive organs.

In contrast to the fight-or-flight response of the sympathetic division, the response of the parasympathetic division has a calming and quieting effect. Rather than a burst of energy, it works to conserve energy while stimulating the digestive system. It causes a decrease in heart rate, metabolism, and bodily functions. The phrase keyed with this subsystem is "rest and digest."

COMMON PATHOLOGY ASSOCIATED WITH THE NERVOUS SYSTEM

Like its endocrine counterpart (see the chapter titled "The Endocrine System"), the nervous system initiates and regulates body functions and ensures its owner of an awareness of the surrounding environment. Nervous system disorders encompass a wide range of complexity and include simple ailments such as headaches and more complex conditions such as Alzheimer's disease. Procedures and tests used to diagnose and treat a variety of nervous system disorders and diseases are described in Table 24-3.

Alzheimer's Disease

Alzheimer's disease is a progressive, degenerative disease that attacks the brain and its cognitive function. More than 5.1 million people are affected by this disease. Of these 5.1 million patients, only approximately 200,000 are under the age of 65. Of the Americans afflicted with this disease, almost two-thirds of the patients are women. Although there isn't a definitive cause, the etiology tends to be centered on genetic predispositions, lifestyle choices (with activity level being a key factor), and the overall environment of the patient.

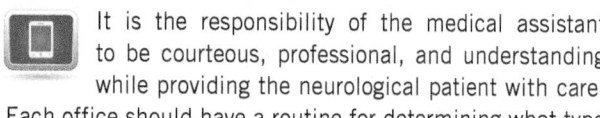

Professionalism   The Workplace

It is the responsibility of the medical assistant to be courteous, professional, and understanding while providing the neurological patient with care. Each office should have a routine for determining what type of care and treatment is necessary for patients afflicted with neurological disorders. Knowing what these tasks are and what is expected before the patient enters the office is paramount to the medical assistant's role.

Signs and Symptoms. An initial symptom is the inability to remember recent events. As the disease begins to progress, the patient may display the inability to rationalize thoughts, speech becomes difficult to understand and follow because of interrupted thought processes, and skills related to reading and writing begin to decline. Personality changes are also common and may include irritability, aggression, agitation, depression, and, at times, violence. This disease continues to wreak havoc on the nervous system to the point where patients become unable to care for themselves, eat, or even speak.

Treatment. During the early stages of Alzheimer's disease, medications are available to slow its progression. Medication must continue throughout the patient's remaining life so as not to forfeit any protection the medication has provided. Recent medical studies suggest that older adults who maintain active lifestyles and engage in mentally stimulating activities may be less prone to develop Alzheimer's disease.

Amyotrophic Lateral Sclerosis

Amyotrophic lateral sclerosis (ALS) has an unknown etiology, although heredity and environmental factors are considered to be associated with the disease. ALS acts by breaking down the motor neurons. This disease is also known as Lou Gehrig's disease, named for the famous New York Yankees baseball player who was afflicted with the disease and forced to retire from the sport.

Signs and Symptoms. As the motor neurons degenerate and die, individuals begin to lose control of voluntary muscle movement, including that of the arms, legs, and trunk. As the disease progresses, more and more muscles become weak and atrophied, resulting in lack of muscular control. Slurred speech, muscle stiffness, and difficulty eating, specifically chewing and swallowing, are common symptoms that are initially displayed. Various forms of ALS may be associated with a loss of intellectual function (dementia) or sensory symptoms.

Treatment. There is no known cure for ALS. Certain medications as well as speech, physical, and respiratory therapy can help to slow the progression of symptoms. The goal is to allow the patient to remain independent as long as possible and maintain a high quality of life.

Bell's Palsy

Bell's palsy is weakness or paralysis of the muscles that control expression on one side of the face, often occurring with sudden onset. It affects the appearance of the face but is not generally considered a serious condition. Bell's palsy is caused

TABLE 24-3 | Procedures and Diagnostic Tests Related to the Nervous System

Procedure/Test	Description
Babinski's Sign	Reflex test developed by John Babinski, a French neurologist, to determine lesions and abnormalities in the nervous system. The Babinski reflex is present or positive when the great toe extends instead of flexes when the lateral sole of the foot is stroked.
Brain Scan	Injection of radioactive isotopes into the circulation to determine the function and abnormality of the brain.
Carotid Endarterectomy	Surgical procedure for removing an obstruction within the carotid artery. It was developed to prevent strokes but is found useful only in severe stenosis with a transient ischemic attack (TIA).
Cerebral Angiogram	X-ray of the blood vessels of the brain after the injection of radiopaque contrast.
Cerebrospinal Fluid Shunts	Surgical creation of an artificial opening to allow for the passage of fluid. Used in the treatment of hydrocephalus.
Cordectomy	Removal of part of the spinal cord.
Craniotomy	Surgical incision into the brain through the cranium.
Cryosurgery	Use of extreme cold to produce areas of destruction in the brain. Used to control bleeding and treat brain tumors.
Echoencephalogram	Recording of the ultrasonic echoes of the brain. Useful in determining abnormal patterns of shifting in the brain.
Electromyogram	Written recording of the contraction of muscles as a result of receiving electrical stimulation.
Laminectomy	Removal of a posterior vertebral arch.
Lumbar Puncture	Puncture with a needle into the lumbar area (usually the fourth intervertebral space) to withdraw cerebrospinal fluid for examination and for the injection of anesthesia.
Nerve Block	Method of regional anesthetic to stop the passage of sensory stimulation along a nerve path, often performed when a patient is experiencing extreme pain.
Positron Emission tomography (PET)	Use of positive radionucleotides to reconstruct brain sections. Measurement can be taken of oxygen and glucose uptake, cerebral blood flow, and blood volume.
Romberg's Sign	Test developed to establish neurological function in which patients are asked to close their eyes and place their feet together. This test for body balance is positive if the patient sways when the eyes are closed.
Spinal Puncture	Puncture with a needle into the spinal cavity to withdraw spinal fluid for microscopic analysis.
Sympathectomy	Excision of a portion of the sympathetic nervous system. Could include nerve or ganglion.
Transcutaneous Electrical Nerve Stimulation (TENS)	Application of a mild electrical stimulation to skin electrodes placed over a painful or injured area, causing interference with the transmission of painful stimuli. Can be used in pain management to interfere with the normal pain mechanism.
Trephination	Process of cutting out a piece of bone in the skull to gain entry into the brain to relieve pressure.
Vagotomy	Surgical incision into the vagus nerve. Medication can be administered into the nerve to prevent its function.

by damage to a facial nerve, one of which runs beneath each ear to the muscles on the same side of the face. It is named for Dr. Charles Bell of Edinburgh, Scotland, who first documented the disorder in 1882. It is also known as facial palsy.

Signs and Symptoms. Bell's palsy is generally characterized by unilateral paralysis of the face. Self-image is a problematic issue associated with the affliction because facial appearance is impacted. Facial drooping and lack of facial expression on the afflicted side are common symptoms. Headaches, changes in taste, excessive drooling, or tearing may also be associated with the disease depending on the extent of nerve damage.

Treatment. Doctors may prescribe corticosteroids within the first few days of onset to reduce swelling and inflammation.

Medications to alleviate patient-specific symptoms may also be used. With the onset of Bell's palsy, paralysis may affect the eyelid's ability to blink. This can cause the eye to become dry and irritated from lack of lubrication. Eye drops, ointments, and eye patches may be prescribed to treat and protect the eye. Most often, Bell's palsy resolves on its own within weeks or months of onset.

Disk Disorders

Disk disorders occur when the intervertebral disks between the spinal vertebrae deteriorate, creating pain and shortening of stature.

Signs and Symptoms. Pain can often be very severe, and sometimes debilitating, with disk disorders. Pain often originates around or near the location of the problematic disk. However, it often spreads to nearby areas. Because the pain can be so severe, decreased mobility of the affected region is also common. This may include neck, back, and leg pain and immobility. Leg weakness and other muscle weakness may occur. Incontinence is also associated with disk disorders.

Treatment. Treatment usually includes bed rest, application of heat or cold, and prescribed muscle relaxers along with analgesics (pain relievers). Physical therapy can be prescribed for a ruptured or slipped disk. Massage therapy, acupuncture, and biofeedback are other therapies used for disk disorders. In serious cases, surgery may also be recommended to alleviate pain and restore mobility.

Encephalitis

Encephalitis is inflammation of the brain often caused by a viral infection such as measles or mumps or viral infections transmitted via insects (mosquito and ticks) such as West Nile virus. Infants and older adults compose the majority of the 1,500 cases per year of encephalitis that occur in the United States.

Signs and Symptoms. Many signs and symptoms are associated with encephalitis, including headache, sudden fever, vomiting, sensitivity to light, stiff neck and back, confusion, drowsiness, clumsiness, and irritability. Emergency care is required should a patient exhibit any of the following: loss of consciousness or decreased responsiveness, seizures, muscle weakness, or impaired judgment. These symptoms may indicate that the disease has taken a life-threatening turn.

Treatment. Those who suffer from encephalitis generally are hospitalized. Their treatments may include antibiotics, antiviral medications, anticonvulsants, steroids to decrease inflammation, and sedatives to control irritability and agitation.

Epilepsy and Seizures

Seizures are disorders associated with misfiring or interference of electrical impulses within the brain. The misfiring occurs when abnormal and often intense bursts of electrical activity are produced within the brain. Epilepsy is thought to afflict approximately 2.2 million people. It is estimated that each year about 48 out of every 100,000 people develop epilepsy. **Epilepsy** is a disorder characterized by recurring seizures. The cause of epilepsy is often unknown. However, it is often the result of another condition, such as head injury, stroke, brain infection, or brain tumor.

Signs and Symptoms. Seizures temporarily interfere with muscle control, movement, speech, vision, or awareness of surroundings. Having seizures is often terrifying, especially if they are severe. Some individuals only have one seizure in a lifetime, whereas others may have repeated episodes.

Treatment. Medication is often used to reduce the occurrence and the severity of seizures. In almost all patients with recurrent seizures or epilepsy, medication must be taken for life. In very severe cases of epilepsy, surgery may be required. Some seizure activity is associated with specific triggers such as sensitivity to light, stress, disrupted sleep patterns, and hormonal fluctuations. Attempting to minimize exposure to or circumstances surrounding these triggers can be helpful.

Headaches

Headaches account for more than ten million visits to a physician each year. Researchers are not exactly sure why headaches occur or which people are more susceptible to them. Likewise, doctors cannot always tell what kind of headache an individual has and, therefore, what kind of medicine would be best. In 1988, the International Headache Society (IHS) developed the criteria most often used to differentiate the various types of headaches from one

Professionalism   The Law

Be aware of the laws in your state regarding driving and neurological disorders. For instance, many states require epileptic individuals to be seizure free for a predetermined period of time before being legally able to drive. These laws are written and enforced to protect the safety of the individual and others around them. It is the physician's ethical (and in some states legal) responsibility to report patients whose driving may be impaired by epilepsy or other seizure disorder and to warn the patient. The medical assistant should also know local laws and be prepared to reinforce the physician's teaching.

another. The criteria are based on clinical features of the headache, including the number of attacks per month, length of time per attack, pain characteristics, and accompanying symptoms. The types of headaches include migraine, tension, cluster, and posttraumatic.

Migraine Headaches

Migraine headaches tend to be more common among women. It is thought that female hormones are responsible for this higher frequency.

Signs and Symptoms. The pain associated with migraine headaches is usually very intense. It is typical for migraine patients to complain of pain on one side of the head, with a focal point behind the eye. In addition to pain, symptoms include sensitivity to light and noise and, possibly, nausea and vomiting. Patients are often able to recognize the onset of a migraine headache because of a pattern of symptoms they have experienced in the past. Some migraine headaches may have an "aura" that accompanies the headache before or during onset. An aura that precedes or occurs during the migraine headache could include tunnel vision, visual disturbances such as a flashing light, and a sensitivity to certain odors.

Treatment. Patients generally opt for over-the-counter medications such as acetaminophen, ibuprofen, and naproxen sodium. When these analgesics fail to help, physicians may recommend prescription medications to relieve the symptoms and prevent the occurrence of future headaches. Patients may be asked to keep a journal of their headaches, documenting days and times as well as symptoms, to help identify triggers that could be avoided to try to reduce the number of occurrences.

Tension Headaches

A tension headache may also be referred to as a muscle-contraction headache, stress headache, psychomyogenic headache, or idiopathic headache. Tension headaches may be episodic or chronic in nature. Many tension headaches have unknown etiology, but they are thought possibly to be caused by stress or fatigue.

Signs and Symptoms. Common symptoms associated with tension headaches include a pressing or squeezing pain on both sides of the head, neck, or even facial areas. Generally, these pressure headaches are not throbbing in nature. Patients may also experience sensitivity to light and sound.

Treatment. A similar course of treatment is indicated for tension headaches as for all headaches. A physician will likely prescribe both prescription and over-the-counter pain relievers. A goal of treatment is to decrease stress through various activities, including yoga, meditation, and biofeedback. It may be necessary for antidepressants and antianxiety medications to be prescribed as well for the overall health of the patient.

Cluster Headaches

Cluster headaches, unlike migraines, are more common in men than women. Those who drink excessively and smoke are at the highest risk of developing these headaches.

Signs and Symptoms. Cluster headaches are defined by a penetrating, intense burst of pain that is commonly felt behind the eyes or temples. A runny nose, tearing eye, or droopy eyelid on the affected side may also be present. Attacks can last from 15 minutes to 3 hours and tend to occur at night or early in the morning. Individuals who suffer from cluster headaches may have multiple episodes a day, and they can occur frequently for weeks and even months at a time.

Treatment. In addition to using the conventional analgesics as well as prescription medications indicated for migraine headaches, those suffering from cluster headaches have sometimes found relief through use of oxygen masks that provide 100 percent pure oxygen. In severe cases, as well as for those who cannot tolerate the side effects of medication, surgical treatment may be an option.

Posttraumatic Headaches

Posttraumatic headaches are often caused by or occur after a traumatic brain injury. It is estimated that approximately 1.7 million traumatic brain injuries occur each year. This type of headache could be caused by brain swelling or shrinkage (as a result of the injury) or the release of chemicals.

Signs and Symptoms. Symptoms of a posttraumatic headache are very similar to those of migraine and tension headaches. General symptoms associated include decreased concentration and memory, sensitivity to both noise and bright light, increased fatigue, dizziness, and personality changes. These symptoms develop 24 to 48 hours after the initial injury; however, they also can develop later. Posttraumatic headaches often resolve within 3 months, though they can last for years.

Treatment. The focus of treatment is to reduce pain and prevent the occurrence of these headaches. A variety of medications may be prescribed depending on the specific symptoms that are present. Pain relievers are most effective in treating immediate symptoms. To reduce the occurrence of headaches, antidepressants, antiseizure medications, and blood pressure pills are commonly used. Nonmedication therapies are also used to reduce symptoms and to prevent headaches. These include nerve stimulation, physical therapy, relaxation techniques, and psychologic support/behavior therapy.

Huntington's Chorea

Huntington's chorea is a progressive degenerative disorder of the basal ganglia that results in uncontrolled bodily movement. It is also referred to as Huntington's disease (HD). It is caused by a genetic mutation that is inherited.

Signs and Symptoms. Generally, the onset of this disease occurs during the patient's mid to late thirties, although it may also develop in juveniles. Other initial symptoms include uncontrolled movements of the hands, feet, and trunk of the body. Initial signs and symptoms of the disease may include changes in physical and emotional patterns, including increased irritability, mood swings, depression, and anger. Involuntary movement, rigidity, problems with balance and coordination, difficulty swallowing, and slurred speech are also common signs and symptoms.

Treatment. The goal of treatment is to control emotional problems and gain control over muscle movements. Antidepressants, mood stabilizers, and antipsychotic drugs are often used. The medication tetrabenazine is specifically approved and used to lessen jerking and movements. There is, at present, no cure for the disorder, and most patients die within 15 years of being diagnosed.

Hydrocephalus

Commonly occurring in infants, this disorder is characterized by an excessive amount of cerebrospinal fluid (CSF) that collects within the ventricles of the brain. This causes the brain to press against the skull. Without proper treatment, this can result in brain damage. There is no specific cause of hydrocephalus; however, causes are thought to include defects in the brain's fluid drainage tubes, complications from premature birth, genetic abnormalities, developmental disorders, and head injuries.

Signs and Symptoms. Varying symptoms occur based on age and severity of the disorder. The most common sign associated with hydrocephalus is an enlarged head. Infants may display irritability, sleepiness, vomiting, and seizures. Older children and adults could display balance problems, coordination and gait disturbance, nausea and vomiting, visual disturbance, drowsiness, and personality changes, including memory loss and irritability.

Treatment. A shunt that is surgically inserted into a ventricle is the only treatment available. This shunt creates an exit through which excessive CSF can drain off the brain and be distributed to the rest of the body, through circulation, to be absorbed.

Meningitis

Meningitis is an infection of the meninges that surround and protect the brain and spinal cord. Similar to encephalitis, meningitis may be caused by a virus or bacterium. Bacterial meningitis, if left untreated, has a high death rate.

Signs and Symptoms. The general characteristics of meningitis include neck stiffness, headache, vomiting, high fever, and chills. Other symptoms may include photosensitivity (sensitivity to light), increased fatigue, decreased desire to eat or drink, and difficulty concentrating.

Treatment. Immediate medical treatment is necessary for a positive outcome, because meningitis can be fatal. Generally, treatment includes antibiotics to treat the bacterial infection, antiinflammatory medications to reduce brain swelling, general analgesics, and anticonvulsants. To prevent the spread of this disease, isolation may be required. Three types of meningococcal vaccinations specifically target bacteria that cause meningitis: *Neisseria meningitidis* (meningococcus), *Streptococcus pneumoniae* (pneumococcus), and *Haemophilus influenzae* type b (Hib). Whereas the Hib vaccine is administered as early as 2 months of age, the meningococcal vaccine is not indicated for patients under 11 years of age.

Multiple Sclerosis

Multiple sclerosis (MS) is a chronic, potentially debilitating disease that affects the brain and spinal cord. There is no known cure. MS is an autoimmune disease in which the body attacks and destroys its own **myelin**, the protective covering, or sheath, that surrounds the nerves of the brain and spinal cord (CNS). The term for the destruction of the myelin is **demyelination**. As the myelin is damaged, scarlike tissue begins to develop and becomes very thick and dense. This dense and thick scarlike tissue is termed sclerosis. An area of sclerotic tissue is known as a lesion, and these lesions can form and develop throughout the CNS. The sclerotic tissue impedes the transmission of nerve impulses, resulting in difficulty with movement, vision, or sensation. MS affects more than 2.3 million people, with women being affected more frequently than men.

Signs and Symptoms. Symptoms may include double vision, dizziness, paralysis, loss of balance, and problems with speech and vision. In addition, symptoms and signs may include depression and emotional changes, pins-and-needles sensations, bladder incontinence, numbness, and either muscle stiffness or uncontrollable tremors. Figure 24-9 lists the multisystem effects of multiple sclerosis.

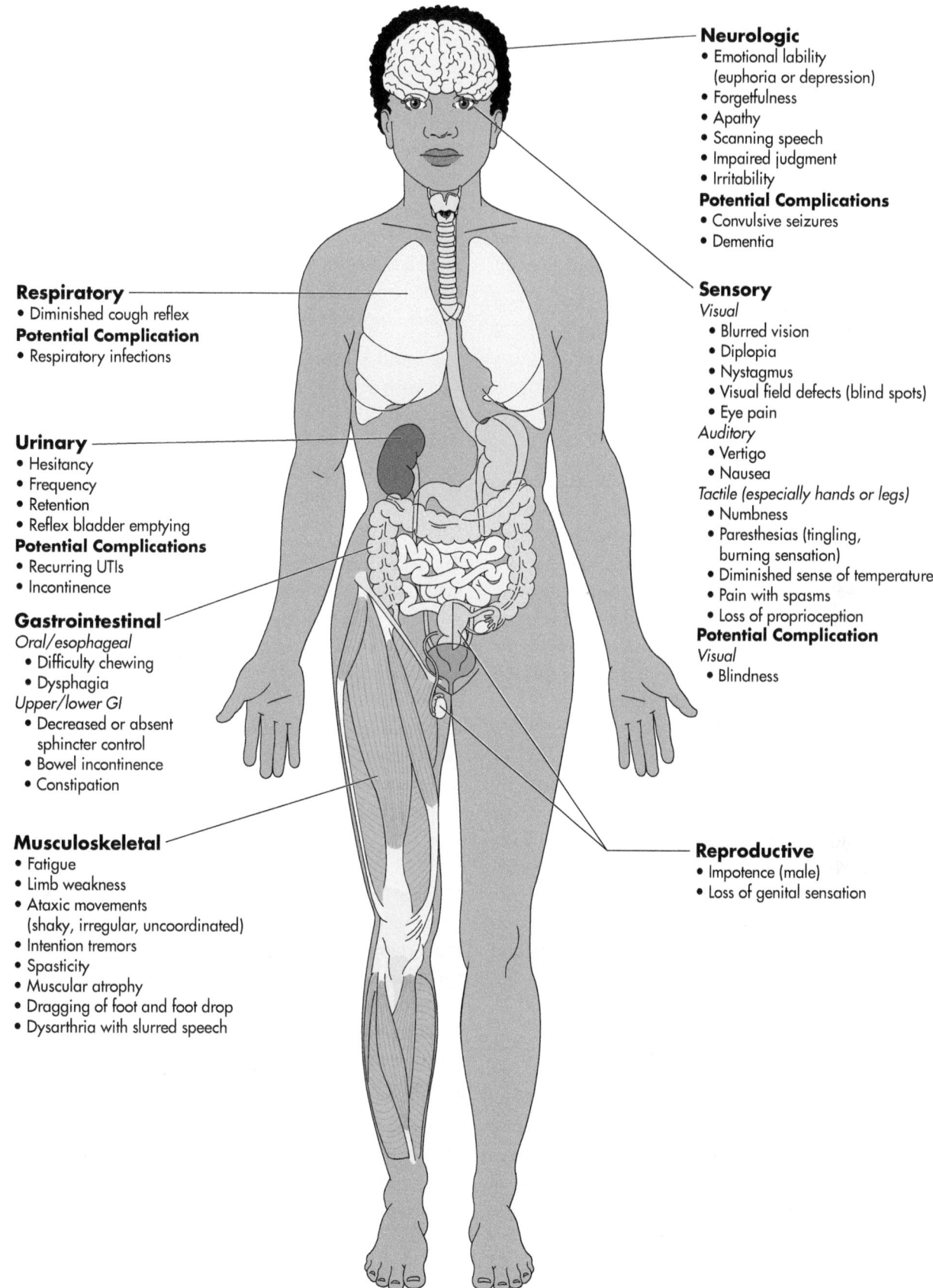

Neurologic
- Emotional lability (euphoria or depression)
- Forgetfulness
- Apathy
- Scanning speech
- Impaired judgment
- Irritability

Potential Complications
- Convulsive seizures
- Dementia

Sensory
Visual
- Blurred vision
- Diplopia
- Nystagmus
- Visual field defects (blind spots)
- Eye pain

Auditory
- Vertigo
- Nausea

Tactile (especially hands or legs)
- Numbness
- Paresthesias (tingling, burning sensation)
- Diminished sense of temperature
- Pain with spasms
- Loss of proprioception

Potential Complication
Visual
- Blindness

Respiratory
- Diminished cough reflex

Potential Complication
- Respiratory infections

Urinary
- Hesitancy
- Frequency
- Retention
- Reflex bladder emptying

Potential Complications
- Recurring UTIs
- Incontinence

Gastrointestinal
Oral/esophageal
- Difficulty chewing
- Dysphagia

Upper/lower GI
- Decreased or absent sphincter control
- Bowel incontinence
- Constipation

Musculoskeletal
- Fatigue
- Limb weakness
- Ataxic movements (shaky, irregular, uncoordinated)
- Intention tremors
- Spasticity
- Muscular atrophy
- Dragging of foot and foot drop
- Dysarthria with slurred speech

Reproductive
- Impotence (male)
- Loss of genital sensation

FIGURE 24-9 Multisystem effects of multiple sclerosis.

Treatment. Treatment of MS depends on the type and severity of the disease and the symptoms present in the patient. Often drug therapy is used to minimize the effects and symptoms, delay the progression of the disease, and improve the overall quality of life.

Neuralgia

Neuralgia is a general term for nerve pain. The causes of neuralgia are varied; however, chemical irritation, trauma (including surgery), inflammation, and infections may all lead to neuralgia.

Signs and Symptoms. The pain associated with neuralgia is usually brief but may be severe. It is often described as a shooting pain along the course of the affected nerve. Patients who have long suffered with diabetes may also suffer from neuralgia.

Treatment. Treatment varies depending on the cause, location, and severity of the pain and other factors. Rest, stretching, and heat are used to aid in pain relief. Mild over-the-counter analgesics such as aspirin, acetaminophen, or ibuprofen may be helpful for mild pain. Other treatments may include the use of anticonvulsants such as Lyrica or Neurontin, narcotic painkillers, nerve blocks, and anesthetic agents that are administered via local injection, or surgical procedures to decrease sensitivity of the nerve.

Parkinson's Disease

Parkinson's disease is a progressive disorder caused by degeneration of the nerve cells in the parts of the brain that control movement. As a result, there is a shortage of the neurotransmitter dopamine, causing the movement impairments that characterize the disease. There is no known cure for Parkinson's disease. Parkinson's disease is considered to be attributed to a combination of genetic factors, aging, and environmental factors.

Signs and Symptoms. Parkinson's typically presents as a tremor of a limb, especially when the body is at rest. The tremor, usually seen in the hand, begins on one side and is localized to one limb. Other common signs include slow movement (bradykinesia) or an inability to move (akinesia), rigid limbs, a shuffling gait, and a stooped posture. Other frequent signs of Parkinson's include reduced facial expression (a symptom termed the "mask") and a soft voice. The disease may also cause depression, personality change, dementia, sleep disturbances, speech impairment, and sexual difficulties. Parkinson's tends to worsen over time.

Treatment. Levodopa (a dopamine-based medication) is commonly used to treat the symptoms of Parkinson's.

Eventually, levodopa must be discontinued because of the side effects caused by the need to regularly increase the dosage amount to control symptoms. Surgical intervention can help to minimize the effects of involuntary motions caused by this disease; however, few patients are eligible for surgical treatment.

Sciatica

Sciatica refers to a pain that runs along the sciatic nerve. It is often caused by inflammation caused by a pinched root or excessive pressure on the sciatic nerve. Sciatica usually occurs on one side of the body.

Signs and Symptoms. The most common symptom associated with sciatica is a sharp pain that runs from the lower back and down the back of the thigh. Pain may be worse during periods of activity as well as at night. Many patients complain of increased pain when the weather changes. Numbness and tingling sensations may also be present with sciatica.

Treatment. Analgesics, antiinflammatories, and steroids are medications commonly used to treat the symptoms of sciatica. Cold or heat therapy may be beneficial. Patients generally are advised to rest and restrict activities that cause pain and discomfort. Gentle stretching exercises as prescribed by a physician or included in physical therapy are also helpful in increasing tolerable movements. In extreme cases, surgical intervention may be necessary. Surgery is most common in instances when sciatica is caused by pressure that is placed on the sciatic nerve from a slipped disk.

Spinal Cord Injuries

Damage, lesions, or a break in the spinal cord can result in paralysis (a lack of mobility and feeling) of the body. It is most common for the paralysis to affect the injured area of the spinal cord and everything below that point. **Quadriplegia** refers to paralysis from approximately the shoulders down. **Paraplegia** refers to paralysis from approximately the waist down. **Hemiplegia** occurs when paralysis affects one side of the body (Figure 24-10).

Signs and Symptoms. Complete immobility from the point of injury and below is the most common sign of paralysis. Many times, sensation and feeling are also lost with the loss of movement. Complications associated with paralysis include pressure sores (decubitus ulcers), blood clots (thrombosis), muscle atrophy, and pneumonia.

Treatment. Treatment is aimed at reducing complications associated with paralysis by effective and careful care of the patient. Physical therapy may also be helpful, especially in

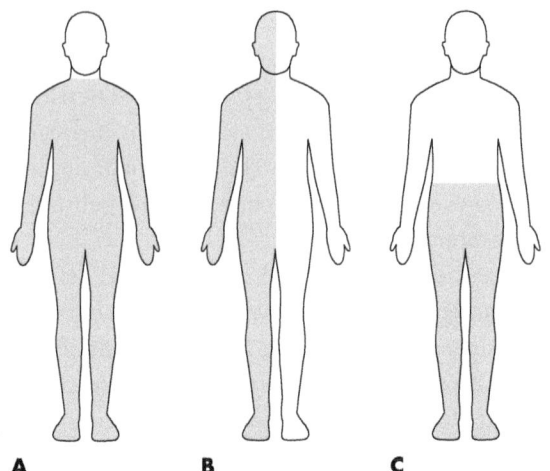

FIGURE 24-10 Types of paralysis: **(A)** quadriplegia; **(B)** hemiplegia; **(C)** paraplegia.

patients who are hemiplegic as a result of complications associated with a stroke.

Stroke

Stroke is the third leading cause of death in the United States. (An older term for stroke, cerebrovascular accident (CVA), may also sometimes be used.) Death occurs to brain tissue when the blood supply to a part of the brain is impaired, either by a clot or by hemorrhage. Brain cells can die when their oxygen supply is interrupted for more than a few minutes, so speed in diagnosis and treatment is extremely important to prevent serious or permanent bodily damage, including death.

Signs and Symptoms. The following symptoms are often sudden and require emergency intervention: numbness or weakness on one side of the body, confusion or trouble speaking, vision disturbances in one or both eyes, dizziness, loss of balance or coordination, and severe headache with no known cause. The headache is described as "the worst headache" of the person's life.

Treatment. As stated, emergency intervention is vital. Physicians will attempt to stabilize the patient's condition by either dissolving blood clots or stopping hemorrhage. Surgery may be necessary, and physicians will administer medications to control the swelling of the brain and control blood pressure. Medications and treatments are given after the incident to reduce the chance of recurrence.

Transient Ischemic Attack

Transient ischemic attacks (TIAs), commonly known as "ministrokes," can last anywhere from a few seconds to hours but generally resolve on their own without treatment. However, they are frequently precursors of a true stroke.

Signs and Symptoms. Temporary sudden weakness, numbness, and change of consciousness are common signs. Signs and symptoms depend on the portion of the brain affected by decreased blood supply.

Treatment. Patients must seek medical attention if they have suffered a TIA. Unfortunately, many people ignore TIAs, because they usually resolve without treatment. However, consulting a physician is important even if the TIA has "gone away" by itself, because, as already noted, TIAs are a sign that a true stroke may soon occur, and preventive measures must be taken. Anticoagulants and aspirin therapy often may be used to reduce the risk of blood clot formation. The following may help in reducing the risk of future TIAs or a stroke: cease smoking, stop overeating and maintain a healthy weight, decrease alcohol consumption, lower blood pressure, and control diabetes.

Traumatic Brain Injuries

Neurological trauma can be devastating, permanent, and even fatal, as discussed in earlier in the sections "Posttraumatic Headaches" and "Spinal Cord Injuries."

Traumatic brain injuries, often referred to as TBI, are the obviously a common result of head injuries. Epidural and subdural hematomas can develop when the head receives a blow. A hematoma is an area of localized swelling that is filled with blood that has usually clotted. An epidural hematoma develops outside the dura mater (between the dura mater and the skull). A subdural hematoma develops beneath the dura mater (between the dura mater and the arachnoid mater). Subdural hematomas can cause pressure on the brain that must be relieved with shunting.

Traumatic brain injuries can result in concussion or contusion. A **concussion** occurs when there is a blow to the head, often as result of sharp jarring impact, that may result in a loss of consciousness. A **contusion** is a more serious injury that results in bruising of the brain. Depressed skull fractures (those in which pieces of the skull are pushed inward) can, of course, cause brain injury.

Signs and Symptoms. Signs and symptoms related to brain trauma vary depending on the injury that causes the trauma. Common symptoms include loss of consciousness, headache, confusion, dizziness, nausea and vomiting, blurred vision, and ringing in the ears. Behavioral, mood, and sleep pattern changes may also be indicative of a more serious trauma to the brain.

Treatment. Treatment depends on the type of trauma. If swelling is present, medications or procedures to reduce swelling and pressure on the brain will be initiated. Pain relievers are often indicated but special caution must be used as some medications (ibuprofen and aspirin) can cause more bleeding. Rehabilitation exercises are usually needed. Medications to suppress seizures, such as benzodiazepines and barbiturates, are frequently prescribed following brain trauma.

SUMMARY

The nervous system is a very complex communication system that affects all functions in the body. The structure and function of the nervous system provide for an efficient system of stimulus recognition and motor reaction for the entire body. The CNS (brain and spinal cord) collects, interprets, and coordinates all sensory input and responses performed by the PNS (peripheral nerves). Nerves do not form a continuous chain but instead fire electrical impulses across synapses through the work of neurotransmitters. The lack of neurotransmitters at the synapse can cause serious disorders. The destruction of the myelin sheath that coats the spinal cord is detrimental to the functioning of the entire system. An intricate fight-or-flight system prepares the body for neurological decisions. However, reaction to chronic stress can fatigue the nervous system.

Because the nervous system is so complex, a disorder can be devastating. Disorders of the nervous system include Alzheimer's disease, amyotrophic lateral sclerosis, Bell's palsy, disk disorders, encephalitis, epilepsy and seizure disorders, headaches, Huntington's chorea, hydrocephalus, meningitis, multiple sclerosis, neuralgia, Parkinson's disease, sciatica, spinal cord injuries, stroke, TIAs, and trauma. Neurological disorders must be recognized and reported to appropriate professionals in a very timely manner to prevent long-lasting disability.

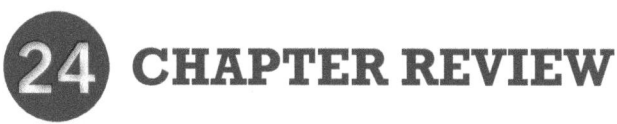

24 CHAPTER REVIEW

COMPETENCY REVIEW

1. Define and spell the terms for this chapter.
2. What are the two main divisions of the nervous system?
3. What are the functions of the nervous system?
4. What is the myelin sheath?
5. What is a neuron?
6. What are the parts of the central nervous system?
7. What are the functions of the hypothalamus?
8. What are the functions of the medulla oblongata?
9. What are three functions of the spinal cord?
10. What are the symptoms of a transient ischemic attack?

PREPARING FOR THE CERTIFICATION EXAM

1. The eighth cranial nerve (acoustic) is responsible for
   a. sense of taste.
   b. sense of smell.
   c. sense of hearing and equilibrium.
   d. sensation in the face and head.
   e. sense of sight.

2. Olfactory senses are those of
   a. taste.
   b. smell.
   c. sight.
   d. touch.
   e. hearing and equilibrium.

3. Measles or mumps may progress into which disease?
   a. Bell's palsy
   b. neuralgia
   c. stroke
   d. meningitis
   e. encephalitis

4. Which of the following is a progressive degenerative disorder?
   a. Huntington's chorea
   b. stroke
   c. TIA
   d. traumatic brain injuries
   e. spinal cord injuries

5. Which word refers to the body being paralyzed from the shoulders down?
   a. quadriplegia
   b. hemiparesis
   c. paraplegia
   d. hemiplegia
   e. paraparesis

6. Bradykinesia, akinesia, and shuffling gait are symptoms of
   a. Alzheimer's disease.
   b. Huntington's chorea.
   c. Bell's palsy.
   d. spina bifida.
   e. Parkinson's disease.

7. Lou Gehrig's disease is another name for which disease?
   a. Alzheimer's disease
   b. Amyotrophic lateral sclerosis
   c. Huntington's chorea
   d. Bell's palsy
   e. Multiple sclerosis

8. A fatty substance that protects nerve fibers is known as
   a. dendrite.
   b. axon.
   c. myelin.
   d. synapse.
   e. ganglia.

9. Which system is sometimes referred to as the "voluntary" nervous system?
   a. central nervous system
   b. peripheral nervous system
   c. autonomic nervous system
   d. somatic nervous system
   e. parasympathetic nervous system

10. Which disease causes the loss of memory?
    a. Bell's palsy
    b. Huntington's chorea
    c. Parkinson's disease
    d. Alzheimer's disease
    e. Lou Gehrig's disease

CRITICAL THINKING

Refer to the case study at the beginning of the chapter and use the information you have learned to answer the following questions.

1. After examining Mrs. Bramatovich, Dr. Miller diagnoses her with Alzheimer's disease in its early stages. Svetlana asks the physician how her mother can be treated. What might Dr. Miller say to Svetlana?
2. Svetlana asks Dr. Miller for information related to Alzheimer's disease. Dr. Miller decides to send Mary Ellen, an RMA, into the room to review a patient education brochure that discusses the progression of the disease. What information should this brochure include?
3. Alzheimer's disease affects memory, reasoning, and problem-solving skills. Which lobe(s) of the brain pertain to these aspects of cognitive functioning?

INTERNET ACTIVITY

Conduct an Internet search to learn about Alzheimer's support groups.

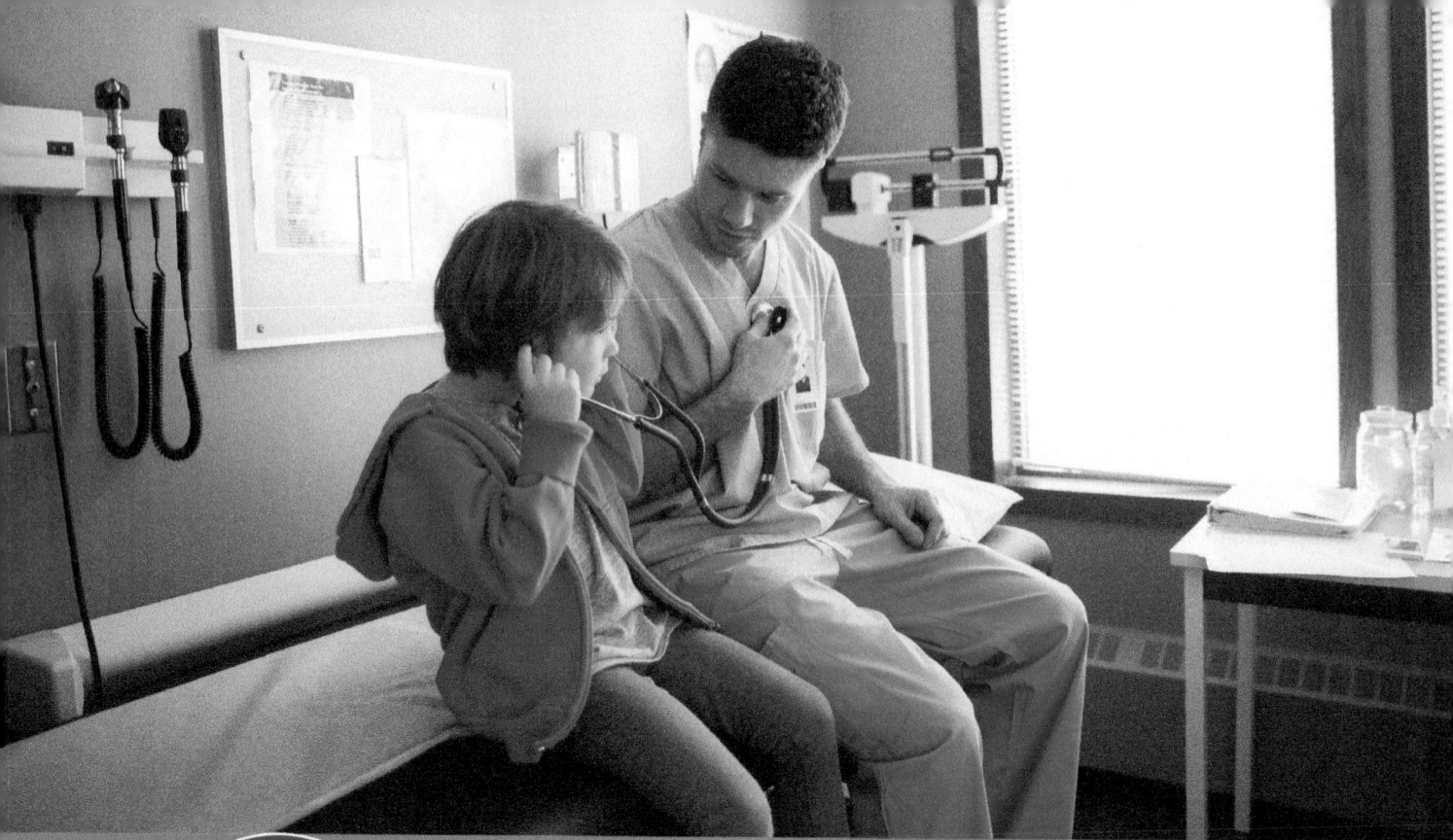

The Special Senses

Learning Objectives

After completing this chapter, you should be able to:

25.1 Define and spell the terms for this chapter.
25.2 List the anatomical structures of the eye.
25.3 Describe the function of the various structures of the eye.
25.4 Describe refractive disorders and other common pathology associated with the eye.
25.5 List the anatomical structures of the ear.
25.6 Describe the function of the various structures of the ear.
25.7 Differentiate between the various types of hearing loss.
25.8 Describe common pathology associated with the ear.
25.9 Explain the anatomy of the nose.
25.10 Describe how the process of smell occurs.
25.11 Describe how the process of taste occurs.
25.12 Explain how the special senses change from childhood to older adulthood.

Case Study

Carmine DiStefano is visiting Dr. Salpega today with his 1½-year-old son, Lucas. Lucas has been very restless and has not been sleeping very well during the past few nights. During the day, he hardly eats and is constantly tugging on his left ear. Mr. DiStefano is concerned because his 5-year-old daughter, Sophia, struggles with chronic otitis media and has recently had tubes placed in her ears. He is certain that Lucas has an ear infection.

Terms to Learn

accommodation	hordeolums	orbit
amblyopia	hyperopia	ossicles
aqueous humor	hypertensive retinopathy	otitis media
astigmatism	impacted cerumen	otosclerosis
audiology	incus	palpebrae
auditory meatus	insufflation	palpebral fissure
blepharitis	iris	papilledema
canthus	labyrinth	pinna
cataract	lacrimal apparatus	presbycusis
cerumen	lacrimal canaliculi	presbyopia
choroid	lacrimal gland	pupil
ciliary body	lacrimal sac	refraction
cochlea	lens	retina
cones	limbus	retinal detachment
conjunctiva	macula lutea	rods
conjunctivitis	macular degeneration	sclera
cornea	malleus	stapes
corneal abrasion	Ménière's disease	strabismus
diabetic retinopathy	myopia	tinnitus
diplopia	myringotomy	tympanic membrane
eustachian tube	nasolacrimal duct	vestibule
fovea centralis retinae	nystagmus (nystaxis)	vitreous chamber
fundus	optic disk	vitreous humor
glaucoma	optic nerve	

The senses are structures and organs that make it possible for us to see, hear, smell, taste, and feel. This chapter presents the five special senses, with particular attention to the organs of seeing and hearing and the disorders that may affect them.

THE EYE AND THE SENSE OF VISION

The eye is a spherical, fluid-filled organ composed of specialized structures that work together to facilitate vision. Light rays pass through the cornea, pupil, lens, and vitreous humor to the retina, where they stimulate sensory receptors. The nervous system plays an integral role in the sense of vision. Nerves in the eye are essential in the function of sight. The nerves of the eye:

- Control the amount of light entering the eye through the pupil
- Focus light on the retina by using the lens
- Transmit the resulting images from the retina to the brain

Anatomy of the Eye

The eye is made up of the eyeball and its internal structures, which perform the complex process of translating light into images, and the external structures that support and protect the eyeball (Figure 25-1).

The Structures of the Eyeball

The eyeball is housed in a cavity in the skull called an **orbit**. The eyeball itself can be divided into two cavities: a front, or anterior, cavity filled with a watery fluid called the **aqueous humor**, and a back, or posterior, section located behind the lens and filled with a very thick fluid in the **vitreous chamber**, called the **vitreous humor**. The surface of the eyeball is made up of three layers: outer, middle, and inner.

The Outer Layer of the Eyeball

The outer layer of the eyeball is composed of the **sclera**, or "white" of the eye. Light is unable to penetrate the sclera. The **cornea** is also found in the outer layer of the eye. The cornea is frequently referred to as the "window" of the eye because it allows the light to enter. The **limbus**, or corneal-scleral junction, is the area of the eye where the cornea and sclera meet.

The Middle Layer of the Eyeball

The middle layer of the eyeball is composed of the following structures:

- **Choroid**—Lines the sclera and absorbs extra light entering the eye.
- **Iris**—Contains the pigment, or eye color, and has

a "hole" in the center called the **pupil**. The muscular tissue that makes up the iris and pupil allows the pupil to constrict and dilate, which is how the pupil controls the amount of light that enters the eye.

- **Lens**—Colorless structure behind the iris, sharpens the focus of light rays onto the retina. The lens is important to a reflexive process called **accommodation**, which adjusts the eye's optical powers to maintain a clear image at various distances.
- **Ciliary body**—Responsible for holding and moving the lens; secretes aqueous humor, which provides nutrients to the cornea, lens, and other tissues.

The Inner Layer of the Eyeball

The innermost layer of the eye is the **retina**, the back of the eyeball, behind the vitreous humor. Photosensitive cells in the retina called **rods** and **cones** translate light rays into nerve impulses that are transmitted to the brain. Rods react to dim light and are used in night vision; cones are sensitive to bright light and are used to see color. The **fovea centralis retinae** contains only cones and is located in the middle of the **macula lutea**, a yellow spot on the back of the eye. The **optic nerve** enters at the **optic disk** and carries incoming information from the eye to the brain. Inflammation at the optic nerve, known as **papilledema**, increases

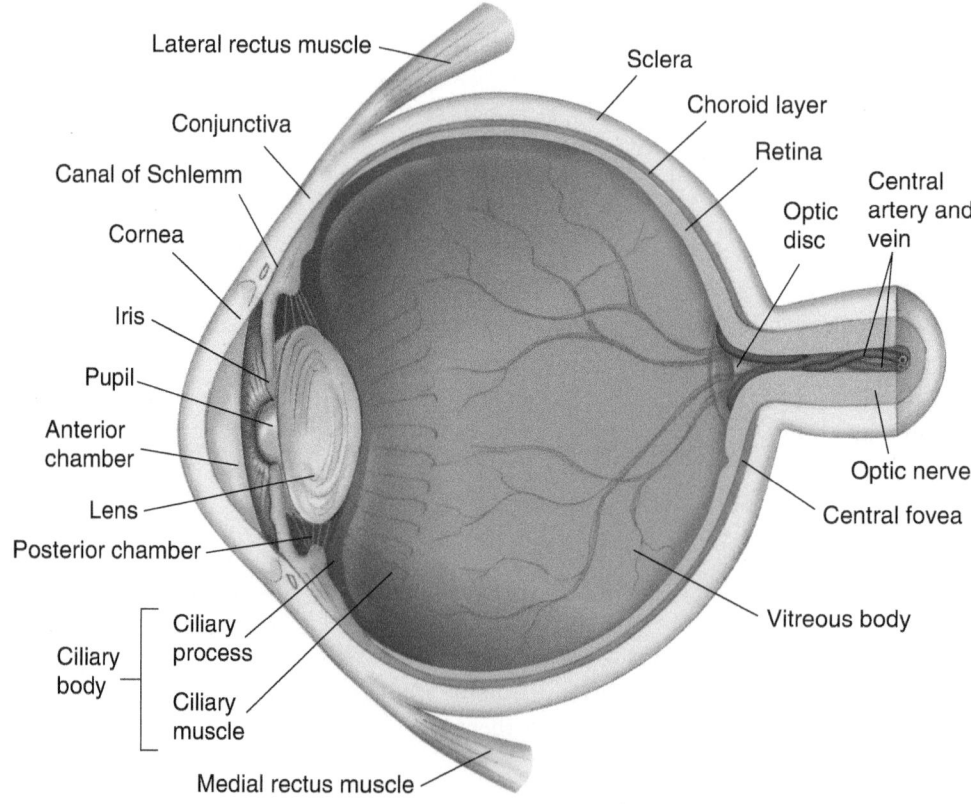

FIGURE 25-1 The eyeball and its anatomical structures.

pressure in the eye and can be caused by multiple factors, including various diseases, increased intracranial pressure, and even frontal lobe tumors.

The External Structures of the Eye

Other important structures of the eye serve the primary functions of protection and support: the eyelids, conjunctiva, lacrimal apparatus, and extrinsic eye muscles.

The eyelids, or **palpebrae**, close over the eyeballs, protecting them from intense light, foreign matter, and impacts. Eyelids are composed of dense connective tissue, muscle, and skin. They also keep the eyes moist by preventing moisture in the mucosal membrane surface of the eye from evaporating. Using its muscular tissue, the eyelid performs the blinking action that helps prevent bacteria and harmful substances from entering the eye. Light enters through the **palpebral fissure**, the opening between the superior and inferior (upper and lower) eyelids. Eyelashes in the margins of the eyelids further protect the eye from foreign matter. The superior and inferior palpebrae meet at the **canthus** at each corner of the eye.

The **conjunctiva** is a mucous membrane that lines the underside of the eyelids and the anterior part of the eyeball. It serves a protective function by helping to keep the eyeball moist and decreasing the opportunity for bacteria to grow.

Tears are a fluid the body produces to cleanse the eyes and keep them moist. Tears are produced, stored, and removed by the structures that make up the **lacrimal apparatus** (Figure 25-2). Above the outer corner of each eye is the **lacrimal gland**, which secretes tears through ducts on the surface of the conjunctiva of the upper lid. At the inner corner of each eye are two ducts, the **lacrimal canaliculi**, which collect and drain the tears into the **lacrimal sac**. The lacrimal sac empties into the **nasolacrimal duct**, which empties into the nasal cavity.

Six short eye muscles connect the eyeball to the orbital cavity. These muscles provide the eyeball with support and enable the eyeball to rotate.

COMMON REFRACTIVE DISORDERS

The most common disorders of the eye are refractive errors, which are characterized by the inability of the eye to focus correctly. They are caused by factors such as aging

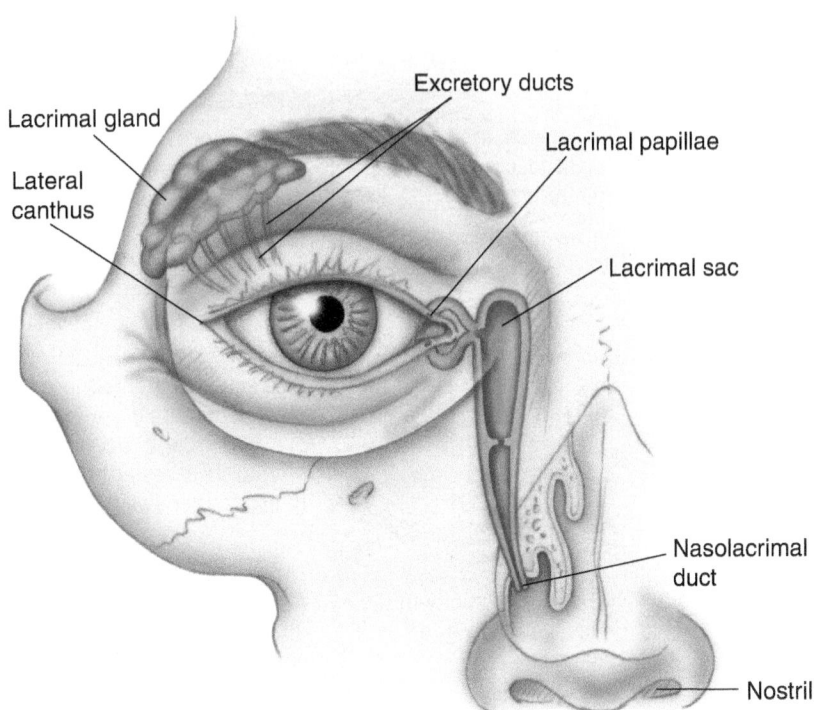

FIGURE 25-2 The lacrimal apparatus.

and changes in the shape of the eyeball and various eye muscles.

Myopia, Hyperopia, and Presbyopia

Refraction problems, the inability to focus correctly, occur because light rays change direction when they pass through the eye. Accommodation, as already noted, is the ability of the lens of the eye to adjust its shape for far and near focus. When the ability to adjust is impaired, the result is some form of difficulty in focusing. **Myopia**, **hyperopia**, and **presbyopia** are all commonly occurring disorders of focus, compared and contrasted in Table 25-1. Focusing difficulties are so common that, it is estimated, 75 percent of people living in the United States wear corrective lenses to fix these disorders.

Astigmatism

Astigmatism is a condition caused by an irregularity in the curvature of the cornea and lens. Usually rounder in shape, a cornea that is more football shaped is often present in those with astigmatism. This irregular shape causes light not to focus on the retina but rather to spread out over an area.

Signs and symptoms. Astigmatism is characterized by blurry near or distant vision. It may be accompanied by squinting and headaches.

TABLE 25-1 | Myopia, Hyperopia, and Presbyopia

Disorder	Structural Abnormality	Signs and Symptoms	Treatment
Myopia	Light focuses in front of the retina.	Also called nearsightedness; objects farther away tend to be blurry and difficult to see. It is easier to see objects that are closer to the eye.	Corrective lenses that help focus light on the retina. Surgical procedures such as radial keratotomy (RK) (surgical incisions are made from the pupil to the periphery of the cornea in a radial pattern) and the Lasik procedure (laser surgery that reshapes and corrects imperfections in the cornea) are also options.
Hyperopia	Light focuses behind the retina.	Also called farsightedness; objects that are close to the eye are harder to decipher and blurred. It is easier to see things farther away.	Corrective lenses that help focus light on the retina. Surgical procedures such as radial keratotomy (RK) (surgical incisions are made from the pupil to the periphery of the cornea in a radial pattern) and the Lasik procedure (laser surgery that reshapes and corrects imperfections in the cornea) are also options.
Presbyopia	A loss of elasticity in the lens; generally a result of aging.	As with hyperopia, there is difficulty focusing and seeing objects that are close. This specific disorder is directly related to the aging process.	Symptoms can be minimized by resting the eyes when reading or working at the computer. Close the eyes for 20–30 seconds every 20 minutes during visual activity. If symptoms persist, corrective lenses or refractive surgeries (like those mentioned above) can be helpful.

Treatment. Treatment generally consists of corrective lenses (glasses or contact lenses) or surgery to reshape the cornea.

Strabismus

Another common refractive disorder is **strabismus**, also called crossed eyes or wall eyes. In this condition, the eyes are misaligned and do not focus on the same image. One or both eyes turn in, out, up, or down. It is caused by abnormal neuromuscular control and weakness in the external ocular muscles of the eye.

Signs and symptoms. Patients with strabismus may experience poor depth perception and double vision, which is also known as **diplopia**.

Treatment. Treatments for strabismus include eyeglasses, eye exercises, wearing a patch over the stronger eye to force the weaker eye to become stronger, and surgery to realign the eyes.

COMMON PATHOLOGY ASSOCIATED WITH THE EYE

Structural irregularities, defects, or underlying disorders of the eye cause blepharoptosis, ectropion, entropion, and exophthalmos. These disorders are outlined in Table 25-2.

Infectious Eye Disorders

Infection and inflammation cause a number of common and often contagious eye disorders, such as blepharitis, conjunctivitis, and hordeolums.

Blepharitis

Blepharitis is an inflammation of the eyelids, particularly near the eyelash hair follicles. It can be caused by skin disorders such as seborrheic dermatitis, rosacea, or lice. It can also be caused by allergies.

Signs and symptoms. Signs and symptoms include redness, itching, and swelling of the eyelids. Burning sensations are common as is the development of crust that covers the eye, sometimes making it difficult to separate the eyelids.

Treatment. Blepharitis is treated with warm wet compresses and ophthalmic antibiotic therapy.

Conjunctivitis

Conjunctivitis is one of the most common and treatable eye infections, affecting both children and adults. Commonly known as pinkeye, this highly contagious condition is an inflammation of the conjunctiva, the tissue that lines the inside of the eyelid. Etiology includes viruses, bacteria, sexually transmitted infections (STIs), allergens, and irritants such as chlorine, dirt, or smoke.

TABLE 25-2 | Structural Irregularity Disorders of the Eye

Disease	Description	Cause	Signs and Symptoms	Treatment
Blepharoptosis	A disorder of the eyelid that occurs when muscles of the eyelid aren't strong enough to raise it.	Can be congenital or acquired as a secondary symptom of another disease such as myasthenia gravis or Horner's syndrome.	Abnormal drooping of one or both eyelids.	Surgery to correct the drooping eyelid.
Ectropion	A disorder that causes the lower eyelid to turn outward.	Can be congenital, or develop as a result of a reaction to a drug, muscle weakness, facial paralysis, and skin lesions.	Eye irritation, excessive tearing of the eye, or excessive dryness of the eye.	Temporary treatment may include eye ointment or drops to protect the cornea; however, permanent treatment requires surgical intervention.
Entropion	A disorder that causes the lower eyelid to turn inward.	Can be congenital, or develop as a result of an eye infection, muscle weakness, or scars from previous surgeries.	• Pain and irritation caused by exposure of the eyeball. • Sensitivity to light, watery eyes, and decreased or impaired vision.	Skin tape that can prevent the inward folding can be a temporary solution, but surgery is usually required for a permanent solution.
Exophthalmos	A disorder that causes the bulging, bug-like appearance of one or both eyes.	Generally, it is caused by hyperthyroidism or Graves disease. An orbital tumor may be the cause of unilateral exophthalmos.	The most distinctive symptom is the outward bulging of one or both eyeballs.	Treatment of the underlying condition is the primary goal. Surgical ablation and radiation are options. Eye drops may be used to keep eyelids lubricated.

Signs and symptoms. Early recognition of signs and symptoms is extremely important. An early symptom is the feeling of a foreign object in the eye, such as a speck of dust or sand. Other common symptoms include redness in the sclera, increased tear production, a thick yellow discharge that crusts over the eyelashes, itchy eyes, burning eyes, blurred vision, and greater sensitivity to light.

Treatment. Early treatment of conjunctivitis is equally important. Cleansing the eyes and applying warm compresses is an effective home remedy for treating pink eye. Over-the-counter eye drops are used to keep eyes lubricated. If the infection is bacterial, or if it is caused by an STI, prescription eye drops may be prescribed. Isolation during the first 24 hours of antibiotic therapy is recommended because of the highly contagious nature of the infection.

Hordeolums

Also known as sties, **hordeolums** are very common and frequently contagious. They are often caused by the *Staphylococcus* bacterium. Sties may accompany blocked or infected eyelid glands or inflamed eyelids. Contaminated fingers that touch the eye area may also cause the infection. Painful hordeolums can also occur under the eyelids (Figure 25-3).

Signs and symptoms. Early signs and symptoms include redness and tenderness followed by itching, swelling, and

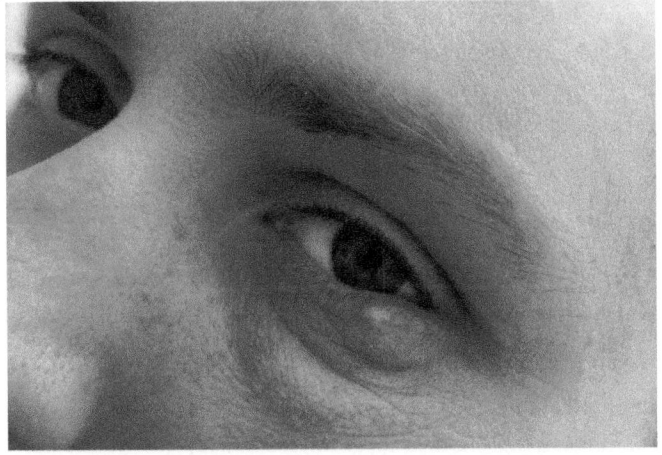

FIGURE 25-3 A hordeolum.

discomfort in the upper or lower eyelid. The stye, or hordeolum, develops as a pus-filled swelling at the base of an eyelash.

Treatment. Hordeolums often resolve on their own. A warm, wet compress applied to the area may help relieve the pain. It is important to tell patients to avoid touching the affected eye, and never to squeeze the hordeolum. Antibiotic creams or ointments may be applied to accelerate healing. In some cases, a physician may need to lance and drain the hordeolum to assist in the healing process; particularly if vision is affected.

Age-Related Eye Disorders

As we age, the muscles and other structures in the eye weaken and vision declines. Eye disorders commonly seen in older adults include cataracts, retinal detachment, and macular degeneration, which is one of the leading causes of blindness in this population.

Cataracts

A **cataract** is a clouding or opacity of the lens that prevents light from entering the eye. Although there is not a clear and specific etiology for all cases, there may be a correlation between the formation of cataracts and smoking, diabetes, use of specific drugs, excessive exposure to sunlight, and the overall aging process of the eye.

Signs and symptoms. As the cataract begins to form and the cloudiness begins to develop, vision begins to decrease. Patients may complain of fuzzy, blurred, or filmy vision. Sufferers may also experience a lack of color intensity as well as seeing halos around lights. Night vision suffers because of the decreased amount of light that is able to enter the eyes. The patient may also experience double vision or problems with bright lights. If left untreated, the cataract may eventually cloud the lens enough to block vision completely.

Treatment. For early or immature cataracts, eyeglasses, magnifying lenses, and stronger lighting may be sufficient. If this is not successful, surgery is the only effective treatment. Cataract removal is a very common surgery; it is also extremely safe and effective, with a cure rate of 90 percent.

Retinal Disorders

Among the disorders that affect the retina, two of the most severe are retinal detachment and macular degeneration. These disorders are fairly rare and primarily age-related.

Retinal Detachment

Retinal detachment occurs when a retina has separated from the underlying choroid layer (a vascular layer of connective tissue between the retina and sclera). Damage may start as small holes or tears and later, if left untreated, develop into full detachment. When such a separation occurs, vision is damaged. However, if the detachment is detected early, it can be repaired and the vision saved. If the retina has already detached, vision can frequently be restored by surgery and laser therapy. Causes of retinal detachment include shrinking of the vitreous that makes the retina tug and possibly tear, inflammatory eye disorders, advanced stages of diabetes, and injury to the eye.

Signs and symptoms. Symptoms of retinal detachment include an increase in floaters (particles that float slowly within the viewer's eyes), or flashes of light in the field of vision. The individual may feel as if a curtain has obscured part of the vision.

Treatment. Early treatment is ideal. Therefore, anyone experiencing the symptoms of retinal detachment should seek professional help as soon as possible. Treatment for small holes or tears is usually laser surgery or cryotherapy (application of intense cold to induce a scar); for retinal detachment, more invasive surgery requiring a hospital stay is generally recommended.

Macular Degeneration

Macular degeneration is the deterioration of the macula, which is the central portion of the retina. It is an incurable disease that affects more than ten million Americans and is one of the leading causes of blindness among people over the age of 55. As with many other eye disorders, there is not a specific etiology for macular degeneration. There are various risk factors associated with age-related macular degeneration. Some of these factors include being Caucasian and having lighter pigmentation, smoking, obesity, a familial history, exposure to sunlight, and gender, as women are more likely to develop macular degeneration.

The two types of macular degeneration are dry and wet. The dry (atrophic) type occurs in 85 to 90 percent of cases. In the dry type, small yellow deposits called drusen form under the macula, causing it to thin and dry out, leading to a loss of central vision. This form of macular degeneration has a slower progression than does the wet type; however, in some cases dry atrophic macular degeneration may develop into wet macular degeneration.

In wet macular degeneration, abnormal new blood vessels grow under the retina and the macula. They may then bleed and leak fluid, which causes the macula to bulge or lift up, impairing or destroying the central vision. Vision loss may be rapid and severe.

Signs and symptoms. Symptoms of dry macular degeneration include a decline in central vision, increasing haziness of overall vision, and a need for brighter illumination for reading and close work. Symptoms of wet macular degeneration include visual distortions and a blurry spot in the central vision.

Treatment. There is no known treatment or cure for dry macular degeneration. If performed early, laser surgery may halt the progression of wet macular degeneration, thus preventing a total loss of vision. Although this outcome cannot be guaranteed, laser surgery is currently the best treatment for wet macular degeneration.

Other Eye Disorders

Pathology related to the eyes and vision may be caused by factors other than those already described. These include amblyopia, corneal abrasions, glaucoma, nystagmus, and retinopathy.

Amblyopia

Amblyopia, or lazy eye, is a disorder often seen in children. Improper development of the nerve pathway from the eye to the brain is the etiology of this disorder. This improperly developed nerve pathway causes the affected eye to send incorrect images to the brain.

Amblyopia may have a hereditary factor. The leading cause of amblyopia is strabismus (crossed eye or wall eye), which was discussed earlier in the chapter. The brain tends to ignore the image from the misaligned eye, and amblyopia develops as the nerve pathway from the affected eye fails to fully develop. It is important to note that not everyone who suffers from strabismus will also suffer from amblyopia, and not all cases of amblyopia are caused by strabismus.

Signs and symptoms. Common symptoms and signs of amblyopia include eyes that appear to turn in or out, decreased vision, and faulty depth perception.

Treatment. Early diagnosis and treatment are essential to a positive and lasting outcome. If not corrected early, the underdevelopment of the nerve from the affected eye tends to become permanent. Treatment for underlying conditions, such as strabismus or refractive disorders, must first be completed. A patch may be worn over the strong eye to force the brain to interpret the images from the afflicted eye to foster development of the nerve pathway from that eye.

Corneal Abrasion

A **corneal abrasion** is a lesion or scratch on the cornea. There are many causes of corneal abrasions. Most result from infection or injury. Other causes include improperly fitting contact lenses and foreign matter becoming stuck in the eyelid.

Signs and symptoms. A corneal abrasion can be very painful and irritating. Other symptoms include blurred vision, excessive tearing, gritty feeling on the cornea, and possibly headache. The patient will be very sensitive to light and will have difficulty opening the affected eye.

Treatment. The usual treatment for corneal abrasion consists of mild analgesics and resting the eyes. If the abrasion becomes infected, antibiotic eye drops or ointments are given.

Glaucoma

Glaucoma affects people of all ages and all races. It is characterized by increased pressure in the eye. Left untreated, the pressure can lead to damage of the optic nerve and eventual blindness. An excessive amount of aqueous humor causes the increased intraocular pressure (IOP) that can lead to glaucoma. Risk factors for developing IOP and glaucoma include age (those over 60 are at higher risk), race (African-Americans are at higher risk), a family history of glaucoma, and those with vascular diseases.

There are two basic types of glaucoma. In open-angle (acute) glaucoma, a blockage gradually develops within the drainage canal from the anterior segment of the eye, slowing the drainage of aqueous humor and causing a gradual buildup of pressure. About 90 percent of glaucoma cases are of this open-angle type. In closed-angle (chronic) glaucoma, which is considered more serious, the space between the iris and the cornea narrows, causing the entrance to the drainage canal to narrow or close completely. In this case, pressure can rise very quickly. Approximately 80,000 people are totally blind as a result of glaucoma, another 250,000 are blind in one eye, and over 1.2 million people have some degree of visual loss.

Signs and symptoms. Open-angle glaucoma is a chronic condition sometimes referred to as primary glaucoma. It is asymptomatic (without symptoms) and is often referred to as the "silent thief" of vison. Eventually the patient may experience tunnel vision. However, once this symptom begins to occur, damage is already severe. Acute, closed-angle glaucoma (also referred to as narrow-angle glaucoma) may present signs and symptoms that include sharp eye pain, decreased hazy vision, and red swollen eyes. A test called tonometry, which measures the intraocular pressure of the eye, is performed on patients when glaucoma is either suspected or the patient is at high risk for developing the disorder.

Treatment. Glaucoma is treated with medications such as eye drops to lower intraocular pressure as well as with laser and conventional surgery.

Professionalism | The Law

Be clear on the rules for driving in your state to help patients who have visual difficulties. A patient who has had recent vision changes and cannot see clearly should be instructed by the physician on local laws and the dangers of driving. The medical assistant should help the patient by providing a list of community resources that provide transportation when necessary. Resources should be readily available and helpful, so the patient can take immediate steps to access them. It is unsafe for patients with limited visual abilities to operate any motorized vehicle. As vision decreases, the patient will need to rely on community resources for activities of daily living.

Nystagmus (Nystaxis)

Nystagmus (nystaxis) is characterized by involuntary, repetitive, rhythmic eye movements. It may be inherited or acquired and usually results in some loss of vision.

Signs and symptoms. Uncontrolled eye movements, which may be lateral, horizontal, or even circular.

Treatment. Treatment must address the underlying cause, which might be a tumor, a lesion, alcohol abuse, or retinal maldevelopment.

Retinopathy

Retinopathy is a disease of the retina that is caused by either recurring or acute damage. Patients with diabetes are prone to **diabetic retinopathy**. Nerve damage can result from **hypertensive retinopathy**, caused by high blood pressure, and can lead to permanent blindness. Sickle cell disease, trauma, and other disorders can cause general retinopathy. Symptoms vary based on the type of retinopathy that is diagnosed, and treatment lies in treating the underlying condition causing the disorder.

THE EAR AND THE SENSE OF HEARING

The ear is the organ responsible for hearing and equilibrium, or balance. Specialized anatomical structures in the ear are sensitive to sound vibrations, gravity, and head movements. The eighth cranial nerve connects these structures to the brain.

Anatomy of the Ear

The ear can be divided into three sections: the external, middle, and inner ears (Figure 25-4). Each section plays a distinct role in the hearing process.

The Outer Ear

The outer ear consists of the following structures:

- **Pinna**, or auricle—The visible portion of the ear outside the head. It funnels sound waves into the auditory canal.

- Auditory canal, or **auditory meatus**—A slightly curved tube, about one inch (2.5 cm) long; receives and carries sound waves from the outer ear to the tympanic membrane; secretes **cerumen**, or earwax.

- **Tympanic membrane**, or eardrum—Separates the outer ear from the middle ear and transmits sound vibrations into the middle ear.

- The **fundus**—The floor of the tympanic cavity.

The Middle Ear

The middle ear is a tiny cavity in the temporal bone of the skull. It contains three small bones, or **ossicles**, whose names describe their shapes: the **malleus** (hammer), **incus** (anvil), and **stapes** (stirrup). The function of the middle ear is to transmit sound vibrations, equalize the air pressure on both sides of the tympanic membrane, and protect the ear from potentially damaging loud noise. Sound vibrations are

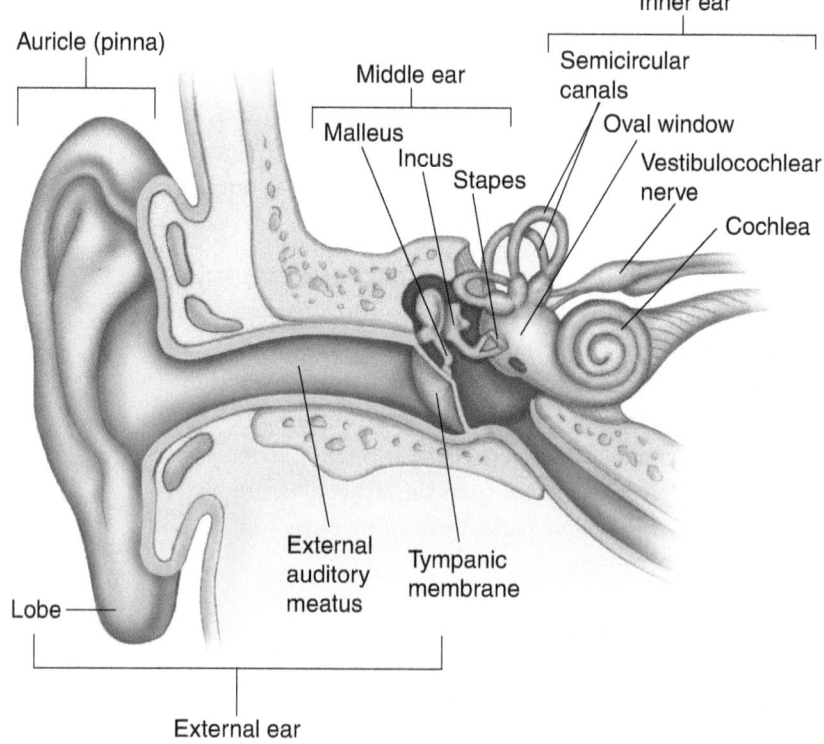

FIGURE 25-4 The ear and its anatomical structures.

transmitted by the ossicles from the tympanic membrane to the oval window and into the inner ear.

The **eustachian tube**, or auditory tube, extends 3 to 4 cm from the middle ear to the nasopharynx. If blocked, the patient may get an infection in the middle ear.

The Inner Ear

The inner ear is a maze of canals within a bony **labyrinth** in the temporal bone. The cochlea, vestibule, and three semicircular canals make up the labyrinth. The bony and membranous labyrinths are separated by a fluid called perilymph. Tiny hair cells in the inner ear function as receptors for hearing and balance.

The **cochlea**, which is the organ of hearing, is a bony spiral structure that resembles a snail's shell (Figure 25-5). Three tubelike channels run the entire length of the spiral; between the upper and lower channels is the cochlear duct. The organ of Corti, located in the cochlear duct, contains nerve endings that transmit sound vibrations received from the stapes to the auditory region of the brain via the eighth cranial nerve.

The **vestibule** is the fundus of the internal auditory meatus (the floor of the internal ear canal). The vestibular system controls the sense of balance. The vestibular nerve is a main division of the acoustic or eighth cranial nerve.

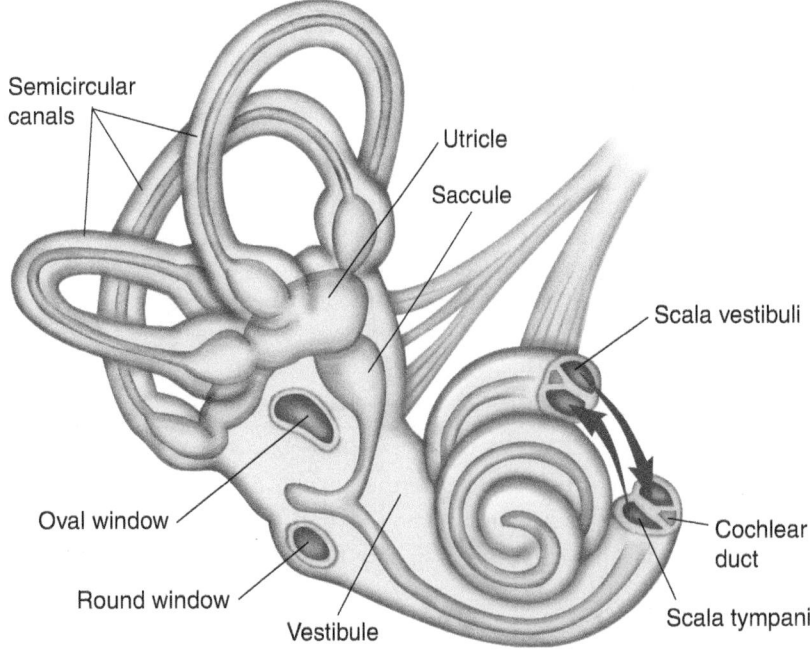

FIGURE 25-5 The cochlea.

HEARING LOSS

Audiology is the study of hearing disorders, including hearing loss. The two most common types of hearing loss are conductive and sensorineural.

- **Conductive hearing loss**—A temporary condition in which sound is not conducted efficiently through the auditory canal to the eardrum and the ossicles in the middle ear. Inner ear infections, swimmer's ear, fluid accumulation within the middle ear, impacted cerumen, and allergies could all be causative factors for this form of hearing loss. Conductive hearing loss can be medically corrected by treating the underlying cause or can be surgically corrected.

- **Sensorineural hearing loss**—Permanent hearing loss caused by damage to the cochlea or to nerve pathways from the inner ear to the brain. Sensorineural hearing loss can be caused by malformation of the auditory structures, head trauma, aging, and exposure to loud noise. Hearing aids can be helpful to those who only have partial hearing loss. In the past, complete hearing loss was generally not a treatable condition and was considered to be permanent. However, new advances in medicine, specifically cochlear implants, are helping to change the outlook for those with this condition.

Professionalism

The professional medical assistant occasionally has days when the physician is running behind and seeing patients later than scheduled. This delay can create anxiety or discomfort for both patients and medical assistants. Explain to patients that the physician is delayed, and give them the option to reschedule. This demonstrates to the patient that the medical office has respect for the patient's time and personal schedule. If the patient chooses to wait, move him to an exam room as quickly as possible. However, keep in mind that some patients might prefer to spend lengthier wait times in a reception area where there are often more options available to pass time, such as television or magazines. When wait times are longer than 15 minutes, use your best discretion for rooming patients or follow the established office protocol. It is also helpful to plan ahead to help maximize the physician's efficiency. Explaining to patients that the physician is providing the same care to other patients that will be provided to them will help to alleviate their frustrations with the delay. If patients do verbalize impatience or even anger, do not take it personally; keep in mind they are simply venting understandable frustration.

Many of the disorders discussed next either involve or result in hearing loss. See "Professionalism: Cultural Considerations" for a brief discussion of sensitivity toward patients with hearing difficulties.

COMMON PATHOLOGY ASSOCIATED WITH THE EAR

Various disorders and diseases can affect all parts of the ear. To help explain and identify these issues, pathology and disorders have been grouped according to the parts of the ear affected: the outer, middle or inner ear.

The Outer Ear

Two of the most common disorders of the outer ear involve impacted cerumen and injury to the tympanic membrane.

Impacted Cerumen

Cerumen is a complex mixture of lipids produced by the sebaceous glands of the auditory canal to lubricate the ear. **Impacted cerumen** is earwax that has accumulated and hardened to the point that it obstructs the auditory canal. It generally affects older adults and is often caused by the patient trying to remove earwax at home by placing external objects into the ear (such as cotton swabs) in an attempt to clean it. When the external object enters the ear canal, rather than fully removing the wax, it actually pushes the cerumen farther into the ear, which makes the buildup worse.

Signs and symptoms. The patient with impacted cerumen may complain of blocked or muffled hearing, a plugged feeling in the ear, and even pain.

Treatment. Treatment includes softening the wax and removing it by flushing the ear with an ear syringe. "Irrigation" is the term used for this procedure in the medical office. Left untreated, impacted cerumen can lead to hearing loss or tinnitus (ringing of the ears).

Ruptured Tympanic Membrane

The tympanic membrane is a thin structure that is vulnerable to injury such as rupture or tearing. These injuries can occur when objects entering the ear perforate the membrane or when unequal air pressure on both sides of the membrane causes a rupture. Commonly known as a ruptured eardrum, this injury can lead to middle ear infections, because the tympanic membrane is no longer intact and providing complete protection of the middle ear.

Signs and symptoms. A sharp, sudden pain in the affected ear may be followed by drainage of fluid. Tinnitus, hearing loss, and vertigo (dizziness) are also common symptoms. In some cases, nausea and vomiting may accompany vertigo.

Treatment. The ruptured membrane is able to heal without any treatment, usually taking a few weeks to fully recover. However, treatment that is usually provided includes antibiotic medications to prevent infection and analgesics to reduce pain. Patients should be instructed not to clean their ears with objects such as swabs but instead to flush the ears with earwax softeners or a room-temperature saline solution. Cold solutions should never be introduced into the ear.

The Middle Ear

Inflammatory disorders are the most common problems that afflict the middle ear. It is not uncommon for the inner ear to also be inflamed because of middle ear disorders. The most common inflammatory disorder affecting the middle ear is otitis media.

Otitis Media

Otitis is an inflammation of any part of the ear. Otitis externa (swimmer's ear) is an inflammation of the outer ear canal, whereas **otitis media** is an inflammation of the middle ear. Otitis media can be caused by viral or bacterial infections, often secondary to sore throats and colds. It occurs in children more frequently than in adults. Any swelling in the tissues that surround the eustachian tube can cause closure, thus decreasing the ability of the ear to drain. Naturally occurring fluids that cannot drain from the ear become a source of infection.

Signs and symptoms. Infants and toddlers with otitis media may tug at the affected ear because they are unable to verbally communicate their discomfort. The child may also be unusually irritable or fussy, have a fever, and have difficulty sleeping. It is not uncommon for fluid drainage from the ear to be present. Drainage as well as exhibiting a loss of balance are more serious than the other symptoms. Older children and adults will complain of pain in their ears, often either sharp or throbbing.

Treatment. The main goal of treatment for otitis media is to eliminate the cause of infection before more serious complications set in. Oral antibiotics help to kill bacteria and eliminate the source of the infection. Decongestants such as pseudoephedrine help reduce swelling by shrinking the blood vessels in the eustachian tubes. A pain reliever may also be prescribed. If the condition is more acute and there is thick effusion and poor eustachian tube function, tubal **insufflation** (introduction of gas, vapor, or powder into the middle ear via the eustachian tube) may be necessary every one to two days. Recurrent ear infections may be treated with **myringotomy**. Myringotomy is a procedure in which a small incision is made and a drainage tube inserted through the tympanic membrane to drain fluid and reduce inner ear pressure.

Otosclerosis

Otosclerosis is a condition characterized by abnormal bone tissue growth around the stapes. This overgrowth of bone prevents the stapes from transmitting sound vibrations to the inner ear. The exact etiology is unknown; however, it is considered to be a hereditary disorder.

Signs and symptoms. The overgrowth causes gradual hearing loss in one or both ears. Some people may also experience tinnitus and dizziness.

Treatment. Mild cases of otosclerosis may be treated with a hearing aid. In more severe cases, surgery may be recommended. During surgery, a portion of the stapes may be removed and replaced with a prosthetic.

The Inner Ear

The inner ear plays a large role in maintaining the body's equilibrium and balance. Many of the disorders specific to the inner ear are characterized by severe dizziness (vertigo), tinnitus, and loss of balance.

Tinnitus

Tinnitus, ringing in the ears, is a symptom that is linked to both hearing loss and other ear ailments. Tinnitus is a very common condition that afflicts approximately 12 million Americans. It can be a persistent and debilitating condition that may be severe enough to interfere with daily life including working and sleeping. Tinnitus may be caused by hearing loss, loud noise, certain medications, and other health problems such as allergies and tumors.

Signs and symptoms. The main symptom of tinnitus is ringing, buzzing, or roaring in one or both ears.

Treatment. A variety of options are available to treat the symptoms of tinnitus, though no cure is available. Maskers are small electronic devices worn like a hearing aid to help mask or drown out the tinnitus through the production of "white noise." Hearing aids have also proven to be helpful by enhancing sounds that need to be heard while lessening the effects of tinnitus. Alternative therapies including relaxation techniques, hypnosis, and acupuncture are being evaluated to help improve quality of life for those who suffer from tinnitus.

Ménière's Disease

Ménière's disease is named after the French physician, Prosper Ménière, who first described the syndrome in 1861. This disease affects a person's balance and hearing. It is believed that changes in fluid volume in the labyrinth of the inner ear cause the symptoms of Ménière's disease. Other possible causes include bacterial or viral infections, environmental factors, and noise pollution.

Signs and symptoms. Four main symptoms present with this disease. They are loss of hearing, pressure in the ear, vertigo, and tinnitus. Other symptoms may include nausea, vomiting, diarrhea, and headaches. Symptoms often occur suddenly, without warning, and they may occur daily or infrequently. Sudden movement may cause symptoms to become worse. Hearing returns after an attack but usually worsens over time.

Treatment. Treatment for Ménière's disease is aimed at controlling symptoms through lifestyle modifications. To combat the excessive fluid pressure in the ear, dietary choices (low-sodium diets) and diuretic drugs to reduce fluid retention are often implemented. Avoiding excessive caffeine and alcohol is also beneficial. Other medications, such as those that control allergies and improve blood circulation (vasodilators) in the inner ear, may be beneficial. Eliminating tobacco use and reducing stress levels may also reduce the severity of symptoms. Currently there is no cure for this disease.

Presbycusis

Presbycusis is a type of hearing loss involving the gradual deterioration of the sensory receptors in the cochlea. Affecting more men than women, one in three people aged 65 to 74 have some form of age-related hearing loss. This number jumps to one out of every two, or 50%, of persons over the age of 75. Factors that lead to presbycusis include simple changes resulting from aging of the ear, prolonged exposure to loud noises, infection, injury, and side effects of certain medications.

Signs and symptoms. Presbycusis generally occurs in both ears, causing problems with hearing both the normal and the high-pitched tones of conversation. Hearing loss is generally gradual.

Treatment. Treatment is generally achieved through the use of a hearing aid. However, if hearing loss is severe enough, cochlear implants may be suggested by a physician.

THE SENSES OF TASTE AND SMELL

The nose is the primary organ for the sense of smell (Figure 25-6). Olfactory cells high in the roof of the nasal cavity respond to changes in volatile chemical concentrations. Once a smell receptor is activated, it sends the information to the brain via the olfactory nerves (Cranial Nerve I).

The sense of taste and the sense of smell function together to create a combined effect that is interpreted by the brain. When you smell something, some of the tiny molecules given off by that object move from the nose down into the mouth region and stimulate the taste buds. In actuality, part of what we refer to as smell is really taste.

Taste buds are microscopic bumps on the tongue, the roof of the mouth, and the walls of the throat. The cells in each

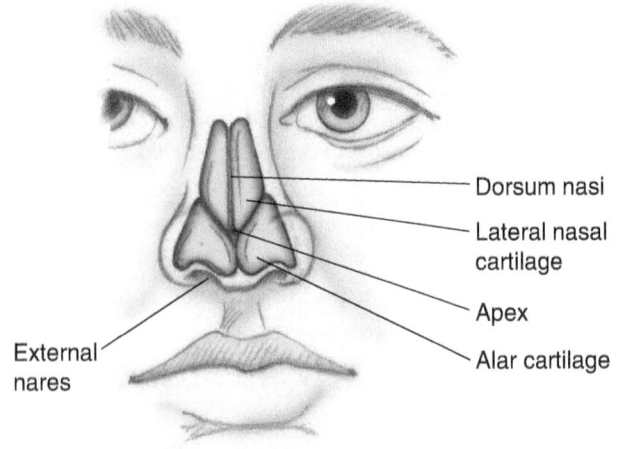

FIGURE 25-6 Nasal cartilage and external structures.

taste bud serve as taste receptors. The four commonly accepted types of taste cells are sweet, sour, salty, and bitter. Recently, a fifth taste cell, umami, was recognized as a savory taste receptor. The word *umami* originates from Japanese and translates as "savory or pleasant."

THE SENSE OF TOUCH

Touch is our oldest, most primitive sense. It is the first sense we experience in the womb and the last one we lose before death. Unlike the other four senses (sight, hearing, smell, and taste), the sense of touch is found over the entire body. It originates in the dermis, the deepest layer of the skin. Nerve endings (receptors) in the dermis transmit information to the spinal cord, which in turn sends messages to the brain, where the feeling is registered.

The more nerve endings there are in a given area of the body, the more sensitive it is. The sides of the tongue, for example, have numerous nerve endings; hence the pain that results from accidentally biting down on the tongue. However, the tongue is not as good at sensing hot or cold, which explains why it is so easy to burn the mouth when eating or drinking something especially hot.

SUMMARY

The special senses of vision, hearing, smell, and taste are extensions of the nervous system, whereas the sense of touch functions all over the body. The eyes are the organs of vision;

the ears are the organs of hearing and balance. Both systems require the collaboration of specialized cells to provide appropriate input to the brain for interpretation. The senses of vision, hearing, taste, and smell are activated through the brain and the nervous system. The sense of touch originates in the dermis, where nerve endings process and transfer information to the spinal cord, and on to the brain. During the aging process, all these systems can decline significantly, greatly affecting the activities and quality of life.

These special senses are also prone to disorders. The position and anatomy of the eye make it vulnerable to problems with fluids, trauma, lens changes, retinal disease, pressure changes, and vascular disorders. Eye problems include refraction disorders, infectious eye disorders, age-related eye disorders, and other generalized disorders.

Because infection and objects can enter the ear, the ear is also vulnerable to disorders. Common problems include impacted cerumen, ruptured tympanic membrane, otitis media, otosclerosis, tinnitus, Ménière's disease, and presbycusis.

The tongue is the sensory organ for the sense of taste. The tongue can detect five different tastes (sweet, sour, salty, bitter, and savory). The skin is the primary organ for the sense of touch. The nose is the primary organ for the olfactory sense (smell).

25 CHAPTER REVIEW

COMPETENCY REVIEW

1. Define and spell the terms for this chapter.
2. What are the four main symptoms of Ménière's disease?
3. What causes refractive errors?
4. What are the five tastes that the tongue can detect?
5. What is the function of the aqueous humor?
6. What are the overall functions of the ear?
7. What are the three ossicles of the ear?
8. What structures make up the bony labyrinth?
9. What is the role of rods and cones in vision?
10. What is the difference between conductive hearing loss and sensorineural hearing loss?

PREPARING FOR THE CERTIFICATION EXAM

1. What is the name of the substance that fills the posterior cavity of the eyeball?
   a. vitreous humor
   b. nasolacrimal fluid
   c. aqueous humor
   d. lacrimal gland
   e. lacrimal fluid

2. The structure of the eye in which the rods and cones determine color perception is called the
   a. pupil.
   b. aqueous humor.
   c. retina.
   d. ciliary body.
   e. choroids.

3. Which of the following is the term for farsightedness, in which the patient cannot focus well on objects close at hand?
   a. myopia
   b. astigmatism
   c. presbyopia
   d. hyperopia
   e. glaucoma

4. A condition of the eye in which the lens clouds over and prevents light from entering is
   a. glaucoma.
   b. cataracts.
   c. retinal detachment.
   d. astigmatism.
   e. corneal ulcers.

5. A highly contagious condition of the eye, also known as a stye, is
   a. corneal abrasion.
   b. astigmatism.
   c. macular degeneration.
   d. conjunctivitis.
   e. hordeolum.

6. This produces, stores, and removes the tears that cleanse and lubricate the eye.
   a. retina
   b. sclera
   c. lacrimal apparatus
   d. conjunctiva
   e. iris

7. The ear bone that is shaped like a stirrup is called the
   a. malleus.
   b. stapes.
   c. incus.
   d. hammer.
   e. anvil.

8. Which of the following is an ear disorder?
   a. blepharitis
   b. glaucoma
   c. strabismus
   d. presbycusis
   e. macular degeneration

9. Which of the following is a condition in which the eyeballs bulge outward?
   a. entropion
   b. ectropion
   c. exophthalmos
   d. eczema
   e. nystagmus

10. Which of the following is *not* a taste that can be detected by the tongue?
   a. bitter
   b. sour
   c. sweet
   d. salty
   e. bittersweet

CRITICAL THINKING

Refer to the case study at the beginning of the chapter and use what you have learned to answer the following questions.

1. When Dr. Salpega sees Lucas, he asks his father if Lucas has had any cough or cold symptoms lately. Why would Dr. Salpega ask this question?
2. Dr. Salpega diagnoses Lucas with acute otitis media. Through some diagnostic assessment, the doctor determines that Lucas has some mild hearing loss. Mr. DiStefano is very concerned about this. He wonders if the hearing loss will be permanent. How will Dr. Salpega likely respond?
3. What is the likely course of treatment for Lucas? Would the doctor want Lucas to follow up? Explain why or why not.

INTERNET ACTIVITY

Conduct an Internet search on Lasik surgery to learn more about the procedure.

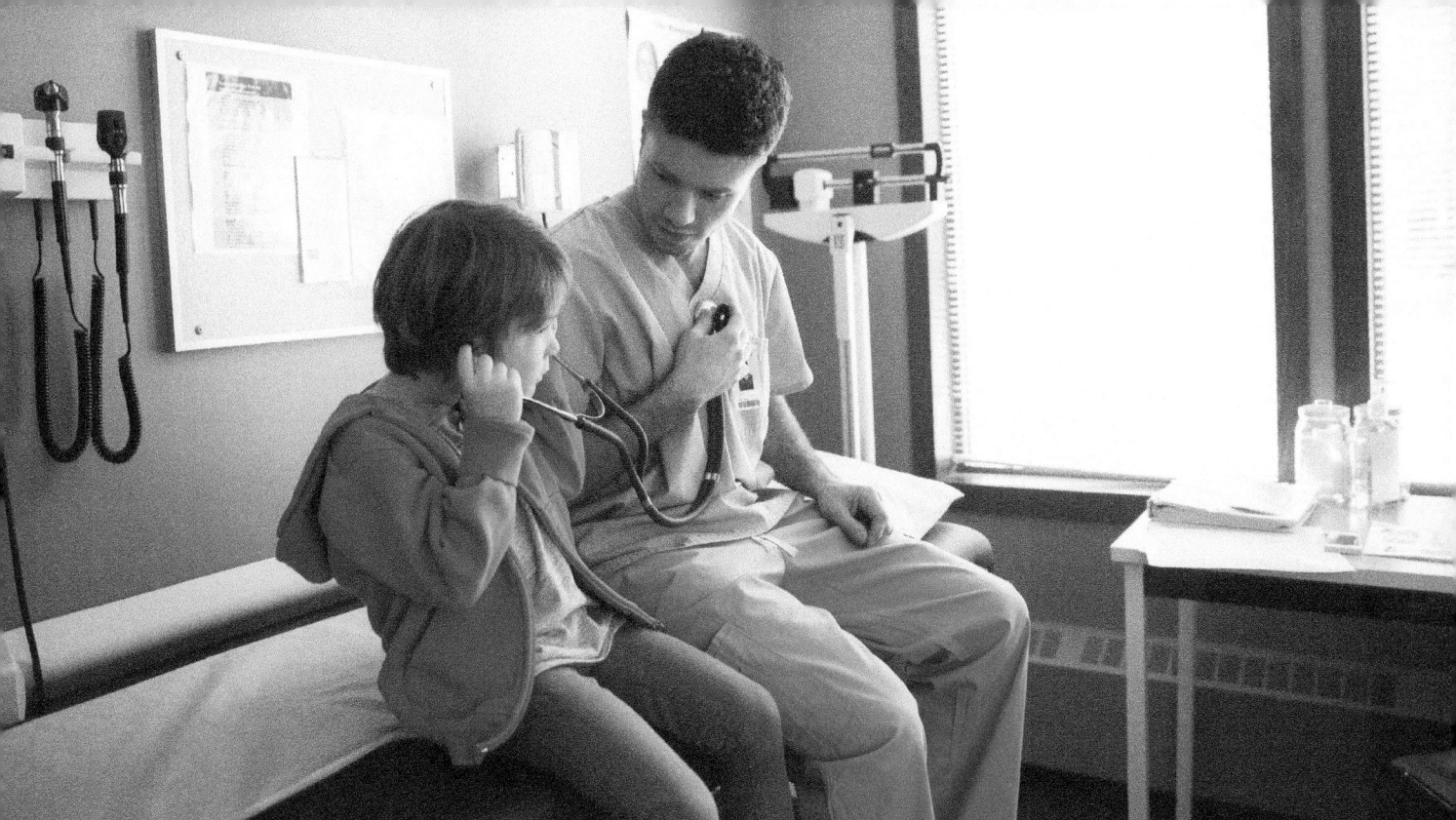

The Cardiovascular System

Learning Objectives

After completing this chapter, you should be able to:

26.1   Define and spell the terms for this chapter.

26.2   Identify the structures that make up the cardiovascular system.

26.3   Explain how the cardiovascular system functions.

26.4   Explain cardiovascular changes between children and the older adult.

26.5   Differentiate between pulmonary and systemic circulation.

26.6   Explain the correlation between blood pressure and pulse pressure.

26.7   Describe the components of blood.

26.8   List the functions of blood.

26.9   Describe common pathology associated with the cardiovascular system.

Jamal Washington has made an appointment to see Dr. Miller at Pearson Physicians Group. He was reluctant to make the appointment and made it only because his wife, Tania, urged him. Now he does not want to go to the doctor. Jamal has been complaining of intense headaches and has had frequent episodes of nosebleeds.

Terms to Learn

agglutination	coronary artery disease (CAD)	occlusion
anemia	cor pulmonale	pericardium
aneurysm	cyanosis	petechiae
angioplasty	diastolic blood pressure	phlebotomy
aorta	dyspnea	plasma
arrhythmia	endocardium	platelets
arteriosclerosis	erythrocytes	prehypertension
atherosclerosis	heart	pulmonary artery
atria	heart murmur	pulmonary vein
atrioventricular (AV) node	hemoglobin	pulse pressure
bicuspid valve	hemophilia	Purkinje fibers
blood pressure	hemostasis	RhoGAM
bradycardia	hypertension (HTN)	septum
bruit	hypotension	sinoatrial (SA) node
buffers	hypoxia	sphygmomanometer
bundle of His	infarction	stroke
cardiac arrest	inferior vena cava	superior vena cava
cardiac tamponade	ischemia	systolic blood pressure
cardiogenic shock	leukemia	tachycardia
carditis	leukocytes	thrombophlebitis
carotid artery	mitral valve	tricuspid valve
congestive heart failure (CHF)	myocardial infarction (MI)	venipuncture
coronary arteries	myocardium	ventricles

The human organism could not live without the powerful cardiovascular system. The heart, never ceasing to beat until death, circulates blood and other important materials through a system of arteries, veins, arterioles, and capillaries.

THE STRUCTURES OF THE CARDIOVASCULAR SYSTEM

The cardiovascular system consists of the heart, the blood vessels, and the blood. In this section, the heart and blood vessels are discussed. Blood is covered later in the chapter.

The Heart

The **heart** is a four-chambered muscular organ. It lies to the left of the chest's midline under the breastbone, or sternum (Figure 26-1). The heart is similar in size and shape to a fist, weighing between 9 and 11 ounces. The apex, or pointed portion of the heart, is at the lowest point of the organ. The heart is composed of three layers (Figure 26-2):

- **Pericardium**—The outer lining, or layer; covers the heart and the large blood vessels attached to it

- **Myocardium**—The middle layer, or heart muscle; is the thickest layer

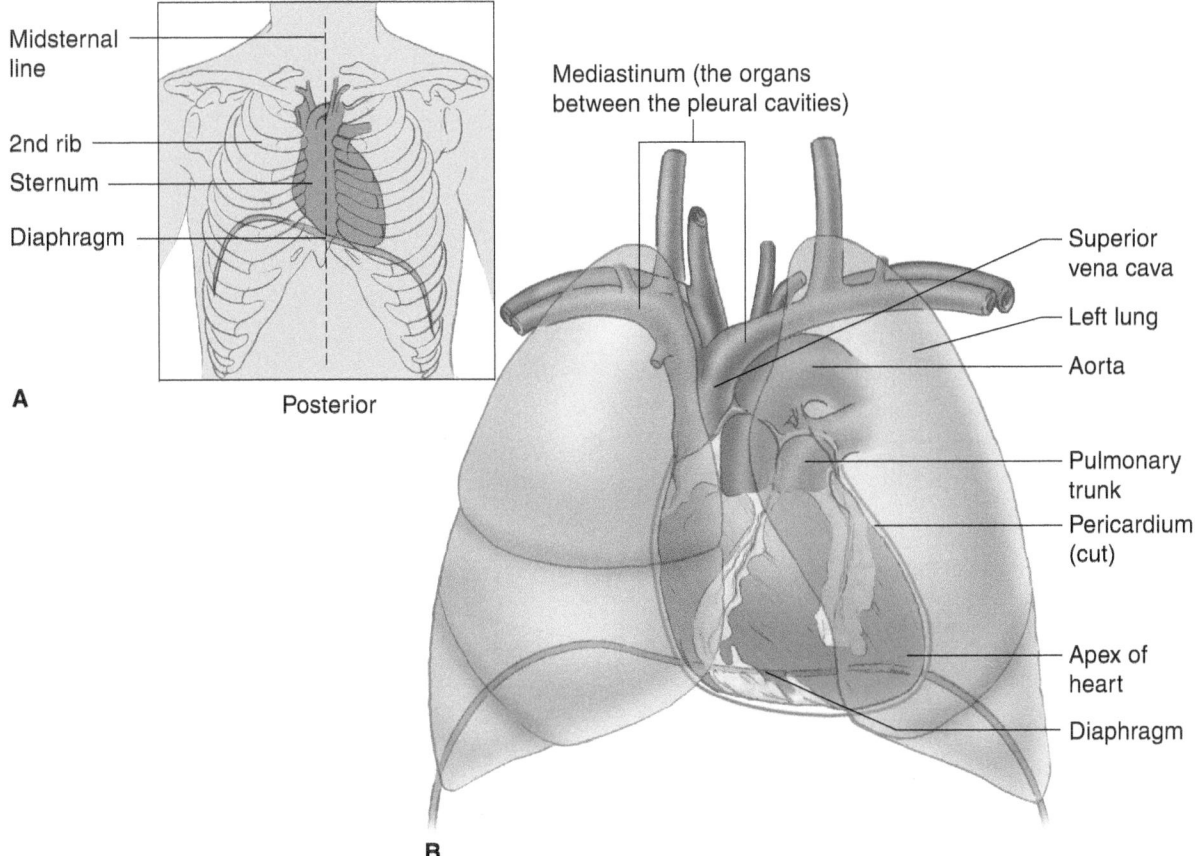

FIGURE 26-1 Location of the heart in the chest cavity.

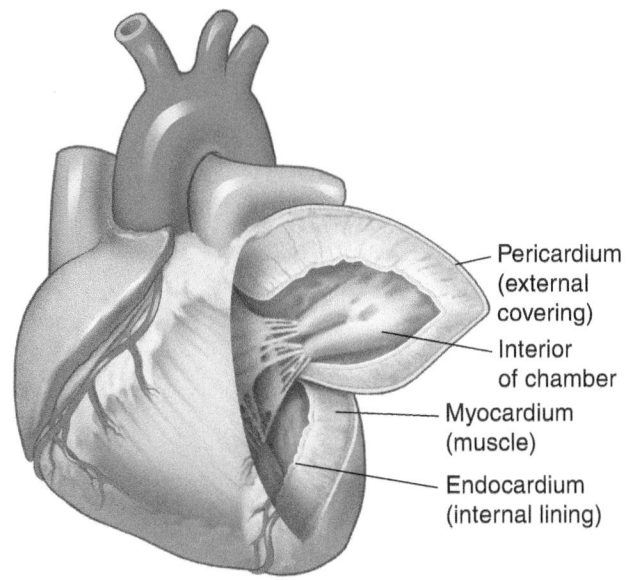

FIGURE 26-2 Linings of the heart.

- **Endocardium**—The innermost lining; is thin and smooth and contains part of the electrical conduction system of the heart

As discussed in the chapter "The Nervous System," the autonomic nervous system controls the heartbeat, which is actually muscular contractions of the heart.

The **septum** is a wall that separates the sides of the heart, creating left and right sides. The right side moves blood from the body to the lungs, and the left side pumps the blood that is returned from the lungs back to the body (Figure 26-3).

The **atria** are the two upper chambers of the heart: the right atrium (singular form of atria) and the left atrium. The **ventricles** are the two lower chambers, also identified as right and left. The atria receive blood from the body or lungs; the ventricles, by contrast, pump blood out to the lungs or body.

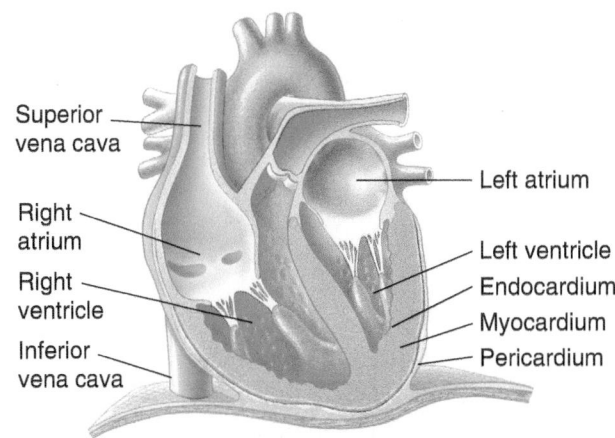

FIGURE 26-3 The heart: interior view of the heart chambers.

Blood Vessels

Some blood vessels carry blood from the heart to the cells of the body, providing the cells with oxygen and nourishment. Other vessels carry away wastes produced by the same cells. Blood vessels vary in size. The largest are arteries and veins, next smaller are arterioles and venules, and the smallest are capillaries.

Arteries and Arterioles

Arteries are the vessels that carry the blood away from the heart (Figure 26-4). High pressure provided by the heartbeat propels the blood forward through the arteries. The largest artery is the aorta, the one that directly exits the heart. From the aorta, arteries divide into smaller and smaller branches as they spread out to all parts of the body. The smallest arteries, called arterioles, connect to the tiny capillaries that make direct contact with individual body cells.

The arteries are thick-walled elastic tubes that expand with pressure from the heartbeat as it pushes blood through them. Between the beats of the heart, the arteries relax. Their constant expansion and relaxation make the arteries easily palpable. When you obtain a patient's pulse rate, it is

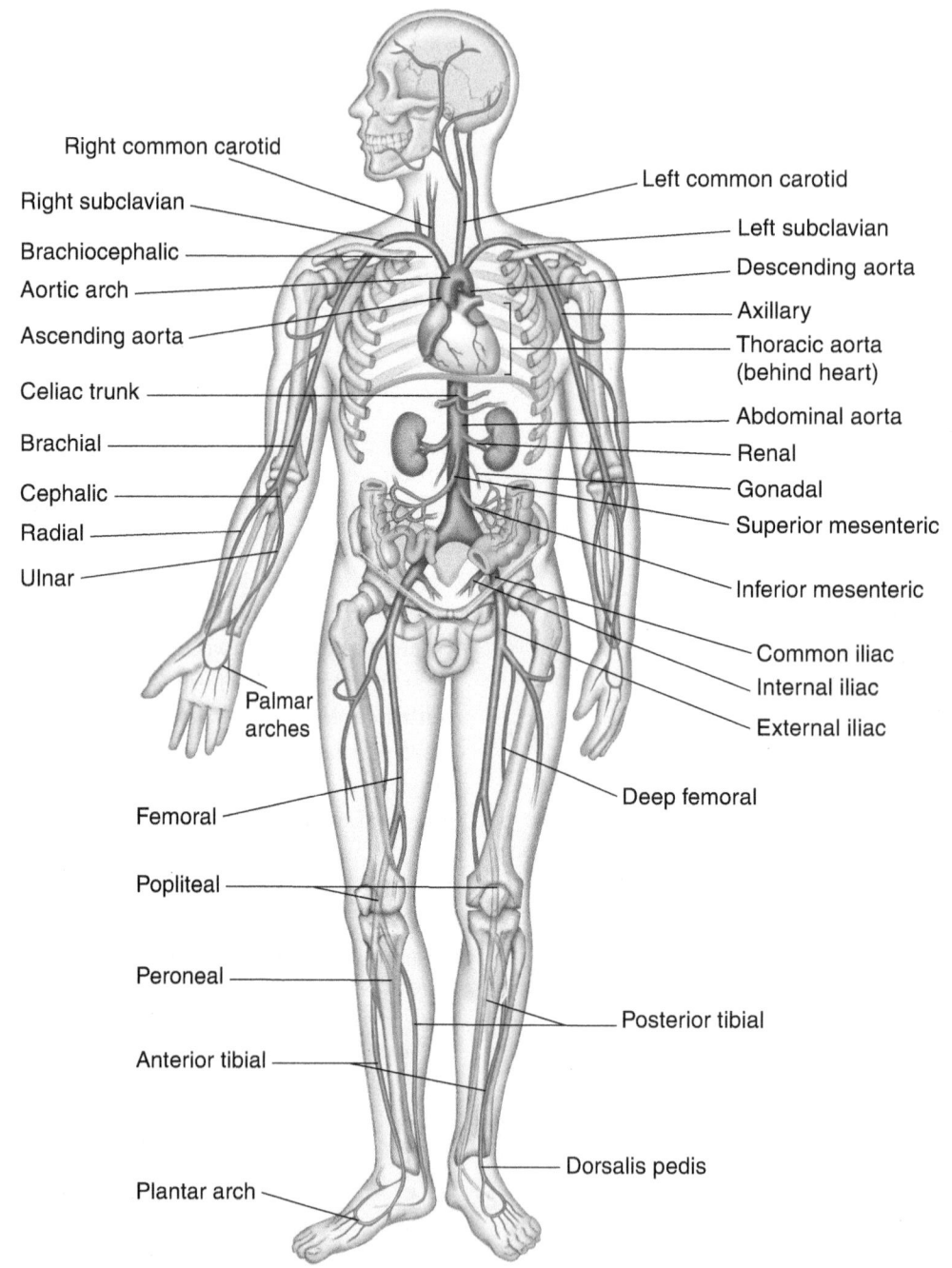

FIGURE 26-4 An overview of the arterial circulation.

usually an artery that you palpate, feeling the expansion and contraction of the artery beneath your fingers. The most common sites for palpating an artery to measure heart rate include the following (Figure 26-5):

- **Radial artery**—In the lateral wrist, just proximal to the thumb
- **Brachial artery**—In the antecubital space of the elbow; also between the biceps and triceps muscles in pediatric and thinner adult patients
- **Carotid artery**—In the lateral neck. Note that a **carotid artery**, located on either side of the neck, is the site most commonly checked for the presence or absence of a pulse, for example in a suspected cardiac arrest.
- **Temporal artery**—In the temple area
- **Femoral artery**—In the groin
- **Popliteal artery**—Behind the knee on the posteromedial (inside rear) aspect

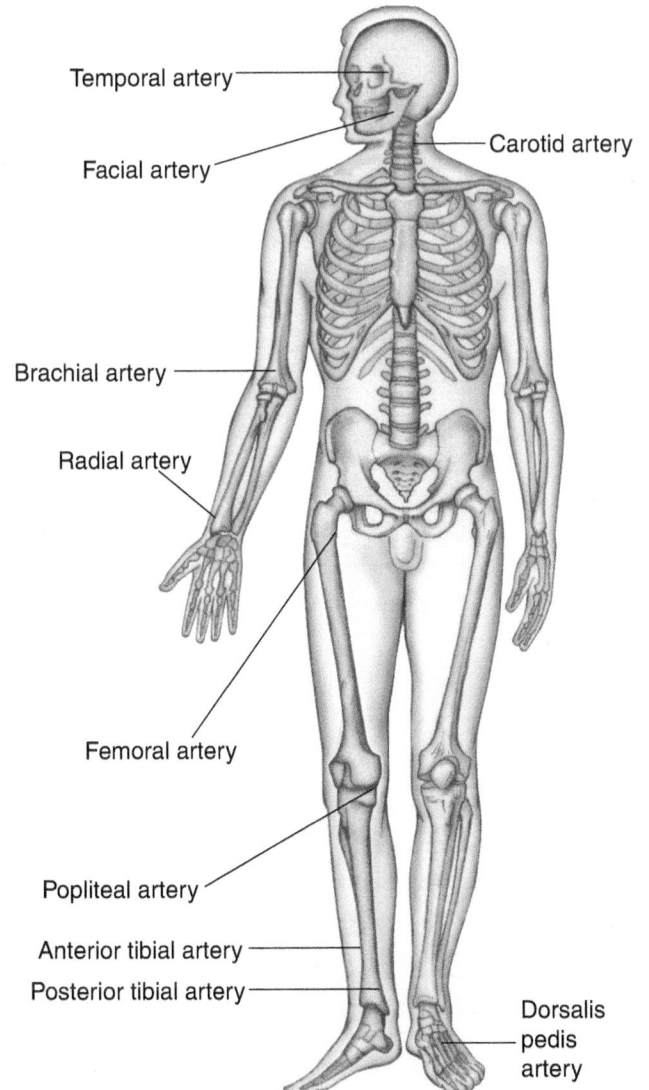

Temporal artery

Facial artery

Carotid artery

Brachial artery

Radial artery

Femoral artery

Popliteal artery

Anterior tibial artery

Posterior tibial artery

Dorsalis pedis artery

FIGURE 26-5 The primary pulse points of the body.

- **Dorsalis pedis artery**—On the upper surface of the foot
- **Anterior tibial artery**—In the ankle medial to (inside) the Achilles tendon

Veins and Venules

Veins are the vessels that transport blood from all parts of the body back to the heart (Figure 26-6). The smallest veins, called venules, branch off from the tiny capillaries and then join to form the full-sized veins. Veins are larger but thinner-walled than arteries, and they contain valves that prevent blood from flowing backward. Like arteries, veins have elastic walls, but the pressure in the veins is significantly lower than in the arteries. The low pressure in the veins is the reason why veins need valves to prevent backflow, in contrast to the high pressure that prevents backflow in the arteries.

Venipuncture, or **phlebotomy**, is the process of removing blood from the veins for examination. It is easier to draw blood from and administer intravenous (IV) medications into veins because they are under less pressure and are more superficial than arteries.

Capillaries

Capillaries are microscopic blood vessels with walls that are just one cell thick. Oxygenated blood travels through the arteries, then to the smaller arterioles, and then to the tiny capillaries within the tissues. Through the extremely thin capillary walls, the blood offloads oxygen and nutrients to the cells and picks up waste material from the cells. The blood then transports carbon dioxide and waste material from the capillaries to the small venules and on to the larger veins that return it to the heart.

Small breaks in the capillaries can lead to **petechiae**, or tiny broken blood vessels that may appear on the surface of the skin.

Vascular System of the Heart

The heart's dense musculature requires its own blood supply. Now, with our general understanding of blood vessels, we can develop an appreciation of the heart's unique vascular system.

The **coronary arteries**, illustrated in Figure 26-7, supply oxygenated blood to the heart. It is important to understand that this is *not* the blood that moves through the chambers of the heart to and from the lungs and the body. This is blood that directly nourishes the heart muscle itself. After nourishing the myocardium (*myo-* means "muscle"; *cardium* means "heart"), the deoxygenated blood is drained into the coronary sinus by the coronary veins and then back into the right atrium for oxygenation. **Occlusion** (blockage) of these

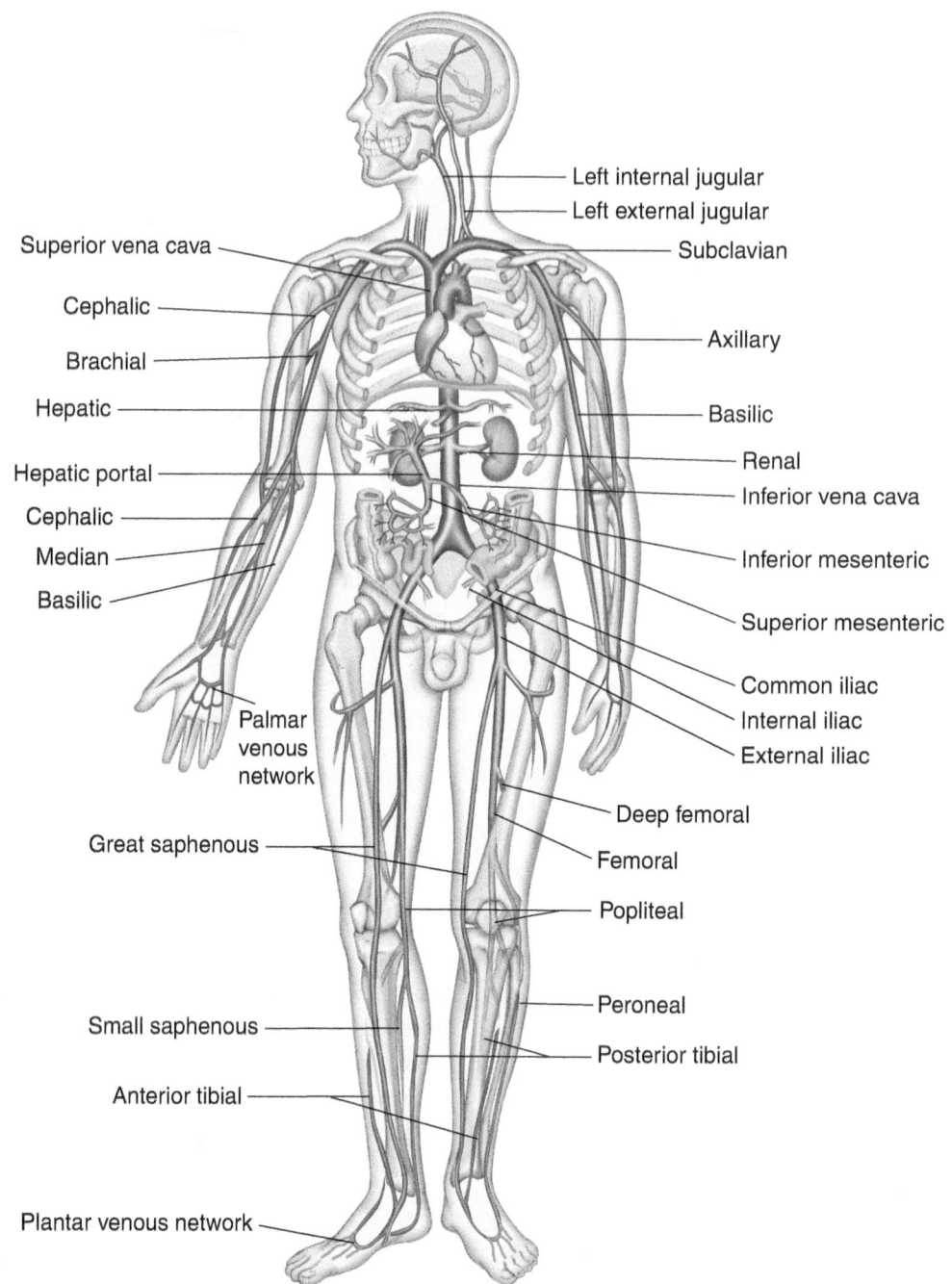

Superior vena cava

Cephalic

Brachial

Hepatic

Hepatic portal

Cephalic

Median

Basilic

Palmar
venous
network

Great saphenous

Small saphenous

Anterior tibial

Plantar venous network

Left internal jugular

Left external jugular

Subclavian

Axillary

Basilic

Renal

Inferior vena cava

Inferior mesenteric

Superior mesenteric

Common iliac

Internal iliac

External iliac

Deep femoral

Femoral

Popliteal

Peroneal

Posterior tibial

FIGURE 26-6 An overview of the venous circulation.

coronary blood vessels deprives the heart muscle of oxygen, causing chest pain.

Permanent damage to the heart muscle, including death of the muscle tissue, can occur if cardiac muscle is deprived of oxygen for a long period of time. Lack of blood flow to the heart muscle is known as myocardial **ischemia**, whereas death of heart muscle is known as a myocardial **infarction** (MI). Cardiac arrest occurs if an occlusion in the heart causes the heart to stop beating (or pumping blood). Occlusion of vessels that supply the heart is the most common cause of

cardiac arrest, but arrest can also be caused by trauma or other medical conditions. The lack of oxygen to the tissues caused by ischemia and infarction is known as **hypoxia**.

HOW THE CARDIOVASCULAR SYSTEM FUNCTIONS

As mentioned earlier, the heart is responsible for the movement of blood through the cardiovascular system and throughout the entire body, providing oxygen and nutrients

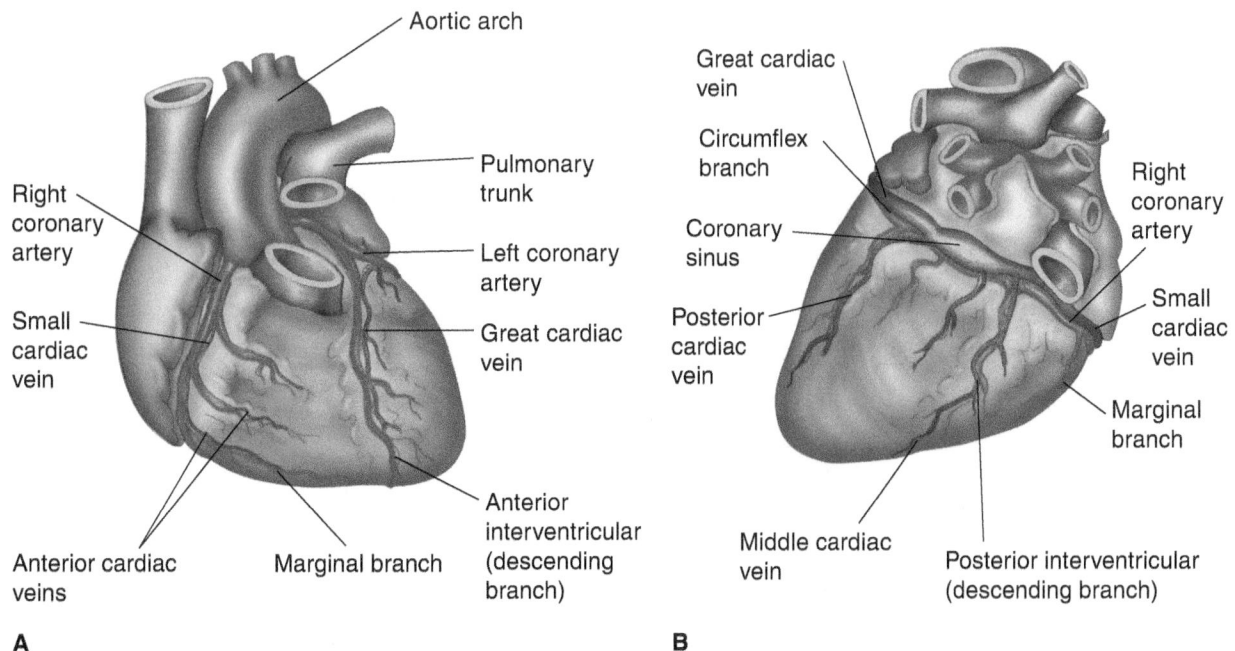

FIGURE 26-7 Coronary circulation: **(A)** coronary vessels portraying the complexity and extent of the coronary circulation; **(B)** coronary vessels that supply the anterior surfaces of the heart.

to cells and removing waste. The following list identifies other functions of the cardiovascular system. These are discussed in greater detail later in the chapter when blood is more closely examined.

- Maintaining fluid balance at a cellular level
- Helping to regulate body temperature
- Protecting the body from infection and illness through the special functions of various types of blood cells

For the cardiovascular system to properly execute its vital functions, it must be able to do two things: initiate and sustain heartbeats, and pump blood throughout the heart and body. The entire process involved in one complete heartbeat is known as the cardiac cycle.

Blood Flow Through the Heart

The mechanical, or pumping, action of the heart occurs with the contraction of the cardiac muscle. During this muscular contraction, an intricate pumping process occurs. First, blood from the body enters the right side of the heart through two large veins. The **superior vena cava** brings blood from the head and upper chest. The **inferior vena cava** brings blood from below the heart.

The right atrium, the smallest of the heart chambers, has the thinnest wall. It receives all the blood delivered to the heart from the body via the superior vena cava and the inferior vena cava. From the right atrium, the heart pumps the blood through a valve into the right ventricle. The valve

that connects the right atrium to the right ventricle is the **tricuspid valve**. (It is called "tricuspid" because this valve has three cusps, or leaves, that close to seal the valve and move apart to open it.)

The right ventricle, which is more muscular than the right atrium, pumps the blood out through the pulmonary valve into the **pulmonary artery**, which carries the blood to the lungs.

Keep in mind that, while the blood was circulating through the body, it was giving up oxygen to nourish the body's cells and, at the same time, accumulating waste and carbon dioxide given off by the cells. So the blood that enters the right atrium and then the right ventricle is deoxygenated blood—blood that contains too much carbon dioxide and not enough oxygen. When the right ventricle pumps this blood to the lungs, there is a gas exchange. The blood passes off its carbon dioxide into the alveoli (air sacs) of the lungs, from which it is exhaled from the body. At the same time, the blood takes on oxygen from the air that has been breathed into those same air sacs of the lungs. So the blood that returns to the heart from the lungs is now oxygenated blood.

The **pulmonary vein** carries the oxygenated blood from the lungs and empties it into the left atrium of the heart. The blood leaves the left atrium through the **bicuspid valve** (a valve with two cusps, which is also called the **mitral valve** because it resembles a bishop's mitre, a hat with two tall flaps).

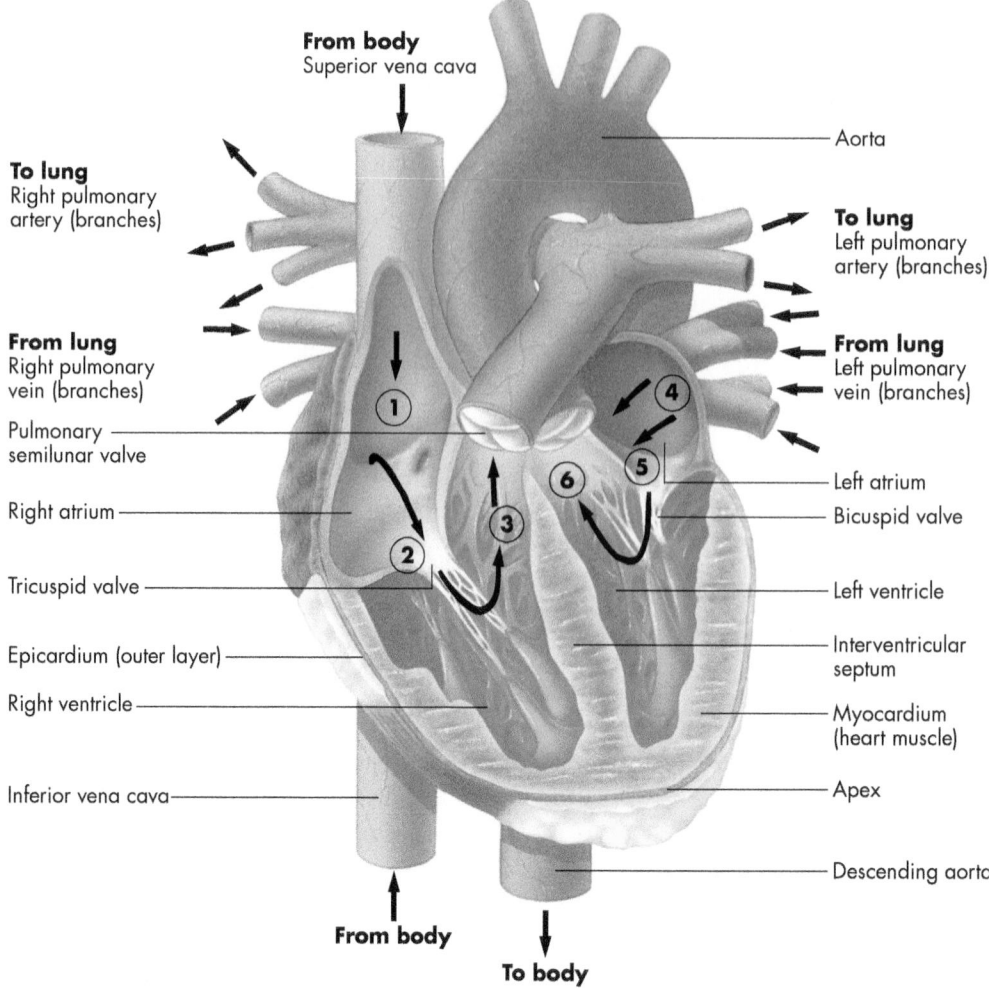

From body
Superior vena cava

To lung
Right pulmonary
artery (branches)

From lung
Right pulmonary
vein (branches)

Pulmonary
semilunar valve

Right atrium

Tricuspid valve

Epicardium (outer layer)

Right ventricle

Inferior vena cava

Aorta

To lung
Left pulmonary
artery (branches)

From lung
Left pulmonary
vein (branches)

Left atrium

Bicuspid valve

Left ventricle

Interventricular
septum

Myocardium
(heart muscle)

Apex

Descending aorta

From body

To body

RIGHT HEART PUMP

1. Deoxygenated blood returns from the upper and lower body to fill the right atrium of the heart creating a pressure against the tricuspid valve.

2. This pressure of the returning blood forces the tricuspid valve open and begins filling the ventricle. The final filling of the ventricle is achieved by the contracting of the right atrium.

3. The right ventricle contracts, increasing the internal pressure. This pressure closes the tricuspid valve and forces open the pulmonary semilunar valve, thus sending blood toward the lung via the pulmonary artery. This blood will become oxygenated as it travels through the capillary beds of the lung and then returns to the left side of the heart.

LEFT HEART PUMP

4. Oxygenated blood returns from the lung via the pulmonary vein and fills the left atrium creating a pressure against the bicuspid valve.

5. This pressure of returning blood forces the bicuspid valve open and begins filling the left ventricle. The final filling of the left ventricle is achieved by the contracting of the left atrium.

6. The left ventricle contracts, increasing internal pressure. This pressure closes the bicuspid valve and forces open the aortic valve causing oxygenated blood to flow through the aorta to deliver oxygen throughout the body.

FIGURE 26-8 The flow of blood through the heart.

After passing through the bicuspid valve, the blood enters the left ventricle. The left ventricle is called the powerhouse chamber. The highly muscular walls of this chamber must forcibly pump the oxygenated blood out from the heart to the farthest reaches of the body. The blood leaves the left ventricle through the aortic valve and enters the **aorta**, the

largest artery in the body. From the aorta, the blood begins its journey through the various arteries that branch off from the aorta to all the different regions of the body. Figure 26-8 shows the flow of blood through the heart.

As the blood makes its way through the chambers of the heart, healthy valves function as gateways, never allowing

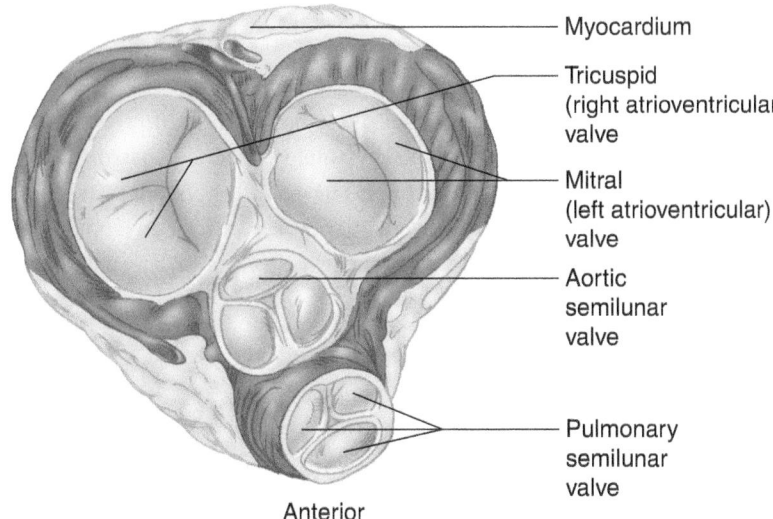

FIGURE 26-9 The valves of the heart.

the blood to flow backward (Figure 26-9). A damaged or diseased valve can allow blood to escape and flow backward through the valve, creating a **heart murmur**, the sound of the backflowing blood as heard through a stethoscope. A heart murmur can sometimes be confused with the sound of turbulent flow in the carotid artery, known as a **bruit**.

Conduction System of the Heart

An electrical conduction system is responsible for initiating the beats that send blood flowing through and from the heart. This cardiac conduction system, controlled by the autonomic nervous system, is responsible not only for creation of the heartbeat but also for its rate and rhythm. Three areas of specialized neuromuscular tissue initiate and sustain the heartbeat. They are the sinoatrial node, the atrioventricular node, and the atrioventricular bundle, also known as the bundle of His. Figure 26-10 shows the conduction system of the heart.

The **sinoatrial (SA) node** is considered the pacemaker of the heart because it initiates the heartbeat. It is located in the upper portion of the wall of the right atrium. The SA node signals the right and left atria to contract by discharging electrical signals. In a healthy adult at rest, the SA node initiates 60 to 80 beats (or contractions) per minute.

The **atrioventricular (AV) node** is located between the atria and ventricles in the endocardium layer of the heart. When the electrical impulse from the SA node reaches this point, the AV node slows down the impulse for a moment to allow the atria time to finish contracting before the ventricles begin their contraction. The AV node senses when the ventricles have filled and then sends an impulse that reaches the bundle of His.

Made up of muscle fibers, the **bundle of His** is also known as the atrioventricular (AV) bundle. The bundle of His is located in the septum of the heart, from which it divides into right and left bundle branches. As the impulse nears the end of the cardiac circuit, it travels from the bundle branches into the Purkinje fibers.

The **Purkinje fibers** are specialized conductive fibers located within the walls of the ventricles. They are responsible for relaying cardiac impulses to the cells of the ventricles, prompting the ventricles to contract.

The Cardiac Cycle

The cardiac cycle consists of all the events that occur during one complete heartbeat. On average, the heart beats about 70 times per minute, although normal adult heart rates can vary from 60 to 110 beats per minute. Various factors can impact the cardiac cycle. Factors

---

Professionalism The Life Span

The Child

- The development of the circulatory system begins with the development of the fetal heart during the first 2 months of gestation, and the newborn's circulation begins to function immediately after birth.
- Children have a smaller circulatory system, and their vital signs are typically different from those of adults. Their blood pressure is typically lower than that of an adult, although their pulse and respiratory rates are higher.

The Older Adult

- Cardiovascular disease in older adults is a real threat. One in four deaths in the United States are related to heart disease.
- Cardiac and other circulatory changes once attributed to aging may be minimized with appropriate lifestyle modifications. Without a healthy lifestyle or modifications, years of sedentary living, poor diet choices, and obesity can contribute to the development of cardiovascular disease.
- Healthy lifestyle choices for overall cardiac health for the older adult include choosing not to smoke, eating a healthy diet rich in vegetables and lean protein, exercise, and maintaining a healthy weight.
- With normal aging, the heart changes: lipofuscin occurs (which is an age-related pigmentation change to the heart), heart valves toughen and become stiffer, and the cells within the heart may begin to slowly degenerate.

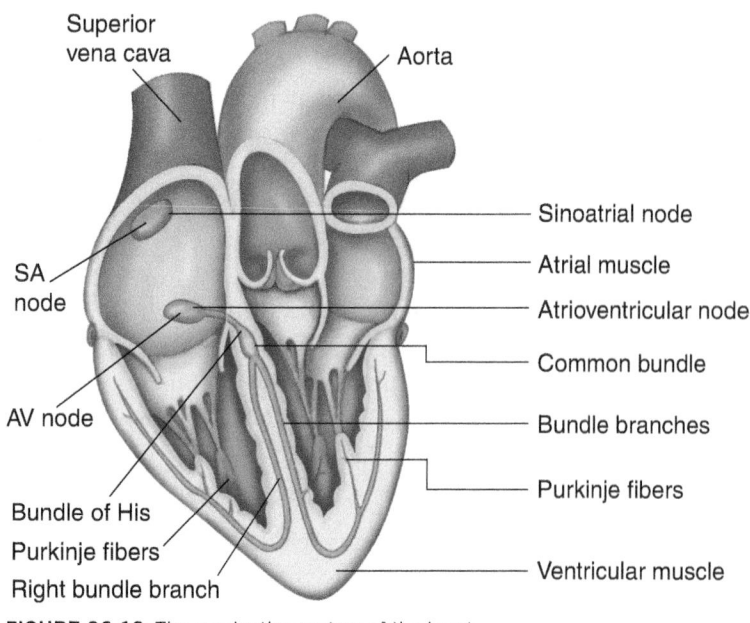

FIGURE 26-10 The conduction system of the heart.

Superior
vena cava

Aorta

SA
node

AV node

Bundle of His
Purkinje fibers
Right bundle branch

Sinoatrial node

Atrial muscle

Atrioventricular node

Common bundle

Bundle branches

Purkinje fibers

Ventricular muscle

that cause the heart rate to increase include exercise, stress, excitement, smoking, and a rise in body temperature.

The cardiac cycle has four distinct phases: atrial diastole, atrial systole, ventricular diastole, and ventricular systole. The term *systole* refers to the contraction phase of the heart and, conversely, *diastole* refers to the relaxation phase of the heart. Figure 26-11 illustrates the systolic and diastolic phases of the heart.

PULMONARY AND SYSTEMIC CIRCULATION

The cardiovascular system can be divided into the pulmonary circulation and the systemic circulation (Figure 26-12).

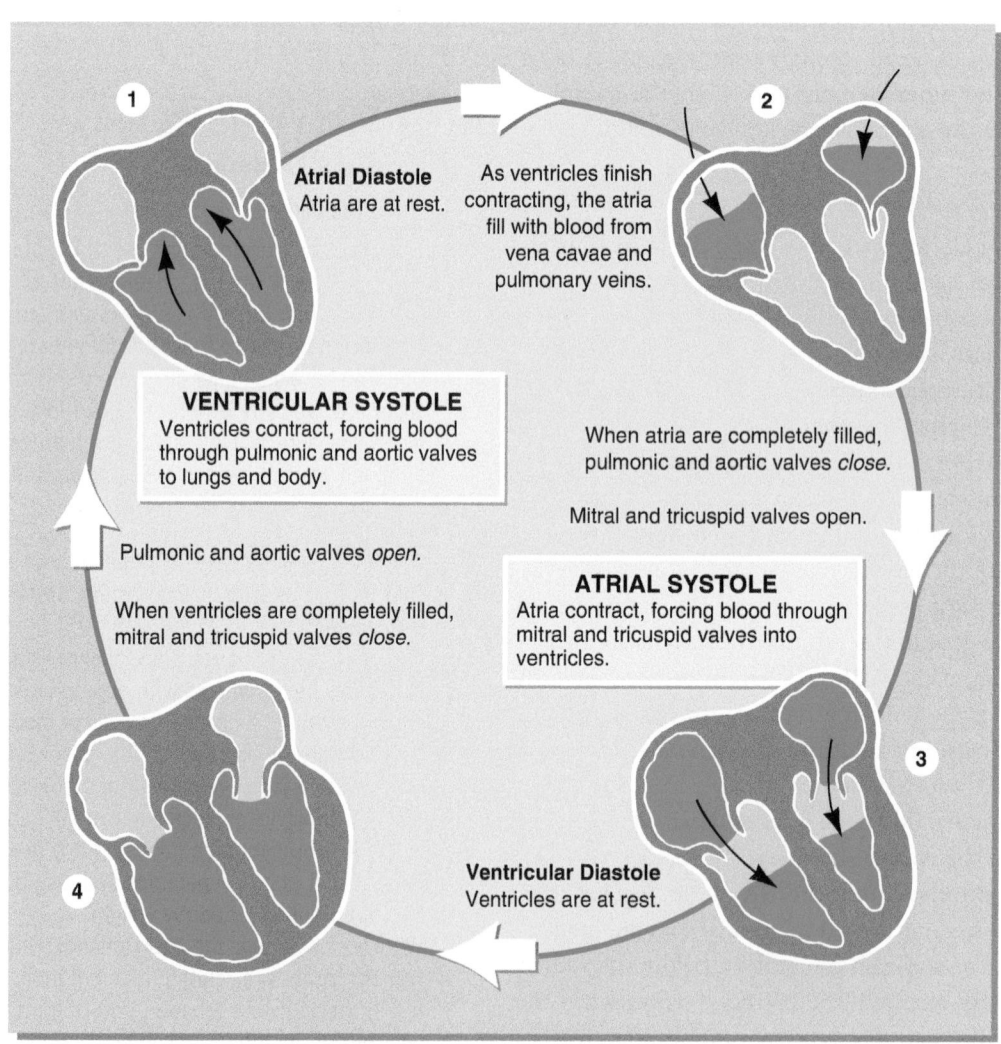

1 Atrial Diastole
Atria are at rest.

2 As ventricles finish contracting, the atria fill with blood from vena cavae and pulmonary veins.

VENTRICULAR SYSTOLE
Ventricles contract, forcing blood through pulmonic and aortic valves to lungs and body.

When atria are completely filled, pulmonic and aortic valves *close*.

Mitral and tricuspid valves open.

Pulmonic and aortic valves *open*.

When ventricles are completely filled, mitral and tricuspid valves *close*.

ATRIAL SYSTOLE
Atria contract, forcing blood through mitral and tricuspid valves into ventricles.

3 Ventricular Diastole
Ventricles are at rest.

4

FIGURE 26-11 The cardiac cycle showing systole and diastole.

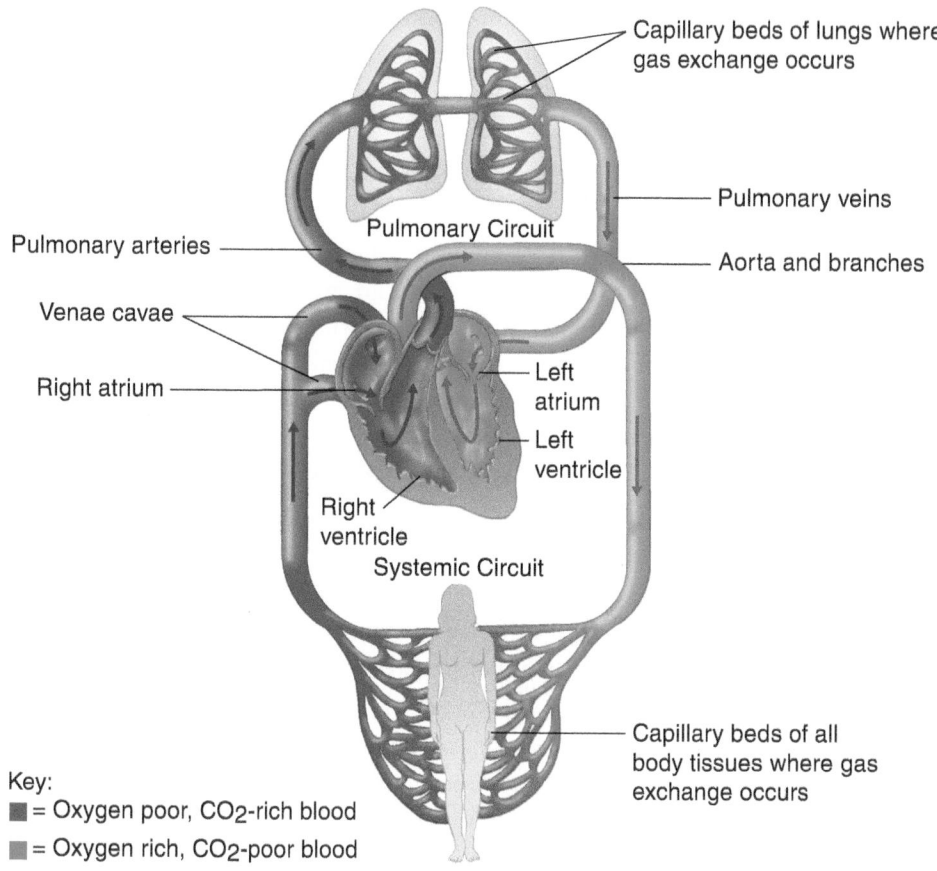

Capillary beds of lungs where gas exchange occurs

Pulmonary Circuit

Pulmonary arteries

Pulmonary veins

Aorta and branches

Venae cavae

Right atrium

Left atrium

Left ventricle

Right ventricle

Systemic Circuit

Capillary beds of all body tissues where gas exchange occurs

Key:
■ = Oxygen poor, CO₂-rich blood
■ = Oxygen rich, CO₂-poor blood

FIGURE 26-12 Systemic and pulmonary circulation.

Pulmonary Circulation

Pulmonary circulation is the route blood takes from the heart to the lungs via the pulmonary artery. It is then returned to the heart via the pulmonary vein. The function of pulmonary circulation is to carry deoxygenated blood from the right side of the heart to the lungs (where it gives off waste carbon dioxide and takes on fresh oxygen) and then to carry the oxygenated blood back to the left side of the heart. The oxygen-rich blood that returns to the left side of the heart from the lungs is then moved out to the cells of the body by the systemic circulation.

Systemic Circulation

Systemic circulation is the route blood takes around the body: It leaves the heart through the aorta; travels through the body via arteries, arterioles, capillaries, venules, and veins; and returns to the heart through the superior and inferior venae cavae. The function of systemic circulation is to deliver oxygenated blood and other nutrients to body cells and to carry carbon dioxide and waste products away from the cells for elimination from the body.

BLOOD PRESSURE

Blood pressure is defined as the force exerted by the blood against the inner walls of the arteries. A person's blood pressure continually changes, depending on activity, temperature, diet, emotional state, posture, physical condition, and medication use.

Blood pressure is usually measured in the brachial artery with a **sphygmomanometer**, an instrument that expresses measurements in terms of millimeters of mercury (mmHg). During ventricular contraction, blood pressure is at its highest in the arteries. The measurement obtained at this point is called the **systolic blood pressure**. By contrast, **diastolic blood pressure** is the measurement obtained when the ventricles relax and blood pressure is at its lowest.

Blood pressure is recorded as a fraction, placing the systolic blood pressure over the diastolic blood pressure. For example, a systolic of 120 mmHg and a diastolic of 80 mmHg would be recorded as 120/80. This blood pressure reading would be verbally expressed as "120 over 80."

The average and healthy resting blood pressure for a young adult is below 120/80.

Pulse Pressure

The **pulse pressure** is the difference between the systolic and diastolic blood pressures. Normal pulse pressure is 30 to 50 points. The pulse pressure is an indication of the tone of the arterial walls. It can be helpful when assessing a patient's risk profile for heart disease. A high pulse pressure may indicate a patient is at risk for developing heart disease. Conversely, a low pulse pressure (often below 40) may indicate a decrease in effective functioning of the heart.

BLOOD

Blood is a type of connective tissue that is composed of blood cells (the formed elements of the blood) and **plasma** (the fluid portion of the blood). Blood (along with the heart and the blood vessels) is one of the three main components of the cardiovascular system.

The amount of blood that circulates in a person's body is known as blood volume. Blood volume levels vary from person to person and depend on factors such as the person's size, level of hydration, and amount of fat tissue. On average, about 5 liters of blood circulates throughout an adult's body.

In adults, the formation of blood cells (a process called hematopoiesis) takes place primarily in the bone marrow.

Composition of Blood

There are three main types of blood cells, also known as the formed elements of blood:

- **Erythrocytes**, or red blood cells
- **Leukocytes**, or white blood cells (There are five types of leukocytes: neutrophils, eosinophils, basophils, lymphocytes, and monocytes.)
- **Platelets**, or thrombocytes

Figure 26-13 shows the formed elements of blood. More information on blood composition is provided in the chapter titled "Hematology."

Red Blood Cells

Red blood cells (RBCs), or **erythrocytes**, are produced in the red bone marrow. Mature red blood cells do not contain nuclei but do contain **hemoglobin**, a red, iron-containing pigment that has the ability to bind oxygen to itself. The function of hemoglobin is to carry oxygen from the lungs to cells throughout the body.

An RBC count refers to the number of red blood cells in 1 microliter of blood. The average range for a healthy adult male is 4.7–6.1 million cells per microliter (mcL). A healthy adult female has 4.2–5.4 million cells/mcL.

White Blood Cells

White blood cells (WBCs), or **leukocytes**, differ from RBCs in that they are usually larger, have a nucleus, lack hemoglobin, and are translucent unless stained (which occurs during laboratory testing). There are not nearly as many leukocytes in the blood as there are erythrocytes. There are normally only 4,000 to 10,000 per microliter (mcL) of blood. WBCs fight infection and, in this function, are important contributors to homeostasis.

The five types of leukocytes are divided into two categories:

- **Granulocytes** have granules in their cytoplasm. Neutrophils, eosinophils, and basophils are granulocytes.
- **Agranulocytes** do not contain granules. Monocytes and lymphocytes are agranulocytes.

A differential WBC count is a type of blood test that is often ordered to measure the number of each of the five types of leukocytes. An increase or decrease in percentages may be indicative of infection or disease.

Blood Platelets

Platelets, or thrombocytes, are fragments of larger cells that have formed in the red bone marrow. They are smaller than erythrocytes and do not have a nucleus. Platelets control the loss of blood through the process of coagulation, or the formation of a clot at the point of injury. A normal platelet count is 150,000 to 400,000 per cubic mm of blood.

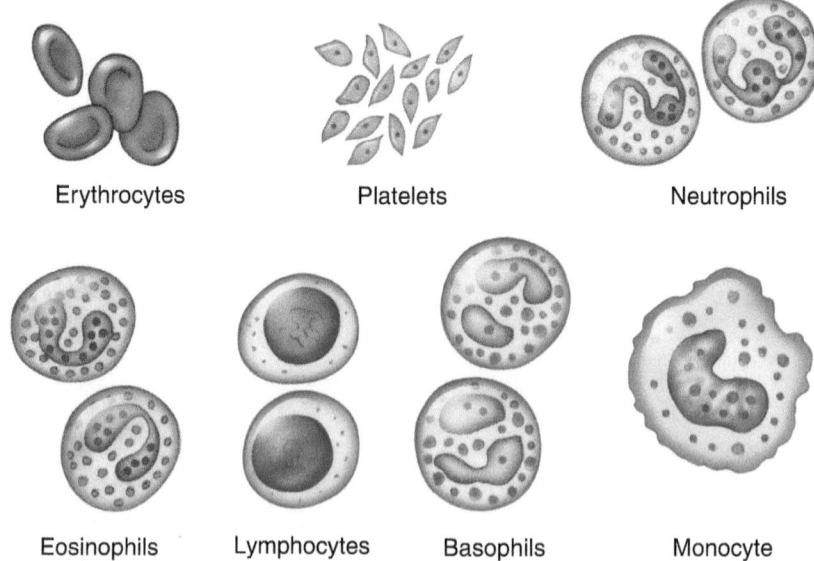

Erythrocytes   Platelets   Neutrophils

Eosinophils   Lymphocytes   Basophils   Monocyte

FIGURE 26-13 The formed elements of blood.

Blood Plasma

Plasma is the liquid portion of the blood. Plasma is 91 percent water. The other 9 percent is a mixture of proteins, nutrients, gases, electrolytes, fats, hormones, enzymes, and waste products. Plasma constitutes about 55 percent of the total volume of whole blood. Albumin, the most abundant protein found in plasma, helps maintain the fluid volume in the blood, thereby controlling blood pressure. Other major proteins found in plasma are fibrinogen and prothrombin (both of which play a role in clot formation), and globulin.

Functions of Blood

It was mentioned earlier that the cardiovascular system has three major functions: transportation, regulation, and defense. Blood is responsible for executing these functions and maintaining a state of balance throughout the body.

Transportation

Blood moves from the heart to all the tissues of the body. It is important to recall that, at the tissue level, gas and nutrient exchange takes place across thin capillary walls between the blood and the individual cells. The blood transports oxygen from the lungs and nutrients from the digestive tract and delivers these to the tissue cells. Various organs and tissues also secrete hormones into the blood, which transports them to other organs and tissues where they serve as signals that influence other metabolic functions. The blood also picks up waste materials from the cells that is later filtered and excreted by the kidneys as well as carbon monoxide that is exhaled from the lungs.

Regulation

Blood helps to regulate body temperature by absorbing heat, mostly from active muscles, and then distributing the heat throughout the body. If the blood is too warm, the heat dissipates from dilated blood vessels in the skin. The dilated vessels cause the skin to become flushed as heat is released. Salts and plasma proteins in the blood act to pull water into the blood vessels (to balance forces that push water out of the vessels) to maintain an adequate liquid content in the blood. In this way, the blood plays a key role in maintaining the body's water–salt balance. Blood also helps the body regulate the pH (acid/alkaline) balance of the body. The blood contains **buffers**, which are mechanisms within the blood that balance the pH level, thus preventing blood from becoming too acidic or too alkaline.

Defense

Leukocytes defend the body against pathogens such as bacteria and viruses. This is accomplished in several ways:

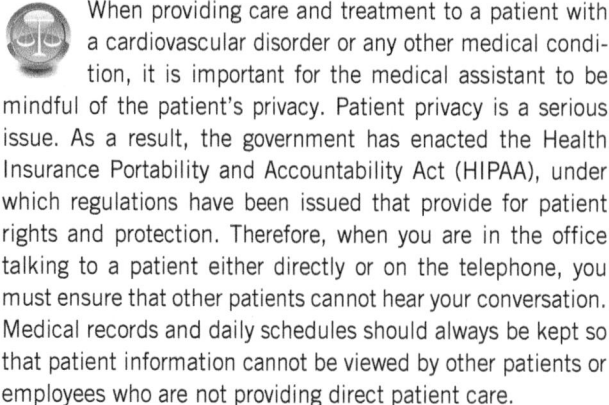

- Neutrophils and monocytes engulf and destroy pathogens. This process is called phagocytosis.

- Lymphocytes secrete antibodies into the blood. Antibodies help to weaken the pathogens, making them vulnerable to destruction.

- When an injury occurs, bleeding is stopped through the formation of clots, which, as noted earlier, are formed from platelets. When a blood vessel breaks, the smooth muscle at the site of the break causes the vessel wall to contract, which in turn causes the blood vessel to spasm. The spasm reduces the amount of blood lost through the break. Platelets begin to attach themselves to both the broken area and to each other to form a "plug" that eventually stops the bleeding. After a period of time, a blood clot forms and replaces the platelet plug.

  The clot is formed in this manner: During the coagulation process, the plasma protein fibrinogen is converted to fibrin. Similar to a glue, the fibrin adheres to the area of the vessel that is broken or damaged. This creates a system that entraps blood cells and platelets. The accumulation of cells and platelets forms a blood clot, which will stop the bleeding until the area has had time to repair. The stoppage of bleeding is termed **hemostasis**.

  Without this clotting capacity and resulting hemostasis, we could bleed to death from even a tiny cut.

BLOOD TYPES

Blood type is based on whether the blood contains or lacks specific antigens and antibodies. Blood type is determined by genetics (Figure 26-14). If an antigen on the surface of a red

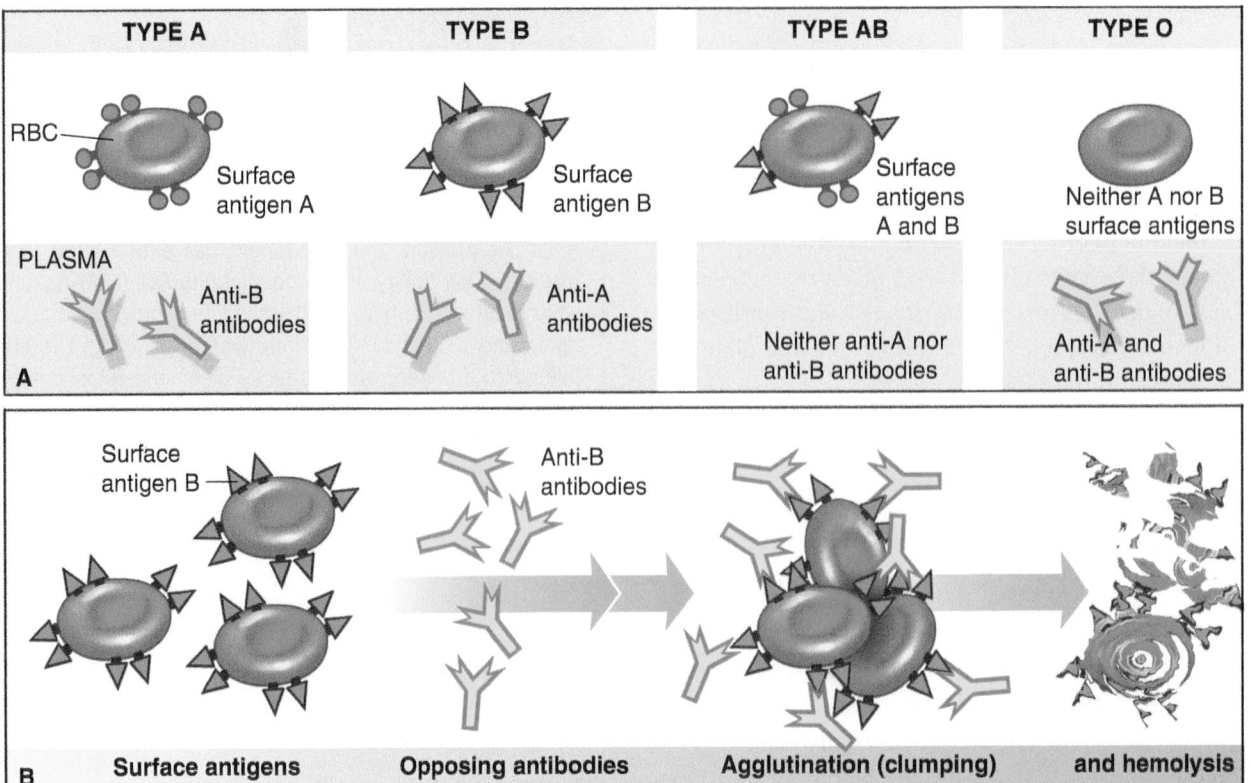

FIGURE 26-14 Blood typing and cross-reactions. The blood type depends on the presence of surface antigens (agglutinogens) on RBC surfaces. **(A)** The plasma antibodies (agglutinins) that will react with foreign surface antigens; **(B)** in a cross-reaction, antibodies that encounter their target antigens lead to agglutination and hemolysis of the affected RBCs.

blood cell binds with antibodies in plasma, **agglutination**, or clumping, occurs The presence of anti-A and anti-B antibodies in the plasma requires that blood be typed and cross-matched for transfusions. If a patient is given the wrong blood type, the new blood may clump with the patient's blood, causing occlusion and shock. For this reason, blood banks carefully type and match blood before it is given to the patient.

The ABO blood group system identifies four blood types (Table 26-1):

- **Type A**—Type A antigen on the surface of the red blood cells and anti-B antibody in the plasma. People with Type A blood can only be given Type A blood.

- **Type B**—Type B antigen on the surface of the red blood cells and anti-A antibody in their plasma; people with Type B blood can only be given Type B blood.

- **Type AB**—Type AB has both A and B antigens on the red blood cell surfaces and neither anti-A nor anti-B antibodies. People with type AB blood are considered universal recipients because the majority of them can receive all ABO blood types given that their plasma lacks antibodies.

- **Type O**—Neither A nor B antigens are found on the red blood cells; however, both anti-A and anti-B antibodies are in the plasma. People with type O blood are considered universal donors because their blood can be administered to most people regardless of the recipient's blood type.

The Rh Factor

The Rh factor is another characteristic of a person's blood (in addition to blood type). The Rh factor is an antigen first discovered on RBCs of the Rhesus monkey (hence the name *Rh*). A person is either Rh positive if they have the Rh antigen or Rh negative if they do not have the Rh antigen.

TABLE 26-1 | Blood Group Identification by Antigen and Antibody

Blood Group	Antigen	Antibody
A	A	anti-B
B	B	anti-A
AB	A and B	neither
O	neither anti-A nor anti-B	anti-A, anti-B

Complications can arise if an Rh-negative individual is given Rh-positive blood. In this scenario, when the Rh-negative person's blood is exposed to the Rh antigen, it will begin to create antibodies in response. Although it isn't a serious concern if given once, consequences arise if the person receives Rh-positive blood a second time. Upon the second exposure, a transfusion reaction occurs in which the antibodies bind to the donor cells, resulting in agglutination and destruction of the donor cells.

The Rh factor plays an important role during pregnancy, so it is vital that a woman know her Rh type. If an Rh-negative female conceives a child with an Rh-positive male, there is a 50–50 chance that the fetus will be Rh-positive. When the blood of an Rh-positive fetus mixes with the mother's Rh-negative blood, the mother will develop antibodies against the fetus's RBCs. Because of the length of time it takes for the mother's body to generate these antibodies, the first Rh-positive fetus generally does not suffer any effect. However, if a second Rh-positive fetus is conceived, the fetus's blood will be attacked by the mother's antibodies almost immediately. This can lead to a serious condition, erythroblastosis fetalis, in which the baby is born severely anemic. The condition can be prevented by giving the drug **RhoGAM** to the Rh-negative mother to inhibit the production of antibodies against the Rh antigen.

COMMON PATHOLOGY ASSOCIATED WITH THE CARDIOVASCULAR SYSTEM

Disorders of the cardiovascular system are very common in the United States. Many result from a combination of lifestyle factors (lack of exercise, smoking, stress, obesity) and genetics. Common tests and procedures used to diagnose and treat cardiovascular disorders are discussed in Table 26-2.

Anemia

Anemia is a condition in which the blood has an abnormally low number of red blood cells. Anemia can also occur if the RBCs do not contain enough hemoglobin or if the hemoglobin that is present is abnormal. Considered the most common dysfunction of RBCs, anemia affects about 3.5 million Americans.

The three most common causes of anemia are (1) decreased production of healthy red cells by the bone marrow, (2) increased hemolysis (erythrocyte destruction), and (3) blood loss from heavy menstrual periods, traumatic injury, or internal bleeding. Vitamin and mineral deficiencies in the diet can also slow the production of hemoglobin.

There are several types of anemia. Some may be inherited, whereas others are brought on by poor nutrition or toxins.

- **Iron-deficiency anemia**—The body needs iron for hemoglobin production. Decreased iron levels, resulting in decreased hemoglobin production, cause a decrease in the capacity of RBCs to transport oxygen.

- **Vitamin-deficiency anemia**—Like iron, vitamin B12 is essential for normal hemoglobin production. However, some individuals do not easily absorb vitamin B12. The result is a vitamin B12 deficiency, a condition known as *pernicious anemia*.

- **Hemolytic anemia**—This type of anemia is caused by the premature destruction of RBCs by antibodies produced by the immune system. This condition is sometimes associated with systemic disorders, such as lupus, or exposure to toxic materials. For instance, lead, copper, and benzene can also lead to the destruction of RBCs, causing hemolytic anemia.

- **Sickle cell anemia**—This form of anemia is one type of sickle cell disease, which is caused by hard, sickled (crescent-shaped) red blood cells. Normal red blood cells are round and flexible and pass easily through the smallest blood vessels to deliver oxygen to the body's tissues. In sickle cell anemia, the rigidity and irregularities of sickled cells create blockages that prevent normal blood flow to the tissues. The African American population is most susceptible to inheriting this serious and often life-threating form of anemia. Sickle cell anemia is one of the few forms of anemia that causes physical pain. Sickle cell disease is also known as hemoglobin S disease.

TABLE 26-2 | Procedures and Diagnostic Tests Related to the Cardiovascular System

Procedure/Test	Description
Aneurysmectomy	Surgical removal of an aneurysm, which is an abnormal dilation of a blood vessel.
Angiography	X-rays taken after the injection of an opaque material (also called contrast) into a blood vessel. They can be performed on the aorta as an aortic angiogram, on the heart as an angiocardiogram, and on the brain as a cerebral angiogram.
Angioplasty	Surgical procedure of altering the structure of a vessel by dilating the vessel using a balloon inside the vessel.
Arterial Blood Gases	Measurement of the amount of oxygen, carbon dioxide, and bicarbonate in the blood, and a pH reading of the blood. Blood gases are measured in emergency situations and provide valuable evaluation of cardiac failure, hemorrhage, and kidney failure.
Artery Graft	A piece of blood vessel that is transplanted from a part of the body to the aorta to repair a defect.
Artificial Pacemaker	Electrical device that substitutes for the natural pacemaker of the heart. It controls the beating of the heart by a series of rhythmic electrical impulses. An external pacemaker has the electrodes on the outside of the body. An internal pacemaker has the electrodes surgically implanted within the chest wall.
Cardiac Catheterization	Passage of thin tube (catheter) through an artery (commonly the femoral artery) and the blood vessels leading into the heart. Radiopaque contrast is injected, and X-rays are taken to view the coronary arteries.
Cardiac Enzyme Analysis	Complex proteins capable of inducing chemical changes within the body. Cardiac enzymes are obtained by blood sample to determine the amount of heart disease or damage.
Cardiac Magnetic Resonance Imaging (MRI)	Noninvasive procedure in which images of the heart and blood vessels are captured for examination to determine effects.
Cardiolysis	Surgical procedure to separate adhesions that involves a resection of the ribs and sternum over the pericardium.
Cardiorrhaphy	Surgical suturing of the heart.
Cardioversion	Converting a cardiac arrhythmia (irregular heart rhythm) to a normal sinus rhythm using a cardioverter to provide countershocks to the heart.
Commissurotomy	Surgical incision to change the size of an opening. For example, in mitral valve commissurotomy, a stenosis or narrowing is corrected by cutting away at the adhesions around the mitral opening.
Coronary Artery Bypass Surgery	Open heart surgery in which a shunt is created to permit blood to travel around the constriction in the coronary vessel(s).
Doppler Ultrasonography	Measurement of sound waves as they bounce off tissues and organs to produce an image. This noninvasive procedure can assist in determining heart and blood vessel damage; it is also called an echocardiogram.
Electrocardiogram (ECG)	Record of the electrical activity of the heart. Useful in the diagnosis of abnormal cardiac rhythm and heart muscle (myocardium) damage. This procedure is explained fully in the chapter on electrocardiography.
Electrolyte Levels	Measurement of blood sodium (Na), potassium (K), and chloride (Cl). Electrolyte balance is important for the heart to function at optimal levels.
Embolectomy	Surgical removal of an embolus or blood clot from a vessel.
Heart Transplantation	Replacement of a diseased or malfunctioning heart with a donor's heart.
Holter Monitor	Portable ECG monitor worn by the patient for a period of a few hours to a few days to assess the heart and pulse activity as the person goes through the activities of daily living. Used to assess a patient who experiences chest pain and unusual heart activity during exercise and normal activities when a cardiogram is inconclusive. This is further discussed in the chapter on electrocardiography.

TABLE 26-2 | Procedures and Diagnostic Tests Related to the Cardiovascular System (*continued*)

Procedure/Test	Description
Lipoproteins	Measurement of blood to determine serum cholesterol and triglyceride levels.
Open Heart Surgery	Surgery that involves the heart, the coronary arteries, or the heart valves. The heart is actually entered by the surgeon.
Percutaneous Balloon Valvuloplasty	Insertion of a balloon catheter through the skin and into a blood vessel across a narrowed, or stenotic, heart valve. When the balloon is inflated, the narrowing or constriction is decreased.
Percutaneous Transluminal Coronary Angioplasty (PTCA)	Method for treating localized coronary artery narrowing. A balloon catheter is inserted through the skin into an artery that leads to a coronary artery and inflated to dilate the narrow blood vessel.
Phleborrhaphy	Suturing of a vein.
Prothrombin Time	Measurement of the time it takes for a sample of blood to coagulate.
Stent	Insertion of a small mesh tube into a weak or narrowed artery. A stent can help improve blood flow as well as prevent an artery from bursting.
Stress Testing (Treadmill Test)	Method for evaluating cardiovascular fitness. The patient is placed on a treadmill or bicycle and then subjected to steadily increasing levels of work. An ECG and oxygen levels are taken while the patient exercises. The test is stopped if abnormalities occur on the ECG.
Valve Replacement	Surgical procedure to excise a diseased heart valve and replace with an artificial valve.
Venography	X-ray of the veins in which the venous flow is traced. Also called phlebography.

- **Aplastic anemia**—This is a condition in which fat cells replace bone marrow and the bone marrow that is present is unable to produce certain types of blood cells. The cause, or etiology, of this condition is unknown. It is one of the most life-threatening forms of anemia, but it is also one of the rarest. Adolescents and young adults are the patient population affected most by this form of anemia. Possible causes of this type of anemia include injury to the bone marrow and exposure to certain chemicals and pesticides.

Signs and Symptoms. The hallmark symptoms of anemia include increased tiredness and fatigue. Other symptoms and signs of anemia include weakness, heart palpitations and tachycardia (rapid heartbeat), shortness of breath, dizziness, headache, pale complexion, tinnitus or ringing in the ears, difficulty concentrating, and interrupted sleep patterns. Fainting is also common among anemic patients. Sickle cell anemia is characterized by pain in the abdomen, joints, and bones. Infections and heart failure may also occur with sickle cell anemia. Signs and symptoms of aplastic anemia can include bleeding in the mucous membranes, infections with high fevers, paleness, and dyspnea.

Treatment. The treatment for anemia depends on the type and cause. In some cases, injections of vitamin B_{12} may be necessary. Oral dietary supplements including iron, folic acid, and vitamin B_{12} have also been effective by helping produce and maintain healthy red blood cells. Elimination of specific medications that suppress the body's immune system may be needed. Blood transfusions, analgesics, and antibiotics may also be required for more serious forms of the disorder.

Aneurysm

Weakened walls of blood vessels may become abnormally wide or may balloon. When this occurs, it is termed an **aneurysm**. Aneurysms may occur in various locations throughout the body. The most common locations include:

- Aorta (aortic aneurysm)
- Brain (cerebral aneurysm)
- Leg (popliteal artery aneurysm)
- Spleen (splenic artery aneurysm)
- Intestine (mesenteric artery aneurysm)

Aneurysms can be congenital or acquired. The exact cause is unknown; however, defective portions of the arterial wall are suspected. Additionally, conditions that may contribute to the formation of aneurysms include hypertension (high blood pressure), high cholesterol, and atherosclerotic disease. Atherosclerotic disease is characterized by narrowing of the arterial walls from increased accumulation of plaque. This is discussed later in this section.

Signs and Symptoms. The signs and symptoms of an aneurysm vary, depending on its location. An aneurysm near the body's surface may be distinguished by a swelling, throbbing mass. Unfortunately, aneurysms within the body or brain often have no symptoms and frequently go undetected until the aneurysm ruptures. A ruptured aneurysm leads to massive internal bleeding and is often fatal. Aneurysms of this type are sometimes discovered when the patient is undergoing an imaging procedure for some other reason.

Treatment. Surgical intervention may be required to repair and prevent rupturing of the vessel. Some people may be candidates for a stent (a mesh tube) placement within the affected vessel to keep it open or to reinforce the vessel wall. A healthy diet and exercise may help prevent certain types of aneurysms. Additionally, maintaining healthy blood pressure and cholesterol levels is beneficial.

Arrhythmia

An **arrhythmia** is an irregular heartbeat caused by a disturbance of the electrical conductivity of the heart. There are many types of arrhythmias. Two general categories are as follows:

- **Tachycardia** is an abnormally rapid heart rate, one that is greater than 100 beats per minute. A heart rate that is too fast may not allow the ventricles of the heart to fill properly, depriving the brain and body of oxygen. Extremely rapid tachycardia can be fatal if not treated immediately. Although the heart rate may be high, the rhythm may be either regular or irregular.

- **Bradycardia** is an abnormally slow heart rate of less than 60 beats per minute. The rhythm may be either regular or irregular.

Although the etiologies of arrhythmias vary, depending on the type, the major contributing factors are heart diseases. These include coronary artery disease (CAD), heart valve disease, problems arising from the SA node (the pacemaker of the heart) or conduction pathways of the heart, heart failure, and infections such as endocarditis.

Signs and Symptoms. Both tachycardia and bradycardia produce similar symptoms, including dizziness, palpitations, shortness of breath, fatigue, weakness, angina (chest pain), and fainting.

Treatment. Arrhythmias can be life threatening, especially when they significantly impact the pumping function of the heart. If the oxygen supply to the brain and major organs is interrupted for more than a few minutes, death can occur. Arrhythmias are often treated with medications. In more serious conditions, a procedure such as cardioversion (applying an electric current to the heart to restore a normal rhythm)

or implantation of a pacemaker (to assist in maintaining a normal rhythm) may be necessary. Many patients can tolerate arrhythmias for years; however, the heart functions much better with a strong, evenly metered rhythm.

Arteriosclerosis

Arteriosclerosis is commonly known, in lay terms, as "hardening of the arteries." It develops when the walls of the arteries become thick and loose elasticity. Eventually, after many years, calcium deposits in the artery walls develop areas that are hard and brittle. Arteries of the brain, kidneys, and upper and lower extremities may be affected.

Signs and Symptoms. Because this disease occurs within the body, its effects cannot be seen and symptoms are usually not felt. Therefore it is not always recognized early or easily. However, a series of signs and symptoms that might seem unrelated at first should alert the individual and the physician. Signs and symptoms that are considered precursors to arteriosclerosis are high blood pressure, recurrent kidney infections, and impaired circulation, particularly to the fingers and toes, caused by peripheral vascular disease.

Treatment. Many prescription medications are available for the treatment of arteriosclerosis. However, the most effective treatments include treating the underlying causes. This is crucial to achieving a desirable long-term outcome.

Atherosclerosis

Atherosclerosis is the hardening and narrowing of the arteries from a buildup of fatty material and plaque within the vessel (Figure 26-15). This condition often results from unhealthy

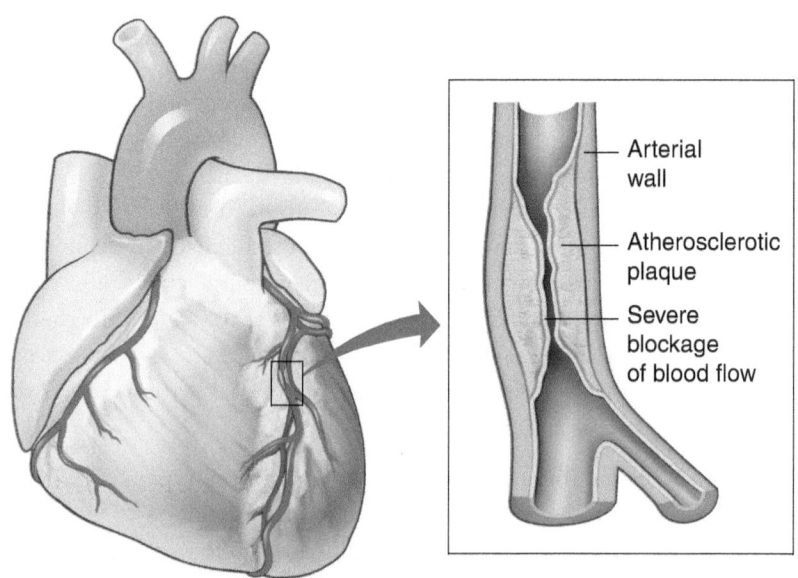

FIGURE 26-15 An atherosclerotic artery.

lifestyle factors including smoking, high cholesterol, excessive alcohol consumption, and a poor diet. There is also a familial link with the disease. Other conditions that often are related to atherosclerosis include diabetes and obesity.

Atherosclerosis is the leading cause of coronary artery disease (CAD). As the coronary arteries become more constricted, the flow of blood within the arteries may slow or even stop. The arteries can narrow to the point of total blockage. Plaque that breaks loose forms an embolus that can move and occlude a narrow vessel, causing death to the tissue and surrounding area supplied by that vessel.

Signs and Symptoms. When the heart needs more oxygen-rich blood than the vessels can supply, angina (chest pain) or other warning symptoms may occur. One of the first recognized symptoms of atherosclerosis is angina during exercise or other exertive activity. Shortness of breath and fatigue may accompany angina. If the blockage is large, angina can occur with little or no activity. With unstable angina, blood flow to the heart is so limited that the individual restricts daily activities because of the risk of chest pain.

Treatment. Typically, angina decreases with rest and oxygen, but unrelieved angina is a common symptom of impending myocardial infarction. Nitroglycerin, a prescription medication that dilates blood vessels and improves the flow of oxygenated blood to the heart, is often prescribed to relieve angina. Prevention and reversal of the disease may be accomplished by making lifestyle changes including avoiding fatty foods, decreasing alcohol consumption, stopping smoking, and engaging in physical exercise. In serious cases, surgical intervention to widen and remove the plaque clogs may be required.

Cardiac Tamponade

Cardiac tamponade, or cardiac compression, is pressure on the heart muscle caused by blood or fluid collecting in the pericardial sac that surrounds the heart. The pressure prevents the ventricles from expanding, making it impossible for the heart to pump enough blood for the body. The etiologies of cardiac tamponade vary, ranging from trauma to the heart to leukemia, heart tumors, radiation to the chest, kidney failure, acute heart attacks, thoracic aneurysm, and other cardiac related disorders.

Signs and Symptoms. Shortness of breath, pale or bluing skin, chest pain, dizziness, drowsiness, anxiety, and the feeling of impending doom are common symptoms of cardiac tamponade.

Treatment. Treatment requires an immediate procedure called pericardiocentesis, which is initiated by inserting a needle into the pericardial sac and removing fluid. Diuretic medications (that decrease body fluid through increased urination) and oxygen therapy may also be used to help reduce the workload of the heart.

Cardiogenic Shock

Cardiogenic shock is a collapse of the cardiovascular system. It is characterized by the inability of the heart to pump enough blood to the body's organs. It is caused by an extremely damaged heart, which may be the result of arrhythmias, ruptured cardiac muscle, or a tear in the septal wall.

Signs and Symptoms. Symptoms and signs of shock include chest pain and pressure, a change in consciousness, rapid breathing and pulse, heavy diaphoresis (perspiration), lightheadedness, and decreased urination.

Treatment. Emergency medical treatment is necessary in this extremely serious situation. Immediate treatment involves controlling and treating the underlying cause. It likely includes medications to restore heart function and normal rhythm, oxygen therapy, and pain medications. Cardiac stenting and catheterization may also be necessary. In some circumstances, heart surgery or the insertion of a pacemaker may be required.

Carditis (Endocarditis, Myocarditis, Pericarditis)

Carditis is an inflammation of the heart. It is more accurately referred to as endocarditis, myocarditis, or pericarditis, depending on the layer of the heart that is affected.

Endocarditis

Endocarditis is an inflammation of the lining of the heart, including the heart valves. It is most commonly caused by a bacterial infection and frequently affects patients with existing abnormal conditions of the heart valves. Endocarditis can also be present at birth.

Signs and Symptoms. Persons who suffer from this life-threatening condition may experience weakness, fever, chills, diaphoresis, **dyspnea** (difficulty breathing), and swelling in the feet and legs.

Treatment. Treatment generally consists of antibiotics given intravenously followed by oral antibiotics over a six-week period. In serious cases, heart valve replacement might be necessary.

Myocarditis

Myocarditis is inflammation of the muscular layer of the heart. Etiologies of myocarditis include viral infection;

however, exposure to bacteria, fungi, and certain drugs, chemicals, and allergens may also lead to its development.

Signs and Symptoms. Signs and symptoms generally resemble those of the flu and include fever, body aches, dyspnea, general fatigue and malaise, fainting, and decreased urine output. However, the most frequent symptom of myocarditis is chest pain.

Treatment. The best treatment for myocarditis is reduction of the inflammation with antiinflammatory medications, antibiotics if necessary, bed rest, and a low-sodium diet. Diuretics may also be prescribed to remove excessive fluid from the body.

Pericarditis

Pericarditis is inflammation of the membrane that surrounds the heart—the pericardium. It is most commonly caused by a viral infection. It may also accompany other diseases such as HIV/AIDS or kidney failure. Less common causes may include bacterial infection, tuberculosis, cancer that has spread to the pericardium, or following heart surgery or injury.

Signs and Symptoms. Symptoms and signs of this deadly condition frequently include sharp, stabbing chest pain, fatigue, fever, and dyspnea, especially while lying down, taking a deep breath, or coughing.

Treatment. Treatment often includes analgesics, diuretics to help reduce the amount of fluid around the heart, and antibiotics or antifungals to treat the infection. Chronic cases may require pericardiocentesis to remove fluid around the heart.

Congestive Heart Failure

Congestive heart failure (CHF), also called just heart failure, is a condition in which the heart is unable to pump sufficient blood to the body's other organs. This can result from several other conditions, including:

- Coronary artery disease
- History of myocardial infarction
- Hypertension
- Diseases or infections of the heart valves
- Primary diseases and infections of the heart muscle itself, such as endocarditis or myocarditis
- Heart defects present at birth

Signs and Symptoms. As the "failing" heart functions less efficiently than it should, exertion causes shortness of breath and general tiredness and fatigue. Some patients have trouble simply walking across a room without becoming out of breath and exhausted. Often swelling, or edema, results, usually in the legs and ankles, but sometimes in other parts of the body including the abdomen. Fluid may collect in the lungs and interfere with breathing, causing shortness of breath that becomes more pronounced when the person is lying down. Heart failure also affects the kidneys' ability to dispose of sodium and water. An increased frequency of urination during the night might be present. Weight gain may occur, and often rapidly, from the increased fluid and resulting edema. Other symptoms of CHF include a cough, decreased appetite, and an irregular pulse.

Treatment. A treatment program for CHF usually consists of rest, proper diet and maintaining a healthy weight, revising daily activities that may aggravate symptoms, oxygen therapy, and medications that help the heart to function more efficiently, including ACE inhibitors, beta blockers, digitalis, diuretics, and vasodilators. When the specific cause of CHF is discovered, it should be treated or, if possible, corrected. For example, some cases can be treated by addressing high blood pressure. If an abnormal heart valve is the cause, the valve can be surgically replaced.

Cor Pulmonale

Cor pulmonale is also known as right-sided heart disease. It is a result of prolonged hypertension of the pulmonary arteries and right ventricle of the heart. Its causes are primarily related to lung disorders such as chronic obstructive pulmonary disease (COPD), cystic fibrosis, chronic blood clots in the lungs, obstructive sleep apnea, and others.

Signs and Symptoms. Pain toward the front of the chest is a common symptom of cor pulmonale, as are frequent fainting episodes during activity. Peripheral swelling of legs and feet and coughing or wheezing may be present.

Treatment. Treatment seeks to relieve the pulmonary problems that precipitate the disease and to control symptoms. Medications that improve pulmonary function are usually prescribed. Other medications such as anticoagulants to thin the blood or antihypertensive medications and diuretics to lower blood pressure may also be prescribed. In severe cases, if medications fail, a lung or heart-lung transplant might be necessary.

Coronary Artery Disease

Coronary artery disease (CAD), also known as coronary heart disease (CHD), is the narrowing of the coronary arteries that supply blood to the heart, which results from a buildup of plaque on the artery walls (generally caused by atherosclerosis, a condition we discussed earlier), resulting in decreased blood flow. Left untreated, this progressive disease raises the risk of myocardial infarction, or heart attack, and possibly sudden death.

CAD is the most common form of heart disease and the leading cause of death in the United States, resulting in the deaths of more than 375,000 Americans each year. According to the American Heart Association, at least two people per minute—men and women—suffer from a CAD-related event, and one person dies from this cause every 40 seconds.

CAD affects people of all races. Lifestyle factors including obesity, unhealthy diet choices, lack of exercise, and stress are possible causes; genetic factors may play a role as well. Other diseases such as hypertension and diabetes also put people at risk for developing CAD. High levels of lipoproteins, or LDL cholesterol, are associated with a higher risk of CAD because this fatty substance is one of the main factors of plaque formation. Risk can be lowered by maintaining a total cholesterol level below 200 mg/dL, an HDL cholesterol (good cholesterol) level above 40 mg/dL, and an LDL cholesterol (bad cholesterol) level less than 100 mg/dL. Daily aerobic exercise, increasing dietary intake of vegetables and whole grain products, weight loss, and smoking cessation are all steps people can take to reach healthier cholesterol levels.

Signs and Symptoms. Shortness of breath and fatigue with exertion and a squeezing sensation of the heart are common symptoms. Edema (swelling) in the ankles may be a sign of CAD, as may a feeling of overall tiredness and weakness.

Treatment. Antihypertensive medications are prescribed to treat high blood pressure if it is an underlying cause of CAD. Nitroglycerin is administered during bouts of angina to help relieve chest pain by working as a vasodilator allowing the blood vessels to open and blood to flow more freely. Aspirin, taken in low doses on a daily basis, is also used to treat

CAD. Additionally, patients are prescribed medications to help lower cholesterol levels and advised to make lifestyle changes (as listed earlier) that will assist in their progress. Diabetic patients are closely monitored and required to take medications to lower their blood sugar levels and ensure that insulin production and effectiveness are optimal.

Heart Attack (Myocardial Infarction) or Cardiac Arrest

A heart attack, or **myocardial infarction (MI)**, occurs when the blood supply to a part of the myocardium has stopped, causing tissue damage or death from oxygen deprivation (Figure 26-16). Coronary artery disease, particularly atherosclerosis (discussed earlier in the chapter) and thrombosis (blood clots), are the main causes of MIs. In a coronary thrombosis, accumulated plaque on artery walls tears loose or ruptures and forms a blood clot that blocks the artery. If the blood supply is cut off, the muscle tissues fed by that artery suffer damage that quickly becomes irreversible, resulting in death of the affected tissue. Depending on the extent of the damage, a patient may suffer disability or death from a heart attack.

A heart attack may or may not lead directly to **cardiac arrest**, the total cessation of heartbeat and breathing. Cardiac arrest may also occur suddenly (known as sudden death) with no prior symptoms of a heart attack.

Heart attack victims can recover if the area of damage to the heart muscle is limited or the infarction is recognized and treated quickly, before the damage becomes irreversible. Even victims of cardiac arrest can sometimes survive if emergency care is initiated within minutes.

Signs and Symptoms. The most common symptom of an MI is chest pain. The chest pain (angina pectoris) is often described as crushing or squeezing, with a feeling of fullness, heaviness, or aching in the center of the chest. This pain may radiate down the left arm or into the neck or back.

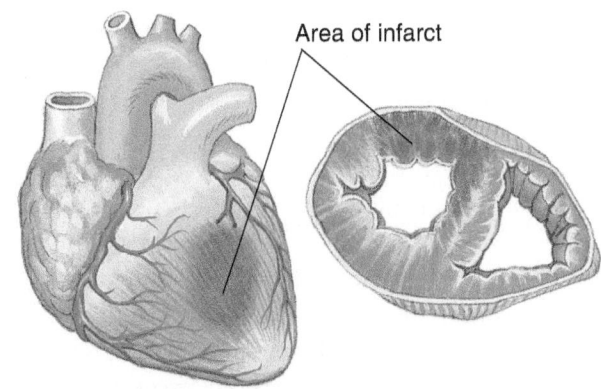

FIGURE 26-16 Cross section of a myocardial infarction.

Men experience chest pain as a symptom of an MI more frequently than do women. It has become clear that women experience different symptoms with a heart attack. A woman is more likely to feel pain in the arms, which may radiate across the shoulders and up into the jaw. Diaphoresis, shortness of breath, nausea, fainting, or dizziness and the overall feeling of impending doom are also common symptoms experienced by women.

Cyanosis, or blue skin, often visible in the lips and around the mouth, is a sign that oxygenated blood is not being perfused (forced through) by the heart.

If any of these symptoms are present for more than two minutes, emergency treatment must be started immediately. Waiting to treat the symptoms permits continuing deterioration of the heart muscle and increases the chances of serious disability or death.

A patient suffering a heart attack may still be conscious or be able to respond to voice or touch, will be breathing, and will have a pulse. Cardiac arrest has occurred if the patient is completely unresponsive, has no pulse, and is not breathing.

Treatment. Treatment for an MI, when administered quickly, can benefit most patients. If the patient is in cardiac arrest, cardiopulmonary resuscitation (CPR) and defibrillation within the first few minutes increase the survival rate. Medical assistants should have training in CPR and defibrillation; however, keep in mind that CPR or defibrillation should not be performed unless the patient is actually in cardiac arrest. Performing CPR or defibrillation on a patient who is having a heart attack but still has a pulse may be harmful. (CPR and defibrillation are discussed in the chapter titled "Assisting with Medical Emergencies.")

Thrombolytics (medications that dissolve clots) can stop some heart attacks in progress. **Angioplasty**, which is surgical vessel repair, is frequently performed to reopen blocked coronary arteries, and stents are used to hold the arteries open, allowing more blood flow. If more conservative measures fail or if the heart attack is too severe, a coronary artery bypass graft (CABG), a form of open heart surgery, will be attempted to bypass the blocked artery using a vein from the leg or arm.

The key to heart attack survival as well as survival of cardiac arrest is immediate intervention. Patients and their caregivers or loved ones must be educated on the warning signs of MI, the signs of cardiac arrest, and the necessity of seeking medical assistance immediately when they or someone they are with has any of these signs or symptoms. After emergency treatment at the scene of the event, transport to a hospital with cardiac care capability must be initiated.

Hemophilia

Hemophilia is a blood-clotting disorder. Its etiology is a genetic defect of the X chromosome. This hereditary deficiency of clotting factors (blood-clotting proteins) primarily affects male children, but in rare circumstances females are also affected. Without these blood-clotting proteins, platelets are unable to form clots to stop bleeding.

Signs and Symptoms. Excessive bleeding, or hemorrhaging (bleeding heavily), is the primary sign of hemophilia. A hemophiliac (a patient with hemophilia) may display signs including excessive nose bleeds, heavy bleeding from a minor cut, and the recurrence of bleeding after it has ceased for a short time. Easily bruising is a sign of internal bleeding as is blood that appears in urine or stool.

Treatment. Hemophilia is treated by transfusing the deficient clotting factor in a process called replacement therapy. Replacing the missing or lacking clotting factors allows the blood to properly coagulate as necessary.

Hypertension

Hypertension (HTN) is high blood pressure. It is the term used when the force of the pumped blood against the arterial walls is too great, causing unhealthy conditions for the body.

Hypertension is caused by congestion in the peripheral arteries. Peripheral artery disease (PAD) occurs when the arteries become diseased and narrowed, causing arteriostenosis. They can also become filled with fatty plaque, giving rise to atherosclerosis. PAD most often affects the arteries of the legs, but it can also affect arteries to the head, arms, and internal organs. When blood does not flow easily through the arteries, blood pressure rises.

It is important to note that a single high blood pressure reading is not enough for a physician to diagnose a patient with hypertension. Blood pressure readings must be consistently high over a period of time in order for a diagnosis of hypertension to be given. By diagnosing the patient with borderline hypertension, or prehypertension (as described in the next section, "Prehypertension"), treatment can be initiated earlier.

Risk factors for HTN include obesity, a sedentary lifestyle, a high salt diet, being of African-American descent, being diabetic, living a high-stress or anxious life, and excessive alcohol consumption. Smoking and family history of hypertension also are risk factors for high blood pressure.

Stages of Hypertension

The American Heart Association has staged hypertension into five categories: normal, prehypertension, stage I, stage II, and hypertensive crisis. Table 26-3 clearly indicates the blood pressure levels for each of these categories.

TABLE 26-3 | Stages of Hypertension

Stage	Blood Pressure Reading
Normal	• Systolic pressure below 120 mmHg AND • Diastolic pressure below 80 mmHg
Prehypertension	• Systolic pressure below between 120–139 mmHg OR • Diastolic pressure between 80–89 mmHg
Stage 1 Hypertension	• Systolic pressure below between 140–159 mmHg OR • Diastolic pressure between 90–99 mmHg
Stage 2 Hypertension	• Systolic pressure that is 160 mmHg or higher OR • Diastolic pressure that is 100 mmHg or higher
Hypertensive Crisis	• Systolic pressure that is higher than 180 mmHg OR • Diastolic pressure that is higher than 110 mmHg

National Committee of the National Institutes of Health National Heart, Lung, and Blood Institute (NHLBI), adults at the upper end of the prehypertension blood pressure range are twice as likely to progress to hypertension as those with lower blood pressure.

Signs and Symptoms. Blood pressure ranging from 120/80 to 139/89 is a sign of prehypertension.

Treatment. The committee report just cited recommends lifestyle changes such as reducing dietary fat and sodium, increasing exercise, and limiting alcohol consumption.

Hypotension

Hypotension, or low blood pressure, is an abnormal condition in which a person's blood pressure is much lower than usual, generally below 90/60 mmHg. If blood pressure drops significantly, blood flow to the heart, brain, and other vital organs becomes inadequate, causing serious complications. Because blood circulation is the way oxygen is transported to the body cells, a sudden, significant drop in blood pressure is a warning that the body is not receiving enough oxygen and is in danger of shutting down.

Causes of hypotension include dehydration, heart failure, heart attack, changes in the heart's rhythm (arrhythmias), anaphylaxis (severe allergic reaction), severe blood loss (shock), certain medications, and drug overdose. A common form of hypotension is orthostatic hypotension, which occurs when there is a sudden change in body position, usually from lying down or sitting to an upright position.

Low blood pressure can also be a sign of a well-conditioned heart in those who get regular aerobic exercise, such as running. In these individuals, the myocardium is able to produce strong contractions to easily pump the blood through the body. Such cases, obviously, do not indicate an emergency situation but rather the normal functioning of a healthy body.

Signs and Symptoms. When the body is getting shortchanged on oxygen because of low blood pressure, normal body functions such as breathing, movement, and brain function can be impaired, and permanent damage can occur. Blurred vision, weakness, confusion, dizziness or fainting, and sleepiness are the most common symptoms of low blood pressure. Blood pressure may drop to life-threatening levels from loss of blood, shock, severe infection, or low body temperature caused by exposure to cold.

Treatment. The goal of emergency treatment for hypotension is to raise blood pressure to a more normal level. This may include the use of vasoconstrictors (medications that cause blood vessels to narrow, or constrict), and increasing fluid and sodium intake. If the patient suffers from

Signs and Symptoms. Hypertension is well known as the "silent killer" because there are very few symptoms, and symptoms that may be present may be easily brushed off by the patient. Some of these symptoms include increased tiredness and fatigue, headaches, and changes in vision. More severe cases of HTN by be indicated by epistaxis (nosebleeds) and blood in the urine.

Treatment. HTN can be controlled in a variety of ways, such as with antihypertensive and diuretic medications as well as dietary and lifestyle changes, including exercise and smoking cessation. If left untreated, hypertension can lead to serious conditions such as kidney failure, stroke, heart attack, eye damage, and peripheral artery disease (which, as noted, may also be a cause of HTN).

Prehypertension

Often a precursor to hypertension, **prehypertension** is a classification of hypertension that is assigned to adults who consistently have blood pressure readings that range from 120/80 to 139/89 mmHg. According to a study by the Joint

orthostatic hypotension, the patient may be instructed to form the habit of changing body position slowly.

Leukemia

Leukemia is a cancer of the bone marrow and blood. Like all cancers, leukemia is caused by uncontrolled growth of abnormal cells, in this case white blood cells (WBCs). Other body tissues are also affected. Leukemia can be acute or chronic.

- **Acute leukemia**—An increased number of nonfunctioning and abnormally developed cells are present in this aggressive form of cancer. The increased number of abnormal cells crowd out the healthy blood cells. Unfortunately, this increases the body's risk of infection and developing anemia. Another characteristic is a lack of platelets, which means that the patient may be at risk for extensive bleeding because of decreased clotting ability.

- **Chronic leukemia**—This form is less aggressive than acute leukemia because the abnormal cells accrue over a longer period of time. The type of leukocyte affected by leukemia provides a more distinct classification of the cancer. Lymphocytic or myeloid leukemia is indicated depending on whether the cancer has struck lymphocytes or myeloid cells, which are bone marrow cells.

Signs and Symptoms. The signs and symptoms of leukemia are broad. They include excessive bruising, fatigue, weakness, dyspnea (breathing difficulty), bleeding of the mucous membranes, bone and joint pain, abdominal pain, weight loss, abdominal bleeding, and enlargement of the lymph nodes, spleen, and/or liver. Anemia and frequent infections are common.

Treatment. Treatment options available for leukemia include chemotherapy, radiation, and bone marrow transplantation. Anticancer drugs are used to kill leukemia cells, and high energy radiation is used to irradiate the cancer cells.

Stroke

A **stroke**, sometimes called a cerebrovascular accident (CVA), occurs when the blood supply to part of the brain is suddenly interrupted. This can occur from blockage of an artery to the brain caused by an embolism (a foreign substance that has been carried to the point of blockage from a distant part of the body) or a thrombus (a fragment of plaque that has broken free of the artery wall). A ruptured artery has the same effect as a blocked artery in depriving an area of the brain of blood flow, oxygen, and nutrients, a condition called ischemia.

Signs and Symptoms. The symptoms and signs of a stroke generally occur suddenly: numbness or weakness on one side of the body, confusion or trouble speaking, vision problems, severe dizziness, loss of balance or coordination, and often a severe headache. The headache is sometimes described as "the worst headache of my life." The National Stroke Association encourages people to be aware of the first signs of stroke so that immediate help may be rendered. They have developed the acronym FAST to assist with recognition of the symptoms:

- **F = Face**—If a stroke is suspected, ask the individual to smile to ascertain if one side of the face droops.
- **A = Arms**—To evaluate balance, ask the individual to hold out both arms. Does one arm drift downward?
- **S = Speech**—The individual should be asked to repeat a simple phrase to assess the speech; look for signs of slurring or strange inflections.
- **T = Time**—If a person demonstrates any of these signs, time is valuable and treatment must be sought immediately by dialing 911. Quick recognition of the signs and prompt hospital treatment may lessen neurological damage.

The patient's first stroke may have been preceded by a transient ischemic attack (TIA), which has the symptoms of a stroke, probably from a temporary artery blockage, but resolves on its own. TIAs are considered to be precursors of stroke.

Treatment. Treatment for stroke is aimed at controlling factors that may place a patient at risk for stroke, or a recurrence of stroke. Risk factors with manageable treatment options include high blood pressure, diabetes, and atrial fibrillation. After a stroke occurs, rehabilitation may be necessary to help the patient with speech and mobility, which are often affected. Medications prevent the formation of thrombi.

Thrombophlebitis

Thrombo means "clot"; *phlebitis* is the inflammation of a vein. **Thrombophlebitis** occurs when a blood clot causes inflammation in one or more veins, typically in the lower extremities (Figure 26-17). On rare occasions, thrombophlebitis can also affect veins in the upper extremities. Superficial thrombophlebitis occurs when the affected vein is near the surface of the skin. A more serious condition is a deep vein thrombosis (DVT), which occurs when the affected vein is deep within a muscle. DVTs may lead to a very serious condition known as pulmonary embolism (PE), which occurs when a dislodged clot travels through the blood vessels to the lungs, where it lodges in and blocks a smaller artery.

Thrombophlebitis can be caused by a genetic clotting disorder or by trauma. It can also be caused by prolonged inactivity such as a long journey in an airplane or automobile, lengthy bed rest following surgery, or as a result of paralysis. Such inactivity decreases blood flow through the

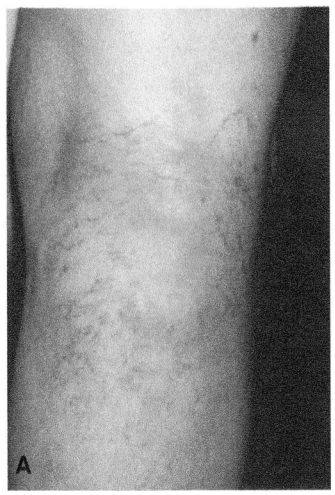
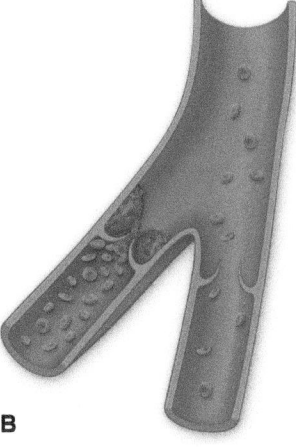

FIGURE 26-17 Examples of thrombophlebitis. **(A)** Superficial thrombophlebitis of the leg. **(B)** Deep venous thrombosis (DVT) commonly affects the veins of the leg.

veins, which may allow a clot to form. Other risk factors include the use of oral contraceptives or hormone replacement therapy. A history of varicose veins can also place someone at higher risk for thrombophlebitis.

Signs and Symptoms. The most common signs and symptoms of thrombophlebitis are redness, swelling, warmth, tenderness, and a dull ache or pain in the affected area. Superficial veins affected often visibly display as a hard and red cord of bulging vein just under the skin. If a deep vein is affected, the leg may become swollen, tender, and painful, particularly when the person stands or walks.

Treatment. For thrombophlebitis in a superficial vein, the physician generally encourages home remedies to alleviate symptoms and resolve the issue. Home remedies include limb elevation, heat application, and the use of NSAIDS (nonsteroidal antiinflammatory drugs) such as aspirin or ibuprofen. Massaging the painful area is never recommended as it could cause the thrombus to break away, forming a traveling embolus. The condition usually subsides within a month.

In more severe cases, as in deep venous thrombosis, an injection of an anticoagulant (blood-thinning) medication often prevents the clot from growing. Additional treatments may include the application of support (compression) stockings to constrict the superficial veins and increase blood flow in the deep veins. Varicose vein ligation or stripping, in which the doctor surgically removes the varicose veins that cause pain or recurrent thrombophlebitis, is also used as treatment. In the most severe cases, a thrombectomy or bypass surgery may be required to remove an acute clot blocking a pelvic or abdominal vein.

Transfusion Incompatibility Reaction

If the wrong type of blood is administered to a patient, a severe transfusion reaction can occur. The two blood types will create an antigen-versus-antibody reaction (as seen in Figure 26-14), and severe agglutination can occur. (We mentioned this kind of transfusion reaction earlier under "The Rh Factor.")

Signs and Symptoms. Signs and symptoms of transfusion incompatibility arise rapidly with collapse of the cardiovascular system. Symptoms of shock, such as confusion, restlessness, and shortness of breath, are dramatic.

Treatment. If an incompatibility reaction occurs, the transfusion of donor blood must be stopped immediately. Normal saline will be infused into the bloodstream intravenously. The physician may order the administration of antihistamines as well as frequent monitoring of vital signs. If the reaction is more aggressive, administration of epinephrine may be needed. Two people, generally advanced health care professionals such as registered nurses, should always double-check the compatibility of the donor blood with the patient's blood type before it is administered.

Valvular Heart Disease

Valvular heart disease is any damage or defect to one of the four valves of the heart: mitral or aortic on the left, tricuspid or pulmonary on the right.

Mitral Stenosis

Mitral stenosis is one of the most common types of valvular heart disease. In this disease, the mitral valve, between the left atrium and ventricle, is unable to fully open. This deficiency prevents proper blood flow and causes a buildup of blood in the left atrium. In turn, this can cause the atrial chamber to swell and lead to other problems, including a backup of blood and body fluid in the lung tissue. (Normally, oxygenated blood flows into the left atrium from the lungs. A blockage of this flow can lead to pulmonary edema, an excess of fluid in the lungs.)

Mitral stenosis can be a congenital condition, and it can occur in adults who suffered episodes of rheumatic fever earlier in their life. It also may be the result of bacterial endocarditis or hypertension or atherosclerosis that has damaged the valve.

Signs and Symptoms. Mitral stenosis can produce a heart murmur that is audible with a stethoscope. Symptoms and signs, which are generally mild, may include increased fatigue, cough, and frequent respiratory infections, discomfort with increased activity including breathing difficulties and chest discomfort, edema of the feet and legs, and heart palpitations.

Treatment. Treatment includes medication to strengthen heart function. However, in mild cases of the disorder, treatment might not be necessary. Short- or long-term antibiotics may be required if bacterial endocarditis is involved. Surgery to replace the damaged valve may be required.

Varicose Veins

Varicose veins are gnarled, enlarged veins, usually superficial veins in the legs. They may be caused by prolonged periods of standing, pregnancy, obesity, or aging.

Varicose veins develop when the valves in the veins malfunction. As a person gets older, the veins tend to lose elasticity and stretch. Blood pools in the veins, which become engorged with deoxygenated blood.

Signs and Symptoms. Symptoms include a feeling of heavy and aching limbs. When severe cases develop and are untreated, the affected veins could rupture and result in varicose ulcers (open sores) on the skin.

Treatment. Treatment for varicose veins falls into two categories: relief of the symptoms and removal of the affected veins (ligation). Symptom relief includes such measures as moderate exercise, avoiding long periods of standing, elevating the legs, and wearing support stockings, which compress the veins and hold them in place. Cosmetic treatments may decrease the size and visibility of the affected veins.

For a summary and additional information on disorders of the cardiovascular system, see Table 26-4.

TABLE 26-4 | Disorders of the Cardiovascular System

Disorder	Description
Angina pectoris	Condition in which there is severe pain with a sensation of constriction around the heart. It is caused by a deficiency of oxygen to the heart muscle.
Angioma	Tumor, usually benign, consisting of blood vessels.
Angiospasm	Spasm or contraction of blood vessels.
Aortic aneurysm	Localized, abnormal dilation of the aorta, causing pressure on the trachea, esophagus, veins, or nerves. This is a result of a weakness in the wall of the blood vessels.
Aortic insufficiency	A failure of the aortic valve to close completely, which results in blood leaking back into the left ventricle and inefficient heart action.
Aortic stenosis	Condition caused by narrowing of the aortic valve.
Arterial embolism	Blood clot moving within an artery. This can occur as a result of arteriosclerosis.
Cardiomyopathy	Disease of the cardiac muscle causing it to weaken and not function properly. It is often a symptom of another cardiovascular disease, and its main symptom is the inability of the heart to pump blood efficiently to the body.
Coronary thrombosis	Blood clot in a coronary vessel of the heart causing the vessel to close completely or partially.
Embolus	A blood clot that moves from one area to another and obstructs a blood vessel.
Fibrillation	Abnormal quivering or contractions of heart fibers. When this occurs within the fibers of the ventricle, arrest and death can occur. Emergency equipment to defibrillate, or convert the heart to a normal beat, is necessary.
Infarct	Area of tissue within an organ or part that undergoes necrosis (death) following the cessation of the blood supply.
Ischemia	A localized and temporary deficiency of blood supply caused by an obstruction to the circulation.
Mitral valve prolapse (MVP)	Common and serious condition in which the cusp of the mitral valve drops back (prolapses) into the left atrium during systole.
Murmur	A soft blowing or rasping sound heard on auscultation of the heart.
Patent ductus arteriosus	Congenital presence of a connection between the pulmonary artery and the aorta that remains after birth. This condition is normal in the fetus.
Phlebitis	Inflammation of a vein.
Reynaud's phenomenon	Intermittent attacks of pallor or cyanosis of the fingers and toes associated with cold or emotional distress. Numbness, pain, and burning may also occur during the attacks. It may be caused by decreased circulation as a result of smoking.

TABLE 26-4 | Disorders of the Cardiovascular System (*continued*)

Disorder	Description
Rheumatic heart disease	Valvular heart disease as a result of having had rheumatic fever.
Tetralogy of Fallot	Combination of four symptoms (tetralogy), resulting in pulmonary stenosis, a septal defect, abnormal blood supply to the aorta, and hypertrophy of the right ventricle. A congenital defect that is present at birth and needs immediate surgery to correct.
Thrombus	A blood clot.

SUMMARY

The cardiovascular system is made up of structures that circulate blood, oxygen, nutrients, and other substances throughout the body. These structures include the heart and the blood vessels. The heart is a muscular pump that moves oxygen- and nutrient-rich blood to the body and carries waste and carbon dioxide back to the lungs for excretion from the body. Arteries carry blood away from the heart to the body. The exchange of oxygen and nutrients for carbon dioxide and waste takes place in the capillaries; then, the veins carry the blood back to the heart and lungs.

Blood pressure keeps the heart functionally pumping blood to all the organs and cells. Blood is connective tissue that circulates through the body. Blood cells include red blood cells (erythrocytes), white blood cells (leukocytes), and clotting cells (platelets). The four blood types are A, B, AB, and O. Being an intricate system, many problems and diseases may arise in the cardiovascular system. Disease can occur in the heart, blood vessels, valves of the heart, or blood cells.

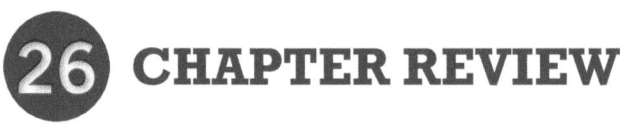

26 CHAPTER REVIEW

COMPETENCY REVIEW

1. Define and spell the terms for this chapter.
2. Name the three major components of the cardiovascular system.
3. Name the three layers of the heart.
4. Name the upper chambers of the heart.
5. Name the lower chambers of the heart.
6. What role do the arteries play in circulation?
7. What role do the veins play in circulation?
8. Name the structure that is considered to be the pacemaker of the heart.
9. Describe how blood pressure is recorded in the patient's chart.
10. Define pulse pressure.

PREPARING FOR THE CERTIFICATION EXAM

1. Which of the following is a valve?
   a. tricuspid
   b. vena cava
   c. sinoatrial node
   d. pacemaker
   e. intraventricular septum

2. Blood enters the left atrium of the heart through the
   a. pulmonary artery.
   b. superior and inferior venae cavae.
   c. pulmonary vein.
   d. descending aorta.
   e. coronary artery.

3. Blood enters the heart through the
   a. right and left atria.
   b. right and left pulmonary arteries.
   c. right and left pulmonary veins.
   d. right and left ventricles.
   e. superior and inferior venae cavae.

4. The muscular layer of the heart is called the
   a. pericardium.
   b. myocardium.
   c. apex.
   d. endocardium.
   e. mediastinum.

5. A common valvular heart disease is
   a. cor pulmonale.
   b. cardiac tamponade.
   c. varicose veins.
   d. mitral stenosis.
   e. anemia.

6. Which of the following is a blood pressure within normal limits?
   a. 90/60
   b. 120/40
   c. 110/80
   d. 130/105
   e. 160/90

7. Tachycardia means
   a. abnormally fast heartbeat.
   b. abnormally slow heartbeat.
   c. abnormally high blood pressure.
   d. abnormally low blood pressure.
   e. normal cardiac function.

8. The artery in the neck where the pulse is taken is the
   a. radial artery.
   b. temporal artery.
   c. carotid artery.
   d. facial artery.
   e. femoral artery.

9. What is the term for right-sided heart disease?
   a. anemia
   b. embolus
   c. coronary artery disease
   d. cor pulmonale
   e. phlebitis

10. What is the term for a clot that travels in blood vessels?
    a. platelets
    b. hemophilia
    c. thrombus
    d. phlebitis
    e. embolus

CRITICAL THINKING

Refer to the case study at the beginning of the chapter and use what you have learned to answer the following questions.

1. David, a CMA (AAMA), obtains Mr. Washington's vital signs after he has escorted him to the examination room. David notes Mr. Washington's vital signs as follows: Wt: 235 lbs, T: 97.6°F, P: 94 bpm, rapid and bounding, BP: 148/92. What can you ascertain from these findings?

2. Mr. Washington is an African American. How does this impact his health status relating to cardiovascular system disorders?

3. What might Dr. Miller suggest to help Mr. Washington take control of his blood pressure?

INTERNET ACTIVITY

Access one of the many "healthy heart" websites, and see what type of education they provide for their readers. What are some good features of the sites you accessed?

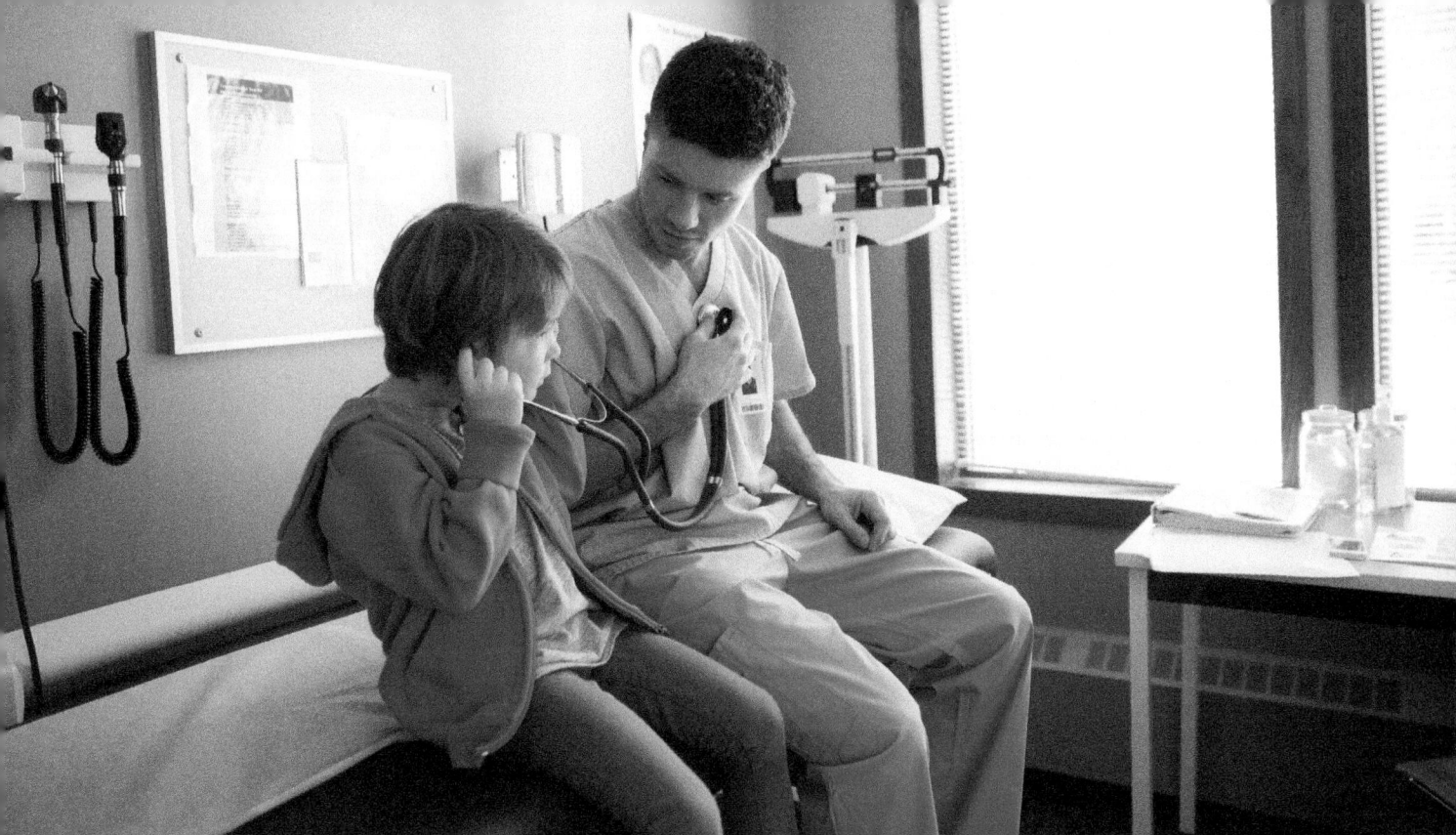

Learning Objectives

After completing this chapter, you should be able to:

27.1 Define and spell the terms for this chapter.

27.2 Identify the structures of the lymphatic system.

27.3 Explain the functions of the immune system.

27.4 Describe how the immune system changes during the life span of a child to an older adult.

27.5 Identify key components to the immune response.

27.6 Differentiate between types of immunity.

27.7 Describe common pathology associated with the immune system.

Rosa Gutierrez, age 49, is being seen today by Dr. Bahjat. She has been suffering from what appears to be a multitude of individual problems including low blood pressure, flulike symptoms, extreme fatigue, and what she describes as "hot and cold flashes." Following a thorough physical exam, which includes a complete blood cell count and an evaluation of her entire treatment history, Rosa is diagnosed with chronic fatigue syndrome. As part of her care, Dr. Bahjat has informed her that she must take an active role in her treatment. This includes getting plenty of rest and being monitored for any additional viral infections.

Terms to Learn

acquired active immunity	chemotherapy	lymphocytes
active immunity	chronic fatigue syndrome (CFS)	medulla
adenoids	complement	metastasis
afferent vessels	cortex	neutrophils
allergen	efferent vessels	oncogenes
allergy	germinal centers	passive immunity
anaphylaxis	immune response	phagocytes
antibodies	immune system	radiation therapy
antibody-mediated response	immunosuppressants	rheumatoid arthritis (RA)
antigen	infectious mononucleosis	systemic lupus erythematosus (SLE)
artificially acquired active immunity	innate immunity	T lymphocytes
asymptomatic	leukocytes	thymus gland
autoimmune diseases	lymph	tonsils
B lymphocytes	lymphatic system	vaccine
cell-mediated response	lymphedema	

The human body is an intricate specimen that is well guarded and protected by a defense system known as the **immune system**. The immune system consists of tissues, organs, and physiological processes that identify abnormal cells, foreign substances (such as bacteria or toxins), and foreign tissues (such as transplanted organs), and defend against those that might be harmful to the body.

FUNCTION AND STRUCTURES OF THE LYMPHATIC SYSTEM

The immune system has several essential elements. One of these is the **lymphatic system**, which is a subsystem of the circulatory system.

Functions of the Lymphatic System

The functions of the lymphatic system are expanded upon throughout the chapter. Although they are complex in nature, the lymphatic system's overall functions can be easily broken down into four distinct parts. It is responsible for:

- Maintaining fluid balance by draining excess fluid from tissues and returning this fluid to the bloodstream
- Acting as a waste removal system for wastes produced by cells
- Working with the digestive system to absorb and transport fatty acids from the digestive tract to the bloodstream
- Defending the body against infectious and other harmful agents

Overview of the Lymphatic System

The lymphatic system (Figure 27-1) is a network of vessels, nodes, and ducts that more or less parallel in function but are separate from the blood vessels of the circulatory system. This system helps maintain fluid balance by removing excess fluid from the spaces between body cells (interstitial spaces). The fluid, called **lymph**, comes from blood plasma that has leaked out from capillaries. Lymph fluid is straw-colored and similar in appearance to plasma. The lymphatic system collects the lymph and returns it to the bloodstream.

The lymphoid tissues of the lymphatic system function as part of the immune system, helping to defend the body against harmful substances.

Lymphatic Pathways

Lymphatic pathways are the structures throughout the lymphatic system that collect and circulate lymph. As noted earlier, lymph is body fluid that comes from plasma (the fluid portion of blood) that has leaked out from the capillaries of the circulatory system. Lymph is highly oxygenated and contains nutrients and small proteins.

Similar to the cardiovascular system, the lymphatic pathways are an intricate system of vessels. The smallest are lymphatic capillaries that join together to form larger lymphatic vessels. The lymphatic vessels transport the lymph to lymph nodes (which are discussed in the next section). From the lymph nodes, lymph is carried away by lymph vessels to lymphatic trunks. Larger than the vessels, the lymphatic trunks circulate the lymph to lymphatic collecting ducts. The two main lymphatic ducts found in the human body are the thoracic duct and the right lymphatic duct. From these two ducts, the lymph empties into the subclavian veins (the veins than run under the right and left clavicle bones). Here, the lymph enters the bloodstream by mixing with the blood that is flowing through the subclavian veins. Figure 27-2 illustrates the lymphatic pathways from smallest to largest structures.

Lymph Nodes

Lymph nodes come in many different sizes and shapes, but most are bean-shaped and about 1 inch long. Covered with a thick fibrous capsule, each node is subdivided into different compartments by inward-pointing trabeculae ("support beams" of tissue that help form a framework). All lymph

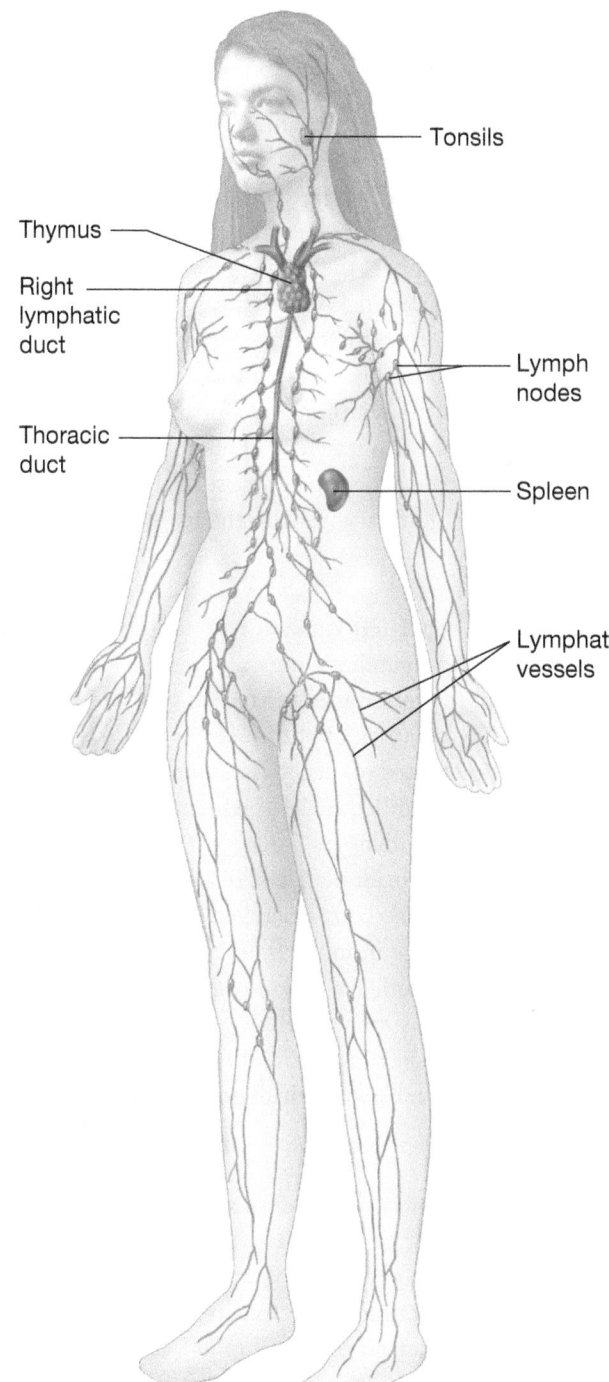

FIGURE 27-1 Components of the lymphatic system.

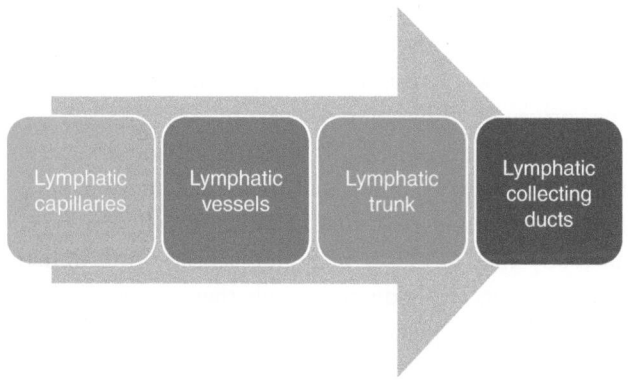

FIGURE 27-2 Structures of the lymphatic pathway from smallest to largest.

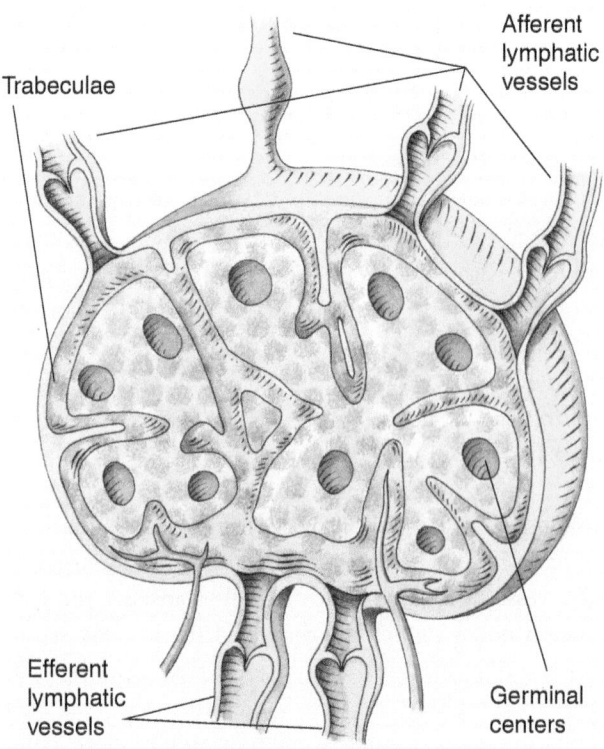

Trabeculae

Afferent
lymphatic
vessels

Efferent
lymphatic
vessels

Germinal
centers

FIGURE 27-3 A cross section of a lymph node.

nodes have multiple (sometimes four or five) **afferent vessels**—vessels that bring lymph into the node. Lymph is circulated out of the node through **efferent vessels**—vessels that carry it away from the node to the rest of the body (Figure 27-3). Each node has two basic parts, an outer **cortex** and an inner **medulla**.

The cortex of the lymph node is populated mainly with lymphocytes, cells that help to initiate the immune response against pathogens (disease-causing organisms). The **germinal centers** in the cortex are the primary locations where B lymphocytes reproduce quite prolifically.

B lymphocytes, also called B cells, are responsible for production of **antibodies**, specialized proteins that lock onto specific **antigens** (receptors on the cells of foreign substances that invade the body). Once an antibody binds with an antigen, it will work to impede the disease-causing process of the antigen or will help to destroy it.

Each unique type of B cell produces only one type of antibody. For example, one B cell will make an antibody that blocks a common-cold virus; another B cell will make an antibody that targets a pneumonia bacterium. When an antigen enters the body, the B cells that produce antibodies against that particular antigen rapidly undergo mitosis and divide, thereby producing large quantities of a specific antibody that will seek out and help destroy the antigen. The antibody may disable the antigen by interfering with its

chemical processes or it may cause the antigen's destruction by attracting scavenger cells that will envelop and actually eat (digest) the enemy antigen. This process is called an **antibody-mediated response** *or humoral immunity.*

In addition to the part of the lymph node cortex that contains B lymphocytes, the rest of the lymph node cortex contains **T lymphocytes**, also called T cells, which are cells that circulate through the lymph nodes, lymphatic ducts, and bloodstream to seek out any infection. T lymphocytes promote immunity through a **cell-mediated response**. This means that, instead of producing antibodies to attack the antigen as B lymphocytes do, T lymphocytes attack directly by binding themselves to the antigens on the cells of the foreign substance.

After their encounter with a pathogen and its antigens, some B and T lymphocytes become memory cells, whose function is to "remember" the pathogen, which enables them to identify and attack quickly if that same pathogen enters the body again. The working partnership of B and T lymphocytes is further discussed in later parts of this chapter.

The medulla of the lymph node is primarily made up of macrophages attached to reticular fibers that are part of the inner structure of the node. The purpose of the macrophages is to engulf and digest pathogens in the lymph.

Spleen

Located in the upper-left quadrant of the abdomen, the spleen is the largest lymphatic organ.

The tissue of the spleen is either of two types: red pulp or white pulp. The majority of the spleen is made up of red pulp, which is composed of special tissues made up of red and white cells and blood-filled cavities, which are also known as sinuses. The red pulp removes damaged red blood cells and also acts as a storage site for platelets. In fact, the spleen stores about 30 percent of the body's platelets. The white pulp of the spleen is where the immune function occurs. The white pulp is composed of both T and B lymphocytes. As the blood enters the spleen, it is monitored by both T and B cells for infectious antigens, creating antibodies, as needed, to fight potentially harmful substances that could cause illness.

Tonsils

The **tonsils** are located in the depressions of the mucous membranes of the throat and pharynx (Figure 27-4). There are three sets: the palatine, the pharyngeal (**adenoids**), and the lingual. The function of the tonsils is to filter bacteria and aid in the formation of white blood cells. When the tonsils are unable to properly filter bacteria and pathogens, they can become enlarged and infected. This often occurs with the streptococcal bacteria and accompanies strep throat.

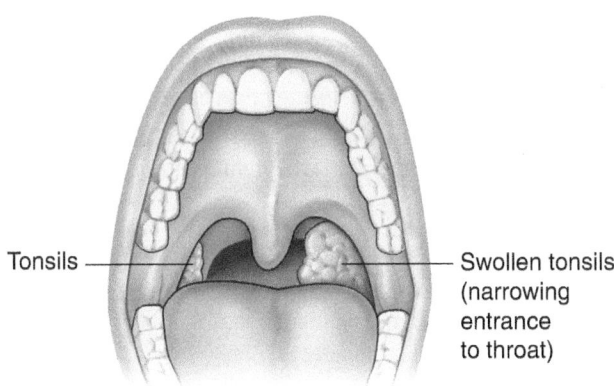

Tonsils ——— Swollen tonsils (narrowing entrance to throat)

FIGURE 27-4 Tonsils—normal and enlarged.

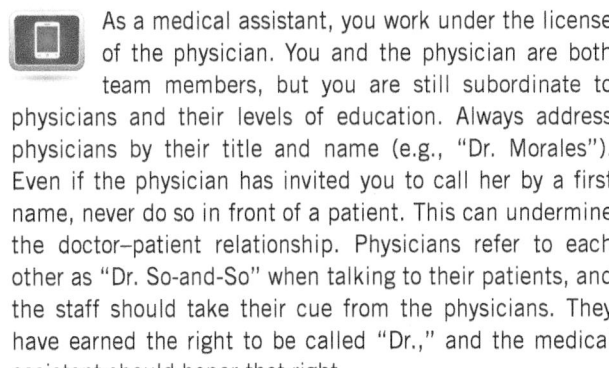
Bone Marrow and Thymus

Bone marrow and the thymus gland are considered to be the primary lymphatic organs because they are where the majority of the body's lymphocytes are produced. Bone marrow contains stem cells that develop into all the cells of the body, including blood cells and the cells of the immune system, in a process called hematopoiesis. The immune system cells produced in the bone marrow either become mature cells of the immune system (B cells and special lymphocytes known as natural killer cells) or they become precursors of cells that will mature in a part of the body other than the bone marrow.

The **thymus gland** is located behind the sternum, in the anterior mediastinum (front of the center section of the chest cavity). The thymus is an endocrine gland, a type of gland that secretes substances into the bloodstream that will be carried throughout the body. The thymus is divided into two distinct compartments, an outer cortex and an internal medulla. Immature lymphoid cells that were created in the bone marrow enter the cortex of the thymus, reproduce and mature, and then move to the medulla, from which they reenter the circulation of the body. The thymus manufactures infection-fighting T cells and helps distinguish normal T cells from those that attack the body's own tissues.

THE IMMUNE RESPONSE AND THE BODY'S DEFENSES

As previously noted, the immune system is the body's defense against infectious organisms and other pathogenic invaders. Through a series of steps called the **immune response**, the cells, tissues, and organs that make up the immune system work together to attack organisms and substances that invade body systems and cause illness and disease.

TABLE 27-1 | Types of Immunoglobulins

Type	Location	Function
IgA	Nose, mouth, digestive tract, ears, eyes, and vagina	Protects external body surfaces from external pathogens.
IgD	Tissue linings of the stomach and chest	Unknown.
IgE	Lungs, skin, and mucous membranes	Triggers allergic reactions and causes the body to react to foreign substances.
IgG	Found in all body fluids, can pass the placenta from mother to fetus, and is the most abundant immunoglobulin in the body	Fights bacterial and viral infections.
IgM	Found in blood and lymph fluid and is the largest immunoglobulin in size	Works in response to infection because it is the first antibody made in a response and initiates other immune system cells to destroy pathogens.

Leukocytes, or white blood cells (WBCs), seek out and destroy harmful organisms. The two types of WBCs are lymphocytes and phagocytes.

Lymphocytes, as already described, enable the body to recognize previous invading organisms/antigens and to produce antibodies in response to the invaders to protect the body.

Phagocytes attack and ingest (engulf, or eat) the invading organism. **Neutrophils** are the most common type of phagocyte. They primarily attack bacteria.

How Immunity Works: Antigens Versus Antibodies

When an antigen is detected, several types of proteins—antibodies/immunoglobulins—work together to recognize and respond to it.

The terms *antibody* and *immunoglobulin* (glycoproteins that function as antibodies) are often used interchangeably. They are found in blood, tissue fluids, and many secretions. Table 27-1 lists common types of immunoglobulins (Ig), their locations within the body, and their purposes.

Once antibodies have been produced by B lymphocytes, they remain in the body, ready to attack and neutralize if the same antigen is presented to the immune system again. Once antibodies have been created to attack a specific antigen (for instance the chicken pox virus), the person cannot get sick from the same antigen again. This is also the reason immunizations, or vaccinations, are given to protect against specific diseases. A vaccine contains either fragments of a disease organism or small amounts of a weakened disease organism. This small amount that is injected is not harmful to the individual receiving the vaccination. Rather, it is just the right amount to stimulate the immune system to develop antibodies that can subsequently recognize and attack the same organism if the body is exposed to it. Although an immunization may not always completely prevent the disease, it will significantly reduce its severity.

Antibodies are singular in their function. Although they are able to recognize an antigen, they are unable to destroy it. This is why they must work with T cells. The T cells destroy antigens that have been tagged by antibodies. T cells also directly destroy infected or abnormally changed cells. The major types of T cells are discussed in Table 27-2.

Antibodies can also activate a part of the immune system called the **complement**. Complement is a made up of a group of proteins that help to destroy infected cells or bacteria or viruses.

Immunosuppressants and Immunity

The immune system provides the body with a powerful and necessary defense against invading organisms. However, there are times when the immune system must be overridden. **Immunosuppressants** are medications that suppress the

TABLE 27-2 | The Types and Functions of the T Cells

T Cell Type	Function
Helper T Cell	These cells encourage the formation and activation of B cells and killer T cells and become activated when they are presented with antigens.
Killer T Cell	Also called cytotoxic T cells, these cells lock onto the antigens that were targeted by helper T cells and destroy them.
Memory T Cell	These cells are able to recall antigens that previously invaded the body. They are able to provide a quicker immune response after a reinvasion.

immune system to keep it from working as efficiently and effectively as it normally would in defending the body. Immunosuppressants are usually given after an organ transplant to prevent rejection of the organ. Rejection of an organ occurs because the body recognizes the transplant as foreign tissue and considers it harmful. Thus, the immune system is activated and the body tries to defend itself by rejecting the transplanted tissue. Though immunosuppressants can help prevent organ rejection, these medications render the patient very vulnerable to illness, because the natural immune process is impeded. Extreme stress can also suppress the immune system.

Types of Immunity

There are three types of immunity: innate, active, and passive.

Innate Immunity

Everyone is born with **innate immunity**, sometimes called natural immunity. This immunity is passed down from parents to children. Part of innate of immunity are the physical barriers to foreign invaders. Examples include the skin, tears, and mucous membranes. As discussed in the chapter titled "The Integumentary System," these work together to protect the body as the first line of defense against pathogens.

Innate immunity also renders many of the viruses and bacteria that affect other species incapable of harming human beings. For example, most viruses that are harmful to pets, such as dogs and cats, are not harmful to humans, and vice versa.

Active Immunity

Active immunity, unlike innate immunity, is not present at birth but rather develops after birth. Active immunity is permanent, meaning that it gives the individual lifelong protection against the disease.

Active immunity occurs in one of two ways: as acquired active immunity or as artificially acquired active immunity. Take a moment and consider chicken pox again. When people are exposed to the chicken pox virus (varicella virus) and develop the disease, they become immune to subsequent exposures to the disease. This is an example of **acquired active immunity**, which develops after exposure to a live pathogen.

Artificially acquired active immunity is induced by a **vaccine**, a substance that contains the antigen and stimulates a primary response against the antigen without causing symptoms of the disease. With the chicken pox example, a child who receives the varicella vaccination has artificially acquired active immunity against chicken pox.

Passive Immunity

Passive immunity is not a permanent form of immunity; it lasts only for a little while. Passive immunity may be either natural or artificial. *Passive natural immunity*, for example, occurs when antibodies are passed to an infant through breast milk. The breastfeeding infant will be temporarily immune to antigens to which the mother has been exposed. This temporary form of immunity helps protect the infant against infection during the its early years. *Passive artificial immunity*, provided by an immunization or vaccine, also is effective for a limited time and then must be renewed. For example, a patient who had previously been vaccinated against tetanus needs a current tetanus shot because of a tetanus infection. This specific type of vaccination is considered to be a booster. Booster vaccinations are needed to maintain immunity after a period of many years has passed since the initial immunization.

COMMON PATHOLOGY ASSOCIATED WITH THE IMMUNE SYSTEM

Immune system disorders occur when the immune response is inappropriate, excessive, or absent. A lack of one or more components of the immune system can result in a number of immunodeficiency disorders.

Sometimes the body begins to attack its own healthy cells and tissue, because it begins to identify these cells as harmful foreign pathogens. This is what occurs with an **autoimmune disease**. Autoimmune diseases can affect different systems of the body. Etiology, signs and symptoms, and treatments vary with each disease. Here are some examples:

- Rheumatoid arthritis is an autoimmune disease that attacks the skeletal system.
- Multiple sclerosis is an autoimmune disease that attacks the nervous system.
- Crohn's disease is an autoimmune disease of the digestive system.
- Glomerulonephritis is an autoimmune disease of the urinary system.

Immune system disorders may occur as the result of an infection or illness. Unfortunately, they are also an unintentional side effects of certain medications (Table 27-3).

Acquired Immunodeficiency Syndrome (AIDS)

Acquired immunodeficiency syndrome (AIDS) is a severe disease of the immune system. It is caused by the human immunodeficiency virus (HIV). AIDS develops as a final stage to HIV infection; therefore, not everyone with HIV has AIDS.

TABLE 27-3 | Disorders of or Associated with the Lymphatic System

Disorder	Description
AIDS-Related Complex (ARC)	A complex of symptoms that appears in the early stages of AIDS. This is a positive test for the virus but has only mild symptoms of weight loss, fatigue, skin rash, and anorexia.
Elephantiasis	Inflammation, obstruction, and destruction of the lymph vessels, which results in enlarged tissues caused by edema.
Epstein-Barr Virus	Virus believed to be the cause of infectious mononucleosis.
Hodgkin's Disease	Lymphatic system disease that can result in solid tumors in any lymphoid tissue.
Lymphadenitis	Inflammation of the lymph glands. Referred to as swollen glands.
Lymphangioma	A benign mass of lymphatic vessels.
Lymphoma	Malignant tumor of the lymph nodes and tissue.
Lymphosarcoma	Malignant disease of the lymphatic tissue.
Mononucleosis	Acute infectious disease with a large number of atypical lymphocytes. Caused by the Epstein-Barr virus. There may be abnormal liver function and spleen enlargement.
Multiple Sclerosis	Autoimmune disorder of the central nervous system in which the myelin sheath of nerves is attacked.
Non-Hodgkin's Lymphoma	Malignant, solid tumors of lymphoid tissue.
Peritonsillar Abscess	Infection of the tissues between the tonsils and the pharynx. Also called quinsy sore throat.
Sarcoidosis	Inflammatory disease of the lymphatic system in which lesions may appear in the liver, skin, lungs, lymph nodes, spleen, eyes, and small bones of the hands and feet.
Splenomegaly	Enlargement of the spleen.
Thymoma	Malignant tumor of the thymus gland.

HIV compromises the immune system, leaving it highly vulnerable to infections and diseases. This occurs as the lymphocytes, mainly T lymphocytes, become destroyed. As a person's lymphocyte count continues to decline, the progression of the disease quickens.

Although the etiology of AIDS and HIV is the actual virus, sources of contracting the virus vary. HIV can be contracted through unprotected sexual intercourse with an infected partner and through blood contact as well as through shared blood circulation between mother and fetus. It can also be transmitted by a breastfeeding mother to her child through breast milk.

Signs and Symptoms. People stricken with HIV can be **asymptomatic** (without any symptoms) for up to 10 years after contracting the virus. Unfortunately, they are able unknowingly to pass along the virus during this time. The progression to full-blown AIDS is diagnosed when a T lymphocyte count is below 200. This is less than one-half of the normal T-cell count of over 400. Fever, weight loss, diarrhea, swollen lymph glands, and ulcers of the skin, mouth, and genitals are common symptoms of AIDS. Meningitis, encephalitis, and yeast infections afflicting the mouth, esophagus, and vagina are also common. Kaposi's sarcoma, which is a skin cancer

marked by red lesions, is frequently seen in AIDS patients. The highly susceptible and deficient immune system makes AIDS patients targets for a multitude of diseases and disorders with varying signs and symptoms.

Treatment. There is currently no cure for HIV and AIDS. As with many autoimmune diseases, treatment is aimed at improving the quality and length of life through symptomatic treatment. Medical advances have included development of medicines that are able to suppress the replication of the virus. These medicines are called antiretroviral drugs. Often multiple forms of these drugs are used in conjunction to form a therapy called highly active antiretroviral therapy (HAART). This form of therapy varies from patient to patient, based on individual needs, and it is very effective if the patient is compliant with taking the medications. After a period of time, some patients become immune to the effects of HAART, and their drug therapy combination must be modified. Scientific research for advanced treatments of HIV continues to increase in hopes that a cure will be found.

Allergies

An **allergy** is an abnormal reaction, or hypersensitivity, to a substance that doesn't normally cause a reaction in most people. An **allergen** is any substance capable of causing an allergic reaction. Most allergic reactions are immune system responses to a "false alarm." When a harmless substance such as dust, mold, pollen, or cat dander is encountered by a person who is allergic to that substance, the immune system overreacts by producing antibodies to attack the allergen.

Allergens enter the body through inhalation, injection, swallowing, or contact with the skin. Almost any substance in the environment can cause an allergic reaction in a sensitive person. Allergic reactions may be localized, such as the red bump caused by a mosquito bite, or may be systemic, such as the red eyes, runny nose, and all-over itchiness of hay fever.

An increase in blood eosinophil levels may occur with allergies. An eosinophil is a granular white blood cell that captures invading microorganisms that cause antibody–antigen reactions and destroys them through phagocytosis (engulfing, or eating).

Anaphylaxis is an extreme, rapidly progressing, and often life-threatening allergic response. For some people this is the response to a bee sting, eating shellfish, or a severe asthma attack. It is sometimes seen in a physician's office after a vaccine or when a medication is first introduced into the patient. For this reason, it is prudent to observe patients for 15 to 30 minutes after any injection.

Signs and Symptoms. The allergic-response interaction of an antigen and antibody causes the release of histamine, which is the substance that produces signs and symptoms of allergies. The symptoms of allergies consist of a local or systemic inflammatory reaction characterized by redness, edema, and heat. Respiratory symptoms include wheezing, sneezing, coughing, and nasal congestion. Allergic conditions include eczema (skin inflammation), allergic rhinitis (irritation of the nasal passages), hay fever, bronchial asthma, urticaria (hives), and food allergies.

During anaphylaxis, the most severe form of allergic response, blood pressure drops, which causes multiple issues, including impeded function of bodily organs. Anaphylaxis also involves swelling in the neck and throat that can cause breathing difficulties. The swelling narrows the airway and can lead to hypoxia (decreased oxygen in the blood) and death. Therefore, it is vital to react quickly to any complaint of swelling or tickling of the throat.

Treatment. Allergies are rarely cured, but many medications, supplements, and other treatment options are available to help relieve symptoms. The treatment for allergies consists of medications, such as the antihistamine diphenhydramine (Benadryl), allergy testing to determine the exact allergen, and desensitization. Desensitizing injections involve administering minute amounts of the allergen into the patient's system over an extended period of time to build and develop a tolerance for the allergen in the patient. Desensitization is necessary if the allergic reactions significantly interfere with the patient's lifestyle or are life threatening. The best strategy for a person with an allergy is to avoid the offending allergen. Reactions to certain airborne allergens may be treated by the use of air filters and dehumidifiers.

Epinephrine is used in the event of anaphylaxis. Epinephrine is a form of adrenaline that surges through the body, causing an increase in blood pressure that counteracts the effects of the allergic reaction. Most patients who suffer from severe allergic reactions are prescribed an EpiPen (containing a single dose of epinephrine) or similar device, which the patient can use to self-administer an injection in the event of an exposure to the harmful allergen (Figure 27-5).

Cancer

Cancer is a collective term for multiple diseases that develop from abnormal cellular activity. Normal body cells grow and, through mitosis, divide. Normal cells automatically stop growing and dividing; eventually they die. Cancer cells are abnormal in form and function. They grow rapidly and keep on growing. Cancer cells do not work on behalf of the body. Instead, they make use of the body's resources at the expense of healthy cells through their uncontrolled growth and reproduction. Cancer cells do not die on their own.

Similar to the way normal cells with the same function come together to form tissues, cancer cells join together to form tumors or masses. Tumors that are cancerous are called malignant tumors. A growing tumor can destroy the normal cells around it and damage the body's healthy tissues. Sometimes cancer cells break away from the original tumor and travel via the bloodstream or lymphatic system to other areas of the body, where they keep growing and form new tumors. This process is called **metastasis**.

Whereas the causes of cancer are relatively unknown, certain risk factors may predispose a person to cancer. These

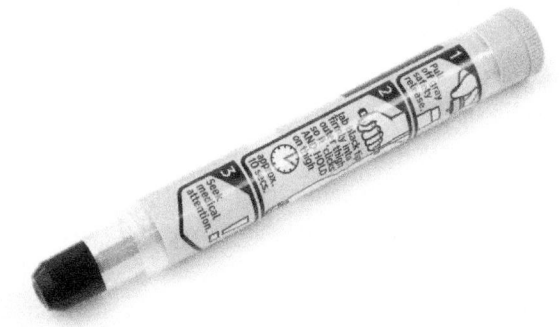

FIGURE 27-5 An EpiPen is used in cases of anaphylactic shock.

include a suppressed immune system; exposure to radiation, tobacco, toxins, or environmental stressors; and some viruses.

Cancer and the Immune System

The immune response is critical to eliminating or controlling cancer. An immune system that is operating at its highest level is alert to destructive cancerous cells and will attack them before the cells have the chance to grow and multiply uncontrollably. A suppressed or impaired immune response fails to respond in a timely manner and becomes overwhelmed by a massive number of corrupted cancer cells that have multiplied rapidly and undetected.

Carcinogens are cancer-causing agents that can transform oncogenes. Examples of carcinogens include tobacco smoke, various chemicals, radiation, and asbestos, to name a few. **Oncogenes** are genes that control cell growth and multiplication and that can produce cancer cells when they come into contact with carcinogens.

Signs and Symptoms. Cancer signs and symptoms are vast and depend on the site of the tumor. Some signs and symptoms common, but not limited, to cancer, include tissues that change color and shape (melanoma), lumps that form (breast cancer, uterine cancer, prostate cancer), shortness of breath (lung cancer), hoarse speech (throat cancer), and depressed organ function (thyroid). Generalized symptoms that often occur with most forms of cancer include extreme fatigue, decreased appetite, unintentional and often rapid weight loss, and fever and chills.

Treatment. Cancer may be treated with surgery, chemotherapy, radiation, or a combination of all three. The choice of treatment generally depends on the type of cancer and the stage of the tumor. Staging of a cancerous tumor indicates the extent of the disease based on the size of the tumor, surrounding lymph node involvement, and if (and how far) it has metastasized throughout the body. These three criteria—tumor, lymph node involvement, and metastasis—are known as the TNM system of staging, or evaluating the extent of a cancer. As a cancer progresses, the stage assigned to the cancer increases. The stages of cancer are as follows:

- **Stage 0**—Early detection indicated by localized cancer cells that are only a few layers deep. This is termed *carcinoma in situ.*

- **Stage I**—Deeper cell layers have been invaded by cancer cells, and some cells may have spread to surrounding tissues.

- **Stage II**—Surrounding tissue has been affected by cancer cells, but the cancer is contained at the primary site of cancer.

- **Stage III**—Cancer cells have spread beyond the primary site to nearby sites.

- **Stage IV**—Cancer cells have metastasized to other body organs, other than the primary site.

Cancer surgery is performed to remove cancerous tissue and perhaps some surrounding tissue. It is commonly used for breast cancer, prostate cancer, colon cancer, and some others. If the cancer has not metastasized, surgery may provide a cure.

In **chemotherapy**, anticancer drugs are used to treat the cancerous growth or tumor. The drugs may be intended to keep the cancer from spreading, slow its growth, kill cancer cells, or relieve symptoms. These medicines are sometimes taken in pill form but more often are given intravenously. Chemotherapy usually is given over a prescribed number of weeks or months. Often, a port-a-cath, a permanent intravenous (IV) catheter, is placed under the skin into one of the larger blood vessels of the upper chest. This method allows the administration of several courses of chemotherapy and other medicines through the catheter without the need to insert a new IV needle each time. The catheter remains under the skin until the cancer treatment is completed. The side effects of chemotherapy can be very intense and include severe nausea, vomiting, diarrhea, hair loss (all over the body), and weight loss.

Chemotherapy may cure some cancers.

Radiation therapy uses high-energy waves, such as X-rays, to damage and destroy cancer cells. This form of treatment causes tumors to shrink and, in some cases, disappear completely. Radiation therapy is one of the most common treatments for cancer. It is often prescribed in the earlier stages of cancer when the chance of cure is greatest.

The most modern form of cancer therapy involves creating mutated defense cells that are "programmed" to specifically target cancer cells. This empowers the body's own immune system to target only cancer cells, rather than also destroying healthy cells. This process is known as immunotherapy.

Professionalism

Patients receiving chemotherapy sometimes notice changes with their sense of smell. Smells can also trigger allergic reactions in patients who have heightened sensitivities. For these reasons as well as others, it is important that the medical assistant not wear strong-smelling perfume, scented body lotions, or aftershave lotion.

JUDGMENT CALL

Although most patients at the family practice office get better, a friendly and much-loved patient has been diagnosed with incurable cancer. How should the medical assistant respond to his questions about death?

Chronic Fatigue Syndrome

Chronic fatigue syndrome (CFS) is a continual sense of tiredness that is not helped by periods of rest or sleep. There is not a definitive etiology of CFS. Many physicians consider CFS to be a shared condition of many preexisting and possibly undiagnosed diseases. Some believe that a defective immune system is the culprit. Other possible conditions that are commonly found in those with CFS include low hormone levels, hypotension (low blood pressure), viral infections, yeast infections, food allergies, and exposure to hazardous chemicals.

Signs and Symptoms. Symptoms include intense and continual fatigue lasting for at least 6 months that is not relieved with rest, lack of energy, depression and anxiety, and sleep disorders. Flulike symptoms including muscle aches, low grade fevers, tender lymph nodes, and headaches may also be associated with CFS.

Treatment. Any treatment regimen for CFS generally begins with a thorough evaluation of the patient's prior treatment history. Medications to treat depression and anxiety may be prescribed. Both the quality and quantity of sleep are important factors that are addressed by a treating physician. A healthy diet, incorporating exercise into daily life, and proper knowledge and implementation of sleep management techniques are helpful. Rest, relaxation, and coping mechanisms for dealing with stress are also an important factor in the

treatment of a patient with CFS. Educating the patient with emphasis on becoming an active participant in the treatment regimen is extremely important in the treatment of CFS.

Infectious Mononucleosis

Infectious mononucleosis is caused by the Epstein-Barr virus (EBV). This specific infection is in the same virus family as herpes. Mononuclear white blood cells multiply in number. The layman's term for this infection, *mono*, is derived from the increase of these mononuclear WBCs. Especially frequent in teens and young adults, this virus is commonly spread through saliva and is often called the *kissing disease*.

Signs and Symptoms. Common signs and symptoms develop after the 4- to 8-week incubation period (the time between exposure and when first symptoms develop). Afflicted patients experience fever, fatigue, sore throat, night sweats, muscle weakness, headaches, and swollen lymph glands.

Treatment. There is no treatment for this virus, so focus is placed on alleviating symptoms. Patients are advised to get plenty of rest. For sore throats, gargling with saltwater or using throat lozenges is helpful. Analgesics (pain relievers) and antipyretics (fever reducers) are also prescribed. Corticosteroids may be prescribed for severe swelling of the throat and/or tonsils. If neglected, mono can lead to liver inflammation (hepatitis) and enlargement of the spleen. Recovery from mono generally takes several weeks. However, for some individuals, it may be several months before they regain their normal energy levels.

Lymphedema

Lymphedema is a condition that derives from a damaged or dysfunctional lymphatic system that results in an accumulation of lymphatic fluid, which causes swelling (Figure 27-6). There are two types of lymphedema; the type is determined

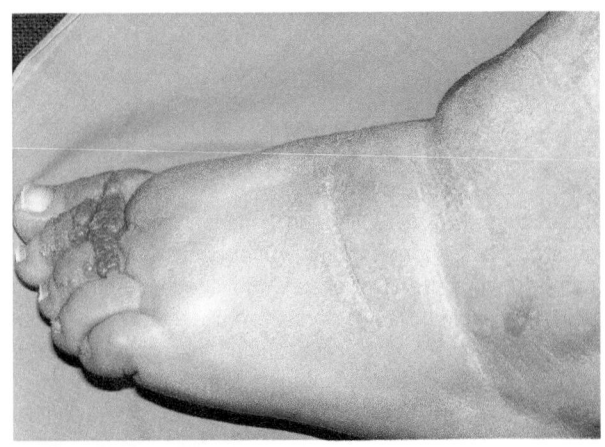

FIGURE 27-6 Chronic lymphedema.

by the specific etiology. The first, primary lymphedema, can be hereditary. It is marked by a developmental disorder of the lymphatic vessels that carry lymph. A fetus's exposure to an infection or injury may cause primary lymphedema; however, more likely causes of this congenital disorder center around difficulties that occur during childbirth.

The other form of lymphedema is termed secondary lymphedema, and its etiology is an interruption of lymphatic flow caused by an obstruction or damage to the lymphatic system.

Causes of secondary lymphedema are multiple as they can stem from anything that could damage or destroy lymphatics, such as surgery, infections, burns, and serious wounds or injuries. Cancer treatments, including surgical removal of lymph nodes and radiation, may also be implicated in this secondary form.

Signs and Symptoms. Swelling at the lymph nodes is the primary sign. Generally, swelling is limited to one arm or one leg as the lymphatic fluid pools in the affected extremity.

Treatment. There are multiple options for increasing the flow of lymphatic fluid; however, curing lymphedema is not possible. Exercises may be encouraged to help with movement and directing the accumulated fluid away from the extremity. Compression stockings and bandages are also used to put pressure on the extremity with the idea of moving the lymph fluid toward the trunk of the body. A specialized massage, called manual lymph drainage, is available for some patients. The massage therapist uses special strokes and movements to circulate the lymph fluid toward healthier lymph nodes. Employing several of these treatments is known as complete decongestive therapy (CDT). However, a patient's overall health must be taken into consideration when employing some of these methods. Those with a history of blood clots, diabetes, and other diseases need specialized consideration for the treatment of

lymphedema. Additionally, blood pressure should not be taken in an extremity with lymphedema.

Rheumatoid Arthritis

Rheumatoid arthritis (RA) is a chronic autoimmune disease. It occurs when the body's immune defenses attack tissue in the joints, leading to pain and degeneration of the articular (joint) cartilage. The disease and its treatment also increase mortality, and patients often have a shorter life expectancy than their healthy peers.

RA causes a great deal of suffering and reduced quality of life, and can pose a major financial burden. Individuals with a family history of RA are four times more likely to develop the disease than others.

Signs and Symptoms. Symptoms include pain, warmth, and stiffness in the joints of the wrists, fingers, knees, feet, and ankles. Pain and stiffness gradually increase as the disease progresses. Morning joint stiffness is a common sign. Over time, the affected joints will have decreased range of motion and may become deformed. Numbness, tingling, and burning sensations may also be felt near the affected joint. Fatigue, poor sleep patterns, and anemia are also common with RA.

Treatment. The treatment of RA is based on medication regimens and educating the patient on how to facilitate daily activities. Drugs are used to treat and reduce the symptoms and to help the patient to function at a more productive level and have a better quality of life. However, because drugs are only effective symptomatically, they do not actually treat or cure the disease. Antiinflammatory medications, rest, and exercises to promote joint strengthening and mobility are used to treat RA. On initial diagnosis, disease-modifying antirheumatic drugs (DMARDs) are often prescribed to patients. Because these drugs have severe side effects, routine blood work to monitor the patient is required for patients taking DMARDs.

Systemic Lupus Erythematosus

Systemic lupus erythematosus (SLE) is another autoimmune disorder. Patients suffering from SLE produce abnormal antibodies in their blood that target tissues within their own body rather than foreign infectious agents. SLE is called a systemic disorder because its effects may appear in many parts of the body—in other words, it is system wide. In addition to the signs and symptoms listed, Figure 27-7 depicts systemic effects, signs, and symptoms of this disease.

Women constitute 90 percent of patients with SLE and are generally diagnosed before menopause. There is a genetic component as well; the risk of developing SLE rises if a close

Systemic lupus erythematosus

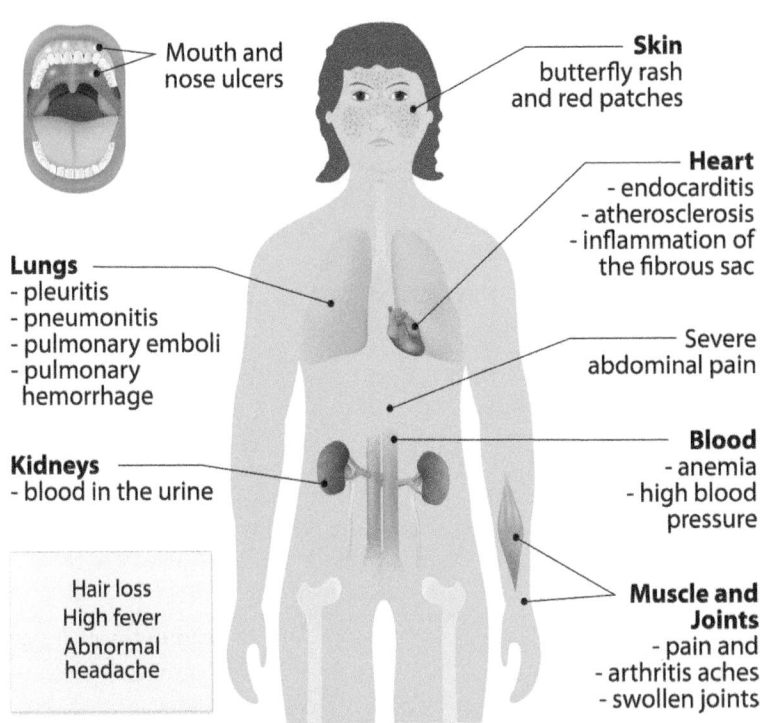

Mouth and nose ulcers

Skin
butterfly rash and red patches

Heart
- endocarditis
- atherosclerosis
- inflammation of the fibrous sac

Lungs
- pleuritis
- pneumonitis
- pulmonary emboli
- pulmonary hemorrhage

Severe abdominal pain

Kidneys
- blood in the urine

Blood
- anemia
- high blood pressure

Hair loss
High fever
Abnormal headache

Muscle and Joints
- pain and aches
- arthritis
- swollen joints

FIGURE 27-7 Systemic effects of SLE.

family member has it. As the exact cause is unknown with this autoimmune disorder, the disease may develop after it has been triggered by a certain incident. Incidents that have been linked to triggering lupus include surgery, illness resulting from infection, pregnancy, and even exposure to sunlight.

Signs and Symptoms. SLE can produce many different signs and symptoms and imitate many other diseases. This can make it difficult to initially diagnose. Many patients with SLE have pain and swelling in the joints. They may also suffer from general fatigue, fever, chills, weight changes (both loss and gain), and headache. Hair loss, mouth sores, and sensitivity to light are also attributed to this disease. One of the most common signs seen in one half of those diagnosed with SLE is the "butterfly" rash. This is a rash that covers the bridge of the nose and the cheeks and it worsens in sunlight.

Round (discoid) lesions that are raised and scaly affect about 20 percent of patients with SLE. This condition is known as discoid lupus erythematosus. If left untreated, these scaly lesions expand and can cause severe scarring.

A condition that may be present with lupus is vasculitis, or inflamed blood vessels, characterized by red marks in any area of the body. Sometimes deep red lumps appear, especially on the leg, where they may develop into ulcers. In some people, the tips of the fingers and toes may develop reddish-purple lesions.

Treatment. Unfortunately, cures are not available for most autoimmune diseases, and SLE is no exception. Treatment is usually aimed at reducing the immune response and controlling symptoms by using drugs such as corticosteroids. SLE is a chronic, lifelong condition with periods of remission and relapse. Antiinflammatory drugs may also be prescribed to alleviate other symptoms.

SUMMARY

The immune system is the body's defense against infectious organisms and other pathogenic invaders. The lymphatic system and other organs, including the spleen, thymus, tonsils, and bone marrow, function together in the immune system. There are three types of immunity: innate, active, and passive. When the immune system is functioning properly, it attacks antigens by forming antibodies. Immune system disorders occur when the immune response is compromised, exaggerated, or absent.

Disorders of the immune system may be inherited, acquired through infection or other illness, or produced as an inadvertent side effect of certain drug treatments. An allergy is an overreaction of the immune system to an allergen. Many cancers appear to have a genetic component, but cancer production is usually a combination of predisposing genetic makeup and environmental carcinogenic factors that trigger the inappropriate immune response. Treatment for cancer includes surgery, radiation, chemotherapy, and measures that boost the correct immune response.

Viral infections can cause infectious mononucleosis. Chronic fatigue syndrome has many possible causes. A dysfunctional immune system may lead to lymphedema. When the immune system inappropriately attacks joints, rheumatoid arthritis results. Systemic lupus erythematosus is an autoimmune disease that causes systemic problems.

27 CHAPTER REVIEW

COMPETENCY REVIEW

1. Define and spell the terms for this chapter.
2. What is the function of leukocytes?
3. Name the lymphatic pathways from smallest to largest.
4. What is the main function of the immune system?
5. Name the structures of the lymphatic system.
6. What is the difference between innate immunity and active immunity?
7. Explain what happens when a person has an allergic reaction.
8. Explain what a carcinogen is, and then provide four examples of carcinogens.
9. Explain how cancerous tumors are staged or evaluated to determine the extent of cancer.
10. List five symptoms of systemic lupus erythematosus.

PREPARING FOR THE CERTIFICATION EXAM

1. Which of the following are foreign substances that invade the body?
   a. neutrophils
   b. lymphocytes
   c. phagocytes
   d. antigens
   e. antibodies

2. An autoimmune disorder in which the myelin sheath of nerves is attacked is
   a. sarcoidosis.
   b. thymoma.
   c. multiple sclerosis.
   d. elephantiasis.
   e. mononucleosis.

3. Immunity conferred to a breast-feeding infant by his mother is
   a. passive immunity.
   b. active immunity.
   c. innate immunity.
   d. vaccination immunity.
   e. immunosuppression.

4. The virus that is known to be the cause of infectious mononucleosis is
   a. allergies.
   b. Epstein-Barr virus.
   c. Hodgkin's disease.
   d. acquired immunodeficiency syndrome.
   e. elephantiasis.

5. Which immune system structure is found in the pharynx?
   a. thymus
   b. bone marrow
   c. spleen
   d. liver
   e. tonsil

6. Which of the following is the usual treatment for systemic lupus erythematosus?
   a. chemotherapy
   b. radiation
   c. surgery
   d. corticosteroidal medications
   e. diet and exercise changes

7. "Surrounding tissue has been affected by cancer cells, but the cancer is contained at the primary site of cancer." This statement defines which stage of cancer?
   a. II
   b. III
   c. IV
   d. V
   e. I

8. All the following are believed to be risk factors that may predispose a patient to cancer *except*
   a. immunosuppression.
   b. bacteria.
   c. radiation.
   d. tobacco.
   e. viruses.

9. Which immunoglobulin is known to fight bacterial and viral infections?
   a. IgA
   b. IgD
   c. IgM
   d. IgE
   e. IgG

10. Which disorder affects the joints, has familial risk factors, and tends to result in a shorter life expectancy?
    a. lymphedema
    b. mononucleosis
    c. rheumatoid arthritis
    d. chronic fatigue syndrome
    e. allergies

CRITICAL THINKING

Refer to the case study at the beginning of the chapter and use what you have learned to answer the following questions.

1. Why was it important to note that Ms. Gutierrez was having many flulike symptoms?
2. For Ms. Gutierrez to be diagnosed with CFS, the physician would review her entire medical history including the duration of current signs and symptoms. How long must symptoms be present for a CFS diagnosis to be made?
3. Why did the physician tell Ms. Gutierrez to get plenty of rest and also decide to monitor her for other viral infections?

INTERNET ACTIVITY

Conduct an Internet search for chronic fatigue syndrome services in your hometown. What resources are available in your area?

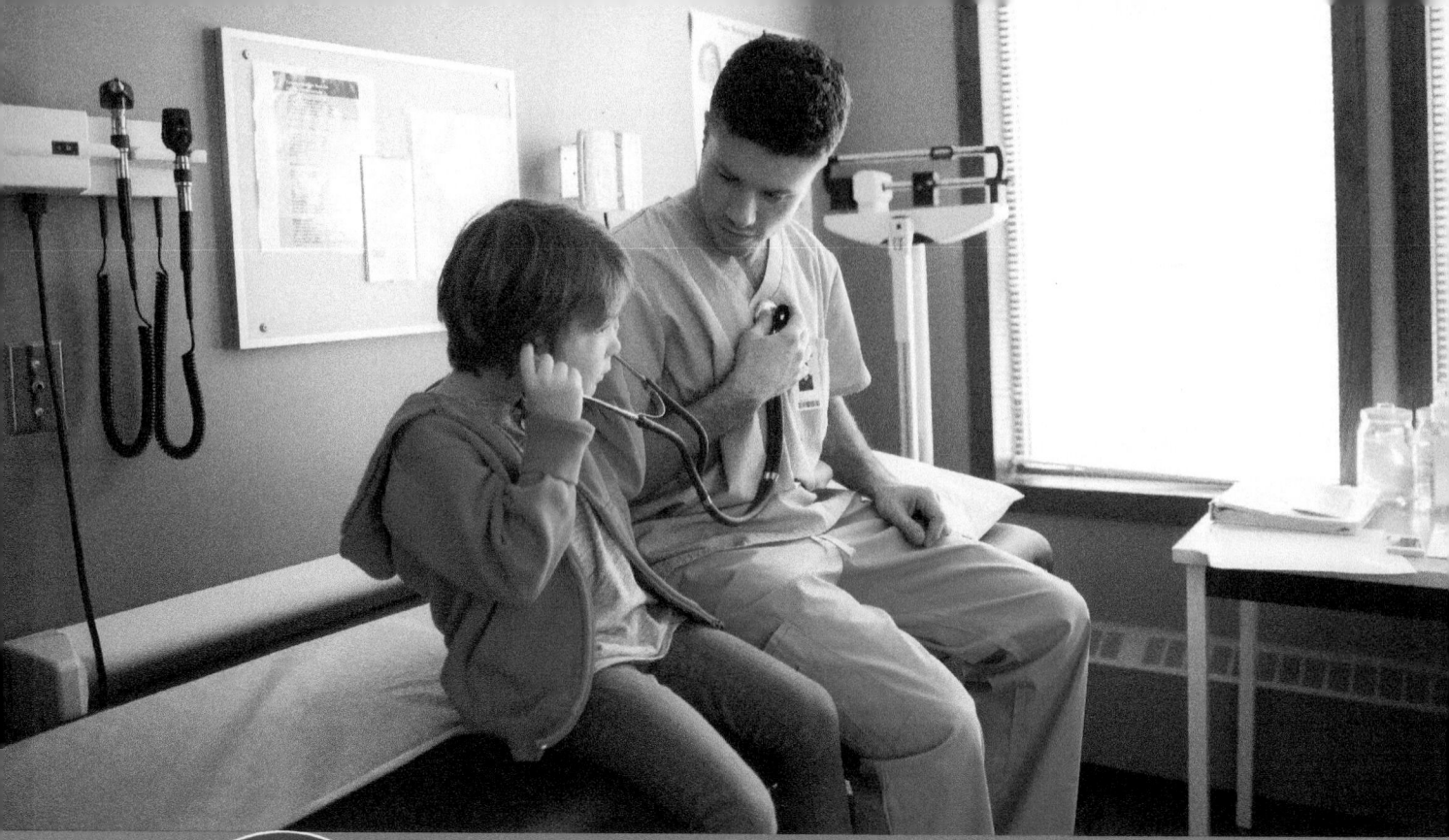

CHAPTER 28

The Respiratory System

Learning Objectives

After completing this chapter, you should be able to:

28.1   Define and spell the terms for this chapter.

28.2   Explain the overall function of the respiratory system.

28.3   List the structures of the respiratory system.

28.4   Describe how the respiratory system changes during the life span of a child to an older adult.

28.5   Detail how the mechanism of breathing occurs.

28.6   Identify common pathology associated with the respiratory system.

Collin McConnley is a 57-year-old businessman who travels 80 percent of his workweek. It is a hot summer day, and he has an appointment with Dr. Miller because he believes that he has the flu. His symptoms include severe headache, high fever, fatigue, and diarrhea.

Terms to Learn

alveoli	epiglottis	pertussis
apnea	expiration	pharynx
arterial blood gases (ABGs)	hay fever	pleura
asphyxia	hemoptysis	pleurisy
asthma	hilum	pneumonia
bronchi	hypoxia	pulmonary edema
bronchitis	influenza	pulmonary embolism (PE)
bronchodilators	inspiration	septum
chronic obstructive pulmonary disease (COPD)	larynx	severe acute respiratory syndrome (SARS)
cilia	Legionnaires' disease	sinusitis
common cold	lung cancer	surfactant
cyanosis	lungs	thorax
diaphragm	nares	trachea
dyspnea	orthopnea	tuberculosis (TB)
emphysema	paranasal sinuses	

The respiratory system is responsible for delivering oxygen to the cells of the body. The cells need oxygen to perform the cellular metabolism that sustains life. The respiratory system plays an equally important role by ridding the body of excess carbon dioxide. Carbon dioxide is a compound of carbon and oxygen that is a waste product of cellular metabolism. Both of these important functions—bringing oxygen to the cells and taking away carbon dioxide waste—occur as a result of breathing, or respiration.

OVERVIEW OF THE RESPIRATORY SYSTEM

When we breathe, an exchange of gases occurs between the **alveoli** (tiny air sacs) of the lungs and the capillaries that surround them. Oxygen from the air that we inhale passes from the alveoli into blood in the capillaries, which carry the oxygen to the body's cells. At the same time, we exhale carbon

dioxide that has been picked up as a waste product of the cells and that passed from the capillaries into the alveoli.

The mouth, nose, trachea, bronchi, bronchioles, and lungs constitute the respiratory tract, the pathway for respiration. Oxygen enters the respiratory system by this path (inhalation), and carbon dioxide exits the system by the same path (exhalation). The actions of inhalation and exhalation are achieved by the alternating contraction and relaxation of the respiratory muscles: the diaphragm, the muscles attached to the ribs (intercostal muscles), and sometimes the muscles of the neck.

STRUCTURES OF THE RESPIRATORY SYSTEM

The respiratory system is made up of structures and organs leading from the nasal passages to the lungs (Figure 28-1). There are two distinct divisions of the respiratory system; the upper respiratory tract and the lower respiratory tract.

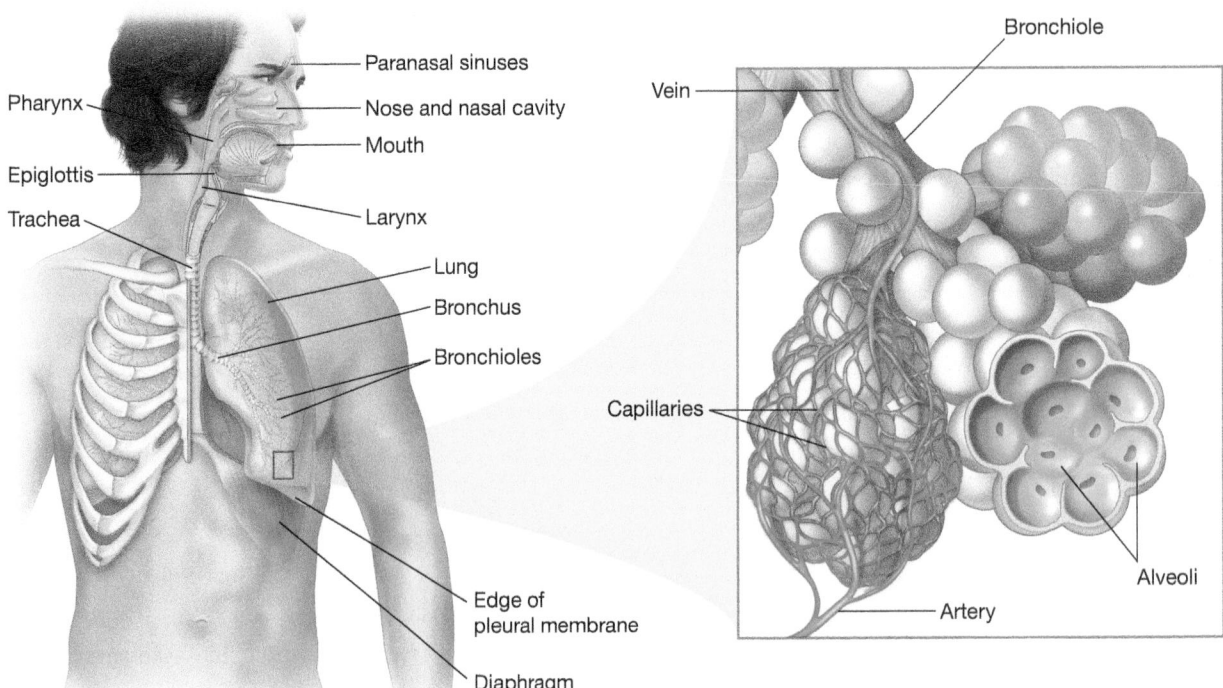

FIGURE 28-1 Structures of the respiratory system.

The nose, mouth, throat (or pharynx), and paranasal sinuses are components of the upper respiratory tract. The lower respiratory tract begins with the larynx, which is commonly known as the voice box. From the larynx, the tract extends to the trachea, and here the tract first splits into the bronchi. The split resembles two branches, similar to that of a tree. The tract farther extends and branches off from the bronchi into much smaller structures called bronchioles. The structural components of the lower respiratory tract end with the lungs, which are described as saclike and spongy.

Nose and Mouth

Air enters the body through the nose or mouth.

The nose, which is the organ of smell, also performs several other functions:

- Serves as a passageway for air
- Warms and moistens inhaled air
- Traps dust, pollen, and other foreign matter with hair-like projections (**cilia**)
- Assists in phonation (production of vocal sounds)

The nose has both external and internal characteristics. The term *nose* itself generally refers to the visible external portion. It is made up of bone and cartilage and is lined with a mucous membrane. The nasal openings that bring air into the nose are known as the **nares**, or nostrils.

Internally, there are two main nasal fossae (cavities). They are separated by a wall of cartilage known as the **septum**. There are three air passageways found on either side of the septum. These passageways are called turbinates, but may also be referred to as conchae:

- Inferior conchae
- Middle conchae
- Superior conchae

These passageways connect (via the eustachian tube) to the middle ear, to the paranasal sinuses, and to the nasolacrimal ducts (tear ducts). The conchae form a "maze" in which air moves around, allowing for warming of the air and removal of foreign particles by the mucus secreted by the mucous membranes (mucosae). The nasal mucosae produce about a quart of mucus per day, which moistens the air moving through the nose and traps pollen, dust, and other foreign matter. The nose is separated from the mouth by the palatine bones of the skull.

The mouth serves just two of the functions of respiration and voice: serving as a passageway for air and assisting in phonation. The mouth does not warm and moisten inhaled air or trap foreign matter as the nose dose.

Paranasal Sinuses

The nose drains the four pairs of **paranasal sinuses**, air cavities in the cranial bones near the nose, which are often

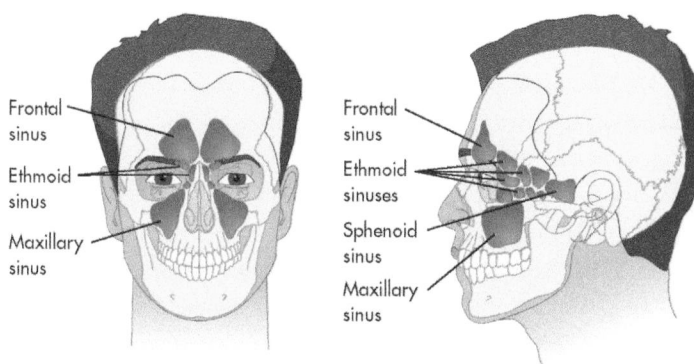

FIGURE 28-2 The four pairs of paranasal sinuses.

simply referred to as "the sinuses" (Figure 28-2). The four pairs of paranasal sinus cavities are:

- Maxillary sinuses over the medial portion on the cheekbones
- Frontal sinuses over the eyebrows
- Ethmoid sinuses in the area between and behind the eyes
- Sphenoid sinuses behind the ethmoid sinuses

The sinuses have important functions. Because they are pockets of air within the bone, they decrease the weight of the skull. Sinuses also aid in phonation and provide protection and insulation.

Pharynx

The **pharynx** is a tube about 5 inches long formed from muscle and membrane that lies behind and connects the nose, the mouth, and the larynx. There are three sections of the pharynx that are all connected with each other:

- **Nasopharynx**—Connects with the nose
- **Oropharynx**—Connects with the mouth
- **Laryngopharynx**—Located behind the larynx

The major function of the pharynx is to serve as a passageway for food to the esophagus and air to the larynx and trachea. The pharynx also plays a role in speech, as do the mouth and nose, by helping to form specific phonetic sounds from the initial sounds produced in the larynx.

Three pairs of tonsils reside in the pharynx:

- **Pharyngeal tonsils (adenoids)**—Located behind the nose and often blamed for snoring, especially in children
- **Palatine tonsils**—Often referred to as simply "the tonsils," located on either side of the throat on the anterior portion of the oropharynx
- **Lingual tonsils**—Located at the base of the tongue

The tonsils are part of the immune system and help in infection control, as was discussed in the chapter titled "The Immune System."

Larynx

The **larynx** (Figure 28-3) is also known as the voice box. It is a muscular, cartilaginous structure lined with mucous membrane and connected to the inferior (lower) end of the pharynx. The larynx has several cartilaginous structures, three of which help protect it from trauma:

- The thyroid cartilage, or Adam's apple, is the largest of the cartilage structures and helps protect the walls of the larynx and the vocal cords. Both men and women have this structure, although the Adam's apple is more prominent in men.
- The epiglottic cartilage, or **epiglottis**, covers the larynx during swallowing so that food is directed down the esophagus to the stomach rather than through the larynx to the trachea and into the lungs.
- The ring-shaped cricoid cartilage, the lowest cartilage in the larynx, wraps around it to protect it from pressure.

The interior of the larynx contains the false and true vocal folds and the glottis, which is the opening between the true vocal folds through which air passes. (Sometimes the glottis is defined as consisting of the space between the folds and the folds themselves.) The larynx functions in the production of vocal sounds. When the vocal cords are long and relaxed, low sounds are produced. Short, tense vocal cords produce higher-pitched notes. (As mentioned earlier, the nose, mouth, pharynx, and bony sinuses impact other aspects of sound production.)

Trachea

The **trachea**, or windpipe (Figure 28-3), is a cartilaginous tube about 1 inch wide and 4.5 inches long that extends from the larynx in the throat to the bronchi in the chest cavity. The cartilage rings in the trachea are C-shaped, with openings at the back bridged by elastic connective tissue. This structure allows the trachea to be flexible, to contract when you cough, and to be pushed inward when a bolus of food passes through the esophagus, which lies behind the trachea. The interior of the trachea is lined with mucous membrane and cilia (hairlike structures) that trap foreign matter. The most important function of the trachea is to serve as an open passageway through which air reaches the lungs.

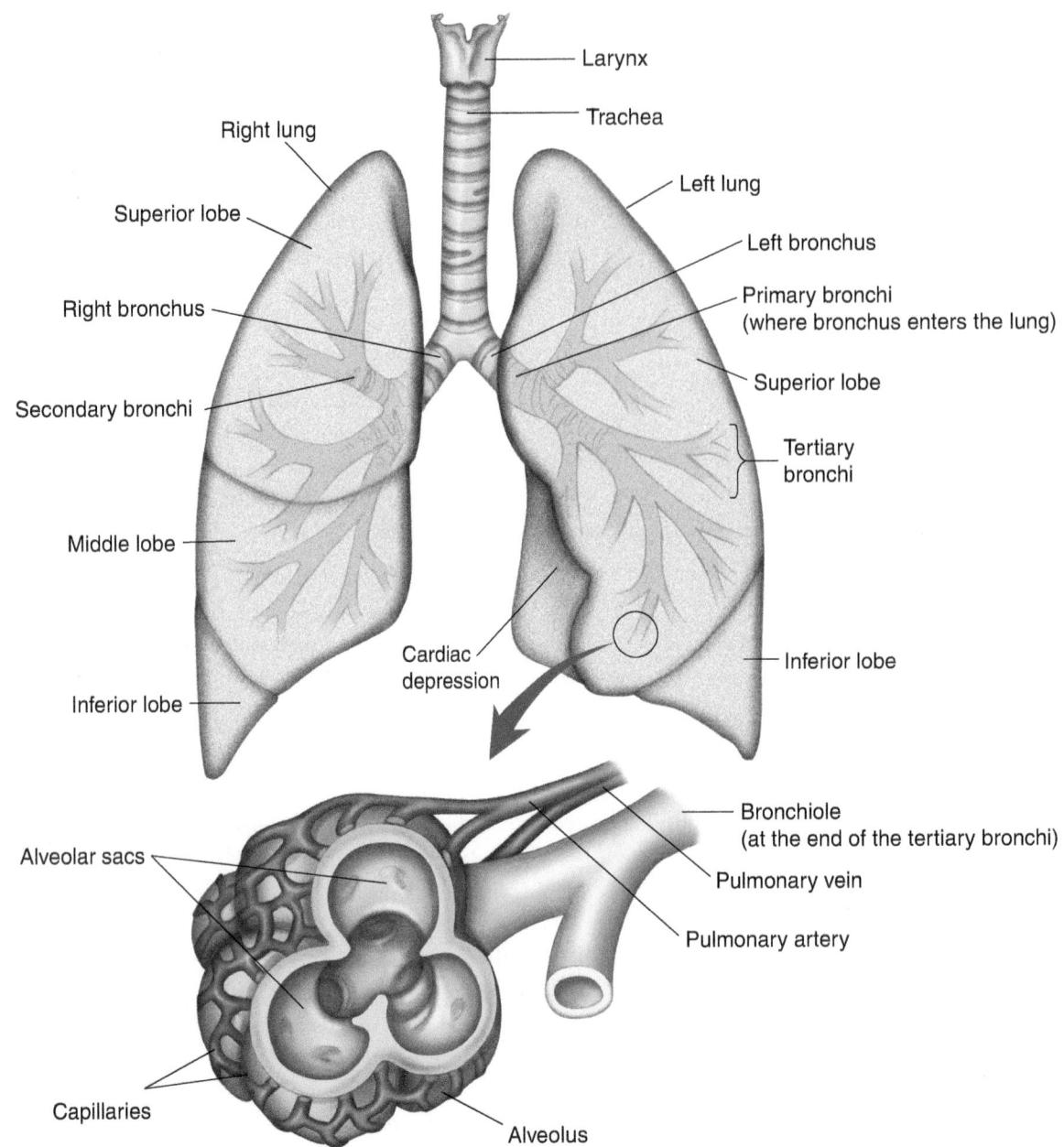

FIGURE 28-3 The larynx, trachea, bronchi, and lungs with an expanded view showing the structures of the alveolus and the pulmonary blood vessels.

Bronchi

The **bronchi** (Figure 28-3) are the two main branches (right bronchus and left bronchus) from the trachea that extend into the lungs. These structures are the passageways for air between the trachea and the lungs. The right bronchus is the wider, shorter branch. The left bronchus is longer but smaller in diameter. After entering the lungs, the bronchi subdivide into the bronchial tree, which continues to branch into smaller and smaller branches.

The right and left bronchi are also called the primary bronchi. The sections that branch off these primary bronchi enter specific lobes of the lungs and are referred to as secondary bronchi. Bronchi that branch from the secondary bronchi are called tertiary bronchi. At the ends of the tertiary bronchi, the smallest components of the bronchial tree—the bronchioles—are formed.

Bronchioles and Alveoli

Bronchioles are composed of a thin layer of epithelium and smooth muscle. These tiny structures are only 1 millimeter (mm) or less in diameter. Eventually, the bronchioles terminate at the alveoli, the small air sacs in the lungs that

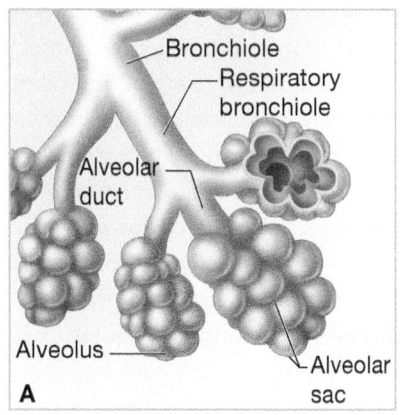
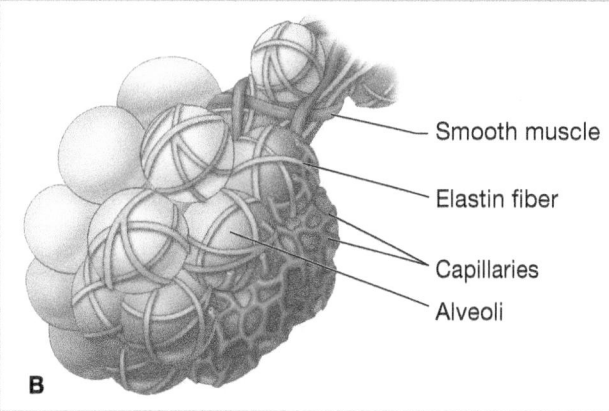

FIGURE 28-4 **(A)** Alveolar sac; **(B)** alveoli with capillaries.

support a network of capillaries where (as described earlier) the exchange of oxygen and carbon dioxide takes place between the air in the alveoli and the blood in the adjoining capillaries (Figure 28-4). The average pair of adult lungs contain about 600 million alveoli.

In healthy individuals, the alveoli resemble small balloons that inflate and deflate as air moves in and out. The cells of the alveoli produce a fatty substance known as **surfactant**. Surfactant reduces the surface tension of the fluid in the wet surfaces of the air-filled sacs, which helps keep them open. Without surfactant, the alveoli would collapse after each breath, making it harder to reinflate with the next breath, thereby increasing the work of breathing, leading to exhaustion and, eventually, an inability to continue breathing.

Lungs

The **lungs** are large, somewhat cone-shaped organs within the chest (review Figure 28-3). At birth the lungs are pinkish in color, but as adulthood approaches they turn a dark, slate-gray. The lungs are porous and spongy in texture and highly elastic. The right lung is made up of three lobes: the superior, middle, and inferior lobes. The left lung has only two—a superior lobe and an inferior lobe—allowing room for the heart, which takes up chest space on the left. Each lung is between 10 and 12 inches in length. The two lungs are separated by the mediastinum, a space behind the breastbone that contains the heart, trachea, esophagus, and blood vessels.

The **hilum** is a wedge-shaped area on the central portion of each lung where the primary bronchus, arteries, veins, and nerves enter and exit the lung. The rounded point at the top of the lung is called the apex, and the wide lowest portion of the lung that rests on the diaphragm is called the base.

The **pleura** (plural *pleurae*) is one of a pair of thin sheets of epithelium that line the inside of the thorax and the outside of the lungs. The pleural space is a tiny area that separates the parietal pleura (covering the inner thoracic cavity and diaphragm) from the visceral pleura (covering the outer surface of the lungs). The pleural space normally contains a small amount of lubricating fluid, which allows the lungs to slide easily over the inner chest as they expand and contract during breathing.

The pleurae are sometimes referred to as pleural membranes.

MECHANISM OF BREATHING

Ventilation is the term for the movement of air to and from the lungs. The two processes of ventilation are inhalation and exhalation (also called inspiration and expiration), which are brought about by the nervous system and the respiratory muscles. The respiratory centers of the brain are located in the medulla oblongata and the pons. The major respiratory muscles are the diaphragm and the internal and external intercostal muscles.

The **diaphragm** is the dome-shaped muscle below the lungs that separates the thoracic cavity from the abdominal cavity. The diaphragm can contract and relax to enlarge and reduce the size of the thoracic cavity. The intercostal muscles are located between the ribs. The external intercostal muscles pull the ribs upward and outward, and the internal intercostal muscles pull the ribs downward and inward. Figure 28-5 illustrates the mechanism of breathing.

Difficulty breathing is known as **dyspnea**. This is a common sign and symptom of many respiratory diseases and disorders. The absence of breathing for more than 19 seconds is termed **apnea**. If a patient has trouble breathing unless a certain position is maintained (such as with head elevated), it is termed **orthopnea**.

Inhalation

Inhalation, or **inspiration**, is an active process that involves a precise sequence of events. First, the nervous system sends

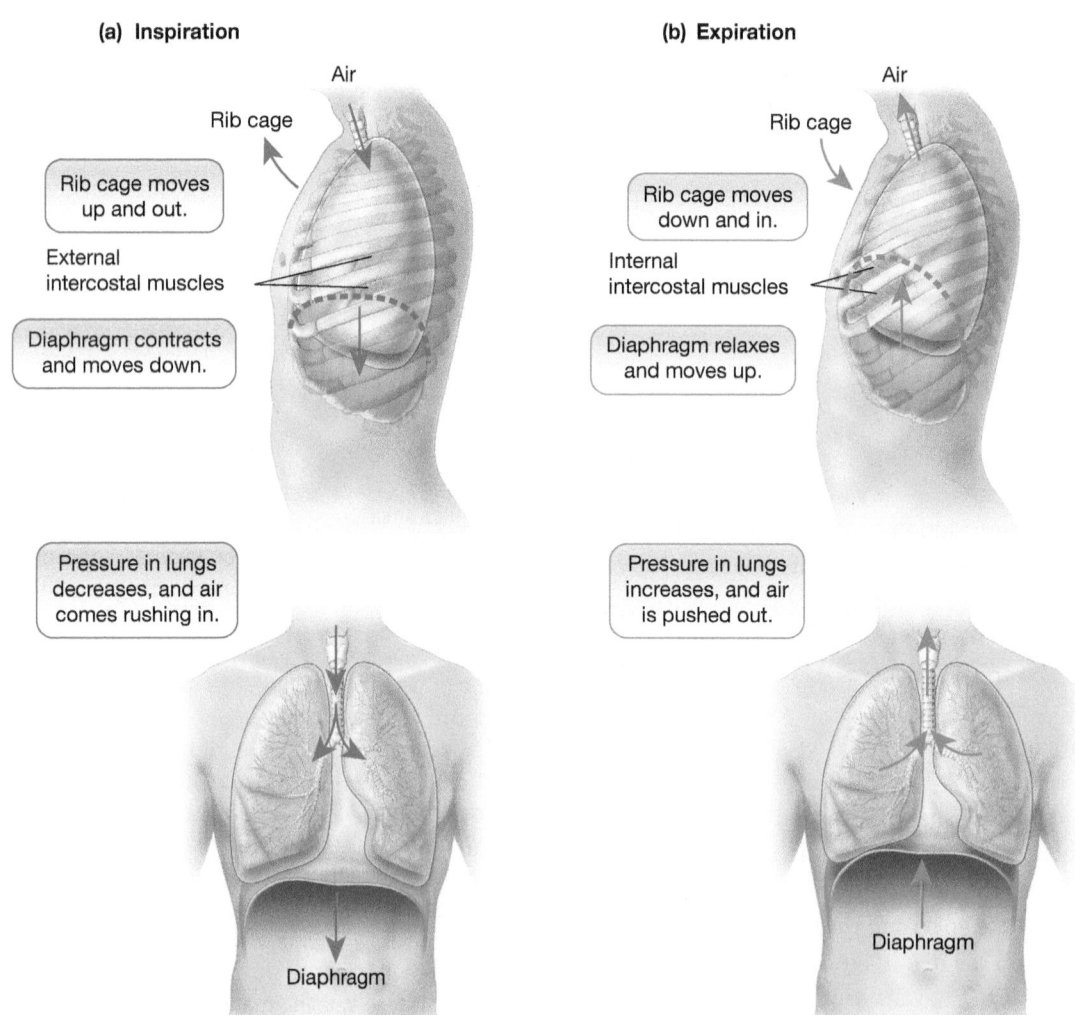

FIGURE 28-5 The process of ventilation: inspiration and expiration.

an impulse to the diaphragm and external intercostal muscles. This causes the diaphragm to contract and flatten, which results in an elongation of the **thorax** (the chest). At the same time, the external intercostal muscles contract to pull the ribs upward and outward, which increases the size of the thorax from the front to the back and from side to side. The increase in the size of the chest cavity reduces pressure within the chest, so that environmental air, which is now under greater pressure, flows into the lungs. Refer, again, to Figure 28-5.

Exhalation

Quiet *exhalation*, or **expiration**, is ordinarily a passive process. During expiration the diaphragm and the intercostal muscles relax and the thorax returns to its resting size and shape. The reduction in the size of the thoracic cavity builds pressure inside the chest cavity until it is greater than environmental air pressure, which causes air to flow out of the lungs. The elastic recoil of lung tissues aids in quiet expiration. Forceful expiration involves the internal intercostals and abdominal muscles.

COMMON PATHOLOGY ASSOCIATED WITH THE RESPIRATORY SYSTEM

Respiratory diseases have a wide range of presentation, from life threatening to mildly irritating. Some diseases are contracted through bacteria, viruses, or injury, whereas others develop as a result of the aging process. In addition to the diseases discussed next, Table 28-1 provides descriptions of some additional respiratory diseases and disorders.

Any lack of oxygen in the body, known as **hypoxia**, can be serious because our bodies require oxygen to survive. It can lead to **asphyxia**, or suffocation. **Arterial blood gases (ABGs)** are drawn by taking blood out of the arteries. If ordered, they must be processed immediately to truly ascertain the level of oxygen and carbon dioxide (CO_2) in the blood, because these gases evaporate quickly.

Asthma

Asthma is a chronic inflammatory disease of the bronchi and is related to the same process that causes allergic reactions. The general etiological factor related to asthma is an allergic reaction, though allergens are the actual offenders. Asthma is typically caused when allergens or other irritating substances cause swelling in the lining of the trachea and bronchial tubes, aggravating sensitive tissues. Common irritants include pet dander, dust mites, cigarette smoke, pollen, and other substances. When exposed to the irritant, tissues within the respiratory tract create mucus in an attempt to trap the offending intruder. The presence of excessive mucus can cause coughing or a sense of struggling to breathe, which, in turn, causes more swelling and more mucus production. A vicious cycle results.

Asthma is commonly seen during childhood, but adult-onset asthma is also common.

Signs and Symptoms. Difficulty breathing, or dyspnea, and cough are classic signs of asthma. Additionally, congestion, wheezing and tightness in the chest may occur, which

TABLE 28-1 | Diseases and Disorders of the Respiratory System

Condition	Description
Atelectasis	A collapse of all or part of the lung; usually caused by blocked airways, deflated alveolar sacs, or increased pressure outside the lung.
Hyperventilation	Rapid, deep breathing that often occurs with panic and anxiety.
Laryngitis	Inflammation of the voice box resulting in a loss of voice, or hoarseness.
Mesothelioma	A cancer that develops on the pleura of the lungs that develops years after exposure to asbestos.
Obstructive Sleep Apnea	Characterized by periods of decreased air flow and breathing cessation during sleep when the airway becomes blocked or narrowed because of the relaxation of throat muscles.
Pneumoconiosis	Known as Black Lung disease, it is caused by inhalation of coal dust, which causes inflammation of the alveolar sacs. Continual inflammation causes scar tissue to develop, which results in a stiffening of the lung tissue.
Pneumothorax	A collapse of the lung caused by a buildup of air between the wall of the chest and the lungs that usually results when the pleura has been punctured allowing air to escape.
Respiratory Distress Syndrome	A breathing disorder, characterized by a lack of necessary oxygen, that usually affects premature infants as a result of their body's inability to produce surfactant.

can cause anxiety in the patient. It is common for the patient's symptoms to be worse in the morning and at night.

Treatment. **Bronchodilators**, which open the bronchial passages, are the treatment of choice when a patient is experiencing an active asthma attack, or episode. Bronchodilators are often administered via an inhaler. Most individuals with asthma carry an inhaler of a beta-2 medication (bronchodilator), either albuterol or pirbuterol.

Long-term, preventive medications include long-acting beta-2 medications such as salmeterol (Serevent); eicosanoid lipid mediators such as leukotrienes (Singulair); and inhaled corticosteroids such as Flovent, Intal, and beclomethasone. These medications do not stop an already occurring asthma episode. Rather, they are taken daily to prevent asthmatic episodes by keeping effective levels of medication within the tissues. In response to a severe asthma attack, a course of treatment with steroids such as prednisone may be prescribed to help reduce the inflammation, speed healing, and reduce complications.

Chronic Obstructive Pulmonary Disease

Chronic obstructive pulmonary disease (COPD) consists primarily of two related diseases: chronic bronchitis and emphysema. Both diseases are characterized by chronic obstruction of the flow of air in and out of the lungs. The obstruction is generally permanent and progressively worsens over time. Air pollution and certain occupational pollutants, such as cadmium and silica, may increase the risk of COPD. Smoking is responsible for 85 to 90 percent of cases in the United States. Smokers also suffer more frequent respiratory symptoms, such as coughing and shortness of breath, and more deterioration in lung function from COPD than nonsmokers. Genetics, including a familial risk for reduced airway and airflow limitations, is also a causative factor for this disorder.

A diagnosis for COPD is established after a medical history of the symptoms and a physical examination detect

signs of COPD. Tests used to make or confirm the diagnosis include chest X-ray, computed tomography (CT or CAT scan) of the chest, pulmonary function tests, and the measurement of oxygen and carbon dioxide levels in the blood.

Signs and Symptoms. Signs and symptoms include shortness of breath and difficulty breathing, particularly with exertion, an increased number of respiratory infections, wheezing, a persistent cough, regular (and sometimes an excessive) production of mucus, fatigue, tightness in the chest, and the inability to catch one's breath.

Treatment. Unfortunately, there is no cure for COPD. The goals of COPD treatment are to prevent further deterioration in lung function, alleviate symptoms, and improve the patient's performance of daily activities and quality of life. Treatment strategies include smoking cessation, bronchodilators to open the airways and decrease airway inflammation, vaccination against influenza and pneumonia, regular oxygen supplementation, and pulmonary rehabilitation. Proper nutrition and minimal exercises—which help to strengthen muscles required for breathing—are both beneficial to COPD patients for overall health.

Bronchitis

Bronchitis is a respiratory disease marked by inflamed mucous membranes in the bronchial passages. As the irritated membrane swells and grows thicker, it narrows the airways of the lungs. The disease occurs in two forms: acute (lasting less than six weeks) and chronic (defined as recurring frequently for more than two years). Chronic bronchitis is considered to be a form of COPD.

Acute bronchitis is generally caused by viral lung infections but can also be caused by bacterial infections. Chronic bronchitis may be caused by repeated attacks of acute bronchitis, which irritate and weaken the bronchial airways over time, and by industrial pollution. Coal miners, grain handlers, metal molders, and others who are continually exposed to fine dust particles often develop chronic bronchitis at higher-than-normal rates. However, the chief cause is heavy, long-term smoking, which results in continual irritation of the bronchial tubes. It also results in excessive mucus production.

Signs and Symptoms. Signs and symptoms of acute bronchitis include a hacking cough; yellow, white, or green phlegm, which usually appears 24 to 48 hours after the cough begins; coughing up blood (**hemoptysis**); low-grade fever and chills; soreness and tightness in the chest; pain below the breastbone during deep breathing; and shortness of breath. Chronic bronchitis is characterized by a persistent cough that produces yellow, white, or green phlegm (for at least three months of the year and for more than two consecutive years) and sometimes wheezing and breathlessness.

Treatment. Conventional treatment for acute bronchitis may consist of simple measures such as getting plenty of rest, drinking lots of fluids, avoiding smoke and fumes, and use of an inhaled bronchodilator and/or cough suppressant. Antibiotics may be prescribed if there is a bacterial infection present. In chronic bronchitis, routine use of inhaled or oral steroids to reduce inflammation of the airways may be implemented, expectorants to thin mucus may be used, and in severe cases supplemental oxygen may be necessary.

Emphysema

Emphysema is a long-term, progressive disease of the lung. As mentioned earlier, along with chronic bronchitis, it is also a form of COPD. The disease attacks the structure of the alveoli in the lungs. Permanent holes develop in the alveolar walls, making them unable to hold their shape properly on exhalation. This decreases the amount of oxygen-rich blood that is able to circulate through the body.

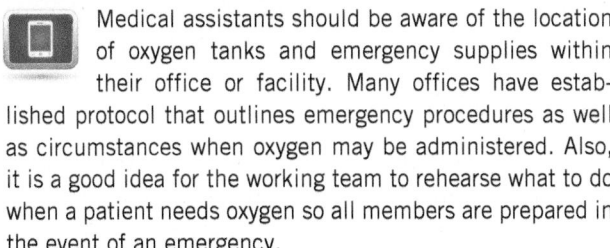

Professionalism   **The Workplace**

Medical assistants should be aware of the location of oxygen tanks and emergency supplies within their office or facility. Many offices have established protocol that outlines emergency procedures as well as circumstances when oxygen may be administered. Also, it is a good idea for the working team to rehearse what to do when a patient needs oxygen so all members are prepared in the event of an emergency.

As with medications, the administration of oxygen must always be ordered by a physician.

Regarding etiology and causative factors related to emphysema, smoking tobacco is by far the most common cause of emphysema—and also the most preventable. Other risk factors include a deficiency of the enzyme alpha-1 antitrypsin, air pollution, airway reactivity, heredity, gender (male), and age.

Signs and Symptoms. Shortness of breath is the most common symptom of emphysema. At times, the shortness of breath is so severe that a person is unable to talk. If severe breathing difficulties persist, the patient's complexion, lips, or nail beds may turn bluish in appearance. This is called **cyanosis** and results from a lack of oxygen in the tissues. Coughing, sometimes caused by the production of mucus, and wheezing may also be symptoms. Rapid heartbeat, decreased cognition, and intolerance for exercise are also common.

Treatment. Treatment for emphysema can take many forms. Smoking cessation is a treatment that most doctors require of patients, as it may halt the progression of the disease and improves lung function to some extent. Bronchodilators are usually the first medications prescribed. Steroids and antibiotics, when infection is present, may also be prescribed. If the patient experiences shortness of breath, oxygen therapy may be given. Patients may undergo pulmonary rehabilitation in which they are taught exercises and techniques to help counter shortness of breath, and possibly enable them to exercise. In very severe cases, surgery to remove a lung may be required.

Common Cold

A **common cold** is a viral infection of the upper respiratory tract. More than 200 viruses can cause a common cold; however, the rhinovirus is the most common culprit. Many cold viruses are highly contagious, because it is transmitted through droplets. It is estimated that infectious droplets can travel 4–6 feet through the air. These droplets can be transmitted through sneezing and coughing, hand-to-hand contact with someone who has a cold, or the use of shared objects, such as utensils, towels, toys, or telephones.

Signs and Symptoms. Because any one of over 200 viruses can cause a common cold, symptoms can vary greatly. Signs and symptoms usually appear one to three days after exposure to a cold virus. They may include a runny or stuffy nose, itchy or sore throat, cough, congestion, slight body aches, mild headache, sneezing, watery eyes, low-grade fever of less than 102°F, and mild fatigue. Nasal discharge may become thicker and turn yellow or green as the cold runs its course. Unlike other viral infections, the common cold is not accompanied by high fever or significant fatigue.

Treatment. There is no cure for the common cold. Antibiotics are useless against cold viruses because they are only effective against bacterial infections. Over-the-counter medications can relieve some symptoms, though they can't shorten the duration of the illness. For fever, sore throat, and headache, mild pain relievers may be helpful. For runny nose and nasal congestion, antihistamines or decongestants may be useful.

Because so many different viruses can cause a common cold, no effective vaccine has been developed. Taking certain precautions can help to slow the spread of cold viruses: washing the hands; scrubbing countertops clean, especially when someone in the household has a cold; sneezing and coughing into tissues and discarding them immediately; and not sharing drinking glasses or other utensils with family members who may be sick.

Hay Fever

Hay fever, sometimes called seasonal allergic rhinitis or pollinosis, is a seasonal allergy in which the mucous membranes of the nose become inflamed. The most likely cause of hay fever is the pollen of trees, plants, and weeds carried by the wind and air. High pollen counts in the air occur with weather changes, particularly exceptionally hot and dry days or cool and wet days. About 50 million Americans experience hay fever symptoms each year.

Signs and Symptoms. Common signs and symptoms of hay fever include repeated and prolonged sneezing; a stuffy and watery nose; redness, swelling, and itching of the eyes; itching of the nose, throat, mouth, and ears; and other ear problems. It is also common for patients to experience impaired senses of smell and taste. At bedtime, patients may experience difficulty breathing and increased coughing from postnasal drip.

Treatment. Hay fever is best controlled by avoiding the substance that causes the reaction. Air filters that are able to purify and remove airborne allergens can be very effective. Antihistamine medication may be prescribed that, as the name suggests, counteracts the histamine that is released by the body during the allergic reaction. In more severe cases, corticosteroids may be taken. Immunotherapy, or allergy shots, are also helpful in these cases by assisting to reduce symptoms in about 85 percent of patients.

Influenza

Influenza, commonly called the flu, is an illness caused by viruses that infect the respiratory tract. Influenza is more severe than other viral infections, having a rapid and quick progression of symptoms, which is usually a recognizable factor. There are three types of the influenza virus: A, B, and C. Typically, influenza Type A is most problematic for humans. These influenza viruses mutate and change over time, making them a continual source of susceptible infection to the body. Because the body is able to defend itself only against a virus it has already been exposed to, viral mutations present new sources for infection to which the body has not been exposed.

It is important to note that gastrointestinal (GI) illness is often mistaken for the flu. Flu is a respiratory condition, not gastrointestinal (although children may have GI symptoms associated with a respiratory flu). GI illnesses are caused by different infectious organisms, not by influenza viruses.

Signs and Symptoms. Typical symptoms of influenza include fever (usually 100°F to 103°F in adults, often higher in children); dry cough, sore throat, and runny or stuffy nose; headache; muscle aches; chills; and extreme fatigue.

Treatment. Antiviral medications can shorten the course of influenza, but only if medication is prescribed and taken within the first two days after the onset of the first symptoms. Medications to treat and alleviate symptoms may be prescribed, including pain relievers (analgesics) and fever reducers (antipyretics). Most people affected by the flu recover completely in one to two weeks, but some people develop serious and potentially life-threatening medical complications such as pneumonia.

The best defense against influenza is an annual influenza vaccination. Because there are many strains of influenza, the three most lethal strains are identified each year. This is accomplished through surveillance-based forecasts that are conducted throughout the year at influenza centers that have been established in 101 different countries. These centers focus on common strains and disease trends to establish which vaccines will be most effective against the most powerful strains for the upcoming influenza season. The patient who receives an influenza vaccination may succumb to other strains of influenza, but the immune system will be more efficient from having developed a defense against the strains in the vaccine. Health care workers, older adults, those who are immunosuppressed, and children have the highest risk of contracting this sometimes fatal disease and should be vaccinated every year.

Legionnaires' Disease

Legionnaires' disease is a type of lung infection caused by breathing in a mist of water that has been contaminated with the *Legionella* bacterium. This bacterium tends to thrive in stagnant water that is found in air conditioning units for large buildings, hot tubs, and showers. The disease came to be known as Legionnaires' disease, or legionellosis, in 1976 after numerous attendees at an American Legion convention became ill in a Philadelphia, Pennsylvania, hotel. The microbe causing the illness was isolated, identified, and named. More than 40 different strains of the *Legionella* bacterium have since been identified.

Legionnaires' disease usually affects middle-aged or older adults and more commonly affects smokers or people with other respiratory problems. The disease is not transmitted via person-to-person contact, but rather through a direct exposure to the bacteria.

Signs and Symptoms. The symptoms of Legionnaires' disease generally start 2 to 10 days after exposure and infection. They include high fever with sweating, severe headache, shortness of breath, a productive cough, fatigue, and muscle aches and pains. In severe cases, other body systems may be affected, leading to diarrhea, vomiting, mental confusion, and kidney and liver damage.

Treatment. Treatment normally consists of administration of antibiotics that will fight the *Legionella* infection. In severe cases, oxygen therapy may be necessary to help with breathing difficulties. Also, fluid and electrolyte replacement might be indicated if the patient is dehydrated because of extreme illness. In the United States, *Legionella* is considered a reportable health condition. Therefore, out of concern for the safety of the general public, health care professionals follow appropriate reporting protocol when their patients are diagnosed with Legionnaires' disease.

Lung Cancer

Lung cancer affects the lung tissue (Figure 28-6). It is the leading cause of cancer deaths in both women and men in the United States and throughout the world. Smoking is the most significant factor in the development of lung cancer. About 90 percent of lung cancers occur in smokers or former smokers. The risk of developing lung cancer is related to the number of cigarettes smoked, the age at which a person started smoking, and how long a person has smoked (or smoked before quitting).

Another cause of lung cancer is secondhand smoke. An estimate from the Centers for Disease Control and Prevention states about 7,300 nonsmokers die each year from secondhand smoke. Other high-risk causes of lung cancer include exposure to asbestos and radon gas, excessive levels of air pollution, arsenic in drinking water, and exposure to certain carcinogens (cancer-causing agents) including cadmium, mustard gas, diesel exhaust, uranium, and coal products, to name a few.

There are two main types of lung cancer: nonsmall cell lung cancer (NSCLC) and small cell lung cancer (SCLC).

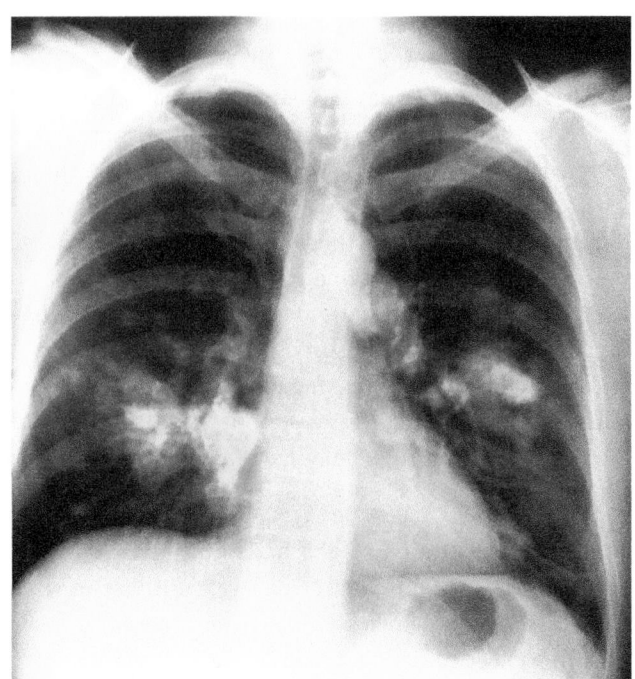

FIGURE 28-6 An X-ray image of lung cancer.

Small cell lung cancer is less common, accounting for only about 10 to 15 percent of total lung cancer cases, but is faster-growing and spreads much more quickly than nonsmall cell lung cancer.

Signs and Symptoms. The early stages of lung cancer can be asymptomatic (without symptoms). As the cancer progresses, patients experience a persistent cough, coughing up blood, shortness of breath, wheezing, chest pain, recurring lung infections (pneumonia or bronchitis), and excessive fatigue. Additionally, many patients experience decreased appetite and weight loss (without trying—that is, weight loss not caused by dieting or other deliberate attempts to lose weight). Symptoms of advanced stage cancer, as evidence of metastasis, includes bone pain, neurological changes, and jaundiced (a yellowish tint) skin or eyes.

Treatment. Treatment depends on the type of lung cancer and the stage at which it is diagnosed. The most widely used therapies for lung cancer are surgery, chemotherapy, and radiation therapy. Surgical treatments may include removal of a lobe of the lung (lobectomy), removal of a small segment of the lung, and the possibility of removing the entire lung (pneumonectomy).

Pertussis

Pertussis, or whooping cough, is a bacterial infection of the upper respiratory tract. It is characterized by intense and uncontrollable coughing spells. It is caused by *Bordetella pertussis*, a highly contagious bacterium that is spread through airborne droplets. A vaccination is available for pertussis that is often first administered when an infant is 2 months old. The infant receives a combination vaccination to protect against pertussis, diphtheria, and tetanus in what is commonly referred to as the DTaP immunization. Even though there is an effective vaccination against pertussis, some people choose not to vaccinate their children for various reasons. If they decide against vaccination, their child may not be able to enter public schools. Because most children have been immunized, pertussis used to be very rare. Recently more cases of pertussis are arising in unvaccinated adults and children. Pertussis is a very serious condition. Infants afflicted with the disease may have permanent disability, and it could be fatal.

Signs and Symptoms. Signs and symptoms include a cough, runny nose, and a low-grade fever. Within two weeks of infection, breathing takes a turn for the worse and becomes difficult. Violent coughing develops that ends in a noise that sounds like a "whoop." However, adults and infants under 6 months of age do not often have the "whooping" sound with their cough. During the intense coughing episodes, some patients may vomit or even lose consciousness for a short period of time. Infants also tend to experience episodes of choking.

Treatment. Antibiotics can be effective if pertussis is diagnosed early on. However, because of the severity of the disease and because decreased oxygen levels are common with the violent coughing spells, many infants and children are hospitalized and monitored. At the hospital, respiratory support including oxygen therapy, oxygen tents with high levels of humidity, IV fluids, and sedatives may be administered to promote healing and relieve symptoms.

Pleurisy

Pleurisy, or pleuritis, is an inflammation of the pleura (membrane that surrounds and protects the lungs). Pleurisy can result from a number of diseases and disorders including lower respiratory infections caused by viruses or bacteria such as pneumonia or tuberculosis; an injury to the chest; a pulmonary embolism; and disorders such as rheumatoid arthritis, lupus, and pancreatitis. Complications from heart surgery may also cause pleurisy.

Signs and Symptoms. The chief symptom of pleurisy is sudden, intense shooting or stabbing chest pain. More often than not, the pain is located directly over the area of inflammation. The pain is most severe with inhalation, whereas holding the breath often provides relief from the pain. Talking, coughing, and sneezing also produce intense pain. In some cases the pain may be referred—that is, felt in other areas, such as the neck, shoulder, or abdomen.

Patients also display distinct respiratory signs including a shallow breathing pattern as a response to the pain. Cyanosis of the patient's lips or nail beds may also occur as a result of severe breathing troubles and decreased oxygen intake.

Treatment. Pleurisy will not be cured unless the underlying disease or disorder is treated. However, pain associated with pleurisy is often treated using two routes. First, overall chest pain associated with breathing is controlled with the use of analgesics and antiinflammatory medicines. Also, codeine-based cough syrups are prescribed to help ease the pain associated with a painful cough. Pneumonia is a concern for patients with pleurisy as they are unable to clear chest congestion because coughing is too painful. When a patient begins to feel relief from pain, it is important for them to practice deep breathing and try to clear congestion by coughing.

Pneumonia

Pneumonia is an inflammation of the lung or lungs. The etiology of pneumonia is various as it can be caused by bacteria, viruses, fungi, or chemical irritants. The most common cause of bacterial pneumonia in the United States is *Streptococcus pneumoniae* (pneumococcus); the influenza virus is the most common cause of viral pneumonia. Individuals with weak immune systems and respiratory disorders are more prone to developing pneumonia.

Signs and Symptoms. Signs and symptoms include chest pain, especially when coughing, increased tiredness and fatigue, a cough that produces green mucus or pus-like sputum, muscle aches, fever, chills, and rapid and labored breathing. Diagnostic procedures including sputum cultures, and chest X-rays may be indicated to confirm diagnosis.

Treatment. Pneumonia is treated with fluids, rest, antibiotics (if the pneumonia is caused by bacteria), and nonprescription drugs for pain relief. Oxygen therapy and respiratory treatments can be administered to thin out and remove secretions as necessary. Cough medicines may be counterproductive, because they may inhibit the patient's ability to cough and expel excessive sputum. Patients suffering from severe pneumonia may require hospitalization for careful monitoring and treatment. Prevention of pneumonia is ideally achieved with the administration of pneumococcal vaccines.

Pulmonary Edema

Pulmonary edema is a condition in which fluid accumulates in the alveoli of lungs. Often it is caused by inadequate pumping of the left ventricle of the heart, as seen with congestive heart failure. Some other causes of pulmonary edema include but are not limited to heart attack, lack of oxygen supply to the heart muscle (ischemia), hypertension, pneumonia, kidney failure, and major injuries. Pulmonary edema can be a chronic condition; however, it can develop suddenly and become life threatening.

Signs and Symptoms. Signs and symptoms of pulmonary edema include shortness of breath brought on by activity; difficulty breathing in positions other than sitting upright; frothy bloody sputum containing pus; increased respirations; cold, clammy, cyanotic skin; leg swelling; decreased alertness; and increased anxiety.

Treatment. The overall treatment goal is to remove excessive fluid from the lungs. Often in severe cases emergency intervention is required. High levels of oxygen will immediately be administered while the patient sits in an upright position. Diuretics (which increase the excretion of water from the body) are often administered. Medications to improve heart function are also prescribed when heart failure is the underlying issue. When pulmonary edema stems from other issues, the underlying cause must be treated to prevent further pulmonary complications.

Pulmonary Embolism

A **pulmonary embolism (PE)** is a blood clot in the lung that occurs when a clot breaks away from the wall of a vein in the leg, pelvis, arm, or, sometimes, the right side of the heart and travels throughout the bloodstream. As it continues through the circulation, eventually it reaches the vessels of the lungs that continually become smaller and smaller. Finally, the clot becomes lodged in a vessel that is so narrow it cannot pass through (Figure 28-7). The wedged clot prevents blood flow to a section of the lung. Deprived of oxygen, that portion of the lung suffers an infarct (necrosis, or death, of the tissue), which is referred to as a pulmonary (or lung) infarct.

The risk of clot formation is higher when a person is immobilized because of illness, injury, or prolonged sitting, such as on an airplane or a long car trip. Immobility allows the blood to pool in the legs, providing an opportunistic environment for blood clot formation. Other factors that contribute to the risk are recent surgery, trauma or injury (especially to the legs), obesity, smoking, hormone replacement therapy and hormonal contraceptives (such as birth control pills), heart disease, burns, and a previous history of blood clots in the legs.

Signs and Symptoms. Shortness of breath is the most common symptom of pulmonary embolism, which is caused by

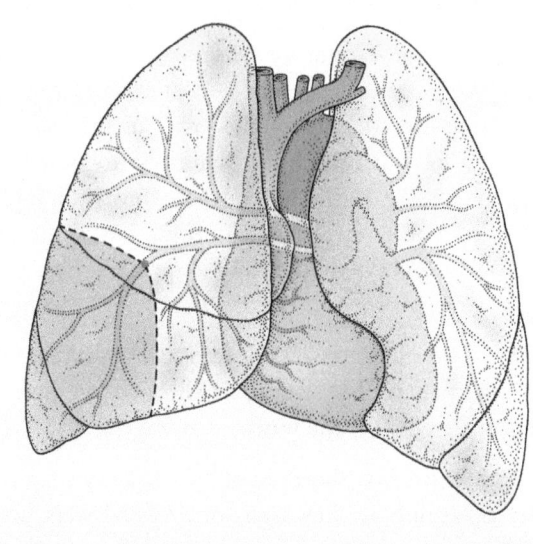

FIGURE 28-7 Pulmonary embolism. The purple shaded section shows the area of the lung that is dying from lack of blood supply caused by the embolism.

the sharp, stabbing pain that occurs when the patient tries to take a deep breath or cough. Other signs and symptoms that accompany a PE include rapid breathing and rapid heart rate; anxiety or apprehension; dry cough or coughing up mucus or blood; sweating; cyanotic lips and/or nailbeds; and low blood pressure resulting in loss of consciousness.

Treatment. Pulmonary emboli can be life threatening and are often treated in emergency care settings. Thrombolytics, which are clot-buster medications, are used to help dissolve the embolus. Blood-thinning medications are administered to prevent the formation of new clots, a process termed anticoagulation therapy. Warfarin and heparin are medications commonly used for this purpose. Oxygen therapy is initiated to assist with breathing. Medications to raise blood pressure levels may also be necessary, depending on the severity of the event.

Severe Acute Respiratory Syndrome

Severe acute respiratory syndrome (SARS) is a recently identified respiratory illness that first infected people in parts of Asia, North America, and Europe in early 2003. This new virus is known as SARS-CoV (severe acute respiratory syndrome coronavirus). It is possible that outbreaks of SARS are seasonal, appearing during winter months. The virus has been found in a catlike wild animal that is eaten as a delicacy in China. This has led experts to believe that SARS first developed in animals rather than humans.

SARS is a highly contagious illness spread via airborne droplets. During extensive research on the disease, it was found that the virus can remain alive for up to six hours after

SARS (severe acute respiratory syndrome) was spread from China to North America by infected persons traveling by airplane. How can we control the entry of microbes into a country? What should China have done to prevent the spread of the disease within and outside China? Should the Chinese government have shared information about SARS with the world immediately in case it spread?

the airborne droplets make contact with a surface. Most patients begin to display symptoms three to ten days after becoming infected with the virus.

Signs and Symptoms. Shortness of breath, a dry cough, and difficulty breathing are key signs of SARS. Fevers greater than 100.4°F, muscle aches, headaches, fatigue, and chills are also common symptoms.

Treatment. Treatment of SARS usually consists of high doses of steroids to reduce inflammation of the lungs and oxygen therapy. More than two-thirds of patients infected with the virus require hospitalization for treatment. A patient with SARS is placed in isolation during treatment to prevent spread of the disease. Antiviral medications are also used, which are not able to cure the disease but help to treat the associated symptoms. In 2004, the World Health Organization (WHO) released a report indicating that about 1 out of 10 people who contract SARS are unable to survive the disease.

Sinusitis

Sinusitis is an infection or inflammation of the mucous membranes that line the inside of the nose and the sinus cavities. When a mucous membrane becomes inflamed, it swells, blocking the drainage of fluid from the sinuses into the nose and throat and causing pressure and pain in the sinuses. Sinuses that do not drain properly are more vulnerable to bacterial and fungal growth.

Sinuses can become blocked during a viral infection such as a cold, and sinus inflammation and infection can develop as a result. Sinusitis also is caused by abnormal tissue growth in the nose (nasal polyps), which hinders drainage; deviated septum; trauma to the face, which could result in blockage and drainage issues; allergies; and bacterial infections.

One key distinction between a cold and sinusitis is that cold symptoms begin to improve within five to seven days. Sinusitis symptoms last longer and worsen after seven days. There are two types of sinusitis: acute (sudden) and chronic (long term). Acute sinusitis clears up within four weeks; chronic sinusitis may last for three months or longer.

Signs and Symptoms. Pain and pressure in the face surrounding the sinus cavities, a stuffy or runny nose, and greenish or yellow nasal discharge are the main symptoms of sinusitis. Sore throat, postnasal drip, and a cough that worsens at night are also common. Other common signs and symptoms, which may seem unusual, include bad breath, tooth pain, and a decreased sense of smell.

Treatment. Medications most commonly used to treat sinusitis include a combination of antibiotics, decongestants, analgesics, corticosteroids, and mucolytics. This combination is used because the goals of treatment are to thin mucus and promote drainage, reduce sinus swelling, alleviate pain and pressure, eliminate infection, and avoid permanent damage to the tissues lining the nose and sinuses. Length of treatment with medications ranges from three days to several weeks or longer. Home remedies to alleviate symptoms include moist heat application to the face, steam baths, increased rest and fluid intake, and using a humidifier in the home to eliminate dry air.

Tuberculosis

Tuberculosis (TB) is a contagious disease caused by the bacterium *Mycobacterium tuberculosis*. The bacteria are spread when infected droplets are inhaled. These infected droplets are expelled from their infected host through talking, laughing, singing, coughing, sneezing, and spitting. TB bacteria are most commonly found in the lungs, where they produce granulomas (granular tumors), but they can be found elsewhere in the body. Individuals who are immunosuppressed, such as those with HIV/AIDS, infants, older adults, diabetics, and individuals receiving chemotherapy have the highest risk of developing TB. Health care workers are often required to be tested for TB, because they are in contact with high-risk population groups. TB is a disease that requires mandatory reporting to local health departments.

TB may be considered inactive in patients who carry the bacteria but do not have signs or symptoms. A patient with inactive TB is not considered to be contagious to others.

Signs and Symptoms. Signs of active tuberculosis include a long lasting cough, hemoptysis, and night sweats. Other signs and symptoms can include fatigue, chills, weakness, pain when coughing and sometimes simply breathing, and loss of appetite (anorexia). Those with advanced TB may have clubbing (enlargement of the ends) of the fingers and toes.

The Purified Protein Derivative (PPD) skin test, also known as the Mantoux tuberculin skin test, is done to check if an individual has ever been exposed to the tuberculosis bacterium and if it is lying dormant; however, this test does not indicate whether the person has an active case of TB. Active TB can be diagnosed only by a chest X-ray and sputum cultures.

Treatment. Treatment of this disease is long term, as it usually takes 9 to 12 months to eradicate the bacteria. The first period requires that the patient take respiratory precautions to prevent the spread of the bacteria; patients may be ordered to practice isolation and stay homebound or hospitalized to prevent the spread of infection. Multidrug therapy is used to kill the bacteria. Four antibiotics that are taken at the same time—usually rifampin, isoniazid, pyrazinamide, and ethambutol—are used to begin eradication of the bacteria.

After the patient shows negative sputum cultures, antibiotic treatment must continue for another four to seven months to prevent the development of multidrug-resistant TB, which is more difficult to treat. The total treatment time is determined by the physician and requires the patient to strictly follow the medications as prescribed for a successful outcome.

SUMMARY

The respiratory system is divided into the upper respiratory system and the lower respiratory system. The upper system includes the nose, paranasal sinuses, and pharynx. The lower respiratory system includes the larynx, trachea, bronchi, bronchioles, alveoli, and lungs. The entire system is lined with mucous membranes and cilia, which serve a protective function. Through the lungs, carbon dioxide is expelled (exhalation) and oxygen is drawn in (inhalation). Multiple disease processes can result from infection and inflammation within the system. Among the often debilitating diseases of the respiratory system are asthma, chronic obstructive pulmonary disease, hay fever, pleurisy, and lung cancer. Microbes cause the common cold, influenza, Legionnaires' disease, pertussis, pneumonia, some sinusitis, severe acute respiratory syndrome, and tuberculosis. Pulmonary edema and pulmonary emboli can also cause severe damage if not promptly and properly treated.

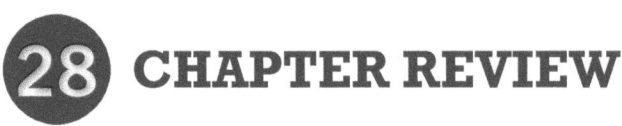

28 CHAPTER REVIEW

COMPETENCY REVIEW

1. Define and spell the terms for this chapter.
2. List the organs of the respiratory system.
3. What is the primary function of the respiratory system?
4. Which two gases are exchanged in the lungs?
5. What are the five functions of the nose?
6. What are the functions of the pharynx?
7. What is the function of the epiglottis?
8. Describe the bronchi. What are the differences between the left and right bronchi?
9. What are the alveoli?
10. Why is immobility a risk factor for developing an embolism?

PREPARING FOR THE CERTIFICATION EXAM

1. What organ is shared by both the respiratory and digestive systems and connects the nose, mouth, and voice box?
   a. pharynx
   b. nares
   c. trachea
   d. bronchi
   e. epiglottis

2. Which of the following breaths per minute would be considered normal for a newborn?
   a. 5
   b. 10
   c. 20
   d. 40
   e. 100

3. Which structure is known as the voice box?
   a. bronchial tube
   b. trachea
   c. larynx
   d. pharynx
   e. epiglottis

4. The function of the larynx is primarily to
   a. aid in swallowing.
   b. aid in speaking.
   c. prevent swallowing.
   d. prevent aspiration.
   e. aid in aspiration.

5. A chronic inflammatory disease caused by allergens or other irritating substances is
   a. asthma.
   b. pneumonia.
   c. cystic fibrosis.
   d. Legionnaires' disease.
   e. tuberculosis.

6. A doctor is required, by law, to report which of the following diseases?
   a. pneumonia
   b. TB

   c. pollinosis
   d. pulmonary edema
   e. pulmonary emboli

7. High fever is a symptom of
   a. sinusitis.
   b. lung cancer.
   c. common cold.
   d. influenza.
   e. pulmonary edema.

8. A PPD test is done to detect which of the following?
   a. cystic fibrosis
   b. emphysema
   c. lung cancer
   d. asthma
   e. tuberculosis

9. Surfactant is produced by
   a. the medulla and pons.
   b. bronchioles.
   c. alveoli.
   d. paranasal sinuses.
   e. the right bronchus.

10. An attack of hay fever is triggered by
    a. touching the infected person.
    b. breathing in an allergen.
    c. breathing in infected droplets.
    d. a casual handshake.
    e. smoking.

CRITICAL THINKING

Refer to the case study at the beginning of the chapter and use what you have learned to answer the following questions.

1. Mr. McConnley has some flulike symptoms. What other respiratory disorder do these symptoms mimic?
2. Dr. Miller asks Mr. McConnley if he has recently stayed at a hotel with an air conditioning system. Why would he be asking this question?
3. Mr. McConnley states that he returned four days ago from a convention in Florida where he both lodged and attended conference meetings at the same hotel. Does this support Dr. Miller's suspicions? Why or why not?

INTERNET ACTIVITY

Conduct an Internet search for COPD services in your hometown, and see what resources are available in your area.

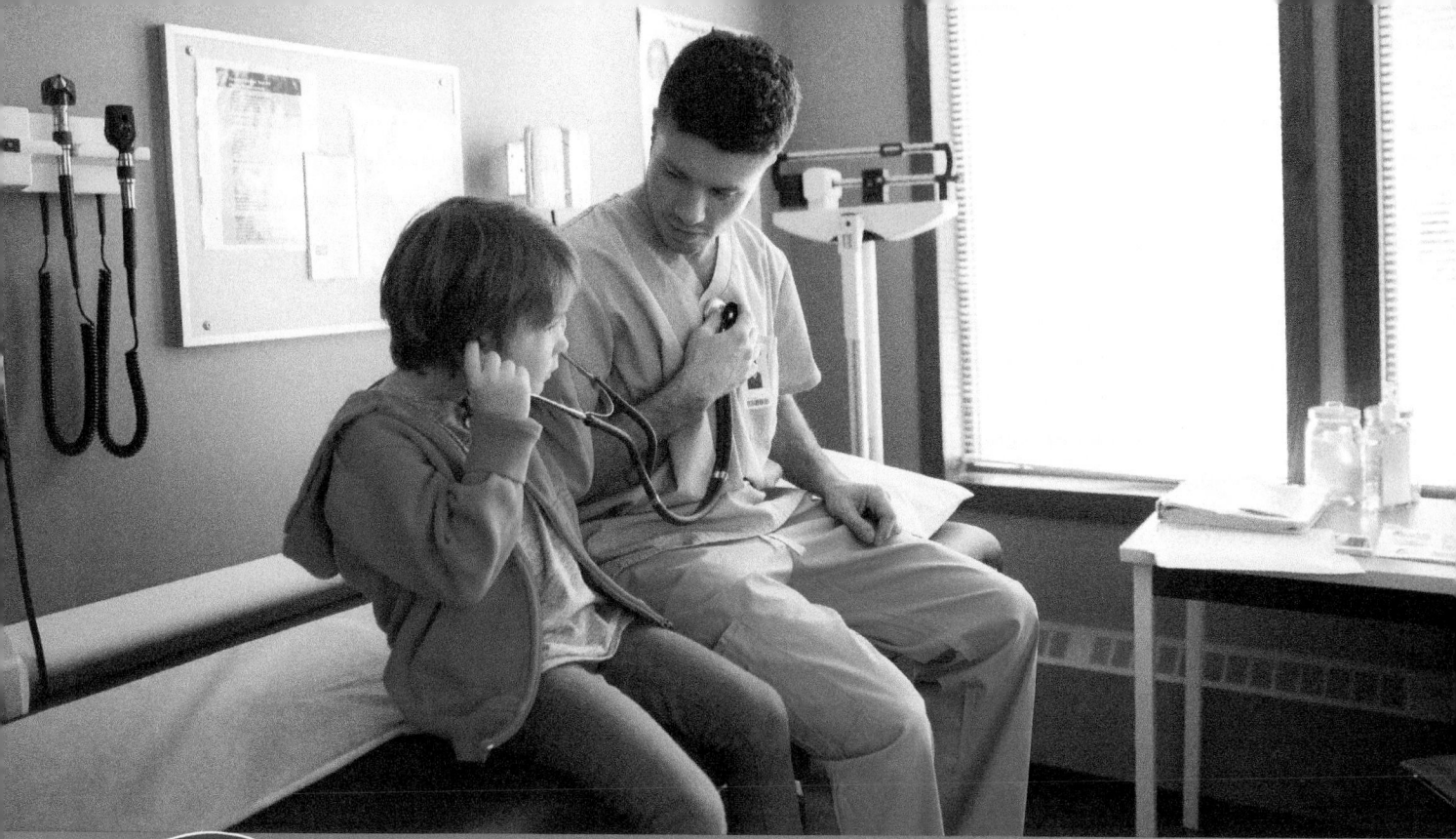

The Digestive System

Learning Objectives

After completing this chapter, you should be able to:

29.1   Define and spell the terms for this chapter.
29.2   List the main functions of the digestive system.
29.3   Identify the primary organs of the digestive system.
29.4   Summarize the function of each primary organ of the digestive system.
29.5   Identify the accessory organs of the digestive system.
29.6   Summarize the function of each accessory organ of the digestive system.
29.7   Identify common pathology associated with the digestive system.
29.8   Describe how the digestive system changes during the life span of a child to an older adult.

Susan Schultz, CMA (AAMA), is working as a clinical medical assistant today with Dr. Penningworth. The doctor's next patient is a new patient, Marshall Raines. Susan immediately notices a yellowish tint to his eyeballs, and because he is wearing shorts, she can see that his legs are slightly swollen and very bruised. She also notices a faint odor of alcohol. When Susan asks Marshall what has brought him to the office, he informs her that he has recently succumbed to alcohol after being sober for three months. Also, for the past few days he "hasn't been feeling right."

Terms to Learn

appendicitis
appendix
bolus
cardiac sphincter
cecum
cementum
cholelithiasis
chyme
cirrhosis
colitis
colon
colorectal cancer
Crohn's disease
dentin
digestive enzymes

diverticulitis
diverticulosis
enamel
esophagus
gallbladder
gastroesophageal reflux disease (GERD)
gingivae
hemorrhoid
hernia
hiatal hernia
inguinal hernia
irritable bowel syndrome (IBS)
large intestine
liver

mastication
oral cancer
pancreas
pancreatic cancer
peptic ulcer disease (PUD)
peristalsis
pharynx
pyloric sphincter
pyloric stenosis
rectum
rugae
salivary glands
small intestine
stomach
ulcerative colitis

The main part of the digestive system is the gastrointestinal tract, which is also known as the alimentary canal. The terms *gastrointestinal tract* and *alimentary canal* are often used interchangeably, as you will find in this chapter. This tract is essentially a long, continuous tube (some 29 feet long in adults) that starts at the mouth, where food and drink enter the body, and ends at the anus, where waste products leave the body. Each of the various organs commonly associated with digestion is described in this chapter, and the organs of digestion are shown in Figure 29-1.

FUNCTIONS AND ORGANS OF THE DIGESTIVE SYSTEM

The digestive system has three main functions: digestion, absorption, and elimination. These functions help to provide the body with nourishment and energy and to maintain homeostasis. The wall of the alimentary canal (think of the rubbery wall around the hollow center of a hose) is composed of four layers—from outermost to innermost the serosa (also called the peritoneum), the muscular layer, the submucosa, and the mucosa. Table 29-1 describes these four layers of the digestive tract wall.

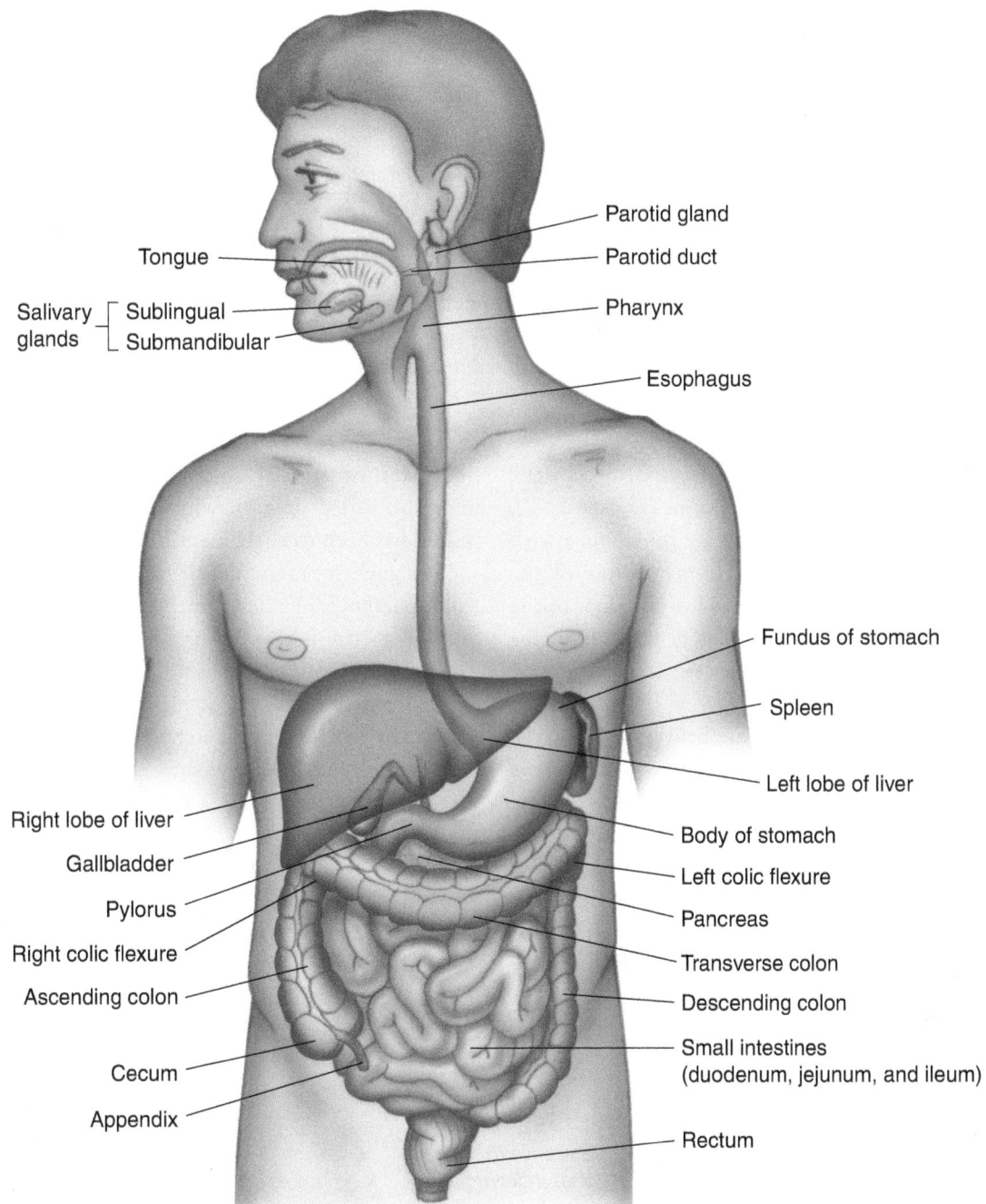

Tongue

Salivary glands
- Sublingual
- Submandibular

Parotid gland

Parotid duct

Pharynx

Esophagus

Fundus of stomach

Spleen

Left lobe of liver

Right lobe of liver

Gallbladder

Pylorus

Right colic flexure

Ascending colon

Cecum

Appendix

Body of stomach

Left colic flexure

Pancreas

Transverse colon

Descending colon

Small intestines
(duodenum, jejunum, and ileum)

Rectum

FIGURE 29-1 The digestive system.

Glands and small cells are found within the mucosal linings throughout the gastrointestinal (GI) tract. These glands and cells are important to food digestion because they produce juices known as **digestive enzymes**. The three main types of digestive enzymes are protease, which helps to digest proteins; amylase, which helps digest carbohydrates; and lipase, which helps digest fats.

Mouth

The digestive process starts a lot sooner than you may realize. The act of chewing food is termed **mastication**. Saliva produced during chewing moistens food and initiates digestion by chemically breaking down food. In the mouth, food is formed into a **bolus** (ball) for swallowing.

TABLE 29-1 | Layers of the Digestive Tract Wall

Layer	Location	Function
Serosa	Outermost layer, also known as the peritoneum	Keeps the outside part of the digestive tract moist by secreting serous fluid and prevents it from sticking to other organs.
Muscular layer	Situated between the serosa and the submucosa	Made up of smooth muscle tissue that, through contraction, is able to move items through the digestive tract.
Submucosa	The second innermost layer	Made of blood vessels, loose connective tissue, and nerves; this layer is the site of nutrient absorption.
Mucosa	The innermost layer of the digestive tract wall	Made up of epithelial tissue, which secretes digestive enzymes and assists in nutrient absorption.

The mouth, also called the oral cavity, is formed by the palate, the lips and cheeks, and the tongue (Figure 29-2). The cheeks form the lateral walls and are continuous with the lips. The hard and soft palates form the roof of the oral cavity, and the tongue is connected to the floor of the cavity by the lingual frenulum, a fold of mucous membrane. The vestibule is the space between the cheeks and the teeth.

Within the oral cavity the teeth are held in place by the **gingivae**, or gums. Three pairs of salivary glands—the parotid, sublingual, and submandibular glands—secrete saliva into the oral cavity.

A mucous membrane covers the skeletal muscle that forms the tongue. The tongue has three distinct sections; the tip, the central body, and the root (the rear portion). Elevations known as papillae cover the tongue; taste buds are found within the papillae. Four types of taste buds receive the tastes: sweet, salty, sour, and bitter. A fifth type of taste receptor, called umami, which is able to decipher savory tastes, has been recently identified.

The posterior margin of the soft palate supports the muscular pharyngeal arches, which function in swallowing and phonation (formation of speech sounds), and the uvula, which is the tissue that looks like a tiny punching bag dangling from the center of the pharyngeal arches. The line formed by the pharyngeal arches and the uvula separates the oral cavity from the pharynx.

Teeth

Humans have two sets of teeth: 20 deciduous teeth (the baby teeth) and 32 permanent teeth (Figure 29-3). The deciduous teeth are smaller than the permanent teeth but generally resemble the permanent teeth, although on a much smaller scale. The set of deciduous teeth includes

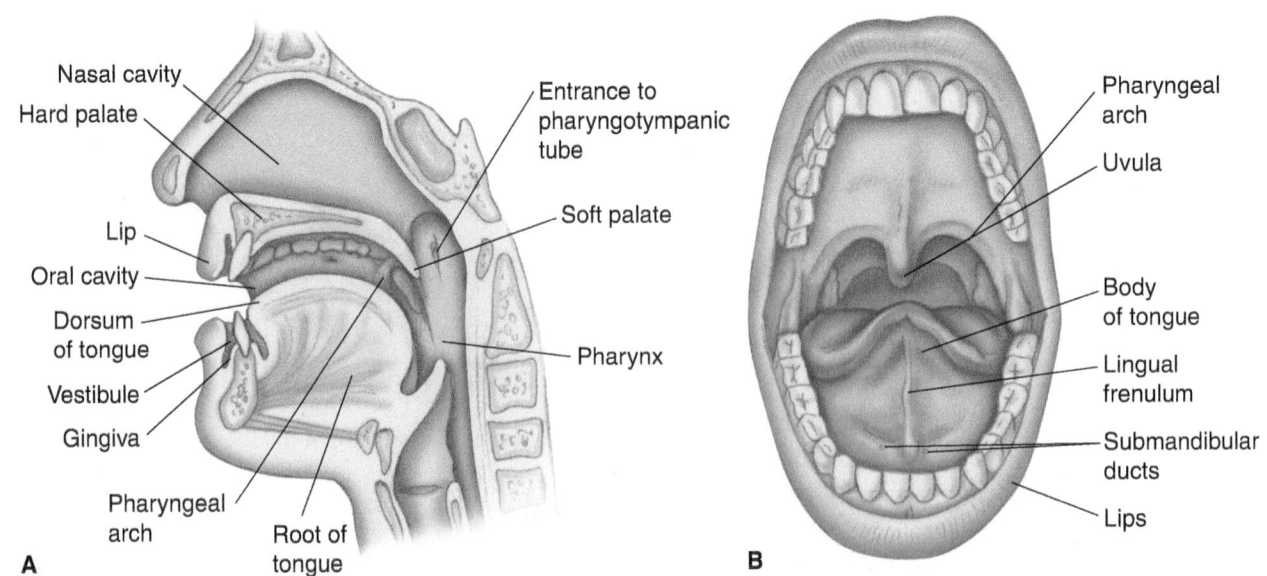

FIGURE 29-2 The oral cavity: **(A)** sagittal section; **(B)** anterior view as seen through the open mouth.

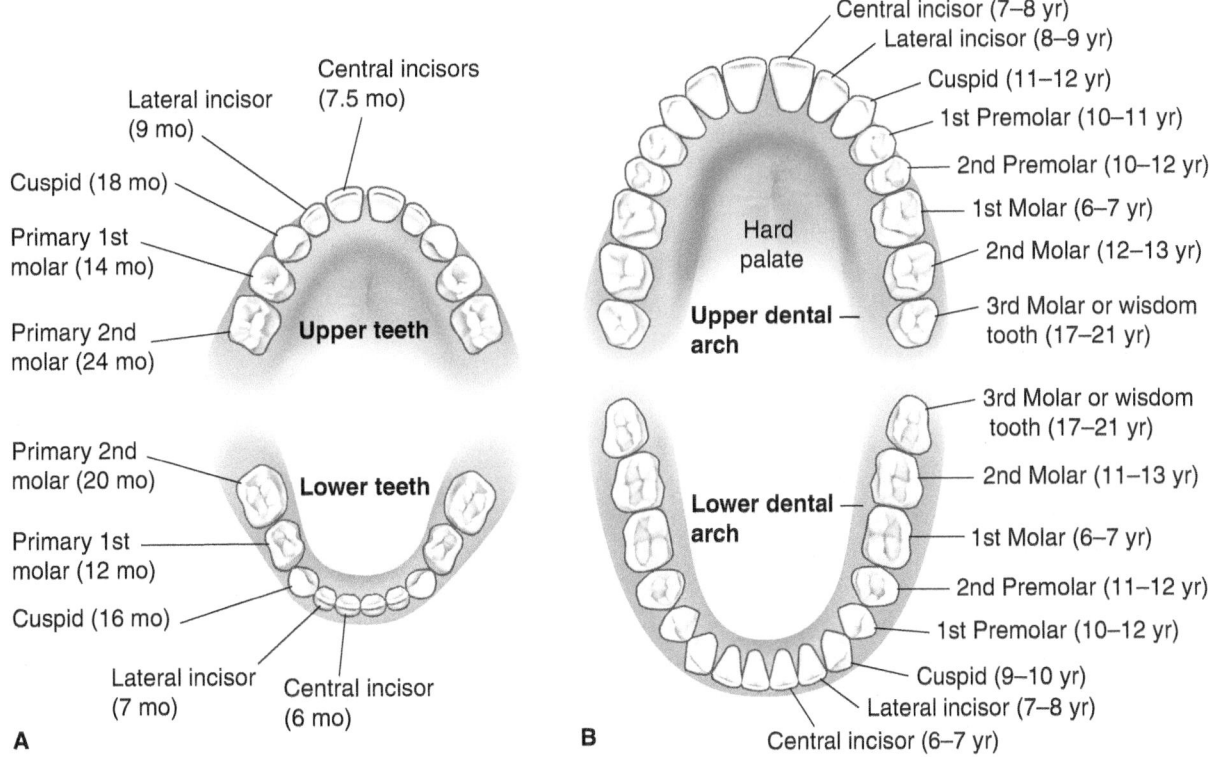

Figure labels (A) - deciduous teeth:

Upper teeth
- Central incisors (7.5 mo)
- Lateral incisor (9 mo)
- Cuspid (18 mo)
- Primary 1st molar (14 mo)
- Primary 2nd molar (24 mo)

Lower teeth
- Primary 2nd molar (20 mo)
- Primary 1st molar (12 mo)
- Cuspid (16 mo)
- Lateral incisor (7 mo)
- Central incisor (6 mo)

Figure labels (B) - permanent teeth:

Upper dental arch
- Central incisor (7–8 yr)
- Lateral incisor (8–9 yr)
- Cuspid (11–12 yr)
- 1st Premolar (10–11 yr)
- 2nd Premolar (10–12 yr)
- 1st Molar (6–7 yr)
- 2nd Molar (12–13 yr)
- 3rd Molar or wisdom tooth (17–21 yr)
- Hard palate

Lower dental arch
- 3rd Molar or wisdom tooth (17–21 yr)
- 2nd Molar (11–13 yr)
- 1st Molar (6–7 yr)
- 2nd Premolar (11–12 yr)
- 1st Premolar (10–12 yr)
- Cuspid (9–10 yr)
- Lateral incisor (7–8 yr)
- Central incisor (6–7 yr)

A   **B**

FIGURE 29-3 Deciduous and permanent teeth: **(A)** deciduous teeth, with the age at eruption given in months; **(B)** permanent teeth, with the age at eruption given in years.

8 incisors, 4 canines (cuspids), and 8 molars. The permanent teeth include 8 incisors, 4 canines, 8 premolars, and 12 molars. The teeth are contained in two dental arches, the superior arch (upper teeth) and the inferior arch (lower teeth). The permanent teeth can be differentiated as follows:

- The incisors are the four front teeth of each dental arch. They have a sharp, cutting edge, used for biting into food. The upper incisors are larger and stronger than the lower ones.

- The canine teeth, or cuspids, have roots that reach deep into the bones of the jaw. The upper canines are also known as the *eye teeth* and are larger than the lower canines. The lower canines are often called the *stomach teeth*.

- The premolar teeth are behind the canine teeth. Also known as *bicuspid teeth*, they are smaller and shorter than the canines. There are four premolars in each arch.

- The molar teeth are the largest teeth in the permanent set and are adapted to grinding and pounding food. An adult has 12 molars, 6 in each arch, posterior to the premolars.

Each tooth consists of three main parts: the crown (the part above the gum); the root (embedded in the gums); and the neck, the portion between the root and the crown (Figure 29-4).

The solid portion of the tooth consists of the following:

- **Dentin**—Calcified, largely mineral tissue that forms the bulk of the tooth

- **Enamel**—Hardest and most compact part of the tooth; covers the exposed part of the crown

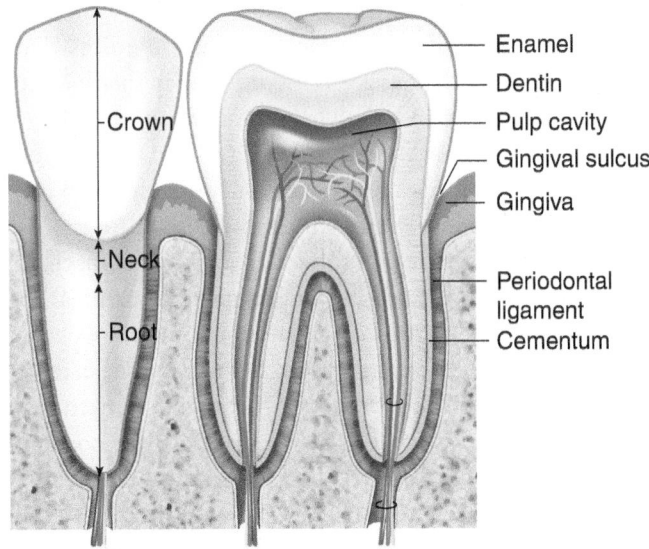

Figure 29-4 labels:
- Crown
- Neck
- Root
- Enamel
- Dentin
- Pulp cavity
- Gingival sulcus
- Gingiva
- Periodontal ligament
- Cementum

FIGURE 29-4 A diagrammatic section through a typical adult tooth.

- **Cementum**—Thin layer of bone that covers the dentin of the root, providing protection and anchoring to the periodontal ligament

The teeth are bound to the bony sockets in the maxillary (upper) and mandible (lower) jawbones by fibers of the periodontal ligament. Deciduous teeth, and then permanent teeth, erupt through the gums during childhood when they are sufficiently calcified to tolerate the stress they will be subjected to later. Review Figure 29-3 and the stages of tooth eruption.

Pharynx

The **pharynx** lies posterior to the mouth and is the beginning of the tubal component of the digestive tract that leads to the stomach. The pharynx is considered to be a part of both the respiratory and the digestive systems because both air and food pass through the pharynx. Once food is swallowed, the bolus, by reflex, passes through the pharynx into the esophagus. The muscular contractions that move the bolus of food into the esophagus also close the larynx to prevent food from entering the trachea, which leads to the bronchi and lungs.

Esophagus

The **esophagus** is a collapsible tube about 10 inches long that starts at the pharynx and ends at the stomach. Food and liquids are carried down the esophagus by the involuntary muscular contractions known as **peristalsis**. These wavelike contractions will continue to move the bolus of food through the entire digestive system.

Stomach

The **stomach** is a large, muscular, saclike organ that can hold 1 to 1.5 liters of food and fluid. Digestion, which began in the mouth, continues in the stomach (Figure 29-5). The stomach secretes hydrochloric acid and gastric juices that convert food into **chyme**, a semiliquid that is then passed into the small intestine for further digestion.

The fundus of the stomach is the upper-rounded portion of the organ. Here, undigested food is stored for up to one hour. The inside of the stomach has **rugae** (also called gastric folds) that allow the inside surface area of the stomach to expand as food is ingested. Two important structures, each a ring of muscle that allows food and liquid to enter or exit the stomach, are the cardiac and pyloric sphincters. The **cardiac sphincter** sits at the superior (upper) part of the stomach just below the esophagus. It opens and closes, allowing food and liquid to enter the stomach. Its counterpart, the **pyloric sphincter**, is situated at the inferior (lower) part near the entrance to the small intestine and facilitates passage of food and liquid out of the stomach.

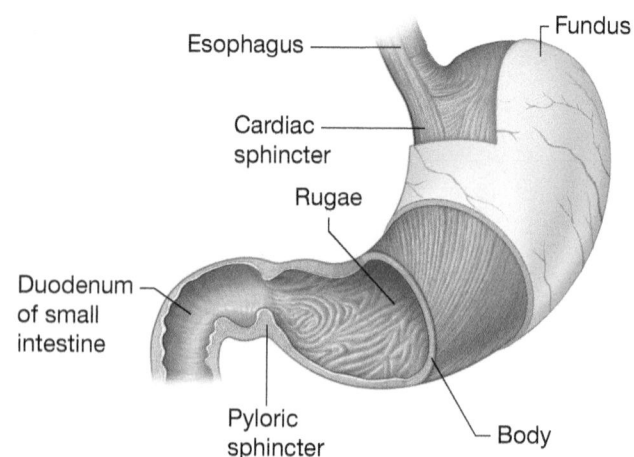

FIGURE 29-5 Stomach.

Small Intestine

The **small intestine** is 21 feet long and about 1 inch in diameter, coiled within the lower abdomen (Figure 29-6). The first 12 inches of the small intestine constitute the duodenum, the next 8 feet of the small intestine make up the jejunum, and the last 12 feet are the ileum.

Digestion continues as the chyme from the stomach enters the small intestine, where it begins to mix with bile secreted by the liver and gallbladder and pancreatic juices secreted by the pancreas.

During this time, nutrient absorption takes place. The microscopic capillaries and lymph vessels that line the walls of the small intestine absorb the nutrients and send them to

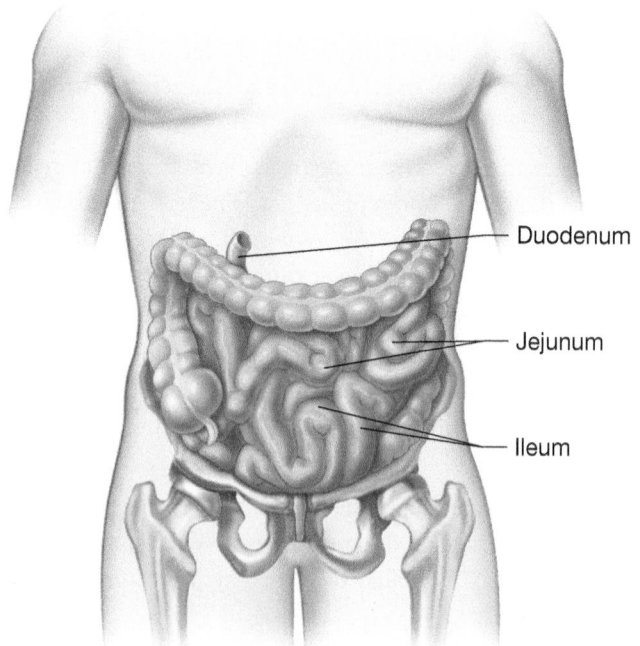

FIGURE 29-6 Small intestine.

the rest of the body's cells by way of the circulatory (cardio-vascular and lymphatic) system.

Large Intestine

The small intestine ends at the ileocecal orifice of the large intestine. At that point, the ileocecal valve connects the ileum of the small intestine to the cecum of the large intestine.

The **large intestine** is about 5 feet long and 2.5 inches in diameter. The functions of the large intestine are to complete digestion and absorption.

The large intestine can be divided into several parts (Figure 29-7):

- The **cecum** is a small pouch about 3 inches long that forms the beginning of the large intestine. It receives fecal (solid) material from the small intestine.

- The **appendix** is a small appendage of the large intestine, attached to the cecum, which is not involved with digestion. In fact, its function in humans, if any, is unknown.

- The **colon** makes up the bulk of the large intestine and is divided into the ascending colon (moves upward on the right side of the abdomen), the transverse colon (moves across the body transversely from right to left), the descending colon (moves downward on the left side of the abdomen), and the sigmoid colon, which leads to the rectum.

- The waste products of digestion are eliminated from the body via the **rectum** (the final portion of the large intestine) and the anus (the external opening of the rectum).

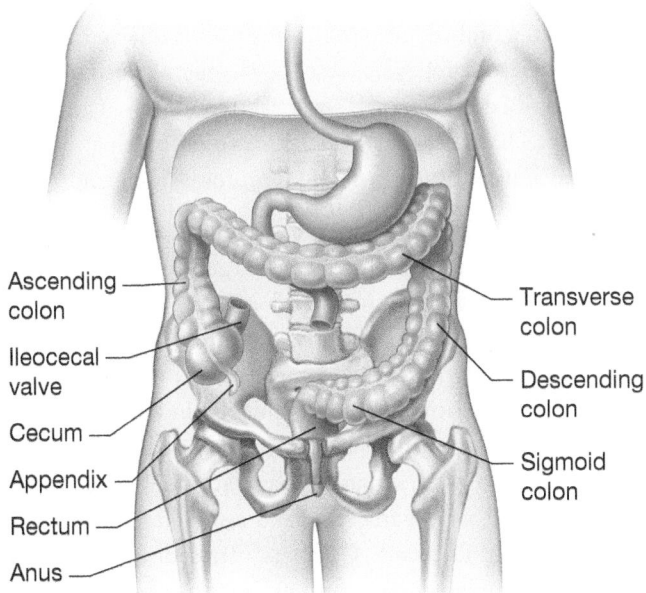

FIGURE 29-7 Large intestine.

Accessory Organs of Digestion

The accessory organs that are important in the role of digestion are the salivary glands, the liver, the gallbladder, and the pancreas (see Figure 29-8). They are not part of the digestive tract but perform functions closely related to it.

Salivary Glands

The **salivary glands** are located in and near the mouth. Saliva is produced by a neurological response to the sight, smell, taste, or mental image of food. There are three pairs of salivary glands. The parotid glands are located on either side of the face, just below the ear. The submandibular glands are located in the floor of the mouth. The sublingual glands are located below the tongue, forward of the submandibular glands. All these glands secrete saliva through ducts (openings) into the mouth. Saliva contains the digestive enzyme amylase, which was discussed earlier in the chapter.

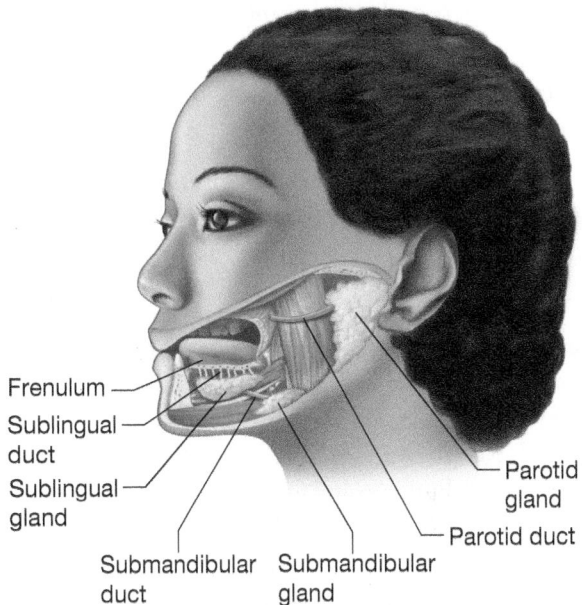

A

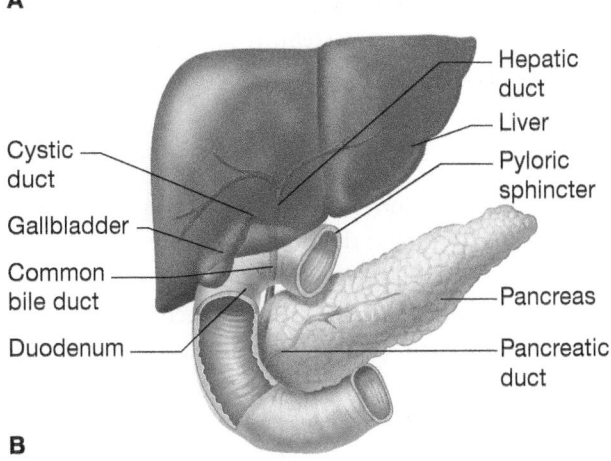

B

FIGURE 29-8 **(A)** Salivary glands; **(B)** gallbladder, liver, and pancreas.

Liver

The **liver** is located in the upper-right quadrant of the abdomen. It is the largest glandular organ and weighs about 3.5 pounds in a healthy, average adult. The liver plays an essential role in the metabolism of carbohydrates, fats, and proteins. In carbohydrate metabolism, it changes glucose to glycogen and stores it for future use (energy the body will need) by the body's cells. To metabolize fat, the liver produces bile, which emulsifies fats (breaks them down into smaller particles to make them more digestible by digestive enzymes) before releasing the products into the bloodstream. In protein metabolism, the liver stores the components of proteins so the body can break down or build up proteins as required.

The liver produces four substances important for body functioning:

- **Bile**—Digestive juice that emulsifies fats
- **Fibrinogen and prothrombin**—Essential for blood clotting
- **Heparin**—Prevents the clotting of blood
- **Blood proteins**—Albumin, gamma globulin

The liver also stores iron and vitamins B_{12}, A, D, E, and K. It produces body heat and detoxifies substances that are potentially harmful to the body, such as drugs and alcohol.

Gallbladder

The **gallbladder** is a membranous sac in which bile is stored and concentrated. Bile stored in the gallbladder is six to ten times more concentrated than bile produced by the liver. Because of its high concentration in the gallbladder, components of bile can build up and form gallstones, possibly causing the gallbladder to become inflamed. (The presence of gallstones in the gallbladder is called **cholelithiasis**.) The removal of the gallbladder is a procedure termed cholecystectomy. Even though the gallbladder is a functioning component of the digestive system, it is not essential and its removal does not usually cause an interruption in the digestive process.

Pancreas

The **pancreas** is an elongated gland, 6 to 9 inches in length, which is situated behind the stomach and secretes pancreatic juice into the small intestine. It contains cells that produce digestive enzymes. It also has cells that secrete the hormones insulin and glucagon, which lower and raise glucose levels in the blood. Because the pancreas produces both digestive enzymes and hormones, it is considered to be a structure of both the digestive and endocrine systems.

COMMON PATHOLOGY ASSOCIATED WITH THE DIGESTIVE SYSTEM

Digestive disorders range from the nonserious, such as the occasional upset stomach, heartburn, or nausea, to the serious and life-threatening, such as colorectal cancer. These disorders involve the gastrointestinal tract as well as the liver, gallbladder, and pancreas. Most digestive disorders and diseases are complex, with subtle symptoms and often unknown causes (see Table 29-2). Some may be genetic or develop from multiple factors such as stress, fatigue, diet, smoking, and alcohol abuse. A thorough medical history and physical examination are crucial for accurate diagnosis. More extensive diagnostic evaluations may be necessary, including laboratory tests, endoscopic procedures, and imaging techniques. Table 29-3 highlights common procedures and tests related to the digestive system.

Appendicitis

Appendicitis is an inflammation of the appendix. The cause of appendicitis is linked to blockage within the appendix, which restricts blood flow and increases pressure. Blockage can occur as a result of fecal obstruction or infections of the digestive system, which cause lymph nodes near the appendix to enlarge, resulting in constriction of the appendix. Anyone can get appendicitis, but it occurs most often between the ages of 10 and 30. The appendix has no known function, and its removal does not seem to cause a change in digestive function.

Signs and Symptoms. Acute pain at the McBurney point (Figure 29-9) on the abdomen is the key symptom. This point is located on the right side of the abdomen, approximately a third of the distance between the right iliac crest (hip) and the umbilicus (navel). This pain is relieved by over-the-counter pain relievers, rest, or change of position. It is often described as sharp and severe and can lead to nausea and vomiting. Diarrhea, abdominal bloating, constipation, and low-grade fever are also possible symptoms of appendicitis.

Treatment. Because there is no effective medical therapy, appendicitis is considered a medical emergency. When a patient arrives in the emergency room and appendicitis is suspected, an appendectomy (removal of the appendix) is almost always performed as it is the only treatment option for appendicitis. Although most patients recover quickly and without problems when treated early, delay in treatment can result in the appendix becoming so inflamed that it ruptures. This leads to severe pain and serious infection and can be fatal. Diagnostic tests including bloodwork, CT scans, ultrasound, and urinalysis may be completed to confirm a diagnosis of appendicitis.

TABLE 29-2 | Disorders and Diseases of the Digestive System

Disorder/Pathology	Description
Anorexia	Loss of appetite that can accompany other conditions such as a gastrointestinal (GI) upset.
Ascites	Collection or accumulation of fluid in the peritoneal cavity.
Bulimia	Eating disorder that is characterized by recurrent binge eating followed by purging of the food with laxatives and vomiting.
Cholecystitis	Inflammation of the gallbladder.
Cholelithiasis	Formation or presence of stones, or calculi, in the gallbladder or common bile duct.
Constipation	Difficult or infrequent defecation; generally two or fewer bowel movements a week at least 25 percent of the time.
Diarrhea	Passing of frequent, watery bowel movements; usually accompanies gastrointestinal (GI) disorders.
Dyspepsia	Indigestion.
Emesis	Vomiting, usually with some force.
Enteritis	Inflammation of only the small intestine.
Esophageal Stricture	Narrowing of the esophagus that makes the flow of foods and fluids difficult.
Fissure	Crack-like split in the rectum or anal canal or roof of mouth.
Fistula	Abnormal tubelike passage from one body cavity to another, or between an organ and the exterior of the body.
Gastritis	Inflammation of the stomach, which can result in pain, tenderness, nausea, and vomiting.
Gastroenteritis	Inflammation of the stomach and small intestine.
Halitosis	Bad or offensive breath, which is often a sign of disease.
Hepatitis	Inflammation of the liver.
Ileitis	Inflammation of the ileum of the small intestine.
Inflammatory Bowel Disease	Ulceration, of unknown origin, of the mucous membranes of the colon; also known as ulcerative colitis.
Intussusception	Result of the intestine slipping or telescoping into another section of intestine just below it; more common in children.
Malabsorption Syndrome	Inadequate absorption of nutrients from the intestinal tract; may be caused by a variety of diseases and disorders, such as infections and pancreatic deficiency.
Peptic Ulcer	Ulcer occurring in the lower portion of the esophagus, stomach, or duodenum thought to be caused by the acid of gastric juices; some now successfully treated with antibiotics.
Pilonidal Cyst	Cyst in the sacrococcygeal region caused by tissue being trapped below the skin.
Polyphagia	Eating excessively.
Polyps	Small tumors that contain a pedicle, or foot-like attachment, in the mucous membranes of the large intestine (colon).
Reflux Esophagitis	Acid from the stomach backing up into the esophagus, causing inflammation and pain.
Regurgitation	Return of fluids and solids from the stomach into the mouth; similar to emesis but without the force.
Volvulus	Condition in which the bowel twists on itself and causes an obstruction; painful and requires immediate surgery.

Procedure/Test	Description
Abdominal Ultrasonography	Ultrasound equipment produces sound waves used to create an image of the abdominal organs.
Air-contrast Barium Enema	Using both barium and air to visualize the colon on X-ray.
Anastomosis	Creating a passageway or opening between two organs or vessels.
Appendectomy	Surgical removal of the appendix.
Barium Enema (Lower GI)	Radiographic examination of the small intestine, large intestine, or colon, in which an enema containing barium is administered to the patient while X-ray pictures are taken.
Barium Swallow (Upper GI)	Barium mixture swallowed while X-ray pictures are taken of the esophagus, stomach, and duodenum. It is used to visualize the upper GI tract. Also called esophagram.
Cholecystectomy	Surgical excision of the gallbladder. Removal of the gallbladder through the laparoscope is most commonly performed, because it has fewer complications than the more invasive abdominal surgery. The laparoscope requires small incisions that are made in the abdominal cavity.
Cholecystogram	Radiopaque contrast given, via the oral route, to the patient that is absorbed and enters the gallbladder. An X-ray is then taken showing the dye contrast.
Choledocholithotomy	Removal of a gallstone through an incision into the bile duct.
Choledocholithotripsy	Crushing of a gallstone in the common bile duct. Commonly called lithotripsy.
Colectomy	Surgical removal of the entire colon.
Colonoscopy	Flexible fiberscope passed through the anus, rectum, and colon is used to examine the upper portion of the colon. Polyps and small growths can be removed during the procedure.
Colostomy	Surgical creation of an opening in a portion of the colon through the abdominal wall to the outside surface.
Diverticulectomy	Surgical removal of a diverticulum.
Endoscopic Retrograde Cholangiopancreatography (ERCP)	Use of an endoscope to X-ray the bile and pancreatic ducts.
Esophagogastrostomy	Surgical connection (anastomosis) of the esophagus and stomach.
Esophagoscopy	The esophagus is visualized by passing a flexible tube down the esophagus. A tissue sample for biopsy may be obtained.
Esophagostomy	Surgical creation of an opening into the esophagus.
Esophagram	As barium is swallowed, the solution is observed (via X-ray) traveling from the mouth into the stomach. Also called a barium swallow.
Exploratory Laparotomy	Abdominal operation for the purpose of examining the abdominal organs and tissues for signs of disease or other abnormalities.
Fistulectomy	Excision of a fistula.
Gastrectomy	Surgical removal of part or all of the stomach.
Gastric Lavage	A sample of gastric contents is obtained by insertion of an orogastric tube through the mouth and into the stomach.
Gastrointestinal Endoscopy	A flexible instrument or scope is passed either through the mouth or anus to facilitate visualization of the GI tract.
Glossectomy	Complete or partial removal of the tongue.
Hemorrhoidectomy	Surgical excision of hemorrhoids from the anorectal area.
Hepatic Lobectomy	Surgical excision of a lobe of the liver.
Ileostomy	Surgical creation of a passageway through the abdominal wall into the ileum. The fecal matter (stool) drains into a bag worn on the abdomen.

TABLE 29-3 | Procedures and Diagnostic Tests Related to the Digestive System (*continued*)

Procedure/Test	Description
Intravenous Cholangiogram	A dye administered to the patient allows for visualization of the bile vessels.
Intravenous Cholecystograph	A dye administered intravenously to the patient allows for visualization of the gallbladder.
Jejunostomy	Surgical creation of a permanent opening into the jejunum.
Lithotripsy	Crushing of a stone located within the gallbladder.
Liver Biopsy	Excision of a small piece of liver tissue for microscopic examination. This is generally used to determine if cancer is present.
Liver Scan	A radioactive substance is administered intravenously to the patient. This substance enters liver cells, and the organ can then be visualized to detect tumors, abscesses, and other liver conditions.
Occult Blood	Test performed on feces to determine the presence of invisible amounts of blood. Positive results may indicate gastrointestinal bleeding.
Ova and Parasites	Test performed on stool to identify ova and parasites. A positive result indicates protozoa infestation.
Proctoplasty	Plastic surgery of the anus and rectum.
Splenectomy	Surgical removal of the spleen.
Stool Culture	Test performed on stool to identify the presence of microorganisms.
Ultrasonography, Gallbladder	Test to visualize the gallbladder by using high-frequency sound waves. It is often used to detect gallbladder inflammation, biliary obstructions, or gallstones.
Ultrasonography, Liver	Test to visualize the liver by using high-frequency sound waves. It is used to detect hepatic tumors, cysts, abscesses, and cirrhosis.
Upper Gastrointestinal Fiberscopy	Direct visualization of the gastric mucosa via flexible fiberscope. Used to detect gastric neoplasm.
Vagotomy	Surgical resection of the vagus nerve in an attempt to decrease the amount of acid secretion into the stomach. This may be used as a treatment for ulcer patients.

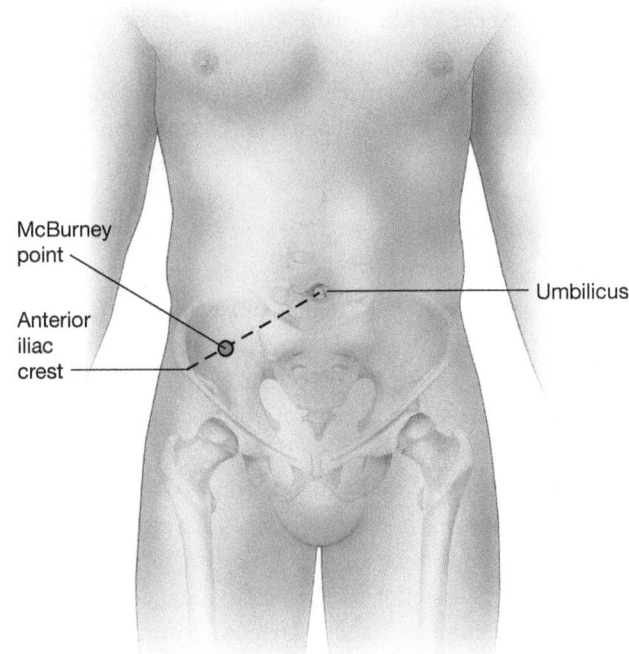

FIGURE 29-9 McBurney point.

Cirrhosis

Cirrhosis is a disease marked by scarring of the tissues of the liver. The scarring is damaging and, in fact, can be life-threatening. When the liver has been in a state of inflammation for an extended period of time (often years), scarring begins to replace healthy liver tissue. This prevents the liver from functioning at its normal capacity.

Multiple factors lead to the inflammation and scarring associated with cirrhosis. In the United States, the major causes of cirrhosis are years of excessive alcohol consumption and certain forms of viral hepatitis (mainly hepatitis B or C). Nonalcoholic fatty liver disease (NAFLD) is a type of cirrhosis caused by excessive amounts of fat stored in the liver. This form of cirrhosis is common in obese patients. Inflammation and blockage of the ducts that transport bile out of the liver is also a cause of cirrhosis that may be related to a problem with the immune system. Autoimmune hepatitis results when the immune system attacks the liver. Sometimes cirrhosis can be caused by an inherited disease, such as cystic fibrosis.

The Child

- Infants may suffer from digestive system disorders including GERD and pyloric stenosis. It is also common for infants and toddlers to have bouts of vomiting and diarrhea. Because of their smaller size, dehydration is more likely to occur during times of illness. Infants, toddlers, and children should be closely monitored and encouraged to increase fluid intake as a precaution. Pedialyte and other electrolyte replacement drinks may be beneficial to prevent dehydration.
- Teeth eruption occurs during infancy, often causing irritability, painful gums, and ear pain.
- Proper nutrition and a healthy diet should be implemented as soon as an infant begins to eat solid foods. This will promote proper growth and enable the digestive system, as well as other bodily systems, to function optimally.

The Older Adult

- Peristalsis becomes weaker and is less effective as the digestive system ages. This causes the movement of food and waste throughout the digestive tract to slow.
- Aging of the teeth and gums, resulting from continual use throughout life, causes tooth surfaces to weaken and wear down. Gums also begin to recede. Periodontal disease is more common among older adults, and some require complete tooth extraction and replacement dentures. Approximately 25 percent of adults aged 60 and older wear full dentures.
- Changes in taste and food preferences are also common as an individual ages. This, along with slowed gastric motor activity, can lead to loss of appetite and decreased fluid intake, which often results in constipation.
- Increased age is also a risk factor for various digestive system diseases and disorders such as cancers, hernias, diverticulosis, and diverticulitis.

Signs and Symptoms. In many cases, signs and symptoms develop only after the disease has progressed. They include fluid buildup in the legs (edema) and abdomen (ascites), fatigue, yellowing of the skin (jaundice), itching, nosebleeds, redness of the palms, easy bruising, weight loss and muscle loss, abdominal pain, frequent infections, and confusion.

Treatment. The patient with cirrhosis must avoid substances that can further damage the liver, especially alcohol and nonsteroidal antiinflammatory drugs. Treatment may also include dietary changes, including a low-fat and low-sodium diet to promote weight loss. Treatment of any underlying conditions (such as hepatitis or alcoholism) is necessary to prevent the progression of the disease. A liver transplant may be considered when liver damage is severe.

Colitis

Colitis is an inflammation of the large intestine. Many disease processes may cause colitis, including acute and chronic infections, primary inflammatory disorders (ulcerative colitis or Crohn's disease), impaired blood flow (ischemic colitis), and history of radiation exposure to the large bowel.

Signs and Symptoms. Signs and symptoms can include abdominal pain, diarrhea, dehydration, fever and chills, abdominal bloating, increased intestinal gas, and bloody stools. Another common symptom is the constant urge to have a bowel movement, a condition known as tenesmus. The disorder may be identified by flexible sigmoidoscopy or colonoscopy. In both tests, a flexible tube is inserted into the rectum and used to evaluate specific areas of the colon. Biopsies taken during these tests may show changes related to inflammation. Other studies, such as barium enema, abdominal CT scan, abdominal MRI, and abdominal X-ray, may be used to identify colitis.

Treatment. Treatment of colitis is directed at treating the underlying cause—infection, inflammation, lack of blood flow, or another cause. When the underlying cause is identified and treated, the symptoms of colitis should begin to lessen and resolve.

Colorectal Cancer

Colorectal cancer is the second-leading cause of cancer-related deaths of both men and women in the United States after lung cancer. When colon and rectal cancer occur together, it is referred to as **colorectal cancer**. When cancer attacks any portion of the large intestine, it is termed colon cancer. If the last 8 to 10 inches of the colon (the rectum) are diseased, it is termed rectal cancer.

Most cases of colon cancer develop when the cells of benign polyps (often called adenomatous polyps) mutate and become cancerous. There isn't an exact known cause related to how or why a person develops the cancerous mutations, though there are a few forms of colon cancer that have genetic ties.

The likelihood of developing colorectal cancer increases with age. Other predisposing factors include a history of inflammatory bowel disease (Crohn's disease or ulcerative colitis), type 2 diabetes, a family history of colorectal cancer, and race and ethnicity, particularly African American or Ashkenazi (Jews of Central or Eastern European descent).

Signs and Symptoms. Because the polyps are small and produce few if any symptoms, regular screening tests are important to help prevent undetected progression to end-stage cancer. If signs and symptoms of cancer do appear, they may include a change in bowel habits, rectal bleeding, bloody stools, long and thin stool, persistent abdominal cramping, gas, abdominal pain, appetite loss and weight loss, and excessive fatigue. Screening tests and dietary changes such as increasing fiber-rich foods and limiting the amount of red meat and processed meats consumed can reduce the risk of developing colon cancer. Lifestyle changes such as increasing physical activity, reducing alcohol consumption, and smoking cessation can also dramatically reduce a person's overall risk of developing colon cancer.

Treatment. The three primary treatment options are surgery, chemotherapy, and radiation. The physician will decide on a treatment based on the stage, size, and location of the cancerous tumor. Surgery is the main treatment for colorectal cancer. The amount of the colon that is removed is determined by the extent to which the cancer has penetrated the wall of the colon and whether it has spread to the lymph nodes or other parts of the body. This information will also determine if chemotherapy or radiation treatments should also be considered. If part of the colon is removed, sometimes the remaining colon is brought to the surface of the abdomen so stool comes out of a colostomy (a stoma, or opening created in the abdominal wall) into an attached receptacle instead of through the rectum. Preventative measures to detect early stages of colon cancer include routine colonoscopy screenings for both men and women after the age of 50.

Crohn's Disease and Ulcerative Colitis

Crohn's disease is a chronic inflammatory disease of the intestines. Usually it causes painful inflammation and ulcerations in both the small and large intestines. However, ulcerations can occur anywhere along the digestive tract from mouth to anus. **Ulcerative colitis** is closely linked to Crohn's disease; however, it affects only the colon. These two conditions, when linked together, are known as inflammatory bowel disease. About 1.4 million Americans suffer from these conditions.

Crohn's disease is not contagious, and the exact cause is unknown. Crohn's disease may have a genetic component, because it tends to be more common in patients within the same family. Crohn's disease also may be caused by environmental factors. Overall, it is classified as an autoimmune disorder because the body attacks the normal and healthy cells of the gastrointestinal tract.

Signs and Symptoms. Common symptoms and signs of Crohn's disease include abdominal pain, urgency and pain with defecation, rectal bleeding, bloody or watery diarrhea, decreased appetite, and weight loss. Patients with Crohn's disease typically experience periods of relapse (worsening of inflammation) followed by periods of remission (reduced inflammation) lasting months to years.

Treatment. There is no cure for Crohn's disease. The goals of treatment are to induce remission, maintain remission, minimize side effects of treatment, and improve quality of life. A large focus is placed on eating a healthy and balanced diet and drinking plenty of fluids as well as limiting dairy products and avoiding high-fiber and high-fat foods, which impact bowel movements. Patients with mild symptoms or whose disease is in remission (symptoms are absent) may not need treatment. Treatment of both Crohn's disease and ulcerative colitis with medications is similar, although not always identical. These medications may include antiinflammatory agents, corticosteroids, antibiotics, and immunomodulators, which are used to weaken the immune system to reduce the severity of autoimmune response. Severe Crohn's disease may lead to a colostomy, either permanently or temporarily. A temporary colostomy bag may be used to allow the colon to rest and heal during times of severe inflammation when recuperation is anticipated.

Diverticulosis and Diverticulitis

Diverticulosis is the condition of having diverticula, small pouches or sacs in the wall of the colon (Figure 29-10). The sigmoid colon is typically where diverticulosis appears. This S-shaped portion of the colon lies in the lower left portion of the abdomen. Diverticulosis is more likely to occur when

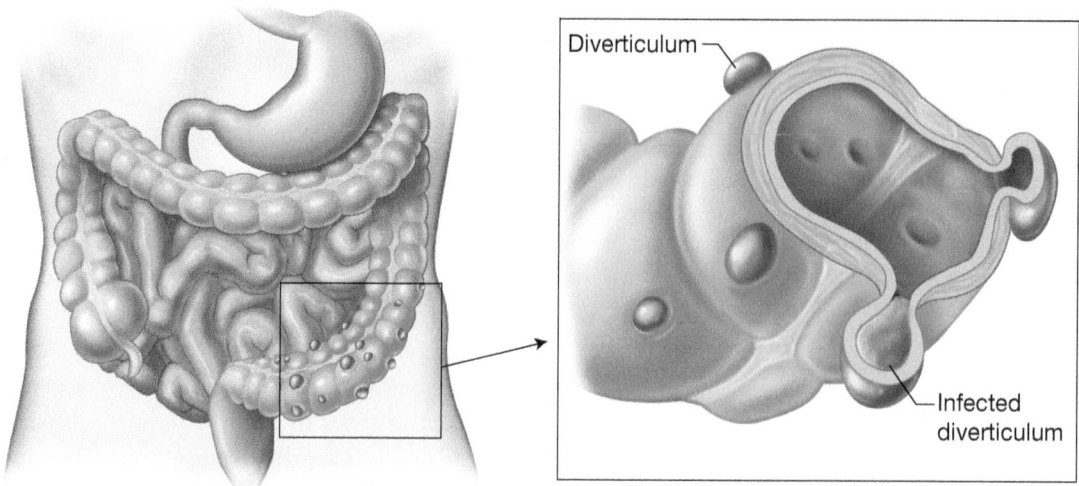

FIGURE 29-10 Colon with diverticulosis. An inflamed or infected diverticulum is called diverticulitis.

the walls of the colon weaken, which naturally happens as a person ages. Constipation as well as the action of trying to push and expel hardened and dry stool causes elevated pressure within the walls of the colon, also resulting in the formation of diverticula.

Diverticulitis is an inflammation or infection of the diverticula. The exact cause of diverticulitis is not known, but the inflammation generally begins when stool becomes stuck within a diverticulum and bacteria form. Infection can lead to complications such as swelling or rupture.

Signs and Symptoms. Most patients with diverticulosis have few or no symptoms; mild symptoms include abdominal cramping and bloating. Signs and symptoms of diverticulitis include pain, fever, chills, cramping, bloating, decreased appetite, constipation, and diarrhea. It is not uncommon for these symptoms to appear suddenly.

Treatment. Preventing the formation of diverticula in the colon is optimal. This can be helped by eating a high-fiber diet, which can help maintain regular bowel habits. Treatment of diverticulitis depends on the severity of the condition and the symptoms. Minor symptoms may be treated with rest and increased fluid intake; the application of heat (as with a heating pad) can also be of comfort. Antibiotics may also be prescribed to treat infection. In serious cases, hospitalization and surgery may be necessary.

Gastroesophageal Reflux Disease

Gastroesophageal reflux disease (GERD) occurs when the cardiac sphincter, sometimes referred to as the lower esophageal sphincter, does not close completely or tightly or when it relaxes. Without proper closure of the sphincter stomach contents, including gastric fluids, move back up into the

esophagus, an action is called reflux. The acidic fluids found in the stomach are very harsh and can be damaging when refluxed into the esophagus, causing inflammation and a condition known as reflux esophagitis.

When not treated, GERD can lead to a variety of other serious conditions, including:

- Barrett's esophagitis, which is a known to be a precancerous condition
- Perforation (tearing) of the esophagus
- Esophageal stricture (abnormal narrowing of the esophagus)
- Esophageal ulcers
- Esophageal cancer

Risk factors for developing GERD include obesity, hiatal hernia (protrusion of part of the stomach into the thorax through a tear in the diaphragm), pregnancy, and smoking. GERD can also be triggered or made worse by many types of prescription medications and over-the-counter pain medications.

Signs and Symptoms. Symptoms include heartburn that is worse when lying down, bending over, and during the night; sore throat; a hoarse voice; a bad taste in the mouth; a sensation of food being stuck behind the breast bone; belching; and regurgitation of food. Some patients with mild cases of GERD are symptom free.

Treatment. Treatment of GERD relies on medications that block the production of hydrochloric acid (the chief digestive acid) and protect the mucosa of the esophagus. Patients may incorporate simple measures such as avoiding foods that cause symptoms, not lying down until at least three hours after eating, losing weight, and sleeping on a bed with the head elevated 6 inches. Over-the-counter antacids may also provide comfort, although only temporarily. If medications and basic treatments do not work, fundoplication, a surgical procedure that tightens the cardiac sphincter and its surrounding tissues, can be performed. Strictures that may result from GERD are treated with dilation, or expansion, of the narrowed area.

Hemorrhoids

A **hemorrhoid** is a dilated, or enlarged, vein in the walls of the anus and sometimes the rectum. Hemorrhoids are sometimes called piles. They are caused by increased pressure in the anus usually because of untreated constipation, but occasionally it is associated with chronic diarrhea. Hemorrhoids are also common after a woman gives birth because of the increased pressure associated with pushing the baby out of the birth canal.

Signs and Symptoms. The major sign is bleeding after defecation, particularly bright red blood on toilet tissue or in the toilet bowl. Itching and pain in the anal region are also common and can be worse with prolonged periods of sitting. If untreated, hemorrhoids can worsen and protrude from the anus. Fissures (cracks or tears in the wall of the rectum) may develop and cause intense discomfort.

Treatment. Treatment is aimed at changing the diet to prevent constipation and avoid further irritation. A patient who is constipated should be instructed to increase fluid intake; increase fiber in the diet; avoid problematic foods such as milk, cheese, and other dairy products; and increase the level of exercise, including walking. The patient should be instructed not to ignore the urge to defecate but to respond in a timely manner, as well as to establish and maintain a daily

routine for defecation. Stool softeners may be used to decrease episodes of constipation. Topical hemorrhoid creams help relieve discomfort from itching and irritation, and corticosteroid creams help reduce swelling and inflammation. Hemorrhoid removal (hemorrhoidectomy) is performed when the patient is in extreme discomfort or has excessive bleeding.

Hernia

A **hernia** is the abnormal protrusion of an organ or part of an organ through a weakness in the wall of the body cavity that contains it. The most common types of abdominal hernias are hiatal hernias and inguinal hernias.

Hiatal Hernia

A **hiatal hernia** develops when a part of the stomach (the upper portion) pushes upward and enters the chest cavity through a weakened esophageal hiatus (an opening in the diaphragm) (Figure 29-11).

The actual hernia is caused, as just mentioned, by a weakened esophageal hiatus, but there are risk factors associated with developing this condition. These include obesity, slouching (poor posture when seated), frequent coughing, straining with constipation, frequent bending over or heavy lifting, heredity, smoking, and congenital defects.

Signs and Symptoms. Some patients with hiatal hernia are asymptomatic. For others, symptoms and signs include belching and hiccups, chest pain or pressure, difficulty swallowing, and coughing. It is common to have both a hiatal hernia and GERD (discussed previously). The reason why hiatal hernia and GERD often occur together is thought to be that the hernia contributes to the weakening of the cardiac sphincter muscle, which in turn allows the reflux of stomach contents into the esophagus. When patients have both of these conditions, heartburn is a very common symptom.

Treatment. Medications used to treat acid reflux are helpful in reducing symptoms caused by excessive gastric acid. Activity changes to reduce symptoms that are suggested include refraining from lifting heavy objects, improving posture, increasing exercise, losing excess weight, and trying to incorporate activity after a meal rather than reclining or lying down. It is also helpful to incorporate dietary restrictions including avoiding chocolate, caffeine, alcohol, and fatty foods. The only cure for a hernia is surgical repair.

Inguinal Hernia

An **inguinal hernia** occurs at a weakened spot on the abdominal wall or groin that allows a portion of the intestine or tissue to push through, causing a round lump, or

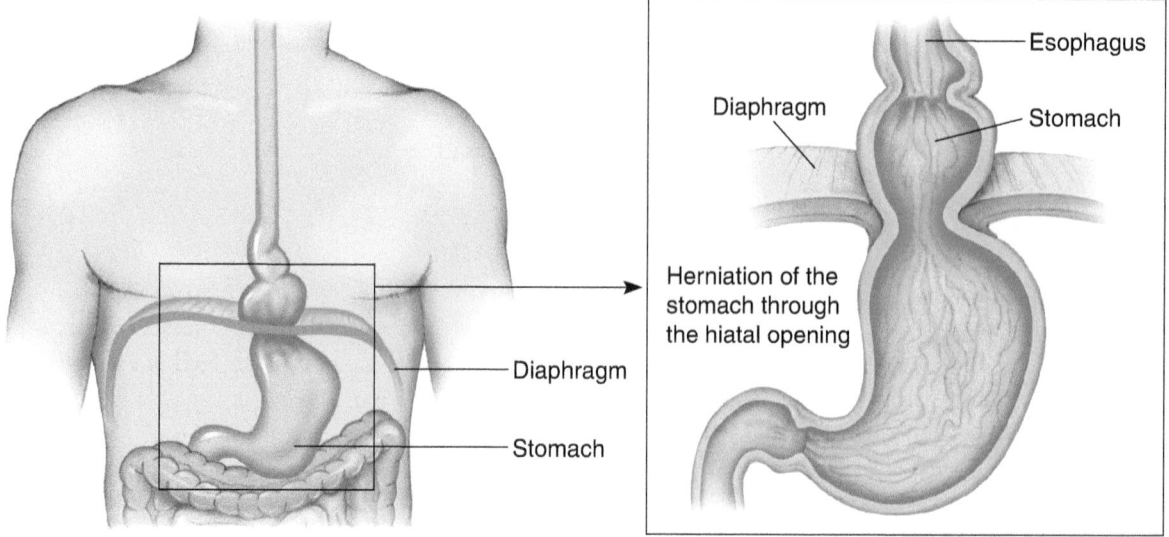

FIGURE 29-11 Hiatal hernia.

bulge, in the scrotum or groin (Figure 29-12). The hernia can be the result of a weakened muscular wall that stems from improper closing of muscular wall openings before birth. In this circumstance, developing a hernia may happen soon after birth of the infant or not until much later in life. An inguinal hernia may also develop suddenly as a result of strenuous activity such as heavy lifting, bending, straining, and even laughing. A common characteristic of inguinal hernias is that the bulge flattens when the patient lies down.

An incarcerated hernia is one that is so blocked or enlarged that it is trapped in the opening it came through and cannot be returned through the opening by manipulation. An incarcerated hernia can worsen to the point of strangulation. A strangulated hernia is one that is so constricted that the blood supply to the intestine is cut off. This is a potentially life-threatening condition.

Signs and Symptoms. Pain and discomfort in the affected area are common and often worsen when the person bends or lifts an object. Other signs and symptoms of an inguinal hernia include tugging or burning sensations and a feeling of heaviness in the area of the hernia, scrotum, or inner thigh. Swelling is also common for both men (in the scrotum) and women (in the labia). Nausea and vomiting, often sudden in onset, may also be present if part of the intestine bulges outside the abdomen and becomes incarcerated.

Treatment. Surgery is the only treatment and cure for inguinal hernia and may be required if the hernia is incarcerated or strangulated. Hernia repair is one of the most common

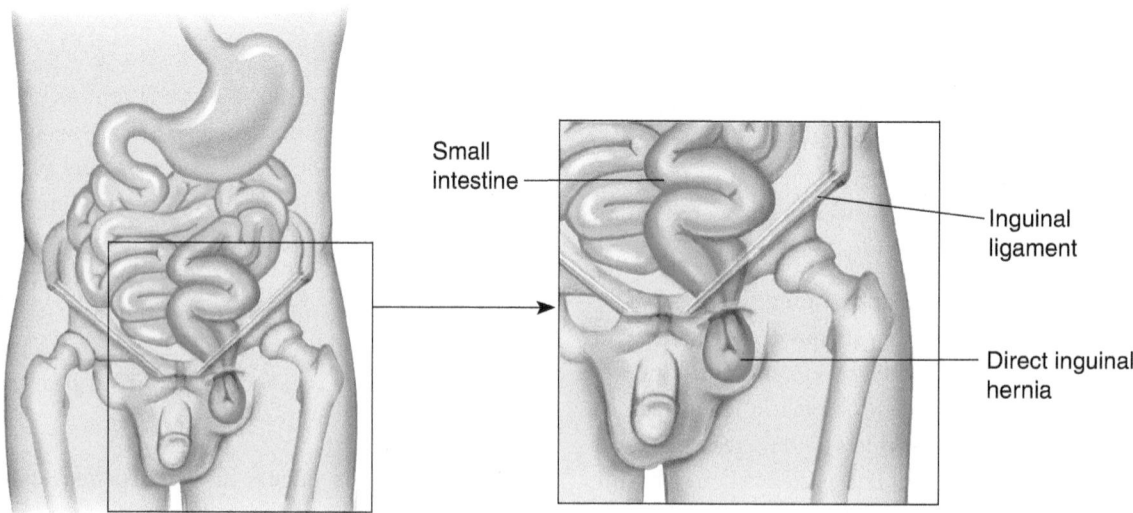

FIGURE 29-12 Inguinal hernia.

surgeries done in the United States. About 750,000 to 1 million people have hernia repairs each year. However, if an inguinal hernia does not cause any symptoms, treatment might not be necessary.

Irritable Bowel Syndrome

Irritable bowel syndrome (IBS) is a common disorder that interferes with normal colon function. It is considered a functional disorder, because it is thought to be a result of activity changes within the colon.

The exact cause of IBS is unclear; however, many factors may contribute to the functional change. A leading factor related to IBS is the impact of stress on the body and colon activity. Although a healthy person can have an upset stomach from a stressful situation, a person with IBS is more greatly impacted. The reason stress impacts the digestive system is the close neurological connection between the brain and the intestines. Postinfectious IBS is another factor related to this disorder in which IBS follows an intestinal infection. In this circumstance, a patient will be affected by IBS only temporarily. Hormonal changes related to the female reproductive cycle have also been shown to be a factor related to IBS. Symptoms related to IBS often worsen during menstruation. Women are twice as likely to suffer from IBS, and although it may occur at any age IBS most often begins in the late teen and early adult years. IBS affects 25 to 55 million Americans.

Signs and Symptoms. Common signs and symptoms associated with IBS include lower abdominal pain as well as cramping, bloating, nausea, and a feeling of gassiness. Changes in bowel function are a significant and troubling symptom, which can range from diarrhea to constipation or alternating between the two. Urgency is another common symptom, which is defined as the uncontrollable urge to defecate. Fecal matter may appear as a mucous-like, sticky fluid. The symptoms of IBS tend to rise and fall in intensity rather than worsen over time. A diagnosis of IBS is often made after a patient has experienced a combination of these symptoms for at least three days a month over a consecutive three-month period.

Treatment. There is no cure for IBS, and much about the condition remains poorly understood. Therefore, focus is placed on controlling symptoms and improving the day to-day quality of life. Dietary and lifestyle changes along with psychologic treatment (to reduce anxiety and stress) are often helpful to eliminate or substantially reduce symptoms. Dietary recommendations include increasing fluid intake, incorporating high-fiber foods into the diet and avoiding problem foods, which often include caffeine, alcohol,

chocolate, and sodas. Lifestyle changes to consider include routine exercise and eating smaller meals throughout the day. Medications may also be prescribed based on the patient's individual needs to treat diarrhea, constipation, and abdominal pain and cramping

Oral Cancer

Oral cancer is a form of cancer that can develop on the lips, on buccal mucosa (the inside of the lips and cheeks), on the gums, under the tongue, and on the front two thirds of the tongue. It can also develop on the hard palate of the mouth and the tissue located behind the wisdom teeth. Over 90 percent of oral cancer cases are linked to abnormal squamous cells that line the mouth.

The etiology of oral cancer is not linked to one specific cause. However, several factors increase the risk of developing it:

- Aging, particularly after 50
- Gender—more men develop oral cancer
- Smoking and heavy alcohol consumption, particularly if combined
- Using chewing tobacco or snuff, or chewing betel nut
- Excessive sun exposure to the lips
- Human papillomavirus (HPV)
- Poor dental hygiene
- Immunosuppressant medications

Signs and Symptoms. The signs and symptoms of oral cancer can be seen and felt quite early. Most commonly, sores, ulcers, irritation, or swelling in the mouth that lasts longer than two weeks should be checked by a doctor or dentist. Velvety red or white patches in the mouth may also indicate a precancerous condition. Other symptoms are a persistent

Professionalism The Workplace

Patients undergoing certain diagnostic testing for digestive disorders may be required to cleanse their bowels. This may be required for colon or sigmoid-oscopies and other procedures. Often, patients are very anxious and apprehensive about this task. It is the responsibility of the medical assistant to provide the patient with both oral and written instruction regarding bowel preparation for certain diagnostic testing. The medical assistant may want to take extra care in discussing these sensitive topics and focus on the positive aspect of how proper test preparation can help provide ideal testing conditions—something both the patient and the physician will appreciate.

sore throat; sores under dentures; a lump in the lip, tongue, or neck; weight loss; unexplained bleeding in the mouth; swollen lymph nodes in the neck; and trouble chewing, swallowing, or speaking.

Treatment. Treatment of oral cancer depends on the extent and stage of the condition when diagnosed. Surgery to remove part or all of the tumor and some surrounding tissue may be required. Radiation and chemotherapy, which interfere with the cancer cells' ability to grow and spread, are other treatment options.

Pancreatic Cancer

The most common type of **pancreatic cancer** is called adenocarcinoma of the pancreas. This cancer develops in the exocrine glands of the pancreas. (Exocrine glands excrete a hormone or substance to target organs through ducts.) The pancreas also has endocrine glands (glands that secrete, not through ducts, but directly into the bloodstream). The endocrine glands of the pancreas can give rise to a completely different type of cancer, a very rare form called pancreatic neuroendocrine carcinoma, or islet cell tumor.

Pancreatic cancer is one of the deadliest of all cancers, because often it is not diagnosed until advanced later stages of the disease. The American Cancer Society states that only 6 percent of pancreatic cancer patients will survive for five years after diagnosis, but most will die within the first year. These statistics reflect the challenge in treating pancreatic cancer and the relative lack of curative options. Risk factors associated with developing pancreatic cancer include obesity, tobacco use, exposure to certain chemicals (some pesticides, dyes, and chemicals), age (the average age of those diagnosed is 71), gender (males are more likely to develop it), race (African Americans are more likely than Caucasians), genetic syndromes and family history, and other health conditions (diabetes, liver cirrhosis, and pancreatitis).

Signs and Symptoms. The signs and symptoms of pancreatic cancer are generally vague and can easily be attributed to other less serious and more common conditions. Unfortunately, signs and symptoms will often not appear until advanced stages. Early signs of this cancer include clay-colored stool, dark urine, and jaundice or yellowing of the skin. Upper abdominal pain or discomfort, weight loss, loss of appetite, nausea, and fatigue are also early indicators of the disease. Other signs and symptoms of pancreatic cancer may include back pain, blood clots, diarrhea, and indigestion.

Treatment. As with other forms of cancer, surgery, chemotherapy, and radiation may be used depending on the type and stage of the cancer. Surgery to completely remove the

cancerous tumor is the only known cure for pancreatic cancer. However, surgery is not an option for all forms of pancreatic cancer. In fact, only 15 to 20 percent of pancreatic cancers can be removed upon diagnosis. The Whipple procedure is the most common surgery performed to remove pancreatic cancer, involving removal of the head of the pancreas, part of the stomach, and a portion of the duodenum. A portion of the pancreas remains to allow for adequate production of digestive enzymes and insulin.

Peptic Ulcer Disease

Peptic ulcer disease (PUD) is characterized by a disruption in the lining of the esophagus, stomach, or duodenum (the upper part of the small intestine). PUD appears most frequently in the duodenum. Ulcers in the stomach are also common. As discussed earlier in the chapter, the stomach produces acid that breaks down food during the digestive process. A mucosal lining protects the stomach and duodenum from the acid. When the lining is damaged, tissue becomes exposed and irritation may cause an ulcer to form (Figure 29-13).

Etiology associated with most cases of PUD is an infection with the bacterium *Helicobacter pylori* (*H. pylori*), which can cause erosion of the stomach mucosa. Additionally, inflammation of the gastric lining is a common causative factor. Inflammation may occur because of an imbalance in secretion of acid and pepsin (an enzyme) as well as from a breakdown in the defenses of the mucosal lining. Inflammation may be aggravated by the use of aspirin or nonsteroidal antiinflammatory drugs (NSAIDs) such as ibuprofen.

Ulcers can be prevented by avoiding alcohol and tobacco and limiting the use of NSAIDs and aspirin. Spicy foods do not cause ulcers but can aggravate symptoms associated with the condition.

Signs and Symptoms. The most common signs and symptoms of PUD are abdominal pain, nausea, vomiting, and weight loss. Esophageal ulcers often cause heartburn and chest pain. Other symptoms include tarry black or maroon stools (indicating the presence of old blood) or bright red blood in the stools (fresh blood), and a burning or gnawing pain in the stomach or the back.

Stomach or gastric ulcers are more common in people over the age of 50. Mild symptoms may be mistaken for indigestion or heartburn. Symptoms and signs may include any or all of the following:

- Pain or a burning sensation (similar to indigestion) in the upper abdomen and sometimes the lower chest
- Pain that is made worse by eating; however, pain from a duodenal ulcer can be worse when the stomach is

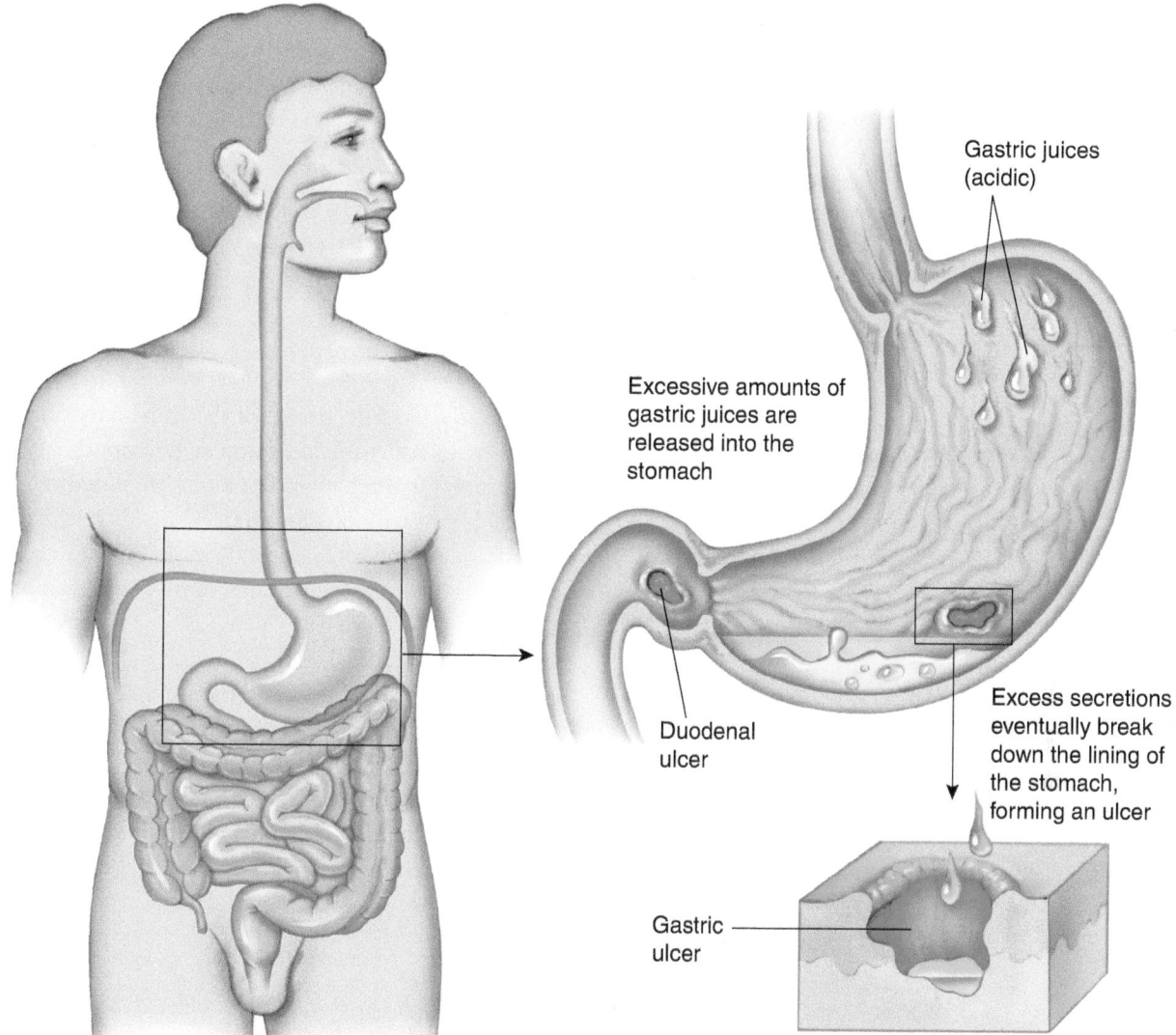

FIGURE 29-13 Peptic ulcer disease (PUD).

empty and is relieved by eating, but then recurs a few hours afterward

- Difficulty swallowing or regurgitation (bringing up swallowed food into the mouth)

- Bloating, retching, and feeling sick, particularly after eating

- Vomiting and nausea

- Loss of appetite and weight loss

The presence of blood in the stool may indicate that an ulcer is bleeding, which points to a more severe condition. Bleeding may mean that an ulcer has eaten its way through the wall of the stomach or duodenum. Also of concern is that the ulcer is blocking the digestive tract, and making it difficult for food to leave the stomach.

Treatment. Treatment of PUD depends on the cause and severity of the ulcer. Tobacco and alcohol should be avoided because they delay healing. Antibiotics may be given to treat *H. pylori* infections. Any medications that may cause or aggravate the condition must be changed. Proton pump inhibitors, such as Prevacid and Protonix, are medications that promote healing and block the production of acid. Medications may be prescribed to protect the stomach by decreasing or stopping the secretion of stomach acids. These are termed histamine (H2) blockers and examples include Zantac and Pepcid. Both proton pump inhibitors and H2 blockers are available by prescription as well as over the counter.

Occasionally, surgery may be required if the ulcer does not respond to medication or to stop a bleeding ulcer that is not responding to other therapies.

Pyloric Stenosis

The pylorus is the connection between the stomach and the duodenum. **Pyloric stenosis** is a condition that develops in

Professionalism | Cultural Considerations

Culture can play a major role in how people eat and view disorders of the digestive system. Hindus, for example, believe in fasting and in eating a specific way. Jews have specific dietary restrictions and customs associated with the preparation and eating of meals, particularly around religious holidays. Other cultures, such as those in the Far East, believe that alternative medicine therapies, such as acupuncture, homeopathy, meditation, and biofeedback, are frequently more useful than Western medicine in treating disorders of the digestive system. It is important for all members of the health care team to always respect a person's beliefs and focus on supporting and treating the patient within the patient's belief system. When asking questions or assisting in a treatment, make sure that the questions are not disrespectful and that your care is directed at the "total" patient, not just the disease.

some infants when the pylorus gradually swells and thickens, interfering with the flow of food into the intestine. This disorder can occur anytime between birth and 6 months of age but most commonly develops about three weeks after birth.

Signs and Symptoms. The main symptom of pyloric stenosis is an infant's repeated vomiting after feeding. The vomiting usually starts gradually and worsens over time. As the pylorus constricts, the vomiting becomes more frequent and more forceful. The infant loses weight, develops symptoms of dehydration, is sleepier than normal, and is very fussy when awake.

Treatment. Pyloric stenosis is always treated with surgery (pyloromyotomy). After surgery, the disorder usually does not develop again.

SUMMARY

The digestive system consists of the alimentary canal, which is tubular in structure and starts at the mouth and ends at the rectum. Its three main functions are digestion, absorption, and elimination. The primary organs of the digestive system are the mouth, pharynx, esophagus, stomach, small intestine, large intestine, and rectum. The accessory organs of digestion are the salivary glands, pancreas, liver, and gallbladder. Disorders of the digestive system involve the organs of the gastrointestinal tract and the accessory organs. Among the diseases of the gastrointestinal system are appendicitis, cirrhosis, colitis, colorectal cancer, Crohn's disease, diverticulitis and diverticulosis, gastroesophageal reflux disease, hemorrhoids, hernias, irritable bowel syndrome, oral cancer, pancreatic cancer, peptic ulcer disease, and pyloric stenosis.

29 CHAPTER REVIEW

COMPETENCY REVIEW

1. Define and spell the terms for this chapter.
2. Name the primary organs associated with digestion.
3. What are the four accessory organs of digestion?
4. What are the three main functions of the digestive system?
5. What is the first portion of the small intestine called?
6. The colon, a part of the large intestine, can be divided into four distinct sections. Name them.
7. What is the function of the gallbladder?
8. What saclike organ converts food into a semiliquid form called chyme?
9. With how many deciduous teeth is a person born?
10. What are the many essential roles of the liver?

PREPARING FOR THE CERTIFICATION EXAM

1. Which of the following is found on the right side of the abdomen?
   a. ascending colon
   b. descending colon
   c. cecum
   d. transverse colon
   e. sigmoid colon

2. The muscle at the most inferior portion of the stomach is the
   a. esophageal sphincter.
   b. pyloric sphincter.
   c. cardiac sphincter.
   d. gallbladder.
   e. fundus.

3. Which vitamin is *not* stored by the liver?
   a. A
   b. K
   c. C
   d. D
   e. E

4. Which of the following structures is a part of the large intestine?
   a. jejunum
   b. ileum
   c. duodenum
   d. pancreas
   e. sigmoid

5. What is a function of the liver?
   a. production of bile
   b. storage of bile
   c. production of pepsin
   d. production of insulin
   e. storage of insulin

6. By what age do most children have all their deciduous teeth?
   a. 6 months
   b. 1 year
   c. 2 years
   d. 3 years
   e. 10 years

7. Which of the following is a disease of the gallbladder?
   a. pancreatitis
   b. cirrhosis
   c. cholecystitis
   d. colitis
   e. stomatitis

8. A chronic disease of the liver is
   a. pancreatitis.
   b. cirrhosis.
   c. cholecystitis.
   d. colitis.
   e. stomatitis.

9. The abbreviation GERD stands for
   a. generalized enteritis recurrent disease.
   b. gastrointestinal reflux disease.
   c. gastrointestinal recurrent disease.
   d. gastroesophageal reflux disease.
   e. gastroesophageal recurrent disease.

10. Which of the following is an adenocarcinoma?
    a. cirrhosis
    b. diverticulosis
    c. pancreatic cancer
    d. oral cancer
    e. GERD

CRITICAL THINKING

Refer to the case study at the beginning of the chapter and use what you have learned to answer the following questions.

1. Dr. Penningworth speaks with Mr. Raines and then excuses himself from the examination room. Meanwhile, Dr. Penningworth tests Susan's knowledge and asks her if she has any idea what might be afflicting Mr. Raines. Based on what is known, what might be Susan's response?

2. Dr. Penningworth asks Mr. Raines how long he has struggled with his addiction to alcohol. Mr. Raines informs him that he has had a drinking problem since he was 18, for more than 28 years. Does this strengthen or weaken your suggestion regarding Susan's response to Dr. Penningworth in the preceding question?

3. Assuming the preceding questions have been answered correctly, which quadrant of Mr. Raines' abdomen would be affected?

INTERNET ACTIVITY

Conduct an Internet search on peptic ulcer disease.

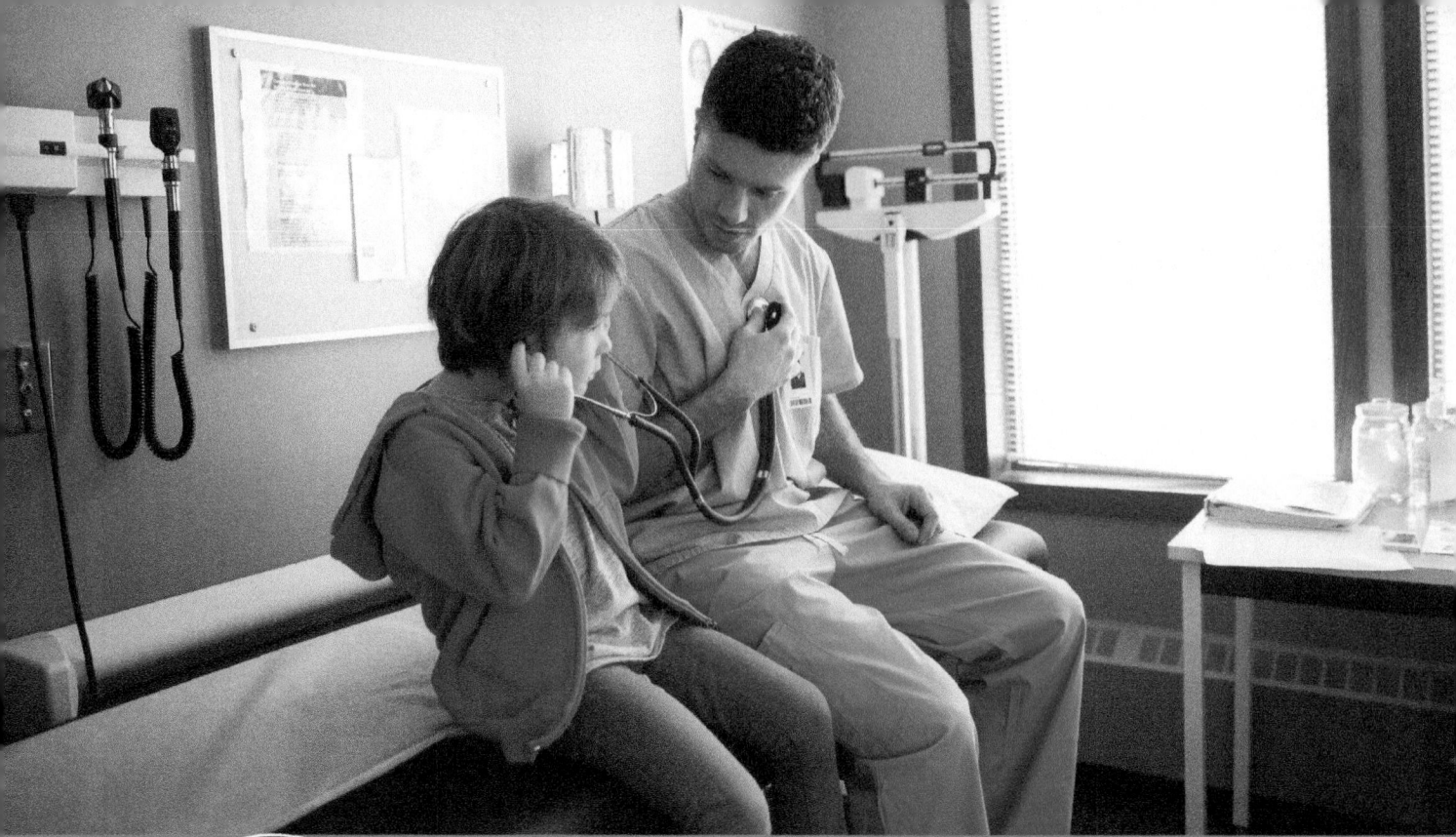

The Urinary System

Learning Objectives

After completing this chapter, you should be able to:

30.1   Define and spell the terms for this chapter.

30.2   Identify the purpose of the urinary system.

30.3   List the structures associated with the urinary system.

30.4   Describe how the urinary system changes during the life span of a child to an older adult.

30.5   Describe the three processes involved with the formation of urine.

30.6   Identify physical characteristics of urine.

30.7   Identify common pathology associated with the urinary system.

Case Study

Martin Wilkinson was seen at the emergency room of Pearson General Hospital. He had complaints of severe right-side flank pain. He did not have a previous history of kidney problems and had no pelvic pain or difficulty urinating. He presented to the ED with the following symptoms: sweating, nausea, and complaints of extreme pain. Mr. Wilkinson is diagnosed with a kidney stone (renal calculus) in the right renal ureter.

Terms to Learn

acute renal failure	incontinence	renal medulla
ascites	kidney stones	renal pelvis
chronic renal failure	kidneys	ureters
cystitis	lithotripsy	urethra
dialysis	micturition	urgency
dysuria	nephrons	urinary bladder
enuresis	polycystic kidney disease (PKD)	urinary meatus
frequency	pyelonephritis	void
glomerulonephritis	renal calculi	
hilum	renal cortex	

The functions of the urinary system are to produce, filter, and excrete urine from the body. This detailed filtration system is vital to maintaining homeostasis, because it removes waste products from the bloodstream. When the filtration system isn't functioning properly, many diseases and disorders can occur. These are discussed later in this chapter. Some organs of the urinary system share structures of the reproductive system, particularly the human genitals. For this reason, the urinary system is also called the genitourinary system.

ORGANS OF THE URINARY SYSTEM

The main organs of the urinary system, which is sometimes called the renal system, are the kidneys. Additional structures within this system help to transport, filter, and store urine. The ureters are responsible for moving urine from the kidneys to the urinary bladder. Here, the urinary bladder stores urine temporarily, similar to a small storage tank. From the urinary bladder, urine exits the body through the urethra during excretion (Figure 30-1). Two sphincters (rings of muscle), an internal involuntary sphincter and an external voluntary sphincter, control the flow of urine through the urethra.

Kidneys

The **kidneys** are a pair of bean-shaped organs located at the back of the abdominal cavity, against the muscles of the

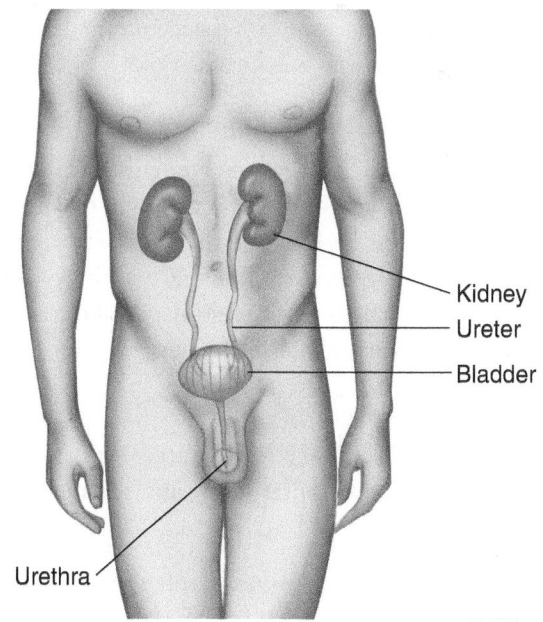

FIGURE 30-1 The urinary system: kidneys, ureters, bladder, and urethra.

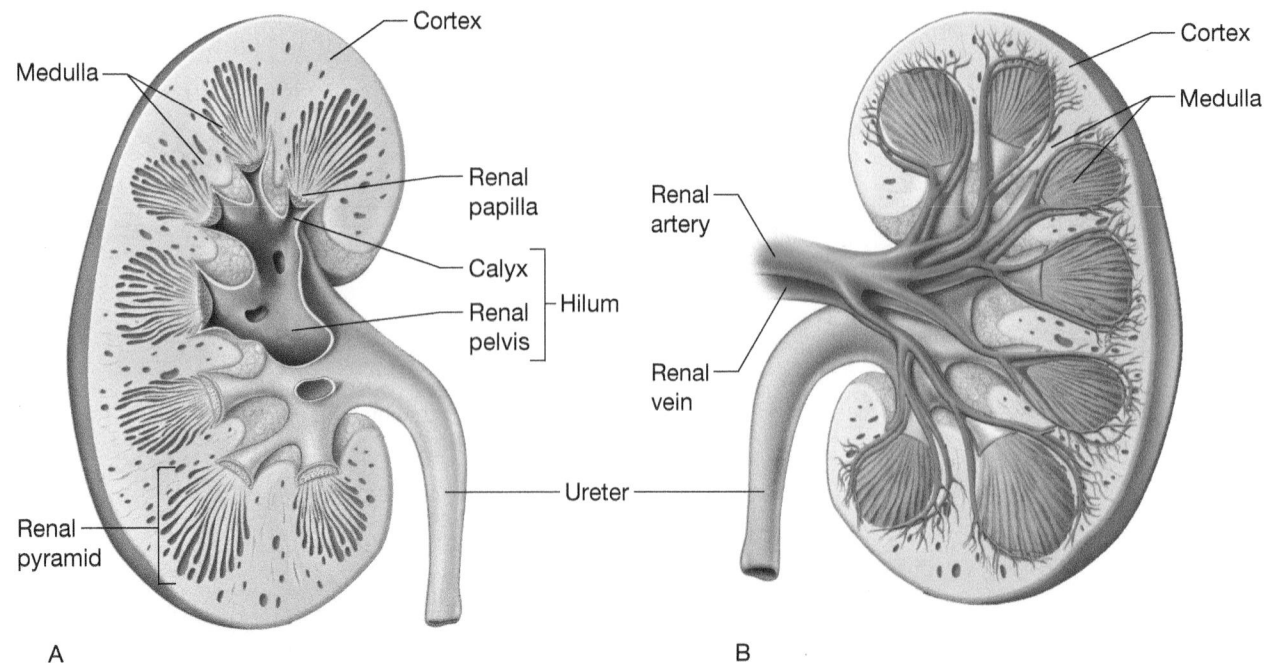

FIGURE 30-2 (A) Sectioned kidney; **(B)** renal artery and vein.

back, and on either side of the spinal column (Figure 30-2). The term *renal* refers to the kidneys.

Each kidney is surrounded by three capsules: the true capsule, the adipose capsule, and the renal fascia.

- **The true capsule**—A smooth fibrous connective membrane that loosely adheres to the surface of the kidney

- **The adipose capsule (perirenal fat)**—Embeds the kidney in fatty tissue, providing a layer of protection

- **The renal fascia**—A sheath of fibrous tissue that anchors the kidney to the surrounding structures and ensures that the normal position is maintained

External Structure of the Kidney

The **hilum** is located on the concave (curved in) border of each kidney. This notch-like area is the point of entry for the renal artery and vein, nerves, and the lymphatic vessels. The hilum is also where the ureter enters the kidney and connects with the **renal pelvis**. The renal pelvis is a small collecting area for urine within the kidney.

Internal Structure of the Kidney

The inside of each kidney is separated into two distinct parts: the **renal cortex** (outer layer) and the **renal medulla** (middle portion).

Renal Cortex. The renal cortex is soft and dense. It is the outermost layer of the internal structure of the kidney. Many veins and tubules are intricately woven within the cortex, giving this structure a granular appearance. Glomeruli (plural of

glomerulus), also found within the cortex, are discussed in detail later in this chapter.

Renal Medulla. The renal medulla is found deep within the cortex and contains cone-like structures called renal pyramids. The widest part of each pyramid lies closest to the renal cortex, and the tip of each pyramid is connected to the renal papilla and calyx. The pyramids are formed, mainly, of tubes to transport urine. The multitude of tubules within the renal pyramid connect to the surface of the papilla, giving it a colander-like appearance. Each of the tiny holes (openings from the tubules) in the papilla allow tiny drops of urine to pass into the calyx. From the calyx, collected urine droplets travel to the renal pelvis.

Nephrons

Nephrons are the functional units of the kidney. There are about a million nephrons in each kidney (Figure 30-3). These microscopic structures have a very important function in maintaining homeostasis within the body. Their function is to help the body maintain fluid balance by regulating the amount of fluid and electrolytes reabsorbed into the blood and the amount excreted in urine.

Each nephron contains a renal corpuscle and a tubule. The renal corpuscle consists of the glomerulus and the Bowman's capsule, which encloses the glomerulus. As blood flows into the glomerulus, the nephron removes waste materials to be discarded via the tubule. The tubule extends from the Bowman's capsule and consists of a proximal convoluted portion, the loop of Henle, and a distal convoluted portion,

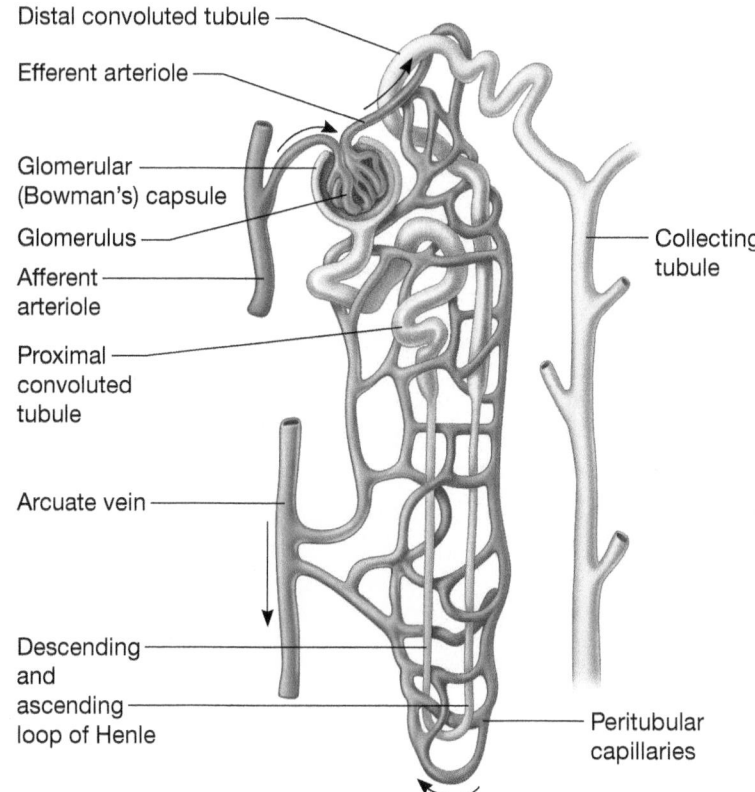

Distal convoluted tubule

Efferent arteriole

Glomerular (Bowman's) capsule

Glomerulus

Afferent arteriole

Proximal convoluted tubule

Arcuate vein

Descending and ascending loop of Henle

Collecting tubule

Peritubular capillaries

FIGURE 30-3 The structure of a nephron.

which opens into a collecting tubule. Multiple nephrons have distal convoluted tubules that all converge to a shared collecting tubule. The connecting tubule transports the discarded waste products (urine) to the renal pelvis, where it is briefly stored and then emptied into the ureters.

Ureters

The **ureters** are two narrow and muscular tubes that carry the newly formed urine from the renal pelvis in each kidney down to the urinary bladder. Each ureter is approximately 8 to 12 inches long. The ureter wall has three layers: an inner coat of mucous membrane, a middle coat of smooth muscle, and an outer layer of fibrous tissue. Small amounts of urine travel through the ureters every 10 to 15 seconds through involuntary muscular contraction and relaxation of the ureter walls.

Urinary Bladder

The **urinary bladder** is a muscular sac in the pelvic cavity that serves as a reservoir for urine. The wall of the bladder is made up of four layers:

- Innermost layer of epithelium—Called urothelium or the transitional cell layer
- Lamina propria—Covers the urothelium and is made of a very thin layer of connective tissue; is also referred to as the submucosa layer

- Muscular propria—A layer of smooth muscle that is responsible for contraction and relaxation of the bladder
- Perivesicle fat—The outermost layer of fatty connective tissue that protects the bladder and separates it from other organs

When the bladder is empty, it feels firm because the walls are thick. As the bladder fills, it stretches and the walls become thinner. The bladder is able to hold approximately 16 ounces (500 milliliters) of urine.

Urethra

The **urethra** is a tube of muscle and membrane extending from the bladder to the **urinary meatus**, the external opening of the urinary system. The male urethra is approximately 20 cm (7 inches) long and has three sections: prostatic, membranous, and penile. In females, the urethra is approximately 3 cm (1.2 inches) long with its external opening situated between the clitoris and the opening of the vagina. In males, the urethra transports both urine and semen and is therefore considered a genitourinary structure. In females, the urethra transports only urine and is therefore considered a urinary structure.

URINE

The formation of urine can be divided into three processes: filtration, reabsorption, and secretion. Figure 30-4 summarizes these processes. Urine consists of 95 percent water and 5 percent solid substances. The average adult feels a need to **void**, or urinate, when the bladder contains 300 to 350 mL of urine, though, as mentioned earlier, it can hold up to 500 mL of urine. The medical term for urination is **micturition**.

Professionalism The Law

Patient privacy is always of utmost concern in every part of the medical field. Never leave a voice mail or answering machine message stating patient testing needs or test results. The only exception is if the patient has expressed in writing that leaving such messages is acceptable. This written permission must be documented in the patient's medical record. Most medical offices and facilities require patients to fill out forms annually, stating their preferred method of contact, persons who are able to receive messages on their behalf, and if detailed voice mail and telephone messages are allowed. By following this procedure, you will avoid violating HIPAA regulations.

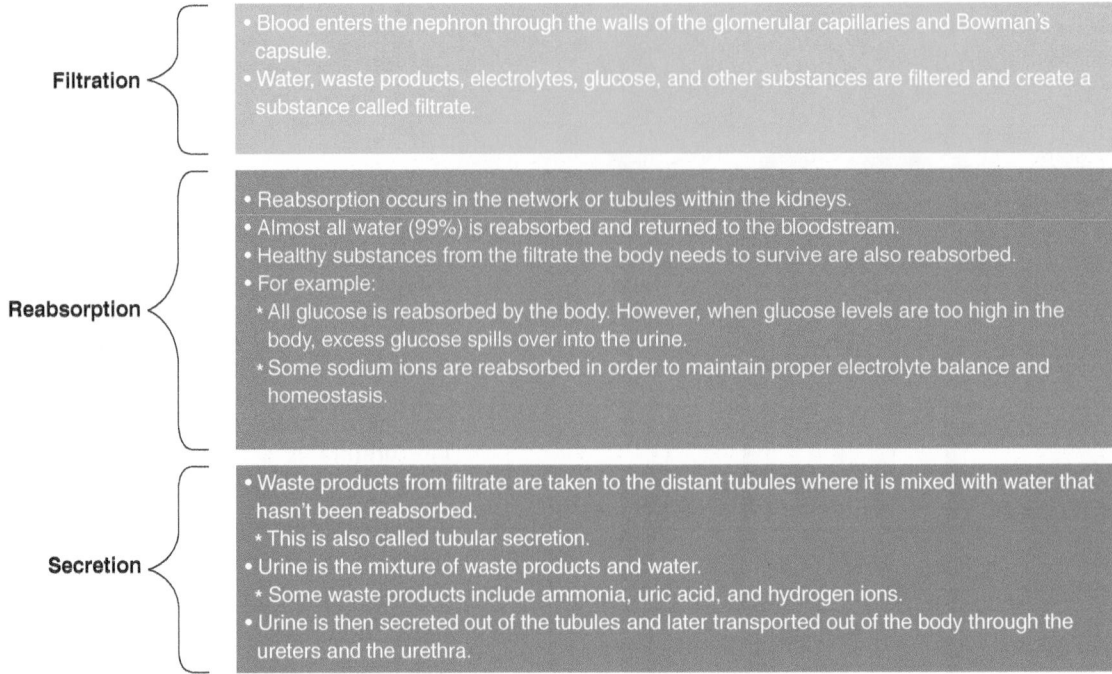

Filtration
- Blood enters the nephron through the walls of the glomerular capillaries and Bowman's capsule.
- Water, waste products, electrolytes, glucose, and other substances are filtered and create a substance called filtrate.

Reabsorption
- Reabsorption occurs in the network or tubules within the kidneys.
- Almost all water (99%) is reabsorbed and returned to the bloodstream.
- Healthy substances from the filtrate the body needs to survive are also reabsorbed.
- For example:
  * All glucose is reabsorbed by the body. However, when glucose levels are too high in the body, excess glucose spills over into the urine.
  * Some sodium ions are reabsorbed in order to maintain proper electrolyte balance and homeostasis.

Secretion
- Waste products from filtrate are taken to the distant tubules where it is mixed with water that hasn't been reabsorbed.
  * This is also called tubular secretion.
- Urine is the mixture of waste products and water.
  * Some waste products include ammonia, uric acid, and hydrogen ions.
- Urine is then secreted out of the tubules and later transported out of the body through the ureters and the urethra.

FIGURE 30-4 The process of urine formation.

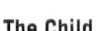

Professionalism The Life Span

The Child
- At about the tenth week of gestation, the kidneys begin forming urine. By the third month of gestation, the fetus actually begins to secrete small quantities of urine. Quantities continue to increase during the rest of fetal development.
- Small children, especially those wearing diapers, are susceptible to urinary tract infections. It is especially important that the diaper area be cleaned regularly and appropriately to prevent this occurrence.
- Bedwetting, also called nocturnal enuresis, frequently occurs while a toddler is potty-training. However, it is an often unspoken problem that can continue into childhood and cause emotional, social, and psychologic issues. About 15 percent of children around the age of 5 continue bedwetting. This decreases to 5 percent of children who are 10 years of age or older.

The Older Adult
- As people age and the blood vessels degenerate, the kidneys begin to lose mass, which leads to decreased urinary system functioning.
- Dehydration can happen more quickly because of a decreased ability to conserve water and sodium.
- A loss of muscle tone in the ureters, bladder, and urethra play a part in incontinence (the inability to voluntarily retain urine), which develops in many older adults.
- Bladder capacity is reduced by as much as 50 percent, causing more frequent trips to the bathroom.

- Urinary tract infections (UTIs) are much more common in older adults. Although symptoms may not seem serious at first, infection can progress quickly and rapidly, leading to further complications that are sometimes fatal.

Physical Characteristics of Urine

The physical characteristics of urine are important to know and understand because deviances from normal ranges could indicate an infection or disease of the urinary system. Typically, 1,000 to 1,500 mL of urine is voided daily, depending on fluid intake. Normal urine is clear (not cloudy), is straw-colored, and has a mildly aromatic odor; it has a slightly acidic pH of about 6 and a specific gravity of 1.003 to 1.030. Specific gravity measures the concentration level of dissolved substances within the urine. Higher amounts of dissolved substances in the urine increase the urine's concentration and specific gravity. Urine that has lesser amounts of dissolved substances is considered to be more diluted. Infants have a smaller range in regard to measured specific gravity because their kidneys aren't as mature and can't produce concentrated urine as effectively.

COMMON PATHOLOGY ASSOCIATED WITH THE URINARY SYSTEM

Compromised kidneys, and even healthy kidneys, can suffer from a variety of conditions that can affect an individual's lifestyle and activities of daily living (Tables 30-1 and 30-2).

TABLE 30-1 | Disorders of the Urinary System

Disorder	Description
Benign Prostatic Hyperplasia	Enlargement of the prostate gland caused by tissue growth, which can cause urinary flow disruption.
Bladder Neck Obstruction	Blockage of the bladder outlet, which inhibits it from opening completely during urination.
Cystocele	A condition that occurs when the vaginal wall weakens, allowing the bladder to droop down into the vaginal space.
Cystolithiasis	The formation of stones in the urinary bladder, similar in formation to kidney stones.
Hypospadias	A congenital birth defect characterized by the opening of the male urethra on the underside of the penis.
Lupus Nephritis	An inflammation of the kidneys caused by systemic lupus erythematosus.
Pyelitis	Inflammation of the renal pelvis often caused by a bacterial infection.
Renal Artery Stenosis	A narrowing of one or both of the renal arteries that carry blood to the kidney; most often it is caused by atherosclerosis.
Renal Colic	Pain caused by a kidney stone; can be excruciating pain and generally requires medical treatment.
Urinary Retention	Inability to start a stream of urine or completely empty the bladder of urine caused by trauma or injury, underlying medical conditions, surgery, and certain medication.
Vesicoureteral Reflux (VUR)	Common in infants and young children, VUR is characterized by urine that backflows from the ureters back into the kidneys, causing urinary tract infections.

TABLE 30-2 | Disorders Related to Urination

Disorder	Description
Anuria	No urine formed by the kidneys and a complete lack of urine excretion.
Dysuria	Painful or difficult urination.
Enuresis	Involuntary discharge of urine after the age by which bladder control should have been established; usually occurs by age 5 years; called bedwetting at night.
Hematuria	A condition of blood in the urine; usually a symptom of a disease process.
Nocturia	Excessive urination during the night; may or may not be abnormal.
Pyuria	Presence of pus in the urine.

Cystitis

Cystitis is an inflammation of the bladder, usually secondary to ascending urinary tract infections (an infection that spreads upward into the urinary tract from the urethral meatus). Cystitis occurs when bacteria infect the lower urinary tract, causing irritation and inflammation.

Urinary tract infections (UTIs) are a common condition that can affect anyone, but particularly sexually active women between the ages of 20 and 50, because sexual activity can introduce bacteria into the urethra. Women are also more frequently affected in large part because of the anatomy of the perineum, the short length of the urethra, and sometimes improper personal hygiene. In men, cystitis is usually secondary to another infection, such as epididymitis, prostatitis, gonorrhea, syphilis, or kidney stones. Other risk factors for developing cystitis include diabetes, pregnancy, urinary retention (inability to empty the bladder), enlarged prostate, bowel incontinence, and aging.

Signs and Symptoms. The most common signs and symptoms of cystitis are **urgency** (the need to void immediately) and **frequency** (the need to void often). Other common symptoms include itching, painful urination, and urine that is dark, cloudy, or blood tinged. Urine may also have a foul odor. Occasionally, if left untreated, the patient may experience chills and fever. In chronic cystitis, **dysuria** (burning or painful urination) may be the only symptom.

Treatment. Antibiotics are used to clear up the infection that is causing cystitis. A urinalysis will indicate if an infection is present, and a culture and sensitivity (C&S) will determine which type of bacteria is causing the infection. Knowing the specific type of bacterial infection allows the physician to prescribe the appropriate antibiotic. Medications may also be used to relieve the sense of burning, pain, or urgency. Increasing fluid intake is also encouraged to promote urination and flushing of the urinary tract.

Glomerulonephritis

Glomerulonephritis, also called glomerular disease, is an inflammation of the kidneys that primarily affects the glomeruli. This disease hinders the kidneys' ability to properly filter waste and fluids from the blood. It can be acute, referring to a sudden attack of inflammation, or chronic, which has gradual onset. Glomerular disease can be the result of a systemic disease, such as lupus or diabetes. It can also be idiopathic, standing alone and not related to another disease—a condition known as primary glomerulonephritis. Glomerulonephritis can lead to kidney failure.

The etiology of glomerulonephritis varies, including infections, autoimmune diseases, inflammation of the blood vessels (vasculitis), and conditions that scar the glomeruli. Chronic glomerulonephritis sometimes develops after a bout of acute glomerulonephritis. It is often difficult to pinpoint the exact etiology, or cause, of the disease.

Signs and Symptoms. Similar to the varying causes of glomerulonephritis, signs and symptoms also vary depending on whether the patient suffers from the acute or chronic form of this disease. Some patients are unaware that there is an issue until a routine urinalysis shows abnormalities. Signs include urine that is dark amber in appearance, caused by the presence of blood in the urine (hematuria). Lesser amounts of blood result in urine that has a pinkish hue. Other signs and symptoms include protein in the urine (proteinuria), which displays as frothy urine; high blood pressure (hypertension); fatigue; joint and muscle aches; fluid retention (edema) throughout the body; abdominal pain; and diarrhea.

Treatment. Treatment options vary depending on the underlying cause. Blood pressure control is imperative, so if the patient is hypertensive, antihypertensives (medications to lower blood pressure) and diuretics (medications to remove excess fluid from the body) will be introduced at the onset of treatment. If the condition is secondary to another disease, it is necessary to treat the primary issue in order resolve the secondary problems associated with glomerulonephritis. Corticosteroids may be used to reduce the inflammation of the renal tissue. Additionally, patients may need to limit sodium, potassium, fluid, and protein intake to reduce excessive kidney function and filtration needs.

Incontinence

Incontinence occurs when the body is unable to control an unpredictable flow of urine. Men and women are both susceptible to incontinence, but it is most common in women who have given birth. Risk factors that are associated with developing various forms of incontinence include gender (females are more prone), age (older individuals are more likely to develop the condition), smoking, obesity (extra body fat causes abdominal pressure), and chronic diseases.

Signs and Symptoms. There are several types of incontinence, and signs and symptoms vary with each:

- **Stress incontinence**—The most common form of incontinence, occurs with sneezing, laughing, and exercise. The involuntary release of urine occurs because of extra pressure within the abdominal cavity that presses on the bladder.

- **Overactive bladder**—Occurs when the muscles of the bladder unexpectedly squeeze because of misfired nerve signals telling the brain that urination is necessary. A sudden, frequent urge to urinate precipitates a leaking or gushing of urine.

- **Urge incontinence**—A condition in which the bladder contracts without warning, and leakage occurs, if the patient is not able to respond to that need to void immediately. Similar to overactive bladder, urge incontinence may be linked to abnormal muscle spasms of the bladder caused by misfiring nerve signals. The spasms can also be related to nerve damage within the bladder caused by a medical condition such as multiple sclerosis, Parkinson's disease, stroke, or injury to the bladder. Other medical conditions such as heightened anxiety, diabetes, and hyperthyroidism also can cause or intensify urge incontinence.

- **Overflow incontinence**—Occurs when a blockage prohibits complete emptying of the bladder. The bladder simply overflows and begins to leak. Causes may include nerve damage, a blocked urethra, or weakened bladder muscles. Men with enlarged prostates may suffer from overflow incontinence.

- **Incontinence while sleeping**—Is known as **enuresis**, or nocturnal enuresis. Although enuresis is common in small children, by the age of 8 years the pituitary gland should be secreting antidiuretic hormone to stop bedwetting at night. Nocturnal enuresis is discussed earlier in this chapter in the "Professionalism: The Life Span" special feature box.

- **Transient incontinence**—A temporary condition that is the result of an acute medical issue such as an infection, delirium, beginning a new medication, decreased mobility, impacted stool, or increased urine output. Normally, this form of incontinence will resolve after the underlying condition has been treated.

Treatment. Incontinence may be diagnosed by a urologist (a physician who specializes in urinary system disorders) or a family physician. Treatment options may include medications such as those that relax the bladder wall and reduce overactive contractions, surgery, and Kegel exercises, which strengthen the pelvic floor. Kegel exercises are performed by squeezing the pelvic muscles that stop urine flow and holding this "squeeze" for 10 seconds and then relaxing for 10 seconds. Enuresis usually responds well to behavior-modification training, but antidiuretic hormone and medications to control the bladder can also be effective.

Kidney Stones

Kidney stones, or **renal calculi**, are formed when the urine contains too much of a certain substance. Several substances may contribute to the formation of renal calculi, including calcium, uric acid, phosphate, and oxalate (a kind of organic acid molecule commonly found in plants and animals, including humans). Most kidney stones are formed by a combination of calcium and oxalate. Excess calcium is absorbed from food and excreted into the urine, where it combines with oxalates to create the stones. Individuals who are prone to this type of stone are advised to control their intake of foods that contain calcium and oxalate. Foods high in calcium include dairy products, leafy dark green vegetables, almonds, and sardines. Foods high in oxalate include beets, chocolate, tea, coffee, cola, nuts, rhubarb, strawberries, wheat bran, and spinach. Certain medications, including calcium supplements, can also increase the likelihood of developing stones.

Renal calculi are formed within the kidney, but when they pass into the ureter, they slow or block urine flow. Because the stones have a rough surface (Figure 30-5), they irritate and scratch the ureters, causing bleeding and intense physical pain. The bleeding and decreased urine flow irritate the kidney and cause spasms.

The exact cause of renal calculi is specific to each individual. Throughout their lifetime, about 10 percent of people in the United States will experience a kidney stone; with men more often afflicted than women. Those with a familial history of calculi, as well as urinary tract infections, kidney disorders, and metabolic disorders, are more likely to be afflicted.

To prevent stone formation, fluid intake should be sufficient to produce at least 2 quarts or at least 1,800 to 2,000 mL of urine each day.

Signs and Symptoms. A person suffering from a kidney stone usually presents with intense lower back, flank, or groin pain along with possible nausea, vomiting, and decreased urine output. Spastic pain in the lower abdomen is also very common. Urinalysis will usually reveal the presence of hematuria.

Treatment. Many kidney stones pass out of the body without intervention by a physician. It is simply a waiting game

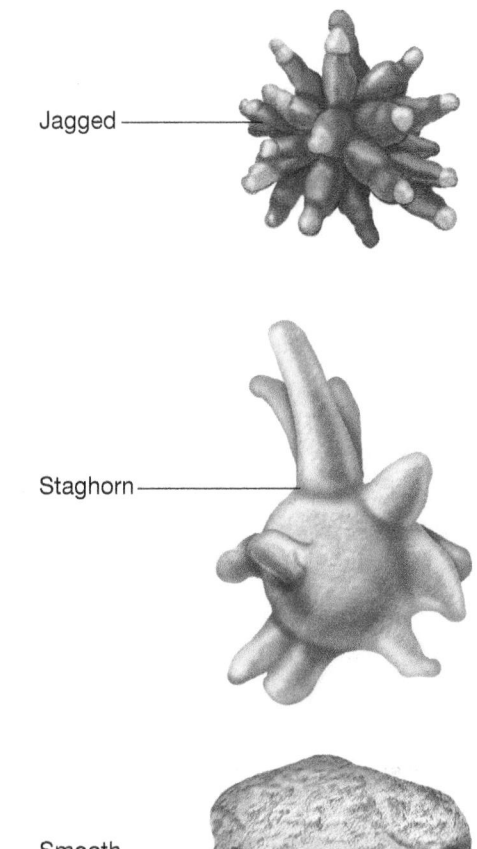
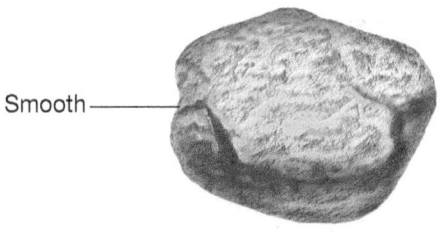

FIGURE 30-5 Types of kidney stones found in an adult.

until the stone passes from the kidney, through the ureter, and out of the urinary meatus. This could occur in a matter of hours, or it could take weeks to completely pass. Stones that cause lasting symptoms or other complications may require treatment, including **lithotripsy**. Lithotripsy involves passing shock waves through the body to break down the physical structure of the stone. Breaking down the stone allows for the smaller pieces to pass more easily through the urinary tract. The two types of lithotripsy are *extracorporeal shock wave lithotripsy* and *percutaneous ultrasonic lithotripsy*. Other procedures require surgical intervention to either retrieve or disintegrate the stone. Stones that do not pass may cause infection or, if they completely block the ureter, hydronephrosis (swelling of the kidney from backup of urine), which can eventually cause kidney damage.

Polycystic Kidney Disease

Polycystic kidney disease (PKD) is a disorder in which multiple (poly) clusters of cysts develop primarily within and on the surface of the kidneys. Cysts (round sacs) contain a fluid similar to water. Cysts are benign, which means noncancerous. It is not uncommon for polycystic conditions to be present in body systems and organs other than the kidneys. The liver and pancreas of the digestive system may develop multiple cysts, as may the reproductive system (ovaries and seminal vesicles). The central nervous system, including membranes that surround the brain are also prone to this condition. Kidneys are the most-often affected organ. PKD is also associated with other disorders including aortic and brain aneurysms and diverticulosis.

More than 12 million people, worldwide, are affected by PKD, which is identified as a congenital condition. The disease varies greatly in its severity, and some complications are preventable. Developing high blood pressure is the greatest risk for people with PKD, but regular checkups can help reduce damage to the kidneys. Kidney failure is also common with PKD.

Signs and Symptoms. Signs and symptoms of polycystic kidney disease include high blood pressure, back or side pain related to enlarged kidneys, abdominal pain particularly over the liver, joint pain, drowsiness, an increase in the size of the abdomen, blood in the urine, excessive night time urination, kidney failure, kidney infections, and headache.

Treatment. Unfortunately, there is no cure for this condition. Treatment is focused on symptom control and minimizing complications of high blood pressure, pain, bladder and kidney infections, blood in the urine, and kidney failure. Cysts that are bleeding, intensely painful, causing a blockage, or infected may need to be drained during a surgical procedure. Because of the multiple number of cysts associated with this disease, complete removal of cysts is not a feasible option.

Professionalism ▶ Cultural Considerations

Be very alert to the modesty requirements of different cultures when discussing urinary tract issues. It is advisable and even required in some medical offices to have a female medical assistant present during examinations of female patients. Female medical assistants should provide patient assistance and education for female patients, and male medical assistants should attend to male patients. Some cultures do not discuss the urinary tract at all, and others may require extensive education and sensitivity to deal with these issues. Be cognizant of patients' body language to help identify issues with which they are uncomfortable.

Pyelonephritis

Pyelonephritis is a urinary tract infection that has progressed to the kidney and renal pelvis. It may have a sudden onset and may progress into a chronic condition. The condition can be caused by either bacteria or viruses; however, most of the time the bacterium *E. coli* is to blame. Other factors that may contribute to the development of pyelonephritis include an indwelling urinary catheter, cystoscopy (visualization of the urinary bladder and urethra with a special telescopic instrument), prostate enlargement, and kidney stones.

Signs and Symptoms. Symptoms and signs of pyelonephritis include back, side, and groin pain; urinary urgency and frequency; pain and burning during urination; fever and chills; nausea and vomiting; concentrated and cloudy urine, which may be foul-smelling; and blood in the urine. It is not uncommon for a patient to exhibit confusion, a symptom most commonly seen with older adult patients.

Treatment. Antibiotics are used to treat pyelonephritis. If it is left untreated, scarring may result that could cause permanent kidney damage.

Renal Failure

Renal failure occurs when the kidney stops functioning properly. The condition inhibits filtration of the blood, which results in an increased buildup of toxins and waste products. Renal failure may be acute or chronic.

Acute Renal Failure

Acute renal failure occurs when there is a change in the filtering function of the kidneys, impairing the kidneys' ability to maintain normal body function. The rapid onset of acute renal failure can occur in a matter of hours, or over the course of two days. It is often caused by a blockage (sometimes because of emboli), toxins, or a sudden loss or decrease of blood flow to the kidneys. Those prone to developing acute renal failure include persons with serious health conditions including liver disease, high blood pressure, heart disease, other kidney diseases, and diabetes.

Signs and Symptoms. The signs and symptoms associated with this disease are numerous. Some of the most common include decreased urine output, resulting in swelling of the legs, feet and ankles; **ascites** (fluid in the abdomen); high blood pressure; nausea and vomiting; seizures; shortness of breath; bloody stools; fatigue; increased bruising; and a metallic taste in the mouth.

Treatment. Treatment is focused on addressing what has caused the renal failure and improving and restoring kidney function. Diuretics to remove excess fluid from the body may

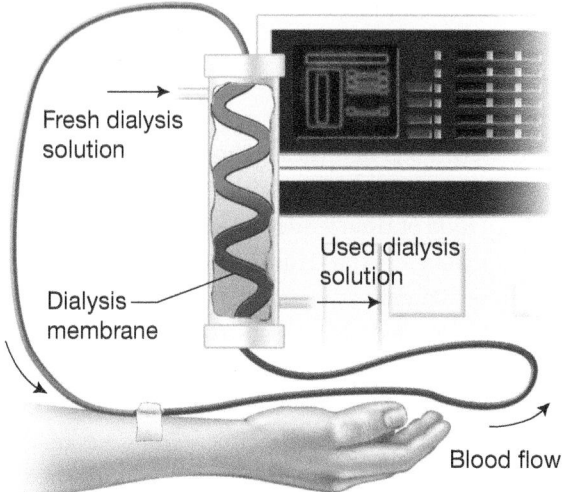

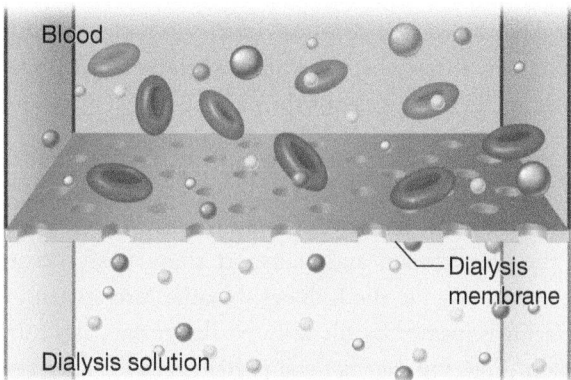

FIGURE 30-6 Dialysis machine showing diffusion of concentrations, which are the same, between the patient's blood and the dialysis solution.

be used, as well as antibiotics to treat or prevent any urinary infections. The patient may require **dialysis** (Figure 30-6). Dialysis uses a filter other than the kidneys to remove toxins and maintain water balance. The two types of dialysis are hemodialysis and peritoneal dialysis. The patient will depend on the dialysis machine until the kidneys are able to be restored to normal function. Dialysis is discussed further in the following section, "Chronic Renal Failure," and in the chapter titled "Assisting with Reproductive and Urinary Specialties."

Chronic Renal Failure

In **chronic renal failure**, there is a gradual and progressive loss of kidney function that transpires over the course of months to years. The final stages of chronic renal failure are referred to as end-stage renal disease (ESRD). As waste and fluid accumulate from lack of filtration, other bodily functions are severely impeded. The affected functions include blood pressure control, red blood cell production, and bone health as it relates to the body's usage of vitamin D. Diabetes and hypertension are the two most common causes of chronic renal failure in the United States.

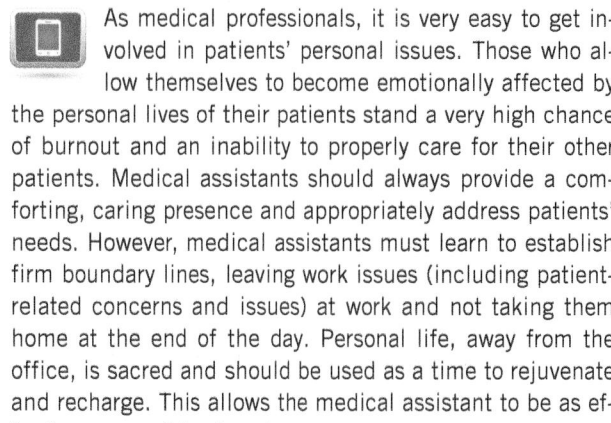

Signs and Symptoms. Symptoms may be mild or nonexistent until at least 10 percent of kidney function is lost. Early signs and symptoms include fatigue, headaches, itchy and dry skin, nausea, and weight loss. End-stage signs and symptoms progress to changes in skin color, bone and nervous system changes, bone pain, weight loss, amenorrhea (cessation of menstrual periods), excessive thirst, frequent hiccups, and low levels of sexual desire and impotence.

Treatment. The treatment goal is to identify, treat, and reverse what is causing the kidneys to fail. Then, treatment focuses on preventing excess fluid volume while the kidneys

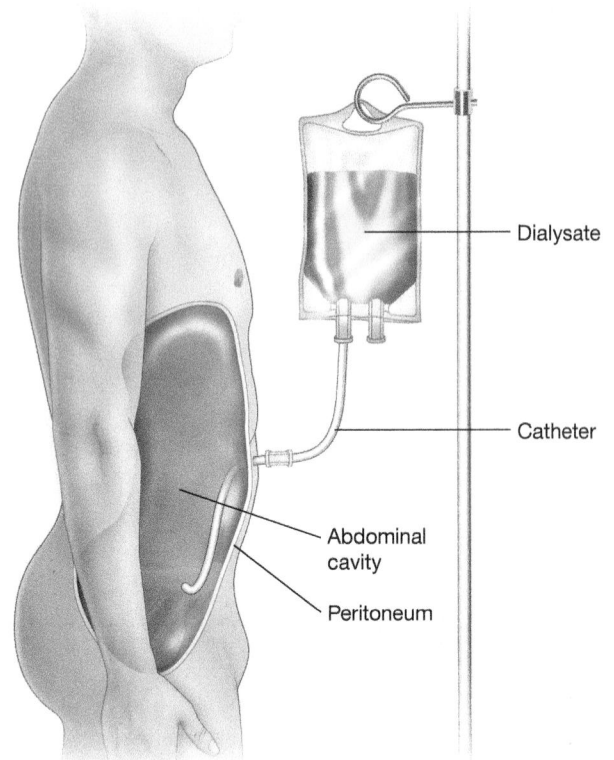

FIGURE 30-7 Peritoneal dialysis.

three times a week for two to three hours at a time for hemodialysis treatments.

Peritoneal dialysis (Figure 30-7) is done through the tissues of the abdomen. Here, dialysate (dialysis fluid) is administered from a catheter and through a permanent tube that is placed within the wall of the abdomen. The fluid is left to absorb for a period of time while abdominal membranes filter dissolved substances and fluids from the blood. These patients can be dialyzed at home or in any environment.

As noted earlier, dialysis is discussed further in the chapter titled "Assisting with Reproductive and Urinary Specialties."

If they qualify, patients may be placed on a list for kidney transplant. Kidney transplant recipients must take antirejection drugs for the rest of their lives to live with the transplanted kidney. Kidney transplants are one of the most common transplant procedures performed in the United States. Dialysis would continue until the patient is able to receive a new kidney or, if a kidney replacement is not performed, for the remainder of the patient's life.

SUMMARY

The function of the urinary system is to extract certain wastes from the bloodstream and transport those wastes as urine outside the body via the kidneys, bladder, ureters, and urethra. Urine is formed by filtration, reabsorption, and tubular secretion. The urinary tract can present many challenges for both the patient and the medical assistant. One of the most common reasons patients come into the medical office is to seek help for a urinary tract infection. Common disorders of the urinary system include cystitis, glomerulonephritis, kidney stones, and pyelonephritis. Incontinence can also pose a problem, both medically and socially. Polycystic kidney disease can severely impair kidney function. Renal failure is the result of acute or chronic kidney problems and is treated with dialysis or kidney transplant.

have a chance to heal and resume their normal function. If normal function cannot be regained, dialysis may be necessary. As noted for acute renal failure, there are two types of dialysis, hemodialysis and peritoneal dialysis.

In hemodialysis, a machine filters and cleans the blood outside the body. A specialized catheter (a shunt) is inserted into the patient's arm or leg. The shunt is accessed with special tubing that carries the blood to the dialysis machine, where it is filtered and cleaned, and then returns the blood to the body. Patients must go to a special dialysis center

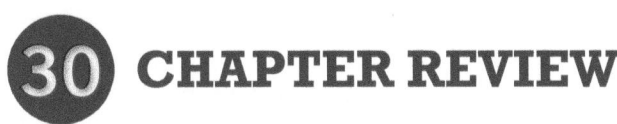

30 CHAPTER REVIEW

COMPETENCY REVIEW

1. Define and spell the terms for this chapter.
2. List the organs of the urinary system.
3. What are the vital functions of the urinary system?
4. Where are the kidneys located?
5. In what portion of the kidney is the medulla located?

6. What is the function of the nephrons?
7. What are the three processes of urine formation?
8. What is the major organ of the urinary system?
9. How is renal failure treated?
10. How much urine is voided daily?

PREPARING FOR THE CERTIFICATION EXAM

1. The part of the urinary tract that collects and holds urine for expulsion is the
   a. ureter.
   b. bladder.
   c. urethra.
   d. meatus.
   e. renal pelvis.

2. The condition in which an individual experiences an involuntary and unpredictable flow of urine while sleeping is
   a. constipation.
   b. anuria.
   c. dysuria.
   d. nocturia.
   e. enuresis.

3. A urinary disease characterized by clusters of noncancerous round sacs of water-like fluid is
   a. pyelonephritis.
   b. glomerulonephritis.
   c. polycystic kidney disease.
   d. cystitis.
   e. renal calculus.

4. Pain caused by a kidney stone is known as
   a. cystitis.
   b. enuresis.
   c. incontinence.
   d. renal colic.
   e. nocturia.

5. The anatomical structure of the urinary system that is responsible for carrying urine from the bladder to outside the pelvis is the
   a. nephron.
   b. ureter.
   c. collecting tubule.
   d. urethra.
   e. renal pelvis.

6. An abnormal condition of stones in the bladder is known as
   a. cholelithiasis.
   b. cystitis.
   c. cystolithiasis.
   d. colitis.
   e. polycystic disease.

7. Which organ is 8 to 12 inches long?
   a. ureter
   b. bladder
   c. urethra
   d. kidney
   e. nephron

8. A normal pH level of urine is
   a. 4.
   b. 5.
   c. 6.
   d. 7.
   e. 8.

9. The average maximum capacity of a bladder is
   a. 100 mL.
   b. 250 mL.
   c. 500 mL.
   d. 1,000 mL.
   e. 1.5 L.

10. End-stage renal disease occurs with what other kidney disease?
    a. chronic renal failure
    b. glomerulonephritis
    c. renal colic
    d. renal calculi
    e. pyelonephritis

CRITICAL THINKING

Refer to the case study at the beginning of the chapter and use what you have learned to answer the following questions.

1. Mr. Wilkinson had a urinalysis performed that showed a substantial amount of blood in his urine. Why is hematuria common with kidney stones?

2. Because of the size and number of kidney stones present, Mr. Wilkinson was unable to pass the kidney stones. Describe a treatment available for Mr. Wilkinson.

3. When Mr. Wilkinson was discharged from the hospital, he was given a list of dietary limitations. What might this list have included?

INTERNET ACTIVITY

Use the Internet to learn about types of incontinence and their treatments.

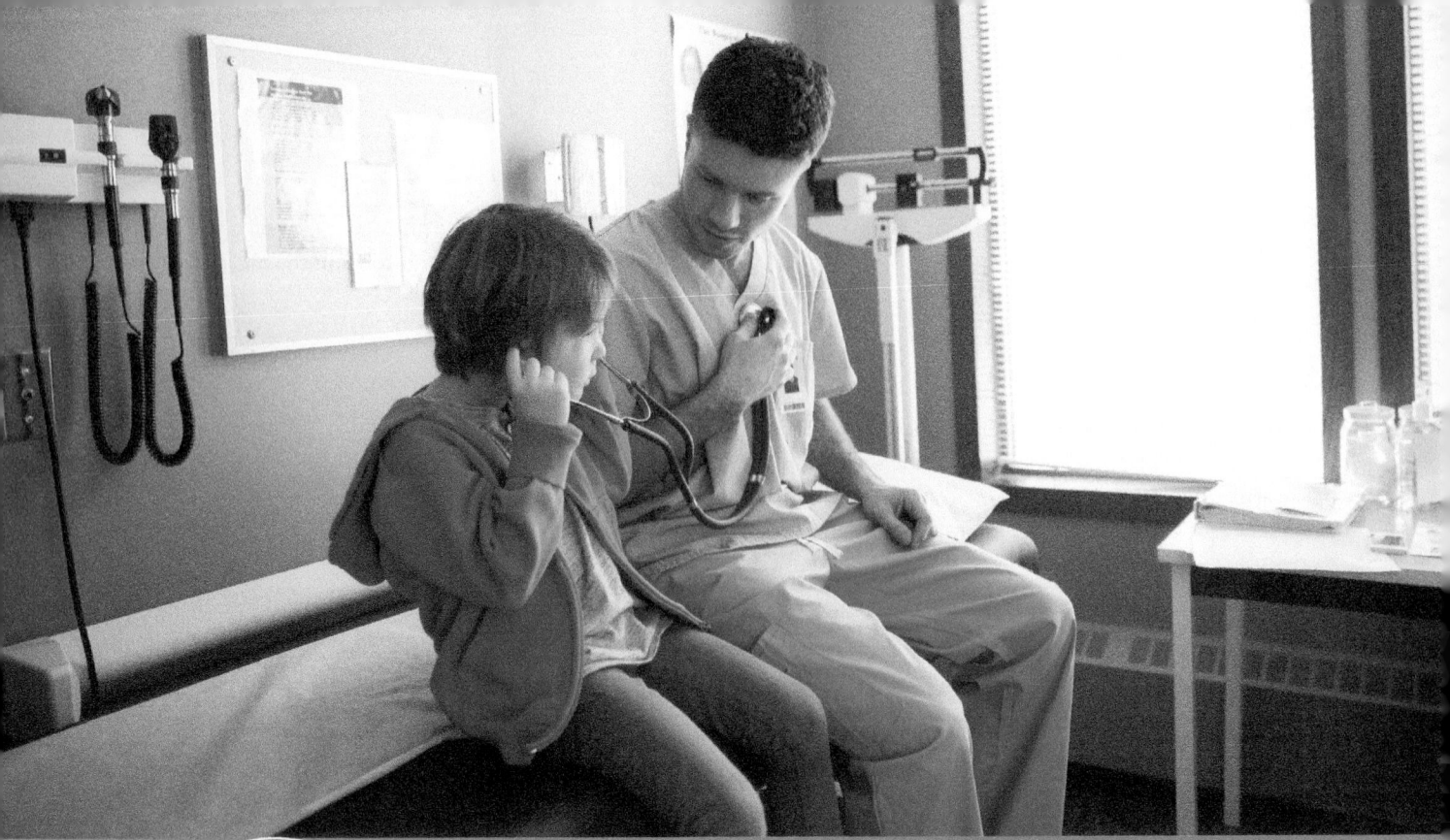

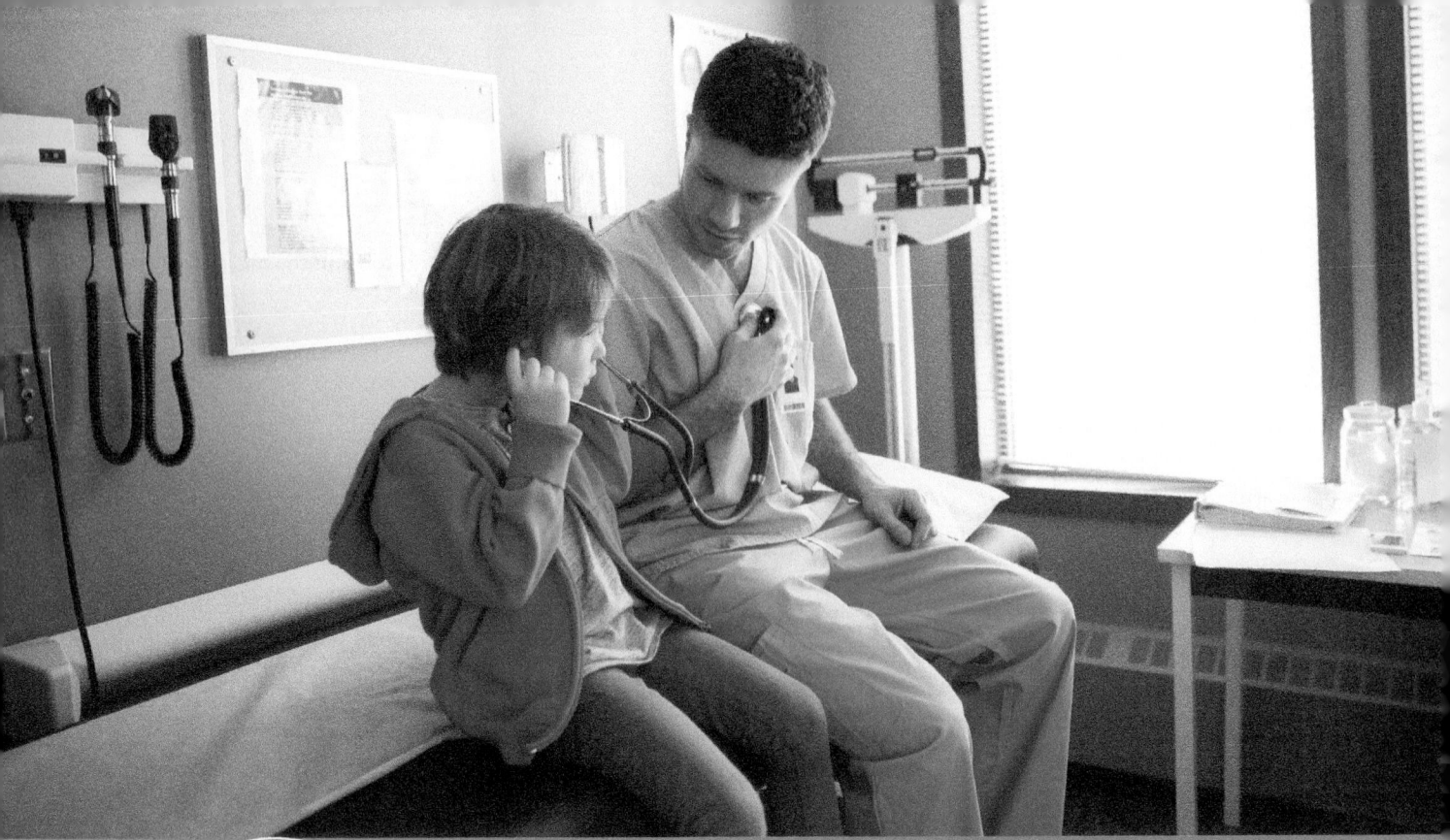

CHAPTER

31

The Endocrine System

Learning Objectives

After completing this chapter, you should be able to:

31.1   Define and spell the terms for this chapter.

31.2   Explain the general function of the endocrine system.

31.3   List the structures of the endocrine system.

31.4   Identify the functions of hormone secretion related to the glands of the endocrine system.

31.5   Describe how the endocrine system changes during the life span of a child to an older adult.

31.6   Describe common pathology associated with the endocrine system.

Rosa Gutierrez was just seen by Dr. Bahjat. Her laboratory tests have come back, and she has been diagnosed with type 2 diabetes. She is a Mexican immigrant who has lived in the United States for the past 31 years. She is very worried about how the disease will affect her life.

Terms to Learn

acromegaly	Hashimoto's thyroiditis	pancreas
Addison's disease	hormones	parathyroid glands
adrenal glands	hypersecretion	pineal gland
cardiomegaly	hyperthyroidism	pituitary gland
Cushing's disease	hyposecretion	placenta
diabetes mellitus	hypothalamus	positive feedback
dwarfism	hypothyroidism	testes
exophthalmos	islets of Langerhans	thymus gland
gestational diabetes	lipolysis	thyroid gland
gigantism	myxedema	type 1 diabetes
goiter	negative feedback	type 2 diabetes
Graves' disease	ovaries	

The human body contains many glands—organs that secrete hormones and other substances. Glands that secrete substances within the body are called endocrine glands. Glands that secrete substances to the outside the body are called exocrine glands. An easy way to remember the difference between endocrine and exocrine glands is to understand the literal translation of their names as shown in Figure 31-1.

Exocrine glands include the salivary glands, sweat glands, and mammary glands. This chapter, however, focuses on the endocrine glands, which together make up the endocrine system.

The endocrine system is an elaborate network of glands that communicate and secrete hormones within the body for the purpose of maintaining homeostasis. Unlike exocrine glands that send their secretions to outer surfaces through ducts, endocrine glands are ductless; they secrete their hormones directly into the bloodstream or surrounding tissues.

The primary glands of the endocrine system are the pituitary, pineal, thyroid, thymus, parathyroid, pancreas, adrenals, ovaries in the female, and testes in the male. These are illustrated in Figure 31-2 and discussed later in the chapter.

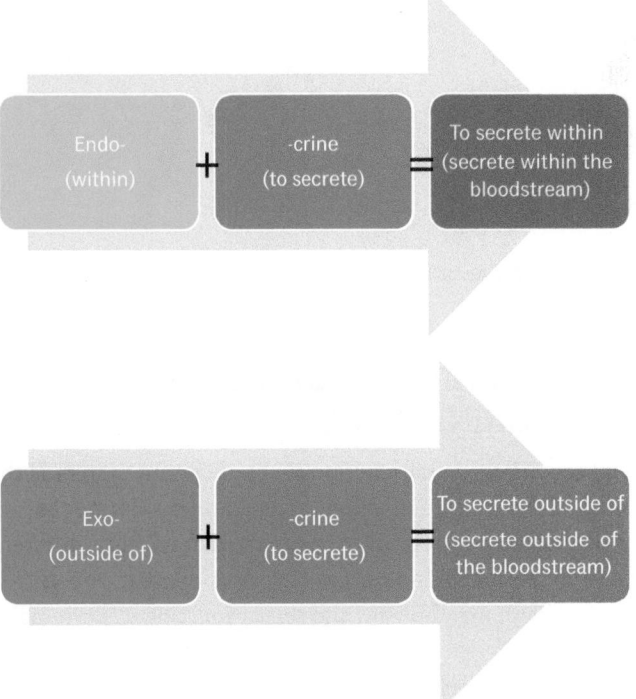

FIGURE 31-1 Explanation of endocrine versus exocrine.

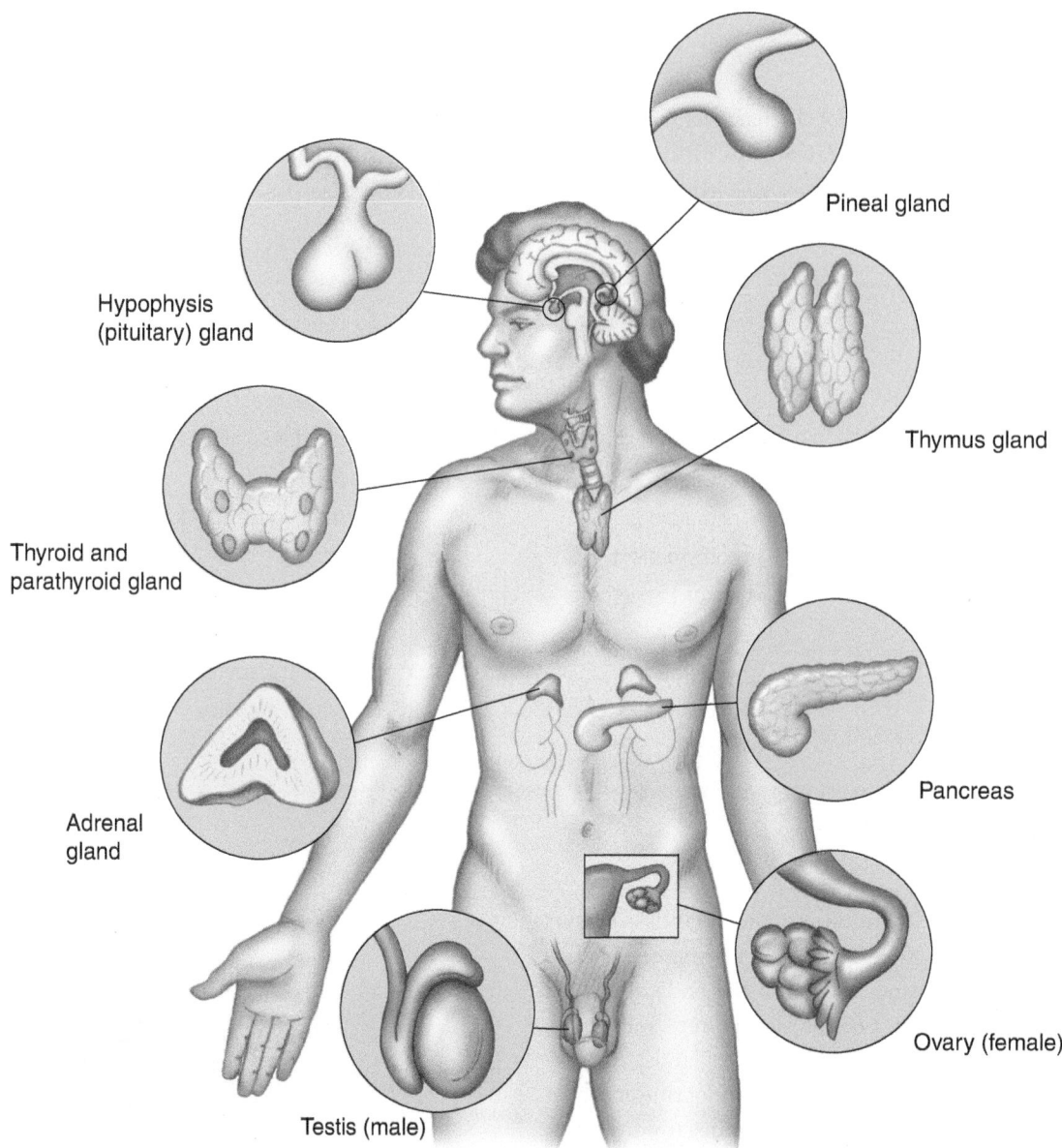

Hypophysis
(pituitary) gland

Pineal gland

Thymus gland

Thyroid and
parathyroid gland

Pancreas

Adrenal
gland

Ovary (female)

Testis (male)

FIGURE 31-2 Examples of endocrine disorders associated with hyper- and hyposecretion.

GENERAL FUNCTION OF THE ENDOCRINE SYSTEM

The general and vital function of the endocrine system is the production and regulation of hormones. **Hormones** are chemical transmitters, or messengers, that regulate different body functions including growth, development, mood, tissue function, metabolism, and sexual function in both males and females.

Many disorders are associated with either the **hypersecretion** (excessive secretion) or the **hyposecretion** (insufficient secretion) of hormones of the endocrine system. Controlling the secretion of specific hormones can help treat many hormonal conditions or disorders. Table 31-1 provides examples

of disorders of the endocrine system associated with hyper- or hyposecretion. These disorders and others are discussed later in the chapter.

The nervous system works closely with the endocrine and exocrine systems to maintain homeostasis. Feedback loops (negative feedback loops and positive feedback loops) are one example of this cooperation between systems. Here is how feedback loops work.

Our bodies are equipped to respond to internal and external stimuli. When the nervous system perceives a harmful change in stimulus, the body responds by creating a *negative feedback loop*. **Negative feedback** means that the body acts to *reverse* the direction of change to regain or maintain homeostasis. For instance, on a hot day your body temperature may rise.

TABLE 31-1 | Examples of Endocrine Disorders Associated with Hyper- and Hyposecretion

	Hormone	Endocrine Gland	Disorder
Hypersecretion	Growth hormone (GH)	Anterior pituitary	Gigantism or acromegaly
	Adrenocorticotropic hormone (ACTH)	Anterior pituitary	Cushing's disease
	T_3 and T_4	Thyroid	Graves' disease
	Parathyroid hormone (PTH)	Parathyroid	Osteoporosis Kidney stones
	Insulin	Pancreas	Hypoglycemia
	Cortisol	Adrenals	Cushing's syndrome
Hyposecretion	Antidiuretic hormone (ADH)	Produced by hypothalamus Stored and secreted by the posterior pituitary	Diabetes insipidus
	Growth hormone (GH)	Anterior pituitary	Dwarfism
	T_3 and T_4	Thyroid	Hashimoto's thyroiditis Goiter
	Parathyroid hormone (PTH)	Parathyroid	Tetany
	Insulin	Pancreas	Diabetes

To counter the rise in body temperature, the nervous system activates the sweat glands of the exocrine system to produce sweat, which helps cool the body and decrease the body's temperature. The body's response to the hot day (an external stimulus) was to produce sweat to cool the body, thus reversing the direction of the change created by the external stimulus.

The other action our bodies may take in response to stimuli is a positive *feedback loop*. **Positive feedback** encourages stimuli to *continue or even accelerate*, which also helps maintain homeostasis. For instance, during childbirth there is an accelerated release of the hormone oxytocin, which is produced in the hypothalamus gland and stored in the pituitary gland for secretion. Oxytocin enables the uterus to contract and the cervix to stretch. In this example, the nervous system has responded to the childbirth process (internal stimuli) by activating production and secretion of oxytocin by the endocrine hypothalamus and pituitary glands. The body will increase the level of oxytocin that is released as needed to enable the birth of the child. After the child has been born, homeostasis is maintained as the body returns to its normal state.

SPECIFIC GLANDS AND THEIR FUNCTIONS

Each gland of the endocrine system has a specific function based on the type of hormone produced and secreted by that gland. Understanding and identifying hormones and their

functions is vital to fully comprehending the intricate workings of the endocrine system.

Hypothalamus

The **hypothalamus** (Figure 31-3) is situated inside the center of the brain, below the thalamus. It is similar in size and shape to an almond. Though it is very small, it is very important to the entire body. The hypothalamus is the connection between the endocrine and nervous systems. One of the main functions of the hypothalamus is to secrete releasing and inhibiting hormones. Releasing hormones start the production and release of other hormones throughout the body, and inhibiting hormones stop the production and release of certain hormones. In that sense, the hypothalamus acts as an on-and-off switch for hormone secretion. Table 31-2 lists these specific hormones.

In addition to releasing and inhibiting hormones, the hypothalamus also produces two specific hormones within the body:

- **Antidiuretic hormone (ADH)** is responsible for increasing water absorption in the blood by the kidneys.

- **Oxytocin** plays a key role in childbirth (as discussed earlier) and also influences our ability to trust and bond with others.

It is important to note that even though these hormones are produced in the hypothalamus, they are stored and released by the pituitary gland.

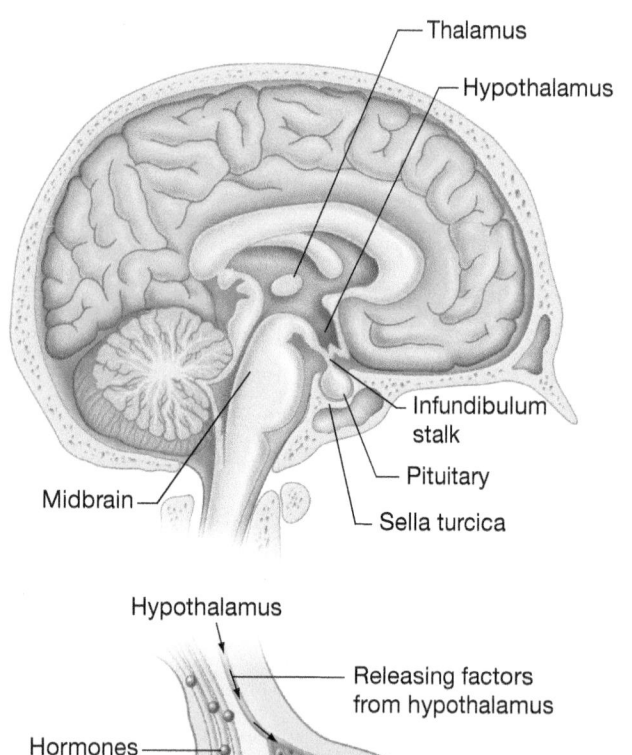

FIGURE 31-3 The hypothalamus and pituitary glands and their relation to the brain.

Pituitary Gland

The **pituitary gland** (Figure 31-3) is a small gland located near the base of the brain in the sella turcica, a small depression of the sphenoid bone. The pituitary is called the "master gland" because it regulates all the other endocrine glands.

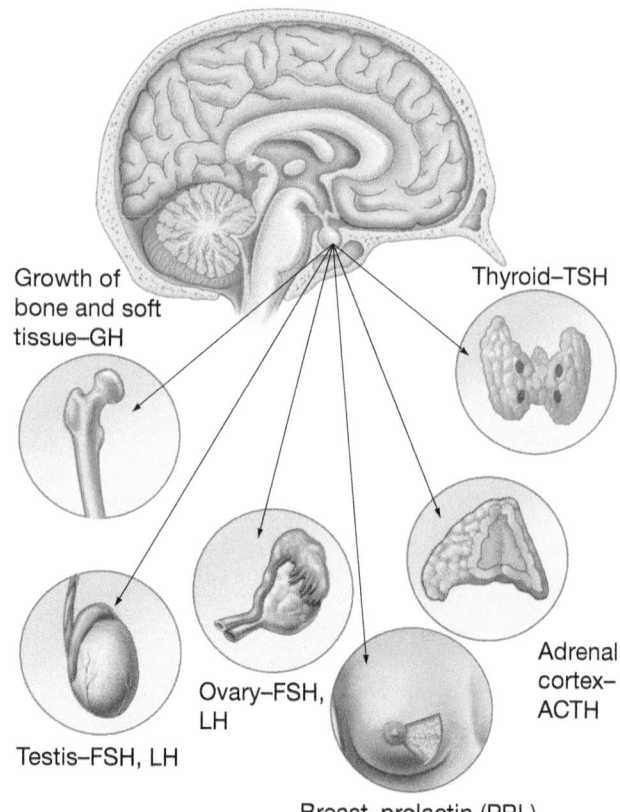

FIGURE 31-4 The anterior pituitary gland and its target organs.

It is attached to the hypothalamus by the infundibulum stalk. The pituitary gland has two lobes, the anterior lobe and the posterior lobe, each with its own particular functions.

Anterior Lobe

The anterior lobe of the pituitary gland is also called the adenohypophysis (Figure 31-4). This portion of the master gland secretes hormones that are responsible for the growth and formation of a number of bodily structures including bones, muscles, and organs. It also is responsible for secreting

TABLE 31-2 | Releasing and Inhibiting Hormones of the Hypothalamus

Hormone	Function
Corticotropin-Releasing Hormone (CRH)	Stimulates the adrenal glands to release corticosteroids.
Gonadotropin-Releasing Hormone (GnRH)	Stimulates the anterior pituitary to release hormones that are essential in proper function of the ovaries and testes.
Growth Hormone–Releasing Hormone (GH-RH) & Growth Hormone–Inhibiting Hormone (GH-IH)	These hormones either prompt or inhibit the release of growth hormones from the anterior pituitary.
Prolactin-Releasing Hormone (PRH) & Prolactin-Inhibiting Hormone (PIH)	PRH stimulates breast milk production, whereas PIH stops the production of breast milk.
Thyrotropin-Releasing Hormone (TRH)	Triggers the release of the thyroid-stimulating hormone, which is produced by the anterior pituitary.

hormones for the growth and development of the thyroid gland, the sex glands, and the adrenal cortex. The hormones produced in the anterior lobe include the following:

- **Growth hormone (GH) (also called somatotrophic hormone)**—Essential for the growth and development of bones, muscles, and other organs in children. In adults, GH enhances bone and muscle mass and promotes the destruction of fats (**lipolysis**). Hyposecretion of this hormone results in dwarfism; conversely, hypersecretion leads to gigantism during early life and acromegaly in adults.

- **Adrenocorticotropic hormone (ACTH)**—Stimulates the adrenal cortex to produce its hormones and is essential for the growth and development of the middle and inner parts of the adrenal cortex.

- **Thyroid-stimulating hormone (TSH)**—Controls the growth and development of the thyroid gland. It also stimulates the production of the hormones of the thyroid glands that are essential in influencing the body's metabolic processes.

- **Follicle-stimulating hormone (FSH)**—Gonadotropic hormone that stimulates the growth of ovarian follicles and eggs in females and the production of sperm in males. It works in conjunction with luteinizing hormone (LH).

- **Luteinizing hormone (LH)**—Gonadotropic hormone that plays an essential role in the maturation process of the ovarian follicles and in stimulating the development of the corpus luteum (progesterone-secreting endocrine tissue) in the female. In the male, LH is responsible for the production of testosterone.

- **Prolactin (PRL) (also known as lactogenic hormone)**—Gonadotropic hormone that stimulates the mammary glands to produce milk after childbirth.

- **Melanocyte-stimulating hormone (MSH)**—Controls skin pigmentation in the epidermis. The deposit of melanin helps protect skin after exposure to sunlight.

Posterior Lobe

The posterior lobe of the pituitary gland, or neurohypophysis, is responsible for storing and secreting the antidiuretic hormone (ADH) and oxytocin (OT), which are produced by the hypothalamus, as discussed earlier in this section.

Pineal Gland

The **pineal gland** is located at the posterior end of the corpus callosum in the brain. It secretes melatonin. Melatonin helps regulate the circadian rhythm, also called the "body clock,"

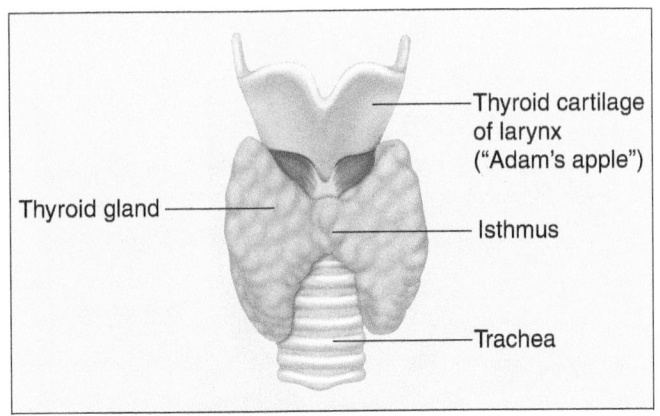

FIGURE 31-5 The thyroid gland.

which is the 24-hour cycle of waking, sleeping, and other daily functions. Melatonin also helps regulate the reproductive cycle by blocking some secretion of the gonadotropins, LH and FSH.

Thyroid Gland

The word *thyroid* is derived from a Greek word meaning "shield-shaped." The **thyroid gland** is the largest of all endocrine glands and it is responsible for the body's metabolism (Figure 31-5). It is located anterior to (or in front of) the trachea, just below the thyroid cartilage. The two lobes of the thyroid give the gland its butterfly-shaped appearance (or shield-shaped, as the Greeks thought). The lobes are connected in the center by a band of tissue called the isthmus. The thyroid gland secretes three hormones: thyroxine (T_4), tri-iodothyronine (T_3), and calcitonin.

- **Thyroxine (T_4) and Tri-iodothyronine (T_3)**—Essential for the maintenance and regulation of the basal metabolic rate (BMR), which is the rate at which the body burns the fuel (food energy) that it consumes. Iodine plays an important role, because the cells of the thyroid gland extract iodine from the blood and incorporate it into the hormones that are produced. The numerals in each of the hormone names, T_3 and T_4, indicate the number of iodine atoms that are necessary for proper function of the hormone. Both hormones are responsible for increasing cellular energy production, protein synthesis, and the repair of tissue damage. Disorders resulting from hyposecretion of thyroxine include cretinism, myxedema, and Hashimoto's thyroiditis. Hypersecretion of T_3 and T_4 results in hyperthyroidism (thyrotoxicosis). Other disorders resulting from hypersecretion of T_3 and T_4 are Graves' disease, exophthalmic goiter, and toxic goiter.

- **Calcitonin**—Influences bone and calcium metabolism. During infancy, a deficiency of calcitonin may result in

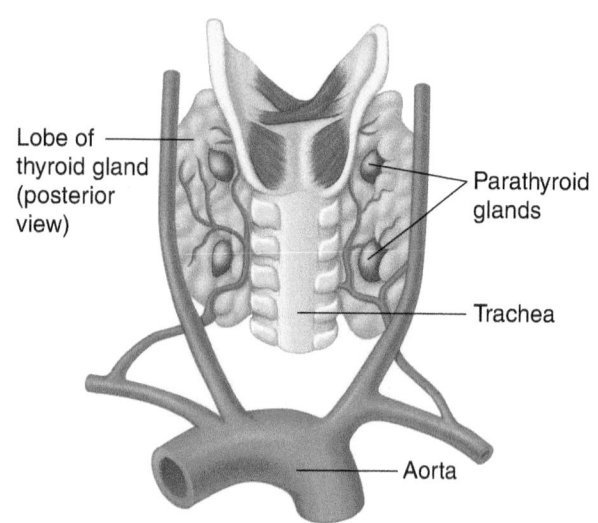

Lobe of thyroid gland (posterior view)

Parathyroid glands

Trachea

Aorta

FIGURE 31-6 The parathyroid glands.

cretinism, with arrested physical and mental development. Myxedema and Hashimoto's thyroiditis also result from hyposecretion of calcitonin and its companion hormones, T_3 and T_4.

Parathyroid Glands

The four **parathyroid glands** are located within the posterior surface of the thyroid gland (Figure 31-6). Even though they are in close proximity to the thyroid gland, they do not share any of its functions. Each of these small glands is about the size and shape of a grain of rice (3 to 5 mm in diameter). They secrete parathyroid hormone (PTH, or parathormone). PTH regulates the amount of calcium that is stored in the bones and the amount of calcium that circulates throughout the bloodstream. Calcium plays an obvious and important role in bone growth and density, but it is also essential to the

process of muscular contraction and the conduction of electricity along the nerve pathways. Hyposecretion of PTH may result in hypoparathyroidism, causing tetany (twitching of muscles or nerves). Hypersecretion of PTH may result in hyperparathyroidism, which may lead to osteoporosis, kidney stones, and hypercalcemia.

Pancreas

The **pancreas** is considered to be both an endocrine and an exocrine gland (Figure 31-7). Its exocrine function is in the secretion of gastric juices to the small intestine via a duct system. Its endocrine function resides in the **islets of Langerhans**, small clusters of cells within the pancreas that secrete hormones directly into the bloodstream.

Three main types of cells make up the islets of Langerhans: alpha, beta, and delta cells. Two additional types of cells within the islets are PP and D1 cells; however, little is known about the purpose of these cells. The alpha, beta, and delta cells play major roles in how the body balances blood sugar levels.

- **Alpha cells**—Secrete the hormone glucagon, which helps break down glycogen into glucose, which increases blood sugar levels.
- **Beta cells**—Create the hormone insulin, which has an action that is adverse to glucagon, lowering blood sugar by allowing the body's cells to absorb glucose from the blood.
- **Delta cells**—Secrete somatostatin, which helps to maintain balance within the bloodstream by suppressing the release of glucagon and insulin when necessary.

A decrease or lack of secretion, as well as hypersecretion, of these hormones results in improper blood glucose levels, which

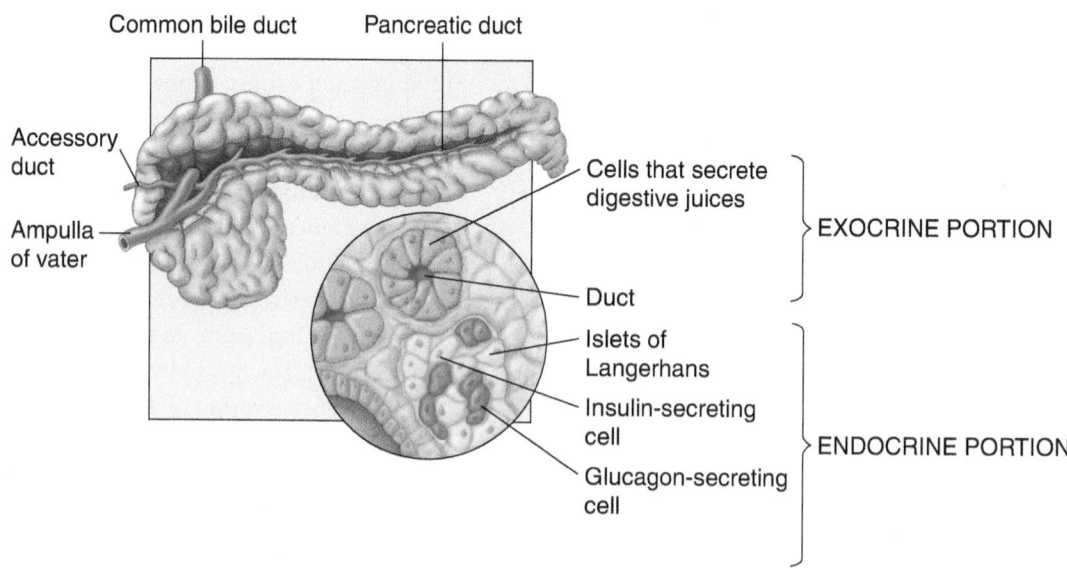

Common bile duct

Pancreatic duct

Accessory duct

Ampulla of vater

Cells that secrete digestive juices

Duct

EXOCRINE PORTION

Islets of Langerhans

Insulin-secreting cell

Glucagon-secreting cell

ENDOCRINE PORTION

FIGURE 31-7 The pancreas, an endocrine and exocrine gland.

can cause multiple issues. For example, a hyposecretion of insulin can cause dangerously high levels of glucose in the blood. In these cases, synthetic insulin can be injected subcutaneously in individuals who do not produce enough insulin. These patients are considered insulin-dependent diabetics who require insulin to help control their blood sugar levels. (Diabetes and its different forms are discussed later in this chapter.)

Adrenal Glands

The **adrenal glands** are located on top of each kidney (Figure 31-8). Each triangular gland consists of an outer portion (cortex) and an inner portion (medulla). These portions serve different functions in hormone production. The adrenal cortex secretes groups of hormones called glucocorticoids (cortisol and corticosterone), mineralocorticoids (aldosterone), and androgens. All these hormones are essential to life. The adrenal medulla synthesizes, secretes, and stores catecholamines. Catecholamines are released into the bloodstream when a person is experiencing physical or emotional stress. High levels of various catecholamines (as measured through a blood test) can indicate rare tumors or that the body is undergoing extreme stress and acute anxiety. Table 31-3 lists the hormones that are secreted by the adrenal glands.

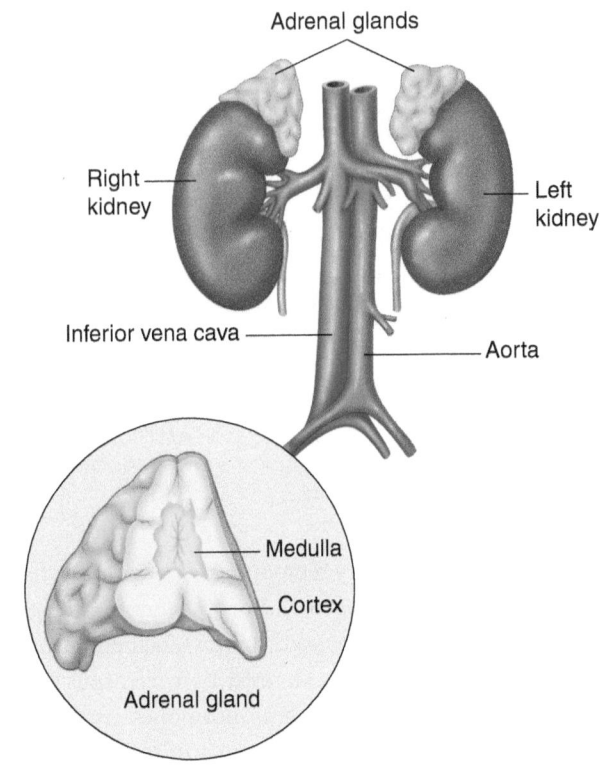

FIGURE 31-8 The adrenal glands.

TABLE 31-3 | Hormones Secreted by the Adrenal Glands

Hormone	Source of Production	Function
Cortisol	Adrenal cortex	• A steroid that is essential in the metabolism of carbohydrates, fats, and protein. • Increases blood sugar levels by stimulating glucose secretion from the liver; transports amino acids for energy storage. • Acts as an antiinflammatory agent.
Corticosterone	Adrenal cortex	• Uses carbohydrates; absorbs glucose. • Allows the liver to form glucose from substances other than carbohydrates (gluconeogenesis).
Aldosterone	Adrenal cortex	• Regulates electrolyte and water balance. • Promotes sodium and chloride retention. • Promotes potassium excretion.
Androgens	Adrenal cortex	• Promote the development of primary and secondary male characteristics. • Main androgens are testosterone and androsterone.
Dopamine	Adrenal medulla	• Elevates blood pressure through vasoconstriction. • Increases cardiac and urine output. • Synthetic dopamine is administered in the treatment of shock.
Epinephrine	Adrenal medulla	• Also known as adrenaline. • Responsible for fight-or-flight response. • Elevates heart rate, blood pressure. • Dilates bronchial tubes. • Synthetic epinephrine is administered during emergencies such as cardiac shock and anaphylaxis.
Norepinephrine	Adrenal medulla	• Causes vasoconstriction. • Elevates heart rate, blood pressure, and cardiac output. • Increases the breakdown of glycogen (glycogenolysis).

TABLE 31-4 | Hormones of the Gastrointestinal Mucosa

Hormone	Primary Location of Secretion	Function
Gastrin	The pyloric area between the stomach and the small intestine	Stimulates gastric acid secretion to aid in the breakdown and digestion of food.
Secretin	Duodenum and jejunum	Stimulates the release of water and bicarbonate from the pancreas to aid digestion.
Cholecystokinin	Duodenum	Activates the gallbladder to release bile and the pancreas to release digestive enzymes when fatty acids are present in the small intestine.
Enterogastrone	Duodenum	Regulates gastric secretions specifically by inhibiting gastric motility and other gastric hormones.

Ovaries

The **ovaries** are the primary reproductive organs of the female body. They produce estrogen and progesterone. Estrogen is the female sex hormone secreted by the Graafian follicles of the ovaries. Progesterone is secreted by the corpus luteum and is a steroid hormone. These hormones promote the growth, development, and maintenance of secondary female sex organs and characteristics, which include sexual desire, body hair growth, breast development, and feminine body features. Other functions of these hormones are preparation of the uterus for pregnancy and promotion of mammary gland development.

Testes

The **testes** are located in the male scrotum and produce the male hormone testosterone, which is essential for the normal growth and development of the male accessory sex organs. Testosterone is necessary for the act of copulation, or sexual intercourse, and developing secondary sexual characteristics in the male including sexual desire, deepening of the voice, body hair growth, and masculine body features.

Placenta

The **placenta** is a spongy structure that joins mother and fetus and provides the blood supply between the two. Present only during pregnancy, it acts as an endocrine gland by producing estrogen, progesterone, and the human chorionic gonadotropin hormone (hCG). HCG is responsible for maintaining a viable and healthy pregnancy by ensuring that the developing fetus is receiving proper amounts of nutrients and calories necessary for proper growth.

Gastrointestinal Mucosa

The mucosal lining of the stomach and small intestine contains endocrine cells that produce specific hormones that facilitate digestion. Hormones secreted by the gastrointestinal mucosa include gastrin, secretin, cholecystokinin (CCK), and enterogastrone. More detail about these hormones can be found in Table 31-4.

Professionalism — The Life Span

The Child

- Most of the structures and glands of the endocrine system develop during the first three months of pregnancy. During pregnancy, the hormones that cross the placental barrier protect the fetus. Because of maternal hormones, both male and female newborns may have swelling of the breasts and genitalia.
- Type 1 diabetes is a common endocrine system disorder of childhood. It is often diagnosed between the ages of 5 and 7 years and also between 11 and 13 years. This childhood-onset disorder is characterized by the lack of the ability to secrete insulin. Unfortunately, because of increased rates of childhood obesity, type 2 diabetes is also becoming a disease that is diagnosed in children. Management of diabetes in children is somewhat challenging, because diet, exercise, and medication must be continually adjusted to meet the changing needs of the growing child. (Type 1 and type 2 diabetes are discussed in more detail later in this chapter.)

The Older Adult

- The number of tissue receptors decreases as the body ages. This diminishes the ability of the body to properly respond to hormones.
- Aging can have a direct influence on the pituitary gland, resulting in decreased size and function. This, in turn, can cause decreased growth hormone function, which can decrease lean muscle and heart function and lead to osteoporosis.
- Aging females begin to experience a decrease in estrogen production as a result of menopause, resulting in increased risk of heart disease and osteoporosis.

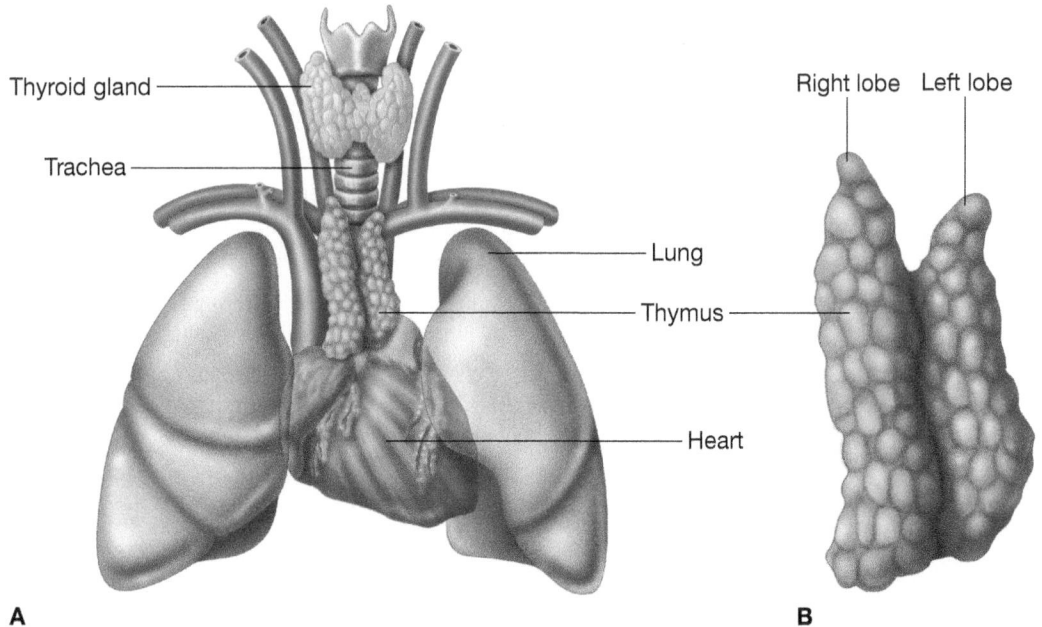

FIGURE 31-9 The thymus gland (A) appearance and position and (B) anatomical structures.

Thymus Gland

The **thymus gland** in the cavity of the mediastinum is both anterior to (in front of) and superior to (above) the heart. The thymus gland is also discussed in the chapter titled "The Immune System" because the gland is comprised of lymphoid tissue, which is an important factor in immune response (Figure 31-9). Having both lymphatic and endocrine functions, the thymus gland secretes two hormones:

- **Thymosin**—Promotes the maturation of T lymphocytes.
- **Thymopoietin**—Influences the production of lymphocyte precursors and aids in their process of becoming T lymphocytes.

COMMON PATHOLOGY ASSOCIATED WITH THE ENDOCRINE SYSTEM

A variety of diseases affect the endocrine system (Table 31-5). Most are treated medically; however, a few surgical options are also appropriate. Table 31-6 lists common procedures and treatments related to the endocrine system.

Acromegaly

Acromegaly is a hormonal disorder that results from the overproduction of growth hormone (GH) by the anterior pituitary gland, many times because of a benign tumor on the gland. Middle-aged adults are most often affected. Left untreated, this disorder can lead to the development of other conditions such as arthritis, diabetes mellitus, hypertension, increased risk of cardiovascular disease, and premature death.

Signs and Symptoms. Acromegaly has many possible signs and symptoms, but it is most commonly characterized by the abnormal growth of the hands and feet. Swelling and excessive growth of the soft tissues of the hands and feet can be noticed when a patient's shoes or rings no longer fit because of growth. Arthritis, carpal tunnel syndrome, and weakness in the hands are common related effects brought on by the abundance of overgrown tissue and bone compressing the structures and nerves within the hands.

Changes that occur to facial features, primarily to the bony structures of the face, are another hallmark feature of acromegaly. The brow and lower jaw become more prominent and protrude, the nasal bone becomes larger, and spacing between the teeth increases. Those with acromegaly may also display signs and symptoms such as a deeper voice (attributed to enlarged sinuses and vocal cords); upper airway obstruction resulting in snoring and sleep apnea; skin changes (thicker and oilier); increased sweating and odor of the skin; and weakness and fatigue. Women may have menstrual and breast changes. Men may experience impotence.

Treatment. Treatment focuses on returning growth hormone levels to a normal range. When a pituitary tumor is involved (which is often the case), it is necessary to relieve pressure on brain tissues caused by the enlarged gland and ensure that the function of the gland is maintained. Treatment options include surgical removal of the tumor, radiation of the tumor if surgery is not an option, and drug therapy to reduce the level of GH production and alleviate symptoms.

TABLE 31-5 | Diseases and Disorders of the Endocrine System

Disorder	Description
Acidosis	Excessive acidity of bodily fluids because of the accumulation of acids, as in diabetic acidosis.
Adenoma	A neoplasm or tumor of a gland, as in a pituitary adenoma.
Cretinism	Congenital condition caused by a deficiency in the secretion of thyroid hormones; may result in arrested physical and mental development.
Cushing's Syndrome	Set of symptoms that result from hypersecretion of the adrenal cortex; may result from a tumor of the adrenal glands; may present symptoms of weakness, edema, excess hair growth, skin discoloration, and osteoporosis.
Diabetes Insipidus (DI)	Disorder caused by the inadequate secretion of antidiuretic hormone (ADH) by the posterior lobe of the pituitary gland; polyuria and polydipsia are symptoms.
Diabetic Retinopathy	Secondary complication of diabetes mellitus (DM); affects the blood vessels of the retina, resulting in visual changes and even blindness.
Goiter	Enlargement of the thyroid gland.
Hashimoto's Thyroiditis	An autoimmune disease that causes thyroid inflammation and hypothyroidism.
Hirsutism	Condition of having an excessive amount of hair on the body; term that describes females who have the adult male pattern of hair growth; can result from hormonal imbalance.
Hypercalcemia	Condition of having an excessive amount of calcium in the blood.
Hyperglycemia	Having an excessive amount of glucose (sugar) in the blood.
Hyperkalemia	Condition of having an excessive amount of potassium in the blood.
Hyperthyroidism	Condition that results from overactivity of the thyroid gland; also called Graves' disease.
Hypoglycemia	Condition of low amount of glucose (sugar) in the blood.
Hypothyroidism	Result of a deficiency in secretion of hormones by the thyroid gland; results in a lowered basal metabolic rate (BMR) with obesity, dry skin, slow pulse, low blood pressure, sluggishness, and goiter; treated with synthetic thyroid hormone.
Ketoacidosis	Acidosis caused by an excess of ketone bodies (waste products); can result in death for the diabetic patient if not reversed.
Myasthenia Gravis	Condition characterized by great muscular weakness and progressive fatigue; may be difficulty in chewing and swallowing and drooping eyelids; if thymoma is causing the problem, can be treated with removal of the thymus gland.
Myxedema	Condition resulting from hypofunction of the thyroid gland and hyposecretion of thyroid hormones; possible symptoms: anemia, slow speech, enlarged tongue and facial features, edematous skin, drowsiness, and mental apathy.
Thyrotoxicosis	Condition that results from overproduction of hormones by the thyroid gland; symptoms: rapid heart action, tremors, enlarged thyroid gland, exophthalmos, and weight loss.
Von Recklinghausen Disease	Excessive production of parathyroid hormone; results in degeneration of the bones.

Addison's Disease

In **Addison's disease**, the cortex of the adrenal gland is damaged, decreasing the production of adrenocortical hormones. Etiology of the disease is far reaching and causes can be linked to infections such as HIV or tuberculosis, an autoimmune attack, tumors (cancerous or benign), or hemorrhage into the glands. The use of anticoagulants (blood thinners) is also linked to the disease. Although this disease is rare, it does not discriminate as it occurs at any age and affects men and women equally.

Signs and Symptoms. Signs and symptoms of Addison's disease include weight loss as a result of decreased appetite; chronic diarrhea, chronic nausea, and vomiting; weakness and lethargy; increased pigmentation of the skin and mucous membranes that produces a patchy appearance; changes in blood pressure and heart rate; paleness; craving of salty foods; and mouth lesions. Most symptoms occur over several months; occasionally, however, they may appear quite suddenly. Addison's disease is diagnosed by blood and urine tests that measure corticosteroid hormone

TABLE 31-6 | Procedures and Diagnostic Tests Related to the Endocrine System

Procedure/Test	Description
17-Hydroxycorticosteroids (17-OHCS)	Test performed on urine to identify adrenocorticosteroid hormones. It is used to determine adrenal cortical function.
17-Ketosteroids (17-KS)	Test performed on urine to determine the amount of 17-KS present. 17-KS is the end product of androgens and is secreted from the adrenal glands and testes. It is used in diagnosing adrenal tumors.
2-Hour Postprandial Glucose Tolerance Test	Blood test to assist in evaluating glucose metabolism. The patient fasts overnight and then eats a high-carbohydrate meal in the morning. A blood sample is then taken 2 hours after the meal.
Basal Metabolic Rate	Somewhat outdated test that is still sometimes performed to measure the energy used when the body is in a state of rest.
Blood Serum Test	Blood test to measure the level of such substances as calcium, electrolytes, testosterone, insulin, and glucose. Used to assist in determining the function of various endocrine glands.
Fasting Blood Sugar	Blood test to measure the amount of glucose circulating throughout the body after fasting for 12 hours.
Glucose Tolerance Test (GTT)	Test to determine the blood sugar level. A measured dose of glucose is given to the patient either orally or intravenously. Blood samples are then drawn at specific intervals to determine the patient's ability to use glucose. This test is often used for diabetic patients to determine their insulin response to glucose and for pregnant women to detect gestational diabetes.
Hemoglobin A1C	Used to provide a clinical picture of a patient's blood glucose levels over a period of 3 months. A normal A1C is below 5.7 percent. The higher the percentage, the higher the patient's average blood glucose level.
Parathyroidectomy	Excision of one or more of the parathyroid glands. This is performed to halt the progress of hyperparathyroidism.
Protein Bound Iodine Test (PBI)	Blood test to measure the concentration of thyroxine (T4) circulating in the bloodstream. The iodine becomes bound to the protein in the blood and can be measured.
Radioactive Iodine Uptake Test (RAIU)	Test in which radioactive iodine is taken orally or intravenously, and the amount of iodine eventually taken into the thyroid gland (uptake) is measured to assist in determining thyroid function.
Radioimmune Assay Test (RIA)	Test used to measure the levels of hormones in the plasma of the blood.
Serum Glucose Test	Blood test performed to assist in determining glucose levels and useful for adjusting medication dosage.
Thymectomy	Surgical removal of the thymus gland.
Thyroid Echogram	Ultrasound examination of the thyroid that can assist in distinguishing a thyroid nodule from a cyst.
Thyroidectomy	Surgical removal of the thyroid gland. The patient is then placed on replacement hormone (thyroid) therapy.
Thyroid Function Tests	Blood tests used to measure the levels of T_3, T_4, and TSH in the bloodstream to assist in determining thyroid function.
Thyroid Scan	Test in which a radioactive element is administered that localizes in the thyroid gland. The gland can then be visualized with a scanning device to detect pathology such as tumors.
Thyroparathyroidectomy	Surgical removal (excision) of the thyroid gland and parathyroid glands.
Total Calcium	Blood test to measure the total amount of calcium to assist in detecting parathyroid and bone disorders.

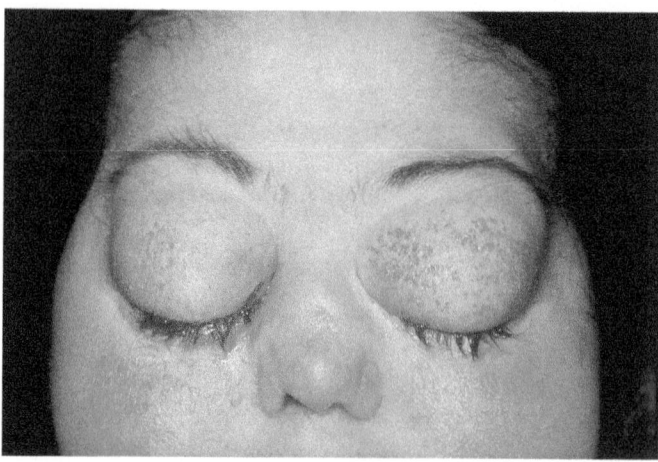

FIGURE 31-10 Facial features of Cushing's syndrome. (*Source:* ©Biophoto Associates/Science Source)

levels, the results of which are very low compared with normal values.

Treatment. Lifelong replacement of adrenocortical hormones and supplemental sodium compose the usual course of treatment for Addison's disease. Patient education focuses on the importance and understanding of this lifelong condition, including the necessity of taking medications as prescribed. Patients may also be required to administer emergency hydrocortisone injections during stressful times. Failure to take necessary medications or missing doses can lead to a life-threatening condition known as adrenal crisis. Because of the severity of this condition, patients are advised to always carry medical identification that states their condition and current and emergency medication dosing requirements.

Cushing's Disease

Cushing's disease is a rare disorder that develops as a result of a tumor growing on the pituitary gland. This tumor results in hypersecretion of adrenocorticotropic hormone (ACTH) into the bloodstream. ACTH stimulates the release of cortisol, so with excessive ACTH secretion, there is also excessive cortisol secretion. Cushing's syndrome is similar to Cushing's disease but differs in etiology. Cushing's syndrome often results from taking too much corticosteroid medication, such as prednisone. The syndrome can also be the result of tumors that develop on the adrenal glands, causing excess secretion of cortisol (Figure 31-10).

Signs and Symptoms. Signs and symptoms of Cushing's disease and Cushing's syndrome are very similar and include muscular weakness, thinning of the skin, easy bruising,

rounding of facial features ("moon face"), weight gain, and fatigue. Acne, backache (during normal activities), and an excess of fat collected between the shoulder blades (buffalo hump) are also telling signs. Women may experience excessive hair growth (face, chest, back, and thighs) as well as irregular menstrual cycles. Men may experience impotence and a decreased sexual desire. Complications of the disease include diabetes, high blood pressure, depression, and osteoporosis. Cushing's disease can cause death if it is not treated.

Treatment. Treatment for Cushing's disease depends on the underlying etiology. Treatment options include surgical removal or radiation of the pituitary tumor. Cushing's syndrome caused by a tumor on the adrenal gland may also be treated with surgery. Medication may be prescribed that blocks the production of cortisol. If Cushing's syndrome is caused by excessive use of corticosteroids, weaning off the medication is ideal. The weaning process requires medical supervision consisting of a gradual decline in dosage.

Diabetes Mellitus

In **diabetes mellitus**, the body is unable to produce enough insulin to properly control blood sugar (glucose) levels or is unable to properly make use of the insulin that is produced. Insulin is a hormone produced by the pancreas that converts sugar and starches into the energy the body needs. The lack of insulin in the body can be caused by a lack of production by the pancreas, the inability of the body's cells to properly use insulin, or a combination of both. There are three types of diabetes; type 1, type 2, and gestational diabetes. Each type has a different etiology.

Type 1 diabetes, formerly known as insulin-dependent diabetes mellitus (IDDM), is typically diagnosed in children, teens, and young adults. This form of diabetes results when the body cannot produce sufficient quantities of insulin or produces no insulin at all. The exact etiology of this form of diabetes is unknown, but it is considered to be linked to a possible autoimmune response where the body attacks the pancreatic cells (beta cells) that produce insulin. Because insulin is the hormone that helps cells absorb glucose from the blood, the result is high levels of blood glucose and insufficient glucose available to the body cells, which need glucose for normal metabolism. Careful monitoring of type 1 diabetes is essential for proper insulin regulation.

Type 2 diabetes, formerly known as non–insulin-dependent diabetes mellitus (NIDDM), is the most common form of the disease and is typically associated with obesity. With type 2 diabetes there is no autoimmune component to the disease. Formerly, this form of diabetes was usually diagnosed later in life; however, increasing rates of childhood and teen obesity are resulting in the diagnosis of type 2 diabetes in earlier years. Type 2 diabetes results from insulin resistance (insulin is present but is ineffective in helping cells absorb glucose from the blood) combined with insulin deficiency that occurs as a person gains weight and the body struggles to make enough insulin to keep blood glucose levels within the ideal, healthy range. A healthy and normal fasting blood glucose level is below 100 mg/dL (milligrams per deciliter). It is estimated that type 2 diabetes accounts for 90 to 95 percent of all of cases of diabetes.

Gestational diabetes is a form of diabetes that develops during pregnancy and results when the body is unable to make and use enough insulin to meet the requirements of both the mother and the growing fetus. It is generally diagnosed around the 24th week of pregnancy. It is very important for the pregnant mother to monitor her blood sugar levels closely and to have routine prenatal care. Most of the time, after the mother gives birth to the baby, diabetes disappears. However, later in life the mother may be at higher risk of developing diabetes mellitus.

Signs and Symptoms. Classic signs and symptoms of diabetes are polyuria (frequent urination), polydipsia (excessive thirst), and polyphagia (excessive hunger). Other symptoms include blurred vision, weakness, weight loss (without trying), lethargy, irritability, dry skin, recurrent infections, abdominal cramps, and vaginal yeast infections in women. Unfortunately, because the signs and symptoms may have a slow onset, a diagnosis may not be made until the patient is very ill.

Treatment. Type 1 diabetes requires lifelong insulin treatment. The most common form of insulin treatment is through the use of daily subcutaneous (in the fatty area under the skin) injections. Some patients are able to use an insulin pump, which is a computerized device that is implanted and delivers insulin to the body when it is needed. The delivery of insulin through a pump can be given in a steady, continual dose (basal insulin) or as a larger, surge dose (bolus). A bolus dose is often administered before meals to be sufficient for carbohydrates that are consumed. (In the body, carbohydrates are turned into glucose.) Pancreatic transplants are also used to treat patients with type 1 diabetes.

Type 2 diabetes treatment begins with diet, exercise, and oral hypoglycemic medications to help control blood sugar levels. Unfortunately, if these methods do not work to control blood glucose levels, as time progresses with the disease, many type 2 diabetics must also administer insulin injections in addition to taking oral medications. Type 2 diabetes may be preventable with modest lifestyle changes, including healthy diet choices, exercise, and weight management. Bariatric (weight loss) surgery has also been helpful for obese diabetic patients. The drastic weight loss can reverse the diagnosis of type 2 diabetes in some instances.

Professionalism — Cultural Considerations

Many ethnic groups are at an especially high risk for developing type 2 diabetes. Take, for instance, the Native American Pima tribe in Arizona. The Pimas have the highest recorded prevalence of diabetes in the world. Latinos and African Americans are also more likely than the Caucasian population to develop the disease. Because food is a major part of any given ethnic group or culture, it can be helpful to have a dietitian who is familiar with the cultural environments of patient groups. The dietitian can consult with the patient regarding diet modifications to fit the practices of the family. Education and reinforcement are necessary in these situations.

Professionalism

One aspect of success as a medical assistant is the attitude you project toward patients, coworkers, and your employer. Professional medical assistants remember that the patients are the reason their profession exists. Maintaining a positive, helpful attitude with patients and with coworkers can make even a difficult day fulfilling. Finding reasons to be thankful for your job and helping patients in all circumstances will help ensure good outcomes for both the medical assistant and the patient. There will always be individuals who are less than pleasant. However, the number of patients who are grateful for the assistance you provide them are far more numerous. Treat all patients the same way, and project a positive, caring attitude toward all.

During pregnancy, as already noted, the patient with gestational diabetes needs to closely monitor her diet and blood sugar levels. Many patients with gestational diabetes meet with an endocrinologist (a physician who specializes in diseases and disorders of the endocrine system) for a treatment plan, which may include daily insulin injections.

Dwarfism

Dwarfism refers to a group of conditions characterized by shorter-than-normal skeletal growth in the arms and legs or the trunk. By definition, those with dwarfism will not be taller than 4 feet 10 inches as a grown adult, and an average height is around 4 feet. Most of the causes of dwarfism are related to genetic disorders and caused by genetic anomalies. Sometimes dwarfism is caused by deficiencies in the growth hormone (GH). More than 200 conditions can cause abnormal skeletal growth and dwarfism.

The most common form of dwarfism is achondroplasia, which is diagnosed at birth. It affects males and females equally and occurs in approximately 1 of every 26-40,000 infants. At least 80 percent of infants born with this condition have parents of average height. The development of motor skills, such as controlling head movements, may be delayed, but intellectual development is normal. People of short stature lead normal, fulfilled lives, achieving high levels of education, career, and personal ambitions.

Signs and Symptoms. The physical characteristics of achondroplasia include disproportionately short arms and legs with a trunk of normal length; bowed legs; reduced joint mobility in the elbow, although loose ligaments make other joints seem overly flexible or double jointed; shortened hands and feet; a large head; a prominent forehead; a flattened bridge of the nose; and crowded teeth (because of a small upper jaw).

Treatment. There is no cure for achondroplasia. In addition to social and family support, treatment focuses on the prevention, management, and treatment of medical complications. Surgery may be performed to relieve pressure on the nervous system, generally at the base of the skull and lower back. Because of smaller jaw structure, the airway is often obstructed; therefore, removing adenoids may be helpful in widening the airway. Dental and orthodontic work may be necessary to correct malocclusion (abnormality in the way the teeth meet) and preserve dental health.

Gigantism

Gigantism is a rare disease that results from excessive secretion of growth hormone (GH) during childhood, before the closure of the bone growth plates. Unlike acromegaly, which is diagnosed in adulthood, gigantism is diagnosed in children.

The cause of excess GH secretion is most often a benign (noncancerous) tumor on the pituitary gland. Gigantism may also be caused by an underlying medical condition such as multiple endocrine neoplasia (abnormal tissue growth).

Signs and Symptoms. Gigantism is characterized by overgrowth of the long bones and very tall stature. Children with gigantism are extremely large for their age. Additional signs and symptoms include delayed puberty, increased sweating, blurred vision, large hands and feet, thick fingers and toes, muscle weakness, and a thickening of facial features.

Treatment. If the underlying cause of gigantism is a pituitary tumor, surgical removal is ideal. However, surgery can be performed only if the edges of the tumor are clearly defined, ensuring complete removal. In other cases, medications that reduce the release or block the effects of GH are prescribed. As a last resort, radiation therapy is also used to reduce GH levels. However, it must be borne in mind that excessive exposure to radiation has serious side effects.

Hyperthyroidism

Hyperthyroidism is characterized by elevated thyroid hormone levels. **Graves' disease**, an autoimmune disorder, is the most common form of hyperthyroidism and tends to affect women more than men. With this autoimmune condition, antibodies produced by the immune system stimulate the thyroid to produce too much thyroxine.

Signs and Symptoms. The symptoms of hyperthyroidism include nervousness, restlessness, heart palpitations, tremors, sweating, frequent bowel movements, menstrual changes, weight loss, and changes in the fingernails and hair (thinning and brittle). Overall itching, clammy skin, hair loss, and high blood pressure are additional signs and symptoms. A condition known as **exophthalmos** is another possible result, in which the eyeballs protrude beyond their normal protective orbit when the tissues behind them swell (Figure 31-11). Hyperthyroidism can lead to a rapid heart rate, atrial fibrillation, and congestive heart failure. Other complications include osteoporosis (weak, brittle bones) and sensitivity to light.

Treatment. Hyperthyroidism is treated with antithyroid medications, radioactive iodine to destroy the thyroid, or surgery (thyroidectomy). If the thyroid is removed or destroyed, lifelong thyroid replacement therapy must be initiated.

Hypothyroidism

In **hypothyroidism** the thyroid produces inadequate amounts of the thyroid hormones. This condition is the complete

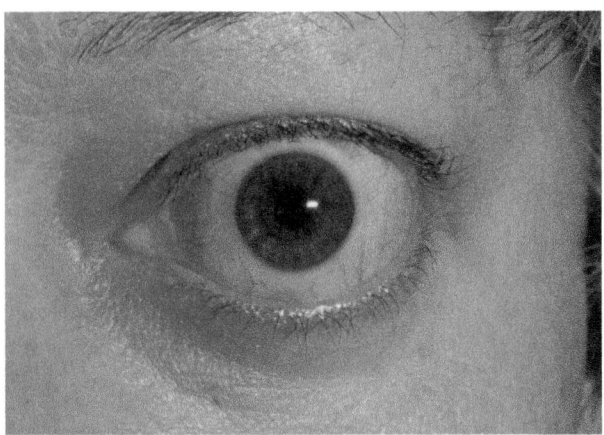

FIGURE 31-11 Exophthalmos.
(*Source:* ©Dr. P. Marazzi/Science Source)

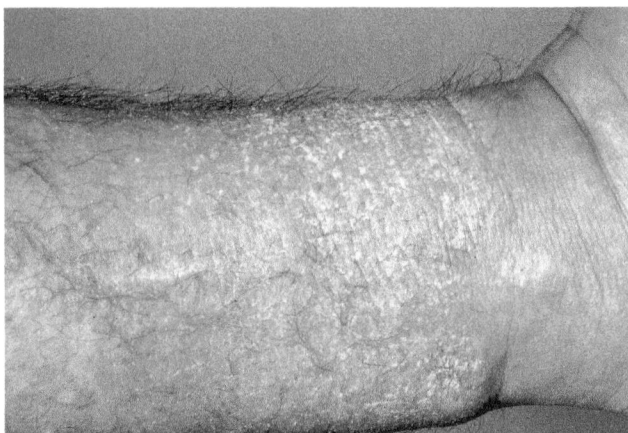

FIGURE 31-13 Dry skin typical of advanced myxedema.
(*Source:* ©Biophoto Associates/Science Source)

opposite of Graves' disease (hyperthyroidism). It is difficult to diagnose hypothyroidism in its early stages because it develops slowly and symptoms are vague. There are approximately seven million cases of this disorder in the United States alone.

The etiology surrounding hypothyroidism involves the thyroid gland becoming overstimulated, resulting in the constant need to compensate and release more thyroid hormones. As this occurs, the thyroid may enlarge and a condition known as a **goiter** develops (see Figure 31-12). The most common cause of a goiter is **Hashimoto's thyroiditis**, an autoimmune inflammation of the thyroid. Untreated hypothyroidism is also associated with a higher risk of heart disease, because of the high levels of low-density lipoproteins (LDL, the "bad" cholesterol) that can develop. **Cardiomegaly** (enlarged heart) can also occur.

Myxedema is a rare, life-threatening condition characterized by tiredness, extreme lethargy, intense cold intolerance, and an eventual loss of consciousness. It occurs when hypothyroidism is left untreated for a long period of time (Figure 31-13).

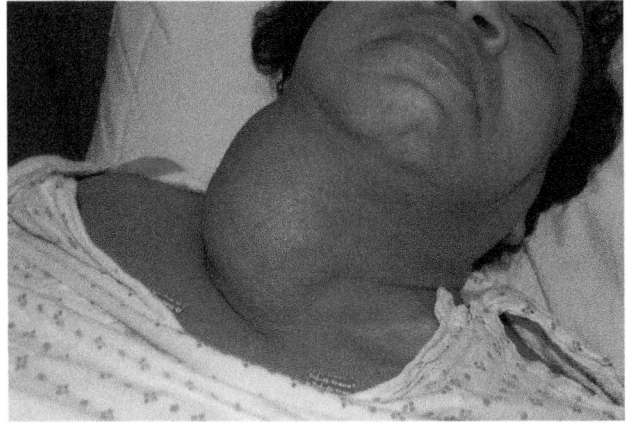

FIGURE 31-12 Goiter.
(*Source:* ©Edward T. Dickinson, MD)

Signs and Symptoms. Initial signs and symptoms tend to be subtle and include fatigue, decreased concentration, intolerance to cold, constipation, loss of appetite, muscle cramping, stiffness, and weight gain. Other symptoms are mood changes, decreased sexual desire, slowed mental function, hair loss, dry skin, and nail changes.

Treatment. Typical treatment for hypothyroidism involves the daily use of a synthetic thyroid hormone, such as levothyroxine (Synthroid, Levothroid). Taken orally, this hormone supplement reduces symptoms, particularly fatigue, weight loss, and increased LDL. This medication must be taken on a routine basis, usually lifelong. A patient's hormone levels are monitored regularly with blood work, and the dosage should be adjusted as necessary.

Professionalism | The Workplace

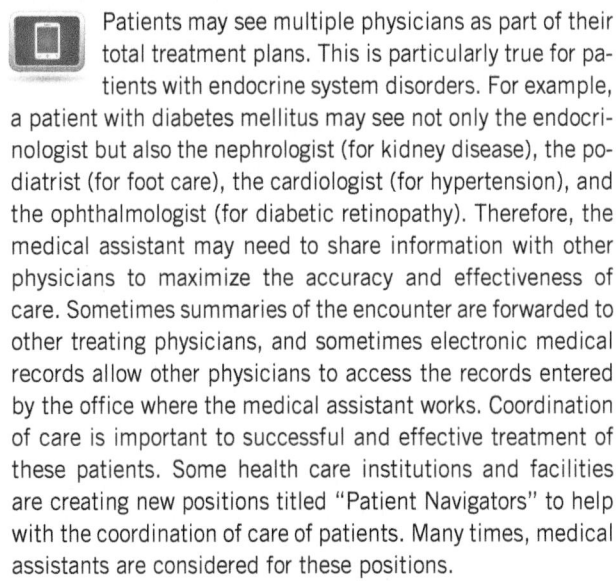

Patients may see multiple physicians as part of their total treatment plans. This is particularly true for patients with endocrine system disorders. For example, a patient with diabetes mellitus may see not only the endocrinologist but also the nephrologist (for kidney disease), the podiatrist (for foot care), the cardiologist (for hypertension), and the ophthalmologist (for diabetic retinopathy). Therefore, the medical assistant may need to share information with other physicians to maximize the accuracy and effectiveness of care. Sometimes summaries of the encounter are forwarded to other treating physicians, and sometimes electronic medical records allow other physicians to access the records entered by the office where the medical assistant works. Coordination of care is important to successful and effective treatment of these patients. Some health care institutions and facilities are creating new positions titled "Patient Navigators" to help with the coordination of care of patients. Many times, medical assistants are considered for these positions.

SUMMARY

The endocrine system releases hormones that keep the body in proper balance, or homeostasis. Working closely with the nervous system, these hormones regulate growth, development, mood, tissue function, metabolism, and sexual function.

The organs of the endocrine system include the hypothalamus gland, pituitary gland, pineal gland, thymus gland, thyroid and parathyroid glands, adrenal glands, pancreas, ovaries, and testes. The anterior lobe of the pituitary gland secretes growth hormone, follicle-stimulating hormone, adrenocorticotropin, thyroid-stimulating hormone, luteinizing hormone, prolactin, and melanocyte-stimulating hormone. The posterior lobe stores and secretes antidiuretic hormone and oxytocin, both of which are produced by the hypothalamus. Melatonin is released by the pineal gland. Thyroxine, tri-iodothyronine, and calcitonin are secreted in the thyroid glands. The parathyroid glands produce parathormone. Insulin and glucagon are secreted by the pancreas. The adrenal cortex secretes cortisol, corticosterone, aldosterone, and androgens. The adrenal medulla secretes dopamine, epinephrine, and norepinephrine. The ovaries secrete estrogens and progesterone. The testes secrete testosterone. The placenta controls pregnancy hormones: human chorionic gonadotropin hormone, estrogen, and progesterone. Secretin is secreted by the gastrointestinal mucosa, and the thymus gland releases thymosin and thymopoietin.

Common disorders of the endocrine system include acromegaly, Addison's disease, Cushing's disease, diabetes mellitus, dwarfism, gigantism, hyperthyroidism, and hypothyroidism.

(31) CHAPTER REVIEW

COMPETENCY REVIEW

1. Define and spell the terms for this chapter.
2. What is the vital function of the endocrine system?
3. Why is the pituitary gland known as the master gland of the body?
4. What hormones are secreted by the thyroid gland?
5. What is the function of insulin?
6. Explain the endocrine and exocrine functions of the pancreas.
7. Name three functions of the hormone epinephrine.
8. Explain the endocrine function of the placenta.
9. What hormones do the ovaries secrete?
10. Name two hormones secreted by the thymus.

PREPARING FOR THE CERTIFICATION EXAM

1. Which of the following organs/structures is/are *not* a component of the endocrine system?
   a. pineal
   b. ovaries
   c. thymus
   d. testes
   e. liver

2. Addison's disease is a result of damage to what structure?
   a. pituitary
   b. adrenal gland
   c. ovary
   d. thyroid
   e. thymus

3. The endocrine gland that is responsible for calcitonin secretion is the
   a. parathyroid.
   b. pancreas.
   c. ovary.
   d. thyroid.
   e. adrenal cortex.

4. A possible disorder that results from the hypersecretion of thyroid hormones is
   a. diabetes insipidus.
   b. diabetes mellitus.
   c. tetany.
   d. exophthalmic goiter.
   e. Addison's disease.

5. A disorder caused by the hypofunction of the thyroid gland is
   a. myasthenia gravis.
   b. myxedema.
   c. Graves' disease.
   d. Cushing's disease.
   e. Addison's disease.

6. Which of the following is *not* one of the cardinal signs of diabetes mellitus?
   a. polypharmacy
   b. polyuria
   c. polyphagia
   d. hyperglycemia
   e. polydipsia

7. Increasing rates of obesity in teens and children are resulting in which disease being diagnosed at a younger age?
   a. type 1 diabetes
   b. Addison's disease
   c. type 2 diabetes
   d. Cushing's disease
   e. gigantism

8. An excessive amount of hair on the body because of a hormone imbalance is known as
   a. Hashimoto's disease.
   b. hirsutism.
   c. myxedema.
   d. von Reckinghausen disease.
   e. myasthenia gravis.

9. Testosterone affects all of the following *except*
   a. sexual desire.
   b. body hair growth.
   c. deepening of voice.
   d. masculine body features.
   e. gastric secretions.

10. Undersecretion of growth hormone (GH) results in
    a. exophthalmos.
    b. dwarfism.
    c. Simmonds disease.
    d. Goiter.
    e. gigantism.

CRITICAL THINKING

Refer to the case study at the beginning of the chapter and use what you have learned to answer the following questions.

1. One of the laboratory tests performed was an FBS (fasting blood sugar) ordered by Dr. Bahjat. Give an example of an abnormal FBS that could be concerning for Dr. Bahjat.

2. List some signs and symptoms that Ms. Gutierrez may have had, which would have indicated to Dr. Bahjat that she should be tested for type 2 diabetes mellitus.

3. How does Ms. Gutierrez's ethnicity play a role in her diagnosis? What should be considered regarding patient education?

INTERNET ACTIVITY

Do an Internet search to learn about support groups for individuals with diabetes. What kind of support is available for people with this disorder?

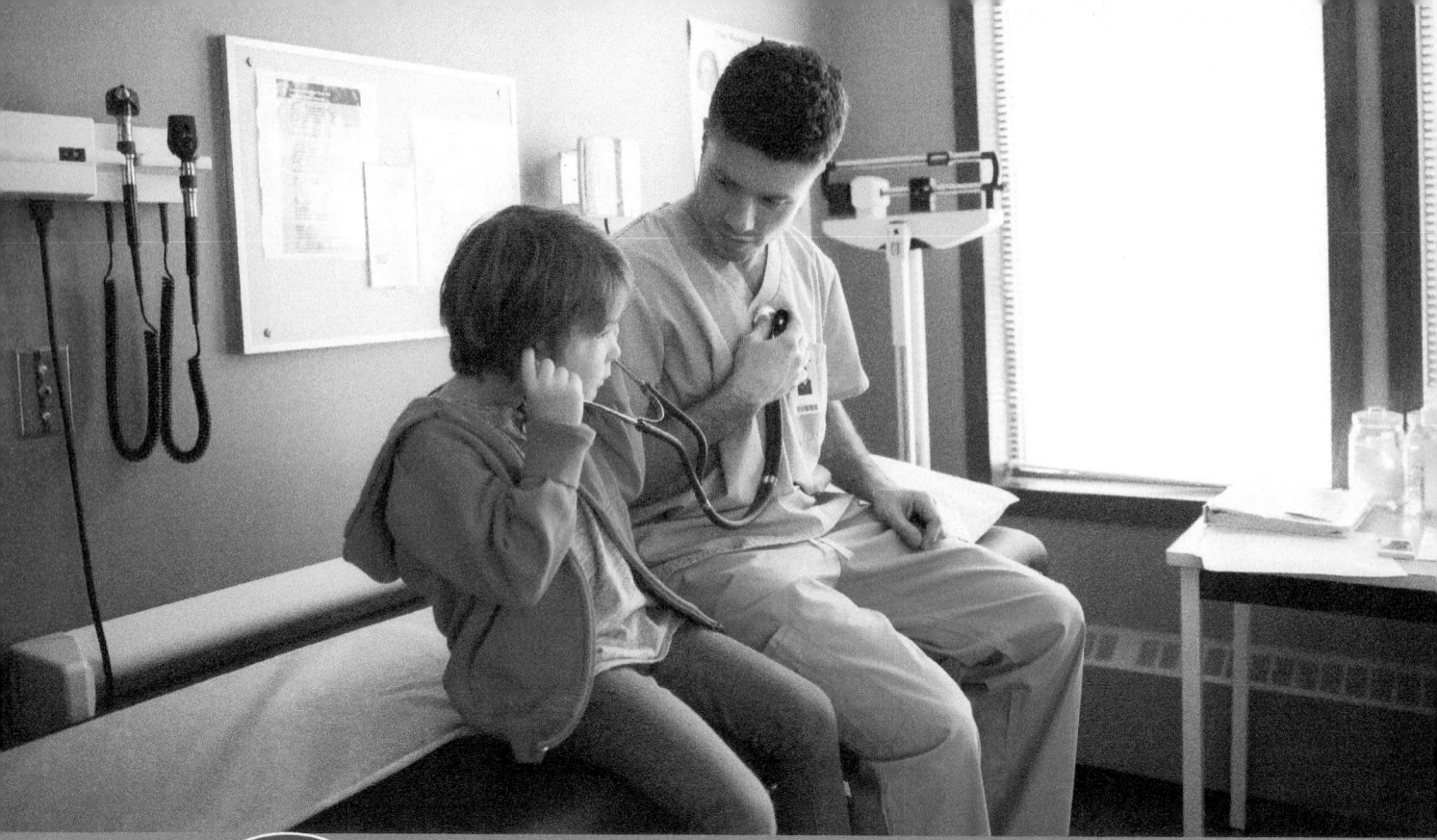

The Reproductive System

Learning Objectives

After completing this chapter, you should be able to:

32.1   Define and spell the terms for this chapter.
32.2   Describe the functions of the various structures of the female reproductive system.
32.3   Explain the four stages of the menstrual cycle.
32.4   Identify milestones that occur with each trimester of pregnancy.
32.5   List the stages that occur during the birthing process.
32.6   Describe common pathology associated with the female reproductive system.
32.7   Describe the functions of the various structures of the male reproductive system.
32.8   Explain how the reproductive system changes throughout the life span from childhood to adulthood.
32.9   Describe common pathology associated with the male reproductive system.

Nabiel Hamsi is a 21-year-old male being seen by Dr. Bahjat. He is being seen in the office today because of a swollen left testicle. Nabiel noticed the swelling a week ago but is now unable to bear the pain. Dr. Bahjat diagnoses Nabiel with epididymitis. During the examination, Dr. Bahjat asks Nabiel if he is sexually active. Nabiel answers, "No, I am waiting until I am married."

Terms to Learn

adhesions	fibrocystic breast disease	premenstrual syndrome (PMS)
benign prostatic hyperplasia (BPH)	flagella	prostate cancer
breast cancer	gestation	prostate gland
bulbourethral glands	hydrocele	salpingo-oophorectomy
cervical cancer	hysterectomy	scrotum
cervicitis	infertility	sexually transmitted disease (STD)
circumcision	menarche	spermatozoa
contraception	menopause	testes
copulation	myomectomy	urethra
dysmenorrhea	ovarian cancer	urethritis
embryonic period	ovarian cysts	uterine cancer
endometriosis	ovaries	uterine fibroids
epididymitis	ovulation	uterus
episiotomy	ovum	vagina
erectile dysfunction (ED)	pelvic inflammatory disease (PID)	vaginitis
fallopian tubes	penis	vulva
fetal period	perineum	

THE FEMALE REPRODUCTIVE SYSTEM

The female reproductive system consists of the primary sex organs, the ovaries, and the accessory sex organs, which include the uterus, fallopian (uterine) tubes, the vagina, the vulva, and the breasts (Figure 32-1). The purpose and function of the female reproductive system is to continue the human species through sexual reproduction.

Ovaries

There are two **ovaries** in the female reproductive system. These oblong, oval-shaped structures flank each side of the uterus, to which they are attached by ovarian ligaments. Figure 32-2 displays these ligaments as well as other structures that are discussed in this section. Each ovary is about 1½ inches long, ¾-inch wide, and ½-inch thick. The ovaries have two functions:

- To produce ova (plural of *ovum*), or eggs
- To produce hormones

The ovaries lie close to the fimbriae of the fallopian tubes. The fimbriae are fingerlike processes that help propel the ovum toward the fallopian tube after it is discharged from the ovary. The fallopian tube is discussed later in the chapter.

The ovary has two distinct microscopic divisions: the cortex (the outer layer) and the medulla (inner layer). The cortex contains small secretory sacs called follicles, which hold the ova in different stages of development: primary, secondary, and Graafian (mature). The ovarian medulla contains connective tissue, nerves, blood, and lymphatic vessels.

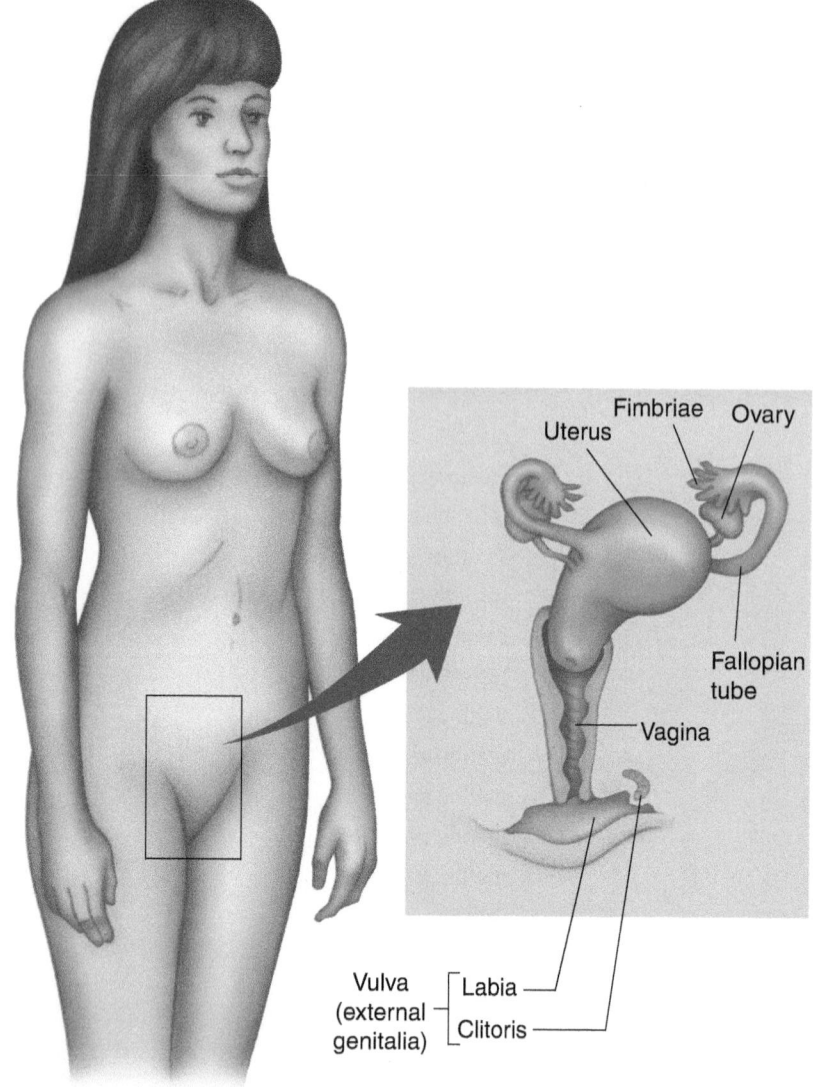

FIGURE 32-1 The female reproductive system.

The anterior lobe of the pituitary gland (a part of the endocrine system as described in the chapter titled "The Endocrine System") controls the production of hormones within the ovary, particularly follicle-stimulating hormone (FSH) and luteinizing hormone (LH). FSH is instrumental in the development of the follicle nurturing the ovum. LH stimulates the development of the corpus luteum, a small mass of cells that develops after the release of the ovum. Each month, a Graafian follicle ruptures on the ovarian cortex, and an ovum is released into the pelvic cavity and into one of the fallopian tubes. This process is known as **ovulation**. In the average woman, more than 400 ova may be produced during the reproductive years.

Two additional hormones produced by the ovaries that are instrumental in the function of the reproductive system are estrogen and progesterone. The follicles secrete estrogen while progesterone is secreted by the corpus luteum. Both these hormones are vital to functions related to pregnancy, breast development, sexual drive, and promoting the growth, development, and maintenance of the secondary female sex characteristics.

Secondary sex characteristics are physical features that are not specific to the function of reproduction but differentiate men from women. Secondary sex characteristics in women include enlarged breasts, less facial hair, functional mammary glands, and smoother skin texture.

Uterus

The **uterus** is a pear-shaped muscular organ with thick walls. It is found in the pelvic cavity above the bladder and anterior to (in front of) the rectum. It has three distinct areas:

- **The upper portion**—Called the body
- **The central portion**—Called the isthmus
- **The neck**—Called the cervix

The fundus is the rounded surface of the uterine body that extends from the internal

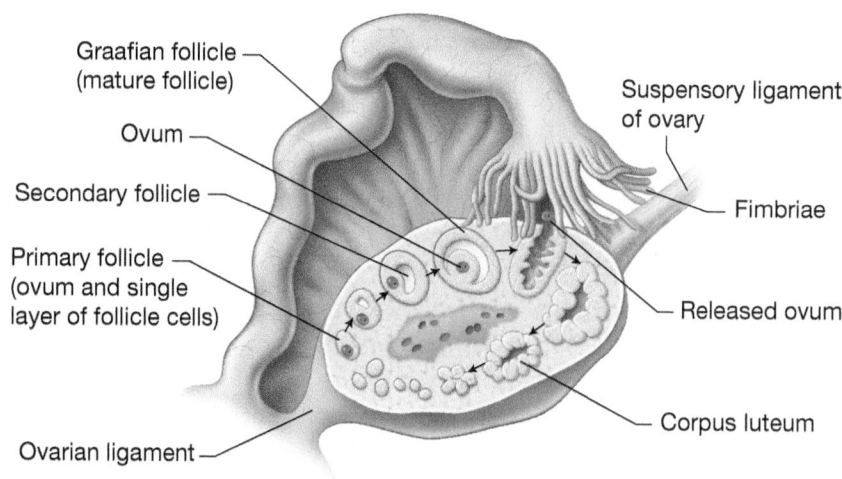

FIGURE 32-2 The ovary.

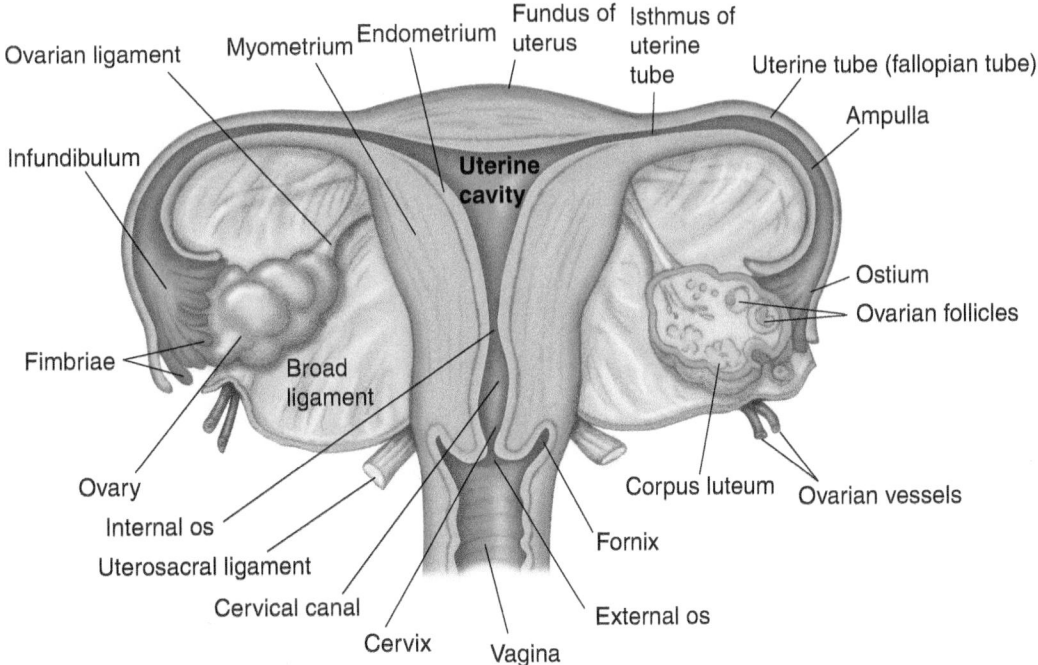

Ovarian ligament — Myometrium — Endometrium — Fundus of uterus — Isthmus of uterine tube — Uterine tube (fallopian tube) — Ampulla — Infundibulum — **Uterine cavity** — Fimbriae — Broad ligament — Ostium — Ovarian follicles — Ovary — Internal os — Uterosacral ligament — Cervical canal — Cervix — Vagina — Corpus luteum — Ovarian vessels — Fornix — External os

FIGURE 32-3 The uterus and associated structures.

os (mouth) of the cervix upward above the fallopian tube (Figure 32-3). A number of ligaments support the uterus and hold it in place: two broad ligaments, two round ligaments, and two uterosacral ligaments.

The walls of the uterus have three defined layers. The innermost surface, the endometrium, has a mucosal lining; the muscular middle layer is the myometrium; the outermost layer is the perimetrium. It is important to note that the endometrium changes because of hormonal response throughout the menstrual cycle. This layer of the uterus is supplied with arterial blood. The primary functions of the uterus include:

- Shedding of the endometrium (in response to hormonal changes) during the monthly menstrual cycle.
- Providing protection and suppling nourishment to a growing fetus during pregnancy.
- Contracting, in a rhythmic pattern, during labor to deliver the fetus from the uterus. The rhythmic contractions occur in the myometrial layer of the uterus.

Fallopian Tubes

The **fallopian tubes** extend along each side of the uterus and curve inward toward each ovary. The two fallopian tubes are sometimes referred to as uterine tubes or oviducts. The main function of these tubes is to serve as pathways for reproductive cells. Within a fallopian tube, the female reproductive cell, the **ovum** or egg, will move from the ovary toward the

uterus; the male reproductive cell, the sperm or **spermatozoa**, moves from the uterus toward the ovary.

Each fallopian tube is about 4½ inches long and ¼-inch wide and is composed of three layers:

- **The serous layer**—Outermost and made of connective tissue
- **The middle layer**—Muscular and made of circular and longitudinal smooth muscle
- **The mucosal layer**—Innermost and consists of simple columnar epithelium

Each fallopian tube has three segments that can be characterized by their shape and position between the uterus and the ovary:

- **Isthmus**—Narrow, constricted portion closest to the uterus
- **Ampulla**—Area where the fallopian tube begins to widen as it extends toward the ovary
- **Ostium**—Funnel-shaped opening with fimbriae (fringelike threads) that project and attach to the ovary

Refer again to Figure 32-3 for a visual representation of these specific structures.

Vagina

The **vagina** is a tube composed of muscle and membranes that extends from the vestibule (discussed next) to the uterus. It is typically 4 to 6 inches in length and is situated between the bladder and the rectum. The hymen, a thin fold of mucousal membrane, partially covers the external opening of the vagina. Typically, when a woman engages in sexual intercourse (**copulation**) for the first time, the hymen is ruptured.

The vagina functions as the female organ of copulation, as the pathway for menstrual discharge, and as the pathway for the birth of a fetus.

Vulva

Five organs (Figure 32-4) make up the external female genitalia known as the **vulva**:

- **Mons pubis**—The rounded area, comprised of a triangular-shaped pad of fatty tissue, that covers the symphysis pubis (where the right and left pubic bones join). After puberty the area is covered in hair.

- **Labia majora**—The two folds of fatty tissue that lie on either side of the vaginal opening.

- **Labia minora**—The two thin folds of skin that enclose the vestibule and are located within the labia majora.

- **Vestibule**—The area between the labia minora. There are four structures in the vestibule: the urethra (the external opening of the urinary system), the vagina, and the two excretory ducts of the Bartholin's glands.

- **Clitoris**—The small organ of erectile tissue that contains a rich supply of sensory nerves.

Between the vulva and the anus is the **perineum**, an external region that is composed of muscle covered with skin. Sometimes, during labor, this area is cut by the physician in an **episiotomy**, a procedure that is performed to prevent tearing of the perineum during childbirth.

Breasts

The breasts, or mammary glands, are rounded structures made of fatty, glandular, and fibrous tissue that protrude from the chest. Each breast has numerous alveolar glands that form 12 to 15 distinct tissue lobes, which are separated by connecting tissue (Figure 32-5). The darkened area of circular skin found in the center of each breast is the areola, and the nipple is the elevated area in the center of

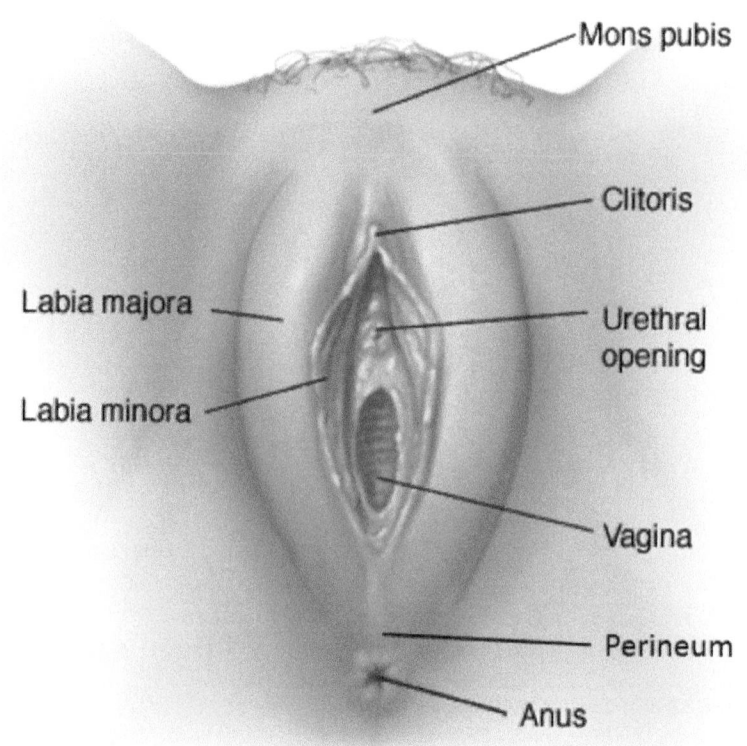

FIGURE 32-4 The structures of the vulva.

the areola. During pregnancy, the areola often becomes darker in color. The areola is supplied with a row of small sebaceous glands that secrete an oil that keeps it resilient. During lactation, milk flows from the lobes of the

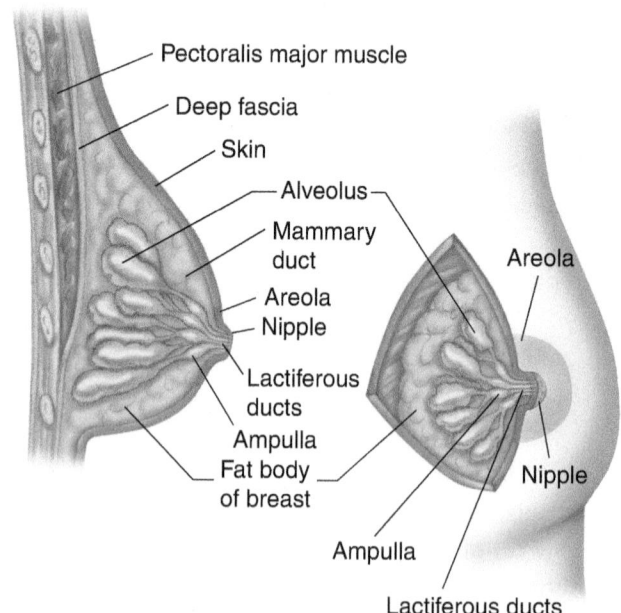

FIGURE 32-5 The breast.

mammary glands through the ampulla, and then through the lactiferous ducts in the nipple to the suckling infant. Prolactin, a hormone produced by the anterior lobe of the pituitary, stimulates the mammary glands to produce milk after childbirth.

THE MENSTRUAL CYCLE

Menarche, the onset of menstrual cycles, occurs at the age of puberty. **Menopause** is the cessation of menstrual cycles that typically occurs in mid-life or later. Typically, a menstrual cycle lasts about 28 days but can vary from 28 to 35 days in the adult female. Hormones, as discussed earlier, control the four phases in the menstrual cycle:

- **Menstruation phase**—Characterized by the discharge of bloody fluid from the uterus as the endometrial layer is shed, caused by decreased estrogen and progesterone levels. The word "period" is a slang term used to describe this phase of the menstrual cycle. The length of this phase averages 4 to 6 days. The first day of the bloody discharge is considered the first day of the menstrual cycle.

- **Follicular phase** (also called the proliferation phase)—Characterized by the endometrial layer beginning to thicken and become vascularized. The ovarian follicle begins to mature because of the release of the follicle-stimulating hormone (FSH). This phase generally spans days 5 to 14 of the menstrual cycle. The cessation of this cycle occurs with the eruption of the Graafian follicle.

- **Ovulation** (also called the ovulatory stage)—Begins on the day the ovum is released from the Graafian follicle, which is triggered by luteinizing hormone. During this phase, the body is preparing for a possible pregnancy by preparing the endometrium to support the early developmental phase of an embryo. This is when a woman is most fertile and able to conceive.

- **Luteal phase**—Characterized by the swelling and continued thickening of the endometrium. In the phase, the corpus luteum in the ovary is developing and secreting progesterone. The progesterone level is at its highest, and the estrogen level begins to decrease. The egg will die if fertilization does not occur during this phase. If the egg dies, the function of the corpus luteum begins to decrease and the levels of both progesterone and estrogen begin to fall. The onset of menstruation marks the end of the luteal phase.

PREGNANCY AND CHILDBIRTH

Pregnancy, or **gestation**, begins with conception and ends with the birthing process. Conception occurs when a spermatozoa fertilizes an ovum during intercourse. As discussed, conception occurs during the ovulation phase (approximately day 14) of the woman's menstrual cycle. Through ejaculation, the semen, containing fluids and more than 40 million sperm cells, is deposited into the woman's vagina. The **flagella** (tail-like projections) of the sperm cause the sex cells to move in a swimming-like fashion from the vagina, through the uterus, and to the fallopian tubes, where they seek a recently released ovum. Only one sperm is able to unite with the egg, resulting in fertilization. Once the ovum has been fertilized, it produces an enzyme that, when released, prevents other sperm from penetrating the ovum.

The ovum and the sperm contain 23 chromosomes each. When they unite, their fusion results in a zygote (fertilized ovum) containing 46 chromosomes. Rapid cellular division begins to occur, and the zygote travels down the fallopian tubes and into the uterus. Here, the zygote implants within the endometrial wall of the uterus. It takes approximately 7 days for the zygote to travel from the fallopian tubes and implant within the wall of the uterus. When implanted, the zygote undergoes cellular changes from within and develops into an embryo.

Prenatal Care

A healthy and problem-free pregnancy is the hope of almost all expectant mothers. It is important for mothers to receive routine prenatal care from their obstetricians (physicians who specialize in pregnancy and childbirth). Although uneventful and stress-free pregnancies are ideal, certain conditions and circumstances may pose challenges. Table 32-1 lists common problems that present during pregnancy. A full-term, healthy pregnancy lasts approximately 40 weeks. These 40 weeks are divided into three trimesters. Each trimester marks specific development changes for both fetus and the mother.

The First Trimester

The first trimester of pregnancy begins with conception and ends around the 12th week of gestation (Figure 32-6). During this time, the growing embryo develops into a fetus. This occurs after the 8th week of pregnancy. The first

TABLE 32-1 | Complications During Pregnancy

Condition	Description
Abruptio Placentae	An emergency condition in which the placenta tears away from the uterine wall after the 20th week of pregnancy; requires immediate birth of the baby.
Breech Presentation	Position of the fetus within the uterus in which the buttocks or feet are presented first for birth rather than the head.
Eclampsia	A condition in which the mother experiences convulsive seizures and coma occurring between the 20th week of pregnancy and the first week postpartum.
Ectopic Pregnancy	A fetus that is abnormally implanted outside the uterine cavity; known as a tubal pregnancy if implanted in a fallopian tube; requires immediate surgery.
Placenta Previa	Condition in which the placenta is attached to the lower portion of the uterus, blocking the birth canal.
Preeclampsia	Toxemia of pregnancy that if untreated can result in true eclampsia; symptoms include hypertension, headaches, albumin in the urine, and edema.
Premature Birth	Childbirth in which the infant (neonate) is born before the 37th week of gestation (pregnancy).
Rh Factor	A condition that can develop in a baby when the mother's blood type is Rh negative and the baby's is Rh positive; the baby's red blood cells can be destroyed as a result of this condition; treatment is early diagnosis and blood transfusion.
Spontaneous Abortion	Loss of a fetus without any artificial aid; also called miscarriage.
Stillbirth	Birth in which the fetus dies before or at the time of birth.

8 weeks of gestation are considered the **embryonic period**. Important changes happen within the embryonic period including:

- **Development of the placenta**—A nourishing organ that facilitates the exchange of oxygen and nutrients between the mother and embryo.

- **Development of the amnion**—A thin and membranous sac that encloses the embryo and serves as a protective barrier.

- **Development of the umbilical cord**—A cordlike structure containing blood vessels that connects the embryo to the placenta; the umbilical vein carries oxygenated blood from the placenta to the embryo, and two umbilical arteries carry deoxygenated blood away from the embryo to the placenta.

- **Development of the yolk sac**—Makes blood cells for the fetus as well as creates cells that will determine the sex of the embryo.

- **External and internal structures are formed**—Including head, arms, hands, legs, and feet.

At the beginning of the 9th week of gestation, the **fetal period** begins and continues until birth. During the fetal period, growth is extremely rapid, and the fetus undergoes a tremendous number of changes. Organs have formed and begin to function, eyelids develop though they are fused shut, and the baby's heartbeat can be heard through ultrasound.

The Second Trimester

The second trimester of pregnancy is marked between weeks 13 and 27 (the end of the 6th month). The mother begins to show signs of pregnancy, including a protruding abdomen. Fetal movements begin to be felt, and there are noticeable periods when the fetus is asleep and awake. During the second trimester, soft hair (lanugo) begins to develop on the shoulders, head, and back of the fetus. Other milestones during this trimester include:

- The baby can make facial expressions and begins sucking the thumb.

Fetal Growth

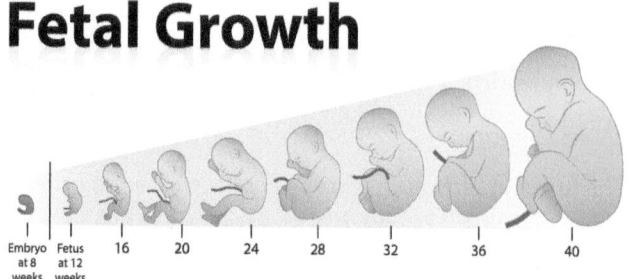

Embryo at 8 weeks | Fetus at 12 weeks | 16 | 20 | 24 | 28 | 32 | 36 | 40

FIGURE 32-6 Embryo and fetus growth from 8 to 40 weeks. (*Source:* Pablofdezr)

- The sex of the baby can be identified.
- The baby can hear the mother's heartbeat and sounds from outside the womb (uterus).
- The brain is growing rapidly, and taste buds are developing.

The Third Trimester

The third trimester of pregnancy lasts from the 28th week of pregnancy to childbirth. Around week 30, the baby has assumed the birthing position (head-down toward cervix). At week 37, the fetus is considered full-term and can be born with very minimal complications because the lungs are fully developed.

The Process of Birth

Hormonal changes are necessary throughout pregnancy to sustain the growth of a developing fetus. Table 32-2 discusses some of the hormonal changes that occur during pregnancy. Hormonal changes at the end of pregnancy allow for childbirth and contractions to begin. A contraction occurs within the muscular wall of the uterus and helps with moving the fetus through the birth canal. When a woman begins the childbirth process, she is said to be in *labor*. The amount of time that a woman labors varies. Generally, labor lasts 12 to 24 hours and, often, shortens with subsequent childbirths. Childbirth occurs in three distinct stages; dilation, expulsion, and the placental stage.

Dilation

Dilation is the first and longest stage of labor. The cervix begins to thin and soften during a process known as effacement. Also during effacement, the cervix begins to dilate, which will allow the fetus to pass through the birth canal. Regular contractions of the uterine wall begin to occur and are timed. The process of cervical dilation is divided into three stages:

- **Latent phase of dilation**—Occurs when contractions are 15 to 20 minutes apart and the cervix dilates up to 4 cm.
- **Active phase of dilation**—Occurs when contractions occur 5 minutes apart and the cervix dilates between 4 and 8 cm. Women are asked to report to the hospital when contractions are 5 minutes apart.

TABLE 32-2 | Hormonal Changes During Pregnancy

Hormone	Function During Pregnancy	Released
Human Chorionic Gonadotropin (HCG)	Produced by embryonic cells during pregnancy, it allows the corpus luteum in the ovary to continue to produce and secrete estrogen and progesterone.	During the first 10 weeks of pregnancy.
Progesterone	Released to help thicken and calm the uterine lining to provide an ideal environment to support the growing fetus.	Increasing levels are released throughout pregnancy to sustain the uterus. Levels start to decline as the body prepares for childbirth.
Estrogen	Works in conjunction with progesterone to thicken the uterine lining. It also stimulates growth of the uterus and increases blood flow between the uterus and the placenta. Estrogen also enlarges milk ducts in preparation for lactation.	Released throughout pregnancy, spikes before childbirth and declines afterward.
Relaxin	Hinders uterine contractions and relaxes the ligaments of the uterus to allow for the growing fetus to expand. It also helps prepare the uterus for childbirth.	Throughout pregnancy with a surge near the end as the body prepares for childbirth.
Oxytocin	Hormone associated with human bonding allowing bonding between mother and child. It also helps stimulate uterine contractions until the baby is born. Also stimulates the ejection of milk from milk glands after childbirth.	Large amounts are released during childbirth.
Lactogen	Secreted by the placenta to stimulate the enlargement of mammary glands.	Secretion begins shortly after implantation, but increases significantly during the late stages of pregnancy.
Prolactin	Secreted by the anterior pituitary gland after childbirth for the production of milk.	Secretion begins after childbirth and ends when breastfeeding ceases.

- **Transitioning phase of dilation**—Generally occurs with the breaking of the amniotic sac, which is often referred to as "water breaking." Contractions become much stronger and are 2 to 3 minutes apart. The cervix dilates 8 to 10 cm.

Expulsion

The expulsion phase of childbirth is the actual birth of the baby. This stage occurs when the cervix is fully dilated at 10 cm. At this point, the fetus begins to travel from the uterus into the vagina through very strong and forceful contractions. The mother experiences strong urges to bear down and push the baby out of the birth canal. The length of this stage can range from several minutes to several hours.

Placental Stage

After the baby is born, the third and final stage of childbirth begins. Also known as the afterbirth, this stage occurs approximately 15 minutes after the birth of the baby. The placenta begins to separate from the uterine wall. Contractions, although much milder, still occur during this phase to allow for the placenta to be expelled from the mother's body (Figure 32-7).

Caesarian Section

A caesarian section is performed when a mother is unable to vaginally deliver a baby. It is often performed to protect the health and safety of the mother or baby. Commonly referred to as a C-section, this surgical procedure allows for birth of the baby through an incision made in the abdominal wall of the mother. C-sections are performed for a variety of reasons including:

- The baby is in a breech position.
- There is a decrease in the supply of oxygen to the placenta before birth (this is an emergency situation).
- The baby is expected to weigh more than 9 pounds.

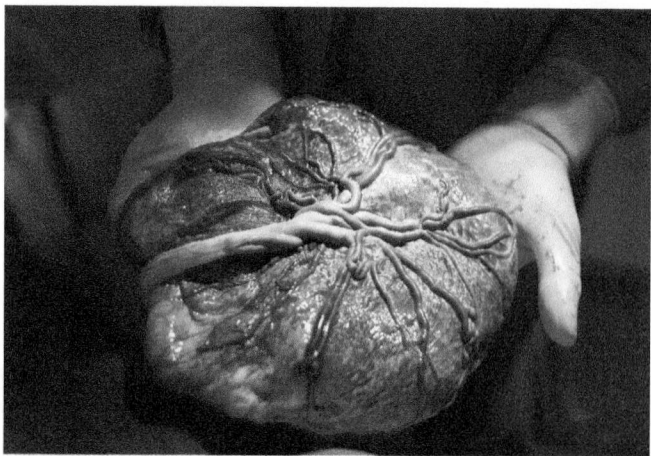

FIGURE 32-7 A doctor showing the placenta after childbirth.

Professionalism

Medical assistants must learn to ask the right questions when interviewing clients for history and medications. Women sometimes do not consider a C-section to be surgery, or they forget that they are using hormone patches and say they are not "on birth control pills." Not including this information in the health history can be harmful to the patient if the physician is unaware and prescribes a medication or treatment procedure that is contraindicated. A professional medical assistant develops and adapts interviewing questions for obtaining complete health history information in a confident and trustworthy manner.

- Maternal health conditions may make vaginal birth unsafe for either the mother or the baby.
- The mother has a previous history of complications during pregnancy or childbirth (may be considered a planned C-section).

It is important for the new mother to exercise caution and receive proper postnatal care, because the healing process from a C-section can be challenging.

Contraception

Contraception, also known as birth control, reduces the risk of an unwanted pregnancy. Various methods of birth control are available. The most common methods include barrier methods, hormonal methods, sterilization, and intrauterine methods. Table 32-3 lists some examples of these methods.

Other methods that are used include coitus interruptus and the rhythm method. Coitus interruptus is also known as "withdrawal"; the male withdraws his penis from the vagina before ejaculation occurs. Great risk is taken with this method, because small amounts of semen may enter the vagina before a complete ejaculation. The rhythm method is based on the idea of periodic abstinence, or refraining from intercourse. This is done by predicting when the female is ovulating and abstaining from sexual intercourse during those times. As with the withdrawal method, risk is being taken because ovulation may not be easily predictable.

Infertility

The term **infertility** is used to describe a situation in which a couple is unable to conceive a child. Primary infertility is diagnosed after 12 consecutive months of trying to conceive without success. Secondary infertility is diagnosed if the couple has had one pregnancy but has been unsuccessful at conceiving for a second time. As with a primary diagnosis, secondary infertility is diagnosed after the couple has

TABLE 32-3 | Methods of Contraception

Method	Form	Description
Mechanical	Male condom	A protective sheath that covers the penis and collects sperm, preventing it from entering the woman's body.
	Female condom	A thin, plastic pouch inserted into the vagina before intercourse that prevents sperm from entering the uterus.
	Diaphragm	A shallow, flexible cup made of latex or soft rubber that is inserted into the vagina before intercourse that prevents sperm from entering the uterus. It is often used with a spermicidal agent.
	Spermicides	Available in jellies, foams, and creams, spermicides are placed near the uterus 30 minutes before intercourse.
Hormonal	Birth control pills	An oral medicine that combines levels of estrogen and progestins to stop ovulation.
	Birth control patch	A thin patch that is applied to the skin; similar to the pill—however, medication is administered transdermally.
	Injectable birth control	An injection of progestin is administered to the buttocks. The most common form is Depo-Provera®.
	Vaginal ring	A ring is inserted around the vagina that delivers doses of estrogen and progestin to stop ovulation. It stays in place for three weeks and is removed during the fourth week of the menstrual cycle.
Intrauterine	Copper IUD	An implantable intrauterine device that delivers small amounts of copper into the uterus. This prevents pregnancy by causing an inflammatory reaction that prevents sperm from reaching and fertilizing an egg. If the egg would become fertilized, the IUD would prevent implantation within the uterine wall.
	Hormonal IUD	An implantable device that releases progestin, which causes a thickening of cervical mucus that doesn't allow the sperm to reach and fertilize an egg. It also thins the uterine wall, making it unable to be implanted if an egg would become fertilized.
Sterilization	Tubal ligation	A surgical procedure that blocks the path of the fallopian tubes to the uterus by either cutting, tying, or sealing the fallopian tubes.
	Vasectomy	A surgical procedure that prohibits sperm from exiting the penis through either cutting, blocking, or closing the vas deferens between the testes and the urethra.

attempted to conceive for 12 consecutive months. A diagnosis of infertility can cause emotional turmoil, because hopeful parents are faced with difficult decisions and harsh realities regarding the outlook for their ideas of family.

Infertility is caused by multiple factors and can be the result of medical issues stemming from either the male or the female. Although infertility in men is not age related, women are most likely to get pregnant early in their childbearing years, particularly in their 20s and early 30s. After the age of 40, conceiving a child becomes more difficult for a woman.

In addition to age, factors affecting infertility in women include:

- Irregular menstrual cycles, lack of menstrual cycles, and lack of ovulation
- Endometriosis
- Polycystic ovarian syndrome (PCOS) and other issues related to hormonal imbalances

- Scarring of the reproductive organs as a result of sexually transmitted diseases
- Structural issues with the reproductive organs, such as an abnormally shaped uterus or cervix

Factors affecting infertility in men include:

- Scarring of the reproductive organs as a result of sexually transmitted diseases
- Impotence and decreased testosterone production
- Low or nonexistent sperm count
- Current or previous diseases, specifically a history of mumps that infected the testes or an inflammation of the testes or epididymis
- The use and overuse of certain drugs or medications, such as prolonged use of anabolic steroids, testosterone replacement therapy, chemotherapy, and certain antifungal medications

A couple hoping to conceive will receive counseling regarding testing options and procedures available to diagnose and pinpoint the cause of the couple's infertility. Various treatment options are available for infertility. The type and extent of treatment depends on the underlying cause. The most common forms of treatment include surgery to repair scarred reproductive organs or to remove endometriosis, hormonal therapies, and medications designed to increase fertility.

COMMON PATHOLOGY ASSOCIATED WITH THE FEMALE REPRODUCTIVE SYSTEM

A wide range of diseases and disorders can affect the female reproductive system. Some of these diseases and disorders include abnormal hormone secretion, breast diseases, sexually transmitted diseases (STDs), cancers of the reproductive organs, inflammations, infections, and others. Many of these disorders frequently affect fertility and the mechanics of reproduction. Table 32-4 lists common disorders and pathology of the female reproductive system.

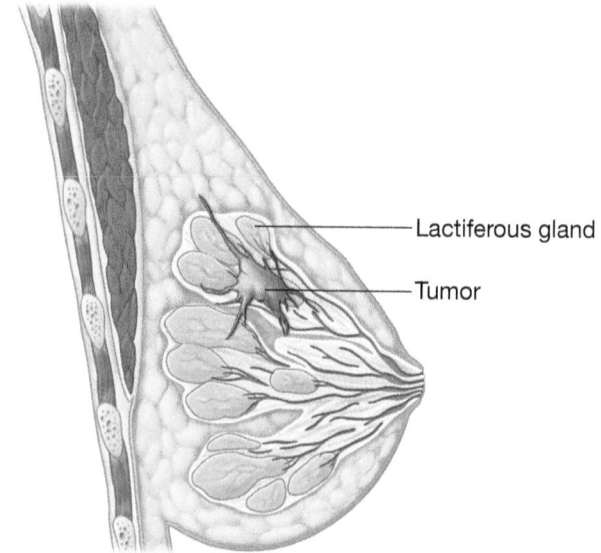

FIGURE 32-8 A cancerous tumor growing within the milk gland.

Breast Cancer

Breast cancer is the development of malignant tumors within the breast tissue (Figure 32-8). Although it affects women primarily, about 1 percent of breast cancers occur

TABLE 32-4 | Disorders of the Female Reproductive System

Disorder	Description
Amenorrhea	An absence of menstruation, which can be the result of many factors, including pregnancy, menopause, and dieting.
Carcinoma in Situ	Malignant tumor that has not extended beyond the original site.
Cervical Polyp	Fibrous or mucous tumor or growth found in the cervix of the uterus; removed surgically because they may become malignant.
Choriocarcinoma	A rare type of cancer of the uterus that may occur following a normal pregnancy or abortion.
Condyloma	A wartlike growth on the external genitalia.
Cystocele	Hernia or outpouching of the bladder that protrudes into the vagina; may cause urinary frequency and urgency.
Endometrial Cancer	Cancer of the endometrial lining of the uterus.
Fibroid tumor	Benign tumor or growth that contains fiberlike tissue; uterine fibroid tumors are the most common tumors in women.
Mastitis	Inflammation of the breast; common during lactation but can occur at any age.
Menorrhagia	Excessive menstrual bleeding (total number of days, amount of blood, or both).
Polycystic Ovarian Syndrome	A condition related to a hormonal imbalance of progesterone and estrogen that results in multiple fluid-filled sacs (cysts) on the ovaries that often cause irregular menstrual cycles.
Prolapsed Uterus	A fallen uterus that can cause the cervix to protrude through the vaginal opening; generally caused by weakened muscles from vaginal birth or as a result of pelvic tumors pressing down.
Salpingitis	Inflammation of the fallopian tube or tubes.
Toxic Shock Syndrome	Rare and sometimes fatal *Staphylococcus* infection that generally occurs in menstruating women.
Vaginitis	Inflammation of the vagina, generally caused by a microorganism.

in men. Not including skin cancers, breast cancer is the most common cancer to afflict women (1 of every 3 cancers diagnosed). It is estimated that 1 out of 8 women will develop invasive breast cancer during their lifetime. The hormone estrogen enables most cancerous tumors of the breast to grow and develop. Therefore, many breast cancers are considered to be highly sensitive to estrogen.

There are two main forms of breast cancer, ductal and lobular. Ductal breast cancer develops in the ducts that transport milk to the nipple. This is the most common form of breast cancer, accounting for about 80 percent of breast cancer cases. Lobular breast cancer develops in the lobules of the breast where milk is produced. The most serious cancers are metastatic cancers, which spread from their origin into other tissues. Common sites of breast cancer metastasis include the lymph nodes under the arm or above the collarbone on the same side as the original cancer. Other common sites of breast cancer metastasis are the brain, the bones, and the liver.

Another type of breast cancer is inflammatory breast cancer. This highly aggressive cancer only accounts for 1 to 5 percent of breast cancer cases. However, because of its rapid progression, it generally isn't diagnosed until stage III or IV, making treatment more challenging.

The exact etiology surrounding breast cancer (and many other forms of cancer) is unknown. However, there are identifiable risk factors that may increase an individual's risk for developing breast cancer. Family history is an important risk factor, particularly if the affected relative developed breast cancer at a young age or is a first-degree relative such as a mother, sister, or daughter. Women who begin menstruating at an early age (before age 12) or experience a late menopause (after age 55) have a higher risk of developing breast cancer. Conversely, having the first menstrual period at a later age or having an early menopause often has a protective effect. Hormonal influences, genetic defects, obesity, increased alcohol intake, and the absence of childbirth or childbirth after the age of 30 are also risk factors in the development of breast cancer.

Signs and Symptoms. Breast cancer in the early stages has no symptoms and is not painful, which is why routine breast examinations are important. A lump or thickening of skin under the arm or above the collarbone that does not go away may indicate the presence of breast cancer. Other possible symptoms are breast discharge, nipple inversion, and changes in the skin overlying the breasts. These symptoms, on their own, can occur normally without cancer as an underlying cause. However, any time these are new developments, they should be evaluated by a physician.

It is important to note that any changes in the skin of the breast such as redness, changes in texture, and puckering also should be evaluated.

Signs and symptoms of inflammatory breast disease include swelling and redness over a third or more of the breast. Burning or tenderness of the breast, rapid growth, or a feeling of heaviness are also symptoms of this rarer form of cancer.

Treatment. Several factors are considered when deciding on a treatment: the type of breast cancer, the stage of the tumor, the size of the breast, and the woman's general health, age, and menstrual status (pre- or postmenopausal).

Surgery is the standard, and often the best, form of therapy for breast cancer. Removal of the lump (lumpectomy) may be performed if the cancer is not in an advanced stage. Complete removal of the breast (mastectomy) may also be performed if the cancer is more advanced or aggressive. Patient preference is a major consideration when determining the treatment for breast cancer. Chemotherapy and radiation are also available forms of treatment. Hormone therapy may also be implemented to block the effects of estrogen. *Tamoxifen* is an example of medication used in hormone therapy for the treatment of breast cancer.

Cervical Cancer

Cervical cancer is the rapid, uncontrolled growth of abnormal cells on the cervix. There is a high cure rate if this form of cancer is detected at an early stage. Regular Pap test screening is the single most important tool for preventing cervical cancer. During a Pap test, abnormal cervical cell changes may be detected and early treatment can be implemented before the development of cancer.

Several factors may contribute to the development of cervical cancer, but most stem from risky sexual activity, including having sexual intercourse at an early age, having multiple sexual partners, or having a partner who has a history of high-risk sexual activity. The majority, about 70 percent, of all cervical cancers result from the human papillomavirus (HPV), which is sexually transmitted. Although some strains of HPV cause genital warts, other strains can lead to the development of cervical cancer. Vaccines are now available to prevent HPV, although there are controversies surrounding its use.

Signs and Symptoms. Abnormal changes in cervical cells rarely cause noticeable signs and symptoms, so, as mentioned before, regular Pap test screening is critical. As cell changes progress to cervical cancer, signs and symptoms may develop. These may include abnormal vaginal bleeding between periods; distinct changes in the menstrual cycle that

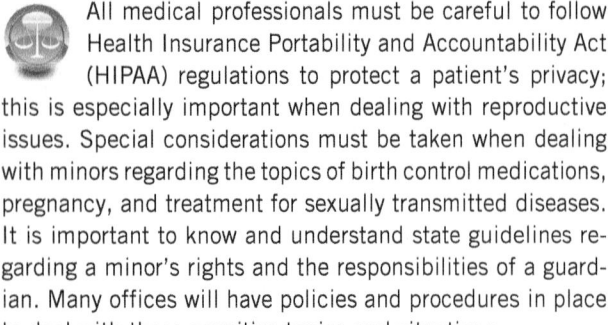
occur without explanation; pain during sexual intercourse; and abnormal vaginal discharge containing mucus that may be tinged with blood. After cervical cancer has progressed, symptoms may include loss of weight (without effort); pain occurring in the pelvis, back, and legs; ureter or kidney blockage resulting in urinary changes; low iron levels (anemia) from abnormal vaginal bleeding; and the development of a fistula (an abnormal opening) between the vagina and bladder or rectum.

Treatment. Cervical cancer detected in its early stages can be cured with treatment and close follow-up. Three types of surgery can be performed to remove abnormal tissues and cells with early detection:

- **Laser therapy**—To remove abnormal tissue
- **Cryotherapy**—To freeze and remove abnormal cells
- **Loop electrosurgical excision procedure (LEEP)**—Uses electricity to remove abnormal tissue

A **hysterectomy** (removal of the uterus) may also be performed if the cancer hasn't spread to surrounding tissues. In advanced forms of cervical cancer, chemotherapy and radiation may be chosen as treatment options. The woman's age, overall health, quality of life, and desire to have children are usually taken into consideration.

Cervicitis

Cervicitis is inflammation of the cervix that is usually caused by an infection. Most cases of cervical infection are caused by sexually transmitted diseases such as herpes, gonorrhea, and chlamydia. Other causes may include allergic reactions to spermicides or latex found in condoms, exposure to chemicals, or devices inserted in the pelvis (such as a diaphragm).

Signs and Symptoms. If signs and symptoms are present, they may include vaginal discharge that is gray or yellow in color and possibly odorous; abnormal vaginal bleeding, which may occur throughout the menstrual cycle, after intercourse, or after menopause; or pain that may be present during urination as well as during intercourse. At times, cervicitis may be asymptomatic (without symptoms) and go unnoticed until a routine Pap test screening.

Treatment. Successful treatment of cervicitis involves addressing the cause of the inflammation, such as treating an underlying sexually transmitted disease. Bacterial or viral causes of infection may be treated with antibiotics and antiviral medications, respectively. When treating cervicitis, it is important for the patient's sexual partner to be treated for infection as well, and abstinence should be maintained throughout the entire course of treatment.

Dysmenorrhea

More than half of all girls and women suffer from some form of **dysmenorrhea**, or painful abdominal cramps during menstruation caused by muscular uterine contractions. Dysmenorrhea is often most simply referred to as "cramps." There are two types of dysmenorrhea. Primary dysmenorrhea occurs when women experience cramping and pain from the onset of their menstrual cycles. Secondary dysmenorrhea occurs when a woman, who hasn't experienced pain or cramping in the past, develops pain and cramping with menstruation because of other pelvic problems such as endometriosis, uterine fibroids, pelvic inflammatory disease, sexually transmitted diseases, or high stress and anxiety levels.

Signs and Symptoms. Dysmenorrhea is generally described as a dull and throbbing pain in the lower abdomen. It is not uncommon for the pain to also be felt in the lower back and thighs. Menstruating women of any age can experience cramps, and although the pain may be only mild for some women, for others the discomfort may be severe enough to significantly interfere with everyday activities. Cramps usually last for two or three days at the beginning of each menstrual period. Some women may also experience nausea and vomiting, diarrhea, irritability, sweating, or dizziness. Some women experience relief from dysmenorrhea after the birth of their first child. This is thought to be attributed to improved blood supply and muscle activity within the uterus.

Treatment. Dysmenorrhea is often treated with the use of nonsteroidal antiinflammatory drugs (NSAIDs) such as ibuprofen, aspirin, or naproxen. Acetaminophen may also be helpful. For more severe pain, prescription-strength NSAIDs may be given. Other treatments to reduce pain and discomfort include the use of heat therapy, such as a heating pad, placed on the abdomen below the belly button; meditation or yoga; light circular massaging of the lower abdomen; and limiting certain dietary foods such as carbohydrates, salt, alcohol, and caffeine. In severe cases of dysmenorrhea, birth control pills may be prescribed to help thin the uterine lining, which decreases the heaviness of the menstrual cycle as well as lessens the uterine contractions associated with cramps.

Endometriosis

Endometriosis occurs when endometrial tissue is found outside the uterus, usually in the pelvis (ovaries and tissues surrounding the pelvis) or abdominal cavity (bowels). Although this tissue reacts to changing levels of estrogen—thickening, breaking down, and bleeding each month—it is not sloughed off with the tissues inside the uterus. Endometriosis can also form scars and **adhesions** (scar-like tissue that forms between two membranous structures), which typically causes daily or monthly cyclic pain.

Etiology surrounding endometriosis is not known. However, there seem to be identifiable risk factors associated with its development. One theoretical risk suggests that having a child later in life may be associated with the disorder. A genetic risk factor is also prevalent as it seems that there is an increased likelihood of development if a first-degree female relative (mother or sister) struggles with endometriosis. Another theory is that during menstruation some of the endometrial tissue backs up through the fallopian tubes into the abdomen. This is called retrograde menstruation.

Signs and Symptoms. Symptoms of endometriosis include infertility, dyspareunia (painful intercourse), heavy menstrual bleeding and very painful cramps, irregular periods, nausea and vomiting, pelvic pain after intercourse or exercise, and dysmenorrhea. Symptoms tend to decrease after menopause, when the involved tissues shrink.

Treatment. Early diagnosis and treatment have been known to prevent or lessen the severity of adhesions by limiting cell and tissue growth. The use of hormone therapy, including high doses of progestin, and oral contraceptives may delay the onset. Treatment with medication focuses on treating the discomfort, such as the use of NSAIDs. Surgery, either conservative or extensive, is generally reserved for women with severe endometriosis. Conservative surgery is aimed at restoring the integrity of the pelvic anatomy by removing and destroying endometrial tissue outside the uterus and removing adhesions. Extensive surgery is performed on women with severe symptoms and no desire to bear children. Typically, a hysterectomy and **salpingo-oophorectomy** (removal of ovaries and fallopian tubes) are performed. After the ovaries are removed, hormonal replacement must be lifelong.

Fibrocystic Breast Disease

Fibrocystic breast disease is a condition that is common, affecting over 60 percent of women. It presents as changes to the breast tissue that are considered to be common and benign. The etiology is not completely clear, but the hormone estrogen seems to play a strong role as the changes in breast tissue tend to occur during ovulation and before menstruation. During menopause the condition often subsides. Diets rich in caffeine, chocolate, and high-fat foods could make symptoms worse, and family history seems to be a prevalent risk factor.

Signs and Symptoms. Symptoms of fibrocystic breast disease may range from mild to severe and frequently include a "cobblestone" consistency in the breast tissue; irregularly shaped and dense breast tissue; breast discomfort that may be persistent or intermittent; and a feeling of fullness in the breasts. Premenstrual tenderness and swelling and nipple sensations, such as itching, may also be present.

Treatment. Treatment of this disorder often involves dietary modifications (eliminating caffeine and eating a lower-fat diet), performing a monthly breast self-exam, and wearing a well-fitted bra that provides good breast support. Oral contraceptives, which often decrease the symptoms, may also be prescribed.

Ovarian Cancer

Ovarian cancer begins with abnormal cell changes in one or both ovaries. Ovarian cancer is classified by the type of cancer and where it originates. When cancer cells begin to grow on the outer covering of the ovary, it is considered to be *epithelial cell cancer*. This is the most common form of ovarian cancer. If the cancer originates in the egg cells found within the ovary, the cancer is termed a *germ cell tumor*. This form of ovarian cancer most often afflicts young women and even children. The final form of ovarian cancer is called *stromal tumor*, and it originates in the ovarian cells that make up the framework and structure of the actual ovary.

Risk factors for developing ovarian cancer include a personal or family history of breast cancer, taking estrogen for more than five years (as in hormone replacement therapy), and having fewer children or having children later in life.

Signs and Symptoms. Ovarian cancer is very difficult to diagnose in its early stages. Most often there are no initial signs and symptoms. Signs and symptoms that do occur may easily be mistaken for those of other common illnesses.

Unfortunately, by the time it is diagnosed, the cancer is usually at an advanced stage.

Early-stage symptoms frequently include mild abdominal discomfort or pain, abdominal swelling, changes in bowel habits, feeling full after a light meal, decreased appetite, nausea and vomiting, chronic fatigue, pain in the lower back or leg, excessive hair growth, abnormal menstrual or vaginal bleeding, more frequent urination, and pain during intercourse.

Treatment. Treatment is based on the type, grade, and stage of the cancer at the time of diagnosis. Treatment may include surgery to remove the affected ovary, which could be either a bilateral or a unilateral salpingo-oophorectomy with or without a hysterectomy. Other treatments may include radiation therapy and chemotherapy. Complementary therapies, such as meditation and supportive therapies, are also encouraged. Alternative therapies, such as traditional Chinese medicines or special diets, are sometimes used; however, their effectiveness has not been scientifically proven.

Ovarian Cysts

Ovarian cysts are pouches filled with liquid or a semisolid material that develops on or within the ovary. Ovarian cysts are not disease related and typically dissolve and disappear on their own. As discussed earlier in the chapter, in the days preceding ovulation a follicle grows in the cortex of the ovary. At the time of expected ovulation, however, the follicle fails to rupture and release an egg. Instead of being reabsorbed, the fluid within the follicle forms a cyst. These are called functional cysts. Most of these cysts are harmless and cause no symptoms. Functional cysts are relatively common and usually disappear within 60 days without treatment. They occur most often during the childbearing years but may occur at any time. Functional ovarian cysts are different from other disease conditions involving ovarian cysts. Other conditions include benign cysts of different types that require treatment; true ovarian tumors, including ovarian cancer; and hormonal conditions such as polycystic ovary syndrome in which the ovary is filled with numerous small fluid-filled cysts.

Signs and Symptoms. Ovarian cysts are often asymptomatic. If symptoms are present, they generally include constant, dull pelvic pain; pelvic pain during movement, with intercourse, or shortly after the beginning or end of a menstrual period; and abdominal bloating or distention.

Treatment. As already noted, functional ovarian cysts generally disappear within 60 days without treatment. Oral contraceptive pills may be prescribed to help establish normal cycles and impede the development of functional ovarian cysts. Ovarian cysts that are not functional may require

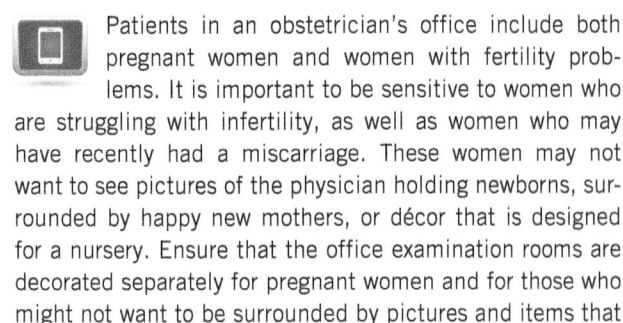

surgical removal for examination. Cysts larger than 6 cm or persisting for longer than six weeks may require surgical removal. If other disorders, such as polycystic ovary disease, are causing the cysts, other medical options may merit exploration.

Pelvic Inflammatory Disease

The most common and serious complication of untreated sexually transmitted diseases (STDs) among women is **pelvic inflammatory disease (PID)**, which is an infection of the upper genital area. It is caused by disease-carrying organisms that migrate upward from the urethra and cervix and infect the uterus, fallopian tubes, and even ovaries. Among the many different organisms that can cause PID, those causing HPV, gonorrhea, and chlamydia are the most common. Other factors, besides STDs, that cause PID may include bacteria entering the body through surgical procedures such as childbirth; endometrial biopsy; abortion; dilation and curettage after miscarriage; and insertion of an intrauterine device. Complications resulting from PID that goes without treatment include infertility, persistent pelvic pain, and ectopic or tubal pregnancies.

Signs and Symptoms. The major signs and symptoms of PID are lower abdominal pain and abnormal vaginal discharge. Other possible symptoms are fever, fatigue, chills, painful intercourse, and irregular menstrual bleeding. Unfortunately, PID can seriously damage reproductive organs without having any symptoms at all.

Treatment. The first goal of treatment for PID is treating the primary source of infection with appropriate antibiotics or other necessary medications. Patients with severe cases may be required to be hospitalized and monitored along with IV antibiotic therapy. When extensive scarring of reproductive organs has occurred, surgery is often indicated.

Premenstrual Syndrome

Premenstrual syndrome (PMS) is also known as premenstrual dysphoric disorder. This common condition is considered to be associated with the increased level of hormones produced during the menstrual cycle. This condition affects approximately 85 percent of menstruating women with risk factors for development that include age (women aged 20-40 are more likely to suffer from the condition), women who have given birth, and a personal or familial history of depression.

Signs and Symptoms. Signs and symptoms of PMS vary greatly and can affect multiple systems of the body (Figure 32-9). Some of the more common signs and symptoms include constipation, diarrhea, nausea, anorexia, appetite cravings, headache, backache, muscular aches, edema, insomnia, clumsiness, malaise, irritability, indecisiveness, mental confusion, and depression.

Treatment. The severity of PMS symptoms may be alleviated by a healthy diet high in vegetables and fruits; low in starches, sugars, sodium, fat, caffeine, and alcohol; and sufficient in vitamins and minerals, especially B vitamins, calcium, and magnesium. Regular aerobic exercise, relaxation therapy, and stress management techniques also may be of benefit. Certain herbal products, such as chasteberry and black cohosh, have been helpful to some women. Medications may be prescribed to aid physical symptoms, including diuretics to reduce fluid retention, antianxiety and antidepressants to help with anxiety and mood disorders, and ibuprofen and acetaminophen to help with aches and pains.

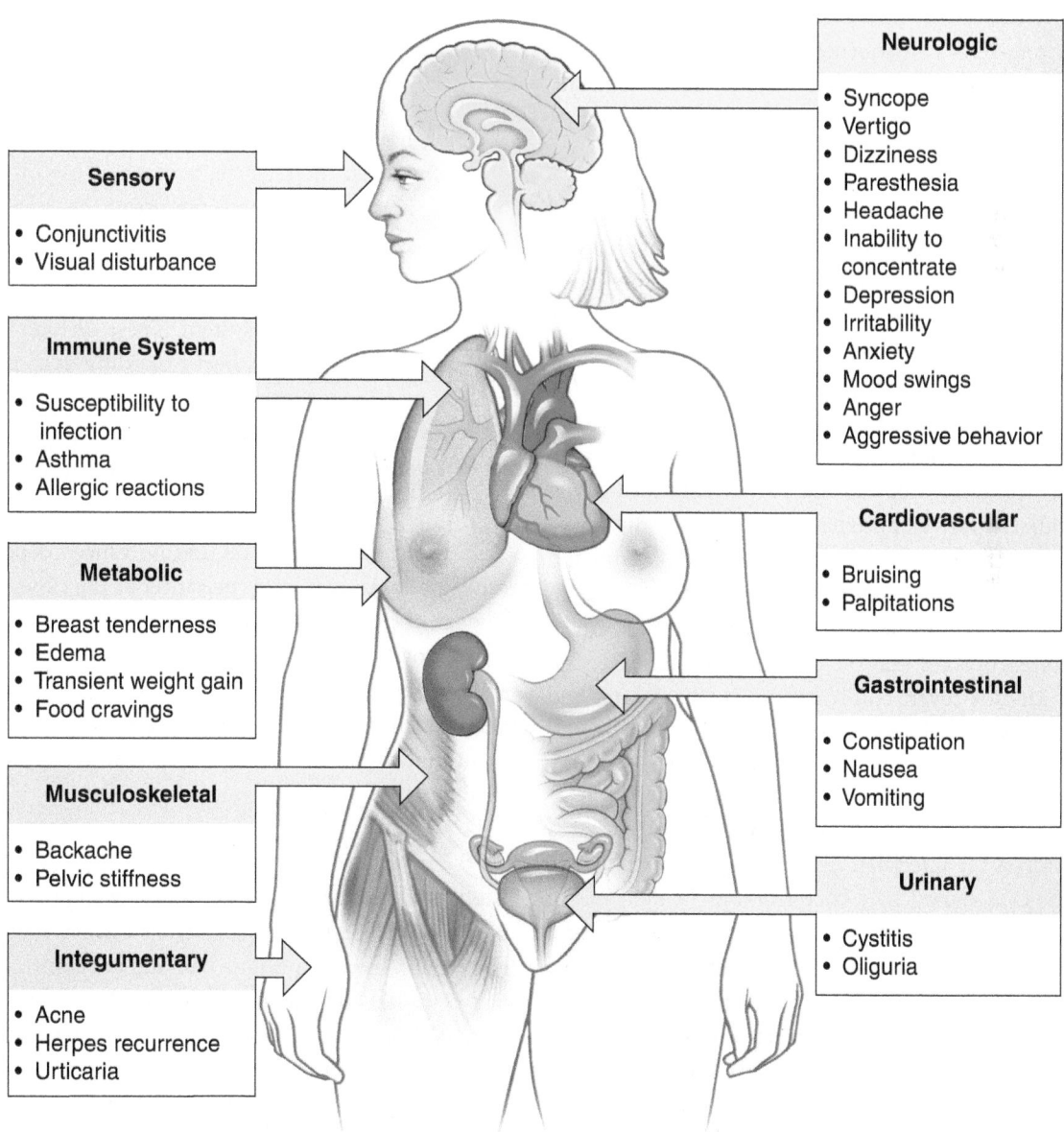

Sensory
- Conjunctivitis
- Visual disturbance

Immune System
- Susceptibility to infection
- Asthma
- Allergic reactions

Metabolic
- Breast tenderness
- Edema
- Transient weight gain
- Food cravings

Musculoskeletal
- Backache
- Pelvic stiffness

Integumentary
- Acne
- Herpes recurrence
- Urticaria

Neurologic
- Syncope
- Vertigo
- Dizziness
- Paresthesia
- Headache
- Inability to concentrate
- Depression
- Irritability
- Anxiety
- Mood swings
- Anger
- Aggressive behavior

Cardiovascular
- Bruising
- Palpitations

Gastrointestinal
- Constipation
- Nausea
- Vomiting

Urinary
- Cystitis
- Oliguria

FIGURE 32-9 Multisystem effects of premenstrual syndrome.

Sexually Transmitted Disease

Sexually transmitted disease (STD) is a general term used to describe more than 20 types of infections that are transmitted by means of sexual contact and the exchange of blood, semen, and other body fluids. The term *venereal disease* is often used, interchangeably, when discussing sexually transmitted diseases and infections.

It is important to note that sexual intercourse is not the only way to acquire an STD. Certain infections can be transmitted simply by having direct contact with a body part that is affected by an STD. In the United States, about 25 percent of the population will experience an STD at some point in their life. The most common STDs in the United States include chlamydia, genital herpes, syphilis, gonorrhea, human papillomavirus (HPV), and HIV infection.

STDs often result in immediate symptoms and health issues, but long-term consequences are also indicated. They can cause birth defects, blindness, bone deformities, brain damage, cancer, heart disease, infertility and other reproductive abnormalities, mental retardation, and death.

Signs and Symptoms. Signs and symptoms vary depending on the type of infection, and the onset of symptoms also varies. Although some symptoms seem to appear immediately after exposure, at other times patients may not realize they have been infected with an STD until much later.

In females, signs and symptoms of STDs that affect the genitals and reproductive organs include bleeding not associated with menstruation, abnormal vaginal discharge with odor, vaginal burning, itching, and pelvic pain during sexual intercourse. Male symptoms include penile discharge and lymph node swelling within the groin area. Painful and burning urination as well as skin rashes are common for both males and females. Skin rashes may present in the form of blisters, bumps, or sores near the mouth or genitals. General symptoms include fever, chills, aching in the joints, and long lasting throat pain and swelling.

Treatment. STDs require medical intervention and treatment, including medication, sometimes antibiotics or antivirals, to address the infection. Antibiotics are only effective when the STD is caused by a bacterium, as in the cases of gonorrhea, chlamydia, and syphilis. Antiviral medications, such as Zovirax, are often prescribed to treat genital herpes, which is caused by a virus (HPV). Specific treatment plans will be discussed with the physician based on the STD, the extent of the infection, and treatments available.

The risk of contracting an STD can be reduced or eliminated by adopting certain personal behaviors. Abstaining from sexual relations or maintaining a mutually monogamous relationship with a partner are legitimate options. Avoiding sexual contact with people who are known to be infected with an STD, whose health status is unknown, who abuse drugs, or who are involved in prostitution are also considered ways of reducing or eliminating altogether the risk of infection with an STD. The use of a condom, which provides a barrier-based protection, can be useful in preventing the spread of STDs. However, they are not always 100 percent effective. See Table 32-5 for more information about STDs.

Uterine Cancer

Uterine cancer (endometrial cancer or adenocarcinoma) generally develops in the glandular tissue of the endometrium. If the cancer is detected and treated early, treatment is usually very successful. There is no one single cause of uterine cancer; however, some factors appear to increase the risk of developing it: age, particularly in women over 50 who are menopausal; obesity; diabetes; polycystic ovarian syndrome (PCOS); having never given birth; history of endometrial polyps; delayed menopause; prolonged use of medications with the hormone estrogen; and use of the drug tamoxifen.

Signs and Symptoms. Many of the signs and symptoms of uterine cancer may be associated with other disorders of the female reproductive system. These include bleeding between menstrual periods, heavy bleeding or spotting during periods or after menopause, and bleeding after intercourse. Other symptoms are cramping pain and pressure in the abdomen, pelvis, back, or legs; difficulty urinating; and discomfort over the pubic area.

Treatment. Treatment of uterine cancer depends on the type, grade, and stage of the cancer at the time of diagnosis. The usual treatment is a total hysterectomy, which includes the removal of the uterus and cervix. The fallopian tubes and ovaries are also usually removed. In addition to surgery, radiation is common in early stages of cancer. Later stages of uterine cancer may require chemotherapy or hormone therapy.

Uterine Fibroids

Uterine fibroids are found within the wall of the uterus (Figure 32-10). They are noncancerous tumors that can vary in size from a seed to a tennis ball and are comprised of tissue and muscle cells. Etiology surrounding the formation of tumors is not exactly known, but hormones, genetic predisposition, and environmental factors seem to be causative factors. Risk factors for developing fibroids include age (common in childbearing years), race (African Americans are most susceptible), having not given birth, and obesity.

TABLE 32-5 | Sexually Transmitted Diseases

Disease	Description
Acquired Immunodeficiency Syndrome (AIDS)	The final stage of infection from the human immunodeficiency virus (HIV); no cure at present.
Candidiasis	A yeastlike infection of the skin and mucous membranes that can result in white plaque on the tongue and vagina.
Chancroid	Highly infectious nonsyphilitic ulcer.
Chlamydia Infection	Genital infection in males and females caused by the bacterium *Chlamydia trachomatis*; can lead to pelvic inflammatory disease (PID) in females and eventual infertility.
Genital Herpes	Painful vesicles on the skin and mucosa that erupt periodically and can be transmitted through the placenta or at birth.
Genital Warts	Growths and elevations on the genitalia of both males and females that can lead to cancer of the cervix in females; currently no cure.
Gonorrhea	Sexually transmitted inflammation of the mucous membranes of either sex; can be passed on to an infant during the birth process.
Hepatitis	Infectious, inflammatory disease of the liver; hepatitis B and C spread by contact with blood and bodily fluids of an infected person.
Syphilis	Infectious, chronic venereal disease that can involve any organ; may exist for years without symptoms.
Trichomoniasis	Genitourinary infection caused by a parasite that is usually asymptomatic (without symptoms) in both males and females; can produce itching and/or burning and a foul-smelling discharge and result in vaginitis in women.

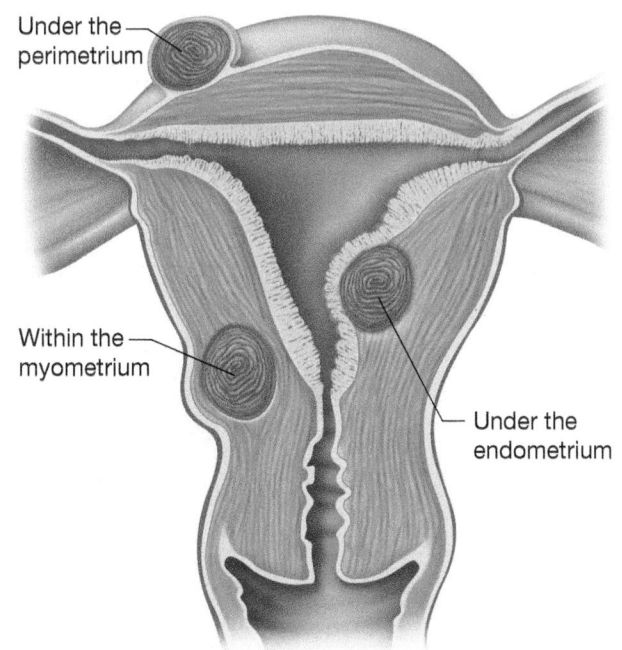

Under the perimetrium

Within the myometrium

Under the endometrium

FIGURE 32-10 Types of uterine fibroids.

Signs and Symptoms. Signs and symptoms of uterine fibroids include heavy bleeding or painful periods, bleeding between periods, feeling of fullness in the pelvic area, frequent urination, pain during sex, lower back pain, and reproductive problems, including infertility and early onset of labor.

Treatment. Patients with mild symptoms may require only over-the-counter medications for relief of pain and inflammation. When these medications are not helpful, a physician may prescribe gonadotropin-releasing hormone agonists (GnRHa), which decrease the size of the fibroids. However, they have multiple side effects including hot flashes, depression, insomnia, decreased libido, and joint pain. Low dose oral contraceptives may slow the growth of fibroids and reduce heavy bleeding with periods. These drugs offer only temporary relief from symptoms, which return as soon the therapy is discontinued.

Various types of surgeries may be used to treat moderate to severe cases of uterine fibroids. A **myomectomy** removes the fibroids without taking any healthy tissue of the uterus. A hysterectomy may also be performed. Endometrial ablation may be performed to remove or destroy the lining of the uterus to control very heavy bleeding. Myolysis may also be performed, which involves electronic freezing of the fibroid through the use of a guided needle that is inserted into the fibroid.

Vaginitis

Vaginitis is an inflammation of the vagina that can be caused by a variety of factors. Infections including bacterial vaginitis, trichomoniasis, and yeast infections are common causes.

Atrophic vaginitis is a condition that is a result of menopause and decreased estrogen levels. Another cause of inflammation is attributed to an imbalance of normal vaginal bacteria, known as normal flora, found within the vagina.

Signs and Symptoms. The signs and symptoms of vaginitis include itching and irritation; vaginal discharge with a marked change in amount, color, or odor; pain and burning during urination; vaginal bleeding; and pain during intercourse.

Treatment. Treatment depends on the type of vaginitis. For bacterial vaginitis, vaginal gels or creams may be prescribed. Yeast infections are usually treated with antifungal creams or suppositories. Trichomoniasis is frequently treated with metronidazole (Flagyl); atrophic vaginitis is treated with estrogen.

THE MALE REPRODUCTIVE SYSTEM

The male reproductive system consists of the testes; various ducts; the urethra; accessory glands, which include the bulbourethral, prostate, and seminal vesicles; and the supporting structures and accessory sex organs, the scrotum and the penis (Figures 32-11 and 32-12). The vital function of the male reproductive system is to provide the sperm cells necessary to fertilize the ovum and perpetuate the species.

External Organs

In the male, the scrotum and the penis are the external organs of reproduction. The **scrotum** is a pouchlike structure situated posterior to (behind) the penis. It is suspended from the perineal region (between the scrotal attachment and the anus) and is divided into two sacs by a septum. Each sac contains one of the two **testes** along with the epididymis, a connecting tube. The tissues of the scrotum have fibers of smooth muscle that contract when not exposed to heat, giving the scrotum a wrinkled appearance. Because the testes are held away from the rest of the body by the scrotum, their temperature is approximately 1 degree lower than that of the human body. This variance in temperature is ideal for the viability of the sperm.

The **penis** is composed of three longitudinal columns of erectile tissue covered with skin. The size and shape of the penis vary; the average erect penis is about 6 to 8 inches in length. Significant enlargement occurs within the columns of erectile tissue when they become engorged with blood, as during sexual stimulation. Two of these columns are the corpora cavernosa that lie along either side of the shaft of the penis. The third column is the corpus spongiosum that surrounds the urethra, the tube through which both urine and semen are expelled from the penis. The corpus spongiosum extends from the portion of the penis closest to the body to the cone-shaped head at the end of the penis. (Review Figure 32-12.) A loose fold of skin known as the prepuce or foreskin covers the penis. Smegma, a lubricating fluid, is produced

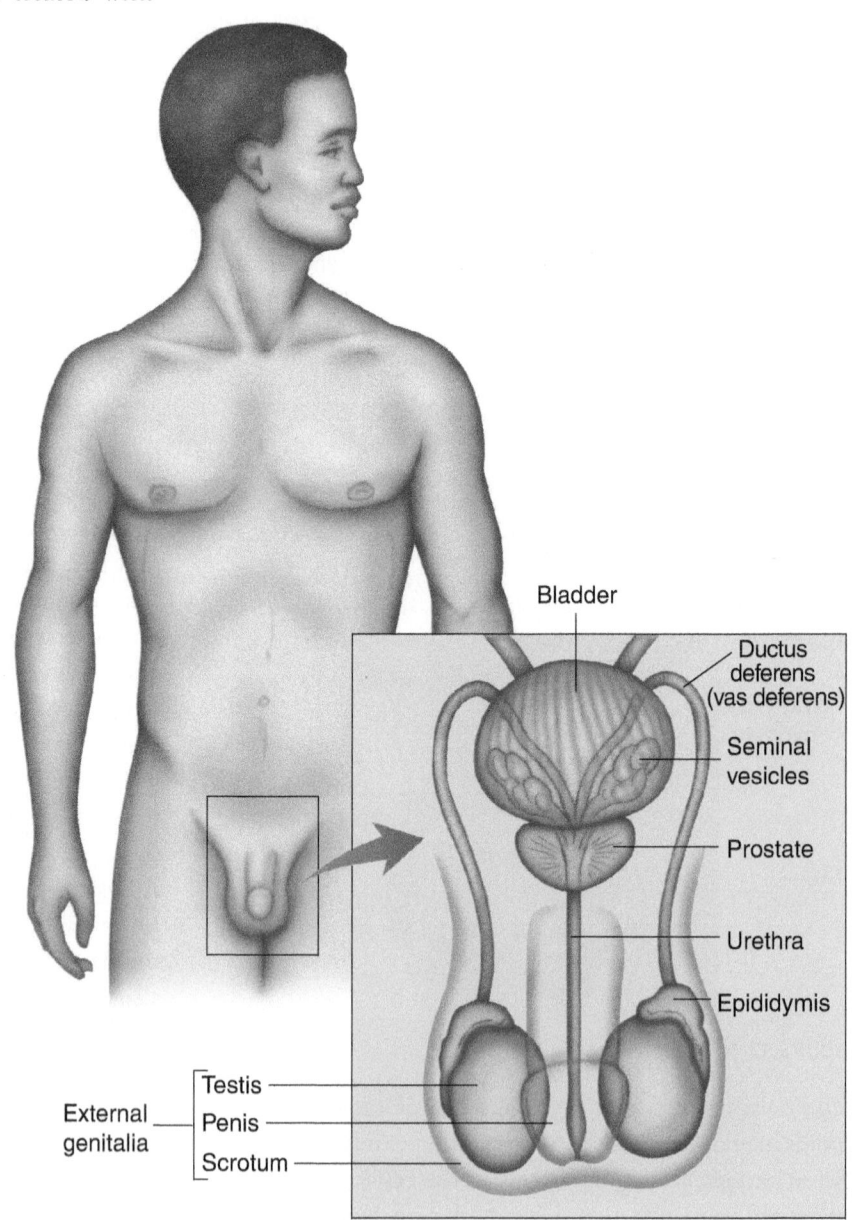

FIGURE 32-11 The male reproductive system.

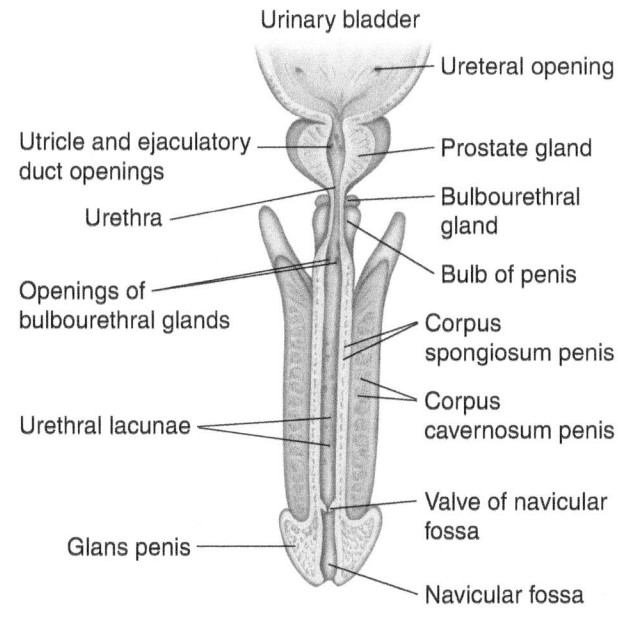

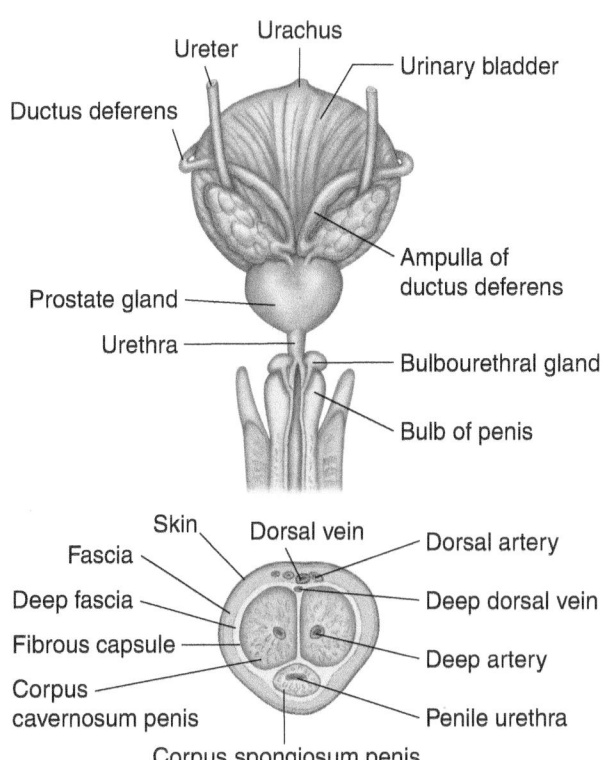

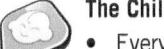

FIGURE 32-12 The structures of the bladder, prostate gland, and penis.

within the glands of the foreskin. During a procedure called **circumcision**, the foreskin is removed. This is often performed for medical, cultural, or religious reasons.

The erectile state in the penis occurs when sexual stimulation, or other factors, causes large quantities of blood from dilated arteries supplying the penis to fill the cavernous spaces in the erectile tissue. When the arteries constrict, as they do after ejaculation, the pressure on the veins in the area is reduced. At this point, the penis is able to return to its normal, nonerect size because more blood is able to leave the penis than enter it. The functions of the penis are to serve as the male organ for intercourse or copulation and, as stated earlier, as the site of the penile urethra through which urine and semen are eliminated from the body.

Internal Organs

The internal organs of the male reproductive system are the testes, the epididymis, the ductus deferens (vas deferens), the seminal vesicles, the prostate gland, the bulbourethral glands, and the urethra. The two oval-shaped organs in the scrotum are called the testes. Fibrous tissues divide the interior of each into about 250 wedge-shaped lobes. The seminiferous tubules are coiled within each lobe and are the site of the development of the spermatozoa (Figure 32-13). Aside from the development of sperm cells, another important function of the testes is the production of testosterone, the

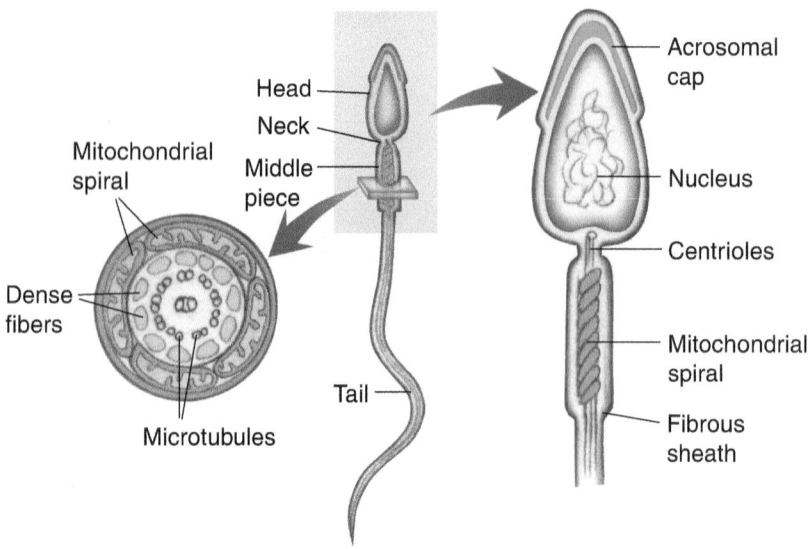

FIGURE 32-13 The basic structure of a spermatozoon (sperm).

male sex hormone. During puberty, testosterone is necessary for the development of chest and abdominal hair, increased facial hair, voice changes (tone and pitch), and other secondary sex characteristics. Testosterone also plays a vital role in the erection process, and thus is necessary for the act of reproduction.

The epididymis is a long, thin coiled tube lying on the upper, rear portion of the testes. Although each epididymis is between 13 and 20 feet in length, it is coiled into a space less than 2 inches in length that ends at the ductus deferens. The function of the epididymis is twofold. First, it is a storage site for the maturation of sperm. Second, it serves as the first part of the pathway through which sperm pass as they travel to the urethra during ejaculation.

Extending upward from the epididymis is the vas deferens, or the ductus deferens. This slim muscular tube is 18 inches in length and serves as the excretory duct of the testes. It is contained within a structure known as the spermatic cord. The spermatic cord also contains arteries, veins, lymphatic vessels, and nerves.

The ejaculatory duct is comprised of two seminal vesicle ducts that merge with the vas deferens. This short tube enters the base of the prostate gland and opens into the prostate portion of the urethra. Within these vesicles, an alkaline fluid is produced that becomes part of the seminal fluid (semen).

JUDGMENT CALL

A 14-year-old female patient calls the office to inquire about birth control options. How would you handle this phone call?

The **prostate gland** lies behind the urinary bladder. Approximately the size of a walnut, it is composed of glandular, connective, and muscular tissue. It wraps around the first inch of the urethra where it exits the urinary bladder. About 1½ inches wide, it is composed of glandular, connective, and muscular tissue. Like the seminal vesicles, the prostate secretes an alkaline fluid that aids in maintaining the viability of the spermatozoa.

The **bulbourethral glands**, or Cowper's glands, are two small, pea-size glands located inferior to the prostate and on either side of the urethra. A tiny duct connects them with the wall of the urethra, where they secrete a mucous secretion into the seminal fluid before ejaculation.

The male **urethra** is approximately 8 inches long and is divided into three sections: prostatic, membranous, and spongy or penile. The urethra extends from the urinary bladder to the penile urethra at the end of the penis. The functions of this orifice, as stated before, are the expulsion of urine and semen from the body.

COMMON PATHOLOGY ASSOCIATED WITH THE MALE REPRODUCTIVE SYSTEM

The male reproductive system has both reproductive and urinary functions, and because of this, it is often referred to as the genitourinary system. Many disorders affect both systems. Conditions range from inflammatory disorders, such as epididymitis, to infectious diseases, such as those classified as STDs, to life-threatening conditions such as prostate and testicular cancer. See Table 32-6 for more information about disorders of the male reproductive system.

Benign Prostatic Hyperplasia

Benign prostatic hyperplasia (BPH) is a condition marked by an enlargement of the prostate. It is also referred to as benign prostatic hypertrophy (Figure 32-14). The etiology of BPH is unknown; however, there is a perceived connection between enlargement of the prostate gland and changes in hormone levels, particularly changes in the level of a powerful androgen known as dihydrotestosterone (DHT) as well as changes in the levels of testosterone and estrogen (which is present in males, in small amounts).

The likelihood of developing BPH increases with age; in fact, by age 75 more than half of all men will have experienced some signs and symptoms related to this disorder. A

TABLE 32-6 | Disorders of the Male Reproductive System

Disorder	Description
Anorchism	A congenital absence of one or both testes.
Aspermia	The lack of, or failure to eject, sperm.
Azoospermia	Absence of sperm in the semen.
Balanitis	Inflammation of the skin covering the glans penis.
Carcinoma of the Testes	Cancer of one or both testes.
Cryptorchidism	Failure of the testes to descend into the scrotal sac before birth (generally descend permanently before age 1 year); may result in sterility; orchidopexy (surgical procedure) may bring the testes down into the scrotum and secure them permanently.
Epispadias	Congenital opening of the male urethra on the dorsal surface of the penis.
Hypospadias	Congenital opening of the male urethra on the underside of the penis.
Impotence	Inability to copulate caused by inability to maintain an erection or to achieve orgasm.
Phimosis	Narrowing of the foreskin over the glans penis that results in difficulty with hygiene; can lead to infection or difficulty with urination; treated with circumcision (surgical removal of foreskin).
Prostatitis	An inflamed condition of the prostate gland that may be the result of infection.
Varicocele	Enlargement of the veins of the spermatic cord that commonly occurs on the left side of adolescent males; seldom needs treatment.

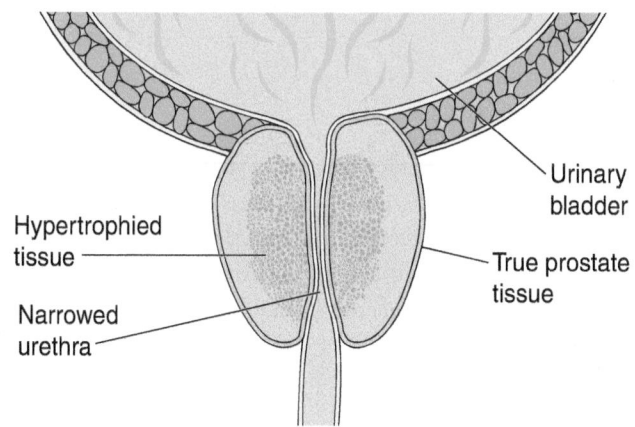

FIGURE 32-14 Benign prostatic hyperplasia.

consequence of BPH is a change in urination patterns. The enlarged prostate, by default, compresses the urethra, which inhibits or limits normal urine flow. When there is an interference with the normal flow of urine from the bladder from any condition related to the prostate gland, it is termed prostatism. One of the most common occurrences is a urinary tract infection (UTI) that develops as a result of urine that is pushed back (retrograde) into the ureters because the normal flow of urine is blocked by the enlarged prostate.

Signs and Symptoms. Symptoms and signs attributed to BPH relate mostly to urinary changes. Specifically, these include urgency; increased nocturia; difficulty in producing a urine stream, which is often weak; straining of the abdomen; urinary retention; recurring UTIs; and a feeling that the bladder is not empty.

Treatment. Treatment for BPH includes drug therapy and surgical procedures. Medications are generally the first line of treatment and work either by reducing the size of the prostate or by relaxing the smooth muscle of the prostate and the bladder neck to improve urine flow and reduce bladder outlet obstruction. If medication is not successful, the physician may choose from a number of surgical options. The goal for surgical intervention is to reduce the size of the prostate and enlarge the urethra to allow for more adequate urine flow, which will reduce symptoms and limit complications associated with BPH.

Epididymitis

Epididymitis is an inflammation or infection of the epididymis. In adult men it is the most common cause of scrotal pain. The most severe pain and swelling are usually associated with the acute form of this condition. Men between the ages of 19 and 35 are most commonly affected.

Epididymitis can be caused by the same organisms that cause some STDs or as a result of prostate surgery. Accumulated urine within the vas deferens, as a result of infection or injury, is also a known cause of the condition. Risk factors for developing epididymitis include urinary tract infections, a recent illness, not being circumcised, a narrowing of the urethra, and recent use of a urethral catheter.

Signs and Symptoms. Epididymitis is characterized by sudden redness and swelling of the scrotum. The inflamed testicle is sore and hardened, and the other testicle is also tender. Chills, groin pain, pain with urination or ejaculation, and acute **urethritis** (inflammation of the urethra) are also common. At times the lymph nodes found within the groin can cause pain in the scrotum. This pain can become increasingly unbearable, sometimes making walking difficult and even impossible.

Treatment. Epididymitis is treated with antibiotic therapy, which should begin as soon as symptoms appear. Left untreated, the condition may cause an abscess to develop or lead to infertility. Pain medications, either prescribed or over-the-counter, may be used as well as antiinflammatory drugs to reduce the swelling. To prevent reinfection, medication must be taken exactly as prescribed, even if symptoms disappear or the patient begins to feel better.

Erectile Dysfunction

Erectile dysfunction (ED) is the inability to achieve or maintain an erection sufficient for sexual intercourse. When the inability to achieve or maintain an erection until ejaculation occurs more than 25 percent of the time, a diagnosis of erectile dysfunction may be made. Lack of blood supply to the penis, inability to retain blood flow, and the inability of the smooth muscle in the penis to relax are all associated with the occurrence of this disorder.

Erectile dysfunction can happen at any age for a number of various reasons. Erections are linked to combined functions of the brain, nerves, hormones, and blood vessels. If there is a disorder or dysfunction with any of these, ED may result. Although the chances of developing ED slightly increase with age, the majority of cases have a physical underlying cause.

Risk factors for ED include hypertension, hyperlipidemia, endocrine disorders such as diabetes or thyroid disease, low testosterone levels, coronary artery disease, peripheral vascular disease, anemia, smoking, alcohol abuse, certain medications, surgical procedures, neurological conditions, anxiety, and feelings of doubt or inadequacy.

ED can affect relationships, and men should discuss the issue with their partners as well as their physicians. A medical evaluation is performed by the physician to explore any underlying causative factors. Many patients are uncomfortable discussing ED because they are embarrassed. Care must be taken by the medical assistant to ensure confidentiality and reassure the patient that medical treatments are available.

Signs and Symptoms. The penis may be able or unable to achieve, but not maintain, an erection.

Treatment. Treatment options are medication therapy, medication changes, urethral and penile injection therapies, and surgery, including penile prosthesis.

Hydrocele

A **hydrocele** is a fluid-filled sac that surrounds one or both testicles. It is noticed by swelling that develops within the scrotal or groin areas. Although it may be unsightly and uncomfortable, this swelling is not painful and generally not dangerous. Most common in newborn infants, a hydrocele can be congenital (present at birth) or acquired (develops after birth). A congenital hydrocele develops when, after the normal process of testicle migration (from the abdomen to the scrotum), the space around the testicles does not close or the closure is delayed. Fluid from the abdominal cavity fills this space, creating the hydrocele.

Signs and Symptoms. The main symptom of a hydrocele is a painless, swollen scrotum or groin area. The scrotum may have a bluish tinge or appear translucent. The amount of swelling may change throughout the day, starting out smaller in the morning and gradually becoming larger. The presence of pain associated with swelling may indicate an inguinal hernia has developed, injury to the testicles has occurred, or another medical condition is present and should be addressed by a physician.

Treatment. Hydroceles generally will dissolve on their own. Medical intervention is initiated if the hydrocele becomes painful or infected. If the hydrocele is related to an inguinal hernia, prompt surgical correction is performed. In other cases, a hydrocelectomy may be performed to correct the issue.

Prostate Cancer

Prostate cancer is a malignant tumor that grows in the prostate gland. The risk of developing prostate cancer increases with age; men under 40 are rarely at risk for this form of cancer. However, prostate cancer is the leading cause of cancer-related death in men aged 75 and over.

In addition to age, other risk factors associated with prostate cancer are a diet high in animal fats, excessive alcohol consumption, a first-degree family history of prostate cancer (a brother or father), exposure to cadmium or Agent Orange (a chemical used during the Vietnam War), and certain occupations such as painters and tire plant workers.

Signs and Symptoms. Prostate cancer can grow slowly for many years, but it occasionally grows quickly and spreads (metastasizes) to other parts of the body. Signs and symptoms may or may not be present. When they are, the most common include dull pain in the lower pelvic area, particularly bone pain in this area; blood in the urine or semen; dribbling when urinating; erectile dysfunction; frequent urination, especially at night; painful urination or ejaculation; smaller stream of urine or urgent need to urinate; and loss of appetite and weight. If the cancer has spread to other parts of the body, there may be persistent bone pain, occasional nerve loss, or loss of bladder function.

Treatment. Treatment for prostate cancer relies heavily on the patient's overall health and his Gleason score. This score is given based on the grades of cancer cells in a prostate biopsy. Cancer cell grades range from 1 to 5 and are assigned based on how quickly the cancer is likely to spread. The sum of the two most prevalent grades of cancer cells are added together to come up with the score. Most prostate cancer patients have a Gleason score of 6 to 7, which is considered an intermediate form of the cancer. Early stages of cancer may be treated with radiation therapy and prostatectomy (surgical removal of the entire prostate and some surrounding tissue). More advanced stages of this cancer may be treated with chemotherapy, additional surgery, and hormone therapy to reduce testosterone levels.

SUMMARY

The reproductive systems of men and women have the purpose of reproducing and continuing the species as well as maintaining secondary sex characteristics for both genders. The organs of the female reproductive system are the uterus, fallopian tubes, ovaries, vagina, vulva, and breasts. A 28-day menstrual cycle prepares the female body for possible impregnation and reproduction. Conception and pregnancy are achieved when the female ovum and the male sperm unite. Pregnancy lasts approximately 40 weeks and is divided into three trimesters. Labor, or childbirth, is also divided into three distinct stages—dilation (the longest stage), expulsion, and placental.

Two reasons why a woman or couple may not conceive are contraception (steps taken deliberately to prevent conception) and infertility. Infertility is a term used to describe couples who have been unsuccessful at attempting to conceive after 12 consecutive months.

Common female reproductive disorders include cancers of the breast, cervix, ovaries, and uterus, as well as cervicitis, dysmenorrhea, endometriosis, fibrocystic breast disease, ovarian cysts, pelvic inflammatory disease, premenstrual syndrome, STDs, and uterine fibroids. Complications of pregnancy include abruptio placentae, breech presentation, eclampsia, ectopic/tubal pregnancy, placenta previa, preeclampsia, premature birth, spontaneous abortion, and stillbirth.

The organs of the male reproductive system include the penis, testes, scrotum, epididymis, ductus deferens, prostate gland, bulbourethral glands, urethra, and seminal vesicles. The male reproductive system produces sperm on a regular basis and does not depend on a reproductive cycle. Many diseases can develop in the reproductive organs.

Common disorders of the male reproductive system include benign prostatic hyperplasia, epididymitis, erectile dysfunction, hydrocele, and prostate cancer.

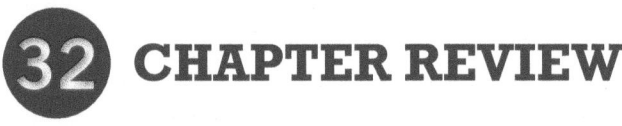

32 CHAPTER REVIEW

COMPETENCY REVIEW

1. Define and spell the terms for this chapter.
2. What are the two functions of the ovaries?
3. What are the three identifiable areas of the uterus?
4. What are the three functions of the vagina?
5. Explain the difference between primary and secondary infertility.
6. What are the two principal hormones, considered to be instrumental, in the female reproductive system?
7. What is the most vital function of the male reproductive system?
8. What are the two functions of the penis?
9. What is the purpose of the prostate gland?
10. List the internal organs of the male reproductive system.

PREPARING FOR THE CERTIFICATION EXAM

1. The triangular-shaped pad of fatty tissue that is rounded over the symphysis pubis is known as
   a. clitoris.
   b. mons pubis.
   c. labia minora.
   d. labia majora.
   e. perineum.

2. Which of the following is *not* a sexually transmitted infection?
   a. syphilis
   b. endometriosis
   c. trichomoniasis
   d. candidiasis
   e. genital warts

3. The fetal period begins at the _____ week of gestation.
   a. 3rd
   b. 6th
   c. 9th
   d. 12th
   e. 15th

4. The lower portion of the uterus is called the
   a. fundus.
   b. corpus.
   c. ovum.
   d. cervix.
   e. vulva.

5. All of the following are pregnancy complications *except*
   a. abruptio placentae
   b. dysmenorrhea.
   c. eclampsia.
   d. preeclampsia.
   e. placenta previa.

6. All of the following are symptoms of premenstrual syndrome *except*
   a. diarrhea.
   b. backache.
   c. mood swings.
   d. depression.
   e. herpes recurrence.

7. Which of the following terms means failure of the testes to descend into the scrotal sac before birth?
   a. epispadias
   b. hypospadias
   c. cryptorchidism
   d. circumcision
   e. anorchism

8. The sterilization of the male reproductive system is done with surgery to what structure?
   a. vas deferens
   b. prostate
   c. penis
   d. scrotum
   e. urethra

9. The ovaries produce
   a. progesterone.
   b. growth hormone.
   c. testosterone.
   d. oxytocin.
   e. prolactin.

10. The hormone that stimulates the uterus to contract is
    a. progesterone.
    b. estrogen.
    c. testosterone.
    d. oxytocin.
    e. prolactin.

CRITICAL THINKING

Refer to the case study at the beginning of the chapter and use what you have learned to answer the following questions.

1. Why would Dr. Bahjat ask Mr. Hamsi if he is sexually active?
2. Dr. Bahjat next asks Mr. Hamsi if he has had any recent injuries. Mr. Hamsi informs him that he was injured in the groin during a soccer game a couple of weeks ago. Could this injury be related to Mr. Hamsi's diagnosis?
3. Because Mr. Hamsi has been in pain for almost two weeks, what possible complications may result from a delay in treatment?

INTERNET ACTIVITY

Conduct an Internet search of the National Breast Cancer Foundation and other breast cancer awareness organizations. Research the following regarding breast cancer: cancer myths, early detection, and up-and-coming research.

Clinical Medical Assisting

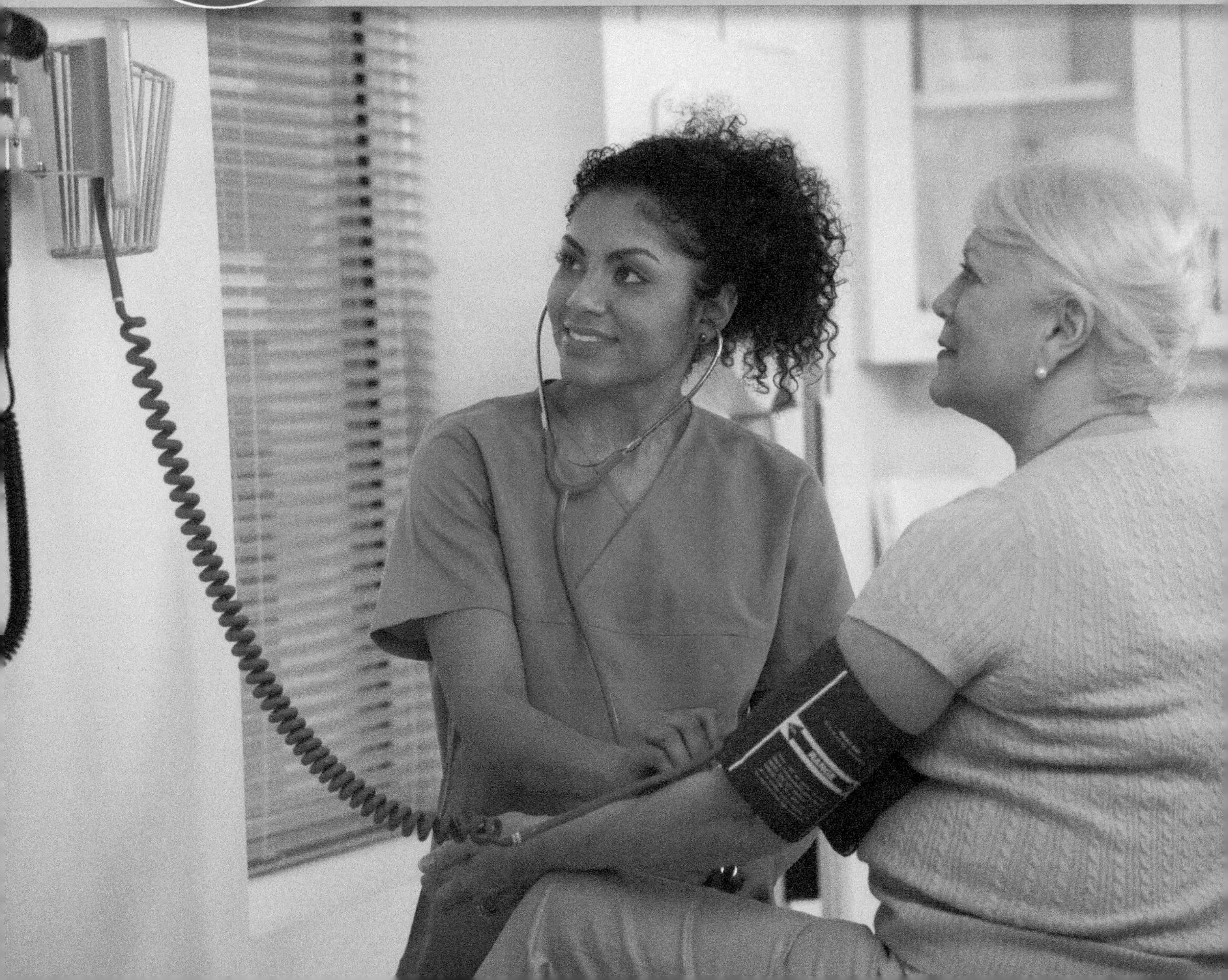

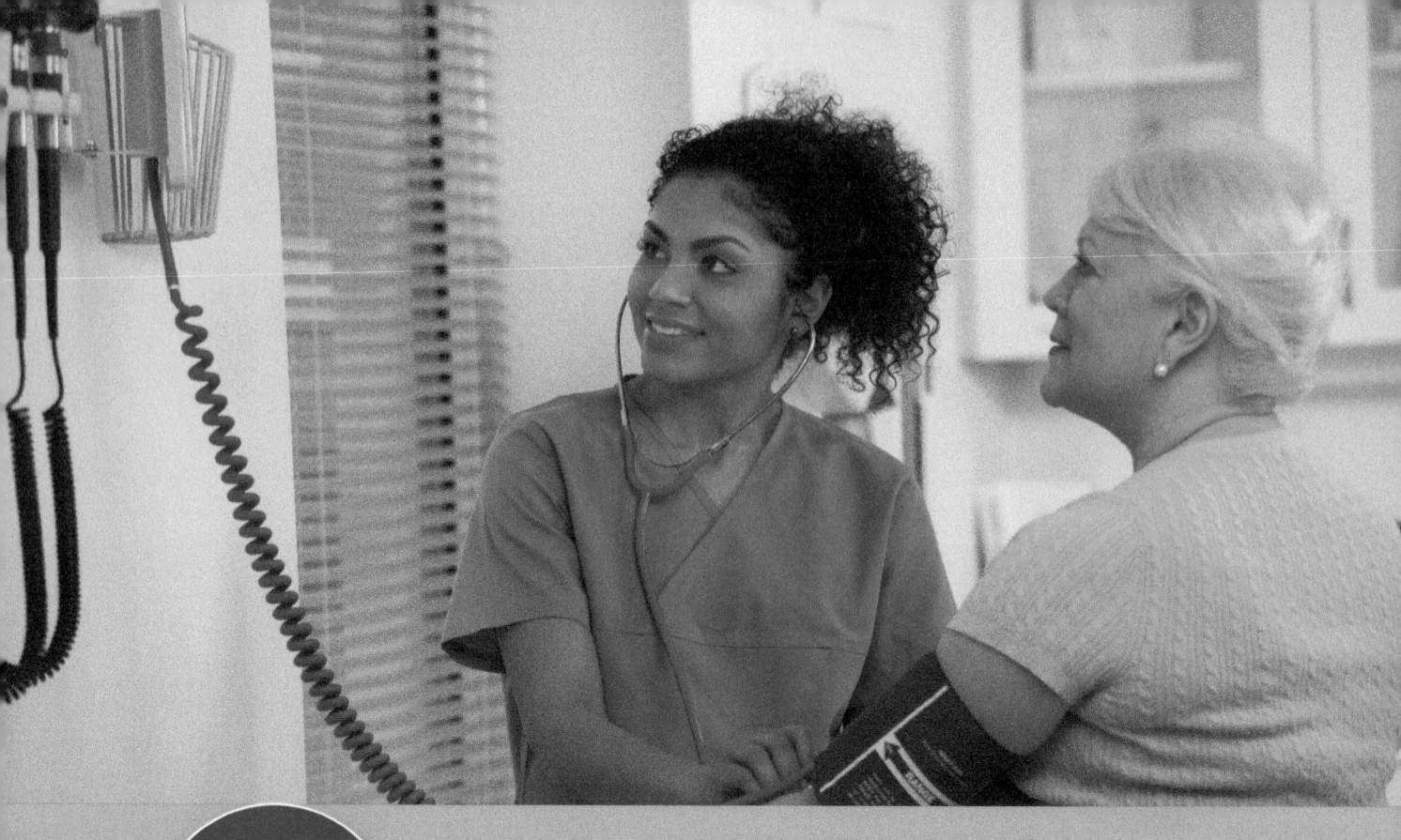

Infection Control

Learning Objectives

After completing this chapter, you should be able to:

33.1 Define and spell the terms for this chapter.

33.2 List types of infectious microorganisms.

33.3 Identify conditions required for bacterial growth.

33.4 Explain the cycle of the chain of infection.

33.5 Describe the body's natural barriers to infection.

33.6 Identify government regulations that impact infection control practices in health care.

33.7 List the three categories of transmission-based precautions, as established by the Centers for Disease Control and Prevention (CDC).

33.8 Describe surgical asepsis.

33.9 Identify types of personal protective equipment.

33.10 Describe methods that can be implemented to control the growth of microorganisms.

Dr. McWalters asks David Dolan, RMA, to perform venipuncture on the 34-year-old female in examination room 4. The physician explains that the patient needs to have routine blood work performed, including a liver function test (LFT), to evaluate the progression of hepatitis B, which the patient was diagnosed with over two years ago.

Terms to Learn

aerobic

airborne precautions

anaerobic

antibodies

antiseptic

asepsis

bactericidal

bloodborne pathogens

contact precautions

direct contact

disinfection

droplet precautions

excreta

immunity

incubation

indirect contact

infectious

medical asepsis

methicillin-resistant *Staphylococcus aureus* (MRSA)

microorganisms

multidrug-resistant organisms (MDROs)

normal flora

opportunistic infections

pathogens

permeable

personal protective equipment (PPE)

phagocytosis

portal of entry

portal of exit

postexposure evaluation

radiation isolation precautions

reservoir host

respiratory hygiene/cough etiquette

safe injection practices

sanitization

standard precautions

sterilization

surgical asepsis

susceptible host

universal precautions

vancomycin-resistant *Enterococci* (VRE)

vancomycin-resistant *Staphylococcus aureus* (VRSA)

Infection control is the process of reducing exposure to pathogens to prevent the spread of disease. **Pathogens**, which are disease-producing organisms, are found everywhere, including on inanimate objects (such as countertops and faucets) and on human skin. In healthy individuals, the immune system provides some measure of resistance to pathogens. However, people who are already suffering from a disease are likely to have a compromised immune system, making them more susceptible to new infections. Therefore, controlling pathogens is especially important in a medical office, where patients with a variety of diseases are constantly coming in and out. These patients can spread pathogens to others, and they are also generally more susceptible to new infections.

As a medical assistant, you must be aware of how easily pathogens can be spread from one person to another or from an inanimate object to a person. **Asepsis** is the state of being free from germs, infection, and any form of microbial life.

Medical assistants must know and understand the theory and practice of asepsis to maintain a healthy environment for patients and medical staff members alike.

MICROORGANISMS AND PATHOGENS

Organisms are systems made up of groups of living cells. **Microorganisms** are organisms that are so small they can be seen only with the aid of a microscope. The sizes of microorganisms (also called microbes) can be expressed in micrometers. A micrometer is one-millionth of a meter or one-thousandth of a millimeter.

Not all microorganisms cause disease; those that do, as noted earlier, are called pathogens. There are numerous types of pathogens, including bacteria, fungi, protozoa, viruses, rickettsiae, and parasites (protozoans, helminths, ectoparasites, and the like) (see Figure 33-1).

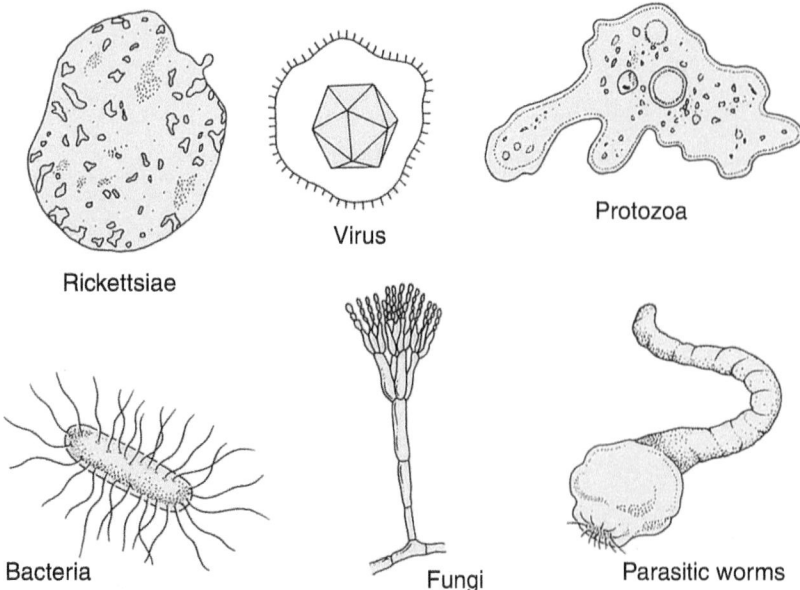

Rickettsiae

Virus

Protozoa

Bacteria

Fungi

Parasitic worms

FIGURE 33-1 Examples of pathogens

The four main types of microoganisms are generally considered to be bacteria, fungi, protozoa, and viruses. The study of each of these types is a separate scientific field:

- **Bacteriology**—the study of bacteria
- **Mycology**—the study of fungi
- **Protozoology**—the study of protozoa
- **Virology**—the study of viruses

As already noted, not all microorganisms are pathogens. Many microorganisms that are not harmful grow and thrive in the human body and may have helpful functions within the body. Microorganisms that are normally found on the skin and in the urinary, gastrointestinal, and respiratory tracts are known as **normal flora**. They do not cause disease under the following conditions:

- If they are not transferred to another part of the body. For example, *Escherichia coli*, a normal bacterium within the colon, aids in food digestion. However, when *E. coli* moves into the bladder or bloodstream, through such poor habits as improper (or lack of) hand hygiene, *E. coli* can cause urinary tract and blood infections.
- If they remain in balance within their environment. For example, when the pH balance of normal flora found within the vagina is altered, a yeast infection may develop.

How Microorganisms Grow

Microorganisms exist everywhere in nature. To grow, they generally require food, moisture, darkness, and a suitable temperature. In addition, some bacteria are **aerobic** (require oxygen to live), and some are **anaerobic** (do not require oxygen to live). Refer to Table 33-1 for the conditions that are necessary for the growth of bacteria. Microorganisms that are capable of producing disease (pathogens) grow best at a body temperature of 98.6°F/37°C, destroy and use human tissue as food, and excrete waste toxins that are absorbed by and may poison the body.

Multidrug-Resistant Microorganisms

One group of microorganisms, **multidrug-resistant organisms (MDROs)**, is of growing concern in health care. These microorganisms are referred to as "super-bugs" because they do not respond to traditional medications and treatments and have developed resistance to antimicrobial drugs. Increased length of hospital stays, increased cost of treatments, and death are associated with these organisms. Common examples include **methicillin-resistant *Staphylococcus aureus* (MRSA)**, **vancomycin-resistant *Staphylococcus aureus* (VRSA)**, and **vancomycin-resistant *Enterococci* (VRE)**.

Methicillin-Resistant Staphylococcus Aureus (MRSA)

Methicillin-resistant *S. aureus*, or MRSA, is an organism that is highly resistant to antibiotics. There are two forms of MRSA: hospital-associated MRSA and community-based MRSA. The first, as the name implies, occurs mostly in health care facilities to individuals with weakened immune

TABLE 33-1	Conditions Required for Bacterial Growth
Condition	**Explanation**
Moisture	Bacteria grow best in moist areas: skin, mucous membranes, wet dressings, wounds, dirty instruments.
Temperature	Bacteria thrive at body temperature (98.6°F). Low temperatures (32°F and below) retard, but do not kill, bacterial growth.
Oxygen	Aerobic bacteria require an oxygen supply to live. Anaerobic bacteria can survive without oxygen.
Darkness	Darkness favors the growth of most bacteria. Some bacteria will die if exposed to direct sunlight or light.

systems. This organism is one of the most common agents responsible for nosocomial infections (infections acquired while in a medical facility), which are discussed later in this chapter.

S. aureus is the causative agent in boils, acne, some forms of septicemia, and pneumonia. Infection may occur from cuts, sores, and through catheters or breathing tubes. Symptoms of *Staphylococcus* (staph) infection include pus formation, fever, swelling, and tenderness around the area of infection. Individuals with weakened immune systems are more susceptible to this type of infection. Serious staph infections may lead to endocarditis (inflammation of the lining of the heart), cellulitis (inflammation of subcutaneous and connective tissue), pneumonia, and toxic shock syndrome.

Diagnosis of *S. aureus* is established by culture from the infected individual. A sensitivity test determines which antibiotics are most effective in killing the organism. If the organism grows in the presence of methicillin, it is classified as MRSA. The physician then prescribes the medication that most readily kills the microorganism.

The best way to avoid contracting or spreading MRSA infection is through the use of good hygiene practices, including handwashing and wearing gloves and other personal protective equipment (PPE) when treating any patient, especially one known or suspected to have a MRSA infection. Using an antiseptic cream and covering any skin breaks with adhesive bandages also will help prevent the spread of MRSA.

Vancomycin-Resistant Enterococci (VRE)

Enterococci are bacteria normally present in human intestines, the female genital tract, and the environment. Most species of *enterococci* are harmless, but some are capable of causing serious infections, which may be treated with vancomycin, an antibiotic often used as a last line of defense; that is, it is an antibiotic generally used after all other antibiotics have failed. Vancomycin-resistant *enterococci* are a strain of these bacteria that has developed a resistance to vancomycin and no longer responds to this drug.

Signs and symptoms of VRE vary, depending on the source of the infection. Skin or wound VRE infections may be present as well as VRE infections of the urinary and gastrointestinal tracts.

VRE is spread by **direct contact** from human to human, usually by caregivers who have not practiced proper hand hygiene. It can also be spread by touching contaminated inanimate objects. To prevent VRE at home or work, always wash hands after using the bathroom and before preparing food. Wash or use alcohol-based hand rubs after contact with persons with VRE.

INFECTIONS

Scientists have determined that microorganisms are capable of multiplying very quickly. If not controlled, germs may spread infection and diseases rapidly from one person to another. As a medical assistant, you will need to understand how infections are spread—the infection process as well as the types of infections that occur.

The Chain of Infection

The sole presence of a pathogenic organism is not enough to cause an infection. Several factors must be in place for infection to occur. These are referred to as the chain of infection:

1. The **reservoir host** begins the chain of infection. The reservoir host is an organism—usually an animal or human—that harbors and nourishes a pathogen. Often, a reservoir host gives a pathogen a "home" for a long time without suffering any ill effects from it. At other times, the reservoir host may become infected by the pathogen. Either way, the reservoir host is the organism that is the source of a pathogen that can then be transferred to another organism that becomes infected by it. The host provides nourishment and sustenance for the pathogen, allowing it to grow. The host, including a human host, generally is not aware that it is harboring a pathogen.

2. For the pathogen to spread to another animal or person, there must be a **portal of exit** from the reservoir host. The means of exit include the respiratory, gastrointestinal, urinary, and reproductive tracts of the body. An open wound is also an excellent portal of exit.

3. Next, there must be a means of transmission for the pathogen to spread to another person. This may be through direct (human to human) contact, either with the infected person or with the discharge or **excreta** (waste products) of the infected person. The transmission can also occur by **indirect contact** (nonhuman to human). Examples include inhaling infected air droplets from a cough or sneeze, or touching a contaminated object. Other methods of transmission through indirect contact are through contaminated food (possibly meat tainted with the bacterium *salmonella*) or insects (such as the transmission of West Nile virus through infected mosquitos).

4. A **portal of entry** into a new host is required. The portal of entry is the means by which a pathogen enters the body. Similar to the portal of exit, these portals include the respiratory, urinary, and reproductive tracts, skin and mucous membranes, or blood.

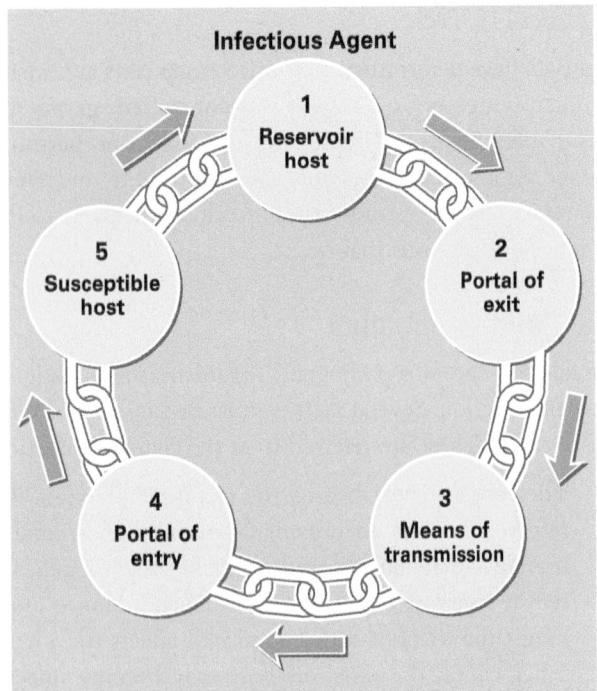

FIGURE 33-2 Chain of infection.

TABLE 33-2 | Stages of the Infection Process

Stage	Description
Invasion	Pathogen enters the body through the portal of entry: respiratory, digestive, reproductive, urinary tracts, and skin.
Multiplication	Reproduction of pathogens.
Incubation	Period may vary from several days to months or years, during which time the disease is developing but no symptoms appear.
Prodromal Period	First, mild signs and symptoms appear; a highly contagious period.
Acute Period	Signs and symptoms are evident and most severe.
Recovery Period	Signs and symptoms begin to subside.

5. A **susceptible host** must be available and capable of being infected by the pathogen. A susceptible host is someone who is unable to fight off the infection. Some situations that lead to susceptibility include poor health, poor hygiene, or poor nutrition. Increased stress levels may also be a factor.

When the susceptible host becomes infected, that person becomes a new reservoir host, and the chain of infection begins again. Figure 33-2 illustrates the chain of infection.

Fortunately, if the chain is broken, infection does not occur. The chain can be broken at various points. For instance, the chain may be broken at the reservoir by using medical asepsis, standard precautions (which are discussed later), and proper hand hygiene to prevent transmission of the pathogen. In fact, attaining medical asepsis through proper hand hygiene is the most important method for decreasing the spread of infections.

The Stages and Types of Infections

Once an infection has begun in the host, it proceeds through specific stages. These stages include invasion by the pathogen, multiplication (reproduction) of the pathogen, an **incubation** period, a prodromal period, an acute period, and, finally, the recovery period. The stages of the infection process are described in Table 33-2.

Additionally, it is important to discuss the various types of infections that may be present. The most common types

of infections are acute, chronic, latent, opportunistic, and nosocomial.

Acute Infections

Many of the common illnesses that afflict the human body are considered acute infections. These may include the common cold and influenza. Acute infections have a rapid transition from invasion of the pathogen to the prodromal period. The body is usually able to rid itself of the virus and recover within three to five weeks of onset.

Chronic Infections

Chronic infections are more serious than acute infections because the effects of the disease-causing pathogen can last for a very long time. In fact, some chronic infections are lifelong. The transition of stages from invasion to the prodromal period varies based on the type of infection. Diseases discussed later in this chapter, including HIV and hepatitis B, are examples of chronic infections.

Latent Infections

A latent infection can be very frustrating to patients because this form of infection is characterized by periods of remission and relapse. Remission is when the disease has been treated and there are no longer any signs or symptoms present. Relapse is when the same infection reoccurs. This is common with viral infections such as those that cause cold sores (herpes simplex virus types I and II) as well as the varicella-zoster virus that can cause chickenpox and later erupt as shingles. The main characteristic of a latent infection is that the virus lies dormant within the body for extended periods of time (often many years). Then, an external or internal factor will trigger the virus to become active within the body again.

Opportunistic Infections

Opportunistic infections are those that occur when the host's immune system has already been impaired by another disease-causing pathogen. The immune system has become weakened and more susceptible to other infections. Patients with severely compromised immune systems, such as those who are being treated for cancer or a patient with HIV, are more likely to suffer from other (opportunistic) infections. Oral thrush (candidiasis) and pneumonia are examples of opportunistic infections that might afflict a compromised immune system but not a healthy one.

Nosocomial Infections

Nosocomial infections are infections acquired while in a medical facility, generally the hospital setting. In fact, nosocomial infections are also called hospital-acquired infections. The pathogens were not in the patient's body when the patient came into the facility but rather were introduced into the body because of poor aseptic technique in the facility. The most common types of nosocomial infections include:

- Bloodstream infections (from improper venipuncture or IV line procedures)
- Urinary tract infections (from improper catheter procedures)
- Surgical site infections (from improper wound care)

In all medical settings, there must be a dedicated emphasis on halting the spread of infection.

The Inflammatory Response to Infection

The body may react to the presence of pathogens, such as bacteria or a virus, with an acute inflammatory process. This process results in the dilation of blood vessels to allow increased blood flow, production of watery fluids and materials (exudates such as pus), and invasion of neutrophils and monocytes into the injured tissues. Neutrophils and monocytes are types of leukocytes (white blood cells) that perform phagocytosis, which means that they engulf ("eat") and destroy disease-causing pathogens.

The signs and symptoms of infection and the inflammatory process may be local (an earache) or systemic (an elevated body temperature). The four cardinal signs of acute inflammation are redness, heat, swelling, and pain. Signs and symptoms may vary according to the part of the body that is affected. Table 33-3 lists signs and symptoms of infection and inflammation.

TABLE 33-3	Signs and Symptoms of Infection and Inflammation	
Cardinal Signs of Inflammation	**Other Signs of Infection**
Redness	Abnormal white blood cell counts: high (leukycytosis) or low (leukopenia). High counts are very common with infection.
Heat	Fever
Swelling (edema)	Increased pulse rate
Pain	Increased respiration rate

THE BODY'S NATURAL BARRIERS

The human body can play both beneficial and harmful roles in infection control and the disease process. Some factors, such as advancing age and genetic predisposition, can be detrimental; other factors, such as a healthy diet and plenty of rest, can work in the body's favor. Antibiotics and other drugs are effective infection fighters, but the body itself provides many defenses against infection.

Prevention and Protection

The human body has several natural barriers to infection. The largest natural barrier to infection is intact skin. The acidity of the skin inhibits bacterial action. Mucous membranes lining the body's orifices and its respiratory, digestive, reproductive, and urinary tracts also assist in repelling microorganisms. The gastrointestinal tract contains hydrochloric acid (HCl), which has a **bactericidal** (bacteria-destroying) action. The lymphatic system and the blood also play key preventive and protective roles.

The Lymphatic System and the Blood

The lymphatic system and the blood produce antibodies to identify and neutralize or destroy disease-causing pathogens that enter the body. As noted earlier, leukocytes (white blood cells) actively fight pathogenic microorganisms through **phagocytosis**, the process of engulfing, digesting, and destroying pathogens. The process of phagocytosis is shown in Figure 33-3.

Antigen–Antibody Reaction

Lymphocytes produce antibodies during the antigen–antibody reaction. **Antibodies**—protein substances produced by lymphocytes in the spleen, lymph nodes and tissue, and the bone marrow—react in response to antigens (foreign substances/pathogens). Antibodies have the ability to neutralize

PHAGOCYTOSIS

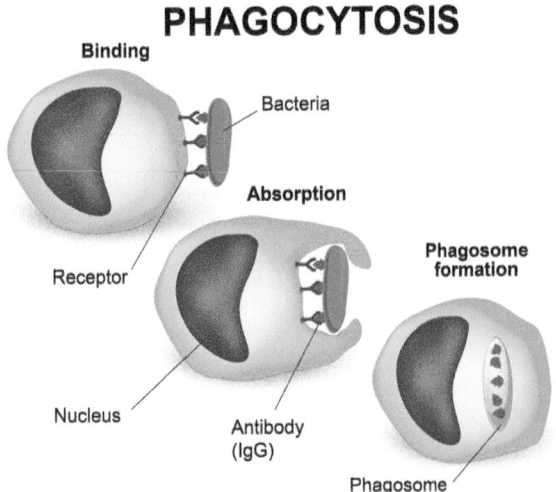

FIGURE 33-3 The process of phagocytosis: a phagocyte engulfing bacteria or other foreign material.

antigens or make them more susceptible to phagocytosis. The antigen–antibody reaction occurs in response to an invasion of antigens.

Immunity

The body has a natural protective mechanism called immunity. **Immunity**, a resistance to disease, is said to have occurred when enough antibodies have been produced to provide protection for weeks, months, or years. Immunity is either innate, active, or passive. Table 33-4 describes the types of immunity.

TABLE 33-4 | Types of Immunity

Type	Description
Innate	Sometimes called natural immunity. It is the body's first line of defense against pathogens including skin, mucous membranes, and tears.
Active	Either acquired or artificially acquired: **Acquired active**—a person is immune to a disease because that person has been previously exposed and has developed appropriate antibodies. **Artificially acquired active**—immunity induced through a vaccine.
Passive Immunity	A temporary form of immunity—such as antibodies that are passed from a mother to an infant through breast milk.

INFECTION CONTROL: PRECAUTIONS AND STANDARDS

Several government agencies have developed guidelines, precautions, and standards to protect patients and health care workers from exposure to pathogens. The guidelines have changed and will continue to evolve as advances are made in what we know about preventing the spread of infection. Although many of these guidelines were first established for health care workers and the care of patients in hospital settings, today these practices are implemented in all medical facilities, including physicians' offices. As a medical assistant, you will need to understand the importance of infection-control guidelines, standards, and precautions as you interact with patients and consistently take the recommended precautions on a daily basis.

Universal Precautions

In the early 1980s, the United States was experiencing an epidemic of the human immunodeficiency virus (HIV) and acquired immunodeficiency syndrome (AIDS), the disease that HIV causes. At the same time, there was increasing awareness of hepatitis, an infection of the liver, especially the B strain of the hepatitis virus (HBV). Table 33-5 discusses forms of hepatitis and HIV, and Box 33-1 provides considerations for caring for a person with HIV or AIDS.

In 1985, the Centers for Disease Control and Prevention (CDC) established **universal precautions** to protect health care workers and patients from HIV, HBV, and other **bloodborne pathogens**. The theory behind universal precautions was simple—treat all blood and bodily fluids as if they are contaminated. Later, the CDC included the precaution that all moist body secretions should be considered contaminated (except sweat). Practices that surrounded universal precautions included proper hand hygiene and the use of gloves when handling blood or performing invasive procedures, such as venipuncture.

Standard Precautions

Standard precautions have been developed by the CDC, which recommends using these precautions when caring for all patients, whatever their diagnosis. As with universal precautions, the guidelines for standard precautions apply to all blood, body fluid secretions, and excretions except sweat, whether blood is visible or not. The original guidelines had to do with handwashing and use of **personal protective equipment (PPE)** such as gloves, gowns, and masks whenever touching or exposed to patients' body fluids. Box 33-2 describes bloodborne pathogen training.

TABLE 33-5 | Hepatitis and HIV/AIDS

Virus	Means of Transmission	Incubation Period	Signs and Symptoms	Vaccination Available
Hepatitis A (HAV)	• Fecal/oral route—such as food contaminated with fecal material. This is the most common means of transmission. • Sexually transmitted.	• 14–50 days, slow onset of symptoms.	• Fever, loss of appetite, jaundice, nausea, vomiting, malaise, dark urine, and whitish stools.	• Vaccination is available for ages 12 months and up.
Hepatitis B (HBV)	• Contact with contaminated body fluids, including blood, semen, and saliva.	• 60–90 days, rapid onset of symptoms.	• Fever, loss of appetite, jaundice, nausea, vomiting, malaise, dark urine, and whitish stools. • 30 percent of individuals have no signs or symptoms. • Can lead to a lifelong infection, scarring of the liver, liver cancer, or liver failure and death.	• Vaccination is available in a series of shots between the ages of birth and 18 years of age. • High-risk groups such as health care workers and public safety workers generally receive the vaccination.
Hepatitis C (HCV)	• Contact with contaminated blood—particularly through the sharing of needles. • Can be passed from mother to baby during the birth process.	• 6–10 weeks.	• About 80 percent of infected individuals do not develop signs and symptoms. • If symptoms do develop, they mimic HAV and HBV.	No vaccine available.
Human Immunodeficiency Virus and Acquired Immunodeficiency Syndrome (HIV and AIDS)	• Sexual contact. • Can be passed from mother to baby. • Contact with contaminated blood.	Varies by individual; in some, the incubation period can be 6 months up to many years.	• HIV virus may develop into acquired immunodeficiency syndrome (AIDS). • Symptoms before the development of AIDS include loss of appetite, weight loss, diarrhea, skin rash, fatigue, night sweats, swollen lymph glands, poor resistance to infection.	No vaccine.

Hand sanitizing is one of the best means of reducing the spread of microorganisms in a health care facility and at home. Hand hygiene recommendations include not wearing artificial fingernails or extenders when having direct contact with high-risk patients. Natural fingernails should be kept short: less than one-quarter inch long.

In 2007, the CDC issued several new elements to be included in standard precautions. These guidelines involve three areas of practice: respiratory hygiene/cough etiquette,

Professionalism The Life Span

Infants, especially those under 3 months of age, and older adults are more prone to infection. Infants' immune systems are underdeveloped, and the immune systems in older adults are slowing down and decreasing in function. In addition, older adults often do not eat nutritionally sound meals, which further weakens their resistance to infection.

BOX 33-1 | Caring for Someone with HIV or AIDS

To protect themselves from infection, health care workers and caregivers should be reminded to do the following:

- Handle all needles with care. Never recap needles or remove needles from syringes. Dispose of all needles in puncture-proof containers out of the reach of children.
- Wear gloves when in contact with blood, blood-tinged body fluids, urine, feces, or vomit.
- Perform hand hygiene after removing gloves.
- Cover with a bandage any cut, open sore, or breaks on exposed skin of either the patient or the caregiver.
- Flush down the toilet all liquid waste containing blood, using care to avoid splashing during pouring. Nonflushable items such as paper towels, sanitary pads and tampons, wound dressings, or items soiled with blood, semen, or vaginal fluid should be enclosed in a plastic bag and tightly sealed. Check with your local health department or physician to determine trash disposal regulations for your area.
- Use a disinfection solution of 1 part bleach to 10 parts water to disinfect such items as floors, showers, tubs, and sinks. Discard the solution in the toilet after using. The application of heat treatment at 132°F (56°C) for 10 minutes can also be implemented.

To protect the person with AIDS from infection:

- If the caregiver has a cold or flu, and no one else is available to care for the AIDS patient, a surgical-type mask should be worn.

- Hands should be washed before touching the AIDS patient.
- Anyone with boils, fever blisters (herpes simplex), or shingles (herpes zoster) should avoid close contact with the patient.
- Gloves should be worn if the caregiver has a rash or sores on the hands.
- Persons living with or caring for an HIV/AIDS patient should have received all the recommended childhood immunizations and booster shots, including the hepatitis vaccine.
- The AIDS patient should not be in the same room with a person who has, or is recovering from, chickenpox or shingles.

The caregiver should also do the following:

- Call the local HIV/AIDS service organization for support.
- Seek the help of clergy, counselors, and other health care professionals to cope with feelings of frustration and stress.
- Be comfortable touching the person with HIV/AIDS.
- Encourage the patient to become involved in his or her own care, and assist the patient in being active as long as possible.
- Freely discuss the disease with the patient.

For more information on HIV or AIDS, write to the CDC National AIDS Clearinghouse, P.O. Box 6003, Rockville, MD 20849-6003; CDC Control and Prevention, 1600 Clifton Road, N.E., Atlanta, GA 30333; or call 1-800-CDC-INFO (1-800-232-4636).

BOX 33-2 | Bloodborne Pathogen Training

Bloodborne pathogen training is required by the Occupational Safety and Health Administration (OSHA) of all employees and students who have the potential for being exposed to bloodborne pathogens. Training includes discussion of pathogens that include, but are not limited to, hepatitis B (HBV), hepatitis C (HCV), and human immunodeficiency virus (HIV). Ways to prevent sharps-related injuries are also discussed, as these injuries may expose workers to bloodborne pathogens. Courses are sometimes developed by employers or presented by consultants. In these courses, health care personnel—including those who do housekeeping—who are at risk for exposure to bloodborne pathogens learn about the risk factors and ways to prevent exposure. A certificate of completion is usually filed in the employee personnel file as evidence of training. For more information, see www.osha.gov/SLTC/bloodbornepathogens/index.html or by contacting OSHA at 1-800-321-OSHA (6742). Your instructor may require you to get bloodborne pathogen training as part of your education. Save your certificate of training to show potential future employers.

safe injection practices, and the use of masks when there is a risk of splashing.

The current complete set of standard precautions, therefore, concern:

1. Hand hygiene, including handwashing with soap and water or the use of alcohol-based hand rubs.

2. Personal protective equipment to include, as appropriate for the situation, gloves, gowns, face masks or shields, protective eyewear, and respirators.

3. **Respiratory hygiene/cough etiquette**—Respiratory hygiene/cough etiquette is designed to reduce the transmission of pathogens from patients, family members, friends, and any other persons entering a health care facility with signs of illness, cough, congestion, or rhinorrhea (runny nose). The guidelines suggest that signs be posted reminding people to cover their mouth or nose when coughing, to dispose of tissues appropriately, to perform hand hygiene after contact with respiratory secretions, to use a mask when appropriate, and whenever possible to provide

at least 3 feet of space between persons with respiratory infections.

4. **Safe injection practices**—Safe injection practices include the use of aseptic technique and the employment of single-use items (needles, syringes, and whenever possible single-dose vials for parenteral medication). No multidose vials should be kept in the immediate treatment area.

5. The use of masks to cover the face and reduce the risk of splash when inserting catheters or when performing procedures involving lumbar puncture.

While practicing standard precautions, it is important to remember that some patients may be latex-sensitive. Before touching a patient while wearing latex gloves, ask if the patient has a history of latex sensitivity. High-risk patients, such as those with congenital defects and indwelling catheters, must always be assessed for latex sensitivity, which can develop after repeated exposures to latex. Patients with allergies to bananas, chestnuts, kiwi, and avocados may have cross-sensitivity to latex. Therefore, it is prudent to ask about those allergies as well. Symptoms to latex sensitivity include contact dermatitis, swelling, itching, and rhinitis (a runny nose) and may, in some cases, include anaphylaxis (a life-threatening allergic reaction).

 Professionalism The Workplace

Wearing excessive jewelry, long fingernails, artificial nails, nail polish, or long hair can harbor microorganisms and cause contamination. Allow your patients and coworkers to view you as someone who maintains immaculate personal hygiene technique and image at all times.

Latex-free gloves, syringes, IV tubing, and solution bags should always be available to meet the needs of the patients and the health care providers.

Standard precautions equipment and examples of situations in which they must be used are found in Box 33-3. Figure 33-4 summarizes standard precautions for all patient care.

Transmission-Based Precautions

The second tier of the 2007 CDC guidelines focuses on infected patients or those suspected of being infected. These guidelines require transmission-based precautions. Transmission-based precautions are used in addition to standard precautions to further interrupt the spread of pathogens. Transmission-based precautions fall into three

---

BOX 33-3 | Summary of Standard Precautions

1. Wear gloves when there is potential for exposure to blood or body fluids, secretions, excretions, or contaminated items. This includes performing routine clinical work, touching mucous membranes and the nonintact skin of patients, and handling tissue and clinical specimens (Figure 33-4).
2. Wear gloves when drawing blood, including finger-stick and heel-stick on infants, and during preparation of blood smears.
3. Wear protective barrier equipment (e.g., face mask, eye shield, or goggles) when there is any risk of splashing, splattering, or aerosolization (becoming airborne in small particles) of potentially infectious body fluids.
4. Change gloves after each patient. Perform hand hygiene before putting on gloves and after removing them.
5. Change gloves if they become contaminated with blood or other body fluids, and discard them in a biohazards collection container.
6. Wash hands and other skin surfaces immediately or as soon as possible if they become contaminated with potentially infectious blood or body fluids.
7. Care for linens and equipment that are contaminated with blood, blood products, body fluids, excretions, and secretions in a manner that avoids contact with your skin

and mucous membranes or cross-contamination to another person.
8. Wear a mask if the patient has an airborne disease. A special mask is recommended if a patient has an active case of tuberculosis.
9. Use care with needles, scalpels, and other sharp instruments to avoid unintentional injury.
10. Dispose of needles and other sharp items in a rigid, puncture-proof sharps container.
11. Do not recap or handle used needles.
12. Store reusable sharp instruments and needles in a puncture-proof container.
13. Avoid the direct mouth-to-mouth resuscitation technique in all but life-threatening situations. Use a mechanical device or mask barrier instead.
14. Use a solution of household bleach (1:10 dilution) to disinfect surfaces (countertops and exam tables) and reusable equipment.
15. Use hazardous waste containers for contaminated materials.

Note: Adapted from Guidelines for Isolation Precaution in Hospitals, developed by the Centers for Disease Control and Prevention and the Hospital Infection Control Practices Advisory Committee, January 2002.

STANDARD PRECAUTIONS
For all patient care

PROCEDURE	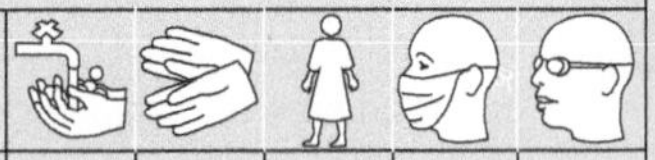				
Talking to patient					
Adjusting IV fluid rate or noninvasive equipment					
Examining patient *without* touching blood, body fluids, mucous membranes	X				
Examining patient *including* contact with blood, body fluids, mucous membranes	X	X			
Drawing blood	X	X			
Inserting venous access	X	X			
Handling soiled waste, linen, other materials	X	X			
Intubation	X	X	X	X	X
Inserting arterial access	X	X	X	X	X
Endoscopy	X	X	X	X	X
Operative and other procedures that produce extensive splattering of blood or body fluids	X	X	X	X	X

FIGURE 33-4 Standard precautions.

categories: airborne precautions, droplet precautions, and contact precautions.

- **Airborne precautions** are designed to reduce the transmission of certain diseases, such as TB, measles, or chickenpox. Airborne precautions are used when patients are infected with pathogens that are transmitted via airborne droplet nuclei (smaller than 5 microns), pathogens that can remain suspended in air and can be widely dispersed throughout a room by air currents. Airborne precautions often involve patient isolation (in a private room if hospitalized) and require use of mask and gown by all health care personnel who come in contact with the patient. When these precautions are used, the risk of transmitting diseases such as TB and chickenpox is reduced. Handwashing and gloves are required as well. Patient transport should be limited, with the patient wearing a mask during transport. All reusable patient care equipment should be cleaned and disinfected before use on another patient. Disposable items

should always be used if available. Special masks (N95 and TB masks) may be used to protect a caregiver from those who have certain microbes that are small enough to enter regular surgical masks. Masks should be changed if they become wet. Check the CDC website (www.cdc.gov) for information about what personal protective equipment (PPE) should be used with patients.

- **Droplet precautions** are used for patients suspected of being infected with organisms spread by droplets during sneezing, coughing, and talking. Some examples are *Haemophilus influenzae* type b, meningitis, pneumonia, pertussis, and streptococcal pneumonia. A mask should be worn if the health care worker is within 3 feet of an infected patient. Gown and gloves are worn if there is a chance of coming into contact with blood or body fluids of suspected patients. Transport of the patient should be limited. All reusable equipment should be cleaned and disinfected.

- **Contact precautions** are specialized precautions used when infections are both difficult to treat and the likelihood of microorganism transmission among patients and health care providers is high. These precautions include isolating patients and wearing gowns and gloves. If there is a chance of coming in contact with body fluids, a mask and protective eyewear should be worn. Health care providers should be aware that some diseases are transmitted by several routes, and all precautions should be taken. Conditions such as intestinal infections, hepatitis, open wounds, respiratory infections, herpes, scabies, and pediculosis are all treated using contact precautions.

- **Radiation isolation precautions**, although not done specifically for infection control, isolate a patient who has received radiation from other people who radioactivity might harm through distance. Those caring for these individuals will usually spend very little time with the patient, stay as far away from the patient as possible, and wear a dosimeter to measure their radiation exposure from the patient.

Bloodborne Pathogen Standard

The Occupational Safety and Health Administration (OSHA) is the main federal agency that enforces safety and health legislation. Much as the CDC developed guidelines regarding the epidemic of HIV and HBV, as well as other bloodborne pathogens such as *Staphylococcus* (staph) and *Streptococcus* (strep), OSHA developed the Bloodborne Pathogen Standard in 1991. The standard was aimed at minimizing exposure of health care workers to harmful bloodborne pathogens. In 2000, the United States Congress passed the Needlestick Safety and Prevention Act, which was created in response to the overwhelming number of exposure incidents each year. In turn, OSHA updated its Bloodborne Pathogen Standard to reflect necessary changes brought about by this new act. Engineered controls like sharps containers must be available to protect health care professionals from accidental sticks from used needles, but fundamentally health care workers must have safe practices with sharps that include using equipment that automatically recaps or retracts, never breaking a needle, and always immediately disposing of used needles in a sharps container like the one shown in Figure 33-5. The OSHA guidelines apply to facilities in which the employees could be "reasonably anticipated" to come into contact with potentially **infectious** materials (materials that can spread infection). An exposure control plan must be implemented in each facility and evaluated yearly, and must include the following:

- An exposure control plan that would reduce occupational exposure that details employee protection measures.
- Use of engineering controls such as availability of gloves (sterile and nonsterile of various sizes), safety needles, disposable cannula, sharps containers, sinks and running water, and biohazard containers. These control measures should be routinely updated for newer and safer devices.
- Employment of work practice controls such as the use of PPE and clothing, proper training, availability of hepatitis B vaccinations, and proper signage and labels.
- Exposure determination indicating job classifications and the possibility of exposure.
- Methods of compliance that document safety measures that would decrease the risk of exposure.
- **Postexposure evaluation**—procedures that would follow in the event of an exposure.

In addition to the exposure control plan, the Bloodborne Pathogen Standard also requires that strict record keeping be enforced including a log of sharps containers and a log of incidents of occupational exposure or illnesses. Routine and documented employee input must also be recorded. The employees (nonmanagerial) are able to provide ideas and recommendations regarding the practices of the office including safety measures, engineering controls, and safer medical devices. Safe housekeeping practices including the use of appropriate containers, bags, and procedures are also a component of the Bloodborne Pathogen Standard. See Procedure 33-1, Disposing of Biohazardous Material.

INFECTION CONTROL: PHYSICAL AND CHEMICAL BARRIERS

Effective physical and chemical barriers can be used to maintain infection control. The development of a nosocomial infection, or health care–associated infection (HAI), is prevented when careful medical and surgical asepsis (sterile equipment and procedures) are maintained.

Medical Asepsis

Medical asepsis refers to the destruction of organisms after they leave the body. (By contrast, surgical asepsis, which we discuss next, refers to the destruction of organisms before they enter the body.) Techniques such as hand hygiene (one of the most effective means of reducing pathogen transmission), using disposable equipment, and wearing gloves can help reduce the transfer of pathogens. Aseptic techniques are the fundamental means of providing a safe environment in medical facilities.

Ordinary hygiene habits of everyday life, such as covering your mouth during a cough or sneeze, are forms of medical asepsis. These ordinary hygiene habits include handwashing when handling food or after using the bathroom. Hand hygiene is considered the first step in infection control because the hands are a primary means of transferring

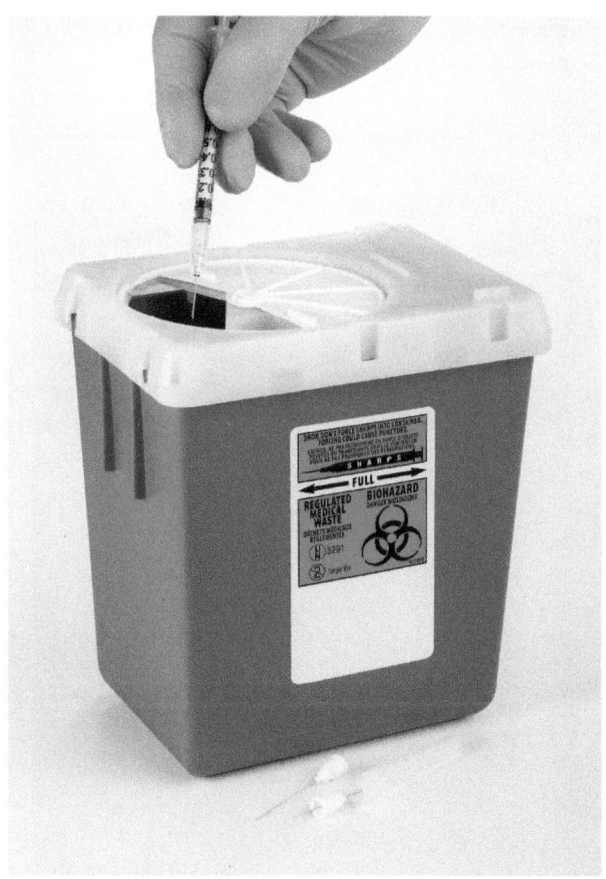

FIGURE 33-5 Sharps containers.

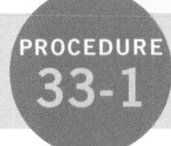

PROCEDURE 33-1   Disposing of Biohazardous Material

Objective ◆ *Properly dispose of biohazardous material.*

EQUIPMENT AND SUPPLIES

Infectious waste container with lid marked appropriately with universal biohazard symbol and label; red disposable plastic liners; gloves

METHOD

1. Check to ensure that the infectious waste container is lined with a red disposal plastic bag.
2. Discard any infectious waste into the infectious waste container.
3. Make sure that all liquid waste is already contained in a closable device or container before putting it into the infectious waste container.
4. Do not put contaminated glass or glass of any kind into the infectious waste bag. Instead, all glass should be placed into a puncture-proof or very highly puncture resistant container for disposal; small glass items can be deposited into a sharps container for disposal.
   a. Needles and syringes should never be recapped and always placed immediately into an appropriately labeled, puncture-proof sharps container after activating the safety device mechanism on the needle or syringe.
5. When the infectious waste container becomes full, close the red trash bag by tying with a securing knot, twist-tying, or otherwise securing it (Figure A).

6. Make sure that the contents of the red bag are completely contained inside the closed bag.
7. Make sure the red bag is not overstuffed so that it cannot be closed, ruptured when handled or lifted, opened, or leak.
   a. If necessary, double-bag the infectious waste bag if there is a small rupture or tear; or when office protocol dictates. Two people should always perform this task to ensure contamination does not occur (Figure B).
8. Do not mix noninfectious trash in the same large bin, container, or dumpster with infectious waste or trash. (Figure C).
9. Closed red bags should be transported from the point of waste generation to a dirty utility room or area and stored in a designated holding area that cannot be accessed by other than authorized staff until they are transported away from the facility. Never store trash in hallways, entrances, corridors, or other areas accessible to and used by the public (Figure D).

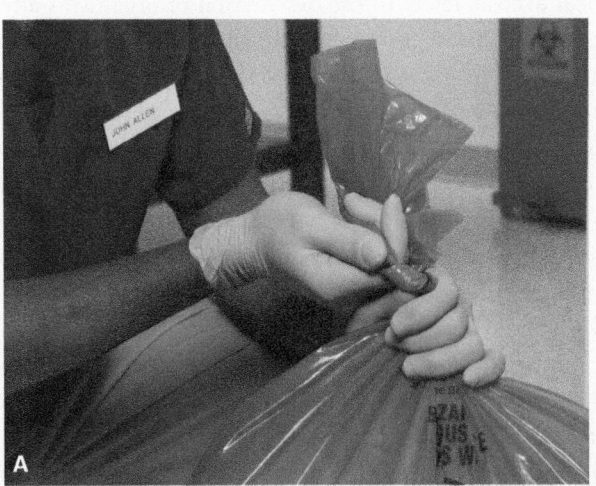

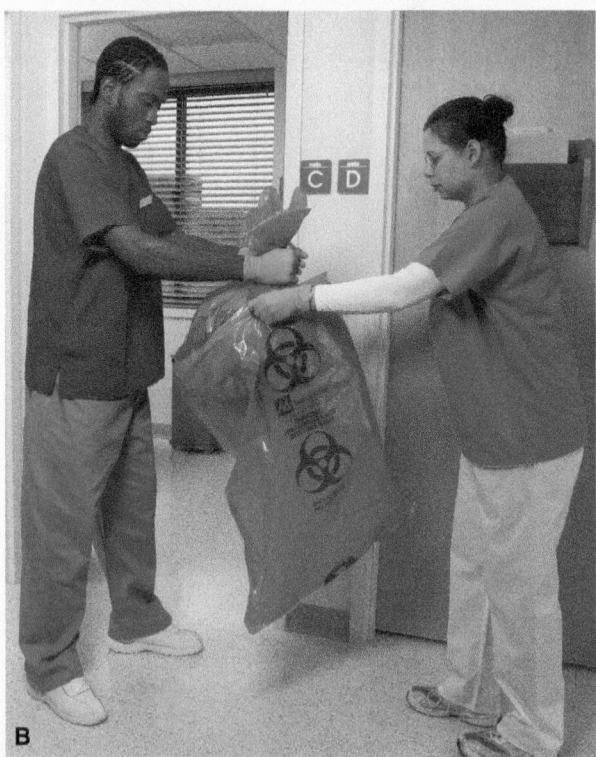

FIGURE A–B (A) Always secure the bag by tying a sturdy knot. **(B)** With a coworker, double bag the infectious waste if necessary.

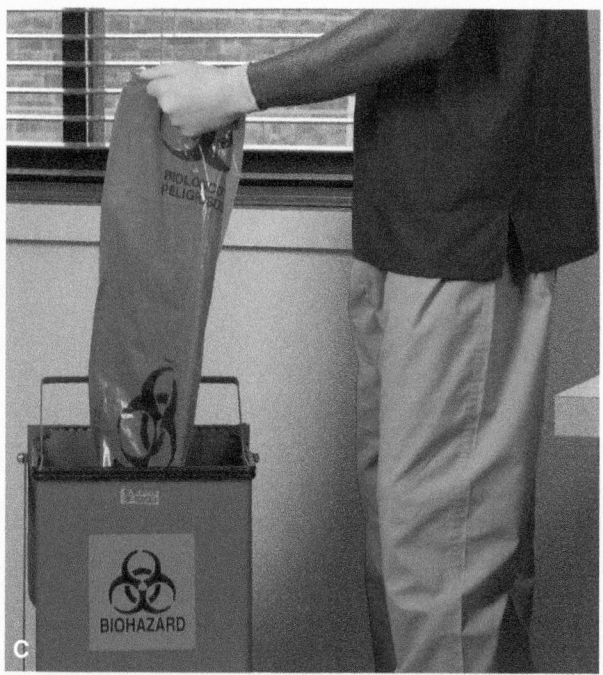
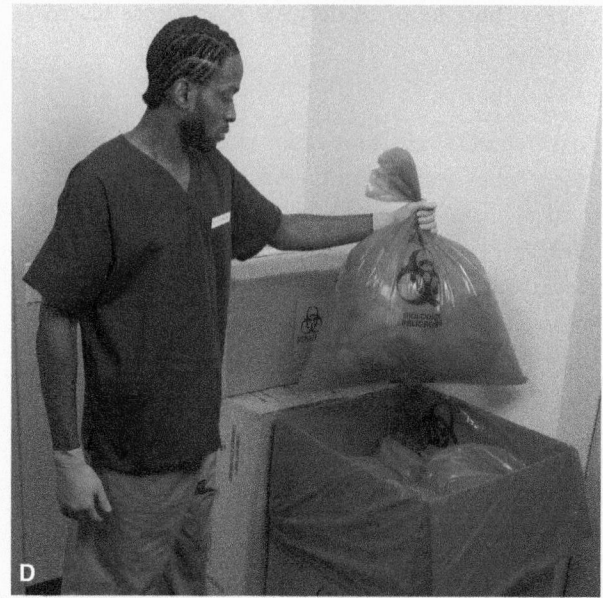

FIGURE C–D **(C)** Place a new biohazard bag in the empty biohazard container. **(D)** Place the properly secured red biohazard bag in the specified area for proper disposal.

infection from the host to the receiver. To keep the skin free of harmful organisms, frequent hand hygiene is necessary—either with soap, friction, and warm running water or with alcohol-based hand sanitizers. Jewelry should be removed before performing hand hygiene or applying gloves.

Situations that should involve medical asepsis include but are not limited to taking oral, aural, and rectal temperatures; obtaining throat or vaginal cultures or smears; performing venipuncture; obtaining urine, stool, or sputum specimens; administering medications; and cleaning treatment rooms.

Preventing infection and causing a break in the chain of infection can be achieved by practicing the following suggested forms of medical asepsis:

- Wash hands before and after any contact with patients or equipment.
- Handle all specimens and materials as though they contain pathogens.
- Use gloves for protection when handling contaminated articles or materials, such as specimens or instruments that have been used during a procedure.
- Do not wear jewelry that can attract and harbor bacteria.
- Use disposable equipment whenever possible, and dispose of all equipment properly after use.

- Clean all nondisposable equipment as soon as possible after patient use, using an approved disinfectant and while wearing appropriate gloves.
- Use only clean or sterile supplies for each patient.
- Use a protective covering over clothes if there is any danger of contaminated materials or supplies coming into contact with them.
- Discard items that fall on the floor if they cannot be cleaned. Any item dropped on the floor must be resterilized or redisinfected before use. All floors are considered contaminated. If in doubt, throw it out!
- Place all wet or damp dressings and bandages in a waterproof bag to protect the persons handling the waste removal.

Medical asepsis relates not only to equipment and instruments but also to other aspects of the facility. Having proper ventilation in all areas of the medical office will assist in decreasing the transfer of microorganisms. All examination rooms, including table surfaces, should be cleaned with an approved disinfectant after each patient contact. Checking and emptying trash cans, replacing sharps containers in a timely manner, and observing for any insect infestation are also means of maintaining medical asepsis.

Some medical offices have one reception area for well patients and another for sick patients. For example, a patient who is returning for a follow-up visit is seated in one area, and a patient with symptoms of the flu is seated in another area. This helps to decrease the chance of cross-contamination.

Hand Hygiene

As we have emphasized throughout this chapter, frequent and diligent hand hygiene provides the first defense against the spread of disease and should be done often. Refer to Procedure 33-2 and Figures A–D for a demonstration of proper handwashing procedure and technique. It is also important to moisturize your hands to prevent cracking or breaks in the skin. Breaks in the skin provide a means of entry for pathogens.

Alcohol-Based Hand Rubs. The CDC has presented some new guidelines concerning the use of alcohol-based (waterless) hand rubs. These rubs have the advantage of not requiring rinsing, and many contain emollients that moisturize and prevent drying of the skin. A disadvantage, however, is that they may be more expensive than hand soaps and may cause stinging if there is an abrasion on the skin.

The CDC guidelines suggest that the alcohol-based hand rubs can be used at the times usually required for handwashing. However, the hands should always be washed with soap and water:

- Every third time hand hygiene is performed
- If they are visibly soiled with dirt or body fluids
- Before eating
- After using the restroom

As with regular handwashing, jewelry should be removed before using the hand rubs. Approximately 2 to 3 ml of the gel should be placed in the palm of the hand and thoroughly spread over the surface of both hands up to ½ inch above the wrist (Figure 33-6). Continue to rub the hands together until dry, approximately 15 to 30 seconds. Waterless hand sanitizers kill 99.9 percent of common microorganisms in 15 seconds. Recent studies indicate, however, that waterless hand sanitizers may not be effective against certain microorganisms, including the norovirus and *Clostridium difficile*, or *C-diff*. Manufacturers' instructions regarding the use of alcohol-based hand rubs should be followed exactly.

PROCEDURE 33-2 Performing Handwashing

Objective ◆ *Perform handwashing procedure without error.*

EQUIPMENT AND SUPPLIES

Soap in liquid soap dispenser; nail cleaner (brush or orange cuticle stick); warm running water; paper towels; waste container

METHOD

1. Remove any jewelry (includes rings with the exception of a plain wedding band). Artificial nails must be removed to maintain infection control practices.
2. Stand at the sink without allowing clothing to touch the sink. Turn on the faucet while holding a paper towel to prevent contamination. Or, if it is available, turn on the water with the foot or knee pedal. Adjust the running water to a moderately warm temperature (Figure A).
3. Wet hands under running water and place liquid soap (1 teaspoon, or about the size of a nickel) into the palm of hand. Work soap into a lather by moving it over the palms, sides, and backs—the entire surface—of both hands for 20 to 30 seconds. Use a circular motion and

friction. Interlace the fingers and move soapy water between them.
4. Keep the hands pointed down with hands and forearms below elbow level during the entire handwashing procedure. Water should always flow from the forearms down, never from the hands up. This also prevents contamination (Figure B).
5. Use nail cleaner (brush or orange cuticle stick) to clean under fingernails at the start of each day and if hands are heavily soiled (Figure C).
6. Rinse hands under running water with fingers pointed down, using care not to touch the sink or faucets.
7. If hands are heavily soiled, reapply soap and wash them again.
8. Rinse hands under running water.
9. Dry hands thoroughly with a paper towel without touching the paper towel dispenser. Discard the paper towel into a trash can that can be opened with a foot pedal.
10. Use a dry paper towel to turn off the faucet if the foot or knee pedal is not available (Figure D).
11. Apply an antibacterial hand lotion to prevent chapping of skin.

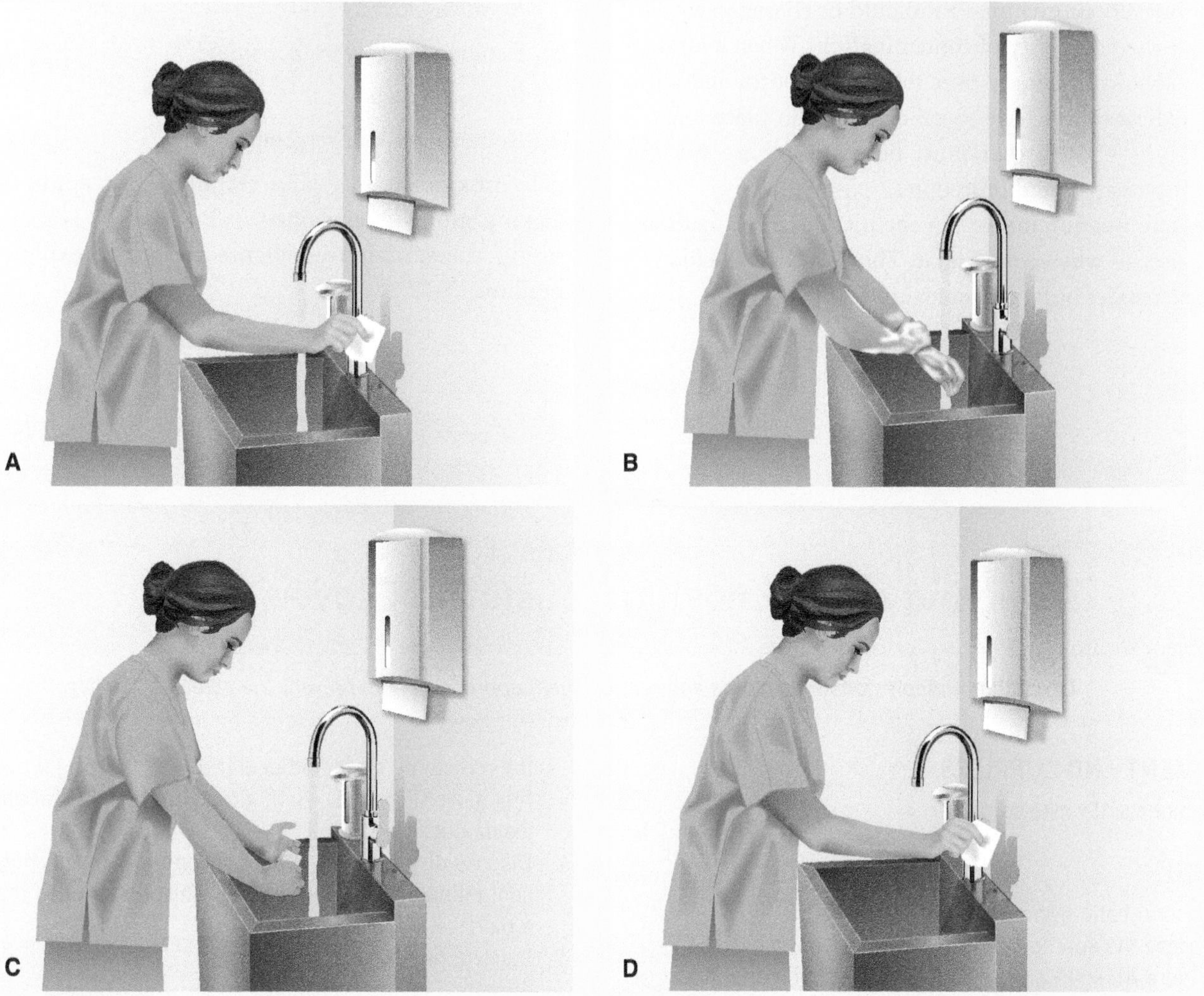

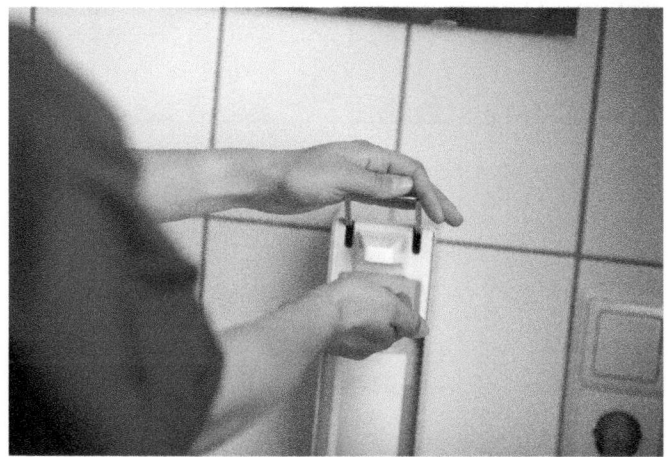

FIGURE A–D **(A)** Turn on the faucet with a paper towel and stand away from the sink so that your clothing is not touching the sink. **(B)** Hands and forearms should always face down below the elbow. **(C)** Use a nail brush or cuticle stick to clean under the fingernails. **(D)** Using a paper towel, turn off the faucet.

FIGURE 33-6 Dispense 2–3 ml of hand sanitizer into the palm of the hand.

Protective Clothing and Personal Protective Equipment

Protective clothing and equipment, such as gowns, gloves, and masks, are worn for two reasons:

1. To protect the patient from any microorganisms that might be present on the health care worker's uniform

2. To protect the health care worker from carrying microorganisms away from the patient

In addition, protective devices, such as gloves and masks, assist in protecting the health care worker from contamination with bloodborne pathogens. Nonsterile gloving technique is used for procedures such as drawing blood and specimen collection. Wearing each piece of PPE will not be needed for every procedure. PPE should be chosen in consideration of the possibility of contamination. When a mask is worn, it should fit snugly over the nose, mouth, and chin. Many medical offices have specific policies in place regarding the type of PPE that must be worn during specific patient interactions and procedures.

If you are wearing more than one piece of PPE, maintain medical asepsis when removing it. The CDC lists the following as the correct order for removing PPE:

1. Remove gloves.
2. Remove goggles or face shield.
3. Remove gown.
4. Remove mask or respirator.

The proper step-by-step technique for applying and removing gloves is explained in Procedure 33-3, and performing transmission-based precautions is explained in Procedure 33-4.

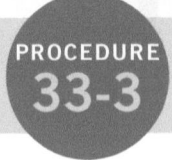

PROCEDURE 33-3 Applying and Removing Nonsterile Gloves

Objective ◆ *Apply nonsterile gloves and remove them appropriately to prevent the spread of pathogens.*

EQUIPMENT AND SUPPLIES

Gloves; biohazard waste container

METHOD

1. Perform hand hygiene (see Procedure 33-2).
2. Choose the appropriate size gloves for your hands (Figure A). Hold a glove at the wrist opening and insert fingers, pulling the glove up to wrist.
3. Apply the second glove in the same manner, checking for holes and other flaws (Figure B). If any flaws are found, discard the gloves and obtain new gloves.
4. To remove gloves, grasp the glove covering your nondominant hand at the palm and pull it away (Figure C).
5. Pull the glove off, and hold it in the palm of the gloved dominant hand (Figure D).
6. While holding the soiled glove in your gloved hand, slide the index finger of the ungloved hand below the cuff of

the remaining glove and peel it down, inverting it over the first glove (Figure E). Both gloves will be in a ball and inside out.

7. Dispose of the gloves in a trash container unless they are contaminated by biohazards, in which case place them in a biohazard container.
8. Perform hand hygiene.

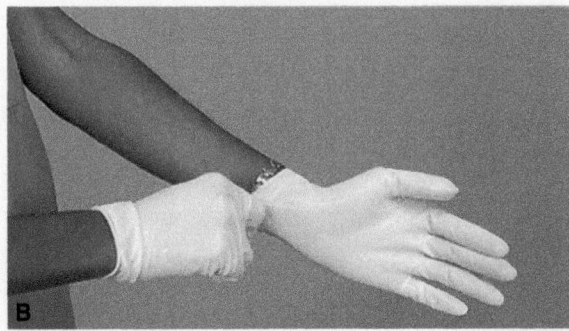

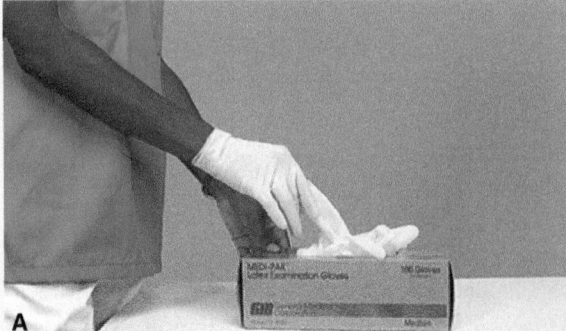

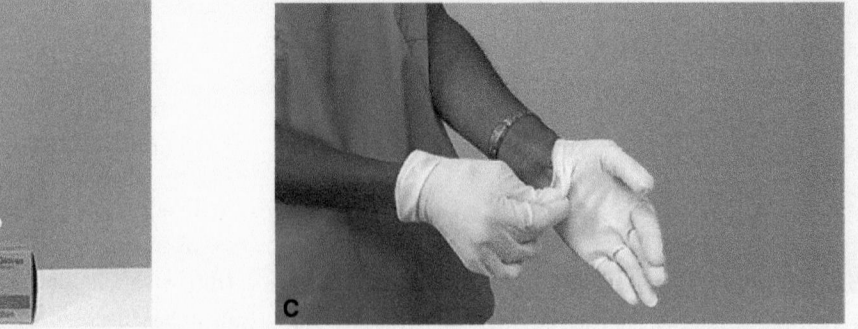

FIGURE A–C (A) Use a clean pair of gloves for each patient contact. **(B)** Grasp the glove just below the cuff. **(C)** Pull glove over the hand while turning the glove inside out.

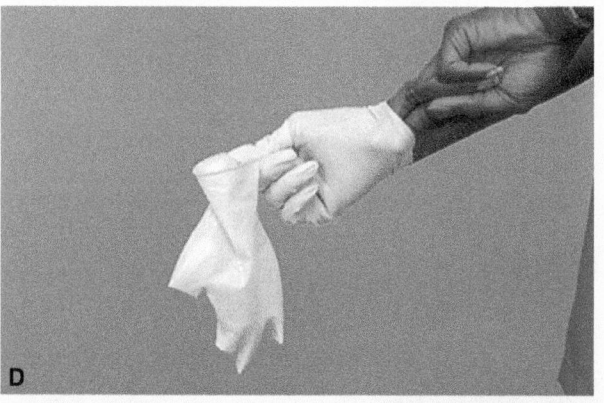
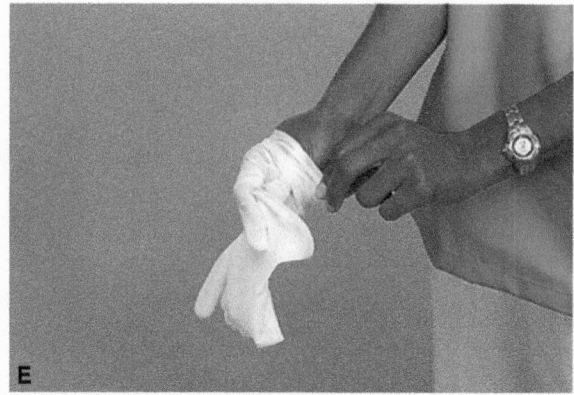

FIGURE D–E (D) Place the ungloved index and middle fingers inside the cuff of the glove, running the cuff downward. **(E)** Pull down the cuff and turn the glove inside out as you remove your hand.

<table>
<tr><td>PROCEDURE
33-4</td><td></td></tr>
</table>

PROCEDURE 33-4

Selecting and Using Personal Protective Equipment (PPE)

Objective ◆ *Select appropriate barrier/personal protective equipment (PPE).*

EQUIPMENT AND SUPPLIES

Disposable gowns, masks, caps, nonsterile gloves, and sterile gloves; sink and running water; paper towels

METHOD

1. Review orders and agency protocols regarding isolation procedures. (Orders depend on whether patient requires isolation for TB, MRSA, radiation, or others.)

Note: Office-based medical assistants may not use transmission-based precautions often, but they should be familiar with the necessary PPE and how to put them on appropriately. Figure A shows examples of four types of PPE.

2. Assemble the necessary protective equipment that is appropriate for the level of isolation necessary based on the patient's diagnosis, signs, or symptoms.
3. Remove lab coat and jewelry.
4. Perform hand hygiene (see Procedure 33-2).
5. Apply the appropriate disposable apparel in the following order:
   a. Apply the cap to cover hair and ears completely.
   b. Apply the gown over uniform or clothing as follows: Hold the gown in front of the body, and place arms through the sleeves. Pull the sleeves on, covering the wrists. Tie the gown securely at the neck and waist.
   c. Apply the mask by placing the top of the mask over the bridge of the nose and pinching the metal strip to

secure a snug fit on the nose, tying it if needed. Apply protective eyewear.
   d. Apply nonsterile gloves, pulling the cuffs of the glove up and over the cuffs of the gown, covering them completely.
6. Enter the isolation room, and perform patient tasks as needed.
7. Exit the isolation room, and immediately remove barrier protections in the following order:
   a. Untie waist of the gown.
   b. Remove gloves (see Procedure 33-3).
   c. Wash hands (see Procedure 33-2).
   d. Untie the neck of the gown. Remove the gown by pulling it down from the shoulders. Turn the gown inside out, and remove arms from the sleeves. The inside of the gown is not contaminated (Figures B and C).
   e. Holding the gown away from the body with contaminated area on the inside, fold and place it in a biohazard container (Figure D).

Note: Most isolation rooms have designated areas and appropriate receptacles near the doorway for immediate removal of protective barriers.

8. Remove protective eyewear.
9. Remove mask and discard in biohazard container.
10. Perform hand hygiene for the final time.

In Figure 33-7, the medical assistant is wearing a mask and other PPE to prevent exposure to airborne droplets from the patient who is coughing.

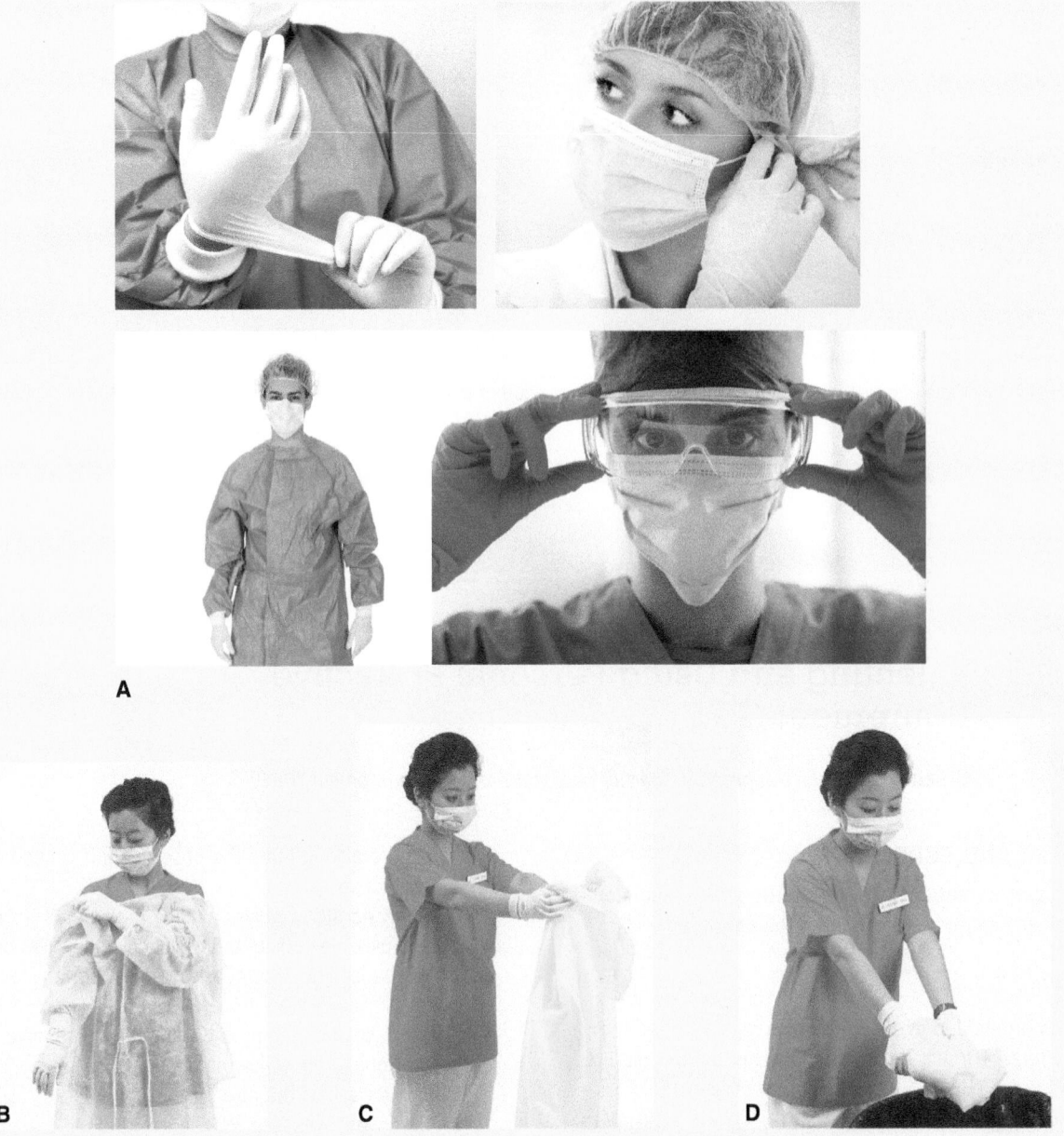

FIGURE A–D **(A)** Examples of personal protective equipment: (top left) gloves; (top right) mask; (bottom left) gown; and (bottom right) face shield (Source: StockPhotoPro). **(B)** Remove gown by pulling it down from the shoulders. **(C)** Turn the gown inside out, and remove arms from sleeves (inside of gown is not contaminated). **(D)** Holding the gown away from the body with contaminated area on the inside, fold and place the gown in a biohazard container.

In Figure 33-7, the medical assistant is wearing a mask and other PPE to prevent exposure to airborne droplets from the patient, who is coughing.

Surgical Asepsis

Surgical asepsis refers to the techniques practiced to maintain a sterile environment. As noted earlier, it involves the destruction of organisms before they enter the body. Surgical asepsis is the practices that are used to control the growth of microorganism and prevention transmission and infection. Three important methods are used to achieve sterility (the absence of microorganisms). These methods for preventing the spread of infectious pathogens in the medical facility include sanitization, disinfection, and sterilization.

Sanitization

Sanitization is a cleaning process that inhibits or inactivates pathogens through the careful cleaning of equipment and instruments to remove debris. This is accomplished by rinsing and scrubbing the instruments with a brush and a detergent with a neutral pH, such as a low-sudsing soap. After the debris has been removed, the items are rinsed in hot

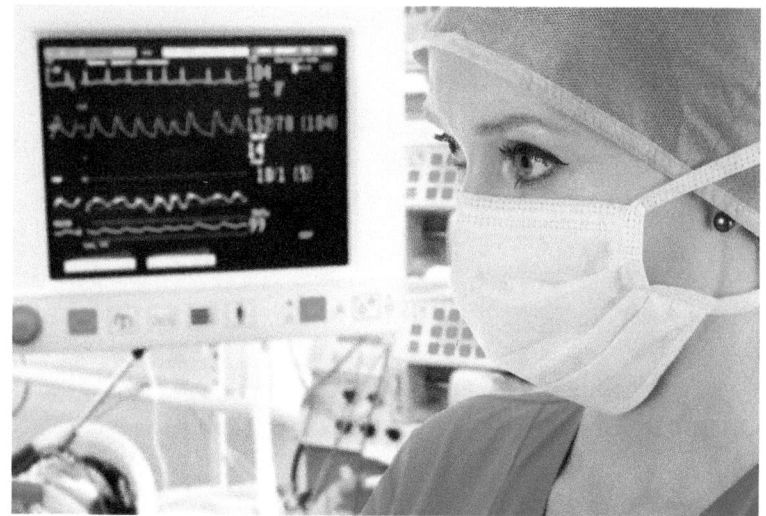

FIGURE 33-7 The mask covers both the mouth and nose to prevent exposure to body fluid and airborne droplets. (*Source:* FotoliaXIV)

Although sanitization cleans items, it does not destroy microorganisms and bacteria. This process can be used for supplies and equipment that do not come into direct contact with the patient or that touch only the skin surface. If a contaminated material cannot be sanitized immediately, then it should be soaked in detergent and water according to the manufacturer's instructions. See Procedure 33-5 for one method of sanitizing instruments.

Ultrasonic Sanitization. Another means of sanitizing equipment is by using ultrasonic technology. In this case, the instruments and equipment are placed into a bath tank in which sound waves vibrate to break up the contamination. The articles are then rinsed thoroughly. Always follow the instructions of the facility procedure manual regarding the proper procedure for sanitizing instruments.

water and air dried. During this process you should protect yourself by wearing thick utility gloves. Instruments and supplies should be separated so that items with sharp or pointy edges (tweezers or scissors) are kept away from other items. Hinged items should be opened completely, and the hinges should be carefully scrubbed with a smaller brush. (Many times a firm toothbrush is sufficient.) After instruments are scrubbed and rinsed in hot water, they are placed on a clean towel for air-drying. The items may also be hand dried to prevent spotting.

Disinfection

Disinfection destroys or inhibits the activity of disease-causing organisms, although it does not always kill spores or certain viruses. The process of disinfection involves soaking items and/or wiping items. Disinfecting agents used include chemical germicides, flowing steam, and boiling water.

Chemical germicides are often used in the medical office for disinfection. A 1:10 bleach solution is also commonly used and is very cost effective. The chemical disinfection process is referred to as a "cold" process, because

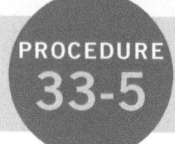

PROCEDURE 33-5

Sanitizing Instruments

Objective ◆ *Clean and sanitize instruments to eliminate any remaining visible contamination.*

EQUIPMENT AND SUPPLIES

Disposable gloves; rubber (utility) gloves; face shield or mask and goggles; plastic brushes (large and small), preferably disposable; disposable towels; sink; running water; container to hold all the instruments; low-sudsing (low-pH) detergent or germicidal agent; biohazard container

Note: Instruments should be rinsed under warm running water immediately after surgery to remove blood, body fluids, and tissue. If it is not possible to clean them immediately, instruments should be submerged in water containing a low-pH detergent.

METHOD

1. Apply both disposable and rubber gloves.
   a. If there is potential of splashing of infectious materials, don face shield or goggles and mask as necessary.
2. Place a low-sudsing (low-pH) detergent or germicidal agent in a large basin with water following manufacturer's instructions.
3. Initially rinse instruments in clear cold water in a sink or other container. Delicate and sharp instruments should be separated from general instruments (Figure A).

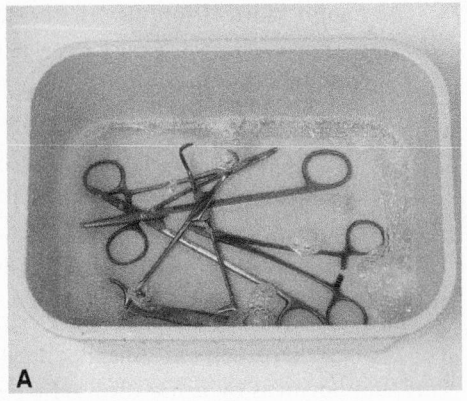 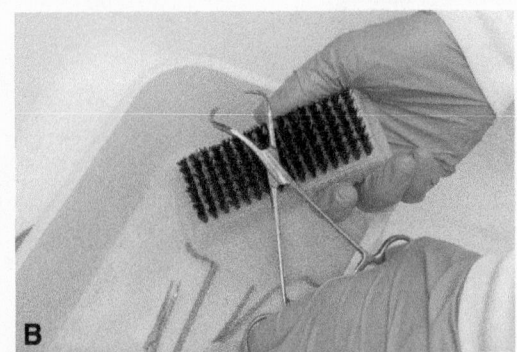

FIGURE A–B (A) Delicate and sharp instruments should be kept separated from others. **(B)** Take extra care to scrub the hinges and screws of equipment as necessary.

4. Scrub each instrument individually with a brush and detergent under running water. Open instruments to thoroughly scrub all serrated edges, crevices, and hinge areas (Figure B).
5. Rinse instruments thoroughly under hot water.
6. After thoroughly rinsing cleaned instruments, roll them in a towel and hand dry them.
7. Check the condition of all instruments for defects or any remaining soil. Take appropriate action, if required.

8. Discard disposable towels and any disposable instruments in the biohazard waste container.
9. Remove utility gloves and disposable gloves (Procedure 33-3), and perform hand hygiene (Procedure 33-2).
10. Place sanitized instruments in the appropriate area for storage, or wrap instrument(s) for sterilization, or place them in an ultrasonic cleaner.
11. If necessary, perform quality assurance reporting in necessary log books regarding sanitization practices.

heat is neither used nor generated. Chemical disinfectants used for soaking and wiping include soap, alcohol, phenol, acid, alkalines (such as bleach), and formaldehyde (Table 33-6).

When performing chemical disinfection, completely immerse contaminated instruments and equipment in a germicidal solution for the period of time stated in the manufacturer's instructions (1 to 10 hours, based on the solution).

TABLE 33-6 | Disinfection Methods

Method	Description and Use
Alcohol (70% Isopropyl)	Used for skin surfaces, equipment such as stethoscopes and thermometers, and table surfaces.
	Causes damage to rubber products, lenses, and plastic. Flammable.
Chlorine (Sodium Hypochlorite or Bleach)	Use in dilution of 1:10 (1 part bleach to 10 parts water).
	Used to eliminate a broad spectrum of microorganisms.
	Has a corrosive effect on instruments, rubber, and plastic products.
	Can cause skin irritation.
	Inexpensive.
Formaldehyde	Used to disinfect and sterilize.
	Dangerous product that is regulated by OSHA—must have clearly marked labels.
Hydrogen Peroxide	Effective disinfectant for use only on nonhuman surfaces and products.
	May damage rubber, plastics, and metals.
Glutaraldehyde	Effective against viruses, bacteria, fungi, and some spores.
	Regulated by OSHA—must have clearly marked labels and be used only in well-ventilated area.
	Must wear gloves and masks when using.

Then rinse in water and dry them. (Instruments are rinsed in distilled water to prevent rust and corrosion.)

Objects that come into contact with mucous membranes, such as vaginal speculums, laryngoscopes, or thermometers, must be disinfected; however, it is ideal if these instruments are sterilized. Instruments and equipment that cannot be soaked, such as scopes, computers, and electrical instruments, should be wiped thoroughly with a germicidal solution. Germicidal solutions must be changed frequently according to the manufacturer's instructions.

Although it is not effective for viruses (such as hepatitis) or for destroying spores, boiling water can be used as a means of disinfection. Stainless steel, glassware, and instruments can be boiled without damage. The articles are submerged in a container filled with cold water. (Distilled water should be used when boiling instruments or stainless steel to prevent sediment or deposits from forming.) The water must completely cover the articles to be disinfected. It is then brought to the boiling point. The water must continue to boil for 20 to 30 minutes for disinfection. When the boiling time has elapsed, the disinfected materials are allowed to cool. To maintain disinfection, they must be touched only with sterile forceps. Using boiling water is generally impractical, so this method is not often used for disinfection.

Antiseptics. It is also necessary to disinfectant a patient's skin before performing invasive procedures, including venipuncture, surgical procedures, and injections. This is accomplished through the use of antiseptics. **Antiseptics** inhibit the growth of microorganisms on skin surfaces. The most commonly used antiseptic is 70 percent isopropyl alcohol. However, it has been found that other antiseptics, such as povidone-iodine solution (Betadine), are safe and are more effective methods of inhibiting microorganisms.

Sterilization

Sterilization is a process that kills all microorganisms, both pathogenic and nonpathogenic. Heat sterilization (produced by an autoclave under steam pressure) can kill spores, bacteria, and other microorganisms. Dry heat is used for sterilizing dense ointments, such as petroleum jelly.

All supplies—including dressings, needles, and instruments that come into contact with internal body tissue or an open wound—must be sterile. Once a sterile article is touched by hands or another unsterile object, it is considered contaminated. Sterile gloves must be used when touching sterilized items. The procedure for applying sterile gloves (as well as nonsterile gloves) is sometimes referred to as donning.

Autoclave. The methods used for sterilization include the autoclave (steam and pressure) and chemical (cold) steriliza-

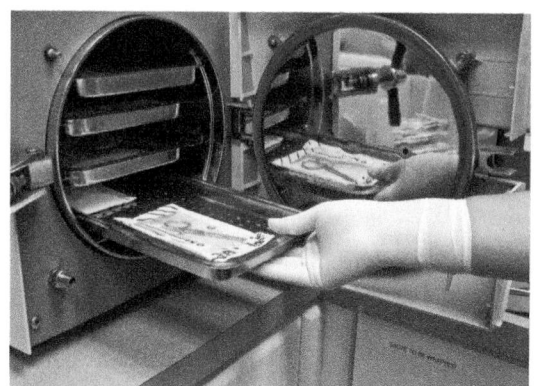

FIGURE 33-8 An autoclave.

tion. Most medical offices use the autoclave for sterilization. Types of autoclaving include steam under pressure, dry heat (320°F for 1 hour), dry gas, and radiation.

The high heat and moisture caused by the steam, which settles on the instruments during the autoclave cycle, causes the cells of the microorganisms to explode, thus killing the microorganisms. This method of sterilization requires 15 pounds of pressure per square inch (PSI) and a temperature of 250°F to 270°F, depending on the manufacturer's recommendations. Heat is actually transferred to the items by way of the steam condensation through the use of distilled water. Steam sterilization of surgical packs is not effective if air pockets are present within them. The autoclave consists of an outer chamber (jacket) that creates a buildup of steam that is forced into an inner chamber. Items that are to be sterilized are placed inside the inner chamber. (Figure 33-8 is an example of an autoclave.)

Depending on the model, an autoclave may have three gauges (some have only one):

1. A jacket pressure gauge to indicate pressure in the outer chamber

2. A chamber pressure gauge to indicate the steam pressure in the inner chamber

3. A temperature gauge to indicate the temperature in the inner chamber in which items are placed

A pump within the autoclave will first remove air from the outer chamber. Once the air is removed from the outer chamber, the pressure level and temperature levels within the autoclave chamber can begin to rise. Therefore, the gauges indicating pressure and temperature must be monitored by the medical assistant. Table 33-7 describes autoclave sterilization time requirements.

Autoclave Maintenance. Always read and follow the manufacturer's instructions for use and maintenance before using any piece of electrical medical equipment. The autoclave

TABLE 33-7 | Sterilization Time Requirements

Time	Article
15 minutes	Glassware
	Metal instruments—open tray or individual wrapping with hinges open
	Syringes (unassembled)
	Needles
20 minutes	Instruments—partial metal in double-thickness wrapper or covered tray
	Rubber products: gloves, tubing, catheters wrapped or unwrapped
	Solutions in a flask (50–100 ml)
30 minutes	Dressings—small packs in paper or muslin
	Solutions in a flask (500–1,000 ml)
	Syringes—unassembled, individually wrapped in gauze
	Syringes—unassembled, individually wrapped in glass tubes
	Needles—individually packaged in paper or glass tubes
	Sutures—wrapped in paper or muslin
	Instrument and treatment trays—wrapped in paper or muslin
	Gauze—loosely packed
60 minutes	Petroleum jelly, 1 oz jar—in dry heat

should be cleansed on a regular basis so that it is free of any materials or lint. The air exhaust valve must also be cleaned and free of lint before each use. It is especially important to follow all manufacturer's instructions regarding how and what items should be used to clean the autoclave.

At various intervals, an outside, independent company should perform regulated checks on the autoclave to ensure proper functioning. The medical office can continue to autoclave items as usual, but usually one item is chosen to be sent to an outside lab where it is checked for sterility. These quality assurance checks are necessary to determine that proper sterilization practices are being upheld.

Autoclave Wrapping Materials and Loading the Autoclave. The wrappings in which the instruments and materials are sterilized must be both **permeable** (allowing steam to pass through) and strong enough to hold together during the steam process. Wrapping materials that are commonly used include heavy paper, muslin, plastic, and stainless steel containers. The wrapping generally consists of two layers of permeable materials. All items must be completely covered with the wrapping material and fastened with autoclave tape, which looks similar to masking tape. Autoclave indicator tape is used to fasten the autoclave package securely. The lines on the tape change color during the autoclaving process and indicate that exposure to the high temperature has occurred (Figure 33-9). However, this is not necessarily

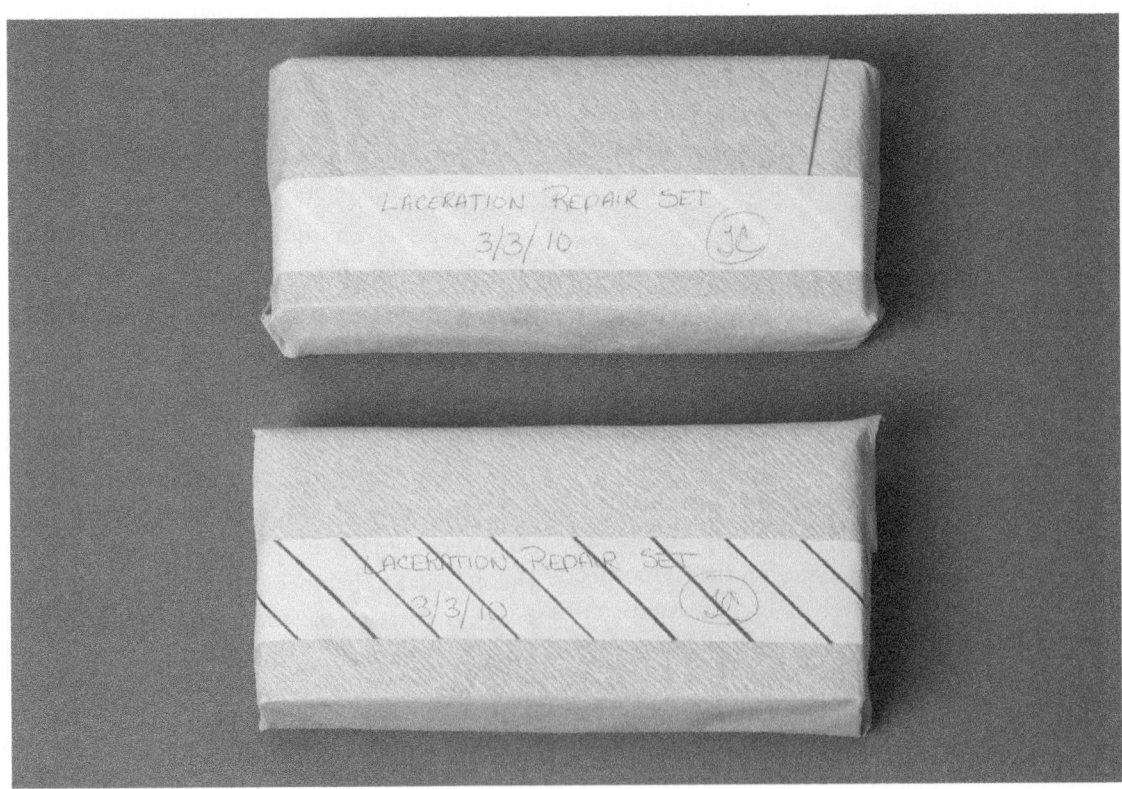

FIGURE 33-9 Top: Autoclave tape before sterilization. Bottom: Autoclave tape after sterilization.

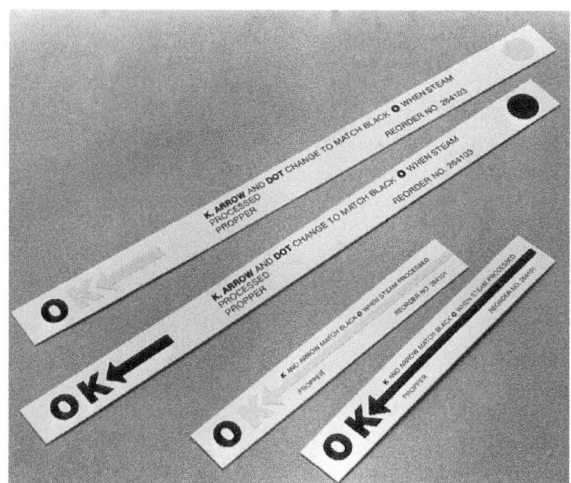

FIGURE 33-10 Sterility check strips.

an indication that the proper time and temperature for sterilization have been reached.

Sterilization indicators are used to signify proper and complete sterilization. Indicators come in a variety of types, including strips (Figure 33-10). The strip is placed inside the wrapper of packages or in the chamber when using open trays. The color changes or dots that appear on an indicator denote that the inner contents have been exposed to the required conditions necessary for sterility: correct temperature, correct time, and exposure to moisture.

Sterilization pouches or bags are often used to hold individual instruments. Small, lightweight instruments are suitable for these pouches. Careful inspection must be made to make sure the bag has not ruptured or been punctured during the autoclave process. The pouches have sterilization indicators both inside and outside the bag.

Each package (whether wrapped or a pouch) should be labeled with the date of sterilization, the items within the packet, and the initials of the individual who prepared the pack. Instruments with hinges should be in the open position, any tubing should be free of any kinks, and syringes should be unassembled before wrapping.

Record Keeping and Quality Control. For quality control, sterilization record keeping should include sterilization logs as well as equipment maintenance and cleaning records. These records would include dates of purchase of equipment, maintenance, cleaning, and quality control checks. Further, biological culture capsules (a special kit that includes a stable vacutainer holder with sterile pack and everything you would need for gathering a sterile culture except the sterile needle) can be purchased to assure sterility in gathering specimens. Indicator strips demonstrate whether the equipment is too old, and date labeling locally shows the length of time the specimen took to be processed.

(Refer to Procedure 33-6 and Figures A–D for how to wrap and label instruments for the autoclave.)

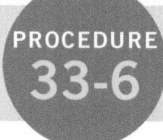

PROCEDURE 33-6

Preparing Items for Autoclaving

Objective ◆ *Wrap and label instruments properly.*

EQUIPMENT AND SUPPLIES

Wrapping material; instrument(s) for autoclaving; sterilization indicator strips; autoclave tape; permanent pen; gloves

Note: Before wrapping instruments for sterilization in the autoclave, it is recommended that instruments be properly sanitized as in Procedure 33-5.

METHOD

1. Wash your hands and don gloves.
2. Place a square of wrapping material on a clean flat surface. Arrange the material so that it appears as a "diamond" shape when you look at it. Be sure the wrapping material is large enough to cover the entire article being wrapped.

   a. According to office policy, it might be necessary to use an additional piece of wrapping material if the material is only single layered.
3. Place the items in the center of the wrapping material.

   a. If hinged items are included, be sure the instrument is in the open position.

   b. If sharp instruments are being autoclaved, place the tip in a piece of gauze to prevent puncture through the material.
4. Place the sterilization indicator strip in the center of the packet.
5. Fold the bottom point of the wrapping material up and over the instruments. Fold a small portion of the point back over so that it can be used to pull back the paper when it is unwrapped (Figure A).

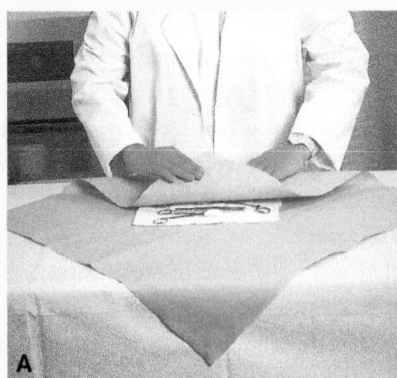
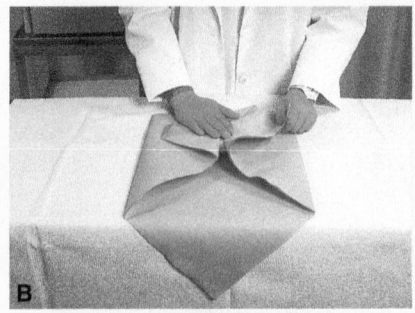
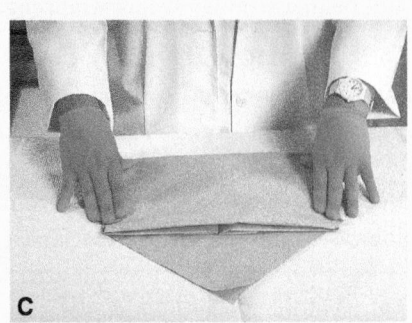
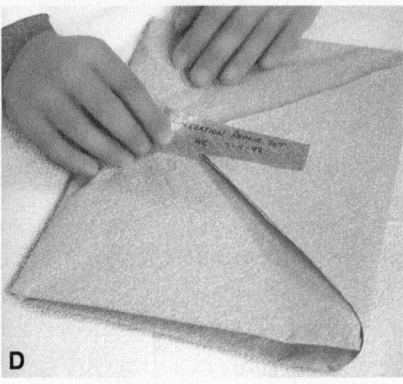

FIGURE A–D (A) Place items (with hinges open) in the center of wrapping material. Fold the bottom up and over the instruments. **(B)** Fold the right side of the paper until it covers the item, and make a small flap. Proceed in the same way with the left side. **(C)** Fold the bottom of the package up toward the top until the top corner remains. **(D)** Use a piece of autoclave tape to secure the package.

6. Fold the right side of the wrapping paper over until it covers the instrument(s). Fold a small portion of the point back over as in the previous step.
7. Fold the left side of the wrapping paper over until it covers the instrument(s). Fold a small portion of the point back over as in the previous step (Figure B).
8. Now fold up the bottom of the package upward until you have reached the top point of the wrapping square (Figure C).
9. Be sure the pack is folded snugly and air pockets are not present.

10. Secure the final point of the package with a piece of autoclave tape (Figure D).
11. Label the package with the name of the item(s) inside, your initials, and the date.
12. If bags are used for the autoclaving procedure, place the item and an indicator strip inside the bag. (If the item has a sharp point, wrap the point in a piece of gauze.)
13. Seal the bag. Label the bag with the name of the item(s) inside, your initials, and the date.

Instruments that will be used immediately can be placed in open perforated trays and left unwrapped. The lid for the tray is placed next to the open tray of instruments inside the autoclave. The lid is immediately placed over the instruments after sterilization. A towel is usually placed under the instruments to absorb moisture during autoclaving.

Containers and jars of supplies should be placed on their sides in order for full sterilization to occur. Solutions should be autoclaved separately, generally in glass containers, because they may boil over during autoclaving.

It is important not to overload or cram items inside the autoclave chamber. Consistent spacing of packages and instruments is vital to allow the steam to properly circulate and penetrate the packages, ensuring complete sterilization.

After the autoclave process is complete, the drying process takes place. This process is almost as important as achieving the correct temperature and pressure during autoclaving. Wetness on items ("wet packs") can cause a break in sterility because moisture will allow bacteria to grow and be transmitted into the inside of the package. Wet packs can be avoided by allowing for a drying period at the end of autoclaving. To do this, open the door of the autoclave ¾ inch (but no more) just before the drying cycle on the autoclave. Run the dry cycle according to the manufacturer's directions.

Autoclaved packages are stored in dry and dust-free shelves or drawers. For easy access, autoclave packs are organized according to the date and type of item(s) visible. The oldest dated packs are placed in front of the stack so that they can be used first. Instruments are considered sterile for 21 to 30 days (21 days in plastic bags, 30 days in muslin). Individual manufacturer's guidelines should be followed concerning when to resanitize and resterilize items. Autoclaved items cannot be reautoclaved in the same packages without washing, rinsing, drying, and rewrapping each item. See Procedure 33-7 for the steps when using an office-size autoclave.

Chemical Gas Sterilization. Gas sterilization removes or kills life through the use of gasses. The most common gas used for sterilization is ethylene oxide (EtO) at low

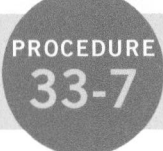

PROCEDURE 33-7 Sterilizing Instruments in an Autoclave

Objective ◆ *Sterilize instruments in an autoclave to prevent the spread of pathogens.*

EQUIPMENT AND SUPPLIES
Autoclave; instruments sanitized and wrapped for autoclaving; distilled water; autoclave directions

METHOD
1. Check the level of water in the autoclave reservoir. Add distilled water as needed to the fill line (Figure A).
2. Load the autoclave:
   a. Trays and packs should be loaded on their sides.
   b. Containers should be loaded on their sides with lids off or ajar.
   c. Mixed loads are loaded with hard objects on bottom racks and softer items on top racks.
   d. Keep large packs 2 to 4 inches apart and smaller packets 1 to 2 inches apart.
3. Read the manufacturer's instructions and follow them exactly. Most autoclaves follow similar protocols.
   a. Turn the control knob to FILL and observe carefully with the door open until the water reaches the chamber fill line.
   b. Turn the knob to autoclave position (Figure B). This shuts off the water. Do not allow the water to overflow.
   c. Close and lock the door.

4. When pressure reaches 15 to 17 pounds per square inch and the temperature reaches 250°F to 270°F, set the timer for the required time. Typical timing is 30 minutes for wrapped trays and packages and 15 minutes for unwrapped items. Always check the manufacturer's suggested times and facility protocol.
5. When timing is complete, turn the control knob to VENT.
6. When the pressure reaches zero, open the chamber door about ¾ inch and allow items in the autoclave to dry completely before removing them (about 30 to 45 minutes).
7. Turn the autoclave knob to OFF.
8. Remove the wrapped items, and check the autoclave tape on the outside for indicated color change. Store in a dry closed cabinet for future use. Unwrapped items must be removed using sterile transfer forceps and must be placed on a sterile field or in a sterile storage area (Figure C).
9. Perform quality assurance measures by recording the activity in the proper log book. Record date, time, and types of items autoclaved in log and initial.

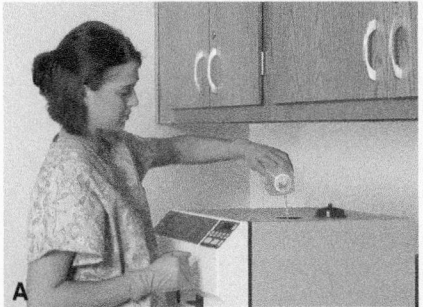
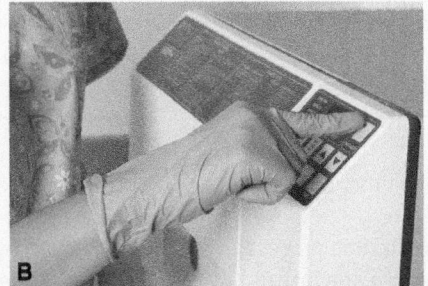
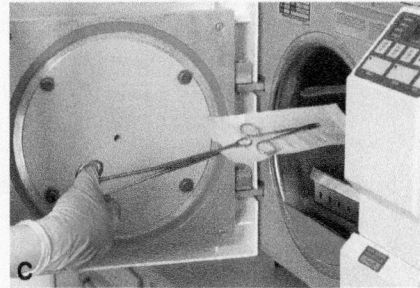

FIGURE A–C (A) Check the water level in the autoclave, and add distilled water as necessary. **(B)** Properly set the autoclave controls according to the manufacturer's instructions. **(C)** Remove instruments and packages to a clean container using sterile transfer forceps.

temperature. It can be used as an ingredient in a mixed gas or as 100 percent EtO. Since the 1950s when chlorofluorocarbon (CFC0) was phased out, alternative technologies that have been used and are cleared by the U.S. Food and Drug Administration (FDA) for medical equipment include 100 percent ETO; ETO with a different stabilizing gas such as carbon dioxide or hydrochlorofluorocarbons (HCFC); immersion in peracetic acid; hydrogen peroxide gas plasma; and ozone. Technologies under development for use in health care facilities, but not cleared by the FDA, include vaporized hydrogen peroxide, vapor phase peracetic acid, gaseous chlorine dioxide, ionizing radiation, or pulsed light.

Chemical Liquid Sterilization. Chemical sterilization uses a chemical that is toxic to the microbes to sterilize objects. The medical assistant may submerge instruments, for example, in liquid chemicals instead of gasses to perform this procedure. Liquid sterilants require much more time to work than dry heat, ultraviolet, or steam sterilization needs. Proper sterilization by chemical liquid can take hours to days to work effectively, as some microbial species form structures called spores, which are very tough and resist killing in a short period of time. Typically, the equipment, such as surgical instruments, must be completely submerged in the liquid sterilant. See Procedure 33-8 for how to perform chemical liquid sterilization.

PROCEDURE 33-8 Sterilizing Instruments Chemically

Objective ◆ *Sterilize heat-sensitive instruments chemically to prevent the spread of pathogens.*

EQUIPMENT AND SUPPLIES

Chemical disinfectant; goggles, disposable gloves, and utility (rubber) gloves; sink; glass or stainless steel container with cover; sterile towels; sterile transfer forceps; sterile basin; sanitized articles

Note: Before anything can be chemically sterilized, it must be sanitized properly as described in Procedure 33-5. Always read and follow the manufacturer's directions on the original container of the chemical agent.

METHOD

1. Sanitize instruments appropriately.
2. Select the type of chemical needed to sterilize the instruments.
3. Read the directions on the original germicidal agent label. If opening the germicide for the first time, write the date on the container and follow directions to properly prepare the chemical agent for initial use.
4. Place the chemical agent in an appropriate container that is large enough to submerge the instrument completely. See Figure A.
5. Cover the container tightly, and record the time, date, and your initials.
6. Do not open the container during the sterilization process.
7. When sterilization timing is complete, remove the instrument from the container using sterile gloves or sterile transfer forceps.

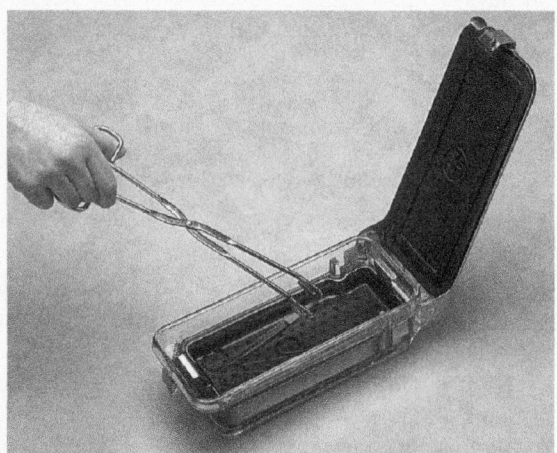

FIGURE A Cold chemical sterilization.

8. Rinse the items thoroughly with sterile water over a sterile basin. Hold the instruments over the basin for a few moments to drain excess sterile water.
9. Dry the instruments thoroughly with a sterile towel, and place onto a sterile field for use.
10. Change the chemical agent every 7 to 14 days, or as recommended by the manufacturer.
11. Remove gloves and perform hand hygiene.
12. Perform quality assurance by recording appropriate information in the appropriate log book.

SUMMARY

Infection control is important not only to health care workers, but to patients as well. The medical assistant is often the first line of defense against the spread of infection in the medical office. A thorough understanding of standard precautions and isolation techniques is important to maintain a safe patient environment. The meticulous attention given to sterilization of all reusable materials and equipment is often the full responsibility of the medical assistant and is a serious responsibility. All who handle bodily fluids and waste products must be trained in safety measures such as standard precautions and the Bloodborne Pathogen Standard. Fines may be imposed for not adhering to OSHA regulations about these precautions. When practicing an aseptic technique, the medical assistant should learn the correct method and then never deviate from it.

33 CHAPTER REVIEW

COMPETENCY REVIEW

1. Define and spell the terms for this chapter.
2. How does the age of a person affect susceptibility to infections?
3. List three natural barriers to infection.
4. List the four cardinal signs of infection.
5. List three examples of body fluids included in standard precautions.
6. A sterilized package has reached its expiration date. What should you do?
7. What solution of household bleach has been found to be effective in destroying HIV?
8. Explain the difference between sanitization and sterilization.
9. List three examples of PPE.
10. Define multidrug-resistant organism (MDRO), and give an example.

PREPARING FOR THE CERTIFICATION EXAM

1. The term *asepsis* means
   a. contaminated.
   b. needs oxygen.
   c. free of pathogens.
   d. soap.
   e. needs sanitizing.

2. Most sterilization indicators operate on what principle?
   a. Color change will revert back when an item is contaminated.
   b. Original color reappears after six weeks.
   c. Color change indicates the package has been properly sealed.
   d. Color change indicates sterilization is complete.
   e. Color change occurs at the beginning of the process.

3. An organism that is infected with a pathogen and is a source of infection to others is
   a. a reservoir host.
   b. a carrier.
   c. an anaerobe.
   d. not an infectious risk to others.
   e. an inanimate object.

4. During which stage of infection are signs and symptoms both evident and severe?
   a. prodromal stage
   b. acute stage
   c. incubation stage
   d. invasion stage
   e. multiplication stage

5. All bacteria require which of the following to grow best?
   a. oxygen
   b. cool temperature
   c. light
   d. sugar
   e. moisture

6. MRSA is a(n)
   a. disinfectant.
   b. type of microorganism.
   c. oxygen source.
   d. physician's credential.
   e. drug.

7. How long is it necessary to wash hands before assisting a new patient?
   a. 1 minute
   b. 6 minutes

c. 2 to 3 minutes
d. 20 to 30 seconds
e. 10 seconds

8. "Treat all bodily fluids as if they were contaminated with harmful pathogens" summarizes which concept?
   a. standard precautions
   b. Bloodborne Pathogen Standard
   c. isolation techniques
   d. universal precautions
   e. none of the above

9. Which of the following PPE and/or protective barrier items would be removed first?
   a. gloves
   b. respirator
   c. gown
   d. goggles
   e. face shield

10. Which process involves the destruction of organisms before they enter the body?
    a. disinfection
    b. sterilization
    c. sanitization
    d. medical asepsis
    e. surgical asepsis

CRITICAL THINKING

Refer to the case study at the beginning of the chapter and use what you have learned to answer the following questions.

1. What type of PPE would David need to wear when performing venipuncture on this patient?

2. Why would the physician include a liver function test as part of the patient's routine blood work?

3. Which particular groups of individuals are encouraged to receive the vaccination to guard against HBV?

ON THE JOB

Emma Brown, 70 years old, is caring for her 78-year-old husband, George Brown. Mr. Brown, a diabetic, has been hospitalized with a recurring infection that may lead to amputation of his right leg. Mr. Brown's physical condition may not be able to withstand another massive leg infection. He has been placed on antibiotics, and his leg is now healing. Mrs. Brown will require instructions on irrigating the leg wound and changing her husband's dressing. When the leg wound was cultured, *E. coli* was present. Mrs. Brown mentioned to the medical assistant that she is concerned about her own health because she has a colostomy.

1. What patient education is required for Mrs. Brown regarding the procedure to be used in caring for her husband?

2. Is it possible that the *E. coli* was transmitted from Mrs. Brown's colostomy site to her husband's leg wound? Explain.

INTERNET ACTIVITY

Conduct an Internet search of published studies detailing infection control rates of health care facilities in your area—research hospitals, nursing homes, urgent care facilities, and health clinics—to determine how well infection control is maintained.

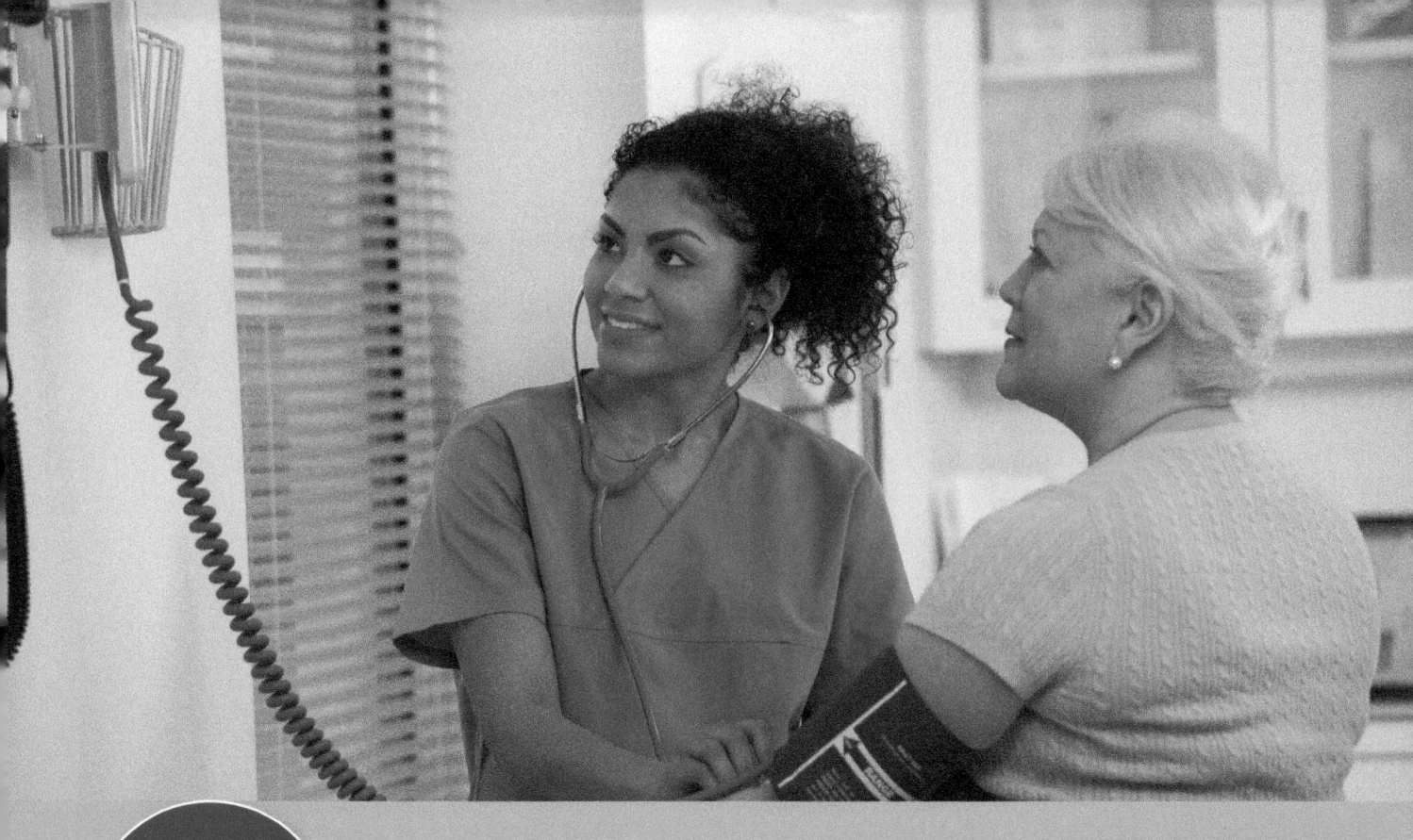

Vital Signs

Learning Objectives

After completing this chapter, you should be able to:

34.1   Define and spell the terms for this chapter.

34.2   Demonstrate weight conversions between pounds and kilograms.

34.3   Identify factors that affect body temperature.

34.4   Demonstrate temperature conversions between Fahrenheit (F) and Celsius (C).

34.5   Describe how to select the proper method to measure body temperature.

34.6   Compare different types of thermometers.

34.7   Describe characteristics of pulse rate.

34.8   List average pulse rates according to age.

34.9   Identify the nine pulse site locations on the human body.

34.10   Describe characteristics of respirations.

34.11   List average respiratory rates according to age.

34.12   Describe the five phases of Korotkoff sounds.

34.13   List average blood pressure readings according to age.

34.14   Identify situations that could cause a variation or error in blood pressure readings.

34.15   Describe pulse oximetry.

Case Study

Elanya Jordan, age 13, is seeing Dr. Salpega for persistent headaches. David Dolan, RMA, obtains her vital signs, which are T: 98.6°F, P: 88 bpm, R: 18 rpm, BP: 118/80. Elanya is 5 feet, 1 inch tall and weighs 104 pounds. Her mother, Mary Ellen, states that she has lost 6 pounds during the past three weeks because she has lost her appetite since the headaches began.

Terms to Learn

afebrile	hyperpyrexia	pulse pressure
anthropometry	hypertension (HTN)	pyrexia
apical	hyperthermia	rate
apnea	hyperventilation	respiratory cycle
arrhythmia	hypotension	rhythm
asymptomatic	hypothermia	sphygmomanometer
bounding pulse	hypoventilation	syncope
bradycardia	intermittent pulse	systolic blood pressure
bradypnea	Korotkoff sounds	tachycardia
cyanosis	manometer	tachypnea
diastolic blood pressure	orthostatic hypotension	thready pulse
dysrhythmia	oxygen saturation	tympanic membrane thermometer
eupnea	pulse deficit	vital signs
febrile	pulse oximeter	volume
frenulum linguae		

In many medical offices, the medical assistant is responsible for taking vital signs. As the name implies, vital signs are able to give quick snapshots regarding how the body is functioning. For example, a body temperature reading that is too high could signify infection within the body, while a blood pressure reading that is too low may be due to low blood volume, nutritional deficiencies, or age. It is important for medical assistants to understand the importance of obtaining accurate vital signs because accuracy is something that physicians expect and patients depend on.

MEASURING WEIGHT AND HEIGHT

Weight and height are two important measurements, even though they are not considered vital signs in the true sense of the term. Weight and height are called anthropometric measurements because they relate to **anthropometry**, which is the science of size, proportion, weight, and height. The majority of physician offices will obtain a weight measurement at each patient visit, whereas a height measurement might only be obtained during an annual physical examination. However, older patients and women may be measured more frequently, for example, to observe for signs of osteoporosis (bone loss).

Weight and height can also provide indications of a person's general health. For example, infants who fail to gain weight, or "fail to thrive," require close supervision of weight gains and losses. If a child has an abnormal growth pattern, this may lead to a diagnosis of a hormonal imbalance. Diabetic patients, pregnant women, patients suffering cardiac problems, patients with fluid retention, and patients suffering from eating disorders, such as anorexia or bulimia, also often require frequent weight monitoring.

Weight

When measuring a patient's weight, it is important to be discreet and provide patients sufficient privacy. Weight can particularly be a sensitive and personal issue for both men and women. Patients can remain fully clothed when obtaining a weight measurement. However, it should be noted in the patient's chart if they have already disrobed and donned a gown for examination before being weighed. Both shoes and outerwear (heavy jackets or coats) should be removed before obtaining weight because they may significantly inflate a person's weight. Patients who cannot stand may be weighed on a chair or bed scale (Figure 34-1). Some patients may refuse to get weighed. When this situation occurs, it is important not to argue with the patient. Rather, make appropriate documentation by simply noting "refused weight" in the patient's medical record and notify the physician. Procedure 34-1 lists the steps for obtaining the weight and height of a patient.

There are many different types of scales that can be used to weigh patients. Scales may be upright scales, balance scales, electronic scales, or digital scales (Figure 34-2). As medical practices and offices evolve with changing technology, it is likely that most scales in medical facilities will be electronic. Scales may be calibrated in either kilograms (metric weight) or pounds.

Although many of these scales are able to change measuring units from kilograms to pounds at the press of a button, the medical assistant must know how to do the correct mathematical conversions. Table 34-1 shows these conversions.

Height

The patient's true height must be measured without shoes. While measuring the patient's height, the patient's weight may also be obtained. When you are measuring height, the patient

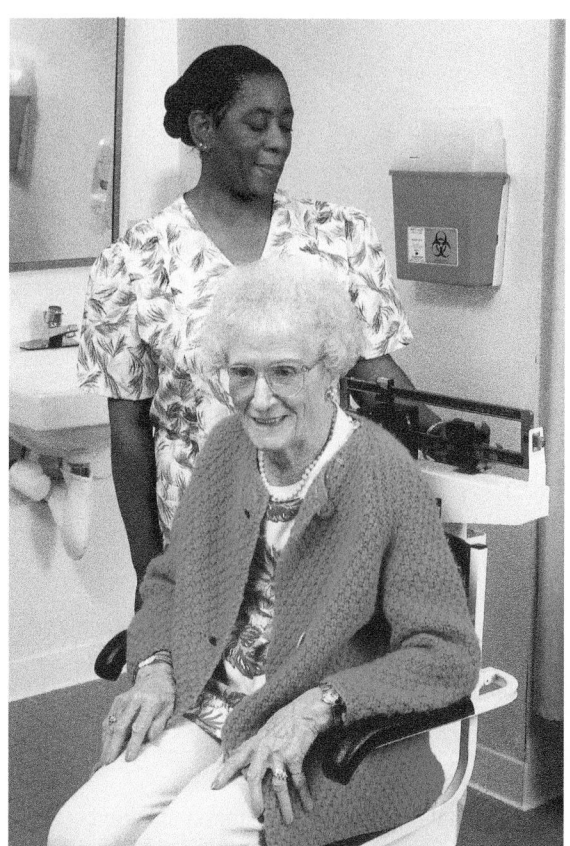

FIGURE 34-1 Patients unable to stand may be weighed using a chair scale.

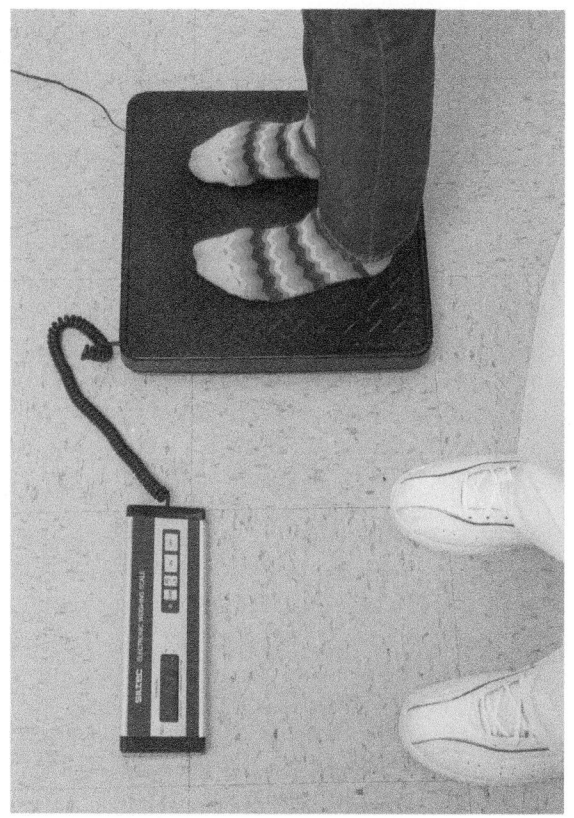

FIGURE 34-2 An electronic scale.

TABLE 34-1 | Converting Pounds and Kilograms

To Convert Kilograms to Pounds (kg to lb)

1 kilogram (kg) = 2.2 pounds (lb)

Multiply the number of kilograms by 2.2 lb
Example: If a patient weighs 64 kilograms, multiply 64 by 2.2.

$$64 \times 2.2 = 140.8 \text{ or } 141 \text{ pounds}$$

To Convert Pounds to Kilograms (lb to kg)

1 pound = 0.45 kilograms

Multiply the number of pounds by 0.45.
Example: If a patient weighs 130 pounds, multiply 130 by 0.45.

$$130 \times 0.45 = 58.5 \text{ or } 59 \text{ kilograms}$$

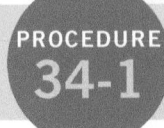

PROCEDURE 34-1

Measuring Adult Weight and Height

Objective ◆ *Obtain height and weight measurements, and perform math conversions.*

EQUIPMENT AND SUPPLIES

Balance scale with bar to measure height; paper towel; pen; patient's medical record

METHOD

1. Perform hand hygiene.
2. Greet and identify the patient.
3. Explain the procedure to the patient.
4. Instruct the patient to remove shoes, and place a paper towel on the scale if the patient is in bare feet.
   a. Heavy objects such as keys or purses should be set aside.
5. Set all the weights to zero. The balance bar pointer should float in the center of the frame.
   a. If the balance bar is not centered at zero, balance the scale by adjusting the small knob at one end until the balance bar pointer floats in the center of the frame. (A coin can be used to make this adjustment.)
6. Assist the patient onto the scale.
7. Ask the patient to stand still while the measurement is being obtained.
8. Move the large weight into the groove closest to the weight you estimate for the patient. (You may refer to the patient's last recorded weight in the medical record.)
   a. If the balance bar pointer touches the bottom of the bar, then move the large weight to the left, one notch.
9. Then move the small weight by tapping it gently until it reaches a point in which the pointer floats in the center of the frame.
10. Leave the weights in place as you proceed to obtain the patient's height.
11. Ask the patient to place his back to the scale, standing erect, and looking straight ahead.
    a. The patient's heels, buttocks, and back of head should be touching the scale.
12. Raise the height bar in a collapsed position making sure the tip is over the patient's head.
13. Open the bar into the horizontal position, and bring it down gently to touch the top of the patient's head. Leave this setting in place (Figure A).
14. Assist the patient in stepping off the scale.
15. Calculate the patient's weight by adding the numbers at the large and small weight groove markings. Record the weight to the nearest ¼ pound.
    a. For example, if the large weight is seated within the 150-pound groove and the small weight

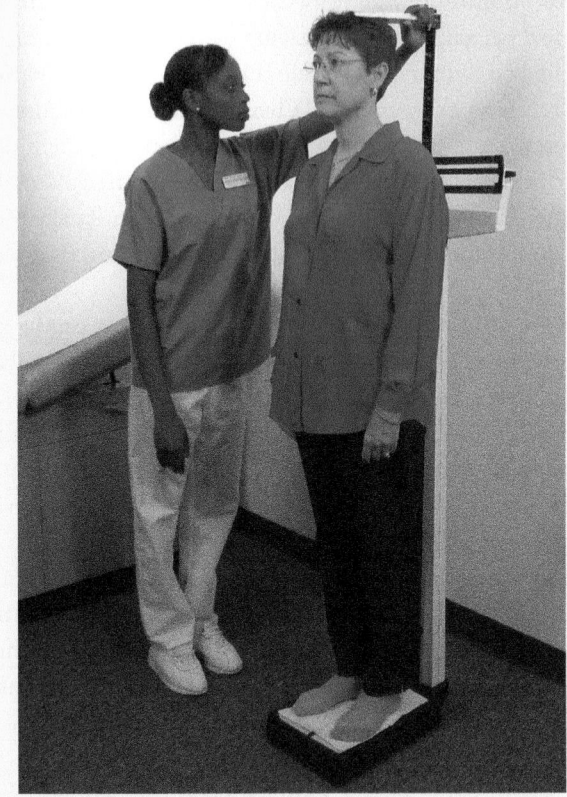

FIGURE A The height bar is gently lowered until it touches the top of the patient's head.

marking is at 23¼ pounds, the total weight is 173¼ pounds.

16. Record this measurement on the patient's record.
17. Read the height as marked behind the movable level of the ruled bar.
    a. Individual medical offices have their own policies about documenting height as feet and inches, total inches, or total centimeters.
18. Record this measurement to the nearest ¼ inch or centimeter, as appropriate, on the patient's record.
19. Return the weights to zero and the height bar to the normal position, and discard the paper towel.
20. Perform hand hygiene.

CHARTING EXAMPLE

2/14/YY 8:00 A.M. wt. 140¼ lbs without shoes;
ht. 5'7" = 67 inches.
....M. King, CMA

stands with heel, buttocks, and back of head touching the measuring stick or bar. The L-shaped arm is raised and then lowered until it rests on the top of the head, not on the top of the hair. The height is then read, and it may be recorded in feet and inches or in centimeters. To convert inches to centimeters, multiply the inches by 2.5. To convert centimeters to inches, divide the centimeters by 2.5.

VITAL SIGNS

A healthy human body is able to self-regulate through homeostasis, which is the body's natural ability to maintain a stable internal environment by correcting abnormal conditions and balancing bodily processes. **Vital signs** are indicators of the body's ability to maintain homeostasis. Temperature (T), pulse (P), respiration (R), and blood pressure (BP) measurements are considered vital signs because they measure some of the body's vital functions and provide necessary information about the patient's physical well-being. Thus, vital signs must be obtained and calculated with the utmost care and accuracy.

Vital signs are routinely measured by medical assistants before physical examinations. Temperature, pulse, respiration, and blood pressure are usually taken in this order. For proper charting of vital signs in the medical record, it is helpful to remember the *T, P, R, BP* sequence and record the results in that order. During some office visits, only one of the vital signs may be measured. For example, only blood pressure may be taken in a patient who is seeing the doctor for a medication check for hypertension.

Although details of standard precautions are not repeated for each procedure in this text, all health care professionals are to adhere to standard precautions in order to maintain infection control while measuring vital signs. As a medical assistant, you are expected to know and continually apply the techniques recommended by the Centers for Disease Control and Prevention (CDC), as discussed in the "Infection Control" chapter.

The remainder of this chapter discusses the physiology of body temperature, pulse rate, respirations, blood pressure, and the body processes that produce these signs. Normal vital sign readings for patients, based on age, are presented. Methods and types of equipment for measuring vital signs are also discussed, along with guidelines and methods for choosing the best equipment for each specific procedure.

TEMPERATURE

When measuring body temperature, use critical thinking skills to execute the task in a way that will achieve the most accurate reading. Take into consideration the patient's age

and health status, and be able to recall normal healthy body temperature ranges in order to identify abnormalities.

Physiology of Body Temperature

Body temperature is regulated by balancing the amount of heat the body produces with the amount of heat the body loses. Body heat is produced as a by-product of metabolism, which is the sum of all biochemical and physiological processes that take place in the body. The hypothalamus, a gland located in the brain, acts as a thermoregulator. It is able to adjust body temperature that results in either increasing or decreasing heat production throughout the day.

Heat can be lost from the body by the following processes:

- **Radiation**—Heat given off from the body and released in the cooler air temperature; 65 percent of the body's heat is released this way

- **Convection**—Dispersion of heat by air currents; 10–15 percent of heat is released through this method

- **Conduction**—Transfer of heat from the body to a cooler source (e.g., when a patient with high fever is placed in cool water)

- **Evaporation**—Heat released from body through respiration (breathing) and sweating

See Figure 34-3 for an example of one way the body can react to increased temperature.

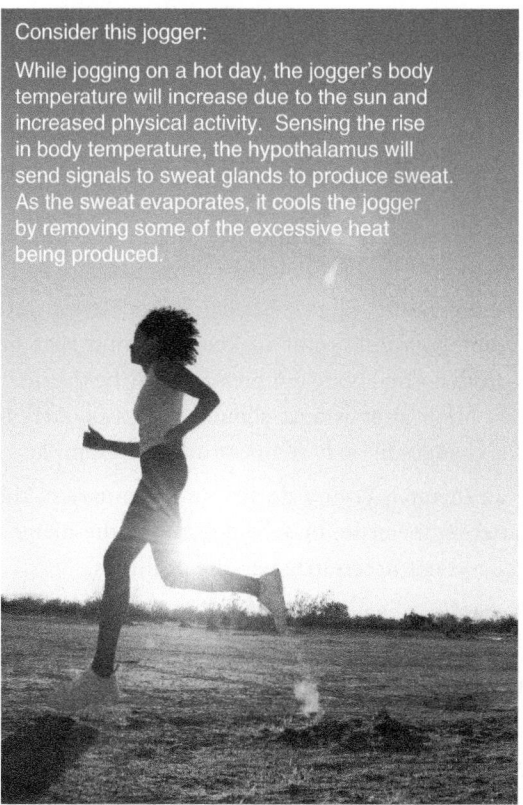

Consider this jogger:

While jogging on a hot day, the jogger's body temperature will increase due to the sun and increased physical activity. Sensing the rise in body temperature, the hypothalamus will send signals to sweat glands to produce sweat. As the sweat evaporates, it cools the jogger by removing some of the excessive heat being produced.

FIGURE 34-3 The hypothalamus helps regulate body temperature.

TABLE 34-2 | Factors Affecting Body Temperature

Time of Day	Body temperature is lower in the morning upon waking, when metabolism is still slow. The body's temperature is lowest between 2:00 A.M. and 6:00 A.M., and the body's highest temperature usually occurs in the evening between 5:00 P.M. and 8:00 P.M. Daily variation in normal temperature can range from 97.6°F to 99.6°F (36.4°C to 37.3°C).
Age	Infants and children normally have a higher body temperature than adults because of immature heat regulation. Children often tend to spike a fever late in the day. Older adults usually have lower-than-normal body temperature.
Gender	Women may experience a slight increase in body temperature at the time of ovulation.
Physical Exercise	Body temperature will rise during exercise as a result of increased muscle contraction and increased blood flow caused by heightened cardiovascular activity.
Emotions	Emotions such as crying and anger can cause an increase in body temperature.
Pregnancy	An increase in metabolism during pregnancy may cause the body temperature to rise.
Environmental Changes	Hot weather can cause serious consequences for older adults whose bodies are less able to regulate body temperature because of decreased metabolic functioning. Exposure to excessively cold temperatures will lower body temperature. Cool environments that may feel fine to a younger adult can cause hypothermia in an older person.
Infection	An elevated temperature may be one of the first signs of an infection. A fever is the body's way of fighting or killing off infectious organisms.
Drugs	Drugs may increase muscular activity or metabolism, which in turn increases temperature. Antipyretic (fever-reducing) drugs such as aspirin lower the above-normal temperature.
Food	The process of eating and digestion may cause a rise in the body temperature. Fasting decreases metabolism, which will lower body temperature.

Temperature: Normal Values and Terms

Body temperature is recorded in either degrees Fahrenheit (F) or degrees Celsius (C). The average body temperature of a healthy person is 98.6°F (37°C). However, there may be a 1- to 2-degree Fahrenheit fluctuation (increase or decrease) throughout the day. For example, temperature is lowest when a person gets up in the morning and will be at its highest in late afternoon. Table 34-2 describes some causes of variations in body temperature. Slight variance in body temperature is normal, but it is important to keep in mind that greater changes from normal body temperature may be the first signs of illness. Medical assistants should always be alert to the causes for changes in body temperature. For example:

- If an infant is crying during an examination, the elevated temperature may be a result of the infant's crying and not necessarily because of illness.

- Acetaminophen or aspirin can lower body temperature. Patients should be asked if they have recently taken any medicine, including over-the-counter medications.

- Older adults, who normally have body temperatures below normal, may be ill even when their temperatures are within a range that would be normal for younger adults.

Fahrenheit and Celsius Conversions

The Fahrenheit (F) scale of temperature measurement is widely used throughout the United States. However, some physicians, hospitals, and medical facilities use the Celsius (or centigrade) (C) scale, which is more commonly used outside the United States. Figure 34-4 shows calibration examples of Fahrenheit and Celsius in non-mercury thermometers. Table 34-3 discusses temperature scale conversion formulas and comparisons.

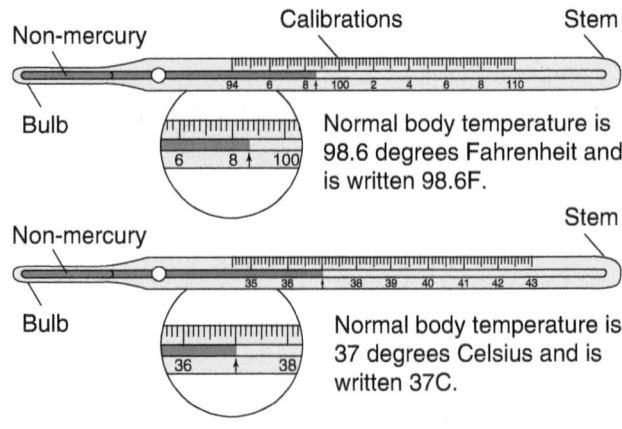

FIGURE 34-4 Fahrenheit and Celsius thermometers.

TABLE 34-3 | Temperature Conversions

- To convert Celsius to Fahrenheit:
  Fahrenheit degrees = (Celsius degrees × 9/5) + 32
- To convert Fahrenheit to Celsius:
  (Fahrenheit degrees − 32) × 5/9

Examples of Celsius and Fahrenheit readings in degrees:

Celsius (C)	Fahrenheit (F)
34.0	95.0
34.5	95.9
36.0	96.8
36.5	97.7
37.0	98.6 (normal oral)
37.5	99.5
38.0	100.4
38.5	101.3
39.0	102.2
39.5	103.1
40.0	104.0
40.5	104.9
41.0	105.8

Abnormal Temperatures
Fever and Hyperthermia

Fever or **pyrexia** is a body temperature above 100.4°F (38°C). When the body is in a feverish state, it is producing more heat than it is losing. A condition caused by fever is termed **febrile**; a condition not caused by fever is termed **afebrile**. For example, a febrile seizure is a seizure caused by fever, whereas an afebrile seizure is caused by something other than a fever, such as a head trauma.

Clinical signs and symptoms of fever include increased heart rate, increased respiratory rate, shivering, chills, decreased appetite, headache, facial flushing (redness to the skin), and sweating. The four most common types of fevers are:

- **Intermittent fever**—Body temperature that alternates between febrile and afebrile states
- **Remittent fever**—Elevated body temperature that remains high throughout the day, fluctuating more than 2 degrees Fahrenheit
- **Relapsing fever**—Febrile periods that last for a couple of days, go away, and then return
- **Constant (continuous) fever**—Elevated body temperatures throughout the day with minimal temperature fluctuation (usually not more than 1 degree Fahrenheit) over a 24-hour period

When the body temperature exceeds 106.7°F (41.5°C), a serious condition known as **hyperpyrexia** or **hyperthermia** develops. Hyperpyrexia is a very high fever resulting from a regulated rise in core body temperature, usually a response to a physiological threat, such as an infection. Hyperpyrexia may lead to serious complications, such as seizures in infants and small children. Hyperthermia, by contrast, is an unregulated rise in core body temperature and is the result of the body's inability to thermoregulate. Hyperthermia may be caused by exposure to high external temperatures, such as being outdoors on a very hot day. As body temperature increases, signs and symptoms of hyperthermia advance in severity. They include muscle cramps, fatigue, loss of coordination, drowsiness, confusion, convulsions, the inability to sweat, and possibly death.

Hypothermia

The reverse of hyperthermia is a below normal body temperature or **hypothermia**. Hypothermia is defined as a body temperature below 95°F (35°C) and is the result of the body losing more heat than it is producing. Hypothermia commonly occurs in cases of environmental exposure to cool or cold temperatures and/or submersion in cold water. In general, a body temperature below 92°F (33.3°C) is considered severe hypothermia and may be life-threatening. Clinical signs of hypothermia are lack of muscle coordination; slurred speech; violent shivering; decreased pulse and respirations; pale, waxy, cool skin; and drowsiness and dazed consciousness progressing to coma and death.

Sites for Measuring Body Temperature

Body temperature can be measured in a variety of ways: oral (mouth); aural (ear) or tympanic membrane (eardrum); axillary (under the arm); rectal (rectum); and temporal artery (forehead). Oral and rectal temperatures measure the body's core temperature and are considered the most accurate. Tympanic membrane, axillary, and temporal artery temperatures are more variable but are acceptable for tracking significant changes.

Professionalism The Law

The medical assistant has an ethical and professional responsibility to use careful, proper techniques when performing procedures to measure vital signs. Incorrect readings could result in a misdiagnosis and serious consequences for the patient. In addition to proper technique, following through with proper documentation is just as critical. Incorrect documentation of vital signs can lead to serious complications for the patient and legal consequences for both the physician and the medical assistant.

TABLE 34-4 | Selecting a Method for Measuring Body Temperature

Method	Advisable	Inadvisable
Oral ("O")	Most adults and children who are able to follow instructions for properly holding the thermometer.	Patients who have had oral surgery, mouth sores, dyspnea; uncooperative patients; patients on oxygen; infants and small children; patients with facial paralysis or nasal obstruction; anyone unable to form an airtight seal around the thermometer.
Rectal ("R")	Infants and small children; patients who have had oral surgery; mouth-breathing patients; unconscious patients.	Active children; fragile newborns; patients with heart conditions (it can stimulate the vagus nerve leading to arrhythmias); those with recent rectal surgery or complaints of diarrhea.
Axillary ("AX")	Small children	Patients who have underarm rash, excessive perspiration, or cannot form an airtight seal around the thermometer.
Tympanic (Aural) ("T")	Small children	Patient with in-the-ear hearing aids, impacted cerumen, earaches, or ear infections.
Temporal Artery ("TA")	Most adults, infants, and small children; patients who have had oral surgery; mouth-breathing patients; unconscious patients.	No restrictions—possibly difficult with combative children or newborns.

Use the guidelines given in Table 34-4 to determine which method to use when measuring a patient's body temperature.

Normal Values

The normal temperature, based on statistical averages, is as follows for each measurement site:

Oral	98.6°F (37°C)
Rectal	99.6°F (37.6°C)
Axillary (under arm)	97.6°F (36.4°C)
Aural (ear)	98.6°F (37°C)
Temporal artery	98.6°F (37°C)

Temperature obtained through the rectal method registers 1°F (or 0.6°C) higher than the oral temperature. Axillary temperatures register 1°F (0.6°C) lower than oral temperatures. Thus, when recording a temperature reading, you must document in the patient's record the body site where the temperature was measured. Temperatures taken rectally are abbreviated with the letter "R" next to the reading, axillary by the abbreviation "AX," tympanic membrane (aural) by "T," or temporal artery with "TA." "O" would indicate an oral measurement, although generally if there is no abbreviation next to a temperature reading, it is assumed the reading was obtained orally.

Oral

The oral method of temperature measurement is most commonly used. Some facilities do not require the designation "O" when documenting this measurement, whereas others do.

When taking oral temperature, insert the thermometer under the tongue on either side of the **frenulum linguae**, which is the longitudinal fold of mucous membrane connecting the tongue to the bottom of the mouth. For an accurate measurement, you must advise the patient not to talk during the procedure and to close the lips tightly around the thermometer. The potential for error with this method is that the patient may not form a tight enough closure around the thermometer, which allows air to enter the mouth and produce a false temperature reading. Ask if the patient either smoked or drank fluids before the appointment. If so, you must wait 15 minutes before obtaining an oral temperature.

Aural (Ear)/Tympanic Membrane

This method uses the tympanic membrane (the eardrum) for temperature measurement. Tympanic membrane thermometers are able to detect heat waves in the ear canal and calculate body temperature from these readings. The aural method is sometimes preferred over the oral method because the space in the external auditory canal is a more tightly closed cavity than the mouth, producing a more accurate measurement. Another benefit of this method of measurement is that it does not come in contact with saliva or mucus, which helps prevent the spread of infection, particularly from a sick patient. However, a tympanic thermometer should not be used if the patient has complaints of ear pain (internal or external) or has impacted cerumen (earwax).

Axillary

The axillary (under the arm) method has proven to be the least accurate of the temperature measurement sites. However, it is the recommended site for small children or for patients unable to properly hold an oral thermometer in their mouths, such as those who have recently had oral surgery, mouth-breathing patients, or when a tympanic membrane thermometer is not available. In axillary temperature readings, the underarm area should be patted dry for an accurate reading because perspiration (sweat) may affect the reading.

Rectal

A rectal body temperature reading is considered to be the most accurate and reliable method. This is because the mucous membrane lining the rectum does not come into contact with air, as it does with the oral and axillary methods, which could interfere with accuracy. The rectal route is advised for unconscious patients, infants and small children, and mouth-breathing patients.

A separate thermometer should be used for rectal readings, and it should be properly labeled "rectal" to prevent it from being used to take an oral temperature. The rectal method should be avoided when there is a danger of rectal wall perforation. Because the rectal method is the most invasive and uncomfortable method for patients, you must show care, sensitivity, and professionalism when you obtain a body temperature by this route.

Temporal Artery

Temporal artery measurement is a newer, noninvasive method of obtaining body temperature. The temporal artery is located close to the skin surface on the forehead and temple area. The temporal thermometer uses an infrared scanning device that detects the temperature of the blood as it is flowing through the temporal artery, which is then recorded as the body temperature. Similar to the tympanic membrane thermometer, it is a fast and fairly accurate method of obtaining body temperature. A number of commercial devices are available to measure the temporal artery temperature.

Types of Thermometers

There are many types of thermometers available for measuring body temperature. However, in 2002, the American Hospital Association (AHA) agreed to eliminate mercury from the health care environment because of the frequency of breakage and the potential danger of mercury. Mercury is toxic and can be harmful to both humans and animals.

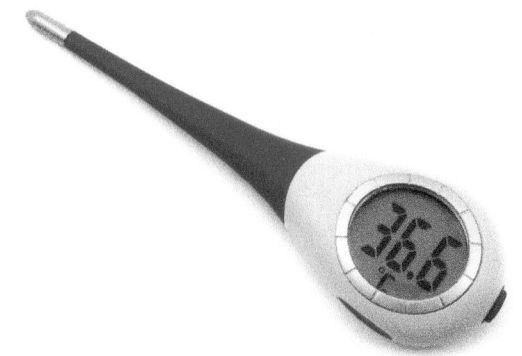

FIGURE 34-5 Electronic digital thermometers are accurate and easy to read.

Electronic or Digital Thermometer

Electronic or digital thermometers are the most commonly used and are accurate, easy to read, sanitary, and fast. They require very minimal cleaning and disinfection. Some electronic thermometers are battery operated with digital windows for easy reading (Figure 34-5). Other types of electric thermometers are charged by plugging them into a base receptacle, which is often mounted on a wall in the patient room.

The electronic thermometer has a metal probe containing a heat sensor that can accurately register body temperature within a few seconds. The electronic thermometer can be used for oral, rectal, and axillary body temperature readings. The metal probes are color coded: blue for both oral and axillary, and red for rectal. The probe is attached to the battery unit by a flexible cord. A nonflexible, plastic disposable probe cover fits over the metal probe to provide each patient with a new and sanitary thermometer.

To use, hold the thermometer in place while the measurement is quickly obtained (Figure 34-6). The unit will emit

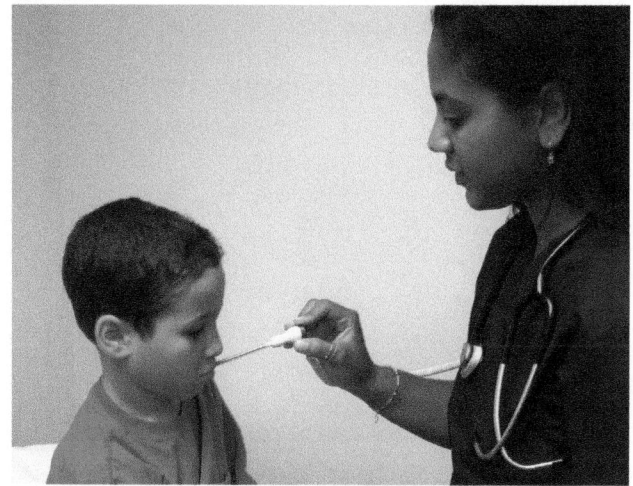

FIGURE 34-6 The medical assistant holds the position of the thermometer while the temperature is being obtained.

a signal, usually a beep, when the temperature has registered. Once the thermometer has been removed from the patient, press the release button to eject the plastic probe cover into a waste container and replace the probe and thermometer unit into the battery-powered storage unit. Procedure 34-2 provides the steps for measuring an oral temperature with an electronic thermometer.

The electronic method is the most widely used method of obtaining a rectal temperature. After lubricating the tip of the probe, insert the rectal probe ½ inch into an adult's

---

PROCEDURE 34-2
Measuring Oral Temperature Using an Electronic Thermometer

Objective ◆ *Perform all steps of the procedure, and provide an accurate temperature reading.*

EQUIPMENT AND SUPPLIES

Electronic thermometer (rechargeable); blue (oral) probe; probe cover; waste container; pen; patient's medical record

METHOD

1. Perform hand hygiene.
2. Assemble equipment, ensuring that the electronic thermometer is properly charged.
3. Greet and identify the patient, and explain the procedure.
4. Attach the correct probe that would be used to measure an oral temperature.
5. Attach a disposable probe cover by inserting the thermometer probe into the disposable tip (probe cover) box, and secure the disposable cover onto the probe (Figure A).
6. Insert the thermometer into the patient's mouth, under the tongue on either side of the frenulum linguae. Instruct the patient to close her mouth, forming a tight seal around the thermometer.
7. When the temperature signal is seen or heard, remove the thermometer from the patient's mouth and read the result displayed on the LED window.
8. Dispose of the probe cover in a waste container (Figure B).
9. Return the thermometer probe to the storage place (Figure C).
10. Return the entire unit to the rechargeable base.
11. Perform hand hygiene.
12. Document the results.

CHARTING EXAMPLE

07/25/YY 4:00 P.M. T: 99.6°FE. Leonard, RMA

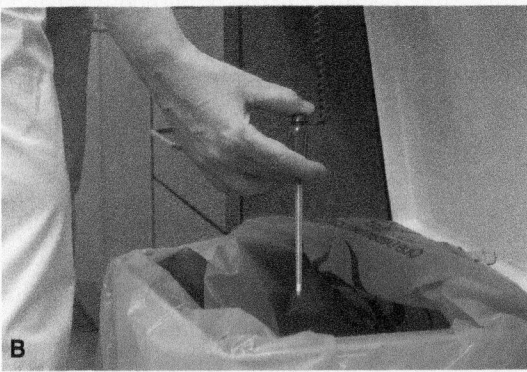

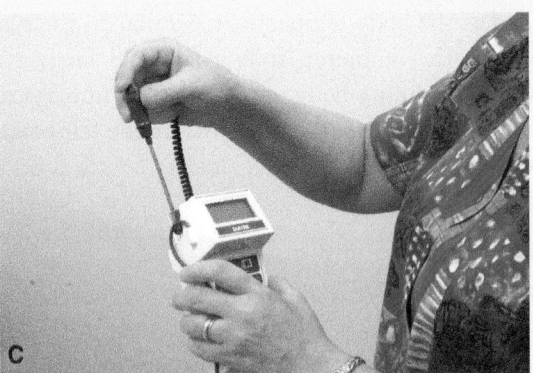

FIGURE A–C (A) Attach a disposable probe cover by inserting the probe into the box and securing a cover. **(B)** Eject the probe cover into the waste container. **(C)** Return the probe to the storage holder.

rectum and ¼ inch into a child's rectum. You may have to angle the probe slightly posteriorly (toward the patient's back) to ensure contact with the rectal mucosa and to prevent tearing of the rectal wall. Procedure 34-3 provides the steps for measuring a rectal temperature with an electronic thermometer.

Electronic thermometers are time saving but expensive. Additionally, the battery-operated thermometers must be calibrated and readjusted to maintain accuracy. It is important to always follow the manufacturer's instructions regarding proper care, use, and storage of electronic thermometers.

Axillary Thermometer

Although it is the least accurate, the axillary area (area under the arm) is considered ideal in some circumstances because it is easily accessible and noninvasive. As mentioned earlier, perspiration can affect the reading, so it is important to pat the armpit to remove wetness. However, do not rub the area because friction from rubbing can generate heat and increase the temperature. The process for measuring axillary temperature is given in Procedure 34-4.

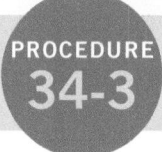

PROCEDURE
34-3

Measuring Rectal Temperature Using an Electronic Thermometer

Objective ◆ *Perform all steps of the procedure, and provide an accurate temperature reading.*

EQUIPMENT AND SUPPLIES

Electronic thermometer; red (rectal) probe; disposable probe cover; disposable gloves; patient's medical record; paper and pen; tissue; water-soluble lubricant; biohazard waste container

METHOD

1. Perform hand hygiene.
2. Don a pair of gloves.
3. Greet and identify the patient.
4. Explain the procedure. If the patient is a child, explain the procedure to both the parent and child.
5. Instruct the patient to remove appropriate clothing so that the rectal area can be accessed.
   a. Excuse yourself from the room while the patient disrobes to ensure patient privacy. Provide a drape or gown, as necessary.
6. Assist the patient onto the exam table, and help assist him into the Sims' position (lying on left side with top leg bent).
7. Because of the delicate nature of the procedure, be mindful of the patient's privacy and adjust draping, as necessary, to provide maximum coverage.
8. Remove the electronic thermometer from the base, and choose the correct probe for a rectal temperature.
9. Attach a disposable probe cover on the thermometer probe.
10. Place a small amount of lubricant on a tissue. Dip the tip of the probe in the lubricant.
11. With one hand, raise the upper buttock to expose the anus or anal opening.
    a. If unable to see the anal opening, ask the patient to bear down slightly. This will expose the opening.

12. With the other hand, gently insert the lubricated thermometer probe ½ inch into the anal canal.
    a. Do not force the thermometer into the anal canal; if any resistance is felt, discontinue the procedure.
13. Hold the thermometer still and in place until the result is signaled.
14. Gently withdraw the thermometer, and dispose of the probe cover by ejecting it into a biohazard container.
15. Make note of the temperature, which will be recorded later.
16. Wipe the anus from front to back to remove any excess lubricant.
17. Assist the patient from the examination table. Instruct the patient to re-dress or don an examination gown. If necessary, provide assistance. If no assistance is needed, excuse yourself from the room to allow the patient privacy.
18. Remove gloves and place in a biohazard waste container.
19. Perform hand hygiene.
20. Record the temperature in the patient's record using (R) to indicate a rectal temperature was obtained.
21. Return the probe to its appropriate storage place, and then return the entire thermometer unit to the rechargeable base.
    a. Perform appropriate sanitization of the thermometer unit according to the manufacturer's instructions or office protocol, possibly by cleaning the unit with a disinfecting wipe.

CHARTING EXAMPLE

2/14/YY 4:00 P.M. T: 99.6°F (R) .... M. King, CMA

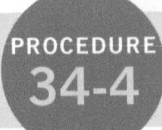

PROCEDURE 34-4 — Measuring Axillary Temperature

Objective ◆ *Perform all steps of the procedure, and provide an accurate temperature reading.*

EQUIPMENT AND SUPPLIES

Electronic thermometer and appropriate probe (blue oral probes are used for axillary temperatures); disposable probe cover; paper and pen; patient's medical record; tissue; waste container

METHOD

1. Perform hand hygiene.
2. Greet and identify the patient.
3. Explain the procedure. If the patient is a child, explain the procedure to both the parent and child.
4. Remove the electronic thermometer from its charging base, select the appropriate probe, and attach a disposable probe cover.
5. Ask the patient to expose the axilla (under the arm).
   a. If the patient is an infant or child, ask the parent to take the child's arm out of clothing to expose axilla.

6. Using a tissue, pat the axilla dry of any perspiration. Do not rub the area.
7. Place the probe with cover into the axillary space.
8. Ask the patient to remain still and to hold the arm tightly next to the body while the temperature registers (Figure A).
9. When the thermometer signals completion, remove the thermometer and discard the probe cover in a waste container.
10. Record the temperature in the patient's medical record, making sure to note that the temperature was obtained via the axillary route (AX) and which side was used (Figure B).
11. Return the thermometer probe to its appropriate storage location, and then return the entire unit to the rechargeable base.
12. Perform hand hygiene.

CHARTING EXAMPLE

2/14/YY 4:00 P.M. T: 97.6°F Lt. (AX) .... M. King, CMA

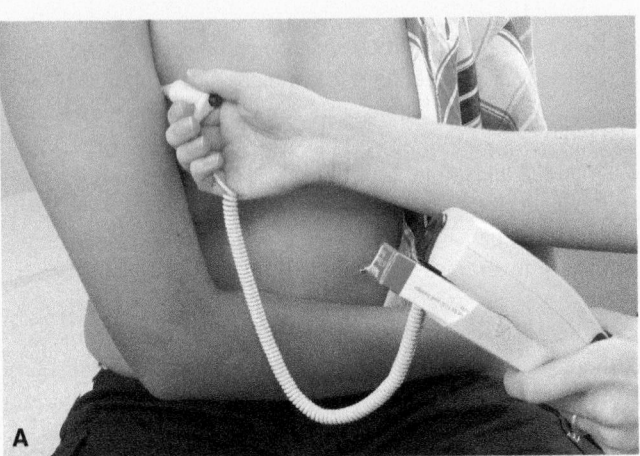

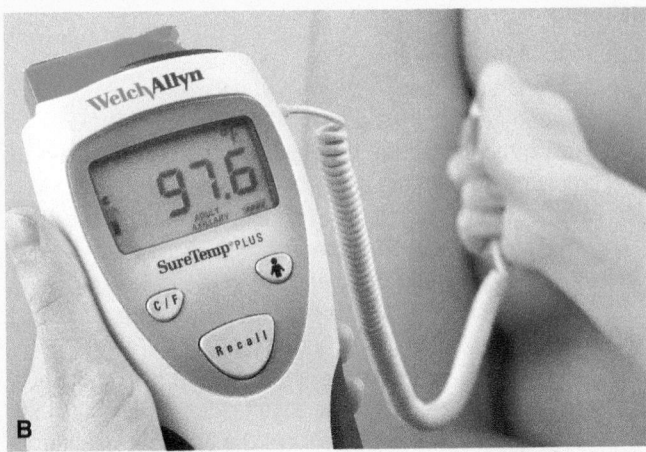

FIGURE A–B (A) The probe is placed in the axillary space while the patient holds his arm tightly to his body. **(B)** Record the body temperature measurement as displayed, indicating (AX) in the patient's medical record.

Tympanic Membrane Thermometer

The **tympanic membrane thermometer**, or aural thermometer, is used for an aural (ear) temperature. As discussed previously, the tympanic membrane thermometer is able to detect the heat waves generated within the external ear canal near the eardrum (tympanic membrane). It is very important to

straighten the ear canal when obtaining a tympanic membrane temperature. This is done by:

• Pulling the outer ear upward and out for patients ages 4 and up; or

• Pulling the ear downward and back for younger patients (ages 3 and under).

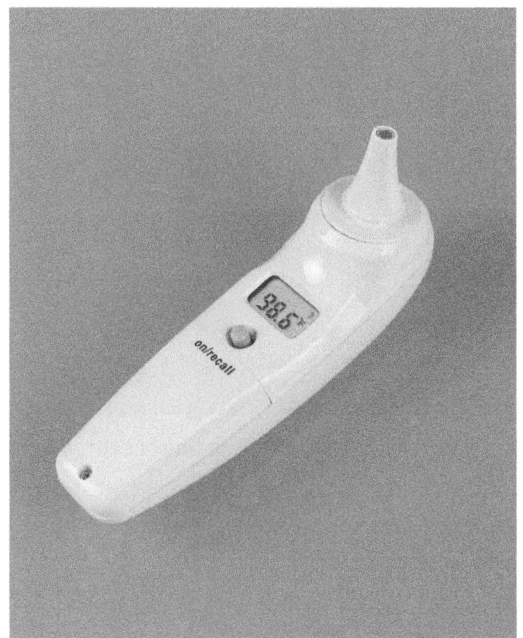

FIGURE 34-7 A tympanic membrane (aural) thermometer.

Figure 34-7 shows an example of a tympanic membrane thermometer. Procedure 34-5 lists the steps required to obtain a temperature reading using a tympanic membrane thermometer.

Disposable Thermometer

There are several types of single-use, disposable thermometers. A chemical disposable thermometer uses liquid dots, heat-sensitive bars, or patches applied to the forehead that change color to indicate body temperature (Figure 34-8). Procedure 34-6 lists the steps to measure body temperature using a heat-sensitive wearable thermometer. When using these unique thermometer devices, hold the thermometer in place for about 15 seconds and read the strip by noting the highest reading among the selection of dots that have changed color. Both the chemical disposable thermometer and the heat-sensitive wearable thermometer are excellent methods when dealing with small children or with large numbers of patients who need to be evaluated in rapid succession.

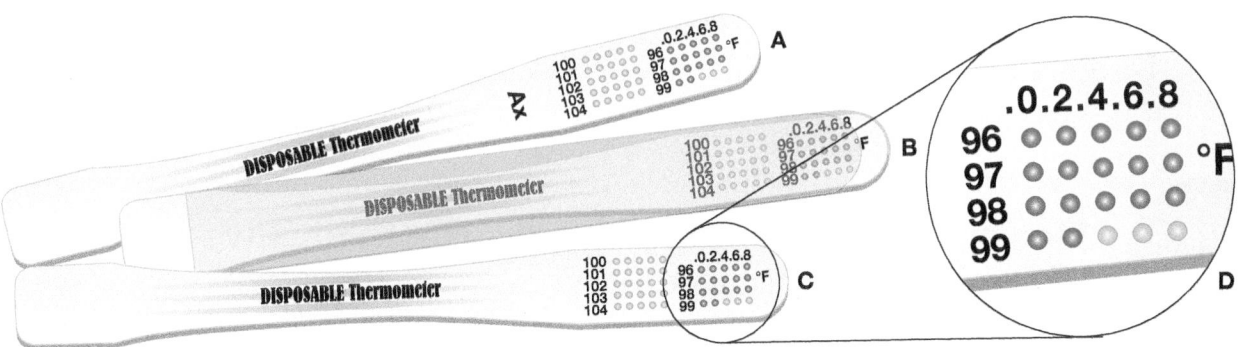

FIGURE 34-8 Disposable thermometers with chemical dots. **(A)** Axillary thermometer (marked "AX"); **(B)** rectal thermometer with plastic cover; **(C)** oral; **(D)** enlargement showing a reading of 99.2°F.

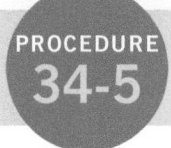

PROCEDURE 34-5

Measuring Temperature Using a Tympanic Membrane (Aural) Thermometer

Objective ◆ *Perform all steps of the procedure, and provide an accurate temperature reading.*

EQUIPMENT AND SUPPLIES

Tympanic membrane thermometer; disposable protective probe cover; paper and pen; patient's medical record; waste container

METHOD

1. Perform hand hygiene.
2. Greet and identify the patient.
3. Explain the procedure to the patient.
4. Remove the thermometer from its base. The display should read "Ready."
5. Attach a disposable probe cover to the earpiece.
6. With one hand, gently pull upward and out on the patient's outer ear if an adult. Pull back and downward if the patient is an infant or child (Figure A).
7. Gently insert the plastic-covered tip of the probe into the ear canal (Figure B).
8. Activate the thermometer by pressing the scan button.
9. Observe the temperature reading in the display window.
10. Gently withdraw the thermometer from the ear canal.

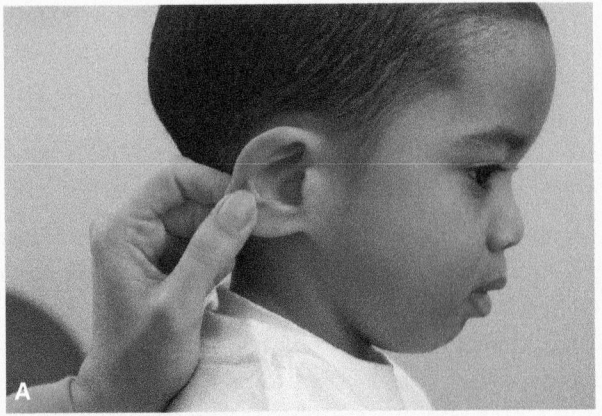
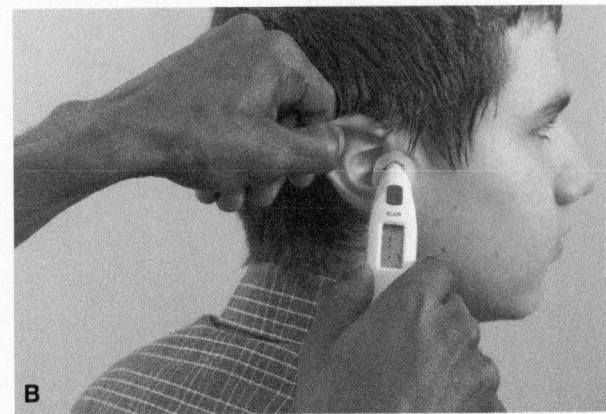

FIGURE A–B (A) Pull the outer ear downward and back for a child age 3 or under. **(B)** Gently insert the probe into the patient's ear canal while pulling the patient's ear (age 4 and up) upward and out.

11. Dispose of the used probe cover into a waste container by pressing the eject button.
12. Record the temperature in the patient's medical record, indicating a tympanic membrane temperature (T) was obtained and which ear was used.

13. Return the tympanic membrane thermometer to its base.
14. Perform hand hygiene.

CHARTING EXAMPLE

10/23/YY 4:00 P.M. T: 99.2°F Rt. (T) .... M. King, CMA (AAMA)

PROCEDURE 34-6

Measuring Temperature Using a Heat-Sensitive Wearable Thermometer

Objective ◆ *Perform all steps of the procedure, and provide an accurate temperature reading.*

EQUIPMENT AND SUPPLIES

Wearable heat-sensitive thermometer (chemical strip, liquid crystal); paper and pen; patient's medical record; tissue; watch with second hand; waste container

METHOD

1. Perform hand hygiene.
2. Greet and identify the patient.
3. Explain the procedure.
4. Dry the patient's forehead by patting it with a tissue. Do not rub the area.
5. Place the thermometer strip on the forehead (Figure A), and begin timing for 15 seconds.
6. After 15 seconds, read the correct temperature by reading the color changes.
7. Record the temperature in the patient's chart indicating the type of thermometer used.
8. Discard the strip in the waste container.
9. Perform hand hygiene.

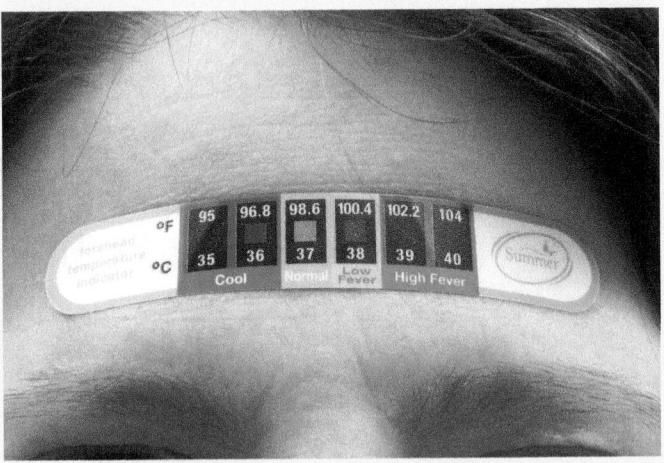

FIGURE A Temperature-sensitive skin tape.

CHARTING EXAMPLE

07/11/YY 9:08 A.M. T: 98.6°F (temp.-sensitive skin tape) ....
.... L. Kenney, RMA

Temporal Artery Thermometer

A temporal artery (TA) thermometer is a scanner that, when stroked gently across the forehead, measures the heat emitted through the skin from the temporal artery, which lies directly below. The instrument actually takes multiple readings per second and selects the most accurate. These devices have been gaining popularity in medical facilities because they are a quick, accurate, and noninvasive method of obtaining body temperature. They are also replacing the tympanic membrane thermometer, which was popular because of its less invasive nature. Temporal artery thermometers have the further advantage of not requiring proper patient positioning, as tympanic membrane thermometers do with the ear canal.

TA temperature is comparable to rectal temperature, about 1 degree Fahrenheit higher than oral temperature, and 2 degrees higher than axillary temperature. TA readings are not affected by factors such as smoking, drinking, or coughing that may interfere with oral measurements.

When measuring a TA temperature, assess the side of the head that is exposed rather than the side covered by hair or resting on a pillow. The latter may cause a higher reading because heat is not allowed to dissipate. Slide the thermometer in a fairly straight line across the forehead, starting at the center of the forehead and moving toward the temple. At this point, the temporal artery is less than 2 millimeters below the surface of the skin. Do not slide the thermometer down the side of the face. Procedure 34-7 lists the steps to measure body temperature using a TA thermometer.

PROCEDURE 34-7

Measuring Temperature Using a Temporal Artery Thermometer

Objective ◆ *Measure body temperature using a temporal thermometer.*

EQUIPMENT AND SUPPLIES
Paper and pen; patient's medical record; alcohol swab; temporal artery thermometer

METHOD
1. Perform hand hygiene.
2. Greet and identify the patient.
3. Explain the procedure.
4. Brush aside the patient's hair, tucking it behind the ear if necessary to keep it out of the way.
5. Remove the cap from the probe of the thermometer, and disinfect the probe by gently wiping it with an alcohol swab.
6. Place the probe flush on the center of the forehead, and depress the red button (Figure A).
7. Keep the button depressed, and slowly slide the probe at the midline across the forehead to one side of the head toward the hairline.
8. Lift the probe from the forehead, and touch it on the neck just behind the earlobe.
9. Release the button, and read the temperature.
10. Record the results in the patient's medical record, indicating the temperature was obtained via a temporal

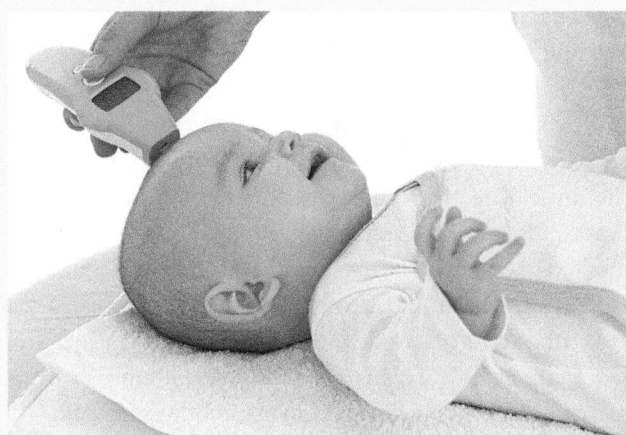

FIGURE A A temporal artery thermometer.

artery (TA) measurement and which side of the forehead.
11. Perform hand hygiene.

CHARTING EXAMPLE
12/18/YY 10:00 A.M. T: 100°F Lt. (TA) .... L. Cohen, CMA

TABLE 34-5 | Factors That Influence Pulse Rate

Exercise	Activity increases pulse rate. Rate may increase 20–30 bpm, based on the intensity of activity.
Age	As age increases, pulse rate decreases. Infants and children have a faster pulse rate than adults.
Gender	Female pulse rate is about 10 bpm higher than a male of the same age.
Size	Pulse rate is proportionate to the size of the body. Heat loss is greater in a small body, resulting in the heart pumping faster to compensate. Larger males have slower pulse rates than smaller males. During sleep and rest, the pulse rate drops.
Physical Condition	Athletes and people in good physical condition have lower pulse rates. The lower rate is a result of a more efficient circulatory system. Pulse rate of 60 or below can be normal for athletes.
Disease Conditions	Pulse rate is increased in certain disease conditions such as thyroid disease, fever, and shock because of increased metabolism.
Medications	Many medications can either raise or lower the pulse rate. Medications such as digoxin are given to regulate the heartbeat. Caffeine and nicotine can increase the heart rate in certain people. Drugs used recreationally, such as cocaine and methamphetamine, increase the pulse rate.
Depression	May lower the pulse rate.
Fear, Anxiety, Anger	May raise the pulse rate.

PULSE

Pulse rate is the number of times the heart beats per minute (bpm). During the cardiac cycle, the pulse is the wave of blood that courses through the body when the left ventricle contracts. After contraction, the heart rests as the cardiac muscle relaxes and the ventricle is filling with blood again. Each pulse beat represents one complete cardiac cycle or one heartbeat: contraction and relaxation.

In a healthy adult, a normal per-minute resting heart rate ranges from 60 to 100 beats a minute. With physical exertion, the muscles require more oxygen, resulting in an increased heart (pulse) rate and respiration (breathing) rate. The general method to calculate the maximum heart rate is to subtract the patient's age from 220. For example, if a patient is 45 years old, subtract 45 from 220 to get that patient's maximum heart rate of 175. This is the maximum number of times a person's heart should beat per minute while exercising.

A resting pulse rate above 100 bpm is considered to be a rapid pulse rate, or **tachycardia**, and a rate below 60 bpm is considered to be a slow pulse rate, or **bradycardia**.

Factors Influencing Pulse Rate

The pulse rate is influenced by numerous factors including exercise, age, gender, body size, physical conditions, disease states, medications, and emotional states, such as depression, fear, anxiety, and anger. Table 34-5 describes factors that influence pulse rate, and Table 34-6 lists average pulse rates based on age.

TABLE 34-6 | Average Pulse Rates by Age

Less than 1 year	120–160 bpm
2–6 years	80–120 bpm
7–10 years	80–100 bpm
11–16 years	70–90 bpm
Adult	60–80 bpm
Older adult	50–65 bpm

Characteristics of Pulse Rate

The following characteristics need to be taken into consideration when taking pulse rates and are often noted in the patient's record:

- **Rate** is the number of pulse beats per minute (bpm).
- **Volume**, or force, refers to the strength of the pulse when the heart contracts. Volume is influenced by the forcefulness of the heartbeat, the condition of the arterial walls, and hydration or dehydration. A variance in intensity of the pulse may indicate heart disease. The most common volume characteristics are:
  - A full or **bounding pulse**, indicating an increase in blood volume.
  - A weak or **thready pulse**, indicating a barely perceptible force or blood volume.

- **Rhythm** refers to the regularity, or equal spacing, of all the beats of the pulse. Normally, the intervals between each heartbeat are of the same duration. A pulse with an irregular rhythm is known as a **dysrhythmia** or **arrhythmia**. The irregular rhythm may be either a set of random irregular beats or a predictable pattern of irregular beats. An **intermittent pulse** occurs when the heart occasionally skips a beat. This is not considered abnormal if it does not happen frequently. Exercise or drinking a caffeine-rich beverage may cause this to occur. However, if arrhythmia occurs on a consistent basis, it may indicate heart disease and should be brought to the attention of the physician. If an irregular pulse is detected, the apical pulse should be assessed. The physician may also order further testing, such as an electrocardiogram (ECG), to further assess the arrhythmia.

Pulse Sites

There are nine areas in the body that allow for easy measurement of the pulse. These pulse sites are at the temporal, carotid, apical, femoral, brachial, radial, popliteal, posterior tibial, and dorsalis pedis arteries (Figure 34-9). Table 34-7 describes these nine common pulse sites, and Figure 34-10A–G illustrates the location of pulse sites on an actual patient. Procedure 34-8 provides the steps for accurately measuring a radial pulse.

Apical Pulse Rate

The **apical** pulse rate is counted at the apex of the heart (the lowest portion of the heart) with the use of a stethoscope that is placed over the apex. This is considered to be a very accurate heart rate and is most often used as the pulse

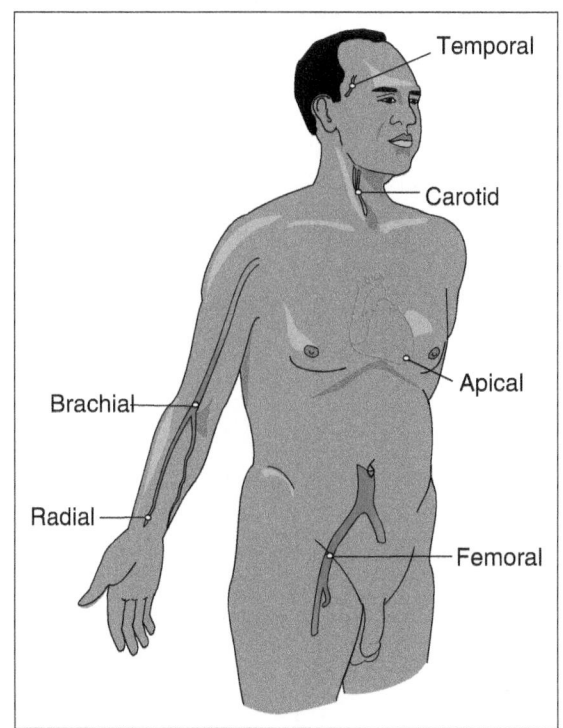

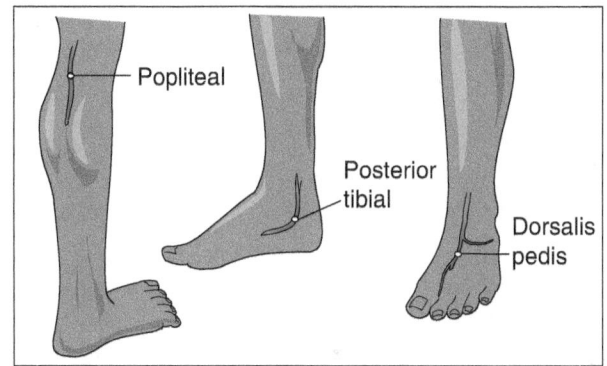

FIGURE 34-9 Nine pulse sites on the human body.

TABLE 34-7 | Location of Common Pulse Sites

Site	Location
Radial	Thumb side of wrist about 1 inch below base of thumb (most frequently used site)
Brachial	Inner (antecubital fossa/space) aspect of the elbow (pulse heard when taking BP)
Carotid	At side of neck between larynx and sternocleidomastoid muscle (pulse used in CPR)
Temporal	At side of head just above the ear
Femoral	In groin where femoral artery passes to leg
Popliteal	Behind the knee; pulse located deeply behind the knee and felt when knee is slightly bent
Posterior Tibial	On medial surface of ankle near ankle bone
Dorsalis Pedis	On top of foot slightly lateral to midline; helps assess adequate blood circulation to the foot
Apical	At apex of heart; left of sternum, 4th or 5th intercostal space below the nipple

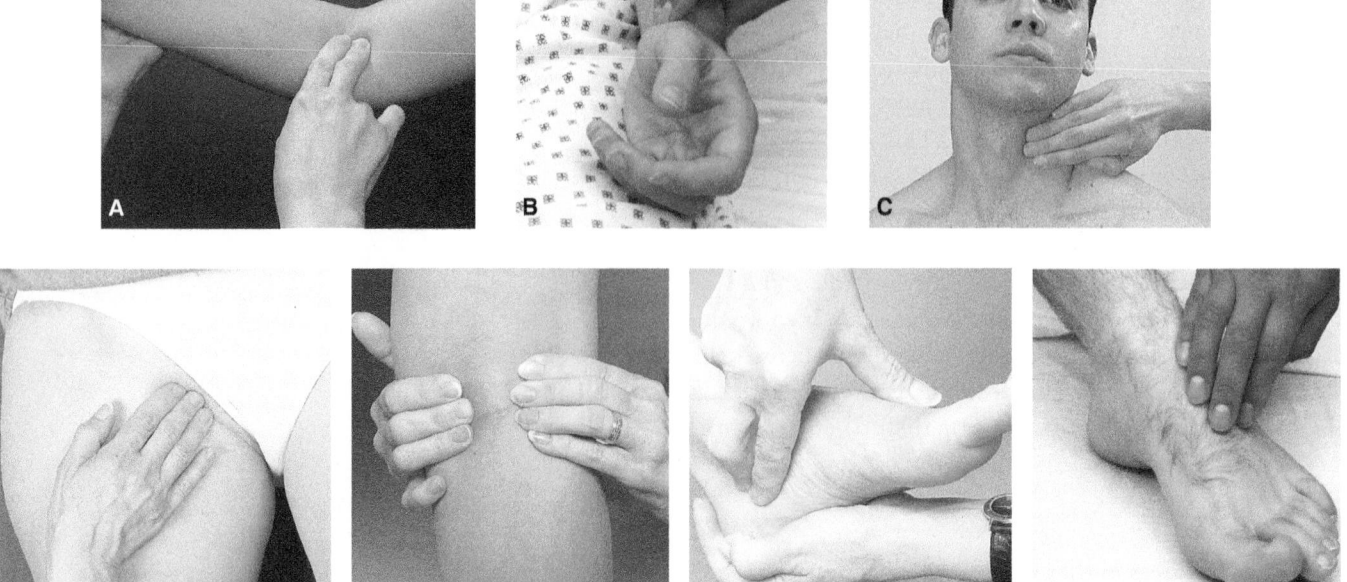

FIGURE 34-10 **(A)** Brachial pulse; **(B)** radial pulse; **(C)** carotid pulse; **(D)** femoral pulse; **(E)** popliteal pulse; **(F)** posterior tibial pulse; **(G)** dorsalis pedis pulse.

PROCEDURE
34-8

Measuring Radial Pulse

Objective ◆ *Perform all steps of the procedure, and provide an accurate radial pulse reading.*

EQUIPMENT AND SUPPLIES

Paper and pen; patient's medical record; watch with second hand

1. Perform hand hygiene.
2. Greet and identify the patient.
3. Explain the procedure.
4. Ask if the patient has recently smoked or performed physical activity. Both of these factors can cause the pulse rate to increase.
5. Ask the patient to sit down and place the arm in a comfortable, supported position. The hand should be at or below chest level with the palm facing up.

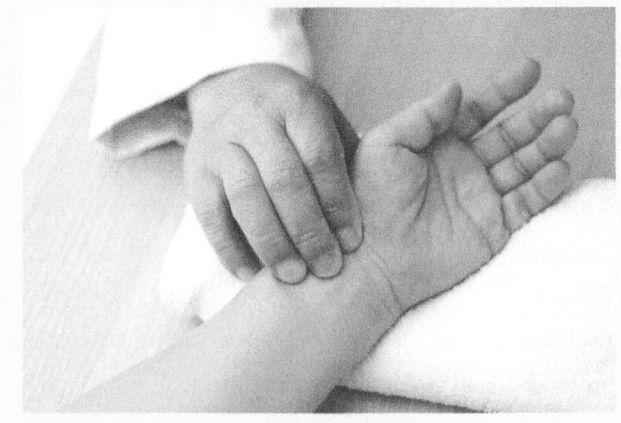

FIGURE A Measuring a patient's radial pulse.

6. Place fingertips on the radial artery on the thumb side of the wrist (Figure A).
   a. Apply enough pressure to feel the pulse. Use caution in pressing too hard because this may collapse the artery and interrupt the pulse.
7. Check the characteristics of the pulse for volume and rhythm.
8. Start counting pulse beats when the second hand on the watch is at 3, 6, 9, or 12.
9. Count the pulse for 1 full minute (60 seconds).
   a. Some medical offices may allow a count for 30 seconds, which is then multiplied by 2. When this is the case, the pulse rate will always be an even number.
10. Perform hand hygiene.
11. Record the pulse beats per minute in the patient's medical record, describing any characteristics or abnormalities in pulse rate.

CHARTING EXAMPLE

2/14/YY 4:00 P.M. P: 72 bpm, regular and strong .... M. King, CMA

measurement in infants and young children. The physician may also request an apical rate be taken when a patient is on heart medications.

Normally, a patient's pulse rates are the same, regardless of the location where they are taken. However, an apical–radial (A-R) pulse rate may be taken to determine if there is a difference between the pulse rates at the two sites. An A-R pulse must be taken for a full minute, rather than a 30-second count multiplied by two, which is common for pulse measurements at other locations. It is most often performed by two people, taking count at the same time. When taking an A-R pulse, have only one person responsible for using the watch. This person will raise one finger or nod the head when counting begins and lower the finger or nod again when a minute has passed. Coordination of timing is imperative when performing this procedure. When only one person is doing the procedure, the apical pulse rate is taken first and then the radial pulse rate.

After the A-R pulse is taken, the radial measurement is subtracted from the apical measurement to determine the **pulse deficit**. The radial pulse should never be greater than the apical pulse. A pulse deficit may indicate that the heart contractions are not strong enough to produce a palpable radial pulse. An A-R pulse will be performed only when ordered by the physician. Refer to Procedure 34-9 for taking an A-R pulse.

PROCEDURE 34-9 Measuring Apical–Radial Pulse (Two Person)

Objective ◆ *Perform all steps of the procedure, and provide an accurate apical–radial pulse reading.*

EQUIPMENT AND SUPPLIES

Stethoscope; alcohol wipe/cotton balls with 70 percent isopropyl alcohol; paper and pen; patient's medical record; watch with second hand

METHOD

1. Perform hand hygiene.
2. Disinfect the stethoscope using an alcohol wipe to cleanse the earpieces and diaphragm of scope.
3. Greet and identify the patient.
4. Explain the procedure. If the patient is a child, explain the procedure to both the parent and child.
5. Uncover the left side of the patient's chest. Provide privacy with a drape, if necessary.
6. The first person will place the earpieces of the stethoscope in her ears, with openings of the ear tips pointing forward.
7. Locate the apex of the patient's heart by palpating to the left fifth intercostal space (between the fifth and sixth ribs) at the midclavicular line, just below the nipple (Figure A).

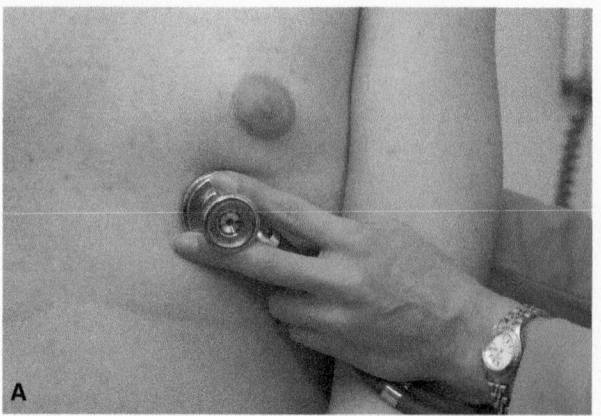
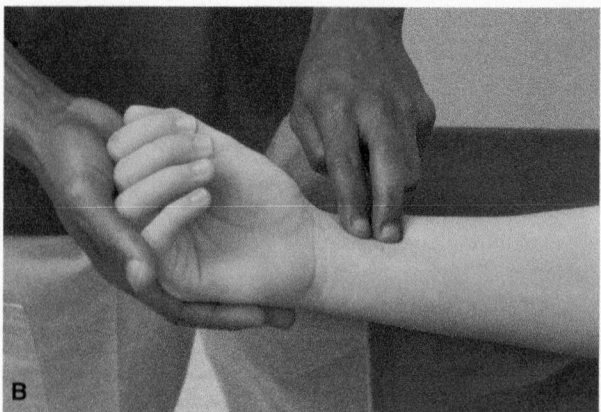
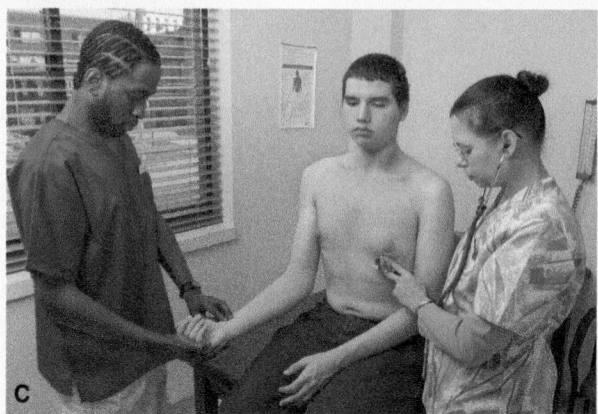

FIGURE A–C (A) The first medical assistant locates the apical pulse. **(B)** The second medical assistant locates the radial pulse. **(C)** One medical assistant takes responsibility for watching the time during the 1 minute of counting.

8. Warm the chest piece by holding it in the palm of the hand before placing onto patient's chest.

9. The second person will locate the radial pulse in the thumb side of the wrist, 1 inch below the base of the thumb (Figure B).

10. The first person places the chest piece of the stethoscope at the apex of the heart. When the heartbeat is heard, a nod is made to indicate to the second person that counting should begin. The count should begin when the second hand is at 3, 6, 9, or 12 (Figure C).

11. Count for 1 full minute (60 seconds), and nod to the second person when time is up and counting should cease.

Note: Both systole and diastole (or "lub/dub") counts as one beat.

12. Remove the stethoscope and earpieces.

13. Record the rate and quality of the heartbeats. Include both apical and radial rates using the designation "AP" and "R," respectively. Calculate the pulse deficit by subtracting the radial pulse rate from the apical pulse rate.

14. Assist the patient with dressing, if necessary, and from the examining table.

15. Wipe the earpieces and chest piece of the stethoscope with alcohol wipes or cotton balls and alcohol.

16. Perform hand hygiene.

CHARTING EXAMPLE

2/14/YY 4:00 P.M. P: 82 (AP), 78 (R); Pulse deficit 4. Quality of beat strong. .... M. King, CMA

RESPIRATION

Respiration, or the act of breathing, is the process of inhaling oxygen into the body and exhaling carbon dioxide. One respiration, also called the **respiratory cycle**, consists of one expiration (exhalation) and one inspiration (inhalation). Respiratory rate is an indicator of how well oxygen is being provided to the tissues of the body. Respirations are counted by watching, listening, or feeling the movement of inspiration and expiration on the patient's back, stomach, or chest. A stethoscope also may be used to assist with counting respirations.

Characteristics of Respiration

Medical assistants often observe and count a patient's respiration rate immediately after the pulse rate has been taken.

Respiration rates should not be measured if the patient has recently experienced exertion, such as climbing stairs or exercising, unless so ordered by the physician. When counting a patient's respiration rate, watch or feel the rise and fall of the chest. Each rise and fall constitutes one complete respiration.

The patient's respiration rate should be measured without the patient knowing. This is because, if patients are aware their rate is being measured, they will often exert control over their breathing rate, either consciously or subconsciously. It is recommended that you count respirations while you appear to be counting the pulse. This will result in a more accurate measurement of the patient's respiratory rate.

In general, the respiratory rate is one-quarter of the pulse rate. However, it is never appropriate to calculate a respiration by dividing the pulse rate by four. Respiration rates must always be counted and measured for one full minute (60 seconds).

When the respiration rate is taken, several characteristics should be noted: rate, rhythm, depth, and the quality or characteristics of breathing. Procedure 34-10 describes how to measure the patient's respiration rate.

Respiratory Rate

Respiratory rate is the number of respirations per minute. The normal respiration rate for healthy adults at rest is 12 to 20 cycles per minute. Children have a more rapid rate of breathing than adults, with an average of 30 to 60 cycles per minute, depending on age. Table 34-8 lists respiratory rates for various age groups. An adult respiratory rate below 12 (**bradypnea**) or above 20 (**tachypnea**) should be considered a

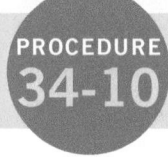

PROCEDURE 34-10 Measuring Respirations

Objective ◆ *Perform all steps of the procedure, and provide an accurate respiration measurement.*

EQUIPMENT AND SUPPLIES
Patient's medical record; watch with sweeping second hand; paper and pen

METHOD
1. Perform hand hygiene.
2. Greet and identify the patient.
3. Assist the patient into a comfortable position.
4. Place your hand on the patient's wrist in position to take the pulse, or place your hand on the patient's chest or back (Figure A).
5. Count each breathing cycle by observing or feeling the rise and fall of the chest, back, or upper abdomen.
6. Count for 1 full minute (60 seconds) using a watch with a second hand. If the rate is atypical or unusual in any way, count respirations again for another minute.
7. Record the respiratory rate in the patient's medical record, noting any abnormality in rate, rhythm, and depth.
8. Perform hand hygiene.

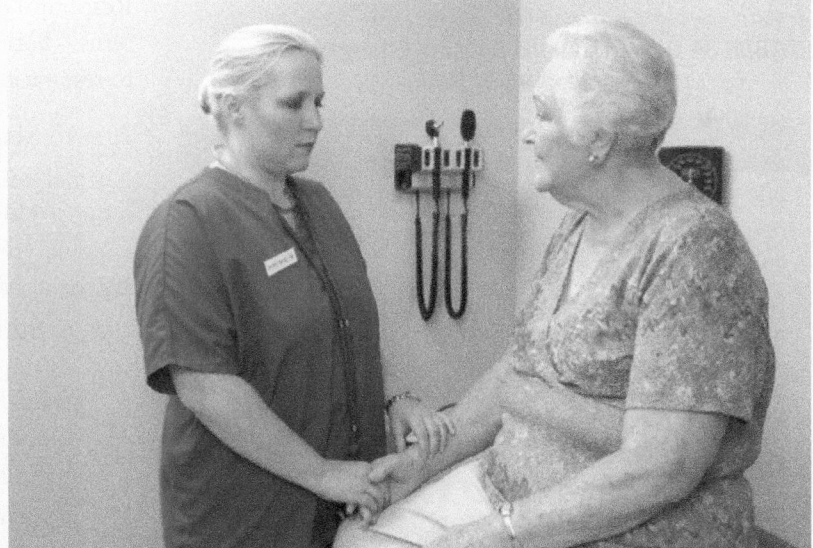

FIGURE A A patient who knows her respirations are being counted may alter her breathing, so the medical assistant counts respirations while appearing to be taking a pulse.

CHARTING EXAMPLE
2/14/YY 4:00 P.M. R: 20 and regular. .... M. King, CMA

TABLE 34-8 | Respiratory Rate Ranges of Various Age Groups

Newborn	30–50
1–2 years old	20–30
3–8 years old	18–26
9–11 years old	16–22
12–Adult	12–20

serious symptom and immediately brought to the physician's attention. Rapid respirations are usually shallow in depth because the lungs are unable to fully expand. **Apnea** means the absence of breathing for a period lasting longer than 19 seconds, and **eupnea** refers to normal breathing.

Many factors may affect the respiratory rate: elevated temperature, age, pain, medications, and some medical conditions. For example, an elevated body temperature in both adults and children can result in an elevated respiratory rate. Extreme pain may also cause respirations to increase. Table 34-9 lists situations that may affect respiratory rate.

Respiratory Rhythm

Respiratory rhythm, similar to pulse rhythm, refers to the regular and equal spacing of breaths. In a regular respiratory rhythm, the cycles of inspiration and expiration have about the same rate and depth. With irregular breathing patterns, the depth and amount of air inhaled and exhaled and the rate of respirations per minute will vary.

When you detect abnormalities in respiratory rhythm, continue assessment and measurement of breathing for 2 to 3 more minutes. This will help establish a more complete pattern of what is happening with the patient's respiratory cycle. Patients with emphysema may not experience difficulty with inhalation but may struggle to fully exhale. Asthma may also cause an irregularity in breathing rhythm.

Respiratory Depth

The depth of respiration is the volume of air that is inhaled and exhaled. It is described as either "shallow" or "deep." Rapid but shallow respirations occur in some disease conditions, such as high fever, shock, and severe pain. **Hyperventilation** refers to deep and rapid respirations, and **hypoventilation** refers to shallow and slow respirations.

When a patient is unable to take in enough oxygen during inhalation, the body becomes deprived of the amount of oxygen needed for proper functioning. If oxygen deprivation continues, the skin around the mouth and nail beds of the hands and feet may appear bluish in color because of the increase of carbon dioxide (CO_2). The resulting condition is called **cyanosis**. In this situation, you must note both the depth of respiration and the signs of cyanosis in the patient's record.

Respiratory Quality

Respiratory quality or character refers to breathing patterns—both normal and abnormal. Labored breathing refers to respirations that require greater effort from the patient.

Breath Sounds

Normal respirations do not usually have any noticeable sounds. However, certain diseases and illnesses can cause irregular respiration sounds. Terms for describing these abnormal breath sounds include the following:

TABLE 34-9 | Situations Causing Changes in Respiratory Rate

Increased Rate	Decreased Rate
Allergic reactions	Certain drugs (e.g., morphine)
Certain drugs (e.g., epinephrine)	Decrease of CO_2 in blood
Disease (e.g., asthma, heart disease)	Disease (stroke, coma)
Exercise	
Excitement/anger	
Fever	
Hemorrhage	
High altitudes	
Nervousness	
Obstruction of air passage	
Pain	
Shock	

- **Stridor**—A shrill, harsh sound, heard more clearly during inspiration but that can occur during expiration. This sound may occur when there is airway blockage, such as in children with croup and patients with laryngeal obstruction.

- **Stertor** (stertorous breathing)—Noisy sounds during inspiration, sounds similar to those heard in snoring.

- **Crackles** (also called rales)—Crackling sounds resembling crushing tissue paper, caused by fluid accumulation in the airways. Crackles can be further defined as coarse or fine. Crackles can be heard with pulmonary edema, asthma, early congestive heart failure, and some types of pneumonia.

- **Rhonchi**—Rattling, whistling, low-pitched sounds made in the throat. Rhonchi can be heard in patients with pneumonia, chronic bronchitis, cystic fibrosis, or COPD (chronic obstructive pulmonary disease).
- **Wheezes**—Sounds similar to rhonchi but more high-pitched, made when airways become obstructed or severely narrowed, as in asthma or COPD.
- **Cheyne-Stokes breathing**—Irregular breathing that may be slow and shallow at first, then faster and deeper, and that may stop for a few seconds before beginning the pattern again. This type of breathing may be seen in certain patients with traumatic brain injury, strokes, and brain tumors.

BLOOD PRESSURE

Blood pressure (BP) is one of the most important vital signs because it aids in diagnosis and treatment, especially for cardiovascular health. Blood pressure readings are almost always taken at every medical visit, even if it is the only vital sign obtained.

Blood Pressure Readings

Blood pressure is the amount of force exerted on the arterial walls while the heart is pumping blood—specifically, when the ventricles contract. Blood pressure is measured by gauging the force of this pressure through two specific readings: systolic and diastolic. **Systolic blood pressure** is the highest pressure that occurs as the left ventricle of the heart is contracting. **Diastolic blood pressure** is the lowest pressure level that occurs when the heart is relaxed and the ventricle is at

rest and refilling with blood. The pulse beat is felt (or heard) at the systolic pressure level and is absent at the diastolic pressure level.

While blood pressure is read in millimeters (mm) of mercury (Hg), or "mmHg," it is not necessary to reference millimeters of mercury when recording blood pressure readings in the patient's medical record. Blood pressure is recorded using just the systolic (highest pressure) reading over the diastolic (lowest pressure), similar to writing a fraction. For example, 120/80 would indicate a systolic pressure of 120 (mmHg) and a diastolic reading of 80 (mmHg). **Pulse pressure** is the difference between the systolic and diastolic readings and calculated by subtracting the diastolic reading from the systolic reading. If the blood pressure is 120/80, the pulse pressure is 40. In general, a pulse pressure that is *greater than 40 mmHg* is considered widened, and one that is *less than 30 mmHg* is considered to be narrowed. A widened pulse pressure may be an indicator for cardiovascular disease and anemia. A narrowed pulse pressure may be an indicator for congestive heart failure (CHF), stroke, or shock. Although pulse pressure is useful in predicting cardiovascular risk in patients, it should not be used alone and depends on various other factors, such as the patient's BP and age.

Measuring blood pressure as a routine part of office visits starts with children ages 5 and over. Readings on younger patients may also be obtained if it is considered medically necessary and ordered by the physician. Often, patients who are newly diagnosed with hypertension will have specialized office visits to routinely evaluate their blood pressure and to see if recommended lifestyle changes and/or medications are effectively lowering blood pressure. These office visits are generally short in length, 15 minutes or less, and are usually scheduled every 3 to 6 months once the patient's blood pressure is stable. Patients with sustained high blood pressure measurements may require more office visits and further diagnostic testing for the presence of other disease conditions to lower the blood pressure. It is important to control a patient's blood

---

Professionalism   The Life Span

As a medical assistant, you will assess vital signs on patients at both ends of the age spectrum. The following are a few considerations to keep in mind when dealing with infants:

- If an infant is crying, all vital signs will be increased. Try to calm the infant by having the parent hold the infant before obtaining the full set of vital signs.
- Always measure the infant's apical pulse when obtaining a pulse rate.
- When assessing the respiratory rate, try to calm the infant. Place your hand on the abdomen to feel inhalation and exhalation.
- When measuring the weight and length of an infant, safety should be your number one priority.

Professionalism   The Workplace

As a medical assistant, you should have your own personal equipment to help you perform your daily job functions. You should have your own stethoscope, which also helps to prevent the spread of infection among coworkers. You should also have a watch with a sweeping second hand so you can accurately count pulse and respiration rates.

pressure because it can lower that person's risk of stroke and heart attack.

Many patients experience "white coat syndrome," which is apprehension about visiting the physician. This apprehension may result in elevated blood pressure readings. Often these same individuals, when tested at home, have readings that are within the normal range. If a patient's blood pressure reading deviates higher from that person's normal range, blood pressure should be tested again before the end of the office visit.

Ideally, blood pressure is measured while the patient is seated in an upright position with both feet flat on the floor. Sitting with legs crossed at the knees can elevate blood pressure readings. If warranted by the patient's condition, blood pressure may be measured while the patient is lying down on an examination table. When this is the case, it should be properly noted in the patient's medical record.

A rise or fall in blood pressure is an indication for many medical conditions. Table 34-10 shows the recommended blood pressure range for healthy adults. Having a systolic above 120 mmHg and a diastolic above 80 mmHg are considered abnormal increases and may lead to **hypertension (HTN)**. As shown in the table, a patient may still have hypertension even if one measurement is low and the other high. This is called isolated hypertension.

Hypertension can be categorized as primary (essential) HTN or secondary HTN. Primary (essential) HTN has no known clear cause but it is thought to result from genetics, poor diet, lack of exercise, or obesity. However, many people who are healthy and frequently exercise may still have primary hypertension. In secondary HTN, the high blood pressure results from another medical condition, such as renal (kidney) or cardiovascular disease, pregnancy, or an endocrine disorder. Patients diagnosed with HTN may often be **asymptomatic** (without any symptoms), which is why it is often called the "silent killer." Other patients, however, may experience headache, blurred vision, and chest pain.

Hypotension is low blood pressure and may be a result of emotional shock, trauma, central nervous system disorders,

or medications. Symptoms of hypotension include dizziness and **syncope** (fainting).

Korotkoff Sounds

Korotkoff sounds, named after the Russian neurologist, Nicolai Korotkoff, are the rhythmic, tapping sounds heard while taking blood pressure as the arterial wall distends under the compression of the cuff. These sounds appear and disappear as the blood pressure cuff is inflated and deflated.

With the blood pressure cuff placed and inflated on the brachial artery, no sound can be heard through the stethoscope because the brachial artery is fully compressed and no blood is flowing through it. As the cuff deflates and air is slowly removed from the cuff, the Korotkoff sounds become audible.

There are five phases of Korotkoff sounds, sometimes denoted as Phase I–V or KI–V. The medical assistant should practice taking blood pressure readings slowly to be able to identify each phase. The systolic pressure is the measurement that is read when the first distinct clear tapping sound is heard as the cuff deflates, which is in Phase I. The diastolic pressure is the pressure measurement at which the last sound is heard, which occurs in either Phase IV or V. Some facilities and physicians measure the diastolic pressure at Phase IV when the sound changes from a clear tapping or thumping sound to a more muffled, softer sound. When the fourth sound is used as the diastolic pressure, three readings are often made: systolic, first diastolic (fourth Korotkoff sound), and second diastolic (last sound). Such a reading might be recorded as 138/86/78. Korotkoff sounds are described in Table 34-11 and Figure 34-11.

Blood Pressure Guidelines

Blood pressure readings can vary among adults, regardless of their health. Because of this, blood pressure ranges have been established to identify normal and abnormal blood pressure measurements. A deviation of 20 to 30 mmHg from the patient's baseline measurement can be a significant indicator of a change in health status for that patient. Average normal blood pressure readings by age are listed in

TABLE 34-10 | Blood Pressure Guidelines

Blood Pressure Category	Systolic (mmHg)		Diastolic (mmHg)
Normal	less than 120	and	less than 80
Prehypertension	120–139	or	80–89
Hypertension	140–179	or	90–109
Hypertensive Crisis (Emergency)	Higher than 180	or	Higher than 110

TABLE 34-11	Five Phases of Korotkoff Sounds
Phase I	This is the first faint sound heard as the cuff is deflated. The number that appears on the blood pressure gauge at that moment is recorded as the systolic pressure reading. The cuff must first be inflated to a level high enough to hear this first sound during relaxation. If the cuff is not inflated high enough and a pulse is heard immediately after deflation, stop the procedure, remove the cuff, wait a couple of minutes, and then start the procedure again, inflating the cuff at least 20 mmHg above the first attempt.
Phase II	The second phase occurs as the cuff continues to be deflated and more blood flows through the artery. This sound has a swishing quality. The cuff has to be slowly deflated to hear this soft sound. An auscultatory gap is said to have occurred if there is a total loss of sound that then reoccurs later. An auscultatory gap can occur in certain cases of heart disease and hypertension and should be reported to the physician.
Phase III	During this phase, the sound will become less muffled and develop a crisp tapping sound as the blood flow moves easily through the artery. If the BP cuff was not inflated enough to hear the Phase I sound, then the Phase III sound may be heard and incorrectly stated as the systolic reading.
Phase IV	This phase is characterized by the sound beginning to fade and become muffled. The American Heart Association, which believes Phase IV is the best indicator of the diastolic pressure, recommends the reading at this phase be recorded as the diastolic pressure for a child.
Phase V	Sound will disappear during this phase. Some physicians may require both Phase IV and Phase V recorded for the diastolic pressure reading.

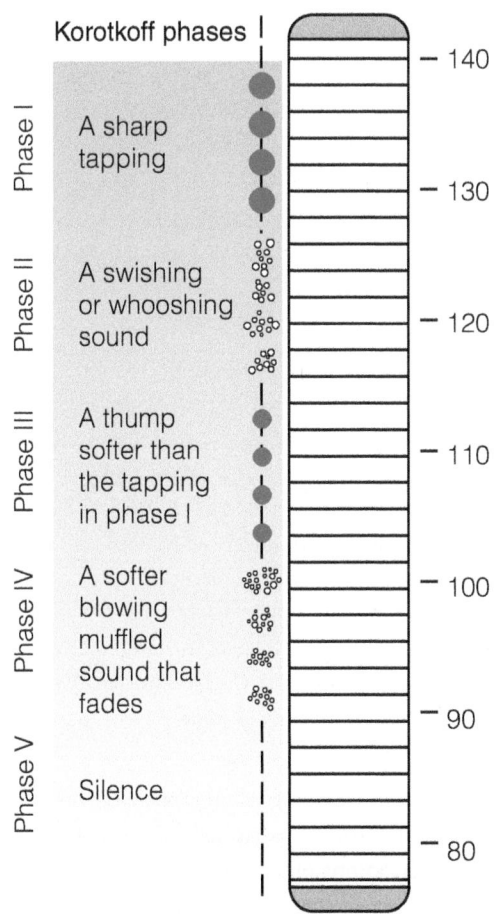

FIGURE 34-11 Phases of the Korotkoff sounds.

Table 34-12. Although an average blood pressure is listed for a newborn, blood pressure readings are not generally taken on infants.

TABLE 34-12	Average Normal Blood Pressure Readings	
Newborn	75/55
6–9 years of age	90/55
10–15 years of age	100/65
16 years to adulthood	118/76
Adult	119/78

Factors Affecting Blood Pressure

Many physiological factors may affect blood pressure, including volume or amount of blood in the arteries, peripheral resistance of the vessels, condition of the heart muscle, and elasticity of vessels. These four factors are discussed in Table 34-13.

In addition, other factors may affect blood pressure, especially gender and age. Women generally have a lower blood pressure than men. Blood pressure is lowest at birth and tends to increase as people age. The time of day can also cause blood pressure variations. For example, blood pressure is usually at its lowest early in the morning and just before waking. Activities such as standing, sitting, or lying down can affect blood pressure. Additionally, the blood pressure reading in the right arm is usually 3 to 4 mmHg higher than in the left arm, so it is often required to document which arm was used for the blood pressure reading. Numerous other situations that can affect blood pressure readings are listed in Table 34-14. Terms

TABLE 34-13 | Physiological Factors Affecting Blood Pressure

Volume of Blood	Increase of blood volume increases the BP. Decrease of blood volume decreases BP. *Example:* Hemorrhage (excessive bleeding) causes volume and BP to drop.
Peripheral Resistance	Relates to the size of the lumen (the cavity or space) within blood vessels and amount of blood flowing through it. *Example:* The smaller the diameter of the lumen, the greater the resistance to blood flow. Fatty cholesterol deposits result in high BP as a result of narrowing of the lumen.
Condition of Heart Muscle	Strength of the heart muscle affects volume of blood flow. The pumping action of the heart and how efficiently it circulates blood affect the BP. *Example:* A weak heart muscle can cause an increase or decrease in BP.
Elasticity of Vessels	The ability of blood vessels to expand and contract decreases with age. *Example:* Nonelastic blood vessels, as in arteriosclerosis, cause an elevated BP.

TABLE 34-14 | Causes of Blood Pressure Variations

Elevated/Increased BP	Lowered/Decreased BP
Anger	Anemia
Certain drug therapies, nicotine, caffeine	Approaching death
Endocrine disorders (hyperthyroidism)	Cancer
Exercise	Certain drug therapies (antihypertensives, narcotics, analgesics, diuretics)
Fear, excitement	Decreased arterial blood volume (hemorrhage)
Heart and liver disease	Decreased arterial BP
Increased arterial BP	Dehydration
Late pregnancy	Massive heart attack
Lying down position with legs elevated	Middle pregnancy
Obesity	Shock
Pain	Starvation
Renal disease	Sudden postural changes
Rigidity of blood vessels	Thyroid and adrenal disorders
Smoking	Time of day (during sleep and early morning)
Stress, anxiety	Weak heart
Taking pressure at the right arm	
Vasoconstriction or narrowing of peripheral blood vessels	

relating to abnormal blood pressure readings are described in Table 34-15.

Blood pressure is commonly measured while the patient is seated; measurements will vary depending on the patient's position. For example, the systolic pressure may be lower and diastolic pressure may be higher if the patient was supine (in a lying-down position). If the patient's arm is lower than the level of the heart, blood pressure measurements will be higher. Thus, when documenting blood pressure, it is important to indicate the patient's position if it is different than the normal seating position.

Orthostatic hypotension (or postural hypotension) refers to a drop in blood pressure that occurs when a patient changes positions from lying down or sitting to standing. Orthostatic hypotension can make you feel dizzy or lightheaded, and maybe even faint, especially if it occurs suddenly. Mild or short-term orthostatic hypotension often does not need treatment or further investigation. However, long-lasting orthostatic hypotension,

TABLE 34-15 | Terms Related to Abnormal Blood Pressure Readings

Benign	Slow-onset elevated blood pressure without symptoms.
Essential	Primary hypertension of unknown cause. It may be genetically determined.
Hypertension	A condition in which the patient's blood pressure is consistently above the norm for that patient's age group. Also called high blood pressure.
Hypotension	Condition of abnormally low blood pressure that may be caused by shock, hemorrhage, and central nervous system (CNS) disorders.
Malignant	Rapidly developing elevated blood pressure that may become fatal if not treated immediately.
Orthostatic (Postural)	A temporary fall in blood pressure caused by a sudden change in body position, such as a patient moving rapidly from a lying to a standing position. Dizziness and blurred vision can also be present.
Renal	Elevated blood pressure as a result of kidney disease.
Secondary	Elevated blood pressure associated with other conditions such as renal disease, pregnancy, arteriosclerosis, and obesity.

especially if a loss of consciousness occurs, may be a sign of a more serious underlying condition.

Although blood pressure is routinely measured at almost every office visit, it is especially important to obtain a measurement in the following patients:

- Patient is on antihypertensive drugs.
- Patient has a history of heart disease, diabetes, kidney disease, stroke, or hypertension.
- Patient (including children) is receiving a complete physical examination.
- Patient is pregnant.
- Patient is receiving preoperative or postoperative care.
- Patient is bleeding or in shock.
- Patient has symptoms of a neurological disorder.
- Patient is experiencing allergic reactions.

As with all vital signs, blood pressure readings should be interpreted in relation to the patient's baseline measurement. This means that the blood pressure reading taken when the patient was not ill should be used as that patient's "normal" measurement. All subsequent readings are then compared with that patient's "normal" baseline reading.

Equipment for Measuring Blood Pressure

Two pieces of equipment are necessary for measuring blood pressure: a sphygmomanometer and a stethoscope. The **sphygmomanometer**, more commonly referred to as a blood pressure cuff, is the instrument used for measuring the pressure that the blood exerts against the walls of the artery (Figure 34-12). The stethoscope is a diagnostic instrument that amplifies sound. It is used to detect sounds produced by blood pressure, as well as the heart and other internal organs such as the stomach.

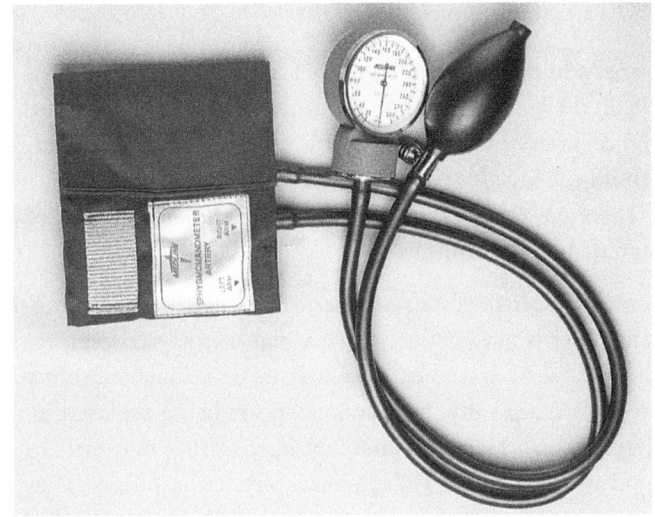

FIGURE 34-12 A portable sphygmomanometer.

Sphygmomanometer

The components of a sphygmomanometer are a manometer, inflatable rubber bladder, cuff, and bulb. The **manometer** is a scale that registers the actual pressure reading. The core of the blood pressure cuff is the rubber bladder, which is inflated and temporarily constricts blood circulation in the arm. A soft material cuff covers the bladder and is placed next to the skin of the patient. The pressure bulb has a thumbscrew attached to a control valve that allows for inflation and deflation of the cuff.

Using the correct-size blood pressure cuff is critical and will ensure a more accurate blood pressure reading. A cuff that is too large may result in a lower reading, and a cuff that is too small may result in a higher reading. Three sizes are available: a small cuff for a child (blood pressure cuffs are not generally used on infants) or a frail or small-limbed adult; a

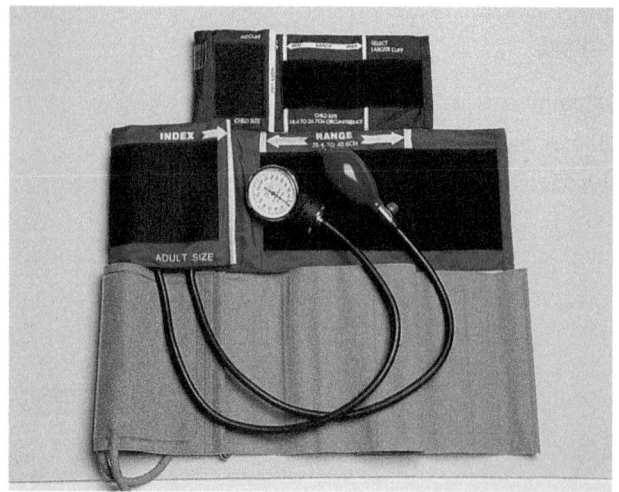

FIGURE 34-13 Three standard sizes of cuffs: a small cuff for a child or frail adult; a normal-size adult cuff; and a large-size cuff to measure blood pressure on the thigh or on the arm of an obese adult.

normal adult size; and a large size for measuring blood pressure on the leg (thigh) or on the arm of a large or obese adult (Figure 34-13). When a leg cuff is used, the popliteal artery (behind the knee) is palpated for a pulse.

There are three types of sphygmomanometers: mercury, aneroid, and electronic.

Mercury Sphygmomanometer. The mercury sphygmomanometer is not as widely used as the aneroid version (Figure 34-14). As stated earlier, mercury is a toxic substance and so mercury sphygmomanometers are being replaced for safety reasons. However, mercury instruments may still be found attached to the walls in many physicians' offices. They contain a column of mercury that rises as the pressure bulb is squeezed and the rubber bladder inflated. A calibrated scale

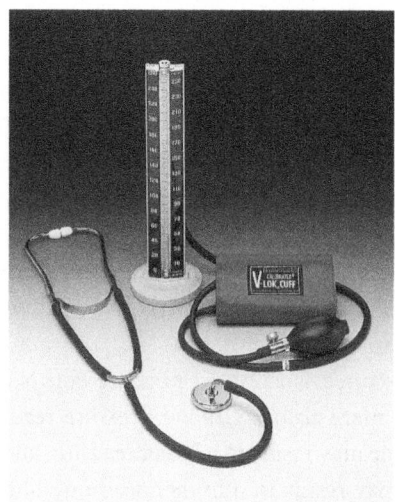

FIGURE 34-14 A portable mercury sphygmomanometer. Mercury versions are being phased out of medical offices and facilities.

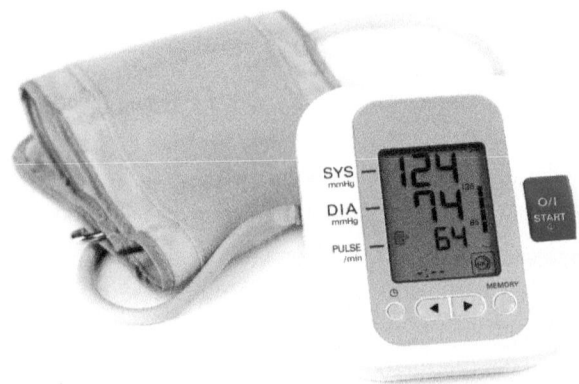

FIGURE 34-15 An electric sphygmomanometer.

runs down both sides of the mercury column. The reading is taken at eye level at the top of the mercury line next to a calibrated scale. This type of instrument must be placed vertically on the wall or on a flat, level surface so that the mercury will rise in a vertical position. Periodic recalibration is necessary to maintain accuracy.

Aneroid Sphygmomanometer. The aneroid sphygmomanometer has a round dial that contains a scale calibrated in millimeters (mm). A needle is attached to the scale to register the reading. The needle must be at zero before starting the procedure. The aneroid sphygmomanometer should be recalibrated for accuracy every year either according to the manufacturer's instructions or by comparing it with a properly calibrated model.

Electronic Sphygmomanometer. The electronic version provides a digital readout on a lighted display. It is easy to use and does not require a stethoscope (Figure 34-15). Many hospitals and outpatient facilities have adopted the electronic sphygmomanometers for their efficiency and accuracy.

Stethoscope

The stethoscope is used to detect sounds produced by blood pressure. This instrument consists of a chest piece containing a diaphragm and/or bell, flexible tubing, binaural, a spring mechanism, and earpieces. The key components of the stethoscope are described in Table 34-16 and shown in Figure 34-16A–B. Besides measuring blood pressure, stethoscopes are used to measure apical pulse, heart sounds, and respiration rates.

Measuring Blood Pressure

Try to ensure that the patient is relaxed before obtaining a blood pressure reading, which will result in a more accurate measurement. After greeting the patient, explain in a calm, quiet manner what the procedure will entail and that the procedure is not painful. To the majority of patients, a blood

TABLE 34-16 | Components of the Stethoscope

Chest Piece	Portion of the instrument that is placed over the site where the sound is to be heard. May consist of a diaphragm or a bell or both.
Diaphragm	A disc-like sound sensor that picks up both low- and high-pitched sound frequencies. More useful for high sounds such as bowel and lung sounds.
Bell	A hollow, curved bell or cup-shaped sound sensor that may have one, two, or three "heads" that are useful in picking up sounds of the cardiovascular system.
Flexible Tubing	Rubber or plastic tubing to carry the sound from the patient to the binaurals. The usual length of tubing is 12 to 14 inches. Some people prefer using longer tubing, up to 22 inches. However, some of the sound clarity is lost as the tubing becomes longer.
Binaurals	Rigid, small metal tubes that connect the tubing to the earpieces.
Spring Mechanism	Flexible external metal spring that holds the binaural steady so that the earpiece will remain in the ear.
Earpieces	Molded plastic tips that attach to the end of the binaurals and are placed in the medical assistant's ears.

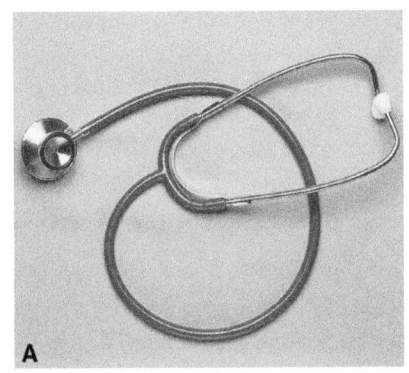 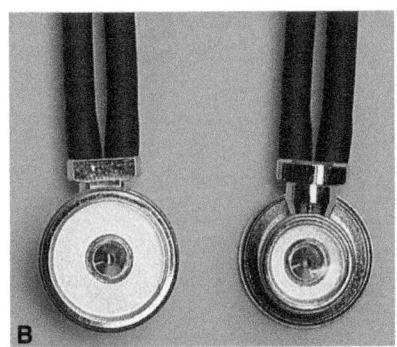

FIGURE 34-16 **(A)** Stethoscope with both a bell and flat disc amplifier. **(B)** Close-up view of a diaphragm amplifier on the left and a bell amplifier on the right.

pressure reading is not a new experience. Ask the patient if he has a history of hypertension and if the patient is aware of his normal blood pressure reading. This will guide you when you have to inflate the cuff (30 mmHg over the normal systolic pressure). It is also beneficial to check the patient's last recorded blood pressure readings from previous visits to serve as a guide.

If this is a new patient visit, a blood pressure reading should be obtained on each arm and recorded in the medical record. Procedure 34-11 lists the procedures for measuring systolic and diastolic blood pressures. Remember to be aware of your office protocol regarding informing patients of their blood pressure readings. Many offices require that the physician discuss the readings with the patient because it is the physician's duty to interpret and discuss results.

Causes of Error in Blood Pressure Measurements

Accuracy is very important in measuring blood pressure. Many diagnosis and treatment plans for a patient are based on a blood pressure assessment. Table 34-17 describes

common causes of errors while taking a patient's blood pressure. It should be noted that one measurement of high blood pressure does not make the diagnosis of hypertension. It usually takes two to three readings at several office visits to diagnose hypertension. Further, abnormal blood pressure measurements are often found with other conditions, such as kidney disease and stress.

OXYGEN SATURATION

For patients with cardiac and pulmonary disorders, it may be necessary to determine the oxygen content of the blood, or **oxygen saturation**. An electronic **pulse oximeter** is a device that can be clipped on the bridge of the nose, forehead, earlobe, or tip of a finger and can determine the oxygen concentration in arterial blood. A pulse oximeter is useful in measuring blood oxygenation even before clinical signs of hypoxia (reduced oxygen in the body tissues) are present. The oximeter measurement, reported as SpO^2 (saturation of peripheral oxygen), can help determine if treatment is

Measuring Blood Pressure

Objective ◆ *Obtain an accurate systolic and diastolic blood pressure reading.*

EQUIPMENT AND SUPPLIES

Sphygmomanometer; stethoscope; 70 percent isopropyl alcohol; alcohol sponges or cotton balls; paper and pen; patient's medical record

METHOD

1. Perform hand hygiene.
2. Assemble the equipment. Using an alcohol wipe or cotton ball with 70 percent isopropyl alcohol, thoroughly cleanse the earpieces, bell, and diaphragm pieces of the stethoscope. Allow the alcohol to dry.
3. Greet and identify the patient, and explain the procedure.
4. Assist the patient into a comfortable position. BP may be taken with the patient in a sitting or supine (lying-down) position.
   a. The patient's arm should be at heart level. If the patient's arm is below heart level, the BP reading may be higher than normal.
   b. Patients should be reminded not to cross their legs or talk during the procedure.
5. Uncover the patient's arm 5 inches above the elbow. If the sleeve becomes constricting when rolled back, ask the patient to slip the arm out of the sleeve.
   a. Never take a BP reading through clothing.
   b. Sleeves that are too tight, when rolled up, will produce an inaccurate result.

6. Locate the brachial artery within the antecubital space (bend in the elbow) by palpating with your fingertips. If the pulse is stronger in one arm than the other, use the arm with the stronger brachial artery pulse.
7. Have the patient straighten the arm with palm up and apply the proper-size cuff of the sphygmomanometer over the brachial artery 1 to 2 inches above the antecubital space (Figure A).
   a. Many cuffs are marked with arrows or circles to be placed over the artery.
   b. Hold the edge of the cuff in place as you wrap the remainder of the cuff tightly around the arm. If the cuff has a Velcro closure, press it into place at the end of the cuff (Figure B).
   c. The manometer should be at eye level for a more accurate reading.
8. With the fingertips of your nondominant hand, palpate the pulse in the radial artery. Then, with your dominant hand, tighten the thumbscrew on the hand bulb and pump air into the cuff quickly and evenly. Pump 20–30 mmHg above the point at which the radial pulse is no longer palpable. Make note of this point. Rapidly deflate the cuff and wait 60 seconds before continuing.

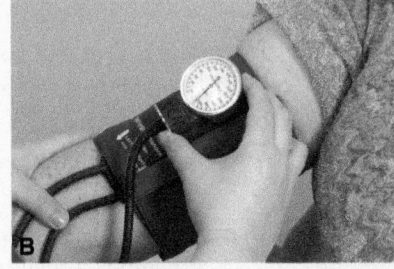

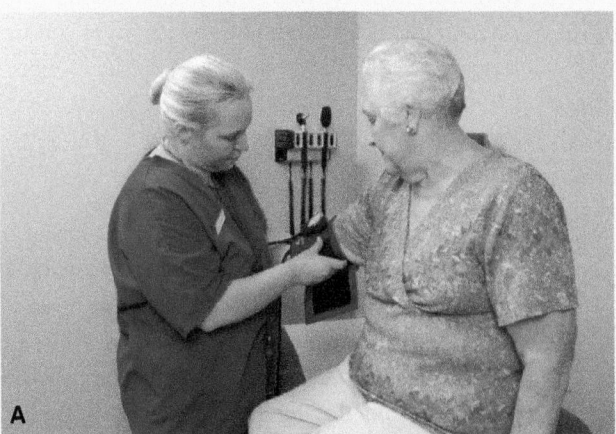

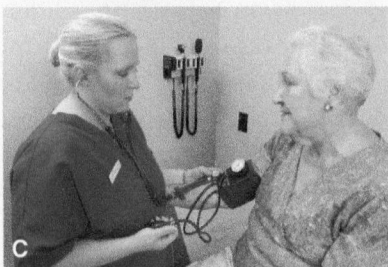

FIGURE A–C (A) Have the patient extend the arm, palm up, and apply the blood pressure cuff over the brachial artery, 1–2 inches above the antecubital space. **(B)** Hold the cuff in place, and wrap the remainder of the cuff tightly around the arm. **(C)** Place the earpieces in your ears and the diaphragm or bell of the stethoscope over the pulsating brachial artery.

9. Place the earpieces in your ears and the diaphragm (or bell) of the stethoscope over the area of the pulsating brachial artery (Figure C).
   a. Hold the diaphragm in place with your nondominant hand, and avoid covering the diaphragm.
   b. The stethoscope tubing should hang freely and not touch the patient or any object during the reading.
10. Close the thumbscrew by turning clockwise with your dominant hand on the hand bulb so no air leaks out. Do not close so tightly that you will have difficulty reopening it with one hand.
11. Pump the cuff to the point where the radial artery pulse is no longer palpable (step 9).
12. Slowly turn the thumbscrew counterclockwise with your dominant hand, allowing the pressure reading to slowly and evenly fall 2 to 3 mmHg at a time.
13. Listen for the point at which the first clear "bump" sound is heard (Phase I). Take note where this occurred on the manometer. This is the systolic pressure.
14. Slowly continue to allow the cuff to deflate. The sounds will change from loud to murmur and then fade away (Phases I, II, III, and IV). Take note where no sound or "bump" is heard on the manometer. This is the diastolic pressure (Phase IV or V).
15. Quickly open the thumbscrew all the way to release the air and deflate the cuff completely.
16. If you are unsure about the BP reading, wait at least a minute or two before attempting to take a second reading.
   a. Never take more than two readings in one arm, because blood stasis may have occurred, resulting in an inaccurate reading and discomfort for the patient.
17. Remove the cuff from the patient's arm.
18. Clean the earpieces and diaphragm or bell of the stethoscope with an alcohol wipe.
19. Perform hand hygiene.
20. Document the patient's BP as a fraction into the patient's medical record, making note of which arm was used and the patient's position.

CHARTING EXAMPLE
2/14/YY 9:00 A.M. B/P: 134/88 left arm, sitting ....
.... M. King, CMA

TABLE 34-17 | Causes of Error in Blood Pressure Readings

Equipment Errors	• Cuff is improper size. The cuff bladder should be 20 percent wider than the diameter of the extremity where the cuff is placed. Large cuffs for obese arms and small cuffs for children should be available in all offices. • Air leaks in the cuff bladder delay the inflation rate and could give a false high reading. Air leaks may also occur along the tubing if it is old or worn. • Sphygmomanometer is not properly calibrated. • Velcro on the cuff may be worn and does not hold.
Procedural Errors	• Patient's arm is not uncovered, and reading is obtained through clothing. • Medical assistant is too far away from manometer to accurately read gauge. • Cuff is improperly applied (too loose or too small). • Cuff is not centered over the brachial artery, 1 to 2 inches above the antecubital space. • End of the cuff is not secured tightly. • Part of stethoscope tubing or chest piece touches the blood pressure cuff while taking the pressure reading. • Failure to locate brachial pulse before placing stethoscope in position. • The rubber bladder in the cuff was not deflated completely before beginning the procedure. • Valve on bulb is not completely closed before beginning to pump air into cuff. • Cuff was not inflated to a level 20 to 30 mmHg above the palpated or previously measured systolic pressure or 200 mmHg. • Deflation occurs too rapidly to accurately determine the sounds. • The arm used for the reading is not at the same level as the heart. • Failure to wait 1 to 2 minutes before taking second reading. • Failure to notice the auscultatory gap.
Patient-Related Errors	• Patient is nervous or anxious, resulting in a false high reading (such as "white coat syndrome"). • Patient's arm is too large for accurate reading with available equipment.

needed. As the medical assistant, you may obtain a pulse oximetry reading as a part of the vital signs or when the patient presents with symptoms indicating respiratory distress. Figure 34-17 shows a pulse oximeter.

Normal oxygen saturation (SpO^2) is 95 to 100 percent. Oxygen treatment and bronchodilators may be initiated when the patient has a SpO2 reading below 90 percent. A reading below 70 percent indicates a life-threatening situation.

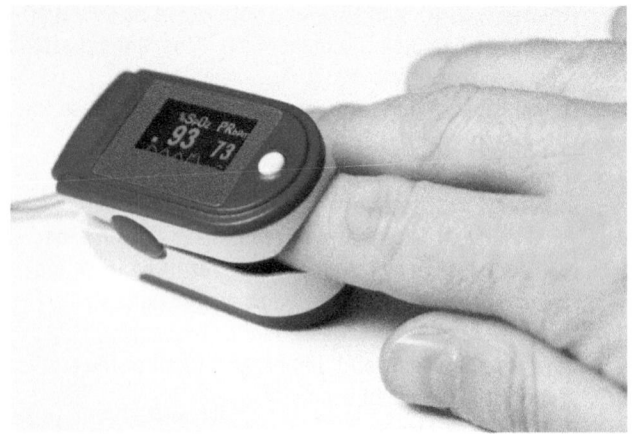

FIGURE 34-17 A pulse oximeter.

Pulse oximeters are selected based on the patient's age, size, and condition. In an adult patient, the fingertip pulse oximeter is generally used. Nail polish should be removed before attaching the pulse oximeter so that the polish does not produce an inaccurate result. See Procedure 34-12 for how to use a pulse oximeter to measure oxygen saturation.

SUMMARY

Vital signs are an important objective indication of the patient's overall physical condition. One vital sign measurement taken alone does not necessarily provide a complete picture. Thus, the medical assistant must be able to skillfully take all vital measurements and be able to assess what she is observing, and whether the observations are considered normal based on the patient's age, gender, and physical condition.

The accuracy of obtaining and recording vital sign measurements is critical for the diagnosis and treatment of the patient. Measurements, such as height and weight, are an

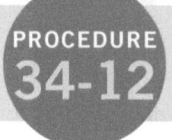

Measuring Oxygen Saturation

Objective ◆ *Attach an oximeter, and measure oxygen saturation of patient.*

EQUIPMENT AND SUPPLIES

Pulse oximeter; nail polish remover; alcohol wipe; patient's medical record

METHOD

1. Perform hand hygiene.
2. Assemble equipment based on the type of sensor that will be used.
3. Warmly greet and identify the patient and explain the procedure.
4. Wipe the selected finger with an alcohol wipe, and allow it to air-dry. Remove nail polish as needed.
   a. If circulation is poor in the patient's hands, select an alternative location, such as the patient's feet, earlobe, or bridge of the nose.
5. Turn on the oximeter device, and verify it is properly functioning.
6. When prompted, attach the device to the patient's finger and wait for the beep (Figure A).
7. After the beep, record the oxygen saturation level in the patient's medical record as SpO_2 and a percentage.
8. If the oxygen saturation level is abnormal, immediately notify the physician of the results.

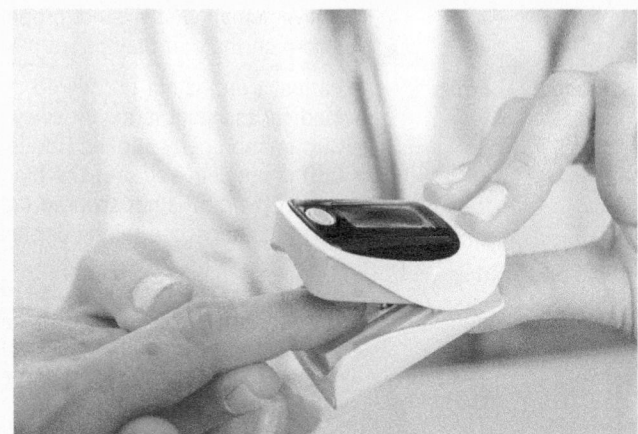

FIGURE A A fingertip oximeter.

9. Perform hand hygiene, and return the oximeter to its storage location.

CHARTING EXAMPLE

11/11/YY 9:15 A.M. HT: 67" WT: 186 lb P: 74 bpm BP: 136/84 SpO_2: 97%............ L. Morton CMA

important part of patient examination. Changes in height and weight can be indicators of a metabolic condition or other diseases that could affect the body. Body temperature is regulated by the hypothalamus, and slight fluctuations in temperature are normal throughout the day. A fever, or increased body temperature, can be indicative of an infection within the body. Pulse rate varies based on the patient's age, with infants having faster pulse rates and adults having slower pulse rates. Various factors can cause the pulse rate to increase or decrease. Medical assistants must be able to accurately measure the rate and quality of a patient's pulse. Respiratory rate is the number of times that a patient breathes (one complete inhalation and exhalation) in a minute. Respiration must also be assessed in regard to quality, specifically the rhythm and depth. Blood pressure measures the amount of force that is placed on the arterial walls during ventricular contraction. High blood pressure (or hypertension) is considered the "silent killer" because it often presents as asymptomatic in the patient. Thus, medical assistants must be able to obtain blood pressure measurement, as well as the other vital sign measurements, with accuracy and competency.

Although important in all aspects of medical assisting work, communication skills are essential when obtaining vital measurements. A positive and empathetic approach when interacting with patients will put the patient at ease and may result in obtaining more valid vital sign measurements.

34 CHAPTER REVIEW

COMPETENCY REVIEW

1. Define and spell the terms for this chapter.
2. Identify the formula for converting pounds to kilograms and vice versa.
3. Name five factors that affect body temperature.
4. Name the four types of fever.
5. What characteristics are considered when assessing respirations?

6. Explain what systolic and diastolic readings are.
7. What is the desirable range for blood pressure in an adult?
8. Name and locate the different pulse sites.
9. Why is hypertension referred to as the silent killer?
10. Explain orthostatic hypotension.

PREPARING FOR THE CERTIFICATION EXAM

1. An abnormally slow pulse rate is
   a. extrasystole.
   b. tachycardia.
   c. thready pulse.
   d. pulse volume.
   e. bradycardia.

2. Systolic pressure of 140 or above is referred to as
   a. bradycardia.
   b. tachycardia.
   c. hypertension.
   d. hypotension.
   e. pulse pressure.

3. Normal pulse rate for an adult is
   a. 12–20.
   b. 40–60.
   c. 60–100.

   d. 90–100.
   e. 100–200.

4. The normal rate of respiration per minute for adults is
   a. 6–10.
   b. 10–13.
   c. 12–20.
   d. 18–22.
   e. 22–28.

5. Although often taken at an office visit, which of the following is *not* considered a vital sign?
   a. weight
   b. respiration
   c. pulse
   d. temperature
   e. blood pressure

6. Which of the Korotkoff sounds represents the systolic pressure?
   a. absence of sound
   b. the muffled sound
   c. the first distinct sound
   d. the change of sound
   e. the light tapping sound

7. The term used to describe difficult or labored breathing is
   a. apnea.
   b. eupnea.
   c. orthopnea.
   d. tachypnea.
   e. dyspnea.

8. If a patient has a normal oral temperature, what is the patient's rectal temperature reading?
   a. 97.6°F
   b. 99.6°F

   c. 30.0°C
   d. 34.0°C
   e. 36.8°C

9. If pulse is taken at the wrist, the artery used is the
   a. temporal.
   b. carotid.
   c. popliteal.
   d. femoral.
   e. radial.

10. An increase in pulse rate may be caused by
    a. fever.
    b. pain relievers.
    c. mental depression.
    d. rest.
    e. chronic disease.

CRITICAL THINKING

Refer to the case study at the beginning of the chapter and use what you have learned to answer the following questions.

1. Elanya's vital signs are almost normal based on her age; however, one vital sign is out of range. Identify the vital sign that is out of range and indicate what it should be, based on Elanya's age.

2. The physician would like to prescribe Elanya a medication for her headaches. The medication dosage is based on body weight in kilograms. What is Elanya's body weight in kilograms?

3. Would the pain that Elanya is experiencing because of her headaches have influence on her vital signs? Explain your answer.

ON THE JOB

Lakisha Smith is working in an OB/GYN clinic affiliated with a major teaching hospital. Her general responsibilities include registering patients, handling phone calls when the receptionist is on a break, escorting patients into the examination room, taking vital signs, running selected laboratory tests, setting up the clinic examination rooms for gynecological examinations, and providing patient education.

The following is the morning's schedule of patients and visitors:

9:00 Adele Bishop	New mother checkup
9:15 Amy Campbell	First OB visit
9:30	
9:45 Maria Lopez	OB patient in last month of pregnancy
10:00 Meg Rivers	Regular OB checkup
10:15 Vanessa Brown	New gynecology patient w/ovarian cyst
10:30	
10:45 Tiffany Baker	Regular OB checkup
11:00 Vern Simmons	Pelvic inflammatory disease
11:15 Latonya Pike	1st visit after miscarriage
11:30 Emma Thompson	Yearly checkup, gynecology patient
12:00 Lunch break	

During the morning, the following occurs:

When Maria Lopez arrives, she tells Lakisha that she has been bleeding since the weekend.

A pharmaceutical representative comes in at 10:00 A.M. and asks to see the doctor.

Supplies are delivered that must be signed for.

Dr. Williams is called away to perform a childbirth at 11:00 A.M.

Vital signs including TPR, BP, and weight are taken for all OB patients.

Urinalysis is performed by another medical assistant assigned to the clinic laboratory.

What are your responses to the following?

1. How should Lakisha handle the pharmaceutical representative?
2. Should Maria Lopez's bleeding be considered an emergency? If so, what is Lakisha's responsibility?
3. Because Dr. Williams was called away for a childbirth, how should the patients be rescheduled? What about the patients who are already in the waiting room?

INTERNET ACTIVITY

Go to the American Heart Association website, and look for dietary guidelines for hypertension.

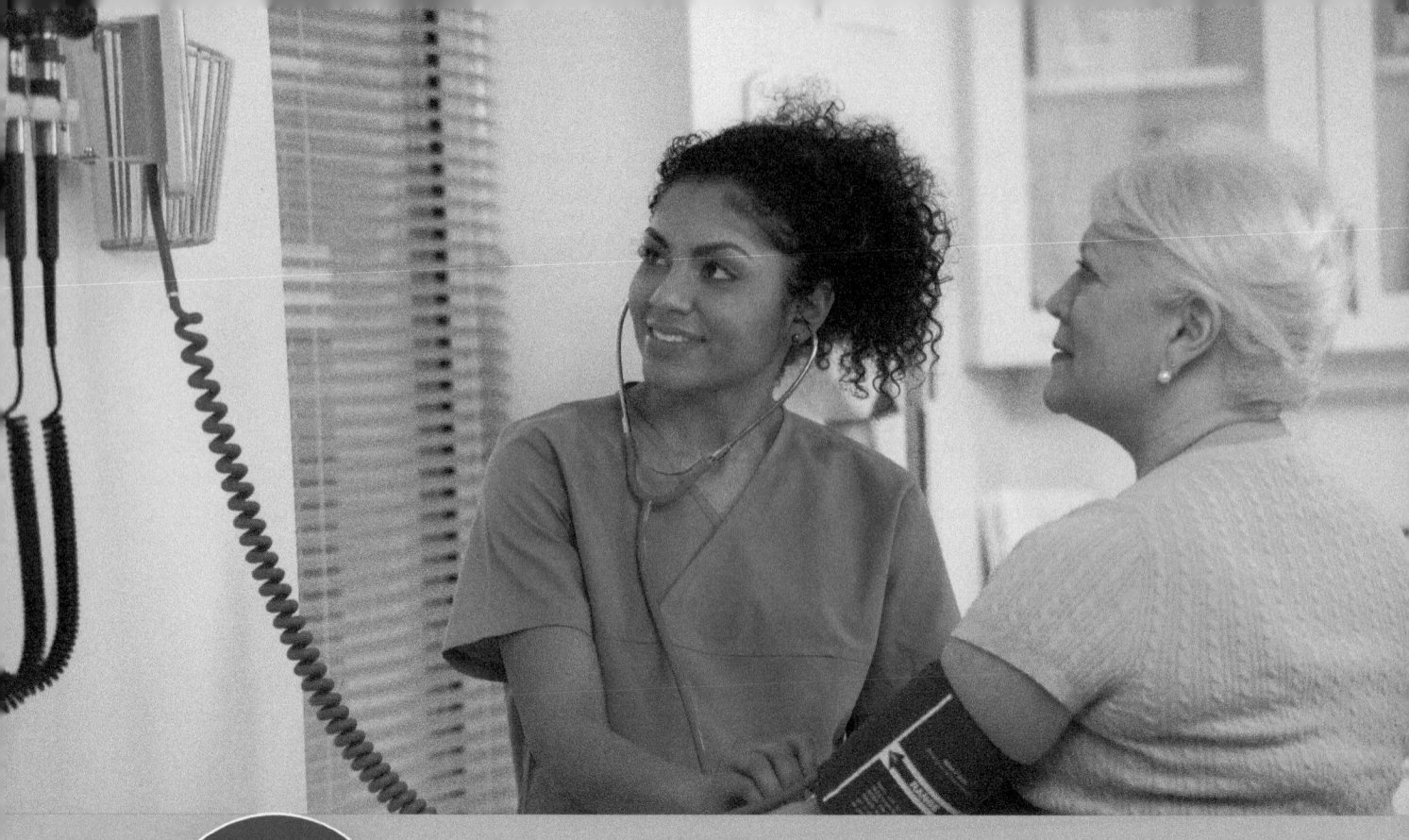

CHAPTER

35

Assisting with Physical Examinations

Learning Objectives

After completing this chapter, you should be able to:

35.1   Define and spell the terms for this chapter.

35.2   Identify key components to preparing an examination room.

35.3   Describe effective communication as it relates to interviewing a patient.

35.4   Outline six topics that should be covered when obtaining patient histories.

35.5   Differentiate between subjective and objective information when obtaining a chief complaint.

35.6   List descriptive terms associated with pain.

35.7   List equipment that is commonly found in an examination room.

35.8   Describe the six main methods of examination used by the physician.

35.9   Explain the medical assistant's role when assisting with a physical examination.

35.10   Describe the types of positions used for patient examinations.

35.11   Identify how a physician conducts a review of systems in sequential order.

Molly McConnley has arrived at Pearson Physicians Group for her appointment with Dr. Miller. The medical assistant, Susan Schultz, CMA (AAMA), escorts Molly to the examination room and asks what brings her to the medical office today. Molly responds by saying, "I am here for my annual physical and Pap test."

Terms to Learn

acute pain	inspection	pinwheel
amplify	intractable pain	present illness (PI)
auscultation	laryngeal mirror	prognosis
bimanual	manipulation	radiating pain
chief complaint (CC)	mensuration	referred pain
chronic pain	objective	reflex hammer
clinical diagnosis	onset	review of systems (ROS)
diagnose	ophthalmoscope	speculum
differential diagnosis	otoscope	subjective
duration	palpation	tuning fork
fenestrated drape	percussion	turgor
frequency	phantom pain	vaginal speculum
goniometer		

One of the key responsibilities of the medical assistant is assisting the physician with a patient's physical exam. The medical assistant's role in the physical exam includes preparing the exam room before the patient visit, taking the patient's medical history, documenting information in the patient's medical record, positioning and draping the patient, assisting the physician during the examination and in any procedures, cleaning the room after the visit, and instrument care.

THE EXAMINATION ROOM

The examination rooms in doctors' offices and other facilities may vary in size, layout, and type of equipment used. For example, an examination room that is used for general examinations will look very different than a room used specifically for procedures, such as sigmoidoscopies or minor surgical procedures. As a medical assistant, you must become familiar with the layouts and equipment of the examination rooms in the offices and facilities where you will be employed.

Preparing the Examination Room

Examination room preparation takes place at the beginning of each day and between patients. At the beginning of the day, check to make sure that the room is adequately stocked with supplies and ensure that the equipment is properly functioning. It is also important that the examination rooms be cleaned properly between patients.

The following is a list of tasks necessary for preparing examination rooms between patients:

- Dispose of used patient gowns and drapes by rolling them into a ball and placing them in the laundry receptacle or in the garbage can if the gown and drapes are disposable. Carefully rolling the items into a ball will help contain the items and keep possible contamination away from your uniform or clothing.
- Clean the examination table with the proper disinfectant, and allow it to dry before placing new paper on the table.
- The paper covering the exam table must be replaced between patient uses. If available, change pillow covers after each patient.

- Disposable equipment used during the previous examination must be discarded in the appropriate containers. Reusable equipment must be taken to the appropriate area for cleaning and disinfection, following standard precautions.
- Focus cleaning on high-touch surfaces: exam bed; blood pressure cuff; stethoscope; wall-mounted ophthalmoscope and otoscope (per manufacturer's instructions); chair and bedside stool; and doorknob.

Proper time management is important in preparing examination rooms. Each room must be thoroughly and efficiently cleaned between patients. However, if a disinfectant is being used, a proper amount of time must pass before bringing patients to the examination room to prevent patients from being exposed to any cleaning chemicals recently used.

No evidence of any other patient should remain when a new patient is taken into an examination room. See Procedure 35-1.

Examination Room Features

Besides the size and layout of examination rooms in different medical offices or facilities, the number of available examination rooms for use by each physician and the equipment found in each room will vary. A standard examination room is most often furnished with an examination table (with stirrups in a practice where pelvic exams are performed), a pillow, a footstool, a supply cupboard, a trash can, biohazardous waste and sharps containers, a rolling stool, and a chair. Sometimes a writing surface and a sink are present. For specialist physicians, diagnostic equipment specific to the practice may also be present. All instruments and equipment to be used during an examination should be readily available for use by the physician. Equipment should be properly stored, and not left on countertops or within reach of the patient. Proper storage both ensures patient safety and avoids the possibility of damaging expensive medical equipment.

PROCEDURE 35-1

Cleaning the Examination Room

Objective ◆ *Clean an examination room to instructor specifications.*

EQUIPMENT AND SUPPLIES

Disinfectant; paper towels; disposable gloves; examination table; pillow; pillow cover; disposable gown; examination table paper

METHOD

1. Perform hand hygiene and don a pair of disposable gloves.
2. Roll the soiled disposable gown into a ball and dispose of it in the appropriate waste container.
3. Roll the soiled examination table paper into a ball and dispose of it in the appropriate waste container.
4. Remove the soiled pillow cover and dispose of it in the appropriate waste container.
5. Remove any other soiled items or equipment from the examination room, discarding them in the appropriate waste containers.
6. Clean the examination table, countertops, and cabinet surfaces with disinfectant and paper towels (Figure A).
7. Dispose of the soiled paper towels in the appropriate waste container.
8. Remove the soiled gloves and dispose of them in the appropriate waste container.

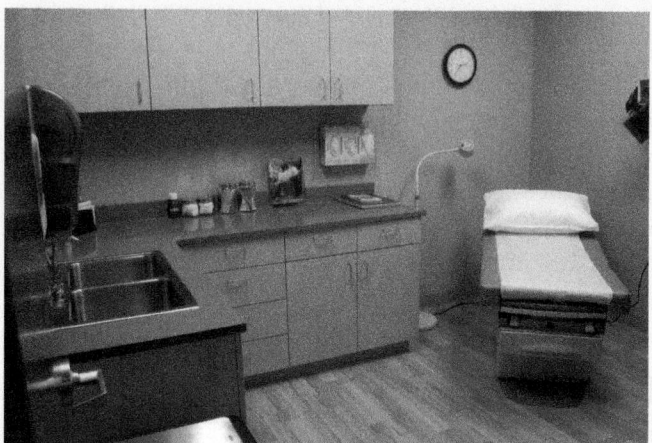

FIGURE A Examination room.

9. Perform hand hygiene.
10. Put clean paper on the examination table.
11. Put a new pillow covering over the pillow.
12. Perform a second check, making sure the examination room is clean and free of clutter and odor.

All examination rooms should be large enough so that the physician, patient, and medical assistant do not feel cramped or confined.

Examination Room Safety

Examination rooms must conform to the standards established by the Americans with Disabilities Act (ADA). These federal standards were designed to make sure that people with disabilities are not discriminated against in public places because of a lack of proper accommodations to meet their needs. These standards address such things as the width of doorways and hallways; placement of door handles, grab bars, and handrails; spatial accommodations for patients in wheelchairs; and floor surfaces. For further information about the ADA Standards for Accessible Design, visit the ADA website: www.ada.gov.

If there are any unsafe situations, they must be addressed immediately. Unsafe situations might include clutter in the hallway or examination room, a spill on the floor, or equipment left lying around where a patient, especially a child, could get hold of it. Clutter, spills, improperly stored equipment, and unsecured electrical cords or cables are unsafe for both patients and medical office staff. As a medical assistant, you must make sure all electrical cords and cables are secured to the floor or wall.

All furniture in the examination room should be checked routinely for proper maintenance. Items such as a broken drawer, a sharp edge on the countertop, or a broken hinge on a door must be immediately reported. If it cannot be repaired right away, you must document the situation in the maintenance log book.

Patient Comfort

A patient's comfort should be of utmost importance. One of the most common patient complaints is about the temperature in the office. Some patients feel too hot; others feel too cold. Most medical offices keep the thermostat around 71°F to 73°F, but a temperature should be decided on by either the office manager or the physicians. In the examination rooms, patients often change into thin, disposable gowns. It is good practice to keep extra drapes or blankets available for patients who may get too cold while waiting in the examination room.

When the patient enters the examination room, it should smell both fresh and clean. Good ventilation can help decrease offensive odors. Offensive odors can come from sweat, urine, feces, vomit, blood, and infectious wounds, as well as from disinfectants recently used to clean the room. If you detect an offensive odor, try to find the source and eliminate it. For instance, if a chair smells from sweat, remove it from the examination room and replace it with a new chair until the soiled chair can be properly cleaned. Items soaked in urine, feces, blood, or infectious waste must be immediately double-bagged and then taken to the designated location where soiled items are stored for either permanent removal or laundering. Once you have eliminated the source of the offensive odor, you can concentrate on removing any of the odor that lingers in the air. Room deodorizer sprays and air fresheners can be useful for these purposes. The examination room can also be left unoccupied until the unpleasant odor dissipates.

Patient Privacy

Patients' privacy should be maintained at all times, especially while they are in the examination room. Before entering an examination room that is occupied by a patient, always knock before entering, announce yourself, and ask for permission to enter. Do not enter the room until the patient has expressed consent. This will help reassure patients that their privacy is respected. For example, if a patient is in the middle of getting dressed and the medical assistant walks into the examination room without permission, the patient may become upset or embarrassed.

Medical assistants should be sure that gowns of all sizes are available for patients who are required to change clothing for an examination or a procedure. Be sure to inform patients where their personal clothing and belongings can be stored during the examination.

Properly draping patients to protect their modesty is important to patients' comfort during an examination. Draping techniques are discussed later in this chapter.

REVIEW OF PATIENT COMMUNICATION AND DOCUMENTATION

Effective communication with patients is always important. This is especially true when you are assisting with physical examinations. A complete and accurate medical record is vital to the management and care of the patient. Thus, all communications and interactions with a patient must be entered in that patient's medical record.

As you gain experience as a medical assistant, you will become more proficient at effectively communicating with patients and at translating those communications into proper documentation in the patients' medical records. You will also learn to recognize which statements by a patient are important to record and what information is important to bring to the attention of the physician.

Effective Communication

The patient interview or intake takes place when you have brought a patient into an examination room and you identify the patient's reason for the office visit. The goal of your interview with the patient is to obtain information about the patient's condition, while establishing a good rapport and a positive relationship.

Although communication techniques were discussed earlier in this book, it is important to review effective communication practices as they relate to the patient interview. Consider these steps when you interview a patient:

- Review the patient's medical record before meeting the patient in order to have an efficient and effective interview.
- Greet the patient by using the patient's last name ("Good morning, Mrs. Jones"), and introduce yourself.
- Maintain a professional and friendly demeanor.
- Make the patient feel as comfortable as possible during the office visit. If you notice apprehension, try an ice-breaker, such as talking about the weather or sports.

Or, pay the patient a sincere compliment ("I really like that sweater you're wearing, Mrs. Jones").

- Be aware of verbal and nonverbal cues as the patient answers questions and describes the reason for the visit.
- Avoid making judgmental responses. Be cautious about facial expressions and body posture when listening to the patient's responses.
- Avoid providing medical assurances ("Everything will be all right"). Treat sensitive topics with respect, and keep in mind the cultural and personal beliefs of the patient.
- Summarize important points the patient has made, giving the patient a chance to correct anything you may have misunderstood.
- Document the interview in the patient's medical record, according to the policy of your facility.

Correct Documentation

As mentioned earlier, the patient's medical record is critical to the office visit. It is a legal document and plays an integral part of the patient's health care. Multiple health care providers and employees access patient records for a variety of reasons: for diagnosing and treating; recording laboratory and other diagnostic test results; documenting phone calls and other interactions between the patient and the medical office; and documenting patient education that has been conducted.

Proper documentation in a patient's medical record also helps ensure continuity of care. It ensures that any health care provider who has authorized access to the medical record will be able to review the record and have a clear and concise picture of the patient's previous health history, current medical status, and treatment plan.

Medical records are legal documents and can be subpoenaed or used as evidence in court, such as for a medical malpractice lawsuit. Thus, it is critical that all pertinent patient information has been accurately documented.

In addition to the following tips, refer to Box 35-1, "The Six C's of Charting," for a summary of charting guidelines:

- Record the date and time of every entry.
- Use medical terminology and abbreviations that are commonly used and accepted by the medical office or facility.
- Use correct spelling and grammar.
- Sign every entry, using either a digital signature for electronic records or a hand-written signature for paper records.

- Accurately document information; record facts, not opinions.

- Document the proper sequence in which events occurred.

- Document appropriate and relevant information concerning patient's health and care given.

- Be concise.

Though many medical offices have transitioned to the use of electronic health records, some medical offices and facilities may still use paper records. When this is the case, consider the following:

- Write legibly.

- Use permanent black ink.

- Correct errors by drawing a single line through the incorrect entry, initialing by it, and then recording the corrected entry.

PATIENT HEALTH HISTORY

A patient's health history can give helpful insight to current health status and condition. The patient history assists the physician in assessing the patient's general well-being, aids in diagnosis, and helps the physician develop a treatment plan for the patient. Figure 35-1 shows an example of a standard patient health history form. These forms may vary according to office preference and specialty. For instance, a cardiologist may have more extensive questions relating to signs and symptoms and family history associated with cardiovascular disorders.

The medical office might have patients fill out health history forms before their appointment either by having them available online or by mailing the form to the patient. Mailing forms and documents is very common, especially to patients who are new to a practice. Alternatively, the medical office might ask the patient to arrive to the appointment early so that the form can be filled out in the office. Either way, the medical assistant is responsible for making sure that the form is completely filled out before the physician sees the patient. Provide additional assistance to those patients who may appear to have difficulty completing the form because of frailty, disability, or illiteracy.

Although the health history form completed by the patient is important, there are multiple additional components to a complete history that should be obtained during the patient's office visit. History that is gathered during the patient's office visit should cover the following six areas:

1. Chief complaint

2. Present illness

3. Past medical history

4. Family medical history

5. Social history

6. Assessment of body systems (review of systems), usually performed by the physician

Physicians' preferences may vary in regard to who should obtain specific information in the patient history. Some physicians may give the medical assistant more responsibility and request that the medical assistant obtain and review multiple components of the patient's history. Other physicians may choose to collect all aspects of the patient's history themselves or may have these components of the patient history obtained by another health care provider, such as the physician's assistant or nurse practitioner. As a medical assistant, you must be flexible and prepared to meet the needs and requests of the physicians in your practice.

Chief Complaint

The **chief complaint (CC)** is the patient's primary reason for making the office visit. It is also referred to as the "presenting problem." The chief complaint usually consists of one or two signs or symptoms the patient has been experiencing and is concerned about.

When documenting the patient's complaints, be aware of the difference between signs and symptoms. Signs are **objective**, meaning that they are observable by others and can be measured, such as weight gain, fever, or a rash. Conversely, symptoms are **subjective**, something the patient experiences but cannot be observed by anyone else, such as dizziness, pain, or feelings of anxiety. A physician has no way of knowing what the patient's symptoms are unless the patient reports them.

The chief complaint should be reported in the medical record in the patient's own words with quotation marks around them—for example, "I'm having trouble sleeping" or "I'm out of breath after climbing only a flight of stairs." It is important to ask *what-when-where* questions to obtain a more complete patient interview.

- *What?* What does it feel like (kind of pain or sensation, how intense)? What makes it worse? What relieves it?

- *When?* When did it start (**onset**)? How long does it last (**duration**)? How often does it happen (**frequency**)?

- *Where?* Where is the symptom located (body part, left or right)?

The medical office and facility where you work will indicate how to record a chief complaint. Some offices might use the abbreviation "*CC*" (chief complaint), and others might prefer "*C/O*" (complains of). Because only the physician is able to diagnose the patient's problems, avoid using diagnostic terms when you record the chief complaint. Here are examples of correct and incorrect documentation of the same patient's chief complaint:

- **Correct documentation:** 10/23/YY Pt. c/o "dying of thirst all the time" and weight loss during past month.

- **Incorrect documentation:** 10/23/YY Pt. experiencing excessive thirst and unusual weight loss indicative of diabetes.

Pearson Physicians Group
123 Michigan Avenue
Parker Heights, IL 30310
(312)-123-1234

Patient Health History

Name: _____   Date: _____

SSN: _____   Birth date: _____

What is the reason for your visit today? (Please describe problem in detail including history of present illness):
_____
_____

Medical History: Please check all that apply to you:

☐ Arthritis	☐ Epilepsy/seizures	☐ Kidney disease	☐ Psychiatric disease
☐ Cancer	☐ Heart problems	☐ Liver disease	☐ Stroke
☐ Depression	☐ Heart surgery	☐ Measles	☐ Thyroid
☐ Diabetes	☐ High blood pressure	☐ Mumps,	☐ Hepatitis
☐ AIDS	☐ Chicken pox	☐ Rheumatic fever	☐ HIV positive
☐ Anemia bleeding disorder	☐ Gall bladder disease	☐ Scarlet fever	☐ Other
☐ Tuberculosis	☐ Typhoid fever		

Please list any medications you are taking with dose and frequency:

Drug	*Dose/Frequency*
_____	_____
_____	_____
_____	_____
_____	_____

Please list any allergies that you have: _____
_____

Please list past surgeries with approximate date: _____
_____

Please describe any serious injuries you have had: _____

FIGURE 35-1 Patient health history form.

Patient Health History

Please check any problems or conditions, that you are experiencing or have experienced.

General Health
- ☐ Good general health
- ☐ Recent weight change
- ☐ Loss of appetite
- ☐ Fatigue
- ☐ Fever/chills

Allergy
- ☐ Drug allergies
- ☐ Food allergies
- ☐ Hay fever
- ☐ Other:

Ears, Nose, Mouth, Throat
- ☐ Difficulty swallowing
- ☐ Earaches
- ☐ Loss of hearing/deafness
- ☐ Loss of smell
- ☐ Loss of taste
- ☐ Painful chewing
- ☐ Ringing in ears
- ☐ Sinus infection
- ☐ Sores in mouth
- ☐ Other:

Skin
- ☐ Rash or itching
- ☐ Sun sensitivity
- ☐ Hair loss
- ☐ Color changes
- ☐ Other:

Genitourinary
- ☐ Blood in urine
- ☐ Female: irregular periods
- ☐ Female: #pregnancies _____
  #miscarriages _____
- ☐ Female: vaginal discharge
- ☐ Kidney stones
- ☐ Male: prostate disease
- ☐ Male: testicle pain
- ☐ Painful or burning urination
- ☐ Sexual difficulty
- ☐ Sexually transmitted disease
- ☐ Urgency with urination
- ☐ Urine retention/incontinence
- ☐ Other:

Gastrointestinal
- ☐ Blood in stools
- ☐ Increasing constipation
- ☐ Nausea
- ☐ Painful bowel movements
- ☐ Persistent diarrhea
- ☐ Stomach or abdominal pain
- ☐ Ulcer
- ☐ Vomiting
- ☐ Other:

Heart and Lungs
- ☐ Pain in chest
- ☐ High blood pressure
- ☐ High cholesterol
- ☐ Irregular heart beat
- ☐ Other:

Muscle/Joints/Bones
- ☐ Back pain
- ☐ Difficulty walking
- ☐ Joint pain
- ☐ Joint stiffness or swelling
- ☐ Muscle pain or tenderness
- ☐ Neck pain

Psychiatric
- ☐ Depression
- ☐ Anxiety
- ☐ Eating disorder
- ☐ Other:

Eyes
- ☐ Blind spots
- ☐ Blurred vision
- ☐ Double vision
- ☐ Loss of vision
- ☐ Glaucoma
- ☐ Injury
- ☐ Pain
- ☐ Other:

Neurological
- ☐ Balance problems
- ☐ Black outs/loss of consciousness
- ☐ Difficulty speaking
- ☐ Difficulty walking
- ☐ Facial drooping
- ☐ Headaches
- ☐ Injury to the brain or spine
- ☐ Light-headed or dizziness
- ☐ Memory loss
- ☐ Mental confusion
- ☐ Migraines
- ☐ Mini stroke
- ☐ Neuropathy
- ☐ Numbness or tingling
- ☐ Paralysis
- ☐ Stroke
- ☐ Tremors
- ☐ Weakness
- ☐ Other:

Pulmonary
- ☐ Asthma
- ☐ Blood in cough
- ☐ Cancer
- ☐ Chronic or frequent cough
- ☐ Emphysema
- ☐ Pneumonia
- ☐ Shortness of breath
- ☐ Other:

Social History:

Do you drink alcohol? ☐ Yes ☐ No If yes, how much/week? _____

Do you smoke? ☐ Yes ☐ No If yes, how many cigarettes/day? _____

Do you consume caffeine? ☐ Yes ☐ No If yes, how many cups/week? _____

Do you use recreational drugs? ☐ Yes ☐ No If yes, what type and frequency? _____

Are you on a special diet? ☐ Yes ☐ No If yes, please describe? _____

Family History: Do you know of any blood relative who has or had:

- ☐ Asthma
- ☐ Aneurysm
- ☐ Brain tumor
- ☐ Cancer, type:
- ☐ Diabetes
- ☐ Epilepsy/seizures

- ☐ Headaches
- ☐ Heart problems
- ☐ High blood pressure
- ☐ Kidney disease
- ☐ Lung disease
- ☐ Migraine

- ☐ Multiple sclerosis
- ☐ Psychiatric disease
- ☐ Stroke
- ☐ Thyroid

FIGURE 35-1 (*continued*)

See Procedure 35-2 for details on documenting chief complaints during a patient interview.

Pain

One of the most common chief complaints from patients is pain. However, no two individuals experience pain in the same way. If the patient says he is in pain, the health care provider must accept this claim because pain is a symptom and, thus, subjective, as discussed earlier. When documenting a patient's description of pain, use the patient's own words. For example, if the patient complains of a "sharp, stabbing pain in my belly," that is how it should be written in the chart.

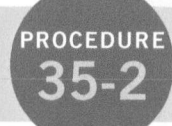

PROCEDURE 35-2

Documenting a Chief Complaint During a Patient Interview

Objective ◆ *Document the chief complaint using correct charting format and abbreviations while interviewing a patient.*

EQUIPMENT AND SUPPLIES

Patient's medical record; patient health history form or progress notes form; pen with black ink

Note: Instructor may provide a variety of patient scenarios for students to role-play for this procedure.

METHOD

1. Gather supplies, including the medical record, patient health history form, or progress notes form.
2. Review briefly the patient's medical history form before greeting the patient.
3. Greet and identify the patient. Introduce yourself, and escort the patient into the examination room.
4. Ask open-ended questions—those that cannot be answered just "yes" or "no"—to gather information about why the patient is being seen today. Maintain eye contact and actively listen to patient responses.
5. Gather information about the present illness by asking questions:
   a. What makes the problem better or worse?
   b. When did it start? When does it occur?
   c. Where does it hurt?
   d. If pain is present, ask the patient to rate the pain on a scale of 0 to 10, with 10 being the greatest.
6. Document the "CC" (chief complaint) and the "PI" (present illness) correctly within the medical record.
   a. Document the CC and PI in the patient's own words whenever possible.
7. Before leaving the room, make sure that the patient is comfortable and ask if there are any questions.
8. Thank the patient and explain that the physician will come in shortly to perform the examination.

CHARTING EXAMPLE

03/03/YY 11:00 A.M. CC: "Pounding headache and Tylenol isn't helping and I've been throwing up for three days." PI: N&V × 3 days. Started after she returned home from a business trip overseas. T: 101°F × 2 days, she states "my body aches all over." .... A. Martinez, CMA

Pain is sometimes difficult to describe. Thus, it is important for medical assistants to have an expansive vocabulary of medical terms in order to be able to accurately describe, or to help the patient describe, the pain. Common terms used to describe pain include:

- Stabbing and sharp
- Cutting or tearing
- Burning, stinging
- Dull or throbbing
- Intermittent or continuous
- Aching, gnawing, nagging
- Unbearable or excruciating

When the patient is discussing pain, the patient's nonverbal cues should also be observed and recorded, such as grimacing, moaning, or grasping a particular body part.

Use of a numerical pain measurement scale can also be useful and is now a common method of evaluating pain. Ask the patient to describe the amount of pain on a scale of 0 to 10, with 0 being no pain and 10 being extreme pain. For children and non–English-speaking patients, picture scales with happy and sad faces should be available. See Figures 35-2 and 35-3 for examples of pain scales.

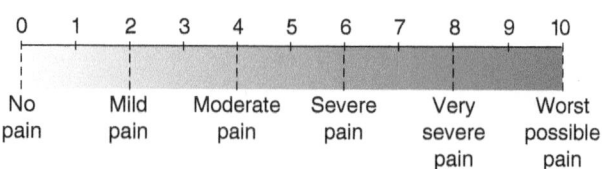

FIGURE 35-2 Numerical pain level chart with word modifiers.

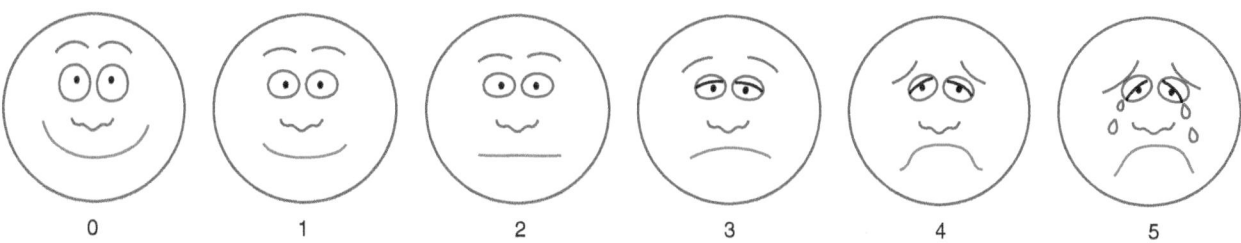

1. Explain to the child that each face is for a person who feels happy because he or she has no pain (hurt, or whatever word the child uses) or feels sad because he or she has some or a lot of pain.

2. Point to the appropriate face and state, "This face...":
   0—"is very happy because he (or she) doesn't hurt at all."
   1—"hurts just a little bit."
   2—"hurts a little more."
   3—"hurts even more."
   4—"hurts a whole lot."
   5—"hurts as much as you can imagine, although you don't have to be crying to feel this bad."

3. Ask the child to choose the face that best describes how he or she feels. Be specific about which pain (e.g., "shot" or incision) and what time (e.g., Now? Earlier before lunch?)

FIGURE 35-3 The Wong/Baker FACES rating scale.

Pain may be acute or chronic. **Acute pain** is pain that begins suddenly and usually lasts only three to six months. It may be caused by trauma or a condition, such as an appendicitis. **Chronic pain** is long-term pain that may interfere with the functions of daily living and usually lasts longer than six months. The medical assistant's job will be to record how the patient describes the pain and its duration. It is the physician's job to decide if it should be considered acute or chronic.

Pain can be further categorized by where it seems to be coming from—from deep in the organs (visceral) or from the surface of the body (superficial). Pain is also described by where it is felt in the body. **Radiating pain** spreads out from a particular area or source. For instance, pain from a heart attack is often felt not only in the chest but also down the left arm and up toward the jaw. **Referred pain** is felt at a site away from the injured or diseased body part. For example, patients with gallbladder disease may complain of pain in the right shoulder. **Intractable pain** is an overwhelming, difficult-to-relieve, or all-consuming pain. It is often defined as pain for which the cause of the pain cannot be removed or treated in the generally accepted course of medical care or after reasonable efforts. **Phantom pain** is a sensation or pain that is felt in a body part that is no longer there, for example, after an amputation.

Present Illness

The **present illness (PI)** provides a more complete, expansive description of the chief complaint. The PI component of the health history must contain a detailed description of the symptom(s), including the onset, duration, and intensity.

Each symptom should be documented as to its relationship to the chief complaint. For example, a patient who came to the office with a chief complaint of "dull aching pain in left side of belly" may add that it happens every time she eats popcorn or nuts and it has occurred monthly for the past six months. This information provides a more comprehensive and detailed picture of the chief complaint.

See Procedure 35-3: Interviewing a New Patient to Obtain Information on Medical History and Preparing for a Physical Examination.

Past Medical History

Past medical history includes all diseases and medical problems the patient has experienced in the past (Figure 35-1). Past illnesses or injuries can still affect the patient's present health. A complete past medical history should include information about the following items:

- Childhood diseases
- Major illnesses
- Injuries
- Hospitalization
- Surgeries
- Allergies
- Immunizations
- Current and past medications (prescription and OTC)
- Last examination

Patients often forget to tell the physician how much aspirin, ibuprofen, or other over-the-counter (OTC) medications they take. Patients may think that OTC medications

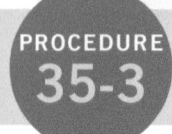

PROCEDURE 35-3

Interviewing a New Patient to Obtain Information on Medical History and Preparing for a Physical Examination

Objective ◆ *Obtain pertinent patient information for a medical history that will assist the physician in establishing a diagnosis and treatment of the present illness (PI). Include CC, past history, social history, and family history.*

EQUIPMENT AND SUPPLIES

Completed medical history form and other new patient documents; clipboard; pens (black and red); gown; drape

Note: This may be performed on a fellow student.

METHOD

1. Identify the patient, greet the patient warmly, and introduce yourself.
2. Escort the patient to a private examination room, and explain that you will be preparing the patient to be seen by the physician.
3. Review the medical history form with the patient. Be sure that all the sections have been appropriately filled out.
   a. Ask for additional information to complete any missing information
4. Speak in a clear voice and avoid using medical terminology when communicating with the patient.
5. Ask why the patient is visiting the medical office today. Using the patient's own words, as appropriate, record this information as the chief complaint (CC).
6. Ask about the patient's present illness (PI) to provide more information about the patient's chief complaint.
   a. Ask the patient open-ended questions.
   b. Observe the patient for any nonverbal signs during the interview.
7. Gather additional information regarding the patient's social and family histories. Information should include education level, occupation, marital status, any disabilities, and substance abuses.

8. Inquire about the patient's allergies and outcome of the allergy, such as hives, a rash, or difficulty breathing. Record allergy information, using red ink if documenting in a paper medical record.
   a. If the patient states she does not have any allergies, record "NKA" (no known allergies), according to the office policy and as appropriate for the method of charting.
9. Include any other information or observations you feel are relevant to the patient's chief complaint or present illness.
   a. This may include illness of other family members at home or the recent loss of a loved one.
10. Record all information using correct charting guidelines, according to the method of charting used in the medical office.
    a. Correct any errors, as necessary. If correcting in a paper medical record, draw one line through the error, enter the correct information, then date and initial the correction.
11. Inform the patient if a gown must be worn and which items of clothing will need to be removed. Provide the patient with a gown, and drape the patient for modesty.
    a. Inform the patient of where clothes may be stored.
12. Ask if the patient has any questions before leaving the examination room, and inform the patient that the physician will be in shortly to perform the examination.
13. Thank the patient and leave the examination room, closing the door behind you to ensure privacy.
14. Place the medical record with completed health history form in the designated location for the physician's review. Inform the physician that the patient is ready to be examined.

should not be reported because they are not prescriptions. Remind patients that all types of medications should be included in their medication list, including vitamins and herbal supplements since they may interfere with prescribed medications or may be toxic if taken too frequently.

Family Medical History

A family history is a record of the health problems of the patient's blood relatives. Often, the family medical history

may be limited to immediate family members, such as parents and siblings, and include information about their current health status, any major health problems, and cause of death and age at death, if applicable. Family medical histories focus on diseases that may be inherited or genetic, such as seizures, heart disease, hypertension, and certain types of cancer.

Social History

Social histories include lifestyle habits or patterns that could affect the health status of the patient. These may include

1. What is your highest level of education?
2. What is your occupation?
3. How long have you done that type of work?
4. Have you been exposed to any toxic or harmful substances such as dust, chemicals, cleaning fluids/fumes, smoke, radiation, pesticides, or paint at work? At home?
5. What do you usually eat for breakfast?
6. Have you gained or lost 10 or more pounds during the past year? Is there a reason?
7. Do you follow a low-fat or low-salt diet?
8. What do you do for exercise? How often do you exercise?
9. How much alcohol do you drink a day? A month? How frequently do you drink? Do you drink liquor, wine, beer, or all of them?
10. Do you smoke cigarettes? Are they filtered? How many packs a day?
11. Do you smoke a pipe or cigars or chew tobacco? If yes, how much and how often?
12. How many cups of coffee do you drink a day? Tea? Soft drinks with caffeine?
13. Have you ever used heroin, cocaine, methamphetamine, or any other recreational drugs? How often and how much?
14. Do you have unusual stress at home or work?
15. What are your hobbies or interests?

smoking, drinking, and the use of recreational drugs. The patient's occupation, marital status, and sexual preferences should also be included. Dietary choices, frequency of exercise, sleep habits, and other health habits may also be inquired, depending on the extent of the intake form. Personal information such as the patient's previous occupation(s), if the patient has had several occupations, and lifelong hobbies or interests may be included if they are relevant to the patient's health status. Box 35-2 provides a list of questions you may ask while obtaining a social history.

EQUIPMENT AND SUPPLIES USED FOR PHYSICAL EXAMINATIONS

In a physical exam, the physician's hands are considered the primary "tool." Other times, special instruments may be necessary, such as an ophthalmoscope, otoscope, reflex hammer, pinwheel, stethoscope, sphygmomanometer, tuning fork, laryngeal mirror, and tape measure. Many items and supplies are generally considered disposable and are replaced as they are used in the exam room. Figure 35-4 shows examples of equipment and supplies often used in a physical examination.

Equipment

The following is a description of the equipment commonly used in a patient examination:

- **Ophthalmoscope**—The **ophthalmoscope** is used to examine the interior of the eye, especially the retina. Light is focused through a magnifying lens onto the inner surfaces of the eye to check for abnormalities. Position the patient in a sitting position with the patient looking straight ahead during this examination.

- **Otoscope**—The **otoscope** is used to examine the ears. The light is focused through the **speculum** to examine the outer ear, the ear canal, and the tympanic membrane (eardrum). A speculum is any instrument used to view a body cavity. The long, pointed speculum on the otoscope is usually disposable and can be replaced with a short, wide nasal speculum for visualization of the lining and the internal structures of the nose.

- **Reflex hammer and pinwheel**—The **reflex hammer** is sometimes called a percussion hammer. It has a hard rubber, triangular head and is used for testing reflexes. This instrument is commonly used to check the patellar reflex of the knee and the reflex of the Achilles tendon (in the ankle) or the elbows. The **pinwheel** has sharp points and is used for testing sensory perception.

- **Stethoscope**—The stethoscope is used to **amplify** sounds in the body, such as the beating of the heart, respirations in the lungs, and bowel sounds in the abdomen. It is made of two earpieces connected by rubber tubing to a chest piece with a bell or diaphragm to amplify sound.

- **Sphygmomanometer**—This instrument is used to measure blood pressure. It may be portable or attached to the wall in the examination room.

- **Tuning fork**—The **tuning fork** is a metal instrument that, when struck, makes a humming vibration that can be heard and felt. The two prongs that extend from the handle are designed to vibrate at a specific frequency. Tuning forks come in different sizes, and each size produces a different pitch level.

- **Laryngeal mirror**—The **laryngeal mirror** or dental mirror is a small mirror attached to a long handle that is used to visualize the larynx. Warming the laryngeal mirror can help prevent fogging. Warming can be done by running warm water over the mirror or by briefly holding the mirror close to the exam light.

Supplies	Purpose
Flashlight or penlight	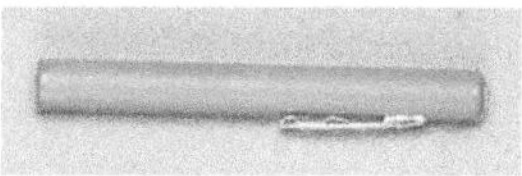 To assist viewing of the pharynx and cervix or to determine the reactions of the pupils of the eye
Laryngeal or dental mirror	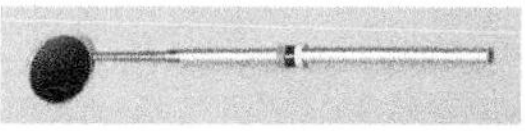 To observe the pharynx and oral cavity
Nasal speculum	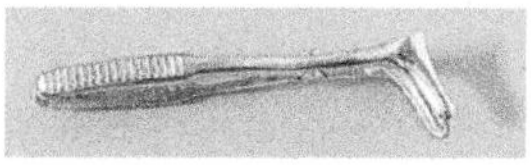 To permit visualization of the lower and middle turbinates; usually, a penlight is used for illumination
Ophthalmoscope	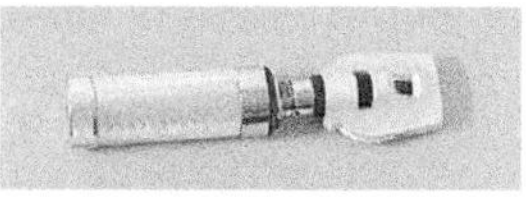 A lighted instrument to visualize the interior of the eye
Otoscope	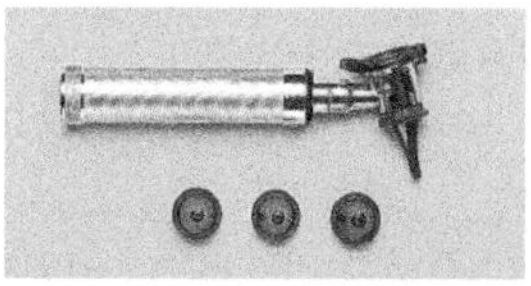 A lighted instrument to visualize the internal and external auditory canal (a nasal speculum may be attached to the otoscope to inspect the nasal cavities)
Percussion (reflex) hammer	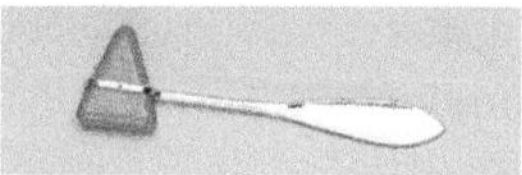 An instrument with a rubber head to test reflexes
Tuning fork	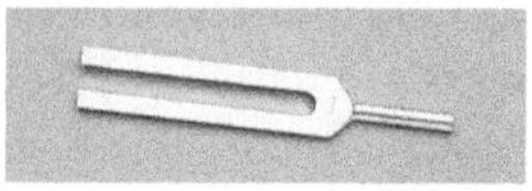 A two-pronged metal instrument used to test hearing acuity and vibratory sense
Vaginal speculum	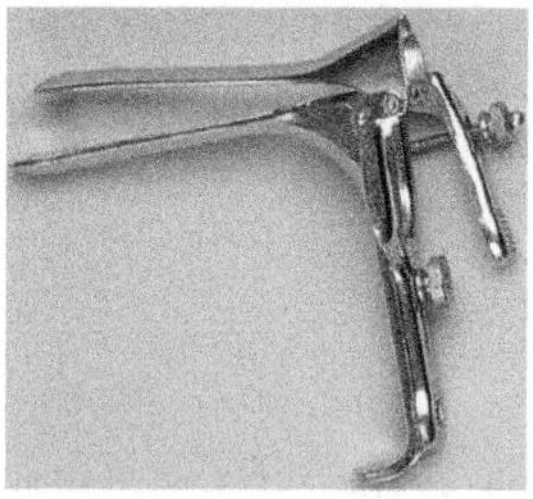 An instrument used to expand the vaginal opening to assess the cervix and the vagina
Cotton applicators	To obtain specimens
Disposable sponges	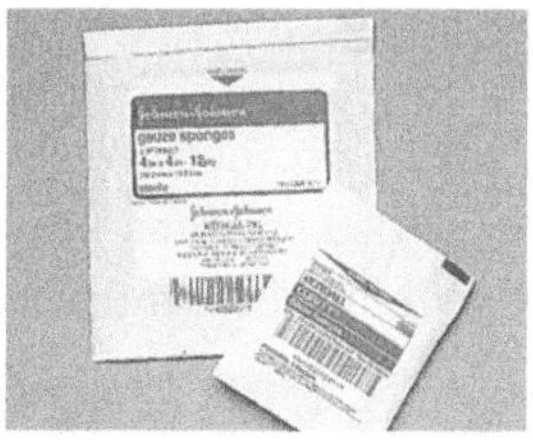 To absorb liquid
Gloves	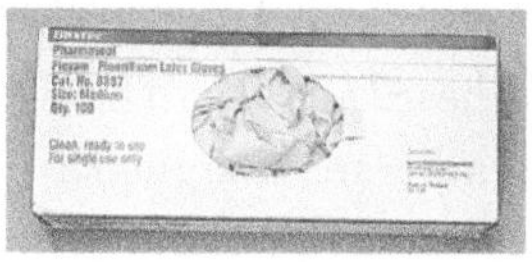 To prevent the spread of disease and infection
Lubricant	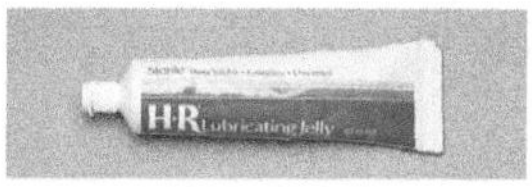 To ease insertion of instruments (e.g., vaginal speculum)
Tongue blades (depressors)	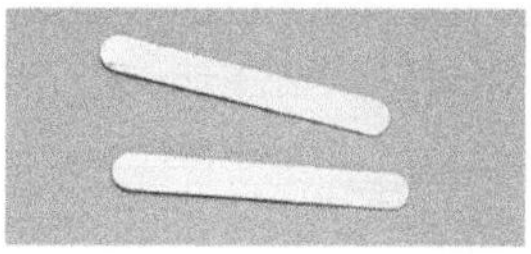 To depress the tongue during assessment of the mouth and pharynx

FIGURE 35-4 Equipment and supplies used during a physical examination.

- **Tape measure**—A tape measure is used to measure the size of a body part, such as the circumference of the chest or head of an infant. It can also be used to measure the length of a cut or lesion. Tape measures are flexible and are calibrated in both inches and centimeters.

Supplies

Supplies are disposable items used for patient examination and treatment. Supplies include examination table paper, paper drapes and gowns, various dressings and bandages, tongue depressors, disposable gloves (both sterile and nonsterile), syringes and needles, and alcohol pads.

Ordering supplies and stocking the exam rooms are important to the efficiency of patient care and for maintaining work flow. Delaying a procedure while you run out of the room to gather supplies, which should have been properly stocked, can put the patient at risk, delay schedules, and be annoying to everyone involved. A good office policy is to maintain an overall supply list for every examination room. Once an item is down to half a box or bottle, a new one should be placed in the exam room as a backup. An inventory system should contain the following information:

- List of supplies used in your facility
- Item numbers for all supply items
- Each supplier's name, address, telephone number, and contact person
- Amount of each supply used monthly
- Reordering frequency

Refer to Table 35-1 for descriptions of additional supplies and equipment commonly needed in examination rooms.

TABLE 35-1 | Typical Examination Room Equipment and Supplies

Equipment/Supply	Use
Alcohol wipes	Disinfect and cleanse skin before injections and phlebotomy.
Balance scale	Obtain the patient's weight and height.
Bandages (small)	Applied after taking blood sample and injections.
Batteries and light bulbs	Extra batteries and lightbulbs are required for lighted equipment such as gooseneck lamps and various scopes.
Betadine (or other topical antiseptic)	Used to disinfect skin before minor surgery.
Biohazard waste container	Closed rigid container with biohazardous labeling and appropriate red waste bags.
Cotton balls (sterile and nonsterile)	Used to apply antiseptic or to clean the skin.
Cotton-tipped swabs (sterile and nonsterile)	Used to clean recessed areas, to apply medications and lubricant, and to obtain specimens from the throat and other orifices.
Drapes	Disposable paper or cloth sheet used to cover patient during examination.
Emesis basin	Kidney-shaped receptacle for body drainage, such as sputum, and for used instruments.
Fixative spray	Used to preserve slides.
Gauze dressings (4 × 4 or 3 × 4)	Applied to dress small wounds.
Gloves (nonsterile disposable)	Worn by all staff to protect against microorganisms and bloodborne pathogens.
Gloves (sterile disposable)	Worn when performing minor surgery and handling sterile materials.
Gooseneck lamp	Movable light used to focus on a body area for increased visibility.
Irrigation syringe	Used to wash cerumen (earwax) out of ear canal or to irrigate wounds.
Lubricant	Water-soluble gel applied to physician's glove, speculum, or rectal thermometer to reduce friction during insertion. Prevents damage to delicate mucous membranes.
Soap dispenser	Used to dispense germicidal soap for handwashing between each patient.
Sphygmomanometer	Instrument used to measure blood pressure.
Tape	Used to secure dressings.
Tape measure	Measure lesions, head circumference, body measurements.
Thermometers of various types	Measure body temperature.
Tissues	Wipe body secretions.
Tongue depressor	Wooden blade used to hold down patient's tongue while examining mouth and throat.
Vaginal speculum	Instrument used to expand vaginal opening to view cervix.

EXAMINATION METHODS USED BY THE PHYSICIAN

As previously stated, the physician's hands are the primary tools used during the physical examination. The ways physicians use their hands vary according to the method of assessment they wish to perform and their medical specialty. The six commonly used methods of physical examination are inspection, palpation, percussion, auscultation, mensuration, and manipulation. All contribute salient information about the patient's general overall health.

Inspection

A physician performs **inspection** by visually examining the exterior surface of the body. At the same time, the physician is examining the patient's general state of health, overall demeanor, mood, grooming, and social interactions. Inspecting some interior portions of the body, such as the throat, eyes, ears, vaginal wall, cervix, and rectum, may require the use of special instruments and equipment. The physician will make note of anything that is unusual in color, size, shape, position, or symmetry of the areas being inspected (Figure 35-5).

Palpation

Palpation is the process of using the hands to feel the organs and other parts of the body to examine for any irregularities. Palpation is used to identify any unusual tenderness, size, shape, and texture on the body. Often, abnormalities and masses in the breasts and abdomen can be discovered through palpation. Figures 35-6A-B shows examples of light palpation using one hand and **bimanual** deep palpation, or using two hands.

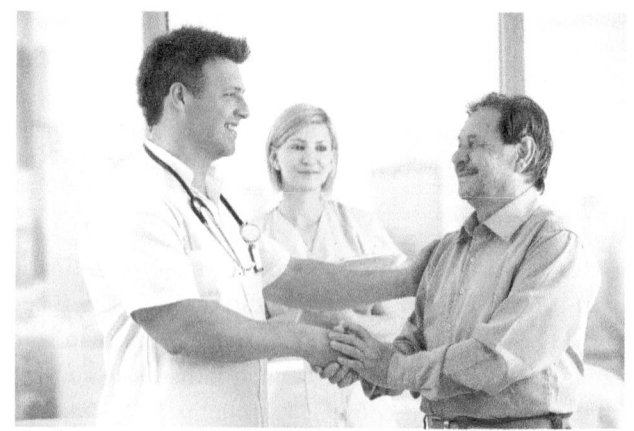

FIGURE 35-5 The physician will begin visual inspection of the patient immediately upon entering the examination room.

Percussion

Percussion is the process of using the fingertips to tap the body with short, sharp blows to gain information about the position and size of the underlying body parts. To percuss,

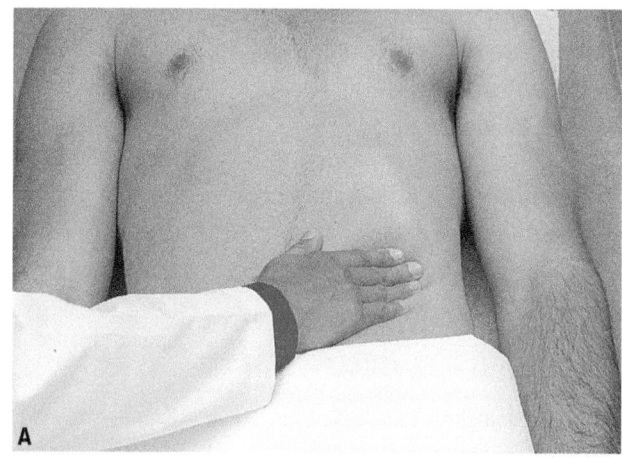

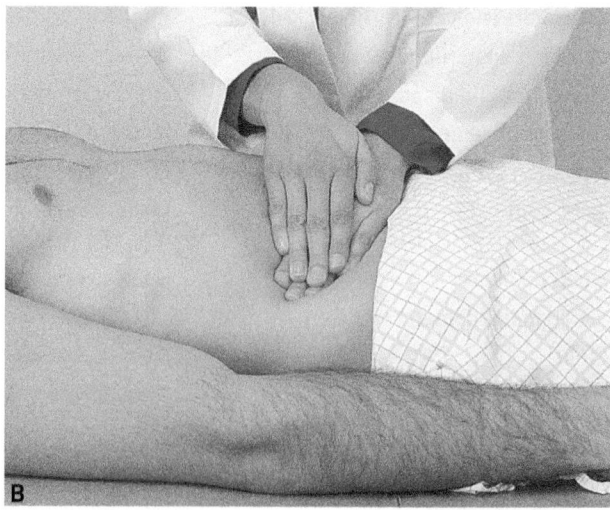

FIGURE 35-6 **(A)** An example of light palpation of the abdomen; **(B)** the physician uses two hands for deep bimanual palpation.

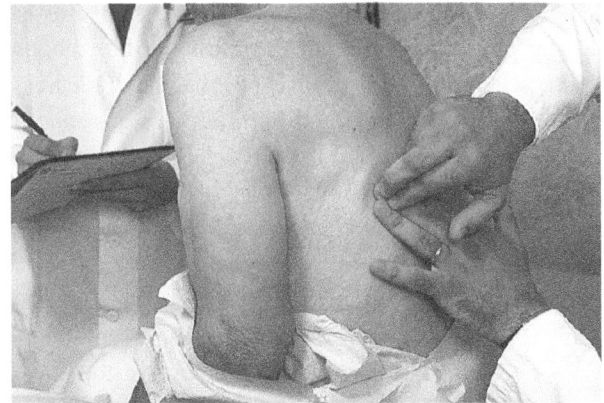

FIGURE 35-7 The physician uses percussion (tapping) to detect sound or vibration.

two fingers of one hand are placed on the patient's skin and then struck with the index and middle finger of the other hand. The physician may percuss the chest wall, back, or abdomen by gentle thumping or tapping, which produces a standard sound or vibrations. An alteration of this sound or vibration aids in determining the presence of air, fluid, or pus in a cavity or a solid mass under the skin. Figure 35-7 illustrates percussion on a patient's back.

Another method of percussion during a physical examination is the physician's use of a percussion or reflex hammer. For example, as part of the neurological test, the physician gently taps the reflex hammer once against the tendon reflex at the bottom of the patella (kneecap) (Figure 35-8). The reaction of the leg (the knee jerk) is an indication of neurological (nervous system) function.

Auscultation

Auscultation is the process of listening to sounds within the body. During auscultation, sounds made by the heart, lungs, stomach, and bowel are assessed for strength and rhythm. The physician differentiates abnormal body sounds from normal ones, as well as the presence and absence of

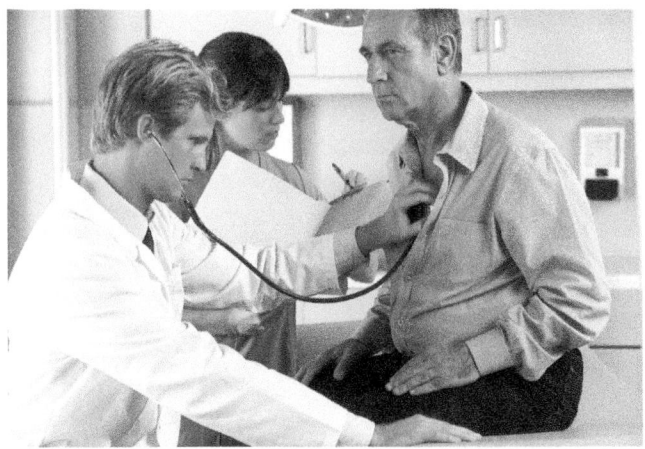

FIGURE 35-9 The physician uses auscultation to listen to a patient's heart.

sounds. These sounds can be heard by either placing the ear directly over the body surface or, more commonly, using a stethoscope to help amplify body sounds (Figure 35-9).

Mensuration

Mensuration is the use of special tools to measure the body or specific body parts. These special tools include a scale, tape measure, and calipers. Scales are used to measure both adult and pediatric weight. Tape measures can be used to measure the length and width of a wound or the circumference of an infant's head or chest. Calipers can be used to determine the amount of body fat (Figure 35-10). A **goniometer** is used to measure the range of motion of a joint (Figure 35-11).

Manipulation

Manipulation is the process of passively assessing the range of motion of a joint. While a physician is manipulating a joint, he or she may also be palpating it for other abnormalities.

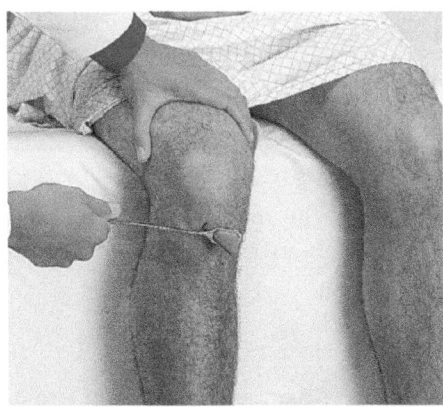

FIGURE 35-8 Testing the patellar reflex with a percussion hammer.

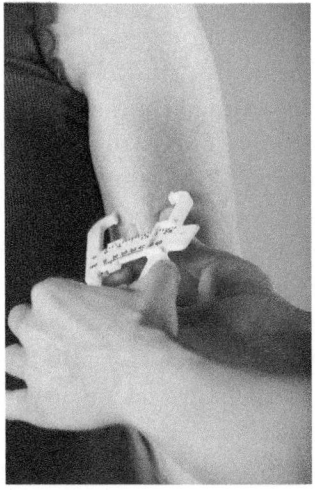

FIGURE 35-10 Calipers are used to measure the body fat on the triceps of a patient.

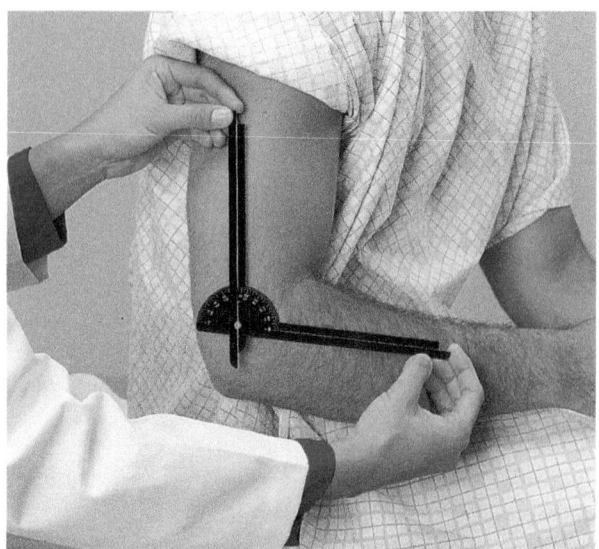

FIGURE 35-11 Mensuration: A goniometer is used to measure the range of motion of a joint.

ADULT EXAMINATION

Routine checkups, illness, urgent visits, and preoperative examinations are all common reasons for medical office visits. Generally, regardless of the type of appointment scheduled, a physical examination is performed by the physician. The medical office visit may vary in the length, extent, and type of exams that will be performed depending on the reason for the visit, what is found during the physical examination, and the specialty of the physician. The purpose of the physical examination is to assess as much of the body as possible to help **diagnose** (determine the cause and nature of a disease or injury) new diseases or to evaluate the effectiveness of established treatment plans from previously diagnosed disorders. The physical examination may also include additional tests and exams, such as blood work and X-rays, to help aid in or confirm an accurate diagnosis.

Patients often have a routine physical examination as part of their annual wellness visit. During these annual visits, it is particularly important for the physician to have the patient's medical records up to date in order to compare the current physical examination results with previous ones. The physician will be looking for weight changes, blood pressure variations, or other conditions that may require more frequent medical visits, treatment, or additional testing.

After all examinations, tests, and procedures are complete, a clinical diagnosis or working diagnosis is made. A **clinical diagnosis** is a preliminary presumptive diagnosis made by the physician based on the health history and physical examination as well as any laboratory results or reports. Sometimes the symptoms a patient presents with can indicate more than one possible diagnosis. If this is the case, the physician has to make a **differential diagnosis**, which is when the physician has to distinguish a particular disease or disorders from others with similar signs and symptoms. Part of the process of the physician's differential diagnosis is to rule out (R/O) diagnoses that may fit some but not all the facts of the case, narrow down the list of possible diagnoses, and eventually determine which is the correct or the most likely diagnosis.

Only the physician may actually diagnose a condition. The medical assistant's role in this process is to assist the physician by obtaining accurate patient information and to perform duties to assist the physician during the examination, as required.

Once the physician makes a diagnosis, although it is sometimes not possible to narrow the possibilities to just one, a **prognosis** is made. A prognosis is a prediction of the course or the outcome of the condition and the probable recovery rate. During the course of the condition, the physician will monitor the patient's progress, and adjust treatment and perhaps the prognosis.

ASSISTING THE PHYSICIAN WITH A PHYSICAL EXAMINATION

The medical assistant provides the physician with essential help during the physical examination. As a medical assistant, you may be asked to help the physician in the following ways:

1. Position and drape the patient for examination. If the patient is an older adult or has a disability, you must help the patient maintain the correct position during the examination.

2. Hand instruments, equipment, and other medical supplies to the physician.

3. Document and label specimens.

4. Offer reassurance and comfort to the patient.

5. Act as a witness to the behavior of the physician and the patient.

6. Carry out treatment plans as directed by the physician, such as providing patient education, applying dressings, and administering medications, depending on individual state laws.

7. Schedule diagnostic tests as ordered by the physician.

Table 35-2 lists the methods and equipment used to examine specific areas or parts of the body during a complete physical examination.

Patient Preparation

As discussed earlier, the medical assistant's role in preparing the patient consists of obtaining the patient's medical

TABLE 35-2 | Body Part, Method of Examination, and Equipment Used During the General Physical Examination

Area	Body Part	Method/Equipment
Head	Skull, hair, scalp	Inspection and palpation
Ears	Ear canals, eardrum	Inspection with otoscope and tuning fork
Eyes	Visual acuity	Vision chart, Snellen eye chart
		Inspection with ophthalmoscope
Nose	Nasal passages	Inspection with otoscope and nasal speculum
Mouth and Throat (Pharynx)	Mucous membranes, lips, gums, teeth, tongue, pharynx	Inspection with laryngeal mirror, flashlight, tongue blade
		Palpation and inspection
Neck	Thyroid gland, trachea, and cervical lymph nodes; carotid artery	Palpation, auscultation, and inspection
Back and Spine	Muscles, spinal cord	Inspection, palpation, and percussion
Chest and Lungs	Heart, lungs	Stethoscope
		Inspection, percussion, palpation, and auscultation
Breasts	Breast tissue, nipples	Palpation and inspection
Heart	Heart sounds, apical pulse	Auscultation with stethoscope
Abdomen	Bowel sounds	Auscultation
	Symmetry	Inspection
	Presence of air, masses, enlargement	Percussion, palpation
	Uterus	Palpation
		Stethoscope
Inguinal Area	Inguinal nodes hernia	Palpation
Genitalia	Female: cervix and vagina	Inspection using vaginal speculum
	Male: penis, scrotum, prostate gland	Palpation
Rectal	Anus	Inspection
	Rectum	Inspection using proctoscope
Legs	Circulation	Inspection
	Pulse sites	Palpation
Musculoskeletal System	Muscle strength	Inspection
	Gait abnormalities	Palpation
Neurological Examination	Reflexes	Percussion hammer, pinwheel

history, acquiring the chief complaint and present illness information, measuring vital signs, obtaining height and weight, and preparing the patient for examination by the physician, which includes providing gowning instructions or assisting the patient onto the examination table. Medical assistants also have to enter all vital signs and other patient information in the patient's medical record, according to the office's charting protocol, before the physician sees the patient.

Prepare the patient for any procedures that will be performed during the examination. Explain the procedures in a caring, simple, and direct manner. Patients are appreciative and usually more cooperative when approached and prepared in this manner. Older adult, frail, and young patients should not be left unattended in the examination room. If you are unable to remain in the room, a family member or another medical assistant should be asked to sit with the patient until the physician is ready to begin the examination.

Ask patients to empty their bladder before undressing. If a urine sample is required, give complete and detailed instructions. (Obtaining urine specimens is discussed in more detail later in this textbook's Urinalysis chapter.) Be sure that patients are able to navigate the office space and find their way back from the bathroom to their examination room. If a specimen collection is being performed, appropriately label all specimen collection containers before giving them to the patient.

The patient needs a gown and a drape for all examinations. Depending on the type of exam, explain to the patient which items of clothing should be removed and instruct the patient to put on the gown with the opening in the front or the back, depending on the examination. For a problem-focused visit or exam, only some clothing items may need to be removed, such as all clothing above the waist. Regardless of the examination, patient gowns and drapes should be provided for the patient's modesty. Depending on the patient's needs, the medical assistant may need to assist the patient with disrobing or with stepping up onto the examination table. Exercise extreme caution when assisting patients on the safety step or step stool, as these items can increase the tendency for falls.

Try to assess the patient's level of anxiety. If the patient seems extremely nervous or agitated, try to put the patient at ease. Report unusual nervousness or behaviors to the physician.

Draping the Patient

Drapes are sheets that are used to protect patient privacy and help keep the patient warm in the examination room. When used properly, they cover all but the body part that is being examined. Respecting and protecting a patient's modesty are important to ensure patient comfort and compliance during the examination. However, the drape must not obstruct the physician's vision or interfere with the examination. Drapes are typically smaller than bed sheets, although they are often made of the same material and often are disposable.

During sterile procedures, sterile drapes must be used to protect the surgical area from contamination. Sterile drapes are also used to provide a sterile surface for instruments, suture materials, and dressings. They also function to protect the patient from blood or drainage during the procedure.

Professionalism | Cultural Considerations

It is very important to be aware of the cultural norms of patients. Many cultures require that only members of the same sex be in the room during an examination or that the husband always be present while a wife is being examined. The patient's wishes should always be respected and never dismissed. If concern arises regarding a patient's cultural norm interfering with an examination, it is important to speak with the physician directly and discretely. Physicians are often well versed in obtaining information and handling difficult situations that arise because of cultural barriers.

Positioning the Patient

As a medical assistant, you will help the physician with the physical examination by positioning the patient. Nine standard positions are used for a variety of medical and surgical examinations and procedures: supine (or supine horizontal recumbent); dorsal recumbent; lithotomy; Fowler's and semi-Fowler's; prone; Sims; knee–chest; Trendelenburg; and proctologic. In addition to these positions, a sitting position and decubitus (lying on one's side) position may be used in certain examinations and procedures.

Medical assistants must be completely familiar with each position. You will need to give patients clear directions on how to assume each position while gently guiding them and protecting their safety. If a patient must turn from back to stomach or vice versa, you should always stand alongside the examination table and have the patient turn toward you to prevent the patient from falling off the examination table.

Procedures 35-4 through 35-10 and Figures 35-12, 35-13, and 35-14 explain and illustrate these positions.

Supine Position. In the supine position, also known as the horizontal recumbent position, patients lie flat on their back with hands at the sides. Be sure that the patient's feet are supported by extending the examination table. This position is used to examine anything on the anterior or ventral (front) surface of the body (head, chest, stomach) and for certain types of X-rays. The patient should be draped from the chest down to the feet. During the examination, you will expose areas, as necessary and as indicated by the physician. The supine position may not be comfortable for patients who have difficulty in breathing or who have lower back problems. For these patients, placing a pillow under the head and under the knees may help alleviate pain and provide more comfort. See Procedure 35-4: Positioning the Patient in the Supine Position.

Dorsal Recumbent Position. In this position, the patient is lying flat on the back with knees bent and feet flat on the examination table. This position relieves strain on the lower back and relaxes abdominal muscles. The dorsal recumbent position is used to inspect the head, neck, chest, vaginal, rectal, and perineal areas. This position can be used for digital (using the gloved fingers) exams of the vagina and rectum. To drape the patient, place the drape at the patient's neck or underarms and cover the body down to the feet. Patients with leg problems may find the dorsal recumbent position uncomfortable, whereas patients with severe arthritis may find this position more tolerable than the lithotomy position, described next. See Procedure 35-5: Positioning the Patient in the Dorsal Recumbent Position.

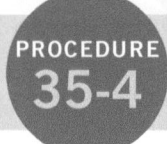

PROCEDURE 35-4 — Positioning the Patient in the Supine Position

Objective ◆ *Assist the patient into supine position for examination of the anterior surface of the body.*

EQUIPMENT AND SUPPLIES

Examination table; gown; drape

METHOD

1. Perform hand hygiene.
2. Greet and identify the patient. Explain that you will be assisting the patient into a position as required for the physical examination.
3. Provide a gown and assist the patient, if necessary.
   a. If the patient does not need assistance with disrobing and gowning, leave the room to maintain the patient's privacy.
   b. Always knock on the exam room door and ask for permission before reentering.
4. Assist the patient onto the examination table.
   a. If a separate step stool is used, stabilize it with your feet as the patient steps up to prevent the stool from sliding.
5. Ask the patient to lie back on the table, and provide an arm of support near the patient's back as the patient lies down. Pull out the foot extension on the examination table.
6. Place a pillow under the patient's head.

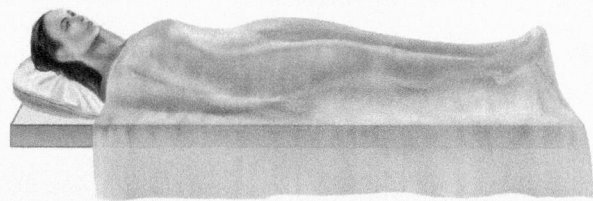

FIGURE A The supine or horizontal dorsal recumbent position.

7. Cover the patient with a drape from the chest to the feet (Figure A).
8. After the examination, assist the patient to a sitting position. Allow and encourage the patient to remain seated to prevent dizziness from the change of position.
9. Push the foot extension into place while supporting the patient's feet.
10. When the patient is stable, assist the patient to a standing position. Hold the patient's arm while she steps down off of the table. Provide assistance with re-dressing, if necessary.
11. After the patient has left, clean the examination room for the next patient following the steps in Procedure 35-1.
12. Perform hand hygiene.

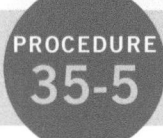

PROCEDURE 35-5 — Positioning the Patient in the Dorsal Recumbent Position

Objective ◆ *Assist the patient into the dorsal recumbent position for examination of the anterior surface of the body or to perform a pelvic examination.*

EQUIPMENT AND SUPPLIES

Examination table; gown; drape

METHOD

1. Perform hand hygiene.
2. Greet and identify the patient. Explain that you will be assisting the patient into a position as required for the physical examination.
3. Provide a gown and assist the patient, if necessary.
   a. If the patient does not need assistance with disrobing and gowning, leave the room to maintain the patient's privacy.
   b. Always knock on the exam room door and ask for permission before reentering.
4. Assist the patient onto the examination table.
   a. If a separate step stool is used, stabilize it with your feet as the patient steps up to prevent the stool from sliding.

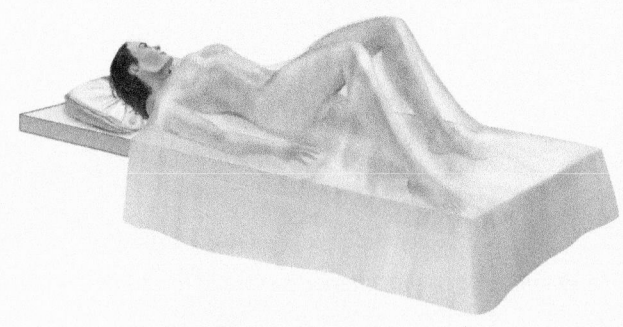

FIGURE A Dorsal recumbent position.

5. Ask the patient to lie back on the table, and provide an arm of support near the patient's back as the patient lies down. Pull out the foot extension on the examination table.
6. Ask the patient to bend the knees and place the feet flat on the table (Figure A). Push in the foot extension.

7. Cover the patient with a drape with the point of the drape between the patient's legs.
8. Place the pillow under the head, if needed to provide additional comfort.
9. Position the light source and a rolling stool in place for the physician.
10. After the procedure is complete, assist the patient to a sitting position using the foot extension to support the patient's feet.
11. Ask the patient to remain seated a few moments to prevent dizziness from the change of positions.
12. When the patient is stable, assist the patient to a standing position and hold the patient's arm while she steps down off the table. Provide assistance with re-dressing if necessary.
13. After the patient has left, clean the examination room for the next patient following the steps in Procedure 35-1.
14. Perform hand hygiene.

Lithotomy Position. The lithotomy position is similar to the dorsal recumbent position, except the patient's feet are placed in stirrups attached to the end and sides of the table. The stirrups must be locked in place to ensure patient safety. Provide additional assistance to patients who may have difficulty placing their feet in the stirrups. After the feet are in place in the stirrups, the patient is instructed to slide down until the buttocks are positioned at the edge of the table. The patient is draped from under the arms to the ankles. This position is used for vaginal examinations, often requiring the use of a **vaginal speculum** (an instrument used to hold open the walls of the vagina) and for obtaining cell samples of the cervix.

It is uncomfortable to maintain this position for any length of time, so the patient's feet should not be placed in stirrups until the physician is in the room and ready to begin the vaginal examination. Patients with severe arthritis or those who are severely obese or at the end of pregnancy may find this position difficult or impossible. If so, the dorsal recumbent position may be used instead if the physician approves. See Procedure 35-6 on how to position the patient in the lithotomy position.

Fowler's Position. In this position the patient sits on the examination table with the head of the table raised to a

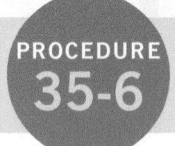

PROCEDURE
35-6

Positioning the Patient in the Lithotomy Position

Objective ◆ *Assist the patient into and out of the lithotomy position for a pelvic examination.*

EQUIPMENT AND SUPPLIES

Examination table with stirrups; gown; drape

METHOD

1. Perform hand hygiene.
2. Greet and identify the patient. Explain that you will be assisting her into a position as required for the physical examination.
3. Provide a gown and assist the patient, if necessary.

   a. If the patient does not need assistance with disrobing and gowning, leave the room to maintain the patient's privacy.
   b. Always knock on the exam room door and ask for permission before reentering.
4. Assist the patient to sit on the end of the table.
5. Cover the patient's legs with a drape.
6. Ask the patient to lie back on the table, and provide an arm of support near the patient's back as she lies down.

7. Position the stirrups level with the height of the table and about 1 foot from the side of the table. Lock the stirrups into place.
8. Ask the patient to slide down on the table until her buttocks are on the edge of the table end.
   a. The patient should not be positioned until the physician is in the room and ready to begin the examination.
9. Once the examination begins, assist the patient to bend her knees and place her feet in the stirrups. Position a drape for privacy with a point between the legs (Figure A).
10. Position the light source and a rolling stool for the physician.
11. Place a pillow under the patient's head as needed for additional comfort.
12. When the examination is complete, pull out the foot extension and help the patient remove her feet from the stirrups. Instruct her to lie with her feet extended out.
13. Ask the patient to slide up on the table, assisting as necessary. Keep the drape in place to ensure privacy.
14. Assist the patient to a sitting position and push in the foot extension. Allow the patient time to adjust to the change in position to prevent dizziness.

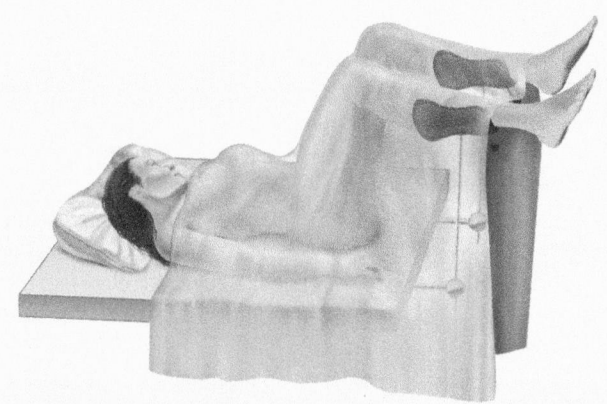

FIGURE A Lithotomy position.

15. When the patient is stable, assist her to a standing position and hold her arm while she steps down off the table. Provide assistance with re-dressing if necessary.
16. After the patient has left, clean the examination room for the next patient following the steps in Procedure 35-1.
17. Perform hand hygiene.

90-degree angle. If able, the patient may be seated on the edge of the table with feet over the edge in an upright position. This position is useful for examinations of the head, neck, and upper body. Patients who have difficulty breathing in the supine position may find this position more comfortable. The drape should be placed over the patient's lap and covering the legs.

Semi-Fowler's Position. The semi-Fowler's position is similar to the Fowler's position, but the head of the table is at a 45-degree angle instead of a 90-degree angle. This position is used for postsurgical exams and patients with breathing difficulties or lower back injuries. The drape should be placed over the patient's lap and covering the legs. See Procedure 35-7.

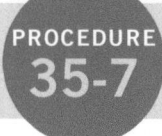

PROCEDURE
35-7

Positioning the Patient in the Fowler's or Semi-Fowler's Position

Objective ◆ *Assist the patient into the Fowler's or Semi-Fowler's position for examination of the upper body and the head.*

EQUIPMENT AND SUPPLIES

Examination table; gown; drape

METHOD

1. Perform hand hygiene.
2. Greet and identify the patient. Explain that you will be assisting the patient into a position as required for the physical examination.

3. Provide a gown and assist the patient, if necessary.
   a. If the patient does not need assistance with disrobing and gowning, leave the room to maintain the patient's privacy.
   b. Always knock on the exam room door and ask for permission before reentering.
4. Assist the patient up the step to sit on the end of the examination table.
   a. Stabilize the step stool as needed.

5. Cover the patient's legs with a drape.
6. Raise the head of the table to a 90-degree angle for Fowler's position (Figure A) and to a 45-degree angle for Semi-Fowler's position (Figure B).
7. Direct and assist the patient to slide back and lean on the raised end of the table.
8. Pull out the foot extension while supporting the patient's feet.
9. Place a pillow under the patient's knees to relieve strain on the lower back. Adjust the drape as needed to ensure privacy.
10. When the examination is complete, push in the foot extension. Ask the patient to remain seated at the end of the table to prevent dizziness.
11. Ask the patient to lean forward, sitting upright, while you support the patient's back and lower the table. Inform the patient before lowering the table.
12. When the patient is stable, assist the patient to a standing position and hold the patient's arm while she steps down off the table. Provide assistance with re-dressing if necessary.
13. After the patient has left, clean the examination room for the next patient, following the steps in Procedure 35-1.
14. Perform hand hygiene.

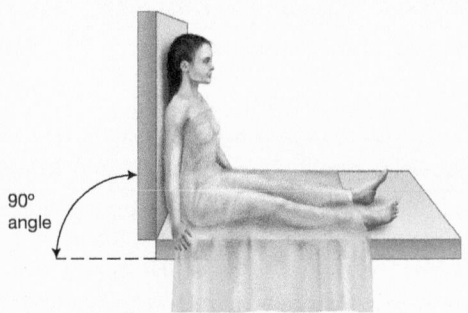

FIGURE A Fowler's position.

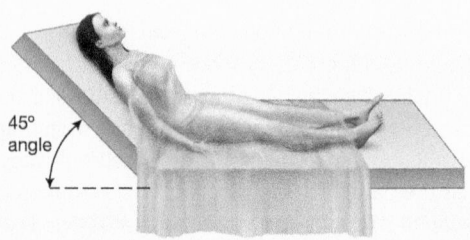

FIGURE B Semi-Fowler's position.

Prone Position. The prone position requires the patient to lie face down, flat on the stomach, with the head turned to the side and arms either alongside the body or crossed under the head. This position is the opposite of the supine position. The drape should cover the patient from upper back to over the feet. This position is used for back exams and certain types of surgery. The prone position should not be used for patients with breathing problems, women in late-term pregnancies, or older adults. In these cases the Sims position may be more appropriate, as described next. See Procedure 35-8.

Sims Position. The Sims, or lateral recumbent, position requires the patient to be placed on the left side with the right leg sharply bent upward and the left leg slightly bent. The right arm is flexed next to the head for support.

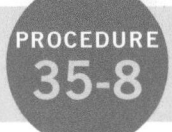

PROCEDURE
35-8

Positioning the Patient in the Prone Position

Objective ◆ *Assist the patient into the prone position for examination of the posterior of the body.*

EQUIPMENT AND SUPPLIES

Examination table; gown; drape

METHOD

1. Perform hand hygiene.
2. Greet and identify the patient. Explain that you will be assisting the patient into a position as required for the physical examination.

3. Provide a gown and assist the patient, if necessary.
   a. If the patient does not need assistance with disrobing and gowning, leave the room to maintain the patient's privacy.
   b. Always knock on the exam room door and ask for permission before reentering.
4. Assist the patient up the step to sit on the end of the examination table.
   a. Stabilize the step stool as needed.

5. Cover the patient's legs with a drape.
6. Ask the patient to lie back on the table, and provide an arm of support near the patient's back as she lies down. Pull out the foot extension.
7. Ask the patient to turn toward you onto her side, then onto the abdomen. Position yourself close to the middle of the side of the table to prevent the patient from falling.
8. Place pillows under the patient's head and feet as needed for comfort. Cover with a drape from the shoulders to the ankles (Figure A).
9. When the examination is complete, ask the patient to turn toward you, turning face up, and then help the patient to a sitting position.
10. Have the patient stay seated a few moments to prevent dizziness from the change in position.
11. When the patient is stable, assist the patient to a standing position and hold the patient's arm while she steps down

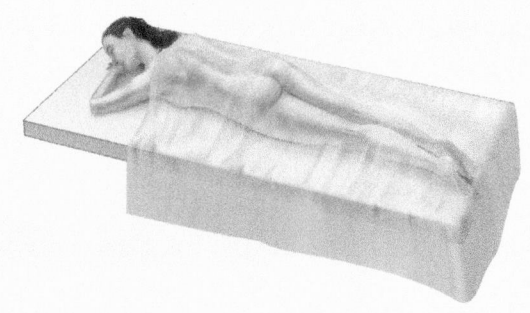

FIGURE A Prone position.

off the table. Provide assistance with re-dressing if necessary.
12. After the patient has left, clean the examination room for the next patient following the steps in Procedure 35-1.
13. Perform hand hygiene.

The patient is draped from under the arm or shoulders to below the knees on an angle. This allows the physician to raise a small section of the drape while keeping the rest of the patient covered. This position is used for rectal exams, taking rectal temperatures, enemas, and perineal and pelvic exams. See Procedure 35-9 for more information on how to position the patient in this position.

Knee–Chest Position. In the knee–chest position, the patient is placed in the prone position and then asked to pull the knees up to a kneeling position with thighs at a 90-degree angle to the table and buttocks in the air. The head is turned to one side, and the arms may be placed under the head or on either side of the head for comfort and support. Most patients need assistance to assume this position

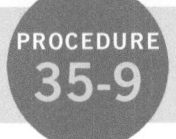

PROCEDURE
35-9

Positioning the Patient in the Sims Position

Objective ◆ *Assist the patient into the Sims position for rectal exams, rectal temperatures, enemas, and perineal and pelvic exams.*

EQUIPMENT AND SUPPLIES

Examination table; gown; drape

METHOD

1. Perform hand hygiene.
2. Greet and identify the patient. Explain that you will be assisting the patient into a position as required for the physical examination.
3. Provide a gown and assist the patient, if necessary.
   a. If the patient does not need assistance with disrobing and gowning, leave the room to maintain the patient's privacy.
   b. Always knock on the exam room door and ask for permission before reentering.

4. Assist the patient up the step to sit on the end of the examination table.
   a. Stabilize the step stool as needed.
5. Cover the patient's legs with a drape.
6. Ask the patient to lie back on the table, and provide an arm of support near the patient's back as she lies down. Pull out the foot extension.
7. Ask the patient to turn onto her left side with the left knee slightly flexed, placing the body weight on the chest.
   a. Position yourself close to the middle of the side of the table to prevent the patient from falling.
8. Ask the patient to flex the right knee to a 90-degree angle. Bend the patient's right arm at the elbow with the hand toward the head. Adjust the drape to cover the patient from the shoulders to the ankles (Figure A).

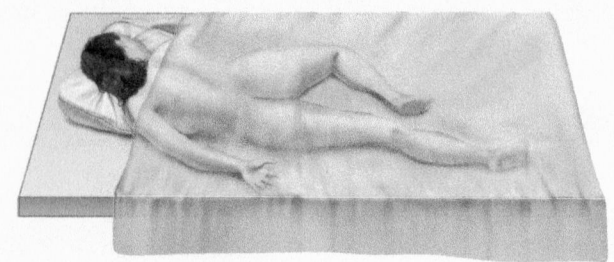

FIGURE A Sims position.

9. When the examination or procedure is complete, ask the patient to turn toward you and onto her back. Assist the patient to a sitting position. Ask the patient to remain seated at the end of the table a few moments to prevent dizziness from the change in position.
10. When the patient is stable, assist the patient to a standing position and hold the patient's arm while she steps down off the table. Provide assistance with redressing, if necessary.
11. After the patient has left, clean the examination room for the next patient following the steps in Procedure 35-1.
12. Perform hand hygiene.

correctly, and they should never be left unattended in this position at any time. It is an uncomfortable and embarrassing position, so the patient should not be made to assume the knee–chest position until necessary during the examination. This position is used for proctologic exams, sigmoidoscopy procedures, and rectal and vaginal exams. The drape should be placed from the upper back at an angle covering the anal area. A **fenestrated drape** (a drape with a precut

opening in the appropriate area) may be used. See Procedure 35-10.

Additionally, many physicians have proctologic tables available for this type of exam. This specialized examination table can be elevated in the middle, which will automatically position the patient with hips bent and the head and feet lowered, making it unnecessary for the patient to assume the knee–chest position.

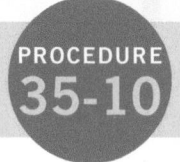

PROCEDURE 35-10

Positioning the Patient in the Knee–Chest Position

Objective ◆ *Assist the patient into the knee–chest position for examination of the rectum, sigmoid colon, or vagina.*

EQUIPMENT AND SUPPLIES

Examination table; gown; drape

METHOD

1. Perform hand hygiene.
2. Greet and identify the patient. Explain that you will be assisting the patient into a position as required for the physical examination.
3. Provide a gown and assist the patient, if necessary.
   a. If the patient does not need assistance with disrobing and gowning, leave the room to maintain the patient's privacy.
   b. Always knock on the exam room door and ask for permission before reentering.
4. Assist the patient up the step to sit on the end of the examination table.
   a. Stabilize the step stool as needed.

5. Cover the patient's legs with a drape.
6. Ask the patient to lie back on the table, and provide an arm of support near the patient's back as she lies down. Pull out the foot extension.
7. Ask the patient to turn toward you onto the abdomen, providing assistance as needed. Position yourself close to the middle of the side of the table to prevent the patient from falling.
8. Assist the patient onto the knees, with hips bent and keeping the chest on the table. Buttocks will be raised in the air, arms bent, head turned to the side, and hands next to the head. The patient may rest her weight on the elbows if it is more comfortable (Figure A).
9. Adjust the drape so the point of the drape is between the patient's legs.
10. When the examination is complete, help the patient to lie flat on her abdomen. When the patient is ready, ask her to turn toward you and then lie on her back. Help the patient

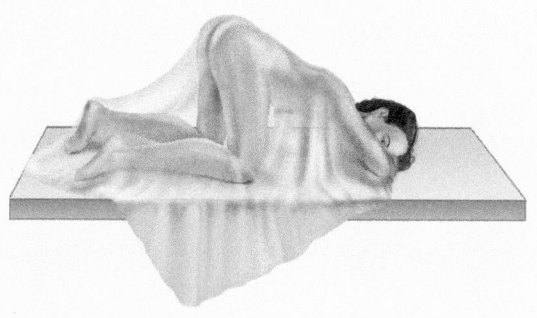

FIGURE A Knee–chest position.

10. to sit up and remain seated a few moments to prevent dizziness from the change of position.
11. When the patient is stable, assist the patient to a standing position and hold the patient's arm while she steps down off the table. Provide assistance with re-dressing if necessary.
12. After the patient has left, clean the examination table for the next patient, following the steps in Procedure 35-1.
13. Perform hand hygiene.

Trendelenburg Position. This position is not normally used in a physician's office except in cases of shock or hypotension (low blood pressure). For this position, the patient may be placed in the supine position, and the end of the table is raised to a 15- to 30-degree angle. This results in the patient's legs being elevated above the patient's head. The patient is draped from underarms to below the knees (Figure 35-12). The effectiveness of the Trendelenburg position in treating shock has been controversial, as some research has shown no effect or even negative effects on patient outcome. However, studies have shown the benefits of using a modified Trendelenburg position, also called the passive leg lift, which is elevating the patient's legs without tilting down of the head. Follow the instructions of the physician in this regard.

Proctologic Position. The proctologic (or jackknife) position is used for proctologic examinations, such as with a sigmoidoscopy. It is similar to the knee–chest position but with a greater bend at the hips. For this position, a special examination table is usually available, as discussed earlier. Patients lie face down with hips at the hinge of the examination table. The table is then tipped downward (Figure 35-13).

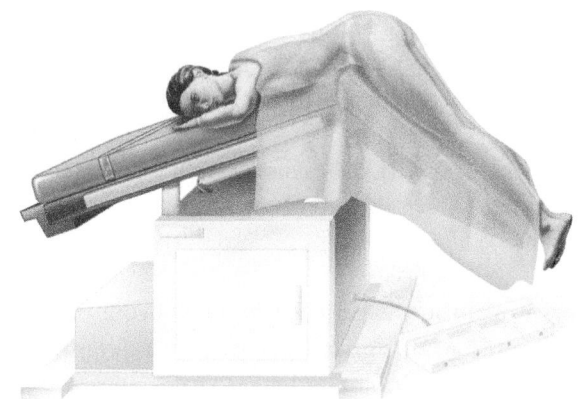

FIGURE 35-13 Proctologic (jackknife) position.

Sitting Position. This position is used to examine the head and chest (anterior and posterior). The patient sits upright with legs over the side of the examination table (Figure 35-14). The sitting position is ideal for patients with breathing problems and for auscultation of the heart and lungs during the physical examination.

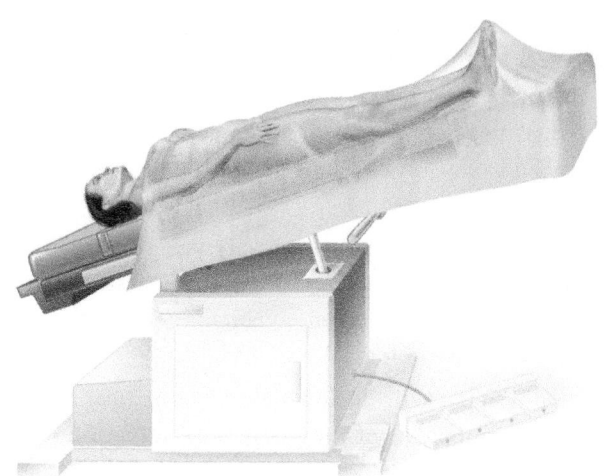

FIGURE 35-12 Trendelenburg position.

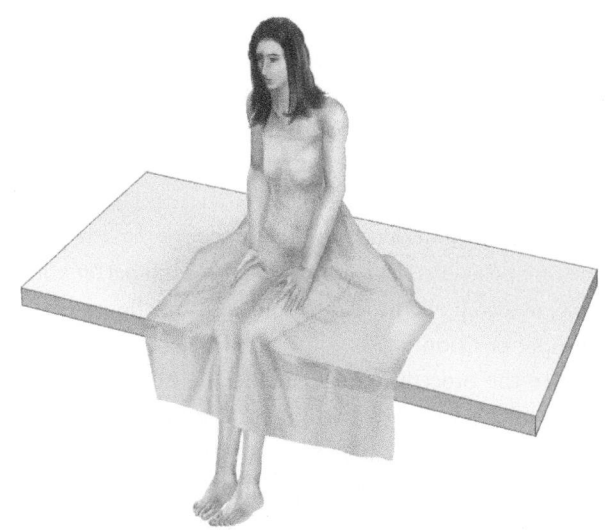

FIGURE 35-14 Sitting position.

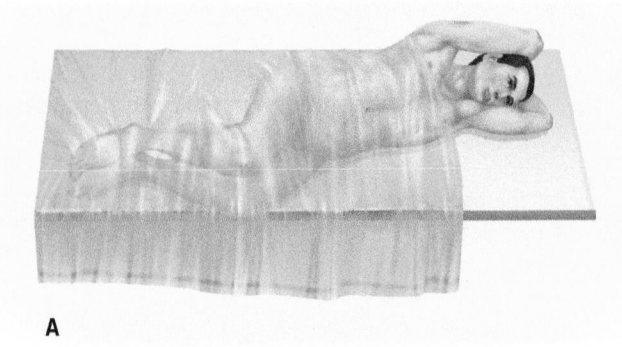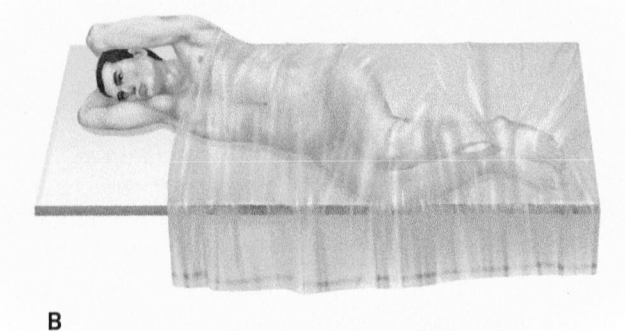

FIGURE 35-15 (A) Left lateral decubitus position (LLDP); **(B)** right lateral decubitus position (RLDP)

Decubitus Position. This position has the patient lying on his side (Figure 35-15A-B). A patient lying on the left side would be in the left lateral decubitus position (LLDP). A patient lying on the right side would be in the right lateral decubitus position (RLDP). This position is commonly used when taking X-rays.

Patient Communication

Always explain to the patient why he is being placed in a specific position. Be sure that the patient is never left in an uncomfortable position any longer than is necessary, and assist the patient when a position change is required. Some of the positions can be both uncomfortable and embarrassing to patients. A medical assistant must be professional at all times, reassuring the patient and minimizing the discomfort and embarrassment as much as possible.

Positions may also be uncomfortable because of the patient's condition. If a patient has low back pain, he may not be able to sit for a long time. If a patient with chronic obstructive pulmonary disease (COPD) is in the supine position and having difficulty breathing, the medical assistant should immediately help the patient to a semi-Fowler's position to allow for better chest and lung expansion. When you are aware of the patient's medical history, you can preemptively take steps to make the patient more comfortable.

The physician will expect you, as the medical assistant, to have the patient in the correct position for a procedure. Thus, you should understand the purpose of placing patients in specific positions. The more you know, the better you will be at explaining the procedure and getting the patient into the proper position.

Before the procedure begins, take the time to explain to the patient the events that will occur. This allows the patient time to prepare as well as ask any questions or voice any concerns. If a certain part of the physical examination may be uncomfortable, let the patient know. For example, if a female patient is having a vaginal exam, explain to the patient that

when the physician inserts the vaginal speculum into the vagina, she might feel some pressure in that area. Effective communication will help establish a sense of trust between the patient and the medical assistant.

Laboratory and Diagnostic Tests

Laboratory and other diagnostic tests may be ordered in addition to the physician's exam. Some of these tests, such as a urinalysis or electrocardiogram (ECG or EKG), may be conducted in the office on the day of the examination, whereas others, such as an X-ray, may be scheduled by appointment at a separate laboratory or diagnostic facility. Table 35-3 gives examples of tests that might be ordered as part of a complete examination.

SEQUENCE OF PROCEDURES IN A COMPLETE PHYSICAL EXAMINATION

Individual physicians may instruct the medical assistant regarding the specific order of a complete physical examination. Typically, the physician will discuss the past medical history, chief complaint (CC), the history of the present illness (PI) first, and then do a **review of systems (ROS)**. A ROS is a complete head-to-toe physical examination that focuses on evaluating all of the patient's body systems. The sequence of the ROS may vary by physician, but a common ROS sequence is:

skin→hair→nails→head→neck→eyes→ears→
nose→mouth→throat→arms→heart→chest→
lungs→breasts→abdomen→genitalia→rectum→
legs→feet→neurological system

The physician will document in the medical record as each ROS component of the physical examination is completed, although the medical assistant may be asked to assist. See Procedure 35-11.

TABLE 35-3 | Laboratory and Diagnostic Tests

Tests	Description
Blood Chemistry Profile	Group (or panel) of chemistry tests that provides overview of patient's body chemistries; less expensive than performing individual tests.
SMA-12 (or Chem 12)	Panel of 12 chemistry tests.
SMAC (or Chem 20)	Panel of 20 tests.
Complete Blood Count (CBC) Including a Differential Count	Includes red blood cell (RBC) count, white blood cell (WBC) count, hemoglobin (Hgb), hematocrit (Hct), RBC indices, platelets, and differential; the differential count indicates characteristics of RBCs, platelets, and types of WBCs.
Electrocardiogram (ECG)	Record of electrical activity of the heart; useful in diagnosis of heart muscle damage causing disruption of electrical activity of the heart and abnormal cardiac rhythm.
Pulmonary Function Test	Determines respiratory function through the use of equipment that measures lung volume and gas exchange.
Sedimentation Rate (Sed Rate, ESR)	Measures the rate at which erythrocytes (RBCs) settle out of blood in one hour; inflammatory conditions cause faster settling because they are heavier, and the sed rate will be higher than normal.
Vital Signs	Measurements of signs of life, which include temperature, pulse, respirations, and blood pressure.
Weight and Height	Anthropometric measurements of the human body.
X-rays	Radiology studies of body parts (e.g., chest and spine).

PROCEDURE 35-11

Assisting with a Complete Physical Examination

Objective ◆ *Assist with a physical examination by preparing the necessary equipment, while observing proper sequencing and ensuring patient safety with limited direction.*

EQUIPMENT AND SUPPLIES

Alcohol swabs; drape; emesis basin; examination table with clean sheet; disposable gloves; laryngeal mirror; lubricant; nasal speculum; ophthalmoscope; otoscope; pillow (with clean cover); reflex hammer; scale with height rod; Snellen chart (vision); sphygmomanometer; stethoscope; tape measure; thermometer; tissues; tongue depressors; tuning fork; urine specimen container

Note: Equipment and supplies will vary, depending on the type and purpose of the examination and personal preferences of the physician.

METHOD

1. Perform hand hygiene.
2. Assemble all equipment in the examining room.
3. Greet and identify the patient. Explain to the patient that the doctor will be performing a physical examination.

4. For comfort and efficiency during the examination, the patient should have an empty bladder. If a urine specimen is needed for the examination, provide the patient with a urine specimen container.
   a. If a urine specimen is not required, simply offer the patient the opportunity to use the restroom. Make sure the patient knows how to find the restroom and then find the way back to the examination room.
5. Obtain the patient's vital signs and measurements (temperature, pulse, respirations, blood pressure, height, and weight).
   a. Immediately document this information in the patient's medical record.
6. Provide the patient with a gown and drape and give instructions on disrobing. Inform the patient as to whether the opening of the gown should be in the front or the

back. Then instruct the patient to sit on the examination table after donning the gown.
   a. Excuse yourself from the room to provide patient privacy while the patient disrobes.
7. After an adequate amount of time has passed, return to the room. Knock on the door, identify yourself, and ask permission to enter the room. Once inside, place the drape over the patient's legs and inquire if there are any questions or concerns.
8. Inform the physician that the patient is ready to be seen.
   a. A female medical assistant should remain in the room if the patient is a female and the physician is a male or if the physician needs assistance. A male medical assistant may be required to remain in the room if the patient is male and the physician is female or if the physician needs assistance.
9. Assist the physician as needed by handing instruments and other supplies needed during the examination.
   a. Pay attention to when you will need to help the patient during positional changes.
10. Use personal protective equipment (PPE), such as gloves, when appropriate.
   a. Use gloves when handling used equipment that may contain biohazardous materials, such as the laryngeal mirror. After they are used, place the mirror and other contaminated equipment in the emesis basin until you can carry them to the decontamination area.
11. As the physician progresses from one section of the body to the next during the ROS, reposition the drape to expose only the portion of the patient's body being examined.
12. If collected, label all specimen slides and containers as soon as possible. Use gloves when handling specimens.

13. When the examination is complete, assist the patient to sit up slowly because some patients may experience dizziness. When removing the patient's legs from stirrups, take both legs down together to prevent strain on hips and back.
14. Assist the patient off the examination table, if necessary.
   a. Ask if the patient requires help dressing. If help is not needed, leave the room to allow the patient to get dressed.
15. Once the patient is dressed, provide the patient with further instructions. For example, you may instruct the patient to head directly to checkout, or the patient might need to remain in the room and await further instructions from the physician.
16. After the patient leaves, clean the examination table for the next patient, following the steps in Procedure 35-1.
17. Resupply the examination room, including replacing soiled linens.
18. Properly document any findings and procedures in the patient's medical record. "CPX" is commonly recognized as the abbreviation for complete physical exam. Most offices are now adopting electronic health records, and documentation is made according to the office policy and software design.

CHARTING EXAMPLE

2/14/YY 3:00 P.M. Ht: 65" Wt: 168# T: 98.4°F (T) P: 82 bpm, strong R: 16, regular BP: 118/78; CPX by Dr. Williams. Pt. referred to clinic lab for CBC, UA, and mammogram. Pt. to return in one week to discuss results. Appointment made for 2/21/YY .... M. King, CMA

Note: The physician will document her own findings from the CPX in the patient's medical record.

As a medical assistant, you need to understand and use correct medical terminology and appropriate medical abbreviations. The proper usage, pronunciation, and spelling of medical terms are also critical to functioning successfully as a medical assistant. If you encounter words you are unsure of, look them up when time permits. Never guess at the meaning. When you are unsure of an abbreviation used in a physician's order, ask the physician or a coworker or look it up. Although many terms and abbreviations are fairly generic and widely used, others are specific to the medical specialty and may be unfamiliar.

Review of Systems

The review of systems will include the following:

- **Skin**—The physician will inspect and palpate the skin. This is an important aspect of the physical examination because it can indicate the patient's nutritional status and level of hydration. The color, temperature, texture, and turgor of the skin are assessed. **Turgor** refers to the resistance of the skin when grasped between fingers. Turgor is decreased in dehydration and increased in edema (swelling).

- **Hair**—The color, texture, distribution, quantity, and growth pattern of the hair are assessed. Certain diseases such as hyperthyroidism can cause alopecia (hair loss). Excessive facial hair in a female (hirsutism) may indicate hormonal imbalance.

- **Nails**—Color, texture, symmetry, shape, and size are assessed for possible circulatory problems, fungal infections, or other infections. Brittle, grooved, or lined nails may indicate local or systemic conditions, such as nutritional deficiencies, endocrine dysfunction, and heart disease.

- **Head**—The shape, size, and symmetry of the head are assessed. The scalp is also assessed for parasites (nits and lice), lesions, flakes, and irritations. The face of a patient reveals much about state of health and stress level. Dark circles under the eyes and a general look of facial fatigue could indicate increased stress. Bruises or other signs of trauma may be indications of physical abuse. During the examination, the physician may ask more specific questions to determine if the patient is experiencing any abuse.

- **Neck**—The neck is assessed for range of motion, pulsations, texture, color, lumps, masses, and swelling. The physician will also assess the carotid pulse, lymph nodes, thyroid gland, and trachea. Asking a patient to swallow while palpating the thyroid gland helps detect lumps or enlargement of the thyroid gland (goiter).

- **Eyes**—Before the physician sees the patient, the medical assistant will test the patient's visual acuity or distance vision by using a Snellen chart. Other vision tests that may be performed are the Jaeger reading card to test for near vision and the Ishihara test book for color vision or color-blindness. The physician will examine visual fields, pupils' reaction to light, eye movement, and the internal and external structures of the eye by using an ophthalmoscope. The color of the sclera (white outer layer of the eye) is evaluated for any discoloration, such as yellowing, which may be a sign of jaundice.

- **Ears**—The physician will examine the internal and external ears for color, size, shape, and position. The physician may use tuning forks or whisper in the patient's ear to assess the patient's hearing. The ear canals are examined with an otoscope for signs of foreign bodies or excess cerumen, or earwax (Figure 35-16).

- **Nose**—The internal and external structures of the nose will be examined for color and symmetry. The physician may use an otoscope with a nasal speculum to view the lining and internal structures of the nose. Red swollen mucosa with yellow to greenish discharge may indicate an infection. The physician may also assess the patient's sense of smell. If drainage is observed, the physician will note the amount, color, and consistency.

- **Mouth**—The physician will assess the lips and inside the mouth for symmetry, moisture, color, and lesions. The tongue's texture, color, size, shape, symmetry, movement, and position will also be assessed. The number of teeth and their color and condition will be noted. Good oral hygiene is important to a patient's overall health. Patients should be reminded to schedule regular dental care and cleaning, usually every six months. Gums should be pink and healthy and not prone to bleeding.

- **Throat**—The physician will begin to assess the patient's throat by asking the patient to say "Ah," which opens the patient's mouth. Using a tongue depressor, the physician can inspect the uvula, tonsils, and throat for color, size, shape, symmetry, and movement. The physician will also check the patient's gag reflex.

- **Arms**—The joints, range of motion, strength, and pulses (brachial and radial) of the arms will be assessed by the physician.

- **Heart**—Using a stethoscope, the physician will auscultate the sounds of the heart, noting the rate, rhythm,

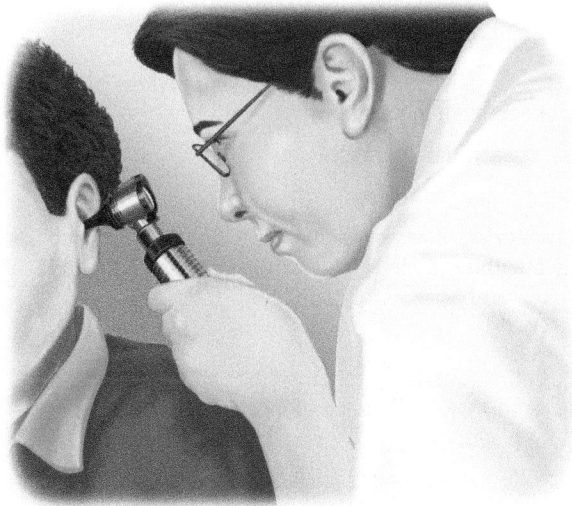
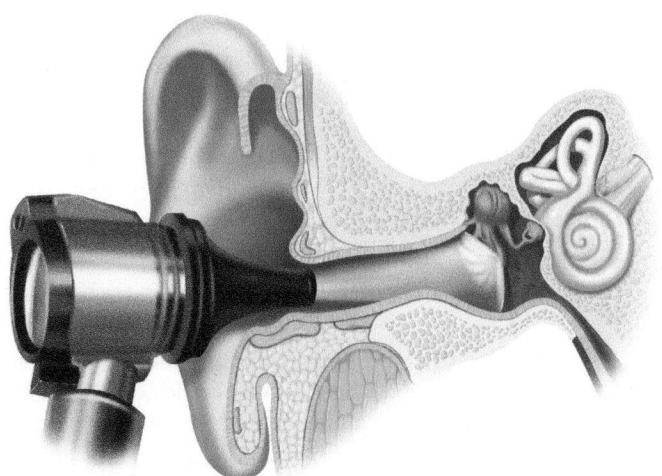

FIGURE 35-16 Inspecting a patient's ear during a physical examination.

pitch, and quality. The physician will then place the stethoscope over various areas of the patient's heart to listen for normal heart sounds. Any murmurs or other abnormalities detected will be noted.

- **Chest**—The chest wall will be assessed for symmetry during inspiration and expiration. It will also be assessed for pain, tenderness, lesions, lumps, and temperature. Postural abnormalities such as scoliosis (curvature of the spine) may be noted as well.

- **Lungs**—Using a stethoscope, the physician will auscultate the patient's breath sounds, noting rate, rhythm, pitch, depth, and location.

- **Breasts**—The physician will assess the breasts of both males and females. The breasts will be assessed for size, shape, symmetry, and texture. Any discharge, lumps, masses, pain, or tenderness will be noted.

- **Abdomen**—The abdomen is assessed for symmetry, texture, temperature, and movement. Using a stethoscope, the physician will auscultate the patient's bowel sounds for frequency, pitch, gurgling, and clicking sounds. The abdomen is visually divided into four quadrants: right and left upper quadrants and right and left lower quadrants. The organs in each quadrant are also percussed and palpated for

signs of masses, position of organs, muscle tone, and pain.

- **Genitalia**—The physician will assess the internal and external genitalia of a female patient. For the male patient, the physician will assess the external genitalia and perform a testicular examination. Any lesion, discharge, odor, and other abnormalities will be noted by the physician.

- **Rectum**—To assess the rectum for lesions or masses, the physician will perform a digital rectal examination. Most physicians require anyone over 40 years of age to have a digital rectal exam for early detection of colorectal cancer. A stool sample may be gathered for occult (hidden) blood at the same time.

- **Legs and feet**—The joints, range of motion, strength, and pulses (popliteal, dorsalis pedis, and posterior tibial) of the legs and feet will be assessed by the physician. Any postural problems will also be noted.

- **Neurological system**—The physician will use a reflex hammer to examine each reflex for the appropriate response. The physician will also observe the patient's gait, facial expressions, speech, movement, and response to sensation.

Table 35-4 presents a summary of the observations made during an ROS. Table 35-5 presents a typical sequence of

TABLE 35-4 | Review of Systems (ROS)

Head	Headaches, sinus pain, masses, alopecia (unusual hair loss), dizziness, injury, or trauma
Eyes	Visual acuity, blurred vision, burning, halo effect, tearing, photophobia (sensitivity to light), discharge, redness, jaundice (yellowing of skin and sclera), known eye diseases, date of last eye exam, prescription glasses, contact lenses
Ears	Tinnitus or ringing in the ears, dizziness, hearing loss, discharge, ear infections, exposure to loud noise on a regular basis
Nose	Allergies, obstruction, sense of smell, pain, discharge
Mouth	Dental work, dentures, gums, sense of taste, teeth, salivation (producing saliva), dryness of mouth, tongue, leukoplakia (white patches, possibly cancerous), gingivitis
Throat	Hoarseness, laryngitis (loss of voice), redness, speech defect, masses, pain
Neck	Tenderness, pain, swelling, difficulty swallowing, enlarged nodes
Respiratory	Dyspnea (labored breathing), cough, asthma, wheezing, allergies, hemoptysis (coughing up blood), chest pain, night sweats, orthopnea (difficulty breathing while lying down), shortness of breath (SOB)
Cardiovascular (CV)	Chest pain, hypertension, peripheral edema, cyanosis, fainting, dizziness, heart murmurs, palpitations, arrhythmias
Gastrointestinal (GI)	Nausea, vomiting, anorexia (loss of appetite), bulimia (eating disorder—binge eating followed by purging), indigestion, diarrhea, constipation, hemorrhoids, presence of blood in stool, number of bowel movements daily, hematemesis (vomiting blood)
Genitourinary (GU)	History of urinary tract infection, frequency, hesitation, oliguria (reduced urine), hematuria (blood in urine), dysuria (difficult or painful urination), renal colic (kidney pain), stones, discharge, nocturia (urination during the night)

TABLE 35-4 | Review of Systems (ROS) (*continued*)

Female Reproductive	Menstrual history, obstetric history, leukorrhea (white discharge), itching, pain, discharge, date of last Pap test, breast self-exam history, sexual habits, menopause symptoms, last mammogram (breast exam)
Male Reproductive	Prostate problems, testicular self-exam, discharge, sexual habits, frequency of urination, decreased stream, nocturia, impotence
Endocrine	Growth and development, goiter, excessive thirst, intolerance to temperature change, hormone therapy, diabetes symptoms, irregular menses, symptoms of thyroid disorders
Skin	Rash, urticaria (hives), texture, moles, infection, redness, jaundice, cyanosis, allergies, dry/oily, acne
Musculoskeletal (MS)	Joint pain, swelling, weakness, stiffness, numbness, muscle pain, fractures, discoloration, edema
Neurological	Fainting, loss of consciousness, headaches, tremor, nervousness, paralysis, pain, memory loss
Psychiatric	Mental health history, emotional stability, depression, stress
General	Weight gain or loss, sleep habits, fatigue, eating habits, smoking, work environment

TABLE 35-5 | Sequence of Physical Examination Procedures

1. **Registration**	Receptionist/medical assistant
2. **History**	Medical assistant
3. **Urine Specimen**	Medical assistant or laboratory technician
4. **Blood Specimen**	Medical assistant or laboratory technician or phlebotomist
5. **Vital Signs**	Medical assistant
6. **Weight and Height**	Medical assistant
7. **Visual Acuity**	Medical assistant
8. **Electrocardiogram**	Medical assistant
9. **X-ray**	X-ray technician (provided X-ray room is available; otherwise X-ray is completed before the patient's visit); some states do allow medical assistants to perform limited radiology with additional education
10. **Preparation of the Patient**	Medical assistant
11. **Review of Systems**	Physician

procedures to be performed and the person responsible for completing the procedure. Guidelines 35-1 lists important guidelines for charting. It is important to remember the steps associated with accurately documenting information in the patient's medical record.

Guidelines 35-1

Charting: Electronic or Paper Medical Records

1. Entries should be concise and complete.
2. Use only accepted medical abbreviations known by the general staff, and correctly spell all medical terms. See Appendix 1 or a medical terminology text for a list of commonly used medical abbreviations.
3. Document all telephone calls, correspondence, and patient interactions relating to the patient in the medical record, and document any action(s) taken.
4. Document all missed appointments.
5. Document any incidences of noncompliance.
6. Document every instance of patient education.
7. Do not record personal opinion, speculations, or judgments.

Charting in Paper Medical Records

1. Double-check to make sure that you have the correct patient chart.
2. Use black ink, and write legibly. Printing is preferred if your handwriting is difficult to read.
3. The patient's name should appear on each page of the record. Many offices have a device that stamps the patient's name and identification number onto the paper.
4. Every entry must be dated and initialed by the person writing in the record. The full name of the person initialing the document should either be in the medical record or on file in the physician's office.
5. Never erase, use a liquid eraser, or in any way remove information from a medical record. If a correction must be made, write the date it was made and your initials beside it.

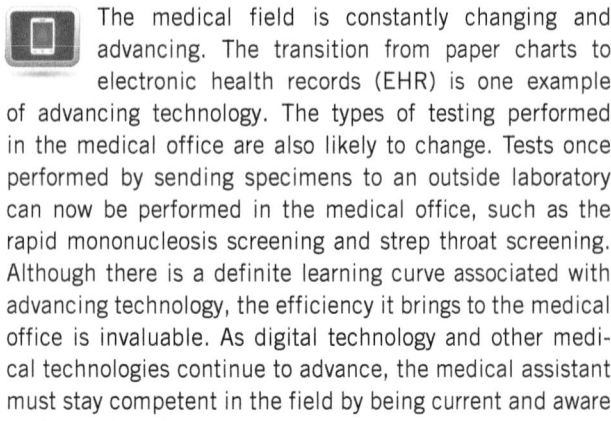

Professionalism | The Workplace

The medical field is constantly changing and advancing. The transition from paper charts to electronic health records (EHR) is one example of advancing technology. The types of testing performed in the medical office are also likely to change. Tests once performed by sending specimens to an outside laboratory can now be performed in the medical office, such as the rapid mononucleosis screening and strep throat screening. Although there is a definite learning curve associated with advancing technology, the efficiency it brings to the medical office is invaluable. As digital technology and other medical technologies continue to advance, the medical assistant must stay competent in the field by being current and aware of these often timesaving trends.

SUMMARY

The medical assistant plays a crucial role in creating a patient's first impression of a physician's office because the medical assistant is often the patient's first contact. The medical assistant has many functions in the medical office, which include preparing the exam room, taking vital signs, conducting the patient interview, documenting in the patient's medical record, and assisting the physician in the physical examination. The most effective medical assistants have the ability to anticipate the physician's needs during the exam, an ability that is acquired with experience.

Patient safety and comfort during the exam are a priority because they allow the physician to complete the examination more efficiently and effectively and obtain the most accurate patient information. The medical assistant's role before, during, and after the examination is to ensure that the medical record, the patient, and the equipment are completely prepared and ready for the physician. Accuracy and thoroughness are imperative to being a successful medical assistant.

35 CHAPTER REVIEW

COMPETENCY REVIEW

1. Define and spell the terms for this chapter.
2. Identify standards of the Americans with Disabilities Act that would pertain to the medical office.
3. Identify five furnishings found in a standard examination room.
4. Identify instruments and equipment used by the physician when completing a physical examination.
5. Explain the difference between signs and symptoms.
6. Discuss the difference between acute and chronic pain.
7. List what you would do to prepare a patient for a physical exam.
8. Identify patient positions used during medical and surgical examinations and procedures.
9. List the six methods used in physical examinations.
10. Identify what information may be collected during a social history.

PREPARING FOR THE CERTIFICATION EXAM

1. The opposite of the prone position is
   a. lithotomy.
   b. Fowler's.
   c. supine.
   d. Sims.
   e. Trendelenburg.

2. To examine a patient vaginally, the patient is usually placed in the
   a. lithotomy position.
   b. Fowler's position.

   c. supine position.
   d. anatomical position.
   e. prone position.

3. Listening to sounds produced through an instrument or with your ear is called
   a. inspection.
   b. auscultation.
   c. percussion.
   d. palpation.
   e. examination.

4. In a common ROS sequence, which would immediately follow the review of the nails?
   a. head
   b. neck
   c. eyes
   d. ears
   e. nose

5. Face down on an examination table with legs out straight is the
   a. supine position.
   b. knee–chest position.
   c. Sims position.
   d. dorsal recumbent position.
   e. prone position.

6. Listening to sounds when the body is struck in a definite manner is called
   a. auscultation.
   b. percussion.
   c. palpation.
   d. mensuration.
   e. manipulation.

7. Distinguishing between two similar diseases by comparing their symptoms is called
   a. physical diagnosis.
   b. laboratory diagnosis.
   c. clinical diagnosis.
   d. differential diagnosis.
   e. radiologic diagnosis.

8. The process of measuring is called
   a. inspection.
   b. palpation.
   c. palpitation.
   d. mensuration.
   e. manipulation.

9. A patient with COPD struggling to breathe in the sitting position should be changed to which position?
   a. lithotomy
   b. dorsal recumbent
   c. semi-Fowler's
   d. knee–chest
   e. prone

10. The instrument used to examine the eyes during a physical examination is the
    a. otoscope.
    b. stethoscope.
    c. proctoscope.
    d. ophthalmoscope.
    e. cystoscope.

CRITICAL THINKING

Refer to the case study at the beginning of the chapter and use what you have learned to answer the following questions.

1. How should Susan record Molly's chief complaint?
2. Susan obtains Molly's vital signs, which are T: 98.8°F, P: 82 bpm, BP: 130/88. Pearson Physicians Group uses the SOAP (subjective, objective, assessment, and plan) method of charting. Which part of the SOAP note would be appropriate to include Molly's vital signs?
3. What should Susan instruct Molly to do before being seen by the physician?

ON THE JOB

Elizabeth Smith, CMA (AAMA), just started working for Coventry Family Practice. Connie Barnaby, RMA, is the clinical manager of the office. Connie is helping Elizabeth during the orientation period of her new job.

1. At the start of the day, Connie asks Elizabeth to make sure all examination rooms are stocked with necessary supplies. What supplies would an examination room typically contain?
2. Connie informs Elizabeth that the first patient of the day is being seen for hemorrhoid pain and itching. Connie asks Elizabeth to assist the patient into the lateral recumbent position. What is another term for the lateral recumbent position, and how would Elizabeth position the patient?

INTERNET ACTIVITY

Perform an Internet search for examples of the various types of EHR systems available for a medical office.

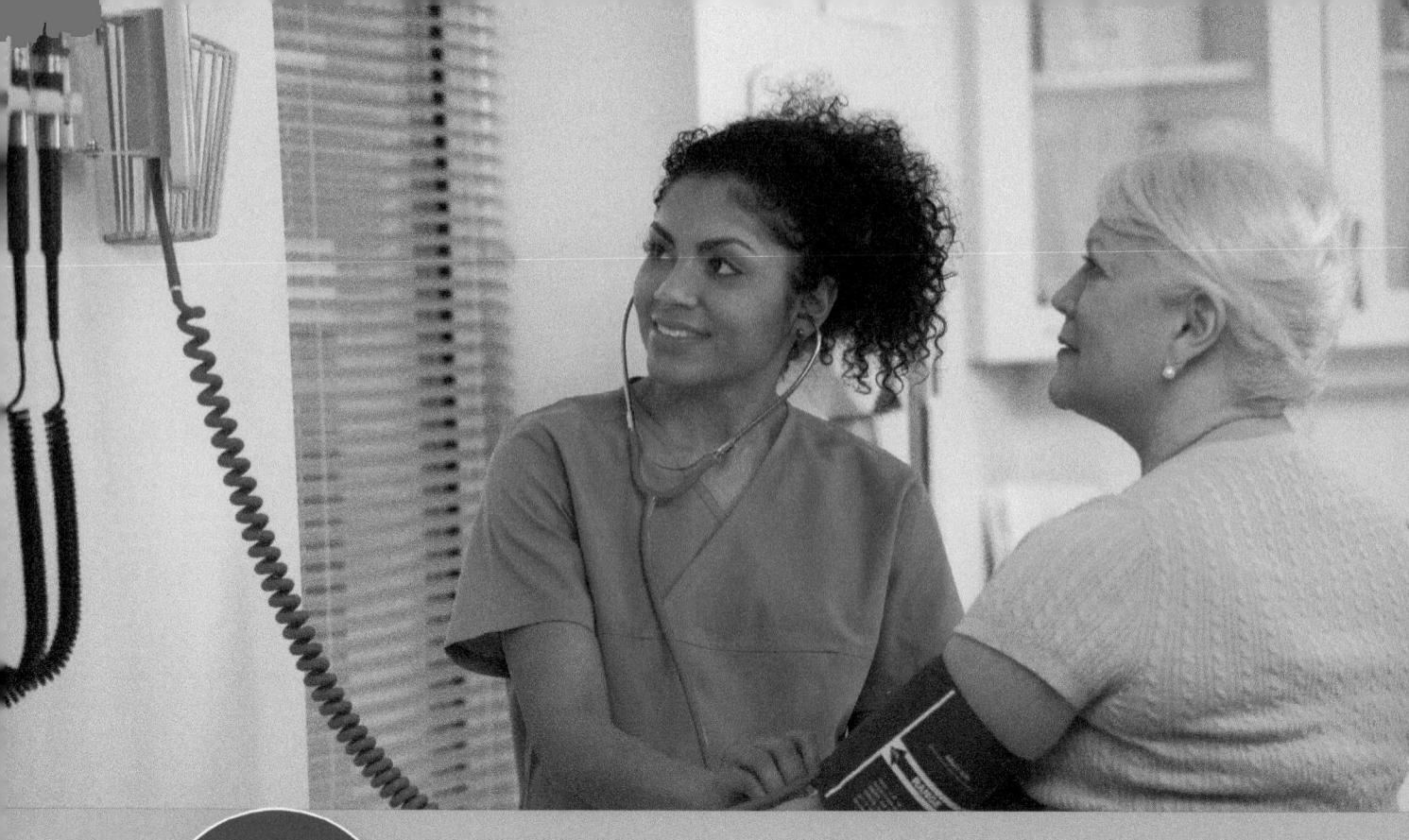

Assisting with Medical Specialties

Learning Objectives

After completing this chapter, you should be able to:

36.1   Define and spell the terms for this chapter.

36.2   List duties of the medical assistant when assisting in the field of allergy and immunology.

36.3   Explain how various forms of allergy testing are performed.

36.4   List duties of the medical assistant when assisting in the field of dermatology.

36.5   Describe different types of dermatological neoplasms.

36.6   List duties of the medical assistant when assisting in the field of cardiology.

36.7   Identify common risk factors associated with cardiovascular disease.

36.8   List duties of the medical assistant when assisting in the field of endocrinology.

36.9   List duties of the medical assistant when assisting in the field of gastroenterology.

36.10 Identify considerations that must be taken when a stool sample must be collected.

36.11 List duties of the medical assistant when assisting in the field of orthopedics.

36.12 List duties of the medical assistant when assisting in the field of neurology.

Benito Salvatore, a 65-year-old business executive, is scheduled to have a sigmoidoscopy with Dr. Bahjat. When David Dolan, RMA, escorts him to the procedure room, Benito confides that he is extremely nervous and is concerned he did not prepare well enough for the procedure.

Terms to Learn

allergist	edema	orthopedist
angina	endocrinologist	polydipsia
arrhythmia	gastroenterologist	polyuria
benign	hematochezia	polyphagia
cardiologist	hemorrhoids	proctologist
colonoscopy	immunologist	psychiatrist
cyanosis	malignant	rheumatologist
debridement	Mohs technician	Romberg test
dermatologist	neurologist	scratch test
desensitizing injections	neurosurgeon	sigmoidoscopy
diaphoresis	occult	wheal
dyspnea	orthopedics	

As a student learning to become a medical assistant, you will be taught a wide range of general procedures and skills that can be used in a variety of medical settings. General administrative skills, such as answering the telephone, scheduling a patient appointment, and performing billing and collections, do not vary significantly from office to office or from specialty to specialty. However, clinical skills and procedures can vary based on the type and specialty of the medical practice and office. Medical assistants must be aware of the various procedures and skills that are unique to each medical specialty.

This chapter discusses the nuances of working as a medical assistant in different medical specialties, specifically allergy and immunology, dermatology, cardiology, endocrinology, gastroenterology, orthopedics, and neurology. Subsequent chapters in this textbook discuss the medical assistant's duties in other specialties, such as urology, gynecology, pulmonology, and radiology.

THE ROLE OF THE MEDICAL ASSISTANT

The medical assistant plays a pivotal role on a medical team and in a physician's office. Some medical assistants may work with primary care and internal medicine physicians; others may work with physician specialists.

Primary care physicians and internal medicine physicians are general practitioners and provide basic diagnosis and treatment of common illnesses and medical conditions and diseases. Primary care and internal medicine physicians are usually a patient's first line of contact for seeking medical treatment. These physicians often refer a patient to a specialist if the patient requires more extensive disease management. A physician specialist is trained and certified in a specific area or field and performs more complex diagnoses and intensive treatments and procedures.

A medical assistant should be prepared to perform the same basic skills and procedures in all types of medical practices and clinics, although specific skills may be used more depending on the practice and specialty. For example, a medical assistant working for a primary care physician might perform one or two electrocardiograms (ECGs) a day. In comparison, a medical assistant working for a cardiologist could perform as many as 10 to 15 ECGs a day.

Although a medical assistant may perform some of the same procedures in multiple medical settings and specialties, other procedures are only performed in a specialist's office and not in a primary care practice; for example, a sigmoidoscopy is usually performed only in a gastroenterology practice.

Regardless of the type of practice, a medical assistant's duties are to assist the physician during examinations and procedures. The medical assistant often has the most exposure to patients during their visit. For example, the medical assistant meets with patients before and after the physician and assists the physician during the patient's visit. In addition, the medical assistant often serves as the "health coach," helping patients understand their diagnosis and treatment and encouraging them to adhere to the treatment plan. Medical assistants may also educate patients about disease prevention and health promotion and maintenance practices, such as weight management, smoking cessation, and healthy eating habits. This topic is further discussed in the chapter titled "Patient Education."

Working as a medical assistant will bring you into contact with a diverse patient population who have various conditions and diseases. Whether the conditions are acute (severe or short-term) or chronic (long lasting or persistent), patients experience a wide range of emotional responses to specialized testing and procedures, including fear, confusion, and frustration. As a result, it is imperative that medical assistants have the ability to communicate effectively and display appropriate sensitivity to help patients in all circumstances.

ASSISTING WITH ALLERGY CARE AND IMMUNOLOGY

An **allergist** or **immunologist** is a physician specialist who is trained in diagnosing, treating, and managing allergies, asthma, and other immune system disorders. A medical assistant working for an allergist/immunologist may perform the following duties:

- Room patients and obtain vital signs and measurements.
- Record the patient's history, including any specialized questionnaires pertaining to the patient's allergy or

immunology history. These questionnaires are usually created by the physicians, who then review the answers obtained by the medical assistant with the patient during the examination.

- Prepare the exam room for specialty procedures, such as those associated with allergy testing.
- Ensure shot room, skin testing room, and exam rooms are clean, prepared, stocked, maintained, and functional at all times.
- Administer allergy injections, such as **desensitizing injections**, to patients and update shot records.
- Provide patient education and support based on the treatment protocol established by the physician.

Medical assistants working in this field should have a working knowledge of some common types of allergies. See Table 36-1 for a brief list of common allergies.

The medical assistant should become familiar with the types of tests the physician may order to help diagnose and identify the allergen. The most common types of allergy tests performed are skin tests (scratch, intradermal, and patch) and the radioallergosorbent test (RAST).

Skin Tests

All of the common types of skin tests—scratch, intradermal, and patch—are usually performed on the patient's back or forearm and allow for the testing of different allergens at the same time. Some medications will interfere with a skin test. Thus, before performing any skin tests, the physician will review the patient's medical chart and history and will advise on which medications to discontinue before the skin test is performed.

Scratch Test

The **scratch test** (also called the prick test) is one of the most common allergy tests and is usually conducted in the allergist's or immunologist's office. In a scratch test, the skin is divided into small squares, which are approximately 1 inch apart. Each square is labeled with a ballpoint pen to indicate which allergen is being used. A drop of allergen is placed on the skin, and then the skin is scratched with a needle or lancet to barely penetrate the skin.

A new needle or lancet must be used for each allergen tested to prevent cross-contamination. After 15 minutes, if the patient is allergic to one (or more) of the allergens, a small, red, itchy bump (**wheal**) develops (Figure 36-1). The patient should be advised to remain in the physician's office for at least 30 minutes after the testing has been completed in case there is a delayed severe allergic reaction to the testing.

TABLE 36-1 | Common Types of Allergies

Allergy	Description
Allergic Rhinitis	Inflammation of the nasal mucosa that results in nasal congestion, rhinorrhea (runny nose), sneezing, and itching of the nose. Seasonal allergic rhinitis, such as hay fever, occurs only during certain seasons of the year. Children suffering from this type of allergy may rub their nose in an upward movement, called the "allergic salute."
Asthma	Condition seen most frequently in childhood. The major symptoms are wheezing, coughing, and dyspnea. Asthmatic attacks may be caused by allergens from the air, food, or drugs. The patient's airway is affected by constriction of the bronchial passages and increased production of mucus. Treatment includes medication and reducing exposure to causative allergens.
Contact Dermatitis	Inflammation and irritation of the skin caused by contact with an irritating substance. Some common irritating substances include soap, perfume, cosmetics, metals or plastics, dyes, and plants, such as poison ivy. Treatment consists of topical and systemic medications to relieve symptoms and removal of the causative allergen.
Eczema	Superficial dermatitis accompanied by papules, vesicles, and crusting. The condition can be acute or chronic.
Urticaria	Also called hives, it is characterized by skin eruptions of pale reddish wheals with severe itching. It is usually associated with a food allergy, stress, or reactions to medications.

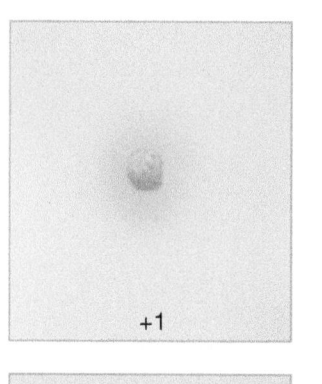
+1

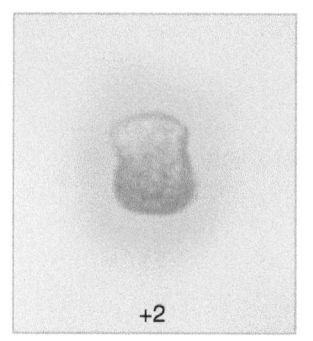
+2

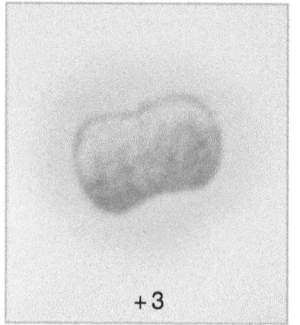
+3

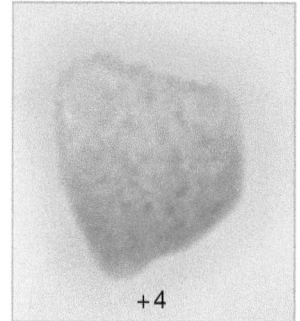
+4

FIGURE 36-1 Wheals are formed in reaction to scratch testing and intradermal testing of allergens.

Scratch testing is an example of a procedure that is more often performed in the specialist's office than the general medicine office. Procedure 36-1 explains how to perform a scratch test.

Intradermal Test

Intradermal allergy testing is performed by injecting 0.01 to 0.02 mL of an allergen extract into the anterior surface of the forearm (Figure 36-2). An intradermal test is considered more accurate than a scratch test. Therefore, it is more commonly performed in specialists' offices for determining allergen sensitivities. Refer to the chapter titled "Administering Medications" for information on performing intradermal injections.

Patch Test

The patch test is noninvasive, consisting of placing a small amount of the allergen onto the anterior forearm or upper back and then covering it with a protective wrap (plastic or specialty paper). Several patch tests can be performed at the same time. Results are read after the patches have remained

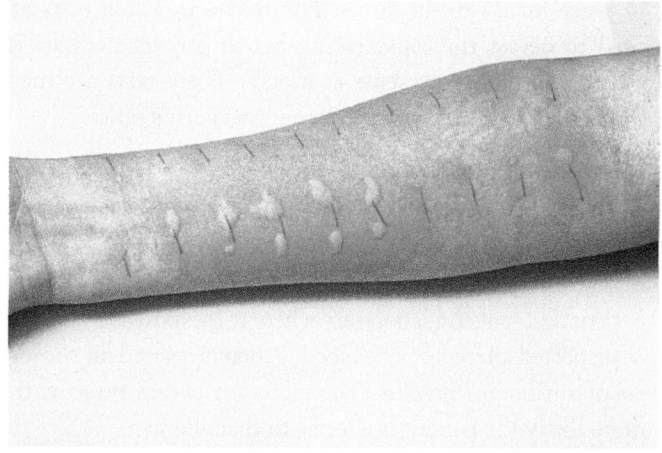

FIGURE 36-2 The patient's forearm shows a number of wheals formed after injection with an allergen. The size of the wheal corresponds to the severity of the allergy to the allergen.

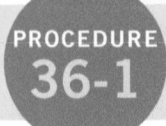

PROCEDURE 36-1

Performing a Scratch Test

Objective ◆ *Identify specific substances (allergens) that cause an allergic reaction in the patient.*

EQUIPMENT AND SUPPLIES

Allergen extracts; control solution; cotton balls; alcohol; disposable sterile needles or lancets; timer; tape; ruler; cold pack or ice bag; patient's medical record; disposable gloves; biohazard waste containers, including a sharps container

METHOD

1. Perform hand hygiene.
2. Warmly greet and identify the patient, introduce yourself, and explain the procedure.
3. Ask the patient to take a seat on the examination table. Provide support and assistance, if necessary.
4. Apply gloves, and swab the test site (either forearm or back) with alcohol and allow it to air-dry.
5. Label the skin surface with adhesive tape in rows about 1½ to 2 inches apart.
6. Place a drop of allergen above or below the correct label. Be consistent with the placement of the allergens to prevent any confusion regarding identifying the allergens.
7. Using a separate sterile lancet or needle for each extract, make a small scratch (no more than 1/8 inch deep) on the skin below each drop.
8. Set the timer for the specified reaction time, usually 10 to 30 minutes.
9. After the specified time period elapses, clean each site with alcohol and a cotton ball. Take special care not to remove labels.
10. Examine and measure each site, and record the results in the patient's record. (Review Figure 36-2, which shows examples of wheals resulting from scratch allergy testing.)
11. Have the physician examine each site and review your measurements.
12. Apply cold packs or ice bag to relieve itching, if necessary.
13. Dispose of used material in the proper waste receptacles.
14. Assist the patient off the examination table, and provide the patient with further instructions, as indicated by the physician.
15. Clean the examination room.
16. Perform hand hygiene.
17. Document information in the patient's medical record.

CHARTING EXAMPLE

03/13/YY 9:05 A.M. Scratch test performed. Admin Rt. Forearm. No positive reactions. Test sites checked by Dr. Rosen.. M. Dennehey, CMA

---

in place for 24 to 48 hours (Figure 36-3). Patch tests are used to detect the causative agents in contact dermatitis, which commonly presents as a rash. These tests are most commonly performed in an allergy specialist's office.

Radioallergosorbent Test

An alternative to the skin tests is blood tests. The radioallergosorbent test (RAST) measures levels of antibodies to particular antigens in the blood. Blood is collected from the patient and sent to a laboratory where it is exposed to a variety of suspected allergens. The blood is then measured for the levels of antibodies present. The more antibodies present, the more likely the patient is allergic to that allergen.

The RAST test may be preferred over skin tests for several reasons. Because the RAST test is performed on blood after it is withdrawn from the patient, it does not directly expose the

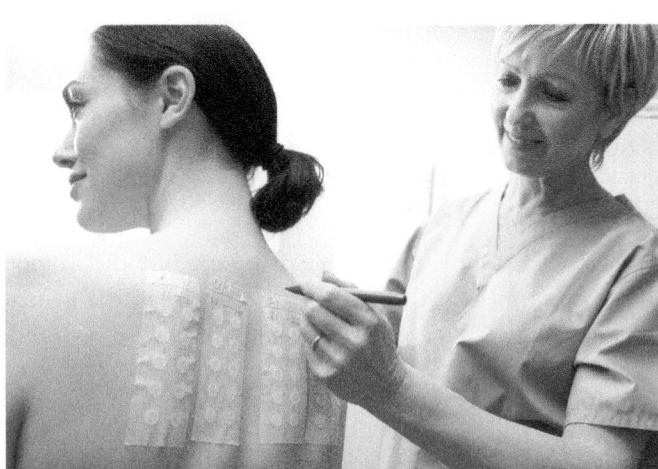

FIGURE 36-3 A medical assistant labels the allergens for a patch test.

patient to any allergens. This is particularly important for patients who are at higher risk if a life-threatening anaphylactic reaction should occur, such as patients with asthma or heart conditions. The RAST test may also be chosen by the physician if patients are unable to stop taking medication a few days before the test, which might be necessary for a skin test. However, the RAST test is more expensive and results may take several days, more time than is required for the scratch or intradermal skin tests. A medical assistant in a primary care office or specialist office can perform the RAST test because it simply requires blood samples to be taken and sent to a laboratory for further testing.

Currently, there are several other blood tests available that may be used instead of the RAST test.

ASSISTING WITH DERMATOLOGY

A **dermatologist** is a physician specialist who is trained in the diagnosis and treatment of disorders of the skin, or integumentary system. A medical assistant who is working for a dermatologist may perform the following duties:

- Room patients and obtain vital signs and measurements.
- Record the patient's history, including any dermatology-related questionnaires established by the physician.
- Prepare the exam room for specialty procedures, such as those associated with performing minor skin surgeries and obtaining skin biopsies.

- Prepare the patient and assist the physician with procedures related to medical and cosmetic dermatology, including laser surgery and chemical peels.
- Assist in the debridement of wounds and obtain wound cultures (Procedure 36-2).
- Provide patient education and support based on the treatment protocol established by the physician.

Once employed by a dermatologist, medical assistants may also have special training to work as a **Mohs technician**, named after the surgeon Frederic E. Mohs, who first developed this type of surgery. A Mohs technician assists the physician who performs the Mohs surgery, which is done to remove cancerous skin lesions and the surrounding layers of skin. During the surgery, the tissue is examined for cancer cells, which will assist the physician in deciding if additional tissue removal is required. Skin cancer is one of the most common forms of cancer in the United States. The Mohs technician plays a critical role in a dermatology practice.

Common Skin Disorders

Medical assistants working in a dermatology practice should have a thorough knowledge of common skin disorders and other diseases associated with the integumentary system. Most skin conditions and diseases are diagnosed, in part, by observing the lesion, which results when the normal surface of the skin is invaded or changed. When information about the chief complaint is entered into the patient's

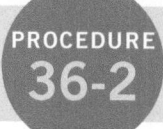

PROCEDURE 36-2 Taking a Wound Culture

Objective ◆ *Obtain a sample from a wound by using a swab technique.*

EQUIPMENT AND SUPPLIES

Gloves; culture tube with sterile swab and transport media; tape for dressing; sterile water for cleansing wound; sterile 4 × 4 gauze dressing; hazardous waste container; bag for soiled dressing; prepared label for culture tube or pen for labeling tube; patient's medical record

METHOD

1. Warmly greet and identify the patient, introduce yourself, and explain the procedure.
2. Assemble equipment, and label the culture tube with the patient's name, date of birth, your initials, and today's date.

3. Perform hand hygiene and don a pair of gloves.
4. Remove the patient's wound dressing. Take note of the amount and type of exudate. Dispose of used dressing materials in a biohazard waste container.
5. Observe the wound for redness, crusting, swelling, and odor.
6. Carefully remove the sterile swab from the culture tube and place it in the wound. Rotate the swab back and forth to obtain a good sample.
   a. Place the swab in the sterile culture tube (Figure A). Crush the ampule of preservative that is found at the bottom of the culture tube, and seal the tube.
   b. Label the tube with the patient's name, date of birth, collection date, and time.

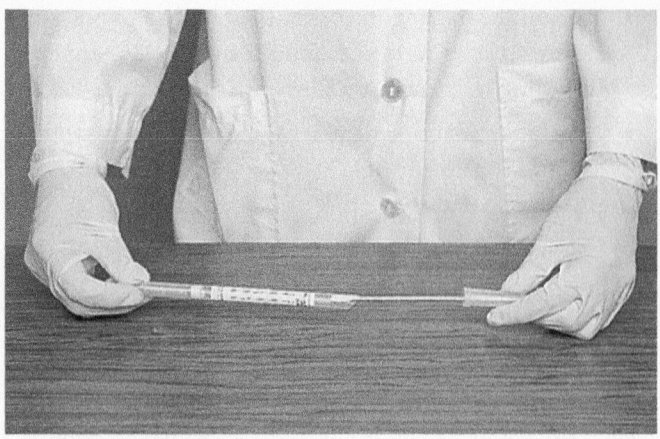

FIGURE A After obtaining the wound culture, push the tip of the swab into the culture medium.

7. Remove and dispose of gloves properly in hazardous waste container. Perform hand hygiene, and apply new sterile gloves.

8. Clean the wound using sterile water and 4 × 4 gauze squares.
9. Apply sterile dressing over the wound.
10. Dispose of used gauze squares in the biohazard waste container.
11. Remove and dispose of gloves properly in the hazardous waste container.
12. Instruct the patient regarding proper wound care. Provide both verbal and written instructions.
13. Document the information in the patient's medical record, including detailed notes regarding the appearance of the wound and any other outstanding observations.

CHARTING EXAMPLE

2/14/YY 3:30 P.M. Small amount of exudate obtained from open wound on L. ankle using sterile swab. Culture tube labeled and sent to lab. Wound cleaned and dressed. Redness surrounded the wound site. No odor noted. Home care instructions given.. M. King, RMA

medical record, it is necessary to include descriptive notes about the lesion's location, shape, color, size, and any other variances of the skin. Neoplasms (tumors) are classified as **malignant** (cancerous) or **benign** (noncancerous). Table 36-2 lists neoplasms that would commonly be seen in a dermatology practice.

Any kind of microorganisms—bacteria, viruses, fungi, and parasites—can invade the skin if its protective barrier is broken. Inflammatory skin disorders result in swelling, redness, pain, and often itching over the affected site. These conditions include cellulitis, decubitus ulcers, psoriasis, acne vulgaris, and scleroderma.

TABLE 36-2 | Dermatological Neoplasms

Benign (Noncancerous) Neoplasms	Description
Dermatofibroma	Fibrous tumor of the skin. It is painless, round, firm, red, and generally found on extremities.
Hemangioma	Benign tumor of dilated vessels.
Keloid	Formation of a scar after an injury or surgery that results in a raised, thickened, red area.
Keratosis	Overgrowth or thickening of cells in the epithelium located in the epidermis of the skin.
Leukoplakia	Change in the mucous membrane that results in thick, white patches on the mucous membrane of the tongue and cheek. It is considered precancerous and is associated with smoking.
Lipoma	Fatty tumor that generally does not metastasize (spread).
Nevus	Pigmented (colored) congenital skin blemish that is usually benign but may become cancerous. Also called a birthmark or mole.
Malignant (Cancerous) Neoplasms	**Description**
Basal Cell Carcinoma	Epithelial tumor of the basal cell layer of the epidermis. A frequent type of skin cancer that rarely metastasizes.
Kaposi's sarcoma	Form of skin cancer frequently seen in acquired immunodeficiency syndrome (AIDS) patients. It consists of brownish-purple papules that spread from the skin.
Malignant Melanoma	Dangerous form of skin cancer caused by an overgrowth of melanin in the skin. It may metastasize.
Squamous Cell Carcinoma	Epidermal cancer that may go into deeper tissue but does not generally metastasize.

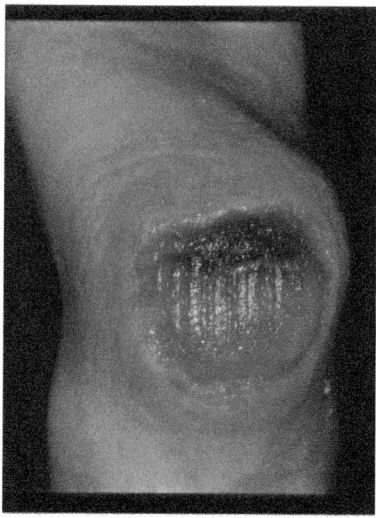

FIGURE 36-4 Decubitus ulcer (bedsore) on a patient's heel.

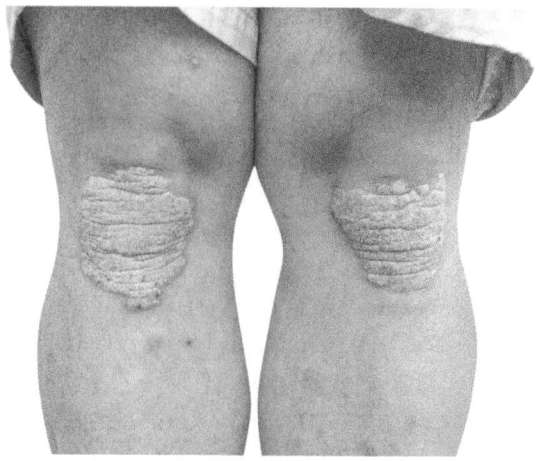

FIGURE 36-5 Bilateral psoriasis on a patient's knees.

- Cellulitis and erysipelas are inflammations of the cellular or connective tissue caused by either the bacteria *Staphylococcus* or *Streptococcus*. Treatment consists of antibiotics and application of warm compresses. Performing a wound culture may be necessary to aid in identifying the causative bacteria. Procedure 36-2 details how to perform a wound culture.

- Decubitus ulcers (bedsores or pressure sores) are open sores caused by prolonged pressure on the skin over bony prominences on the body, causing a decrease or lack of blood flow. The most commonly affected areas are the heels, elbows, hips, and lower spine (Figure 36-4). Patients most at risk are those who are bedridden or who lie in one position for too long. Treatment consists of relieving the pressure through frequent changing of positions, exercising the patient, and thorough cleansing of the wound and use of topical antibiotics. Deep ulcers may require surgical **debridement** (removal of dead tissue).

- Psoriasis is a chronic inflammatory condition consisting of distinct red or pink lesions covered with silver scaling, often referred to as plaques. The most common sites for psoriasis are the scalp, elbows, and knees, but it can be found throughout the body (Figure 36-5). Psoriasis is thought to be an autoimmune disease and is not contagious. Treatment consists of topical ointments and, in some severe cases, ultraviolet light therapy.

- Acne vulgaris is an inflammatory disease of the sebaceous glands and hair follicles that results in papules and pustules, commonly referred to as "pimples" or "zits." It may affect people of all ages, but mainly occurs in adolescents. Treatment consists of thorough cleansing of the skin and systemic and topical antibiotics in severe cases.

- Scleroderma is a chronic, progressive autoimmune disease that affects the connective tissue of the skin, blood vessels, and other organs. Scleroderma may result in hardening or tightening of the skin, which may limit movement in the affected areas; exaggerated responses to cold temperatures; and numbness or pain in affected areas.

ASSISTING WITH CARDIOLOGY

A **cardiologist** is a physician specialist who is trained in the diagnosis, treatment, and management of cardiovascular diseases and disorders. A medical assistant who is working for a cardiologist may perform the following duties:

- Room patients and obtain vital signs and measurements.

- Record the patient's history, including any cardiology-related questionnaires established by the physician.

- Schedule cardiovascular testing in both inpatient and outpatient facilities.

- Provide patient education and support based on the treatment protocol established by the physician for cardiovascular-related diseases and disorders.

- Perform electrocardiograms and Holter monitoring, providing patient education as necessary.

Electrocardiograms (ECGs) and Holter monitoring are the two common tests that medical assistants perform in a cardiovascular office. Both tests are used to monitor and record the heart's electric activity and are often used to diagnose heart disorders, especially in regard to its rhythm and rate.

An ECG is able to record a patient's heart activity for only a short period of time while the patient is hooked up to the machine. A Holter monitor, however, is a small, portable device that the patient wears usually for 24 to 48 hours that records the heart's activity while the patient is performing daily activities. The Holter monitor is beneficial because some patients have heart rhythm issues during sleep or physical activities, which the Holter monitor would be able to record but not the ECG. A more detailed discussion and instruction on how to perform an ECG can be found in the chapter titled "Electrocardiology."

Cardiovascular Diseases, Procedures, and Diagnostic Tests

Cardiovascular disease is the most frequent cause of illness and death in the United States, regardless of gender. For this reason, many of the patients you will manage will have heart disease, regardless of the type of clinic or specialty where you are employed. Thus it is important that you are able to recognize the signs and symptoms of cardiac diseases and disorders.

The causes of cardiovascular diseases and disorders are varied but include poor circulation, defective heart valves, conduction defects, and blood clots in the heart or blood vessels. The most common signs and symptoms of cardiovascular disorders include:

- **Angina**—Chest pain (crushing or stabbing type of pain)
- **Arrhythmia**—Irregular heartbeat
- **Cyanosis**—Bluish skin color caused by lack of oxygen in the tissues
- **Diaphoresis**—Excessive sweating
- **Dyspnea**—Difficulty breathing
- **Edema**—Swelling, particularly of the extremities

It is the responsibility of the medical assistant to schedule diagnostic tests and procedures for patients. Therefore, a medical assistant must also be able to explain diagnostic procedures and tests associated with the cardiovascular system to the patient and provide appropriate pretesting instructions.

Risk Factors for Cardiovascular Disease

As a medical assistant, you must understand the risk factors associated with cardiovascular disease to recognize at-risk patients and provide proper patient education. Patients with multiple risk factors are at risk not only for heart attack but also for pulmonary embolism caused by a blood clot traveling to a lung, stroke caused by a blood clot traveling to the brain, or stroke caused by plaque buildup

within cerebral arteries. Evidence indicates that cardiac changes that were once associated with aging and thus thought to be unavoidable can be modified by lifestyle changes and personal habits. A competent medical assistant will recognize risk factors for cardiovascular disease:

- Obesity
- High blood pressure
- High cholesterol
- Smoking
- Diets high in fat and sodium
- High stress levels
- Inactive or sedentary lifestyles
- Diabetes

Thus, medical assistants must play an active role in patient education by serving as a "patient coach" to help patients reduce or eliminate these risk factors and promote good cardiovascular health. Furthermore, the physician may recommend routine tests to monitor these risk factors—for example, an annual physical examination, periodic tests for blood lipid levels, and checks of the patient's blood pressure at every visit.

The National Institute of Health's National Cholesterol Education Program has published guidelines that recommend more aggressive treatment, such as drug therapy for individuals with moderately high to high risk of a heart attack. Research indicates that the more you lower low-density lipids (LDL or "bad" cholesterol), the less likely you are to have a heart attack. For very high-risk patients, such as those with heart disease, hypertension, or diabetes, the recommended goal is to have an LDL below 100 mg/dL. In moderate risk patients, the recommended goal is an LDL under 130 mg/dL.

ASSISTING WITH ENDOCRINOLOGY

An endocrinologist is a physician specialist who is trained in the diagnosis, treatment, and management of diseases and disorders associated with the endocrine system. There are two types of glands in the endocrine system: exocrine glands and endocrine glands. Exocrine glands secrete hormones into ducts that carry the hormones to various parts of the body for short-term but faster effects. Conversely, endocrine glands secrete hormones directly into the bloodstream without ducts, causing a longer-lasting but delayed effect. An endocrinologist diagnoses, treats, and manages patients affected by disorders involving both endocrine and exocrine glands.

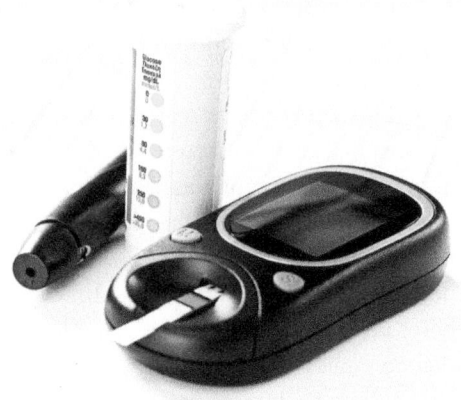

FIGURE 36-6 The medical assistant provides patient education regarding the daily use of diabetic glucose monitoring equipment.

A medical assistant who is working for an endocrinologist may perform the following duties:

- Room patients and obtain vital signs and measurements.

- Record the patient's medical history and complete endocrine system–related questionnaires established by the physician.

- Perform frequent venipuncture. Many endocrine system diseases are diagnosed and treated based on monitoring hormone levels through blood tests.

- Perform glucose monitoring and education related to proper use of glucose monitoring equipment, including glucometers, test strips, and lancets (Figure 36-6).

- Provide patient education and support based on the treatment protocol established by the physician for endocrine system–related diseases and disorders (Figure 36-7). This is particularly true for newly diagnosed

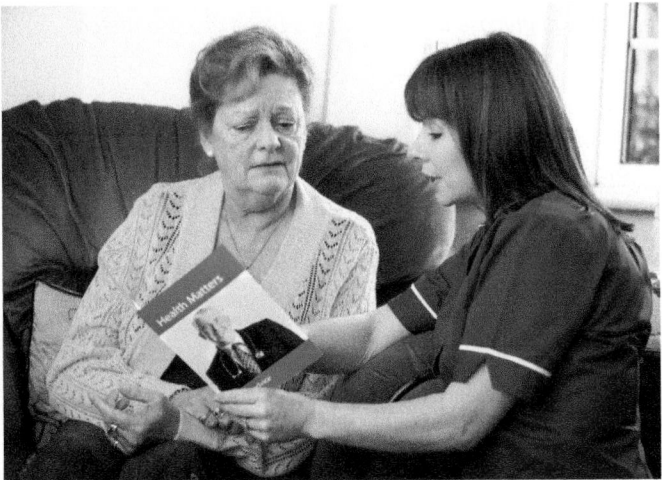

FIGURE 36-7 Using educational materials, the medical assistant discusses lifestyle changes with a diabetic patient.

diabetic patients who require extensive education and "coaching" regarding diet and lifestyle changes. Often, these patients are referred to a dietitian who has extensive training in working with diabetic patients, such as a Certified Diabetes Educator (CDE).

- Assist the physician by helping maintain accurate medication records. Many endocrine system disorders require multiple medications to maintain appropriate hormone levels.

- Similar to other specialties, the medical assistant will provide patient instruction and information regarding routinely scheduled diagnostic tests and procedures.

Hormones

The medical assistant working in the endocrinology practice must have a proper understanding of hormones and their functions. Hormones are chemical messengers produced by the endocrine glands and transported to target tissue by the bloodstream. Hormones transfer information and instructions from one set of cells to another to cause a specific action. For example, hormones are able to regulate growth and metabolism, sexual development, mood, and metabolism and help maintain homeostasis (the body's ability to keep its functions within normal ranges). Each hormone targets specific cells in the body. For example, the pituitary gland produces prolactin, a hormone that targets the breast tissue to stimulate milk production.

Medical assistants will also recognize that the majority of endocrine disorders are a result of hormonal imbalances. The under- or overproduction of even a small amount of a hormone can have drastic consequences for the patient. For instance, the underproduction of growth hormone (GH) from the pituitary gland in a child can result in dwarfism. In this condition, the body has normal proportions but attains a height of only 3 to 4 feet. Conversely, overproduction of GH in a child can result in gigantism, in which the person may grow to a height of 8 feet.

Treatments Using Hormones

Many conditions are treated with hormones, many of which are manufactured synthetically in laboratories. For example, diabetes mellitus is treated with insulin, a hormone naturally produced by the body but now able to be produced synthetically. Steroids, another type of hormone naturally produced in the body, can be produced synthetically and commonly used as antiinflammatory agents in diseases. Synthetic thyroid hormones are used to treat disorders of the thyroid, including hypothyroidism.

The medical assistant will work closely with the endocrinologist to help closely monitor patients who use hormones as treatment to ensure that safe and sufficient treatment dosage levels are maintained.

Diabetes Mellitus

According to the Centers for Disease Control and Prevention's National Diabetes Statistic Report, more than 29 million people or 9.3 percent of the U.S. population have diabetes mellitus (DM). Thus, it is one of the most common diseases a medical assistant will encounter. Although diabetes is often treated by endocrinologists, the patient usually presents to a primary care physician's office with the initial signs and symptoms indicative of the disease.

Diabetes mellitus is characterized by hyperglycemia (too much glucose/sugar in the blood), which results from a lack of insulin or a resistance to the effects of insulin. Insulin is a hormone that is produced and released from the pancreas. The primary function of insulin is to assist in transporting glucose from the blood into the body's cells. Glucose is critical to producing energy and maintaining body function. When levels of glucose in the blood are too high, insulin can also signal the excess glucose to be transported from the blood to the liver for storage.

Without proper production and use of insulin, the patient will continue to be in a hyperglycemic state, which may result in excessive thirst (**polydipsia**), excessive urination (**polyuria**), and excessive hunger (**polyphagia**)—the primary symptoms of DM. Patients with DM may also experience rapid weight loss, fatigue, itching, and skin infections.

If DM remains untreated, life-threatening conditions can result, such as stroke, cardiovascular disease, nerve damage, amputations as a result of infection, blindness caused by retinal damage, kidney damage, and diabetic coma. Although there are various types of diabetes, insulin-dependent (type 1) and noninsulin dependent (type 2) diabetes are the most common. A more detailed discussion of diabetes and the different types can be found in the chapter titled "The Endocrine System."

A critical part of managing diabetes is routine and frequent monitoring of blood glucose levels. Patients with diabetes may be required to test weekly or even several times a day using a blood glucose meter (also called a glucometer). Monitoring blood glucose fluctuations helps guide the physician in managing the patient. Whenever possible, blood glucose meters should be assigned to an individual person and not be shared. If a blood glucose meter must be shared, the device should be cleaned and disinfected after every use. Procedure 36-3 provides the steps for performing and coaching patients on blood glucose monitoring using a blood glucose meter.

PROCEDURE 36-3

Performing and Educating the Patient Regarding Blood Glucose Monitoring

Objective ◆ *Demonstrate how to monitor a patient's blood glucose level by using a blood glucose meter.*

EQUIPMENT AND SUPPLIES

Blood glucose meter (glucometer); a test strip; lancet; gauze or cotton balls; disposable gloves; bandage; patient's medical record

METHOD

1. Perform hand hygiene. If the patient is doing self-testing, recommend using warm water during the hand washing to help blood flow. Dry hands completely.
2. Prepare the equipment and supplies. If you are performing the blood glucose check, gloves should be worn.
   a. Turn on the meter and remove a test strip from its container. Blood glucose meters vary by manufacturer, and the manual may need to be referenced.
   b. Place a test strip into the meter, ensuring that the metal end is fully inserted.
3. Select a site, such as the middle or ring fingertip. Because frequent testing will be required, recommend to the patient to use different fingertips for each test.
4. Puncture the finger using the lancet. Use the side of the fingertip because it will be less painful than the fleshy pad.
5. Touch a drop of blood from the fingertip to the exposed end of the test strip.
   a. Avoid touching the test strip to the skin to prevent contamination.
   b. If the drop of blood is slow to come out, lower the hand or gently squeeze the finger to stimulate blood flow.

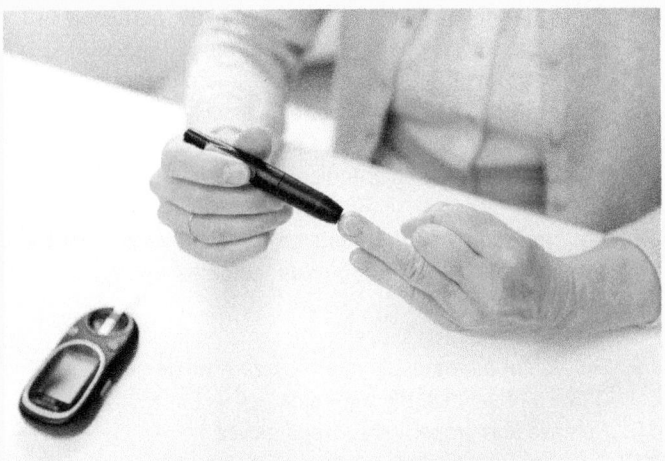

FIGURE A A blood glucose meter (glucometer) may be used to monitor a patient's blood glucose levels.

6. Within several seconds, the meter will provide the results, which should be documented in the patient's medical record or the patient's logbook.
7. Properly discard the used lancet. The test strip can be disposed of in the trash.
8. Use a gauze or cotton ball to apply pressure to the fingertip to stop the bleeding. Use a bandage, if necessary.
9. Perform hand hygiene.

CHARTING EXAMPLE

1/16/YY 10:20 A.M. Assisted patient in performing self-check with blood glucose meter. Lt. ring finger. 100 mg/dL, last meal was 8am. Finger was pink, warm, and puncture site did not need bandage. Patient was comfortable, did not have questions about procedure..K. Bruce, CCMA

ASSISTING WITH GASTROENTEROLOGY

A **gastroenterologist** is a physician specialist who is trained in the diagnosis, treatment, and management of diseases related to the digestive system and its associated structures. The gastrointestinal (GI) or digestive system stores and digests food, eliminates waste, and converts food to energy and nutrients to help the body function. The GI system includes the mouth, esophagus, stomach, small and large intestines, anus, rectum, and accessory organs (liver, gallbladder, and pancreas). A subspecialty of gastroenterology is proctology. A **proctologist** treats disorders of the rectum and anus.

Because the GI system involves many organs, similar symptoms may be present in a number of digestive disorders and conditions. A patient who sees a gastroenterologist is usually referred by the primary care physician because of specific symptoms or symptoms that require more thorough diagnostic examination. A medical assistant who is working for a gastroenterologist or proctologist may perform the following duties:

- Room patients and obtain vital signs and measurements.
- Record the patient's medical history and complete gastrointestinal system–related questionnaires established by the physician.
- Instruct patients regarding the proper method of obtaining stool samples and perform testing on the samples obtained. (Procedure 36-4 outlines steps for testing stool samples.)

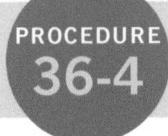

PROCEDURE 36-4

Testing for Occult Blood

Objective ◆ *Test stool samples for occult blood.*

EQUIPMENT AND SUPPLIES

Three occult blood slides; applicators; envelope; timer; pen; gloves; color developer; patient's medical record

Note: Many test kits are available on the market. Each one has its own set of directions, color developer, slides, and control monitors. The test kit directions should be followed exactly.

METHOD

1. Perform hand hygiene and don gloves.
2. Place a paper towel on the area to hold the slides.
3. Verify the patient's name and date of birth against the patient's medical record. Verify that the dates on the occult blood slides are from three different dates.
4. Check the expiration date on the color developer.

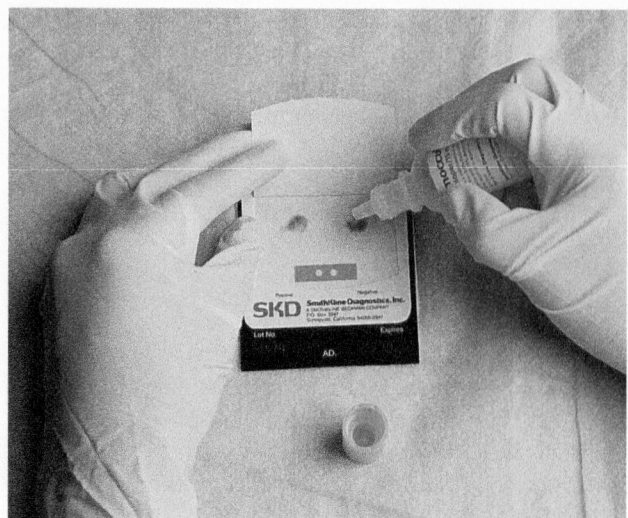

FIGURE A Open the back flap of the slide, and apply two drops of color developing fluid over each box.

5. Open the window flap on the back of slide, and apply two drops of the developer to Box A and Box B (Figure A).
6. Immediately set the timer for result interpretation according to manufacturer's instructions, usually 30–60 seconds.
    a. A negative result will have no color change. Any amount of blue color indicates a positive result for occult blood.
7. Perform quality control tests on the positive and negative controls on each card or as indicated by the manufacturer.
8. Test the remaining slides in the same manner.
9. Dispose of all materials in a biohazard waste container. Clean and sanitize the work area.
10. Remove and properly dispose of gloves.
11. Perform hand hygiene.
12. Document the results in the patient's record.

CHARTING EXAMPLE

03/21/YY 10:30 A.M. 3 occult blood rec'd. All tested neg. for occult blood. Dr. Chang notified of results. Pt. notified per Dr. Chang...B. Negri, CM

- Prepare the examination room, and assist with specialized procedures, such as sigmoidoscopies (Procedure 36-5).

- Provide patients with clear and concise instructions regarding proper preparation for gastrointestinal procedures, such as a colonoscopy (Procedure 36-6). Many of the procedures associated with the gastrointestinal system involve endoscopy (looking into an opening of the body with a flexible tube with a light and camera). Proper patient preparation is important to obtain valid results.

- Provide patient coaching and support based on the treatment protocol established by the physician.

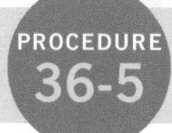

PROCEDURE 36-5

Assisting with a Sigmoidoscopy

Objective ◆ *Assist the physician during the sigmoidoscopic examination by positioning the patient, handling all equipment and biopsy material, and providing support for the patient throughout the procedure.*

EQUIPMENT AND SUPPLIES

Sigmoidoscope (metal or plastic) with obturator; rectal speculum; insufflator; suction equipment; sterile specimen container with preservative; sterile biopsy forceps; cotton applicators (long); lubricating jelly; basin of warm water; patient drape; gloves; patient gown; small towel or examination table pad; tissue; biohazard waste container; patient medical record; cleaning supplies for disinfection; patient's medical record

METHOD

1. Perform hand hygiene.

2. Prepare the equipment and supplies.
    a. Check that all lights and lightbulbs in equipment are properly functioning.
    b. Prepare a basin of warm water to receive used instruments.
    c. Test the suction equipment.
    d. Place the obturator within the sigmoidoscope.
3. Warmly greet and identify the patient, introduce yourself, and explain the steps of the procedure.
4. Verify that the patient has followed the enema and diet instructions.

5. Verify that the patient has signed an informed consent form for the procedure and for the biopsy of samples that may be obtained.

6. Ask the patient to undress, put on a patient gown with the opening in the back, and empty the bladder.
   a. Direct the patient to the location of the restroom.
   b. Allow the patient to privately undress and don a gown. Before reentering the examination room, knock on the door and wait for permission to enter.

7. Assist the patient into the Sims', lateral, or knee–chest position or onto the proctology table. Drape the patient and place a towel or disposable examination pad under the perineal area.

8. Inform the physician that the patient is ready, and don a pair of gloves when the physician is prepared to begin the procedure.

9. Place lubricant on the physician's gloved fingers for a digital examination, which is initially performed.

10. If a metal scope is being used, place it in a basin of warm water before it will be inserted into the patient. Lubricate the tip of the scope.

11. Attach the inflation bulb (for air inflation during the procedure) and attach the light source. Turn the scope on just before the physician is ready to use it.

12. Remind the patient to take deep breaths and relax the abdominal muscles. Observe the patient for any undue reactions or signs of discomfort.

13. Assist the physician by handing instruments and equipment as they are needed, such as suction and cotton-tipped applicators. Place used equipment, including suction tubing, into the basin of water.

14. Assist with biopsy by holding open specimen containers to receive specimen, while maintaining sterility of the container.

15. After the procedure is completed, clean around the patient's anal opening with tissue. Discard the tissue in a biohazard waste container.

16. Remove and dispose of gloves properly in hazardous waste container.

17. Perform hand hygiene.

18. Slowly assist the patient to a sitting position.

19. Inform the patient that she may re-dress, providing assistance as needed. If assistance is not needed, exit the examination room to provide patient privacy.

20. Label the specimen container with the patient's name and date of birth, date and time of collection, source of the specimen, and patient ID number.

21. Apply gloves, and clean and sterilize the equipment according to manufacturer's instructions and office protocol.

22. Disinfect the examination table and clean the examination room.

23. Remove and properly dispose of gloves.

24. Perform hand hygiene.

25. Document the procedure in the patient's medical record. The physician will document the results of the procedure.

CHARTING EXAMPLE

2/14/YY 9:00 a.m. Assisted physician with sigmoidoscopy. Two samples were sent to lab for biopsy. No dizziness or discomfort noted by the patient after procedure....................M. King, CMA

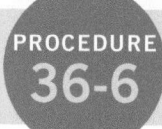

PROCEDURE 36-6

Instructing and Preparing a Patient for a Colonoscopy

Objective ◆ *Instruct the patient on how to empty and clean the colon in preparation for a colonoscopy procedure.*

EQUIPMENT AND SUPPLIES

Two (2) tablets of 5 mg. bisacodyl (Dulcolax) laxative formula; one (1) 8.3 oz. bottle MiraLAX; 64 oz. clear liquid (sports drink); written instructions on bowel prep; patient's medical record

Note: If the physician prescribes a prepared bowel cleansing solution from a pharmacy, the patient should follow those instructions.

METHOD

1. Warmly greet and identify the patient, introduce yourself, and explain the procedure.

2. Reserve enough time during the appointment to instruct the patient on preparing for the procedure and to answer any questions.

3. Provide the patient the written instructions from the physician on how to prepare for the procedure.

4. Review the patient's medical history, and inform the physician of any changes, including any new medication.

5. Seven days before the procedure, instruct the patient to stop taking any fiber or iron supplements.

6. One day before the procedure, the patient should begin a "clear liquid" diet, such as water, apple juice, coffee or tea with no milk, and sports drinks.
   a. Any colored liquids, especially red or purple, should be avoided because they may affect the physician's ability to see during the procedure.
   b. A list of food and liquid items that can be consumed should be included in the written instructions provided by the physician.
7. Instruct the patient to take two tablets of bisacodyl (Dulcolax) at 12:00 P.M. the day before.
8. Instruct the patient to mix 8.3 oz. of MiraLAX with 64 oz. of sports drink at 4:00 P.M. the day before.
   a. The patient should drink one 8 oz. glass of the mixture every 15 minutes until half the mixture (32 oz.) is gone.
   b. If the patient is experiencing nausea or vomiting, instruct the patient to drink water and increase the interval to 30–45 minutes between drinking the solution.
9. Instruct the patient to drink the remainder of the mixture, drinking 8 oz. every 15 minutes at 8:00 P.M. the day before.

   a. If the colonoscopy is scheduled late in the day, the patient should drink the first 32 oz. at 8:00 P.M. the night before and the second 32 oz. at 7:00 A.M. the morning of the procedure.
10. Inform the patient that the stool should be a clear, yellow liquid and not formed.
    a. Recommend to the patient to be near a toilet because diarrhea may occur and may be sudden.
11. The patient should stop drinking any fluids at least four hours before the procedure.
12. Ensure that the patient has made arrangements for someone to drive him home after the procedure because the patient may be drowsy from the sedation.
13. Document that the patient was provided written and verbal instruction to prepare for the procedure in the patient's medical record.

CHARTING EXAMPLE

1/6/YY 3:15 P.M. Provided written and verbal prep instruction for colonoscopy, scheduled for 1/20. Pt's wife will drive home after procedure. Pt. had no other questions.....A. Johnson, RMA

Many of the examinations associated with the digestive system may be uncomfortable and embarrassing for the patient, such as a digital rectal examination or colonoscopy. The medical assistant must be prepared to comfort and reassure the patient before, during, and after procedures. Patients have the right to privacy, and every effort must be made to properly drape the patient throughout the procedures to prevent unnecessary exposure.

Also, as the medical assistant, you must pay attention to details when obtaining chief complaints and symptoms from patients. Patients may complain about bloating, constipation, diarrhea, and vomiting. If the patient has pain, ask the patient to describe or point to where the pain is located. Be aware that pain may be referred (felt somewhere other than the organ in which it originates). For example, gallbladder pain may be felt in the upper right back or shoulder, not necessarily in the abdomen (Figure 36-8). The patient may also complain about having blood in the stool (**hematochezia**) and will require further tests to determine the source of the bleeding. Blood in the stool may have many causes, such as **hemorrhoids** (swollen blood vessels in the rectum), polyps, or colorectal cancer.

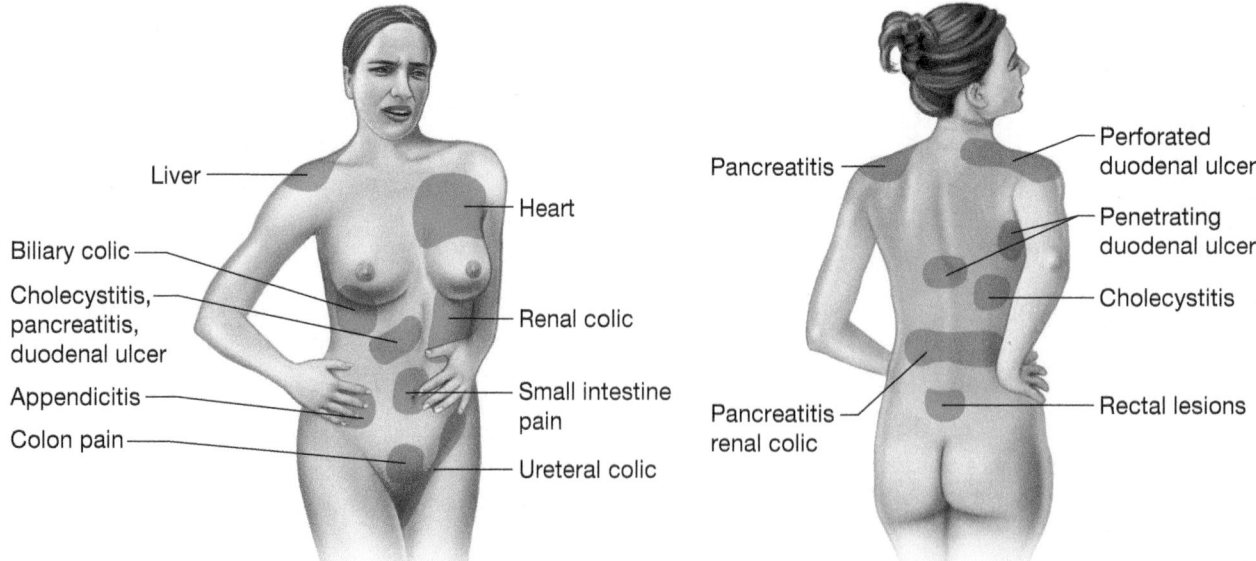

FIGURE 36-8 Examples of sites of referred abdominal pain.

If you are called on to provide a patient with information about a condition, the information presented must be appropriate to the ability of the patient to comprehend the information. Once the instructions are provided, documentation is required. What would you do if a patient refused to follow the instructions and was noncompliant?

Testing for Occult Blood

One of the early signs of colorectal cancers may be bleeding into the GI tract, which often presents in the stool. Sometimes blood can be easily seen in the stool. Other times it is either in such a small amount or has darkened with time so that it is no longer visible. Thus, a chemical test is required to detect the blood. A fecal occult blood test (FOBT), sometimes referred to as a fecal guaiac test, may be requested by the physician to check a patient's stool for **occult** (hidden) blood.

In an FOBT, a patient's stool is tested using special kits that contain cards on which the stool sample is placed. The patient's stool can be tested either at home or in the medical office. Home testing requires three different samples, whereas a one-time sample is performed by the medical assistant in the medical office.

For home testing, the patient will be given a testing kit with three cards for specimens that will need to be tested on three separate days. The patient will also be given applicator sticks that will be used to apply small amounts of stool onto the appropriate sections of the card (Figure 36-9). It is also recommended to include disposable gloves for the patient to

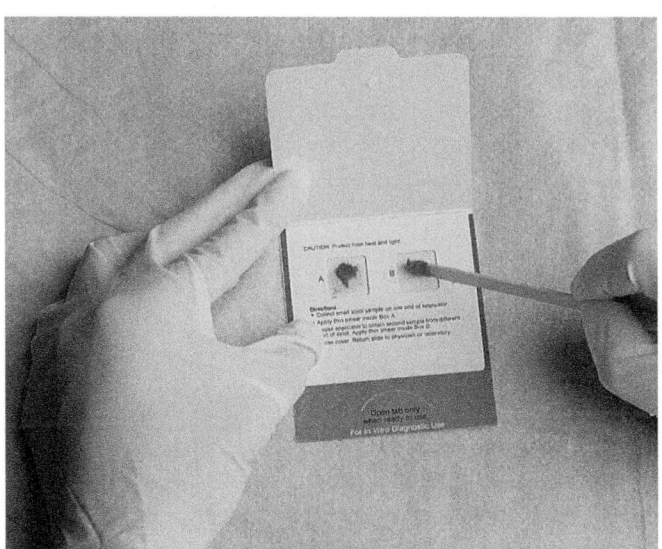

FIGURE 36-9 Instruct the patient to use an applicator to apply a small amount of stool in the appropriate boxes on the test slide.

wear while preparing the slides. Once all three samples have been obtained, the slides are placed in an envelope and returned to the medical office for testing.

Patient preparation is necessary for collecting stool samples at home. Patients are often given written instructions to follow, but the medical assistant should also discuss the instructions with the patient to be sure they are understood. These instructions should detail how to collect three separate stool samples. The steps they will need to follow begin two days before collecting the first stool specimen and continue until all three samples have been obtained.

To help ensure valid results, the FOBT instructions for the patient usually include these general guidelines:

- Drink plenty of fluids.
- Do not collect samples during menses.
- Avoid red meats, liver, and processed meats.
- Avoid turnips, broccoli, cauliflower, and melons.
- Avoid aspirin, iron supplements, and large doses of vitamin C for seven days before collecting specimens, unless otherwise instructed by physician.
- Eat a high-fiber diet.
- Store slides at room temperature away from sun and heat.

For testing in a medical office, FOBTs are commonly performed in both primary care offices and gastroenterology practices. If the patient has a positive FOBT, the physician may need to perform an additional procedure, such as a sigmoidoscopy or colonoscopy (discussed next) to view the interior of the patient's GI tract. Procedure 36-4 provides the steps for testing stool samples for occult blood.

Sigmoidoscopy

A **sigmoidoscopy**, also called a proctoscopic or proctosigmoidoscopic examination, is an examination of the interior of the sigmoid colon for diagnostic purposes. The sigmoid is the part of the large intestine that is closest to the rectum and anus.

The sigmoidoscope is a rigid or flexible metal or plastic instrument with a light source and magnification lens. The flexible sigmoidoscope is more widely used by physicians than the rigid sigmoidoscope since it allows the physician to see farther into the colon and view the mucous membranes of the intestines, and it is more comfortable for the patient. Figure 36-10 shows a flexible sigmoidoscope with parts labeled. A sigmoidoscopy may be performed to detect polyps, ulcerations, colon cancer, or to investigate the source of bleeding in the lower intestinal tract. For this procedure, the

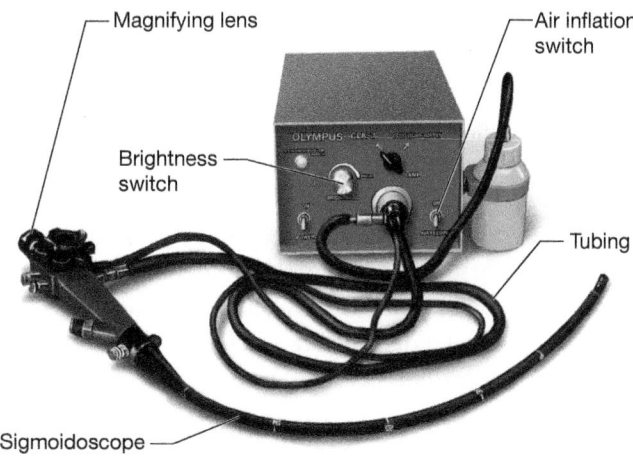

FIGURE 36-10 The parts of a flexible sigmoidoscope.

patient may be placed in the Sims' position or on a proctoscopic examination table (Figure 36-11).

A sigmoidoscopy is scheduled in advance to allow for adequate patient preparation. The medical assistant plays an important role in preparing the patient for the procedure. For example, patients will be instructed to empty their bowels and bladder before coming in for the procedure. The physician may ask the patient to use a commercially prepared enema preparation before the examination. Patients should also be advised to drink plenty of clear liquids and eat sparingly the day before the examination. Some physicians ask the patient to refrain from eating raw fruits and vegetables, grains, and dairy products a few days before the examination to allow the colon to be more easily viewed.

It is critical that the patient follow the preparation instructions. Provide the patient with written instructions, usually

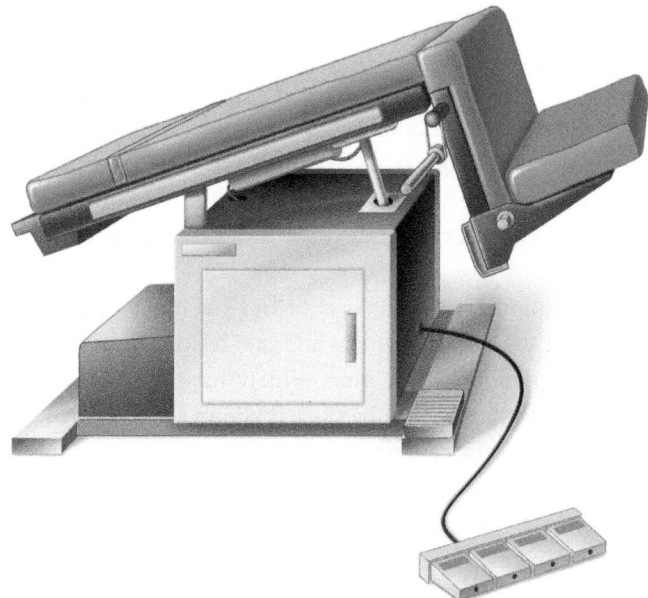

FIGURE 36-11 Proctoscopic examination table.

in a step-by-step format, to ensure compliance. Discuss the instructions with the patient to be sure they are understood. Improper bowel preparation may result in the need to reschedule the procedure, which could cause further anxiety for the patient and a delay in diagnosis. The patient also needs to sign an informed consent form to allow for both the procedure and any biopsy of samples that may be obtained.

During the procedure, the medical assistant plays an important role. A sigmoidoscopy can be physically uncomfortable and may cause anxiety for patients. Even though the procedure may last only a few minutes, the patient needs encouragement throughout the procedure. The medical assistant can reduce the physical discomfort for patients by instructing them to concentrate on deep breathing through the mouth while relaxing the abdominal muscles. The physician may take several biopsy samples during the procedure, requiring that labeled specimen containers be part of every sigmoidoscopy setup. After the procedure, it is helpful to inform patients that they might experience flatulence (gas) as a result of the air introduced into the colon during the procedure. Procedure 36-5 provides the steps for assisting with a sigmoidoscopy.

Colonoscopy

Sometimes the physician needs to see more of the large intestine and will perform a **colonoscopy** instead of a sigmoidoscopy. Colonoscopy procedures are performed in a medical office or, more often, in a hospital outpatient setting because an intravenous (IV) sedative is administered before the procedure. The American Cancer Society recommends all individuals over the age of 50 with average risk have a colonoscopy every 10 years to screen for cancer. A colonoscopy should be performed more frequently for patients with increased or higher risk of colorectal cancer, such as those having a family history of polyps or cancer.

The medical assistant working for a gastroenterologist or an outpatient testing center may assist with the actual procedure, whereas a medical assistant working for a primary care physician may be responsible only for scheduling the test and helping to prepare the patient for the procedure.

Professionalism

Some of the procedures associated with the GI system may be uncomfortable or embarrassing for patients. All patients must be treated with dignity and respect. Their privacy must be maintained by appropriate draping and privacy while dressing and undressing. A caring attitude is important in every patient interaction.

Once the patient is admitted to the outpatient clinic or the hospital, an IV line will be inserted in the patient's hand or arm. The patient's blood pressure, heart rate, and respiration rate are monitored during the test. Through the IV line, fluids and anesthetic agents are given to sedate and numb the patient during the procedure. Most patients sleep during the test and feel little discomfort.

Similar to a sigmoidoscope, a colonoscope is a long black flexible tube with a camera and a light at the end. The physician gently pumps air and sterile water or saline through the scope into the colon to inflate it, which allows the physician to view the entire lining. During the procedure, a biopsy (small sample of tissue) may be taken or polyps may be removed. After the colonoscopy, the patient may feel some bloating or cramping.

As in a sigmoidoscopy, before a colonoscopy, the colon must be completely empty and cleansed so that the physician can see any abnormal areas. If the patient's colon is not completely emptied and cleaned, the physician may miss any abnormalities. The physician should have specific written instruction or a packet of information that can be provided to the patient on how to prepare for the colonoscopy. As with the sigmoidoscopy, the patient needs to follow preparation steps at home several days before the procedure.

The medical assistant needs to thoroughly review the written instructions on preparing for a colonoscopy with the patient and answer any questions the patient may have. If the instructions are not carefully followed and the patient's colon has not been emptied and cleaned, the procedure must be rescheduled. Procedure 36-6 outlines how to prepare a patient for an outpatient colonoscopy procedure.

ASSISTING WITH ORTHOPEDICS

An **orthopedist** is a physician who specializes in **orthopedics**, which is the medical field concerned with the diagnosis and treatment of conditions related to the musculoskeletal system (bones and muscles). In addition to the orthopedist, several other physicians work on the musculoskeletal system. Osteopathic physicians, also called osteopaths, are Doctors of Osteopathic Medicine (DO). They are degreed as physicians and diagnose and treat diseases and disorders similar to physicians with the credentials of MD (Medical Doctor). However, osteopathic physicians also receive specialized training in musculoskeletal manipulation, which may affect the condition of other body systems. Another physician specialist who deals with musculoskeletal disorders is a **rheumatologist**, who specializes in managing patients with joint inflammations and patients with autoimmune disorders, such as rheumatoid arthritis and lupus.

A medical assistant's training is comprehensive enough to permit employment in any of the specialties just mentioned. A medical assistant who is working for an orthopedist may perform the following duties:

- Room patients, and obtain vital signs and measurements.
- Record the patient's medical history, and complete appropriate forms and documentation relating to the patient's orthopedic condition.
- Schedule appropriate diagnostic tests and procedures related to the musculoskeletal system, and provide the patient with information specific to each test.
- Work closely with other allied health professionals, such as physical therapists and occupational therapists, which may be a part of the patient's health care treatment and management team.
- Provide patient education and support based on the treatment protocol established by the physician.
- Apply therapeutic modalities as necessary, such as the application of heat and cold compresses.
- Perform or obtain X-rays and other diagnostic images to aid the physician in diagnosis and treatment of the patient's condition (Figures 36-12A and 36-12B). Many orthopedists and osteopaths have X-ray equipment in or associated with their offices. Some states require medical assistants who perform X-rays to receive additional training and be registered as X-ray technicians.

Caring for Patients with Musculoskeletal Problems

There are 206 bones and over 600 muscles in the body. Muscles account for approximately 50 percent of the body's weight. In addition to bones and muscles, the musculoskeletal system includes all the connective tissue, such as tendons, ligaments, and cartilage, which is necessary for proper functioning of this complex system. The functions of the musculoskeletal system are to provide movement, protect internal organs, produce blood cells of all types, and store minerals, such as calcium. In your career as a medical assistant, regardless of which specialty you work in, you will encounter patients with musculoskeletal conditions.

The signs and symptoms that may present with a musculoskeletal disorder are numerous and may vary widely. Some of these symptoms may be debilitating and may significantly impact the patient's quality of life. For example, a young woman suffering from rheumatoid arthritis may be so disabled and in so much pain she cannot work or care for

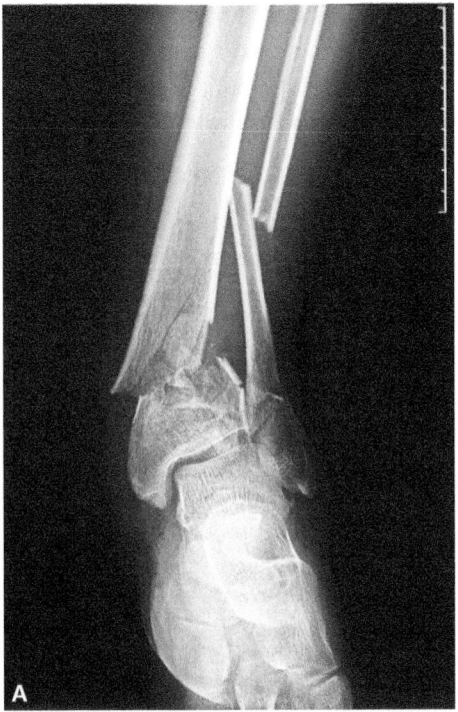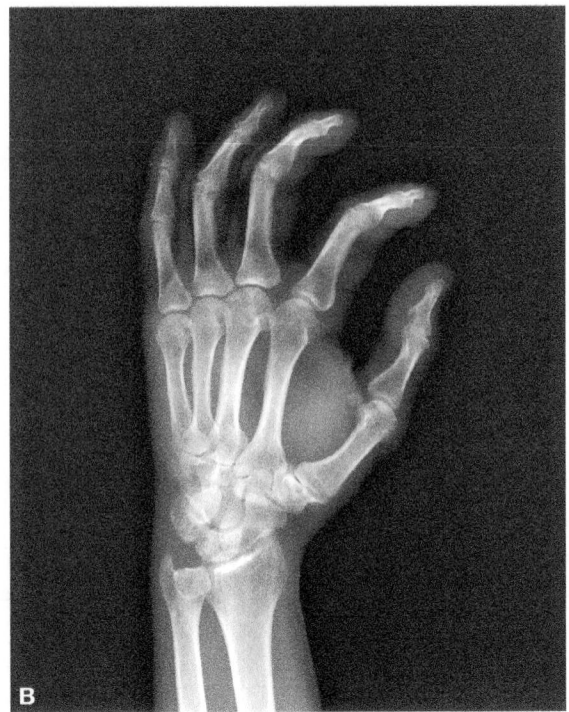

FIGURE 36-12 **(A)** An X-ray of a fractured tibia and fibula; **(B)** an X-ray of arthritic joints of the wrist and hand.

herself. Also consider the older adult patient who falls and fractures a hip, requiring a total hip replacement (THR), or the young child who suffers from muscle weakness and lack of motor control from muscular dystrophy.

The medical assistant's role includes listening carefully to the patient's description of the problem and engaging in open-ended questions to provide a clearer picture of their problem:

- When did it start?
- What were you doing before the problem started?
- What was done to alleviate the problem?
- What are your most pressing current concerns?

When documenting in the patient's medical records, carefully note the location of the pain, and ask the patient to quantify it on a scale of 0 to 10, with 10 being the greatest amount of pain.

Offer to assist the patient to the examining room, and provide a wheelchair, if necessary. Once in the examining room, make any accommodations necessary to ensure that the patient is comfortable. This may include providing a blanket for warmth or an extra pillow to support the injured part.

When evaluating muscle strength, recall that it should be equal on both sides of the body. For instance, if you ask a patient to squeeze your hands, the amount of pressure the patient exerts with each hand should be equal. Observe the patient's gait (manner of walking or posture) and the range of motion of the affected area. These are important clues that the medical

assistant must relay to the physician to help make an accurate diagnosis.

ASSISTING WITH NEUROLOGY

A **neurologist** specializes in treating and diagnosing conditions of the nervous system, which includes the brain, spinal cord, and associated nerves throughout the body. If an invasive procedure is required, a **neurosurgeon** will perform the surgical procedures on the nervous system. A **psychiatrist** is a physician who specializes in diagnosing and treating mental health and emotional problems that may affect behavior.

A medical assistant may work for any of these physicians and may perform the following duties:

- Room patients, and obtain vital signs and measurements.
- Record the patient's medical history, and complete appropriate forms and documentation relating to the patient's needs.
- Schedule appropriate diagnostic tests and procedures related to the nervous system, and provide the patient with information specific to prepare for each test. Many types of tests and procedures may be ordered as follow-ups to the initial neurological examination. Prepare the examination room and assist the physician with the neurological examination.
- Provide patient education and support based on the treatment protocol established by the physician.

Assisting with Neurological Examinations

Patients with nervous system conditions exhibit many different types of symptoms. The major areas of a neurological examination focus on the patient's reflex response, motor response, muscle tone, speech patterns, coordination, sensory response, gait, and mental status and behavior.

If, as a medical assistant, you notice inappropriate responses or changes in grooming habits of a patient, the physician should be made aware of your observations. Your role in the neurological examination is to ensure necessary supplies are ready for use by the physician, to provide support and encouragement to patients, and to assist in positioning the patients as needed. The following supplies and equipment should be prepared and ready for the physician to use during the neurological examination:

- Otoscope
- Ophthalmoscope
- Percussion hammer
- Penlight
- Tuning fork
- Cotton ball
- Safety pin
- Tongue depressor
- Small vials containing hot and cold liquids, vials with different scents, and vials with different tasting liquids, per the physician's order

The medical assistant may also be asked to check the patient's pupils. The pupils of the eyes often display signs relevant to the functioning of the brain and nervous system. This is why evaluating a patient's pupils is so important. This straightforward noninvasive procedure is simple and quick and checks the pupils for the following:

- Equal size
- Equal dilation in both eyes in darkness or dim light
- Rapid constriction to light in both eyes
- Equal reaction to light
- Accommodation to objects near or far

When the pupil exam is normal, it should be documented in the patient's medical records as PERRLA, for Pupils Equal, Round, Reactive to Light and Accommodation. Procedure 36-7 lists the steps for evaluating a patient's pupils. Procedure 36-8 lists the steps for assisting in all aspects of the neurological examination.

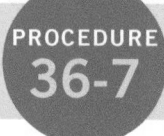

PROCEDURE 36-7 Performing a Pupil Check on a Patient

Objective ◆ *Check patient's pupils for size, dilation, constriction, accommodation, and equal reaction to light.*

EQUIPMENT AND SUPPLIES
Penlight or small flashlight; patient's medical record; pen

METHOD

1. Warmly greet and identify the patient, introduce yourself, and explain procedure. Partially darken the room because the procedure checks for the patient's response to light changes.
2. Ask the patient to look straight ahead. Using a penlight or flashlight, approach from the side and shine light on one pupil at a time.
   a. Observe for constriction (narrowing) of the pupil. Figure A shows variations in pupil diameters in millimeters.
   b. Shine the light on the pupil again and observe the other pupil for constriction.

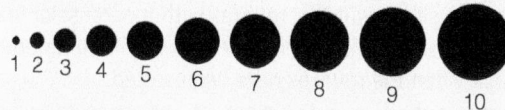

FIGURE A This figure shows the variations in pupil sizes in millimeters.

3. Hold open the eyes by gently separating the eyelids (lightly grasping near the brow bone and below the eye socket), and observe the pupils for size. They should be equal in size.
4. Hold an object (penlight or pen) about 10 cm (4 in.) from the bridge of the patient's nose. Ask the patient to look at the top of the object and then at a different object on the wall across the room, forcing the patient to shift focus. Observe for pupil response. (Pupils should constrict when looking at a close object and dilate when looking across the room.)
5. Move the pen toward the patient's nose. Pupils should converge (come together) toward the patient's nose.

6. Observe the pupils for shape. They should be equal or similar in shape.
7. Next, explain to the patient what other tests will be performed.
8. Document the results in the patient's medical record. When the pupil exam is normal, it should be documented as PERRLA. If the pupil exam is abnormal, document the results observed.

CHARTING EXAMPLE

03/21/YY 11:00 A.M. T: 99°; P: 82 bpm; R: 18; BP 168/80; HT 68"; WT 182 lb; PERRLA..............T. Blardo, RMA

PROCEDURE 36-8
Assisting with a Neurologic Examination

Objective ◆ *Assist the physician with a neurological screening examination.*

EQUIPMENT AND SUPPLIES

Percussion hammer; safety pin; tongue depressor; Mayo tray; penlight; cotton ball; tuning fork; neurological wheel; ophthalmoscope; otoscope; hot and cold water; materials with different odors; patient's medical record

METHOD

1. Perform hand hygiene.
2. Assemble equipment on the Mayo tray and cover the tray.
3. Warmly greet and identify the patient, introduce yourself, and explain the procedure.
4. Evaluate the patient's mental status while taking a medical history. Pay attention to responses, memory, coherence of thought, overall mood, and awareness.
5. Perform a visual acuity test, if ordered.
6. Assist the patient onto the examination table and drape as needed for comfort.
   a. Some physicians may request that the patient undress and wear a patient gown. If so, provide assistance or privacy as necessary.
7. The physician will test reflexes with a percussion hammer. Be prepared to hand the physician the hammer and take it back when the reflexes have been tested.
8. Sensory abilities and skin sensations are tested using a safety pin, neurological wheel, and cotton ball and the patient's recognition of simple objects by touch (key, pen, coin). Be ready and alert to provide these items to the physician when necessary.
9. The physician will check the patient's coordination by having the patient touch the finger to the nose (Figure A), touch the heel to the shin, and move the heel down the opposite shin.
10. The physician may want to evaluate gait or to have the patient perform the **Romberg test** (patient closes eyes and stands with feet together without swaying). Assist the

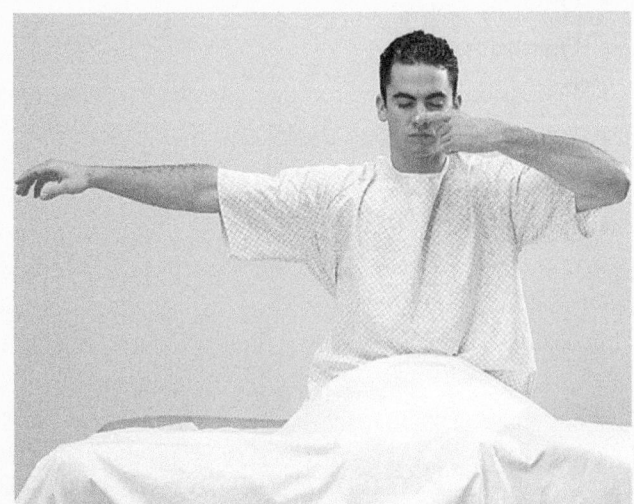

FIGURE A To check coordination, patients may be asked to close their eyes and touch a finger to their nose with each hand.

patient off the table and support the patient in case the patient falls while performing these tests.
11. When the neurological exam is completed and the physician is finished, assist the patient off the examination table and allow the patient to re-dress. Assist and provide privacy as needed.
12. After the patient leaves the examination room, clean the examination room and disinfect the items used during the exam according to office protocol.
13. Perform hand hygiene.
14. Document information in the patient's record. The physician will document the results of the neurological examination.

CHARTING EXAMPLE

03/21/YY 11:00 A.M. Assisted Dr. Young with neurological screening. Scheduled pt. to see Dr. Black, neurologist on 04/04/YY at 11:00 A.M.......................................C. Negri, CMA

Professionalism   The Life Span

 Alzheimer's disease is a progressive, chronic disorder of the nervous system. It is named for Alois Alzheimer, a German neurologist. This disorder affects people usually between the ages of 40 and 80 and is characterized by dementia, which is a general term for a decline in mental ability that prevents an individual from performing daily activities. People with dementia may present with many different symptoms. The most common are progressive memory loss, difficulty in communicating or finding words, poor coordination and movement, disorientation, difficulty completing complex tasks, and agitation and other behavioral issues. Although dementia may be present in other conditions, such as strokes, Alzheimer's disease accounts for 60 to 80 percent of cases of dementia. As a medical assistant, you need to show patience and understanding when dealing with patients with dementia.

Professionalism   The Workplace

 Every health care facility depends on cooperation among employees. If a colleague is extra busy and you have a few minutes, offer to help clean up an examination room, escort a patient to the checkout desk, or set up for an upcoming examination. Use initiative and show dedication as a medical assistant. Show your peers and supervisors that you are a valuable asset to the working team.

SUMMARY

The topics presented in this chapter describe the medical assistant's role in a variety of medical specialty areas. No single physician's practice will represent every procedure found within this chapter. However, because the profession of medical assisting is for the multiskilled individual, the medical assistant is expected to have a general knowledge of the subspecialties of medicine.

Much of the clinical role of the medical assistant involves assisting with procedures related to the body systems, including digestive, integumentary (skin/dermatology), musculoskeletal (orthopedics), endocrine, cardiovascular, and nervous systems. In each of these areas, the medical assistant serves as a critical member of the medical team and provides a helping hand to the physician through proper patient care and execution of specialized procedures. The medical assistant also works to ensure that the patient's needs, including privacy and education, and coaching, are met. No matter what the task requires, the hallmark of a good medical assistant should be careful attention to detail and respect for the rights of the patient.

36 CHAPTER REVIEW

COMPETENCY REVIEW

1. Define and spell the terms for this chapter.
2. List four types of allergy test used to determine a patient's sensitivities.
3. Explain why a physician would order a wound culture.
4. Discuss why it is important for patients to properly comply with bowel preparation before digestive diagnostic testing, such as a sigmoidoscopy or colonoscopy.
5. Why is it important for a patient with diabetes to routinely monitor her glucose levels?
6. List the guidelines patients should follow when preparing to obtain stool samples for occult blood.
7. Identify five risk factors for developing cardiovascular diseases.
8. Explain the difference between a physician who has the MD credential and one who has a DO credential.
9. What instruments should you have ready before a neurological examination?
10. What does PERRLA stand for?

PREPARING FOR THE CERTIFICATION EXAM

1. Testing a patient's gait would test for which body system?
   a. digestive
   b. integumentary
   c. cardiovascular
   d. nervous
   e. endocrine

2. Diabetes mellitus is the result of the impaired action of what hormone?
   a. thyroxine
   b. insulin
   c. adrenaline
   d. glucagon
   e. testosterone

3. To test a patient for allergies, the physician would order a
   a. fasting blood glucose.
   b. lumbar puncture.
   c. neurological evaluation.
   d. RAST test.
   e. colonoscopy.

4. Before a stool sample is collected for occult blood, fiber and iron supplements should be avoided for
   a. 12 hours before collection.
   b. 24 hours before collection.
   c. 48 hours before collection.
   d. three days before collection.
   e. seven days before collection.

5. Orthopedics pertains to the
   a. endocrine system.
   b. nervous system.
   c. integumentary system.
   d. musculoskeletal system.
   e. digestive system.

6. All of the following are common symptom of cardiovascular disease *except*
   a. dyspnea.
   b. polydipsia.
   c. angina.
   d. diaphoresis.
   e. cyanosis.

7. The Romberg test is used to evaluate the
   a. nervous system.
   b. skeletal system.
   c. digestive system.
   d. endocrine system.
   e. integumentary system.

8. Which of the following is *not* taken into consideration when evaluating pupils?
   a. equal dilation
   b. equal reaction to light
   c. accommodation to objects near or far
   d. ability to consciously adjust pupil size
   e. rapid constriction to light

9. Which of the following is *not* a complication of diabetes?
   a. heart disease
   b. blindness
   c. skin hardening
   d. kidney damage
   e. nerve damage

10. An occult blood test is performed using which type of sample from the patient?
    a. blood
    b. serum
    c. skin
    d. saliva
    e. feces

CRITICAL THINKING

Refer to the case study at the beginning of the chapter and use what you have learned to answer the following questions.

1. Mr. Salvatore expressed concern regarding his preparation for the procedure. What instructions should Mr. Salvatore have been given regarding proper preparation?

2. What can David do to help Mr. Salvatore's comfort level during the procedure?

3. Mr. Salvatore becomes increasingly anxious when he is informed that biopsy samples are going to be obtained during the procedure. How should David respond to Mr. Salvatore's anxiety?

ON THE JOB

Shelia Meyer, a medical assistant in Dr. Ryan's large cardiovascular practice, is taking the medical history of Edna Helm, an obese older adult woman with congestive heart disease. Edna states, "I'm always short of breath, and I perspire all the time. I guess I'm gaining weight, but the funny thing is that only my legs seem heavier. My heart is pounding when I lie down at night; it even seems to stop sometimes. I've even started to wear red nail polish to hide the funny blue color of my nails."

Edna gives Shelia a copy of her medical history from an out-of-state physician. The medical history indicates that she has had the following tests and procedures:

Conditions	Tests
Positive Babinski sign	Holter monitor testing
Allergic rhinitis	Radioimmunoassay test
Aortic insufficiency	Protein bound iodine test
Ascites	Glucose tolerance test
Gastritis	
Osteoarthritis	

Surgical Procedures

Basal cell carcinoma removed in 1992

Sebaceous cyst removed in 1982

Meniscectomy in 1978

Rhytidectomy in 1970

1. Considering Edna's chief complaint, identify at least three medical terms that could be used to describe her signs and symptoms.

2. Using your textbook, medical dictionary, or Internet resources, define at least five of the items from Edna's medical history information.

INTERNET ACTIVITY

Radiologists are considered allied health professionals. Perform an Internet search, and discover the types of facilities where radiologists are normally employed, their duties, educational requirements, employment opportunities, and licensure, certification, or registration requirements.

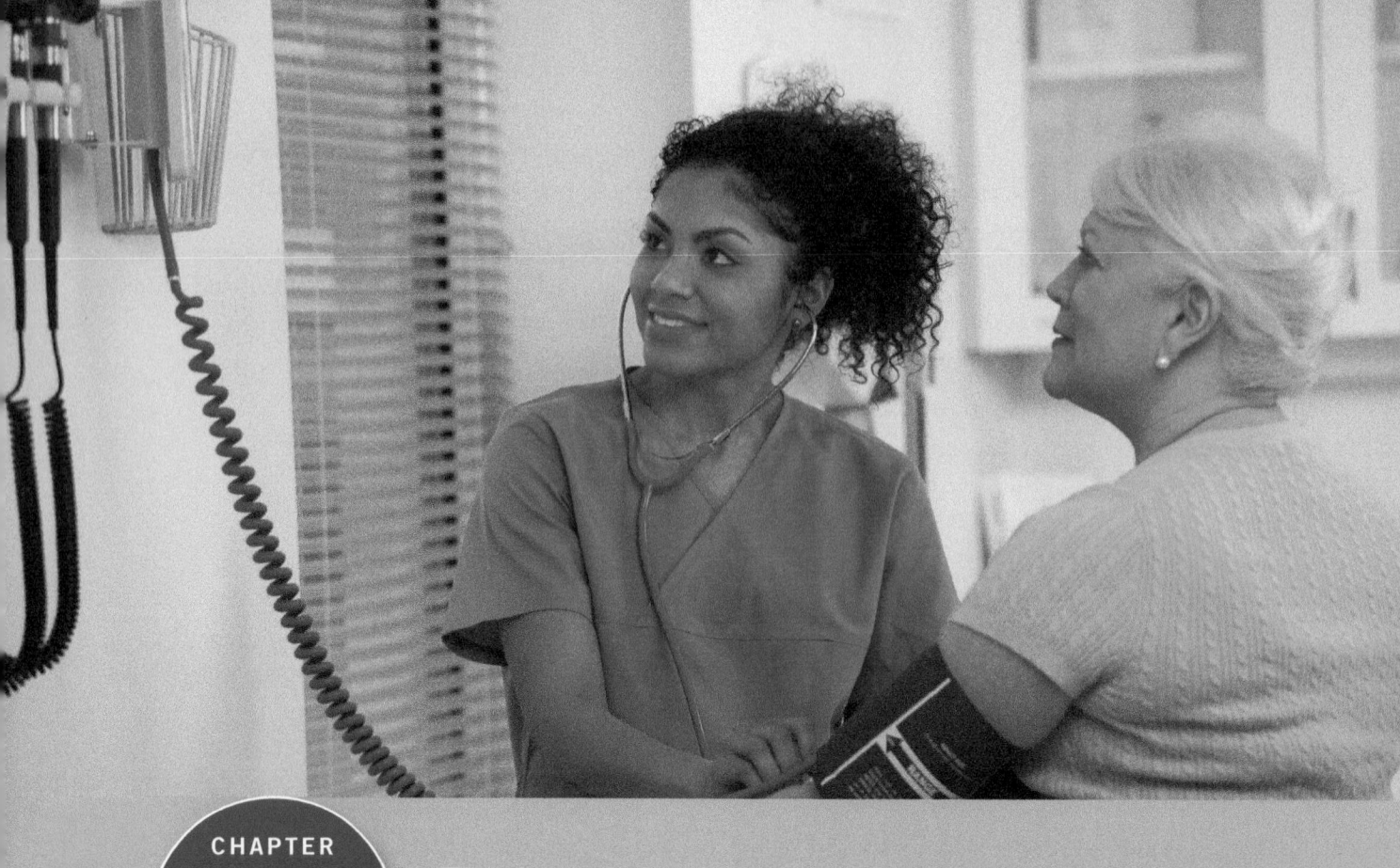

CHAPTER 37

Assisting with Reproductive Specialties

Learning Objectives

After completing this chapter, you should be able to:

37.1   Define and spell the terms for this chapter.

37.2   Explain how a medical assistant assists a physician during gynecological appointments.

37.3   Describe components related to prenatal care appointments.

37.4   Describe the postpartum visit.

37.5   List various methods of contraception.

37.6   Identify medical issues common to the male reproductive system.

37.7   Outline items that would be discussed with patients regarding the prevention of sexually transmitted infections.

37.8   Describe types of sexually transmitted infections.

Case Study

Sonja Lufti is being seen by Dr. McWalters for her first prenatal visit. Sonja's last menstrual period was January 14. This is the third time that Sonja has been pregnant. She has one 5-year-old son and had a miscarriage at 14 weeks of pregnancy two years ago.

Terms to Learn

abortions	external genitalia	oxytocin
abruptio placentae	fetal heart tone (FHT)	para
amenorrhea	fundal height	parturition
carcinoma in situ	fundus	pelvic inflammatory disease (PID)
chancre	gravida	placenta previa
chorionic villus sampling (CVS)	human papillomaviruses (HPVs)	preeclampsia
dilation	intrauterine device (IUD)	puerperium
dysplasia	lochia	quickening
eclampsia	menarche	vasectomy
ectopic pregnancy	nocturia	viability
effacement		

In this chapter, we explore assisting with special examinations related to the reproductive systems of both males and females. In addition, we discuss sexually transmitted infections (STIs) and their effects on both sexes. You will learn how, as a medical assistant, not only to assist in several of these specialized procedures but also to instruct and coach patients on cancer screening, prenatal care, and STI prevention.

The main function of the male and female reproductive systems is to produce offspring to continue the human species. The reproductive system includes both internal and external organs in males and females. The male reproductive system includes the scrotum, testes, spermatic ducts, sex glands, and penis. These organs work together to produce sperm and the other components in semen to help in the fertilization of an ovum (egg) in the female. The female reproductive system includes the ovaries, fallopian tubes, uterus, vagina, vulva, mammary glands, and breasts. These organs are involved in the production and transportation of the ova and the production of sex hormones necessary to sustain the pregnancy. The female reproductive system also supports the development of the fetus. For a more detailed review of the reproductive systems, see the chapter titled "The Reproductive System."

FEMALE REPRODUCTIVE MEDICAL ISSUES

Gynecology is the branch of medicine that deals with the health and with the diseases and disorders of the female reproductive system. The practice of gynecology is closely related to the medical specialty of obstetrics, which is the branch of medicine concerned with the care of women during pregnancy, childbirth, and the period of time immediately after childbirth.

An examination of the female reproductive system includes both invasive and noninvasive procedures to determine the condition of both the external and the internal reproductive organs. Several of the examinations performed are part of a patient's routine health screening, such as a breast and pelvic examination and a Papanicolaou (Pap) test. A medical assistant working in an obstetrics and gynecology (OB/GYN) office should be prepared to assist in these and a number of other more specialized procedures that will be discussed in this chapter.

Assisting the Obstetrics and Gynecology Patient

Patients in an OB/GYN practice may include a wide range of ages and present with a variety of symptoms and conditions.

As a medical assistant, you may encounter a teenager having her first pelvic examination, a first-time mother, a mother with seven children, a perimenopausal female, a middle-aged menopausal female, and an older postmenopausal female. All of these patients are in distinct life stages, and thus their emotional and physical needs will differ.

An important job responsibility of the medical assistant is to take a thorough patient history to identify the patient's problems and provide information to aid the physician with diagnosis and treatment. However, one of the challenges you may face in taking the patient history is that some patients may feel shame or embarrassment about the reason for their visit and may withhold important health information, particularly information regarding sexual behavior and sexually transmitted infections (STIs). Thus, it is imperative throughout your interaction with the patient that you provide a nonjudgmental environment in which the patient can feel comfortable about sharing her feelings, concerns, and discomfort.

The Breast Examination

After skin cancer, breast cancer is the most common cancer in women in the United States with one in eight women (12 percent) being affected. Fortunately, according to the National Cancer Institute, the incidence (new cases) of breast cancer has not risen but has been stable over the past 10 years. Additionally, the mortality, or death rate, from breast cancer has decreased over that same period of time. The American Cancer Society reports that the death rates from breast cancer in the United States have dropped 34 percent since 1990. This decrease in breast cancer death rates is believed to be largely because of cancer screening and early detection methods such as breast self-examinations (BSE), clinical breast examinations (CBE), mammograms, and magnetic resonance imaging (MRI).

Although there are no studies to show that BSE or CBE reduces the rate of breast cancer, the American Cancer Society recommends that women should be familiar with how their breasts normally look and feel to be able to identify any abnormalities they may see or feel, such as a nodule (swelling or lump), dimpling of the skin, or bleeding.

If BSE is recommended by the physician, the medical assistant may have the responsibility of explaining and demonstrating the correct procedure for the BSE. The physician may advise the patient to perform the BSE every month, usually one week after the menstrual period ends. Menopausal women may be advised to examine their breasts on the same day each month. Some patients may feel more knowledgeable than others about how to perform a BSE. For this reason, as the medical assistant, you should be prepared to teach a patient how to perform one. Also, advise the patient that any abnormalities or changes need to be immediately reported to their physician. Procedure 37-1 provides guidance on how to instruct patients on performing a BSE.

Often during the routine pelvic examination, which is discussed later in the chapter, the physician may also perform

---

PROCEDURE 37-1 Instructing a Patient on Breast Self-Examination

Objective ◆ *Instruct the patient how to do breast self-examination (BSE).*

EQUIPMENT AND SUPPLIES
Breast model (if available); pamphlets on breast self-examination; patient's medical record

METHOD
1. Perform hand hygiene.
2. Assemble equipment, if available.
3. Warmly greet and identify the patient and introduce yourself.
4. Explain to the patient that the procedure should be performed once a month and in three of the following different positions each month.

In the shower (Figure A):
- Raise the right arm, and use the left hand to examine the right breast. Then raise the left arm, and use the right hand to examine the left breast.
- Flatten the fingertips and check the breast tissue and underarm tissue, gently feeling for any lumps or thickening. Wet skin will allow hands to move more easily over the breast tissue.

In front of a mirror (Figure B):
- With arms at the side of body, inspect the breasts for any irregularity in shape.

- Look for swelling, dimpling, puckering, or lumps on the skin or changes in the nipples, such as retracting. Gently squeeze both nipples and look for any discharge.
- Raise the arms over the head and look for size, shape, and contour changes in each breast.
- With palms resting on hips, flex chest muscles to observe for any obvious differences in breasts. It is common for breasts to be slightly different in size.

Lying down (Figure C):
- To examine the right breast, place a pillow or folded towel behind the right shoulder and place the right hand behind the head. Examine the right breast with the left hand, and the left breast with the right hand.
- Using the hand with flattened fingers, gently press the breast tissue using small circular motions starting at the outermost top of the breast in the 12:00 position toward the nipple (Figure D). An up-and-down motion can also be used, as long as all breast tissue is systematically examined. Cover all the breast tissue, feeling for lumps or any abnormal changes in breast tissue. Gently squeeze the nipple of each breast between the thumb and index finger, and note any lumps or discharge.
- Repeat the procedure for the left breast.

With the arm resting on a firm surface (Figure E):
- Use the same circular motion to examine the underarm area. Repeat the procedure for the other underarm area.

5. Use the breast model to explain the correct application of fingertips (Figure F). Recommend to the patient to pick the same time of the month to minimize any breast changes because of hormone fluctuations that occur throughout the month.
   a. Premenopausal women should test one week after the end of their menstrual period.
6. Instruct the patient to immediately report any abnormalities to the physician.
7. Perform hand hygiene.
8. Document the information in the patient's medical record.

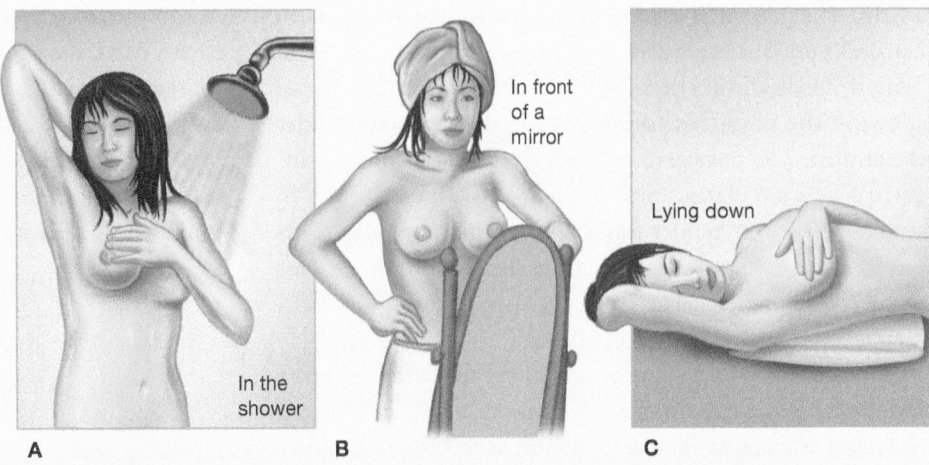

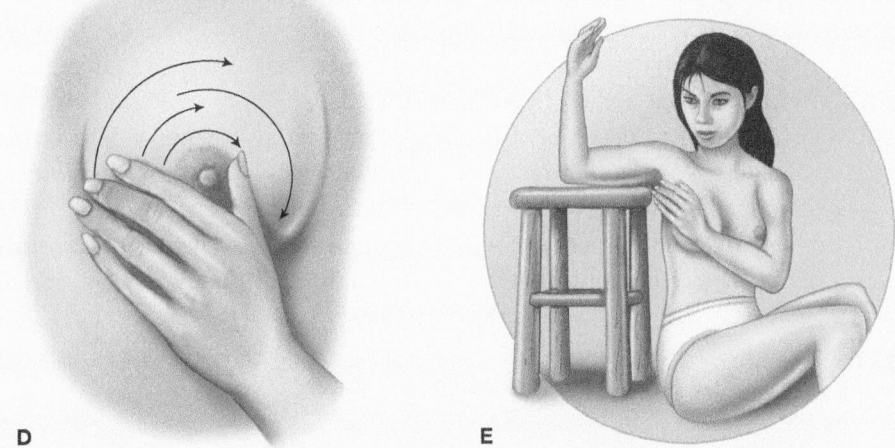

FIGURE A–E **(A)** In the shower; **(B)** in front of a mirror; **(C)** lying down; **(D)** in concentric circles; **(E)** with arm raised.

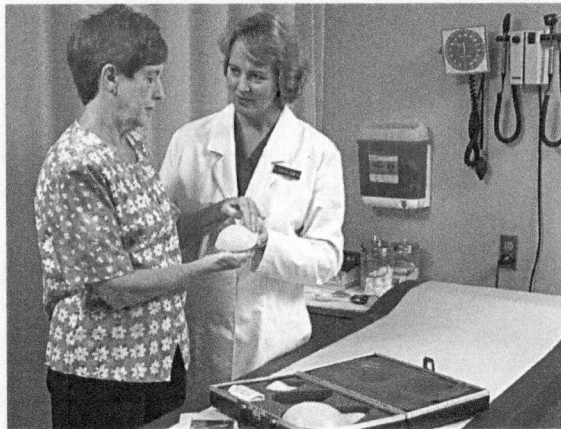

FIGURE F A medical assistant uses a breast model to instruct a patient on proper technique for performing self-examination of the breasts.

CHARTING EXAMPLE

2/14/YY 2:00 P.M. Breast self-exam explained to patient using breast model. Pt demonstrated procedure satisfactorily.............
....M. King, CMA

a CBE. The patient is asked to lie in the supine position (on her back) for this examination. The patient places her hand behind her head on the side that is being examined first, allowing the physician to examine the lymph nodes under the armpit. The physician palpates the breast using the fingertips in a circular fashion around all the breast tissue to search for lumps, tenderness, or inflammation. Any dimpling, puckering, or cracking of the skin around the breast or bleeding or discharge from the nipple must be documented in the patient's medical record.

A more effective test for breast cancer screening than the SBE or CBE is a mammography, a specialized imaging tool that uses X-rays to look deep within the breast. Regular health screening with a mammography exam, or mammogram, can often detect breast cancer in its early stages and before any signs or symptoms are present. Further, if the cancer can be found early, the treatment is likely to be less aggressive and the cancer is more likely to be curable.

Another test used to detect breast cancer is magnetic resonance imaging (MRI), an imaging tool that uses magnetic fields and radio waves to take pictures inside the body. It is more sensitive and more effective in detecting breast cancer than a mammography. However, an MRI is not recommended to be used as a screening tool for breast cancer. An MRI should be used in combination with a mammogram, especially in women who are at high-risk for developing breast cancer. Box 37-1 provides a summary of risk factors for developing breast cancer.

The American Cancer Society recommends the following guidelines for breast cancer screening:

- Women with average risk and who are 45 to 54 years of age should begin having routine mammograms. Beginning at age 55 and with a history of normal mammograms, it is recommended that women get mammograms every two years.

- Women with higher than average risk should get an MRI and a mammogram every year.

The Pelvic Examination

A pelvic examination allows the physician to visually and manually assess a patient's reproductive organs. A pelvic examination is a procedure that is usually performed as part of a routine physical examination for the female. It can also be performed if a patient complains of having symptoms, such as unusual vaginal discharge or pelvic pain. Although some primary care and internal medicine physicians may perform a

---

BOX 37-1 | Risk Factors for Developing Breast Cancer

Gender—Females develop breast cancer 100 times more frequently than males, most likely because of the effects of estrogen and progesterone, which can promote breast cancer cell growth.

Aging—Risk increases with age: Only one in eight invasive breast cancers are found in women younger than 45, whereas about two in three occur in women age 55 or over.

Genetic factors—Five to 10 percent of breast cancer cases are believed to be hereditary, where a gene defect or mutation is inherited from one or both parents. Genetic tests can now be performed to look for these specific genetic mutations, which allows for early detection and intervention.

Family history—Risk is higher if a blood relative developed breast cancer, especially if the cancer occurred at an early age. Occurrence in mother, sister, or daughter doubles a woman's risk.

Personal history of breast cancer—Women with cancer in one breast have an increased risk of developing it in another part of the same breast or the other breast.

Race and ethnicity—White women are slightly more likely to develop breast cancer, but African-American women are more likely to die from it. Women of other racial and ethnic groups have some of the lowest rates, with Asian women having the lowest rates of breast cancer.

Dense breast tissue—Women with dense breasts have a higher risk of breast cancer than women with breasts that have more fatty (less dense) tissue. Dense breast tissue also can make mammograms harder to read. Breast density is affected by age, menopausal status, the use of hormone replacement therapy (HRT), pregnancy, and genetics.

Certain benign breast conditions—Women with certain benign breast conditions may also be at higher risk for breast cancer development.

Lobular carcinoma in situ (LCIS)—Women with this condition have abnormal cells that form in the lobules or milk glands in the breast. Although not a true cancer, LCIS increases a woman's risk of developing invasive breast cancer.

Menstrual periods—Women who started menstruating before age 12 or went through menopause after age 55 have a slightly higher risk of developing cancer. This may be caused by increased lifetime exposure to estrogens and progesterone.

Previous chest radiation—Women who, as children, received chest radiation therapy for other cancers, such as Hodgkin's disease, have significantly greater risk for developing breast cancer.

Diethylstilbestrol (DES) exposure—From the 1940s through the 1960s, many women took the drug DES in the hopes of preventing miscarriage of pregnancies. These women and their daughters have been found to have a greater risk of developing breast cancer.

pelvic examination on their patients, other physicians prefer that their patients see a gynecologist for the examination.

The medical assistant will begin the gynecologic examination by taking a thorough history from the patient. Even though a patient may be seen for a specific gynecological problem, the gynecologic history must include an evaluation of the patient's overall health. You should ask the patient about her menstrual cycle, past pregnancies, and any discomfort during sexual intercourse. You should have knowledge of the various diseases and disorders affecting the reproductive system and be able to recognize the signs and symptoms of sexually transmitted infections (STIs), which are further discussed later in this chapter. During the interview, you should also ask the patient about her relationship status and screen for any signs of violence or abuse in the relationship. All observations and information must be documented in the patient's medical records.

For legal reasons, a female medical assistant must be present to assist with a gynecologic examination. The pelvic examination begins with an examination of the **external genitalia** (vagina, labia majora and minora, and clitoris) for swelling, redness, or ulcerations. The vaginal speculum is then inserted into the vagina to inspect the cervix for color, lacerations, nodules, or discharge. The size of the speculum selected depends on the sexual maturity and physical state of the patient. Vaginal specula may be either metal, requiring sanitization and sterilization after each use, or disposable and meant for single use only. Some specula may even have an attached lighting system to help the physician view the inside of the vaginal canal. Warming the speculum in warm water or keeping it warm in a drawer equipped with a heating pad will make the examination more comfortable for the patient. (Figure 37-1 illustrates the speculum and the manual pelvic examination for females.) The patient may need reassurance, especially if it is her first gynecologic examination.

Pap Test and Cervical Cancer

During the pelvic examination, the physician may also perform a Pap test to screen for abnormal or precancerous cells in the cervix. Named for Greek physician George Papanicolaou, the Pap test is one of the most common screening tools for cancer and has reduced cervical cancer incidence (new cases) and mortality (death) rates in the United States by more than 80 percent.

The most common risk factor for cervical cancer is an infection by **human papillomaviruses (HPVs)**, which is a group of more than a hundred related viruses. Some of these viruses may also cause papillomas or genital warts. HPV is spread by sexual contact, and women who become sexually active at an early age and those who have multiple partners are at higher risk of infection from HPV.

Four types of HPV are responsible for the majority of cervical cancer cases and for genital warts. Type HPV 6 and HPV 11 cause most cases of genital warts but seldom result in cervical cancer. HPV 16 and HPV 18 are responsible for more than 70 percent of all cases of cervical cancer.

The Pap test looks for changes in cervical cells caused by HPV infection. In addition to the Pap test, an HPV test may be done to look for the virus by finding genes (DNA) from HPV in the cells. The HPV test is used along with the Pap test as a part of screening and rarely used as a screening test by itself, because it can only detect the virus, not cancer cells. The American Cancer Society recommends women follow these guidelines for cervical cancer screening:

- After 21 years of age, all women should begin having a Pap test. From age 21 to 29, a Pap test should be performed every three years, unless there is an abnormal Pap test.

- After 30 years of age, women should be co-tested with the Pap test and an HPV test every five years until the age of 65.

- After 65 years of age, a woman who has had regular screening in the past 10 years should stop cervical cancer screening unless there have been abnormal results.

- Women who have had a total hysterectomy do not need cervical cancer screening unless they have a history of precancerous cells or cervical cancer.

Women who have been vaccinated against HPV should still follow the above guidelines.

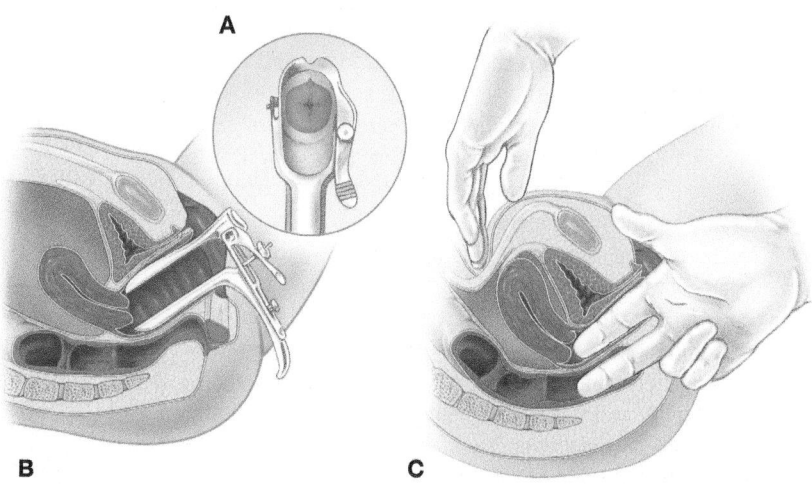

FIGURE 37-1 (A) and **(B)** Pelvic examination of female using a vaginal speculum; **(C)** a bimanual examination.

Your professional development should include an awareness of domestic violence and types of abuse that may be affecting your patients. Violence in the home may include different types of abuse, such as physical, sexual, emotional, mental, and financial. Children, women, and older adults are the most vulnerable populations for abuse. Domestic violence and abuse occurs in every community, regardless of age, socioeconomic status, ethnicity, religion, and sexual orientation.

As a medical assistant, you are often the first person to encounter the patient during a visit and must be prepared to ask about domestic violence and abuse as well as to observe signs of abuse. Signs of domestic violence and abuse include bruising, possibly in various stages of healing; burns; welts; bite marks; dislocations; and fractures. Patients may not be able to explain the injury, or the explanation may not fit the injury. Alternatively, the patient may present with injuries on multiple visits over the course of several months or years. Elder abuse may take many forms, such as neglect, poor hygiene, poor nutrition, bruises and sores, and being overly concerned about money. Signs of child abuse or neglect may be bruising, welts, or burns that cannot sufficiently be explained or in unusual locations, such as the torso, neck, back, and thighs. Children suffering from abuse or neglect may also present with speech disorders, seem withdrawn or antisocial, have poor nutrition, or lack medical and dental care.

When asking about domestic violence or abuse, you must make every effort to establish a safe and secure environment to help the patient feel comfortable in discussing these issues. Some physician offices may include questions about domestic violence and abuse in the patient intake form or questionnaire. Any findings of domestic violence or abuse must be documented in the patient's medical record, and any concerns should be immediately brought to the physician.

Although laws vary from state to state, most states have enacted mandatory reporting laws, which require the reporting of specified injuries and wounds and suspected domestic violence or abuse for individuals being treated by a health care professional. In addition, there are federal laws that protect against elder and child abuse. Every physician's office should have a protocol on how to report suspected abuse and to whom to report it.

As the medical assistant, take the initiative and prepare a folder containing names and numbers of local women's shelters, counseling centers, and domestic violence hotlines. Additionally, you should have the contact information for state agencies and the Department of Health, the Department of Aging, and the Department of Children and Family Services. All of these agencies have printed material and guidelines to help you understand and report your suspicions of abuse.

Although there is currently no cure for HPV infection, there are ways to treat the warts and abnormal cell growth that HPV causes. In 2006, the United States Food and Drug Administration (FDA) approved the use of a new vaccine, Gardasil®, to prevent infection from the four types of HPV: 6, 11, 16, and 18. In 2014, the FDA approved Gardasil® 9, which prevents an additional five HPV viruses (HPV 31, 33, 45, 52, and 58) that are responsible for 20 percent of cervical cancer. Both Gardasil® vaccines are given in a series of three injections over a six-month period. The second injection is two months after the first, and the third injection is six months after the first. It is recommended that the vaccine be given before a female becomes sexually active and as early as 9 years of age in females. Vaccination is also recommended for females age 13 through 26 years and for males age 13 through 21 years who have not been previously vaccinated or who have not completed the three-dose series. Cervarix® is another available vaccine for cervical cancer, approved in 2009, and protects against HPV 16 and HPV 18.

Regardless of whether the patient has been vaccinated, every woman should undergo a routine Pap test to be screened for cervical cancer.

Pap Test Procedure

As already noted, the Pap test is a screening procedure that examines cells from the vaginal and cervical mucosa to check for precancerous or abnormal cells. A thin scraping of these exfoliated cells is taken from the cervix, vagina, and endocervical canal using a cervical spatula and cervical brush or broom. Two methods of Pap specimen preparation are currently being used. In the conventional "dry" method, the physician places samples or "smears" on glass microscope slides. The medical assistant labels the slides C, V, E (cervix, vaginal, and endocervical canal) based on the source of the cells, then sprays the slides with a fixative to preserve the cells. The newer "liquid" method has the samples collected in a similar fashion as with the "dry" method, but instead of being placed on slides, the samples are placed in vials of liquid preservative. The "liquid" method is now more commonly used because it permits co-testing for both the Pap test and HPV test.

With either method of collection, the properly labeled samples are then sent to a laboratory for examination. When sending the samples, the laboratory requisition form has a specific field that requires the medical assistant to enter the first day of the patient's last menstrual period (LMP). In some cases, the cytologist needs this information to make an accurate evaluation and to provide a maturation index (MI). An MI provides a hormonal evaluation of the patient that may assist in evaluating causes of infertility, menopausal or postmenopausal bleeding, or **amenorrhea** (absence of menstrual periods). Upon receiving the samples, the cytologist prepares, stains, examines, and evaluates the samples for evidence of infection, **dysplasia** (abnormal cells), or cancerous cells.

Before scheduling a patient for a Pap test, the medical assistant should advise her of the following:

- Do not douche 24 to 48 hours before the examination. Doing so may wash away cervical cells that should be obtained during a Pap smear.
- Avoid sexual intercourse for at least 48 hours before the examination.

Do not schedule the Pap test for a time when the patient may be menstruating. It should be scheduled at least five days after the last day of menstruation.

After collecting the specimens, the physician performs a bimanual pelvic examination by inserting a gloved, lubricated finger into the vagina and simultaneously palpating the lower abdomen. By this method, the physician can detect the size, shape, and position of the uterus and ovaries and can identify any lumps or other abnormalities. A digital rectal examination (DRE) may follow in which the physician inserts a lubricated, gloved finger into the rectum to check for hemorrhoids, polyps, or other abnormalities of the organs of the lower pelvis.

The medical assistant should be ready to assist the physician by providing new gloves before each procedure, lubricating the physician's gloved finger, and assisting in handing the physician any supplies or equipment needed during the procedures. The medical assistant should also monitor the patient's comfort level and try to reduce her anxiety during the procedures. Procedure 37-2 lists the steps for assisting with a pelvic examination and a Pap test.

PROCEDURE 37-2

Assisting with a Pelvic Examination and Pap Test

Objective ◆ *Set up and assist with a gynecologic examination, including collecting dry or liquid-based prep method Pap smear.*

EQUIPMENT AND SUPPLIES

Vaginal speculum; water-soluble lubricant; cotton-tipped applicator; patient drape; Pap smear materials: Dry Prep—cervical spatula brush, glass slides, fixative spray or liquid slide holder, identification label; Liquid-Based Prep—plastic cervical spatula, broom or brush, cytology medium transport vial, identification label; laboratory request form; cleansing tissue; gloves; container for contaminated vaginal speculum; gooseneck lamp; biohazard waste container; patient's medical record

METHOD

For dry prep collection:

1. Perform hand hygiene.
2. Assemble equipment, label the slides, and complete the laboratory form.
3. Warmly greet and identify the patient, introduce yourself, and explain the procedure.
4. Direct the patient to the bathroom to empty her bladder.
5. Ask the patient to remove her clothing and put on the gown with the opening in front.
6. Drape the patient appropriately, and assist her into the supine position (on her back) for breast and abdominal examination.

7. When the physician is ready to collect the Pap specimen, assist and instruct the patient to assume the dorsal lithotomy position with her buttocks at the edge of the table, knees flexed, and feet in the stirrups. Knees should be relaxed and rotated outward. Expose the genitalia by moving the drape away from this area while it still covers the legs.
8. Adjust the gooseneck lamp and place the physician's stool in the proper position at the end of examination table.
9. Assist the physician with the following procedures (Figure A, B, C):
   - Apply gloves.
   - Hand gloves and equipment to the physician when needed. Place lubricant onto the speculum as the physician holds it.
   - Hold the microscopic slides as the physician smears the slides. Mark the slides: C for cervical, V for vaginal, and E for endocervical.
   - Spray fixative from about 6 inches away from the slide.
   - Place the slide into a container with the appropriate label.
10. Hold the receptacle as the physician places the contaminated speculum into it. Set the container into the sink for later cleaning.

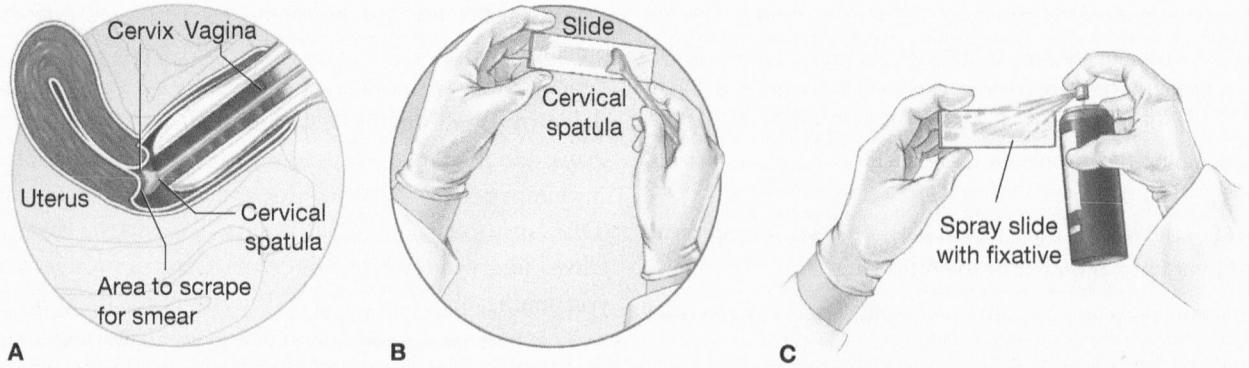

FIGURE A–C **(A)** Female reproductive organs showing the location for obtaining a scraping for a Pap smear; **(B)** making a Pap smear; **(C)** spraying slide with fixative.

11. Apply lubricant to the physician's gloved finger in preparation for the manual examination.
12. Properly dispose of gloves in a hazardous waste container and perform hand hygiene.
13. Assist the patient in sitting up by (a) helping her move back on the table, (b) taking her feet out of the stirrups, and (c) helping her to a sitting position.
14. Sanitize and sterilize equipment as needed.
15. Perform hand hygiene.
16. Prepare the Pap specimen to be sent to the laboratory.

For liquid-based prep collection:
17. Follow steps 1–8 above.

18. Open the vial of liquid preservative and hold for the physician to place both the plastic spatula and either a brush or broom containing the specimen in the vial.
19. Rinse the broom vigorously by pushing it to the bottom of the vial 10 times.
20. Use the spatula to scrape cells from the broom and swirl both in the vial to mix before removing.
21. Label the vial, and dispose of hazardous waste appropriately.
22. Proceed through steps 11–16 above.
23. The physician may chart the procedure or will delegate charting to the medical assistant and will review and sign after the medical assistant.

Grading of Pap Specimens

If a Pap test is positive or has cervical dysplasia (abnormal cells), the patient is determined to have squamous intraepithelial lesion (SIL), which is not diagnostic of precancer or cancer but requires further tests. The physician may then recommend performing a full evaluation with a colposcopy procedure. A colposcopy uses a specialized instrument, called a colposcope, to view the cervix, vagina, and vulva, and it allows for a biopsy (sample of tissue) from the cervix to be taken (Figure 37-2).

Once the cervical biopsy is found to have dysplasia, the patient is now determined to have cervical intraepithelial neoplasia (CIN), which is considered precancerous. A grading system for CIN describes the amount of cervical dysplasia. CIN I (1) is mild (low-grade) dysplasia, CIN II (2) is moderate to moderately severe dysplasia, and CIN III (3) indicates **carcinoma in situ (CIS)**, which is considered early stage cancer.

Prenatal Care

Prenatal care is health care provided to pregnant women before childbirth that includes a series of visits and specific tests to monitor and promote the health of both mother and

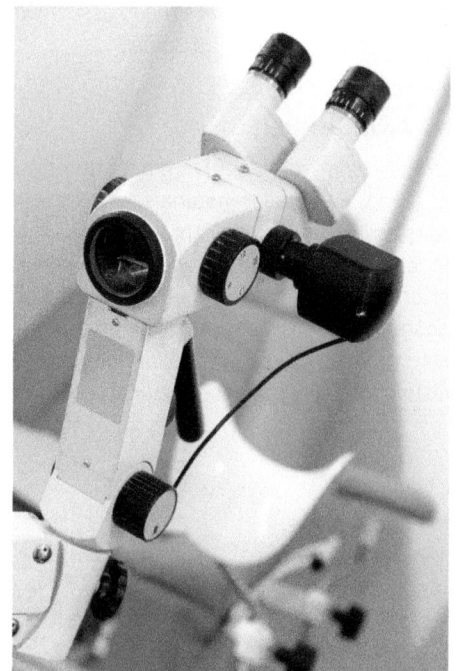

FIGURE 37-2 A colposcope.

fetus. (Postnatal or postpartum care covers the time period from the birth of the infant to the mother's six-week postnatal follow-up appointment.)

Many health practitioners recommend that any woman considering or wishing to become pregnant visit or call her health care provider to discuss her preconception health. The U.S. Department of Health and Human Services's Office of Women's Health recommends that women take the following measures before becoming pregnant:

- Take 400 to 800 micrograms (or 0.4 to 0.8 milligrams) of folic acid every day for at least three months to lower the risk of birth defects, such as spina bifida, which affects the brain and spine. Folic acid can be taken as a vitamin supplement or can be found in some foods.

- Women should stop smoking and drinking alcohol, which may result in birth defects and miscarriages.

- Discuss with the physician any over-the-counter (OTC) or prescription medication that is currently being taken, including dietary and herbal supplements. Physicians may allow some medications to be taken during the pregnancy if failure to take the prescribed treatment would hinder the health of the mother.

- Do not use illicit drugs. Avoid contact with any toxic substances or materials at work and at home. Stay away from chemicals and cat or rodent feces.

A normal, full-term pregnancy lasts 40 weeks that are divided into three trimesters, or stages, of approximately three months each. The first trimester includes the period of time from implantation of the embryo in the uterus through the 14th week. This is the most critical stage of fetal life because most of the major organ systems are developing during this period. It is also the period when the embryo is fastest growing and most vulnerable to substances that may cause birth defects, such as bacterial and viral infections, drugs, alcohol, and other chemical substances. After the eighth week, the embryo is referred to as a fetus.

The second trimester begins at the end of the 14th week and continues to the end of the sixth month. During this period, refinement of all the organs takes place, and fetal movement (**quickening**) may be felt. The baby's sex can be determined in the second trimester.

The third trimester is the period from the end of the sixth month to birth and is marked by an increase in the size and weight of the fetus. During this stage, the fetus usually assumes a head-down position. The fetus is said to have reached the age of **viability** (able to sustain life independently) at seven months.

First Prenatal Visit

The first prenatal visit usually takes place after the patient has missed at least two menstrual cycles (periods). This visit requires more time than follow-up visits because a full history and prenatal assessment must be done. In addition, a complete physical examination and pelvic examination, including a Pap test, must be performed. Blood tests are ordered at this visit, which include a complete blood count (CBC) test, an ABO/Rh test, a serology test for syphilis, a rubella titer, and a blood culture and complete urine analysis (UA), if necessary. These test results provide a baseline to compare with results obtained throughout the pregnancy to help monitor the health of the mother and fetus.

The **fundal height** measurement is taken on the initial visit and is used as a guideline for all subsequent visits. Fundal height is measured from the top of the mother's pubic symphysis (joint between the pubic bones) to the **fundus** (top of the uterus) using a nonstretchable tape measure. During pregnancy, the uterus enlarges and rises into the abdominal cavity, with the fundal height increasing each month.

Prenatal History

The prenatal history includes recording menstrual history, including the patient's **menarche** (onset of menstruation), menstrual interval cycle, duration of menses, amount of flow, any menstrual cycle problems, and any types of currently or previously used contraception.

Past obstetrical history is another important component of the prenatal history to be documented in the patient's medical records. This includes **gravida** (total number of pregnancies), **para** (births after 20 weeks of gestation, regardless of whether the infant is born dead or alive), and **abortions** (number of fetuses that did not reach the age of viability, usually under 20 weeks gestation). This information should be charted using Roman numerals. For example, a woman pregnant for the first time would be gravida I, para 0. A woman pregnant at the current visit, who delivered a single child during her first pregnancy, delivered twins on her second pregnancy, and had one miscarriage would be charted as follows: gravida IV, para III, abs I.

After the patient's past history is obtained, it is important to gather the present pregnancy history. The patient should be asked the following questions:

- Do you have any preexisting conditions? Heart disease, kidney disease, and diabetes are especially important.

- Do you have any symptoms, such as morning sickness, fatigue, headaches, vaginal bleeding, discharge, or breast changes?

- Are you taking any prescriptions, over-the-counter medications, vitamins, or herbal supplements?

- Do you drink, smoke, or use recreational drugs? If so, what and how much?

- Are you employed, a student, married, divorced, or single?

More often than not, the question most patients ask during their first prenatal visit is the expected date of childbirth. A gestation calculator may be used to predict the estimated date of childbirth (EDD). Another method to calculate EDD is to use Naegele's rule, applying the following formula:

LMP (last menstrual period) + 7 days − 3 months + 1 year = EDD

Example: LMP was June 10, 2017
  Add 7 days (= 17)
  Subtract 3 months from June (= March)
  Add 1 year (= 2018)
  Thus, the EDD is March 17, 2018.

Prenatal Patient Education

The initial prenatal visit affords an opportunity to provide the patient with information about what to expect during each stage of pregnancy, nutritional guidelines, vitamin and mineral requirements, and substances to be avoided. Pamphlets and brochures should be available in the reception room and examining room. At this visit, the physician will order blood tests and other diagnostic procedures, such as an ultrasound, to be completed at a later date. As the medical assistant, be sure to remind patients of the importance of prenatal visits when you schedule the procedures and follow-up visits.

Follow-up Prenatal Visits

The patient will return for a follow-up visit every four weeks through the 28th week. Then she will return every two weeks up to the 36th week, and then every week until childbirth. These return visits offer another opportunity for the medical assistant to educate the patient on the importance of maintaining her follow-up visit schedule, reinforce proper nutritional guidelines, and answer any questions the patient may have.

The Medical Assistant's Role in Follow-up Prenatal Visits

On each subsequent visit, the medical assistant's responsibilities include but are not limited to:

- Setting up the examining room
- Obtaining a urine specimen from the patient
- Weighing the patient
- Obtaining the patient's blood pressure
- Asking the patient if she has any problems or issues
- Charting all information in the patient's medical record
- Assisting the patient onto the examining table
- Draping the patient appropriately

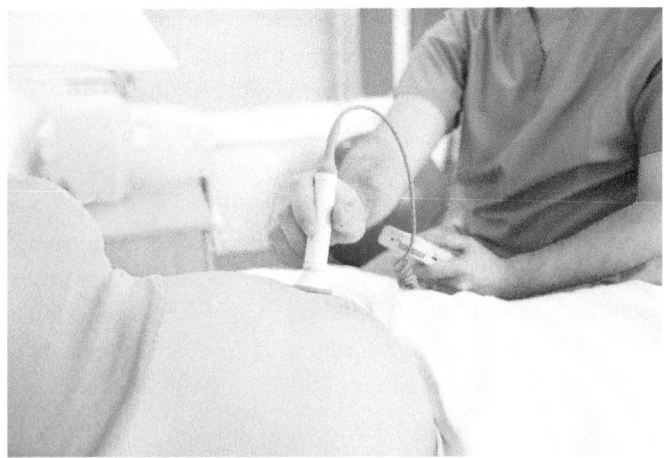

FIGURE 37-3 Listening to the fetal heartbeat with a Doppler device.

The physician will review the findings, ask the patient to recline so the fundal height can be measured, check for signs of edema (swelling), use a fetoscope (also called Pinard horn or fetal stethoscope) to listen to the fetal heartbeat, and answer any questions the patient may have. At 10 to 12 weeks, the **fetal heart tone (FHT)** is audible with the use of a Doppler fetal monitor (Figure 37-3). The normal FHT is 120 to 160 beats per minute. If fetal distress is indicated by an extremely rapid or slow heart rate, the physician may order fetal stress tests to evaluate the condition of the fetus. The results of these measurements must be recorded in the patient's medical record.

Closer to the date of birth, the patient will attend classes on preparing for childbirth and breast-feeding. Classes are usually given at the facility chosen for childbirth. The physician will also discuss childbirth options with the patient, such as location of the birth (hospital, birthing center, or home birth) and type of birth (vaginal or Cesarean). Notes about this conversation will also be entered in the medical record.

Screening Tests

Later in the pregnancy, the medical assistant may need to schedule additional screening tests for the patient. Some tests will be routine and others will be needed based on the patient's age, personal or family history, or the results of routine tests already performed. Some screening and diagnostic tests to monitor the fetus's health are:

- The carrier test is a genetic test recommended if there is a family history of certain diseases, such as cystic fibrosis or hemophilia. It can be performed on the mother and father and done before or during the pregnancy. However, genetic disorders can occur in families with no history of genetic disorders.

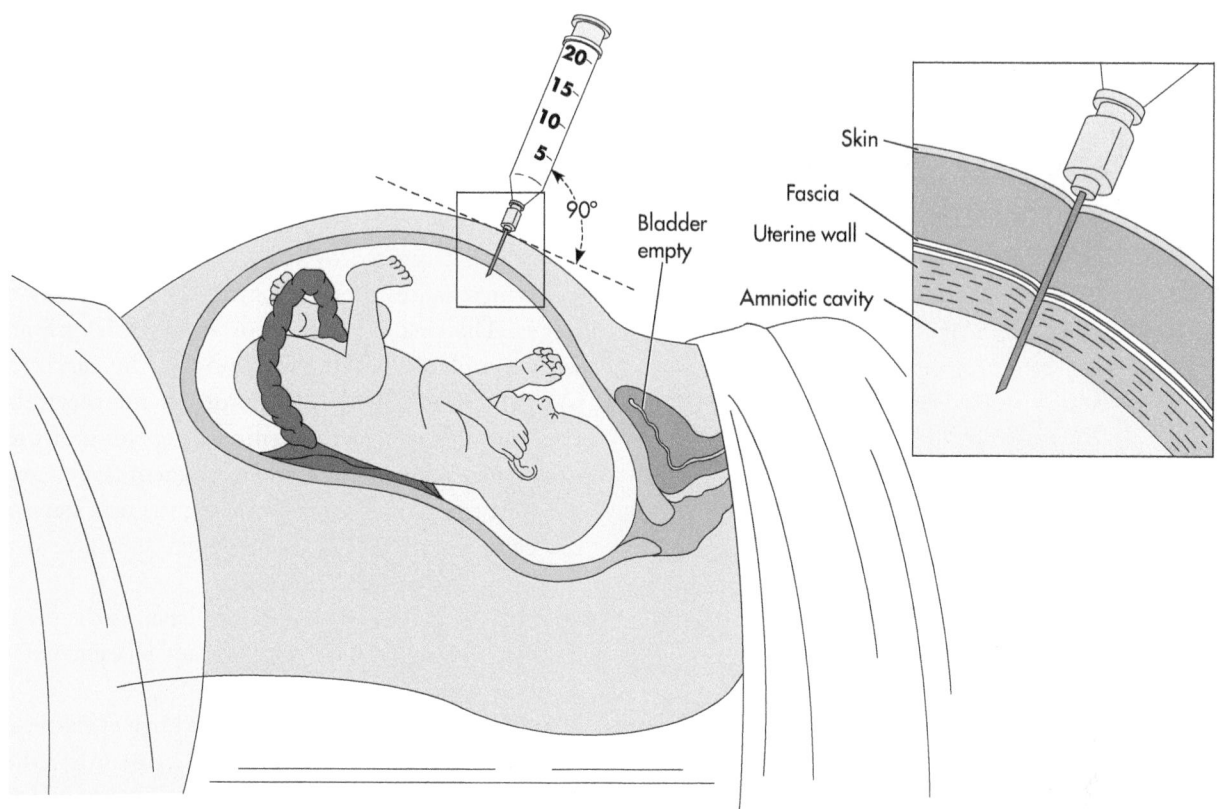

FIGURE 37-4 Amniocentesis. The patient is examined with ultrasound to determine the placental site and to locate the fluid. When the needle is in place within the amniotic cavity, amniotic fluid is withdrawn.

Labels in figure: 90°; Bladder empty; Skin; Fascia; Uterine wall; Amniotic cavity

- **Chorionic villus sampling (CVS)** is a procedure in which a small sample of cells is taken from the placenta and examined for chromosomal abnormalities. It is performed between 10 and 13 weeks of pregnancy, which is sooner than an amniocentesis. There is some risk to the fetus with this test, such as possible miscarriage and infection.

- Nuchal translucency screening is a special ultrasound test of the fetus to screen for the risk of Down syndrome and other chromosomal abnormalities. The ultrasound is performed between 11 and 14 weeks and measures the thickness of the fluid buildup at the back of the fetus's neck. If this area is thicker than normal, it can be an early sign of Down syndrome or other chromosomal abnormalities.

- Alpha-fetoprotein (AFP) test is a blood test taken between the 15th and 18th week of pregnancy to detect neural tube defects, which are birth defects of the brain, spine, or spinal cord.

- Amniocentesis is performed between weeks 15 and 20. It involves using a fine needle to take a sample of amniotic fluid from the sac around the fetus (Figure 37-4). The amniotic fluid contains fetal cells, which will be cultured, grown in a laboratory, and screened to

detect chromosomal defects, such as Down syndrome. Amniocentesis is also used to assess fetal sex, maturity, and development. It is recommended that women over age 35 and women who have a family history of genetic defects have this test.

- Ultrasound is used to determine the age, growth rate, position of the fetus, and obvious birth defects. It is generally performed at 16 to 20 weeks and is generally painless. A vaginal ultrasound may be done to examine the fetus more closely. Ultrasounds can also be performed to determine the fetus's sex, usually by the 20th week. Figure 37-5 shows an ultrasonogram of a male fetus.

- Glucose tolerance testing is performed between 24 and 28 weeks of pregnancy to test for gestational diabetes. After fasting, the patient is given a specific dose of glucose, and blood is taken one hour later. If the patient has a positive test or elevated blood glucose levels, the physician will recommend a more comprehensive three-hour glucose tolerance test. To prevent complications, the patient's glucose will be carefully monitored. The patient may be advised to eat a diet low in fat, moderate in carbohydrates, and high in fiber and to exercise regularly. Insulin may be needed

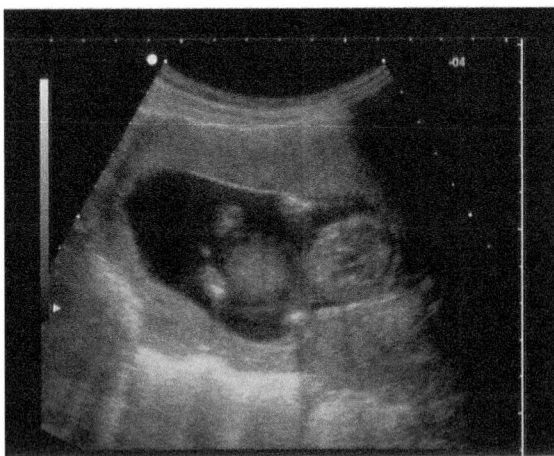

FIGURE 37-5 Ultrasonogram showing a male fetus.

if diet and exercise are not sufficient to lower blood glucose levels. In most situations, the gestational diabetes resolves once the baby is delivered, but women who develop gestational diabetes are at higher risk of developing diabetes later in life.

- The high blood glucose levels in women with gestational diabetes may cross the placenta, which may result in a pregnancy complication such as a larger than normal infant (macrosomia) for gestational age. This may require the infant be born early or via Cesarean section (C-section). Gestational diabetes generally does not cause birth defects in infants, and infants born from women with gestational diabetes do not have higher than normal risk of developing diabetes later in life.

- Group B *Streptococcus* (GBS) is a part of the body's normal flora, commonly found in the urinary and reproductive system. GBS does not normally cause illness in the mother, but it may be passed to the baby during birth. Between 1 and 2 percent of infants may be infected, and the infection may be life threatening. A vaginal culture at 35 to 37 weeks is recommended. A patient who tests positive will be treated with antibiotics during labor to prevent fetal infection.

Professionalism The Life Span

In the field of obstetrics, the medical assistant deals with pregnant women of varying ages. Pregnancy in both the teen years and pregnancy beyond age 35 pose greater risks. Teen mothers and mothers who do not have access to prenatal care have an increased risk for premature and low birth weight babies. Women over the age of 35 are at increased risk of having babies with chromosomal abnormalities, such as Down syndrome.

Childbirth

Parturition, or birth, occurs anytime from week 37 to 42 under normal circumstances. Birth before 37 weeks is considered a preterm or premature birth and can lead to serious health issues and complications for the baby, such as infections and respiratory issues.

Labor is triggered by the release of the hormone **oxytocin**, which causes uterine contraction and occurs in three stages. The first stage of labor varies in length and ends with complete **dilation** (widening of the cervix) (Figure 37-6A) and **effacement** (thinning of the cervical walls). Dilation measures the widening or opening of the cervix from 0 to 10 centimeters, and effacement is often expressed in percentages. For example, during the first stage of labor, the cervix may be 3–4 centimeters and have 0 percent effacement.

Stage two, the pushing stage of labor, is the period from complete dilation (10 centimeters) and effacement (100 percent) through the birth of the fetus.

Stage three is the period from the birth of the fetus to the expulsion of the placenta (Figure 37-6B). After the birth, the placenta will become separated from the uterine wall and be expelled through the vaginal canal (Figure 37-6C).

Postpartum Visit

The **puerperium** is a span of usually six weeks after childbirth during which the patient's body slowly returns to its prepregnant state. The uterus shrinks, or involutes, and healing of the birth canal takes place. During this time, the patient experiences **lochia**, which is vaginal discharge from the uterus that may occur after childbirth. This discharge consists of blood, tissue, mucus, and white blood cells, and indicates the healing occurring in the uterus. Lochia begins as bright red until about the fourth day, then becomes brownish red by the tenth day, and finally becomes yellow-white. The patient should be instructed to call the physician if, at any time, the discharge becomes bloody or foul smelling because these may be signs of infection or more serious bleeding. During the puerperium, the patient should be encouraged to eat balanced meals, continue taking vitamins, and avoid lifting heavy objects.

A postpartum visit should be scheduled approximately six weeks after childbirth to evaluate overall health status of the patient. The postpartum visit includes measuring height, weight, and vital signs; performing pelvic and breast examinations; a rectal examination to detect hemorrhoids; and testing hemoglobin and hematocrit levels for anemia.

Menstruation should resume after about eight weeks in the nonnursing mother and six months in the nursing

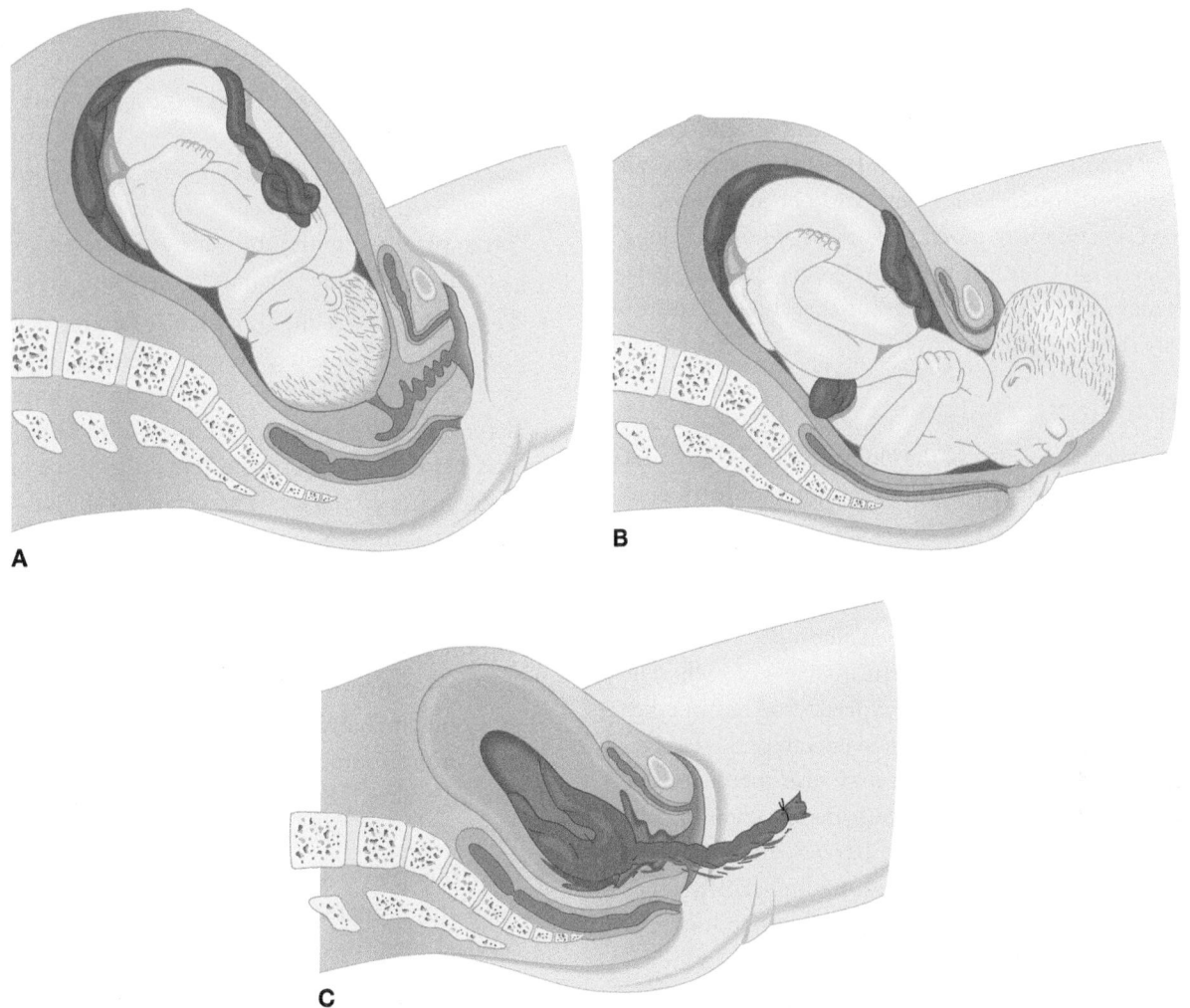

FIGURE 37-6 The stages of labor: **(A)** dilation stage: uterine contractions cause dilation of the cervix; **(B)** expulsion stage: birth, or expulsion, of the baby; **(C)** placental stage: expulsion of the placenta.

mother. Information about contraceptive methods may be provided, if desired by the patient.

Complications During Pregnancy

Placenta previa is a complication in which the placenta develops in the lower portion of the uterus, blocking the opening in the cervix. During labor, the cervix is unable to completely dilate and efface, resulting in maternal hemorrhage and oxygen deprivation for the fetus. Both can be life threatening. An ultrasound examination can detect the placental placement, and a scheduled C-section may be required to avoid an emergency situation.

Abruptio placentae is a complication that occurs when the placenta tears away from the uterine wall, resulting in hemorrhage and fetal distress. Abruptio placentae occurs secondary to trauma, such as a fall, or because of vascular insufficiency resulting from hypertension or preeclampsia. If the abruption is mild and the pregnancy is 34 weeks or less, the mother may be hospitalized for close monitoring until birth is possible.

If the pregnancy is more than 34 weeks or the abruption is severe, an emergency C-section may be required.

Hypertension during pregnancy (gestational hypertension) occurs in roughly 10 percent of pregnancies. If hypertension is present along with signs of damage to another system, such as the kidneys, the patient may be diagnosed with **preeclampsia**. Preeclampsia develops in approximately 5 percent of pregnant women and usually occurs after the 20th week of pregnancy. Although the cause of preeclampsia is not definitively known, it is believed that blood vessel spasms in the placenta may elevate blood pressure. The blood flow to the placenta can be compromised and lead to organ damage in the fetus and even fetal death.

Symptoms of preeclampsia in the patient may include agitation and confusion, changes in mental status, decreased urine output, headaches, nausea and vomiting, pain in the upper right quadrant, shortness of breath, sudden weight gain, swelling of the face or hands, and visual impairment. There are no known ways to prevent preeclampsia. Treatment for preeclampsia includes medication and bed rest with close monitoring. The only cure for preeclampsia is birth of the baby.

If preeclampsia is not controlled and seizures develop, the patient is diagnosed with **eclampsia**. Because eclampsia can have serious consequences for both mother and baby, an emergency C-section is required, regardless of how far along the pregnancy is. Thus, all pregnant women should have good prenatal care and closely monitor their blood pressure throughout their pregnancy.

Methods of Contraception

Because the average woman in the United States is fertile for about half her life, it is fairly safe to assume that birth control will be a consideration for her at some point in her life. The chance of a woman becoming pregnant without any form of contraception is 85 percent. Thus, it is important for the medical assistant to have an understanding of the various methods of birth control and the effectiveness of each. The patient will choose the most appropriate method for her based on physical condition, cost, side effects, and effectiveness. Cultural or religious beliefs may also influence the method of birth control the patient ultimately chooses.

Contraceptive methods include barrier methods, hormonal methods, implantable devices, natural family planning/rhythm method, coitus interruptus or withdrawal of the penis during intercourse, and sterilization. A newer contraceptive method is the emergency contraception pill, commonly referred to as "the morning-after" pill.

Barrier Methods

Barrier contraceptive methods work by preventing sperm from reaching the egg. Barrier methods include the following:

- **Spermicides**—Substances that inactivate or kill sperm on contact. They are available in foam, gel, cream, tablet, and suppository forms. They can be used alone (70 percent effectiveness rate) but are more effective when used with other barrier methods, such as condoms, diaphragms, cervical caps, shields, or sponges.

- **Male condom**—Worn over the penis during intercourse to prevent the sperm from entering the vagina. It is inexpensive, easy to use, and available without prescription. Condoms also provide a measure of protection from sexually transmitted infections (STIs). Condoms have an effectiveness rate of about 85 percent.

- **Female condom**—A polyurethane sheath that lines the vagina with an inner ring that fits over the cervix and an outer ring that permits entrance of the penis.

The sheath is removed after ejaculation. It has an effectiveness rate of about 80 percent.

- **Diaphragm**—A flexible dome of rubber that fits over the cervix and prevents the entry of sperm. An examination and physician's prescription are needed. It can be inserted six hours before intercourse and must be left in place six hours afterward. It is effective about 88 percent of the time when used correctly.

- **Cervical cap**—A small, reusable, flexible device that fits over the cervix and prevents the entry of sperm. It is obtained by prescription and requires a physician to determine the size needed. It must be in place 30 minutes before intercourse and remain in place for six to eight hours afterward. The cervical cap has an effectiveness of about 84 percent. It is found to be less effective in women who have had vaginal deliveries in whom there is an effectiveness rate of 68 percent.

- **Shield**—A reusable, one-size-fits-all, cup-shaped device that fits over the cervix and is held in place by suction and the vaginal wall. It must be left in place for a minimum of eight hours after intercourse and is effective about 85 percent of the time when used correctly.

- **Contraceptive sponge**—A piece of polyurethane foam impregnated with spermicide that blocks the cervical opening. It can be inserted up to 24 hours before intercourse and must remain in place six hours afterward. The contraceptive sponge has the same issue as the cervical cap where the effectiveness rate differs based on whether the woman has had a vaginal birth. Its effectiveness rate is 84 percent in women before vaginal birth and 76 percent in women after vaginal birth.

Hormonal Methods

Hormonal methods of birth control are based on using hormones to change the levels of female hormones in the body to prevent ovulation or implantation of the fertilized ovum. They include birth control pills, emergency contraception, hormonal implants, hormone injections, the "minipill," hormone patches, and the vaginal ring. These methods are easy to use and very effective:

- **Birth control pills** ("the pill")—Also known as oral contraceptives, are the most widely used method of contraception, and usually contain a combination of the hormones estrogen and progestin. They are contraindicated in women who smoke, are over age 35, or have had a history of blood clots, high blood pressure, breast cancer, liver disease, or advanced diabetes. The pill has a 92 percent effectiveness rate. It does not protect against STIs. Side effects include headache, nausea, bloating, depression, and decreased sex drive.

- **Emergency contraceptives**—Include the "morning-after pill" and copper IUD. The morning-after pill consists of a series of pills containing estrogen and progestin that prevents the possibility of implantation of an egg for up to three to five days after unprotected sex. Its effectiveness rate is 89 percent at day three and becomes less effective as time passes. The copper IUD (Para Guard) is an intrauterine device that is placed in the uterus for long-term birth control, as well as an emergency contraceptive. It has a 99 percent effectiveness rate even if placed five days after unprotected sex. Both methods of emergency contraceptives may be used in unwanted pregnancies, such as in cases of rape and sexual abuse.

- **Implanon**—An implantable, matchstick-size contraceptive device that was approved in 2006 by the FDA. It may be left in place for up to three years. It is said to be 99 percent effective. Implants may also stop menstruation but may cause irregular bleeding, breast soreness, and acne.

- **Injection** (Depo-Provera)—Is highly effective at 97 percent. One injection is given every three months within the first five days of the menstrual cycle. Weight gain, irregular bleeding, and delayed return of menstrual cycle after stopping use are common side effects.

- **Progestin-only pill**—Also known as "the minipill," it is taken daily and is safe for nursing mothers. Effectiveness is 92 percent, comparable to other hormonal methods. However, it may cause breakthrough bleeding.

- **Skin patch**—An adhesive square that slowly releases estrogen and progestin through the skin to the bloodstream. It is 98 percent effective.

- **Vaginal ring**—Inserted into the vagina and contains estrogen and progestin. It is used for the first three weeks of the menstrual cycle and removed for the fourth week for menstruation. It is 92 percent effective and has side effects similar to other hormonal methods.

Intrauterine Devices

An **intrauterine device (IUD)** is a small device with progestin that is placed in the uterus by the physician. IUDs are very effective, up to 99 percent. However, in some cases they may cause pain, bleeding, and infection. See Figure 37-7 for examples of IUDs.

Natural Family Planning

Natural family planning, also known as the rhythm method, but more recently called fertility awareness–based birth control, is based on avoiding intercourse around the time of ovulation. It relies on the woman having a relatively predictable and normal menstrual cycle. Other fertility awareness–based practices include measurement of basal body temperature, keeping an accurate menstruation calendar, and being aware of the viscosity of cervical mucus. The effectiveness of this method varies greatly from 80 to 98 percent because of human error and the need for the individual to be disciplined in charting and monitoring her menstrual cycle.

Coitus Interruptus

Coitus interruptus is the withdrawal of the male's penis before ejaculating into the vagina. The effectiveness rate varies widely between 73 and 96 percent because it greatly depends on self-control. Thus, it is an unreliable form of birth control, especially because sperm may be released even before a male ejaculates (preejaculate).

Sterilization

Women are fertile for about 40 years of their adult lives, whereas healthy men are fertile throughout most of their adult lives. Since the 1960s, sterilization has become more common as a permanent method of birth control. Several methods are available for women, including Essure coils and tubal ligation. The sterilization method for a male requires vasectomy, which is discussed in the male reproductive system section of this chapter.

- **Essure**—A permanent method of birth control in which the physician places tiny metal coils in the fallopian tubes. Over time, scar tissue forms over these coils and blocks the tubes, thus preventing sperm from reaching the ovum. It does not require surgical incision, unlike tubal ligation. This method is 99 percent effective. Side effects and risks are few.

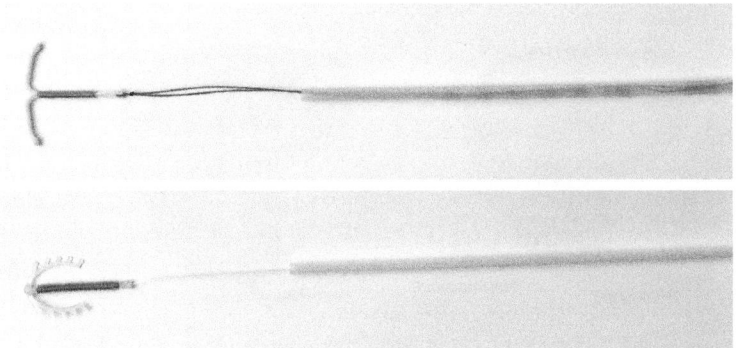

FIGURE 37-7 Examples of intrauterine devices.

- **Tubal ligation**—A permanent method of birth control and is effective 99 percent of the time. A small incision is made near the navel, and a laparoscope is inserted. Instruments are inserted through the laparoscope to seal the tubes by cauterizing (burning) or closing them with clips or rings.

MALE REPRODUCTIVE MEDICAL ISSUES

The male reproductive system combines reproductive and urinary functions. The major male organs of reproduction are located outside the body in the scrotum and penis. The scrotum (scrotal sac) contains two testes and the seminal ducts. The penis contains the urethra, which carries both urine and sperm to the outside of the body. The internal organs of reproduction are the seminal vesicles, ejaculatory duct, bulbourethral gland, and prostate gland. To review these systems, see the chapters titled "The Urinary System" and "The Reproductive System."

Prostate Conditions

The prostate is a walnut-sized gland located between the bladder and the penis. It produces the seminal fluid that contains sperm. The prostate gland also surrounds the urethra, which carries urine from the bladder and out of the body. As men age, the prostate gland enlarges, pressing on the urethra, and eventually restricting the flow of urine. This enlargement of the prostate gland is called benign prostatic hyperplasia (BPH) and is one of the most common conditions in men over 50 years old (Figure 37-8). Restricted urinary flow can result in urinary retention, interruption of the urine stream, and difficulty starting to urinate. Medications and other nonsurgical treatments are available that

Benign Prostatic Hyperplasia

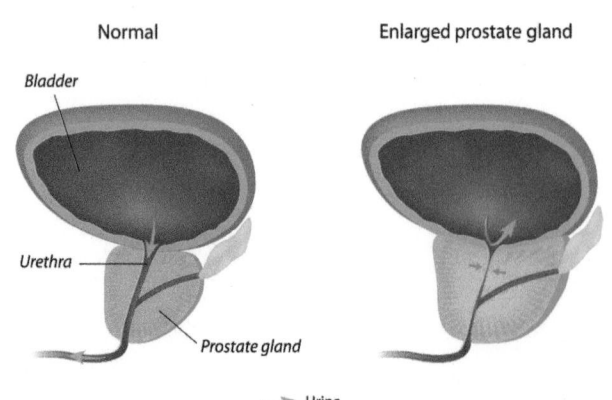

FIGURE 37-8 Benign prostatic hyperplasia.

may relieve the symptoms in some men. BPH is not cancer and does not seem to increase a male's risk of getting prostate cancer. However, the early symptoms of BPH are similar to those of prostate cancer.

Prostate cancer is a slow-growing, malignant tumor of the prostate gland affecting one in seven men in the United States. It is the second most common form of cancer in men. Prostate cancer may metastasize (spread) to the adjacent urinary tract and male reproductive organs as well as to the lymph nodes and bones. Because of its slow rate of growth, prostate cancer can be detected and treated in its early stages. The cause of prostate cancer is not known, but age, heredity, and a high-fat diet increase the risk of developing it. Symptoms include weak stream of urine, blood in the urine, erectile dysfunction, **nocturia** (frequency of urination at night), and pelvic or back pain.

Prostate cancer screening includes a digital rectal examination (DRE) and a protein-specific antigen (PSA) blood test. A DRE has long been used to diagnose prostate cancer. Abnormal prostate findings from a DRE include nodules, asymmetry, or hardening. DREs are not very sensitive and should not be used alone when screening for prostate cancer. Another screening tool for prostate cancer is the PSA test, which is a blood test that measures protein released by the prostate. The blood level of PSA is often elevated in men with prostate cancer. Thus, men who report prostate symptoms often undergo PSA testing (along with a DRE) to help the physician determine the nature of the problem.

According to the American Cancer Society, recommendations regarding screening for prostatic cancer depend on the results of the PSA blood test:

- Men who choose to be tested who have a PSA of less than 2.5 ng/mL may only need to be retested every two years.

- Screening should be done yearly for men whose PSA level is 2.5 ng/mL or higher.

PSA results of under 4 ng/mL are considered normal. However, caution should be used when interpreting PSA levels because very high levels may not mean prostate cancer, and very low levels may not mean the individual is cancerfree. A number of noncancerous conditions can cause the PSA level to rise.

However, if PSA levels are elevated and continue to be elevated, the physician may recommend an additional test, such as a transrectal ultrasound, X-ray, or cystoscopy. A prostate biopsy may also be needed. During this procedure, multiple samples of prostate tissue are collected by inserting hollow needles into the prostate and then withdrawing them. If the biopsy is positive for abnormal or cancer cells, further tests may be required, such as an MRI or a bone scan to detect possible spread of the cancer.

Treatments for prostate cancer vary from watching and waiting with regular checkups, to surgery, radiation, hormone therapy, and chemotherapy. However, prostate cancer has one of the highest survival rates with more than 90 percent surviving past 15 years after being diagnosed.

Circumcision

Circumcision is the surgical removal of the foreskin, which covers the tip of the penis. In the United States, it has been customary for most newborn male babies to have this procedure performed in the hospital shortly after birth. More than 80 percent of males are circumcised in the United States. However, the circumcision rate of newborns has been declining over the past several decades. This may be because of changing racial and ethnic demographics and a growing number of families who lack or have limited health insurance and, thus, have less access to the surgical procedure.

Studies about the benefits of circumcision conflict, so the American Academy of Family Physicians and the American Academy of Pediatrics do not currently recommend routine circumcision for all male newborns, but recommend leaving the decision up to the parents. Circumcision is believed to have some health benefits, however, including:

- Promoting cleanliness and easier hygiene
- Decreased risk of urinary tract infections (UTI)
- Decreased risk of sexually transmitted infections
- Decreased risk of penile cancer

Complications from circumcision are bleeding and infection. Also, some studies have found that circumcision may decrease sensitivity during sex and may reduce a male's overall sexual satisfaction.

Most circumcision procedures are quick and safe. One of the more common procedures uses the Plastibell, which is a plastic device slipped between the penis and the foreskin to circumcise a male. A cut in the foreskin usually is required

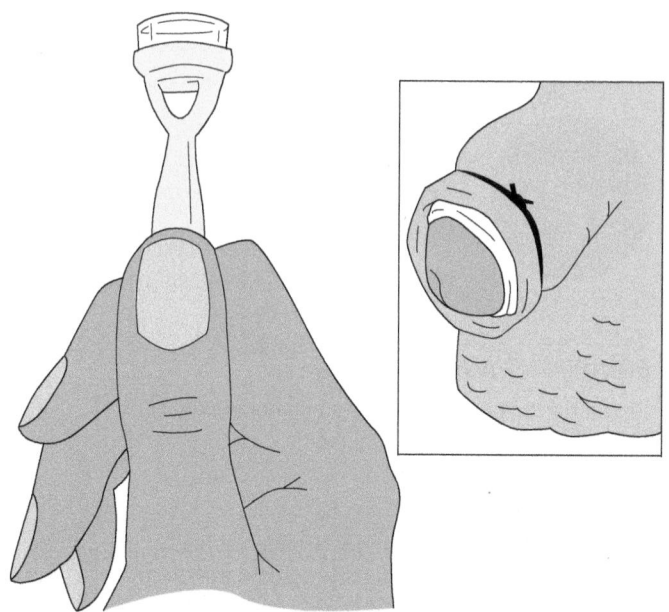

FIGURE 37-9 Circumcision using the Plastibell. The bell is fitted over the glans penis, and a suture is tied around the bell's rim. The excess prepuce (foreskin) is cut away. The device is left in place for three to four days until healing occurs. it may be allowed to fall off or is removed after eight days.

before the device can be placed. Sterile string is tied around the device and over the foreskin to cut off the blood supply. Foreskin tissue is trimmed off, and the end of the bell is removed, leaving the ring tied in place. Figure 37-9 shows a circumcision using the Plastibell device.

Testicular Examination

Testicular cancer is largely a disease of young and middle-aged men, with the average age of 33 at the time of diagnosis. Testicular cancer is not very common. The mortality or death rate from testicular cancer is very low, and it can be successfully treated with early detection from cancer screening.

Some men in the early stages of testicular cancer may experience symptoms that make them seek medical attention, such as a lump on the testicle. The testicle may also be swollen or larger than normal without a lump. Other men may not have any symptoms and are not aware something is wrong until the cancer has grown or metastasized.

Most doctors agree that screening for testicular cancer should be part of a general physical exam. In addition, a regular testicular self-exam to check for lumps or other abnormalities may be done monthly after puberty. Men with risk factors, such as an undescended testicle, previous testicular cancer, or a family member who has had this cancer, should be encouraged to perform a monthly self-exam. Procedure 37-3 and Figures A–D describe how to instruct a patient on performing a testicular self-examination.

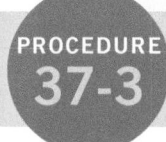

Instructing a Patient on Testicular Self-Examination

Objective ◆ *Instruct a male patient how to correctly perform a testicular self-examination.*

EQUIPMENT AND SUPPLIES

Instruction sheet; testicular examination model or illustration; patient's medical record

METHOD

1. Identify the patient and introduce yourself.
2. Explain to the patient that he should perform the examination in the shower or right after a warm shower, which causes the scrotal tissue to relax.
3. Using the testicular model or an illustration, explain that he should place his middle and index fingers underneath the scrotum and thumb on top and use a gentle motion to roll the testes between the fingers.
   a. Indicate on the model or illustration the location of the epididymis, a soft tubular cord behind the testis, which stores and carries sperm. The patient should know what the epididymis feels like so he does not confuse it with a lump (Figures A–D).
4. The entire procedure should be repeated on the second testicle.
5. Encourage the patient to immediately report to his physician any lumps or thickening found during an examination.
6. Document in the patient's medical record.

CHARTING EXAMPLE

09/11/YY 3:30 P.M. Pt. given verbal and written instruction on testicular self-examination. Pt. verbalized understanding...........
....J. Holloran, RMA

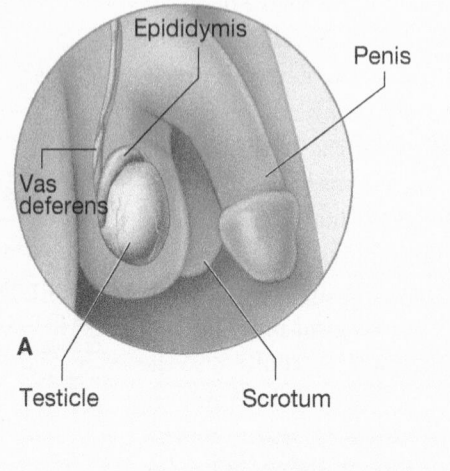
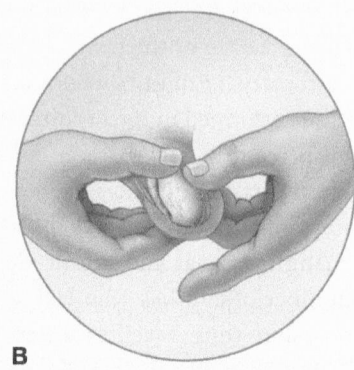
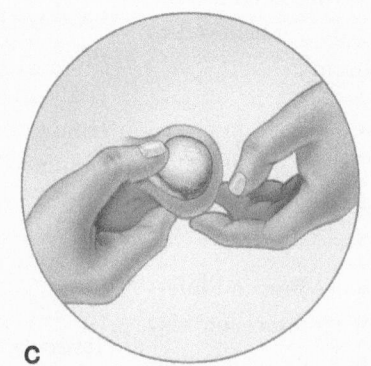
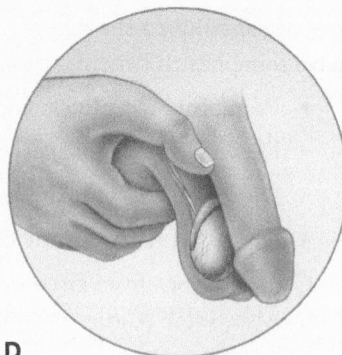

FIGURE A–D Testicular self-examination: **(A)** male reproductive system; **(B)** begin by examining the testicles; **(C)** next examine the cord behind the testicles (epididymis); **(D)** continue by gently feeling the tube that runs from the epididymis (vas deferens).

Vasectomy

Vasectomy is a widely performed surgery to render the male sterile (Figure 37-10). It involves cutting the vas deferens and tying off the ends to prevent sperm from being transported out of the testes. This is a brief procedure performed in the urologist's office with little or no discomfort to the patient. The patient can return home immediately after the procedure and resume work and regular activities the next day. After a vasectomy, the man can still achieve an orgasm and can ejaculate but without sperm in the semen.

Birth control methods should still be used for six to eight weeks after the procedure or until a post-vasectomy sample can be done to confirm the absence of sperm. In some cases, the vasectomy can be reversed, but it should be considered a permanent form of birth control.

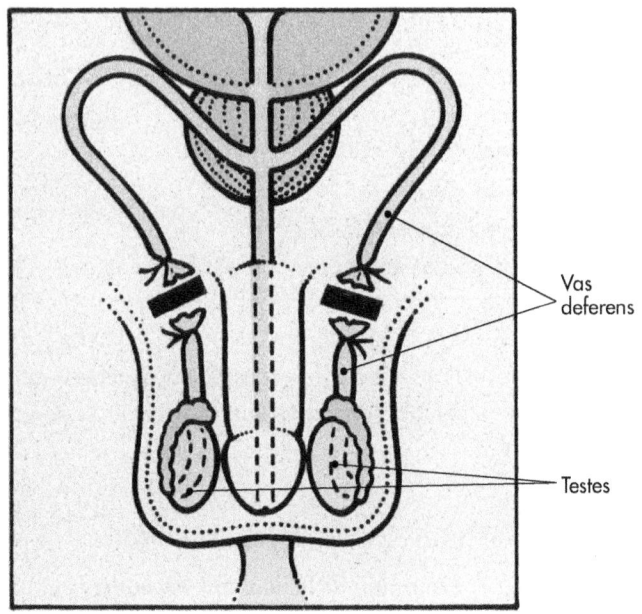

FIGURE 37-10 Illustration of a vasectomy.

SEXUALLY TRANSMITTED INFECTIONS (STIs)

Sexually transmitted infections (STIs) can occur in males and females of any age and are transmitted by sexual contact from person-to-person or mother-to-child. STIs caused by bacteria are generally treated successfully with antibiotics. Recently, antibiotic-resistant strains of organisms that cause gonorrhea and syphilis have developed, making it more difficult to treat these infections. Viral STIs, such as herpes, genital warts, hepatitis, and HIV, are incurable at this time although the symptoms can be reduced with treatment. Thus, prevention must play a key role when discussing STIs with patients.

In both males and females, most patients with an STI usually seek medical attention when they have symptoms, such as sores, discharge, itching, and pain. If the infection is left untreated, women may develop pelvic inflammatory disease (PID), which causes abdominal pain, fever, malaise, scarring in the reproductive organs, ectopic pregnancies, and infertility. See Box 37-2 for information on infertility caused by chlamydia infection and treatment of infertility with in vitro fertilization. Men may have profuse discharge from the penis, swelling and pain in the testicles, and painful urination.

Individuals infected with an STI may not have any symptoms at all, especially early in the disease. For example, most people who have HIV have no symptoms for many years before symptoms appear. Symptoms from gonorrhea may not appear in females until two months after exposure. Genital warts may not appear until five months after exposure.

Certain examinations and some laboratory procedures can identify the organism from the STI. However, no diagnostic tests are completely accurate. Patients may have the disease but test negative until later in the cycle of the disease when more bacteria or viruses can be detected, such as with HIV.

 Professionalism

Patients' rights to privacy are an important part of your professional demeanor. This is critical to remember when dealing with patients with STIs. Patients may often be reluctant to provide information, particularly at first. Professionals should avoid any office gossip and maintain the trust and confidentiality of their patients.

BOX 37-2 | Infertility and In Vitro Fertilization

In vitro fertilization (IVF) is one method of treating infertility in those who are unable, or have a diminished capacity, to conceive. There are many causes of infertility, and selecting the correct treatment depends on determining whether the cause is functional or a result of infection.

Repeated infections of sexually transmitted diseases, such as chlamydia, are often asymptomatic yet may cause scarring and occlusion (blockage) of the fallopian tube. When this happens, the ovum released during ovulation is unable to make its way to the uterus through the fallopian tube. Normally, conception occurs in the upper third of the fallopian tube, and the zygote (fertilized ovum) then moves down the tube to implant into the uterus. If the fallopian tube is blocked or scarred, as with PID, conception and implantation cannot take place. Many women are unaware that they have ever had a chlamydia infection, and, when

they decide it is time to conceive, they may discover it is impossible.

IVF is fertilization outside the body, usually occurring in a Petri dish in the laboratory. A woman who wishes to conceive may be given follicle-stimulating hormone (FSH) to stimulate the release of more than one ovum. The ova are then removed through laparoscopic surgery and put into the Petri dish. Sperm, from either the husband or a sperm donor, is added to the Petri dish. After fertilization and cleavage (cell division of the zygote) have taken place, the zygote is then placed in the woman's uterus.

Since the birth of the "first test tube baby" in 1978, thousands of babies have been born through in vitro fertilization. It is not always successful, however, and it may be necessary to repeat this procedure several times before achieving a successful result. Each attempt is very costly and may take an emotional toll on the patient.

STI Education

Treating and preventing the spread of STIs begins with proper education and identifying sexual partners who may have been exposed. Committing to a monogamous (one-partner) relationship significantly reduces the chance of being infected. However, the only foolproof means of preventing STIs is complete abstinence from sexual activity.

If individuals are going to be sexually active, there are strategies that will reduce the chance of exposure to STIs:

- Use a barrier device (condom) with spermicide during every act of sexual intercourse.
- Limit the number of sexual partners.
- Know your sexual partners and their history of sexual partners.
- Seek prompt diagnosis of any suspected STI.
- Complete all courses of medication and comply with follow-up testing.
- Cooperate in tracing sexual contacts.

Educating patients about STIs and their causes, symptoms, and treatments is very important. Often the medical assistant is the individual with whom the patient feels most comfortable discussing personal and embarrassing problems. The medical assistant should feel comfortable with the facts about STIs and their mode of transmission, and be able to discuss them in an empathetic, nonjudgmental manner. Brochures and pamphlets should be readily available and accessible in your office. Patients may feel more comfortable picking up these reading materials when they can review them in the privacy of their own home rather than asking questions in the office. It is important for the medical assistant to follow up afterward and see if the patient has any questions.

Confidentiality is extremely important when dealing with sensitive information such as testing positive for an STI. Many states require a post-treatment follow-up for certain diseases. Therefore, the medical assistant's role in patient compliance is vital.

Reporting STIs

Identifying partners of infected patients is one way to stop the spread of STIs and protect the health of unsuspecting people. In your role as a medical assistant, you should be aware of the legal requirements of reporting patients with STIs to the proper state and national agencies. For example, in all 50 states, confirmed cases of HIV/AIDS are reportable conditions by either statute or administrative act. Other STIs, such as gonorrhea and syphilis, are also reportable

diseases in most states. As a medical assistant, you need to be aware of your legal responsibilities in whichever state you are employed in.

Types of Sexually Transmitted Infections

The following are common STIs you may encounter in your patient population as a medical assistant.

Bacterial Vaginosis

Bacterial vaginosis (BV), the cause of which is unknown, is the most common vaginal infection in women of childbearing age. Certain behaviors, such as having multiple partners and douching, may increase the risk of contracting this infection. BV may occur when the normal balance of "good" and "bad" bacteria has been disrupted. Symptoms include thin gray or white discharge with an unpleasant "fishy" odor. Having BV also increases susceptibility to other STIs. Treatment is especially important for pregnant women; if left untreated, it may cause premature birth or low birth weight in the infant. Treatment includes metronidazole or clindamycin.

Chlamydia Infection

Chlamydia infection is caused by the bacterium *Chlamydia trachomatis*. It is the most frequently reported bacterial infection in the United States. In 2014, a total of 1,441,789 chlamydia infections were reported in the United States, although underreporting is an issue because many individuals are asymptomatic. Chlamydia infection in males is characterized by urethritis and epididymitis, whereas there may be no initial symptoms in females. Because of the lack of symptoms, there may be a delay in seeking treatment, which may lead to pelvic inflammatory disease (PID). Women with PID have an increased risk of ectopic pregnancies and sterility. Infants born to infected mothers may develop conjunctivitis or pneumonia.

Chlamydia infections can be successfully treated with azithromycin or doxycycline. Persons with chlamydia should abstain from sexual activity for seven days after single-dose antibiotics or until completion of a seven-day course of antibiotics to prevent spreading the infection to partners. Repeat infection with chlamydia is common. Women and men with chlamydia should be retested about three months after treatment of an initial infection regardless of whether they believe that their sex partners were successfully treated. The Centers for Disease Control and Prevention (CDC) recommends yearly testing for chlamydia for all pregnant women, sexually active women 25 years or younger, and women who are at risk from having multiple partners.

Genital Herpes

Herpes is a common contagious viral infection caused by herpes simplex virus type 1 (HSV-1) and type 2 (HSV-2). HSV-1 herpes is associated with cold sore lesions, and HSV-2 causes most cases of genital herpes. However, HSV-1 may also be transmitted to the genitals through oral/genital sex. The CDC estimates that 776,000 people in the United States get new herpes infections each year. In the United States, 15.5 percent of persons aged 14 to 49 years have HSV-2 infection. But the overall prevalence of genital herpes is likely higher because of the increasing number of genital herpes infections being caused by HSV-1.

Sores from genital herpes usually appear as one or more blisters on or around the genitals, rectum, or mouth. The blisters may break and leave painful sores that may take weeks to heal. These symptoms are sometimes referred to as "having an outbreak." The initial outbreak may also be accompanied by flu-like symptoms such as fever, body aches, or swollen glands. Repeat outbreaks of genital herpes are common, especially during the first year after infection. However, repeat outbreaks are usually shorter and less severe than the first outbreak. Although the infection can stay in the body for the rest of an individual's life, the number of outbreaks tends to decrease over a period of years.

Currently, there is no known cure for herpes, but antiviral medications may lessen the duration of symptoms. The lesions are usually self-limiting but reoccur during stressful situations. Recently, new treatments have reduced the severity of the reoccurrences or the risk of contracting genital herpes. Abstinence and careful use of condoms help to eliminate or reduce the risk of contracting genital herpes.

Genital Human Papillomavirus Infection

Human papillomavirus (HPV) infection is a common STI caused by more than 100 related strains of the virus. Most genital warts are caused by two types of HPV—types 6 and

11. They are passed from one person to another by skin-to-skin contact, usually during sex.

Genital warts, or condylomas, are found in clusters on the external sexual organs of both males and females. Internally, genital warts may be found in the female's vagina and cervix, and in the male's anus and rectum. Though the patient may not have visible signs of warts, HPV can be discovered in the female by a Pap test. It may take several months to several years after contact for the person to show signs of infection. Genital warts also increase a female's risk of developing cervical cancer.

There is no cure for genital warts, although the warts usually resolve on their own. If the patient prefers a quicker solution, the physician can remove the genital warts with various treatments, such as cryotherapy (freezing), cauterization (burning), or surgically with a laser.

Gonorrhea

Gonorrhea is an STI caused by the organism *Neisseria gonorrhoeae*, a bacterium that grows well in warm, moist conditions. It can grow in the vagina, fallopian tubes, and uterus in the female and in the urethra, mouth, and anus in the male. The eyes may be affected in both males and females. The rate of infection is high in the United States and is increasing after declining or remaining stable since 2006. It is estimated by the CDC that the rate of infection is about 120 infections per 100,000 people. It is estimated that only about half of the gonorrheal infections are reported to state departments of health, however.

In males, gonorrhea is characterized by penile discharge, clear at first and then becoming thick and milky. Men may also complain of burning, itching, and pain with urination. Females are often asymptomatic, but may develop a yellowish-green discharge. Other symptoms that may be experienced by both sexes include sore throat, swollen glands, anal discharge, and fever.

If left untreated, gonorrhea may lead to PID in women, infertility in both males and females, and, in rare situations, spread to the blood or joints (gonococcal arthritis). Untreated gonococcal infection in pregnancy has been linked to miscarriages, premature birth, and low birth weight infants. Gonorrhea can also infect an infant during childbirth as the infant passes through the birth canal. The infant can develop eye infections, which may lead to blindness. Gonorrhea can cause devastating problems in both the mother and her baby, so it is important to accurately identify the infection, treat with effective antibiotics, and closely follow up to make sure that the infection has been cured.

Tests for gonorrhea can be diagnosed by smear and Gram stain. Many people who have gonorrhea also have chlamydia and must be treated for both infections. Treatment includes large doses of penicillin or tetracycline with follow-up examinations because antibiotic-resistant strains of the bacteria may complicate treatment. Condoms, abstinence, and long-term monogamous relationships greatly reduce the risk of infection.

Human Immunodeficiency Virus

Human immunodeficiency virus (HIV) causes acquired immunodeficiency syndrome (AIDS), the final stage of HIV infection. It can take years and even decades to reach the AIDS stage. At this point, the immune system—specifically the infection-fighting white blood cells known as T-cells or CD4 cells—is destroyed, allowing opportunistic infections to attack the body and eventually cause death. According to the CDC, more than 1.2 million people in the United States are living with HIV infection, and almost one in eight (12.8 percent) are unaware of their infection.

There are many misconceptions about how HIV is transmitted. HIV cannot survive outside the body. It is not spread by any type of casual contact or day-to-day activities, such as shaking hands, kissing, or sitting on toilet seats. It cannot be transmitted by mosquitoes. HIV can be spread by having oral, vaginal, or anal sex with someone infected with HIV; sharing needles or syringes with someone infected with HIV; and being exposed as a fetus or infant to HIV before or during birth or breast-feeding. It also can be spread through blood infected with the virus, by means such as receiving a blood transfusion. However, since 1985, all donated blood supplies are tested for HIV.

Preventing HIV transmission depends on responsible sex, knowing one's sexual partners, avoiding illegal drug use, using condoms with lubricant during every instance of sexual intercourse, getting tested, and having one's partner or partners tested. A variety of HIV tests are available, including those performed in a clinic and laboratories and those available as at-home HIV tests.

Lymphogranuloma Venereum

Lymphogranuloma venereum (LGV) is an STI caused by three strains of the *Chlamydia trachomatis* bacterium. Although it is less common than other types of STIs, it is difficult to diagnose because the symptoms are similar to those of other conditions. LGV may cause papules (small, solid pimples) on the genitals, swollen lymph glands, rectal ulcers, pain, bleeding, and discharge. It can be mistaken for ulcerative STIs, such as syphilis and genital herpes. If left untreated, LGV may cause lymphatic obstruction and genital elephantiasis (massive swelling of the scrotum). Diagnosis is mainly based on clinical findings. Treatment includes use of doxycycline, erythromycin, or azithromycin.

Pelvic Inflammatory Disease

Pelvic inflammatory disease (PID) is inflammation of the vagina, cervix, uterus, and fallopian tubes. It may be caused by a number of untreated STIs, resulting in pregnancy complications and even sterility. PID may cause scar issue to develop in the fallopian tubes, which then blocks the movement of the ovum in the tubes. If the tubes are completely blocked, sperm cannot reach the ovum to cause fertilization. If partially blocked, a fertilized ovum may begin to grow in the fallopian tube rather than in the uterus, causing an **ectopic pregnancy**. An ectopic pregnancy can rupture the fallopian tube, causing severe pain or even death. PID can also result in blood clots, peritonitis, and even death if untreated.

PID is diagnosed by clinical symptoms and by an ultrasound of the abdomen. Because PID symptoms are similar to those of other abdominal conditions, such as appendicitis, diverticulitis, and ulcerative colitis, a thorough history and diagnostic tests are necessary. PID can be cured with antibiotics. However, treatment does not correct any damage already done to the reproductive organs, such as scar tissue development in the fallopian tubes.

Syphilis

Syphilis is an STI caused by the bacterium *Treponema pallidum*. The CDC reports that the rate of syphilis has increased every year since 2001. In 2014, more than 20,000 cases of syphilis were reported in the United States, a 15 percent increase from the previous year. The rise in the syphilis rate is primarily attributed to increasing numbers of men who have sex with men (often referred to as MSM). As in recent years, MSM accounted for the majority of syphilis cases in 2014. In the United States, the highest rates of syphilis in 2014 were observed in men aged 20–29 years, men in the West and in the South, and black men. However, during 2013–2014, the rate increased in both men (14.4 percent) and women (22.7 percent).

Syphilis infection can be divided into three stages: primary stage, secondary stage, and latent or late stage. The signs and symptoms of syphilis are similar to those of other diseases and, thus, syphilis is often called the "great imitator." However, the signs and symptoms of syphilis may not appear for years in an infected person. During the first (primary) stage of syphilis, a single or sometimes multiple **chancres** (sores or ulcers) occur about three to six weeks after exposure (Figure 37-11). Chancres are usually firm, round, and painless, and may go unnoticed. Chancres may occur on

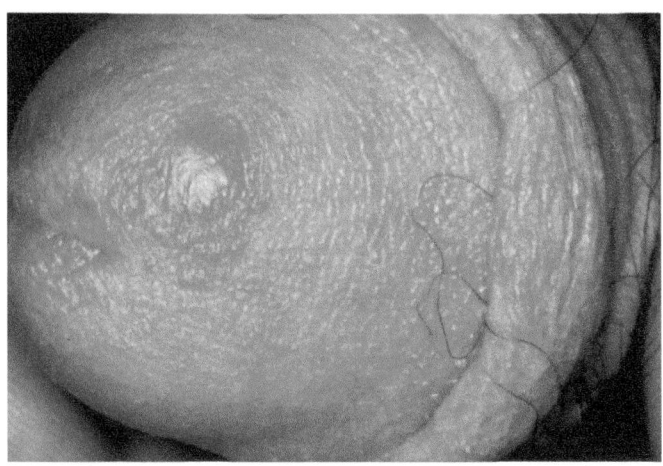

FIGURE 37-11 Syphilitic chancre.

the genitals, anus, rectum, mouth, and lips. Chancres may heal without treatment, but, without treatment, the disease will progress to the next stage even though the chancres have healed.

In the next, or secondary, stage of syphilis infection, the patient may present with a skin rash, especially on the palms of the hands and the soles of the feet; fever; swollen glands; weight loss; and fatigue. The signs and symptoms of the secondary stage may also disappear, even without treatment.

The latent, or late, stage in syphilis occurs 10 to 20 years after the first two stages have disappeared. However, if no treatment has been provided, the person will still be infected with syphilis for years without any signs or symptoms. Symptoms of late stage syphilis may include poor muscle coordination and movement, paralysis, dementia, blindness, damage to the internal organs, and death.

Syphilis may be transmitted to a newborn by an infected mother during pregnancy (congenital syphilis). An infected baby maybe born without signs or symptoms of the disease, but, if not treated immediately, the baby may be stillborn (fetal death after 20 weeks of pregnancy) or may develop serious problems within a few weeks after birth, such as cataracts, deafness, developmental delays, seizures, and death. Thus, it is recommended that all women be tested for syphilis during pregnancy.

There are several methods of testing for syphilis. One method is for the physician to scrape a small amount of cells from the chancre. The cells are examined using dark-field microscopy to visualize the bacteria. Although this is a

highly accurate test, it is not commonly performed because of its technological difficulty. The diagnosis of syphilis is more commonly made by blood tests to detect antibodies made against the bacteria (VDRL and RPR tests). If there is nervous system involvement, such as in the latent stage, the physician may confirm syphilitic infection by collecting a sample of cerebrospinal fluid (CSF) through a lumbar puncture (spinal tap).

Treatment of syphilis is fairly simple. In the primary stage, a single large dose of penicillin may cure the patient. Additional treatments with penicillin may be necessary for those who have had syphilis longer than a year. A person with syphilis is also at a higher risk of sexually contracting HIV infection. Responsible sexual behavior and proper hygiene after sexual contact reduce the chances of contracting syphilis. Some cases of penicillin-resistant syphilis have been reported.

Trichomoniasis

Trichomoniasis is a protozoal (one-celled organism) infection caused by the organism *Trichomonas vaginalis*, resulting in an infection of the lower genitourinary tract. Trichomoniasis in females causes a white or yellow foamy vaginal discharge with a foul odor. The male is usually asymptomatic except for urethral itching. Diagnosis can be made by obtaining a sample of vaginal secretions and preparing a slide with normal saline. Microscopic examination will reveal the oval-shaped *Trichomonas* parasite with four hair-like flagella whipping across the field. Treatment for both males and females is an oral course of antibiotics, such as metronidazole or tinidazole.

SUMMARY

The topics covered in this chapter include the medical specialties for the male and female reproductive systems, pregnancy and childbirth, methods of contraception, cancer screenings, and STIs. These topics are presented to ensure that medical assistants are up to date on information critical to the health of their patients. It is the responsibility of the medical assistant to be empathetic and nonjudgmental when discussing sensitive issues with patients and to be certain that HIPAA regulations regarding privacy are carefully followed.

37 CHAPTER REVIEW

COMPETENCY REVIEW

1. Define and spell the terms for this chapter.
2. Develop a brochure instructing female patients how to do a breast self-examination and male patients how to do a testicular self-examination.
3. List three specific types of histories obtained when taking a female's prenatal history.

4. According to state laws, some STIs must be reported to both state and national agencies. Identify STIs that require reporting in all 50 states.
5. Identify sterilization methods for both males and females.

PREPARING FOR THE CERTIFICATION EXAM

1. Health care workers who acquire HIV from occupational exposure are at greatest danger from
   a. unprotected personal care.
   b. contaminated blood in an open wound.
   c. accidental needlesticks.
   d. using clean gloves with each patient.
   e. not washing hands.

2. Using Naegele's rule, the due date for childbirth for a woman who had her last menstrual period on 10/4/2017 is
   a. 4/11/2018.
   b. 7/4/2018.
   c. 7/11/2018.
   d. 10/4/2018.

3. An exam tray that includes gloves, speculum, three glass slides, fixative, and sterile culture swabs with containers is ready for what type of examination?
   a. rectal
   b. pelvic
   c. gastroenterology
   d. neurological
   e. urological

4. The causative agent of syphilis is
   a. *Treponema pallidum.*
   b. *Streptococcus pyogenes.*
   c. *Staphylococcus aureus.*
   d. *Trichomonas vaginalis.*
   e. herpes simplex type 2.

5. All of the following are symptoms or complications from PID *except*
   a. peritonitis.
   b. ectopic pregnancies.
   c. infertility.
   d. blood clots.
   e. ulcerative colitis.

6. The STI that is caused by a protozoan is
   a. gonorrhea.
   b. chlamydia.
   c. candidiasis.
   d. trichomoniasis.
   e. genital warts.

7. Barrier methods of contraception include all of the following *except*
   a. morning-after pill.
   b. contraceptive sponge.
   c. condom.
   d. cervical cap.
   e. diaphragm.

8. All of the following are prenatal screening tests *except*
   a. amniocentesis.
   b. digital record exam.
   c. glucose tolerance test.
   d. ABO/Rh blood test.
   e. ultrasound.

9. Vasectomy involves the severing and tying off of the
   a. fallopian tubes.
   b. scrotum.
   c. urethra.
   d. vas deferens.
   e. epididymis.

10. All of the following are risk factors for breast cancer *except*
    a. aging.
    b. family history of breast cancer.
    c. fatty breast tissue.
    d. early menarche.
    e. smoking.

914 UNIT 4 Clinical Medical Assisting

CRITICAL THINKING

Refer to the case study at the beginning of the chapter and use what you have learned to answer the following questions.

1. Determine Mrs. Lufti's EDD based on her LMP.

2. How would Mrs. Lufti's past obstetrical history be recorded in the prenatal record?

3. What should Mrs. Lufti expect to have completed during her first prenatal visit with Dr. McWalters?

ON THE JOB

A young male patient has an appointment but refuses to speak to you, the medical assistant, about his problem. He indicates that it is a "very personal matter." After asking some questions, you surmise that he has symptoms of an STI. What should you do? How should you respond to him?

INTERNET ACTIVITY

Look up online the newest statistics related to HIV/AIDS worldwide. Find the website in your state dealing with reportable STIs.

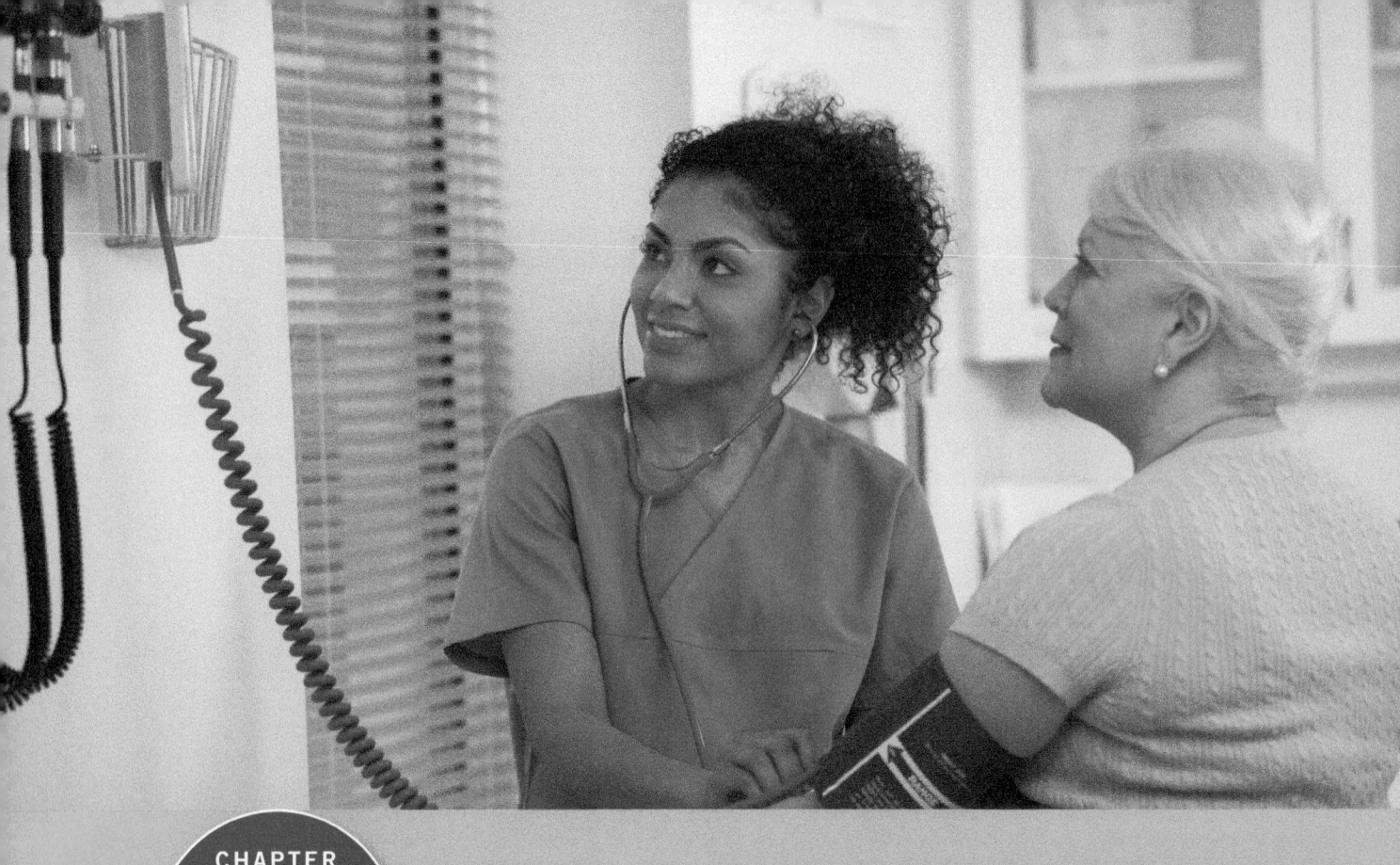

CHAPTER 38

Assisting with Care of the Eye, Ear, Nose, and Throat

Learning Objectives

After completing this chapter, you should be able to:

38.1 Define and spell the terms for this chapter.

38.2 Describe tests used to assess visual acuity.

38.3 Outline steps taken when performing eye irrigation.

38.4 Explain the technique for instilling eye medication.

38.5 Identify adaptations that can be made to assist a patient with visual impairment during a medical office visit.

38.6 Describe procedures that a medical assistant may perform related to ear care.

38.7 Explain how an audiometer is used for hearing assessment.

38.8 Identify adaptations that can be made to assist a patient with hearing impairment during a medical office visit.

Kyle Schultz is a 9-year-old boy whose parents are concerned that he is having trouble seeing the blackboard in school. Kyle is shy and will not ask the teacher to change his seat. Kyle's parents have both worn glasses since their teens. Samra Belkovich is working with Dr. Miller. Dr. Miller asks Samra to perform a Snellen eye exam. The results are 20/80 in the right eye and 20/60 in the left eye. After Dr. Miller reviews the results, he orders a further eye exam that requires instillation of eyedrops in both eyes to dilate the pupils. Kyle does not want to have this procedure done.

Terms to Learn

acuity	irrigate	otorhinolaryngologist (ENT)
astigmatism	Ishihara test	otoscope
audiogram	lavage	presbycusis
audiometer	myopia	presbyopia
cerumen	myringa	pure tone audiometry
conduction hearing loss	ophthalmologist	sensorineural hearing loss
cornea	ophthalmology	Snellen chart
decibel	ophthalmoscope	speculum
electronystagmograph (ENG)	optician	strabismus
frequencies	optometrist	tympanometry
hearing acuity	organ of Corti	tympanum
hyperopia	otology	visual acuity
instill		

Special examinations and procedures related to specific body systems are commonly performed in the medical office. In this chapter, we consider examinations and procedures related to the eye, ear, nose, and throat. Although some information in this chapter was presented in the "Special Senses" chapter, it is important to review as it pertains to the discussion of eye and ear care. The role of the medical assistant is to assist the physician during special examinations and procedures and to instruct the patient before, during, and after procedures. You will learn the procedures to perform visual and auditory **acuity** (sharpness) testing; to **instill**, or put in, eye and ear medications; and to **irrigate** or rinse both eyes and ears. Keep in mind that you are representing the physician and that you play an important role in setting a positive tone and atmosphere in the office. All patients should be treated with respect during all phases of the procedures.

Special instruments are used for examinations of these body systems. The **otoscope** is used to examine the **tympanum**, or **myringa** (medical terms for the eardrum), for signs of infection and inflammation. The **ophthalmoscope** is used to view inner parts of the eye. The physician positions the ophthalmoscope so light penetrates the pupil of the patient's eye and then screens for retinal damage and vascular problems. The care and maintenance of the otoscope and the ophthalmoscope are routine tasks performed by the medical assistant. These instruments use batteries that must be recharged on a regular basis. The tiny bulbs used in both instruments must be replaced occasionally.

Most physicians use disposable ear and nasal specula to examine the tympanic membrane and nose. A **speculum** (*specula,* pl.) is any instrument that holds open a body cavity to permit inspection. Monitoring supplies for the examining room, including disposable specula, is a routine task performed by the medical assistant.

STUDY AND CARE OF THE EYE

The eye is the organ of sight. The branch of medical science that deals with the structure, function, and diseases of the eye is **ophthalmology**. An **ophthalmologist** is a medical doctor who can perform eye examinations and eye surgery and prescribe medications, eyeglasses, and contact lenses. An **optometrist** is a doctor of optometry, not a medical doctor, who can perform eye examinations, prescribe medications, and write prescriptions for eyeglasses and contact lenses. An **optician** is a technician who specializes in grinding lenses and preparing eyeglasses and contact lenses. (See the chapter titled "Special Senses" to review the structure and function of the eye.)

Eye Examination

A number of complex tests are used to diagnose and treat vision problems, many of which are done in the office of specialists, such as ophthalmologists. In primary care and pediatric offices, routine screening examinations for vision problems are performed as part of physical examinations.

Before every eye examination, the overall appearance of the eye is evaluated for symptoms such as redness, puslike discharge, and excessive tearing. In addition, the physician evaluates the status of the patient's pupils and ability to focus on objects at different distances. PERRLA is an acronym that stands for "Pupils Equal, Round, Reactive to Light and Accommodation." Normally the pupils of the eyes are the same size and change or accommodate when a beam of light is focused on the eye and is then removed. Injuries to the brain may result in the patient having pupils of unequal size.

Visual Acuity and Refractive Errors

Normal **visual acuity**, or clarity of vision, is referred to as 20/20 vision, which means the eye should see an object 20 feet away clearly. Errors of refraction occur when the eyeball is either too long or too short, the lens loses its elasticity, or the lens or cornea has an irregular curvature. The **cornea** is the clear, transparent covering of the eye. Refractive errors include myopia, hyperopia, presbyopia, astigmatism, and strabismus.

Myopia, or nearsightedness, means that the eye sees near objects well but distant objects appear blurry. This occurs either because the eyeball is too long or because the lens is too thick and light rays do not reach the retina at the back of the eye but, instead, focus in front of the retina. The shape of the eyeball and lens is hereditary. The myopic eye requires a concave lens to correct vision. **Hyperopia**, or farsightedness, means that the eyes see distant objects well, but near objects are blurry. In this case, the eyeball is too short or the lens too thin. Light rays focus behind, rather than on, the retina. The hyperopic eye requires a convex lens to correct the visual

defect. **Presbyopia** is the term associated with farsightedness that occurs with aging. The lens loses its elasticity, and glasses are needed for reading. **Astigmatism** is a refractive disorder in which irregularities in the curvature of the cornea cause light not to focus on the retina but to spread out over an area, causing overall blurring of vision. Images may be clear in the center of the field and blurry at the outer edges of the visual field. Figure 38-1 shows how lenses correct visual problems.

Strabismus is an eye disorder caused by weakness in the external eye muscles, often resulting in the eyes looking in different directions. Normally, the eyes focus on a subject in coordination; otherwise double vision occurs. Children with strabismus may appear "cross-eyed" or "wall-eyed" and may need to wear a patch over the "good" eye to strengthen the weaker eye. You may need to teach the patient basic eye exercises as part of the treatment plan. It is important that treatment begin at an early age to prevent permanent damage to the eye. If the patch and exercise plan are ineffective, surgery on the eye muscle may be necessary.

Assessing Visual Acuity

As noted previously, visual acuity testing is frequently performed in a variety of medical settings. Performing these tests is usually the task of the medical assistant. These may include acuity testing, near vision acuity testing, and testing for color blindness.

Distance Vision Acuity

Distance acuity is measured using the **Snellen chart**. Snellen charts place the largest symbols on the top line, and each line after is of decreasing size. A person with normal vision would be able to read the top line at 200 feet. To the right of each line is a ratio indicating what a person with normal vision could read at decreasing distances of 100, 70, 50, 40, 30, and 20 feet. A result of 20/20 vision means that a person with normal distance acuity could read that line at a distance of 20 feet.

The abbreviation for the right eye is OD (oculus dexter); for the left eye it is OS (oculus sinister). The abbreviation for both eyes is OU (oculus uterque). These abbreviations are often used; however, the Institute for Safe Medication Practices (ISMP) recommends that the complete words for right and left eye must be used to avoid error or misinterpretation.

Because the purpose of the test is to measure vision, not literacy, for preschool children and patients who are illiterate or have a language barrier, the Snellen E, the Landolt C, or pictorial charts are used. Figure 38-2 shows different types of Snellen eye charts.

If you are unsure if the patient has the ability to recognize the Snellen eye chart letters, you should verify it by using a

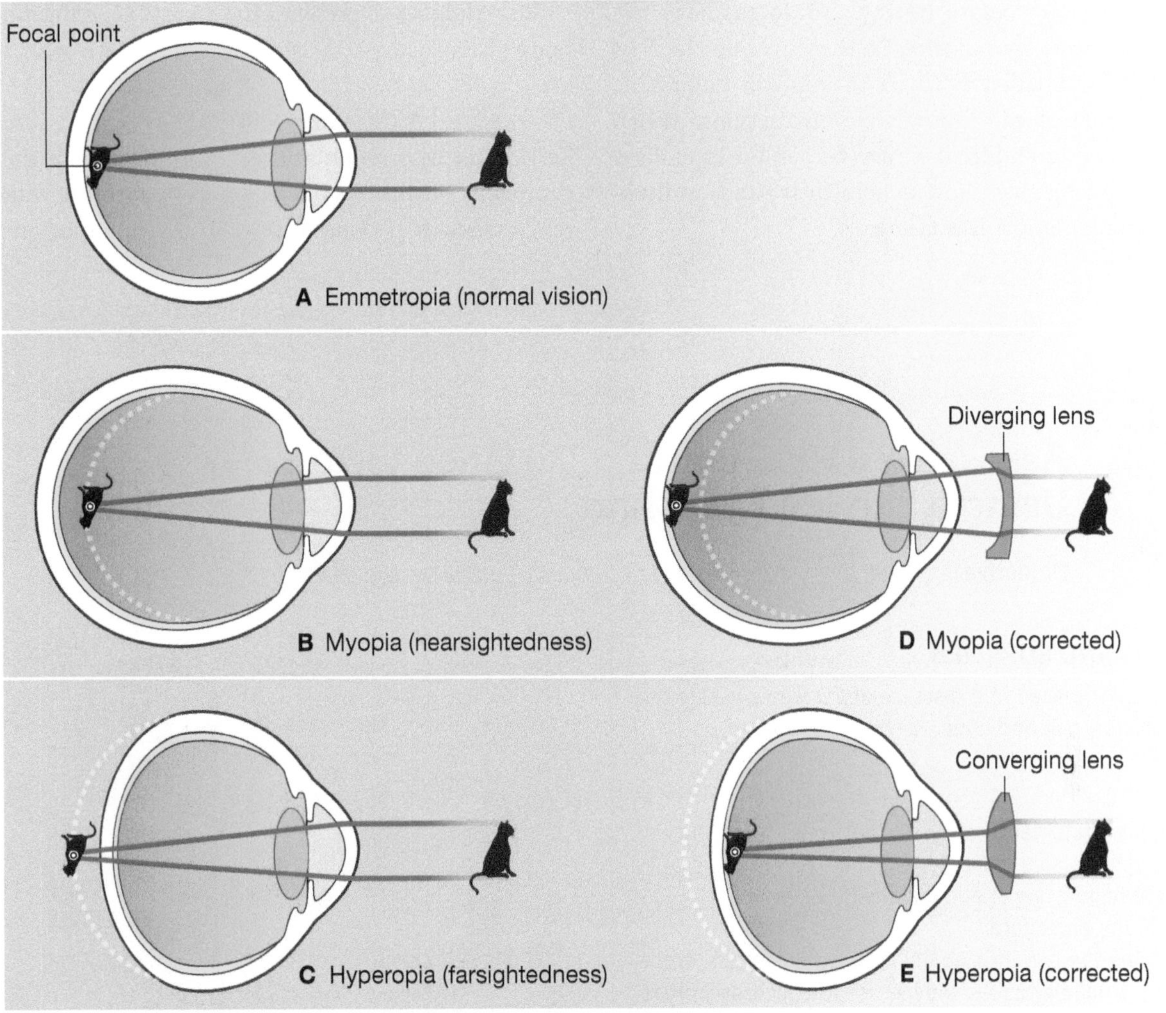

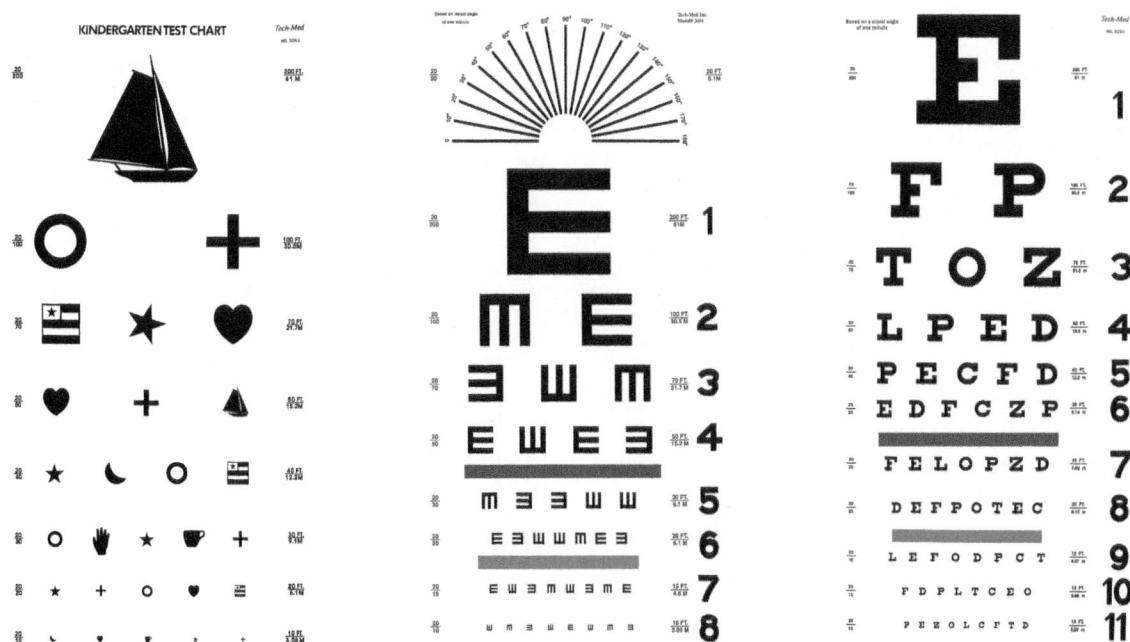

FIGURE 38-1 How lenses correct visual problems: **(A)** emmetropia; **(B)** myopia; **(C)** hyperopia; **(D)** corrected myopia; **(E)** corrected hyperopia.

FIGURE 38-2 Different types of Snellen eye charts.

demonstration chart before testing. To do so, have the patient demonstrate by pointing in the direction the E is pointing on the Snellen E Chart so you can determine whether the patient can follow your instructions. When dealing with young children, it may be helpful to make a game of it, showing them how to hold their hands to illustrate which direction the E is facing.

Procedure 38-1 presents the steps for performing a distance vision acuity test using the Snellen eye chart.

Near Vision Acuity

Testing for near vision acuity should be done if the patient complains of difficulty reading or performing other close-range tasks. It is done to test for hyperopia or presbyopia.

PROCEDURE 38-1 — Assessing and Recording Distance Vision Acuity Using a Snellen Eye Chart

Objective ◆ *Screen a patient for distance acuity using a Snellen eye chart.*

EQUIPMENT AND SUPPLIES

Snellen eye chart placed at a distance of 20 feet; eye shield or occluder; pointer; pen and paper; alcohol and gauze

METHOD

1. Assemble equipment.
2. Review physician's order.
3. Perform hand hygiene and identify the patient.
4. Explain the procedure.
5. Determine the patient's ability to recognize letters. If the patient is unable to read letters, use the necessary chart to accommodate the patient's abilities.
6. Place the patient 20 feet from the chart, either seated or standing, as long as the Snellen eye chart is at eye level (Figure A).
7. Follow office policy regarding testing with or without corrective lenses.
8. Following office policies regarding which eye to test first, have the patient cover the other eye with a cup or occluder. The occluder should be held in such a way so as not to interfere with the normal position of a patient's glasses.
9. Instruct the patient to keep both eyes open even though one eye is covered. Have the patient read the lines with both eyes first at a distance of 20 feet.
10. Use a pointer and point to letters or appropriate symbols in random order.
11. Starting with the 20/70 line, ask the patient to identify each line and proceed down the chart to the last line the patient can read without error. Observe for signs of squinting or tilting of the head, which indicate difficulty identifying letters.
12. Record the ratio numbers adjacent to the line the patient can read without error. If there is an error, note it (e.g., "Right eye 20/40—1"; or "Right eye 20/40—1 with correction," meaning glasses were worn during testing). ISMP

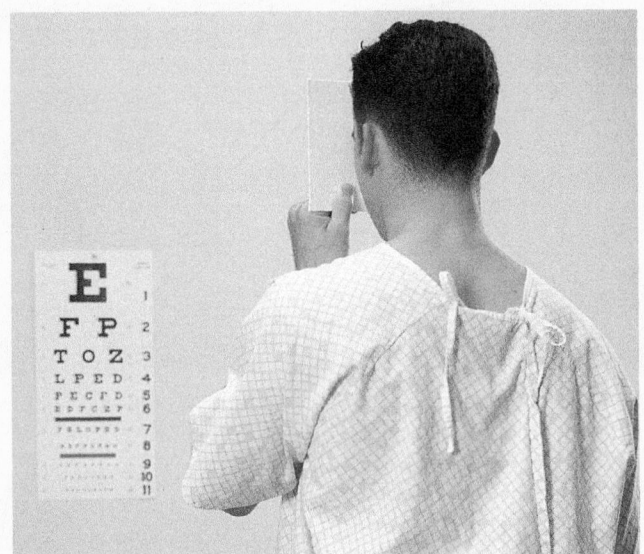

FIGURE A Test of distance vision using the Snellen eye chart.

recommends using words instead of abbreviations for eye designations to avoid misinterpretation. In many cases, the patient is allowed to make no more than two errors per line when acuity is being assessed. However, it is important to follow office policy in such instances.

13. Repeat the procedure with the other eye and record the result, noting any unusual symptoms such as squinting or blinking excessively.
14. Clean the occluder with gauze and alcohol.
15. Remove gloves and perform hand hygiene.
16. Document the results accurately.

CHARTING EXAMPLE

2/14/YY 4:00 P.M. Snellen eye test. Rt eye 20/30. Lt eye 20/30. Both eyes 20/30..........................M. King, CMA (AAMA)

The lens of the eye loses its elasticity with age and cannot change from viewing distant objects to close work as readily as before. Close work appears blurry, and the individual tends to hold the book or newspaper farther away to make it appear clearer.

Testing for near vision acuity is done by using the Jaeger card. The patient reads a card held at normal reading distance (14 to 16 inches). The card has a series of paragraphs decreasing in size of print with a number above each. The number one (J1) is above the paragraph with the smallest text, and as the text becomes larger the number increases. Paragraph J2 represents 20/20 vision. The patient's result is the number above the last paragraph that can be read easily. This test should always be performed in a well-lit room. Office policies differ on whether to have patients wear corrective lenses during the test and whether to test each eye individually or both eyes together. As a medical assistant, you will follow the policy of your facility. Procedure 38-2 presents the steps to perform a near vision acuity test.

Color Vision Impairment

Color vision impairment is the inability to distinctly differentiate colors of the spectrum. Defects in color vision are either congenital (patient was born with the defect), inherited, or acquired through disease or injury. Congenital color blindness is more prevalent in males. It is important to test for color vision defects because changes in color vision may indicate diseases of the retina, optic nerve, or thyroid.

The ability to distinguish colors depends on the cones of the retina, which react to light and permit us to see shades of red, green, and blue. The inability to see any colors is rare and is most likely caused by a defect or absence of the cones in the retina. The most common type of color vision defect, which is inherited, is the inability to distinguish red and green. Other types of color blindness prevent patients from distinguishing shades of various colors.

The **Ishihara test** is printed in either card or booklet form with a single color-dot illustration containing a number or curved lines and shapes. For instance, a person with normal color vision would be able to see the green number 27 on

---

PROCEDURE 38-2

Assessing and Recording Near Vision Acuity Using a Jaeger Card

Objective ◆ *Screen near vision acuity using the Jaeger system.*

EQUIPMENT AND SUPPLIES
Jaeger near vision acuity chart; paper and pen

METHOD
1. Perform hand hygiene.
2. Review physician's order.
3. Assemble equipment.
4. Identify the patient and introduce yourself.
5. Explain the procedure.
6. In a well-lit room, have the patient hold the Jaeger card at a distance of 14 to 16 inches.
7. Ask the patient to read aloud, with both eyes open, the smallest paragraph or line possible without error (Figure A).
8. Document the results accurately, noting any unusual symptoms, such as squinting.

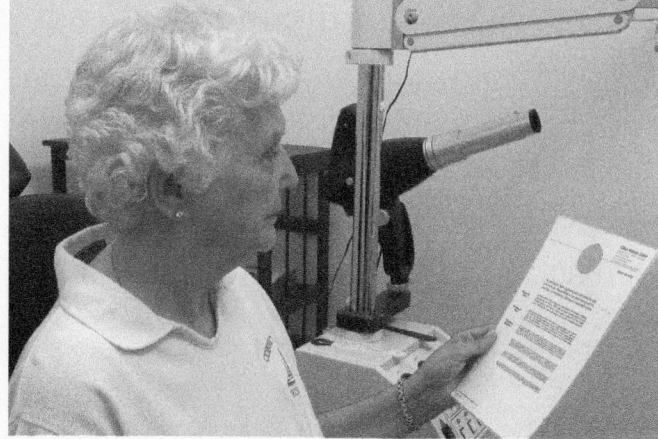

FIGURE A A patient using a near vision acuity card.

CHARTING EXAMPLE
09/11/YY Pt performed near vision acuity screening reading without error—J2...L. Mckay, RMA

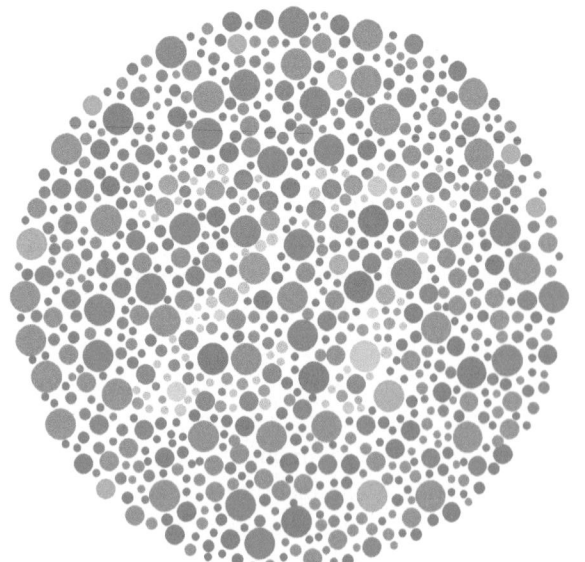

FIGURE 38-3 One page of color vision chart.

the red-orange background in Figure 38-3. The patient is shown 14 color plates or pages and must correctly identify 10 of them to be considered to have color vision within normal limits. The Ishihara booklet or cards should be stored out of direct light to prevent fading of the color plates. Procedure 38-3 presents the steps to perform a screening for color vision acuity using the Ishihara test.

Contrast Sensitivity

Contrast sensitivity measures the patient's ability to distinguish faint differences in shades of gray. Several new testing procedures and instruments are used to test for contrast sensitivity, such as the Vistech Consultant system and the Pelli-Robson chart. To perform a procedure for contrast sensitivity, adhere to the manufacturer's directions and observe the usual procedural steps for appropriate patient care, such as hand hygiene and correct documentation. It has been determined that contrast sensitivity is affected by most major eye conditions, such as macular degeneration, cataracts, glaucoma, and diabetic retinopathy. Figure 38-4 shows a Pelli-Robson chart for testing contrast sensitivity.

Intraocular Pressure and Visual Field Tests

Intraocular pressure is measured through tonometry in millimeters of mercury (mm Hg). Normal eye pressure has historically been considered to be less than 21 mm Hg, but this normal upper limit may vary in different populations. Ocular hypertension is a risk factor for glaucoma. The test is sometimes performed by numbing the surface of the eye with drops. A fine strip of paper stained with orange dye is held to the side of the eye. The dye stains the front of the eye to help with the exam. The patient sits in front of the slit-lamp and rests his chin on a platform. The tonometer is then

---

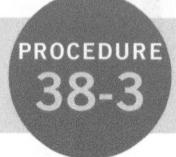

PROCEDURE 38-3

Assessing and Recording Color Vision Acuity Using the Ishihara Test

Objective ◆ *Screen a patient for color vision defects.*

EQUIPMENT AND SUPPLIES

Ishihara screening book/cards; paper and pen

METHOD

1. Perform hand hygiene.
2. Review the physician's order.
3. Assemble equipment.
4. Identify the patient and introduce yourself.
5. Explain the procedure.
6. Have the patient assume a comfortable position, and ask the patient to keep both eyes open.
7. In a well-lit room, have the patient identify, at a distance of 30 inches, the number that is formed by the colored dots on each card or page within three seconds per page or card.

8. If the patient is unable to identify the numbers, have the patient trace the number with a finger.
9. Score each plate as it is read. (Figure 38-3 is an example of one color plate.) If the patient is able to identify the number, then record the number seen after the plate number (e.g., Plate 1:7). If the patient is unable to identify a number on a plate, record the plate number and mark an X next to it.
10. Note any unusual symptoms.
11. Document the results accurately.

CHARTING EXAMPLE

2/14/YY 3:00 P.M. Ishihara eye chart normal..............M. King, CMA (AAMA)

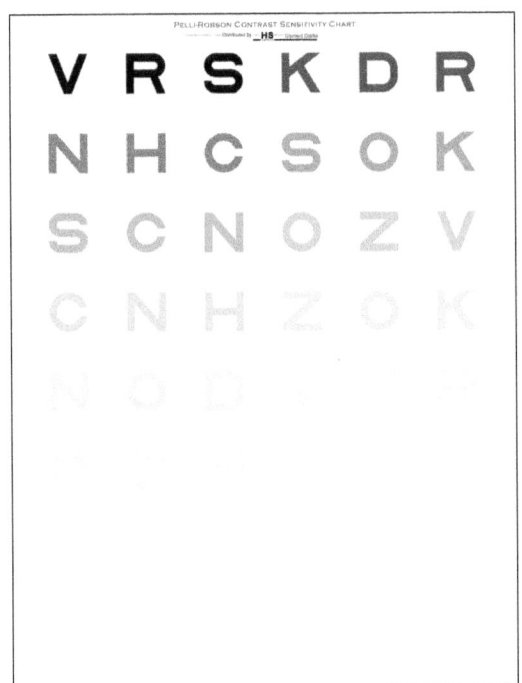

FIGURE 38-4 Pelli-Robson contrast sensitivity chart.

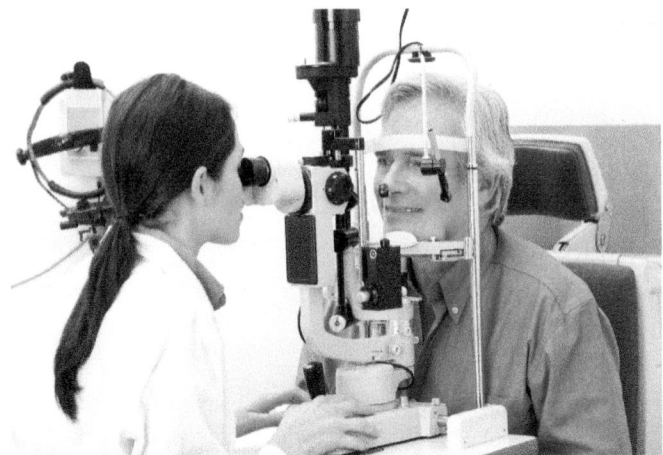

FIGURE 38-5 Patient having glaucoma test.

moved so the tip is just touching the cornea. Blue light is used so the orange will glow green. The health care provider looks through the eyepiece and adjusts a dial to read the pressure. An alternative method is to have the patient stare into the examining device. The provider shines a light into the patient's eye to line up the instrument and delivers a puff of air toward the eye. The machine then measures the eye pressure by looking at how the light reflections change as the air hits the eye.

Visual field tests, known as perimetry tests, measure the central and peripheral vision of the patient to determine if the patient might have glaucoma, retinal disease, possible optic nerve disease, or ptosis. All perimeter tests measure sensitivity to stimuli at multiple locations in the visual field, though multiple variables define the perimeter. Currently, standard automated perimetry or white-on-white perimetry is the most common form of visual field testing. Here, a white stimulus is projected on a white background to determine the threshold values. Trained perimetrists can either use kinetic (dynamic) or static testing. Either a stimulus is moved from an unseen area into view or is kept static. The test is done one-on-one with the health care provider facing the patient. In the kinetic test, the provider moves a finger in four quadrants and asks the patient to state when the finger is visualized. The tests can also be done by automated equipment, which provides more reproducible, sensitive, and quantitative results and can be done by a trained medical assistant in most cases. To do the test, the patient looks inside a dome-shaped instrument called a perimeter. While the patient stares at the center of the perimeter, the instrument flashes lights. The patient should press a button whenever a flashing light is seen. The equipment records the spot of each flash and whether the button was depressed when the light flash occurred. At the end of the test, a printout documents any vision deficits of peripheral vision, which can be an early sign of glaucoma. Figure 38-5 shows a patient being tested for glaucoma.

Irrigation of the Eye

Irrigation or **lavage** (rinsing) of the eye is necessary to remove foreign substances or chemicals. Eye irrigation requires the use of sterile technique and equipment. As with any procedure you perform as a medical assistant, you must first explain the procedure to the patient and answer any questions. Never try to remove a foreign object from the eye using an applicator stick because this may cause corneal abrasions. Procedure 38-4 presents steps for irrigating the eye.

Instillation of Eye Medications

Instilling (putting in) eye medications may be one of your duties. Only ophthalmic or optic medications can be used in the eye, and they must be sterile. It is important that you reinforce the need to maintain the sterility of sterile medications with your patients. Encourage them to discard eye medications when the prescribed treatment time has been completed. In addition, instruct them that eye medications should never be shared with others or even used in the other eye if treatment is needed. The danger of contamination is great. Procedure 38-5 provides the steps for performing instillation of eye medication.

Eye Safety Guidelines

Patients should be made aware of some general safety guidelines to protect their sight. Regular physical examinations

Irrigating the Eye

Objective ◆ *Cleanse or irrigate the eye.*

EQUIPMENT AND SUPPLIES

Nonsterile gloves; sterile basin; kidney-shaped emesis basin; sterile solution; sterile irrigating syringe; sterile gauze; towel; tissues; pen and patient's chart

METHOD

1. Identify the patient and explain the procedure.
2. Review the physician's order.
3. Assemble the equipment. Check the label of the irrigating solution three times to ensure it is the correct solution and concentration ordered by the physician. Check the expiration date on the label to make sure the solution has not expired. The solution should be brought to room temperature by wrapping the bottle in a dry heating pad or standing the bottle in a warm water bath.
4. Perform hand hygiene and apply gloves.
5. Ask which position the patient would prefer, sitting or lying down.
6. Place a towel over the patient's shoulder. If both eyes are to be irrigated, then two separate sets of equipment must be used to prevent cross-infection.
7. Pour irrigating solution into the sterile basin, and withdraw the solution directly from the basin, using the syringe.
8. Ask the patient to tilt the head to the affected side, if seated, and hold the kidney-shaped emesis basin against the cheek below the eye to catch run-off fluid.
9. Open the patient's eye using the index finger and thumb of the nondominant hand.
10. Hold a tissue on the patient's cheekbone below the lower lid and pull down and expose the conjunctiva.
11. Hold the syringe ½ inch from the eye (Figure A).

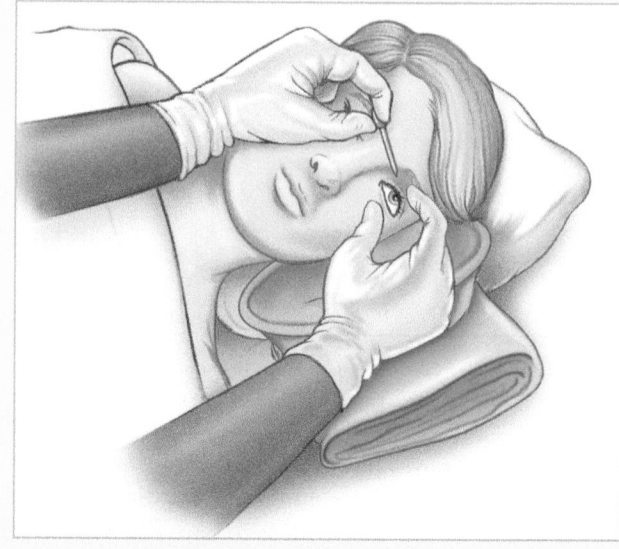

FIGURE A Irrigation of the eye.

12. Gently irrigate from inner to outer canthus (corner of eye), aiming at the lower conjunctiva.
13. Continue irrigating until the solution is used up.
14. Dry the area around the eye with sterile gauze.
15. Dispose of the equipment properly.
16. Perform hand hygiene.
17. Document information in the patient's chart in the appropriate manner.

CHARTING EXAMPLE

09/13/YY 10:00 A.M. Rt eye irrigated with 50 mL of 100°F normal saline. Eye sl. Red Pt. says "eye feels fine."
....E. Zandri, CMA (AAMA)

on a yearly basis may discover conditions or diseases, such as diabetes or hypertension, that impact their vision. An eye examination every one to two years is important to monitor changing conditions in the patient's vision. Encourage patients to wear sunglasses to protect eyes from ultraviolet rays, which can damage the cornea. For minor eye problems, tell patients to avoid rubbing and apply cold compresses. Advise patients to wear protective eyewear when using tools or machinery that can cause flying objects. Make patients

aware that when chemicals splash in the eye, they should flood the eye with water for 20 minutes and seek immediate medical attention. Remind patients of the importance of maintaining the sterility of optic medications.

Changes in the Aging Eye

The eye ages just like the rest of the body. Because these changes may impair vision, care must be taken to instruct older adults on safety issues. Decreasing depth perception

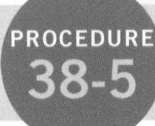

PROCEDURE 38-5 | Instilling Eye Medication

Objective ◆ *Instill eye medication following the physician's orders.*

EQUIPMENT AND SUPPLIES
Sterile medication; sterile eyedropper (if needed); tissues; sterile gauze squares; nonsterile gloves; drape or towel

METHOD

1. Perform hand hygiene.
2. Check the physician's orders.
3. Identify the patient, introduce yourself, and explain the procedure.
4. Check the name of the medication, expiration date, and concentration three times.
5. Ask if the patient has any known allergies to the medication.
6. Give the patient a tissue to blot cheeks.
7. Put on gloves.
8. Position the patient with head tilted back and looking up.
9. Pull down the lower eyelid, exposing the conjunctiva (Figure A).
10. Place the dropper about ½ inch above the eyeball with the dominant hand. Insert the proper number of drops to the center of the conjunctiva, or if ointment is used, apply as a thin strip from inner to outer canthus.
11. Do not touch the dropper or ointment tube to the eye.
12. Ask the patient to gently close the eye and rotate the eyeball.
13. Using sterile gauze, dry the excess medication from the inner canthus to the outer canthus.

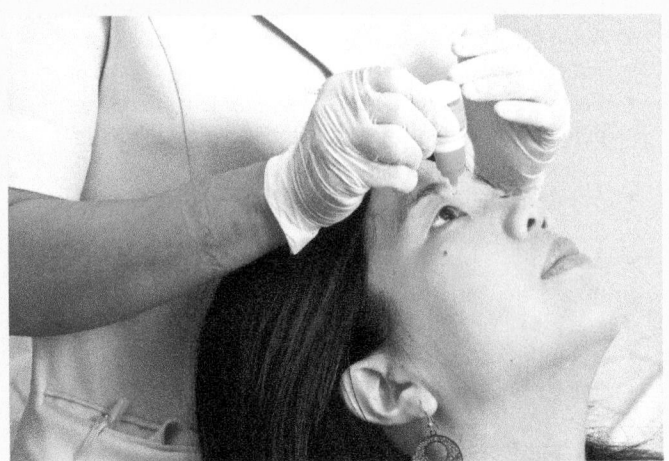

FIGURE A Instilling eye medication.

14. Explain to the patient that vision may be blurry.
15. Clean the area and dispose of unused medication.
16. Remove gloves and perform hand hygiene.
17. Document the procedure appropriately.

CHARTING EXAMPLE
09/12/YY 9:00 A.M. Instilled 2 gtt of 1 percent atropine sulfate to both eyes. Pt. complained of "stinging and blurry vision for a few minutes."..L.McKay, RMA

---

and difficulty seeing at night make them more vulnerable to falling. "Professionalism: The Life Span" lists some changes that occur in the structure and function of the eye with age.

Assisting the Visually Impaired Patient

Blindness occurs from accident, birth defect, injury, or disease. Some people are totally blind and have been blind since birth. Their frame of reference to the world depends on descriptions from others. Some individuals can sense light and dark but may not be able to discern anything else. Others have some vision but cannot read. To be declared legally blind, a person must only be able to see at 20 feet what a normal person would see at 200 feet. Those who have lost their sense of sight need special training and education. Special equipment may be needed to help the visually impaired person to function more adequately. Additionally, service

Professionalism | The Life Span

Changes in Structure and Function of the Eye with Age
- Eyelids droop because of decrease in amount of fatty tissue in the lids.
- Tears decrease both in quantity and quality.
- Cornea develops a ring of fat around it.
- Whites of eyes may develop brown spots.
- Conjunctiva becomes thinner and drier.
- Irises become smaller, and less light enters eye.
- Retinal changes may make vision fuzzy.
- Night vision may be impaired.
- Eyes become more sensitive to glare.
- Depth vision is diminished.
- Floaters or wavy lines or spots may appear in visual field.
- Lenses lose elasticity and impair ability to focus.

Professionalism   The Workplace

Assisting the Visually Impaired Patient to Prepare for a Physical Examination
- Call the patient by name and identify yourself.
- Face the patient and speak clearly.
- Ask if the patient needs assistance and offer your arm to the patient.
- Guide the patient to the examining room.
- Explain specifically what you would like the patient to do.
- Again offer your assistance to help the patient disrobe, put on a gown, sit on the examination table, and so on.
- Describe what will be happening, how long the procedure will take, and what level of discomfort the patient is likely to experience.
- Ask if the patient would like you to remain in the room until the physician arrives.
- After the examination is complete, offer your assistance to help the patient get off the examination table, dress, and speak with the physician.
- Ask if the patient has any questions or concerns.
- Relay any concerns to the physician.
- Offer your arm to escort the patient from the examination room.
- Locate the patient's coat and belongings.
- Ask if the patient would like you to arrange for transportation.
- Speak to the patient with respect and empathy.

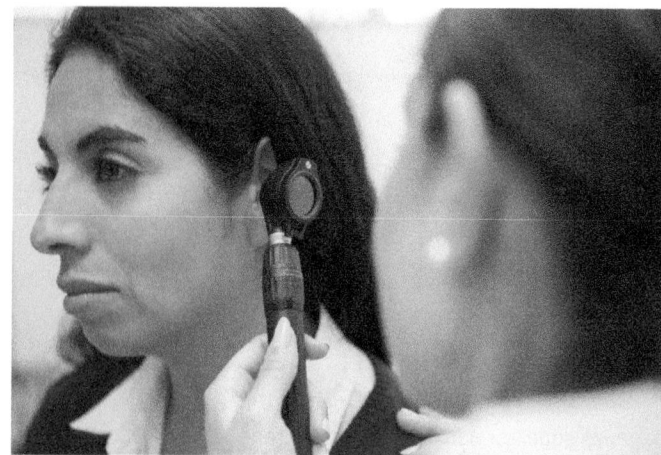

FIGURE 38-6 Examination of the ear using an otoscope.

lighted instrument with a small, disposable speculum that is inserted into the ear canal to examine the tympanic membrane. Figure 38-6 shows a physician performing an ear examination using an otoscope. A healthy eardrum should be pearly gray and concave. An infected eardrum appears reddened, swollen, and bulging. See Box 38-1 for an explanation of ear infections in children.

Irrigation of the Ear

Irrigation of the ear is necessary to remove impacted **cerumen** (earwax) or a foreign matter from the ear. Figure 38-7 shows irrigation of the ear. Patients may be apprehensive about the discomfort of the procedure, and it is your responsibility to put them at ease as much as possible. Procedure 38-6 outlines steps for irrigating the patient's ear.

Instillation of Ear Medications

Instilling ear medication is also commonly performed by medical assistants. You may also be required to instruct a

animals can help those who are visually impaired. Blindness is a devastating impairment, both physically and psychologically. As a medical assistant, you should keep a list of local resources for people with disabilities to best serve those with impairments.

STUDY AND CARE OF THE EAR

The study of hearing is known as **otology**. Physicians who specialize in the ear are otologists or **otorhinolaryngologists (ENT)** (ear, nose, and throat) doctors. Every physical examination includes an examination of the nose, throat, and ears. In patients, infections that affect the throat or nose may also affect the ear.

The ear is the organ of hearing and balance. Most parts of the ear are internal and are protected by the temporal bone of the skull. For a review of the structures and function of the ear, see the chapter titled "Special Senses."

Ear Examination

The instruments used in the office for ear examinations are the otoscope, tuning fork, and audiometer. The otoscope is a

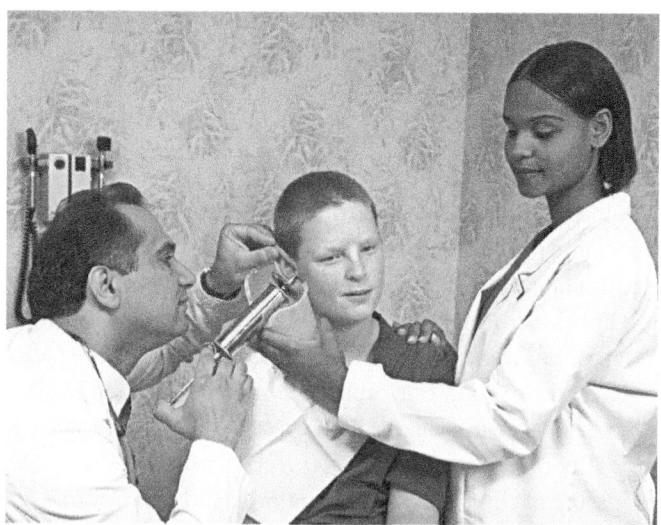

FIGURE 38-7 Ear irrigation.

BOX 38-1 | Otitis Media in Children

Otitis media—middle ear infection or inflammation—is the most frequent ear problem in the pediatric patient, particularly those under 6 years of age. The several types of otitis media are acute otitis, recurring otitis, otitis media with effusion (fluid buildup in middle ear), and chronic otitis media.

Because young children lack the ability to explain how they feel, it is important to know the symptoms of earaches in children. In an upper respiratory infection, whether viral or bacterial, organisms may spread from the mucous membranes of the nose and throat through the eustachian tube, or auditory tube, which connects the nasopharynx and the middle ear. Allergies may also cause fluid buildup in the middle ear. When excess fluid or pus builds up in the middle ear, sound waves cannot be transmitted as easily and pressure on the tympanic membrane is increased. The eardrum will become reddened and inflamed and bulging or convex. It may even rupture. In addition, ear pain can be intense. Signs that an infant or small child has an ear infection are pulling on an ear, redness of the external ear, drainage from an ear, fever, crying, crankiness, and unsteadiness.

Treatment in the case of infection is usually antibiotics; if allergy related, an antihistamine is prescribed. An analgesic to reduce fever and discomfort may also be necessary. Children who have frequent ear infections, regardless of the cause, run the risk of hearing impairment from scarring of the eardrum. Scar tissue renders the tympanic membrane less flexible to incoming sound waves. In addition, chronic ear infections can lead to ossification of the tiny ear bones: The bones become fused together and cannot transmit sound waves effectively, leading to a form of conductive hearing loss.

Surgical treatments for children with reoccurring ear infection are a myringotomy, or cutting of the eardrum to release pressure, and insertion of a small plastic tube to permit drainage of the middle ear. After several months to a year, the tubes will fall out unassisted. When tubes are placed in the ear, it is important to keep water from entering the ear canal. For this reason, earplugs should be used while shampooing and swimming.

PROCEDURE 38-6 Irrigating the Ear

Objective ◆ *Irrigate ear following the physician's orders.*

EQUIPMENT AND SUPPLIES

Gloves; ear syringe; sterile basin; kidney-shaped emesis basin; warm irrigation solution per physician's order; towels; cotton balls, patient's medical record

METHOD

1. Check the physician's orders.
2. Perform hand hygiene.
3. Assemble the equipment.
4. Check the name, concentration, and expiration date of the irrigating solution three times.
5. Identify the patient, and explain the procedure.
6. Apply gloves.
7. Have the patient sit with the affected ear tilted slightly downward.
8. Place a towel over the patient's shoulder, and ask the patient to hold the kidney-shaped emesis basin against the neck below the ear to catch run-off fluid.
9. Clean the external ear with a moistened cotton ball.
10. Pour the warmed solution into a sterile basin and fill the syringe with 50 mL of solution.
11. For adults, pull the earlobe up and back to straighten the ear canal; for children under 3 years, pull the earlobe down and back to straighten the ear canal.
12. Expel air from the syringe and insert the tip into the ear canal; aim the stream of flow toward the roof of the canal (Figure A).
13. Repeat until the return from the ear is clear.
14. Remove the basin, dry the outer ear, and remove the towel.
15. Give the patient cotton balls to wipe any external drainage.
16. Instruct the patient about home care if needed. Ask if the patient has any questions.
17. Dispose of any waste material properly.
18. Perform hand hygiene.
19. Document the procedure in the patient's medical record, noting the type of drainage and any patient symptoms such as pain or dizziness.

CHARTING EXAMPLE

2/14/YY 11:00 A.M. Ear irrigation to both ears. Cerumen plug removed from right ear. No pain or dizziness experienced. Patient remained lying on right side for 15 minutes......M. King, CMA (AAMA)

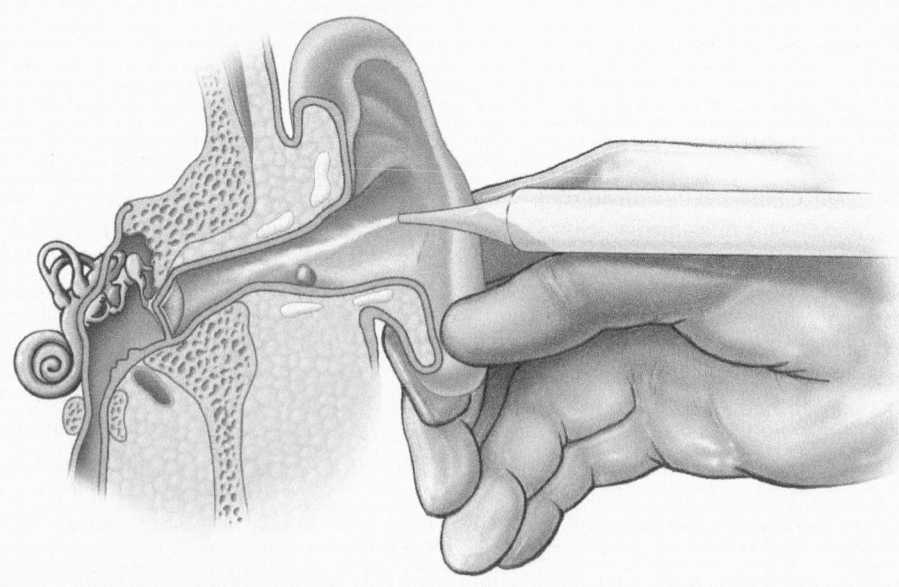

FIGURE A Irrigating the ear to remove a foreign body.

patient how to administer eardrops. You may instruct the patient to use the same steps that you would use performing instillation of medications in the office. Provide the patient with a printed list of instructions, and review the guidelines in the office. Ask the patient to demonstrate the steps before leaving the office to ensure that the patient understands the procedure. Procedure 38-7 provides the steps for performing instillation of eardrops.

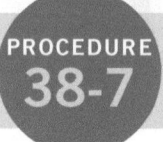

PROCEDURE 38-7 Instilling Ear Medication

Objective ◆ *Instill ear medication as ordered by physician.*

EQUIPMENT AND SUPPLIES

Otic drops in dropper bottle; cotton balls; nonsterile gloves; patient's medical record

METHOD

1. Check the physician's orders.
2. Assemble the equipment.
3. Identify the patient, and explain the procedure.
4. Check the medication label three times for the correct name, expiration date, and concentration.
5. If the medication is cold, warm it by rolling the bottle between the palms.
6. Perform hand hygiene and don gloves.
7. Have the patient tilt the head away from the affected ear or lie down with the affected ear facing up.
8. Pull the earlobe up and back for an adult (Figure A), or down and back for a child (Figure B).
9. Place the dropper in the ear canal without touching the sides of the canal (Figure C).
10. Instill the appropriate number of eardrops along the side of the canal.
11. Instruct the patient to remain in the same position for three to five minutes.
12. Give instructions for home care if needed. Ask if the patient has any questions.
13. Dispose of the equipment and clean the area.
14. Remove gloves and perform hand hygiene.
15. Document the procedure appropriately in the patient's medical record.

CHARTING EXAMPLE

09/11/YY 7:00 P.M. 2 drops Neosporin solution instilled in Rt ear. Pt verbally confirmed instruction for home instillation 2× days for 7 days..C. Lynch, RMA

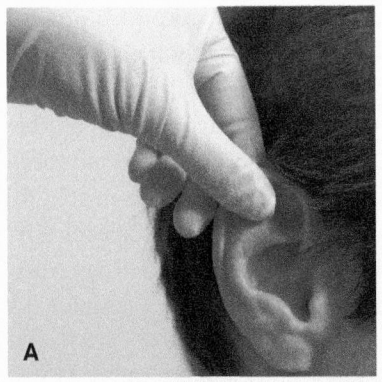 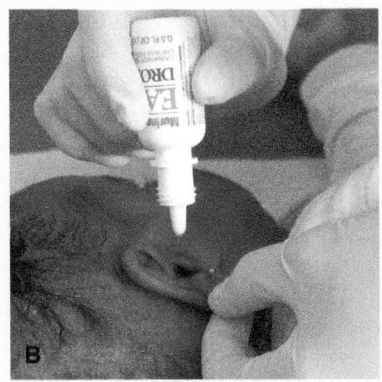 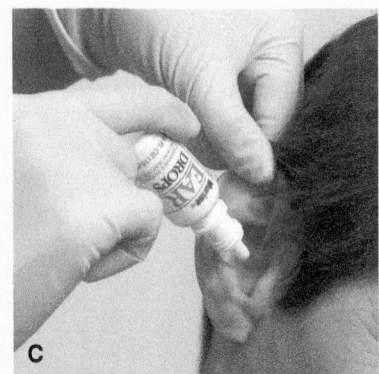

FIGURE A–C (A) Straightening the ear canal of an adult by pulling the ear up and back; **(B)** straightening the ear canal of an infant by pulling the ear down and back; **(C)** instilling eardrops.

Hearing Acuity

Hearing is essential in the process of learning to talk because speech is based on imitation of sounds and mimicking the way words are used to communicate. As with vision, there are many degrees of hearing loss. Various forms of hearing impairments fall into one of two main categories: sensorineural hearing loss and conduction hearing loss.

Sensorineural hearing loss—nerve damage—results from damage to the organ of Corti or damage to the auditory nerve. The **organ of Corti**, located in the cochlea (part of the inner ear), contains hairlike fibers that convert the waves of sound that travel through the ear to electrical impulses that are then sent to the brain via the auditory nerve. When the sound waves reach the inner ear but are unable to be converted into electrical impulses, damage to the organ of Corti is present. If the waves are converted to impulses but are not transmitted to the brain, the damage is to the auditory nerve. Nerve deafness can be hereditary or may be caused by loud noises or viral infections.

Conduction hearing loss is caused by obstruction of sound waves; thus, the sound waves never reach the organ of Corti. Foreign material or excess cerumen in the external ear canal, calcification of the bones in the middle ear, infection or fluid buildup in the middle ear, or a combination of these problems may cause conduction hearing loss.

A number of tests are used to evaluate **hearing acuity** (sharpness of hearing). The abbreviations AD (auris dextra) for right ear, AS (auris sinistra) for left ear, and AU (aurus uterque) for both ears are used when charting results involving ears. However, it is recommended that whole words for right and left ear be used to avoid error or misinterpretation. Tests for speech and word recognition can distinguish whether there is actual hearing loss or problems with the Wernicke center of the brain that produces speech and the Broca center that understands speech. A whisper test, in which the provider whispers quietly behind the patient, is an easy way to determine need for more in-depth testing of hearing acuity.

Hearing Assessment

A tuning fork is a metal, forked-shaped instrument that produces vibrations when struck (Figure 38-8). The vibrating instrument is then held near the patient's ear or placed on various locations on the head to give a rough hearing assessment.

An **audiometer** (Figure 38-9) is an electronic instrument that measures more precisely the **frequencies** or the number of fluctuations per second of energy in the form of sound waves. The intensity of the sound or **decibel** that patients hear is evaluated as well. When the patient indicates the ability to hear a sound, a recording is made. The **audiogram**, which is a record of patient responses, is then used by the physician to evaluate the patient's hearing. A person with normal hearing should hear all frequencies up to 15 decibels under normal conditions. **Pure tone audiometry** is performed

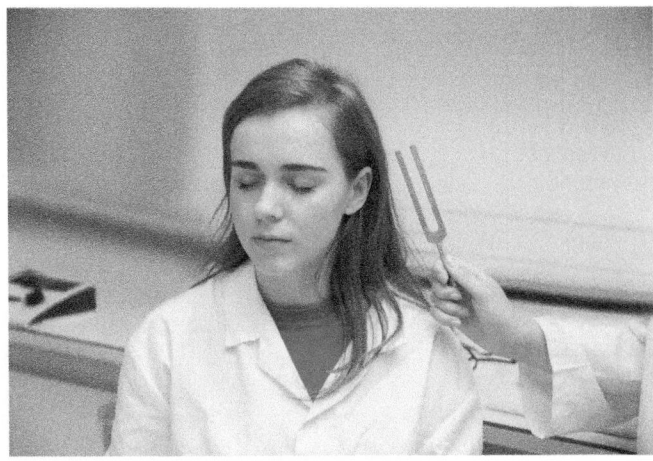

FIGURE 38-8 Testing hearing acuity using a tuning fork.
(*Source:* wavebreakmedia)

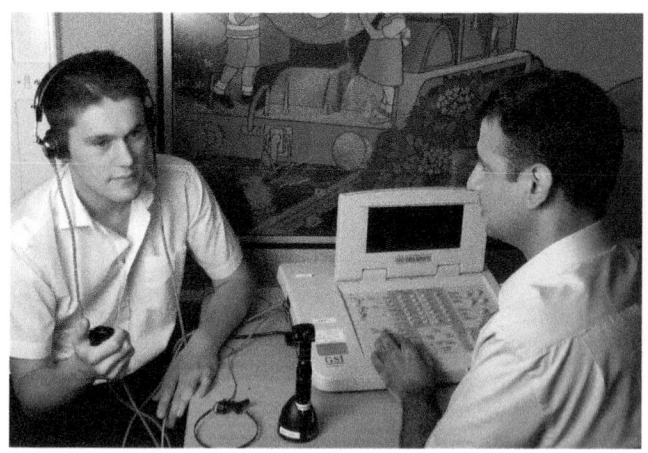
FIGURE 38-9 Audiometer.

in a soundproof room with the patient usually wearing headphones, and indicating when tones are heard by raising a hand on the side where the tone is heard. Prolonged exposure to loud noise over 85 decibels can cause temporary or permanent hearing loss. Figure 38-10 illustrates the decibel levels in various locations and associated with various conditions.

Many varieties of audiometers are in use today. Although most audiometers function in a similar way, it is important to follow the instructions provided by the manufacturer. Sales representatives often give in-service demonstrations to staff when an instrument is purchased. A procedure document should be drawn up based on the manufacturer's specifications for audiometer use and should be included in the office policies and procedures manual.

See Box 38-2 for information about allied health professionals who are ophthalmic assistants or audiologists.

As a medical assistant, you may be asked to perform an audiometer test and may do so if you have undergone the proper training. The physician will interpret the results and inform the patient of the outcome. You are not permitted to release results to a patient unless you have been specifically instructed to do so by the physician. Procedure 38-8 describes the steps for performing an audiometric test on a patient.

Additional Diagnostic Tests Related to the Ear

Tympanometry, a diagnostic test, is used to measure the ability of the myringa to move, thereby estimating the pressure in the middle ear. If the middle ear is filled with fluid, the tympanic membrane will be more rigid. A probe-type device is inserted in the ear canal, creating only mild discomfort at most, and the device measures the eardrum's response to loud tones. For accurate results, it is vital that the patient not move, talk, or swallow during the test, which lasts about two minutes. A printout of the results is produced for the physician to evaluate.

The **electronystagmograph (ENG)** is a special examination that evaluates balance through measurement of the movement of the eyes. ENG is used to evaluate patients with vertigo (a false sense of spinning or motion that can cause dizziness) and other disorders that affect hearing and vision. Electrodes are placed above and below the eye to record electrical activity. By measuring electrical changes in the

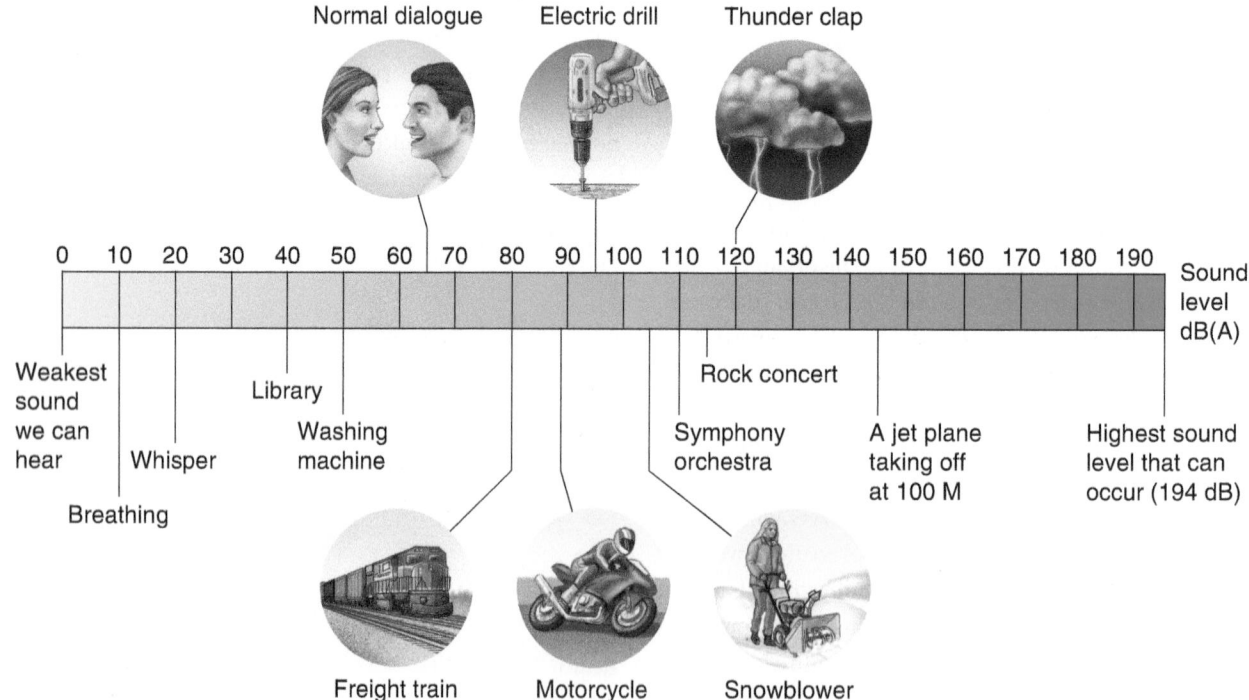

FIGURE 38-10 This illustration shows the decibel level in various locations and associated with different conditions.

BOX 38-2 | Other Professionals in Health Care

Your occupation as a medical assistant will often bring you into contact with other allied health professionals. To improve communication with other health care workers, it is important that you understand the duties and training of other members of the allied health team. Ophthalmic assistants work under the supervision of an ophthalmologist and work in offices or clinics. Although some ophthalmologists hire medical assistants and train them on the job to perform the functions necessary in their office, others only hire an ophthalmic assistant (OA). There are specific programs of training for the OA, as there are for the medical assistant. The OA must have a high school diploma or equivalency and attend a clinical program approved by a review committee of ophthalmic medical personnel. An OA's duties include conducting acuity testing, tonometry, adjusting glasses, assisting during surgical procedures, and administering some eye medications. In addition, the OA may be trained in the use and care of more highly technical instruments. OA students who pass a national certification examination earn the title of certified ophthalmic assistant (COA). For information on this field, contact the Joint Commission on Allied Health Personnel in Ophthalmology, 2025 Woodlane Drive, St. Paul, MN 55125-2995, (800) 232-3937.

Another health professional you may encounter is the audiologist. An audiologist is an allied health professional who performs diagnostic hearing tests, assesses patient's hearing, fits hearing aids, teaches proper use of the hearing aid, and rehabilitates clients with hearing loss.

PROCEDURE 38-8 | Assisting with Audiometry

Objective ◆ *Perform audiometric test without error.*

EQUIPMENT AND SUPPLIES

Audiometer with headphones; quiet room or small, enclosed cubicle; patient's record; pen

METHOD

1. Check the physician's orders.
2. Perform hand hygiene.
3. Prepare the equipment.
4. Test the equipment and make sure the power is on.
5. Identify the patient, and explain the procedure.
6. Establish a signal response that the patient will give if no automatic button is available; nodding head and holding up a finger are acceptable signals (Figure A).
7. Have the patient assume a comfortable position.
8. Place headphones over the patient's ears.
9. Begin with low frequency and watch the patient for indication that the sound is heard; push the button to record if the machine does not do it automatically.
10. Gradually increase the frequency until the test is completed in the first ear.
11. Proceed to the other ear and repeat the entire procedure.
12. Remove the headphones.
13. Clean the equipment following the manufacturer's instructions.

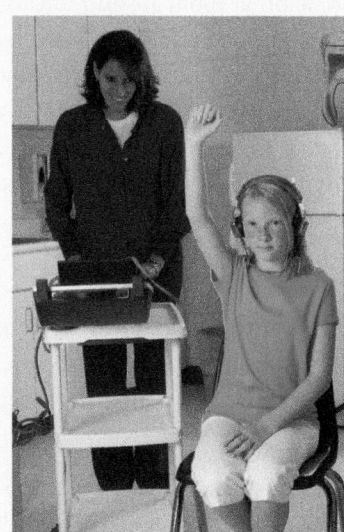

FIGURE A Performing a hearing test on a child.

14. Perform hand hygiene.
15. Document the procedure appropriately.

CHARTING EXAMPLE

2/14/YY 9:00 A.M. Audiometry test administered in both ears. Results given to Dr. Williams.................M. King, CMA (AAMA)

electrical field in the eye, an ENG can detect nystagmus (involuntary rapid eye movement) in response to stimuli.

There are several different types of ENG examinations. In the water caloric test, warm or cool water is placed into the ear canal so that it touches the tympanic membrane. Air can also be used in this procedure instead of water for patients who have a damaged eardrum. A normal response to the stimuli means no nystagmus. If nystagmus does not occur on stimulation, a problem may exist within the ear, nerves associated with the ear, or certain parts of the brain.

Assisting the Hearing-Impaired Patient

It is important to provide for the comfort level of the hearing-impaired patient as much as possible in your office setting. Accommodations such as having available telephones with hearing amplifiers demonstrate that your care is patient-centered. It is important not to lose patience with the patient who is having difficulty hearing your instructions. Remember to face the patient when speaking, not to speak with shadows or hands over your face, and to speak clearly without raising your voice.

Presbycusis is a decline in hearing acuity and a normal part of aging. Older adult patients may be reluctant to admit that they are having hearing problems, but the family will frequently volunteer the information. Signs like speaking louder, turning up the radio or television, and not hearing what is said from another room are all indications that hearing loss has occurred. As a medical assistant, you must handle these situations with delicacy. Your responsibility is to act in the patient's best interest and speak to the physician about your concerns. Other signs of aging are narrowing of the ear canal, dryness of earwax, lessened flexibility of the eardrum, and sclerosis of the ear bones.

Ear Safety Guidelines

Remind patients never to put anything in the ear canal. Earwax is a protective substance produced by the body to prevent foreign objects and substances from getting to the

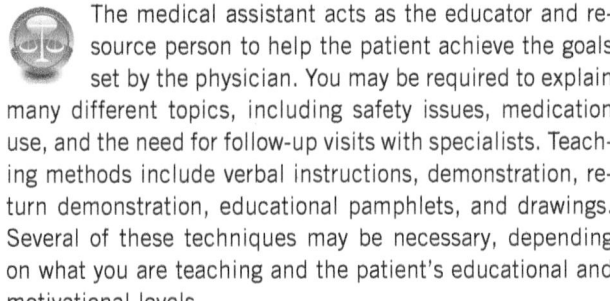

Professionalism   The Law

The medical assistant acts as the educator and resource person to help the patient achieve the goals set by the physician. You may be required to explain many different topics, including safety issues, medication use, and the need for follow-up visits with specialists. Teaching methods include verbal instructions, demonstration, return demonstration, educational pamphlets, and drawings. Several of these techniques may be necessary, depending on what you are teaching and the patient's educational and motivational levels.

For example, the correct use of optic or otic medication ordered by the physician is very important. The patient must be made to understand that the label must be read carefully. You must explain that otic medications are for the ear, and optic medications are for the eye. It is important to stress this point because the words are easy to confuse. The sterility of these medications is critical. Furthermore, you need to reinforce with the patient or family members the fact that these medications should be discarded properly once the course of treatment is concluded. The danger of cross-contamination is great. Patients should be made aware of signs and symptoms related to the eye and ear. They may not connect the symptoms appearing in eyes or ears as being related to other systemic conditions. Always perform only those functions within your scope of practice.

eardrum. Attempting to remove earwax is a dangerous habit and could cause perforation of the tympanic membrane.

Patients must understand the connection between repetitive exposure to loud noise and deafness. Young people who listen to loud music on earphones or at concerts are particularly susceptible to this danger. Workers who must engage in duties that require them to be exposed to loud noise should wear protective ear gear.

Patients who are hearing impaired and cannot use devices such as hearing aids may need other strategies to help increase

Professionalism   Cultural Considerations

Though many hearing-impaired patients are able to read lips, some patients bring along interpreters to assist with the appointment. When working with a patient via an interpreter, you should always direct your questions toward the patient. Consider learning a few common sign language signs, such as alphabetic letters and the sign for "Thank you."

Professionalism

The safety of patients is your responsibility when they are under your care. Patients with diminished visual or hearing capacities need extra care to avoid accidents and injuries. Always ask hearing or visually impaired patients if they need assistance. Offer your arm to ensure their safety, and never allow them to leave immediately after a procedure requiring anesthesia.

their awareness of their surroundings at home. Devices such as doorbells that light up when rung, telephone amplifiers, and close-captioned television are accommodations that help the hearing impaired. Specially trained service animals can also aid patients with hearing impairment.

EXAMINATION AND TREATMENT OF THE NOSE AND THROAT

Examination of the nose and throat is part of a physical examination and is considered routine in most offices. The physician will use a nasal speculum to inspect the mucous lining of the nose for signs of irritation and infection. The physician will use a tongue depressor to examine the throat for signs of infection, enlarged tonsils, and abnormalities of the tongue or oral cavity. If signs of infection are present in the throat, a throat culture may be ordered to determine the infecting agent. An appropriate antibiotic will then be ordered for the patient. The most common cause of throat infection is the *Streptococcus* bacteria, group A. When untreated, this organism can cause secondary infections and possibly serious damage to the kidney, heart, and other organs. Signs and symptoms of nasal problems include nosebleeds or epistaxis, reduced sense of smell, congestion, and allergic rhinitis (inflammation of the lining of the nose). See Procedure 38-9 for steps to assist with instilling nasal medication.

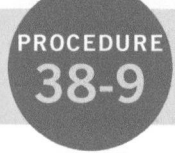

PROCEDURE 38-9

Instilling Nasal Medications

Objective ◆ *Instill nasal medication as ordered by the physician.*

EQUIPMENT AND SUPPLIES

Physician's order; patient's record; nasal medication; sterile medicine dropper; tissues; gloves

METHOD

1. Check physician's orders
2. Perform hand hygiene.
3. Assemble the equipment.
4. Identify the patient and explain the procedure.
5. Position the patient with head lower than the shoulders to instill medication into the ethmoid and sphenoid sinuses.

To instill medication into the maxillary and frontal sinuses, have the patient assume the same back-lying position with the head turned toward the side to be treated (Figures A and B). Place patient in a supine position with a pillow under the neck to lower the head below the shoulders. Make the patient as comfortable as possible.

6. Check the medication three times for correct name, dosage, and expiration date. Draw the medication into a dropper, and hold it over the center of the affected nostril, taking care not to touch the dropper to the inside of the nostril.

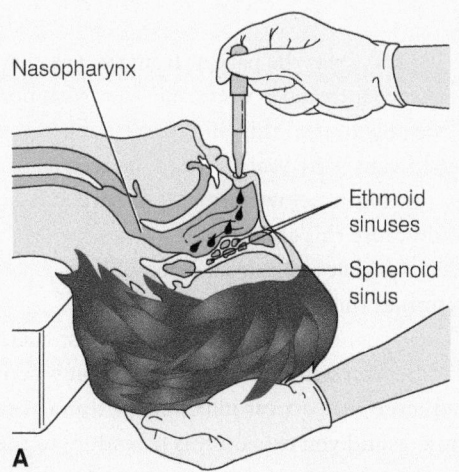
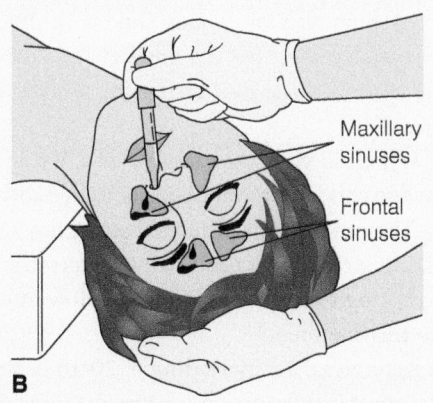

FIGURE A–B (A) Instilling nosedrops into the ethmoid and sphenoid sinuses; **(B)** instilling nosedrops into the maxillary and frontal sinuses.

7. Administer the medication. Repeat in the other nostril if ordered.
8. Tell the patient to stay in that position for five minutes to prevent medication from running out of the nostril.
9. Provide tissues for the patient to wipe excess from the skin.
10. Discard the dropper in the biohazard waste container, recap the medication, and return it to the storage place.
11. Clean the area and remove gloves.
12. Provide home instruction if needed. Verify patient understanding.
13. Perform hand hygiene.
14. Document the procedure in the patient's record.

CHARTING EXAMPLE

09/13/YY 9:00 A.M. Afrin nasal drops 3 gtt per nostril instilled per Dr. Schwartz...N. Lynch, RMA

SUMMARY

In this chapter, we considered signs and symptoms of disorders of the eye, ear, nose, and throat. As a multiskilled health care professional, you will be expected to assist with or perform a number of technical functions while you aid the physician. The procedures in this chapter deal with irrigating the eye and ear and instilling medications in the eye, ear, and nose. You may need to swab the nose or take a throat culture. You will be expected to be able to accomplish these tasks independently and without error. In addition, you will be asked to assess both visual and hearing acuity using the procedures provided in this chapter. Dealing with special needs patients, such as children, older adults, patients with dementia, or those who are illiterate, requires extra skills. Knowing the changes in vision, hearing, and smelling that occur with age enables you to be more sensitive to these patients. Educating the patient to perform certain technical skills, such as administering eye and ear medications at home, is an important factor in treatment. As a patient advocate, you can encourage eye and ear safety suggestions. To care for the patient holistically, the medical assistant must become aware of local resources for people with sensory impairments. At all times, it is your responsibility to provide the most respectful and empathetic care for the patient.

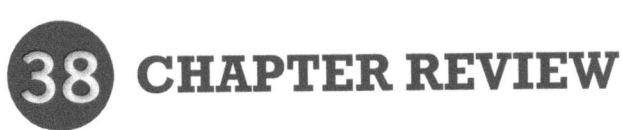

38 CHAPTER REVIEW

COMPETENCY REVIEW

1. Define and spell the terms for this chapter.
2. Develop a teaching plan for a young child with strabismus.
3. What are several precautions the medical assistant should take in the office to assist the hearing-impaired older adult patient?
4. During a well-child visit, the caregiver of a 5-year-old explains that the child often complains of itchy ears because of earwax. The caregiver then states that she has found relief by itching the child's ear canal with cotton swabs while attempting to remove the ear wax. How might you respond to this comment?
5. A patient has a visual acuity reading of 20/10 in the left eye. Using this information, answer the following questions:

   a. How far was the patient from the eye chart?
   b. At what distance would a person with normal acuity be able to read this line?
6. Mrs. Evans is 81 years old and has a contrast sensitivity test result below normal. List several conditions that could cause this abnormal result.
7. Identify what a physician is looking for when he or she examines the throat.
8. The mother of a 2-year-old boy has just been informed that her son will require a myringotomy because he has had more than six ear infections within the past year. How would you explain this procedure to the mother?

PREPARING FOR THE CERTIFICATION EXAM

1. On the Snellen eye chart, the symbol on the top line can be read by people with normal vision at a distance of
   a. 100 feet.
   b. 200 feet.
   c. 150 feet.
   d. 20 feet.
   e. 50 feet.

2. An illuminated instrument used to examine the ear is an
   a. ophthalmoscope.
   b. anoscope.
   c. otoscope.
   d. cystoscope.
   e. sigmoidoscope.

3. To measure intraocular pressure, the instrument used is the
   a. eye spud.
   b. ophthalmoscope.
   c. probe.
   d. tonometer.
   e. otoscope.

4. Infection of the ear involving fluid buildup behind the eardrum is
   a. otitis externa.
   b. otitis media.
   c. pruritus.
   d. ossicles.
   e. rhinitis.

5. Hearing loss associated with age is
   a. myopia.
   b. myringa.
   c. presbyopia.
   d. presbycusis.
   e. anacusis.

6. Ear irrigations are performed
   a. daily.
   b. to remove cerumen and foreign matter.
   c. as part of every physical examination.
   d. to relieve conjunctivitis.
   e. to relieve retinitis.

7. What chart is used to measure near vision acuity?
   a. Snellen
   b. Pelli-Robson
   c. Jaeger
   d. Ishihara
   e. nomogram

8. Impaired color vision
   a. is a factor of old age.
   b. is hereditary.
   c. is more common in females.
   d. is correctable with surgery.
   e. improves over time.

9. To straighten the ear canal of a child under 3 years, you would
   a. pull the earlobe down and back.
   b. pull the ear lobe up and back.
   c. leave the ear lobe untouched.
   d. straighten the ear drum.
   e. ask the parent to do it.

10. The term used to describe someone who is nearsighted is
    a. emmetropic.
    b. hyperopic.
    c. myopic.
    d. presbyopic.
    e. astigmatic.

CRITICAL THINKING

Refer to the case study at the beginning of the chapter and use what you have learned to answer the following questions.

1. What do Kyle's results of the Snellen examination mean?
2. What could you say to Kyle to help put him at ease about the eyedrops he needs to receive?
3. Dr. Miller writes a prescription for corrective lenses for Kyle. After Dr. Miller leaves the room, Kyle says, "I will never wear glasses because my friends will make fun of me." What would you say to Kyle?

ON THE JOB

Agnes Jones, the medical assistant in a busy ENT office, is asked to transcribe the following ophthalmology report for the physician:

Reason for consultation—Evaluation of progressive loss of vision in right eye.

History of present illness—Patient has noted a gradual deterioration of vision and increasing photophobia over the past year, particularly in the right eye. She states that it feels like there is a film over her right eye. She denies any change of vision in her left eye.

Results of physical examination—Visual acuity test showed no changes in this patient's long-standing hyperopia. The eye muscles function properly, and there is no evidence of conjunctivitis or nystagmus. The pupils react properly to light. Intraocular pressure is within normal limits (WNL). Ophthalmoscopy after application of mydriatic drops revealed presence of a large, opaque cataract forming in the right eye. There is no evidence of retinopathy, macular degeneration, or keratitis.

1. The results of the physical exam state that the patient's pupils react properly to light. What does this mean?
2. This patient wears corrective lenses for which condition?
3. The patient history states that she does not have nystagmus or conjunctivitis. Explain these two conditions.

INTERNET ACTIVITY

LASIK surgery is a popular eye procedure. Research it on the Internet. If you were a candidate for this procedure, would you have it done? Why, or why not? How will the information you obtain help you in dealing with patients?

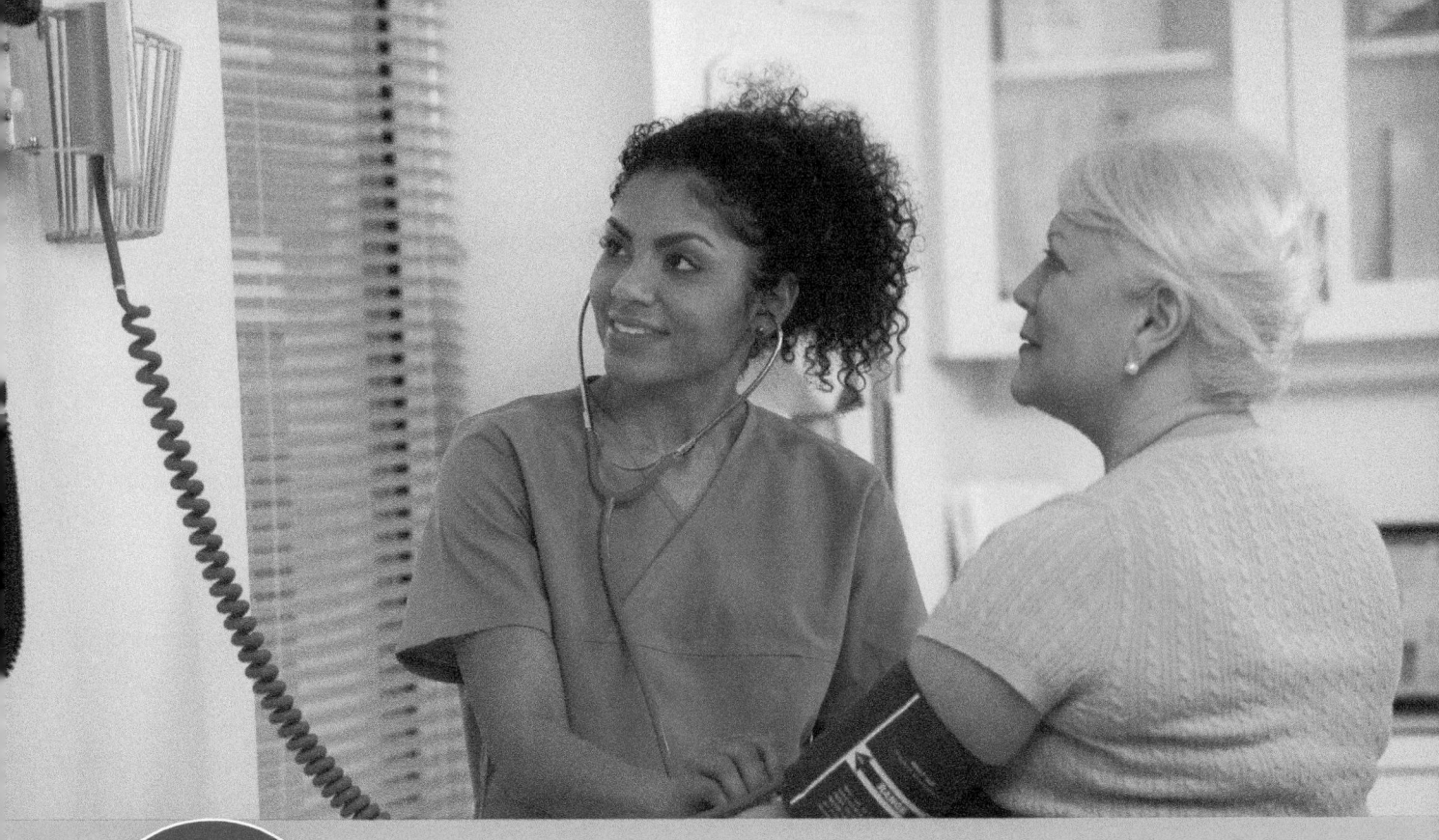

Assisting with Life Span Specialties: Pediatrics

Learning Objectives

After completing this chapter, you should be able to:

39.1   Define and spell the terms for this chapter.

39.2   Identify communication adaptations that are helpful with pediatric patients.

39.3   List considerations that must be taken regarding the pediatric office environment.

39.4   List developmental milestones in children.

39.5   Describe how measurements are obtained during a pediatric office visit.

39.6   Identify baseline vital sign ranges based on a child's age.

39.7   Explain the process of collecting a pediatric urine specimen.

39.8   List diseases common among pediatric patients.

39.9   Describe emotional changes that occur during puberty.

39.10   Compare the signs and symptoms of eating disorders.

Keyla Jefferson, age 6 months, is being seen by Dr. Penningworth for a well-child check. Dr. Penningworth is concerned about Keyla's size and developmental delays. He diagnoses her with failure to thrive as her weight measurement places her in the second percentile on the growth chart.

Terms to Learn

adolescence	failure to thrive (FTT)	purging
amenorrhea	febrile seizures	respiratory syncytial virus (RSV)
anorexia nervosa	genitalia	rhinovirus
BRAT diet	hydrocephalus	sleep apnea
bronchiolitis	meatus	stridor
bulimia nervosa	microencephaly	sudden infant death syndrome (SIDS)
croup	myringotomy	tonsillectomy
excoriation	pediatrician	

As a medical assistant, you will need to have an understanding of the unique circumstances and considerations involved with the pediatric patient population. In the medical office, pediatric visits include routine well-child checkups as well as sick-child visits. In this chapter, we discuss measurements that are taken during well-child visits, including height, weight, head and chest circumference, and vital signs. In addition, the chapter reviews childhood diseases and disorders. Health considerations for adolescents are given special attention as well.

ASSISTING IN PEDIATRICS

Pediatrics is the branch of medicine that deals with the development and care of children and the diagnosis and treatment of childhood illnesses. A **pediatrician** is a physician who specializes in the treatment of newborns, infants, children, and adolescents. Pediatricians treat patients from birth to 20 years of age. When patients reach age 20, they will transfer their routine health care to a primary care physician. Primary care physicians may also care for pediatric patients. Pediatricians may have subspecialties in the fields of pediatric surgery and pediatric oncology (cancer diagnosis and care).

Communicating with Pediatric Patients

Communication is an essential component of patient care. Communicating with the pediatric population presents special challenges. For example, infants are unable to verbalize their feelings and needs, and toddlers and young adolescents are in the process of developing their communication skills. For some medical assistants, the field of pediatrics is ideal. These are individuals who enjoy working with children, are good at dealing with the communication challenges, and have a lot of patience. Children generally have a way of sensing and relating to those who are comfortable being around them.

To save time and work quickly, medical staff often try to establish the needs of the pediatric patient by talking to the parent or guardian who is accompanying the child. It is necessary to communicate with parents and guardians because they are responsible for the care of the child, able to explain the child's needs, and able to make health care decisions for the child. However, the medical assistant must try to establish a positive connection with the young patient. Establishing trust and good rapport with a child goes a long way toward having a more cooperative patient. Additionally, these early encounters in children's lives will help shape and develop their perception of going to a doctor's office, interacting with medical personnel, and experiencing new and sometimes intimidating or scary procedures.

Consider the following suggestions when communicating with the pediatric patient:

- **Smile**—All individuals, especially infants and children, are receptive to a warm and friendly smile. Be sincere and warmly greet and welcome young patients and their parents or guardians to the medical office.

- **Communicate at their eye level**—When talking with pediatric patients, move down to their level to communicate: Sit in a chair next to them; crouch down and talk to them in the hallway when you introduce yourself. Do not attempt to communicate while towering over the child. This creates both physical and emotional barriers to communication, as a towering position indicates a domineering role.

- **Speak gently and calmly**—It isn't necessary to use "baby talk" when communicating with pediatric patients, particularly toddlers and older children. The tone of your voice will set the mood for the appointment. If you speak with a calm and gentle spirit, the child may be more apt to comply with requests (stepping on a scale or donning a gown). Patience is important because a hurried manner and sharp voice can immediately cause a child to become guarded and put up walls that can halt all progress that has been made.

- **Never lie**—Medical personnel often decide it is best to lie, or fib, to get a patient to comply. Although it is done without malice and with hopeful intentions, false statements do nothing but break trust. For example, pediatric patients require multiple injections, often during the same office visit. "Don't worry, this won't hurt a bit" is often said to calm an apprehensive toddler or child. However, injections do pinch, and sometimes the fluid that is injected burns or tingles. Children must be reassured that though the procedure may not feel good, it will be over quickly.

- **Take time for role-play**—Medical offices are often rushed, and medical assistants move quickly from room to room addressing patient needs according to the physician's orders. Nevertheless, one of the most helpful things a medical assistant can do is take some extra time to facilitate a role-play situation with the child. For example, allow the toddler or older child to handle a safe and nonbreakable piece of medical equipment and pretend to use it on a stuffed animal or a doll (Figure 39-1). This "play time" will help put the child at ease and facilitate a cooperative interaction.

Role-playing is also a tool that you can use to help you prepare to deal with situations when your pediatric patients may be upset and resistant to care. Box 39-1 presents two scenarios you and your classmates can use to anticipate and practice possible ways to calm and provide emotional support to an infant or child who is agitated or frightened.

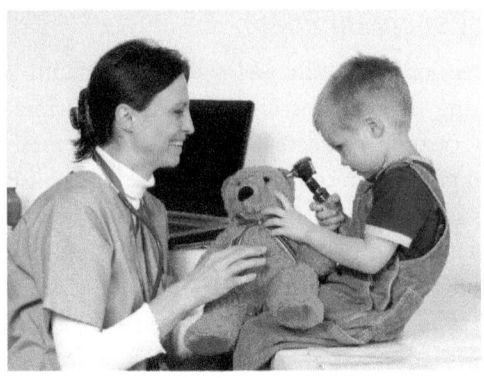

FIGURE 39-1 Supervised role-play can help a child feel more at ease during office visits.

JUDGMENT CALL

Mason Teriberry is 4 years old and is being seen today for a well-child visit. He has a lot of anxiety when he visits the doctor's office. Today, he is scheduled to have one vaccination. Sarah Teriberry, Mason's mother, keeps telling Mason that the injection won't hurt and that it will be a little "tickle." She says to you, "Go ahead and tell Mason it will just be a little tickle." How would you handle her request?

BOX 39-1 | Role-Play Scenarios

Consider the following scenarios. Role-play the scenarios with a classmate, and consider appropriate ways to handle each situation.

Scenario A: An infant is screaming and crying in the reception room. The new mother is obviously frazzled and trying to calm the screaming child. Other patients are becoming bothered by the incessant screaming. As a medical assistant, what would you do and say to the mother?

Scenario B: Alton Cranfield is a 4-year-old patient who is extremely sensitive to touch. He doesn't like *strangers* and is scared of the medical office. As a medical assistant, what can you say to Alton, and what can you do to help improve his experience in the office?

THE PEDIATRIC OFFICE

Factors of prime importance in a pediatric office include ensuring the safety of infants and children and maintaining a healthy environment for these young patients. Filling out the vast numbers of forms encountered in pediatrics (school physical, sports, and health insurance forms) correctly and in a timely fashion is also significant.

Office Reception Room

The reception room in a pediatric office should be bright, welcoming, and interesting to the child. Primary colors, popular cartoon characters, and animal themes are often found in pediatric reception areas. Toys and books should be made available to entertain children while they wait. These toys should be stored and separated according to the appropriate age group they are intended for. The most practical and safest toys are easy-to-clean, plastic toys without tiny pieces or sharp edges.

Although the reception area is the ideal waiting space for healthy children, children with contagious infections should, if possible, be brought directly to an examination room to avoid spreading the infection to other patients and their families. Some offices have separate reception areas for sick children.

Routinely throughout the day, and most certainly at the end of the day, toys should be picked up and put away as needed to prevent falls. Sanitizing toys should be done at the end of each day.

Patient Safety

Once the child enters the medical office, that child's safety is your prime concern. Children should never be left alone on an examination table, scale, toilet, or other place that could pose possible danger for falling or other injury. Always place a protective hand on infants at all times to protect them from rolling or falling.

Carrying an Infant

When carrying an infant, it is helpful to mimic the way the caregiver holds the child; this position is most likely

Professionalism The Workplace

In some states, caregivers other than parents must obtain signed legal permission to bring a pediatric patient into a medical facility for treatment. Because pediatrics deals with the treatment of minors (those under age 18 who are unable to make their own medical decisions), it is important to know the laws that pertain to the treatment of minors in your state. The medical office may have policies and procedures in place that specifically address the treatment of minor patients.

preferred by the infant. Three positions are most often used for carrying an infant: the cradle hold, the football hold, and the shoulder or upright hold. These are shown in Figure 39-2 A–C. Supporting the infant's head should always be foremost in your mind. Until about age 1, an infant often lacks strong and developed neck muscles, which are necessary to support her own head, and neck injuries can occur without proper support. The head must be supported, especially when you are holding the infant upright.

Wrapping an Infant

At times, it may be necessary to restrict the movements of the infant or small child so a procedure or evaluation can be performed. A small sheet or receiving blanket may be used to wrap or swaddle the child, binding the arms to the sides. To restrain movement of the head, hold your hands on either side of the head, but avoid sealing off the ears or touching the fontanel (soft spot) on the baby's head.

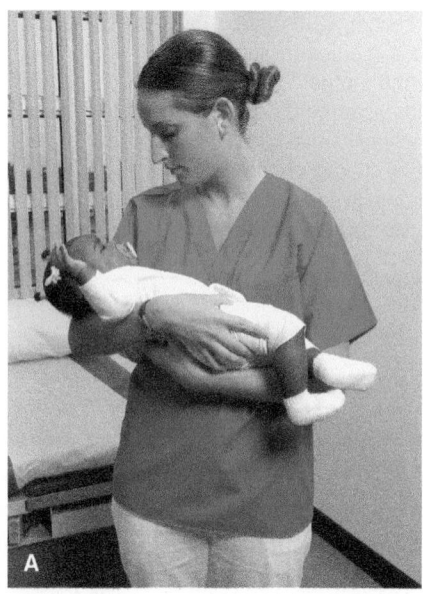
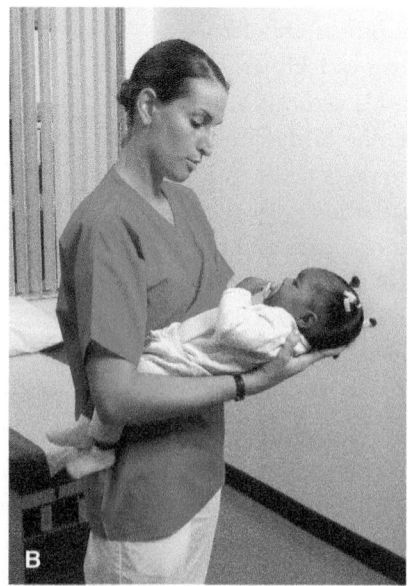
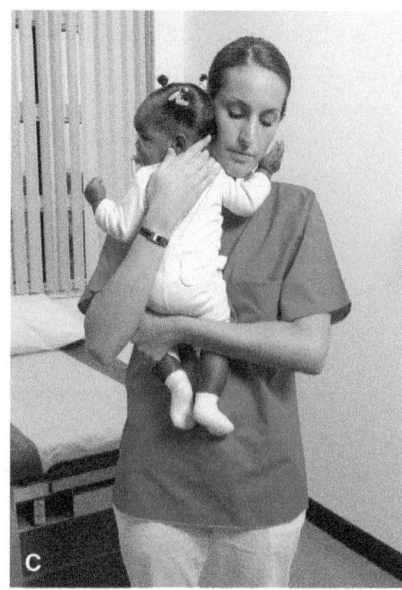

FIGURE 39-2 (A) The cradle hold; **(B)** the football hold; **(C)** the shoulder (or upright) hold.

THE PEDIATRIC PATIENT

Growth and development refer to changes that occur as the child grows and matures. Growth patterns provide valuable information regarding the physical progress of the child. Development refers to the motor, mental, and social progress that the child achieves. Children mature at different rates; however, the stages they pass through are consistent, as are the age ranges for specific stages of development.

The pediatrician looks for markers to detect abnormalities in growth and in social, emotional, and intellectual development. The earlier a problem is detected, the better the outcome may be for the child as appropriate intervention and support services may be used. Information from each office visit is compared with national standards and charts. It is important for you, the medical assistant, to understand the stages of growth and development in your role as a health care provider. Some pediatric offices train the medical assistant to perform a checklist, asking the parent or guardian if specific developmental markers have been achieved. Table 39-1 is a checklist of physical, mental, and

TABLE 39-1 | Checklist of Developmental Milestones: Birth to 5 Years

Age	Developmental Check
Birth to 1 Month	Generally helpless, dependent on parent/caregiver, soothed by rocking motions and soothing sounds.
1–2 Months	Raises head from surface when lying on stomach; pays attention to someone's face in his line of vision; moves arms and legs in energetic manner; likes to be held.
2–3 Months	Smiles and recognizes voices; coos and makes other vocal sounds; rolls partially to the side when lying on back; is startled by loud sounds.
3–4 Months	Eyes follow moving object; able to hold head erect; grasps objects in hands; babbles; laughs out loud; rolls from stomach to back; recognizes bottle and familiar faces.
4–5 Months	Reaches for and holds objects; stands firmly when held; stretches out arms to be picked up; likes to play peek-a-boo; turns toward sound of a voice; tracks moving objects easily.
5–6 Months	Turns from back to stomach; turns toward sounds; sits with a little support; reaches for objects that are out of reach; listens to own voice; crows and squeals; reaches for and grasps objects and brings them to mouth; holds, sucks, bites, and begins chewing.
6–7 Months	Transfers an object from one hand to the other; sits for a few minutes on her own (but not unattended); pats and smiles at image in mirror; creeps, pulling body with arms and leg kicks; shy at first with strangers; distinguishes emotions by voice tones.
7–8 Months	Sits steadily for five minutes; crawls on hands and knees; grasps things with thumb and first two fingers; likes to be near parent or caregiver; fears strangers.
8–9 Months	Says mama or dada; responds to own name; can stand for a short time holding onto support; can pick up small objects; responds to no.
9–12 Months	Pulls self up at side of crib or playpen; drinks from a cup when it is held; walks around holding onto furniture; waves bye-bye; repeats a few words; eats solid foods; eats with fingers.
12–15 Months	Walks by self; pulls toys while walking; shows wants by pointing and gesturing; scribbles on paper after shown; begins to use a spoon; cooperates with dressing; dumps out toys from container and replaces them.
15–18 Months	Builds a tower with blocks; likes to climb and take things apart; can say six words; tries to put on own shoes; drinks from a cup held in both hands; follows one-step directions; throws a ball; points to objects or pictures when they are named.
18 Months to 2 Years	Runs, walks up and down stairs using alternate feet; says at least 50 to 200 words; sometimes uses two-word sentences; points to objects in a book; undresses with help; capable of bowel control.
2–3 Years	Can repeat two numbers in a row; knows sex; dresses self except for buttoning; can copy a circle; can follow commands of on, under, or behind (stand on the rug); knows most parts of the body; jumps, lifting both feet off the ground; can build tower of nine blocks; can name a color; stays dry during the day and night.
4–5 Years	Can repeat a simple six-word sentence; can wash hands and face without help; can copy a cross; can stand on one foot; can catch a tossed ball; can skip; follows three commands.

Note: If a child is late doing several activities in a time period, seek further evaluation. A child born prematurely will be delayed by the number of months born early.

TABLE 39-2 | Apgar Scoring

Sign	0	1	2
Heart Rate	Absent	Slow (less than 100)	Over 100
Respiratory Effort	Absent	Slow, irregular	Good crying
Muscle Tone	Flaccid	Some flexion of extremities	Active motion
Reflex Irritability	No response	Cry	Vigorous
Color	Blue, pale	Body pink, extremities blue	Completely pink

social developmental milestones children achieve during their first five years.

Apgar Scoring

Immediately after birth, the newborn is assessed using the Apgar scoring system. This is a method of evaluating a newborn's condition at one and five minutes after birth. The higher the Apgar score, the healthier the newborn. If a newborn scores less than 7 at five minutes after birth, the child must be evaluated every five minutes for 20 more minutes. Generally, 9 is the highest Apgar score because most babies have some bluing to their extremities. Table 39-2 illustrates Apgar scoring.

- Newborns scoring 7–10 are considered out of immediate danger.
- Newborns scoring 4–6 are considered moderately depressed.
- Newborns scoring 0–3 are severely depressed.

PEDIATRIC OFFICE VISITS AND PROCEDURES

Pediatric office visits are divided into well-child visits and sick-child visits as described in the following sections.

Well-Child Visits

During well-child visits, growth and development are measured, immunizations are given, and health information is provided. Well-child visits are scheduled routinely after birth: 1 month, 2 months, 4 months, 6 months, 9 months, 12 months, 15 months, 18 months, 24 months, and then on a yearly basis.

Growth

The average infant weighs about 7 pounds at birth. By 6 months, that weight has doubled, and usually by age 1 the child's length has doubled and weight tripled. The child will not experience a similar growth spurt until puberty. By 3 years old, the child reaches half her adult height. From ages 5 to 10, the child grows 2 to 3 inches and gains 3 to 5 pounds yearly. Infants and small children grow from the top down, with the head growing considerably in the first four months. Adult proportions will not be reached until about 12 years. See Figure 39-3 A–E for examples of developmental growth stages in children.

Failure to Thrive

When an infant is unable to gain a sufficient amount of weight, according to the standardized baby growth charts, it is called **failure to thrive (FTT)**. Children have irregular

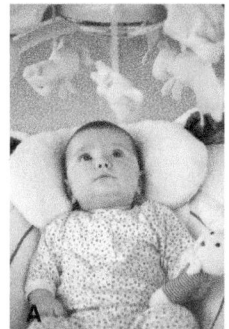 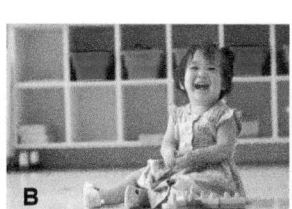 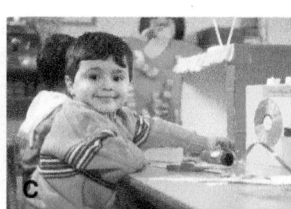 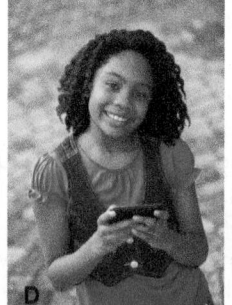 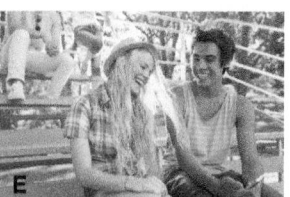

FIGURE 39-3 (A) Infant: 4 weeks to 1 year; **(B)** toddler: 1–3 years; **(C)** preschool: 3–6 years; **(D)** school age (late childhood): 6–12 years, or to puberty; **(E)** adolescence: 12 years or puberty to the beginning of adulthood.

growth patterns; however, if an infant's growth is considerably under the goal for age, normal development could be affected. Failure-to-thrive syndrome is diagnosed when an infant's weight falls under the third percentile on the growth charts.

The most frequent cause of FTT is inadequate nutrition. FTT may occur as a result of medical problems such as endocrine, neurological, and gastroenterological issues.

Other causes could be cleft palate, which affects the ability to suck well during eating, and malabsorption disease, which prevents food from being absorbed normally. In addition, insufficient stimulation and lack of nurturing can cause failure to thrive. Social problems such as abuse, poverty, and drug or alcohol dependence can affect the parents' ability to care for and nourish the child.

Measurements

When the child arrives for a well-child visit, the physical examination follows a similar pattern as an adult examination. The physician will examine the patient from head to toe.

Vital Signs

In your role as a medical assistant, you will obtain temperature, pulse, respirations, and—depending on the age of the child—blood pressure measurements. Procedure 39-1 describes steps for measuring pediatric vital signs, including

---

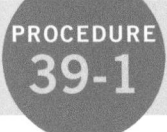

PROCEDURE 39-1

Measuring and Recording Pediatric Vital Signs

Objective ◆ *Perform all steps of obtaining pediatric vital signs, and provide accurate readings according to the instructor's guidelines.*

EQUIPMENT AND SUPPLIES

Gloves; tympanic thermometer; electronic thermometer with blue and red probes; lubricating gel; watch with second hand; pediatric stethoscope; pediatric blood pressure cuff; patient's medical record

METHOD

1. Gather the appropriate equipment.
2. Warmly greet and ask the parent or guardian to identify the patient, introduce yourself, and explain the procedures to the parent.
3. Speak calmly and reassuringly to the child; this will help to gain trust and rapport with the child.
4. Perform hand hygiene.
5. Explain how the parent or guardian can assist you in holding the infant patient while vital signs are obtained.

OBTAIN TEMPERATURE WITH TYMPANIC THERMOMETER AS FOLLOWS

1. Remove the thermometer from the base, and note that it reads "Ready."
2. Attach the disposable probe cover to the earpiece.
3. Gently pull the patient's earlobe downward and out to straighten the ear canal.
4. Insert the probe into the ear canal.
5. Press the scan button.
6. Observe the temperature reading.
7. Gently withdraw the thermometer, and eject the probe cover into a waste container.

8. Record the temperature reading using "T" to indicate the temperature reading was obtained via the tympanic membrane route.
9. Return the thermometer to the charging base.

OBTAIN TEMPERATURE READING USING AXILLARY METHOD AS FOLLOWS

1. Remove the electronic thermometer from the charging base and attach the blue probe, which can be used for oral and axillary temperatures.
2. Attach a disposable probe cover, and make sure that the thermometer is turned on and ready to take a temperature.
3. Place the thermometer in the infant's axilla (armpit), and hold the infant's arm across the chest, causing a tight seal in the axillary region (Figure A). Hold this position until the thermometer beeps, indicating the temperature has been successfully obtained.

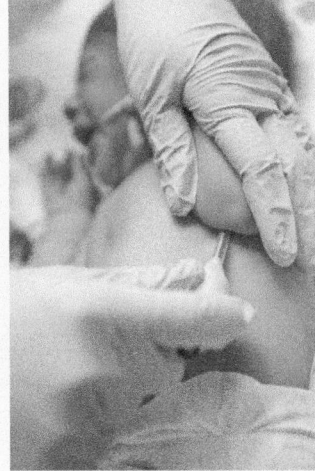

FIGURE A Hold the infant's arm to ensure a tight seal in the axillary region. This will allow for the most accurate axillary temperature.

4. Read the thermometer; then record the reading with "AX" to indicate that the axillary method was used.
5. Dispose of the probe cover in a waste container, and return the electronic thermometer unit to the charging base.

OBTAIN TEMPERATURE READING RECTALLY BY USING A DIGITAL THERMOMETER WITH RED PROBE (RECTAL USE)

1. Remove the electronic digital thermometer from the charging base and attach the red probe, used for obtaining rectal body temperatures.
2. Perform hand hygiene and don gloves.
3. Attach the disposable probe cover.
4. Lubricate the tip of the thermometer to assist with insertion of the tip into the rectum.
5. Place the infant in the supine position and pull the feet up to expose the rectal area.
6. Insert the thermometer ¼ inch into the rectum and hold in place with hand to prevent expelling (Figure B).
7. Hold the infant securely to restrict movement and maintain the thermometer's position until the beeping sound indicates the body temperature has been obtained.
   a. Make a mental note of the patient's body temperature after the thermometer beeps. You will record this number after a few additional steps have been completed.
8. Gently remove the thermometer and wipe off excessive lubricant (from front to back) from the infant's rectum.
9. Dispose of the probe cover into a waste container. Remove and discard gloves. Perform hand hygiene.
10. Record the reading in the patient's medical record using "R" to indicate the rectal method used.

MEASURE HEART RATE/PULSE BY APICAL MEASUREMENT AS FOLLOWS

1. Place the stethoscope on the child's chest at the midpoint between the sternum and the left nipple (Figure C).

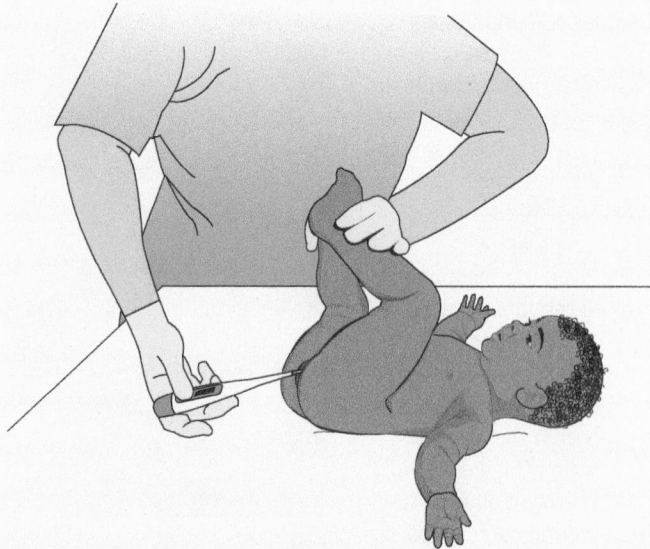

FIGURE B Obtaining a body temperature rectally.

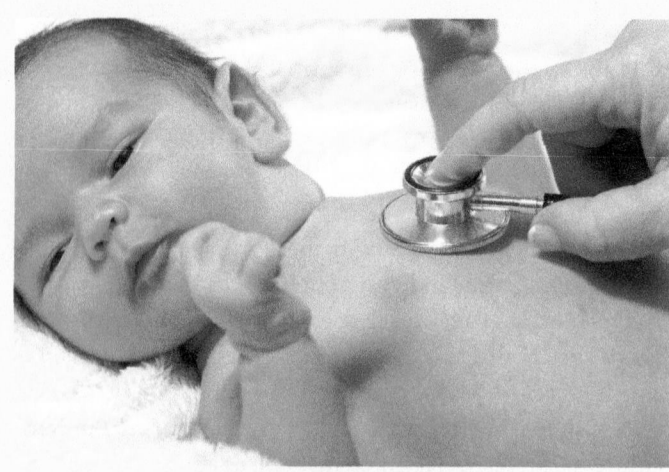

FIGURE C Measuring the apical pulse of an infant.

2. Listen for the "lub-dub" of the apical pulse.
3. Count the apical pulse for one full minute. Each lub-dub represents one complete beat.
4. Record the apical pulse using "AP" before the pulse measurement to indicate the apical reading was obtained.

MEASURE INFANT RESPIRATIONS FOR ONE FULL MINUTE AS FOLLOWS

1. Following the count of the apical pulse, remove the stethoscope from your ears.
2. With the infant in the same position, place your hand gently on the child's chest.
3. One complete respiration includes the rise and fall of the chest. Count respirations for one full minute.
4. Record the results in the patient's medical record.

MEASURE THE INFANT'S BLOOD PRESSURE USING A PEDIATRIC CUFF AND STETHOSCOPE AS FOLLOWS

1. Obtain a blood pressure reading on the child if the patient is age 5 or older, or if the physician indicates that BP measurement should be obtained.
2. Choose the correct-size cuff and wrap it securely around the upper arm, above the antecubital space.
3. Feel for the brachial pulse.
4. Place the stethoscope earpieces in your ears and place the diaphragm or bell (whichever allows you to hear the best) of the stethoscope near the brachial pulse.
5. Tighten the valve of the pump and inflate the cuff until the pulse is no longer heard.
6. Release the valve slowly, listening for systolic and diastolic sounds.
7. Record the results.

CHARTING EXAMPLE

4/10/YY T: 99°F (T), AP: 118 bpm, R: 48, BP: 80/62..............
....M. King, CMA (AAMA)

temperature (rectal, aural, and axillary methods), apical pulse, respiration, and blood pressure using a pediatric cuff. Although all the procedures are similar to performing vital signs on an adult, it is essential to use pediatric equipment.

Temperature. In children under age 5 years, temperature should be measured via the tympanic membrane, temporal artery or axillary routes. The procedures for measuring body temperature in young children are the same as they are in adults; the major difference is keeping the child still and calm during the procedure. Some medical offices prefer to measure an infant's body temperature rectally. To do so, place the infant in the supine position and place your nondominant hand securely under the baby's bent knees. With the other hand, insert the thermometer into the rectum and hold it securely in place. This will prevent the thermometer from being inserted too far as well as prevent the infant from expelling it. Take note and ensure that the proper thermometer is being used when obtaining a rectal body temperature.

Table 39-3 provides the normal pulse, respiration, and blood pressure values based on age for children from birth to adolescence. Normal body temperature is dependent on the method used, as with adult body temperatures. The normal values are as follows:

- Oral 98.6°F/37°C
- Aural 98.6°F/37°C
- Axillary 97.6°F/36.4°C
- Rectal 99.6°F/37.6°C

Pulse Rate. In children under age 2 years, pulse rate is measured using the apical pulse; placing the stethoscope on the left side of the chest to the right of the nipple and counting for one full minute.

Respirations. Respirations are easy to count because of visible rise and fall of the chest in a small child. The younger the child, the higher the respiratory rate will be.

Blood Pressure. Most pediatricians do not require routine blood pressure measurement unless the child has a cardiovascular or kidney disorder. Some physicians require blood pressure readings on every patient regardless of age, and others monitor blood pressure once a year after age 5 years. It is important to be aware of the policies of the office where you are working.

The blood pressure reading for a child will be lower than that of an adult. A blood pressure cuff measuring no wider than two-thirds of the child's upper arm must be used. In addition, a pediatric stethoscope has a smaller bell that makes it easier to place over the brachial artery.

Weight, Height, and Head and Chest Circumference

Infants and children are weighed and measured at each office visit.

Weight and Height. Infants should be weighed either without a diaper or with a completely clean diaper to ensure that the most accurate weight is obtained. If the infant is wearing a diaper during measurement, it should be noted in the medical record. The length of an infant is measured on the examining table until the child can stand reasonably still on the adult scale. Weight and height are measured without shoes. Procedure 39-2 lists the steps for measuring an infant's weight and height.

Circumference of the Head. Measurement of the circumference of the head is also part of each well-child office visit until age 6 years. Procedure 39-3 provides the steps to measure the circumference of a baby's head. Rapid growth of the head may indicate **hydrocephalus**, which is excessive fluid around the brain that may lead to brain damage. Head growth that falls below the normal percentile may indicate **microencephaly**. This condition may be caused by a premature closing of the fontanel, constricting brain growth and leading to mental retardation. Normal head circumference at birth should be between 12.5 and 14.5 inches (31.75–36.83 cm).

TABLE 39-3 | Baseline Respiration, Pulse, and Blood Pressure Values from Birth to Adolescence

Age	Respirations	Pulse	Systolic BP mmHg	Diastolic BP mmHg
Infants	30–60	100–160	74–100	50–70
Toddlers	24–39	90–150	80–112	50–80
Preschoolers	22–34	80–139	82–110	50–78
School Age	18–30	75–120	84–120	54–80
Adolescents	12–16	60–100	100 + age	30–39 minus the age

Note: Pulse and respirations are taken for one full minute. The apical pulse is used with a child under age 2 years.

Measuring and Recording the Weight and Length of an Infant

Objective ◆ *Obtain the weight and length (height) of an infant.*

EQUIPMENT AND SUPPLIES

Baby scale; patient's medical record; small towel or protector for scale; tape measure

METHOD

1. Warmly greet the parent/guardian and patient. Introduce yourself and ask the parent/guardian to verify the patient's full name and date of birth.
   a. Have the infant remain with the parent or caregiver while you prepare the equipment and explain the procedure.
2. Perform hand hygiene.
3. Place a towel or paper protector on the baby scale.
4. Balance the scale by placing all the weights to the far left side. Turn the bolt at the right edge of the scale until the balance bar pointer is at the middle of the balance bar.
5. Ask the parent to undress the infant, and provide assistance if necessary.
   a. Follow office protocol regarding whether the infant should be diaperless or wearing a clean diaper.
6. Gently lay the infant on the scale. Always use one hand to guard the infant until the weights are adjusted.
   a. Never leave an infant unattended on a scale, for any reason.
7. Keeping one hand hovering over (but not pressing on) the infant's body as a safety precaution, move the large pound weight into the groove closest to the weight estimated for the baby. Move the smaller ounce weight by tapping it gently until it reaches a point at which the pointer floats in the center of the frame. See Figure A for an example of an electronic baby scale.
8. Inform the caregiver that the infant can be diapered. Keep the weights in place and remain with the infant, with a protective hand guarding, until the caregiver picks up the infant for diapering.
9. When the infant has been removed from the scale, document the weight in the patient's medical record. Return the scale weights to the zero point, or turn off the electronic scale.

CONTINUE WITH LENGTH

10. Gently place the infant on the papered examination table. It is best, and preferred, to have two people cooperate to measure the length of an infant. The parent or caregiver can assist by holding the infant's head still.

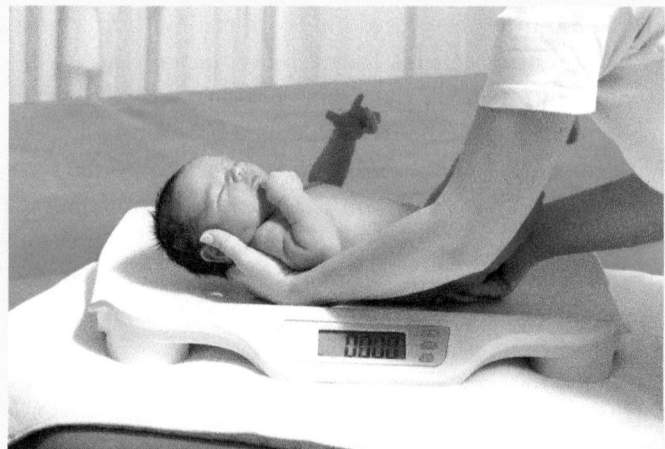

FIGURE A Electronic baby scale.

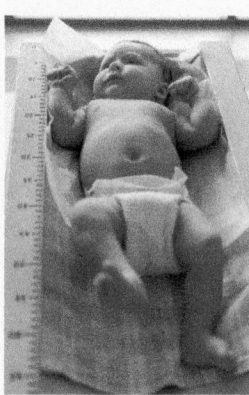

FIGURE B Measuring the length of an infant from the top of the head to the base of the heels.

11. Make pencil marks on the examination table paper at the top of the child's head and at the bottom of the feet at the heels. When the child is removed, measure the area between the two marks. Or, holding the tape measure with one hand, place the tape at the top of the side of the infant's head. Stretch the infant out full length as you pull the tape measure down to the bottom of the feet (Figure B).
    a. If you are using a table with a measure bar, place the infant's head at one end of the table with the soles of the feet touching the footboard so that the toes are pointing toward the ceiling.
12. Note the infant's length in inches and fractions of an inch, and write it on the paper covering the exam table or on a

scrap piece of paper so that it is not forgotten while the infant is tended to.
13. Inform the parent or caregiver that he or she may re-dress (if allowed before an examination) and hold the infant while waiting for the physician to perform the examination.
14. When the infant is safely being cared for by the parent or caregiver, document the length measurement in the patient's medical record.

a. If allowed by medical office protocol, inform the parent/caregiver of the patient's measurements.
15. Perform hand hygiene.

CHARTING EXAMPLE

2/14/YY Wt: 16 lb 3 oz, length: 30 ¼ inches...............M. King, CMA (AAMA)

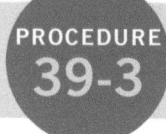

PROCEDURE 39-3 · Measuring and Recording Head Circumference

Objective ◆ *Measure the head circumference of an infant or small child.*

EQUIPMENT AND SUPPLIES

Flexible tape measure (no elasticity); patient's medical record; growth chart and pen (if an electronic medical record is not being used)

METHOD

1. Warmly greet the parent/caregiver and patient. Ask the parent/caregiver to identify the patient's full name and date of birth.
2. Smile and speak gently with the infant or child to establish a positive rapport.
3. Explain the procedure to the parent or caregiver and the small child.
4. Perform hand hygiene.
5. Position the infant on the examination table or have the caregiver hold the infant. If measuring a small child, ask the child to "please sit nice and tall and look straight ahead."
6. Hold the end of tape (0 inches) on the forehead over the patient's eyebrows. Bring the tape around the head and above the ears to meet in front (Figure A).
7. Measure with accuracy to the nearest fraction of an inch or centimeter.
   a. If there is any doubt about the measurement, repeat the procedure.

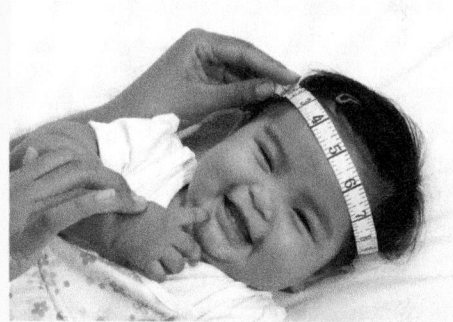

FIGURE A Measuring the head circumference of an infant.

8. Thank the small child for helping, or inform the parent/caregiver of an infant that the child may now be held.
9. Document the measurement in the patient's medical record, and (if necessary) record it on the growth chart.
10. Perform hand hygiene.

CHARTING EXAMPLE

2/10/YY Head circumference 42.5 cm......................................
....M. King, CMA (AAMA)

Generally, the head and chest circumferences are equal sometime between ages 1 and 2.

Circumference of the Chest. Chest circumference measurement is not normally performed at each office or well-child

visit. It may be performed if the physician suspects over- or underdevelopment of the heart or lungs. Calcification of the rib cage causing constriction of the growth of organs could also be a causative consideration for obtaining chest measurements. To measure the chest circumference, wrap a

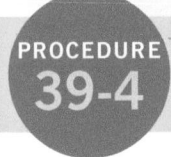

PROCEDURE 39-4 Measuring and Recording Chest Circumference

Objective ◆ *Measure the circumference of a child's chest.*

EQUIPMENT AND SUPPLIES

Nonelastic tape measure; examination table; patient's medical record

STEPS

1. Warmly greet the parent/caregiver and patient. Ask the parent/caregiver to identify the patient's full name and date of birth.
2. Talk to the patient soothingly to gain trust and establish a positive rapport.
3. Perform hand hygiene.
4. Position the child on the examination table in a supine position. If over 2 years of age, the child may sit upright on the table for this procedure.
5. Place the end of the tape (0) in the center of the child's chest in line with the child's nipples and slip the tape under the child's body and under the armpits. Bring it completely around to meet the other end of the tape (Figure A).
6. Take a measurement to the nearest 0.01 of a centimeter or to the nearest ½ inch.

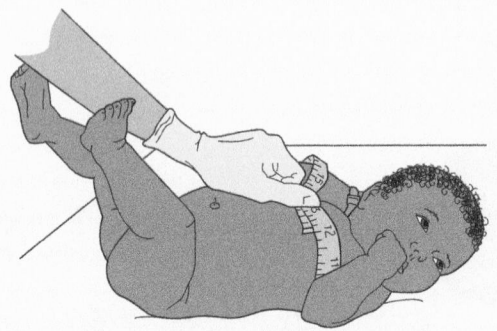

FIGURE A Measuring the chest circumference of an infant.

7. Return the child to the parent/caregiver's care before recording the results.
8. Perform hand hygiene after the measurement has been documented.

CHARTING EXAMPLE

05/25/YY Well-child visit, age 13 months. Chest circum.: 18.25"...A. Rashid, RMA

---

measuring tape around the chest at nipple level and read the measurement during the resting phase between respirations as described in Procedure 39-4.

Growth Charts

We have been discussing child measurement during each well-child visit. These vital measurements are plotted on a growth chart. A copy of the National Center for Health Statistics growth chart, with the plotted measurements, is part of every child's permanent medical record. Individual growth charts are available for boys and girls ages birth to 36 months and 2 to 20 years (Figure 39-4). It is important to be sure that the correct growth chart is chosen for each patient.

After the measurements are obtained, the medical assistant charts the information in both the medical record and the growth chart. A growth percentile is obtained when the values are accurately plotted on the growth chart. When done manually (as when an office uses paper medical records), the plotting

of measurements requires skill and precision. However, today, many practices use electronic health records. A benefit of the electronic health record is that once measurements are entered, the software program automatically calculates the child's growth and percentile range. The percentile is used to identify children with growth or nutritional abnormalities.

Procedure 39-5 lists the steps necessary to manually calculate the growth percentiles.

Sick-Child Visits

During a sick-child visit, the ill child is brought in for examination to diagnose and recommend treatment for an illness. Pediatric offices have time blocked off in the daily schedule to allow for sick-child visits, even though many of the daily appointments are allotted for well-child visits.

It is unfortunate, but children develop sicknesses quite often. This is because their young bodies do not have a fully developed immune system. When they are exposed to new

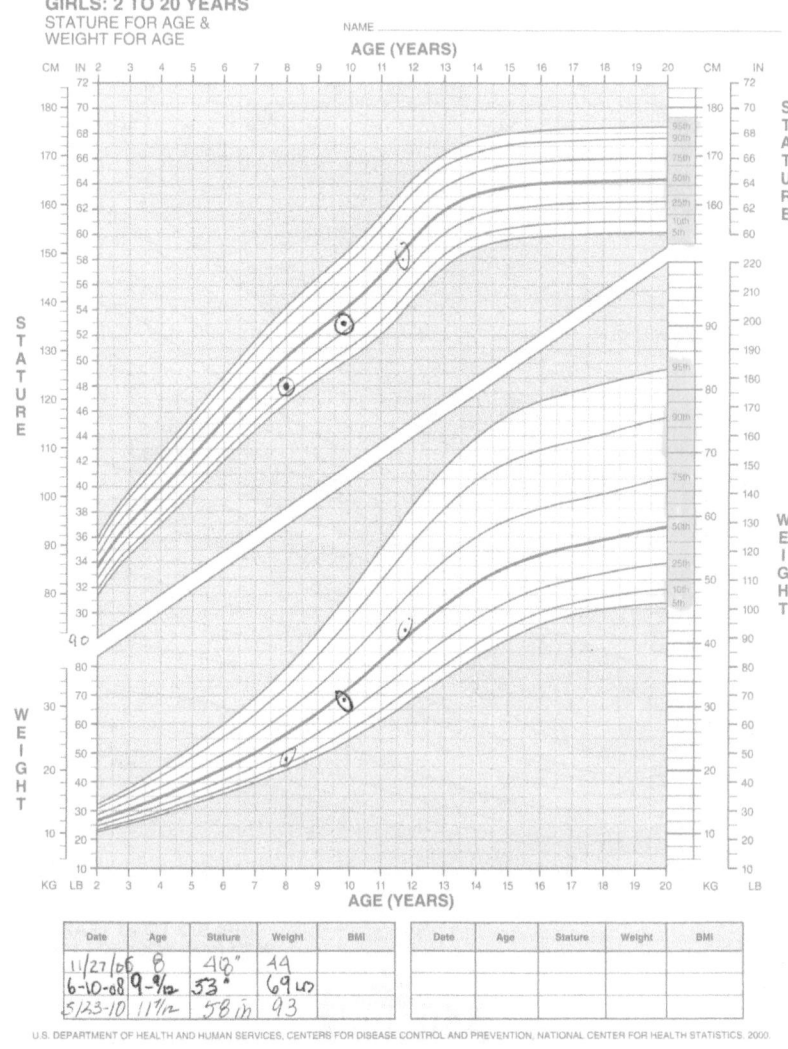

GIRLS: 2 TO 20 YEARS
STATURE FOR AGE &
WEIGHT FOR AGE

NAME

Date	Age	Stature	Weight	BMI		Date	Age	Stature	Weight	BMI
11/27/06	6	48"	44							
6-10-08	9-9/12	53"	69 40							
5/23-10	11 9/12	58 in	93							

U.S. DEPARTMENT OF HEALTH AND HUMAN SERVICES, CENTERS FOR DISEASE CONTROL AND PREVENTION, NATIONAL CENTER FOR HEALTH STATISTICS. 2000.

FIGURE 39-4 This pediatric growth chart tracks the height and weight for girls ages 2–20.

germs, particularly when the child enters a public day care or school system, the child tends to contract infections more readily from the increased degree of exposure. For this reason, it is important to teach children (as early as possible) about the importance of breaking the cycle of infection—particularly the importance of hand washing and covering their nose and mouth when they cough or sneeze.

When a caregiver brings a sick child into the office, it is helpful to place the patient in an examination room as quickly as possible. This helps reduce the possibility of spreading infection among the vulnerable population in the office reception room. As mentioned earlier, some offices have separate reception areas for sick children.

Collecting a Urine Sample

Based on the patient's symptoms, the physician may request a urine sample. If the child is toilet trained and over 2 to 3 years old, it is easiest and recommended that the parent or caregiver collect the specimen after she has been provided instructions regarding proper cleansing of the genital area. Sometimes, the urine sample container may be given to the parent/caregiver before the designated appointment time and a urine sample is brought from home and then tested in the office.

The instructions are the same as those for cleansing before attaching a urine collection device, which is explained in Procedure 39-6. If

PROCEDURE 39-5

Documenting a Growth Chart

Objective ◆ *Plot the age, weight, and height of a patient, and obtain correct percentiles.*

EQUIPMENT AND SUPPLIES

Patient's record with weight and height values; pen; growth chart; ruler or straight edge

METHOD

1. Select the proper growth chart for the patient, based on age and gender. See Figure A for an example.
2. Assume the patient is a female age 18 months. Locate the child's age in the horizontal axis at the bottom of the

chart. Draw an imaginary vertical line on the chart, using a ruler or straight edge.

3. Assume the patient's length is 33". Draw an imaginary horizontal line on the chart that intersects with the patient's age (it should intersect at the straight edge of the ruler).
4. Find the point at which the two imaginary lines intersect on the graph; then place a dot there.
5. Assume the patient's weight is 27.5 lb. Draw an imaginary horizontal line on the chart that intersects with the patient's age (it should intersect at the straight edge of the ruler).

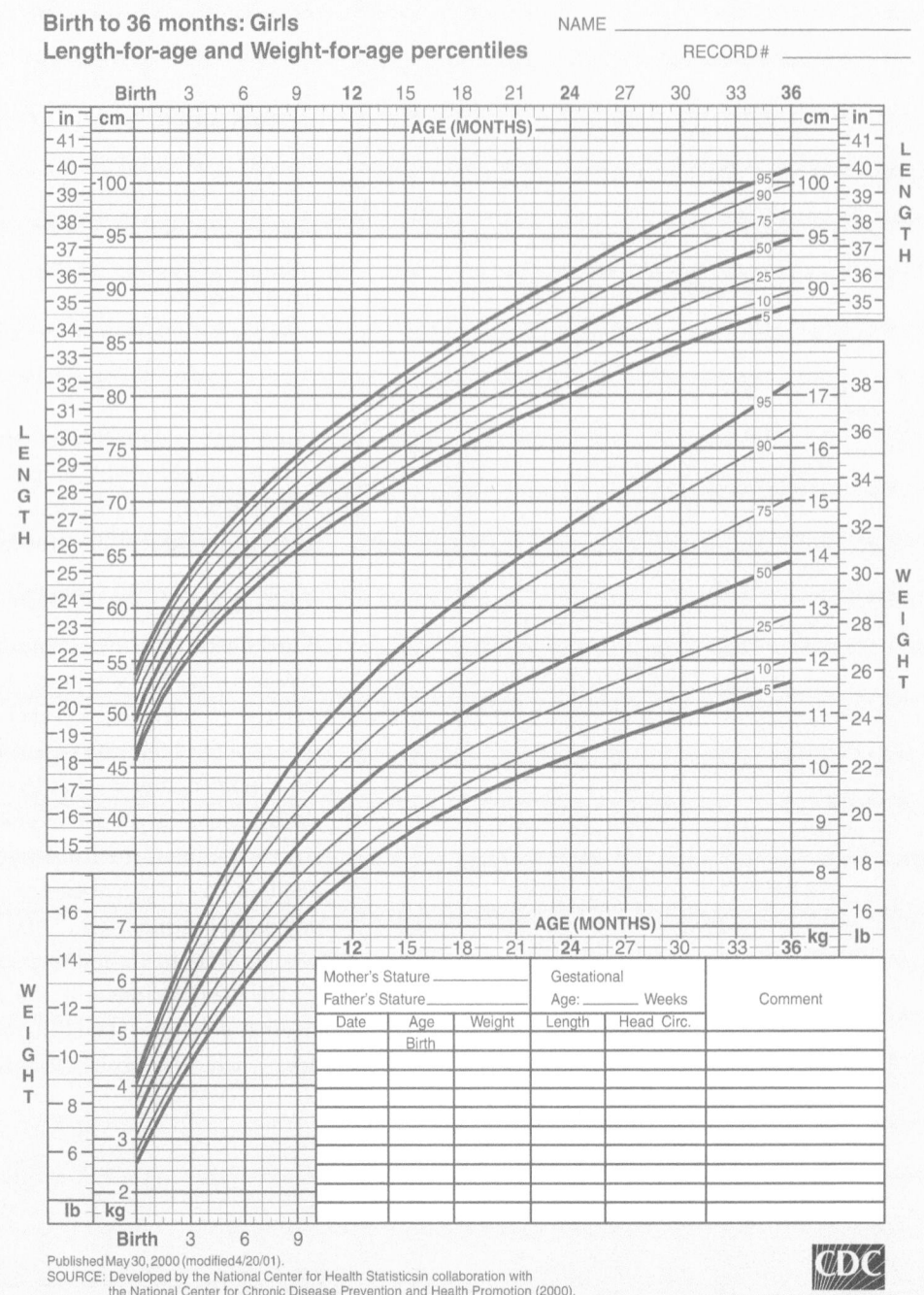

Birth to 36 months: Girls
Length-for-age and Weight-for-age percentiles

NAME _____

RECORD# _____

AGE (MONTHS)

Published May 30, 2000 (modified 4/20/01).
SOURCE: Developed by the National Center for Health Statistics in collaboration with
the National Center for Chronic Disease Prevention and Health Promotion (2000).
http://www.cdc.gov/growthcharts

FIGURE A Pediatric growth chart for girls ages birth to 36 months.

6. Find the point at which the two imaginary lines intersect on the graph; then place a dot there.

   Note: You will now have two dots on the horizontal line of the chart that corresponds with the patient's age.

7. Follow the curved line closest to the dot upward; then read the percentile located on the right side of the chart.

8. If the dot you placed falls between two curved lines, extrapolate or estimate the percentile that falls between the two closest percentile lines.

- For example, if the dot you placed based on the correct age and weight was halfway between the 10 and 25 percentile lines, the difference between 25 and 10 is 15, and half of 15 is 7.5. Therefore, the percentile would be 17.5. The child would weigh more than 17.5 percent of the children his or her age, which is below normal.

9. Record the results in the patient's medical record.

CHARTING EXAMPLE

05/25/YY Length 33 inches—90th percentile, Wt. 27.5 lb—90th percentile................................A. McGrath, CMA (AAMA)

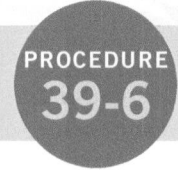

PROCEDURE 39-6 — Applying a Pediatric Urine Collection Device

Objective ◆ *Apply a urinary collection device.*

EQUIPMENT AND SUPPLIES

Pediatric urine collection bag; laboratory specimen container with label; pen; antiseptic wipes; gloves; biohazard waste container; patient's medical record

METHOD

1. Assemble all equipment and label the laboratory specimen container with the patient's name, date of birth, and today's date.
2. Warmly greet and introduce yourself to the patient and the parent/caregiver. Ask the caregiver to verify the patient's full name and date of birth, and explain the procedure to the caregiver.
3. Perform hand hygiene and don gloves.
4. Ask the parent or caregiver to place the infant on the examination table in a supine position; then remove the diaper.
5. Gently cleanse the **genitalia** (reproductive organ) area with antiseptic wipes (not alcohol wipes). Explain the importance of this delicate step to the caregiver, indicating that the lack of or improper cleansing could cause the test results to be compromised.
   Male: Cleanse the urinary **meatus** (urinary tract opening) with a circular motion, starting at the opening and progressing outward. Repeat with a clean wipe if the infant is uncircumcised, retracting the foreskin to clean the meatus. When finished cleaning, replace the foreskin to the normal position.
   Female: Hold the labia open with your nondominant hand, cleanse the labia from the front to the back, wiping in one directional motion. Discard the wipe, and repeat with a new wipe.
   Note: Make sure the area is dry before attempting to apply the urine collection device.
6. Unfold the collection device and remove the upper portion of paper protecting the adhesive surface. Apply to the mons pubis and press to secure. Continue removing paper and applying to perineum, securing the device and ensuring that it isn't sticking to the infant's leg (Figures A and B).
7. Offer water or suggest that the parent try to get the infant to drink fluids to increase the likelihood the child will produce a urine specimen.
8. When a sufficient urine sample is collected, remove the bag, wipe down the area to which the bag was attached, and

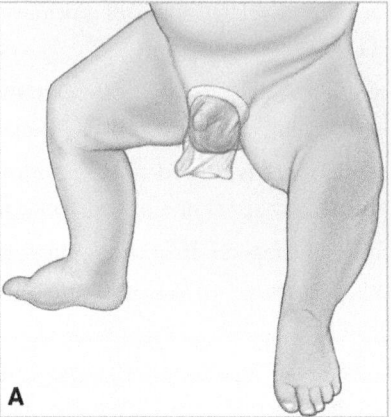

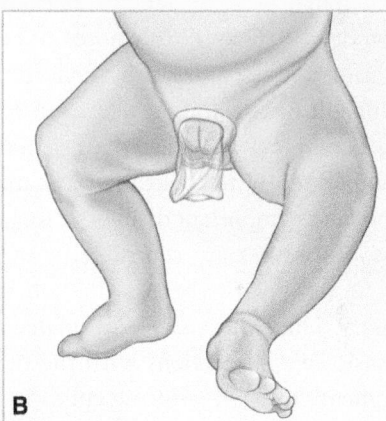

FIGURE A-B Applying a urine collection device **(A)** on a male and **(B)** on a female patient.

re-diaper the infant. It may be advisable to have the parent/caregiver re-diaper the infant, based on office protocol.
9. Pour the sample into a labeled laboratory specimen container and handle according to office policy.
10. Dispose of all used equipment in a biohazard waste container.
11. Remove gloves and perform hand hygiene.
12. Document the procedure; specific details are encouraged.

CHARTING EXAMPLE

1/10/YY 9:00 A.M. Pedi urine bag attached
9:25 A.M. No spec obtained
10:00 A.M. Pt is given juice by her mother to facilitate a urine collection, will recheck at 11:00 A.M..............
....M. King, CMA (AAMA)

the child is too ill or too young, a pediatric urine collection device should be applied as soon as possible to increase the possibility of collecting a sample. When collecting a urine sample, ask the parent or caregiver specific questions to uncover other urinary tract–related problems, such as the following:

- Have there been any changes in the amount of urine produced recently?
- Does the child complain of burning, itching, or pain during urination (symptomatic of a urinary tract infection [UTI])?
- Does the child have persistent diaper rash (caused by diarrhea or a change in urine composition)?
- Has the child reverted to bed-wetting or loss of bladder control (caused by stress or a urinary tract infection)?
- Is the child in diapers? If so, how many diapers does the child wet each day (to determine hydration or dehydration)?

A positive response to any of the preceding questions could be indicative of urinary tract problems. The physician, after examination, may order the medical assistant to apply a urine collection device. As previously noted, Procedure 39-6 lists the steps necessary to apply a urine collection device on a child who is unable or unwilling to urinate into a container. In some cases, a child may be catheterized to obtain a specimen. Urine samples reflect the health status of many systems in the body and are an important diagnostic tool.

After these procedures are complete, your duty is to remain ready to assist with the examination in whatever manner necessary. Once the visit is completed, be sure to review the physician's instructions with the caregiver and take a few moments to bond with the child. Remember to document any results.

PEDIATRIC DISEASES AND DISORDERS

Children experience frequent colds, gastrointestinal upsets, and other fairly routine conditions, which are seen in a pediatric practice. The following section discusses some of the most common ailments that afflict the pediatric patient population.

Upper Respiratory Diseases and Disorders

The common cold can be caused by more than 200 varieties of **rhinovirus**. It is highly contagious and usually resolves after about a week. In infants and children, low-grade fever, nasal congestion, and coughing may be present. During their first two years, children may have six to ten colds a

year. Again, this incidence may increase if a child is in public day care systems. Many pediatricians no longer recommend the use of decongestants and cough medications because recent studies demonstrate that they have little or no effect in children. Treatment may include over-the-counter (OTC) medicines to reduce fever as well as saline nose drops to ease breathing from stuffy noses and facilitate breathing with less discomfort. If the cold lingers, it is possible for a secondary infection to develop. Secondary infections, such as strep throat or otitis media (ear infection), may result from colds and may require treatment with antibiotics.

Most upper respiratory infections are spread easily by droplets from the nose, throat, or contaminated items handled by the infected person. Prevention is the best approach when dealing with upper respiratory infections. As discussed earlier, children should be reminded to cover their nose and mouth when sneezing, as well as taught about the importance of hand washing. Hand washing is the best defense to ward off upper respiratory infections.

Strep Throat

Strep throat is caused by group A betahemolytic *Streptococcus pyogenes*. These highly infectious bacteria may lead to other problems when left untreated, such as scarlet fever and rheumatic fever, which can damage heart valves. The pediatrician may order a throat culture to confirm that strep is the causative agent before prescribing an antibiotic. Many offices perform these tests on site with the use of rapid strep testing. Rapid strep testing is discussed in more detail in the chapter titled "Microbiology."

Strep throat is treated with antibiotics, which are often administered in a liquid form to young patients. Caregivers should be reminded that children must finish the entire antibiotic prescription to prevent relapse, even if the child's symptoms improve before the course of the antibiotic is finished. Failure to do so may result in a bacterial recurrence that is resistant to an antibiotic. A child who has recurring strep throat infections may be a candidate for a **tonsillectomy** (surgical removal of the tonsils). When this is a possibility, the child is often referred to an otolaryngologist, more commonly called an ENT (ears, nose, and throat) specialist.

Otitis Media

Otitis media is an infection of the middle ear caused by cold, allergies, or other respiratory infections. Fluid accumulates, which applies pressure to the eardrum, causing pain, irritability, and sometimes fever. Treatment of otitis media consists of decongestants, analgesics, and sometimes antibiotics. Repeated infections can lead to damage to the eardrum and loss of hearing. Children with chronic ear infections may require a **myringotomy**. During this procedure, an incision is made into the eardrum and a tube inserted through the eardrum to permit drainage of fluid. Again, the pediatric patient would be referred to an ENT specialist for this procedure.

Croup

Croup is an inflammation of the larynx and trachea, which leads to a distinctive barking cough and hoarseness. There are two types of croup: spasmodic and viral. Both types of croup begin with a cold. Spasmodic croup begins suddenly at night with the distinct "seal-bark" type of cough, but viral croup develops more slowly, with swelling, increased mucus secretions, and **stridor**. Stridor is a high-pitched sound heard during respiration caused by obstruction of the airway. Croup is most commonly treated at home. Sitting the child in a steamy bathroom, with the door closed, for 15 to 20 minutes can help restore normal breathing. Afterward, a cool steam vaporizer or humidifier in the child's room adds moisture to the air and may help breathing. Exposing the child to cool moist night air is also frequently effective. If breathing is extremely labored, emergency medical help may be needed.

Bronchiolitis

Bronchiolitis is an inflammation of the bronchioles and is more common in children under 2 years old who have upper respiratory tract infections. Children with asthma and those exposed to secondhand smoke are at higher risk. Symptoms of bronchiolitis include cold-like symptoms such as nasal and chest congestion and low-grade fever. Treatments are the same as those used to treat colds. If excessive coughing is present, using a cool steam vaporizer or humidifier may help add moisture to the air and reduce coughing.

Respiratory Syncytial Virus

Respiratory syncytial virus (RSV) is a common, highly contagious virus that affects the upper and lower respiratory tract. It normally occurs in winter and early spring and is the most common cause of bronchiolitis. RSV can spread by contact with upper respiratory secretions. By age 3 years, most children have had a bout of RSV. When very young children or children with compromised immune systems are affected, they may need hospitalization for intravenous fluids because of dehydration, bronchodilators to open the airway passages, and oxygen therapy. Confirmation of RSV is done by a throat swab or sputum culture that tests positive for the presence of viral antibodies. Infants and children at high risk for serious complications, should RSV be contracted, may be eligible to receive a medicine to help protect them from the virus. The medicine, though not considered a vaccine, is administered monthly during cold and flu season.

Asthma

Asthma is the most common chronic disease in children, affecting one in seven children usually before the age of 4. Inflammation and spasms of the bronchi, increased mucus secretions, and narrowing of the airways make it difficult to exhale and inhale for the asthmatic patient. Symptoms include wheezing, shortness of breath, tightness in the chest, difficulty speaking, and anxiety. The cause for asthma is unknown. However, triggers such as allergies, exposure to pollutants, cigarette smoke, cold viruses, and strenuous exercise may bring on an asthma attack.

Children who experience two or more asthma attacks per week should be seen by a specialist. Inhalers or nebulizers may be necessary to improve breathing during attacks. If attacks occur more frequently than twice a week, daily anti-inflammatory medications will most likely be prescribed to prevent and lessen attacks. All asthmatic patients should be given an asthma treatment plan that has been developed by the physician. This provides the caregiver with information regarding how to handle and treat each stage of an attack, culminating in emergency treatment at a hospital if necessary. Bronchodilators are administered either by inhaler or nebulizers. A peak flow meter may be used to measure the capacity of the child's ability to exhale forcefully. If specific allergens are identified, then removing the offending allergens from the child's environment is helpful.

Gastrointestinal Disorders

Children are often affected by gastrointestinal disorders. Some of the most common include diarrhea and colic.

Diarrhea

Diarrhea may be caused by bacterial, viral, and parasitic infections; food allergies; and medications. Infants and children may have diarrhea with no apparent cause. However, if diarrhea persists for more than two days, the child may need to be seen in the office.

Diarrhea in infants and small children can rapidly lead to dehydration. Dehydration can trigger an imbalance of electrolytes that could cause lethargy and hyperventilation. Acidosis and death can also occur if left untreated. The signs of dehydration are vital for both you, the medical assistant, and the caregiver to recognize. They are listed in Box 39-2. In addition to dehydration, diarrhea may cause **excoriation**, or painful chafing or rawness of the skin in the diaper area (as with a severe diaper rash). Other symptoms include cramping, weakness, fever, and irritability. Pediatricians often recommend the **BRAT diet**, consisting of bananas, rice, applesauce, and toast. The infant or child should avoid dairy products until diarrhea subsides. As symptoms subside and the child improves, food and dairy products may be slowly reintroduced to the diet.

Colic

Colic is severe gastrointestinal pain occurring in both breast-fed and formula-fed infants. The cause of colic is unknown, although some suspect reflux or immaturity of the digestive system to be a factor. Colic does not have lasting effects and usually disappears by age 4 months. Symptoms include intense crying, irritability, fussiness, distended abdomen, and gas. Parents and caregivers often feel frustrated, angry, at fault, and exhausted when dealing with a colicky infant. In your work as a medical assistant, your ability to empathize with the caregiver can ease frustration. There is no specific treatment for colic. Caregivers often attempt a trial-and-error approach to feedings, how to hold the baby, and soothing remedies like rocking and patting the baby's back. OTC gas relief drops, such as Mylicon®, can be helpful to aid the discomfort of the infant. Some babies find relief being held in the football position: lying on their bellies along the parent's arm or leg.

Other Disorders

Other conditions and disorders that pediatric patients are inclined to be diagnosed with are discussed in this section. These disorders vary in their etiology, prognosis, and treatment.

Autism

Autism is a disorder that is marked by the brain's abnormal development of social and communication skills. It is often noticed and diagnosed by 3 years of age and is more prevalent in males than in females. There are various forms diagnosed within the autism spectrum disorder. According to the Centers for Disease Control and Prevention (CDC), 1 in 68 children in the United States were affected by an autism spectrum disorder in 2014. This is a 30 percent increase from the 1 in 88 statistic released by the CDC in 2012.

Etiology is unknown, but genetics may play a role, as autism may tend to be more prevalent among family members. Other possible causes include exposure to toxic chemicals during pregnancy, pesticides, flame-retardant chemicals, prenatal or postnatal viruses, and exposure to heavy metals such as mercury. There is no link between autism and immunizations according to the latest CDC research.

Symptoms of autism and autism spectrum disorders are varied and may include the following:

- Failure to make eye contact
- Engaging in repetitive behavior
- Delayed language skills
- Preference for solitary activities
- Upset by changes in routine
- Indifference to people

No cure has yet been found for autism, but research indicates that early intervention by specialists can be beneficial. The earlier autism is diagnosed with interventions designed to meet the child's needs, the better the prognosis is for the child throughout his lifetime.

Sudden Infant Death Syndrome

Sudden infant death syndrome (SIDS) is the death of an apparently healthy infant, usually before age 1 year, with no known cause. SIDS usually occurs during sleep and is a leading cause of death in children within the first year of life. The highest number of deaths occurs between 1 and 4 months of age. SIDS happens more frequently in winter and is more prevalent among boys. The most probable causes proposed are immature waking centers in the brain leading to **sleep apnea**, abnormal regulation of breathing, abnormal heart rates, and lack of airway control. Sleep apnea involves periods of a complete absence of breathing during sleep.

Factors that increase the risk of SIDS are low birth weight, premature birth, a family history of SIDS, putting the child to sleep on her stomach, births from very young mothers, and prenatal exposure to alcohol, drugs, or smoking. Possible prevention techniques include having the infant sleep on her back or in a side position for at least the first six months, and using apnea monitors.

The loss of a child to SIDS is particularly difficult because parents often feel that they were at fault. Support groups and therapy may help devastated parents begin their healing process. Numerous SIDS associations have local and national chapters that can provide valuable information and help.

Febrile Seizures

Febrile seizures are suffered by some children with high fevers following a rapid spike in body temperature. Seizures can involve jerking arms and legs, loss of consciousness, and stiffening of the child's body. After a seizure, the child may be sleepy and have a headache. Watching a child have a febrile seizure is alarming for parents and caregivers; however, there is no lasting effect on the child, and these specific seizures are not associated with epilepsy. During the seizure, the child should be placed on his side in an area free of sharp objects. Do not put anything in the child's mouth or attempt to restrain the child. The only treatment involved for febrile seizures is to reduce the fever, often with OTC medications or a cool bath.

Obesity

Obesity is defined as being 20 percent above the patient's ideal weight with a body mass index over 30. Body mass index (BMI) is a measurement of body weight relative to height and is associated with the amount of body fat. BMI is calculated using the following formula:

$$BMI = weight (lb)/[height (in.)]^2 \times 703$$

A BMI of 25 to 27 means a child is overweight. Childhood obesity is an epidemic leading to multiple lifelong complications and other diseases if intervention is not obtained. Genetic tendencies, family patterns of overeating, poor food choices, and lack of exercise cause children to be obese. Very few children are obese as a result of endocrine disorders. More than 35 percent (or one-third) of adults in the United States are considered obese. It is estimated that 18 percent of children in the United States over age 5 years are obese. Obesity carries serious consequences to health in the short and long terms (e.g., early development of type 2 diabetes) and may cause damage to a child's self-esteem. A medical assistant will provide support, encouragement, and physician-approved educational materials, as well as serve as a link to community resources for the family dealing with an obese child.

Fifth Disease

Fifth disease, or erythema infectiosum, is a mildly contagious viral disease that occurs during spring. It affects children over 2 years old. It is caused by parvovirus B19. Symptoms, which last about a week, include reddened cheeks, fever, and a lacy rash on the chest, abdomen, arms, and legs. If Fifth disease is contracted during pregnancy, the fetus may suffer damage or die in utero. Therefore, it is important for children who are diagnosed with Fifth disease not to come in contact with pregnant women.

Roseola

Roseola is a common early childhood viral infection. It is characterized by a sudden high fever, which can last about four days, followed by a rash of tiny pink spots on the head and trunk. Treatment includes reducing the child's fever (generally with acetaminophen) and sponging the body with lukewarm water.

Hand, Foot, and Mouth Disease

Hand, foot, and mouth disease is another mild viral infection common among pediatric patients. The virus causes blisters to appear in the mouth, on hands, and on feet. It commonly occurs in summer and early fall, and generally affects children up to age 4 years, but can afflict older children as well. It is commonly spread in day care or nursery schools. It is usually caused by the Coxsackievirus and is spread by the fecal–oral route, saliva, or direct contact with blisters. In addition to blistering, symptoms include fever and loss of appetite. Treatments include reducing fever with OTC medications, rinsing the mouth with warm salty water, and increasing fluid intake. Hand washing, especially after diaper changes, washing and disinfecting toys, and disinfecting surfaces possibly contaminated by infected children help prevent reinfection.

ADOLESCENCE AND PUBERTY

Adolescence is the transition period between puberty and adulthood. It is divided into stages:

- Early adolescence—ages 12 to 14 years
- Middle adolescence—ages 15 to 17 years

Adolescence is a time of dramatic physical, emotional, and social changes. These changes bring with them choices and decisions that teens need to make on their own. During this time, teens derive an incredible amount of self-worth from physical appearance. This, in addition to peer pressure, has caused an increased number of eating disorders among adolescents.

Early Adolescence

Puberty marks the beginning of the development of secondary sexual characteristics: body hair, breasts, menstrual cycles, beard, voice changes, and muscle development. Adolescents begin to make their own choices regarding courses of study, sports, and friends. Peer pressure to use drugs, have sex, and drink alcohol increases. In urban areas, the threat of violence may be endured on a daily basis. Loosening of parental ties creates sources of conflict for both parents and teens. Eating disorders, depression, and family crises may be prevalent in this age group.

Medical assistants need to display empathy and compassion for this patient population. Young adolescents may pose difficulties in the medical office—being aloof, distant, or uncooperative. However, it is best for the MA to remember the time in his life when he was the same age and facing new (and sometimes scary) changes.

Emotional Changes

Socially, early adolescents become very concerned with body image, clothes, and how friends view them. They become more self-centered, moody, less affectionate toward parents, and more influenced by peer groups. Teens waver between having great expectations for themselves and experiencing total lack of confidence in their abilities. Risk taking is common among this group of teens, as they seek thrills of trying new and sometimes prohibited activities.

Middle Adolescence

Developmentally, girls are physically mature during middle adolescence. Boys may still be maturing. Body image is important, and often the primary concern, to these teens. Eating disorders may continue to develop among females and even males. Middle teens may be developing more individual opinions and a definite, unique personality. As middle adolescents grow during these years, they develop a clearer sense of identity; thus, they may not be as strongly influenced by their peers. Teens may start to assert independence, begin driving, and find employment.

Emotional Changes

During the middle teen years, conflicts with parents may decrease; these adolescents exhibit greater independence and a greater interest in the opposite sex. Middle teens spend more time with peers and less with parents and develop a greater capacity to develop more caring relationships. Acceptance by peers is incredibly important during this period of time, and middle teens thrive on positive affirmations and encouragement from both family and friends. They have a greater sense of right and wrong, more concern for the future, and better work habits. Some teens experience depression, which can lead to problems in all areas of their lives. See Box 39-3 for tips on parenting adolescents.

Eating Disorders

Eating disorders are prevalent among adolescents and teens. According to the National Association of Anorexia Nervosa and Associated Disorders, 95 percent of those with eating

> ### BOX 39-3 | Parenting Tips for Teen Years
>
> - Be honest and answer questions directly.
> - Take an interest in your children's friends and school activities.
> - Have family meal times as often as possible.
> - Respect the opinions of adolescents.
> - Encourage a healthy lifestyle, including proper nutrition and exercise.
> - Set clear-cut rules—and stick to them.
> - Know where your son or daughter is at all times, and be sure a responsible parent or guardian is present.
> - Talk about sex and drugs, and really listen to their questions and thoughts.

disorders are between the ages of 12 and 25. These disorders are categorized into four main types: anorexia nervosa, bulimia nervosa, binge eating disorder, and other specified feeding or eating disorders (OSFED), which was previously known as eating disorders not otherwise specified (EDNOS). Eating disorders are marked by extreme problems with eating behavior. The urge to eat smaller or, in some cases, larger amounts of food spins out of control.

Although females suffer more frequently than males, eating disorders in males are present in 5 to 15 percent of all patients with eating disorders. The National Institute of Mental Health (NIMH) reports that binge eating affects males and females equally. Some medical and psychological treatments, including family counseling, are effective for some eating disorders; however, no specific treatment is available for chronic cases.

Anorexia Nervosa

Anorexia nervosa is associated with a distorted sense of body image and the persistent quest for thinness, at times to the point of emaciation. Some anorexic patients lose weight by stringent dieting, or **purging** (by vomiting or taking laxatives, enemas, or diuretics). These patients often have coexisting psychiatric or physical illnesses. Signs of anorexia nervosa include the following:

- Extreme weight loss
- Excessively dry skin and brittle hair
- **Amenorrhea** (absence of menses)
- Low vital signs (particularly pulse and blood pressure)
- Fatigue
- Osteopenia or osteoporosis
- Electrolyte imbalance

Some patients recover after one episode, others have relapses, and still others have a chronic form that leads to health deterioration and, in some cases, death. Treatment includes psychotherapy, including family therapy or intensive inpatient or outpatient therapy. Antidepressant or anti-anxiety medications are also commonly used. Anorexia nervosa remains a difficult condition to treat because of the psychological link to the disease.

Bulimia Nervosa

Bulimia nervosa patients have behaviors characterized by binge eating and then using self-induced vomiting, laxatives, or diuretics (sometimes all three) to rid themselves of the large amounts of calories consumed. These patients commonly appear to be within the normal weight range for their age. Bulimic patients are secretive about their condition and often deny any problem with food. Episodes of binging and purging may occur several times a week. These patients generally have coexisting conditions such as depression, anxiety, and substance abuse problems. Bulimic patients exhibit some of the following symptoms:

- Chronic sore throat from vomiting stomach acids
- Worn enamel on teeth from stomach acids
- Dehydration
- Gastrointestinal reflux disorder (GERD)
- Intestinal irritation from laxative use
- Swollen neck glands

Treatment for bulimic patients includes nutritional and psychological counseling, treatment with fluoxetine (Prozac) or other antidepressants, appetite suppressants, and behavioral modification.

Binge Eating Disorder

In 2013, binge eating disorder (BED) was included as an official diagnosis in the *Diagnostic and Statistical Manual of Mental Disorders*, Fifth Edition (DSM-5). Before its inclusion, it was diagnosed as an eating disorder not otherwise specified (EDNOS). This eating disorder is characterized by binge eating episodes that happen all throughout the day, without preference to daytime or nighttime binging. The disorder is often associated with feelings of shame, guilt, depression, and other coexisting psychological disorders. Treatment is much the same as treatment for bulimia, including psychotherapy, antidepressants, behavior modification techniques, and the possible use of appetite suppressants.

Other Specified Feeding or Eating Disorder

Other specified feeding or eating disorder (OSFED) is a newer diagnosis that replaced the more commonly known eating disorders not otherwise specified (EDNOS). This eating disorder diagnosis is assigned to individuals who have eating disorders that cause significant levels of distress but don't qualify or meet all of the criteria for an exact eating disorder diagnosis. Within this category, there are five distinct subtypes of OSFEDs. These subtypes are atypical anorexia nervosa, bulimia nervosa, binge eating disorder, purging disorder, and night eating syndrome.

SUMMARY

The medical assistant should be prepared to function competently with pediatric patients of all ages. Medical assistants need an understanding of how to appropriately communicate with pediatric patients to develop a positive relationship with the child. Medical assistants should also be aware of childhood growth and development and diseases and disorders that are unique to the pediatric patient population. As a medical assistant, you must be able to accurately perform such procedures as obtaining vital signs on children, measuring children's height and weight, and assisting with all phases of the sick- and well-child examinations. Sensitive issues of suicide, eating disorders, and developmental problems should be handled with understanding, empathy, and an overall safeguarding of the patient's rights. Having contact information regarding community resources readily available to assist parents and caregivers is a vital part of the medical assistant's responsibility.

(39) CHAPTER REVIEW

COMPETENCY REVIEW

1. Define and spell the terms for this chapter.
2. List three important considerations regarding communicating with a pediatric patient.
3. Name three common carrying holds for an infant.
4. Describe the difference between well-child and sick-child visits.
5. Discuss how head circumference is measured.
6. Identify factors that are considered to contribute to the childhood obesity epidemic.
7. Explain how electronic health records (EHRs) change the medical assistant's role in the use of growth charts.
8. Describe the BRAT diet and when it is used.
9. Identify five risk factors for sudden infant death syndrome (SIDS).
10. Discuss why eating disorders are prevalent among adolescents and teens.

PREPARING FOR THE CERTIFICATION EXAM

1. The average infant doubles in weight
   a. at 3 months.
   b. at 3 years.
   c. at 1 year.
   d. at 6 months.
   e. at 2 years.

2. The Apgar scale is
   a. used to evaluate newborns.
   b. used to evaluate preteens.
   c. used to measure weight.
   d. a component of measuring body mass index.
   e. used to evaluate brain function.

3. Conditions such as microencephaly or hydrocephalus are evaluated by
   a. diameter of the infant's chest.
   b. the length of the infant.
   c. the weight of the infant.
   d. the size of the infant's limbs.
   e. the circumference of the infant's head.

4. A normal 10- to 12-month-old
   a. prefers to play alone.
   b. can wave bye-bye.
   c. cannot sit up.
   d. cannot say any words.
   e. can repeat two numbers in a row.

5. To reduce spread of infection in a pediatric waiting room,
   a. see well patients only on specific days.
   b. make ill patients wait in a hallway.
   c. place ill patients in an examination room as soon as possible.
   d. spray room with air freshener.
   e. raise heat to reduce germs.

6. Symptoms of dehydration in infants include
    a. bright and vibrant eyes.
    b. dry skin and loss of elasticity of skin.
    c. increased urine output.
    d. being energetic and alert.
    e. overproduction of tears.

7. The respiratory rate of an infant
    a. is lower than that of an adult.
    b. is the same as that of an adult.
    c. does not need to be measured until puberty.
    d. is higher than that of an adult.
    e. is measured by the parent.

8. Bulimia nervosa is an eating disorder that
    a. affects only males.
    b. is characterized by binging and purging.
    c. is curable with antibiotic medication.

    d. is characterized by extreme weight loss in all patients.
    e. is uncommon in adolescents and teens.

9. _____ leads to a distinctive barking cough and hoarseness.
    a. RSV
    b. Asthma
    c. Bronchiolitis
    d. SIDS
    e. Croup

10. An infant who scores under the third percentile on growth charts
    a. may be suffering from failure to thrive (FTT).
    b. may be gravely ill.
    c. must be reported to authorities.
    d. will reach normal weight at a year.
    e. may suffer from Fifth disease.

CRITICAL THINKING

Refer to the case study at the beginning of the chapter and use what you have learned to answer the following questions.

1. What is failure to thrive, and what problems could it cause the child?

2. What are some common causes of FTT in newborns and infants?
3. At age 6 months, what developmental skills should Keyla have mastered?

ON THE JOB

Sara, a 14-year-old, has come to the office for her school physical. She is very remote, moody, and unwilling to answer any questions you ask her as part of her physical exam. She seems to have changed a great deal in the past year, and is thinner, more unkempt, and lethargic. You notice also that her mother is constantly badgering her and rolling her eyes in exasperation at her lack of cooperation.

1. What could you do to facilitate the examination and improve communication with Sara?
2. What possible problems could Sara be experiencing?
3. What should you do about the concerns that you have for Sara?

INTERNET ACTIVITY

Research a childhood disease or disorder that interests you.

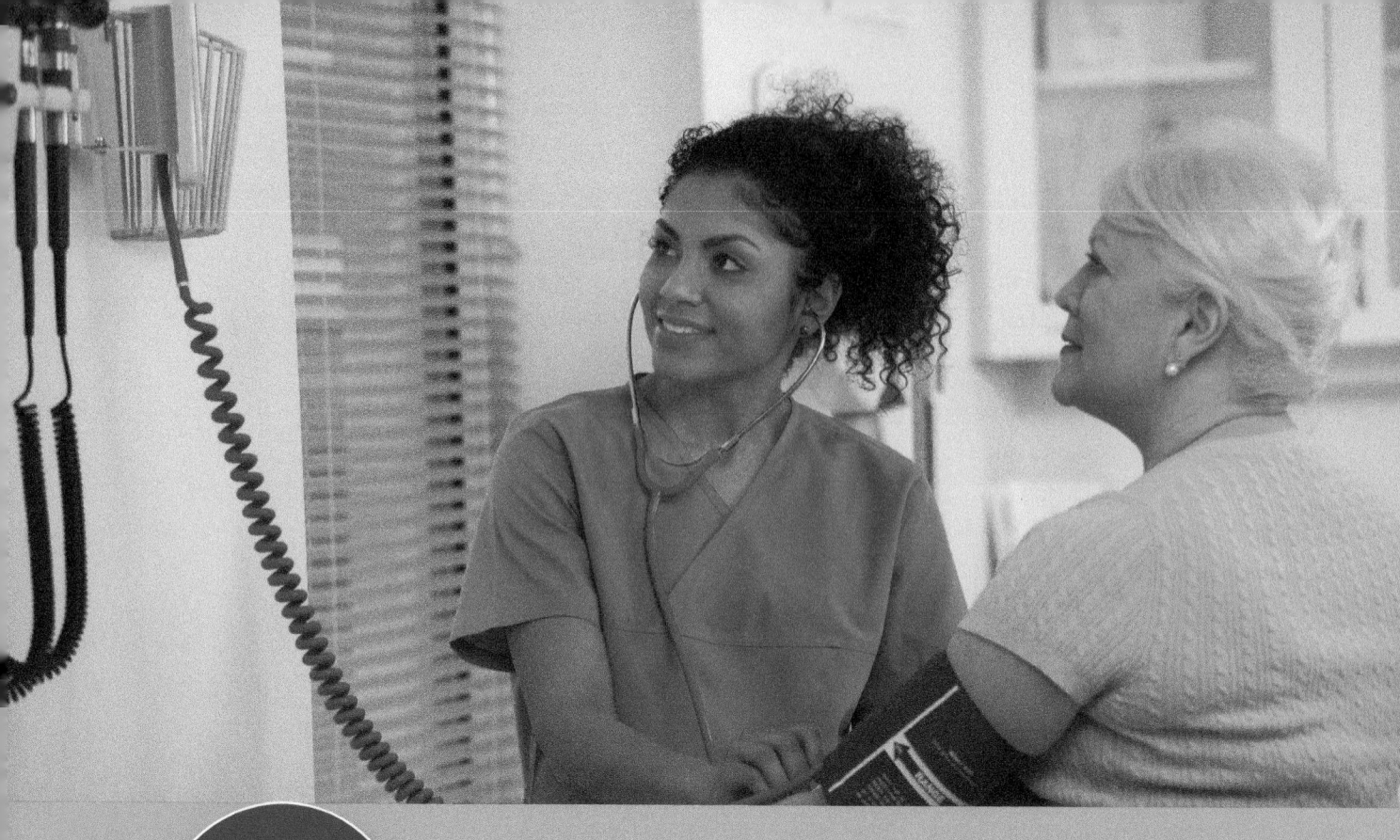

Assisting with Life Span Specialties: Geriatrics

Learning Objectives

After completing this chapter, you should be able to:

40.1 Define and spell the terms for this chapter.

40.2 Identify communication adaptations that are helpful with geriatric patients.

40.3 Explain how the aging population is impacting health care in the United States.

40.4 Describe how the aging process affects each system of the body.

40.5 Outline the cognitive changes that occur during the aging process.

40.6 Identify medicolegal issues of aging patients.

40.7 List six safety measures to recommend to caregivers of aging patients.

Shandra Wilkinson, an RMA at Pearson Physicians Group, is assigned to work with Dr. Penningworth today. The doctor's next patient is Sylvia Jordan, age 76, who is in the office for her annual physical. As Shandra escorts her to the examination room, Ms. Jordan confides that her husband of 54 years passed away seven months ago.

Terms to Learn

acute confusion	extended-care facilities	Medicare
advance directive	geriatrician	Medigap policy
ageism	geriatrics	osteoporosis
assisted-living facilities	gerontology	respite care
chronic confusion	long-term memory	sensory memory
cognitive ability	Medicaid	short-term memory

Geriatrics is the field of medicine specializing in the treatment and care of older adults. This term is derived from the Greek word *geras*, which means "old age," and from the word *iatrikos*, which means "physician." Geriatrics as a medical specialty began in the early 1900s. Dr. Ignatz L. Nascher wrote the first textbook geared toward this population in 1914, in which the term *geriatrics* was first used. A **geriatrician** is a physician who diagnoses and treats diseases and conditions that predominantly affect older adults, such as osteoarthritis, congestive heart failure, arthritis, emphysema, strokes, and Alzheimer's disease.

The United States is experiencing considerable growth in its older populations, largely because of the baby boomer generation, which is further discussed later in this chapter. **Gerontology**, the scientific study of the process of aging and its effects on people, will become even more important because of the widespread effect of the older adult population on health care and the health care community. Although there is no absolute definition of who or what is geriatric, the term generally refers to a person who is 65 years of age or older.

THE MEDICAL ASSISTANT'S ROLE IN GERIATRICS

As a medical assistant, you may work in a medical office or specialty that provides medical care to the geriatric population or a general practice that treats patients of every age.

This chapter covers differences you may encounter and should be aware of when providing care to older adults.

Surprisingly, older adults generally have fewer acute illnesses than younger adults. However, when older adults do become acutely ill, their recovery is much longer than that of a younger person. Chronic illness is the predominant issue for the geriatric population, and they generally take more prescription and over-the-counter (OTC) medications than younger populations. When the geriatric patient is seen in the medical office, it is often the medical assistant who is responsible for reviewing the medication list and verifying the dosages taken. It is necessary to allot extra time for a patient with extensive medication history. Rushing or hurrying through this step of patient care can result in obtaining inaccurate information or missing critical information—both of which could be detrimental to the patient's overall treatment plan.

Working with and providing care to the geriatric population requires special considerations. As a medical assistant, you will need to consider ways to support their physical and emotional needs during the medical visit. As a part of the body's aging process, which is discussed later in this chapter, patients may have decreased mobility and instability. You may need to provide additional assistance while escorting patients to the examination room or provide extra care when assisting them on or off the examination table.

Some of the physical problems associated with aging may cause patients to lose aspects of their independence. For instance, they may no longer be able to drive, take care of

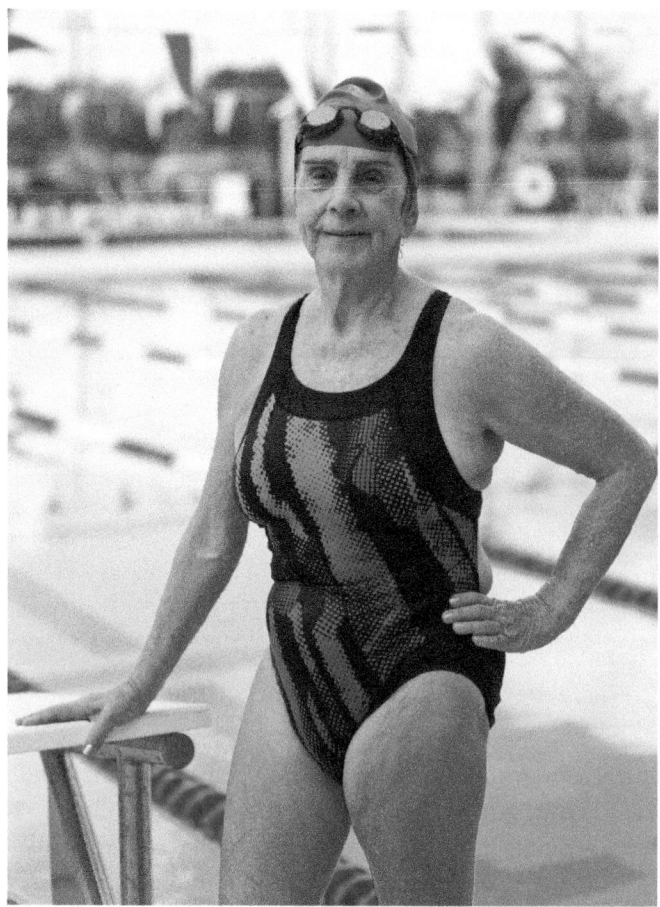

FIGURE 40-1 Many older adults have active lives well into their eighties and beyond.

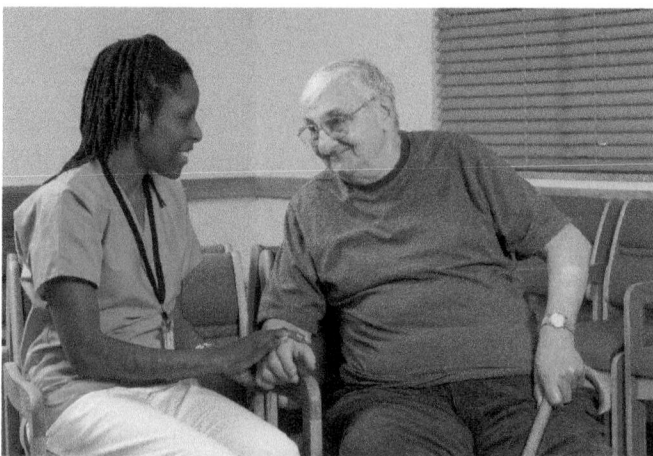

FIGURE 40-2 Effective communication skills are essential to the medical assistant's career.

certain household chores, feed or wash themselves, or live independently. However, keep in mind that older people vary widely in their state of physical and mental health. It is important not to assume or stereotype your older adult patient. Some patients will be quite ill, frail, or mentally disoriented at a relatively early age, whereas others will remain active and healthy into their eighties and beyond (Figure 40-1).

Effective Communication

It is critical to have a calm, relaxed, and respectful communication and interaction with the geriatric patient (Figure 40-2). As with all patients, effective communication is more likely to result in older patients adhering to treatment, expressing greater satisfaction with their treatment, and having better health outcomes. When communicating with geriatric patients, follow the basic principles of patient communication:

1. **Do not be hurried**—Not only will rushing through your tasks increase the risk for errors, it will also send a message of unimportance to the geriatric patient. All patients, regardless of their age, should be made to feel that ensuring their care and well-being is the most important task you are undertaking while working with them in the medical office. Allow extra time for older patients to follow directions and respond to questions. Do not finish sentences for older patients or ignore a patient by talking about him in front of family members or caregivers.

2. **Speak clearly and slowly**—Just as physically rushing is not acceptable, neither is rushing your speech and verbal communication. When you are providing instructions or asking questions, always speak slowly (though not so slowly as to cause offense) with clear enunciation. The words you use and information you are conveying should be clear and concise.

3. **Make eye contact**—Many geriatric patients consider eye contact a form of respect and confidence. This is important to consider because proper respect is of tremendous importance to many people in this age group. When you make eye contact, your disposition should be friendly and polite.

4. **Avoid pet names**—Establish respect right away by using formal language. Avoid using pet names, such as "sweetie," "honey," or "dear." Although these may be intended as affectionate or friendly terms, people of all ages, including and especially the geriatric demographic, may perceive it as disrespectful, demeaning, and patronizing. Patients may feel that they are being talked to as children rather than as competent adults.

Procedure 40-1 lists the proper steps to take when communicating with older adults.

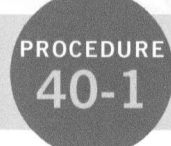

Communicating Effectively with the Older Adult Patient

Objective ◆ *Communicate effectively with an older adult patient in preparation for a physical examination.*

EQUIPMENT AND SUPPLIES

Patient's medical record; pen and paper; patient history form; examination table; gown and drapes; physical examination equipment, as needed

METHOD

1. When entering the reception area to call the patient back to the examination area, have a cheerful disposition and welcoming smile on your face.
2. Different offices may have different policies about how to address patients, whether by their first or last name. Follow the policy of your practice.
   a. Calling patients by their first name in the reception area—for example, "Jerry, we are ready to see you now"—protects their privacy by not revealing their last name. However, calling patients by their first name in the reception area or elsewhere may be considered disrespectful or rude, even though it is meant to protect privacy. The policy of your office may be to summon the patient this way: "Mr. Brown, we are ready to see you now."
3. Introduce yourself. Be sincere and polite. From this point on, address the patient using the title, "Mr.," "Mrs.," or "Miss." For example, "Hello, Mr. Timmons. My name is Robin. It's nice to see you this morning."
4. Escort the patient to the examination room. If the patient is using a walker or a cane, walk closely to the patient and offer assistance, if needed (Figure A).
5. Build rapport with the patient by making small talk while walking in the hallway or preparing items in the examination room. The tone of your voice must be sincere, not seemingly forced. You might say, "How are you this morning?" or "Are you dealing with this cold weather okay?"
6. Explain that you will be preparing the patient to see the physician for a physical examination or whatever procedure will be performed. Let the patient know what will be done and if anything will be expected of the patient during the appointment. For instance, "Mr. Timmons, before you see the doctor, I am going to gather some information about your health history and check your height and weight, as well as your blood pressure. After that, the doctor would like a urine sample for routine testing. I'll show you to the bathroom once we get to that point. Does that sound okay to you?"

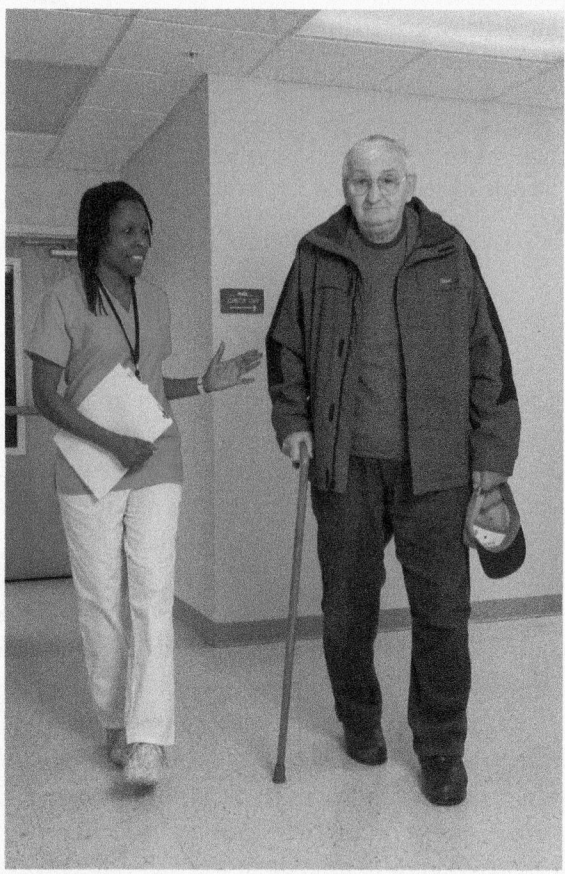

FIGURE A The medical assistant should provide assistance while promoting independence in patients.

7. Observe the patient for cues to indicate whether your remarks have or have not been understood.
   a. If it appears that the patient does not comprehend, paraphrase. Use other words and simple gestures.
8. Allow enough time for the patient to comprehend the information and ask any questions before continuing.
9. Observe the patient's overall physical ability to comply with your requests as you progress with preparing the patient for the examination or procedure.
10. Offer any assistance if it appears the patient needs it. However, allow the patient to do as much as possible independently.
11. Ask the patient to be seated while you begin to gather information for the patient history. If you think the patient would be unsteady sitting on the examination table for an

extended period of time, allow the patient to answer questions while seated in a chair in the examination room.

12. While taking the patient history, speak respectfully, and convey a feeling of warmth and empathy. If the patient's responses to questions become too lengthy, gently interrupt and bring the patient back to the subject.
    a. Never assume the patient is incapable of understanding you because she is old.

13. If answers to some of your questions seem incorrect or inappropriate, do not correct the patient. Gently distract the patient with another topic and proceed with your examination preparations.

14. If the patient exhibits mental confusion in regard to some of your questions, do not press the patient for immediate answers. Inform the physician and make note of questions that need clarification. A caregiver or family member may be able to help with these answers at a later time.

15. Do not leave the patient unattended if the patient is physically unstable or appears confused. Remember that relaxed body language, pleasant facial expressions, a gentle touch, and being personable are most important in caring for patients who are confused.

16. Document information appropriately in the patient's medical record. Keep in mind that opinions are never to be included, only objective information and observable facts.

CHARTING EXAMPLE

03/18/YY 11:00 A.M. While preparing the Pt. for his exam, he seemed confused about questions about previous surgeries. I assisted in helping remove his shirt and put on examination gown because he seemed unsteady. Overall, Pt. appeared cheerful..M. King, CMA

THE AGING POPULATION

Every culture has its own traditions in the way it views and treats older adults. Depending on cultural norms and beliefs, aging can be seen as undesirable and the older adult as a burden, or the older adult may be seen as a highly respected person with vast life experiences and wisdom.

In the United States, traditions and attitudes toward older adults have changed, in part because of our changing economic and social structures. Historically, older generations lived with their children or other relatives, and often relied on them economically until they died. However, the economic crisis of the Great Depression in the 1930s resulted in widespread unemployment, loss of savings and investments, and economic instability. As a result, individuals and families were forced to migrate to seek new job opportunities, often fragmenting and displacing families. This exposed the fragile and precarious nature of old age and emphasized the need for the government to create a system to address the economic, social, and health care needs of the geriatric population—a "safety net" for older adults.

As a response, the United States government enacted federal laws to provide services to older adults and others in need. One of these laws was the Social Security Act of 1935, which established a system of federal benefits to assist marginalized groups, including older adults. Later, the Social Security Act was amended to include the Older Americans Act (OAA). The intent of the OAA was to provide support and services to older adults that included in-home services, nutrition programs (e.g., meals on wheels, senior center group meals), and health promotion and disease prevention services.

In 1965, 30 years later, two amendments were made to the Social Security Act to meet the growing needs of the aging population as well as low-income individuals and families:

- **Medicare**—a medical insurance program to meet the needs of Americans aged 65 and older, as well as others with special health conditions, and administered by the federal government.

- **Medicaid**—a medical insurance program to finance health care for low-income individuals or those close to the public assistance level. This program is financed and administered by state governments with federal matching funds.

Retired and older adults living on limited incomes may be eligible for both Medicare and Medicaid.

In addition to the federally and state funded and administered insurance plans, Medicare and Medicaid, several private companies, such as the American Association of Retired Persons (AARP), offer a Medicare supplement insurance policy, commonly referred to as a **Medigap policy**. A Medigap policy helps offset some of the health care costs that Medicare does not cover, such as copayments, coinsurance, and deductibles.

In the United States today, many Americans are still working and enjoying an active social life well into their seventies, eighties, and nineties. Some older adults continue to thrive by finding new part-time or full-time jobs and careers, going back to school, and exploring new hobbies and activities (Figure 40-3). Box 40-1 lists some well-known people who were successful in their later years. As the number of older adults continues to increase, more attention must be given to the needs of the geriatric population in the

Patients from various cultures may have different views and beliefs about diseases, health care, and their own need for care. For example, some may be very private and may find the probing questions health care providers must ask inappropriate and rude. Patients may also follow traditional health practices that are a part of their culture before seeking help from a medical professional. Members of certain cultures may view their health status as God's will. Some consider good health as a reward for living well and taking care of their bodies, whereas being ill is a punishment for not living appropriately or having sinned.

As a medical assistant, you should not view the traditions of other ethnic or cultural groups as wrong or misguided; they merely may be different from your own. Patients should never be made to feel that their religious beliefs and cultural practices are undervalued, ridiculous, or not respected. An appreciation and respect for patients' cultural values and beliefs will help you better understand patients' behaviors and choices and, hopefully, improve their health outcomes.

BOX 40-1 | Success Later in Life

- Harlan Sanders, better known as Colonel Sanders, started Kentucky Fried Chicken when he was 65 years old.
- Laura Ingalls Wilder was 65 when she began writing the "Little House" series.
- Eleanor Roosevelt, wife of President Franklin D. Roosevelt, chaired the United Nations Commission on Human Rights from age 62 to 67 and wrote her autobiography at age 74.
- Nelson Mandela became president of South Africa at age 75 after 27 years in prison and winning the country's first multiracial election. He served as president until age 80.
- Benjamin Franklin was 81 when he signed the United States Constitution.
- Frank Lloyd Wright designed the Guggenheim Museum in New York City at age 91.
- Anna Mary Robertson ("Grandma") Moses, an American artist, started painting at age 75. She published her autobiography at age 91. In 1960, the Governor of New York proclaimed "Grandma Moses Day" on her one-hundredth birthday.

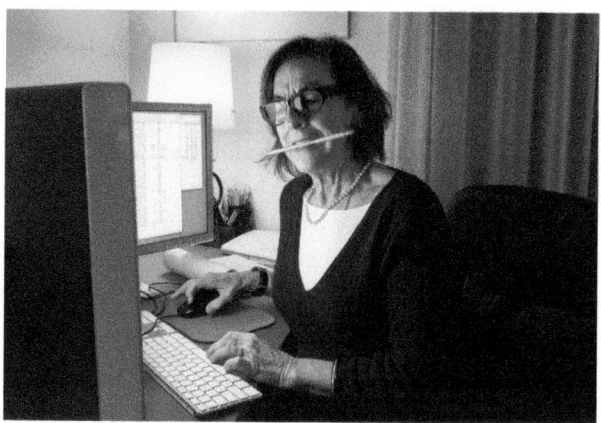

FIGURE 40-3 Many seniors pursue new careers, education, and hobbies well beyond what used to be considered retirement age—like this woman immersed in Internet research.

areas of health care, living conditions, and ensuring a high quality of life.

Life Expectancy

According to the United States Census Bureau, the country will experience a significant rate of growth in its older population. By 2050, the estimated population of older adults (ages 65 and over) will be more than 83.7 million, double what it was in 2012, and will comprise 20 percent of the population. Life expectancy is also increasing (Table 40-1) as a result of better living conditions and nutritional and medical advances,

new medications, and, most important, changes in health behaviors, such as quitting or never smoking and reducing obesity. Thanks in part to these advances, older adults are not only living longer, they are living healthier lives.

TABLE 40-1 | Life Expectancy at Birth for Men and Women

Birth Year	Life Expectancy (in years)
1900	47.3
1940	62.9
1950	68.2
1960	69.7
1970	70.8
1980	73.7
1990	75.4
1995	75.8
2000	76.8
2005	77.4
2010	78.3*
2015	78.9*
2020	79.5*

*Represents calculated projections.
Source: Centers for Disease Control and Prevention, National Center for Health Statistics, U.S. Census Bureau, National Vital Statistics Reports, 2012, *57*(14), Table 104.

As the population ages, older adults will require more health care resources as well as long-term care housing and services. Most older people try to live independently and in their own homes for as long as possible; others may not be able to live as independently and may require more and earlier support and services on a daily and/or long-term basis. Fortunately, a variety of housing options and types of care are available for older adults and their families. The nature of the options and services older adults may choose depends on individual needs, such as current living conditions and lifestyle choices, support services available, and cost. Many housing options for older adults provide room and board, social and recreational activities, and help with personal care and other activities of daily living (ADL), such as bathing or showering, dressing, eating, taking medications, and using the toilet.

There are variations in what these housing options are called and how they are licensed in individual states, but the following summarizes the types of housing options that are commonly available to older adults and the services they generally offer:

- **Assisted-living facilities**—These are group settings designed for residents who cannot live independently but do not require 24-hour care. These facilities offer a range of on-site support services, some social activities, and help with ADL, but no or limited medical care services.
- **Extended-care facilities**—These are facilities that provide 24-hour specialized care for residents who require a high level of medical care and assistance for complex medical conditions and/or treatment. Facilities in this category may include convalescent care, nursing or skilled nursing centers, and long-term care facilities. Residents typically share a room and are served meals in a central dining area unless they are too ill to participate. Many extended-care facilities have a separate wing or unit for residents with Alzheimer's disease or other types of dementia because these residents require specially trained staff and living environments that are secured or locked down to prevent residents from wandering off.

The Baby Boomer Generation

After World War II, when thousands of military personnel returned home, there was a significant increase in the birth rate, with more babies being born in 1946 than ever before: 3.4 million, 20 percent more than in the previous year. This was the beginning of the so-called "baby boom," with increased birth rates continuing for several more years. Individuals born between 1946 and 1964 are called "baby boomers." By the end of the "boom," almost 77 million babies had been born, comprising almost 40 percent of the nation's population at that time.

The oldest of the baby boom babies became senior citizens in 2011, and, every year for the following 19 years, roughly 3 million baby boomers will reach retirement age. By 2029, all surviving baby boomers will have reached senior citizen status. As a result, this boom in the aging population is drastically changing society, public policy, and health care.

Considerations for the Baby Boomer Generation

The baby boomers have several characteristics that tend to affect health care and your role as a medical assistant. The baby boomer generation in the United States generally had fewer children than previous generations or waited longer than previous generations to start a family. As a result, many baby boomers do not have the financial safety net and family support from grown children as previous generations.

Baby boomers are also often referred to as the "sandwich generation." Many boomers are facing the reality of caring for both aging parents and young children at the same time, and so are "sandwiched" between these generations and "sandwiched" between retirement and caregiving. Further, the baby boomers have not necessarily done as well as their parents in regard to education and financial stability.

The economic hardship many baby boomers are experiencing or will experience, combined with advancing age and deterioration of health, will mean an increased strain on government resources for health care and prescription drug assistance. As a medical assistant, you must be aware of the life circumstances of older patients, which may lead to stress and anxiety, and the health care decisions these patients may make.

THE AGING PROCESS: PHYSICAL CHANGES

The aging process is continuous, beginning at birth and ending at death. This process is not an illness but rather a normal part of life, progressing at different rates for each person. Factors that affect how the body ages include genetics, lifestyle choices, occupational hazards, nutritional choices, access to health care services, and an individual's physical and social environment.

Ageism is defined as a form of prejudice or discrimination against an individual or individuals because of their age. For most people, aging is not easy—physically, mentally, or emotionally. The older adult population faces further challenges because of the stereotypes and misconceptions many in society harbor about them. Your goal as a medical assistant

TABLE 40-2 | Physical Changes of Aging

Body System	Physical Changes
Integumentary	Hair loses color and becomes thinner; skin dries, becomes less elastic, and wrinkles develop; skin tears easily; skin bruises easily (senile purpura); fingernails and toenails thicken; reduced amount of sweat; increased sensitivity to cold; age spots more common.
Nervous	Problems with balance; temperature regulation becomes inconsistent; deep sleep is shortened; more awakening during the night; brain cells lost, but intelligence remains intact unless pathological condition present; decreased sensitivity of nerve receptors for heat, cold, pain, and pressure.
Sensory	More difficult to see close objects; night vision may decrease; cataracts (clouding of the lens) more common; peripheral vision and depth perception diminish; hearing diminishes; smell and taste receptors less sensitive.
Musculoskeletal	Less muscle strength; less flexibility; slower movements; arthritis and osteoporosis more common; body posture becomes stooped.
Respiratory	Breathing capacity lessens.
Urinary	Kidneys decrease in size; urine production less efficient; complete emptying of the bladder is more difficult; stress incontinence may develop.
Digestive	Primary taste sensations of salty, sweet, and sour decrease and appetite often decreases; constipation increases; flatulence increases; movement of food through the digestive tract slows.
Cardiovascular	Blood vessels less elastic and more narrowed; heart may not pump as efficiently; decrease in cardiac output and circulation.
Endocrine	Decrease in estrogen and progesterone; hot flashes; nervous feelings; higher levels of parathyroid hormone and thyroid-stimulating hormone; weight gain; insulin production less efficient; diabetes mellitus more likely.
Reproductive	*Females:* ovulation and menstruation cease; vaginal walls thinner and drier. *Males:* scrotum less firm; prostate gland may enlarge.

should be to view the aging adult as an individual. Provide each person the best possible health care, casting aside any preconceived thoughts or assumptions related to age.

Understanding the effects that the aging process has on the human body as a whole and on individual body systems will help foster a better awareness of the needs of the aging population. This awareness will help increase the respect and empathy with which care is provided to the individual older patient.

Physical Changes

Physical changes of aging for each body system are presented in Table 40-2. During the medical visit, document and report your observations to the physician if you notice new problems in the older patient to ensure immediate evaluation. Table 40-3 lists some diseases common in the older population.

Integumentary System

Integumentary system changes in older adults are often obvious. The skin becomes less elastic, drier, and more fragile. Advancing age is evidenced by wrinkles and sagging as well as "age spots" or "liver spots" in areas that have had excessive exposure to the sun.

Make sure the examining room is at the proper temperature and that sufficient coverings (drapes and blankets) are available to make the patient comfortable. Observe the patient's skin as you prepare the patient for the examination. Since pain receptors diminish with age, older patients may not be aware of an injury, particularly on parts of the body they are unable to see. Because adhesive bandages may damage the skin and cause chafing or wearing off during removal, select a type of bandage that will cause the least discomfort when it is removed.

Diabetes mellitus, a problem for many older adults, may impede the body's ability to heal. As a result, it is important to examine the patient's fingernails and toenails because the patient may not be able to keep them properly trimmed, resulting in cuts and infection. The patient may need to see a podiatrist (foot specialist) or have a specially trained nurse trim toenails to reduce chance of infection. It is common to ask older patients, particularly those diagnosed with diabetes,

TABLE 40-3 | Diseases Common to Older Adults

Disease/Condition	Explanation
Alzheimer's Disease and Other Dementias	Brain disorders that lead to progressive loss of memory and other cognitive functions.
Aortic Aneurysm	Dilation of the wall of the aorta that can rupture and lead to death if left untreated.
Atrophic Urethritis and Vaginitis	Thinning of the tissue of the urethra and vagina that can lead to burning with urination and painful intercourse.
Benign Prostatic Hyperplasia	Enlargement of the prostate gland, which blocks the flow of urine.
Cataracts	Clouding in the lens of the eye that impacts vision.
Chronic Lymphocytic Leukemia	A type of leukemia that usually has a long phase with little growth or progression (indolent phase) but may cause fever, fatigue, weight loss, night sweats, and abdominal pain.
Decubitus Ulcers (Bedsores)	Breakdown of skin from prolonged pressure on the same spot, often from remaining in the same position for a prolonged period of time.
Diabetes Mellitus Type 2	A type of diabetes usually associated with older age and obesity.
Glaucoma	Elevation of the pressure in one of the chambers of the eye that can decrease vision and lead to blindness, usually begins in middle age.
Heart Failure	Condition caused by various factors that damage the muscle of the heart. Some of these conditions include myocardial infarction, coronary artery disease, and cardiomyopathy.
Hypothyroidism	Thyroid gland is underactive and does not produce enough thyroid hormone, can eventually result in anemia, low body temperature, mental confusion, and heart failure.
Osteoarthritis	Degeneration of the cartilage that lines the joints, usually begins in middle age.
Osteoporosis	Loss of calcium from the bones that makes them fragile and leads to fractures.
Parkinson's Disease	Slow, progressive degenerative brain disease that leads to tremor, muscle rigidity, difficulty moving, and instability.
Pneumonia	Lung inflammation often caused by a viral or a bacterial infection.
Shingles (Herpes Zoster)	A reactivation of the dormant chickenpox virus that causes skin rash and nerve pain.
Stroke	A blockage or bleeding of a blood vessel in the brain that leads to weakness, loss of sensation, difficulty talking, or other neurological problems.
Urinary Incontinence	Inability to control urine flow.

to remove their shoes and socks in preparation for the physical examination.

Nervous System

With advanced age, nervous system function begins to slow and reaction times are delayed. (Cognitive ability and dementia are discussed later in this chapter.) Slower responses to changes in balance can make the older patient more prone to falls and injuries. Some older adults may also present with muscle tremors, also called essential or "senile tremors," particularly in the hands, which are associated with degeneration of part of the motor portion of the nervous system.

Offer your arm to patients when walking, and assist them on and off the examination table. Make sure the step stool is secure as patients get on and off the examination table. If you use a beam scale in your office, assist patients on and off the platform and provide wall-mount handgrips for additional support. The platform on this type of scale moves in multiple directions and can make patients lose their balance.

Sleep cycles are also affected by the aging of the brain. As people age, they tend to have a harder time falling asleep and more trouble staying asleep than when they were younger. Older adults may also have more fragmented sleep, meaning they wake up more often in the middle of the night and get less restful sleep. Some older adults take frequent naps during the day, which can affect their ability to sleep restfully at night, but can also make up for loss of sleep at night. Ask patients how they are sleeping, how many hours they sleep, and if they feel rested. Always make appropriate documentation in the patient's medical record regarding changes in the patient's overall sleep pattern.

Sensory Systems

Sensory changes in the eyes, ears, nose, and mouth affect older adults' ability to react to the world. Presbycusis (impairment of hearing associated with aging, especially with high-pitched sounds) and presbyopia (inability to focus on objects at close range) reduce older adults' ability to interact with the environment around them. As older patients prepare for their examination, inquire about hearing and visual abilities. If applicable, ask if their hearing aid is functioning, whether eyeglasses are helping them to see, and, if they still drive, how they react to the glare of lights at night.

Without being condescending, speak clearly and slowly enough so patients can understand you. Be aware that these questions and this subject may be sensitive to patients because they may be seen as calling their independence into question. Because most older adults dread losing their independence, they may be hesitant to answer these questions honestly, so be alert for both verbal and nonverbal communication cues, such as hesitation in answering these questions.

The senses of taste and smell begin to decline with age, especially after the age of 70. In fact, more than 75 percent of people over the age of 80 have reported major impairment of the sense of smell, which may result in the patient's decreased appetite and interest in food. In addition, older adults are sometimes called "tea and toasters," meaning that, instead of eating a nutritious, balanced meal, they will have just tea and toast or crackers during the day. This may result in poor nutrition and weight loss.

As another consequence of dulled senses, older adults may also over-salt or over-season their food to compensate for the reduction in taste and smell. Consuming too much salt in the presence of other disorders or dietary factors may have negative effects on kidney function, blood pressure, and cognition, especially in older patients. Proper eating can also be hindered by poor oral hygiene and side effects of certain medications. Engage older patients in a discussion of favorite foods and what they normally eat each day. Observe their teeth and oral hygiene and ask if they regularly visit a dentist. If they wear dentures, check that the dentures fit properly.

Musculoskeletal System

Aging of the musculoskeletal system is characterized by a decrease in muscle strength and muscle tissue, a loss of flexibility, and bone mass loss. Older adults will experience a steady reduction in physical strength, with the most rapid decline occurring after age 50. The cartilage surface of joints can also deteriorate, thus limiting joint movement or making moving painful. As they age, older adults may tend to stoop forward, with head tilted backward and hips, knees, and elbows flexed. This can lead to gait and stability problems,

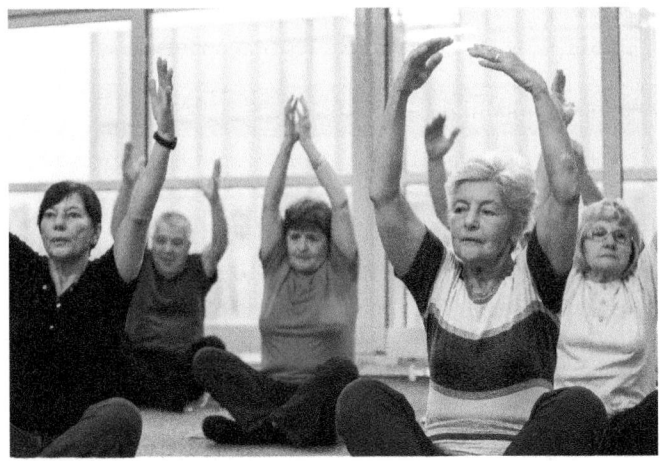

FIGURE 40-4 Group fitness activities geared toward senior citizens can improve their physical strength and promote socialization.

which increases the risk of falling and sustaining fractures. It is helpful to provide information about exercises to increase upper body strength that older adults can perform at home while seated (upper body strength is needed to help get up if you have fallen). You may also provide information about exercise classes that are appropriate for their age and ability. Often, local senior centers offer special exercise sessions, which may help improve strength as well as provide an environment for socializing (Figure 40-4).

Older adults are also at higher risk of bone fractures as a result of decreased bone density and mass. A condition known as **osteoporosis**, which means "porous bone," is the most common cause of bone loss in older adults. In osteoporosis, the bone is unable to rebuild or replace the bone loss that normally occurs, resulting in the bone having less density or mass (Figure 40-5). The bone becomes weak and brittle and may break from minor falls or trauma or even

OSTEOPOROSIS

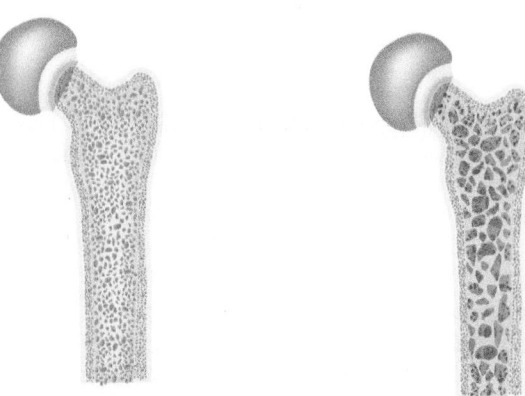

Normal Bone   Bone with Osteoporosis

FIGURE 40-5 Osteoporosis means "porous bone." Shown here a normal hip bone and a hip bone with osteoporosis. *(tigatelu)*

TABLE 40-4 | Risk Factors for Osteoporosis

Uncontrollable Risk Factors	Controllable Risk Factors
• Being over age 50 • Being female • Menopause or post menopause • Family history of osteoporosis • Low body weight or being small and thin • History of broken bones or height loss	• Not getting enough calcium and vitamin D • Not eating enough fruits and vegetables • Getting too much protein, sodium, and caffeine • Having an inactive lifestyle • Smoking • Drinking too much alcohol • Losing weight • Use of certain medications (e.g., corticosteroids)

simple actions, such as sneezing or bumping into furniture. The most commonly broken bones in osteoporosis are those of the hip, spine, and wrist.

Although osteoporosis can affect both sexes, women have four times the risk, especially white, Asian, and post-menopausal women. Bone loss begins after the age of 30 with symptoms commonly presenting after age 45 in women and age 55 in men. Bone loss in osteoporosis is often called "silent" because bone loss is gradual and often occurs without symptoms. People may not know that they have osteoporosis until a sudden strain, bump, or fall causes a bone to break, resulting in a trip to the hospital, surgery, and possibly a disabling condition or complications.

Fortunately, osteoporosis can often be prevented and treated if diagnosed early. The U.S. Preventive Services Task Force recommends screening for osteoporosis in women aged 65 years and older and in younger women who are at risk of fractures comparable to a 65-year-old white woman with no additional risk factors. There are a variety of factors—both controllable and uncontrollable—that put an individual at risk for developing osteoporosis. Table 40-4 lists the various risk factors for osteoporosis. Currently, there are no recommendations for men to be screened because of a lack of scientific evidence to support its benefit.

Several types of bone density screening tests use imaging to help diagnose osteoporosis. These screening tests are normally noninvasive and painless. Table 40-5 describes the different types of bone density screening tests.

Healthy lifestyle choices such as proper diet, exercise, and medications can help prevent further bone loss and reduce the risk of fractures. Encourage older patients to eat proper amounts of dairy products to supply the body's calcium need. Discuss safety issues at home that can put the older patient at risk and steps to minimize the risk such as removing furniture and area rugs. Speak to older patients about how they bathe: Do they have grab rails and chairs in the tub or shower area? Encourage them to use assistive devices as needed, such as a cane, walker, and bedside commode (portable toilet). If patients who need them do not have these assistive devices, check the office policy or discuss with the physician about prescribing them. Review safety concerns with caregivers and family members.

TABLE 40-5 | Screening Tests for Osteoporosis

Test	Description
Dual-energy X-ray absorptiometry (DXA)	Considered the most useful and reliable bone density test. DXA is a specialized kind of X-ray that provides precise measurements of bone density at specific bone sites (spine, hip, and forearm) with minimal radiation. DXA is the best at predicting who will have an osteoporotic fracture, at identifying who should be treated for osteoporosis, and at monitoring response to treatment.
Quantitative computerized tomography (QCT)	This is a type of computed tomography (CT) that provides accurate measures of bone density in the spine. Although this test may be an alternative to DXA, it is seldom used because it is expensive and requires a higher radiation dose.
Ultrasonography (US)	Ultrasound can be used to measure the bone density of the heel. This may be useful to determine a person's risk of fracture. However, it is used less frequently than DXA because of a lack of guidelines for diagnosing osteoporosis or estimating fracture risk. In areas that do not have access to DXA, ultrasound is an acceptable way to measure bone density.

Respiratory System

Respiratory system changes are characterized by loss of elasticity in the alveoli and lungs, leading to a reduction in gas exchange. In addition, as the respiratory muscles become weaker, it becomes more difficult to move air into and out of the lungs. Stridor, or breathing with a high-pitched sound, may also be observed. Inactivity in older adults, combined with reduced pulmonary function, make them more prone to pneumonia.

Provide videos and written materials on breathing exercises to help older patients with strengthening respiratory muscles and increasing their depth of breathing. Any activity that increases endurance, such as jogging or swimming laps, is beneficial in protecting older adults from respiratory infections and improving the oxygen supply to all body systems.

Urinary System

Urinary system changes that can occur with aging result in decreased kidney mass and renal function. There is a decline in blood flow to the kidneys, a decrease in the ability to concentrate urine, and a decrease in the reabsorption of glucose. The kidneys' slower rate of waste removal may affect the excretion of drugs from the body. As a result, drugs may stay longer in the system in older adults, who generally take a higher number of drugs than younger people, resulting in a higher risk for drug toxicity.

Older adults have decreased bladder storage capacity and an inability to empty the bladder completely, placing them at higher risk for urinary tract infections (UTIs). Increased frequency of urination and increased urgency may both become problems for many older adults. Urgency may make them feel reluctant to leave home for fear they may embarrass themselves by not making it to the bathroom in time. Nocturia (urinating during the night) may also be common in older adults, causing a disruption of sleep and making some patients tired and irritable. If the patient gets up to void during the night, the path to the bathroom should be kept clear of furniture or other obstacles, and a light should be kept on at night to prevent falls.

Professionalism **The Life Span**

Keep a small supply of adult-size absorbable undergarments or disposable incontinence pads available in your office for patient use. If you notice your patient is in need of these items, you can discreetly offer them so that the patient will be more comfortable and able to concentrate on the conversation with the health care provider.

Some patients may feel that reducing fluid intake is the way to cope with urination problems; however, this can lead to dehydration, electrolyte imbalance, and increased risk of constipation, blood clots, and UTIs. It is important to stress to the patient that a sufficient intake of water and other fluids is critical to maintain homeostasis in the body.

Digestive System

With age, the passage of food through the digestive tract is slower with less absorption of food, minerals, and vitamins and an increase in constipation and flatulence. Because liver function also slows with age, it takes longer for drugs and alcohol to be absorbed. This may cause older patients to increase their drug dose or drink more alcohol, causing an increased risk of adverse drug interactions and toxicity.

Esophageal motility is decreased and the esophagus tends to become slightly more dilated, which may increase the chances for aspiration. Encourage patients to be upright while eating or make sure the head of the bed is elevated, if they are unable to get out of bed.

Proper nutritional education can be helpful, especially in making healthy food and beverage choices from all five food groups. Provide patients with a brochure to take home that shows a diagram of foods in each food group, as well as appropriate portion sizes and amounts to eat within each group. If it is obvious that an older patient is struggling with nutrition issues, a consultation with a registered dietitian may need to be scheduled.

Cardiovascular System

Age-related cardiovascular changes increase the risk of disease and disorders in older patients. Lifestyle habits such as smoking, high-fat diets, and lack of exercise also take a toll on the cardiovascular system. Cardiac output and the amount of oxygen supplied to organs of the body decrease as a result of the aging heart muscle and other conditions, such as hypertension.

Orthostatic hypotension may occur in some older patients. Orthostatic hypotension is a 20 to 30 mmHg drop in blood pressure that is associated with dizziness and fainting when changing positions, commonly from lying down or sitting to a standing position. Dizziness can increase an older patient's risk of falling and injury. The medical assistant should help the patient understand why this may happen and emphasize the importance of slow and controlled movements, assisted by holding on to stable objects to prevent or decrease dizziness and increase stability.

Endocrine System

Endocrine system aging is characterized by decreasing levels of estrogen, thyroid hypofunction, and insulin resistance. The decrease of estrogen in females ends menstrual cycles, decreases vaginal secretions, and may lead to hot flashes, night sweats, and sleep disturbances. Thyroid hypofunction can lead to patients being overweight, fatigued, and confused, which may be mistaken for dementia. As noted earlier, many older adults develop diabetes mellitus and need nutrition counseling, daily monitoring of blood sugar levels, and lifestyle changes. Older patients should have routine blood work performed to screen for endocrine system dysfunctions.

Reproductive System

Despite popular belief, people's sexual activity patterns and libido tend to be consistent over their life span, including during old age. However, older patients may find it difficult and embarrassing to discuss anything related to sex and sexual matters. Specifically, male patients may struggle with erectile dysfunction and find it difficult to discuss this topic with the medical assistant. For female patients, problems may include vaginal dryness and inelasticity, preventing intercourse or making it painful. Sexual health should be discussed with patients, regardless of age. The medical assistant must be ready to discuss these issues comfortably and without judgment. Written materials for the patient to read at home are important educational tools and may be helpful in beginning the conversation.

THE AGING PROCESS: MENTAL CHANGES

Mental deterioration is not a normal part of aging, contrary to what many people think. However, the risk for certain changes in mental functioning increases with age.

Mental health is the capacity to cope effectively with life changes, manage life's stresses, and achieve a state of emotional balance. Brain function slows with aging; however, many factors may have an impact on a patient's mental status. To maintain good mental health, individuals must participate in activities they find interesting and engage in regular social interactions. For optimal mental health, older adults should have a sense of self-worth and feel they are of value to society.

Cognitive Ability

Cognitive ability, or the ability to think clearly, reason, and perceive, is affected by many factors. The psychologic status of the mind is altered by overall health, genetics, social

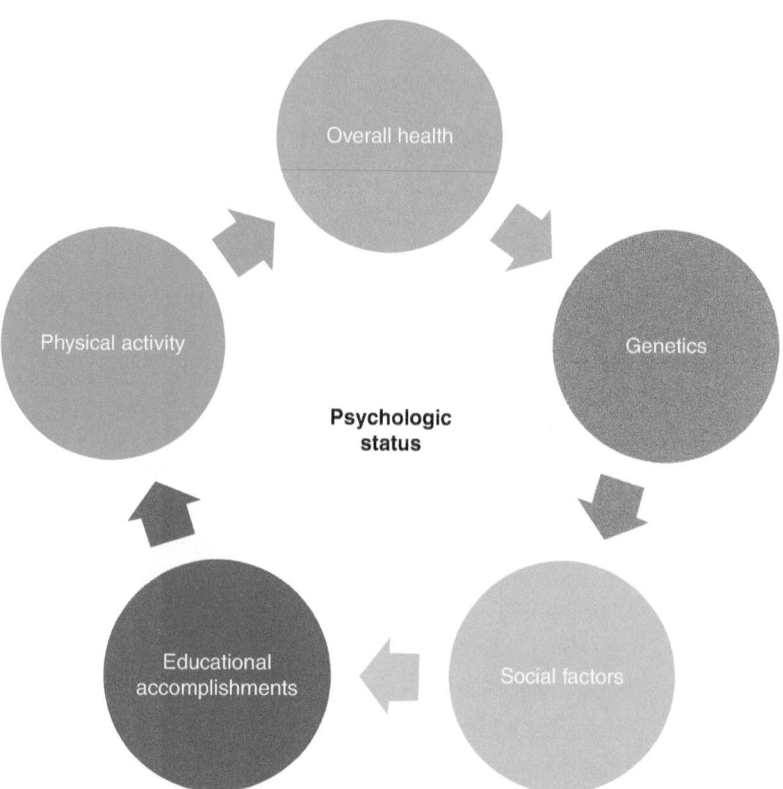

FIGURE 40-6 A patient's cognitive ability depends on psychologic status, which is influenced by multiple factors.

factors, educational accomplishment, and physical activity (Figure 40-6). Normal aging does not reduce cognitive ability. Basic intelligence is unchanged throughout the life span, as are the abilities for verbal comprehension, arithmetic operations, and problem solving. Learning is not altered by aging. However, with increasing age, more time may be needed for problem solving. Keeping the brain active with mentally challenging work, taking some interesting courses, and even engaging in games, puzzles, and other types of mental stimulation help maintain memory retrieval (Figure 40-7).

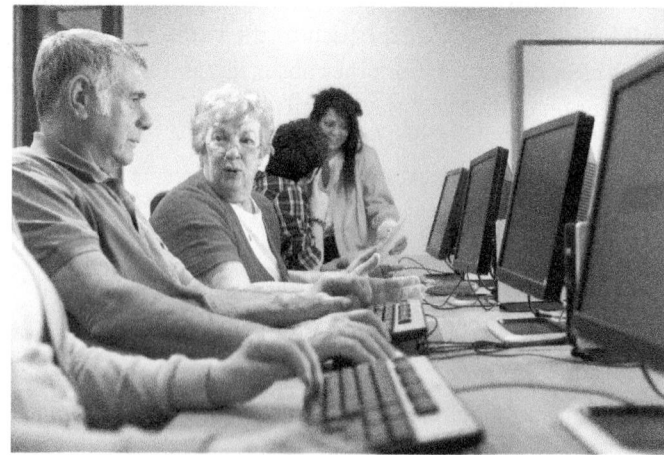

FIGURE 40-7 Taking an interesting course can help keep your brain active. These seniors are taking a class in information technology (IT).

Normally, an individual's personality does not change with age unless there is a pathological problem or a life event has altered the individual's attitude, such as retirement, loss of independence, or loss of a spouse.

Memory

Memory may be altered with age. There are three types of memory: **short-term memory** (things that can be recalled for about 30 seconds or so but, if not repeated multiple times, will fade from memory, such as the name of a one-time acquaintance at a party); **long-term memory** (memories that have been activated multiple times and committed to the brain); and **sensory memory** (information gained through the senses and lasting a few seconds). Aging does not mean that a loss of memory in older adults is inevitable, although the ability to retrieve information from long-term memory may be slower with age.

Sleep is equally important to memory. Studies have shown that memories and information are consolidated during sleep and that insufficient physical rest delays the brain's response time. Activities, such as knitting and crocheting, stimulate the brain. In addition, physical exercise increases oxygen flow and helps maintain blood supply to the brain, improving memory function. The expression "use it or lose it" could apply to the brain, as well as other muscles. Medical assistants should encourage patients to exercise both their physical body and their mind.

It is important to assist the patient who has true memory loss to remain as active and self-sufficient as long as possible. Tips to assist these patients could include placing notes in specific locations to trigger memory, such as a note by the door prompting individuals to remember their keys. You might also recommend safety precautions, such as an audible device that chimes if a window is left open or a stove with automatic shut-off burners.

Although there are many types of memory loss, people with memory loss often struggle in four common areas: (1) recalling the distant past; (2) processing new information; (3) remembering people's names; and (4) separating fact from fiction. The following are suggestions that may aid the patient dealing with memory loss:

- **Recalling distant memories**—Caregivers can review the patient's souvenirs, pictures, and movies. Looking at pictures and memorabilia often helps jog a patient's distant memory.

- **Retaining new information**—Keep new information short, and repeat it frequently. If the information has more than three steps, break those steps into smaller segments so they can be learned individually. Provide patients with written instructions if multiple steps are necessary for daily patient care.

- **Remembering people's names**—Consistently reintroduce yourself and your intentions (e.g., when you leave the examination room and come back, when the caregiver at home steps away, or any time there is a lapse in visual contact).

- **Separating fact from fiction**—It is important to correct the patient in a nonthreatening manner if there is an obvious error. For instance, a patient might say he does not take any medications despite there being a documented list in the patient's medical record.

Effect of Medications on Mental Abilities

Sometimes a medication may impair mental abilities, especially if the medication is taken in the wrong amount, at the wrong time, or if a dosage is missed. More than half of older patients take five or more medications a week, which include both prescription and OTC preparations, such as vitamin and mineral supplements and herbal products.

The following guidelines can help the patient be more careful and compliant with daily medications:

- Provide the patient with a pill organizer. Pill organizers are divided into days of the week, and some have compartments that are further divided into morning, afternoon, evening, and bedtime (Figure 40-8).

- Provide a printed list of medications the patient is currently taking. As discussed earlier in the chapter, it is vitally important that you thoroughly review the patient's medication list at each appointment. With the advance of electronic medical records, tracking and monitoring patients' medication lists has become a much easier task. A simple click of the "print" button at the end of the patient appointment will provide the patient with the most updated list of medications, including dosages and frequency of administration.

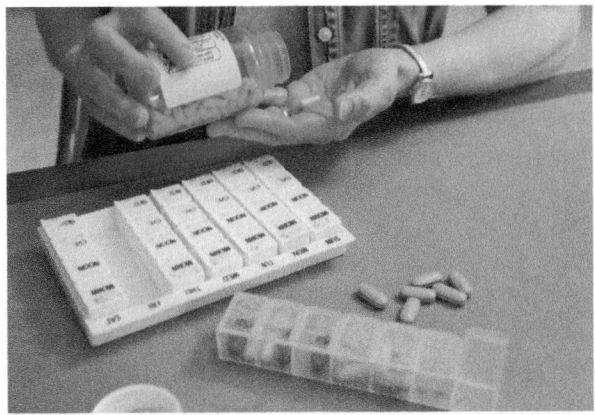

FIGURE 40-8 Pill organizers can help reduce confusion and ensure that medications are taken at the appropriate times on the correct days.

- Explain why the patient is taking each of the medications. It is helpful to include this information on the printed medication list as well.
- Provide verbal and written warnings about possible food and drug interactions.

Caregivers should be provided with these aids if the patient is not competent.

Confusion

Confusion is a term used by physicians and health care providers to indicate that the patient cannot easily follow a conversation, answer questions appropriately, understand where she is, remember important facts, or make appropriate safety judgments. Confusion is not a normal consequence of aging. Confusion is a broad term that can mean an acute or chronic condition. **Acute confusion** is a form of confusion with symptoms lasting less than three months. **Chronic confusion** is characterized by symptoms persisting longer than three months.

Confusion can be further divided into three categories:

- **Systemic confusion**—occurs when normal brain functions or the metabolic processes of the brain are interrupted by factors that are reversible, such as spikes or drops in blood glucose.
- **Mechanical confusion**—occurs when a sudden physiological change in the brain's functioning takes place, such as a stroke or traumatic injury.
- **Psychosocial/environmental confusion**—occurs with a sudden change of the environment, such as the loss of a life partner or a move to a different residential setting.

If confusion is demonstrated by a patient, the cause must be determined. However, pinpointing the exact cause may

---

JUDGMENT CALL

Joseph Rowe, 87 years old, arrives for his appointment with Dr. Black. He needs assistance with walking in the hallway because he is unsteady on his feet. He admits that he forgot his glasses at home and "needs some extra help today." His daughter, Sylvia, usually brings him to all of his appointments, but she is not with him today. When asked how Mr. Rowe is getting home today after his appointment, he replies, "I'm driving myself, of course. That's how I got here in the first place."

You immediately think that perhaps Mr. Rowe should not be driving himself home, but what can you do about it? How might you handle this situation?

---

be difficult and may only be determined by ruling out or eliminating other possible causes.

The most common cause of acute-onset confusion in older adults is a UTI. In general, older adults do not present with the typical symptoms of a UTI, such as urinary frequency, burning, and difficulty emptying the bladder. Often, acute mental confusion is the first and only symptom. The confusion will resolve without lasting, permanent damage as soon as the infection has been treated. Family members of the confused individual will often be relieved at the quick diagnosis and recovery but also alarmed by the onset of symptoms.

Sundowner Syndrome

Sundowner syndrome is a term used to describe the type of confusion occurring in patients with Alzheimer's or other forms of dementia after sundown or at night. (Alzheimer's and dementia are both discussed later in this chapter.) It tends to be present more often in those with cognitive impairments. Factors that may increase the incidence of sundowner syndrome include disruption of routine, such as a hospital admission, unfamiliar surroundings, a disturbance in sleep patterns, use of restraints, or excessive sensory stimulation (leaving lights on all night or excessive noise). In the morning, symptoms of confusion subside. Surrounding the patient with familiar objects, establishing a routine, and controlling room lighting, temperature, and noise level may relieve the problem.

Depression

Depression is one of the most common reasons for a medical visit. Depression is defined by the American Medical Association as "an abnormal and persistent mood characterized by sadness, melancholy, slowed mental processes, and changes in eating and sleeping habits." Medical depression is confirmed if these five symptoms have been present daily for at least two weeks.

Depression is often overlooked in older adults or misdiagnosed as part of another problem, such as dementia. Life changes may also overwhelm the aging person, causing depression that can worsen with some medication interactions.

Many medical providers use the geriatric depression scale (GDS) form to aid in the diagnosis of depression (Box 40-2). Developed in 1982 by J. A. Yesavage and others, the GDS is often used as part of a comprehensive geriatric assessment because of its ease of use and established validity and reliability. However, the results of the GDS test should not be used as the sole basis of a diagnosis of depression. If the results of the GDS questions indicate possible depression, the physician then usually refers the patient for a comprehensive psychiatric diagnostic workup.

BOX 40-2 | Geriatric Depression (Mood Assessment) Scale

1. Are you basically satisfied with your life?
2. Have you dropped many of your activities and interests?
3. Do you feel that your life is empty?
4. Do you often get bored?
5. Are you hopeful about the future?
6. Are you bothered by thoughts you can't get out of your head?
7. Are you in good spirits most of the time?
8. Are you afraid that something bad is going to happen to you?
9. Do you feel happy most of the time?
10. Do you often feel helpless?
11. Do you often get restless and fidgety?
12. Do you prefer to stay at home, rather than going out and doing new things?
13. Do you frequently worry about the future?
14. Do you feel you have more problems with memory than most?
15. Do you think it is wonderful to be alive now?
16. Do you often feel downhearted and blue?
17. Do you feel pretty worthless the way you are now?
18. Do you worry a lot about the past?
19. Do you find life very exciting?
20. Is it hard for you to get started on new projects?
21. Do you feel full of energy?
22. Do you feel that your situation is hopeless?
23. Do you think that most people are better off than you are?
24. Do you frequently get upset over little things?
25. Do you frequently feel like crying?
26. Do you have trouble concentrating?
27. Do you enjoy getting up in the morning?
28. Do you prefer to avoid social gatherings?
29. Is it easy for you to make decisions?
30. Is your mind as clear as it used to be?

This is the original scoring for the scale: One point for each of these answers. Cutoff: normal-0–9; mild depressives-10–19; severe depressives-20–30.

1. no	6. yes	11. yes	16. yes	21. no	26. yes
2. yes	7. no	12. yes	17. yes	22. yes	27. no
3. yes	8. yes	13. yes	18. yes	23. yes	28. yes
4. yes	9. no	14. yes	19. no	24. yes	29. no
5. no	10. yes	15. no	20. yes	25. yes	30. no

http://www.stanford.edu/~yesavage/GDS.english.long.html

It is beneficial to maintain a good rapport with older patients so they feel comfortable enough to speak to you. You can detect changes in their mental state, making you a more valuable member of the patient's health care team.

Dementia

Dementia is not a specific disease, but describes a syndrome marked by progressive loss of memory and decline in mental abilities that interferes with daily life. It can occur at any age, but more frequently it is found in older adults. Although dementia may affect people of all ages, more than 7 percent of people over age 65 are diagnosed with dementia. The onset is usually slow and progressive and, because behavioral changes are subtle at first, it may be difficult to detect and diagnose. Like confusion, dementia is not a normal consequence of aging. However, dementia is usually irreversible unless caused by a treatable condition such as electrolyte imbalance or thyroid dysfunction.

Dementia differs from normal age-related forgetfulness. An older person may misplace keys or fail to remember a person's name, whereas a dementia patient forgets what keys are used for or fails to recognize another individual at all. There are more than 70 types of dementia, of which the following are the most common causes:

- Alzheimer's disease
- Stroke
- Parkinson's disease
- Brain tumor
- HIV/AIDS
- Multiple sclerosis
- Drug and alcohol abuse.

Alzheimer's disease accounts for 60 to 80 percent of all cases of dementia.

Professionalism The Workplace

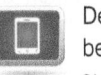

Dealing with a dementia patient in the office can be challenging. The patient must be kept in safe surroundings with someone always observing the patient's activities. Following a simple routine within the office may be helpful. Always tell patients what you are going to do and what to expect next, although they may not always comprehend your information. Sometimes using tactics of diversion and distraction, such as directing attention to something else, works to relieve tension. Keep in mind that the dementia patient cannot control impulses. Allow the patient to maintain dignity, knowing that no one really knows what is going on in the patient's mind. On the other hand, the patient may be uncooperative and maybe even violent. In this case, the physician must decide whatever precautions must be taken when dealing this patient.

Signs and Symptoms of Dementia

In patients with dementia, symptoms gradually worsen at different rates over a period of time. The first sign of dementia is usually forgetfulness regarding recent events or places. The patient has difficulty learning new information and may ask repetitive questions. The patient may forget what he or she is doing while in the middle of the task. The patient may forget the correct words for everyday objects, have difficulty with time orientation, and misplace items or put them in an inappropriate place. Often, the patient will show a lack of emotion or have mood swings, and will demonstrate lack of initiative or show disinterest in something he previously loved to do. As dementia progresses, patients become unable to follow conversations, unable to perform activities of daily living, and eventually become bedridden as brain function continues to deteriorate. Dementia can eventually lead to death.

Treatment for Dementia

Treatment for dementia depends on the cause. If there is an underlying disease or disorder, it must first be treated. Medications such as antipsychotics, mood stabilizers, and stimulants may be used to treat behavior-related issues associated with dementia.

Alzheimer's Disease

Alzheimer's disease (AD) is a progressive disorder of the central nervous system that eventually destroys mental capacities. It occurs more frequently in older adults and accounts for the majority of cases of dementia. There is no definitive cause for this disease, although genetic factors do play a role, particularly if a brother, sister, or parent suffered from AD. Abnormal changes in the brain of patients with AD have been found, such as plaques (deposits of protein fragments) and tangles (twisted protein fibers) that may be damaging and killing nerve cells in the brain.

In the United States, there are more than 5 million people with AD, almost all of them over the age of 65 and almost two-thirds of them women. The number of Americans with Alzheimer's disease and other dementias will grow each year as the size and proportion of the U.S. population age 65 and older continue to increase. The cost of caring for people with AD and other dementias is more than $226 billion and may reach $1.1 trillion as the older adult population increases.

Signs and Symptoms of Alzheimer's Disease

AD can have a devastating effect on family members as well as on the patient. One of the first signs of AD is loss of memory. Although there is a normal loss of some memory as people age (forgetting dates, names, and telephone numbers), the memory loss with AD is profound. As the disease progresses, a patient may not remember where home is or who family members are. The toll of caring for a family member with AD can be emotionally, physically, and financially devastating.

Medical assistants must recognize the symptoms of AD and other forms of dementia so they may be proactive in providing assistance to patients and caregivers. Box 40-3 lists some of the common warning signs of AD.

There are three general stages of AD: mild (early-stage); moderate (middle-stage); and severe (late-stage). Because

---

BOX 40-3 | Alzheimer's Warning Signs

1. Memory loss that disrupts daily life. Forgetting recently learned information is one of the most common early signs of AD. A person begins to forget more often and is unable to recall the information later.
    What's normal? Forgetting names or appointments occasionally.
2. Difficulty performing familiar tasks. People with AD may often find it hard to plan or complete everyday tasks. Individuals may lose track of the steps involved in preparing a meal, placing a telephone call, or playing a game.
    What's normal? Occasionally forgetting why you came into a room or what you planned to say.
3. Problems with language. People with AD often forget simple words or substitute unusual words, making their speech or writing hard to understand. For example, they may be unable to find or ask for a toothbrush, and instead ask for "that thing for my mouth."
    What's normal? Sometimes having trouble finding the right word.
4. Disorientation to time and place. People with AD can become lost in their own neighborhood, forget where they are and how they got there, and not know how to get back home.
    What's normal? Forgetting the day of the week or where you were going.
5. Poor or decreased judgment. Those with AD may dress inappropriately, wearing several layers on a warm day or little clothing in the cold. They may show poor judgment, like giving away large sums of money to telemarketers.
    What's normal? Making a questionable or debatable decision from time to time.
6. Problems with abstract thinking or problem solving. Someone with AD may have unusual difficulty performing complex mental tasks, like forgetting what numbers are for and how they should be used.
    What's normal? Finding it challenging to balance a checkbook.

BOX 40-3 | Alzheimer's Warning Signs (*continued*)

7. Misplacing things. A person with AD may put things in unusual places: an iron in the freezer or a wristwatch in the sugar bowl.

   What's normal? Misplacing keys or a wallet temporarily.

8. Difficulty with spatial and visual relationships. Someone with AD may have difficulty in judging distance and determining color or contrast. They may pass a mirror and think someone else is in the room.

   What's normal? Vision changes caused by cataracts or glaucoma.

9. Changes in mood. The mood of people with AD can change dramatically. They may become extremely confused, suspicious, fearful, or dependent on a family member.

   What's normal? People's mood can change, but is there a pathological problem causing the change?

10. Loss of initiative. A person with AD may become very passive, sitting in front of the TV for hours, sleeping more than usual, or not wanting to do usual activities.

    What's normal? Sometimes feeling weary of work or social obligations.

Someone with Alzheimer's Disease Symptoms

Forgets entire experiences

Rarely remembers later

Is gradually unable to follow written/spoken directions

Is gradually unable to use notes as reminders

Is gradually unable to care for self

Someone with Normal Age-Related Memory Changes

Forgets part of an experience

Often remembers later

Is usually able to follow written/spoken directions

Is usually able to use notes as reminders

Is usually able to care for self

Source: © 2009 Alzheimer's Association. All rights reserved. *This is an official publication of the Alzheimer's Association but may be distributed by unaffiliated organizations and individuals. Such distribution does not constitute an endorsement of these parties or their activities by the Alzheimer's Association.*

AD affects people in different ways, each patient experiences symptoms or progress differently. Table 40-6 describes the different stages of AD.

Diagnosis of AD is made by ruling out or eliminating other causes of dementia. A patient who is suspected of having AD should have a complete physical examination, a

TABLE 40-6 | Stages of Alzheimer's Disease (AD)

Stage	Description
Mid-AD **(early-stage)**	• Problems coming up with the right word or name • Trouble remembering names when introduced to new people • Having greater difficulty performing tasks in social or work settings • Forgetting material that has just been read • Losing or misplacing a valuable object • Increasing trouble with planning or organizing
Moderate AD **(middle-stage)**	• Forgetfulness of events or about own personal history • Feeling moody or withdrawn, especially in socially or mentally challenging situations • Being unable to recall their own address or telephone number or the high school or college from which they graduated • Confusion about where they are or what day it is • The need for help choosing proper clothing for the season or the occasion • Trouble controlling bladder and bowels in some individuals • Changes in sleep patterns, such as sleeping during the day and becoming restless at night • An increased risk of wandering and becoming lost • Personality and behavioral changes, including suspiciousness and delusions or compulsive, repetitive behavior like hand wringing or tissue shredding
Severe AD **(late-stage)**	• Require full-time, around-the-clock assistance with daily personal care • Lose awareness of recent experiences as well as of their surroundings • Require high levels of assistance with daily activities and personal care • Experience changes in physical abilities, including the ability to walk, sit and, eventually, swallow • Have increasing difficulty communicating • Become vulnerable to infections, especially pneumonia

blood profile, a thorough medical and family history, an MRI, and a PET scan. After possible causes are ruled out, such as thyroid and medication, the patient should be given the Mini Mental Status Exam (MMSE), a frequently used screening tool that evaluates the patient's mental status. The MMSE requires 5 to 10 minutes and consists of a series of tasks to evaluate the patient's recall, writing, and math skills. If the patient scores lower than expected for the patient's age, more extensive testing should be ordered. A significant portion of the AD and dementia diagnosis depends on symptoms often reported by family members or caregivers.

Initially, dementia patients may try to cover up forgetfulness or inabilities and may be unwilling to accept that they are having difficulties. This display of denial is understandable, because patients may fear the diagnosis and prognosis, loss of independence, and the emotional toll that will be placed on their family members.

Treatment for Alzheimer's Disease

Although there has been much advancement in our understanding of AD through research, there is currently no cure. There is also no treatment to recover any of the mental functions that have already been lost with AD and to prevent the loss of more functions in this progressive disease. However, there are medications that have been able to reduce the symptoms, such as memory loss and confusion, for a period of time. Two main classes of drugs are used in managing AD: cholinesterase inhibitors (Aricept, Exelon, Razadyne) and memantine (Namenda).

Patients with AD should not drink alcohol, which can worsen the symptoms of AD. Some depressed AD patients may benefit by taking antidepressants in the early stages. Creating a soothing home environment, avoiding criticism, and avoiding constantly correcting errors may help reduce the stress for AD patients (Figure 40-9).

Community resources can assist patients and caregivers in getting support and help to deal with the complex circumstances caused by Alzheimer's disease. Support groups can often help the caregivers establish contact with others in a similar situation, and can provide coping strategies that have worked for others with family members who have AD. Many caregivers provide 24-hour care with no outside help for extended periods. This often leads to caregiver burnout and, in some cases, may result in elder abuse. Helping caregivers obtain **respite care**, which is a temporary relief to individuals or families caring for a family member with AD (or other chronic condition), allows time for relaxation and can be of great assistance. Respite care can help caregivers relieve the extraordinary

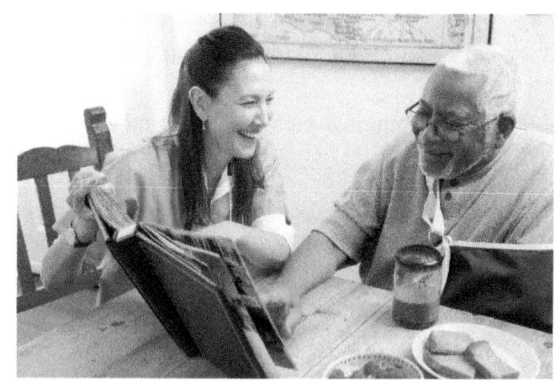

FIGURE 40-9 Soothing environments and familiar objects can help reduce behavioral problems with some dementia patients.

demands of this disease. Refer to Box 40-4 for a list of elder care resource phone numbers.

LEGAL AND MEDICAL DECISIONS

Caregivers with older family members who are progressively declining will ultimately face difficult decisions, such as when to take away car keys for safety reasons, when to speak about advance directives, what to do with a living will once it is written, when to take over decision making, and when to place the family member in a long-term-care facility. It is the professional responsibility of physicians and family lawyers to provide guidance to caregivers and family members when having to make these difficult decisions.

Advance Directives

An **advance directive**, or Advance Health Care Directive or living will, provides guidelines or directives formulated by the patient, while the patient is still competent to do so, that express desires about terminal care. An advance directive should detail whether the person wants to be resuscitated if he stops breathing; whether artificial life support should be used; and whether a feeding tube should be inserted.

The matter of creating an advance directive should not be taken lightly. Patients and family members should be aware that they need to specify which directives they wish to choose if the patient, for example, degrades into a persistent vegetative state. Besides resuscitation, other directives may include:

- Withholding medication, with the exception of pain relief
- Withholding food and hydration, particularly if nutrition is the only factor that would keep the patient alive
- Desire for organ donation
- Desire for autopsy

BOX 40-4 | Elder Care Resource Phone Numbers

Emergency (Paramedics, Fire, Police): 911
AARP: 213-380-1800
AMC Cancer Information Center: 800-525-3777
AT&T TDD Hearing Impaired: 800-735-2929
Amyotrophic Lateral Sclerosis (ALS) Association:
    800-782-4747
Alzheimer's Association 24-Hour Help Line: 800-262-3900
Alzheimer's Disease and Related Disorders Center:
    800-621-0379
American Cancer Society: 800-227-2345
American Council of the Blind: 800-424-8666
American Diabetes Association: 800-232-3472
American Dietetic Association Consumer Nutrition
    Hotline: 800-366-1655
American Heart Association: 800-242-8721
American Kidney Fund: 800-638-8299
American Liver Foundation: 800-223-0179
American Mental Health Foundation: 800-443-5959
American Paralysis Association: 800-225-0292
American Parkinson's Disease Association: 800-223-2732

American Speech and Hearing Association: 800-638-8255
Arthritis Foundation: 800-283-7800 or 213-954-5750
Asthma and Allergy Foundation of America: 800-727-8462
Cancer Information Service: 800-422-6237
Captioned Films for the Deaf (Voice/TDD): 800-237-6213
Elder Abuse Hotline: 800-992-1660
Eldercare Information and Referral: 800-662-1998
MedicAlert Foundation International: 800-825-3785
Medicare Hotline: 800-638-6833
Medicare/Medicaid Fraud Hotline: 800-368-5779
National Alliance for the Mentally III: 800-950-6264
National Hearing Aid Society Hotline: 800-521-5247
Random House Audiobooks: 800-733-3000
Recorded Books: 800-638-1304
Recordings for the Blind: 800-499-5525
Simon Foundation for Continence: 800-237-4666
Social Security Administration: 800-772-1213
Social Services/In-Home Services: 800-555-5555
Suicide Prevention Center 24-Hour Hotline: 800-273-8255

Patients who do not wish to be resuscitated in the case of respiratory or cardiac arrest may state this within a broader advance directive or in a separate legal document called a Do Not Resuscitate (DNR) order. Patients and families may incorrectly assume that when they have a DNR order written, it covers all life-sustaining treatments. Providing families and patients with information in advance may be very helpful.

An advance directive should also include a Durable Power of Attorney (DPOA), which names the patient's health care representative, also called an agent, who can make medical decisions and carry out the patient's advance directive wishes if the patient becomes unable to make or communicate her choices.

Refer to Box 40-5 for a sample advance directive. The U.S. Living Will Registry website is a comprehensive resource that patients and their caregivers or family members can use to create advance directives: www.uslivingwillregistry.com.

The patient's physician and lawyer should be included in advising, drafting, and executing a legal advance directive and making sure that the patient's physician and the hospital the patient is likely to go to have copies of the directive on file. In most states, however, unless the physician writes a specific order restating what the patient has expressed in the advance directive, a directive is not binding on the medical staff and facility where the patient may be hospitalized.

HIPAA Authorization

The Health Information Portability and Accountability Act (HIPAA) mandates keeping a patient's health information and records private. Unless the patient authorizes in writing for someone else to receive that information, it is illegal for any health care provider to share any details with anyone about the patient's health. HIPAA authorization is a simple document that permits the physician to share necessary information about the patient with designated individuals.

SAFETY GUIDELINES FOR THE OLDER ADULT POPULATION

Some older adults must rely on others for care and living accommodations, which may make safety issues a primary concern. Patients and caregivers should be aware of safety risks and develop a plan to eliminate or reduce those risks.

Older adults may be faced with increased risk of injury and may have a reduced capacity to protect themselves. The risk for personal injury increases after the age of 65. The normal aging processes and declining health place older adults at risk for falling, sustaining fractures, and other injuries. Early identification and addressing of health problems, as well as the use of assistive devices, can help reduce safety risks. Confusion, disorientation, decreased memory, and poor judgment decrease the ability of older adults to reduce hazards to their health and safety.

BOX 40-5 | Sample Advance Directive

LIVING WILL

If you do not wish to prepare a living will, strike through this entire part and initial here _____.

My name is: _____   My birth date is: _____/_____/_____
                              (Please Print)

1. **If I am unable to make or communicate health care decisions, I desire that my life not be prolonged by life-prolonging measures in the following situations** (you may initial <u>any or all</u> of these choices):

    _____ (initial)   I have a condition that cannot be cured and that will result in my death within a relatively short period of time.

    _____ (initial)   I become unconscious and my doctors determine that, to a high degree of medical certainty, I will never regain my consciousness.

    _____ (initial)   I suffer from advanced dementia or any other condition which results in the substantial loss of my ability to think, and my doctors determine that, to a high degree of medical certainty, this is not going to get better.

2. _____ **(initial) Even though I do not want my life prolonged by other life-prolonging measures in the situations I have initialed in section 1 above, I DO want to receive tube feeding in those situations** (initial here <u>only</u> if you **DO** want tube feeding in those situations).

3. **I wish to be made as comfortable as possible.** I want my health care providers to keep me as clean, comfortable, and free of pain as possible, even though this care may hasten my death.

4. **My health care providers may rely on this living will to withhold or discontinue life-prolonging measures in the situations I have initialed above.**

5. **If I have appointed a health care agent in Part A of this advance directive or a similar document, and that health care agent gives instructions that differ from the desires expressed in this living will, then:** (NOTE: initial **ONLY ONE** of the two choices below):

    _____ (initial)   **Follow this living will.** My health care agent cannot make decisions that are different from what I have stated in this living will.

    _____ (initial)   **Follow health care agent:** My health care agent has the authority to make decisions that are different from what I have indicated in this living will.

BOX 40-5 | Sample Advance Directive (*continued*)

COMPLETING THIS DOCUMENT
(Wait Until Two Witnesses and a Notary Public are Present Before You Sign!)

1. Your Signature

I am mentally alert and competent, and I am fully informed about the contents of this document.

Date: _____

Signature: _____

2. Signatures of Witnesses

I hereby state that the person named above, _____, being of sound mind, signed (or directed another to sign on the person's behalf) the foregoing document in my presence. I am not related to the person by blood or marriage, and I would not be entitled to any portion of the estate of the person under any existing will or codicil of the person or as an heir under the law, if the person died on this date without a will. I am not the person's attending physician. I am not a licensed health care provider or mental health treatment provider who is (1) an employee of the person's attending physician or mental health treatment provider, (2) an employee of the health facility in which the person is a patient, or (3) an employee of a nursing home or any adult care home where the person resides. I do not have any claim against the person or the estate of the person.

Date: _____ Signature of Witness: _____

Date: _____ Signature of Witness: _____

3. Notarization

_____ COUNTY, _____ STATE

Sworn to (or affirmed) and subscribed before me this day by

_____ (*type/print name of signer*)

_____ (*type/print name of witness*)

_____ (*type/print name of witness*)

Date: _____   _____

(*Official Seal*)   Signature of Notary Public

_____, Notary Public

Printed or typed name

My commission expires: _____

Environmental risks in the following areas should be identified and corrected:

- **Bathroom**—A small light in the bathroom, such as a night light, should be left on at all times. This will help illuminate pathways and walls in order to see light switches during the night. Tub and showers should have nonstick surfaces underfoot and grab bars and chairs for support while bathing. Toilets and nearby walls should have grab bars for assisting the patient on and off the toilet. If the toilet is low, a raised seat attachment may be needed.

- **Electrical cords**—Electrical cords should not be present in traffic flow areas. Minimize the number of devices plugged into an outlet because overloaded electrical outlets may cause fire.

- **Emergency numbers**—Emergency numbers, including those of police and fire departments, close relatives, or friends, should be near each phone or be put on automatic dial. The numbers should be posted in a font large enough for individuals to read, especially if the patient has vision problems.

- **Floor wax**—Highly polished floors increase the risk of falling; thus, floor wax should be avoided.

- **Furniture**—Furniture for older adults should be sturdy with good armrests to lend support for standing. Rooms stuffed with furniture and clutter increase a patient's risk of falling.

- **Lighting**—Provide adequate lighting and reduce glare. Several smaller areas of light are better in a room than one overhead light that may produce glare.

- **Rugs**—All area rugs should be removed or taped down to prevent tripping hazards, especially for patients who use walkers and canes.

Professionalism

Professional development hinges on becoming a lifelong learner. Keeping current in your field of medical assisting is crucial to maintaining your certification and becoming a better health care provider. To become a lifelong learner, you must seek out groups or facilities that provide continuing education unit (CEU) credits for attending seminars, such as at hospitals; local, state, and national medical assisting associations; state medical societies; nursing associations; and community colleges. Besides attending seminars, you can subscribe to professional journals and health magazines. Learning how to search the Internet and reading specific health care websites, such as the Centers for Disease Control and Prevention (CDC) or the National Institutes of Health (NIH), will provide valuable information and keep you current on a vast array of medical topics.

SUMMARY

The medical assistant should be prepared to function competently with geriatric patients. People suffer from many common diseases, regardless of age, but some diseases are more common or more severe in the older adult population.

With the growing number of people in the geriatric population, the medical assistant must be able to understand the aging process and how it affects these patients. In addition, to provide good health care, effective and appropriate communication is key. Understanding the special challenges older men and women face and having the tools and skills to help them overcome or mitigate them will make you a valuable asset to any medical practice.

40 CHAPTER REVIEW

COMPETENCY REVIEW

1. Define and spell the terms for this chapter.
2. Identify ways the medical assistant can support the physical needs of a patient in the medical office.
3. List four components of effective communication with older patients.
4. Explain why pet names should not be used to address patients.

5. How do Medicare and Medicaid help provide for the older adult population?
6. Discuss how the increase in life expectancy will impact health care.
7. Describe how aging affects the musculoskeletal system and ways patients can prevent degeneration.

8. List four common struggles for people who suffer from memory loss.

9. Identify three diseases that could lead to dementia.

10. Explain why respite care is so important for the caregivers of patients with dementia and Alzheimer's disease.

PREPARING FOR THE CERTIFICATION EXAM

1. When communicating with older adults, all of the following principles should be used *except*
   a. Speak clearly and slowly
   b. Make eye contact
   c. Express warmth by affectionately addressing the patient
   d. Refer to the patient as "Mr.," "Mrs.," or "Miss"
   e. Repeat questions or comment, if necessary

2. What is the most common form of dementia?
   a. Alzheimer's disease
   b. brain tumor
   c. HIV/AIDS
   d. stroke
   e. drug and alcohol abuse

3. All of the following diseases are common in older adults *except*
   a. diabetes.
   b. Alzheimer's disease.
   c. stroke.
   d. chickenpox.
   e. osteoporosis.

4. In what year was Medicare established?
   a. 1953
   b. 1935
   c. 1965
   d. 1956
   e. 1955

5. DNR stands for
   a. Do Not Revive.
   b. Do Not Repeat.
   c. Do Not Restrict.
   d. Do Not Resuscitate.
   e. Do Not Reevaluate.

6. In the reproductive system, all of the following are more common in older adults than in younger people *except*
   a. erectile dysfunction.
   b. enlarged prostate.
   c. decreased elasticity of the vagina.
   d. decrease in libido.
   e. vaginal dryness.

7. Which of the following is *not* a warning sign of Alzheimer's disease?
   a. poor judgment
   b. misplacing items
   c. increased sleep
   d. change in personality
   e. loss of initiative

8. The most common cause of acute-onset confusion in the older adult is
   a. diabetes.
   b. Alzheimer's disease.
   c. Varicella virus.
   d. sundowner syndrome.
   e. UTI.

9. The baby boomer generation includes people born in what years?
   a. 1940–1958
   b. 1946–1964
   c. 1950–1968
   d. 1956–1974
   e. 1935–1953

10. A type of confusion that occurs in some older patients at night is referred to as
    a. cognitive effect.
    b. confusion.
    c. sundowner syndrome.
    d. depression.
    e. dementia.

CRITICAL THINKING

Refer to the case study at the beginning of the chapter and use what you have learned to answer the following questions.

1. As Shandra obtains Ms. Jordan's weight, she notes that she has lost 15 pounds since her last physical examination over a year ago and now weighs only 113 pounds. She appears very frail in her 5'3" frame. What should Shandra do, and what might be the causes for Ms. Jordan's weight loss?

2. The physician would like Ms. Jordan to return to the office for nutritional education. She requested that her son, Lewis, accompany her to the visit. What type of patient education materials might Shandra want to prepare before the office visit with Ms. Jordan and her son?

ON THE JOB

Olive Johnson is a 62-year-old practicing lawyer and a patient of Dr. O'Brien. She is coming in today for an annual physical examination. On arrival, she seems cheerful, talkative, and cooperative as usual. After you place her in the examination room and give her instructions about obtaining a urine sample and where to have the gown opening, she seems confused and frustrated. She is unable to open the gown properly and mistakes the door to the hallway for the bathroom door. After directing her to the bathroom, you can hear her crying from the other side of the door.

1. How should you handle the situation?
2. How and when should you inform Dr. O'Brien about Ms. Johnson's behavior?
3. What tests do you think Dr. O'Brien might order?

INTERNET ACTIVITY

Select your own ethnic group or one in which you are interested (Greek, Irish, Chinese, etc.), and perform an Internet search for issues related to aging in that group using the search term *elderly*.

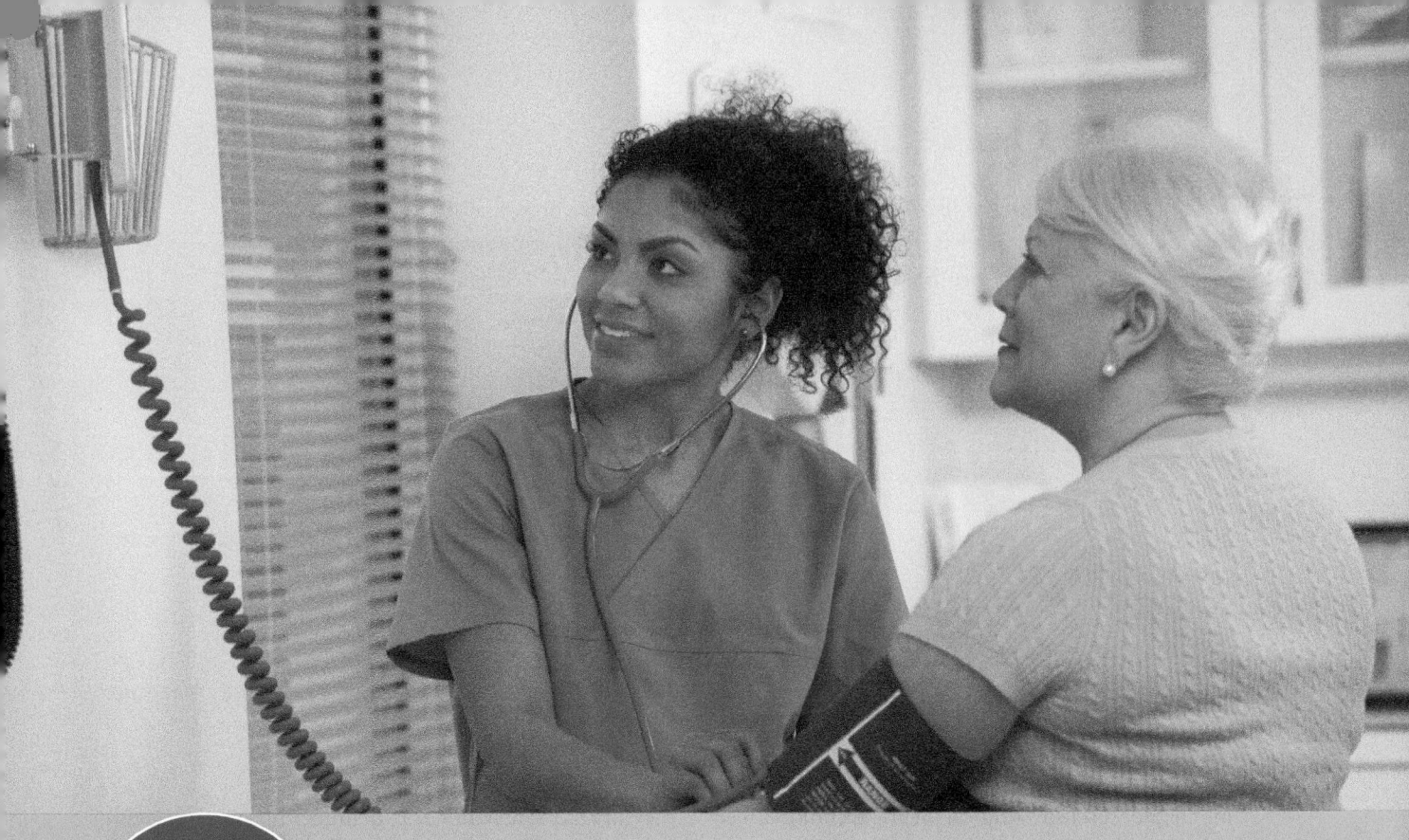

Assisting with Minor Surgery

Learning Objectives

After completing this chapter, you should be able to:

41.1   Define and spell the terms for this chapter.

41.2   Differentiate between types of ambulatory surgery.

41.3   List guidelines for surgical aseptic technique.

41.4   Outline the differences between medical and surgical asepsis.

41.5   Describe the types of instruments commonly used during ambulatory surgery.

41.6   List details pertaining to the use of specific types of suture materials.

41.7   Identify guidelines for handling instruments.

41.8   Describe the steps to prepare a patient for minor surgery.

41.9   Outline specific considerations related to postoperative patient care.

41.10 Explain the medical assistant's role as it pertains to assisting with various types of surgical procedures performed in a physician's office.

Today, Shandra Wilkinson, RMA, is working with Dr. Penningworth at Pearson Physicians Group. Dr. Penningworth has instructed Shandra to prepare examination room 4 for an I & D of a sebaceous cyst. He will be performing the I & D on Carmen DiStefano, a 32-year-old male who presented to the office with pain and discomfort surrounding the cyst.

Terms to Learn

ambulatory surgery	eschar	outpatient surgery
anesthesia	evisceration	scrub assistant
biopsy	hyfrecator	sterile field
cryosurgery	incisions	surgical scrub
debridement	invasive procedure	
dehiscence	Mayo stand	

This chapter discusses surgical aseptic technique, also known as sterile technique. Procedures requiring sterile technique, such as minor surgical procedures, suture insertion and removal, breast **biopsy** (microscopic examination of tissue to detect cancerous cells), incision and drainage, removal of growths, and wound treatment are included. Strict adherence to aseptic technique is necessary when assisting with these procedures. It is important to always remember that an item is either sterile or nonsterile. If there is any doubt about sterility, assume it is nonsterile.

THE MEDICAL ASSISTANT'S ROLE IN MINOR SURGERY

Medical assistants perform many duties related to minor surgery (Figure 41-1). Before surgery you will perform administrative duties, such as completing insurance forms, obtaining consent forms, and meeting with the patient to answer questions related to the procedure. Before beginning the surgery, the provider will expect the medical assistant to have set up the sterile field with the instruments and equipment necessary for the specific procedure that is about to be performed. During the procedure, the health care provider may ask the medical assistant to add items to the sterile field and, if properly scrubbed and wearing sterile gloves, even hand sterile instruments to the provider. On completion of the procedure, your duties will include providing postoperative instructions to the patient, such as proper wound care. Other duties will include cleaning the procedure room after

the surgery, sanitizing and disinfecting or autoclaving the instruments used, and restocking supplies as needed.

Setting Up the Sterile Field Before Surgery

A surgical setup for a typical minor surgical procedure includes the following:

- Local anesthetic materials
- 3 mL syringe with needle(s)
- Alcohol sponges to cleanse vial top
- Sterile gloves for surgeon
- 4 × 4 and 2 × 2 gauze sponges
- No. 3 scalpel blades and handle, extra scalpel blades (Nos. 10, 11, and 15)
- Curved iris scissors

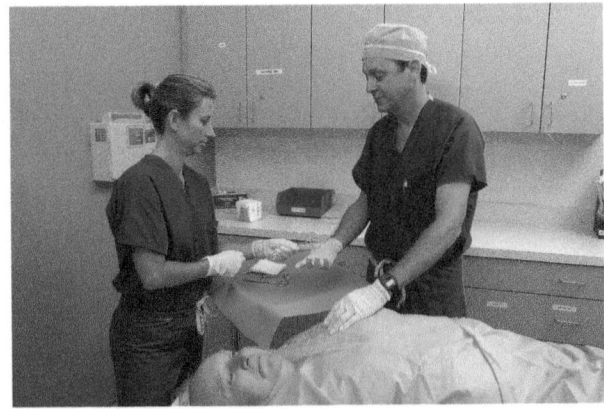

FIGURE 41-1 A medical assistant assists with minor surgery performed in the medical office.

- Tissue forceps
- Straight and curved mosquito forceps
- Straight and curved Kelly forceps
- Towel forceps
- Sterile drape towels
- Needle holder with mounted needle and suture materials
- Sterile specimen container with preservative solution

Additional Supplies That May Be Needed During Surgery

Other surgical supplies may be needed during a procedure. Wound drains such as a rubber Penrose drain may be inserted at the end of a procedure to remove excess fluid. Other packing materials, such as sterile petroleum jelly, saturated gauze squares, or sterilized Iodoform gauze strips of varying lengths, may also be used to pack wounds. Additional sterile syringes may be necessary to irrigate the wound, or extra sterile gauze squares may be needed to absorb blood from a surgical area. In preparation for minor surgery and before the procedure begins, check the supply inventory thoroughly.

AMBULATORY SURGERY

Ambulatory surgery is surgery performed on a person who is admitted and discharged from a surgical facility on the same day. This includes outpatient surgery in a hospital setting, a surgicenter, or a medical office. Because ambulatory surgery is on the increase, the medical assistant is increasingly called on to assist the physician with surgical procedures in the office.

Ambulatory surgery, with its option for surgical procedures performed outside the hospital setting, has resulted in a cost savings to the consumer and to the insurer. Hospitalization is not required unless an unexpected complication occurs. The patient is able to return home after a brief recovery time. The disadvantage to this type of surgery is the short time the health care team has for assessing the patient's postoperative condition. It is important for each ambulatory facility to develop a consistent follow-up procedure to track the patient's condition after leaving.

Outpatient surgery is generally limited to procedures requiring less than 60 minutes to perform. Today, many surgeries are performed in free-standing surgicenters or surgical centers that are part of a hospital complex.

Surgeries can be categorized as follows:

- **Elective**—Considered medically necessary but can be performed when the patient wishes (e.g., removal of benign growths)
- **Emergency**—Required immediately to save a life (e.g., hemorrhage) or prevent further injury or infection

- **Optional**—May not be medically necessary, but the patient wishes to have it performed (e.g., cosmetic surgery, vasectomy)
- **Outpatient**—Does not require an overnight stay in a hospital
- **Urgent**—To be performed as soon as possible but is not an immediate or acute emergency (e.g., cancer surgery)

PRINCIPLES OF SURGICAL ASEPSIS

Surgical asepsis, or sterile technique, is used when sterility of supplies and the immediate environment are required, as in surgical procedures. Sterile technique results in the killing of all microorganisms and spores. It is necessary during any **invasive procedure** (a procedure in which the body is entered), such as when administering an injection, making a surgical incision, or working with an open wound.

Open tissues provide an excellent reservoir (host) for infection. Infections can delay the healing process, cause permanent harm or death to a patient, and result in additional medical costs. Sterile technique prevents microorganisms from being introduced into the body, thereby decreasing the risk of infection.

Both medical asepsis and surgical asepsis have the overall purpose of decreasing the risk of infection. Medical asepsis is a reduction in the number of microorganisms, such as when you wipe a countertop with disinfectant. Medical asepsis results in a "clean" approach in which materials can be handled with clean hands or nonsterile gloves. Surgical asepsis means a complete absence of microorganisms and spores. Surgical asepsis requires a sterile handwashing or scrub, sterile gloves, and sterile technique when handling materials. A way to remember the difference is to recall "Clean for clean" and "Sterile for sterile." For example, use clean hands when applying a clean bandage to unbroken skin. Use sterile procedure when handling sterile materials, such as using sterile gloves when touching sterile instruments. See Table 41-1 for a comparison of medical and surgical asepsis.

TABLE 41-1 | Surgical Asepsis and Medical Asepsis

Surgical Asepsis	Medical Asepsis
Sterile technique used	Clean technique used
Absence of microorganisms	Controls microorganisms
Surgical scrub performed	Basic hand hygiene procedure used
Sterile equipment and supplies required	Clean equipment and supplies
Sterile field	Clean field

Surgical Asepsis

A STERILE ITEM CAN ONLY TOUCH ANOTHER STERILE ITEM

- If a sterile item touches a nonsterile item, it is contaminated.
- If a clean item touches a sterile item, it is contaminated.
- A sterile packet that is torn, wet, or punctured is contaminated.
- A sterile packet is contaminated after the date on the packet.
- If unsure of sterility, consider the item contaminated.
- Skin is always considered contaminated. It cannot be sterilized, only disinfected.

A STERILE ITEM ON A STERILE FIELD MUST BE WITHIN YOUR FIELD OF VISION AND ABOVE YOUR WAIST

- If you cannot see an item, it is contaminated.
- If items or your hands are below your waist, they are contaminated.
- If you turn your back on a sterile field, it is contaminated.
- If you leave a sterile field unattended, it is contaminated.

AIRBORNE MICROORGANISMS CONTAMINATE STERILE FIELDS

- Do not place sterile fields in a draft.
- Avoid extra movements near the sterile field.
- Do not talk, cough, sneeze, or laugh over a sterile field.
- Wear a mask if you need to talk during a procedure.
- Do not reach over a sterile field.
- Avoid spills on a sterile field. A wet field is contaminated.

THE EDGES OF A STERILE FIELD ARE CONTAMINATED

- If an item touches any part of the 1-inch border around the sterile field, it is contaminated.

STERILE GLOVES MUST ONLY TOUCH STERILE ITEMS

- Do not touch the outside of sterile gloves with bare hands.
- Sterile gloves are contaminated if punctured. Remove and dispose of the item and gloves, rescrub, and reglove.

STERILE PACKETS MAY BE TOUCHED ON THE OUTSIDE WITH BARE HANDS

- Outer wrappings are considered contaminated.
- Open sterile packets away from you to avoid contaminating the packet by touching your clothing.
- Never rewrap an unused sterile packet. The unused items must be resanitized, rewrapped, and reautoclaved.

BE HONEST IF YOU MAKE AN ERROR OR SUSPECT YOU HAVE MADE AN ERROR

- Remove the contaminated item and correct the error.
- Report contamination to your superior.

Guidelines for Surgical Asepsis

When practicing surgical asepsis, follow the guidelines presented here or those used in your office. Guidelines 41-1 provides some rules for surgical asepsis. Refer to this list of key points often as you read through this chapter. They are the ground rules for establishing a sterile field.

The purpose of personal protective equipment (PPE) is to protect the patient and health care worker from exposure to pathogenic organisms. See the chapter on infection control for more information about PPE. Remember that nonsterile scrub suits should not be worn home. All personnel should change to street clothes before leaving a medical facility.

Surgical Scrubs and Sterile Gloving

In the "Infection Control" chapter, medical asepsis and hand hygiene were introduced. Performing hand hygiene is the number-one way to prevent spreading infection. In this chapter, you will learn the procedure for surgical asepsis or a **surgical scrub**. A surgical scrub removes microorganisms more effectively than regular handwashing. It is necessary that the hands be as free from microorganisms as possible in the event that sterile gloves are punctured during a procedure. Procedure 41-1 and Figures A–G demonstrate the steps and rationale for performing surgical hand hygiene. Figure 41-2 shows a medical assistant in PPE, including

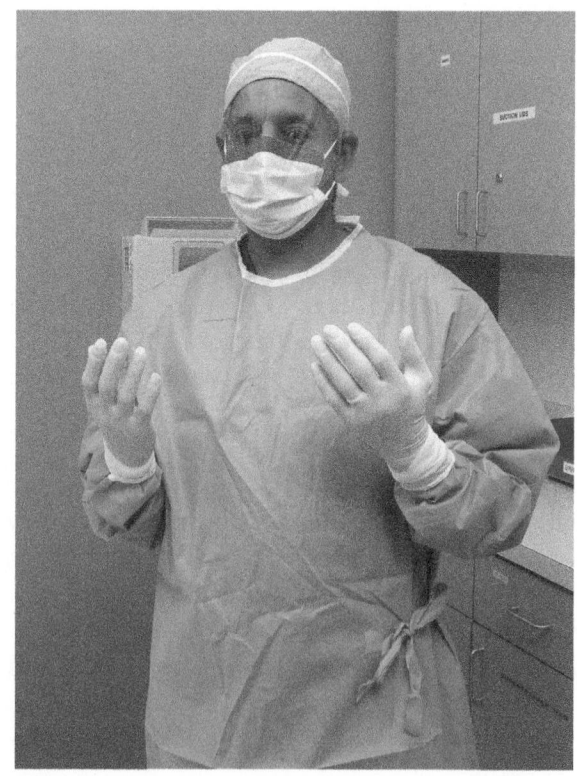

FIGURE 41-2 A medical assistant wearing PPE—gown, face shield, and gloves.

Performing Sterile Scrub/Surgical Hand Hygiene

Objective ◆ *Perform a surgical scrub on hands and arms using the correct procedure for the appropriate length of time.*

EQUIPMENT AND SUPPLIES

Cuticle stick; germicidal dispenser soap (not bar soap); sterile scrub brush; sterile towel pack (with two to three sterile paper or cloth towels); sterile gloves (prepackaged); running water (foot pedal preferable)

METHOD

1. Remove all jewelry. With a nail file, remove any gross dirt from beneath fingernails before scrubbing.
   Rationale: Microorganisms can accumulate in crevices of rings or watches and under fingernails.
2. Assemble equipment.
3. Stand at the sink without allowing your body to touch it.
4. Remove your lab coat. Roll up your sleeves above the elbows. Keep your hands and arms above waist level at all times.
5. Regulate running water temperature to warm, not hot.

6. Place hands under running water with hands pointed upward. Allow water to run from fingertips to elbows.
7. Apply a circle of soap from the dispenser and lather well.
8. Vigorously scrub your hands and wrists with a scrub brush (Figure A). Wash thoroughly between fingers. Scrub under fingernails. Scrub toward the elbows using five minutes on each hand (Figures B and C).
9. Raise hands, bending at the elbow, and place them under running water to rinse off soap (Figure D). Allow water to flow from fingertips to elbows (Figure E).
10. If performing a second lather and scrub is the policy in your facility, use three minutes for each hand.
11. Using a sterile towel (if possible), pat hands dry moving from fingertips to wrists, and then to elbows. Hands should still be held above the elbows (Figure F).
12. Turn off the faucet with a fresh towel if foot lever is not available (Figure G).
13. Glove immediately. Keep hands above waist and folded together until the procedure begins.

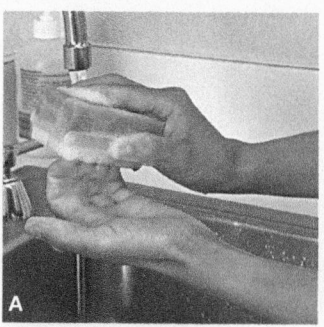
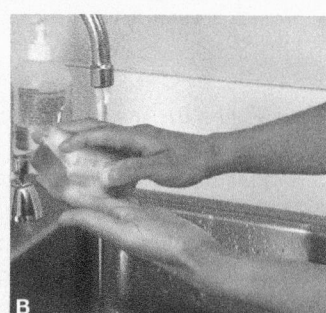
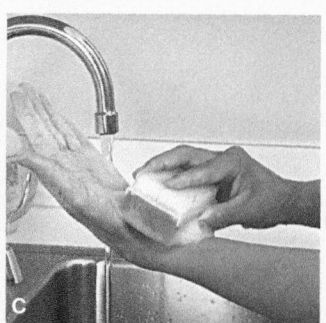
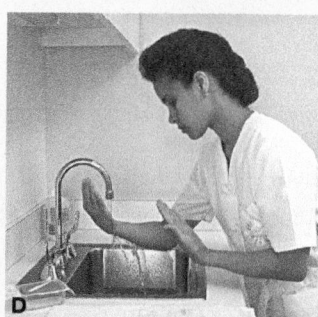
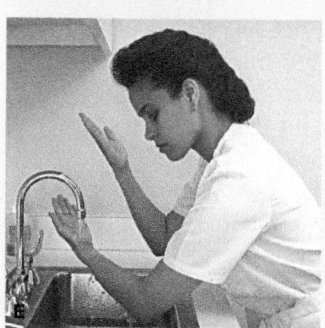
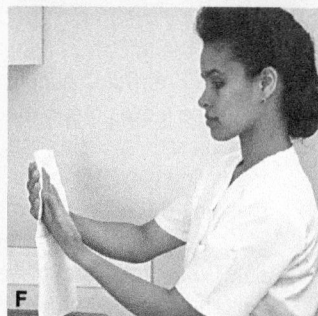
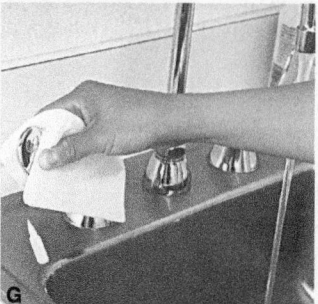

FIGURE A–G Performing sterile scrub/surgical hand hygiene.

face shield, gown, and gloves, preparing to assist with a surgical procedure. PPE provides a barrier between infectious or hazardous material and the wearer. Remember that if a sterile glove is punctured or if you touch the outside of the glove with your hand, the glove is considered nonsterile and must be replaced after you perform another surgical scrub. Procedure 41-2 lists the steps for surgical gloving and glove removal.

Sterile Packaging

Sterile packages (packets) are prepared for use in surgery. Each one may contain either a single instrument or piece of equipment or several items packed together. These packets are then autoclaved with sterilization indicators and dated. Sterile packs may be purchased from a medical supply company or packaged by the medical assistant in the office. To prepare sterile packets, you must know the names and uses of instruments routinely used in minor surgery (discussed later in this chapter). Review the

"Infection Control" chapter for packaging and autoclaving procedures.

Sterile packets are used for various procedures. For example, all the instruments needed for a procedure, such as a biopsy, are packaged together in a tray and autoclaved.

When you assist the physician or surgeon with a procedure, set up the specific tray or instruments before the procedure begins. The packets are set up on a **Mayo stand**, a small portable table with enough room to hold an instrument tray. For some procedures, you may need to use more than one Mayo stand. After you open the sterile packet, the inside of its wrapper becomes the **sterile field** (a specific area free of all microorganisms that will be the work area for a surgical procedure). However, the outer, 1-inch border all around the open wrapper is considered contaminated. If the field becomes wet, it is contaminated, and you must open a new packet. If the physician wants an additional instrument while performing a procedure, you will open a sterile packet and drop the instrument carefully onto the sterile field.

PROCEDURE 41-2

Donning and Removing Surgical Gloves

Objective ◆ *Apply sterile gloves without a break in sterile technique.*

Note: This procedure follows a surgical hand scrub.

EQUIPMENT AND SUPPLIES

Double-wrapped sterile glove pack

METHOD

1. Assemble equipment and check the tape or seal for expiration date and condition of pack.
2. Place the pack on a flat surface at waist height with the cuffed end of the gloves toward you.
3. Open the outside wrapper by touching only the outside of the pack. Leave the opened wrapper in place to provide a sterile work field.
4. Open the inner wrapper without reaching over the pack or touching the inside of the wrapper. Pull inner wrapper edges to each side without touching the inside of the pack (Figure A).
5. Using the thumb and fingers of your left hand (if you are right-handed), pick up the glove on the right side of the pack by grasping the folded inside edge of the cuff

(Figure B). The glove can be dangled slightly off the sterile packing material for easier insertion.
6. Pull the glove onto the right hand using only the thumb and fingers of the left hand (Figure C). Do not allow fingers to touch the rest of the glove.
7. Place the fingers of the right-gloved hand under the cuff of the left glove and pull onto the left hand and up over the left wrist (Figure D).
8. With the gloved right hand, place your fingers under the cuff of the left glove and pull up over the left wrist (Figure E). The thumb should not touch the cuff.
9. After the gloves are in place, the fingers can be adjusted, if necessary, by using the gloved hands.
10. Removing gloves (Figures F–H): Remove the first glove by grasping the edge of that glove (with fingers of the other gloved hand) and pull the first glove over the hand inside out. Discard the first glove into the proper biohazard waste container. Remove the other glove by grasping the edge of the cuff with your fingers (from the ungloved hand) and pull the second glove down over the hand, inside out. Discard the gloves appropriately.

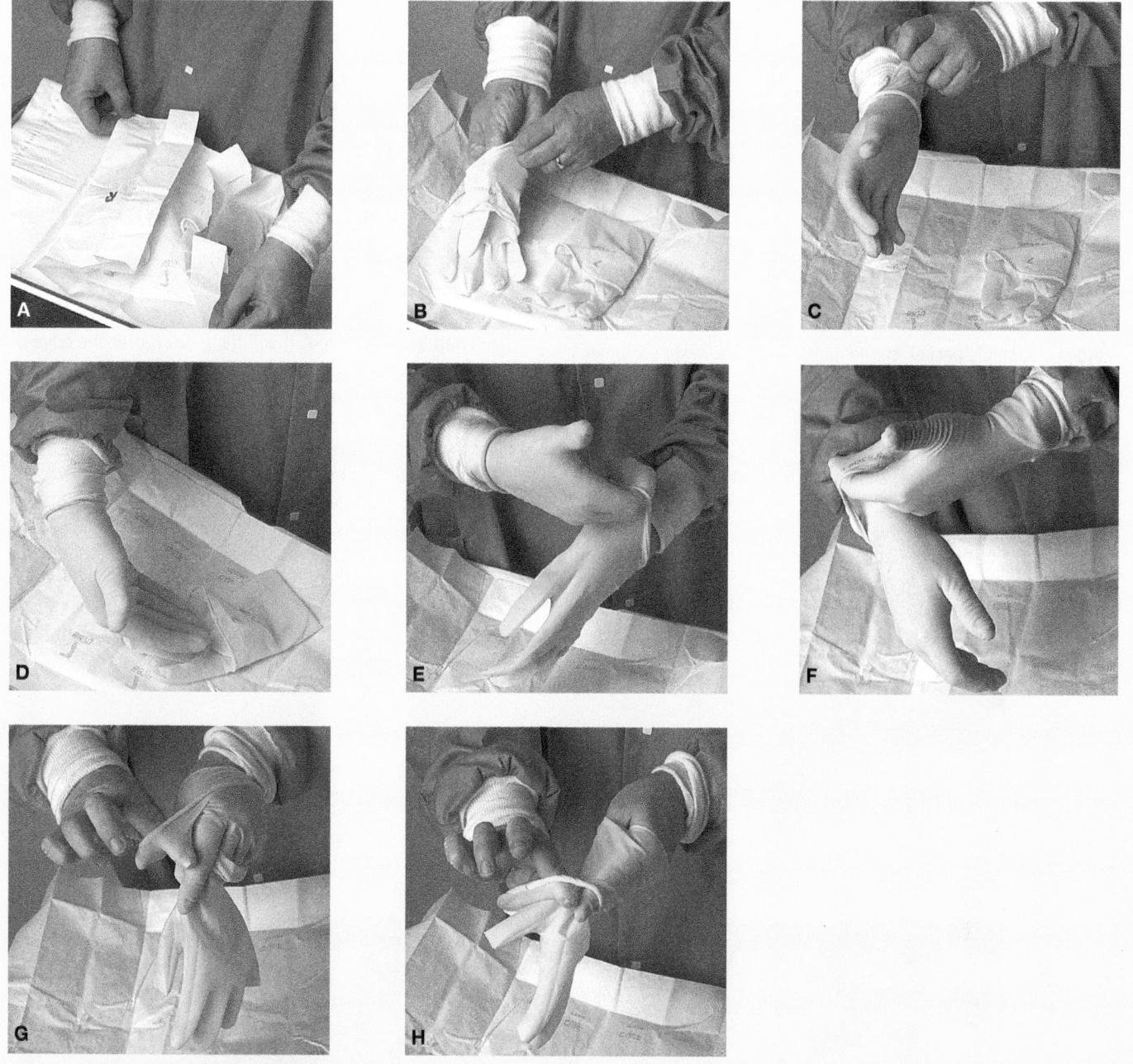

FIGURE A–H Sterile gloving and glove removal technique.

Procedure 41-3 and Figures A–F show the steps and rationale for preparing a sterile field. Procedure 41-4 shows how to perform within a sterile field. Figure A illustrates dropping a sterile item onto a sterile field.

Sterile Transfer

To place instruments and supplies onto a sterile field or to move them around on the sterile field, you must put on sterile gloves or use transfer forceps. In Procedure 41-4, Figure B illustrates the steps and rationale for transferring

sterile objects using transfer forceps. Remember not to reach across the sterile field or turn your back on the field unless it is covered with a sterile towel.

SURGICAL INSTRUMENTS

Surgical instruments have been developed over centuries to meet specific needs during an operation such as cutting, suturing, or grasping. In some cases, an instrument developed by a surgeon bears the name of the surgeon—for

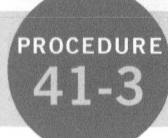

PROCEDURE
41-3

Preparing a Sterile Field

Objective ◆ *Open a sterile packet (pack), and use it to set up a sterile field without a break in sterile technique.*

EQUIPMENT AND SUPPLIES

Mayo stand; sterile packet; sterile transfer forceps; waste container

METHOD

1. Perform hand hygiene.
2. Assemble equipment. Adjust the Mayo stand to the correct height.
3. Place the packet on the Mayo stand with the folded edge on top. Position the packet on the stand so that the top flap will fold away from you.
4. Remove the tape or fastener and check the sterilization indicator and date. Discard in a waste container.
5. Pull the corner of the pack that is tucked under and lay this flap away from you. It will hang down over the edge of the Mayo stand (Figures A and B).
6. With both hands, pull the next two flaps to each side (Figures C and D). The packet will still be covered with the last layer of the outer wrapper.
7. Grasp the corner of the last flap, without reaching over the sterile field, and open the flap toward your body without touching it (Figures E and F).
8. The inside of this outer wrapper is now your sterile field. If you need to arrange items within this field, use sterile forceps. If an inner packet must be opened with an instrument setup, then someone wearing sterile gloves must open it.

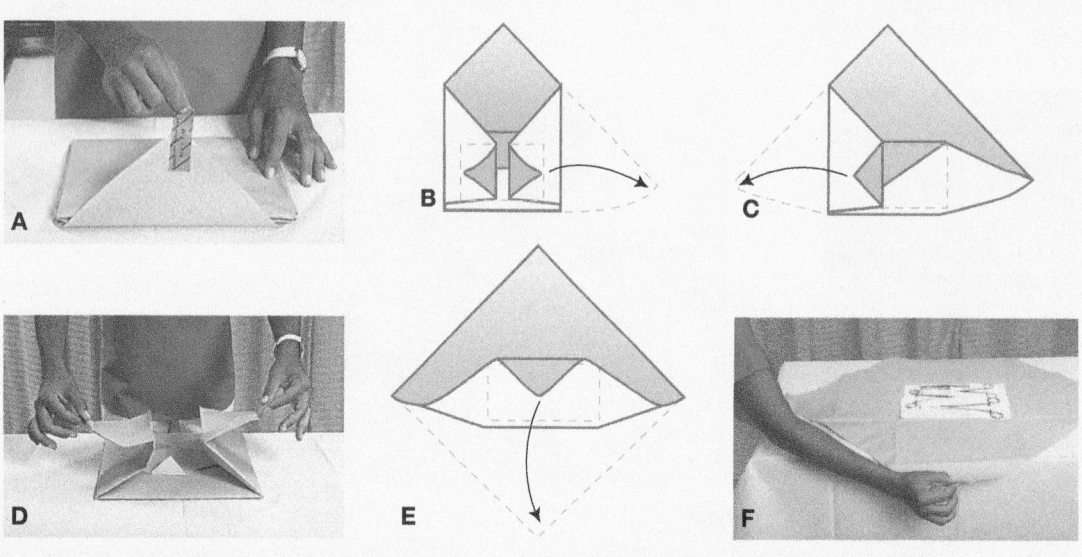

FIGURE A–F Preparing a sterile field.

example, Kelly forceps, Halstead mosquito clamp, and Bozeman uterine forceps.

Instruments Used in Minor Surgery in an Office

The general classification of instruments is based on their use: cutting, dissecting, grasping, clamping, dilating, probing, visualizing, or suturing. Specific instruments are related to individual specialties, such as gynecology; urology; orthopedics; ear, nose, and throat; proctology; obstetrics;

and neurology. A minor surgical setup includes a standard group of instruments, such as scalpel, blades, scissors, hemostat, and suture materials. Instruments are usually made of steel and treated to be rust and heat resistant, stainproof, and durable. However, sometimes disposable instruments (such as disposable vaginal specula) are used for convenience.

You must be able to identify common instruments used in your facility. Some physicians use the full name of the

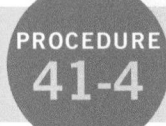

PROCEDURE 41-4

Performing Within a Sterile Field

Objectives ◆ *Place (drop) a sterile item onto a sterile field or into a gloved hand without contaminating the packet or the field, transfer items using transfer forceps, and pour sterile fluid into a sterile basin on a sterile field without spilling the solution or contaminating the field.*

EQUIPMENT AND SUPPLIES

Sterile pack (containing, for example, prepackaged items such as a specimen container or needle and syringe in a pull-apart packet); sterile transfer forceps in a forceps container with a sterilant solution, such as Cidex; Mayo stand; sterile 4 × 4 gauze package; transfer forceps; sterile solution; sterile basin; waste container

METHOD

1. Assemble equipment; check the expiration date of packet, sterile solution, and solution basin; and check the sealed condition of packet.
2. Locate the edge on the prepackaged item and pull apart by using the thumb and forefinger of each hand. Do not let your fingers touch the inside of the packet. Rationale: The inside of the packet is sterile and the outside is considered contaminated.
3. Pull the packet apart by securely placing the remaining three fingers of each hand against the outside of the packet on each side. The wrapper edges will be pulled back and away from the sterile item.
4. Holding the item securely about 8 to 10 inches from the sterile field, gently drop the packet contents inside the sterile field (Figure A). Instead of having you drop the

item, the physician may wish to remove the item directly from the packet by grasping it firmly with a gloved hand. Rationale: Nonsterile hands and arms should not be placed over the sterile field.
5. Discard the paper wrapper in a waste container.
6. Grasp forceps handles firmly without separating the tips and remove vertically from the container. Remove vertically to avoid dripping solution onto the exposed contaminated portion of forceps.
7. Holding forceps vertically with tips down, gently tap tips together to drop excess solution onto dry sterile 4 × 4 gauze or touch the sterile 4 × 4 gauze to dry the tips.
8. Pick up the sterile item to be transferred by holding transfer forceps vertically with tips down. Do not touch the sterile field. Grasp the article to be transferred firmly at its midsection.
9. Place the sterile item within the sterile field (Figure B).
10. Place forceps back into the container without touching the sides of the container.
11. Set up the sterile basin on the Mayo tray using the inside of the wrapper to create a sterile field.
12. Remove the cap of the solution and place it on a clean surface with the outer edge down (inside facing up). Avoid touching the inner surface of the cap, which is considered sterile.
13. Check the label on the bottle before pouring the solution.

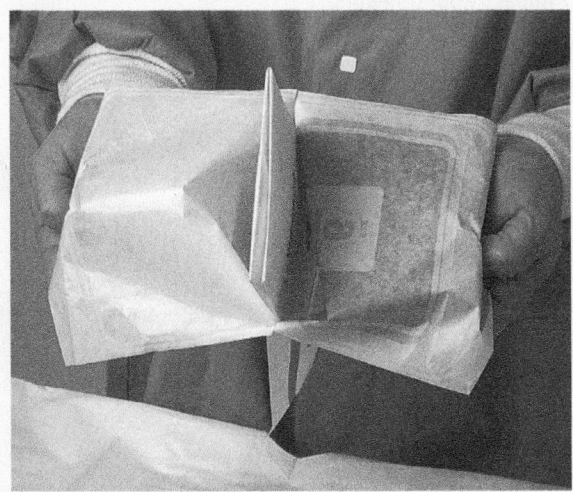

FIGURE A Dropping a sterile supply onto a sterile field.

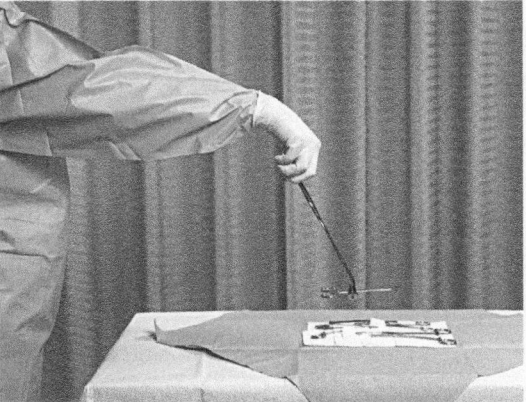

FIGURE B Proper technique to handle sterile equipment with transfer forceps in a sterile field.

CHAPTER 41 Assisting with Minor Surgery   **993**

14. Pour a small amount of the liquid into a waste container for discarding. This will dislodge any bacteria that may have collected on the edge of the bottle after opening it.
15. Pour the bottle with the label held against the palm (Figure C). This protects the label from drips that can destroy the name of the solution.
16. Hold the bottle about 6 inches above the basin and pour slowly to avoid splashing.
17. Replace the lid immediately after using.
18. Clean and sterilize the forceps and container in the autoclave. Change the solution.

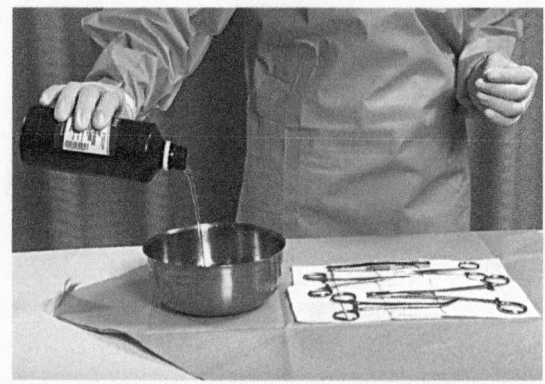

FIGURE C Pouring sterile solution into a sterile container.

instrument—for example, Pederson vaginal speculum—and others refer to it simply as a vaginal speculum. The following tips will help you identify instruments.

- Categorize the instrument by its use: to cut, probe, grasp, clamp, retract, dilate, or other.
- Examine the parts of the instrument, and ask yourself the following questions:
  - What type of handles does it have (e.g., ring, serrated)?
  - What type of tip does it have (e.g., pointed, blunt, teeth, no teeth, serrated)?
  - What type of closure does it have (e.g., spring, box-lock with a screw, ratchet)?
  - What type of edges does it have?
  - How long is it (may indicate for which body part it is used)?
  - Whose name does it bear, or what is it usually called?

Each time you encounter an instrument you are unfamiliar with, answer the preceding questions to determine its characteristics and remember the name.

Cutting Instruments

Scalpels or knives are used to make **incisions**, which are surgical cuts into tissue. They are small, curved instruments that are made to fit easily into the surgeon's hand. Figure 41-3 illustrates a scalpel and a variety of blades. A scalpel blade must be inserted into the scalpel handle. Blades come in various sizes depending on the type of incision and tissue.

Dissecting Instruments

Scissors are the most common tool for dissecting or cutting tissue. For example, scissors are used for **debridement** (removal of dead tissue around wound edges using sterile technique) or to cut sutures (thread;

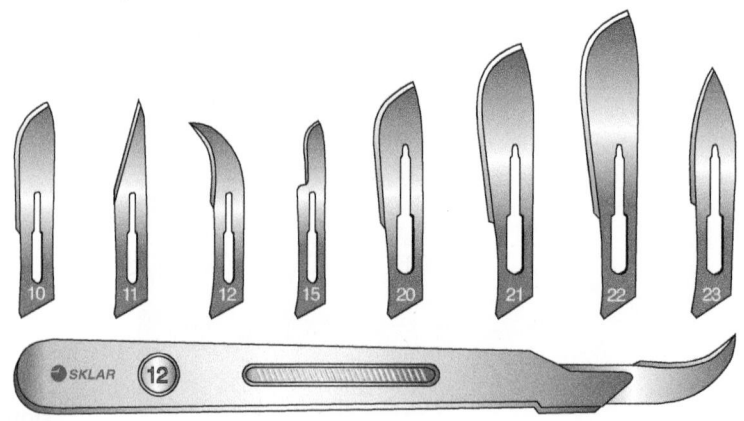

FIGURE 41-3 A scalpel and a variety of blades.

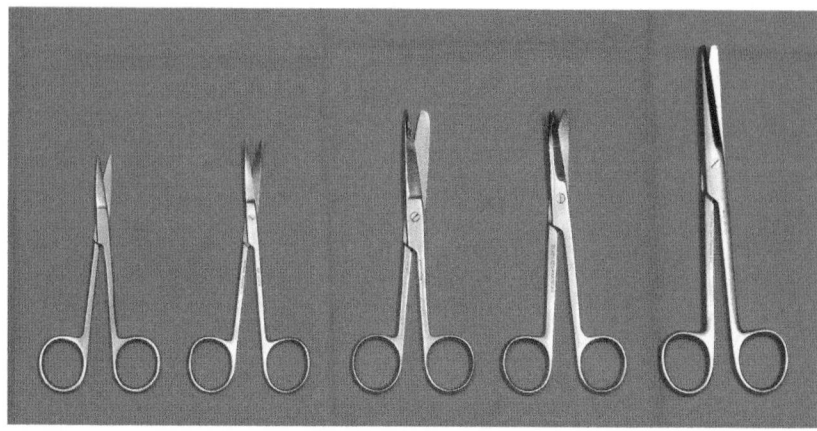

FIGURE 41-4 A variety of types of scissors.

stitches). Scissors have two blades with sharp edges that come together when the handles are drawn together.

The tips of scissors vary greatly to perform a variety of functions. Some scissors have blunt tips that can slide under bandages and dressings to cut without damaging the skin. Metzenbaum scissors are short, curved, and blunt and intended for use on and to prevent piercing of delicate tissue. Operating scissors or suture scissors are used to cut suture material during surgery; they have a hook on one edge that fits under the suture for ease in suture removal. Dissecting scissors are also called straight or Mayo scissors. Operating scissors are straight or curved with a combination of blades, such as sharp/sharp (s/s), blunt/blunt (b/b), and sharp/blunt (s/b). Bandage scissors have a blunt tip and a blunt flat edge to allow it to fit easily under a bandage for cutting. Figure 41-4 illustrates a variety of scissors.

Grasping and Clamping Instruments

Forceps are used to grasp tissue or objects (Figure 41-5). One type of forceps is a two-pronged instrument that has a spring-type handle used to clamp together tightly to prevent

slipping. Another type of closure mechanism is a ratchet closure or clasp. The ratchet clasp allows the forceps to close with differing degrees of tightness. Forceps often have serrations or teethlike edges that prevent tissue slipping out of the forceps.

Types of Forceps. The following are several widely used types of forceps:

- *Tissue forceps* have teeth and are used to grasp tissue.
- *Thumb forceps* are two-pronged with serrated tips to hold tissue.
- *Splinter forceps* are used to grasp foreign bodies.
- *Needle holder forceps* are used to grasp needles during suturing.
- *Hemostats* are applied to blood vessels to hold vessels until they can be sutured (Figure 41-6).

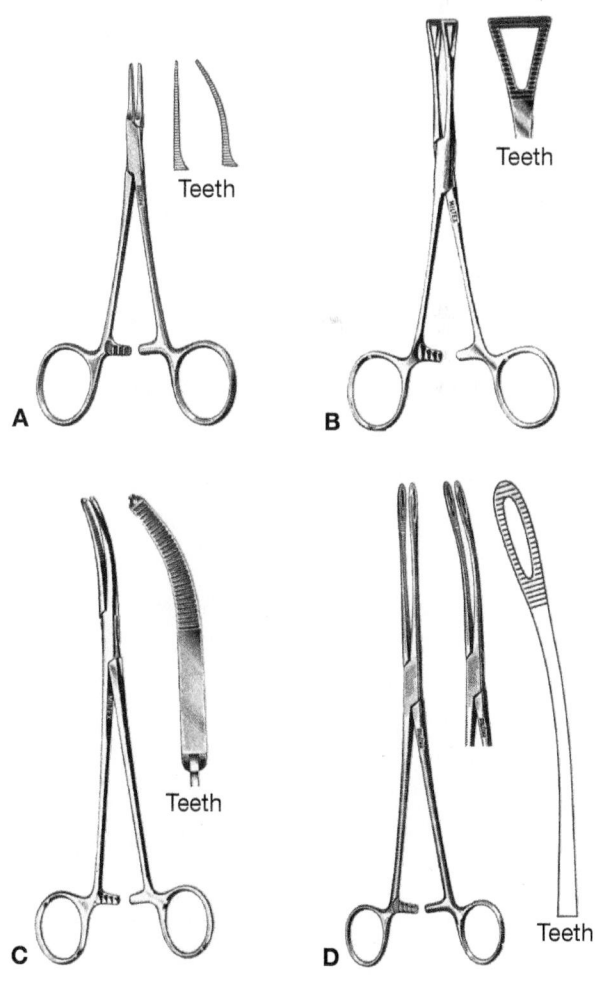

FIGURE 41-6 Hemostats: **(A)** mosquito forceps; **(B)** Pennington hemostatic forceps; **(C)** curved forceps; **(D)** sponge forceps.

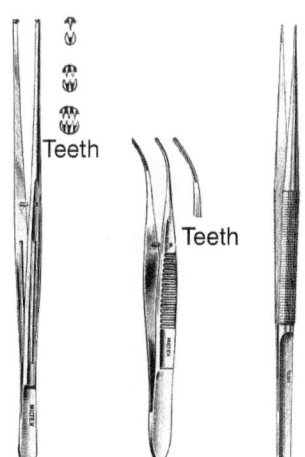

FIGURE 41-5 Types of forceps.

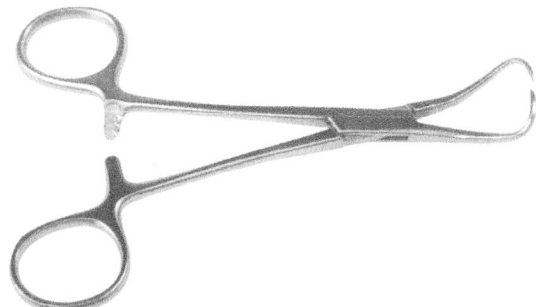

FIGURE 41-7 Towel clamp.

- *Sponge forceps* are used for holding sponges during surgery.

- *Towel clamps* are used to hold together the edges of sterile drapes (Figure 41-7).

Probing and Dilating Instruments

Instruments used to enter body cavities for probing or dilating purposes include the following:

- **Scope**—Usually lighted, it is inserted into a body cavity or vessel to visualize the internal structures. Figure 41-8 shows different sizes of laryngoscopes that are used to look at a patient's voice box or larynx. An obturator is placed inside a scope to guide it into a cavity or canal and then removed during visualization of the surgical site. Some obturators have a point used to puncture tissue.

- **Speculum**—Unlighted instrument with movable parts that when inserted into a cavity, such as the nasal

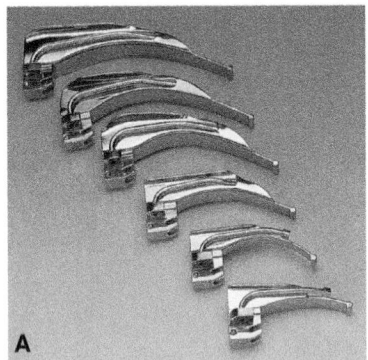

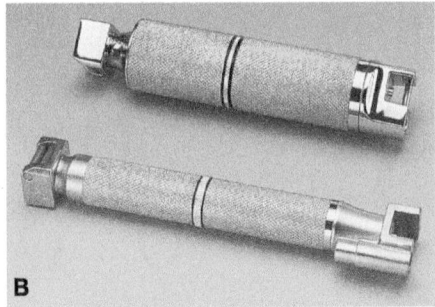

FIGURE 41-8 Laryngoscopes: **(A)** scopes; **(B)** handles.

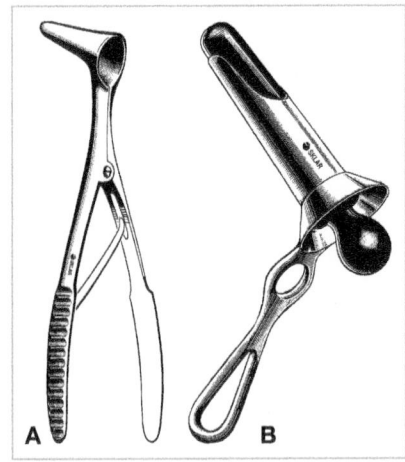

FIGURE 41-9 Specula: **(A)** Vienna nasal speculum; **(B)** Ives-Fanster rectal speculum.

cavity or rectum, can be spread apart for ease of visualization and tissue sample removal (Figure 41-9).

- **Probe**—Used to explore wounds and cavities usually with a curved, blunt point to facilitate insertion (Figure 41-10).

- **Retractor**—Used to hold back the edge of a surgical incision (Figure 41-11).

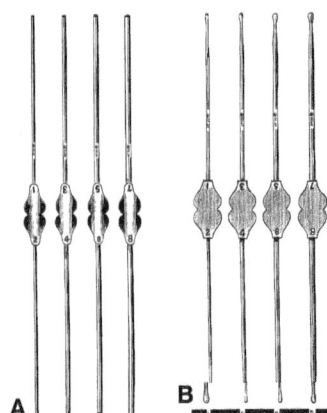

FIGURE 41-10 Lachrymal probes: **(A)** Bowman; **(B)** Williams.

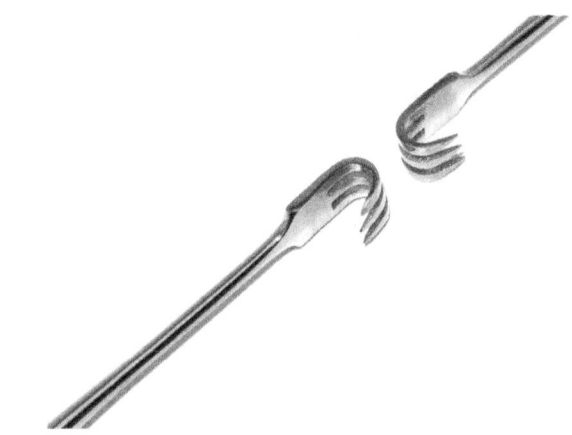

FIGURE 41-11 Retractors.

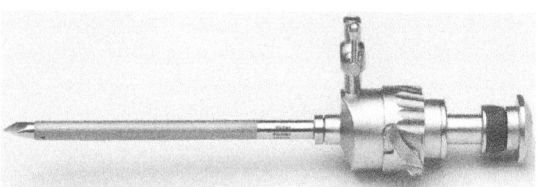

FIGURE 41-12 Trocar.

- **Trocar**—Used to withdraw fluids from cavities. It consists of a cannula (outer tube) and a sharp stylet that is withdrawn after the trocar is inserted (Figure 41-12).
- **Punch**—Used to remove tissue for examination and biopsy.

Specialized instruments are used for disciplines, such as gynecology and obstetrics (Figure 41-13), urology (Figure 41-14), and orthopedics (Figure 41-15).

Suture Materials and Needles

Suture (thread) materials are used to bring together or approximate a surgical incision or wound until healing takes place. Suture materials are added to the surgical tray setup when they are needed for a procedure. Sutures come either with or without an attached needle. The package label will indicate type, size, and length of the suture material. Suture types include absorbable and nonabsorbable.

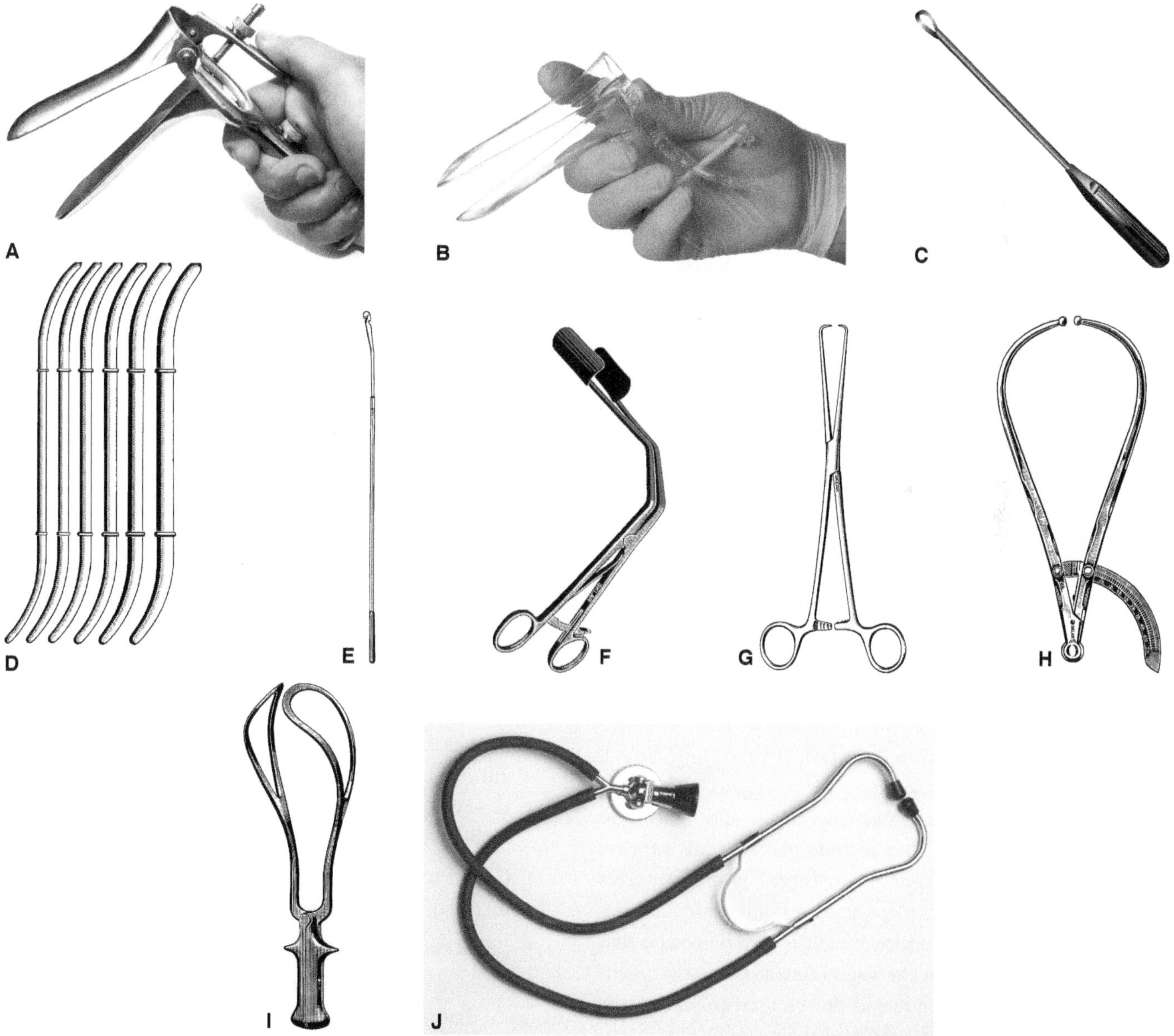

FIGURE 41-13 Gynecological instruments: **(A)** metal vaginal speculum; **(B)** disposable vaginal speculum; **(C)** uterine curette; **(D)** uterine dilators; **(E)** IUD extractor forceps; **(F)** lateral vaginal retractor; **(G)** Schroeder uterine tenaculum forceps; **(H)** Martin pelvimeter; **(I)** De Lee OB forceps; **(J)** Bowles obstetrical stethoscope.

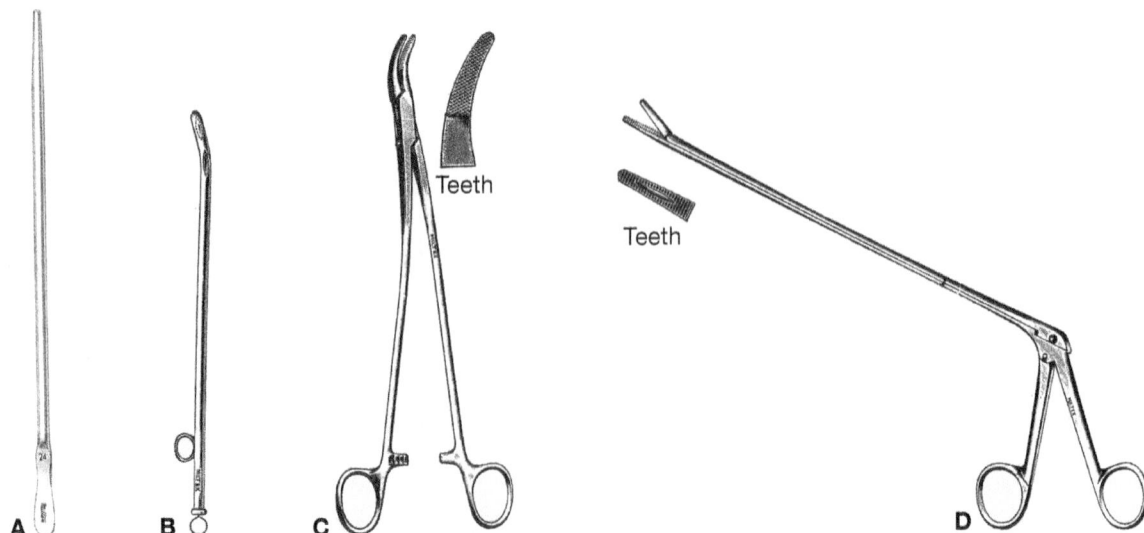

FIGURE 41-14 Urological instruments: **(A)** sound; **(B)** female catheter; **(C)** needle holder; **(D)** urethral forceps.

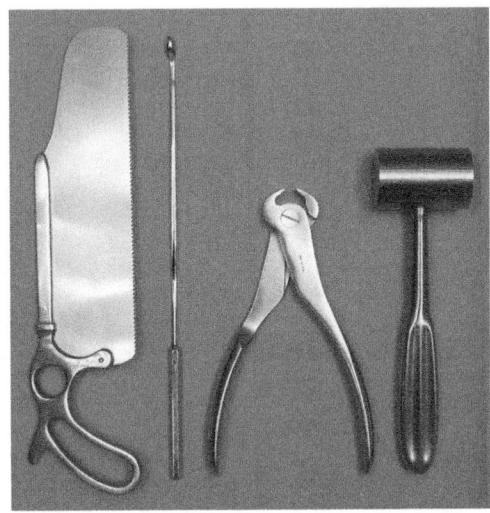

FIGURE 41-15 Orthopedic instruments.

Absorbable Sutures. Absorbable sutures are digested by tissue enzymes and absorbed by the body tissues. They do not have to be removed. Absorption usually occurs 5 to 20 days after insertion. This type of suture, such as surgical catgut (made from sheep's intestinal lining), or Vicryl, a synthetic material, is used for internal organs such as the bladder and intestines, subcutaneous tissue, and ligating or tying off blood vessels. They include plain catgut, surgical catgut, and chromic catgut. Plain catgut is used in areas where rapid healing takes place, such as highly vascular areas of the lips and tongue. Surgical catgut is used on tissues that are fast healing, such as the vaginal area. Chromic catgut has a slower absorption rate and can be used to hold tissue together longer, such as for muscle repair.

Nonabsorbable Sutures. Nonabsorbable sutures are used on skin surfaces where they can easily be removed after an incision heals. This type of suture material, such as nylon, cotton, silk, Dacron, and stainless steel, is not absorbed by the body. Black silk is the most commonly used nonabsorbable suture.

Suture Material. Suture materials vary and are selected based on how they are used.

- Silk suture, although the most expensive, is also considered the most dependable. An all-purpose suture, it is widely used and easy to tie.

- Nylon suture has elasticity and strength that make it ideal for use in joints and for skin closure. The disadvantage is the difficulty in forming a tight knot.

- Polyester suture is the second strongest of all the standard suture material, and steel is the strongest.

- Polyester is used in ophthalmic, cardiovascular, and facial surgery, all of which require a strong, unbreakable suture because a broken suture could result in permanent damage to the patient.

- Steel is used in staples, as well as nonabsorbable suture wire that is composed of 316L stainless steel, and is the most widely used suture material in major surgery. It is the strongest of all suture material.

- Cotton suture, with less strength than other suture materials, is no longer widely used.

- Linen suture is created from natural flax fiber.

The size of the suture material, which is measured by the gauge or diameter, is stated in terms of 0s, decreasing in size with the number of zeros. For example, 0 is the thickest and 6-0 (000000) is the smallest. Sizes 2-0 through 6-0 are most commonly used. Delicate tissue, on areas such as the face and

TABLE 41-2 | Suture Use, Size, and Type of Material

Use	Gauge	Type of Material
Blood vessels	3-0 to 0	chromic gut
	3-0	cotton
	3-0 to 0	silk
Eyelid	6-0 to 4-0	silk
	6-0 to 5-0	polyester
Fascial	2-0 to 0	chromic gut
	2-0 to 0	silk
	2-0 to 0	cotton
Muscle	3-0 to 0	plain gut
	3-0 to 0	chromic gut
	3-0 to 0	silk
Skin	6-0 to 2-0	Nylon
	5-0 to 3-0	polyethylene
	5-0 to 2-0	stainless steel

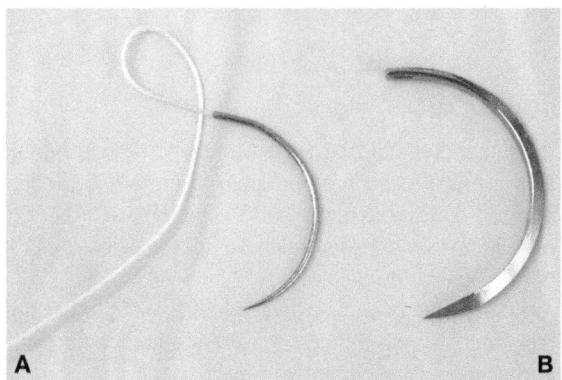

FIGURE 41-17 Surgical needle shapes: (A) taper point; (B) cutting point.

This type of needle has an eye that is threaded with the suture material. The suture material thickness doubles when threaded through the needle because it enters the eye from one side and comes out the other.

Curved needles allow the surgeon to go in and out of a tissue when there is not enough room to maneuver a straight needle. This type of needle requires a needle holder.

A swaged needle and suture materials are combined in one length. This offers the advantage of the suture material not slipping off the needle because it is attached. A swaged needle pack contains a label indicating the gauge, type of needle point (cutting or noncutting), and type and length of the suture material.

Other Wound Closure Materials. Other materials used for wound closure include sterile tapes such as Steri-Strips (Figure 41-18), staples, and skin adhesives such as Dermabond. Sterile tapes are nonallergenic and available in a variety of widths. They are used instead of sutures when not much tension will

neck, would be sutured with 5-0 to 6-0 suture material. These fine sutures would leave less scarring. Heavier sutures, such as 2-0, would be used for the chest or abdomen. The physician determines the type and gauge of sutures to be used. Table 41-2 summarizes suture uses, sizes, and types. Figure 41-16 illustrates different suture material.

Suture Needles. Suture needles are available in differing shapes depending on where they are used (Figure 41-17). Needles have either a sharp cutting point used for tissues that provide some resistance, such as skin, or a round noncutting point used for more flexible tissue such as peritoneum. They are available in three shapes: straight, curved, or swaged.

The straight needle is used when the needle is pushed and pulled through the tissue without the use of a needle holder.

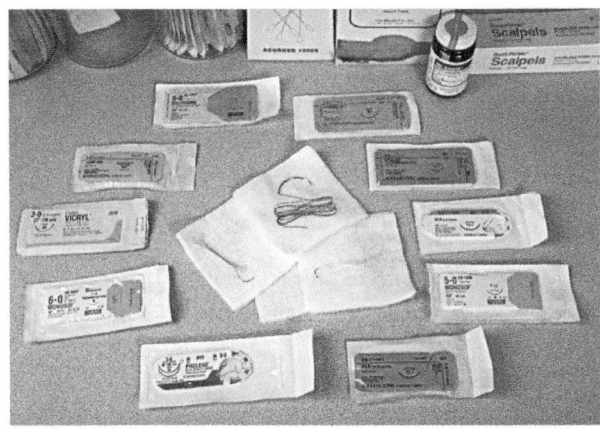

FIGURE 41-16 Types of suture material.

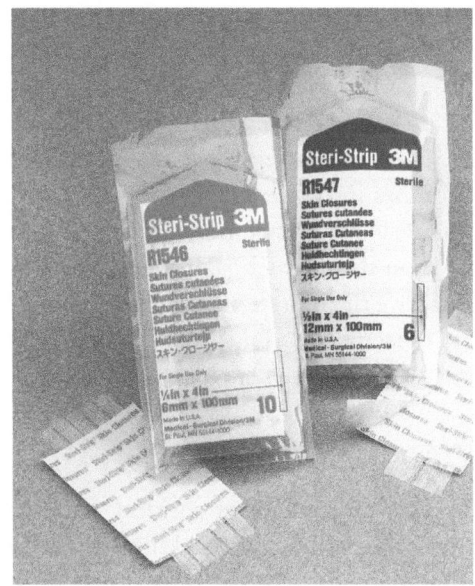

FIGURE 41-18 Steri-Strips from 3M.

be applied to a wound, such as on a small facial cut. Skin adhesives are composed of cyanoacrylate adhesives that react with water to create an instant, strong, flexible bond. The composition of skin adhesives is similar to Superglue and can be used to close lacerations or small surgical incisions. Staples are made of stainless steel and applied with a surgical stapler.

Guidelines for Handling and Care of Instruments

Surgical instruments are expensive and may be delicate. They require special care and attention. In some instances, there might not be a duplicate of an instrument. Even slight damage to an instrument can result in malfunction at a critical time during surgery. Instruments may be disposable, in which case care must be taken to dispose of them in sharps containers or biohazardous containers as necessary. However, if the practice uses instruments that are reusable, care must be taken to presoak used instruments in an appropriate solution, gently clean them of debris, lubricate them if needed, and then autoclave them to sterilize them. Store instruments according to office policy. Guidelines 41-2 provides guidelines for handling instruments.

SURGICAL ASSISTING

The medical assistant's role in surgical assisting varies depending on the type of practice and the needs of the physician. For example, an eye surgeon who performs a large number of outpatient cataract operations may employ a

full-time **scrub assistant**, scrub technician (scrub tech), or operating technician (OR tech) who will apply sterile gloves and hand instruments to the surgeon. In this case, the medical assistant might act as the nonsterile assistant, who positions the patient, uses transfer forceps to bring additional supplies as needed, holds the vial of local anesthetic while the surgeon draws up the correct dosage into a syringe, and applies dressings. Anyone not in sterile attire and assisting with a procedure can be described as a nonsterile assistant. This person may also be referred to as a floating assistant, circulating assistant, circulator, or floater.

In many practices, the medical assistant will scrub, apply sterile gloves, and act as the only assistant for the surgeon. A good assistant can help the procedure flow smoothly. The exact surgical tray setup and sequence of passing instruments vary depending on the procedure and the surgeon's preferences.

A good assistant anticipates the needs of the physician, uses care in handing instruments efficiently, uses care that injury does not occur, and accounts for all materials and instruments used during the procedure. The assistant must maintain an accurate count of absorbent sponges used for cleaning out the wound site during surgery to ensure that all sponges are removed before the patient's wound is closed.

Scrub Assistant

The scrub assistant performs all procedures in sterile protective clothing using sterile technique. The scrub assistant's responsibilities include arranging the surgical tray to meet the operating physician's preferences, handing instruments, swabbing (sponging) bodily fluids away from the operative site, retracting the incision area, and cutting suture materials. See Guidelines 41-3 for guidelines on sterile technique for scrub assistants. To become competent as a scrub assistant, practice reaching for an instrument with your eyes closed. This is similar to the conditions under which the physician works because he or she does not look up from the operative site when reaching for instruments.

Instruments should be passed to the physician firmly and by the handle first. An instrument should remain in your grasp until you feel confident that the physician has a firm grip on it. Figure 41-19 illustrates a medical assistant using proper technique when passing instruments to the physician. In Procedure 41-4, Figure C shows the steps for transferring sterile solutions onto a sterile field. All the preceding procedures are vital for you to master to properly assist the physician with minor surgery, as described in Procedure 41-5.

Floating Assistant

The floating assistant performs nonsterile duties during a surgical procedure and thus "floats" between the operating

Sterile Techniques for Scrub Assistants

- Always be aware of where your hands are, because they should never touch a nonsterile area. Immediately re-glove if sterility is broken.
- Arrange the surgical tray for efficiency, closing all instruments that were left open during the autoclave process.
- Close all instruments before passing them. Protect the surgeon from injury by handing needles with the point away from the surgeon, paying close attention to where scalpel blades and scissors' points are in relation to the surgeon's hands.
- Anticipate the surgeon's needs by memorizing the types of instruments used in a procedure and the order they are most often used. An index card with a list of the preferences for each procedure is useful for this purpose.
- Do not release your grip on the instrument until you feel the surgeon take it away. This prevents an instrument from falling to the floor and being damaged. In addition, you may not have a duplicate of that particular instrument on your tray, and that will cause a delay in the procedure.
- Place the instrument with a firm "slap" into the surgeon's extended hand. Because the surgeon may not look up from the surgical site when his hand is extended, do not look away from the instrument until you feel it being taken from you. The handles should be placed into the surgeon's hands first.
- If asked to provide retraction to open the incision area for better visualization, follow directions from the surgeon regarding the amount of pull needed. Move slowly and deliberately when retracting. Do not make abrupt, forceful moves.
- If sutures are used to close the wound, be prepared to cut the suture material. The surgeon will pull both ends of the suture material together away from the wound. Cut both ends at the same time 1/8 to 1/5 inch above the knot.
- Many requests for assistance will not be verbalized by the surgeon. It is important to pay attention and anticipate what instruments or assistance will be required next.

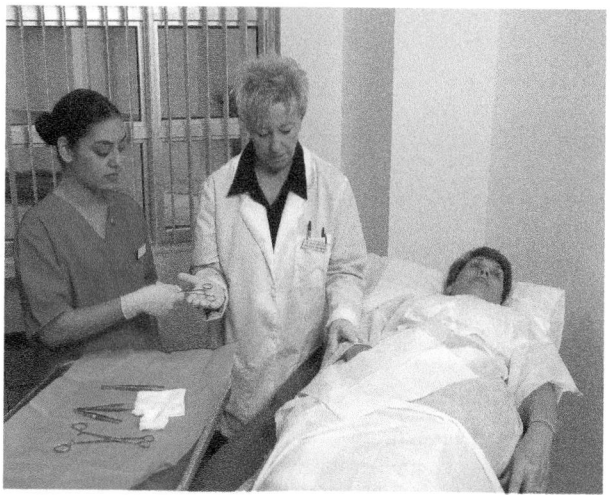

FIGURE 41-19 A medical assistant using the proper technique when passing instruments to the physician.

Floating Assistant Techniques During Surgery

- Immediately report any unusual observations about the patient to the operating physician.
- Use care not to touch the physician during any assisting because this will contaminate the physician and cause a delay in the procedure while the physician regloves (and regowns if necessary).
- Provide additional medications such as local anesthetics that are needed during the procedure. When providing medication during the procedure, follow the correct procedure to identify the medication, clean the top of the vial/bottle with alcohol, hold the vial/bottle upside down so that the physician can insert a sterile needle into the vial without touching the contaminated outer surface, and keep the label in plain view for the physician to read. Hold the vial firmly with both hands at your shoulder height to allow the physician easy access and withdrawal. Do not place the vial in front of your face. Note that the physician will have to use some force when inserting the needle into the vial.
- Because the floating assistant is not sterile, this person must perform all lighting adjustments, patient repositioning, chart notations made during the procedure, requisition forms, and specimen container labeling.
- The floating assistant can place additional sterile materials and instruments onto the sterile field by opening the packet without touching the sterile inside and gently dropping them into the sterile field on the Mayo stand. The sterile scrub assistant or physician may remove them from the inside of the packet as the floating assistant firmly holds on to the outside.
- When holding a container to receive a specimen, tilt the container slightly so the physician can place the specimen inside without touching the rim of the container.

table, supplies, and equipment. One of the major roles of the floating assistant is to monitor the patient by taking vital signs every 5 to 10 minutes. Other duties include providing additional sterile equipment, opening sterile packets, adding sterile equipment to the field, and performing the necessary counts of supplies used, such as gauze squares. Other guidelines for proper floating technique during surgery are listed in Guidelines 41-4.

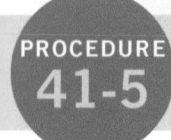
Assisting with Minor Surgery

Objective ◆ *Prepare all materials and equipment for immediate use in a surgical procedure using sterile technique.*

EQUIPMENT AND SUPPLIES

Mayo stand; side stand; transfer forceps and container; sharps container; waste container/plastic bag; biohazard waste container; anesthetic; alcohol swab; sterile specimen container, depending on type of surgery; sterile pack (two pairs sterile gloves, towel pack, 4 × 4 sponge pack, patient drape, needle pack, and suture materials); instrument pack(s), including towel clamp pack; syringe pack; two sterile basin packs

METHOD

1. Perform hand hygiene.
2. Open sterile tray packs on the Mayo stand and side stand. Use the sterile wrapper to create a sterile field. The wrapper will hang over the edges of the tray.
3. Use sterile transfer forceps to move instruments on the tray or to place equipment from packets. Materials in peel-away packets should be flipped onto the tray.
4. Open the sterile needle and syringe unit and drop gently onto the sterile field. Use care not to reach over the sterile field.
5. Open the sterile drape packs and towel clamp packs.
6. Open a set of sterile gloves for the physician.
7. After the tray is ready with all equipment open and arranged, pull the edge of the sterile towel across the tray, using sterile transfer forceps. The sterile towel will provide a protective covering for the sterile tray until the procedure begins. The medical assistant should not leave the room once the tray is set up (Figure A).
8. When the physician has donned the sterile gloves, remove the sterile towel covering the tray of instruments.
9. Remove the towel by standing to one side and grasping the two distal corners, then lifting the towel toward you so that you do not reach over the unprotected sterile field.

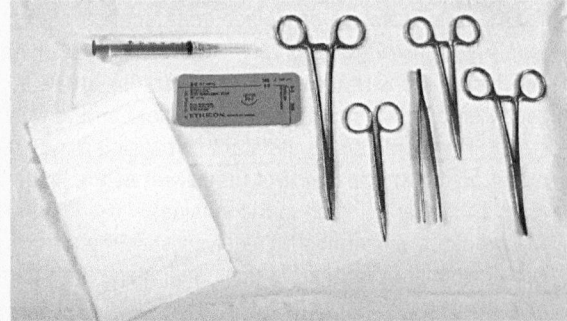

FIGURE A Sterile instrument setup.

10. Cleanse the vial of anesthetic with a sterile alcohol swab and hold it upside down in the palm of your hand with the label facing toward the physician. Hold it steady while the physician draws up the anesthetic.
11. Stand to one side of the patient and assist the physician as requested. Provide additional supplies as needed. If you assist by handing instruments directly to the physician, you must perform a surgical scrub and wear a sterile gown and gloves.
12. Hold all containers for specimens, drainage, or contaminated 4 × 4s. Wear nonsterile gloves to protect yourself from contact with drainage.
13. Collect and place all soiled instruments in a basin out of the patient's view.
14. Place all soiled gauze sponges (4 × 4s) and dressings in a plastic bag. Do not allow wet items to remain on a sterile field.
15. Immediately label all specimens as they are obtained. Close all specimen containers tightly.
16. Periodically reassure the patient by quietly asking how he is doing. Do not touch the patient with soiled gloves.
17. When the procedure is complete, wash your hands before assisting the patient. The patient will often be moved to a recovery area so the surgical area can be cleaned. To dispose of soiled dressings, use the following steps:
    a. Remove gloves.
    b. Place one hand into the empty plastic bag.
    c. Using the hand covered with the plastic bag, pick up all the soiled materials. With the other hand, pull the outside of the bag over the soiled dressings.
    d. Dispose of the bag in a biohazard waste container.
    e. Perform hand hygiene and document the procedure.
18. Allow the patient to rest and recover from the anesthetic. Periodically check the patient's vital signs according to your office policy.
19. Provide clear oral and written postoperative instructions for the patient. Make sure the patient is stable before he leaves the office.
20. Send the specimen(s) to the laboratory with a requisition slip.
21. Clean, sanitize, and sterilize the instruments. Clean and sanitize the room in preparation for the next patient.
22. Perform hand hygiene.

CHARTING EXAMPLE

11/8/20YY 9:00 A.M. The physician will chart the details of the surgical procedure... J. Wall, RMA

PREPARING THE PATIENT FOR MINOR SURGERY

The medical assistant is often responsible for providing instructions to the patient before and after minor surgery. Preoperative and postoperative instructions can be presented in a variety of formats, including one-on-one discussion, videotapes, brochures, pamphlets, and models. These instructions must be reinforced through one or more telephone reminders. It is especially important to provide postoperative instructions in a variety of formats because the patient may not be fully alert right after surgery. Family members should be included in these explanations whenever practical.

Patient Instructions

Box 41-1 provides guidelines for preoperative and postoperative instructions. For purposes of efficiency, some preoperative patient preparation can take place before the patient arrives for the procedure. For example, patient education with an explanation of the procedure, preoperative and postoperative instructions, and laboratory testing can take place up to a week before the actual procedure.

Preoperative instructions might include an explanation of what laboratory testing is needed and when it is to be done, food and fluid restrictions, directions for special bathing/skin cleansing preparations or cleansing enemas, and restrictions on bedtime sedative use. If a patient cannot safely drive home after a procedure, be sure to say that she may need to bring a friend or family member to provide safe transportation home.

Postoperatively, patients should have a clear understanding of what to expect during recovery and how to care for the surgical incision at home. If the patient has had anesthesia, you must ensure that the patient is able to safely drive home, has someone to drive her, or is using public transportation.

(Check this at the time of the surgery even though you may have given this instruction earlier.) Clear instructions about postoperative medications should be given in writing as well as verbally to the patient and possibly to family members, if appropriate. Further, the patient should be instructed about whether a return visit to the office will be necessary and when that should be scheduled.

Informed Consent

Although informed consent was discussed in depth in the chapter titled "Medical Law and Ethics," it is important to re-emphasize it here as it pertains to minor surgery. The physician must provide the patient with an honest, thorough explanation of the surgical procedure, including the benefits and risks. (Informed consent is explained in more detail in the chapter titled "Medical Law and Ethics.") Any invasive procedure with a scalpel, scissors, or other device requires written permission (consent) from the patient. Procedures in which a body cavity is entered for the purposes of visualization, though no incision is made, such as a bronchoscopy, cystoscopy, and colonoscopy, also require written consent. The procedure, with all the risks involved, must be explained by the physician. Every attempt must be made to determine if the patient actually understands the explanation given by the physician. The medical assistant can witness the patient's signing the consent form.

Positioning and Draping

Before the surgical procedure, ask the patient to remove all clothing and put on a patient gown with the ties at the back, unless otherwise instructed. Have the patient void before assisting him onto the operating table, and place the patient in the proper position for the procedure. Every attempt should be made to ensure the patient's comfort because the patient may have to remain in one position for

---

BOX 41-1 | Preoperative and Postoperative Patient Instructions

PREOPERATIVE INSTRUCTIONS

- Explain the procedure verbally and provide printed materials.
- Be honest about the level of discomfort expected.
- Advise the patient on the length of the procedure.
- Explain what type of clothing to wear for the procedure.
- Schedule preoperative diagnostic tests—blood, X-ray, etc.
- Describe what at-home preparations the patient will need, such as fasting, and for how long.
- Explain that someone must accompany the patient.
- Inform the patient how long he will be out of work.
- Confirm the informed consent form has been signed.
- Answer any questions.
- Measure vital signs.

POSTOPERATIVE INSTRUCTIONS

- Provide verbal and written instructions for follow-up care.
- Explain when the patient should notify the physician of possible postoperative problems, such as fever, bleeding, swelling, or other symptoms.
- Schedule a follow-up visit, if required.

an extended period of time. General guidelines for positioning and draping are discussed in the chapter titled "Assisting with Physical Examination."

Anesthesia

Anesthesia, medication that causes the partial or complete loss of sensation, is used to block the pain of surgery. Anesthesia can also relax muscles, produce amnesia, calm anxiety, and cause sleep. Medical assistants do not administer anesthetics, but they should be familiar with them and their effects.

The two types of anesthetics are general and local (conduction).

General Anesthesia

A general anesthetic depresses the central nervous system (CNS) to cause unconsciousness. It is usually administered through inhalation or intravenous (IV) injection. Inhaled anesthetics are generally in the form of gases or volatile liquids. In many cases, these are administered after a patient has received a sedative or narcotic to relieve pain or a tranquilizer to relieve anxiety. Sedatives and narcotics are usually administered intramuscularly before surgery. In some cases, they are administered by IV immediately before the general anesthetic is given.

Anesthetics are hypnotic sedatives that produce anesthesia, or sleep, when given in large doses, such as sodium pentothal. Precautions to be taken when administering a general anesthetic include the following:

- Administering the anesthetic only to a patient on an empty stomach to prevent vomiting and possible aspiration of vomitus into lungs resulting in pneumonia.

- Cautioning patients not to drive or engage in other activity that could result in harm from impaired consciousness. General anesthetics can interfere with the patient's alertness for 12 to 24 hours after the surgery.

- Advising patients to avoid alcohol and depressant drugs for two to three days before the surgery and one day after the surgery.

Local Anesthesia

Local anesthetics provide a loss of sensation in a particular area of the body without overall loss of consciousness. A local anesthetic is also referred to as a conduction anesthetic. The conduction of pain transmission by way of the nervous system is blocked. The following are examples of this type of anesthetic:

- **Topical and local infiltration**—Acts on nerve endings

- **Nerve block**—Affects pain transmission along a single nerve

- **Regional, spinal, epidural, or saddle block**—Affects a group of nerves

A local infiltration anesthetic is injected directly into the tissue that will be operated on. Examples of a local are lidocaine hydrochloride (Xylocaine) and procaine hydrochloride (Novocaine). This type of anesthetic is used for such procedures as removal of skin growths, skin suturing, and dental surgery. Local anesthesia takes from 5 to 15 minutes to become effective and lasts from one to three hours. During longer procedures, additional injections of anesthetic may have to be administered when the first dosage wears off.

Epinephrine, a vasoconstrictor that causes superficial blood vessels to narrow, is often added to the local anesthetic when the physician is operating on the face and head. The addition of epinephrine allows for better visualization of the surgical site because it diminishes bleeding. Epinephrine causes local anesthetics to be absorbed by the body more slowly and gives them a longer-lasting effect. Clearly mark anesthetics that have been prepared with the addition of epinephrine. Patients with heart problems could have a reaction to epinephrine that causes tachycardia or other irregularities.

Nerve blocks are administered by injection into a nerve adjacent to the operative site. This type of anesthetic is used for surgery on hands, fingers, and toes.

Topical anesthetics are local pain control medications that are applied to the skin and produce a numbing effect. These can be applied by drop, spray, or swab. They are commonly used in eye procedures. An example of a spray anesthetic is ethyl chloride, which produces a freezing effect on the skin. Benzocaine (Solarcaine) is another example of a topical anesthetic.

Administering Anesthesia

Only physicians or anesthesiologists can administer an anesthetic, and only they must chart the administration. Either the medical assistant or the physician will draw up the local anesthetic. (The correct procedure for drawing up medication is discussed in the chapter titled "Administering Medications.") The medication vial must be correctly identified and then wiped with an alcohol sponge. If the medical assistant draws up the medication, then the medical assistant must present both the syringe and the vial to the physician so that the physician can read the label. The anesthetic will be injected into the patient's prepared skin by the physician before the physician has donned gloves. This syringe is not placed onto the sterile field because it has been contaminated by the medical assistant's ungloved hands.

If the physician prefers to draw up the anesthetic, it can be done using a sterile syringe after the physician has applied gloves. The medical assistant will hold the vial securely while the physician withdraws the anesthetic without contaminating the needle. The outside of the vial cannot be touched by the physician's sterile gloved hand. This syringe can then be placed onto the sterile field.

Some physicians prefer to change the needle after drawing up the local anesthetic. For example, they may draw up the drug using a 21-gauge needle and then administer the solution using a 23-gauge or 25-gauge needle.

Preparation of the Patient's Skin

Although skin cannot be sterilized, it can be cleaned using medical aseptic technique. Careful cleansing of the skin before performing a surgical procedure reduces the number of microorganisms on the skin. This decreases the chance of carrying infection-producing microorganisms through the skin during the invasive procedure (incision into skin or entrance of a probe).

In some situations, the physician may order the surgical site to be shaved because bacteria can reside in hair. See Procedure 41-6 and Figure A for skin preparation and shaving instructions. Care must be taken to avoid scraping or cutting the skin during the shaving process. The physician will order either a wet shave (moistening the skin with soap and water) or dry shave (Figure B). Some physicians feel that shaving the skin presents more risk of skin injury and prefer only to have the patient's skin cleansed carefully.

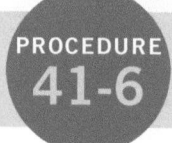

PROCEDURE
41-6

Preparing the Patient's Skin for Surgical Procedures

Objective ◆ *Prepare the patient's skin for a surgical procedure using a sterile scrub and shave.*

EQUIPMENT AND SUPPLIES

Antiseptic germicidal soap; sterile saline; antiseptic such as Betadine; eight sterile applicators; Mayo tray; waste receptacle (may be included in sterile pack); biohazard waste container; plastic bag for soiled dressings; sterile pack (sterile gloves, three to four towel packs, sterile basin pack with three basins, patient drape, 4 × 4 gauze sponge pack with 12 to 24 sponges, shave preparation kit)

METHOD

1. Perform hand hygiene.
2. Assemble equipment by placing packs on a Mayo stand or side tray and opening outer wraps from all packs.
3. Identify the patient and explain the procedure.

4. Have the patient remove appropriate clothing and put on gowning. Ask the patient to void, if necessary.
5. Position and drape the patient to provide exposure of the operative site.
6. Unwrap the basin pack. Pour germicidal soap solution into one basin, sterile saline into the second basin, and antiseptic into the third.
7. Wash hands using sterile scrub, and apply sterile gloves.
8. Drape the skin with two towels placed 3 to 5 inches above and below the surgical site.
9. With a sterile gauze or sponge, apply soapy solution to the patient's skin. Use a circular motion starting at the site of the proposed incision and move outward (Figure A). Pass

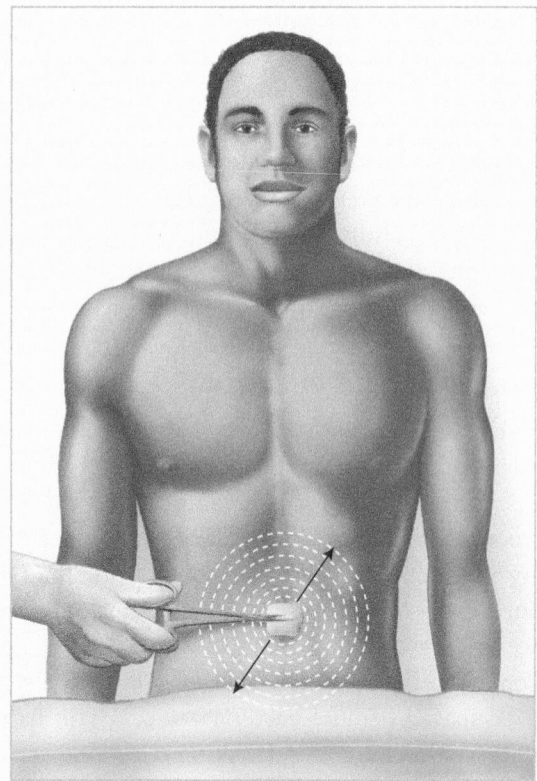

FIGURE A Preparing the patient's skin at the surgical site.

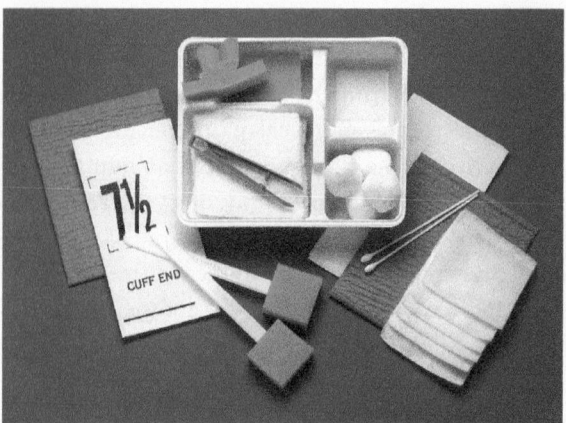

FIGURE B Dry skin prep tray.

over each skin area only once. Place each used sponge into a waste receptacle immediately.

10. Take a fresh sterile gauze or sponge for each cleansing wipe. Repeat this process until the area is completely washed. The last area cleansed will be the outer edges.

11. Rinse using sterile saline on a clean gauze or sponge. Pat dry with a dry gauze only on the area that has been washed. Avoid touching any other skin area.

If shaving is ordered, then proceed with the following steps:

1. Apply soap solution to the site area. Remove the razor from the shave preparation pack. Pull the skin taut and shave the surgical site in the same direction as the hair is growing. Rinse with a saline solution using the single-pass, circular motion as before and pat it dry.

2. Reapply soap solution to the area and repeat the preceding process according to your office policy (around five minutes).

3. Pat the entire area dry with the third sterile towel.

4. Apply the antiseptic solution using two cotton applicators together in the same single-pass, circular motion.

5. Cover the prepared surgical site with the remaining sterile towel.

6. Properly dispose of gloves and soiled materials in a biohazard waste container.

Instructions for a dry shave Some physicians prefer that the patient receive a dry shave. To remove hair, electric clippers are preferred to razor blades because they lessen the likelihood of accidental nicks in the skin.

1. Clip the hair as short as possible with scissors.

2. Apply firm traction to the skin with the nondominant hand.

3. Remove hair in the direction of hair growth. Never shave against the grain, as this will cause unnecessary irritation to the skin and increase the likelihood of nicks.

CHARTING EXAMPLE

3/12/YY 11:00 A.M. Pt arrived for removal and biopsy of growth on outer aspect of left forearm. Surgical site prepared using Betadine. No cuts or lesions noted..........................J. Wall, RMA

POSTOPERATIVE PATIENT CARE

Postoperative care includes monitoring the patient during recovery from anesthesia, wound care, applying dressings, and communicating patient instructions. Patient education addresses more about instructing patients on home care of wounds.

Recovery from Anesthesia

Topical and other local anesthetics take effect either immediately or within a few minutes. Their effects wear off quickly.

The use of large amounts of local anesthetic, beyond normal dosages, is not recommended and may result in an adverse reaction in patients. Some patients are allergic to anesthetics and may slip into anaphylactic shock, which requires emergency treatment (see the chapter titled "Assisting with Medical Emergencies"). An emergency tray or cart stocked with drugs used to counteract shock should always be available in the office. Many facilities require employees to have current CPR certification.

To prevent choking on food or burning the mouth, the patient treated in the mouth or throat with a local anesthetic

TABLE 41-3 | Local Anesthetics

Anesthetic Agent	Use
Benzocaine	Topical use only
Chloroprocaine	Nerve block, epidural
Lidocaine (Xylocaine)	Infiltration or topical
Mepivacaine	Infiltration nerve block
Procaine (Novacaine)	Infiltration; seldom used now
Tetracaine	Infiltration, topical nerve block, spinal

should be advised not to eat until the effects of the anesthetic wear off. Table 41-3 contains examples of local anesthetics. Patients must be observed carefully after surgery for signs of adverse reaction to the anesthetic, bleeding, and circulatory problems. The patient's vital signs (blood pressure, temperature, pulse, and respiration) should be monitored immediately after surgery and then every 15 minutes for the first hour. Never give fluids to a patient who is not fully alert. This can result in choking. Oral medications for pain, nausea, and vomiting have to be withheld until the patient is fully recovered from anesthesia. Medications may be given by injection until recovery occurs.

Excessive disorientation and inability to revive within a normal recovery time should be reported immediately to the physician. Observe the patient for nausea and vomiting. The physician may order medications to counteract nausea and vomiting.

Types of Wounds

The skin acts as a protective barrier and is the body's first line of defense. Any break in the skin, whether from injury or a surgical incision, is referred to as a wound. A surgical procedure requiring an incision through the skin is considered an invasive procedure because a wound is created when the skin is entered. Wounds cause blood vessels to rupture and blood to seep into tissues, which results in skin color changes. Typically, skin coloration changes from erythema in a fresh wound to a greenish yellow color during the healing process, which involves oxidation of blood pigments. There are four types of wound classification:

- **Abrasion**—Outer layers of skin are rubbed away because of scraping; will generally heal without scarring.

- **Incision**—Smooth cut resulting from a surgical scalpel or sharp material, such as razor or glass; may result in excessive bleeding and scarring if deep.

- **Laceration**—Edges are torn in an irregular shape; can cause profuse bleeding and scarring.

- **Puncture**—Made by a sharp, pointed instrument such as a bullet, needle, nail, or splinter; external bleeding is usually minimal, but infection may occur because of penetration with a contaminated object, and there may be scarring.

Wounds are also briefly discussed in the next chapter, "Assisting with Medical Emergencies and Emergency Preparedness."

The Healing Process

Wounds pass through various stages of healing, including inflammation, as the body starts to fight off potential infection. Inflammation is the body's protective response to trauma and invasion by microorganisms; it is generally localized around the site of trauma or infection. Signs of inflammation are redness (erythema), swelling, warmth, and pain. Wounds go through three phases before healing or restoration of structure and function take place:

- **Inflammatory phase (3 days)**—Blood clot forms to stop bleeding and plug the opening of a wound; **eschar** or scab forms to keep out microorganisms.

- **Proliferating phase (3 to 21 days)**—Fibrin threads extend across the opening of a wound and pull edges together; cells multiply to repair the wound.

- **Maturation phase (21 days to 2 years)**—Tissue cells strengthen and tighten the wound closure, form a scar; scar eventually fades and thins.

Wound Complications

Wound complications include infection (signs of inflammation, purulent or puslike drainage, fever); hemorrhage or bleeding; **dehiscence** (separation of wound edges); and **evisceration** (separation of wound edges and protrusion of abdominal organs). Uneven or ragged-edged wounds and large wounds take more time to heal. Without proper wound care, infection will set in. Infection is the result of wound contamination during or after the injury or surgical procedure. Drainage occurs as fluid and cells escape from the tissues during the inflammatory phase of wound healing. The amount and type of drainage observed on a dressing should be charted. The following are types of wound drainage:

- **Serous drainage**—Clear, watery drainage, such as the fluid in a blister.

- **Sanguineous drainage**—Bloody (bright red is fresh blood, dark red is older blood); the amount and color of sanguineous drainage is important.

- **Serosanguineous drainage**—Thin watery drainage tinged with blood.

- **Purulent drainage**—Thick puslike drainage that is green, yellow, or brown.

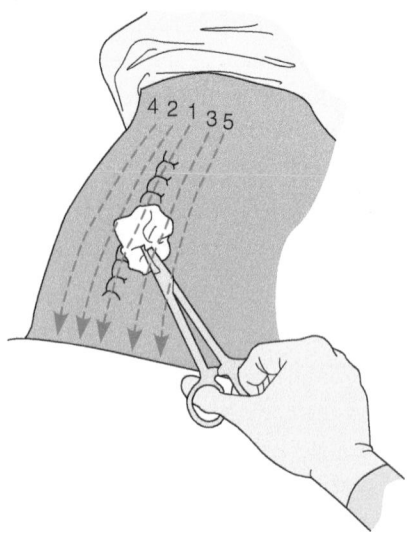

FIGURE 41-20 Cleanse a linear wound by using a new sterile gauze pad for each stroke, beginning next to the wound and working from the top to the bottom of the wound area.

Cleansing a Wound

A wound must be cleaned before a sterile dressing can be applied. The physician will indicate which of the many products available for wound cleansing is preferred. Warm water and soap are used to remove surface dirt from around the wound area.

To clean a wound using a sterile gauze or swab, work from the clean area near the wound outward to less clean areas. This will prevent dragging more microorganisms into the wound. Wipe in one direction and then discard the sterile swab or gauze. Cleanse a linear wound from top to bottom with one stroke per sterile gauze or swab (Figure 41-20). Use a new sterile gauze or swab for each stroke. Work outward from the wound in parallel lines. To cleanse an open wound, such as a pressure ulcer, work in circles, half or full, beginning in the center and working outward (Figure 41-21).

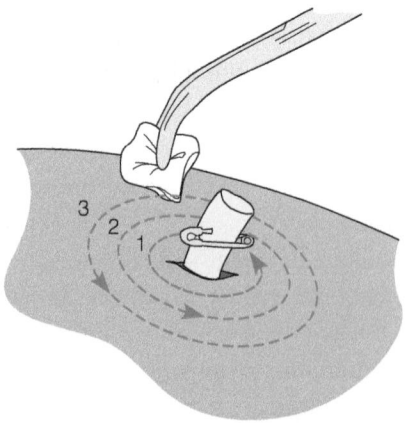

FIGURE 41-21 To cleanse an open wound, begin close to the wound and work outward in full or half circles.

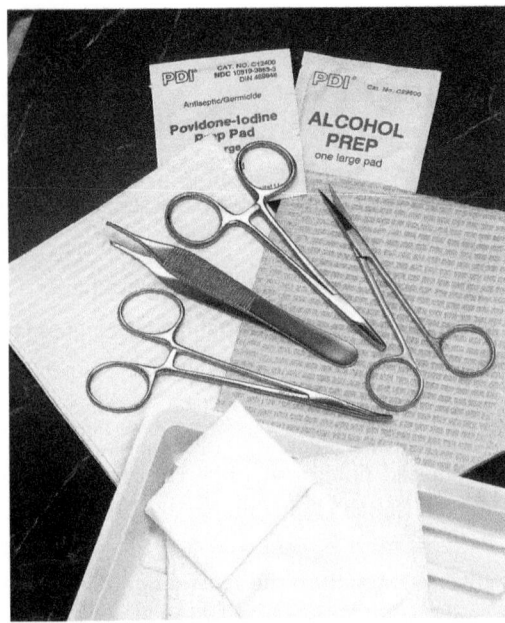

FIGURE 41-22 Wound closure kit.

Always clean at least 1 inch beyond the edge of the dressing to be applied. If no dressing is to be applied, clean 2 inches beyond the edges of the wound. Use a new gauze pad for each circle.

The size and shape of the dressing needed depend on the size, location, and amount of drainage from the wound. Sterile 4 × 4 gauze pads ("four by fours") are used for most dressings. If drainage is expected from the wound, a prepared dressing, such as Telfa, may be used to prevent the dressing from sticking to the wound. See Figure 41-22 for an example of a wound closure kit.

Each patient should be asked how long it has been since she received a tetanus shot. In the event that the shot was not received within the previous 10 years, the physician should be informed. Procedure 41-7 describes how to perform wound care.

Sutures

As already discussed, a suture is a thread used to sew together body tissues. Sutures used to attach tissues beneath the skin are often made of an absorbable material that disappears in several days. Skin sutures, by contrast, are made of nonabsorbable materials such as silk, cotton, linen, wire, nylon, and Dacron (polyester fiber). Silver wire clips or staples are also available. Sutures or staples are inserted by the surgeon at the end of a procedure to hold tissues in alignment during the healing process. The steps necessary to assist with suturing are given in Procedure 41-8. Sutures generally remain in place five or six days and then have to be removed if they are nonabsorbable. If sutures remain in the body too long, they

Performing Wound Care and Changing a Dressing

Objective ◆ *Cleanse a wound and change a wound dressing using sterile technique.*

EQUIPMENT AND SUPPLIES

Disposable gloves; antiseptic solution; solution container; prepackaged dressing pack; thumb forceps; sterile cotton balls; sterile gloves; sterile dressing; adhesive tape; scissors, if necessary for tape; waste container/plastic bag; biohazard waste container; Mayo stand or side tray

METHOD

1. Perform hand hygiene.
2. Assemble equipment using the Mayo stand.
3. Explain the procedure to the patient.
4. Assist the patient into a comfortable position with the area to be dressed resting on a support, such as an examination table.
5. Apply nonsterile gloves.
6. Prepare the sterile field, using aseptic technique and a prepackaged dressing packet. Employ sterile transfer forceps to place additional sterile items on the sterile field.
7. Remove the dressing from the wound by using gloved hands or forceps to loosen the tape; then pull the dressing from both sides toward the wound (Figure A). Inspect the wound for signs of infection and inflammation. Note any discharge by its type, amount, and color (Figure B).
8. Dispose of the soiled dressing in a biohazard waste container. Be careful not to pass the soiled dressing over the sterile field during this step. The dressing should not touch the outside of the biohazard container or its edges (Figure C).
9. Discard gloves and contaminated forceps properly. Place disposable gloves and forceps in a biohazardous waste container. Reusable forceps are placed in the basin for later cleaning.
10. Pour the antiseptic onto several cotton balls in a sterile bowl until they are moist but not saturated.
11. Perform handwashing.
12. Open sterile gloves and apply properly.
13. Cleanse the wound by using sterile forceps to hold the cotton while moving from top to bottom of the wound once. Use a new cotton ball with antiseptic for each wipe. Move from the inside of the wound to the outside edges.
14. Pick up the sterile dressing with gloved hands and place over the wound.
15. Discard gloves and forceps.
16. Apply adhesive tape to hold the dressing in place. Do not apply too tightly as to restrict circulation. The strips of tape should be long enough to hold the dressing in place. Do not wrap the tape entirely around an extremity or completely cover the dressing.
17. Instruct the patient on dressing care, and to schedule a follow-up appointment to see the physician.
18. Chart the procedure, including the date, time, location, and condition of the wound and the instructions given to the patient.

CHARTING EXAMPLE

2/14/YY 11:00 A.M. Dressing change on right anterior forearm. Moderate amount of serous drainage with slight erythema surrounding wound. Incision healing well with edges aligned. Cleansed with Betadine. Sterile dressing applied. Pt. instructed on wound care...M. King, CMA (AAMA)

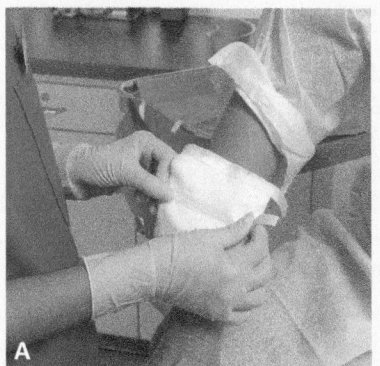
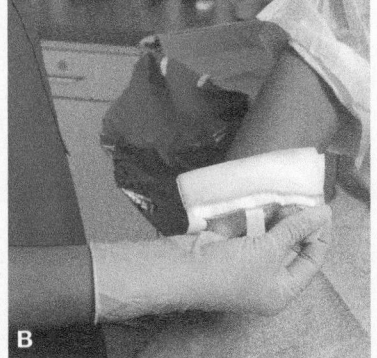
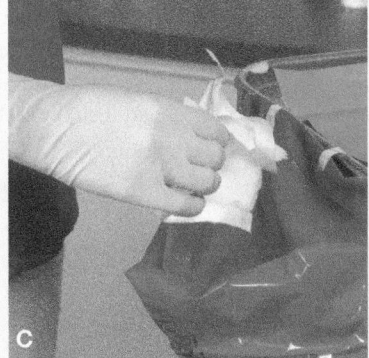

FIGURE A–C Wound dressing **(A)** removal; **(B)** inspection; and **(C)** disposal.

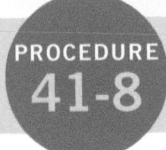

Assisting with Suturing

Objective ◆ *Assist with suture repair of an incision or laceration using sterile technique.*

EQUIPMENT AND SUPPLIES

Mayo stand; side stand; anesthetic; sterile transfer forceps; sterile saline; waste container/plastic bag; biohazard waste container; sharps container; sterile gloves (two pairs); sterile pack(s) (patient drape, towel pack with four towels, 4 × 4 gauze sponge pack); scalpel blades pack (Nos. 10 and 15); needle and syringe pack; suture and needle pack (according to physician's preference); two sterile basins; suture pack (scalpel handle, needle holder, thumb forceps, two scissors, three hemostats)

METHOD

1. Use a sterile scrub and gloving procedure.
2. Stand across from the physician.
3. Place two sponges ready for the physician near the wound site.
4. Assist by using additional sponges to keep the wound dry.
5. Pass instruments, such as scissors, to the physician using a firm snap of the handle into the physician's hand without letting go until the physician has a firm grasp.
6. The blade is placed into the scalpel using a hemostat.
7. Hand the scalpel to the physician with blade edge down to avoid cutting the physician.
8. Continue to use sponges to keep the wound free of drainage.
9. Pass all instruments to the physician as requested. Try to anticipate the next instruments that the physician may need, such as another hemostat or scissors for cutting a suture.
10. Pass the toothed forceps to the physician if laceration edges need to be grasped.
11. Mount the needle into the needle holder and pass as one unit to the physician, using care to keep the suture within the sterile field. Pass the needle holder with the needle pointing outward. Hold the suture with the other hand, and do not let go of it until the physician sees it.
12. Using the suture scissors, prepare to cut the suture as directed by the physician (usually ⅛ to ¼ inch from the knot).

13. Sponge the closed wound once with a sponge and discard.
14. Repeat this step with each suture.
15. Apply a layer of sterile dressing over the wound, such as a sterile gauze pad. You may use forceps if preferred. The sterile dressing should extend a minimum of 2 inches past all edges of the wound.
16. Apply a second layer of gauze over the wound site.
17. Add a final third layer of wound dressing, such as a SurgiPad.
18. Secure the edges of the dressing with paper tape or similar product. Some physicians prefer the wound be covered with a clear, waterproof membrane such as Telfa. Paper tape is often used because it contains a less intense adhesive, lowering the risk for adverse skin reactions.
19. After they are used, place all soiled instruments on the sterile field if they will be used again; discard others in the instrument basin.
20. When the procedure is complete, remove your gloves and perform hand hygiene before assisting the patient.
21. Allow the patient to rest and recover from the anesthetic. Periodically check the patient's vital signs according to your office policy.
22. Provide clear oral and written postoperative instructions for the patient. Make sure the patient is stable before he leaves the office.
23. Clean, sanitize, and sterilize the instruments. Clean and sanitize the room in preparation for the next patient.
24. Perform hand hygiene.

CHARTING EXAMPLE

2/14/YY 1:00 P.M. Cleansed wound with antiseptic. Assisted physician with suturing wound. Instructed on wound care, signs and symptoms of infection, and given follow-up appointment............
....M. King, CMA (AAMA)
The physician will chart the details of the surgical procedure.

---

can cause skin irritation and infection. The suture acts as a wick to carry bacteria through the skin and into the subcutaneous tissues. Suture removal times differ depending on the site:

- Facial sutures may be removed after only 24 to 48 hours to prevent scarring.

- Head and neck sutures remain in place for three to five days.
- Abdominal sutures remain in place for five to seven days.
- Sutures over weight-bearing joints and large bones may remain seven to ten days.

The medical assistant prepares the patient for suture or staple removal by taking off the dressing, if one is present. Each edge of the dressing is removed by pulling toward the suture line. If the dressing is adhering to the suture line, then a small amount of sterile saline or hydrogen peroxide can be used to moisten the dressing to ease removal.

In some office practices and in some states, medical assistants are permitted to remove sutures. Explain the procedure to the patient, reminding her that there may be a pulling sensation. Then thoroughly cleanse the skin with an antiseptic such as alcohol or Betadine solution. After opening the sterile suture packet (Figure 41-23) and creating a sterile field with the wrapper, gently pick up the knot of the suture using a thumb forceps. Then cut the suture with suture scissors below the knot as close to the skin as possible. Remove the suture by pulling the long remaining suture out. Never pull suture material that is outside the skin through the skin, which might pull infection-causing microorganisms through the skin along with it. Very little of the suture is actually pulled through the skin. (Procedure 41-9 and Figure A illustrate the steps to remove sutures. Removal of staples is also described.)

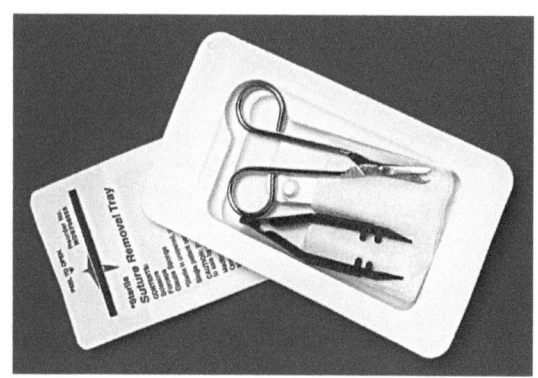

FIGURE 41-23 Disposable suture removal set.

Sterile Dressing

A dressing is the application of a sterile covering over a surgical site or wound using surgical asepsis. A patient who has sustained an injury or undergone a surgical procedure may need to schedule an appointment to remove the old dressing and apply a new sterile dressing. Review Procedure 41-7 and Figures A–C, which demonstrate the steps for changing a sterile dressing.

PROCEDURE 41-9

Removing Sutures and Staples

Objective ◆ *Remove sutures and staples using sterile technique, following the physician's order.*

EQUIPMENT AND SUPPLIES

Suture removal pack (suture scissors, sterile gauze squares, thumb forceps, skin antiseptic, sterile gloves, bandages, biohazard waste container)

METHOD
Removal of sutures

1. Perform hand hygiene.
2. Assemble equipment and check the expiration date on the pack.
3. Identify the patient.
4. Explain the procedure to the patient, and assist the patient into a comfortable position.
5. Perform hand hygiene.
6. Remove the old dressing using the proper technique.
7. Perform hand hygiene.
8. Open a suture or staple removal pack using the proper technique.
9. Apply sterile gloves using the proper technique.

10. Cleanse the wound as needed.
11. Place a gauze square next to the wound for placement of sutures or staples as they are removed.
12. Grasp the knot of the suture with thumb forceps and lift gently (Figure A).
13. Insert the suture scissors and cut the suture at skin level. Pull out the suture.
14. Place the cut suture on the gauze.
15. Repeat these steps until all sutures are removed.
16. Count sutures to make sure that all have been removed.

Removal of staples
1–10. Perform steps 1 through 10 above.
11. Place the lower tips of a sterile staple remover under the staple.
12. Squeeze the handles together until they are completely closed. (Pressing the handles together causes the staple to bend in the middle and pulls the edges of the staple out of the skin.) Do not lift the staple remover when squeezing the handles.

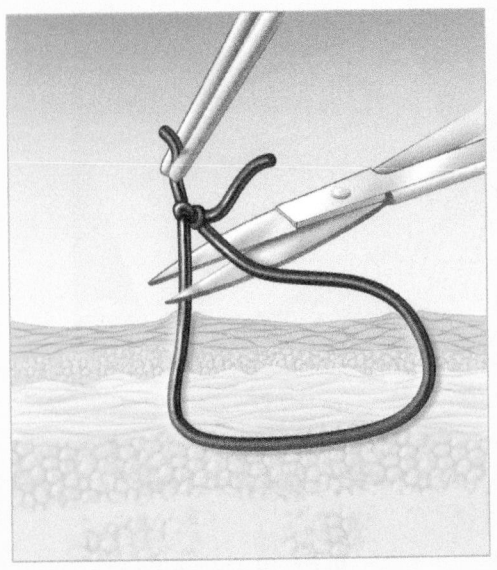 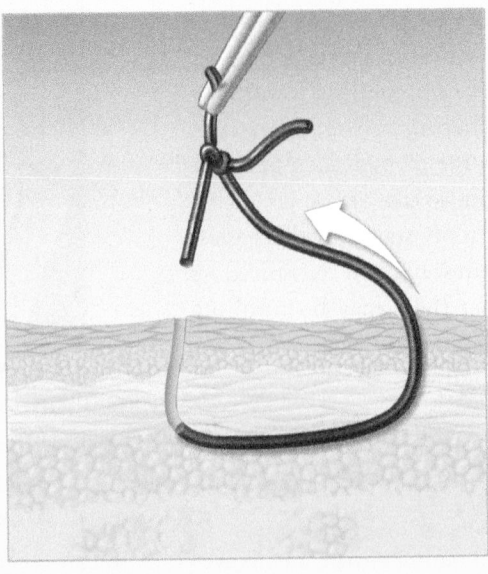

FIGURE A Removal of sutures.

Closing steps for removal of sutures or staples

16. Clean the wound with antiseptic and allow it to dry.
17. Dress the wound as ordered.
18. Properly dispose of equipment and supplies.
19. Remove gloves and perform hand hygiene.
20. Instruct the patient on wound care.
21. Document the procedure, including condition of the wound, number of sutures or staples removed, and patient instructions on wound care.

13. When both ends of the staple are visible, gently move the staple away from the incision site.
14. Hold the staple remover over a disposable container, release the staple remover handles, and release the staple.
15. Place the staple on the gauze, repeat these steps until all staples are removed, and count the number of staples to ensure all have been removed.

CHARTING EXAMPLE

2/14/YY 11:00 A.M. Removed sutures and cleansed wound with antiseptic. Wound healing well. Pt. instructed on wound care...M. King, CMA (AAMA)

Bandaging the Wound

After the wound is dressed, the physician may instruct you to apply a bandage to hold the dressing in place. Bandages may be gauze, fabric, or elasticized and need not be sterile (Figure 41-24). Bandages are available in various sizes, lengths, and shapes. Some bandages are self-adhering and easier to apply to awkward areas. Elastic bandages are used to support an injured part and reduce swelling. Care must be taken not to bandage too tightly and restrict circulation. Procedure 41-10 and Figures A–C show the steps for applying a bandage to a patient's forearm.

SURGICAL PROCEDURES PERFORMED IN THE MEDICAL OFFICE

Many minor surgical procedures can be performed efficiently in the physician's office. This saves the patient the time and expense of having to go into an ambulatory surgical facility or a hospital. The basic surgical setup is the standard setup with the addition of specific instruments for each procedure. Some minor procedures performed in the medical office include biopsy, cautery, colposcopy,

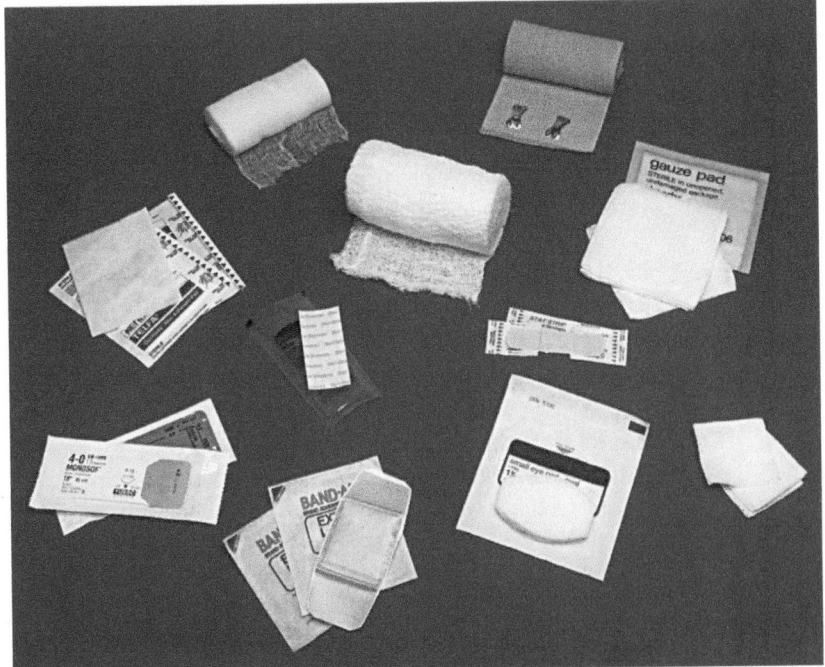

FIGURE 41-24 Various types of bandages.

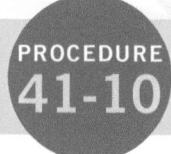

PROCEDURE 41-10

Applying a Bandage over a Sterile Dressing

Objective ◆ *Apply a bandage to the forearm.*

EQUIPMENT AND SUPPLIES

Nonsterile gloves; bandage material prescribed by physician or office procedures; bandage scissors; tape

METHOD

1. Identify the patient.
2. Perform hand hygiene.
3. Apply nonsterile gloves.
4. Explain the procedure.
5. Hold a bandage against the skin with your nondominant hand 1 inch below the dressing.
6. Wrap the bandage around the wrist two to three times to secure (Figure A).
7. Wrap the forearm from distal (part farthest away from the body) to proximal (closest to the body) with overlapping spiral turns (Figure B).

8. Check that the bandage is not restricting blood flow.
9. Continue wrapping to at least 1 inch above the dressing (Figure C).
10. Wrap two more times to secure the bandage; then cut.
11. Tape the cut end to the bandage; do not tape the end to the patient's skin.
12. Check again for any blood flow restriction.
13. Remove gloves.
14. Perform hand hygiene.
15. Explain home care to the patient.
16. Document the procedure accurately.

CHARTING EXAMPLE

1/18/YY 9:30 A.M. Applied bandage to sterile dressing. Pt instructed on home care for dressing.......M. King, CMA (AAMA)

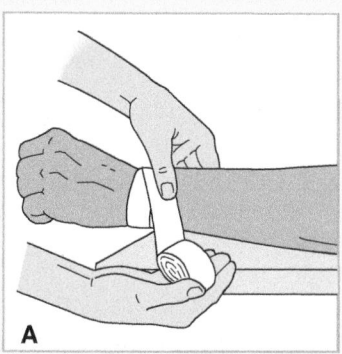
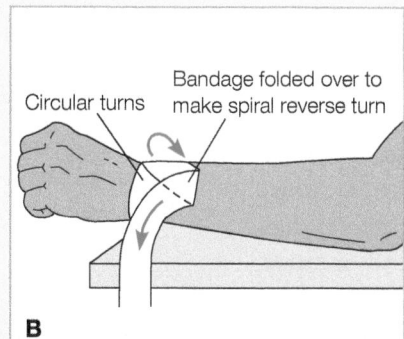
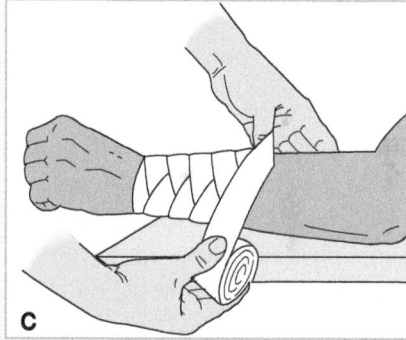

Circular turns

Bandage folded over to make spiral reverse turn

A   **B**   **C**

FIGURE A–C Bandaging a forearm.

cryosurgery, laser surgery, endocervical curettage, endoscopic procedures, suture removal, removal of foreign bodies, incision and drainage, vasectomy, and removal of growths and tumors.

The medical assistant does not administer these procedures but must understand them and their effects in order to assist the physician and the patient. A brief description of some procedures follows.

Electrosurgery

Electrosurgery is the application of high-frequency electrical currents. These currents are used to heat tissue to cut,

destroy, or remove it in very specific areas and patterns. Electrosurgery is most often performed in dermatological, gynecological, cardiac, ocular, ENT, and orthopedic surgical procedures. Because of the risk of accidental burning with electrosurgery, it is important to follow strict safety precautions, which include inspecting the equipment before use, using only as the manufacturer directs, ensuring that the equipment is properly working, and avoiding the use of alcohol prep on skin before using electrocautery. Be sure not to touch the cautery device to dry gauze, drapes, or other flammable objects. Ensure fire extinguishers and sprinkler

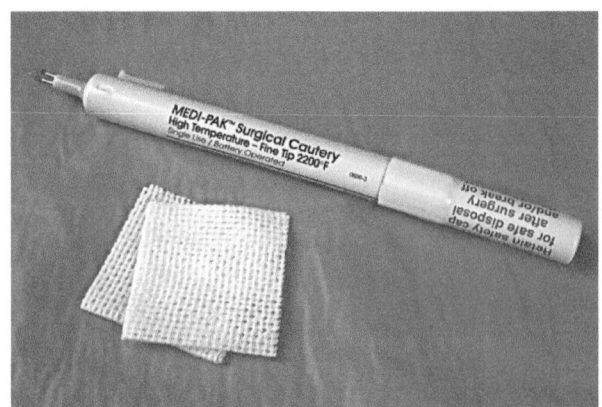

FIGURE 41-25 A disposable cautery unit.

systems are in working order. See Figure 41-25 for a photo of a disposable cautery unit.

Five types of currents are used in electrosurgery:

- **Electrocoagulation**—Destroys tissues and controls bleeding by coagulation.

- **Electrodesiccation**—Destroys tissue by creating a spark gap when the probe is inserted into unwanted tissue.

- **Electrofulguration**—Destroys tissue with a spark emitted from the tip of a probe positioned a short distance away from the unwanted tissue.

- **Electrosection**—Uses electric current to incise and excise the tissue.

- **Electrocautery (or cautery)**—Uses high-frequency, alternating electric current to destroy, cut, or remove tissue. Electrocautery is also used to coagulate small blood vessels, thereby reducing bleeding and cell loss. Some physicians have a **hyfrecator**, which is a miniature electrocautery unit (Figure 41-26).

In some offices, either the electrosurgical unit (ESU) or the ultrasonic surgical unit (USU) is taking the place of

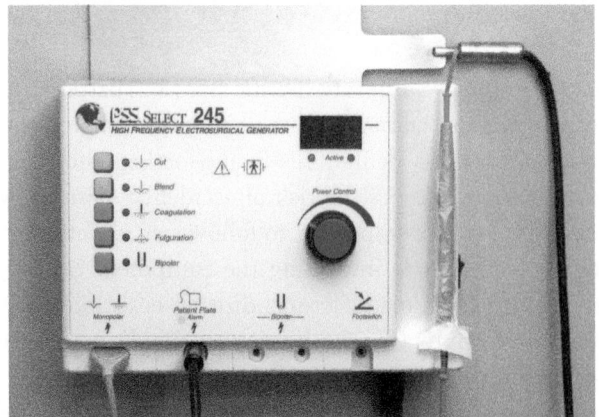

FIGURE 41-26 A hyfrecator, an electrocautery unit.

electrocautery. The ESU is able to provide a more controlled, less damaging form of electric current through the use of a variety of attachments. For example, an incision can be made using ESU with a small electrode blade. The blade cauterizes as it cuts, thus minimizing bleeding. Other attachments can be used to coagulate and suction. The USU uses high-frequency sound waves to break apart calcified or sclerosed tissue that can be removed in small segments. Some models have the ability to suction as they break apart and dissolve body calcifications.

In some forms of electrosurgery, a local anesthetic may be administered.

Laser Surgery

The term *laser* is an acronym for **L**ight **A**mplification by **S**timulated **E**mission of **R**adiation. A laser emits an intense beam of light and originally was used to treat diseases of the retina. Today laser surgery is used to treat a wide variety of diseases and conditions, including vascular, neurological, orthopedic, and dermatologic problems. Laser surgery has the advantage of promoting quick healing and not destroying surrounding tissue. A medical assistant may need extra training to assist with laser surgery. When a room is to be used for laser surgery, it is important to shut out any stray light rays, post OSHA's laser warning sign, and make sure everyone, including the patient, is wearing safety goggles. As with electrocautery, there is some risk of fire as well, so be sure that equipment is working correctly and that flammable objects do not catch fire. After surgery is complete, the wound should be cleaned with antiseptic and dressed with a sterile dressing.

Colposcopy

Colposcopy is an examination of the vagina and cervix performed using a colposcope, a lighted instrument, with the patient in the lithotomy position. The colposcope allows the physician to observe the tissues of this area in great detail through light and magnification. Abnormal areas of tissue or cells can then be removed for biopsy to detect cancer. In some cases, cryosurgery using freezing temperatures to destroy cells is then applied.

Colposcopy is performed in the following cases:

- When an abnormal tissue development is observed by the physician during a routine pelvic examination

- When a Papanicolaou (Pap) smear result is in the abnormal range

- For magnified visualization

- To obtain a biopsy specimen

If the physician is unable to visualize the entire cervical canal during the colposcopy, she may perform an endocervical curettage (ECC) to scrape endocervical cells from inside the cervical canal. These cells are then sent for further testing to determine any abnormality. Abnormal cell growth can be a sign of a precancerous condition that, if untreated, could lead to the development of cancer.

The patient may experience slight bleeding after a colposcopy if a biopsy is taken. In such cases, provide a perineal pad for the patient with instructions for home care. The patient should receive instructions to call the physician if abnormal pain or bleeding is experienced after this procedure.

Endoscopy

An endoscope is an instrument used to look into a hollow organ or body cavity. An endoscope is used to examine the larynx, bladder, colon, sigmoid colon, stomach, abdomen, and some joints. Some attachments are used with some endoscopes, such as a light source, suction, a monitor, and a video recorder. Great care must be taken with these sensitive instruments. In most instances, the patient will need preparation before the examination—for example, fasting, taking a laxative, or administering an enema.

Figure 41-27 is an example of a flexible colonoscope with monitor and video recorder.

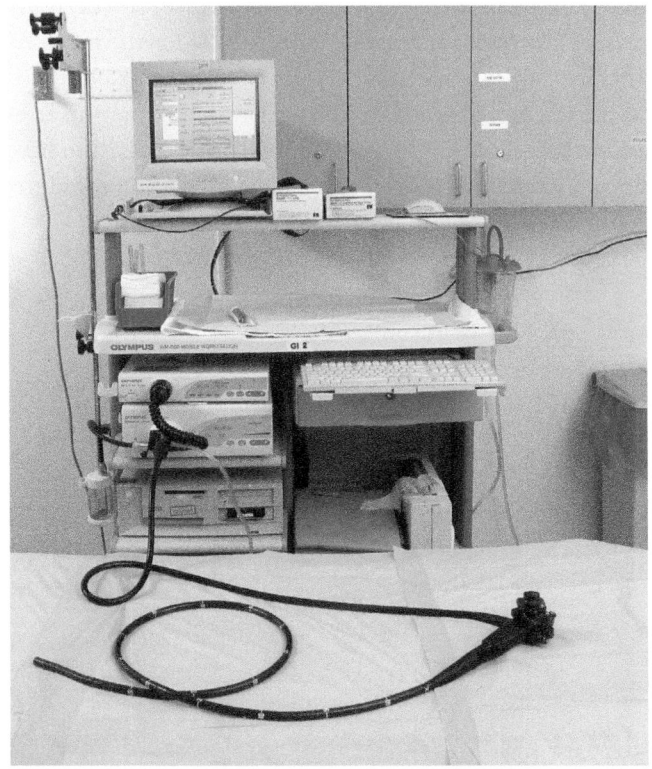

FIGURE 41-27 A flexible colonoscope with monitor and video recorder.

Cryosurgery

Cryosurgery is the use of subfreezing temperatures to destroy tissue. This procedure is also known as cryocautery, rooted in the term *cautery*, which refers to a destruction of tissue.

One example of cryosurgery is the treatment of cervical erosion and chronic cervicitis. With the patient in the lithotomy position, the colposcope is used to magnify the surface of the cervix. Then a probe capable of reaching subfreezing temperatures is placed within the colposcope to destroy abnormal cells. The patient may experience mild cramping and a watery discharge after the procedure. The physician may advise her to take a mild analgesic, such as acetaminophen (Tylenol). The patient should be advised against using a tampon for at least a month because it could irritate sensitive tissues. Additional instruction should include details on reporting any unusual pain or foul discharge, abstaining from sexual intercourse for one month, douching, and scheduling a follow-up visit.

The probe used in cryosurgery must be sterilized according to manufacturer's instructions immediately after use.

Endometrial Biopsy (EMB)

An endometrial biopsy (EMB) consists of using a curette or suction tool to remove uterine tissue for testing. EMB is performed for a variety of reasons:

- To detect precancerous and cancerous conditions of the endometrial lining of the uterus
- To detect inflammatory conditions
- To determine if polyps are present
- To assess abnormal uterine bleeding
- To assess the effects of hormonal therapy
- To screen for early detection of endometrial cancer (particularly if risk factors are present)

An EMB is performed with the patient in the lithotomy position. The physician performs a bimanual examination of the uterus and administers a local anesthetic. A uterine curette is sounded into the uterus, indicating depth and direction, after the anesthetic has taken effect. The specimen is taken by means of a curette or with a suction device to aspirate a specimen. The specimen is sent to the laboratory in a container containing a 10 percent formalin preservative solution.

Provide a perineal pad for the patient with instructions for home care. The patient should receive instructions to call the physician if abnormal pain or bleeding occurs after this procedure. The patient may experience mild cramping for which the physician may advise her to take a mild analgesic. She should be advised against using a tampon, douching, or having sexual intercourse for at least 72 hours.

Incision and Drainage

The incision and drainage (I & D) procedure is performed to relieve the buildup of purulent (pus) material as a result of infection. The purulent discharge may be cultured to determine what microorganism is causing the infection and, thus, what antibiotic would be effective. The procedure is performed using sterile surgical technique, keeping in mind that the purulent material may be highly infectious. All soiled dressings and 4 × 4s immediately should be placed in a plastic waste container and then disposed of properly using OSHA guidelines.

A tray setup for an I & D includes the following:

- Scalpel handle and blades (No. 11)
- Curved iris scissors
- Tissue forceps
- Kelly hemostat
- Retractor
- Thumb dressing forceps
- 4 × 4 gauze squares

Removal of Foreign Bodies and Growths

A foreign body can include a variety of materials from a small splinter or fishhook to a large object, such as an arrow that is embedded in tissue. Splinter forceps are needed on an instrument tray for foreign body removal.

Growths include tumors, warts, moles, and cysts. The most frequent growth removal procedure in the medical office is for cysts, which are enclosed fluid-filled sacs. Some growths are sent to the laboratory for biopsy testing depending on the physician's instructions. The removal of a foreign body or neoplasm (new growth) requires a surgical setup that includes the following:

- Thumb dressing forceps
- Retractor
- Scalpel handle and blades (Nos. 10 and 15)
- Curved tissue scissors
- Tissue forceps
- Hemostats
- Blunt probe
- Splinter forceps
- Needle holder
- Suture materials and needles
- Sterile 4 × 4 gauze

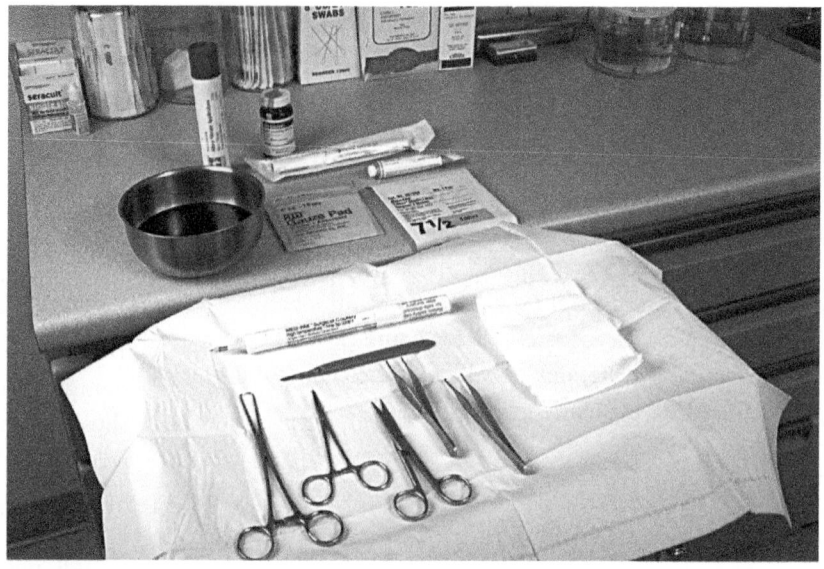

FIGURE 41-28 Surgical tray set up for a biopsy procedure.

Figure 41-28 shows a surgical tray for biopsy removal. Figure 41-29 shows a medical assistant holding a specimen container so the physician can place the biopsy specimen into it without touching the rim or outside of the container and the contaminating tissue.

Vasectomy

The vasectomy procedure, tying and cutting of the vas deferens, on the male patient is a surgical procedure that is now commonly performed in the urologist's office. A vasectomy provides a permanent form of birth control for the male. As with any surgical procedure, a consent form must be signed and placed in the patient's record before beginning this irreversible procedure. The patient should be instructed to have someone available to drive him home after the procedure.

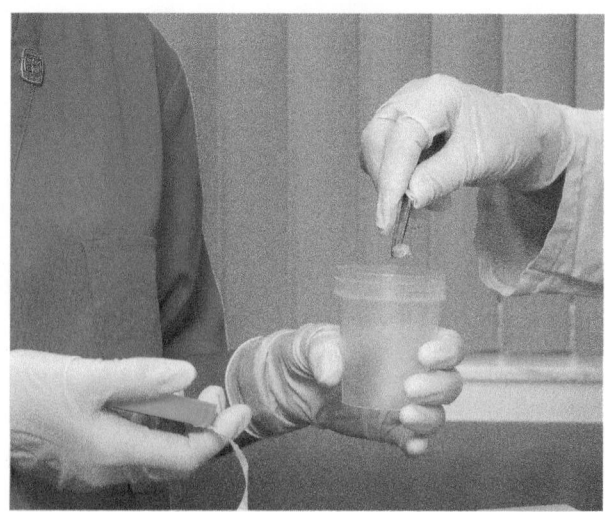

FIGURE 41-29 A medical assistant holds a specimen container to receive a biopsy sample.

Professionalism

If, as a medical assistant, you find assisting with minor surgery fascinating, you may wish to pursue additional training to become a surgical technologist. A surgical technologist, also known as a surgical technician or operating technician, works in an operating room as a member of the surgical team. An operating technician's duties include, but are not limited to, the following:

- Set up the operating room
- Set up surgical instruments and supplies
- Prepare the patient for surgery
- Drape the incision site
- Assist physicians and nurses to don PPE
- Measure vital signs
- Pass instruments
- Operate suction machines and lights
- Prepare specimens for the laboratory
- Dress the patient's wound
- Restock operating room supplies

About 130 programs for surgical technologists are recognized by the Committee on Accreditation of Allied Health Education Programs (CAAHEP). Programs average one to two years in length. After completion of the program, you may take a national certification examination. For further information, contact the Association of Surgical Technologists, 7108-C South Alton Way, Englewood, CO 80112.

The patient will be uncomfortable for a short period of time (two to three days). He should be given detailed instructions on home care including activity level and sexual intercourse. The instructions may vary somewhat from one urologist to another. A typical vasectomy tray includes the following:

- Scalpel handle and blade (No. 15)
- Dressing forceps
- Towel clamp
- Straight and curved mosquito forceps
- Curved tissue scissors
- Tissue forceps
- Retractor
- Needle holder and suture material
- Suture scissors

SUMMARY

Along with a thorough knowledge of gowning, gloving, and surgical hand hygiene, assisting with surgery involves maintaining aseptic technique, setting up sterile instrument trays, passing equipment to the physician, packaging and surgical setup, and preparing the patient for the procedure. Assisting with surgical procedures carries with it a grave responsibility for maintaining absolute sterile technique. The medical assistant incorporates a variety of clinical skills when assisting with a surgical procedure.

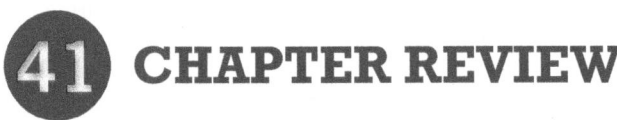

41 CHAPTER REVIEW

COMPETENCY REVIEW

1. Define and spell the items for this chapter.
2. Explain the difference between elective surgery and optional surgery.
3. Describe a sterile field, including how one is created and how it could become contaminated.
4. Explain how the size of suture material is measured.
5. Samaria is working as a floating assistant at the outpatient surgical center where she is employed. What are some of her job duties as a floating assistant?
6. Because of an error with a clinical supplies order, Dr. Henderson's practice has run out of suture removal packs. Dr. Henderson's medical assistant, Brad, must gather all the necessary supplies for a suture removal that is being performed on the patient in exam room #1. What items must Brad gather and prepare for this procedure?

PREPARING FOR THE CERTIFICATION EXAM

1. Which of the following is *never* considered an outpatient surgery?
   a. elective
   b. urgent
   c. optional
   d. organ transplant
   e. tonsillectomy

2. Head and neck sutures remain in place for
   a. 4–7 days.
   b. 1–2 days.
   c. 3–5 days.
   d. 8–10 days.
   e. 12–14 days.

3. Which of the following is not used to categorize instruments?
   a. cutting
   b. probing
   c. grasping
   d. clamp
   e. cover

4. _____ are used to grasp foreign bodies.
   a. Splinter forceps
   b. Tissue forceps
   c. Thumb forceps
   d. Sponge forceps
   e. Addison forceps

5. A _____ is used to remove tissue for examination and biopsy to detect cancerous cells.
   a. speculum
   b. trocar
   c. punch
   d. probe
   e. hemostat

6. The most expensive suture material is
   a. nylon.
   b. silk.
   c. polyester.
   d. cotton.
   e. linen.

7. If you were to assist in suturing an eyelid, which gauge of silk would you choose?
   a. 3-0
   b. 5-0
   c. 2-0
   d. 7-0
   e. 8-0

8. _____ anesthesia is specifically injected into a nerve adjacent to the operative site. This type of anesthetic is used for surgery on hands, fingers, and toes.
   a. Local
   b. General
   c. Nerve block
   d. Topical
   e. Spinal

9. Which of the following is an anesthetic?
   a. Ethyl chloride
   b. Procaine (Novacaine)
   c. Tetracaine
   d. Chloroprocaine
   e. Epinephrine

10. This type of wound has edges that are torn in an irregular shape and can cause profuse bleeding and scarring.
    a. puncture
    b. laceration
    c. incision
    d. abrasion
    e. contusion

CRITICAL THINKING

Refer to the case study at the beginning of the chapter and use what you have learned to answer the following questions.

1. What is an I & D, and why is it usually performed?
2. What supplies would Shandra need to gather to have the examination room ready for the I & D to be performed by Dr. Penningworth?

3. Dr. Penningworth informs Shandra that the patient has had the cyst for a significant amount of time and would like to send a sample, which will be collected during the procedure, to the laboratory. What type of sample will likely be collected, and why would the physician want to send it to the laboratory for testing?

ON THE JOB

Victor Krenz is assisting Dr. Connors with the fifth cataract surgery for the day. The patient is Kathy Wall, a patient with diabetes, whose condition has been stable enough for her to undergo a surgical procedure. Victor has performed a six-minute surgical scrub on his hands before each of the five procedures. Dr. Connors indicates that he is in a hurry to get back to his office for a heavy afternoon schedule of patients. After both Dr. Connors and Victor are scrubbed, gowned, and ready to begin the operation, Victor feels a slight prick on the tip of his gloved finger as he moves the sterile syringe and needle on the tray. Dr. Connors, who does not notice the accidental needlestick to Victor's glove, states again that he is in a hurry to finish this procedure. Victor knows that it will delay the surgery if he has to change gloves. He also knows that his hands have had a surgical scrub five times that morning and that they are clean.

1. Can Victor justify not changing into new gloves?
2. What could happen to Ms. Wall as a result of Victor's needlestick?
3. How should Victor handle this situation?

INTERNET ACTIVITY

Research the Internet for the newest information about using laser surgery to reduce or remove facial wrinkles. After examining the information, do you think you would elect laser surgery to remove wrinkles? Would you recommend this procedure to others?

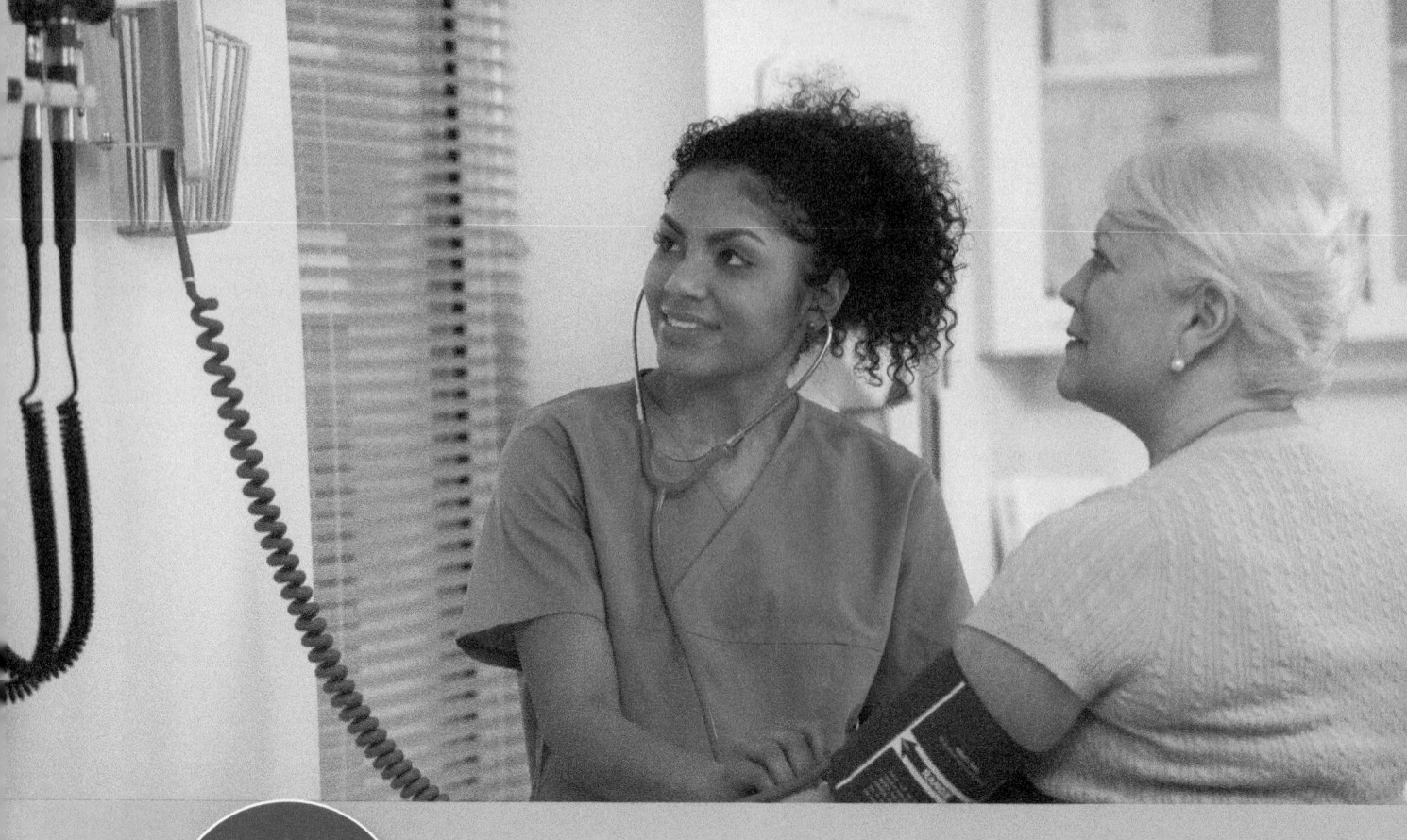

Assisting with Medical Emergencies and Emergency Preparedness

Learning Objectives

After completing this chapter, you should be able to:

42.1   Define and spell the terms for this chapter.

42.2   Identify types of resources related to emergency care.

42.3   Outline the steps of primary assessment.

42.4   List items commonly found on an emergency crash cart.

42.5   Describe the principles of cardiopulmonary resuscitation.

42.6   Explain how to provide first aid to a person with an obstructed airway.

42.7   Describe the symptoms of different types of respiratory distress.

42.8   Explain how to provide first aid to a person in shock.

42.9   Explain how to provide first aid to a person with a diabetic emergency.

42.10 Explain how to provide first aid to a person who is bleeding.

42.11 Explain how to provide first aid to a person with a wound.

42.12 Explain how to provide first aid to a person with a burn.

42.13 Explain how to provide first aid to a person with temperature-related emergencies.

42.14 Explain how to provide first aid to a person having a seizure.

42.15 Explain how to provide first aid to a person who has syncope.

42.16 Explain how to provide first aid to a person with a musculoskeletal injury.

42.17 List the elements of an emergency plan in response to an emergency.

42.18 Describe the importance of participating in a mock exposure event.

It is a very busy day at Pearson Physicians Group. The examination rooms are full, and three patients are still in the reception area waiting to be seen. Many of the patients have been discussing the odd weather patterns of alternating rain and hail. Lewis Jordan, RMA, is working on medical billing in the front office when he notices that the weather has finally calmed down. Within minutes, Lewis hears a fire siren and an emergency broadcast on the radio station announcing a tornado warning. Everyone within the listening area is advised to take immediate cover.

Terms to Learn

algorithm	first responders	intubate
anaphylactic shock	heat exhaustion	patent
bandage	hyperglycemia	primary assessment
crash cart	hyperthermia	Rule of Nines
dressing	hypoglycemia	stat
emergency kit	hypothermia	triage

This chapter presents a number of medical emergencies. The physician must be notified immediately of any emergency that occurs in the medical office. In some cases, you will need to call 911 to access the Emergency Medical Services (EMS) system. To ensure every patient's safety until additional medical help arrives, medical assistants are cautioned not to perform procedures outside their scope of practice while providing the emergency care they are trained to provide.

EMERGENCY RESOURCES

People with a medical emergency have several options about where to seek care, depending on the nature and severity of their emergency.

- **Medical office: conditions that pose no immediate danger to life or limb.** During normal office hours, minor emergencies, such as a twisted ankle or a moderate nosebleed, may be handled in a medical office. Some physician group practices may have an emergency clinic where emergency service is provided both during and after office hours.

- **Freestanding clinics or urgent care centers: conditions that need to be treated quickly but that are not life threatening.** Freestanding clinics or urgent care centers provide emergency care during regular hours until late in the evening and often on weekends. However, many of these facilities do not offer critical-care intervention for life-threatening conditions.

- **Hospital emergency departments: most emergencies, including those that are life threatening.** Hospitals usually have 24-hour emergency departments (EDs) that are open seven days a week. These "24-7 EDs" can handle most emergencies and arrange transport of patients to critical-care trauma centers.

- **Critical-care centers: life-threatening conditions that require specialized critical care.** Critical-care centers, such as trauma, cardiac, burn, and surgical centers, have specialty-trained physicians, surgeons, anesthesiologists, and other critical-care staff on duty at all times.

As a medical assistant, you should be aware of the emergency care options available in your community. It is prudent to have a list of these centers prepared before an emergency happens and placed in the reception area so patients can be appropriately redirected to a venue that can best serve them if they call or come in for advice. Further, the practice's voice messaging system should instruct patients who call with an emergency to hang up and dial 911 to prevent patients from leaving messages or waiting to speak to someone in the doctor's office rather than acting quickly and appropriately in an emergency.

Emergency Medical Services

Emergency Medical Services (EMS) was established to provide prehospital emergency care and safe and prompt transportation from any location, including a medical office, to a hospital or other appropriate facility. It is often said that EMS brings the emergency department to the patient.

There are four nationally recognized levels of EMS practitioner:

- An *Emergency Medical Responder (EMR)* can provide immediate basic life-saving care while awaiting response from a higher-level EMS practitioner.

- An *Emergency Medical Technician (EMT)* can provide basic emergency medical care, administration of a few specific medications, and transport to a hospital or other appropriate facility for definitive care.

- An *Advanced Emergency Medical Technician (AEMT)* can provide basic emergency medical care, some advanced care, administration of a somewhat broader range of medications, and transport.

- A *Paramedic* can provide all the care that an EMT or AEMT can provide plus a broad range of advanced emergency care, a much broader variety of medications, and transport.

The term **first responder** is sometimes used to mean what is now called the Emergency Medical Responder (EMR) (often a policeman or firefighter trained as an EMR) and is sometimes used to mean any EMS practitioner at any level of training who is first to respond to an emergency.

Paramedics and AEMTs are trained to use advanced airway devices to **intubate**, which may involve inserting a breathing tube into the trachea, and they may start an intravenous (IV) line in seconds. They carry ample oxygen supplies and an assortment of emergency medications, and they are able to perform other invasive procedures.

The following summarizes the roles played by EMS:

- Provide on-the-scene intervention and treatment.

- Prepare the patient with injuries, trauma, or illness for transport.

- Transport the patient to the emergency facility. Emergency transportation is accomplished by ambulance, helicopter, or fixed-wing aircraft.

- Transfer the patient to medical personnel at the receiving facility (Figure 42-1).

EMS personnel are accustomed to working with other health care professionals. An EMT or Paramedic may ask the office staff for all the pertinent patient information, including information about patient complaints, immediate and

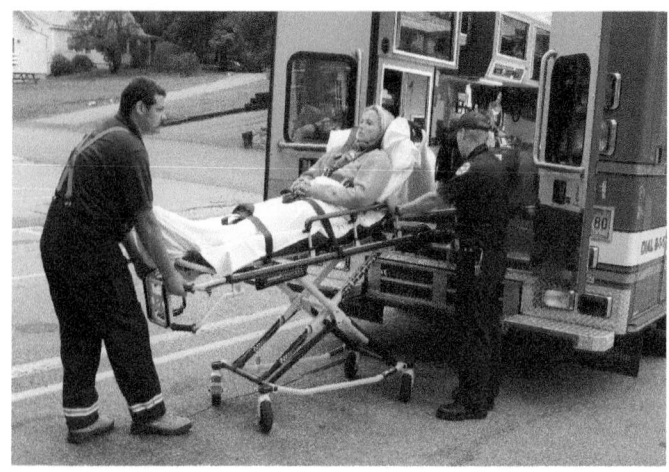

FIGURE 42-1 EMS personnel respond to emergencies and transport patients to the hospital.

overall history, medications taken and allergies, and care that has been administered up to the point of the EMS responders' arrival. EMS personnel will make sure this information accompanies the patient to the hospital and may transmit the information by radio from the ambulance to the hospital so hospital personnel can prepare for the patient's arrival. Thus, this communication between you and EMS personnel is vital for the patient's continuity of care.

Specialized Resources

Apart from emergency response teams, the medical assistant will occasionally need to consult with specialists in such areas as poison control, pediatrics, trauma, and burns. Some consultations will be under emergency conditions, so make sure the specialists' telephone numbers are displayed prominently near the phones in the office to be readily accessible.

Good Samaritan Laws

A health care professional who volunteers in an emergency situation in which duty is not owed a victim is generally protected by various state laws that hold the medical professional not legally liable when rendering first aid. These laws are often referred to as Good Samaritan laws.

Once a health care professional has decided to provide care, that health care professional is committed to rendering such care according to the scope of his license, certification, or training given the resources available at the scene. In an emergency situation in which the health care professional has begun to provide care to the patient, he must remain with the patient, as long as the scene is safe, until relieved by another health care professional with an equal or higher level of training. It is important that health care professionals be aware of the laws in their own state and remember that they must meet the standard of care within their license, certification, or training.

GUIDELINES FOR PROVIDING EMERGENCY CARE

Medical assistants and other staff members must stay up to date on the emergency plans of the office, facility, and community. These plans should be reviewed with personnel of the practice on a regularly scheduled basis.

For major or catastrophic events, local law enforcement and emergency management agencies direct rescue, treatment, and transportation efforts. In such an emergency or disaster, health care professionals are expected to provide care with whatever limited resources are available, so those patients who have little hope of survival may not be treated. Patients with very severe injuries may be diverted to trauma centers. Treatment of patients with mild or non–life-threatening injuries will be deferred until after life-threatening but survivable injuries have been treated.

Medical assistants need to be able to handle emergencies in three types of situations. The most common is on the telephone, when a patient or patient's relative calls to ask for advice for an emergency that is occurring outside the office. Another type is when an emergency occurs near the doctor's office, and someone brings the patient to the office. The third is when an emergency occurs in the office setting.

In an emergency, the medical assistant must be able to look at someone or listen to her on the phone and quickly decide whether that person is ill or injured and does or does not require emergency care. The medical assistant may ask the physician for advice anytime the physician is in the office or may decide to activate EMS by calling 911. Sometimes a decision tree, or map of what action to take in certain circumstances, is created by the physician for the medical assistant to use for **triage**, which refers to assessing and prioritizing the emergency care needed by patients.

In some states, triage is not within the scope of practice of the medical assistant. In these states, the medical assistant should not work alone in the medical office but should assist the physician during emergencies.

Primary Screening and Assessment

Every patient contact by a medical professional begins with a few questions and a basic patient examination, the **primary assessment**. When the patient presents with an emergency, the primary assessment is critically important for the medical assistant, whose role is to organize the process of caring for patients and to maintain control of an emergency situation. The steps of primary assessment include the following:

Professionalism The Law

As a medical assistant, you have three primary legal responsibilities in an emergency. The first is a duty to act within your scope of practice. Even though we all feel a little intimidated by the thought of an emergency, you are a medical professional and must act. You are accountable to yourself, your employer, and the public for actions that fall within the scope of your medical training and certification.

Your second legal responsibility is to ensure and document the constant emergency readiness of the office in which you work. You not only need to check your equipment when you come to work every day or as deemed by your employer (an ethical responsibility), but you need to be able to prove that you did so (a legal responsibility). That means documentation, by means of timed, dated, and signed logs as required by your office. When a piece of equipment that you were supposed to check, but did not, fails, you may be held wholly or partly legally responsible.

Your third legal responsibility, which you share with others in your workplace, is to do all you can to prevent emergencies—for example, by creating emergency preparedness plans. Educating patients and their families about their own safety is also part of emergency prevention.

1. Determine the patient's name, approximate age, and gender.

    When you ask patients their name, they must quickly go through an extensive neurological process to give a simple appropriate answer. They must be able to do the following:
    - Hear you.
    - Localize the sound of your voice, using both ears and both eyes.
    - Look at you with a symmetrical gaze, and focus on you with both eyes.
    - Reason that you are a caregiver, and then process the meaning of your words, hopefully in your own language (but maybe not).
    - Remember their name, and formulate a meaningful response.
    - Answer in coherent speech and with a symmetrical face.

    During that brief period of time, you may learn a lot about a patient's mental function by observing other details, such as facial expressions and body language.

2. Determine the patient's need for intervention.

    A patient who cannot be aroused or who cannot stay awake deserves serious concern. Does the patient

TABLE 42-1 | Emergency Intervention

Life-Threatening: Immediate Intervention	Not Life-Threatening: Immediate Intervention	Not Life-Threatening: Intervention as Soon as Possible
• Extreme shortness of breath (airway or breathing problems) • Cardiac arrest • Severe, uncontrolled bleeding • Head injuries • Poisoning • Open chest or abdominal wounds • Shock • Severe burns, including face, hands, feet, and genitals • Potential neck injuries	• Decreased levels of consciousness • Chest pain • Seizures • Major or multiple fractures • Neck injuries • Severe eye injuries • Burns not on face, hands, feet, or genitals	• Severe vomiting and diarrhea, especially in the very young and in older adults • Minor injuries • Sprains • Strains • Simple fractures

seem too weak to stand up? Does the skin color seem very pale or red or perhaps blue? Is the patient very sweaty for no apparent reason (such as hot weather or recent exercise)? Is the patient bleeding uncontrollably or struggling to breathe? Table 42-1 lists various conditions, signs, and symptoms categorized by severity and need for immediate intervention or intervention as soon as possible.

3. Obtain the history of the event.

The immediate history can reveal a lot about the nature of a problem. For instance, a patient who feels "dizzy" on awakening in the morning with a cold is a lot different from a patient who feels the same way after several episodes of dark-colored, foul-smelling diarrhea. Although these patients have the same complaint (dizziness), their histories differ. By itself, the first patient's history suggests an ear infection, whereas the second patient's history points to gastrointestinal bleeding. Another example is a caller who describes where his terrible headache is located and then loses consciousness. The data reported in the patient's history would prompt the initial decisions and actions of an entire team of people who would then care for that patient.

Past medical history is also important in emergency situations. The best way to gather the past medical history is to use a checklist, whether mental or written. The questions you ask may depend on your employer's standard procedures, but should probably be the same for every patient, regardless of the complaint. Specifically, you might ask if the patient has:

• Heart problems (Has the patient ever had a heart attack or a diagnosed heart disease?)

• Lung problems (Does the patient have both lungs?)
• Asthma or allergies
• Kidney problems (Does the patient have both kidneys?)
• Diabetes (Does the patient take insulin? Has the patient had insulin today and, if so, when?)
• High or low blood pressure (Which?)
• Seizures
• Fainting spells
• Pregnancy, if possible (OB/GYN history? Last menstrual period?)
• Previous similar events (When, treatment, outcome?)

4. Gather medication information.

A medication list can provide information regarding medical history. Also, many medical conditions are caused by interactions among medications or by a patient's reaction to one or more of them. It is important to ask the patient both the name of each drug and the dosage taken.

5. Identify the patient's allergies.

Many caregivers underestimate the importance of allergies. People can go into **anaphylactic shock**, a severe allergic reaction that causes respiratory distress from swelling of the upper airways. This condition must be treated immediately. (Anaphylactic shock is discussed in more detail later in this chapter.) Thousands of patients experience anaphylactic reactions to medications that are dispensed every day. Many wear some kind of identifying jewelry as a reminder, in the form of bracelets, wristbands, or necklaces. Usually, they are keenly aware of their allergies, but it happens sometimes during a medical crisis that people either forget about their allergies or become unable to

It is necessary to consider the age and body structure of a patient whom you are treating in a medical emergency. Just as there are specific guidelines for administering CPR to a child, there are factors to take into consideration when performing an emergency intervention on an older adult. As discussed in the chapter titled "Assisting with Life Span Specialties: Geriatrics," the aging body undergoes various systemic changes. For example, as patients enter their seventies and eighties, their skeletal structure is likely to be frailer than that of patients who are in their twenties and thirties. Keep this in mind when performing emergency interventions such as abdominal thrusts, chest compressions, and CPR. The amount of force necessary to achieve the desired effect may not be as great in older adults. (However, do not withhold such interventions, as needed, because you fear injuring the patient. The life-saving imperative outweighs the possibility of skeletal injury.)

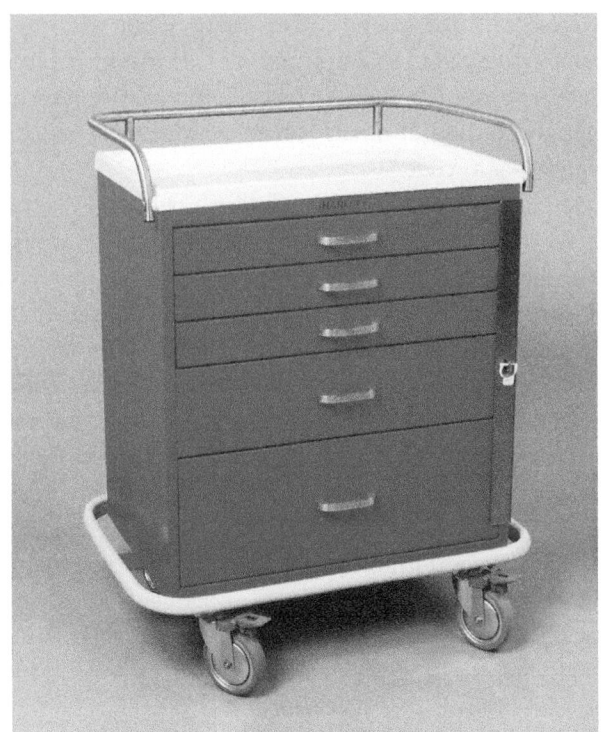

FIGURE 42-2 Emergency crash cart.

communicate about them. Check for warning tags and jewelry during the patient examination, even if a patient denies having any allergies.

6. Take the vital signs.

With the patient's permission, take vital signs. Take the patient's temperature; then count respirations for about 30 seconds and multiply by 2. Then spend 30 seconds checking the pulse and multiply by 2, followed by taking the blood pressure. Record these readings on the chart. If the patient has a potentially serious complaint, or if anything in the vitals or the patient's appearance concerns you, terminate the physical examination and notify the physician immediately. If the physician is unavailable, call 911. Have the patient lie down on the examination table, and make the patient comfortable. Oxygen may need to be administered, as ordered by the physician.

OFFICE EMERGENCY CRASH KIT

Every doctor's office has an **emergency kit** or box (sometimes called a **crash cart**) that contains all supplies that may be needed during an emergency and that is instantly accessible to anyone in the office (Figure 42-2). A crash cart resembles a large roll-around toolbox with drawers that can store emergency medications, intubation equipment, needles and syringes, assorted small instruments, a resuscitator, a heart monitor-defibrillator, an oxygen supply, and airway and suction devices. The emergency medical or drug box is kept on

or close to the crash cart. Table 42-2 lists some of the drugs that may be stocked in an emergency medical box.

The physicians in each office determine which drugs are appropriate for the practice, as established by emergency **algorithms**, sequences of actions to perform tasks. It is best if these algorithms are created before the emergency and frequently rehearsed with staff to ensure that all are trained on how to perform as a team in sequence during an emergency. These algorithms provide decision trees so that depending on whether the answer to a question is yes or no, you proceed to the next question in the algorithm until you have found the action needed for the specific situation. For example, if the patient is not breathing, then opening an airway is paramount. If the patient is breathing, then looking for other injuries will be the next action.

TABLE 42-2 | Drugs Commonly Stocked in an Emergency Medical Box	
• Activated charcoal	• Local anesthetics
• Atropine	• Nitroglycerin
• Diphenhydramine	• Normal saline
• Epinephrine	• Phenobarbital and
• Furosemide	diazepam
• Instant glucose	• Sodium bicarbonate
• Insulin	• Solu-Cortef
• Lidocaine	• Verapamil

A crash cart may contain items that are not within the scope of practice for a medical assistant. However, a physician or nurse may use them. In a small office, a crash cart can be brought to the side of any patient within moments of an emergency, or a "code."

Emergency supplies must be checked routinely. The cart must be restocked after every use and maintained at least once a month on a regular basis, with expiration dates checked, for two reasons. First, emergency medications tend not to get used often, and they expire. The same is true of the batteries that power monitor-defibrillators, laryngoscopes, and suction devices. When these items do get used, someone who is not currently dealing with the aftermath of the emergency must double-check them. Second, being able to use emergency equipment under pressure in an emergency situation requires comfortable, hands-on familiarity with the equipment. When emergencies are infrequent, as in most physicians' offices, familiarity can only come from handling the equipment during frequent maintenance checks. Mock practice sessions can also help medical assistants become more familiar with the equipment and how to use it.

Finally, crash cart supplies must include a checklist that names every drug container and every piece of equipment the cart contains. (The physician decides what equipment and supplies should be stocked in the emergency cart.) The checklist should provide space for a daily date and signature, and someone in the office should be specifically accountable for maintaining the cart. However, all persons who are likely to use the cart must check it personally as well, for the sake of their own performance.

MEDICAL EMERGENCIES

The following sections of this chapter describe medical emergencies that may be seen in the medical office and treatments that should be initiated by the medical assistant.

Cardiopulmonary Resuscitation and Automated External Defibrillation

Respiratory arrest and cardiac arrest may be caused by an occluded airway, electrocution, shock, drowning, heart attack, trauma, anaphylaxis, drugs, poisoning, or traumatic head or chest injury. Intervention must be immediate if resuscitation is to be successful. Basic life support guidelines should be followed for respiratory arrest, cardiac arrest, or an obstructed airway.

For individuals experiencing loss of consciousness with no breathing or no normal breathing (gasps of air known as agonal breathing), follow the cardiopulmonary resuscitation

(CPR) protocol. These guidelines vary somewhat according to age group. The adult guidelines include adolescents, who are defined as those who have gone through puberty. Signs of puberty include chest or underarm hair in males and breast development in females. A child is defined as 1 year of age to puberty. Infant guidelines should be applied to patients less than 1 year of age. Table 42-3 lists the standards for CPR recently established by the American Heart Association (AHA) and American Red Cross (ARC).

Because we assume that there is probably more than one person in the medical office with professional-level CPR certification, we will primarily focus on two-rescuer, professional-level CPR standards. However, if you are alone when you find an unresponsive adult patient who is not breathing or who has agonal breathing, you should shout out for help immediately after checking to confirm the patient's unresponsiveness and lack of normal breathing. If someone responds, instruct that person to activate the emergency response system, which is 911 if outside a hospital setting, get an automated external defibrillator (AED), if available, and immediately return to assist you. (If that person is not trained in two-person CPR, he should bring someone who is.)

If someone has responded to your shout for help, while that person calls 911 or activates the emergency response system and retrieves the AED, you should work alone to check for a pulse. If there is no pulse, immediately begin the CPR protocol with chest compressions.

If, however, no one has responded to your shout for help, and if the patient is an adult, before performing CPR you should first leave the patient to call 911 or activate the emergency response system and get an AED. When you return to the patient, then check for a pulse and, if it is absent, immediately begin the CPR protocol with chest compressions.

If an infant or child is unresponsive and not breathing or not breathing normally (agonal breathing), and you are working alone, you should provide five cycles (approximately two minutes) of CPR first, before you leave the patient to activate the emergency response system and get an AED. The reason for first providing five cycles of CPR in the infant or child is that the cardiac arrest is likely caused by an airway obstruction or a ventilation or hypoxia issue and not from a cardiac cause as is likely in the adult patient.

The sequence of actions is critical. Early access to EMS is important. Access is initiated by calling 911 or activating the emergency response system as soon as you have determined that the adult patient is unresponsive and not breathing or not breathing normally (or after five cycles of CPR for the infant or child).

TABLE 42-3 | Adult, Child, and Infant CPR Standards

Conscious Choking	Abdominal thrusts for adult or child over 1 year of age. Five back slaps, then five chest thrusts (same as chest compressions) for an infant (less than 1 year of age). Continue the sequence for the adult, child, or infant until the obstruction is relieved or the patient becomes unconscious.
Unconscious Choking	Activate emergency response system, lower the patient to the ground or onto a hard surface, initiate CPR beginning with chest compressions (do not check for a pulse). Before ventilation, open the airway and inspect for an obstruction. If the obstruction is seen and can be removed, remove it with your fingers. If no object is seen, attempt to deliver two breaths and continue with CPR until the obstruction is relieved or EMS arrives on the scene. Use this sequence for adults, children, and infants.
Rescue Breaths	Deliver the breath over one second with enough volume to cause the chest to rise. Do not overventilate with too much volume, too fast, or with too much pressure.
Chest Compression to Ventilation Ratio for a Single Rescuer	30 compressions: two ventilations for the adult, child, and infant.
Chest Compression to Ventilation Ratio for Two Rescuers	30 compressions: two ventilations for the adult, 15 compressions: two ventilations for the child and infant.
Chest Compression Rate	At least 100–120/minute for the adult, child, and infant.
Chest Compression Hand Position	Center of the chest on the lower half of the sternum for the adult and child. Two fingers in the center of the chest just below the nipple line for one-rescuer infant chest compressions. Both hands encircling the chest with both thumbs on the center of the chest just below the nipple line, with hands supporting the back, for two-rescuer infant chest compressions.
AED	Use adult defibrillation pads on any patient 8 years of age or older. Use child defibrillation pads on any child less than 8 years of age. If no child pads are available, adult defibrillation pads should be used on children and infants. Deliver one shock if advised and then continue CPR until advised—approximately two minutes (or five cycles).
Anaphylaxis	Assist person with use of prescribed auto injector.
Asthma	Assist person with use of prescribed inhaler.

Professionalism

As a medical assistant, you are responsible for upholding the highest professional standards. You should obtain and always maintain professional-level CPR certification from either the American Heart Association (AHA) or the American Red Cross (ARC). Your employer may require it.

The Chain of Survival, established by the AHA, illustrates the key factors affecting survival of a cardiac arrest. The Chain of Survival has five steps: (1) immediate recognition of the emergency and activation of EMS; (2) early CPR; (3) rapid defibrillation; (4) effective advanced life support; and (5) integrated post-cardiac-arrest care.

If a cardiac arrest occurs in the medical office, medical assistants with CPR training will perform the first three of the five steps of the Chain of Survival.

Immediate initiation of chest compressions (or as promptly as possible given the scenarios just discussed) is imperative to a patient's survival. Thus, the initial sequence followed for CPR is to provide circulation support by chest compressions, followed by opening the airway and providing ventilations. This sequence is referred to as CAB: Circulation, Airway, Breathing.

One-Person and Two-Person CPR Sequence for an Adult Patient

The sequence for CPR for an adult patient (anyone beyond puberty) is as follows:

1. Tap the patient's shoulder and ask, "Are you okay?" If there is no response, check for breathing. If the patient is unresponsive and there is no breathing or no normal breathing (agonal breathing), shout for someone to activate the emergency response system by dialing 911.

2. Check for a carotid pulse for at least 5 seconds but no more than 10 seconds. If a pulse is not found within 10 seconds, initiate CPR by immediately beginning chest compressions (CAB sequence).

3. Begin chest compressions by positioning yourself at the patient's side. The patient should be in a supine (face up) position and on a hard or firm surface. If the patient is in a prone (face down) or lateral (on the side) position, logroll him into a supine position. If a spinal injury is suspected, try to keep the patient's head and neck in line with the navel when doing the logroll. Place the heel of one hand on the center of the patient's chest on the lower half of the sternum (breast bone). Place the heel of your other hand on top of your first hand with your fingers interlaced. Straighten your arms and get up on your knees until your shoulders are directly over your hands (Figure 42-3).

4. According to the AHA, you should "push hard and fast." Push hard so that each compression is delivered at a depth of at least 2 inches but not to exceed 2.4 inches (5–6.1 cm). Make sure that at the end of each compression, you allow the chest to recoil completely without taking your hands completely off the patient's chest. This is vitally important to facilitating blood flow. By not allowing the chest to recoil completely, you will impede the flow of blood to the heart and brain. Push fast by delivering the compressions in a smooth motion at a rate of at least 100–120 compressions per minute (30 compressions should be delivered in 18 seconds or less). Do not interrupt compressions or minimize the time and number of interruptions. The more interruptions, the more poorly the blood flows to the brain and heart. Provide 30 compressions.

5. After the first rescuer provides the first 30 compressions, the second rescuer will open the airway with a head-tilt, chin-lift by placing the palm of one hand on the forehead and two or three fingers of the other

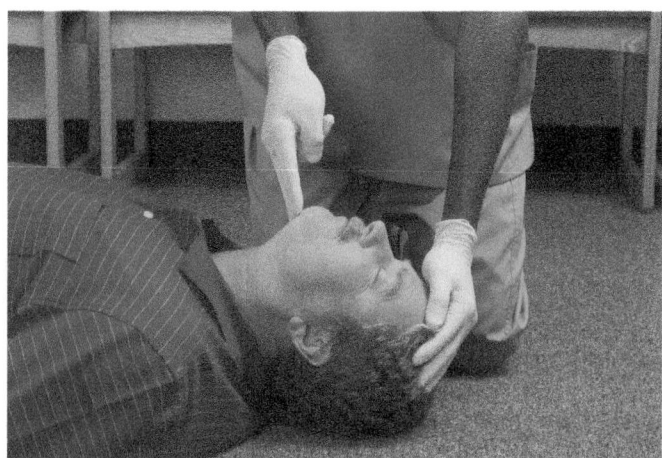

FIGURE 42-4 Head-tilt, chin-lift maneuver.

hand under the bony part of the lower jawbone near the chin. The second rescuer will then gently tilt the head backward and lift the jaw forward (Figure 42-4). If a spinal injury is suspected, a jaw-thrust maneuver must be used to open the airway (Figure 42-5). If the jaw thrust fails to open the airway, switch to a head-tilt, chin-lift. When you do the head-tilt, chin-lift, or jaw-thrust maneuver, the tongue is lifted forward and the airway opened.

6. To deliver ventilations, pinch the patient's nose shut, seal your lips tightly around the patient's mouth, and slowly deliver two breaths, each lasting one second. It is recommended that mouth-to-mask or bag-valve mask devices be used initially, if available, or to replace mouth-to-mouth as quickly as possible. You will know the artificial ventilation is effective if the patient's chest rises with each delivered breath. For a patient with a tracheotomy, it may be necessary to close the mouth and nose and administer breaths to the tracheotomy.

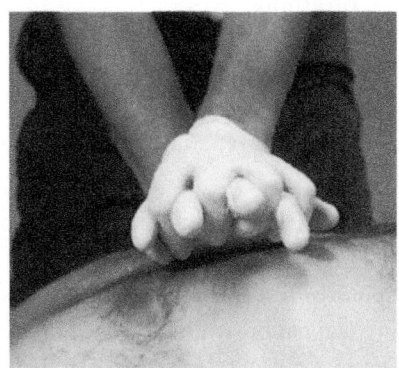

FIGURE 42-3 Position of hands for chest compression on an adult.

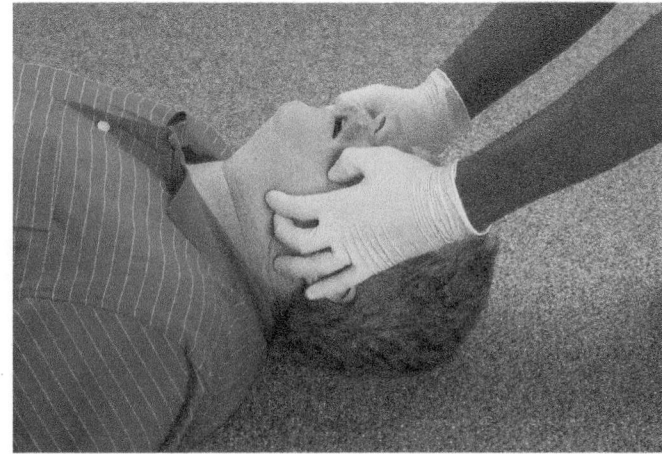

FIGURE 42-5 Jaw-thrust maneuver.

7. Continue to deliver cycles of 30 compressions and two breaths. Switch duties between the rescuers every five cycles or approximately every two minutes. Chest compressions should not be interrupted for more than five seconds to switch compressors. As soon as an automated external defibrillator (AED) becomes available, power-on the device and apply the proper defibrillation pads (adult or pediatric) and follow the prompts.

Procedure 42-1 details the procedures for one- and two-person adult rescue breathing and CPR.

One-Person and Two-Person CPR Sequence for a Child from 1 Year of Age to Puberty

1. Assess for responsiveness by tapping the child's shoulder. If the child is unresponsive and there is no breathing or agonal (gasping) breathing, have someone activate the emergency response system and get an AED.

2. Check the femoral or carotid pulse for at least 5 seconds but no more than 10 seconds. If you do not definitely feel a pulse or the heart rate is less than 60/minute with signs of poor perfusion, begin CPR by initiating chest compressions (CAB sequence).

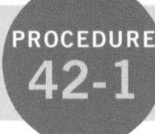

PROCEDURE
42-1

Performing Adult Rescue Breathing and One- and Two-Rescuer CPR

Objective ◆ *Administer rescue breathing for an adult and one- and two-rescuer CPR for an adult correctly, within the time frames designated.*

EQUIPMENT AND SUPPLIES

Approved mannequin; gloves; ventilation mask; mouth guard

METHOD

Note: All medical assistants should obtain and maintain professional-level CPR certification (which includes performance of two-person CPR). Medical offices often have more than one employee with professional-level CPR certification. If, as a medical assistant, you are alone with a patient who needs CPR, shout for help. If someone comes right away—and while you begin one-person CPR—that second person can call 911 to activate EMS response and can also retrieve the office defibrillator. If that or another person in the office has professional-level CPR certification, the two of you can then continue with two-person CPR and defibrillation until EMS arrives.

The first set of instructions below, for one-rescuer CPR, assumes you will be working alone. The second set of instructions, for two-rescuer CPR, assumes that a second person with professional-level CPR certification will be available to work with you.

ONE-RESCUER ADULT CPR

1. Assess the patient and determine if help is needed. Shout "Are you okay?" while gently tapping the patient's shoulders.
2. If you determine that the adult patient is unresponsive and not breathing or not breathing normally (agonal breathing), *activate EMS immediately* by calling 911; then get an AED if available (or shout for another office employee to call 911 and get the AED).
3. Check a carotid pulse (Figure A) for no less than 5 seconds but no longer than 10 seconds. If there is definitely no pulse, begin chest compressions. Kneel at the patient's

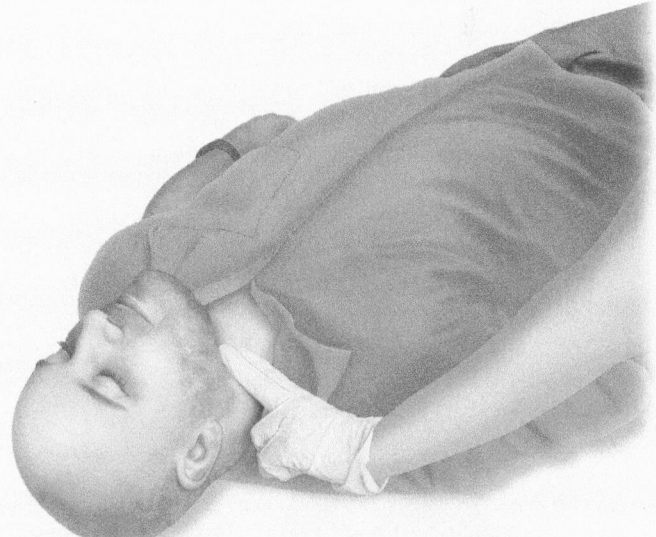

FIGURE A Assess circulation by feeling for carotid pulse.

side. Place your hand in the center of the chest on the lower half of the sternum.
4. Place your other hand on top of the first hand on the chest, interlock your fingers, and be sure to lift your fingers off the chest using only the heels of your hands to administer compressions.
5. Kneel next to the patient and keep your shoulders directly over your hands. Compress the chest at least 2 inches but not to exceed 2.4 inches, and allow the chest to completely recoil after each compression (Figure B). Do not lift your hands completely off the chest.
6. Continue to compress the chest a total of 30 times at a rate of at least 100–120 compressions/minute.

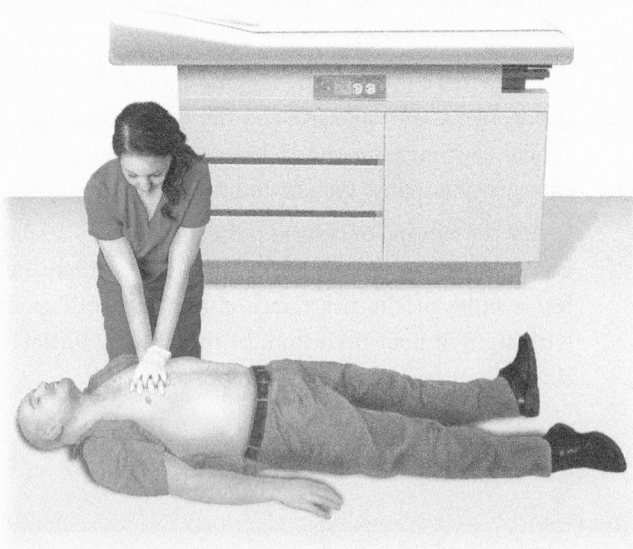

FIGURE B Rescuer working alone delivers chest compressions.

7. After 30 compressions are delivered, perform a head-tilt, chin-lift, or, if spine injury is suspected, a jaw-thrust maneuver to open the airway. Administer two breaths with each delivered over one second, preferably using a mouth-to-mask protective device (Figure C).

   Continue chest compressions and ventilations.

8. Apply the AED as soon as it becomes available. (See Procedure 42-3 regarding defibrillator use.)

9. Repeat this sequence until a pulse has been restored or until EMS arrives.

10. If breathing is absent, but a pulse has been restored, administer two rescue breaths, preferably using a mouth to-mask device. If your breaths do not cause the chest to rise, reestablish the head-tilt, chin-lift, or jaw-thrust

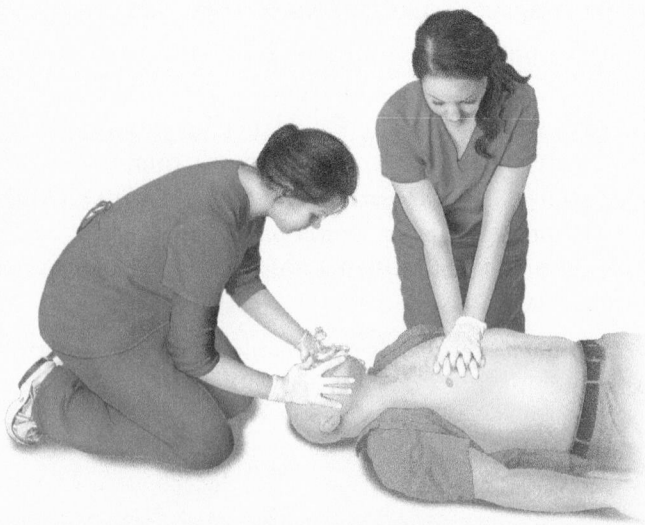

FIGURE D First rescuer continues chest compressions as second rescuer takes a position above the patient's head.

maneuver. If you suspect choking, look in the patient's mouth and remove an object if you see one. If you see no obstruction, continue with rescue breathing. Check the pulse every two minutes. If an obstruction is present, perform the steps for an obstructed airway.

11. Wash your hands and document the incident in the patient's chart.

TWO-RESCUER ADULT CPR

1. Follow the steps just described for one-rescuer adult CPR until a second rescuer certified in professional-level CPR can join you.

2. Continue performing chest compressions while the second rescuer positions herself by kneeling above the patient's head (Figure D). After you have completed a cycle of 30 compressions, the second rescuer will administer two breaths, as described in the steps for one-rescuer CPR (Figure E).

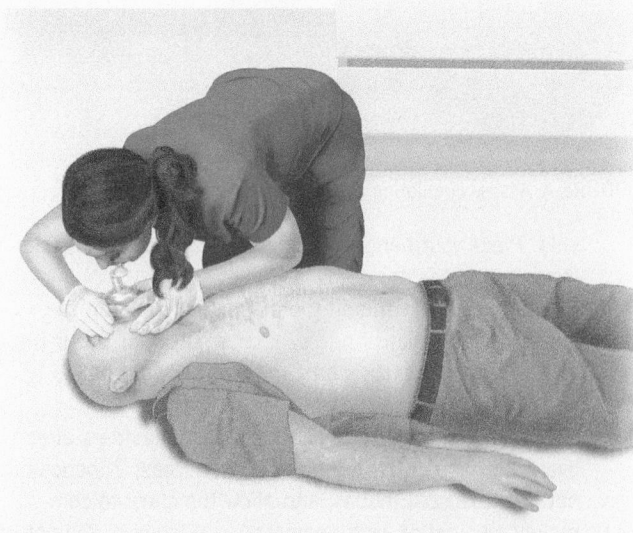

FIGURE C Rescuer working alone delivers ventilations through a mouth-to-mask protective device.

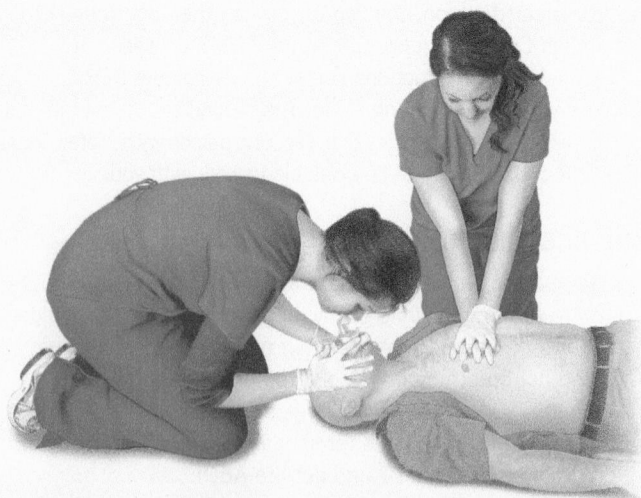

FIGURE E First rescuer rests but does not remove hands from the patient's chest while the second rescuer administers two ventilations.

3. Switch positions with the second rescuer every five cycles (approximately every two minutes), the ventilator taking over chest compressions while the compressor takes over ventilations.

4. Repeat this sequence until a pulse has been restored or until EMS arrives.

5. If breathing is absent, but a pulse has been restored, administer two rescue breaths as described in step 10 for one-rescuer CPR.

6. Wash your hands and document the incident in the patient's chart.

CHARTING EXAMPLE

08/05/YY 7:30 P.M. Patient found collapsed in bathroom and unresponsive. 911 call placed and CPR started. EMS arrived in approximately six minutes and took over care. Patient was transferred to Deaconess Medical Center...............................
....V. Nagle, RMA

---

3. Depending on the size of the child and your strength, you can provide chest compressions using both hands or the heel of one hand for smaller children (Figure 42-6). Until the second rescuer arrives back at the patient's side, use a ratio of 30 compressions to two ventilations. Once the second rescuer arrives, switch to a ratio of 15 compressions to two ventilations. Compress at a rate of at least 100–120/minute and at least ⅓ the depth of the chest, or approximately 2 inches. As in the adult, allow the child's chest to completely recoil after each compression. Provide 15 compressions.

4. The second rescuer will open the airway using a head tilt, chin-lift, or jaw-thrust maneuver. Deliver two slow ventilations over one second and watch for chest rise with each ventilation.

5. When the AED becomes available, power-on the AED, apply pediatric defibrillation pads, if available, and follow the prompts. (Use adult pads if pediatric pads are not available.)

6. Push hard and push fast while delivering 15 compressions followed by two breaths.

One-Person and Two-Person CPR Sequence for an Infant Less Than 1 Year of Age

1. Assess the infant for responsiveness. You can flick the sole of the foot to assess for any response if the infant does not seem to be responsive. If the infant is unresponsive and has no breathing or agonal (gasping) breathing, have someone activate the emergency response and get an AED.

2. Check the infant's brachial pulse for at least 5 seconds but no longer than 10 seconds. If there is definitely no pulse or if the heart rate is less than 60/minute with signs of poor perfusion, begin CPR by initiating chest compressions. If a second rescuer is immediately available, use a 15 compression to two ventilation ratio. However, if the second rescuer has not yet returned, immediately initiate CPR using a 30 compression to two ventilation ratio until the second rescuer arrives back at the patient's side. If one rescuer is providing CPR, use the two-finger compressions technique; however, if two rescuers are providing CPR, the two thumb-encircling hands techniques should be used to deliver the chest compressions (Figure 42-7). Push hard enough to compress the chest at least ⅓ the anterior-posterior diameter, which is approximately 1½ inches in the infant. The compressions should be delivered at a rate of at least 100–120 compressions/minute. Deliver 15 compressions.

3. The second rescuer should open the airway by placing the infant's head and neck in a neutral position. Use a chin lift and ventilate by using a mouth-to-mask device or an infant bag-valve-mask device. If mouth-to-mouth is required, place your mouth over the nose and mouth of the infant. If chest rise is not present, slightly extend the head and neck until the airway is open. Do not hyperextend the head and neck because this may collapse the trachea and obstruct the airway. Ensure that the chest rises with each delivered ventilation. Administer two ventilations after each 15 compressions when performing two-rescuer CPR.

4. Apply the AED using pediatric defibrillation pads, if available, as soon as it becomes available. Turn on the device and follow the prompts.

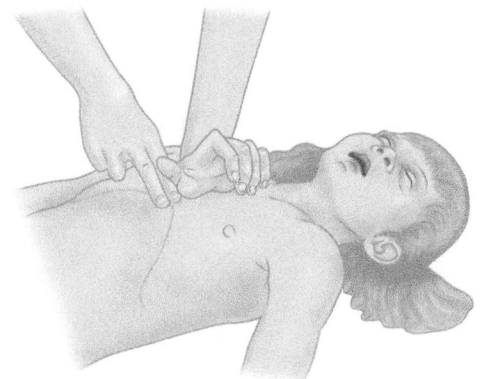

FIGURE 42-6 Compressions for a child.

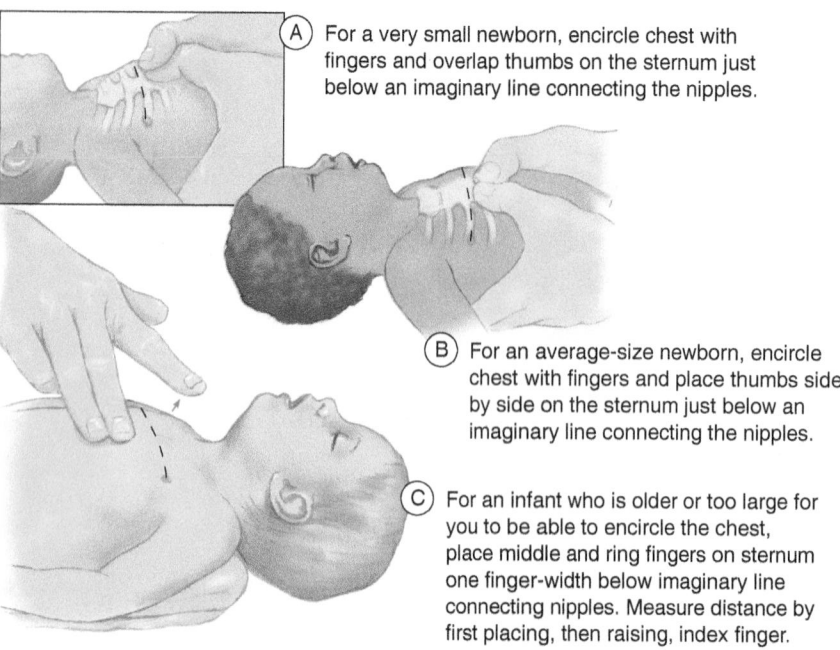

(A) For a very small newborn, encircle chest with fingers and overlap thumbs on the sternum just below an imaginary line connecting the nipples.

(B) For an average-size newborn, encircle chest with fingers and place thumbs side by side on the sternum just below an imaginary line connecting the nipples.

(C) For an infant who is older or too large for you to be able to encircle the chest, place middle and ring fingers on sternum one finger-width below imaginary line connecting nipples. Measure distance by first placing, then raising, index finger.

FIGURE 42-7 Compressions for an infant.

Rescue Breathing

If a patient of any age has a pulse but is not spontaneously breathing, provide rescue breaths until EMS arrives. An adult should be ventilated once every five to six seconds (10 to 12 breaths/minute), whereas a child or infant should be ventilated every three to five seconds (12 to 20 breaths/minute). Each ventilation should be delivered over one second. Check the pulse every two minutes. During ventilation, if an infant's heart rate decreases to less than 60 bpm with signs of poor perfusion, begin CPR by initiating chest compressions. Ensure that the airway is open and ventilations are being delivered adequately because bradycardia in infants most often results from an occluded airway, inadequate ventilation, or hypoxia (lack of adequate oxygen in the body tissues).

With an adult, child, or infant, place the palm of one hand on the forehead and two or three fingers under the lower jawbone to gently tilt the head backward (review Figure 42-4). If cervical or other spinal injuries are suspected, a jaw-thrust maneuver must be used to open the airway (review Figure 42-5). When the airway is opened, the patient may begin spontaneous breathing because the tongue is lifted and is no longer occluding the oropharynx. If a pulse is present but spontaneous breathing is not present, continue rescue breathing until EMS arrives.

Procedure 42-2 details the procedures for one- and two-person infant rescue breathing.

Defibrillation

Automated external defibrillation (AED) is highly effective when provided immediately after or within minutes of cardiac arrest. Most cardiac arrests in adults are related to fatal electrical arrhythmias of the heart that are sometimes converted (corrected) with defibrillation. The automated external defibrillator (AED) gives verbal prompts to the rescuer or rescue team that are easy and safe to follow. AEDs are applied to adults, children, and infants. It is recommended that child-size defibrillator pads and pediatric attenuator cables be used in children less than 8 years of age. Adult defibrillation pads and cables are used for any patient older than 8 years of age. If no child defibrillator pads or pediatric cables are available, an adult AED should be applied to the patient regardless of age, including children less than 8 years and infants.

Procedure 42-3 explains the use of an AED.

Obstructed Airway

An obstructed airway prevents the movement of air into or out of the respiratory tract. Certain conditions, such as anaphylaxis or croup, can cause a blockage from swelling of the upper airway tissue, but foreign objects are the cause of most obstructions. With small children, the obstruction is usually from food or small toys. With adults, an obstructed airway may be the result of the following:

- Not chewing large pieces of food properly
- Talking too excitedly or laughing too much while eating
- Drinking alcohol before and during eating
- Choking on body or extraneous fluids, such as vomit or blood

As a medical assistant, you should know how to respond to the following choking scenarios:

- **Partial airway obstruction with good air exchange**—The patient is conscious, is capable of moving air through the upper airway, and is able to produce a strong and forceful cough. This is also known as a mild airway obstruction.
- **Partial airway obstruction with poor air exchange**—The patient is conscious but is not moving adequate air and does not have the ability to produce a strong cough. This is also known as a moderate airway obstruction.
- **Total airway obstruction**—The patient is unable to speak or cough and is not moving any air. This is also known as a severe airway obstruction.

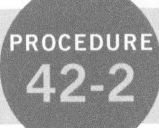

PROCEDURE 42-2

Performing Infant Rescue Breathing

Objective ◆ *Administer rescue breathing for an infant correctly and within the designated time frame.*

EQUIPMENT AND SUPPLIES

Approved mannequin; gloves; ventilation mask; mouth guard

METHOD

1. Assess for responsiveness and breathing. Never shake an infant.
2. If you determine that the infant is not breathing or not breathing normally but has a pulse, perform rescue breathing. *Immediately* activate EMS by calling 911.
3. Carefully place the patient in a supine position. If a spine injury is suspected, keep the head and neck in line with the navel.
4. With the palm of one hand, tilt the patient's head back. With two to three fingers of the other hand, lift the lower jaw forward to open the airway (Figure A).
5. If possible, place a face mask for mouth-to-mask ventilation over the patient's mouth and nose (Figure B). If two rescuers are present, one may cradle the infant in a supine position while the other administers ventilations (Figure C). Administer two rescue breaths. If your breaths do not cause the chest to rise, reestablish the head-tilt, chin-lift, or jaw-thrust maneuver. If you suspect choking, look in the patient's mouth and remove an object if you see one. If you see no obstruction, continue with rescue breathing. If an obstruction is present, perform the steps for an obstructed airway.
6. Once the obstruction is clear, begin rescue breathing by administering one breath every three to five seconds or 12 to 20 breaths every minute.

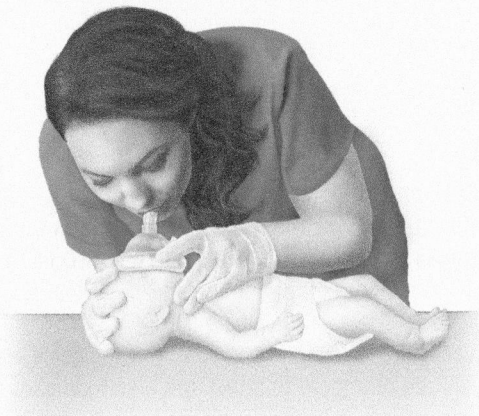

FIGURE B Cover the infant's mouth and nose with the mouth-to-mask device before delivering ventilations.

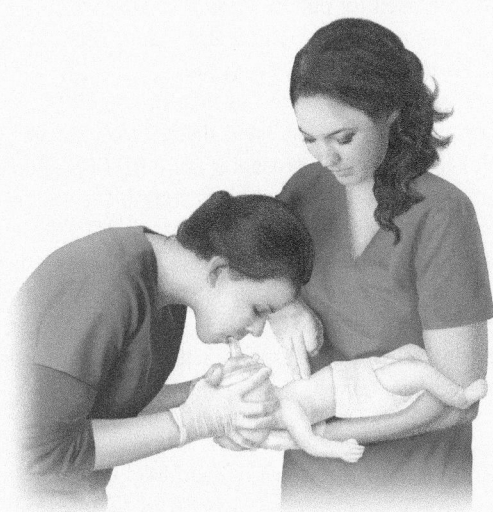

FIGURE C If two rescuers are present, one may cradle the infant in a supine position while the other delivers ventilations.

7. Continue breaths until the infant recovers or EMS arrives.
8. Wash hands and document the incident in the patient's chart.

CHARTING EXAMPLE

10/09/YY 9:45 A.M. 10-month-old patient choked in exam room and was not responsive when physician and medical assistant arrived. Called 911 and EMS activated as directed by the physician. Infant rescue breathing was initiated by the physician until EMS arrived. Patient transported to Walters Creek General Hospital................................M. Cowan, CMA (AAMA)

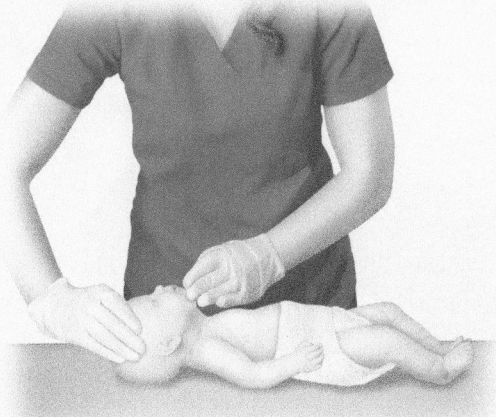

FIGURE A For infant rescue breathing, gently open the airway.

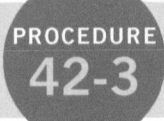

PROCEDURE 42-3

Demonstrating the Use of an Automated External Defibrillator

Objective ◆ *Use an automated external defibrillator (AED) correctly within the time frame designated by the instructor.*

EQUIPMENT AND SUPPLIES

AED machine; patient chart

METHOD

1. Place the AED (Figure A) next to the patient's left ear. This position allows the rescuers clear access to the chest and airway for continued CPR while the AED is being set up. (One provider may continue one-person CPR while the other sets up the AED) (Figure B).
2. Turn the AED on (Figure C) and follow the voice prompts.
3. You will be prompted to attach the electrode pads to the patient's chest, following the diagram provided for correct placement (Figure D). Use adult-size electrode pads on patients 8 years of age and older. Child-size electrode pads are used for patients less than 8 years of age. (Use adult-size pads on a patient less than 8 years of age if child-size pads are not available.)
4. Next, you will be directed to clear the patient to allow the machine to analyze the heart rhythm to determine if a shockable rhythm is present (Figure E). CPR should cease while the machine is analyzing, and no one should be in contact with the patient for any reason.
5. If a shockable rhythm is present, the AED will automatically begin a charging sequence and warn rescuers to stand back and not to touch the patient. The voice prompt will then tell you to press the SHOCK button to administer the electrical current to the patient (Figure F).

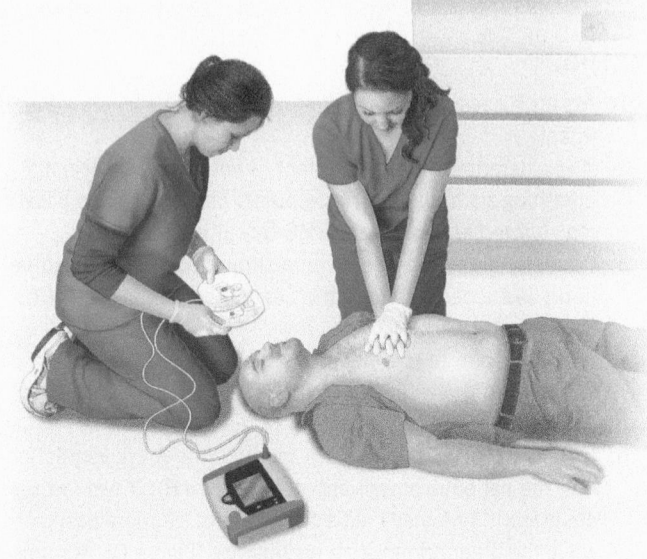

FIGURE B One rescuer continues chest compressions while a second rescuer sets up the AED.

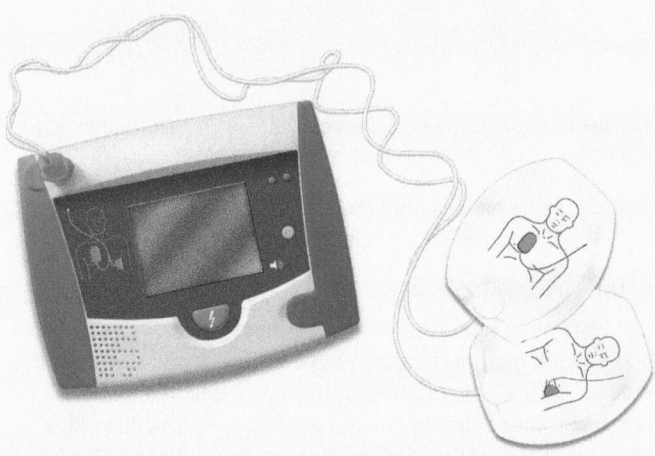

FIGURE A Place the AED next to the patient's ear in order not to interfere with continuing chest compressions and ventilations.

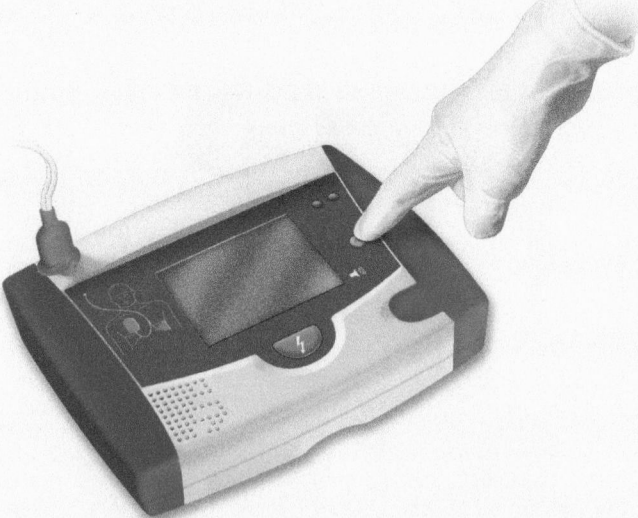

FIGURE C Press the "on" button of the AED to hear instructions.

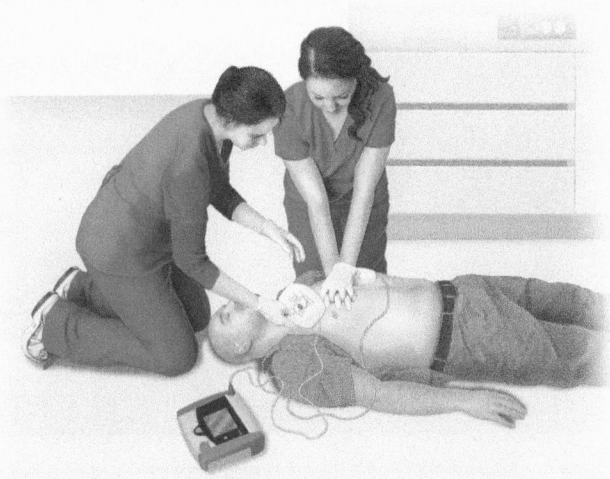

FIGURE D Rescuer two applies the AED pads while rescuer one continues chest compressions.

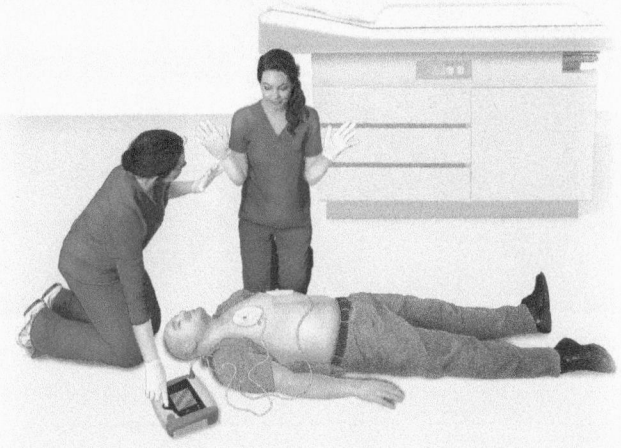

FIGURE E Rescuer one commands "CLEAR" before AED analyzes the heart rhythm. No one must touch the patient during analysis or shock delivery.

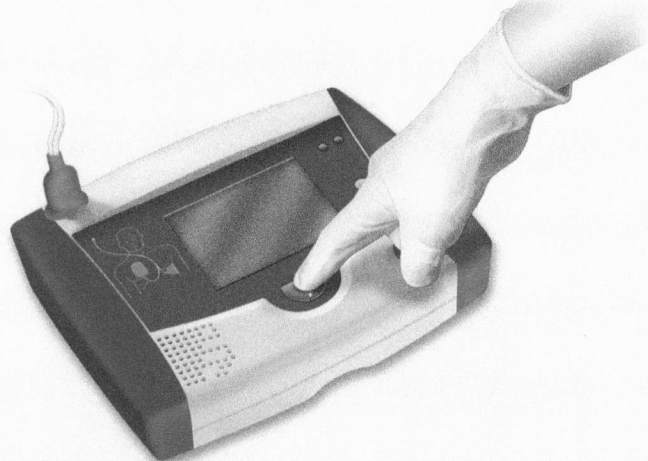

FIGURE F If advised by the AED, press the "SHOCK" button.

6. If the machine indicates "No shock is advised," continue CPR beginning with chest compressions. After two minutes, the AED will prompt you to stand clear and will reanalyze the rhythm. Repeat step 5 if a shockable rhythm is present or continue CPR beginning with chest compressions. Repeat this sequence until advanced medical personnel arrive or the patient regains a pulse.

CHARTING EXAMPLE

11/25/YY 3:30 P.M. Patient found in stairwell, unresponsive, with absence of pulse and respirations. 911 protocol initiated with two-rescuer CPR. Third rescuer initiated AED response, and patient was analyzed for shockable rhythm. CPR and AED shocks administered a total of eight cycles before advanced medical support arrived. Patient released to EMS care and transferred to Sacred Heart Medical Center...............................
....M. Cowan, CMA (AAMA)

The conscious choking adult may use the universal choking sign—crossing the hands at the throat—to signal for help (Figure 42-8).

A partial airway obstruction will allow some air to flow past the obstruction in the upper airway, which may produce a high-pitched noise on inhalation and exhalation. The patient may still be able to cough and expel the foreign object. Any time the patient can speak or cry, air is moving in and out of the airway. For example, if a phone call comes into the medical office and the caller says, "My child is not breathing," and you hear the child crying in the background, the airway is not obstructed.

As a rescuer, ask the choking patient, "Are you choking?" If the patient cannot speak, and responds by nodding yes,

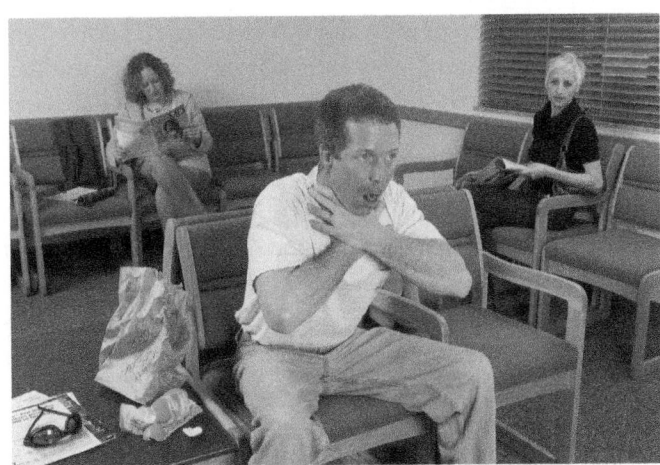

FIGURE 42-8 The universal choking sign.

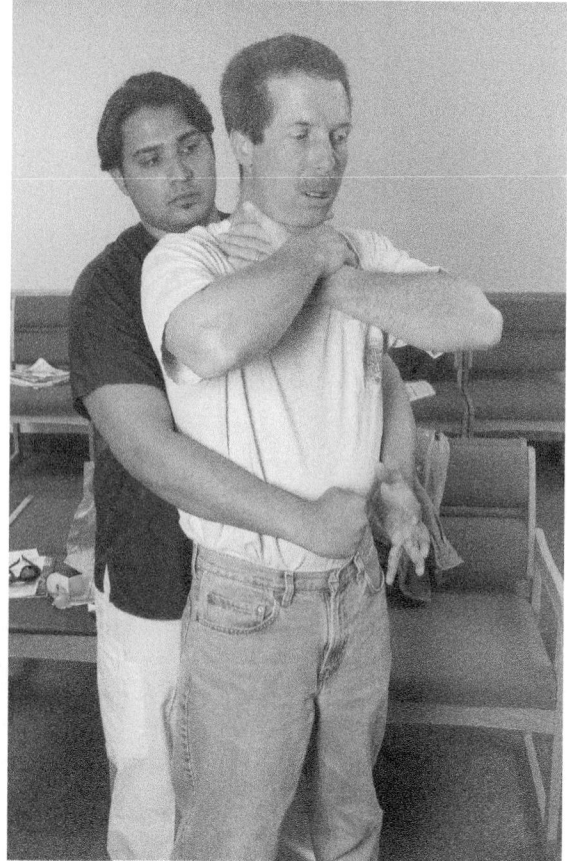

FIGURE 42-9 Abdominal thrusts are delivered with a firm thrust into the patient's abdomen with an upward movement.

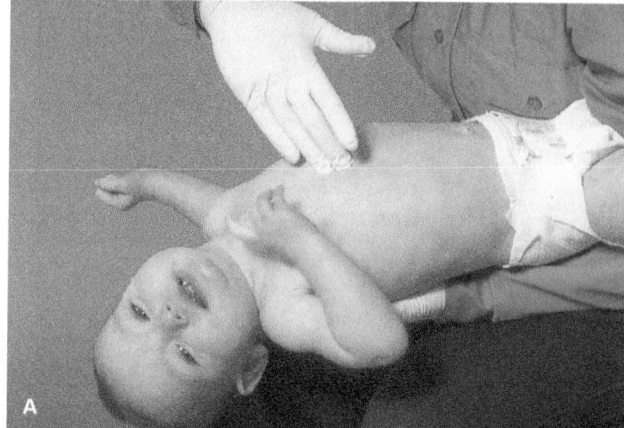

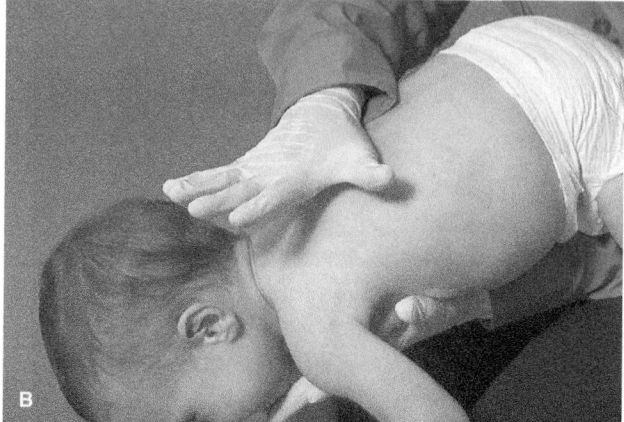

FIGURE 42-10 To clear an obstructed airway in an infant (A) use chest thrusts followed by (B) back blows.

the airway is obstructed and immediate intervention is required.

For the Still-Conscious Patient. Request permission to assist the patient, and perform the abdominal thrusts for the still-conscious adult or child (Figure 42-9) and chest thrusts and back slaps for the infant (Figure 42-10).

To perform the abdominal thrusts, stand behind the patient and put your arms around the abdomen between the xiphoid process (pointed extension at the bottom of the sternum) and the umbilicus (navel). Make a fist with one hand, with the thumb turned into the fist. Wrap your other hand around the fisted hand and pull the fisted hand in and up toward the diaphragm. This force against the diaphragm may be sufficient to loosen the foreign object and propel it out of the airway. If the patient becomes unconscious, ease him to the floor to prevent any additional injuries and proceed with the technique described in the next section for unconscious obstructed airway. Procedure 42-4 explains how to respond to an adult with an obstructed airway.

For a very obese patient or a visibly pregnant woman, provide chest thrusts to the center of the chest over the

lower half of the sternum in place of abdominal thrusts. If an obese or visibly pregnant patient is unconscious, perform CPR with the additional step of inspecting the airway, as described next.

For the Unconscious Patient. If the patient becomes unconscious, activate the emergency response system, lower the patient to the ground or onto a hard surface, and initiate CPR beginning with chest compressions (Figure 42-11—do not check for a pulse). Before performing ventilation, open the airway and inspect for an obstruction. If you can see the obstruction and it can be removed, remove it with your fingers. If you don't see an object, attempt to deliver two breaths and continue with CPR until the obstruction is relieved or EMS arrives on the scene. Use this sequence for adults, children, and infants.

Respiratory Distress

Respiratory distress may be a reaction to a long-term debilitating disease, such as chronic obstructive pulmonary disease (COPD), or to an emergency situation, such as anaphylactic response to medication. It also can be the result of other

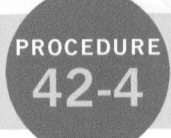

Responding to an Adult with an Obstructed Airway

Objective ◆ *Administer abdominal thrusts to an adult correctly, within the time frame designated.*

EQUIPMENT AND SUPPLIES

Approved mannequin; gloves; ventilation mask with one-way valve for unconscious patient

METHOD

1. Once it has been established that the patient is choking, with no air exchange, direct someone to call 911 and shout, "Are you choking?" If the answer is yes—as indicated by a head nod—tell the patient you are going to begin emergency treatment.
2. Stand behind the patient with your feet slightly apart, placing one foot between the patient's feet and one to the outside. This stance will give you greater stability, and if the patient should pass out, you can safely guide the patient to the ground by sliding him or her down your thigh.
3. Place the index finger of one hand at the person's navel or belt buckle to mark that spot. If the patient is an obviously pregnant woman or is obese, perform chest thrusts (see step 7).
4. Make a fist with your other hand and place it, thumb side to patient, above your other hand.
5. Place your marking hand over your curled fist and begin to give quick inward and upward thrusts (review Figure 42-9).
6. There is no set number of thrusts to give to an adult who remains conscious. Continue to give thrusts until the object is removed or the patient becomes unconscious.

7. If the patient is an obviously pregnant woman or is obese, help the patient to lie on the ground in a supine position and perform chest thrusts.
8. If the patient becomes unconscious, gently lower him or her to the ground.
9. Activate EMS and put on gloves.
10. Immediately begin CPR with 30 chest compressions followed by two rescue breaths, using a ventilation mask. Before administering the rescue breaths, open the airway with the head-tilt, chin-lift maneuver (review Figure 42-4). Look for a foreign body in the patient's mouth and remove it if it is visible. Blind finger sweeps are no longer recommended and should not be performed.
11. Continue with cycles of 30 compressions and two rescue breaths until the foreign body is expelled or advanced medical personnel arrive to relieve you. Check for the foreign object each time the airway is opened to deliver the rescue breaths.
12. Wash hands and document the event in the patient's chart.

CHARTING EXAMPLE

10/25/YY 11:30 A.M. Jason Jones exhibited signs of choking at lunch. Jason grabbed his throat and was unable to cough or make noise. Tina Muller, RMA, alerted the physician and placed a call to 911. Abdominal thrusts were given until the piece of apple was expelled. EMS arrived and checked Jason for signs of throat irritation and swelling.................J. Walker, CMA (AAMA)

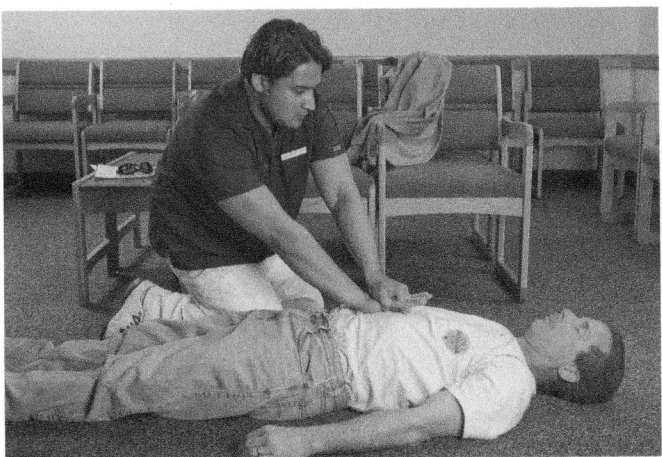

FIGURE 42-11 Deliver chest compressions to the supine unconscious patient.

disease processes, including obstructive conditions, such as asthma, chronic bronchitis, and emphysema, pneumonia, and acute pulmonary edema. Conscious control is usually not a factor in respiratory distress. Being unable to get enough oxygen causes extreme anxiety, and the medical staff should be prepared to give the patient emotional support. Signs and symptoms vary, depending on the cause. One of the most serious conditions is an occluded airway that causes the patient to grasp at the neck and attempt to cough. Unconsciousness soon follows, then cardiac arrest. Other conditions of respiratory distress may cause signs and symptoms such as the following:

• Acute anxiety with gasping breaths

• Bradypnea (abnormally slow breathing, fewer than eight breaths per minute)

- Cyanosis
- Failure of the chest to rise and fall
- Nasal flaring
- Pursing of the lips
- Noisy breathing (snoring, gurgling, wheezing, rattling, or stridor)
- Tachypnea (abnormally rapid breathing, more than 24 breaths per minute)

If respiratory distress is severe or results from a change in a known diagnosis, the patient may need follow-up with an emergency facility or a medical specialist.

Asthma Attack

Patients presenting with coughing, wheezing, shortness of breath, and chest tightness may have asthma. Short-acting Beta2 agonists in inhalers work well for acute asthma attacks, and corticosteroids work well for long-acting treatment. The physician may ask the medical assistant to administer oxygen to the patient.

Shortness of Breath

Any individual experiencing shortness of breath (SOB) needs immediate intervention. A **patent**, or unobstructed, airway is necessary to support life. If the person can speak, air is moving in and out. Ask the patient about the onset for difficult breathing and what activity caused it. This information helps to identify the problem. The patient experiencing SOB may be gasping for air, looking pale or cyanotic, and exhibiting nasal flaring and extreme anxiety (Figure 42-12). Usually the patient sits in an upright position and may be quite weak. If the airway is partially obstructed, the patient may cough in an attempt to clear the passages. If the patient is not in a sitting position, help her to a sitting position with support to the back. Call out for assistance.

Hyperventilation

Hyperventilation is quick, shallow breathing or rapid, deep breathing that results in decreasing carbon dioxide in the blood, dilation of blood vessels, and lowered blood pressure. The patient feels faint or light-headed and may experience any of the following:

- Chest tightness
- Cardiac palpitations
- Rapid pulse
- Deep sighing breaths
- Anxiety

Inform the physician and encourage the patient to breathe slowly and as deeply as possible. This condition can generally be resolved quickly and without further intervention.

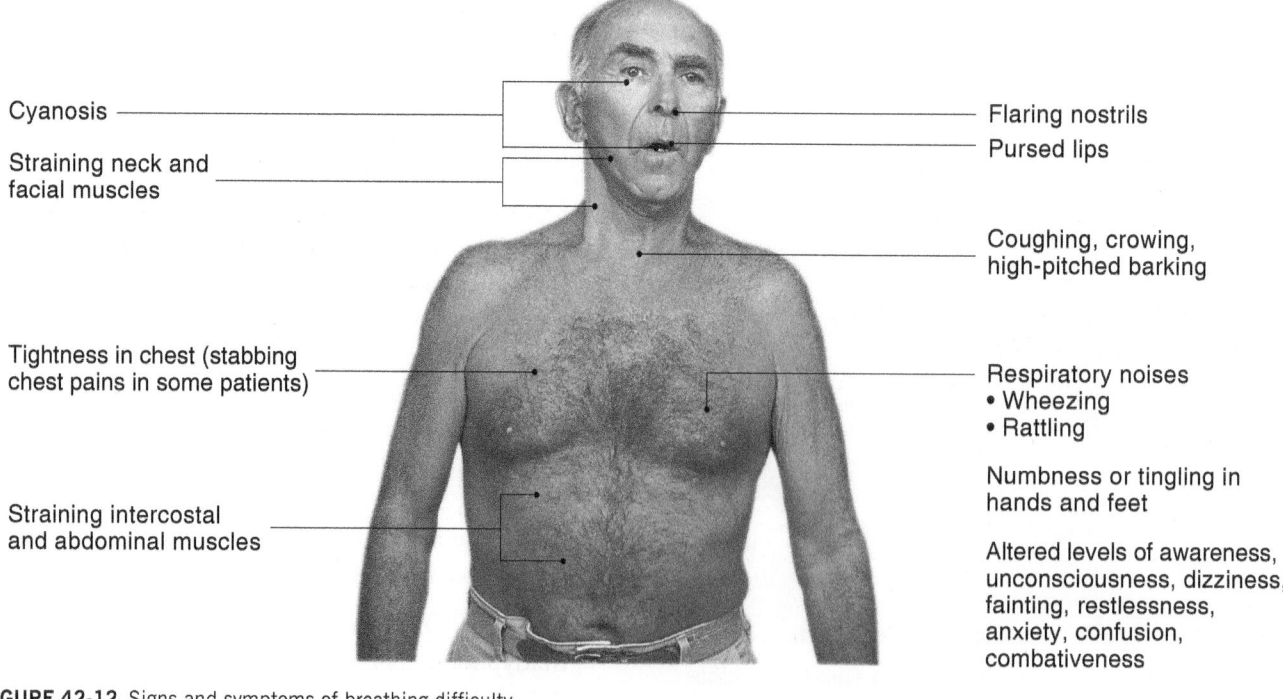

Cyanosis

Straining neck and facial muscles

Tightness in chest (stabbing chest pains in some patients)

Straining intercostal and abdominal muscles

Flaring nostrils
Pursed lips

Coughing, crowing, high-pitched barking

Respiratory noises
• Wheezing
• Rattling

Numbness or tingling in hands and feet

Altered levels of awareness, unconsciousness, dizziness, fainting, restlessness, anxiety, confusion, combativeness

FIGURE 42-12 Signs and symptoms of breathing difficulty.

Chronic Obstructive Pulmonary Disease

Asthma, chronic bronchitis, and emphysema are types of chronic obstructive pulmonary disease (COPD). Air is trapped in the lungs, and the patient is unable to expel all the carbon dioxide from the alveoli. Although each condition has specific signs and symptoms, they share many of the same problems. A person with COPD has SOB and a rapid heart rate and experiences weakness. Asthma may also be characterized by audible wheezes, diaphoresis, and tightness in the chest. Inform the physician in all cases and, if ordered, administer oxygen. Depending on the situation, the physician may order administration of medications, delivery of oxygen, or transport to an emergency facility by EMS.

Pulmonary Edema

Fluid accumulation in the lung tissue and alveoli results in a condition known as pulmonary edema. The patient presents with difficulty breathing, wheezing sounds, cyanosis, rapid heartbeat, distended neck veins, extreme anxiety, and orthopnea. Inform the physician. Place the patient in a sitting position with knees bent or dangling, which helps to trap venous blood and reduce the volume for the heart to pump. Administer supplemental oxygen if ordered and available. Call EMS for transport to an emergency facility.

Chest Pain

Heart attacks are the leading cause of death for both men and women. The patient experiencing chest pain may display various signs and symptoms. The primary complaint will be pain in the middle or left side of the chest, described as sharp, stabbing, crushing, squeezing, or aching. The pain may radiate to the left arm, to the back, or up the neck. Sometimes the pain is brought on by exertion, but other times onset is sudden and unexplained. Other symptoms are nausea, weakness, SOB, apprehension, and the feeling of impending doom. The skin may be clammy, moist, pale, or cyanotic. Denial is common, as the individual tries to explain the pain as heartburn or indigestion.

The first intervention is to have the individual stop what he is doing and sit down, with the feet elevated if possible. Immediately request help from a coworker. Ask the coworker to stay with the patient while you inform the physician of the situation. If instructed by the physician, or if a physician is unavailable, call EMS. If oxygen is available, administer it according to office protocol by nasal cannula at 6 to 8 liters per minute (L/min) until the physician or emergency personnel arrive. Assess heart rate and blood pressure. If the patient has previously been diagnosed with angina and has nitroglycerin tablets, insert one tablet under the tongue (Figure 42-13). If the pain is not relieved within five minutes,

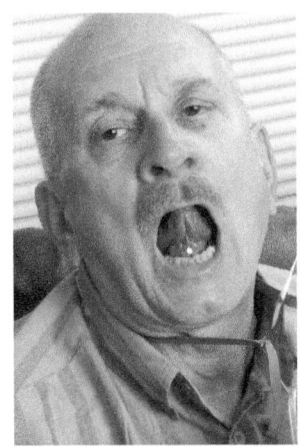

FIGURE 42-13 Nitroglycerin is administered sublingually.

inform the physician or EMS on the scene. Have the patient chew 162 to 325 mg of uncoated aspirin.

Do the following if a patient calls on the telephone complaining of chest pain:

- Keep the caller on the line while asking for help from another office staff member.

- Write down the caller's name and location. (If someone is calling for the patient, ask the caller for the patient's name and location.)

- Follow office protocol regarding assisting patients with chest pain. Offices often want all patients calling with chest pain sent to the emergency department. If this is the case, call EMS for the patient and remain on the phone with the caller until EMS has arrived. Your protocol may include instructing the patient to chew an uncoated aspirin tablet immediately.

Shock

Shock, the collapse of the cardiovascular system, is caused by insufficient cardiac output. Blood supply and nourishment (oxygen and nutrients, including glucose) to the tissue and perfusion to the organs are inadequate. Untreated shock can progress very rapidly to death.

Causes, Signs, and Symptoms of Shock

Shock may be the result of many insults to the body, including anaphylaxis, cardiac failure, hemorrhage, extreme emotional upset, respiratory distress, neurological collapse, severe metabolic insult, and sepsis. Some of the signs and symptoms that may occur after the initial crisis are listed in Table 42-4.

Anaphylactic Shock

Anaphylactic shock, as mentioned previously in this chapter, is a severe allergic reaction to a foreign substance. Examples

TABLE 42-4 | Signs and Symptoms of Shock Following a Crisis Situation

• Weakness	• Cool skin
• Rapid heartbeat	• Clammy skin
• Thirst	• Cyanosis
• Nausea	• Confusion
• Dizziness	• Disorientation
• Restlessness	• Unresponsiveness
• Pallor	• Shallow breathing

of foreign substances that may trigger allergic reactions include medications, bug bites, and latex gloves. Inform the physician immediately and call EMS. The physician may order epinephrine with or without an antihistamine. An IV may also be started. Prevention is the most important factor in anaphylactic shock. Always ask the patient about allergies to any medication before administering it, and record this information on the front of the chart in red. After administering medication, ask the patient to wait 20 minutes before leaving the office and observe for any potential reactions. In offices where antibiotics and allergy injections are given on a regular basis, you must be alert to possible reactions and prepared with an emergency drug box for rapid intervention.

Assisting Patients in Shock

Patients go into shock for varied reasons, including blood loss, infection, and pain. The most common signs of shock include pale, gray, or bluish skin; moist, cool skin; dilated pupils; a weak, rapid pulse; shallow, rapid respirations; and extreme thirst. Regardless of the cause, immediate, aggressive intervention is required to stop the progression of the condition and the possible death of the patient.

When a patient exhibits signs of shock, ensure that the patient has an open airway and proper circulation. Encourage the patient to lie down. Next, cover the patient with blankets for warmth and keep him calm until emergency personnel arrive. The medical assistant should inform the physician, call EMS for further assessment and transport, monitor the patient's vital signs, and provide emotional support. Procedure 42-5 describes how to perform first aid for a person in shock.

Most emergency treatments for shock patients need to be administered by a physician or emergency personnel. Oxygen may be administered, if ordered and available, by trained personnel. Table 42-5 lists types of shock and recommended treatments.

Diabetic Emergencies

A patient with diabetes may exhibit signs of either **hypoglycemia** (low blood sugar level) or **hyperglycemia** (high blood

---

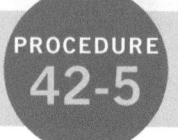

PROCEDURE 42-5   Performing First Aid for a Person in Shock

Objective ◆ *Administer first aid for a person in shock correctly, within the time frame designated by the instructor.*

EQUIPMENT AND SUPPLIES

Blanket; examining table

METHOD

1. Assist the patient to a supine position.
2. If the patient complains of cold or the room is cold, apply a blanket.
3. Loosen tight clothing.
4. Encourage the patient to keep still and remain calm.
5. If the patient vomits or bleeds from the mouth, turn on her side to prevent choking, unless you suspect spinal damage.
6. Perform CPR if needed.
7. Wash hands and document in the patient's chart.

CHARTING EXAMPLE

6/25/YY 11:30 A.M. Jason Blevins exhibited signs of shock after car accident in parking lot. Clover Bolgiano, RMA, alerted the physician and placed a call to 911. Patient was assisted to examination table, with feet elevated. Blanket applied. Patient remained calm under supervision of physician and Clover Bolgiano until EMS arrived and took Jason to the hospital..
....J. Walker, CMA (AAMA)

TABLE 42-5 | Treatment for Shock in the Medical Office

Cause	Treatment
Anaphylactic Shock	Epinephrine
Cardiogenic Shock	IV dopamine, immediate transport to the emergency department
Hemorrhagic Shock	Stop bleeding, replace volume, immediate transport to the emergency department
Hypovolemic Shock	Replace volume
Insulin Shock	Sugar given to patient by any means tolerated
Neurogenic Shock	IV dopamine, immediate transport to the emergency department
Poisoning	Consult the poison control center for treatment specific to the poison
Respiratory Shock	Intubation and immediate transport to the emergency department
Sepsis	Fluids, IV norepinephrine and immediate transport to the emergency department

sugar level). Both conditions may cause the rapid onset of altered levels of consciousness. The greater risk for a patient is hypoglycemia. Hypoglycemia, in which blood sugar falls below 70 mg per deciliter (mg/dL), may be the result of a skipped meal, vomiting after taking diabetic medications, excessive exercise, or an unknown reason. A patient may appear to be intoxicated (slurred speech, balance disturbances, and uncharacteristic behavior), have cold clammy skin, and be anxious or combative.

Intervention must be immediate and consists of some form of glucose administration. If the patient is conscious, ask about the last intake of food and diabetic medication. If the patient is able to swallow, glucose paste may be placed inside the mouth behind the lip and along the cheek, or the patient may drink orange juice with added sugar. If the patient is unconscious, IV glucose is administered.

The person experiencing hypoglycemia is in grave danger when the blood glucose drops below 40 mg/dL. The brain requires glucose to survive, and brain cells begin dying unless glucose is administered promptly. If possible, blood glucose levels should be checked with a blood glucose monitor. Contact EMS if a physician is not available to administer IV glucose. If there is doubt about whether the patient is hypoglycemic or hyperglycemic, glucose may be administered. It will raise the glucose 25 to 50 points, but this rise can be reversed with an insulin injection as soon as an elevated

glucose level is diagnosed. The hyperglycemic patient may progress to an unconscious state, reversible with insulin. The physician orders the amount and administration route of the insulin.

Whether the patient is hypoglycemic or hyperglycemic, keep her as warm and comfortable as possible on an examination table until the physician arrives. Procedure 42-6 demonstrates how to perform first aid for diabetic shock or coma.

Bleeding

Bleeding can be external or internal. External bleeding occurs when the skin is broken. Internal bleeding occurs with tissue damage and intact skin. Bleeding can originate from any of the three types of blood vessels: arteries, veins, and capillaries. Internal bleeding is unlikely to be diagnosed in the medical office and requires advanced interventions to correct. External bleeding can be controlled if it occurs in the medical office.

Arterial bleeding is usually copious, rapid, and bright red. The blood often spurts, echoing the heartbeat. Arterial bleeding must be brought under control as soon as possible. Apply pressure directly over the wound and elevate the injured part higher than the heart to help control bleeding.

Venous blood flows more slowly, is darker in color, and can usually be controlled by direct pressure. Blood from capillaries oozes rather than flows and can also be halted with direct pressure. Bleeding from the scalp or face is often copious because of the many blood vessels in those areas.

Direct pressure is applied by placing a sterile dressing over the wound and holding it in place with a gloved hand (Figure 42-14). A pressure bandage may be wrapped around the injured part to maintain pressure on the site. If blood seeps through, reinforce the bandage by applying more dressings and bandages over it. Do not remove the original dressing.

Exercise caution if a fracture is suspected, especially a facial or skull fracture that could be exacerbated by pressure. EMS should be activated if bleeding cannot be controlled or if head injuries or extremity fractures are suspected.

Epistaxis

Nontraumatic epistaxis (nosebleed not caused by an injury) may be messy and embarrassing, but it is usually a benign (not life threatening) occurrence. Nosebleeds tend to occur most commonly in dry weather or in dusty conditions and are usually easy to treat.

A nosebleed that occurs after a head injury and does not stop should be considered a serious emergency until proven otherwise. Even if there is no history of trauma, at least three other circumstances should worry a caregiver about

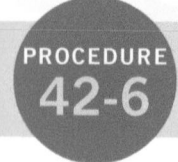

Performing First Aid for Diabetic Shock/Diabetic Coma

Objective ◆ *Administer first aid for a patient in diabetic shock, within the time frame designated by the instructor.*

EQUIPMENT AND SUPPLIES

Two glucose tablets; ½ cup fruit juice, ½ cup sugary soda, cup of milk, 1 tablespoon sugar, 1 tablespoon honey, 5–6 hard candies, or ¼ cup raisins

METHOD

1. Identify signs and symptoms of diabetic shock in the patient.
2. Assist the patient to a sitting position.
3. Offer the patient a glucose tablet to put under the tongue or one of these to drink: fruit juice, sugary soda, or milk or sugar cube, honey, candy, or raisins to eat if the case is mild and the patient is alert.
4. Check vital signs.
5. Assess blood sugar.
6. Monitor the patient for the time frame designated by the instructor (representing time that may elapse before arrival of the physician or of EMS if a physician is not available).
7. Wash hands and document in the patient's chart.

CHARTING EXAMPLE

3/14/YY 9:30 A.M. Carmen Spears presented with confusion, headache, shaking hands, and rapid heart rate (101). Assessed blood sugar through glucometer as 40. Administered ½ cup of orange juice. Vital signs 130/90 BP right arm, 86 pulse, 20 respirations, 98.8 temperature. Second blood sugar after 30 minutes was 89.....................................J. Walker, CMA (AAMA)

---

persistent nosebleeds. One is high blood pressure, especially in a patient who has recently changed or stopped taking medicines for the condition. Another is a clotting disorder of some kind. The third is a patient history of nosebleeds that have caused shock in the past.

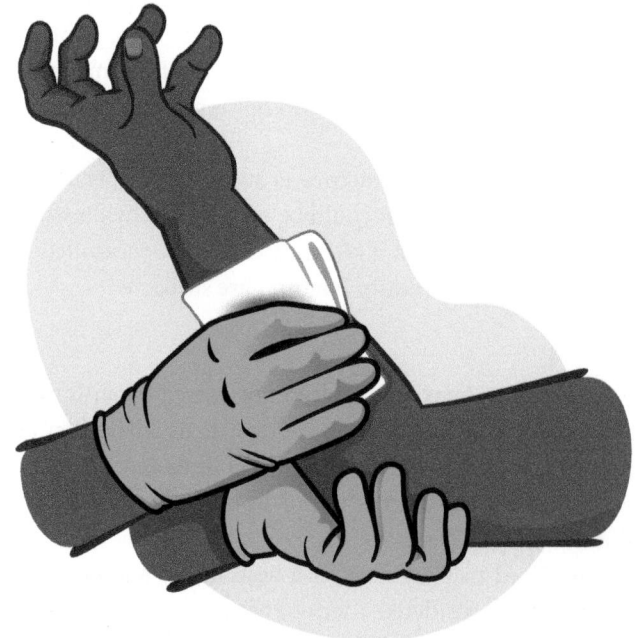

FIGURE 42-14 Apply direct pressure to the patient's wound.

Nosebleeds severe enough to cause changes in a patient's vital signs are rare, but they do occur. If the patient's vital signs are normal in the absence of trauma, the patient should be seated upright. If the vital signs are compromised, the patient should lie on the affected side and may need oxygen.

Bleeding from both nostrils is likely to be more serious than bleeding from just one nostril. If the blood emerges from both nostrils, its origin is not in the nose but somewhere above it, and it requires the immediate attention of a physician or **stat** (immediate) transport to an emergency department.

A nosebleed that emanates from one nostril is easily treated by a physician. To stop it, the physician will grasp a facial tissue by one corner and twist that corner firmly into a cone shape about 4 inches long. The physician then inserts the pack deeply into the patient's affected nostril, while continuing to twist it and until the nostril is firmly packed. Then a washcloth is placed over the patient's upper face, and the patient is instructed to hold a chemical cold pack against the washcloth so it fits the bridge of the nose like a saddle.

Bleeding should stop after only a few minutes, at which time the packing can be removed. If bleeding does not stop, electrocautery may be necessary. The physician may be able to perform this treatment in the office, or the patient may require transport to an emergency department.

If trauma is a possible factor in the medical office, the physician may not attempt to pack the nose or stop bleeding. In this case, the physician will order immediate contact of 911 and anticipate transport to the emergency department. The physician may insert an oral airway if the patient is unresponsive. (Do not use a nasal airway in a patient with this type of condition.) Place the patient on oxygen by non-rebreather mask, and monitor the patient carefully for changes in status.

Open Wounds

Open wounds are seldom life threatening, unless they penetrate the head, chest, throat, or abdomen. These cases are serious emergencies that warrant EMS transport to an emergency department. Most soft tissue injuries are uncomplicated. They typically require irrigation, debridement (or surgical trimming of damaged tissue), sutures, and antibiotics. Wounds that involve important structures such as nerve or muscle tissue, the genitalia, the eyes, and possibly the hands require specialized care and will probably be referred.

You may see some industrial soft tissue injuries that appear quite dramatic but that will probably heal well after office treatment. The one thing that you, as a medical assistant, can almost always control is bleeding.

Abrasions

An abrasion occurs when the outer layer of skin is scraped away, exposing the underlying tissue. Common types of abrasions include friction burns, rug burns, road rashes, and scrapes. Bleeding is usually in the form of oozing, and the injury is quite painful because nerve endings are exposed or damaged. As with all open wounds, the area is cleansed and any debris removed. Depending on the physician's choice, antibacterial ointment may be applied to the area and covered with a sterile dressing. Large areas of abraded tissue may require burn treatment.

Lacerations and Incisions

A laceration is an open wound in which the skin and underlying tissue are torn. It usually has jagged edges that may interfere with the healing process. When vessels are torn, bleeding results and must be controlled by direct pressure, pressure on pressure points, or eventual suturing or application of Steri-Strips. Cleanse the laceration with soap and water or an antiseptic solution, removing all debris and foreign matter. If bleeding is severe, a physician should direct the cleansing process. For minor lacerations, after cleansing, the edges of the wound are approximated and then held together with a small dressing, such as a Band-Aid, Steri-Strip, or sterile butterfly. Lacerations over a joint may

require joint immobilization for a few days while healing progresses.

An incision, which is a type of laceration, is a cut with smooth edges made with a knife or other sharp object. It is treated in the same manner as any other laceration. If the wound is deep or extensive, the physician usually performs a surgical intervention consisting of debridement, bleeding control, and trimming away of the jagged wound edges. If there is damage to underlying tissue, such as a tendon or ligament, further surgical intervention is required.

Avulsions and Amputations

An avulsion is the tearing away of skin or tissue. Avulsions usually occur on limbs and appendages, including fingers, toes, hands, arms, feet, legs, nose, and penis. The body part may become entangled in machinery or be injured in a motor vehicle accident or a confrontation with an animal. Cleanse minor avulsion wounds with soap and water and return any skin flap to its normal position. Apply direct pressure to control bleeding; then apply a dressing when bleeding is controlled.

If the body part has been amputated (completely separated from the body) and recovered, cleanse the dismembered part with sterile saline. Wrap it with moist, sterile gauze, seal it in a plastic bag, and place the plastic bag in a cooler with an ice pack or ice in the bottom. Do not place the bag containing the amputated part directly on the ice or ice pack to avoid freezing the tissue. Prompt medical attention and preservation of the body part enhance the chances for successful reattachment. Cover the wound or stump with a sterile dressing until advanced treatment can be provided.

Puncture Wounds

A puncture wound results from a pointed foreign body penetrating the skin and tissue. Often the wound edges close, trapping pathogens and debris in the tissue. Depending on the nature of the pointed object, cleansing may consist of simply soaking the area or may require invasive irrigation. After cleansing, a dressing is applied. Bleeding from a puncture wound is usually minimal.

Impaled Objects

A patient who has been impaled by an object such as a large piece of glass or sharp metal requires special treatment. The general rule is to leave the object in place until it can be safely removed by trained personnel. Stabilizing the object is critical to preventing further damage. Control bleeding and stabilize the impaled object with a bulky dressing held in place with tape or other bandages. Splint the area to prevent movement. For a small penetrating object, a small paper cup may be used. Make a hole in the bottom of the cup, place it over the object with the lip of the cup against the skin, and secure it with bandages.

Soft Tissue Injuries

Soft tissue trauma involves both the skin and underlying tissue. Abrasions, incisions, lacerations, and puncture wounds are easily identified as open-wound skin injuries. Avulsions, amputations, and burns are considered soft tissue injuries because underlying tissues as well as skin are involved. Contusions (bruises) are closed soft tissue wounds in which the skin is not broken. Damage to the underlying tissue may involve subcutaneous tissues, blood vessels, nerves, muscles, ligaments, and tendons. The tearing of small blood vessels results in bleeding into the tissue and discoloration of the area. Swelling may exert pressure on nerve endings, creating pain. Crush injuries result when force is applied to the tissue. Depending on the area involved, the crush may be similar to pinching of tissue or so severe as to involve organs and bones.

For soft tissue injuries, elevating the body part above the heart and applying cold are often the only interventions needed. With a more severe injury, the body part should be immobilized. Monitoring vital signs and observing skin color, temperature, and moisture are essential to deciding whether more extensive intervention is needed.

Wound Care Pointers

Following is a list of concepts that relate to dressing wounds:

- A **dressing** is a sterile covering placed directly over a wound to absorb blood and other body fluids, prevent contamination, and protect the wound from further trauma. Dressings come in many commercially

available forms: sterile and nonsterile gauze (2 × 2s, 4 × 4s), compress (bulky sterile dressing to help control bleeding), occlusive (creates an airtight seal), petroleum (sterile gauze covered with petroleum that prevents the wound from sticking), and premedicated and packed dressings (medicated gauze for application over a wound, or strips to pack into the wound).

- A **bandage** is a strip of binding material used to hold a dressing in place. Commonly used dressings are roller gauze (e.g., Kerlix and Kling) and elastic bandages (e.g., Ace and Coban). A dressing or compress prefastened to a bandage is called a bandage compress (e.g., a Band-Aid). A pressure dressing is a compress held in place by an elastic bandage. All of these devices come in various widths. Choose the type and size that fit the wound. Bandage types depend on where the injury is located.

Circular bandage turns are used to hold and secure a dressing in place. A figure-eight bandage is used for holding a dressing in place, bandaging joints, and providing immobilization of the area. A spiral turn is used to cover cylindrical (round) body parts such as the forehead. A reverse spiral turn is used for covering cone-shaped body parts such as the lower leg and forearm.

Simple direct pressure (as discussed) with a dressing (bulky if needed) will usually stop bleeding from a soft tissue injury. Once the direct pressure is determined to be sufficient, keep the dressing in place with a bandage as ordered by the physician. The priority is to prevent infection by dressing the wound properly. That always begins with cleansing. Cleanse the wound from the center outward, beginning with vigorous irrigation using a disinfecting solution prescribed by the physician. Wipe the edges of the wound in all directions away from the wound with sterile gauze, then cover with a sterile dressing and fasten the dressing in place. The use or nonuse of antibacterial ointments or creams should be specified by the physician. Procedure 42-7 describes the application of a pressure bandage.

Figure 42-15 provides a classification of open wounds for injuries. Open soft tissue wounds can be superficial (penetrating only the skin) or deep (penetrating the fascia, or connective layer beneath the skin, and other structures that lie deeper still). Once bleeding is controlled and the wound dressed, obtain a complete set of vital signs and allow patients to remain in the supine position or the position that brings greatest comfort while you take the time to document in the chart. Watch for signs of shock and treat as needed. Next, get patients into a sitting position and make

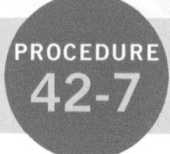

PROCEDURE 42-7

Applying a Pressure Bandage to Control Bleeding

Objective ◆ *Apply a pressure dressing.*

EQUIPMENT AND SUPPLIES

Dressing supplies or makeshift materials; gloves and other available PPE

METHOD

1. Escort the patient immediately to an examination room.
2. Perform hand hygiene.
3. Put on disposable gloves.
4. Under the physician's supervision, apply direct pressure with a dressing placed on the open wound. If possible, elevate the affected part.
5. After assessment, the physician will decide if EMS should be contacted.
6. Apply additional dressings as needed. Do not remove the original dressing.
7. Apply pressure to pressure points as necessary and with the physician's supervision.
8. If bleeding is controlled, anchor the dressing to maintain pressure.
9. If the physician orders, prepare the patient for transport to an emergency care facility.
10. Dispose of waste in a biohazard waste container.
11. Remove and discard gloves.
12. Perform hand hygiene and document the procedure in the patient's chart.

CHARTING EXAMPLE

08/31/YY 8:00 A.M. Pt came to office with 6" laceration to right forearm. Injury occurred from fight with 7-year-old brother when patient fell into glass patio door. Bleeding profusely. Physician called to examination room. B/P 96/60 P 100, regular but weak. R 26. Pt appears very nervous. Pt transported to ED to further control bleeding and take to surgery. Pt is alert and talking to parents................................S. Porter, CMA (AAMA)

---

sure they are not dizzy and that they understand their home care instructions. When a patient is ready, provide assistance to a standing position, again ensuring stability before allowing the patient to leave. If there are signs of shock, notify the physician immediately and do not leave patients alone. If instructed by your physician, contact EMS.

Burns

A burn injury occurs when an area of tissue is destroyed by the action of physical heat, chemical activity, high electrical current, or heavy exposure to radiation. The severity of a burn depends on the amount and depth of tissue injury. Survival depends on those factors and the amount of surface area that is destroyed. Destruction of skin surface is an important consideration because of all the skin functions that are lost: insulation, regulation of fluids, sensation, and protection from infection. All of these are crucial to life.

If directed by a physician, the medical assistant may help stop

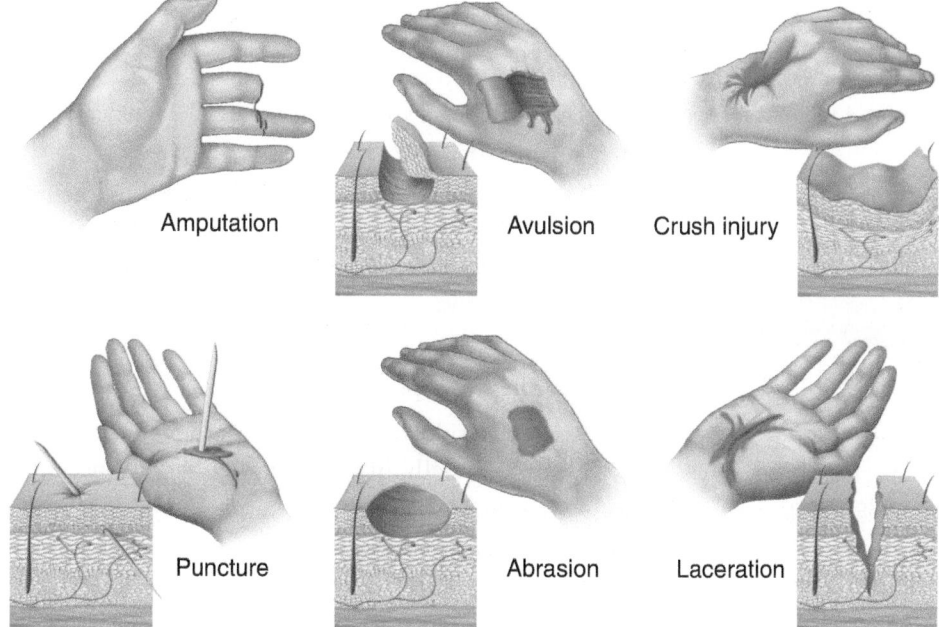

FIGURE 42-15 Classification of open injuries.

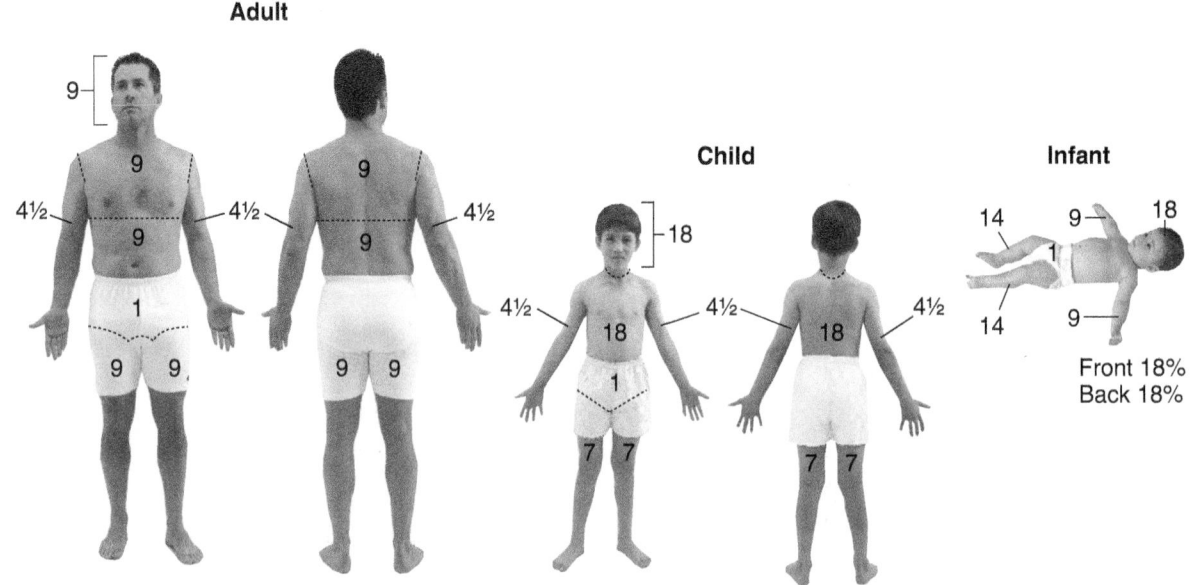

Adult

9

9

4½   4½   4½

9   9

1

9   9   9   9

Child

18

4½   18   4½   18   4½

1

7   7   7   7

Infant

14   9   18

1

14   9

Front 18%
Back 18%

Note: Each arm totals 9% (front of arm 4½%, back of arm 4½%)

FIGURE 42-16 Rule of Nine for burns.

the burning and remove any metal jewelry from the burn patient.

Classification of Burns

Burns are classified in two basic ways: by surface area and by depth. The **Rule of Nines** is a useful tool for estimating body surface area (Figure 42-16). For an adult, each of the following areas represents 9 percent of the body surface: head and neck, each upper extremity, chest, abdomen, upper back, lower back and buttocks, the front of each lower extremity, and the back of each lower extremity. These make up 99 percent of the body's surface. The remaining 1 percent is assigned to the genital region.

In the Rule of Nines, the percentages are modified for infants and young children, whose heads are much larger in relationship to the rest of the body.

Table 42-6 gives you a basic idea of burn severity by depth.

TABLE 42-6 | Classification of Burns

Classification	Characteristics
Superficial Burn (First Degree)	Reddening, swelling of epidermis (like a mild sunburn)
Partial Thickness Burn (Second Degree)	Reddening, swelling of epidermis and outer dermis; blisters noted
Full Thickness Burn (Third Degree)	Charring of all layers of skin and at least some deeper structures
Full Thickness Burn (Fourth Degree)	Underlying muscle, tendons, ligaments and bone are damaged; very often fatal

Superficial and partial thickness burns are extremely painful, even those involving very small areas. Full thickness burns tend not to be painful immediately because, along with the entire dermis, this kind of burn destroys sensory nerve endings. The edges of the burn are likely to be very painful partial thickness burns, however.

Full thickness burns disrupt all the normal functions of skin, including its self-regenerative properties and its ability to resist infection. Full thickness burns are profound injuries, even if they involve only a small amount of surface area.

Certain special considerations can also help determine the seriousness of a burn:

- The mortality of serious burns is higher for older patients and for very young patients.

- The mortality is higher if the patient was burned in a closed area (partly because of the possibility of carbon monoxide poisoning and partly because of the possibility of airway burns).

- Burns of the genitalia are always considered serious, regardless of depth.

- Always consider the possibility of other injuries besides burns, especially in a patient who was burned in an auto or industrial accident.

- Patients with chemical burns should have the area irrigated immediately with large amounts of water. If the burns resulted from an alkali substance, irrigation should be continued for a minimum of 20 minutes.

Contact EMS as soon as you encounter such a patient to be sure that you have access to the proper resources as early as possible if you are dealing with a hazardous substance that cannot be rendered harmless.

- Electrical burns serious enough to leave marks on the body are considered serious burns because of the probability of internal injuries. (Electrocution by lightning is always considered serious until proven otherwise.)

Extremely severe full thickness burns are sometimes called fourth degree burns. These burns are frequently fatal because they damage underlying muscles, tendons, ligaments, and even bone. Burns that may be called fifth and sixth degree burns are not compatible with life and are usually diagnosed on autopsy. Burns of this severity are regarded as stand-alone admission criteria by trauma centers and burn centers in most places.

Treatment of Burns

Treatment for superficial burns involving less than 10 percent of the body surface includes pain relief by applying cool water. Cool water instantly relieves pain, but it is not appropriate for larger surface areas. Damaged skin may not be able to regulate body temperature, so the use of cooling measures over large surface areas can cause hypothermia. Analgesic (pain-relieving) creams and ointments are appropriate for use on superficial burns only if ordered by the physician.

Cool water can also be used to soothe partial thickness burns involving small surface areas as long as there are no broken blisters. Partial thickness burns should never be treated with creams or ointments because of the risk of breaking blisters and the resulting potential for infection.

Burns of any kind that involve broken skin may need to be debrided (have dead or damaged tissue removed) by a physician. Full thickness burns of any size warrant treatment at a trauma center or burn center.

Burns should be dressed with dry sterile dressings, and pain should be managed with injectable analgesics as ordered by the physician. If Paramedics transport the patient, they will start an IV and administer analgesics by that route if the physician has not already done so.

Upper airway burns are a dire emergency and always warrant prompt intubation by the physician or EMS with the largest tube that can be inserted. The burned epiglottis can swell quickly and make intubation very difficult or impossible at a later time. If the patient sounds even slightly hoarse or complains of difficulty breathing; if you notice singed nasal hairs, eyebrows, or eyelashes; or if you detect stridor in any burn patient, suspect airway burns and notify the physician right away. Administer oxygen as ordered by the physician.

Large surface-area burns should be dressed with dry sterile sheets that are wrapped entirely around the patient's body. These patients should be promptly transported to a trauma center or burn center. All burn patients should be monitored for signs of shock, especially in the case of large surface-area involvement.

Heat- and Cold-Related Emergencies

Heat Exhaustion

Heat exhaustion, which is an extreme fatigue caused by heat, occurs as the result of sodium and water depletion from the body. Strenuous activity often precedes heat exhaustion because the individual becomes overheated and perspires profusely. The skin is moist, pale, and cool, and body temperature is normal. The individual may complain of headache, muscle cramps, weakness, dizziness, and nausea. The patient should be moved to a cooler environment and encouraged to lie down. Apply cool compresses and give sips of water if the individual is conscious. Heat exhaustion can usually be prevented by taking salt pills and drinking lots of water before, during, and after strenuous activities in a warm environment.

Hyperthermia

Prolonged exposure to extremely hot temperatures often results in an elevated body temperature, or **hyperthermia**. The loss of water and salt through perspiration leads to a state of mild shock. If the body's cooling mechanisms fail, heat exhaustion can progress into heat stroke. An individual experiencing heat stroke usually fails to perspire and has a body temperature of 105°F or higher. The skin is dry, red, and hot to the touch. Headache, shortness of breath, nausea or vomiting, dizziness, weakness, and dry mouth are common symptoms. At the onset, the pulse is rapid, but it gradually slows and becomes weak. The blood pressure begins to drop. Mental confusion may appear, possibly accompanied by irritability and hysterical behavior. In some cases the patient collapses. If the individual remains exposed to heat, brain cells begin to die. Permanent brain damage or even death may eventually result. The patient must be removed from the environment immediately. Loosen the clothing and cool the body down as quickly as possible by pouring cool water over the patient or sponging with a cool, wet cloth. If heat stroke is suspected, after the initial emergency treatment, EMS should be contacted to transport the patient to an emergency facility where vital signs and cardiac status can be monitored. The patient should not be left alone and should be assessed by a physician as promptly as possible.

Hypothermia

The patient with **hypothermia** is also at great risk. Hypothermia results from prolonged exposure to cold or cold water and can cause the core temperature to drop below 95°F. The patient shivers and experiences numbness and tingling throughout the body. The skin becomes very cool to the touch and is pale with a blue or ashy tinge. Respirations are slow and shallow, and the patient becomes disoriented and eventually unconscious as body functions and organs slow down to the point of complete shutdown.

Treatment involves removing any cold, wet clothing and wrapping the patient in warm blankets. Heat packs may be used but not directly on the skin. Once the patient is conscious, offer sips of warm liquid. When possible, the patient should be transported to a treatment facility for assessment by a physician.

Seizures

Seizures, or convulsions, are produced by disorganized electrical activity in the brain and are characterized by involuntary muscle contractions that alternate between the contraction and relaxation of muscles. In some cases the convulsions are generalized, involving the entire body, or localized and limited to a specific area of the body. Convulsions can result from a number of problems or combinations of problems.

By themselves, convulsions are not life threatening, but the muscle spasms that come with full-body seizures can restrict breathing. Seizure patients may also bite their tongues, causing bleeding and swelling, which can obstruct the airway. Finally, seizure patients are sometimes injured when their convulsions cause them to fall.

Once a seizure stops, especially a full-body seizure, it is normal for a patient to remain unconscious for as long as 15 minutes. During that time, most patients cannot control their secretions—for example, urine—the way they would in normal sleep.

A medical assistant can do two important things for a seizing patient. First, prevent injuries. Keep the patient from falling, and prevent the head from striking anything until the seizure stops. Second, pay close attention to what the patient is experiencing so you can describe it later. Observations will eventually be very important to the patient's neurologist. If breathing seems adequate, note the patient's response, apply oxygen as ordered, and place the patient on the left side to allow any secretions to drain. Listen for noise in the airway, and be prepared to assist the patient by moving any furniture or objects away from him. Never place anything in the mouth of a seizing patient.

You must immediately notify your physician. If the physician is not available, contact EMS and anticipate transport. Continue to assess the patient until EMS personnel arrive, and communicate your findings to them. Procedure 42-8 describes how to perform first aid for a patient having a seizure.

Fainting

Many serious disorders cause unresponsiveness. Fainting, or syncope, is the sudden loss of consciousness. Sometimes it is preceded by vertigo, the sensation of feeling dizzy or that

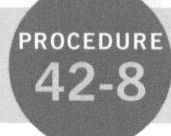

PROCEDURE 42-8

Performing First Aid for a Patient Having a Seizure

Objective ◆ *Administer first aid for a patient having a seizure, in the time frame designated by the instructor.*

EQUIPMENT AND SUPPLIES

None

METHOD

1. Identify that the patient is having a seizure.
2. Assist the patient to the floor, protecting the head and assuring no hard or sharp objects nearby can injure her.
3. Loosen clothing around the neck.
4. After seizure, lay the patient on her side, and monitor and reassure the patient.
5. If the seizure lasts more than five minutes, call 911.

6. Wash hands and document in the patient's chart.

CHARTING EXAMPLE

2/28/XX 3:30 P.M. Heidi Haldeman began seizing while sitting in examining room. Assisted patient to the floor, protecting the head from trauma. Loosened collar and monitored patient. Post-seizure, patient began to vomit, so turned her on her side and offered emesis basin. Reassured and reoriented patient. Seizure lasted two minutes. Afterwards, patient complained of soreness and fatigue but was oriented x 3...............M. Jimenez, RMA.

the room is spinning. It seems to be caused by a brief interruption in the body's ability to control the brain's circulation. Fainting often occurs just after a patient has received an emotional shock of some kind. The patient usually collapses and becomes unresponsive but, within a minute, should awaken and return to normal function. Patients seldom become incontinent or have seizures as a result of simple fainting but may be injured in the course of a fall.

There is always a reason for unresponsiveness, and determining the reason is, of course, important. However, early in your contact with any unconscious patient, your first concern should be to take care of the ABCs (airway, breathing, and circulation). A patient who suddenly becomes unresponsive may be experiencing arrhythmia such as ventricular fibrillation or ventricular tachycardia. If a patient has fainted and there is no response, provide oxygen if the physician orders this. Check the ABCs and call for help. If the patient is breathing well but will not wake up, place him on his left side and contact your physician. If your physician is not available, contact EMS. While you await their arrival, try to get a good set of vital signs and if possible obtain a blood sugar reading. Procedure 42-9 illustrates how to assist a patient with syncope.

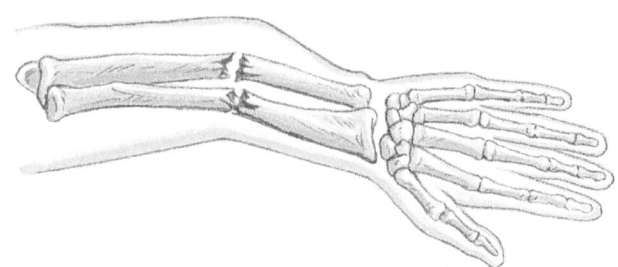

FIGURE 42-17 A closed fracture.

Musculoskeletal Injuries

Musculoskeletal injuries involve bones, muscles, tendons, and ligaments and include fractures, dislocations, sprains, and strains. Definitive diagnosis is made by X-ray, but these injuries must be considered fractured bones until determined to be otherwise. Therefore, the affected part must be immobilized.

Fractures

In a closed or simple fracture, the bone is broken but does not penetrate the skin (Figure 42-17). In an open or compound fracture, the bone pierces the skin, or the skin is torn

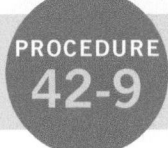

PROCEDURE
42-9

Responding to a Patient with Syncope

Objective ◆ *Correctly care for a patient with syncope, within the time limit set by the instructor.*

EQUIPMENT AND SUPPLIES
Blanket; small stool or box; ½ cup of orange juice; glucometer

METHOD
1. Identify signs of syncope.
2. Assist the patient to a supine position.
3. Elevate legs.
4. Loosen tight clothing and apply a blanket if the physician directs.
5. Assess the patient for respirations, heart rate, chest pain, and consciousness.
6. If any of the following is present and the physician directs, call 911: blue lips or face, irregular or slow heart rate, chest pain, difficulty breathing, is difficult to awaken, or acts confused.

7. If none of the above are present, assess blood sugar and treat for hypoglycemia if appropriate.
8. Wash hands and document in the patient's chart.

CHARTING EXAMPLE
1/16/XX 9:30 A.M. Chester Tyler was found on the floor of the examining room. Assisted patient to supine position and loosened collar. Applied blanket and elevated feet. Patient's pulse was irregular and 55, and he was difficult to awaken. 911 immediately called. Physician and Jenny Erkfitz CMA (AAMA) remained with patient until EMS arrived five minutes later and took patient to hospital..............................C. Glidewell, RMA

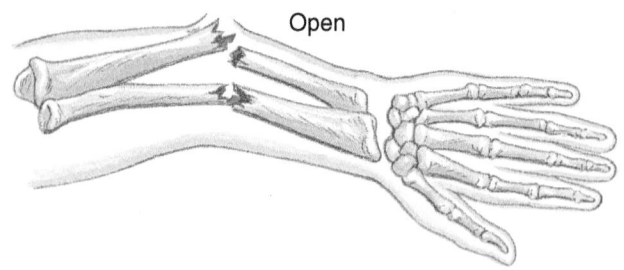

FIGURE 42-18 An open fracture.

open by the bone or by an external force (Figure 42-18). Fractures may also involve single or multiple breaks in the bone. Bone breaks can be complete, twisted, or splintered.

The affected part is immobilized and examined for impaired circulation to the distal aspect. The location of the fracture and the possible presence of heavy bleeding or bruising are also determined. Knowing the cause of the injury is very helpful in this assessment. A fracture may occur in any bone. Procedure 42-10 shows the steps to perform first aid for a patient with a fracture.

Special precautions must be taken for suspected fractures of the spinal column or skull. For any injury caused by sudden acceleration and deceleration, the cervical spine must be immobilized. Other injuries to the spinal column require extreme caution when moving the patient. The best response is to call 911. Allow EMS professionals to stabilize the cervical spine with a cervical collar; then logroll the patient onto a spine board for transport to a facility where X-rays can be taken to determine the extent of the injury.

Suspected fractures of the thigh (femur) and pelvis are always severe and dangerous injuries that require immobilization and transport and are best handled by the EMS.

In open or compound fractures, the soft tissue injury must be tended. Cover the open wound with a sterile, saline-moistened dressing; then place a sterile occlusive dressing over that. Generally, the tissue must be surgically cleaned and debrided.

Splint Application

Fractures of long bones require immobilization by splinting to prevent joint movement above and below the fracture. In addition to preventing additional damage to the bone and surrounding soft tissue, the splint helps to relieve pain and allows safe movement of the injured part. Another comfort measure is the application of cold, usually after splinting, to prevent swelling.

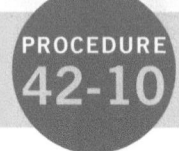

PROCEDURE
42-10

Performing First Aid for a Patient with a Fracture

Objective ◆ *Perform first aid for a patient with a fractured arm, within the time period established by the instructor.*

EQUIPMENT AND SUPPLIES

Sling; arm splint; gauze; tape; ice pack

METHOD

1. Identify the patient and introduce yourself.
2. Obtain vital signs.
3. Examine the injury, without straightening the arm, for bleeding, bruising, or protruding bones.
4. If the bone has broken through the skin, wrap in gauze and apply pressure to stop bleeding and get emergency help.
5. If the bone has not broken through the skin, apply a padded arm splint under the ulna and radius, and secure the splint by wrapping dressings or material around the arm and splint. Place ties above and below the suspected fracture and then along the arm to secure.

6. Assess circulation distal to the wound.
7. Elevate the arm and place in a sling.
8. Apply ice for 20 minutes.
9. If the physician requests, send to the patient to the hospital for X-ray and possible casting.
10. Wash hands and document in the patient's chart.

CHARTING EXAMPLE

9/30/XX 2:30 P.M. Charlton Parker presented with a possible fracture after a soccer injury at school. Mother administered Tylenol 480 mg for pain en route to office. Bone has not broken through skin, but patient complains of pain. Secured arm in arm board and sling. Applied ice and instructed mother to remove ice after 20 minutes. Referred to Radiology at Blue Ridge Hospital for radiograph by physician......C. Glidewell RMA

Sprains, Strains, and Dislocations

A *sprain* occurs when muscles, tendons, or ligaments are torn. It may be the result of trauma or cumulative overuse of the joint. A *strain*, often called a pulled muscle, occurs when a muscle or tendon is overextended by stretching. The patient complains of pain and may be unable to use the joint. In the lower extremities, weight bearing is painful and sometimes impossible. In a *dislocation*, the bone is actually pulled away from the joint, stretching or tearing the ligaments and tendons. A deformity is generally noted. Dislocations must be reduced and the bone reinserted into the joint. The injured body parts should be immobilized to prevent additional damage and reduce pain. Applications of cold also help with the pain and slow edema. The physician assesses the injury and usually orders radiographs to eliminate the possibility of fracture and diagnose sprain, strain, or dislocation. Table 42-7 describes first aid for some emergencies sometimes seen in medical offices.

Planning for Medical Emergencies in the Office

It is important for the physician and staff in a medical office to develop a plan for medical emergencies that can occur in the office, in order for all staff to be prepared. Procedure 42-11 shows how to develop a medical emergency plan policy for a medical office.

EMERGENCY PREPAREDNESS

The medical assistant should be knowledgeable in the area of emergency preparedness. This includes knowing how to respond in the event of a human-caused disaster, such as a terrorist event, and to a natural disaster, such as a hurricane. Remaining calm in the event of an emergency is paramount to the success of handling it. Through proper education, preparedness, and simulation, a medical assistant can play a key role in emergency response.

Earthquakes

Because earthquakes can happen at any time, and without any warning, the medical assistant must know how to respond to this type of emergency. One of the first steps to preventing injury during an earthquake is to prepare before an earthquake happens. Advance preparation may save lives as well as prevent injuries. According to the Federal Emergency Management Agency (FEMA), six steps are involved

---

TABLE 42-7 | Response to Emergencies

Emergency	Response
Poisoning	If you suspect poisoning because the patient states that she ingested a poison or has lost consciousness with a poison nearby, or is vomiting profusely, gather information about potential poisons by asking about the scene and circumstances. Encourage family to call, or call the National Poison Control Center at (800) 222-1222 and follow their instructions. Instructions may be to go to emergency room, ingest milk, hydrate with water, etc. It depends on the suspected poison and amount.
Stroke	If you suspect stroke, ask the patient to smile (F)—does one side of the face droop? Ask the patient to raise both arms (A)—does one arm drift downwards? Ask the patient to repeat a simple phrase (S)—does the speech seem slurred or strange? And (T) if you observe any of these signs, call 911 immediately. Immediate transportation to the hospital gives the patient access to thrombolytic (clot-dissolving) drugs that can greatly reduce damage.
Animal Bite	If the bite is minor and barely breaks the skin, wash with soap and water and apply an antibiotic and bandage. For a deeper wound, rabies is possible. Apply pressure with a clean dry cloth, and have the patient seen by a physician for possible treatment for rabies or tetanus. Also refer to a physician if you see signs of infection.
Insect Bite	For a mild bite, get to an area safe from further bites. If needed, remove the stinger with a credit card or similar device. Wash with soap and water. Apply a cool compress. Apply hydrocortisone, pramoxine, or lidocaine to help control pain. Use creams such as calamine lotion or those containing colloidal oatmeal or baking soda to help soothe itchy skin. Treat for pain with a mild pain reliever like Tylenol. For more serious bites such as a scorpion sting, a bite on a child, or a bite that leads to anaphylaxis, contact 911. You may need to administer an epinephrine autoinjector for an allergic reaction. Hold the autoinjector against the thigh, and inject as indicated on instructions. Loosen tight clothing, cover with a blanket as needed, and monitor the patient. Do not give the patient anything to eat or drink. If vomiting or bleeding occurs, turn on the side. Perform CPR if needed.
Concussion	If concussion is suspected, have the person stop the activity and rest. Apply ice as needed. For pain, use Tylenol, aspirin, or ibuprofen. Monitor for at least 24 hours. Notify physician if: a headache gets worse, vomiting continues, drowsiness or dizziness increases, patient experiences increased confusion, or if a child will not nurse or eat or stop crying.

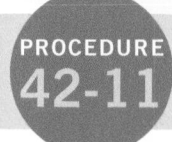

PROCEDURE 42-11

Creating a Medical Emergency Plan

Objective ◆ *Create a medical emergency plan.*

EQUIPMENT AND SUPPLIES

Pen; paper; emergency kit composed of water, canned food, can opener, snacks, personal hygiene products, first aid kit, trash bag, gloves, battery-powered radio, flashlight, extra batteries, whistle, tools, protective masks, diapers, powdered milk, formula, baby wipes, and crash cart

METHOD

1. Develop an emergency kit using the above-listed supplies and any others you desire, explaining what each supply might be used for in an emergency.
2. Document a policy that would cover the actions needed in each of the following situations that might occur in the medical office:
   a. Choking
   b. Lack of pulse
   c. Shortness of breath
   d. Shock
   e. Bleeding
   f. Epistaxis
   g. Superficial burn
   h. Hyperthermia
   i. Seizures
   j. Fainting
3. Determine the best location to store your medical emergency policy and kit.
4. Develop a memorandum to the physician stating that you have developed the medical emergency plan.

DOCUMENTATION

12/6/YY 1:30 P.M. Medical emergency plan developed and posted at the reception desk on bright yellow paper. Medical emergency kit inventoried and stored in lowest drawer of receptionist's desk.............................M. Schuknecht CMA (AAMA).

---

in planning ahead for an earthquake as well as other emergency situations:

1. Check for hazards around the facility.
   - Make sure shelves are fastened securely to walls.
   - Keep large or heavy objects on lower shelves.
   - Store any breakable items in low, closed cabinets equipped with locks.
   - Do not hang heavy items on walls above where patients will sit or lie.
   - Secure overhead light fixtures.
   - Repair any defective electrical wiring or leaky gas connections.
   - Strap water heaters to wall studs and bolt them to the floor.
   - Repair any deep cracks in ceilings or foundations.
   - Store all flammable products on the bottom shelves of closed cabinets with locks.
2. Identify safe places indoors and outdoors.
   - Under sturdy furniture
   - Against an inside wall
   - Away from glass that could shatter
   - Away from bookcases or furniture that could fall over
   - In the open, away from buildings, trees, telephone or electrical lines, overpasses, or elevated expressways
3. Educate yourself and your coworkers.
   - Contact the local EMS office or ARC chapter for information.
   - Teach all staff members how and when to turn off gas, electricity, and water.
4. Have disaster supplies on hand (Figure 42-19).
   - Flashlight and extra batteries
   - Portable battery-operated radio and extra batteries
   - First-aid kit and manual
   - Emergency food and water
   - Extra blankets
5. Develop an emergency communication plan.
   - In case staff members are separated from one another during an earthquake, have a plan in place for reuniting after the disaster.

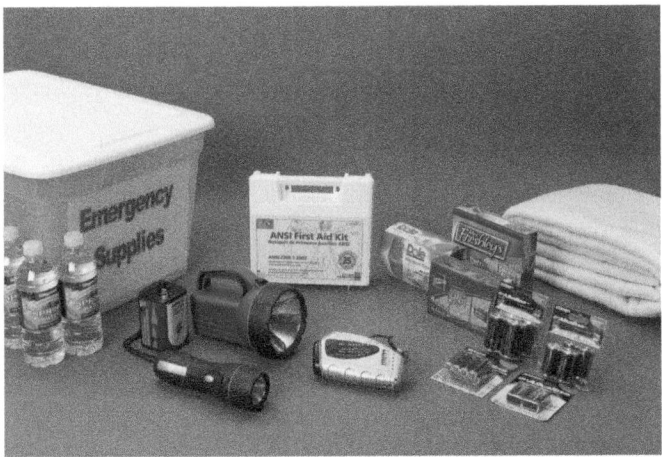

FIGURE 42-19 Every medical office should keep emergency supplies in a waterproof container.

- Define the expectations of each staff member: Who will escort patients from the building? Who will check the treatment rooms?

6. Help your community get ready.
   - Provide literature for patients on how to prepare for an earthquake.

Tornadoes

According to FEMA, tornadoes are the most violent storms occurring in nature. Tornadoes are very erratic can strike with very little or no warning. The warning signs of a tornado include thunderstorms with heavy rain and large hail; dark, almost greenish-colored skies; and dark, low-lying clouds. Many people have related the sound of a tornado to that of a freight train.

Often, tornado watches and warnings are issued before a tornado touches down. A tornado watch indicates that the weather conditions are right for a tornado and a tornado is possible, whereas a tornado warning indicates that a tornado has been sighted and all persons are to take shelter immediately.

It is important to designate a safe area within the office should a tornado watch occur during working hours. This often will be the basement of a building or the lowest level of a structure. If a basement is not available, it is advisable to seek shelter in a closet or interior hallway. Above all else, stay away from windows, doors, and outside walls. Avoid elevators and use the stairs to reach the lowest level of the facility.

Before the occurrence of a tornado (or an earthquake, hurricane, or other natural disaster), it is important to educate yourself, fellow office staff, and the community about safety precautions. The role that a medical assistant plays in the event of a natural disaster is discussed toward the end of this chapter.

Hurricanes

Hurricanes can strike with little warning, although most allow for some advance warning, giving the medical office staff time to prepare. If the office is in the path of a hurricane, the windows may need to be secured; this can be done using permanent storm shutters or ⅝-inch plywood cut to fit and ready to install. Trees and shrubs around the office should be well trimmed. Secure rain gutters and clean clogged ones. If the medical office is to be evacuated before a hurricane, the medical assistant should listen to the radio or television for information and instructions provided by local emergency management personnel. During the hurricane, the medical assistant should listen to the radio or television for additional information.

Floods

FEMA declares floods to be the most common hazard in the United States. Some floods can develop over days of rainy weather; others may be in the form of flash floods and may come on very quickly. The medical assistant should be aware of the flood dangers that exist in the local area. During a flood, the medical assistant should listen to the radio for information. In the event of a flash flood, the medical assistant should move to higher ground. If there is time before evacuating, the medical assistant should disconnect any electrical equipment and shut off utilities at their main valves. When evacuating, the medical assistant should be careful not to walk through moving water. As little as 6 inches of moving water can make a person fall.

Fires

Because more than 4,000 Americans die and more than 25,000 are injured in fires each year, the medical assistant should be prepared to respond to this type of disaster. Fire spreads quickly, and typically no time is available to gather belongings or make a telephone call. In just two minutes, a fire can become life threatening, and in five minutes a fire can engulf a building. Heat and smoke from fire are often more dangerous than the flames.

The medical office should be equipped with properly working smoke alarms. These should be placed on every level of the building and in every room, either on the ceiling or high on the walls. Every smoke alarm should be tested and cleaned once per month. The batteries in every alarm should be replaced at least once per year, and every individual alarm should be replaced once every 10 years.

The medical assistant should know the escape routes to use in the event of a fire. Staff members should practice those escape routes. If the office is located above the first level, escape ladders may be used.

Any flammable items must be stored in well-ventilated areas, and care must be taken in placing any items near a heat source or heating vent. Any defective wiring must be repaired to avoid a fire hazard. Fire extinguishers should be located throughout the office, and staff should be trained in their use.

During a fire, the medical assistant should be aware that if a person's clothes are on fire, that person should stop, drop, and roll until the fire is extinguished. Running makes the fire burn faster.

When escaping a fire, the medical assistant should check closed doors for heat before opening. This is done by using the back of the hand to feel the top of the door, the doorknob, and the crack between the door and the door frame before opening the door. If the door is hot, it should not be opened, and another route of escape should be sought. If the door is cool, it should be opened slowly. The medical assistant should crawl low under any smoke on the way to the exit and close doors as they are passed through to delay the spread of fire. Once out of the building, the medical assistant should not attempt to reenter until or unless the fire department declares that action to be safe. (Review the chapter titled "The Office Environment," which discusses basic fire safety within the medical office.)

Terrorism

In the event of a terrorist attack, the medical assistant should be aware of the steps to take in each of the following types of emergencies.

Explosions

In the event of a bomb threat, the medical assistant should try to obtain as much information from the caller as possible. The following questions should be asked:

1. When is the bomb going to explode?
2. Where is the bomb right now?
3. What does it look like?
4. What kind of bomb is it?
5. What will cause it to explode?

Any information obtained should be immediately provided to the police, and their instructions should be followed. If an explosion has occurred, the medical assistant should respond by following the steps as if an earthquake or fire has occurred.

Biological Threats

Bioterrorism is defined as the deliberate release of bacteria, viruses, or other agents that can cause illness and death in humans, animals, or plants with the intent to intimidate or coerce a government or civilian population to further political or social objectives. Biological agents can be spread through air, water, or food. Some biological agents are difficult to detect; thus, if a terrorist spreads the agent, its effects may not be felt for several hours or days.

Biological terrorism agents are classified by the Centers for Disease Control and Prevention (CDC) into categories A, B, and C, with A being the agents of highest risk. Terrorists seek agents that are easily transmitted, with high morbidity and mortality, to cause lengthy illness and incite panic— preferably with a long incubation period and nonspecific signs and symptoms. These are the agents that are classified as Category A.

Since the terrorist attacks on the United States on September 11, 2001, the awareness of possible additional terrorist attacks has been on the minds of Americans. The term *agents of mass destruction* is all too familiar as well. The CDC Special Pathogens Branch and the CDC National Center for Preparedness, Detection, and Control of Infectious Diseases (NCPDCID) monitor outbreaks of the category illnesses. Their goals include developing rapid diagnostic tests, gathering information, and offering assistance in control and prevention during outbreaks. Each of the Category A agents is briefly discussed in the following paragraphs. Although not a Category A agent, sarin is also discussed because it has been used recently for bioterrorism. For more information, see the CDC website.

Anthrax. Anthrax is a disease caused by the spore-forming organism *Bacillus anthracis*. This acute infectious disease can be passed from animal to human by contact with animal hair or waste. This disease can attack the lungs, skin, and gastrointestinal tract, causing signs and symptoms from respiratory distress to coma. In 2001, anthrax was spread in the United States through the U.S. Postal Service system, causing 22 cases of anthrax infection. The first signs and symptoms of anthrax contracted through inhalation are the same as for the flu. Respiratory anthrax is the most severe, with half the cases ending in death. Penicillin, tetracycline, and erythromycin are antibiotics of choice for treatment.

Professionalism

Professionalism is not just appearance and good grooming, although they are very important aspects of becoming a professional. Learning by observing and challenging yourself on a daily basis give you the experience you need to become a seasoned medical assistant. Remember to continue updating your skills and education frequently.

Contaminated materials should be incinerated. The CDC and other government agencies are developing plans for an anthrax attack with training and education programs for health care providers, public service personnel, and media. A vaccine to prevent anthrax has been developed but is not yet available for the general public.

Botulism. Botulism is a paralytic condition caused by the neurotoxin produced by the spore-forming bacteria *Clostridium botulinum*. The three types of botulism are food-borne botulism, wound botulism, and infant botulism. Food-borne botulism is caused by eating foods containing the toxin. Improperly prepared canned foods are often a source. Wound botulism is caused by a wound infected with *C. botulinum*. Infant botulism is caused by consumption of spores that grow and release toxins. All forms may be fatal and should be considered a medical emergency.

Botulinum toxin is one of the most poisonous substances known. One gram of toxin evenly dispersed and inhaled would kill more than a million people. It is the first biological toxin to be licensed in the United States for treatment of disease. It is used to treat conditions such as eyelid spasms, dystonia (abnormal, repetitive muscle movements), and strabismus (crossed eyes). A weakened form of the botulinum toxin (Botox) is widely used to reduce facial wrinkles.

The CDC reports that cases of botulism are rare in the United States. Most of these cases are infant botulism. The signs and symptoms of food-borne illness appear as early as six hours and as long as 10 days after eating contaminated food. Double vision, slurred speech, difficulty breathing, and paralysis caused by the toxin occur unless treated. Recovery may take weeks and necessitate use of a ventilator. Food-borne and wound types may respond to horse antitoxin if given early enough. Human antitoxin is available from the state of California Public Health Department for treatment of infant botulism.

Plague. Plague, an infectious disease that affects humans and animals, has several forms. All forms of the plague are caused by the bacterium *Yersinia pestis*, which is found in rodents and their fleas in the United States and many other areas of the world. A person may develop one form or may develop a combination of pneumonic plague, which affects the lungs; bubonic plague, which affects the lymph glands and causes swelling; and septicemic plague, which occurs when the organism enters the bloodstream. Signs and symptoms include fever, chills, and pneumonia, and if not treated, death can occur in a matter of a few days. Wearing a mask and early treatment with antibiotics such as gentamycin or tetracycline within 24 hours are suggested.

Sarin. Although sarin is not a Class A agent, it was used for bioterrorism in Japan in 1994 and 1995 and Syria in 2013. Sarin is a human-made nerve agent, similar to insecticides (insect killers) called organophosphates. Also known as GB, sarin is a clear, colorless, and tasteless liquid that has no odor in its pure form. Sarin can evaporate into a vapor (gas) and spread easily into the environment. Victims can be exposed through inhalation, contact, water, or food. Damage depends on the amount of sarin a patient was exposed to, how the patient was exposed, and the length of the exposure.

Signs and symptoms of sarin exposure present immediately and include fatigue, watery eyes, eye pain, pinpoint pupils, blurry vision, runny nose, drooling, excessive sweating, rapid breathing, cough, chest tightness, nausea, vomiting, abdominal pain, diarrhea, confusion, drowsiness, headache, weakness, increased urination, and changes in heart rate. Exposure to large amounts of sarin can cause loss of consciousness, convulsions, paralysis, and respiratory failure leading to death.

Treatment for sarin exposure includes removing the victim from the area where sarin exists, washing the body thoroughly, and providing access to sarin-free air.

Smallpox. Smallpox is caused by the *Variola* virus. It causes an acute, contagious disease that can be quickly spread from person to person. Signs and symptoms of smallpox include fever, macules, papules, vesicles, pustules, and crusts.

Smallpox outbreaks have been occurring for thousands of years according to historians. The CDC reported that the last case of smallpox in the United States occurred in 1949, and the last case in the world was in Somalia in 1977. Until 1972, smallpox vaccinations were recommended for the general public. Eventually, it seemed that smallpox had been eradicated because no new cases have been reported. Recently, there has been the possibility of heightened danger of the use of the *Variola major* virus as a bioterrorism weapon.

According to the CDC, as of 2004 the United States has enough vaccine stockpiles to inoculate every citizen in the event of a smallpox emergency. Vaccinations are available and have been given to military personnel and to medical personnel who might come into contact with the virus.

Tularemia. Tularemia is a serious illness caused by the bacterium *Francisella tularensis*. This organism is found in rabbits and rodents. The signs and symptoms of tularemia include fever, chills, headache, cough, weakness, and diarrhea.

Tularemia is spread by the bite of a tick or flea infected with the organism; by contact with an infected animal carcass, food, or water contaminated with *F. tularensis*; or by inhaling the organism. It is not spread from person to person and can be treated with antibiotics. To protect against tulare-mia, practice good personal hygiene and handwashing, and use insect repellent containing N,N-diethyl-meta-toluamide (DEET).

Viral Hemorrhagic Fevers. Viral hemorrhagic fevers are a group of illnesses caused by several different groups of viruses. These viruses have a number of similar features, such as the following:

- They are RNA viruses.
- They must live in either an animal or insect host (ticks, mosquitoes, certain types of rats, mice).
- They are usually restricted to areas where the hosts live.
- Humans can transmit viruses to one another but are not natural hosts.
- There are no vaccines or cures for the most part, with a few exceptions.

Some examples of VHFs are Ebola-hemorrhagic fever and Lassa fever. The signs and symptoms vary but include fever, fatigue, and loss of muscle strength; bleeding under the skin and from the mouth, eyes, and ears; delirium; and coma. Death is possible. Precautions include controlling rodent populations, proper cleaning of rodent nests and droppings, good personal hygiene, isolation of affected people, and use of PPE.

Preparation for a Biological Attack. Weapons of mass destruction are by nature indiscriminate and prolonged in destruction. To prepare for a biological attack, the medical facility may have a high efficiency particulate air (HEPA) filter installed. In the event of a biological attack, the medical assistant should be prepared to move away from the con-taminant quickly, wash with soap and water, contact author-ities, listen to the radio for instructions, and remove and bag clothing if contaminated.

Nuclear Blast

In the event of a nuclear attack, the medical assistant should take cover as quickly as possible, below ground if the build-ing has a basement. The medical assistant should remain in a safe location, listening to the radio for instructions. The medical assistant should not look at the flash or fireball but should lie flat on the ground with the head covered and seek shelter as quickly as possible.

Mock Environmental Exposures

Medical assistants can play a vital role in the event of an environmental emergency. It is helpful to be prepared for

such events by understanding how to help patients and pro-vide assistance to other health care providers. Organizations within the community, colleges, and hospitals may offer mock environmental exposure events. These events provide real-life scenarios and situations that may arise during times of disaster. Examples of mock environmental events include a tornado site with injured patients, an exposure to a bio-logical chemical, or treating injured patients of flash floods or hurricanes. The role of the medical assistant varies in every situation; however, overall, medical assistants may be able to provide assistance in numerous ways:

- Aiding in evacuation plans
- Triaging patients to determine which patients require immediate attention
- Assisting in first-aid response for wounded individuals
- Administering tetanus and other vaccines under the direction of a physician
- Facilitating order and organization in the midst of chaos
- Implementing and following through on an environ-mental exposure safety plan

Procedure 42-12 lists the steps to create an environmen-tal exposure plan. Staff should frequently practice a variety of potential disaster scenarios to be prepared for an environ-mental emergency.

Community Resources

It is vital for the medical assistant to be aware of community resources before a disaster. Good sources of information are found through the U.S. Department of Homeland Security (www.ready.gov), the ARC (www.redcross.org), and FEMA (www.fema.gov). Through these resources, the medical assis-tants can develop personal emergency kits for use at home, office emergency kits for use at work, and community

Developing an Environmental Exposure Safety Plan

Objective ◆ *Develop an environmental exposure plan that can be used in all hazards.*

EQUIPMENT AND SUPPLIES

Pen; paper; computer; copy machine; various emergency supplies; waterproof containers; flashlights; batteries; bottles of water; nonperishable food; duct tape; plastic sheeting; masks; bandages; alcohol wipes; blankets; gloves; tweezers; scissors; self-powered radio; assorted medications; map of a hypothetical medical office; hypothetical staff chart

METHOD

1. Create an emergency kit that can be used by your office in the event of an environmental emergency. Supplies may include flashlights, batteries, bottles of water, nonperishable food, manual can opener, bandages, alcohol wipes, blankets, vinyl or latex gloves, tweezers, scissors, self-powered radio, and medications (ibuprofen, acetaminophen, antihistamines, antibiotic ointment, tetanus vaccines, etc.).
2. Enclose the kit in a waterproof container.
3. Place the kit in a safe area, such as a medicine closet or storage closet.
4. Create evacuation plans for every room in the sample medical office that has been given to you.
5. Create a delineation chart that outlines responsibilities of office staff members in the event of an environmental emergency.
6. Create a list of safety zones that can be used in the event of an emergency (e.g., a safety zone in the event of a tornado, an outdoor safety zone in the event of a fire, a safety zone in the event of a flood).
7. Document development of the policy for the physician.

DOCUMENTATION

2/16/YY 10:00 A.M. Developed Environmental Exposure Plan and placed information in red folder on receptionist's desk.
....S. Porter CMA (AAMA)

survival kits. The medical assistant may also consider volunteering to serve on the local Medical Reserve Corps (https://mrc.hhs.gov/), ARC Disaster Services (www.redcross.org), and Community Emergency Response Teams (https://www.fema.gov/community-emergency-response-teams). The Department of Homeland Security stated the best way to prepare for a disaster is to get a kit, make a plan, be informed, and get involved!

SUMMARY

Each team member must know what procedures to follow in a medical emergency. As a medical assistant, you will need advanced training in CPR, AED, and treating specialty office emergencies, such as allergic reactions. Patients may experience fainting, seizures, anaphylactic shock, and other conditions when visiting the medical office for other health reasons. Contacting the physician and EMS, if necessary, is part of office protocol. Good Samaritan laws were established to encourage health care professionals to volunteer in emergencies without fear of financial liability. It is important that health care professionals render emergency care according to the scope of license, certification, or training until relieved by another health professional. EMS may be called for on-the-scene care, stabilization of the patient, and transport to the appropriate emergency department for further assessment and treatment. Equipment is kept for medical emergencies in the medical office. Medical assistants must have an understanding of the various facets of emergency preparedness. Students are encouraged to create an environmental exposure control plan as well as participate in mock environmental exposure scenarios.

42 CHAPTER REVIEW

COMPETENCY REVIEW

1. Define and spell the terms for this chapter.
2. List the four recognized levels of EMS responders and identify which responder is able to provide the most advanced level of care for patients.
3. Identify the signs, symptoms, and treatment options for a patient with diabetic shock.
4. Explain the Rule of Nines and what it is used to assess.
5. Identify when it is appropriate to use abdominal thrusts in a patient with an obstructed airway.
6. Describe how strains differ from sprains.
7. Identify supplies that are needed to create an emergency kit for the medical office to use in the event of an environmental emergency.

PREPARING FOR THE CERTIFICATION EXAM

1. Which of the following is not a role of EMS?
   a. provide on-the-scene intervention and treatment
   b. prepare the patient for transport
   c. diagnose patients
   d. administer emergency medications
   e. intubate a patient

2. Who decides the equipment and supplies to have stocked on a crash cart?
   a. medical office manager
   b. certified medical assistant
   c. clinical supervisor
   d. physician
   e. malpractice insurance company

3. When assessing an unconscious infant for responsiveness, you should
   a. flick the soles of the feet.
   b. gently shake the shoulders.
   c. ask the parent for assistance.
   d. shout the infant's name.
   e. wait to activate EMS until a physician directs you to do so.

4. A(n) _____ is an example of an abrasion.
   a. avulsion
   b. amputation
   c. friction burn
   d. puncture
   e. laceration

5. A severe allergic reaction to a substance is known as
   a. metabolic shock.
   b. anaphylactic shock.
   c. hypoallergenic shock.
   d. neurological collapse.
   e. sepsis.

6. Hypoglycemia is present when a patient's blood sugar is
   a. above 120 mg/dL.
   b. between 80 and 90 mg/dL.
   c. below 200 mg/dL.
   d. above 300 mg/dL.
   e. below 70 mg/dL.

7. Arterial bleeding is
   a. slow and bright red.
   b. rapid and dark red.
   c. slow and dark red.
   d. rapid and bright red.
   e. pulsating and dark red.

8. Hyperthermia occurs when a person's body temperature reaches
   a. 105°F.
   b. 95°F.
   c. 109°F.
   d. 89°F.
   e. 103°F.

9. Syncope is another term for
   a. vomiting.
   b. a blood infection.
   c. fainting.
   d. dizziness.
   e. respiratory distress.

10. FEMA declares this disaster to be the most common hazard in the United States:
    a. hurricane.
    b. flood.
    c. tornado.
    d. earthquake.
    e. bioterrorism.

CRITICAL THINKING

Refer to the case study at the beginning of the chapter and use what you have learned to answer the following questions.

1. What should be Lewis's immediate concern and action on hearing the emergency tornado warning announcement?

2. How can Lewis assist in ensuring the safety of the patients and staff members of the medical office?

3. How could Lewis and the other staff members of Pearson Physicians Group prepare for natural disasters, such as the tornado?

ON THE JOB

Mary Ann, a medical assistant, works in a busy primary care office operated by two physicians, Dr. Johnson and Dr. Laskar. It is Saturday, so the staff consists of just Mary Ann, Dr. Johnson, and another medical assistant named Valerie. On Saturdays, the office is only open until 1:00 P.M., but it is already 11:00 A.M. and the office has been extremely busy. Valerie has not had time to do her morning checks yet, and the reception room is full of crying children.

As Mary Ann is looking over the schedule, she hears a commotion out front, followed by sudden quiet, and then Valerie's call for help. When Mary Ann gets to the reception room, there is a worried-looking man bent over a 35-year-old woman who is supine on the floor. She appears to be awake, but her eyes are closed and she is grimacing. She seems very short of breath. Her face is profusely diaphoretic and pale. "She had some indigestion last night when she went to bed," the man says, "and she did not sleep much last night. This morning when she got up to go to the bathroom, she stated she was very nauseated."

When asked, the lady responds with her name and says she is having some really sharp pain in her right lower abdomen. She points to it with one finger. Dr. Johnson is notified immediately to further evaluate the woman. As instructed, Mary Ann and Valerie help the woman into a wheelchair and wheel her into an examining room. She immediately complains of dizziness and increased pain, and now her breathing becomes extremely labored. She cannot seem to talk at all in response to questions.

1. Given her deteriorating state, what action should you take?

2. What kind of additional information should you try to find out about her medical history?

3. What should you do when EMS arrives at the office to transport the patient?

INTERNET ACTIVITY

Find a website for the poison control center. What types of information does the center have that you might be able to share with your pediatric patients, for educational purposes, to help remind them not to consume unknown substances or items that could poison them?

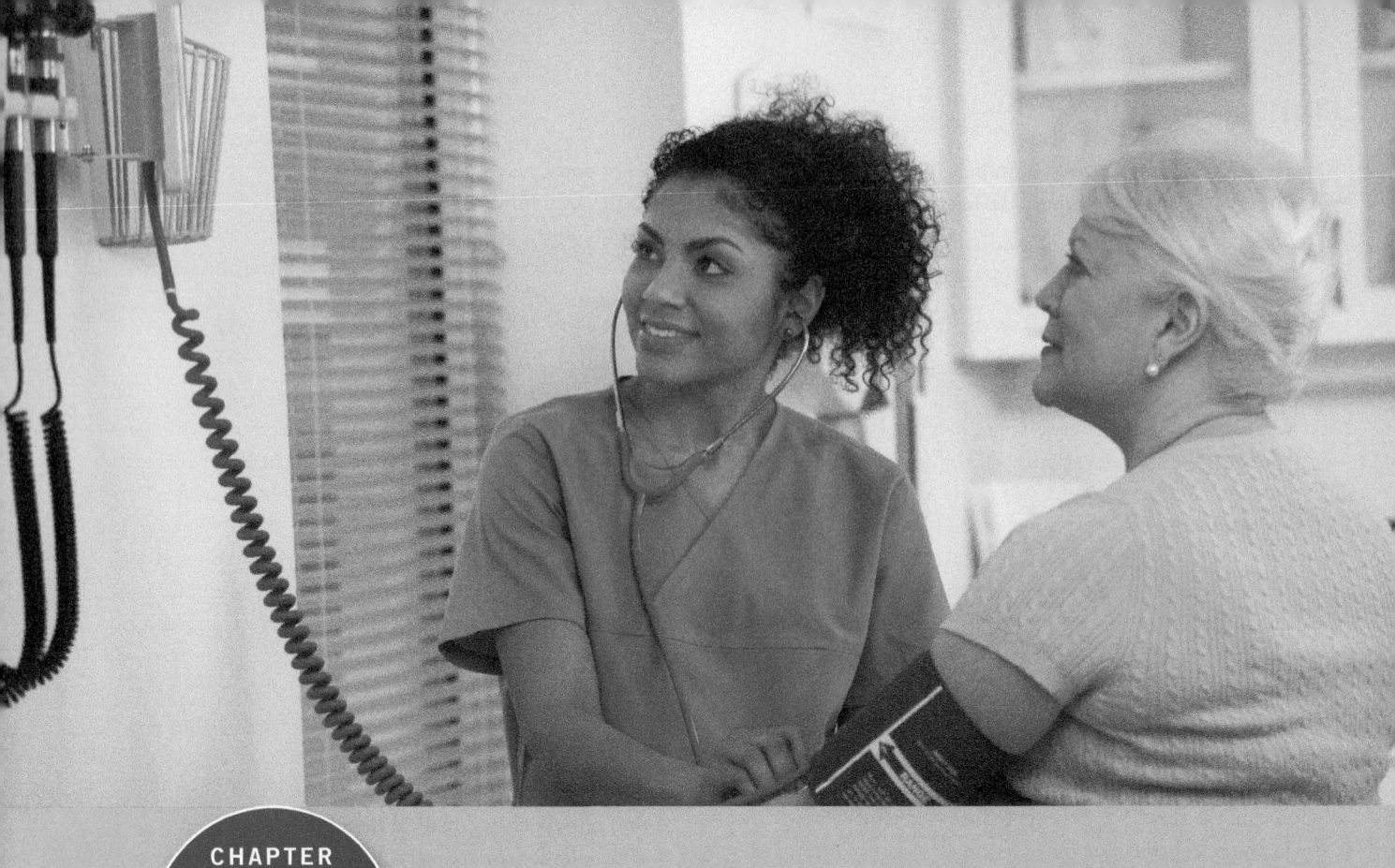

Learning Objectives

After completing this chapter, you should be able to:

43.1 Define and spell the terms for this chapter.

43.2 Explain the role of the clinical laboratory in patient care.

43.3 Describe the roles of three types of clinical laboratories.

43.4 Explain the role of a medical assistant in the physician's office laboratory.

43.5 Explain how tables and graphs are used in health care.

43.6 Identify quality assurance practices.

43.7 Summarize laboratory safety regulations.

43.8 List CLIA-waived tests that are associated with common diseases.

43.9 Describe the uses of laboratory equipment commonly found in a physician's office laboratory.

43.10 Identify the parts of a microscope.

43.11 Demonstrate how to use a microscope.

Susan Schultz, CMA (AAMA), is working in the clinical lab of Pearson Physicians Group. Dr. Miller has sent Ravi Patel back to the clinical laboratory with a lab requisition for a urinalysis and blood glucose screening. He also has asked Ravi to schedule an appointment to come back to the office to have a two-hour postprandial glucose test performed.

Terms to Learn

autoclave	flow sheet	postprandial (PP)
automated analyzer	hemolyzed	practitioner
calibration devices	icteric	qualitative test
centrifuge	incubator	quality assurance (QA)
Certificate of Waiver Tests (WTs) or CLIA-Waived Tests	laboratory requisition form	quality control (QC)
	nonfasting	quantitative test
Clinical Laboratory Improvement Amendments (CLIA)	objectives	quantity not sufficient (QNS)
	oculars	reference laboratory
compound microscope	outside laboratory	resolution
control solutions	photometer	specimen
fasting	physician's office laboratory (POL)	turnaround time

Most of us have had laboratory tests performed at one time or another on samples of blood, urine, or tissue. Clinical laboratory tests provide part of the framework on which physicians base their diagnoses and monitor patients' health. Medical assistants may be actively involved in the collection and processing of some tests, or they may simply transfer samples or refer patients to local laboratories for others. In either case, it is important for you, as a medical assistant, to have a basic understanding of the laboratory and to understand the implications of laboratory results.

THE ROLE OF THE CLINICAL LABORATORY IN PATIENT CARE

Clinical laboratory test results provide clues to assist with proper diagnosis, treatment, and evaluation. They are an essential part of patient care and may be helpful in the following ways:

- To screen for disease
- To confirm a condition suspected by the physician
- To rule out a condition

- To establish a baseline level before medication administration
- To monitor effectiveness of medication or treatment
- To assess the progress of disease

Because people are unique individuals and disease does not always progress according to textbook descriptions, laboratory data should be used in conjunction with other clinical findings to provide quality care. Relying on laboratory results alone to diagnose or treat a patient is unwise.

Laboratory tests fall generally into two categories: qualitative tests and quantitative tests. A **qualitative test** result is typically positive or negative for the presence of a specific substance. An example of this is a pregnancy test, which determines if the hormone HCG is present. A **quantitative test** gives a numerical value, such as a glucose level of 82 mg/dL. Quantitative values may vary from facility to facility because differing procedures, product manufacturers, techniques, and equipment may be used at each. Therefore, test results that are considered normal at one lab may be considered abnormal at another lab. This is why normal reference ranges may vary from book to book and lab to lab. Always determine the normal ranges associated with the specific laboratory and test before evaluation of results.

TYPES OF CLINICAL LABORATORIES

There are three types of clinical laboratories in which tests of varying levels of complexity are performed. They are the outside laboratory, the reference laboratory, and the physician's office laboratory (POL).

Outside Laboratory

The **outside laboratory**, either a hospital-based or an independent laboratory, handles specimens collected from many types of facilities and performs tests ranging from simple to very complex. For example, the laboratory of a local hospital in your town may perform Pap tests on specimens collected in gynecologists' offices. Or a physician may have a contract with a managed care company that requires all specimens to be tested at a specific laboratory named in its contract. A patient may go to a laboratory to have blood drawn or a specimen taken with the test results to be sent to the referring physician. A medical assistant may be employed in one of these laboratories as a phlebotomist (one who performs a blood draw) or as an administrative assistant.

Some physicians choose simply to refer a patient to an outside lab, and others prefer to have the specimen collected in the office and transferred to an outside lab. In this instance, outside laboratories typically provide supplies and forms for specimen collection and transport. Most offer a directory with instructions for proper handling and transport of specimens. When these instructions are available, always consult them to determine how much of a specimen to collect, which container to use, and how to prepare the specimen for transport. Keep in mind that the medical assistant is also responsible for requesting additional supplies to replenish the inventory on hand.

Reference Laboratory

The **reference laboratory** may be associated with a teaching hospital or a medical school, or it may be independently owned. This type of laboratory handles tests that are more complex than those usually handled by an outside laboratory as well as tests that are infrequently requested. Tests performed on a regular basis at a reference lab may provide more accurate results than tests performed only a few times a year in an outside laboratory.

Physician's Office Laboratory

A **physician's office laboratory (POL)** is a laboratory in which some of the tests that the physician orders are performed right in the office. In the POL, the doctor has the advantage of receiving the results more rapidly than if tests are done outside the office. **Turnaround time** is how long it takes for the test to be performed and the results generated, sent back for physician review, and added to the patient's chart. Disadvantages to the POL are that in-house testing may require more employees and the purchase of expensive equipment. This is the laboratory environment that medical assistants are particularly suited to, although they are limited to performing only Clinical Laboratory Improvement Amendments (CLIA)–waived tests (to be described later in the chapter).

The physician's office laboratory generally occupies a separate room or work area that is well lighted and adequately ventilated. Most have a refrigerator that is clearly labeled for storage of (potentially infectious) specimens only. A supply of personal protective equipment, including gloves, masks, gowns, and protective eyewear, is essential. A sharps container and a biohazardous waste receptacle should be within easy reach. Handwashing facilities and an eyewash station are also important.

THE MEDICAL ASSISTANT'S ROLE IN THE CLINICAL LABORATORY

Medical assistants are particularly suited to working in POLs and clinical laboratories because of their cross-training in administrative and clinical areas. For medical assistants working in a laboratory, training in phlebotomy and basic knowledge of laboratory testing is essential. In addition, training in administrative duties helps medical assistants to perform the many administrative tasks required in a laboratory. Medical assistants' patient-oriented training helps them to be empathetic caregivers.

Whether you work as a medical assistant in a laboratory or in other areas of a medical practice, a fundamental understanding of basic lab methods and techniques helps you understand the nature and importance of specific tests. This includes an understanding of why specific tests are done, how to prepare a patient for a test, conditions that may render a test inaccurate, and how to evaluate the results.

Medical assistants may play any of several key roles in a clinical laboratory. Depending on their level of involvement in the laboratory, these roles may include managing records, teaching patients, managing specimens, and performing quality assurance.

Record Management

Methods of lab test record management vary, depending on where a sample is collected and where it is tested. The first priority is to make sure that the physician's order is clearly recorded and the proper lab forms are completed. In-house collection and processing must be charted. Results should be evaluated and carefully documented.

A **laboratory requisition form** is a form that provides essential information about the test that is ordered, how results will be reported, and information for billing and coding. As a medical assistant, you will need to complete a requisition if you are not performing the tests right away. See Procedure 43-1 for instructions on completing a laboratory requisition and preparing a specimen for transport to an outside lab. The requisition will be transported with specimens that are collected at the physician's office and sent out for testing. Alternatively, the requisition will go with the patient who is required to travel to a laboratory for collection and testing. If the physician wants the results immediately for a medical intervention, then the requisition must be labeled STAT (immediately) and processed accordingly. Box 43-1 lists the information necessary to complete a requisition form. Figure 43-1 is an example of a laboratory test requisition. Be sure to use the laboratory requisition slip designed specifically for the laboratory that will receive it because the physician's office may send specimens to several different testing sites and thus will have several different requisition forms on hand.

With POL testing, it is imperative that accurate results are properly recorded as soon as possible. This may prevent confusion and inaccuracies that could lead to the wrong patient diagnosis or treatment. The medical assistant will also document specimen collection in narrative notes. A good

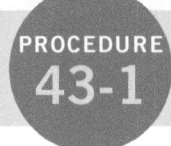

PROCEDURE 43-1   Completing a Laboratory Requisition Form

Objective ◆ *Complete a laboratory requisition form for testing as ordered by the physician, obtain the required specimen(s), and prepare specimen(s) for transport to an outside laboratory.*

EQUIPMENT AND SUPPLIES
Physician's order for laboratory tests; patient's record; pen; laboratory requisition form; gloves; specimen container; laboratory logbook; biohazard waste container

METHOD
1. Check the patient's record for orders for specific lab tests.
2. Verify which lab will be doing the testing and locate its required requisition form (Figure 43-1).
3. Complete the patient demographic section.
4. Complete the section requiring the physician's name, address, phone number, and account number.
5. Complete the patient's insurance and billing information.
6. Mark each box to indicate each test ordered by the physician. If a test is ordered that is not listed on the requisition, write in the name of the test on the lines provided.
7. Indicate the type and source of the specimen to be tested.
8. Enter the patient's diagnosis on the requisition as needed. If no diagnosis has been made, then code the patient's symptoms.
9. Complete the patient authorization to release and assign the benefits as needed.
10. Assemble the equipment and supplies needed to obtain the specimen.
11. Perform hand hygiene and apply gloves.

12. Obtain the specimen required after explaining the procedure to the patient.
13. Label the specimen with the patient's name, date, physician's name, time of collection, and other information required by the facility.
14. Initial the laboratory requisition, and complete the date and time the specimen was obtained.
15. Process the specimens, and if they are not to be sent out until later in the day, store them according to laboratory policies and procedures manual requirements.
16. Attach the laboratory requisition securely to the specimen before sending.
17. Remove gloves; dispose of them in the biohazard waste container only if the gloves are contaminated with blood or bodily fluids. Otherwise they can be disposed of in an ordinary waste can. Perform hand hygiene.
18. Document the patient's record.
19. Record the specimen in the laboratory logbook, indicating date, time of collection, type and source of the specimen, tests ordered, where samples were sent, and the date they were sent.

CHARTING EXAMPLE
08/04/YY 8:00 A.M. Venous blood sample for STAT CBC sent to Memorial Lab at 8:40 A.M. Lab will call back with results.
....R. Patel, CMA (AAMA)

BOX 43-1 | Laboratory Requisition Information

- Physician's name address, phone number, and account number
- Patient's full name, address, phone number
- Patient's age, sex, date of birth (DOB)
- Patient's complete insurance information
- All relevant diagnostic codes
- Diagnosis, if possible
- Source of specimen
- If **fasting** or **nonfasting** specimen
- Date and collection time
- Specific tests requested per physician's orders, including five-digit procedure code
- Patient's present medications
- If request is STAT or regular

note states the test ordered, the method of collection, the patient's response, and either results (if tested at the patient's side) or where the specimen was sent. For example:

12/05/YY 7:45 A.M. CBC ordered. Stick X1 in left antecubital via aseptic technique. Pt. tolerated well and denies discomfort. Prepared for pickup by ABC Lab.

H. Mills, RMA

Paper Versus Electronic Documentation

Because federal law in 2014 mandated that all paper charts be converted to electronic records, medical assistants should become familiar with how to use electronic records. For outside testing, when paper forms are used, a form will be completed to send with the patient or specimen going to an outside lab. The results may be faxed, couriered, mailed, or

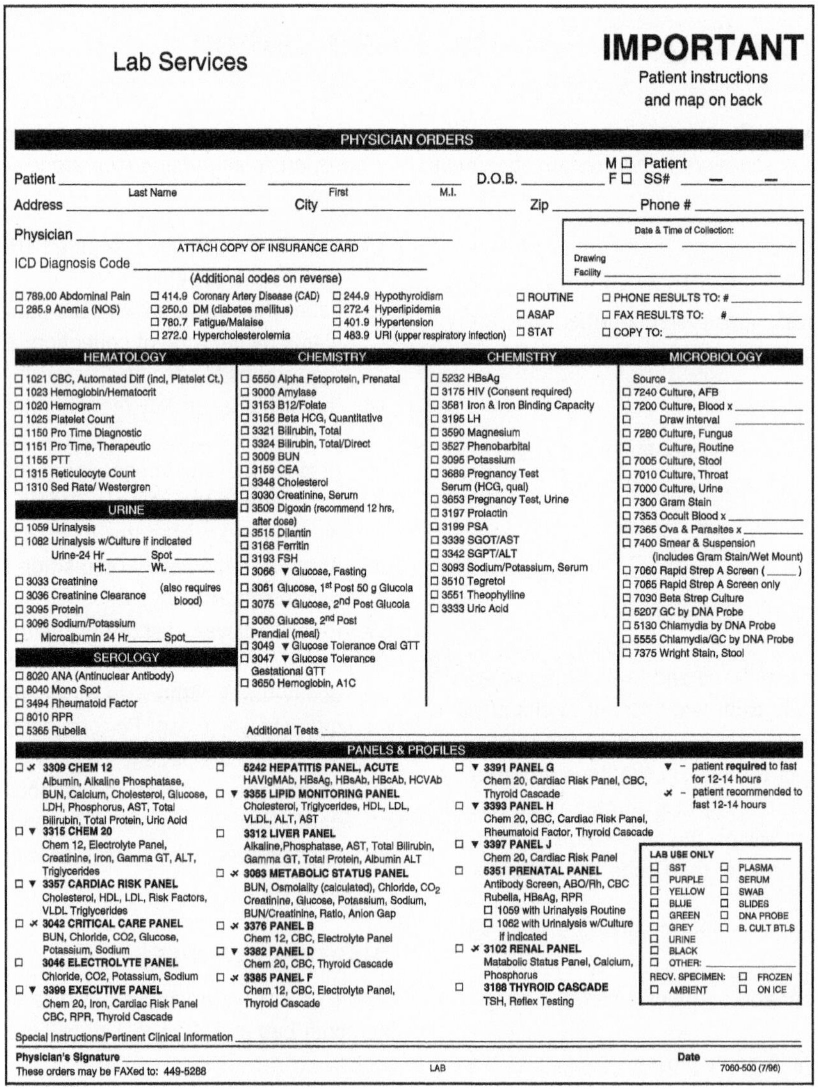

Lab Services

IMPORTANT
Patient instructions
and map on back

PHYSICIAN ORDERS

Patient ______ (Last Name) ______ (First) ___ (M.I.) D.O.B. ______ M ☐ F ☐ Patient SS# ___ – ___ – ___
Address ______ City ______ Zip ______ Phone # ______
Physician ______
ATTACH COPY OF INSURANCE CARD
ICD Diagnosis Code ______
(Additional codes on reverse)

Date & Time of Collection: ______ ______
Drawing Facility ______

☐ 789.00 Abdominal Pain
☐ 285.9 Anemia (NOS)
☐ 414.9 Coronary Artery Disease (CAD)
☐ 250.0 DM (diabetes mellitus)
☐ 780.7 Fatigue/Malaise
☐ 272.0 Hypercholesterolemia
☐ 244.9 Hypothyroidism
☐ 272.4 Hyperlipidemia
☐ 401.9 Hypertension
☐ 483.9 URI (upper respiratory infection)
☐ ROUTINE
☐ ASAP
☐ STAT
☐ PHONE RESULTS TO: # ______
☐ FAX RESULTS TO: # ______
☐ COPY TO: ______

HEMATOLOGY
☐ 1021 CBC, Automated Diff (incl, Platelet Ct.)
☐ 1023 Hemoglobin/Hematocrit
☐ 1020 Hemogram
☐ 1025 Platelet Count
☐ 1150 Pro Time Diagnostic
☐ 1151 Pro Time, Therapeutic
☐ 1155 PTT
☐ 1315 Reticulocyte Count
☐ 1310 Sed Rate/ Westergren

URINE
☐ 1059 Urinalysis
☐ 1062 Urinalysis w/Culture if indicated
Urine-24 Hr ______ Spot ______
Ht. ______ Wt. ______
☐ 3033 Creatinine
☐ 3036 Creatinine Clearance (also requires blood)
☐ 3095 Protein
☐ 3096 Sodium/Potassium
☐ Microalbumin 24 Hr ______ Spot ______

SEROLOGY
☐ 8020 ANA (Antinuclear Antibody)
☐ 8040 Mono Spot
☐ 3494 Rheumatoid Factor
☐ 8010 RPR
☐ 5365 Rubella

CHEMISTRY
☐ 5550 Alpha Fetoprotein, Prenatal
☐ 3000 Amylase
☐ 3153 B12/Folate
☐ 3156 Beta HCG, Quantitative
☐ 3321 Bilirubin, Total
☐ 3324 Bilirubin, Total/Direct
☐ 3009 BUN
☐ 3159 CEA
☐ 3348 Cholesterol
☐ 3030 Creatinine, Serum
☐ 3509 Digoxin (recommend 12 hrs, after dose)
☐ 3515 Dilantin
☐ 3168 Ferritin
☐ 3193 FSH
☐ 3066 ▼ Glucose, Fasting
☐ 3061 Glucose, 1st Post 50 g Glucola
☐ 3075 ▼ Glucose, 2nd Post Glucola
☐ 3060 Glucose, 2nd Post Prandial (meal)
☐ 3049 ▼ Glucose Tolerance Oral GTT
☐ 3047 ▼ Glucose Tolerance Gestational GTT
☐ 3650 Hemoglobin, A1C

CHEMISTRY
☐ 5232 HBsAg
☐ 3175 HIV (Consent required)
☐ 3581 Iron & Iron Binding Capacity
☐ 3195 LH
☐ 3590 Magnesium
☐ 3527 Phenobarbital
☐ 3095 Potassium
☐ 3689 Pregnancy Test Serum (HCG, qual)
☐ 3653 Pregnancy Test, Urine
☐ 3197 Prolactin
☐ 3199 PSA
☐ 3339 SGOT/AST
☐ 3342 SGPT/ALT
☐ 3093 Sodium/Potassium, Serum
☐ 3510 Tegretol
☐ 3551 Theophylline
☐ 3333 Uric Acid

MICROBIOLOGY
Source ______
☐ 7240 Culture, AFB
☐ 7200 Culture, Blood x ______
☐ Draw interval ______
☐ 7280 Culture, Fungus
☐ Culture, Routine
☐ 7005 Culture, Stool
☐ 7010 Culture, Throat
☐ 7000 Culture, Urine
☐ 7300 Gram Stain
☐ 7353 Occult Blood x ______
☐ 7365 Ova & Parasites x ______
☐ 7400 Smear & Suspension (includes Gram Stain/Wet Mount)
☐ 7060 Rapid Strep A Screen (______)
☐ 7065 Rapid Strep A Screen only
☐ 7030 Beta Strep Culture
☐ 5207 GC by DNA Probe
☐ 5130 Chlamydia by DNA Probe
☐ 5555 Chlamydia/GC by DNA Probe
☐ 7375 Wright Stain, Stool

Additional Tests ______

PANELS & PROFILES
☐ ✗ **3309 CHEM 12** Albumin, Alkaline Phosphatase, BUN, Calcium, Cholesterol, Glucose, LDH, Phosphorus, AST, Total Bilirubin, Total Protein, Uric Acid
☐ ▼ **3315 CHEM 20** Chem 12, Electrolyte Panel, Creatinine, Iron, Gamma GT, ALT, Triglycerides
☐ ▼ **3357 CARDIAC RISK PANEL** Cholesterol, HDL, LDL, Risk Factors, VLDL Triglycerides
☐ ✗ **3042 CRITICAL CARE PANEL** BUN, Chloride, CO2, Glucose, Potassium, Sodium
☐ **3046 ELECTROLYTE PANEL** Chloride, CO2, Potassium, Sodium
☐ ▼ **3399 EXECUTIVE PANEL** Chem 20, Iron, Cardiac Risk Panel CBC, RPR, Thyroid Cascade
☐ **5242 HEPATITIS PANEL, ACUTE** HAVIgMAb, HBsAg, HBsAb, HBcAb, HCVAb
☐ ▼ **3355 LIPID MONITORING PANEL** Cholesterol, Triglycerides, HDL, LDL, VLDL, ALT, AST
☐ **3312 LIVER PANEL** Alkaline,Phosphatase, AST, Total Bilirubin, Gamma GT, Total Protein, Albumin ALT
☐ ✗ **3063 METABOLIC STATUS PANEL** BUN, Osmolality (calculated), Chloride, CO_2 Creatinine, Glucose, Potassium, Sodium, BUN/Creatinine, Ratio, Anion Gap
☐ ✗ **3376 PANEL B** Chem 12, CBC, Electrolyte Panel
☐ ▼ **3382 PANEL D** Chem 20, CBC, Thyroid Cascade
☐ ✗ **3385 PANEL F** Chem 12, CBC, Electrolyte Panel, Thyroid Cascade
☐ ▼ **3391 PANEL G** Chem 20, Cardiac Risk Panel, CBC, Thyroid Cascade
☐ ▼ **3393 PANEL H** Chem 20, CBC, Cardiac Risk Panel, Rheumatoid Factor, Thyroid Cascade
☐ ▼ **3397 PANEL J** Chem 20, Cardiac Risk Panel
☐ **5351 PRENATAL PANEL** Antibody Screen, ABO/Rh, CBC Rubella, HBsAg, RPR
☐ 1059 with Urinalysis Routine
☐ 1062 with Urinalysis w/Culture if indicated
☐ ✗ **3102 RENAL PANEL** Matabolic Status Panel, Calcium, Phosphorus
☐ **3188 THYROID CASCADE** TSH, Reflex Testing

▼ – patient **required** to fast for 12-14 hours
✗ – patient recommended to fast 12-14 hours

LAB USE ONLY ______
☐ SST ☐ PLASMA
☐ PURPLE ☐ SERUM
☐ YELLOW ☐ SWAB
☐ BLUE ☐ SLIDES
☐ GREEN ☐ DNA PROBE
☐ GREY ☐ B. CULT BTLS
☐ URINE
☐ BLACK
☐ OTHER: ______
RECV. SPECIMEN: ☐ FROZEN
☐ AMBIENT ☐ ON ICE

Special Instructions/Pertinent Clinical Information ______
Physician's Signature ______ **Date** ______
These orders may be FAXed to: 449-5288 LAB 7060-500 (7/96)

FIGURE 43-1 Laboratory requisition slip.

called in. If a result is flagged as high priority, always bring it to the immediate attention of the **practitioner**. All documentation is either written in or added to the patient's paper chart.

With electronic health records (EHRs), many offices can communicate with outside labs through the computer. In this case, lab orders are either submitted electronically or printed out and sent with a patient or specimen. Test results are immediately accessible, and abnormal results are often highlighted or marked for easier identification. The medical care practitioner simply reviews and signs electronically. The medical assistant then saves the report to the patient's EHR.

Flowcharts, Tables, and Graphs

It is a medical assistant's responsibility to ensure that the physician or practitioner evaluates and signs all results. Flowcharts, tables, and graphs can facilitate the interpretation of data, as well as being useful to share with patients when educating them on trends in their health. For example, a chart, table, or graph of blood sugars can demonstrate to both the physician and the patient the need for changes in diet or medication.

After the physician has evaluated the laboratory results, signed the results, and reviewed the flowcharts, tables, or graphs that are often generated by EHR software, the physician can best make a judgment for plan of the care for the patient. Only then should the result be filed or entered into the patient's record.

Many physicians prefer to use **flow sheets**, which are charts used to evaluate a patient's progress and response to treatment over time. See Figure 43-2 for a sample flow sheet. This is particularly useful for tests such as PT/INR (Coumadin/warfarin), glucose, hemoglobin A1C (average blood glucose), lipid, and liver panels. As new results are added to the patient's record, the data should be added to the flow sheet as well. With electronic documentation, at the click of a button, flow sheets can be generated to visualize the changes that occur from test to test. See Figure 43-3 for an example of a chart derived from a flow sheet. Procedure 43-2 describes how to enter lab test results on a flow sheet.

Patient Preparation

Various tests require different types of patient preparation. For example, a fasting specimen means that the patient must not consume anything other than water for a prescribed

number of hours before collecting the specimen. For many tests, the fasting period is at least eight hours before the specimen collection. **Postprandial (PP)**, or post cibum (pc), means "after a meal." A fasting blood glucose would be drawn after the patient has abstained from eating for at least eight hours, but the patient can have water or black coffee because hydration facilitates venipuncture drawing. A two-hour PP or pc glucose means that the patient eats a prescribed amount of food for a meal and a blood glucose level is drawn exactly two hours after completion of the meal. Timing of specimen collections is important in testing to assess the highest level of medication in the patient's system (peak) or the low point (trough) and thus to determine the correct dose to be administered.

PT/INR/Coumadin (warfarin) flow sheet

Patient: Carole Smith
DOB: 05/02/1970
Physician: Leonnard Sweezey

Date/Time	Results: INR	Results: PT	Current coumadin dose	Physician notified	Dose change	Next test date:	MA signature
12/01/2015 8AM	2.7	11	2 mg QD	8:30 AM	No	01/01/16	H. Mills, RMA
1/01/2016 8AM	2.6	12	2 mg QD	8:30 AM	No	02/01/16	H. Mills, RMA
2/01/2016 8AM	2.5	13	2 mg QD	8:30 AM	No	03/01/16	H. Mills, RMA
3/01/2016 8AM	1.9	14	2 mg QD	8:30 AM	Increase to 3 mg	03/15/16	H. Mills, RMA

Normal prothrombin time (PT) 10-13 seconds
INR Range (determined by the physician, based on individual's condition): 2.5-3.5
Condition: Mechanical Heart Valve

FIGURE 43-2 A sample flow sheet.

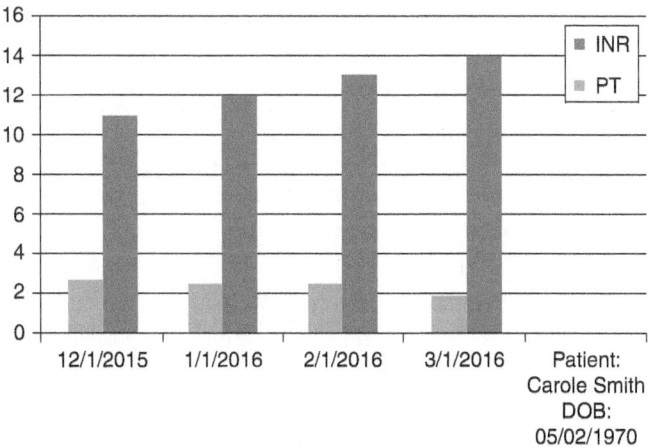

FIGURE 43-3 Lab results displayed on a chart.

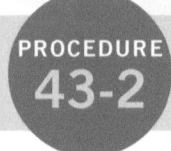

PROCEDURE 43-2 Maintaining Lab Test Results Using Flow Sheets

Objective ◆ *Maintain lab test results using flow sheets, within time specified by instructor.*

EQUIPMENT AND SUPPLIES
Flow sheet; lab test results; pen

METHOD

1. Obtain a blank flow sheet and complete the patient information as indicated at the top of the sheet. This information can be obtained from the patient's medical record.
2. Gather laboratory test results, which will be entered on the flow sheet. Examples of tests used for flow sheets include PT/INR, hemoglobin A1C, lipid and liver panels.
3. Confirm that the laboratory test results match the patient medical record you are using.
4. Carefully chart the test results on the flow sheet. Pay strict attention when entering the data, ensuring that spelling is accurate and numbers are not transposed. Refer to the example shown in Figure 43-3.
5. When all information has been entered, review and compare the information on the flow sheet against the test results, double-checking for any errors.
6. Attach the flow sheet to the laboratory test results with a paper clip and give to the physician for review.

Medical assistants are responsible for educating the patient about laboratory tests and procedures. This includes explaining what tests are ordered, how they will be useful, how a specimen will be collected, and when results will be available. Special preparations should also be explained. This may include dietary or medication restrictions, activity limitations, time requirements, or special directions. It is always best to provide a written copy of the instructions for the patient to take home as well. However, simply giving instructions is not enough. A patient who understands why restrictions or procedures are in place is more likely to be compliant than one who is told what to do but not why. Explain to the patient that results may be inaccurate if directions are not properly followed, which might require retesting.

Follow office protocol regarding reporting results to patients. Some offices don't typically notify a patient unless there is a problem that needs to be addressed, but others routinely notify patients about all results. Many medical practitioners prefer to speak personally to the patient about results that are significantly abnormal; the medical assistant simply sets up an appointment for the patient to discuss results in person or makes the chart available for the physician to make a call. Other physicians routinely expect medical assistants to contact patients for them, relaying new orders or instructions.

Specimen Management

A **specimen** is a small sample taken from the body. This can include urine, feces, sputum, blood, and other body tissues or secretions. Of these, urine and blood are the most commonly obtained specimens for laboratory testing. It is vital to properly collect and preserve a specimen to ensure that it truly represents the patient's body functions. Otherwise, inaccurate test results are likely, which may alter the patient's diagnosis and treatment.

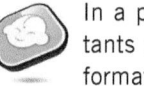 **Professionalism**   The Life Span

In a physician's office, laboratory medical assistants are usually the caregivers who provide information to the patient regarding preparation for laboratory tests. With some geriatric patients, extra time may be required to be certain they comprehend. If there is any doubt in your mind, ask to speak with the legally appointed person in charge of the patient's health care decisions.

You must be very clear about the preparation required for a test and never assume that because the patient has had the test before she will know what to do. It is always better to give the patient instructions in writing whenever possible. A period of fasting or a special diet may be required before a test. The decision to have the patient abstain from medications is made by the doctor, who will inform the patient which medications should or should not be taken. It is helpful to testing laboratory personnel to know what medications the patient is taking so they may be alert to possible test interference from certain drugs.

In a POL, specimens are generally processed for in-house testing according to office policy, though some may be prepared for transportation to an outside lab. As a medical assistant, you should perform CLIA-waived tests precisely according to manufacturer's instructions after checking expiration dates. If specimens are sent to an outside lab, you must determine the specific requirements of the lab being used. Each lab has its own policies regarding which specimen containers to use and how much to collect. Some specimens need to be refrigerated, spun, or have chemicals added to them. Some labs schedule routine pickups, but others may require specific contact to pick up a specimen. In Procedure 43-1, review the steps to correctly complete a laboratory requisition and prepare a specimen for transportation to an outside laboratory.

Complications of specimen collection may occur. If there is difficulty drawing blood, the cells may hemolyze, or burst. Accidental contamination or collection in the wrong container can be a problem. Exposure to heat or direct sunlight may cause damage. If less than the required amount of a specimen is collected, testing may not be possible; in this case, a lab report will read **QNS (quantity not sufficient)**. Incomplete or incorrectly handled specimens may require retesting.

To avoid collecting a specimen from the wrong patient, proper identification is important. This is performed in a three-step process. First, check the chart to verify the order. Then, during introductions, ask the patient to state his full name and date of birth. The reason that the patient must state, rather than verify, this information is to prevent miscommunication, especially if there is a language barrier or the patient has difficulty hearing. Finally, compare the information the patient has given with the chart to verify that this is the right patient. Always compare both the name and the date of birth in case more than one person with that name has a file in the same office.

Properly labeling specimens is essential. Typically, this includes using two identifiers (such as name and date of birth), as well as the date and time collected. To prevent cross contamination and mislabeling of specimens, a label should never be placed on a removable lid, and a specimen should always be sealed and labeled before walking away from a sample. If the patient wasn't supposed to eat before the test and forgot, label the specimen as **nonfasting** and check with the physician to determine if the test should still be run.

In many activities in the medical facility, no one but you knows whether you have followed the proper procedure. Whether you wash your hands each and every time you go to a new patient, whether you change gloves as required,

JUDGMENT CALL

Dr. Jorge orders STAT blood tests on Sally Myers. You draw the patient's blood and leave the vial on the counter while you assist the patient to the restroom. When you return, you realize that you forgot to label the container of blood. Another medical assistant is already set up in the room. She is drawing blood on someone else, so she is too busy to notice.

What problem or problems could arise as a result of this situation? What is the best way to proceed?

whether you perform a test procedure correctly, whether you write down the correct test results, whether you actually perform controls as required are all up to you. Your integrity, honesty, and reliability are on the line every day. Always follow the Code of Ethics and the Medical Assistant Creed.

QUALITY ASSURANCE

As a medical assistant, you are responsible for carrying out **quality assurance (QA)** procedures, which involve planned and systematic activities to ensure that requirements are met and results are accurate. A quality assurance program is a written program that includes mechanisms to evaluate laboratory procedures and policies, identify and correct problems, and ensure reliable and prompt reporting of results and testing by competent individuals.

Professionalism   The Law

Circumstances may arise that require a specimen be obtained from a patient that may have medicolegal implications. Specimen collection in cases of rape; child, spousal, or elder abuse; or drug or alcohol abuse could have important implications for the outcome of a legal case in a court of law. Proving a chain of custody is vital for the specimen to be considered valid. The term *chain of custody* refers to a specific set of procedures used to collect, process, test, and report results on a specimen. A chain-of-custody form must be signed at each step of processing to prove that the chain of custody was unbroken. Blood alcohol collection kits may be required in certain states for alcohol levels to be considered as evidence in court. Each testing facility should have in its policies and procedures manual chain-of-custody procedures for all types of specimens. Clinical laboratory personnel may be subpoenaed to testify in court about specimens they have collected.

Steps for Quality Assurance in the Laboratory

Most offices and laboratories have a policies and procedures manual with a set of routine checklists to follow. A basic quality assurance (QA) checklist generally begins with keeping the lab and patient areas clean and providing clear patient instructions. It includes restocking supplies to ensure that the correct materials are available. Checking storage instructions and expiration dates for all reagents and test kits is important before storage and before use. QA involves routinely reviewing procedure manuals, testing protocols, and following the most recent manufacturer's instructions for correct test performance. Scheduling or performing routine equipment maintenance, including calibrations to assure accuracy of results, should always be properly documented. Laboratory refrigerators should be properly labeled for restricted use and should have a thermometer that is both checked and recorded daily. When opening a new stock container of multiuse reagents, chemicals, or test strips, you should date and initial the container. Reagents, chemicals, and test strips must be stored and the temperatures indicated on their labels. You should also be able to identify assigned lab values and compare them to the specimen result.

Maintenance

All laboratory equipment must be maintained on a regular basis according to manufacturers' instructions. A written record of the maintenance performed must be readily available. In addition, a record of each piece of equipment with model and serial numbers, date of purchase, and manufacturers' inserts should be available when repair is necessary or the laboratory is being inspected.

Documentation

Documentation of testing records and performance logs is important for QA. Without a written record of a test result, control result, maintenance performed, or temperature recorded, you have no proof of activity. The end result is the same as if you did not perform the procedure. If it is not written down in the appropriate place, you did not do it.

Documentation of tests to ensure the accuracy of the equipment is as vital as documentation of actual patient test outcomes. It is crucial to also document daily equipment maintenance and which reagents, chemicals, and test strips were stored.

Quality Control

Whereas quality assurance focuses on processes to ensure quality, **quality control (QC)** is focused on physical proof that results are accurate. This is accomplished by routinely performing mock tests, using one of two predetermined methods: calibration or control solutions.

Some machines require evaluation by **calibration devices**, which are specially prepared test strips or cartridges that are designed to produce a predetermined result. Other tests are evaluated by using regular testing materials but, instead of adding a patient sample, a provided control solution is added in its place. **Control solutions** are chemicals that produce an expected result; they are usually purchased from or provided by the manufacturer of the testing equipment. In either case, the result should fall within the acceptable range listed on the calibration device or control solution bottle. Box 43-2 and Procedure 43-3 explain the process of using a control solution to perform quality control measures.

Abnormal quality control results should always be investigated. Things that may cause abnormal results include

---

BOX 43-2 | Using Controls to Monitor Results

As a professional in health care, you must comprehend the importance of patient test results and control samples. What would you do if the control sample results were correct according to the manufacturer's value sheet but the patient test results were very abnormal compared with the reference values of your facility? For example, imagine a patient's fasting glucose level is 47 mg/dL when tested. The reference range in your facility is 70 to 100 mg/dL. The control tests were 55 mg/dL and 132 mg/dL, which were in range according to the manufacturer.

- If a result seems incongruous to you, it should not be reported without retesting.
- The test and controls should be repeated.

- The original specimen should be examined to ascertain that the specimen was not **hemolyzed** (red cells burst, causing serum to be a cherry-red color) or **icteric** (bilious yellow-green color). If either problem exists, a new specimen may be required and the test repeated.
- The results from previous tests on this patient should be examined. Is there a pattern among previous test results?
- The patient's results should be flagged and brought to the attention of the supervisor or physician if test and control results were the same as the first test results.
- A protocol should be in place in your POL that establishes the appropriate steps to follow when a result is flagged.
- A small portion of the original specimen may be sent to an outside laboratory for testing to compare results.

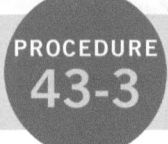

Performing Quality Control Measures for a Glucometer

Objective ◆ *Determine the effectiveness of a glucometer through quality control testing.*

EQUIPMENT AND SUPPLIES

Glucometer, testing strips, and control solutions; wax paper; pen; lab coat; quality control log

METHOD

1. Assemble the equipment and supplies. Check the expiration and discard dates for the control solutions and test strips. Make sure the test strip is dry, clean, and intact.
2. Hold the test strip with the gray end facing up, and insert into the orange port at the front of the meter.
3. The machine will automatically turn on. Once the test strip and the drop of blood appear on the screen, wait for the blood drop to flash.
4. Before opening, gently rock the control bottle to mix the solution evenly.
5. Squeeze a small drop of the control solution onto a piece of wax paper and recap the solution. Do not apply the solution directly onto the test strip.
6. Immediately touch the tip of the test strip to the drop of control solution. Hold it in place until the machine beeps.
7. Compare the test result with the control range printed on the bottom of the test strip bottle label. If the result falls outside the specified range, consult the manufacturer's instructions for the error codes and symbols chart. Compare the code or symbol that appears on the screen. Repeat the test, if necessary.
8. Record the results in the quality control log.
9. Remove the test strip and dispose.
10. Repeat the above steps with a different control solution, as required.

Note: Several different types of glucometers and testing instruments may be used to perform similar tests. It is critical to follow the manufacturer's instructions for the testing equipment provided.

CHARTING EXAMPLE

Glucometer Calibration and Quality Control Log							
Date	Time	Test Strip Lot#	Exp. Date	Low Control Results	High Control Results	MA's Initials	Comments/ Corrective Actions

Name: <u>Helen Mills. MA(AMT)</u> Initials: HM

---

user error, impaired quality or outdated materials, or a malfunctioning machine. In this case, try retesting with newly opened materials or asking a coworker to perform a quality control test. If results remain abnormal, the machine is not considered accurate and should be serviced or repaired and retested before using on patients. Quality control tests are performed according to manufacturer's requirements and lab policy, often daily. Results are recorded in a quality control log, which is evaluated after each use.

The CLIA 1992 standards mandate that written policies and procedures must be in place for a comprehensive quality control program that will "evaluate the ongoing and overall quality of the testing process." To this end, the laboratory is required to do the following:

- Evaluate the effectiveness of its policies and procedures.
- Identify and correct problems.
- Ensure reliable and prompt test results.

- Ensure the competence and adequacy of staff.

- Take corrective action if errors are found.

- Integrate corrective procedures into future policies and procedures.

- Document employee training, and assess competency yearly after the first year.

- Maintain the identity and integrity of patient samples during the entire testing process.

- Be subject to inspection every two years if performing moderate- or high-complexity tests.

LABORATORY SAFETY REGULATIONS

Although laboratory safety guidelines are briefly discussed in the chapter titled, "The Office Environment," it is important to review in depth in our discussion of the clinical laboratory. Several agencies and committees set and review safety guidelines affecting clinical laboratories. In 1970, Congress established the Occupational Safety and Health Administration (OSHA) within the U.S. Department of Labor to ensure that all employers provide a safe work environment free of hazards that may cause serious injury or death. OSHA enforces the Centers for Disease Control and Prevention's (CDC's) Standard Precautions in health care. Other agencies include the Clinical Laboratory Standards Institute (CLSI), previously known as the National Committee for Clinical Laboratory Standards (NCCLS); the Environmental Protection Agency (EPA); and the College of American Pathologists (CAP). It is important that medical assistants have a working knowledge of the guidelines and regulations of these agencies and keep up to date on changes to provide better health care.

OSHA Regulations

In 1970, Congress established OSHA within the U.S. Department of Labor to create safeguards covering nearly every employee in the United States. Two programs of standards under the OSHA umbrella particularly impact the clinical laboratory. They cover exposure to chemical hazards and bloodborne pathogens. Both are discussed in some detail in the chapter titled "Infection Control," so they are only briefly considered here. OSHA develops and implements specific guidelines governing particular fields and requires adherence. If no specific guidelines exist, then the "general duty clause" must be followed, which means that all employers must provide a safe work environment free of hazards that may cause serious injury or death.

OSHA enforces CDC precautions. In 1996, the CDC developed and published specific guidelines for isolation precautions in hospitals, and these were termed standard precautions. Focusing on limiting direct contact with body fluids, standard precautions combine major features of the CDC's universal precautions and body substance isolation precautions into one set of recommendations. Copies of these general guidelines can be obtained from the CDC website: www.cdc.gov.

Clinical Laboratory Improvement Amendments

In 1988, Congress enacted the **Clinical Laboratory Improvement Amendments (CLIA)** as developed by the Centers for Medicare & Medicaid Services (CMS) in response to widespread concern over the accuracy of laboratory tests. These federal regulatory standards mandate that all laboratories that test human specimens must be regulated to help ensure accurate patient test results. Since their enactment in 1988, the CLIA have been kept current through periodic amendments and updates.

CLIA divides laboratories into three categories: waived, moderate complexity, and high complexity (Box 43-3). Each category specifies the types of tests that may be performed. Medical assistants are qualified to perform only waived testing.

Some tests, known as CLIA-waived tests, do not require extensive training and so are able to be performed at home with basic instructions or in a POL. They frequently come in a boxed test kit set that contains several tests and the materials needed to properly use them. Many **automated analyzers**

BOX 43-3 | Categories of CLIA Tests

- *Waived Tests*—Simple procedures approved for home use and POL or POC testing. Common examples include:
  Dipstick urine testing or table testing
  Fecal occult blood testing
  Ovulation testing
  Urine pregnancy testing
  Erythrocyte sedimentation rate (nonautomated)
  Hemoglobin testing with CLIA-waived analyzer
  Spun hematocrit
  Blood glucose using FDA-approved glucose analyzer
  Rapid *Streptococcus* testing
- *Moderate-Complexity Tests/Level I Tests*
  75 percent of tests performed daily using automated analyzers for chemistry and hematology
  Microscopic analysis of urine sediment
- *High-Complexity Tests/Level II Tests*
  All tests in the field of cytogenetics, cytology, histopathology, and histocompatibility

are now CLIA-waived, too, as a result of the advancements of technology. An automated analyzer is typically a small or handheld machine that processes a specimen with single-use reagent test strips or cassettes. Results are displayed quickly, proving an advantage for a patient who may need to be treated right away.

Information regarding state laboratory regulations may be obtained from state health departments. A facility is required to have a Certificate of Waiver from the CMS so that its employees can legally perform simple tests used to prevent, diagnose, or treat a disorder or disease. These tests are referred to as **Certificate of Waiver Tests (WTs)** or **CLIA-Waived Tests**. They are the least complex and present the least risk if performed incorrectly. Some examples of these tests are indicated in Box 43-3. Many of these tests have been approved by the U.S. Food and Drug Administration (FDA) for home use. These are the only laboratory tests that a medical assistant may perform without further training; they may be performed only in a laboratory that has been granted a Certificate of Waiver. Although other types of testing are discussed in this text book, anything that is not CLIA-waived is for demonstration purposes only and does not qualify the medical assistant to perform that test in the laboratory. Table 43-1 lists some CLIA-waived tests and the diseases for which they test.

To maintain CLIA-waived status, facilities must permit on-site inspections, as requested. During an inspection, evaluators will determine if necessary standards are being met. A significant issue of discovery is when manufacturer's instructions are either missing, outdated, or not followed to the letter. This is a concern because the only CLIA

requirement for performing waived testing is to follow the manufacturer's instructions. Improper testing can lead to inaccurate results, which may result in incorrect diagnosis or treatment. Therefore, if modified even the slightest bit, tests are no longer considered waived tests and become subject to the more stringent CLIA requirements. Box 43-4 lists the critical steps to follow.

A POL must apply to perform WTs and then may not perform the more complex tests from Level I or Level II (such as those listed in Box 43-3). Approved tests are considered exempt from complying with CLIA 1988 standards and are thus termed CLIA-waived or Waived Tests (WT). However, quality assurance and quality control methods should still be observed. The laboratories that perform WTs may be subject to random inspections and investigation if test results are questioned or complaints are made against the laboratory. A Certificate of Waiver is given to laboratories that perform only low-complexity tests.

A POL qualified to perform moderate-complexity and waived tests receives a Certificate of Provider-Performed Microscopy (PPM). A medical assistant employed in a facility with a PPM certificate can perform moderate-complexity tests with further training and under the supervision of a laboratory professional or physician.

LABORATORY EQUIPMENT

Clinical laboratories use a wide array of equipment. A POL, however, requires less equipment for clinical laboratory testing than does an outside or reference laboratory. An autoclave, centrifuge, photometer, incubator, microscope, and measuring devices are generally found in most POLs.

Autoclave

The **autoclave** is used to sterilize equipment or instruments that are used on patients or in certain test procedures. It

TABLE 43-1 | Selected CLIA-Waived Tests and Diseases/Conditions

CLIA-Waived Test	Disease/condition
Cholesterol (HDL, LDL, VLDL)	Lipidemia
Helicobacter pylori	Gastric Ulcer
HCG	Pregnancy
HIV antibody	HIV, AIDS
Influenza	Influenza infection
Prothombin time	Clotting disorders
Strep	Strep throat infection
Urine dipstick	Glucose/ketones—diabetes, RBC/WBC/nitrates—urinary tract infection, protein—kidney disease, pH-acid-base disorders

provides high-pressure, saturated steam that is capable of sterilizing metal objects.

Centrifuge

The **centrifuge** is an instrument used to separate specimens into component layers. It works by spinning samples at high speed, which allows lighter components to float to the top and heavier components to sink to the bottom. It can be used to separate urine so urine sediment can be examined under the microscope or to separate whole blood from plasma for chemical testing. A micro centrifuge is used to separate whole blood samples into layers to measure patient hematocrit.

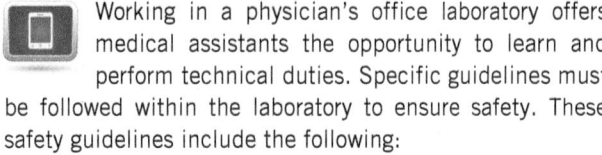

Working in a physician's office laboratory offers medical assistants the opportunity to learn and perform technical duties. Specific guidelines must be followed within the laboratory to ensure safety. These safety guidelines include the following:

1. Wear appropriate personal protective equipment (PPE) in the lab only. Do not wear lab coats, masks, and gloves outside the lab.
2. Avoid hand-to-mouth contact or hands touching the eyes, nose, or ears while in the lab.
   a. No pens or pencils placed in mouth or behind the ears.
   b. No food or drink in lab or lab refrigerator.
   c. Never apply cosmetics, such as lipstick or lip balm, or handle contact lenses while in the lab.
3. Dress appropriately.
   a. Never wear long chains, dangling earrings, or bracelets.
   b. Always tie back hair.
   c. Keep fingernails short, well-manicured, with no polish or artificial nails.
   d. Wear comfortable, sturdy shoes with nonslip soles—no sandals, open-toed shoes, or heels.
4. Do not draw material up through a pipette using suction from the mouth.
5. Do not store caustic material above eye level.
6. Locate fire extinguishers in the lab, and know how to use them.
7. Be sure hands are dry when transferring reagent bottles.
8. Keep a first-aid manual and supplies available.
9. Avoid inhaling any chemical substance that might cause injury to nasal membranes or lungs.
10. Never use chipped, broken, or cracked glassware.
11. Follow written cleanup policies and procedures for spills.
12. Discard contaminated material in appropriate containers.

Photometer

A **photometer** is an instrument that measures light intensity. A glucometer is a type of handheld photometer that is used to test glucose levels in patients.

Incubator

An **incubator** is used to maintain a specific temperature to achieve a specific result. For example, incubators that mimic body temperature are used in POLs to encourage growth of throat and urine cultures. Once the culture has grown sufficiently, identification of the infecting organism can be made.

Microscope

Microscopes are frequently used in the medical office to examine urine sediment, vaginal and bacteriological smears, and differential smears, which categorize types of white cells in a sample. This optical instrument magnifies structures unseen by the naked eye for the purpose of counting, naming, or differentiating. Figure 43-4 shows an example of a **compound microscope**. A compound microscope achieves maximum magnification by using two sets of lenses: **oculars** (eyepiece lenses) and **objectives** (lenses at the bottom near the sample). The **resolution** of a microscope refers to the ability to distinguish clearly between two adjacent but distinct objects. Better microscopes have better resolution.

Parts of the Microscope

The following are the components of a microscope:

1. One or multiple eyepieces (monocular or binocular) with magnification imprinted on them
2. Body tube (directional light source)
3. Arm (used in carrying the microscope)
4. Revolving nosepiece (holds objectives and rotates for selection)
5. Objectives (magnification imprinted on each objective: 10, low-power setting; 40, high dry setting; and 100, oil immersion setting (settings are described in the next section)
6. Stage
7. Mechanical stage (movable device that holds slide)
8. Mechanical stage adjustments (two knobs that control vertical/horizontal movement of slide)
9. Coarse and fine adjustment knobs (small knob atop larger knob that adjusts stage up and down for focusing)
10. Condenser (lens system used to increase light for sharper focus)
11. Condenser adjustment knob

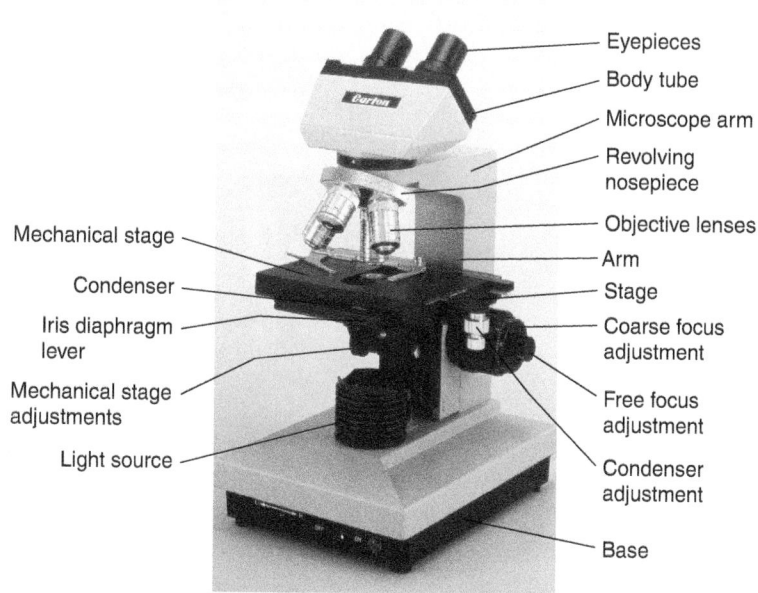

FIGURE 43-4 A compound microscope.

objective, 10×, is used to view epithelial cells, such as skin scrapings; the high dry setting, 40×, is used for urine RBCs (red blood cells), WBCs (white blood cells), or blood RBCs; the oil immersion setting, 100×, is for differential blood smears (stained with Wright's stain) or bacteria slides (stained with Gram stain). Microscopic work on the high dry setting is done with a cover glass on the specimen.

Care of the Microscope

Microscopes are delicate instruments that last for many years if maintained properly. Guidelines 43-1 lists the rules for the proper care and maintenance of a microscope. Procedure 43-4 lists the methods for properly using, cleaning, and storing a microscope.

12. Light source (illuminator set in base)

13. Iris diaphragm lever

14. Base (holds illuminator, rheostat, and microscope upright and is used while carrying microscope)

Using the Microscope.

The magnification of an object is calculated by multiplying the objective magnification by the eyepiece magnification. On low power, magnification would be 10 (the objective) times 10 (the eyepiece), equaling magnification of 100 times the size of the sample.

It is important to use the correct lens for the type of microscopic work to be done. For example, the low-power

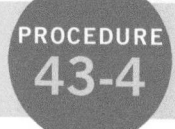

PROCEDURE 43-4

Using and Cleaning a Microscope

Objective ◆ *Observe a slide under 10x, 40x, and oil immersion properly, and clean and store microscope correctly.*

EQUIPMENT AND SUPPLIES

Binocular compound microscope; specimen slide; lens paper; lens cleaner; dust cover for microscope

METHOD

1. Always carry the microscope with one hand on the arm and one hand under the base.

2. Make sure the stage is in the down position before starting.
3. Clean objectives with lens paper starting with 10x and ending with oil immersion (Figure A).
4. Turn on the light and rotate the nosepiece until 10x objective is directly over the slide (Figure B). Place the prepared slide on the stage (Figure C).

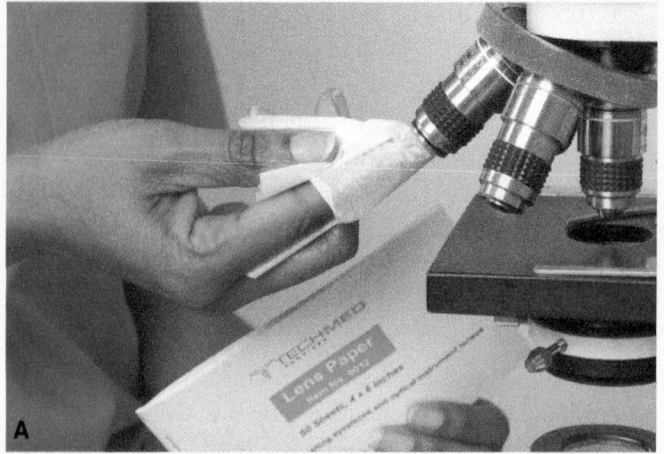

FIGURE A Clean the objective lens.

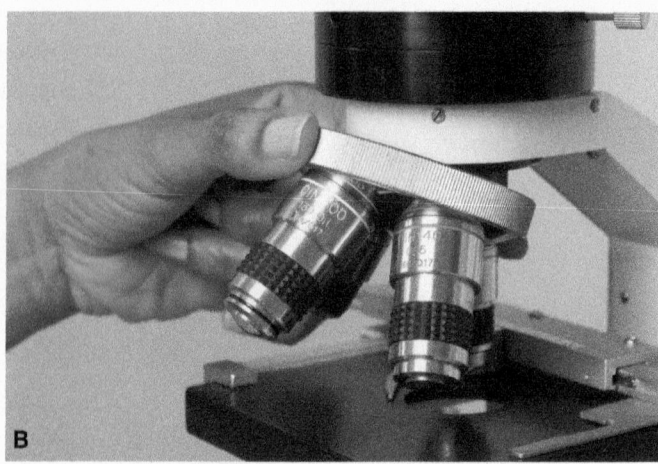

FIGURE B Rotate the nosepiece.

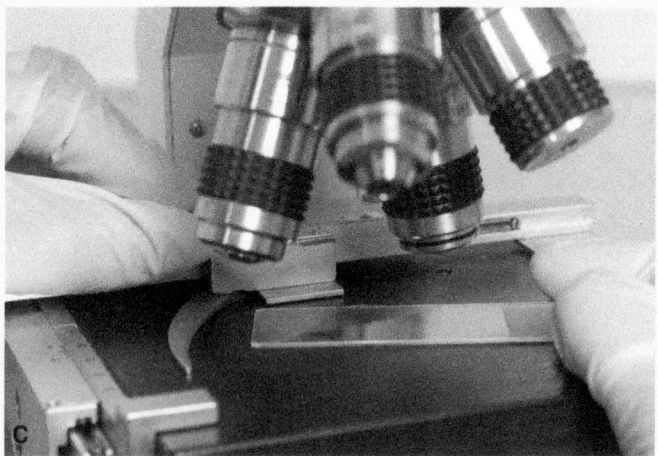

FIGURE C Place the slide on the stage.

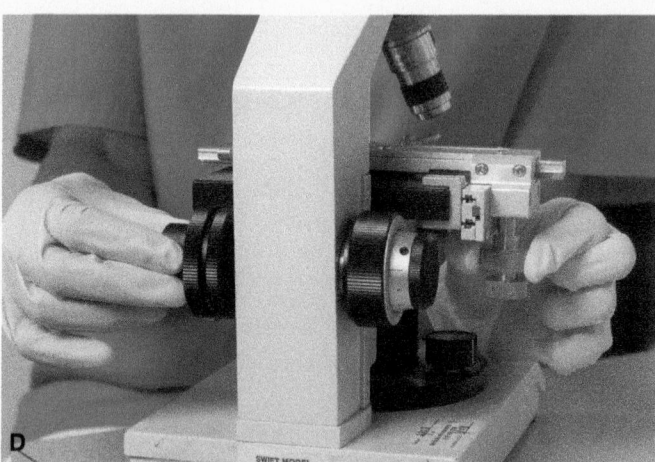

FIGURE D Fine focus with the adjustment knob while moving the slide slightly with the mechanical slide controls.

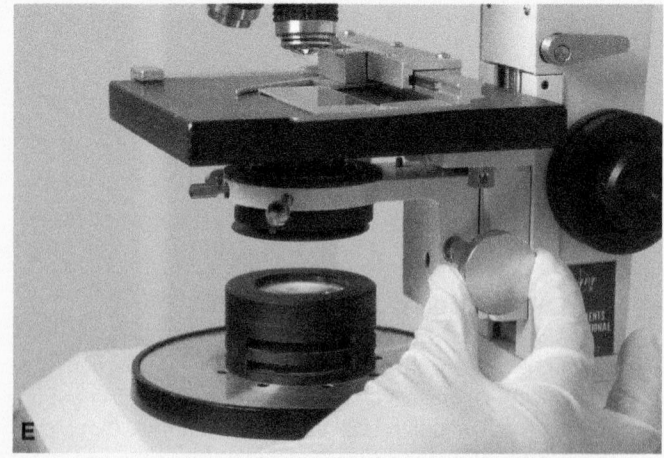

FIGURE E The condenser height control is on the left, and the diaphragm control is on the right.

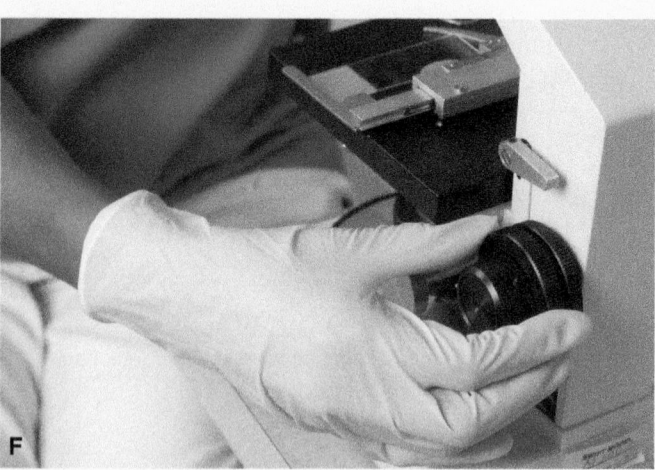

FIGURE F The mechanical stage control moves the slide up and down and back and forth.

5. Use the coarse adjustment knob to raise the stage until the objective is close to the slide on the stage.
6. Look through the eyepiece and adjust the coarse focus knob until the microscope field is seen (a round circle of bright light).
7. Use the fine adjustment knob for a clearer image (Figure D).
8. Open the diaphragm and, if necessary, adjust the rheostat to focus.
9. Raise or lower the condenser to alter light refraction. The condenser is usually lowered when using 10× power (Figure E).
10. Observe the slide.
11. Change the objective to 40× and readjust as needed (Figure F). Move the objective and place a drop of oil on the slide before completing the turn to oil immersion lens.
12. When focusing and examination are complete, lower the stage before removing the slide.
13. Turn off the light.
14. Clean the eyepieces and objectives with lens paper. Clean the oil immersion lens with lens cleaner.

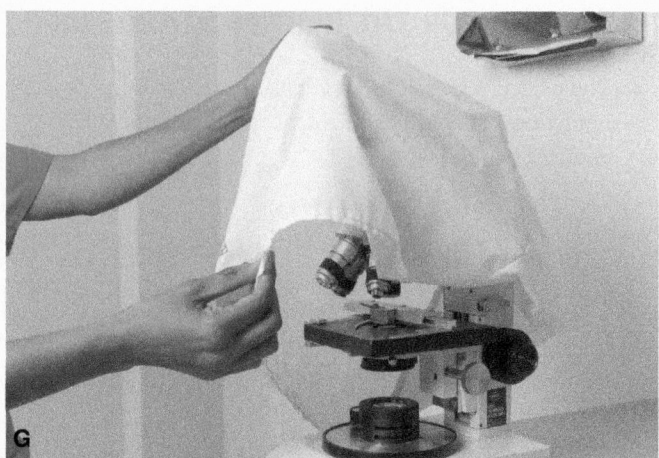

FIGURE G After cleaning, always store the microscope with its protective cover.

15. Unplug the electrical cord and wrap it around the base.
16. Cover the microscope with a dust cover (Figure G).
17. Clean the slide and store.

SUMMARY

In this chapter, we examined the role of the clinical laboratory in health care. We discussed different types of laboratories, the types of clinical laboratory departments, and categories of laboratory personnel. We considered OSHA and CLIA guidelines and laboratory safety issues. The medical assistant has an important role in laboratory testing. It is up to the medical assistant to secure the integrity of the specimen and ensure the proper processing, handling, transporting, and recording of test results. We discussed quality assurance and quality control and their roles in ensuring accurate test results. We covered the microscope, its parts, and how to use it in the POL. We introduced other types of equipment, such as the incubator, glassware, centrifuge, photometer, and microscope.

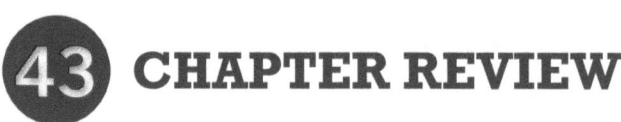

43 CHAPTER REVIEW

COMPETENCY REVIEW

1. Define and spell the terms for this chapter.
2. Define quality assurance, and explain why it is important to the clinical laboratory.
3. Explain the role of the clinical laboratory in patient care.
4. Explain the role of the medical assistant in the clinical laboratory.
5. Define CLIA-waived testing and provide examples of common CLIA-waived tests that a medical assistant would perform in the physician's office laboratory.
6. Explain how flow sheets are used in the medical care setting.

PREPARING FOR THE CERTIFICATION EXAM

1. The federal regulations for clinical laboratories specifying guidelines for quality control, qualified personnel, and quality assurance are
   a. OSHA.
   b. DEA.
   c. CDC.
   d. NIH.
   e. CLIA 1988.

2. All of the following are true of laboratory refrigerators *except*
   a. They should be labeled for restricted use.
   b. Thermometers should be checked daily.
   c. Drinks may be stored there, but not food.
   d. Thermometer temperature readings should be recorded daily.
   e. Proper documentation of temperature readings are a component of a quality assurance program.

3. A qualitative test is one that
   a. tests for the presence or absence of a substance.
   b. tests for all substances in a sample.
   c. tests for the presence and amount of a substance in a sample.
   d. is performed only by trained technicians.
   e. is only performed at home.

4. Which of the following is not a critical step in CLIA testing?
   a. Always adhere to expiration dates.
   b. Perform quality control testing four times a year.
   c. Use only recommended storage requirements.
   d. Keep manufacturer's instructions in an easily accessible area.
   e. Be aware of federal, state, and local regulations.

5. Which of the following answers is a correct safety rule in the laboratory?
   a. It is unnecessary to supervise new laboratory personnel.
   b. Hands must be thoroughly washed frequently.
   c. Eating and drinking are acceptable in a laboratory.
   d. Gloves are unnecessary when working with patients' samples.
   e. Smoking is permitted in the laboratory.

6. What are typical roles that a medical assistant may assume in a clinical laboratory?
   a. record management
   b. patient teaching
   c. specimen management
   d. quality assurance and control
   e. all of the above

7. Which component of the microscope is used for carrying?
   a. arm
   b. revolving nosepiece
   c. stage
   d. body tube
   e. none of the above

8. QNS stands for
   a. quality not sufficient.
   b. quantity not standard.
   c. quality not satisfactory.
   d. quantity not sufficient.
   e. quantity not satisfactory.

9. When evaluating test results from an outside facility, the medical assistant should always check reference values for the laboratory being used. Quantitative test results that are considered normal at one lab may be considered abnormal at another lab because
   a. procedures may be performed differently at different facilities (venous versus capillary).
   b. results for different product manufacturers may vary.
   c. policies for techniques may vary slightly.
   d. different equipment may be used at each site.
   e. all of the above.

10. A control
   a. is another word for reagent.
   b. never needs to be performed when doing lab tests.
   c. is similar to the testing specimen with a known value.
   d. never needs diluting.
   e. is another word for a standard.

CRITICAL THINKING

Refer to the case study at the beginning of the chapter and use what you have learned to answer the following questions.

1. What is the clinical laboratory at Pearson Physicians Group required to have in order to perform laboratory tests, even if they are considered simple? How is it obtained?
2. Mr. Patel questions why he needs to come back for the two-hour postprandial blood glucose test. What should Susan tell him?

3. Susan performs a dipstick urinalysis on Mr. Patel's urine sample. After she discards the urine sample, she realizes that the reagent strip she used came from an expired package. How could this situation have been avoided? What should Susan tell the patient?

ON THE JOB

Carmel Lopez has been working in a busy internal medicine office mainly performing clinical procedures. She often performs Certificate of Waiver tests and has helped train new medical assistants to perform them correctly. Carmel observes Rachel not bothering to run the controls that came with a test kit necessary to perform a waived test. Rachel has worked in the office longer than Carmel.

1. Why are controls important when performing a test?
2. What should Carmel do? What should Carmel do if Rachel reacts in a negative way?
3. How would you handle this situation?
4. How might a patient be affected by Rachel's actions?

INTERNET ACTIVITY

Imagine your supervisor asks you to research the Clinical Laboratory Improvement Amendments of 1988 and 1992 and make a short presentation. Do the research and prepare a report.

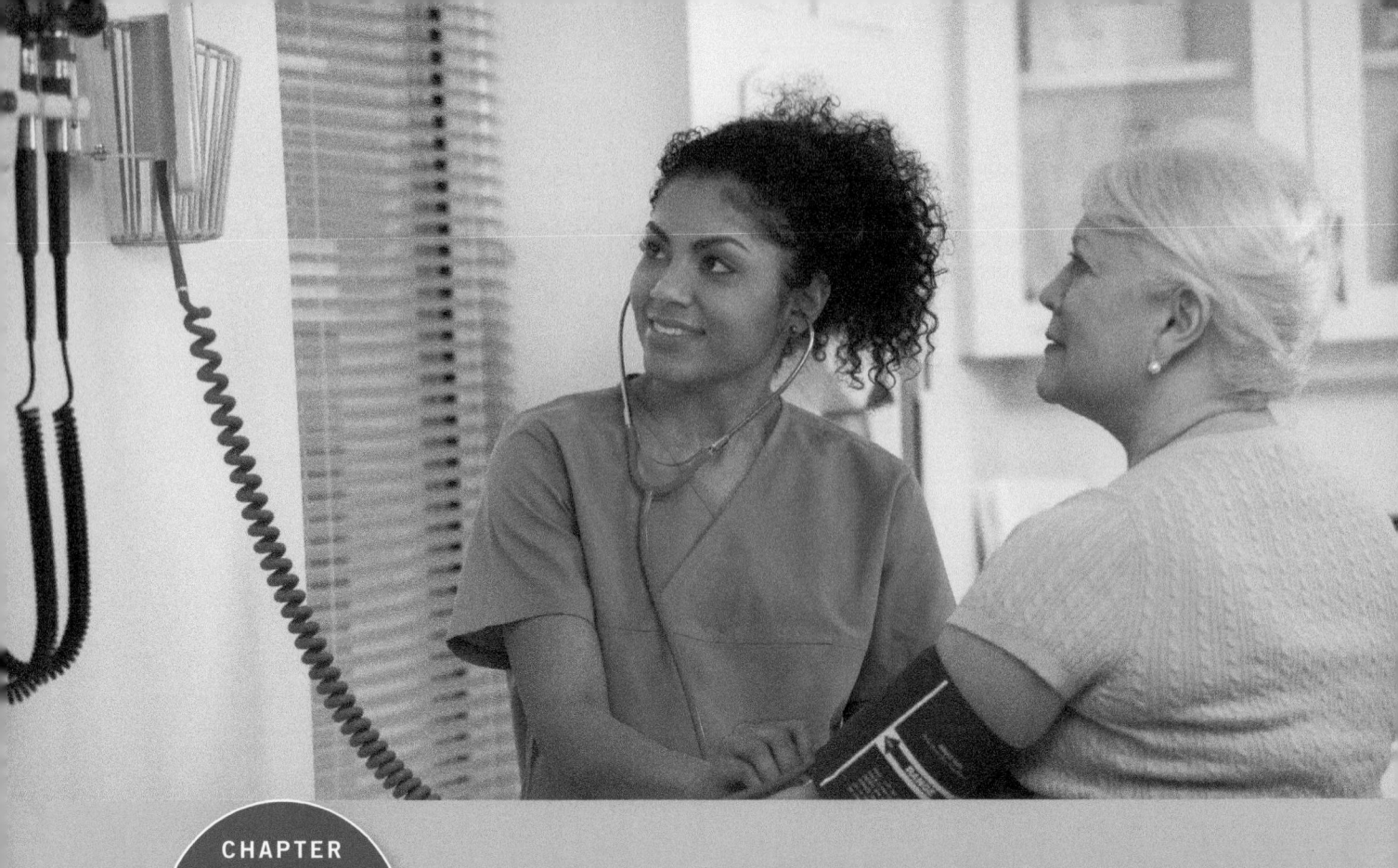

Microbiology

Learning Objectives

After completing this chapter, you should be able to:

44.1   Define and spell the terms for this chapter.

44.2   Explain the medical assistant's role in microbiology.

44.3   List criteria for classifying microorganisms.

44.4   Describe the characteristics of different types of microorganisms.

44.5   Explain the steps involved with diagnosing an infection.

44.6   List the guidelines for specimen collection.

44.7   Describe different types of specimens that may be collected by a medical assistant.

44.8   Differentiate between culture and inoculating media.

44.9   Explain methods for preparing a specimen for direct examination under a microscope.

It has been a very busy day at Pearson Physicians Group. David Dolan, RMA, has been working with Dr. Penningworth's patients. The next patient David leads to an examination room is 12-year-old Marc Gutierrez. He is accompanied by his mother and is complaining of a sore throat.

Terms to Learn

acid-fast stain	feces	necrotizing fasciitis
agar	fixed	normal flora
agglutination	fungus	organelles
candidiasis	inoculated	sequela
colony	lawn technique	serology
culture	microbiology	smear
culture and sensitivity (C&S) test	microorganisms	spore
culture media	methicillin-resistant *Staphylococcus aureus* (MRSA)	sputum
Culturette™ system	moniliasis	steatorrhea
enteritis	morphology	swabs
exudates	mycology	viable
facultative anaerobes		wet mount

The field of **microbiology** is the fascinating study of living organisms too small to be seen with the naked eye (**microorganisms**). Antonie van Leeuwenhoek's invention of the microscope in 1674 allowed humankind to observe for the first time a variety of microbes. Louis Pasteur, the father of microbiology, developed methods for culturing and identifying microbes in the laboratory. The study of microorganisms has greatly advanced the field of medicine and currently allows individuals to live longer, healthier lives. To successfully treat a patient, it is important to first discover the exact cause of the problem. By evaluating body fluid samples, an offending microorganism may be identified so that the most effective medication or treatment can be prescribed.

We are surrounded by microorganisms. Yet, not all bacteria are bad. Bacteria in the environment help us to decompose and recycle waste. **Normal flora** on our bodies consist of beneficial bacteria that help us resist pathogens. However, a bacterium that is harmless in one area may be pathogenic in another, especially in large amounts or in an area that is normally sterile. It is important to understand differences between microorganisms and learn which can be harmful to effectively help patients to recover from illness.

This chapter covers the characteristics of microorganisms, how they are identified, and the diseases some pathogens cause.

ROLE OF THE MEDICAL ASSISTANT IN MICROBIOLOGY

Medical assistants frequently come in contact with blood and body fluids. This may occur while collecting or preparing specimens for testing or simply while assisting in patient care. Some specimens that medical assistants might collect include urine, stool, blood, drainage, and wound samples. Preparation of the specimens can affect the results, so it is vital to follow procedures strictly, including storage and transportation requirements. The temperature at which a specimen is stored can affect the results of the test. Observing standard precautions is a significant priority to prevent contamination and the spread of infection. Safety must come above all else. Through an understanding the basic concepts of microbiology, the importance of prevention becomes easier to understand and accomplish. Of course, it is also the role of the medical assistant to assist the physician and educate the patient in relation to obtaining specimens.

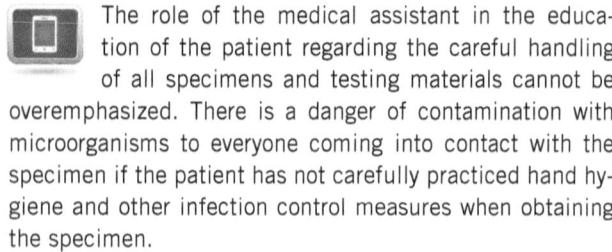
CLASSIFICATIONS OF MICROORGANISMS

Although medical assistants are not responsible for identifying and naming specific microorganisms, it is important to understand how they are classified and named. There are many types of microorganisms, and we know already that they are categorized by their ability to cause disease as either pathogens or nonpathogens. Most microbes are nonpathogenic (98 to 99 percent); only 1 to 2 percent are pathogenic.

Naming Microorganisms

Scientists use a binomial system to name all living organisms—animals, plants, bacteria, fungi, and protozoa. Just as we each have two names—a first name and a last name—each organism has two names: the genus (always capitalized) and the species (lowercase). For example, the organism that causes strep throat is known as *Streptococcus pyogenes* (literally, "a chain of round bacteria that produce pus"). The convention is to spell out the entire name at first mention and then abbreviate with the initial of the genus followed by the species name (e.g., *S. pyogenes*). Although you are not expected to learn all the genus and species names, understanding the system of nomenclature is necessary when you receive laboratory reports over the phone or read a patient's chart.

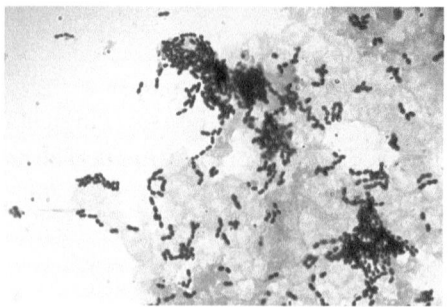

FIGURE 44-1 Gram-positive *S. pyogenes* bacteria in chains.

Retention of Dyes

Although many types of microorganisms are classified by their major structural differences, bacteria are also characterized by their reactions to certain stains. A stain is a dye used in coloring microorganisms to make them visible under a microscope. The Gram stain, named for Dr. Hans C. J. Gram, a Danish physician, is a commonly used method of staining bacteria. A Gram-positive bacterium retains the violet color of the stain used in the staining of the microorganism. Some of the more common Gram-positive bacteria are *Staphylococcus aureus* and *Streptococcus pneumoniae*. Figure 44-1 shows Gram-positive streptococci.

A Gram-negative bacterium has the pink color of the counterstain used in Gram's method of staining microorganisms. A few of the most common Gram-negative bacteria are *Escherichia coli*, *Neisseria gonorrhoeae*, and *Salmonella typhimurium*. Figure 44-2 shows Gram-negative *N. gonorrhoeae*. Some organisms do not stain well with Gram stain and require a special stain, such as the **acid-fast stain** used for the organism that causes tuberculosis.

Use of Oxygen

Bacteria also can be categorized by whether they survive in an oxygen-rich environment (aerobes), die in the presence of oxygen (anaerobes), or are anaerobes that are flexible and can live with some oxygen (**facultative anaerobes**). Successful culturing requires an understanding of the oxygen requirements

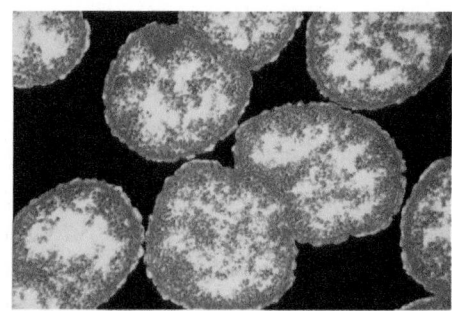

FIGURE 44-2 Gram-negative *N. gonorrhoeae*.

of bacteria. If the ultimate goal is to grow and identify a sample of the organism that is causing disease in a patient, then we must provide proper oxygen, moisture, nutrition, and temperature in the laboratory setting.

Other Identifying Characteristics

Differences such as cell structure and the presence or absence of **organelles** (small structures in the cytoplasm of a cell) are used to classify organisms. If they are capable of movement, their means of motility is unique to specific categories of microorganisms. They may possess flagella (long whiplike extensions of the cytoplasm) or cilia (fine hairlike extensions). For example, *Trichomonas vaginalis*, the protozoan that is responsible for one type of vaginitis, has four flagella at one end that produce the characteristic circular whiplike movement seen in wet preparations and microscopic examinations of infected individuals' urine. Bacteria are also categorized by their ability to hemolyze (burst) red blood cells in the blood **agar** (a medium for growing bacterial **cultures** that contains whole blood).

Biochemical analysis, often done on semiautomated analyzers, provides the microbiologist with information that assists in identification of certain pathogens, such as enteric organisms (those that live in the intestines).

TYPES OF MICROORGANISMS

Although we briefly presented information about microorganisms in the chapter titled "Infection Control," it is important to expand on this information to fully understand microbiology. Microbes are divided into groups based on shared special characteristics. Bacteria, viruses, protozoa, fungi, parasites, and other organisms that share similar characteristics are discussed next. Table 44-1 provides a list of microorganisms, including descriptions and examples of each.

Bacteria

Bacteria (singular bacterium) are small, unicellular microorganisms that are capable of rapid reproduction. Although their mere presence is not necessarily harmful, the overgrowth of bacteria can cause an imbalance and lead to disease or pathology. Most bacteria thrive in a warm, dark, moist environment. Because the human body is capable of providing this atmosphere upon entry, bacteria can easily thrive and grow. Their reproductive ability explains how some infections become overwhelming in a short period of time and can be dangerous. For example, one *Escherichia coli* organism, the most common cause of urinary tract infections (UTIs), reproduces in about 30 minutes. By the end of a

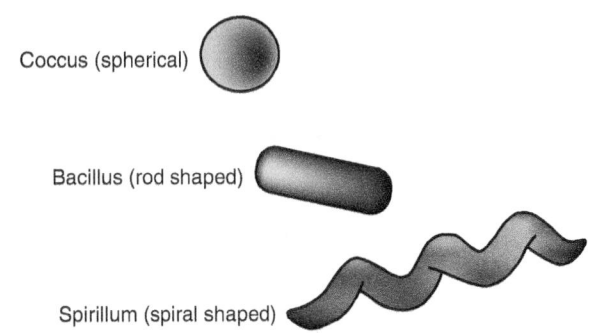

FIGURE 44-3 Bacteria may be named for their morphology (shape): coccus (spherical), bacillus (rod shaped), or spirillum (spiral shaped).

24-hour period, this one *Escherichia coli* (*E. coli*) cell will have produced an enormous number of cells capable of creating an infection if they have been introduced into the bladder.

Bacteria may be named for their **morphology** (shape): cocci (spherical), bacilli (rod-shaped), or spirilla (spiral-shaped) (Figure 44-3).

Cocci

Cocci (singular *coccus*) are round bacteria that are arranged in various configurations. *Staphylococci* are found in grapelike clusters, *Streptococci* in chains, and *Diplococci* in pairs (Figure 44-4).

Staphylococci. *Staphylococci* are Gram-positive, grapelike clusters of *cocci*, some of which are pathogenic. Nonpathogenic *Staphylococci* are found on our skin and in many of our body orifices or openings. *S. aureus*, or staph, is the major pathogen of this genus and may be found as normal flora in the nose and on the skin. It causes infection especially when resistance is lowered by a break in the skin or in the mucous membranes. *S. aureus* produces infections such as impetigo in children and is associated with infection of wound sites and surgical incisions. It causes pus-producing abscesses such

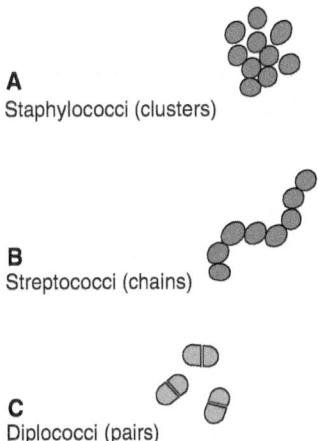

FIGURE 44-4 Configurations of *cocci*: **(A)** *Staphylococci*; **(B)** *Streptococci*; **(C)** *Diplococci*.

TABLE 44-1 | Classes of Microorganisms with Descriptions and Examples

Microorganism	Description	Example
Bacteria	Most numerous of all microorganisms	(See *Cocci*, *Bacilli*, and *Spirilla* entries)
	Unicellular	
	Some are pathogenic to humans	
	Identified by shape and appearance	
• *Cocci*	Three types of spherical bacteria	
1. *Staphylococci*	Form grapelike clusters of pus-producing organisms	Boils, pimples, acne, osteomyelitis
2. *Streptococci*	Form chains of cells	Rheumatic heart disease, scarlet fever, strep throat
3. *Diplococci*	Form pairs of cells	Pneumonia, gonorrhea, and meningitis
• *Bacilli*	Rod-shaped bacteria	Gram-positive *Bacilli*: tetanus, diphtheria, gas gangrene
		Gram-negative *Bacilli*: *E. coli* (UTI), *Bordetella pertussis* (whooping cough)
• *Vibrios*	Curved rod-shaped bacteria	Cholera
• *Spirilla*	Spiral-shaped organisms	Syphilis
• *Rickettsia*	Spherical, rod-shaped, or threadlike bacteria	Rocky Mountain spotted fever
	Visible under a standard microscope	
	Susceptible to antibiotics	
	Transmitted by insects (ticks, fleas)	
Fungi	Parasitic and some nonparasitic plants and molds	*Histoplasma capsulatum* (histoplasmosis), *Tinea pedis* (athlete's foot), *Candida albicans* (yeast infection), and *Tinea spp.* (ringworm)
	Depend on other life forms for their nutrition, such as dead or decaying organic material	
	Reproduction method is budding	
	Yeast is a typical fungus	
	Feed on antibiotics and flourish on antibiotic therapy	
	The Latin word *fungus* means "mushroom"	
Protozoa	One-celled organism	Trichomoniasis (caused by *Trichomonas vaginalis*), amoebic dysentery, and malaria
	Both parasitic and nonparasitic	
	Can move with cilia or false feet	
	Typically 2–200 mm in size	
Viruses	Smallest of microorganisms	Herpes virus, HIV, ARC, AIDS, common cold, influenza virus, smallpox, hepatitis A, hepatitis B, mumps, shingles
	Can only be seen with electron microscope	
	Can only multiply within a living cell (host)	
	Difficult to kill with chemotherapy because they become resistant to the drug	
	Can be destroyed by heat (autoclave sterilization) but generally not by chemical disinfection	
	More viruses than any other category of microbial agents	
	Feed on antibiotics and flourish on antibiotic therapy	

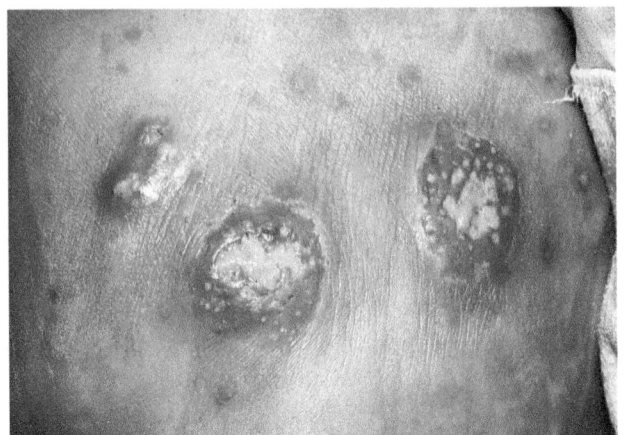

FIGURE 44-5 Carbuncles caused by *S. aureus*.

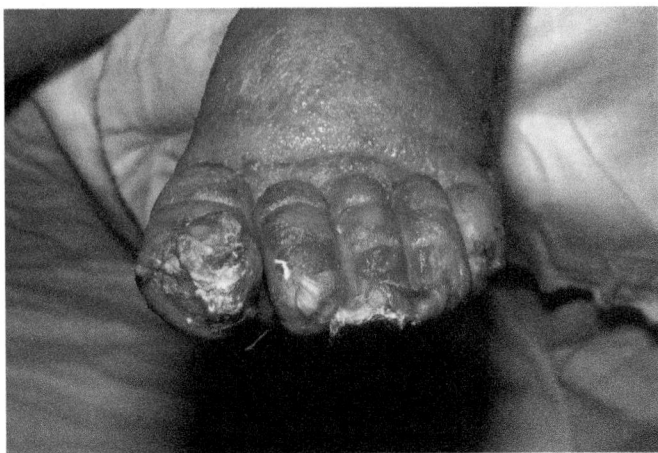

FIGURE 44-6 A patient with necrotizing fasciitis to the feet, caused by group A beta-hemolytic strep.

as boils, carbuncles, and folliculitis. Figure 44-5 shows an example of carbuncles.

S. aureus is a common cause of nosocomial infections (infections that are acquired in hospitals) and may also cause pneumonia, meningitis, and septicemia in individuals with reduced resistance. Toxic shock syndrome is also caused by this virulent organism. *S. aureus* produces one type of **enteritis** (food poisoning) that occurs within a few hours of eating improperly refrigerated food contaminated with the toxin produced by the bacteria. This toxin causes nausea, vomiting, diarrhea, and abdominal cramping. *S. aureus* is coagulase positive, meaning it produces an enzyme that can be used to help differentiate *S. aureus* from other species of this organism.

Because of increased reliance on treatment with antibiotics to treat low-level infections today, superbugs (various microorganisms that are mutating to produce antibiotic-resistant forms) are becoming common. Of particular interest is **methicillin-resistant Staphylococcus aureus (MRSA)**. This form of *S. aureus* produces an enzyme the makes the organism resistant to penicillins and cephalosporins normally used for treatment and renders these antibiotics ineffective. Similarly, vancomycin-resistant enterococci (VRE) and carbapenem-resistant enterobacteriaceae (CRE) are becoming more prevalent. Tests are available to indicate the presence or absence of these organisms and help determine the most favorable treatment. The problem of antibiotic resistance is a major concern for health care providers and is being experienced worldwide. Additional information on this topic is found later in this chapter.

Streptococci. *Streptococci* are round, Gram-positive bacteria arranged in chains, some of which are nonpathogenic, but others are dangerous to humans. Streptococcal organisms are part of the normal flora of the upper respiratory tract and skin. As previously mentioned, one classification of streptococcal organisms is based on the type of hemolysis the organisms cause on blood agar plates. In addition, *Streptococci* can be

classified serologically with antisera specific for antigens in cell walls and specific for each group (A–H and K–V). Identification of the specific group of strep organisms is important in epidemiology, the study of outbreaks of infections.

Group A beta-hemolytic *S. pyogenes* causes a variety of diseases varying from mild such as strep throat to life threatening such as **necrotizing fasciitis** (severe infection as a result of destruction of subcutaneous tissue and fascia, with a 30 percent mortality rate—Figure 44-6). This organism also causes other infections, including pneumonia, tonsillitis, scarlet fever, rheumatic fever, acute glomerulonephritis, and bacterial endocarditis, as well as abscesses, wound infections, and bacteremia.

Commercial kits are available for rapid detection of group A beta-hemolytic strep in the office or laboratory setting. Any negative test should be followed up by a culture that includes bacitracin sensitivity. Sensitivity to the antibiotic bacitracin is a useful tool to separate group A beta-hemolytic strep from other strep organisms. The information about rapid strep tests and the procedure for a throat culture with bacitracin are covered later in this chapter. Figure 44-7 shows a model of *Streptococci*.

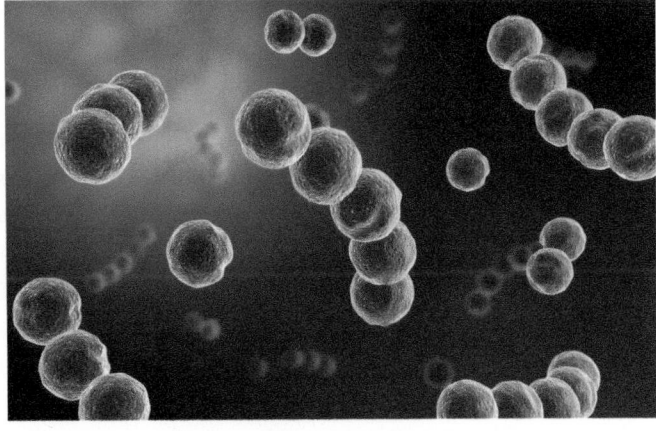

FIGURE 44-7 *Streptococci*: Individual bacteria that have a rounded shape and have clumped together to form a chain.

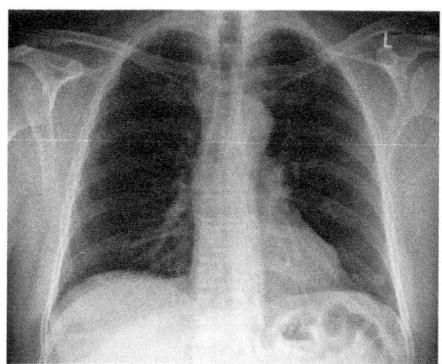

FIGURE 44-8 An X-ray showing pneumonia.

S. pneumoniae (also called *Pneumococcus* or *Diplococcus pneumoniae*) frequently are found as normal flora in the throat. However, it is the frequent cause of bacterial pneumonia (Figure 44-8), particularly in the older population, and in middle ear infections in children and meningitis in older children and adults.

Diplococci. *Diplococci* occur in pairs. Some *Diplococci* are Gram-positive, such as *S. pneumoniae*, which causes bacterial pneumonia. Others such as *N. gonorrhoeae* and *Neisseria meningitidis* are Gram-negative, the former causing gonorrhea, a sexually transmitted infection, and the latter causing a form of bacterial meningitis and septicemia. Meningococcal meningitis has a high mortality rate and requires immediate treatment. Injected vaccinations introduce a weakened form, allowing the body time to learn how to defeat it so that, when a true infection later occurs, it can be easily destroyed by the defense mechanisms already in place. A vaccine for meningococcal meningitis is now available that is recommended for students entering high school or college, those joining the armed services, and other individuals who may be at high risk (Figure 44-9).

Although these diplococcal organisms are pathogenic, many of the *Diplococci*, both Gram-negative and Gram-positive, are normally found in areas such as the upper respiratory tract.

Bacilli

Rod-shaped *Bacilli* (singular *Bacillus*) may be pathogenic or nonpathogenic. Some *Bacilli* are Gram-positive, and others are Gram-negative. Figure 44-10 illustrates *Bacilli*. Various *Bacilli* form chains of different lengths. Figure 44-11 shows *Diplobacillus* (a chain of two rods) and *Streptobacillus* (a longer chain). *Bacilli* are responsible for a wide variety of illnesses, including gastroenteritis, UTIs, whooping cough, tetanus, botulism, tuberculosis, and pneumonia.

Gram-Negative *Bacilli*. Enterobacteriaceae are a large family of Gram-negative *Bacilli* found mainly in the intestinal

tract; however, many of them cause infections in other body locations. One type, *E. coli*, is most frequently associated with UTIs. Another is the group of *Salmonella* organisms. *Salmonella* organisms are a major cause of foodborne illnesses worldwide. They can be classified serologically to differentiate which among the thousands of members of this pathogenic group are causing the outbreak of disease. Most frequently, outbreaks of food poisoning are caused either by *Salmonella enteritidis* or *S. typhimurium*. Symptoms of enteric food poisoning include rapid onset, abdominal pain, nausea, diarrhea, and in some children even death. Contaminated food such as raw eggs, chicken, or beef is the usual route of transmission.

Typhoid fever is caused by *S. typhimurium* and is frequently found in Third World countries and natural disaster areas where proper sanitation is lacking. Another member of the genus of Gram-negative *Bacilli* is a group of *Shigella* organisms that causes bacillary dysentery, characterized by frequent blood-, pus-, or mucus-containing stools. This bacillary dysentery results from inadequate sanitary conditions.

Another Gram-negative *Bacillus* not a member of the previously mentioned group is *Helicobacter pylori*, which was discovered in the early 1980s. This organism is found in about half of the human population and causes no symptoms in most individuals. It was discovered that *H. pylori* is the causative agent of peptic ulcers and a risk factor in gastric malignancy in some infected persons. The organism is responsive to a number of antibiotics, including tetracycline. The discovery of *H. pylori* led to major breakthroughs in ulcer treatment. Previously it was believed peptic ulcers were caused by anxiety or increased acid production, and treatments were generally ineffective.

Gram-Positive *Bacilli*. Gram-positive *Bacilli* may be found in chains or singly and are spore forming or non–spore forming. A **spore** is a thick-walled reproductive cell produced by some organisms that is capable of withstanding unfavorable environmental conditions. Notable in this group are *Clostridium botulinum*, which causes botulism, and *Clostridium tetani*, which causes tetanus. Tetanus immunizations are given to protect from the extremely potent neurotoxin produced by *C. tetani*. Tetanus is a disease resulting from a cut or injury associated with contaminated soil such as from a rusty farm implement. Botulism is a severe, possibly fatal form of food poisoning caused by the powerful neurotoxin produced by the anaerobe *C. botulinum*; it is associated with improper canning processes and its potential use as a bioterrorism agent.

Vibrio/Vibrios. *Vibrios* are comma-shaped *Bacilli*. The main pathogen is *Vibrio cholerae*, whose enterotoxin causes

Meningococcal Vaccines

What You Need to Know

1 What is meningococcal disease?

Meningococcal disease is a serious bacterial illness. It is a leading cause of bacterial meningitis in children 2 through 18 years old in the United States. Meningitis is an infection of the covering of the brain and the spinal cord.

Meningococcal disease also causes blood infections.

About 1,000–1,200 people get meningococcal disease each year in the U.S. Even when they are treated with antibiotics, 10–15% of these people die. Of those who live, another 11%–19% lose their arms or legs, have problems with their nervous systems, become deaf, or suffer seizures or strokes.

Anyone can get meningococcal disease. But it is most common in infants less than one year of age and people 16–21 years. Children with certain medical conditions, such as lack of a spleen, have an increased risk of getting meningococcal disease. College freshmen living in dorms are also at increased risk.

Meningococcal infections can be treated with drugs such as penicillin. Still, many people who get the disease die from it, and many others are affected for life. This is why preventing the disease through use of meningococcal vaccine is important for people at highest risk.

2 Meningococcal vaccine

There are two kinds of meningococcal vaccine in the U.S.:

- Meningococcal conjugate vaccine (**MCV4**) is the preferred vaccine for people 55 years of age and younger.

- Meningococcal polysaccharide vaccine (**MPSV4**) has been available since the 1970s. It is the only meningococcal vaccine licensed for people older than 55.

Both vaccines can prevent 4 types of meningococcal disease, including 2 of the 3 types most common in the United States and a type that causes epidemics in Africa. There are other types of meningococcal disease; the vaccines do not protect against these.

3 Who should get meningococcal vaccine and when?

Routine vaccination

Two doses of MCV4 are recommended for adolescents 11 through 18 years of age: the first dose at 11 or 12 years of age, with a booster dose at age 16.

Adolescents in this age group with HIV infection should get three doses: 2 doses 2 months apart at 11 or 12 years, plus a booster at age 16.

If the first dose (or series) is given between 13 and 15 years of age, the booster should be given between 16 and 18. If the first dose (or series) is given after the 16th birthday, a booster is not needed.

Other people at increased risk

- College freshmen living in dormitories.

- Laboratory personnel who are routinely exposed to meningococcal bacteria.

- U.S. military recruits.

- Anyone traveling to, or living in, a part of the world where meningococcal disease is common, such as parts of Africa.

- Anyone who has a damaged spleen, or whose spleen has been removed.

- Anyone who has persistent complement component deficiency (an immune system disorder).

- People who might have been exposed to meningitis during an outbreak.

Children between 9 and 23 months of age, and anyone else with certain medical conditions need 2 doses for adequate protection. Ask your doctor about the number and timing of doses, and the need for booster doses.

MCV4 is the preferred vaccine for people in these groups who are 9 months through 55 years of age. MPSV4 can be used for adults older than 55.

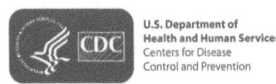

U.S. Department of Health and Human Services Centers for Disease Control and Prevention

FIGURE 44-9 A vaccine for meningococcal meningitis is now available.

cholera. Cholera is characterized by profuse watery stools, vomiting, leg cramps, dehydration, and shock. It is caused by ingesting drinking water or eating shellfish from water contaminated with infected urine, feces, or vomitus. Cholera is common in Asiatic countries, and travelers to these areas can be vaccinated for protection; however, travelers still should boil all drinking water and avoid uncooked foods. Figure 44-12 illustrates a *Vibrio*.

Spirilla

Spirilla (singular *Spirillum*), or spirochetes as they are also known, are spiral-shaped or corkscrew-shaped organisms. Technically, they are rods that are twisted in various shapes; however, they are classified as a separate phylum of bacteria. As with other shapes of bacteria, some are nonpathogenic and are found in certain areas of the body, and others, such as *Treponema pallidum*, cause the sexually transmitted infection

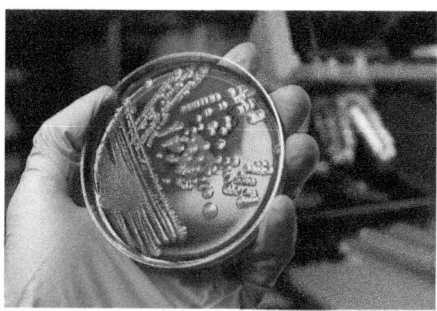

FIGURE 44-10 *Bacilli.*

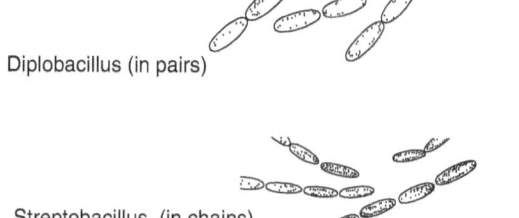

Diplobacillus (in pairs)

Streptobacillus (in chains)

FIGURE 44-11 *Diplobacillus* (a chain of two rods) and *Streptobacillus* (a longer chain).

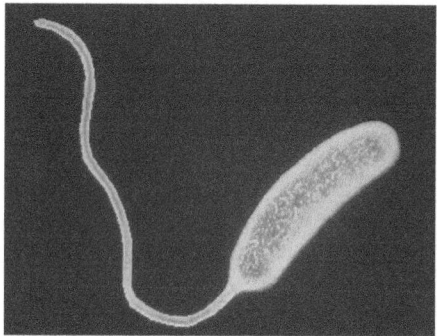

FIGURE 44-12 *Vibrio.*

syphilis. *Borrelia burgdorferi* was discovered in the mid-1970s to be the causative agent of Lyme disease. Lyme disease is a deer tick–borne disease named after a town in Connecticut that was investigating a cluster of juvenile arthritis cases. Ticks are infected by feeding on deer or rodents, which are natural hosts for the organism. The infected tick then bites a human and transmits the organism. This tick is so tiny that many people are unaware of the bite until the characteristic expanding rash is discovered, followed after a period of time by fever, muscle pain, headache, and fatigue. Immunoassay tests exist to aid in the diagnosis of Lyme disease. Figure 44-13 is an illustration of *Spirilla.*

Special Categories of Bacteria

Some types of bacteria do not fall clearly into any of the previously mentioned groups. These are *Mycobacteria, Rickettsia, Mycoplasma,* and *Chlamydia. Mycobacteria* have a different

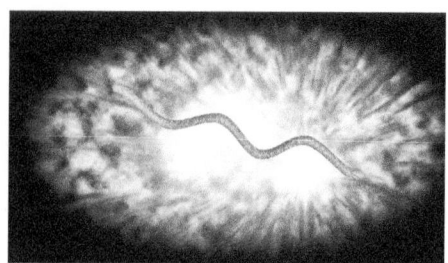

FIGURE 44-13 *Spirilla* bacteria. (*Ezume Images*)

type of material in the cell wall and can only be stained with an acid-fast stain. Two members of this genus are fairly well known.

Mycobacterium tuberculosis is the causative agent of tuberculosis, and *Mycobacterium leprae* is the cause of leprosy. These organisms do not stain well with a Gram stain. In a positive slide for acid-fast *Bacilli* (AFB), the slender *Bacilli* will appear pink with an acid-fast stain.

Rickettsia, Chlamydia, and *Mycoplasma* are very tiny bacteria in the size range of viruses. *Rickettsia* are bacterial parasites that live in ticks and mites and transmit the disease when they bite humans. Rocky Mountain spotted fever and typhus are both rickettsial diseases. *Chlamydia* is also an obligate parasite, but it does not live in arthropod hosts. *Chlamydia* must invade living cells to reproduce. *Chlamydia trachomatis* is an STI (sexually transmitted infection) that may be a silent inhabitant of the vagina or cause mild burning sensations and discharge. After repeated infections, this organism may cause scarring in the fallopian tubes, making conception difficult. *Rickettsia* and *Chlamydia* cannot be grown on artificial media. Tissue cultures or serological testing must be done for identification.

Mycoplasma were thought to be viruses at one time, but they are very tiny bacteria lacking a rigid cell wall. They cause *Mycoplasma* pneumonia and a type of venereal disease.

Viruses

Although potent, a virus is the smallest known infectious organism and requires the use of an electron microscope for visualization. A virus, a simpler form of life than a cell, is parasitic, depending on living cells of other organisms for growth. When a virus enters a cell, it may immediately cause a disease, such as influenza, or it may remain dormant for days or even years. Figure 44-14 shows an example of an influenza virus. For instance, herpes zoster may cause an outbreak of chickenpox within 7 to 14 days of exposure. Yet, HIV can lie dormant for a long period of time, sometimes years, before any symptoms are noted.

Viruses cause many common diseases, such as colds, chickenpox, mumps, infectious mononucleosis, and warts.

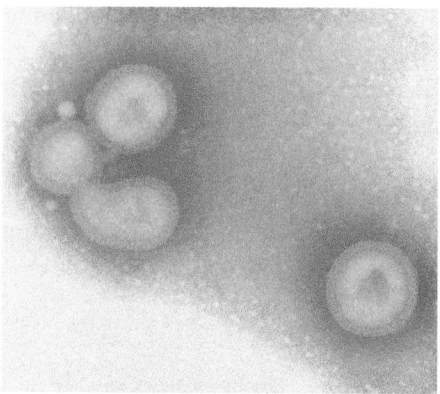

FIGURE 44-14 Influenza virus.

Other illnesses caused by viruses are hepatitis, measles, encephalitis, and herpes. Fortunately, vaccines are available to protect people from diseases such as polio, German measles, measles, hepatitis B, mumps, and chickenpox.

Protozoa

Although they are single-celled parasites, protozoa (singular protozoan) are usually larger than bacteria. Most protozoa live in the soil and receive nourishment from dead or decaying organic material. Lack of proper sanitation can lead to rapid spread of infections. Some protozoa are pathogenic and may cause diseases such as trichomoniasis (a type of STI caused by *T. vaginalis*), or malaria, which is transmitted by the bite of an infected *Anopheles* mosquito. The organism inhabits the red blood cells (RBCs) in the affected individual. Figure 44-15 models malaria protozoa.

Fungi

The study of fungi (singular **fungus**) is known as **mycology**. Fungi are present in soil, water, and air. Fungi are unable to

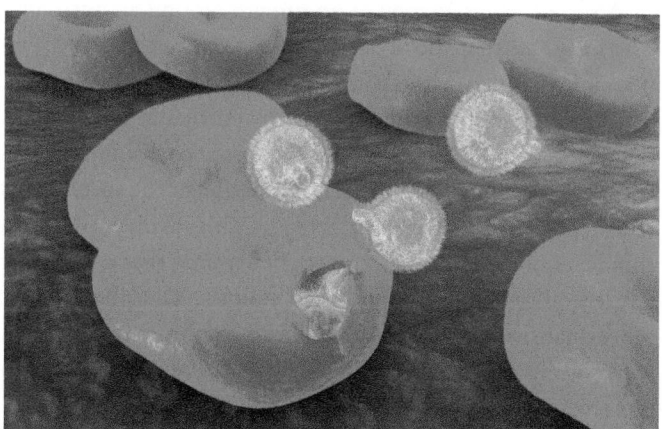

FIGURE 44-15 Model of malaria protozoa in a red blood cell. New parasites are produced and mature in the RBC, then push their way out of the cell.

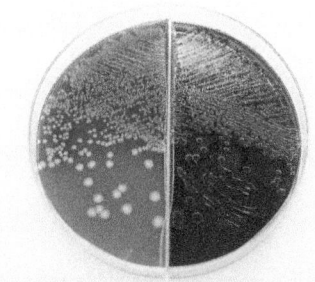

FIGURE 44-16 Mold is growing on red/green agar in a divided Petri dish.

make their own food, so they feed on other life forms. Included in this classification are yeasts and molds. In our environment we encounter fungi in the forms of mushrooms and penicillin molds on stale bread. *Penicillium* mold was discovered by Alexander Fleming, and its antibiotic properties changed modern medical treatment. Penicillin is now synthetically produced. Figure 44-16 shows an example of a mold.

Yeasts are single-celled fungi that reproduce by budding. Those fungi that produce spores are molds. Most fungi are not pathogenic and cause few diseases in humans. Of those that do, most will produce only superficial infections, such as athlete's foot (*Tinea pedis*) or ringworm. A few do produce life-threatening illnesses when they invade the internal organs of the body.

Candida albicans is the causative agent of the yeast infection known as **moniliasis**, **candidiasis**, or thrush. Individuals with compromised immune systems or those who have been on long-term antibiotic therapy may develop severe infections. In these cases, the normal flora that protect the openings of the body cavities are killed by the antibiotic therapy and allow fungi a fertile environment in which to reproduce. This type of infection is referred to as a superinfection. As anyone who has endured the unpleasantness of athlete's foot knows, it takes a long time and persistence to get rid of a fungal infection. Fungal infections are resistant to antibiotics and must be treated with antifungal agents.

Parasites

As previously noted, a parasite receives nourishment from another organism. As a result of this activity, the host organism becomes diseased. Parasites may be single celled, such as *Chlamydia*, or multicellular, such as pinworms.

Examples of parasites include worms and insects:

- **Worms (helminths)**—A person may ingest the egg or an immature form of the worm, or the worm may penetrate the skin. Some of the worms that infect people are flatworms, roundworms, tapeworms, and pinworms. Figure 44-17 shows a female roundworm.

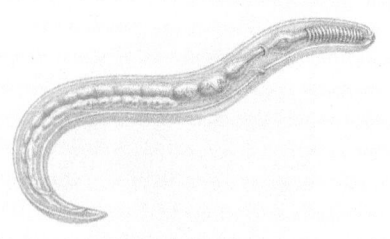

FIGURE 44-17 Female roundworm. Roundworms have long, cylindrical bodies with a tough covering. Eggs laid by the females are excreted in the feces of infected people.

Roundworms, flatworms, and tapeworms inhabit the intestines. Tapeworms, for instance, may grow to be many feet in length. The stool or **feces** of the patient can be inspected for the presence of ova and mature forms of the worm. The procedure for collecting stool for ova and parasites (O&P) is covered later in this chapter.

- Insects—Insects may bite, burrow under, or attach to the skin of a human. An example of a disease occurring by attachment of an insect is Lyme disease, caused by a tick-transmitted spirochete. Lyme disease has been documented in many parts of North America and has an incubation period of 3 to 32 days. Figure 44-18 shows a deer tick.

With early detection of Lyme disease and treatment with antibiotics, many patients have complete recovery. Arthritis may be a **sequela** (long-lasting effect) of Lyme disease. Cardiac conduction abnormalities, aseptic meningitis, and Bell's palsy may also be associated conditions.

Scabies and lice infestations are additional examples of insect parasites. Both are transmitted by direct contact with bedding or clothing and cause severe itching.

Refer to Table 44-2 for some examples of pathogenic microorganisms, their location in the body, and diseases they produce.

Medication-Resistant Microorganisms

Medication resistance occurs when a patient does not complete the full course of treatment and the surviving organism

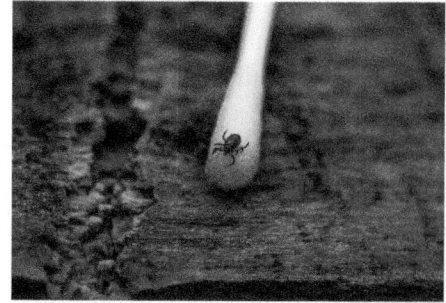

FIGURE 44-18 A deer tick can cause Lyme disease. *(puhimec)*

learns to live in the toxic environment, rendering that medication ineffective. This is a significant problem because it becomes increasingly difficult to treat that patient. Furthermore, the newly resistant organism may spread to others. Health care costs and the wellness of the population are quite dramatically impacted by these superbugs. Proper and consistent hand and personal hygiene are critically important in decreasing the prevalence of these difficult microorganisms.

DIAGNOSING INFECTION

When a patient comes to the office with an apparent infection, exactly what steps are taken to diagnose and begin treatment of the infection? First, the patient is examined and the usual procedures are followed, including gathering information, such as patient identification, vital signs, chief complaint, and present illness. If the infection is one that can be diagnosed on sight by the physician, such as chickenpox, further testing will not be necessary. For an open infected wound, the site should be measured, described, and charted, including information about drainage, odor, and level of patient discomfort.

Next, specimens are collected and labeled and prepared safely for transportation to ensure any organisms remain alive and safety issues are observed. A culture of the specimen may be necessary, in which case a swab of the specimen is streaked on appropriate culture medium in such a way as to allow individual colonies of microorganisms to develop. This permits easier identification. A second culture plate may be heavily **inoculated** (microorganisms placed on or in media) to be tested for antibiotic sensitivity. Certain microorganisms are sensitive to specific antibiotics and resistant to others. The culture plates are incubated at 37C° for 24 hours to allow the organisms to grow.

After 24 hours, a zone of no growth around an antibiotic disk indicates that the organism is sensitive to that drug, and if it is used to treat the patient, it should work in the same way. If the patient is allergic to that particular medication, then the antibiotic with the next largest zone of inhibition is chosen for treatment. If direct examination of the specimen is required, then a direct smear is made. This involves placing a thin layer of the specimen material on a slide that is properly labeled, allowed to dry, and then stained. The physician or other qualified personnel will examine it for microorganisms, considering their morphology and stain reactions (Gram-positive or Gram-negative). In some cases, a presumptive diagnosis can be made and treatment determined.

Preparation of a **wet mount** may be necessary in cases where the organisms, if present, must be kept alive to

TABLE 44-2 | Pathogenic Microorganisms and Resulting Diseases

Body Location	Pathogen	Disease
Respiratory System	*Streptococcus pyogenes*	Strep throat, scarlet fever
	Corynebacterium diphtheriae	Diphtheria
	Mycobacterium tuberculosis	Tuberculosis
	Haemophilus influenzae type B	Influenza
	Streptococcus pneumoniae	Pneumonia
Central Nervous System	*Neisseria meningitidis*	Meningitis
	Polioviruses	Poliomyelitis
	Rabies virus	Rabies
Genitourinary System	Herpes simplex viruses 1 and 2	Genital herpes
	Candida albicans (fungus)	Vaginitis
	Chlamydia trachomatis	Vaginitis
	Escherichia coli	Urinary tract infection
Integumentary System	*Staphylococcus aureus*	Boils, carbuncles
	Varicella zoster virus	Chickenpox
		Scabies
		Lice
Gastrointestinal System	Hepatitis A, B, and C viruses	Hepatitis A, B, and C
	Salmonella enteritidis	Food poisoning
	Escherichia coli	*E. coli* diarrhea
Circulatory System and Blood, Immune System	*Streptococcus pyogenes, Staphylococcus aureus*	Septicemia, endocarditis
	Plasmodium falciparum, P. vivax, P. malariae, P. ovale	Malaria
	Human immunodeficiency virus	HIV/AIDS
	Epstein-Barr virus	Infectious mononucleosis
	Borrelia burgdorferi	Lyme disease
Tissue	*Streptococcus pyogenes*	Necrotizing fasciitis

observe for motility and morphology. A wet mount is a preparation in a liquid that will preserve motility of the microbe. The ultimate goal of all these steps is to select the most favorable treatment that will restore the patient to a healthy condition. A more detailed discussion of the preceding steps follows.

SPECIMEN COLLECTION AND PROCESSING

Specimens for microbiology must be collected according to protocols established by the microbiology department of the laboratory performing the testing. One of the first priorities of quality control (QC) is proper specimen collection. No shortcuts may be taken in the collection process. Any incorrect steps could result in a contaminated or altered specimen, delayed diagnosis, and postponed or possibly harmful treatment. Sources of contamination might include microbes

that could be on swabs, surfaces, hands of medical assistants, or vectors other than cultured from the patient.

Guidelines 44-1 provides guidelines for specimen collection. Keep in mind when dealing with microbiological specimens that they are living organisms and must have proper conditions to survive but not to multiply.

Collection Devices

Sterile **swabs** are frequently used in collection of specimens. The shafts and the tips of swabs vary in terms of the type of material used. They are wrapped in a sterile wrapper or container to preserve sterility. Figure 44-19 shows examples of sterile swabs of various types. Cotton swabs are used less frequently today because certain microbes are inhibited by the natural ingredients in cotton. Polyester and rayon are used for the tips; wood, plastic, or wire is used for the shaft. Swabs also vary in size of tip and flexibility of the shaft to permit collection in difficult-to-reach areas. After a swab is

Specimen Collection

The basic rules for specimen collection are:

1. Confirm the identity of the patient by asking the patient to state his name and spell it, if necessary.
2. Screen the patient to determine if pretest preparation was followed.
3. Collect specimen before beginning antibiotic treatment.
4. Collect sufficient quantity of material for testing.
5. Use only appropriate collection technique by observing proper cleaning and aseptic procedures to control contamination.
6. Use only sterile containers.
7. Select the proper containers for collection that comply with the reference laboratory's or outside laboratory's requirements.
8. Ensure that the collection container is tightly closed and appropriately sealed to avoid leakage and contamination of the specimen and any surface with which the container may come in contact.
9. Label the specimen accurately at the time of collection with the following information:
    a. Patient's full name
    b. Date
    c. Time of collection
    d. Type of specimen
    e. Antibiotic treatment in use, if any
    f. Your initials
10. Fill out the requisition form for the reference lab and double-check that the information matches the label.
11. Deliver the specimen promptly to the laboratory and document it. Otherwise, maintain proper storage until the specimen can be picked up or transported appropriately.

Note: *Cerebrospinal fluid always requires immediate delivery.*

FIGURE 44-19 Examples of sterile swabs (removed from protective wrappers).

collected, it is placed in a sterile container that may or may not contain culture media.

Culture Tubes and Other Collection Devices

The **Culturette™ system** is composed of a disposable, clear plastic tube; a sterile, cotton-tipped applicator swab inside the tube; and a sealed plastic vial of medium (broth containing nourishment for bacteria and a preservative). This system is used to obtain many types of specimens, from sites ranging from the throat, nose, or eyes to wounds and the genital or urethral areas. Throat samples can be taken for tests like strep tests. Nasal samples are used for rapid tests such as influenza. Genital swabs are used to sample endocervical cells for Pap smears, to check for cervical cancer, or to check the vagina for bacterial vaginosis. It is important that these types of specimens, collected in Culturettes, be transported immediately so that microorganisms remain **viable** (capable of living) when they reach the laboratory. Commercially available swab collection and transportation units are widely used. Some of these units contain two sterile swabs, one for culturing and one for preparing the direct smear. A **smear** is a thin layer of microorganisms spread on a glass slide for identification purposes. (Figure 44-20 demonstrates a variety of collection devices, including a swab and Culturette in the lower left of the photograph.) Specimens such as **exudates** (wound drainage material made of serum, white blood cells, and fibrin) may be collected with Culturette units. Collection devices also are available for anaerobic cultures. Sterile containers are available for urine, stool, blood, and cerebrospinal fluid. Fluids drained from body cavities may require larger sterile containers.

Specimen Preservation

If possible, obtain specimens before antibiotics or other antimicrobial agents are administered. Collect specimens from the area where the microorganisms are most likely to be found and then store them in leak-proof containers, sealed tightly. Deliver the specimen to the laboratory promptly, usually within an hour, for best results. If the specimen cannot be processed immediately, most specimens can be stored in a refrigerator for up to several hours, except cerebral spinal fluid and blood.

Specimens for *Neisseria gonorrhoeae* isolation *must* be submitted on appropriate isolation plates (Martin-Lewis or Neigon agar plates). Do not refrigerate inoculated plates. All stool specimens being examined for ova or parasites require preservation in a formalin fixative and PVA or equivalent immediately after collection. Soft and liquid stools require PVA fixative to maintain the integrity of the trophozoites

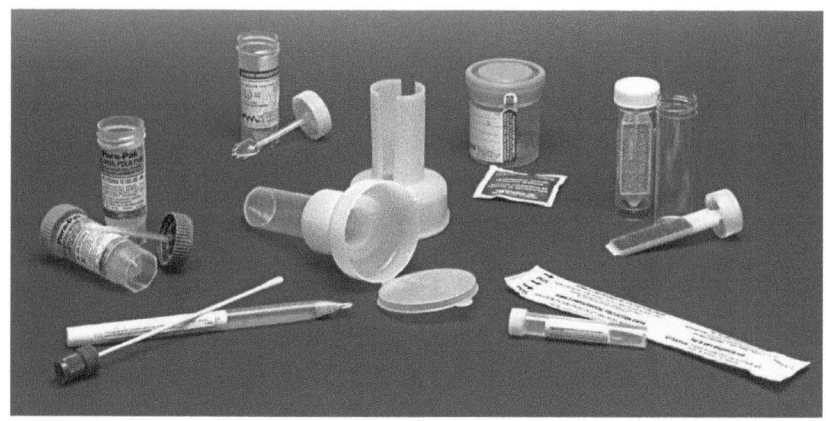

FIGURE 44-20 Examples of specimen collection containers for stool, urine, and swabs for wounds or secretions.

for the performance of the trichrome stain, and you must order ova and parasites with trichrome stain.

For mycobacterial (TB) culture, it is recommended to collect three sputum specimens for acid-fast smears and culture in patients with clinical and chest X-ray findings compatible with tuberculosis. These three samples should be collected at 8–24 hour intervals (24 hours when possible) and should include at least one first morning specimen.

For blood cultures, draw two to three separate sets within a 24-hour period, spaced as far apart as possible (a minimum of 30 minutes between sets). If sepsis is suspected, draw two separate sets before antimicrobial therapy is started; spaced a minimum of 30 minutes apart. For bacterial endocarditis, draw three separate sets before therapy. For fever of unknown origin (FUO), draw two separate sets initially, then two sets the next day just before the expected fever spike. Except as noted above for FUO, wait at least 72 hours from the time of first set for identification and sensitivity results before obtaining additional cultures. If cultures are still negative after 72 hours and the clinical condition warrants, draw a maximum of three more blood cultures over the next 24 hours. Wait another 72 hours for results.

Guidelines 44-2 discusses how to instruct a patient in collecting a stool specimen.

TYPES OF SPECIMENS

Pathogens can be observed in specimens of blood, feces, cerebrospinal fluid, mucus, urine, sputum, wounds, tissue, and exudates of other body substances. The following paragraphs discuss these types of specimens and information for obtaining them.

Throat

One of the most frequently requested specimens in a physician's office laboratory (POL) is the throat swab or culture.

Based on signs and symptoms the patient presents with, such as upper respiratory infection, sore throat, or sinus infection, the physician will order a throat culture to identify the pathogen involved and begin treatment. Confirmation of *Streptococcus pyogenes* is important because of its virulence and possible complications. When you are performing a throat culture, it is important not to touch the inside of the mouth or the tongue with the swab to avoid contaminating it. Procedure 44-1 lists the steps for correctly obtaining a throat culture.

If the culture is to be done in house, then it is streaked as mentioned previously. A bacitracin antibiotic disk will be placed on the culture plate in the area with the heaviest inoculation. A zone of no growth around the disk is presumptive evidence that the pathogen is group A beta-hemolytic strep. Other strep organisms are not sensitive to bacitracin. Bacitracin is not used to treat strep throat, only as a differentiating antibiotic. Broad-spectrum antibiotics such as penicillin, ampicillin, and erythromycin are used to treat strep. If strep is suspected, an antigen–antibody test for strep may be ordered. These types of tests are discussed later in the chapter.

Nasal swabs are sometimes requested, and care should be taken to label the swabs "Right" and "Left" to identify from which nostril the specimen was taken. Smaller sterile swabs with thinner, more flexible shafts are generally used for obtaining nasal specimen.

Guidelines 44-2

Instructing the Patient in Collecting a Stool Specimen

When instructing a patient to collect a stool specimen at home, ensure the patient has the following:

- Sterile specimen container with lid (for culture or ova and parasite testing)
- Biohazard transport bag
- Bedpan or other container for the collection of stool

Instruct the patient as follows:

1. Capture stool in container for stool.
2. Place only stool in the specimen container and close lid tightly.
3. Wash hands.
4. Label with name and time of collection, and place in biohazard bag.
5. Bring stool specimen to laboratory immediately. Refrigerate if it is not possible to drop off at laboratory within two hours.

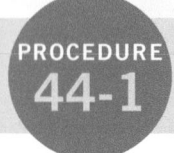

PROCEDURE 44-1

Performing a Throat Swab for Culture

Objective ◆ *Collect a throat or nasopharyngeal culture without contaminating the specimen.*

EQUIPMENT AND SUPPLIES

Culturette system; laboratory requisition; tongue depressor; gloves; biohazard waste container

Note: Follow standard precautions and safety guidelines when working with body fluid samples. Use care to avoid splashing or spilling body fluids. Wipe up all spills using guidelines established by OSHA.

METHOD

1. Assemble equipment and Culturette system.
2. Identify the patient and explain the procedure.
3. Perform hand hygiene and apply gloves.
4. Position the patient facing a light source, and have the patient open the mouth as wide as possible (Figure A). The gag reflex may be diminished if the patient says "Aaaah."
5. Remove the sterile swab from the Culturette.
6. Depress the tongue, insert the swab, and roll it firmly across the back of the patient's throat or nasopharyngeal area where infected. Be careful not to contaminate the swab on the teeth, lips, tongue, or inside of the cheeks. Avoid touching the uvula to prevent gagging.
7. Insert the swab into a plastic vial. Crush the internal vial of transport medium, making sure that the swab is saturated.

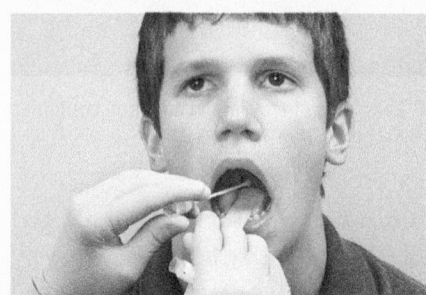

FIGURE A Swab the posterior pharynx between the tonsils.

8. Place the transport medium in labeled mailing or transporting envelope and staple shut if necessary. If being evaluated in the POL, immediately inoculate the culture plate, and apply a bacitracin disk according to office procedure.
9. Remove and dispose of gloves.
10. Perform hand hygiene.
11. Document the procedure in the patient's record.

CHARTING EXAMPLE

2/14/YY 9:00 A.M. Throat culture obtained. Specimen labeled and sent to outside lab. (Specify name of the lab.)....................
....M. King, CMA (AAMA)

Sputum

To obtain a **sputum** (mucous substance expelled by coughing or clearing the bronchi) specimen, the patient must be carefully instructed to cough deeply and spit up the coughed material into a sterile container. Explain to the patient that this should not be saliva from the mouth. Often it is possible to obtain a good sputum specimen if the patient is reminded to try to collect it on rising in the morning (in a sterile container provided by the POL). The purpose for obtaining a sputum specimen is to isolate and diagnose diseases such as streptococcal pneumonia, influenza, and tuberculosis. Refer to Procedure 44-2 for directions on obtaining a sputum specimen.

Urine

Urinalysis is discussed the chapter titled "Urinalysis"; however, obtaining a urine culture is an important procedure in this chapter on microbiology. A urine specimen for culture must be either a catheterized specimen or a clean-catch midstream sample (CCMS). Both methods provide sterile samples. Any other type of urine specimen (one for routine analysis, for example) would be contaminated by organisms in the container or on the hands or genitals of the patient. See Procedure 45-1 in the chapter titled "Urinalysis" for collection of a clean-catch midstream urine specimen from both male and female patients.

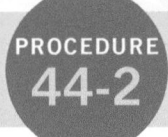

PROCEDURE 44-2

Obtaining a Sputum Specimen for Culture

Objective ◆ *Collect a sputum specimen without contaminating the specimen.*

EQUIPMENT AND SUPPLIES

Sterile labeled sputum container with lid; lab requisition form; gloves; biohazard waste container

Note: Follow standard precautions and safety guidelines when working with body fluid samples. Use care to avoid splashing or spilling body fluids. Wipe up all spills using the guidelines established by OSHA.

METHOD

1. Identify the patient.
2. Explain the procedure and give written instructions that the patient can take home, if necessary. Explain that the patient should breathe in or out deeply two to four times and perform a few low, deep coughs to raise sputum. This avoids getting only saliva. The first morning specimen, collected before eating or drinking, usually provides the best sample.
   a. Cough deeply and expel fluid into center of container and close lid immediately (Figures A and B).
   b. Make sure no other fluids, such as tears, nasal mucus, or saliva, find their way into the cup.
   c. Fit the lid securely; then write the time and date the specimen was obtained.
   d. Bring the specimen into the physician's office as soon as possible, or place it in a refrigerator for no longer than two hours.
3. Perform hand hygiene and apply gloves.
4. Label the transport envelope with information, staple it shut, and transport sample immediately.
5. Remove and dispose of gloves and perform hand hygiene.
6. Document the procedure in the patient's record.

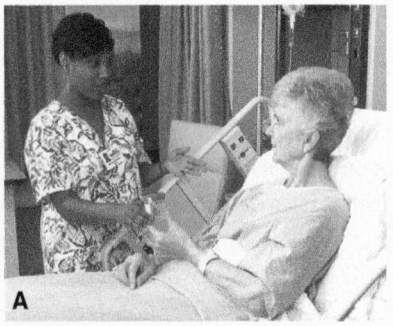

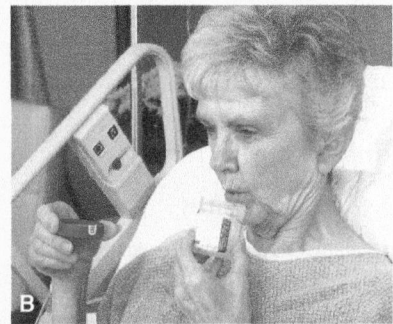

FIGURE A, B (A) Instruct the patient to cough deeply to bring up sputum; **(B)** instruct the patient to obtain 1 to 2 teaspoons of sputum; then close and seal the container with the lid.

CHARTING EXAMPLE

2/14/YY 10:30 a.m. Sputum specimen collected. Labeled and sent to outside lab. (Specify name of the lab.)........................
....M. King, CMA (AAMA)

Stool

Stool, or feces (waste product from the bowel), may be tested for bacterial, parasitic, or protozoal infections; for the presence of occult blood; and for excessive amounts of fat (**steatorrhea**). The collection of stool specimens varies with the type of test ordered. Discussing stool sample collection is often embarrassing to both patient and medical assistant; however, correct collection is critical to an accurate result. Fecal specimens must be free of urine, water from the toilet, and toilet tissue.

Stool Culture

To detect bacteria or viruses, a small amount of feces is needed. The collection containers must be sterile, and aseptic technique must be used in the collection process. Once collected, the stool must be sent immediately to the testing facility. Sterile collection devices are available. Sheets of special paper, coverings for the toilet, and bedpans can be used to collect specimens. Sterile tongue depressors or applicator sticks can be used to transfer a small amount of stool to a sterile container for transport to the laboratory or office. In the office, a sterile bedpan may be used, or a sterile pan may be placed over the bowl of the toilet. The sample is transferred to a sterile specimen container and sent to the lab for testing.

Occult Blood

A stool specimen is required to test for occult or hidden blood that may indicate bleeding in the gastrointestinal tract. Often the patient is given the test units to take home and collect the specimen. Directions are provided on each test unit; however, you should review the instructions each time they are given to a patient. Patients are instructed to write their name, date, and doctor's name on the label of the collection unit. Using one of the wooden spatulas provided, they are to collect a small amount of stool and place it in one of the circles on the back of the booklet, obtain another sample from a different area of the stool, and place this sample on the other circle. Patients should close the unit and take it or mail it to the doctor's office or the laboratory as requested. See the procedure on testing for occult blood in the chapter titled "Assisting with Medical Specialties."

For more accurate results, patients should be instructed to refrain from consuming vitamin C and red meat for three days before testing because those substances may cause false positives. Also, it is important to check the expiration date of any test kit before giving it to the patient.

Stool for Ova and Parasites

The presence of microbial organisms, such as ova and parasites (O&P), may be determined by testing feces or stool. The presence of ova (eggs) or other forms of a parasite indicate parasitic infestation. Identification of the parasite aids in selecting the correct treatment. Commercial kits are available that provide containers for fresh stool specimens and two additional vials for preserved specimens: one containing formalin and the other containing polyvinyl alcohol.

The patient should be instructed to mix portions of stool in each vial and seal. If O&P are suspected, three specimen collections will be requested. The specimen is usually obtained in the early morning. The patient should be instructed to defecate into a stool specimen container or into a bedpan, if available, placed over the toilet. The stool specimen samples should be taken from several different parts of the stool because O&P may be in one portion of the stool and not another.

Collecting Pinworm Specimens. One examination for ova and parasites may be performed in the office. The pinworm (*Enterobius vermicularis*) is a common parasite that inhabits the lower gastrointestinal tract with mature pinworms migrating out of the anus at night, causing intense itching. Transmission is by the fecal–oral route or by ingesting eggs with hand-to-mouth transmission. Adult worms mate in the colon, and the female migrates out of the anus at night to lay eggs. The eggs stick to the anal area, pajamas, and other items of clothing. Collection of a specimen should be done first thing in the morning before a bowel movement or bathing to detect ova or worms. The collection of a pinworm specimen can be done in the office or at home by touching the anus with the sticky side of a piece of tape, then affixing it to a microscope slide.

Medications are available for treatment, and reexamination is recommended after a cycle of medication has been completed. In addition, parents and other infected individuals must be told to observe strict personal hygiene, including laundering of all bedding and underclothing on a regular basis. It may be necessary to examine other family members and playmates for signs of infection if reinfestation occurs.

Wound Specimens

Sterile swabs are used to obtain a specimen from a wound, abscess, or incision to test for pathogenic microorganisms (Figure 44-21). The procedure is similar to obtaining a throat

Professionalism   The Life Span

Throat cultures are not pleasant for the patient. Children often rebel at the idea of a throat culture. Using a soothing voice and calm manner helps. The procedure should be done quickly without touching the tongue or inside of cheeks. A tongue depressor is used to hold the tongue down and avoid the uvula because touching it will cause gagging. Explain that the procedure will take only a few seconds, and give the patient an example of what "a few seconds" means, such as "Saying the ABCs lasts a few seconds."

The procedure should be done with the child lying down. The parent, caregiver, or another medical assistant can assist. If the child refuses to open her mouth, squeeze the nostrils shut, and the patient will open the mouth. Once the swab is removed, place it at once in its plastic covering, taking care not to touch the outside of the covering. Console the child afterward, and be sure to compliment good behavior.

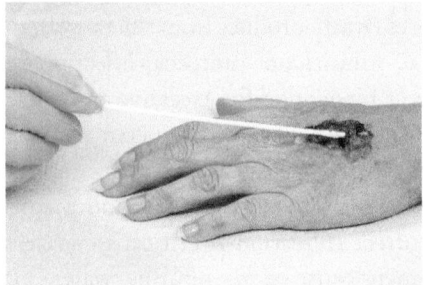

FIGURE 44-21 Swab the inside of the wound.

culture. Several specimens may be necessary from different locations. Be certain to label the source of each specimen.

Other Types of Specimens

Cerebrospinal fluid (CSF) is always treated as a stat procedure. The procedure to collect CSF is uncomfortable for the patient, and the specimen must be handled with care. Usually three tubes are collected under sterile conditions and sent for testing. The **culture and sensitivity (C&S) test**, performed to determine what organisms are growing and what effectively kills them, should be performed before chemical and other tests using the second of the three tubes. (See Box 44-1 for more information on sensitivity testing.) The first and third tubes are more likely to be contaminated because of the entry and removal processes of collection.

Blood and CSF under normal conditions are free of any type of microorganisms. Commercially available containers containing a broth media are widely used to grow cultures to test for septicemia or bacteremia.

MICROBIOLOGY EQUIPMENT AND PROCEDURES

The equipment and supplies necessary in a microbiology laboratory vary with the size and type of facility. A typical POL has a microscope, incubator, autoclave, refrigerator, biohazard waste containers, and a variety of specimen collection devices and containers (all of which are discussed in other chapters). Inoculation equipment (equipment for implanting microorganisms into a culture medium), such as loop, needle, and incineration equipment and culture media, are also necessary to process microbiology specimens.

Inoculating Equipment

A loop is a long instrument with a small loop on the end designed to pick up fluids and transfer them to culture media. Specifically calibrated loops for urine cultures are available that allow for the transfer of 1 μL (microliter) of urine to a culture plate. This precise amount of urine allows for quantitative evaluation of the number of microorganisms to evaluate whether a UTI is present. Inoculating loops and needles (a needle is a long, straight instrument with a pointed end used to sample individual colonies of microorganisms) may be purchased in sterile, prewrapped packages or may be made of metal for sterilization and reuse. After a prewrapped sterile loop or needle is used, it is discarded in a biohazard waste container. A metal loop or needle requires incineration before and after use to ensure sterility; Bunsen burners requiring a natural gas supply or electric incinerators are used.

Culture Media

Once a specimen has been obtained, it must be inoculated onto a medium that will enhance the growth of the microorganism. The most common types of **culture media** are broth and agar. A culture is the propagation of microorganisms or living cells in a special media that enhances their growth. Some types of media contain special dyes or ingredients that will enhance the growth of one type of bacteria while retarding growth of others to enable easier identification. The microbiologist observes the culture for the presence and the appearance of a **colony**, or group of living organisms, then examines a sample of the specimen under a microscope for morphology and staining properties. Each bit of information about the nature of the microorganism assists in identification and diagnosis.

All media should be inspected for contamination before use to ensure the integrity of the culturing process. Media may be solid like a slant (agar in a tube placed in a tilted position to harden), semisolid like agar, or liquid like broth. Media will either inhibit or encourage the growth of certain pathogens and are classified as supportive, selective, differential, or enrichment:

- **Supportive**—Used to grow a wide variety of organisms
- **Selective**—Encourages growth of some organisms and restricts growth of others (e.g., vaginal and stool cultures). Figure 44-22 shows an example of a fecal culture growing on selective media.
- **Differential**—Includes dyes or chemicals that give organisms a different appearance (e.g., differentiate *Staphylococci*)
- **Enrichment**—Contains special organic substances needed to encourage growth of organisms that are fastidious (fussy) (e.g., gonorrhea organisms)

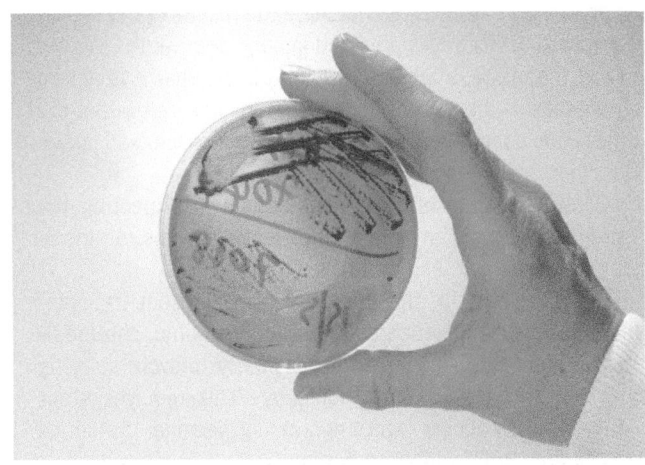

FIGURE 44-22 Petri dish containing fecal bacteria cultures.

TABLE 44-3 | Culture Media and Isolates

Common Culture Media	Isolates
Blood agar	Most bacteria
Chocolate agar	*Neisseria, Haemophilus*
Eosin-methylene blue (EMB)	Gram-negative bacteria
MacConkey agar	Gram-negative bacteria
Thioglycollate broth	Anaerobic microorganisms
Gram-negative (BN) broth	Fecal microorganisms

Inoculating Media

Pathogens are identified by growing cultures (propagating microorganisms) taken from the specimen. Colonies of bacteria can be grown only on certain media. Pathogens are often identified by the manner in which they grow on a particular medium. An example of this is *Streptococci* bacteria that cause strep throat. Mucus swabbed from a sore throat inoculated on a medium that contains blood will produce pinpoint-size colonies that have a transparent ring around each, which is the result of hemolysis or bursting of red blood cells by the *Streptococci* in the surrounding medium. Table 44-3 lists common culture media and microorganisms that can be isolated on each.

The main goal in growing cultures is to separate pathogenic colonies of organisms from colonies of normal flora

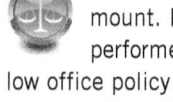

Professionalism   The Law

Confidentiality regarding any patient testing is paramount. Results of testing are confidential, whether performed in the POL or an outside laboratory. Follow office policy concerning who is or is not allowed to give results to the patient. If you call the patient at home and get an answering machine, do not leave the results of the test as a message. State your name and facility, and ask the patient to call the office, after assuring the patient that it is not an emergency. If the patient does not return your call within the time limits considered appropriate for your office, call again. Document calls made to your patients.

Careful labeling of specimens assists in protecting the patient and physician from an incorrect diagnosis. An incorrect diagnosis can lead to delayed treatment.

Because many of the microorganisms present in specimens taken in the office setting are pathogenic, the medical assistant has an ethical responsibility to avoid carrying the microbes outside the laboratory. This requires strict adherence to policies regarding wearing personal protective equipment (PPE) and hand hygiene.

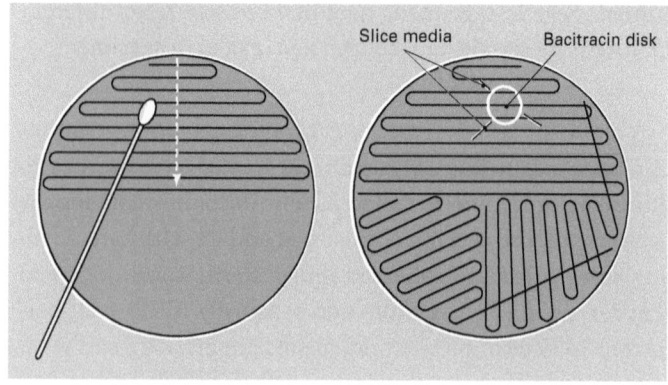

FIGURE 44-23 Swabbing a Petri dish to spread apart colonies. Bacitracin disk is used to prove the presence or absence of *S. pyogenes*.

(Figure 44-23). To isolate colonies, the agar must be inoculated properly. The specimen is transferred by rubbing the swab across one small area of the agar near the edge. Next, a wire inoculating loop is sterilized in a Bunsen burner flame or electric incinerator, cooled, and used to streak through the area already inoculated and onto an unmarked area of the agar in a zigzag motion. This procedure is repeated twice more to inoculate the remaining two sections of the agar. This is called quadrant streaking to isolate colonies and is illustrated in Figure 44-24.

After inoculation, the lid or top of the Petri dish is replaced and the agar plate inverted and placed into an incubator upside-down (Figure 44-25). The inversion of the agar plate allows moisture to collect on the lid of the Petri dish and not on the culture itself. The culture is allowed to grow in the incubator at 37°C for a 24-, 48-, or 72-hour period. Fungi take longer to grow and may need to grow at slightly lower temperatures.

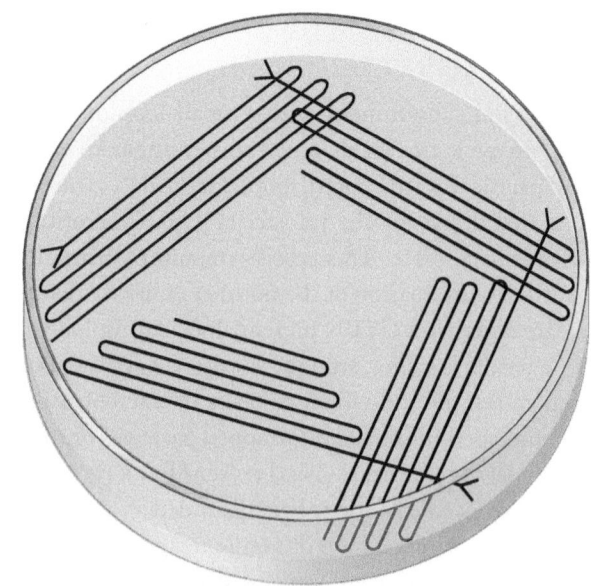

FIGURE 44-24 Quadrant streaking.

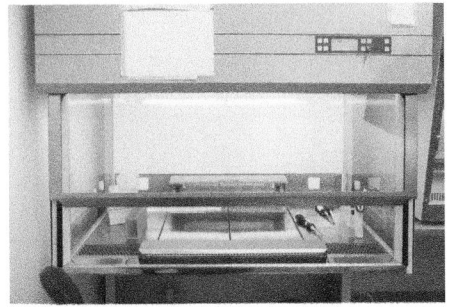

FIGURE 44-25 An incubation chamber. *(WavebreakmediaMicro)*

A secondary culture can be obtained by selecting an isolated colony from the initial agar plate and placing it on another media plate using a sterile loop or needle. This provides a pure culture, a colony containing only one type of organism. Identification of the organism is made by using the pure culture to prepare and stain a slide and by performing various biochemical tests.

Instruments such as Vitek and Autobac use automated technology to facilitate organism identification. The BAC-T Screen Bacteruria-Pyuria Detection Device is an automated system that immediately determines if significant numbers of bacteria are present in a urine specimen, avoiding the 24- to 48-hour wait for complete growth and identification. All the tests mentioned are performed by medical laboratory specialists.

Direct Examination

Two methods are used to prepare a specimen for direct examination under the microscope: the direct smear and the wet mount preparation. These methods allow the physician to obtain information quickly in the office and thus start treatment immediately.

Direct Smear

A direct smear may be from a swab of the specimen or from a colony on a culture plate (Procedure 44-3). The smear from a specimen is made after the culture is inoculated to prevent contamination of the media because slides are not usually sterile. The swab is rolled carefully across the slide so all areas of the swab touch the slide. The slide is labeled by placing the patient's name and specimen type on the

---

BOX 44-1 | Sensitivity Testing

Once the physician or laboratory specialist identifies the pathogenic organism on the culture, it is necessary to determine which antibiotics will be effective in killing these bacteria. This method of detection is called sensitivity testing. A new Petri dish with Mueller-Hinton agar is prepared with the pure culture specimen, using overlapping strokes in a technique called the **lawn technique** or colony count (Figure 44-26). Several disks, each soaked in a different antibiotic, are placed on top of the inoculated agar. The lid of the Petri dish is replaced, inverted, and placed in the incubator for 24 hours (Figure 44-27). After 24 hours, the organism will have grown all over except around those disks that inhibit its growth. These zones around the disks are measured to determine the susceptibility of the organism to each particular antibiotic disk. The disk with the largest, clearest area around it has the most effective medication. After the best antibiotic is identified, the patient is given that medication.

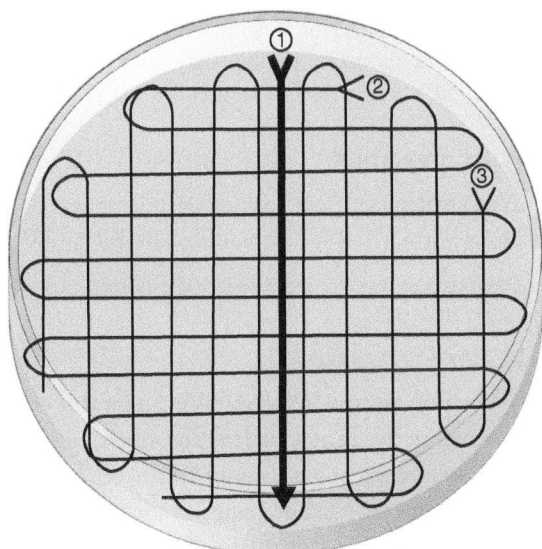

FIGURE 44-26 Lawn spread or colony count streaking.

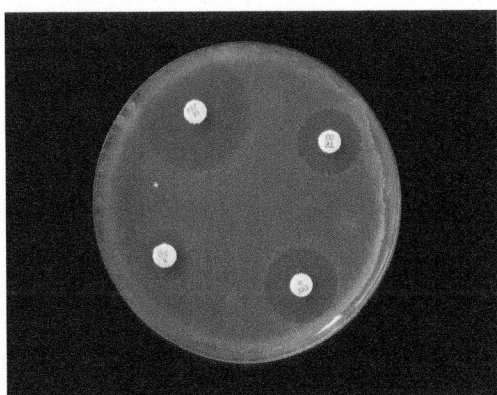

FIGURE 44-27 Paper disks containing various antibiotics are placed on a bacterial culture. If the bacteria are sensitive to that particular antibiotic drug, a large clear zone of inhibition or no growth will appear around that particular disk.

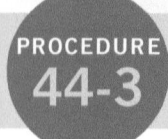

PROCEDURE 44-3 Preparing a Smear

Objective ◆ *Prepare a smear for microscopic examination.*

EQUIPMENT AND SUPPLIES

Frosted slides; specimen from Culturette applicator or inoculating loop; Bunsen burner; inoculating loop (or swab); microscope; oil immersion; gloves; biohazard waste container

Note: Follow standard precautions and safety guidelines when working with body fluid samples. Use care to avoid splashing or spilling body fluids. Wipe up all spills using guidelines established by OSHA.

METHOD

1. Perform hand hygiene and apply gloves.
2. Assemble equipment.
3. Label a clean slide with the patient's name, date, and type of specimen.
4. Collect a specimen sample. To transfer a swabbed specimen to a slide, roll the swab over the entire slide (Figures A–C). To transfer a specimen from a culture medium, use a sterile needle or loop to pick up the material from one type of colony, place it in a drop of sterile saline on the slide, and spread it gently over two-thirds of the slide.
5. Allow the slide to air-dry for 20 to 30 minutes.

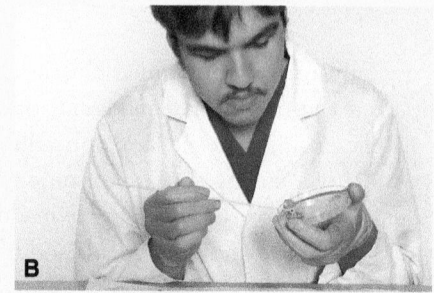
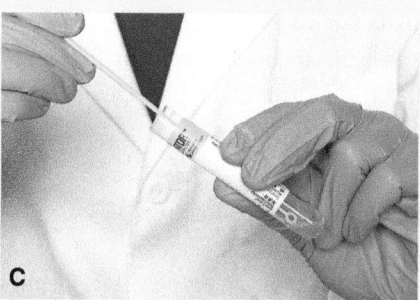

FIGURE B–C (B) Using a loop to pick up a microbial specimen to spread on slide; **(C)** using a loop to obtain a sample of material from a liquid media.

6. Hold the slide with thumb forceps and pass the slide over the Bunsen burner flame. This heat fixes the specimen to the slide in the process known as smear fixation. Let the slide cool. If open flame is unavailable, flood the dry smear with methanol and let it dry to fix the slide.
7. The slide is then ready to be stained.

CHARTING EXAMPLE

11/16/YY Direct smear from abscess RT thigh prepared for staining...M. King, CMA (AAMA)

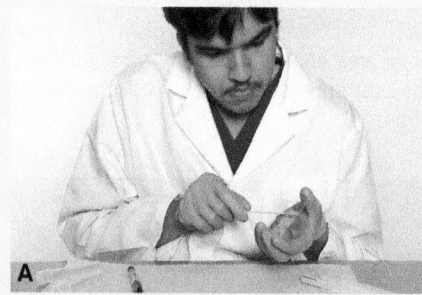

FIGURE A Roll and turn the swab across the slide.

frosted end of the slide. The smear air-dries; do not wave it in the air, which could spread microorganisms. The slide must be **fixed** to ensure that the specimen material remains on the slide during the staining process. It is fixed by passing the clear underneath part of the slide through an open flame three to four times or flooding the slide with methanol and letting it dry. These steps must be done before any staining procedure.

Wet Mount Preparation

Wet mount preparation involves taking a sample either from a colony or directly from a patient specimen, placing it on a frosted slide, and adding a drop of sterile normal saline and a cover slip. A wet mount preparation such as this allows the physician to observe the motility of the organism and what types of cytoplasmic extensions the organisms have (cilia, flagella). These observations render important identifying

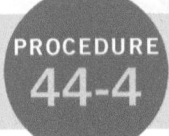

PROCEDURE 44-4   Preparing a Wet Mount Slide

Objective ◆ *Prepare a wet mount slide for microscopic examination.*

EQUIPMENT AND SUPPLIES

Clean, dry slide, frosted; cover slip; saline; specimen from a Culturette applicator or swab; paper/pen; microscope; gloves

Note: Follow standard precautions and safety guidelines when working with body fluid samples. Use care to avoid splashing or spilling body fluids. Wipe up all spills using guidelines established by OSHA.

METHOD

1. Perform hand hygiene and apply gloves.
2. Label dry slide with the patient's name and date.
3. Inoculate the dry slide by rolling a swab containing the specimen across the surface.
4. Place a drop of saline solution on top of the specimen.
5. Place the cover slip on top of the smeared slide.

   Note: The following steps would be performed by a physician or laboratory specialist (Figure A).

6. Observe the wet mount slide immediately under the microscope.
7. Special stains may be used to enhance characteristics.
8. Note what is observed, remove the slide, and dispose of it properly.
9. Remove gloves and perform hand hygiene.
10. Chart the findings on the patient's record.

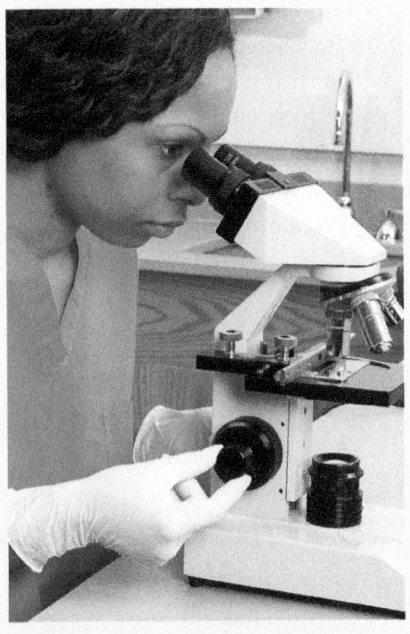

FIGURE A A medical technician examining a wet mount.

CHARTING EXAMPLE

11/16/YY Wet mount prepared from vaginal swab for physician to examine..M. King, CMA (AAMA)

information. Refer to Procedure 44-4 for instructions on the preparation of a wet mount slide.

In the POL, a wet mount for fungus often is performed using potassium hydroxide (KOH). Fungus is often difficult to see on direct preparation because keratin from the body, particularly nails, hair, and skin, often obscures the fungal structures. Potassium hydroxide dissolves the keratin, allowing visualization of any fungi present, such as yeast that causes vaginitis (Figure 44-28). To prepare a KOH mount, a specimen is suspended in 1 drop of 10 percent potassium hydroxide and a cover slip is applied. Allow the specimen to sit at room temperature for 30 minutes to dissolve the keratin. The slide will be examined by the physician or laboratory specialist for evidence of fungi in the wet mount.

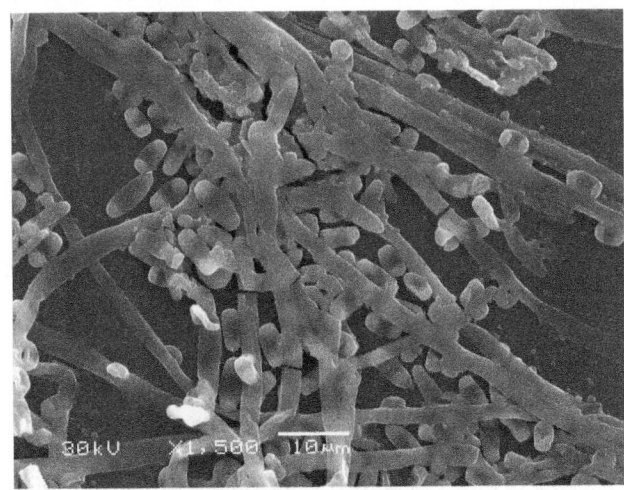

FIGURE 44-28 Example of fungi.

Staining Specimens

The use of stained smears in microbiology is extensive. The color and shape (morphology) of microorganisms on smears can be observed, for example, in vaginal and nasopharyngeal specimens. Although a medical assistant is not trained to perform Gram staining in the medical setting, it is important to know how to prepare a smear and have a general knowledge of the Gram stain and why it is used. Because several colors are used, the Gram stain differentiates, or separates, bacteria into two groups: Gram-positive and Gram-negative. Different bacteria stain differently, depending on the compounds in their walls. Gram-positive bacteria retain the crystal violet-blue color, and Gram-negative bacteria retain only the pink safranine color. Thus, Gram-positive (violet) bacteria can be distinguished from Gram-negative (pink) bacteria. Precautions must be taken in Gram staining in that temperature, age of specimen, or length of incubation could cause a change in Gram-positive bacteria. Gram stains must always be accompanied by culture for microorganism identification.

Procedure 44-5 and Figures A–F list the steps needed to perform a Gram stain correctly. Particular attention must be paid to the timing of the various steps. Crystal violet is poured on a fixed smear for one minute. The stain is washed off with water, and iodine is applied for one minute. The iodine is washed off, and the decolorizer is used to wash for 15 seconds. (Care must be taken not to decolorize too long because it will make the slide difficult to evaluate.) Next, safranine is applied to the slide for 30 seconds, followed by washing the slide and wiping off the back side of the slide to remove excess stain, then standing it upright to dry.

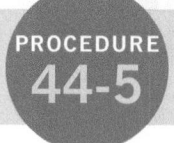

PROCEDURE 44-5   Performing a Gram Stain

Objective ◆ *Prepare a slide for a Gram stain to differentiate a Gram-positive organism from a Gram-negative organism.*

EQUIPMENT AND SUPPLIES

Gram-stain kit with decolorizer; culture specimen; slides; Bunsen burner or methanol; staining rack; water wash bottle; water; immersion oil; stopwatch; gloves; slide stand; paper towels; biohazard waste container

Note: Follow standard precautions and safety guidelines when working with body fluid samples. Use care to avoid splashing or spilling body fluids. Wipe up all spills using guidelines established by OSHA.

METHOD

1. Perform hand hygiene and apply gloves.
2. Assemble equipment.
3. Make a smear, label it, air-dry the smear, and use heat or methanol to fix.
4. Place the slide on a staining rack, smear side up.
5. Pour crystal violet solution all over the slide; let it stand one minute (Figure A).
6. Tilt the slide to drain the excess crystal violet stain and rinse with water (Figure B).
7. Pour Gram's iodine stain all over the slide; let it stand one minute (Figure C).
8. Tilt the slide to drain excess iodine and rinse with water.
9. Gently pour decolorizer with alcohol-acetone all over the slide for 15 seconds or until the color blue stops running (Figure D).
10. Rinse with water.
11. Pour safranine stain all over the slide, and let it stand for 30 seconds (Figure E).
12. Tilt the slide to drain the excess safranine and rinse with water. Wipe the back of the slide (Figure F).
13. Stand the slide on end on a paper towel or in a slide drying rack, and air-dry.

    Note: Examination of a Gram-stained slide is beyond the scope of practice of the medical assistant. It should be performed by a physician or laboratory specialist.

14. Examine under the microscope, using oil immersion lens and oil.

CHARTING EXAMPLE

11/16/YY Gram stain of spec. from abscess of RT thigh prepared for physician to examine...............M. King, CMA (AAMA)

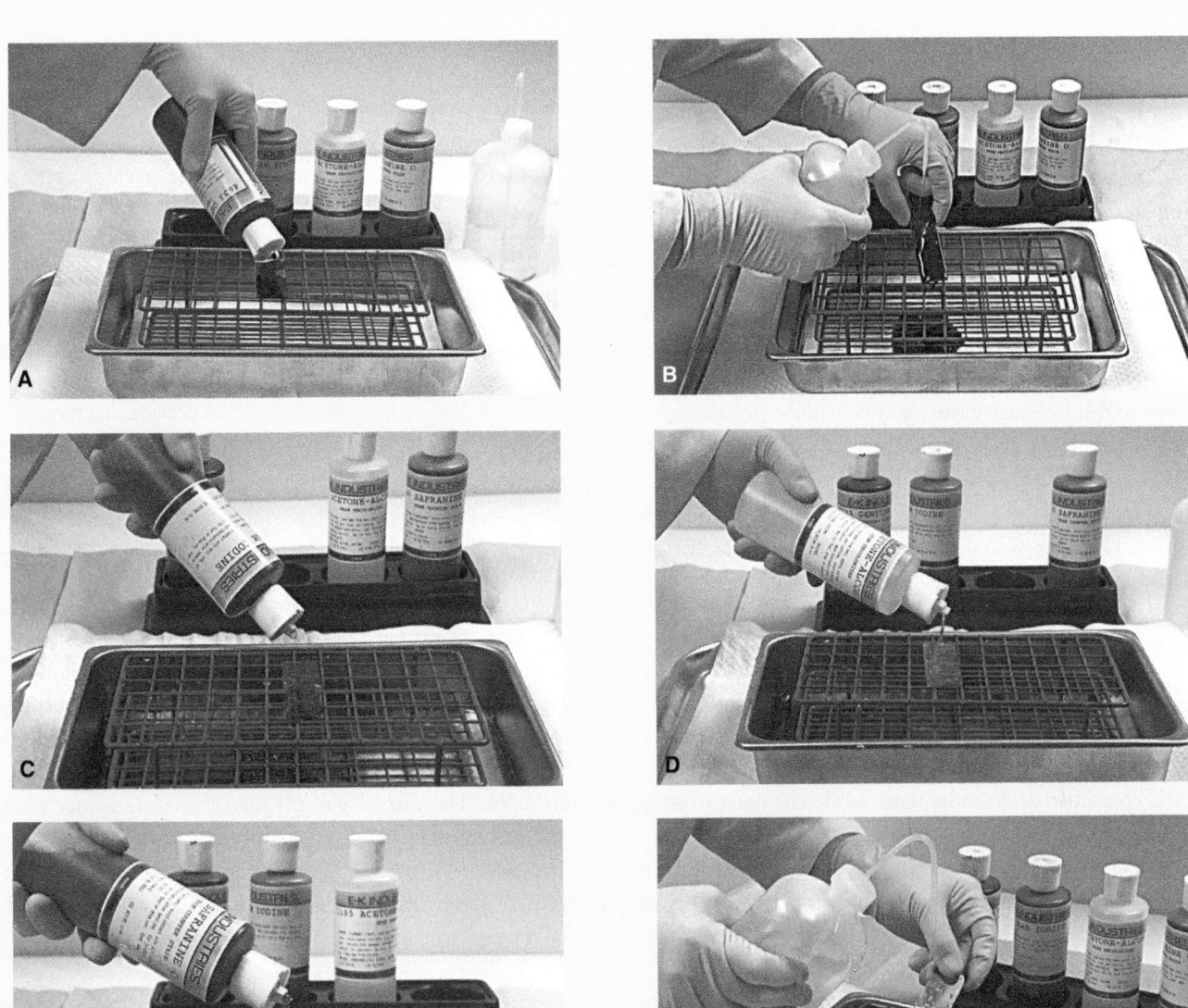

FIGURE A–F (A) Pour crystal violet stain over the entire slide and let stand for one minute; **(B)** tilt the slide to drain excess and rinse with water; **(C)** pour Gram's iodine stain over the entire slide and let stand for one minute; **(D)** gently pour decolorizer with alcohol-acetone all over the slide for 15 seconds or until blue color stops running; **(E)** pour safranine stain over the entire slide and let stand for 30 seconds; **(F)** rinse with water and wipe back of the slide.

The staining properties, shape, and size of the organisms can sometimes be used to identify pathogens in specimen samples. As previously noted, *Bacilli* are rod-shaped microorganisms found singly or in groups. *Cocci* are round microorganisms found singly, in pairs (*Diplococci*), in strings (*Streptococci*), or in clusters (*Staphylococci*). *Spirilla,* curved or spiral rods, can be arranged singly or in strands. Some bacteria can produce resistant spores under adverse environmental conditions. Spores can lie dormant for thousands of years and, when conditions are right, can revert back to active form. This trait makes it difficult to destroy these pathogenic bacteria.

Serology Testing

Serology is the study of the antigen and antibody reactions of the body's immune system. The body's ability to recognize a foreign substance (antigen) and produce an antibody against it is the immune response. Antibodies are specific for a particular antigen. For example, polio antibody is specific for polio only.

This antigen–antibody reaction is a frequently used testing tool. It is used to test for pregnancy, rheumatoid arthritis, mononucleosis, and strep, among other conditions. This testing is serological because it studies or tests the serum component of the blood. These testing kits contain all the equipment and supplies necessary and assist the medical assistant in ensuring that reagents are fresh and quality control is maintained. The kits standardize testing, thus ensuring accuracy, precision, and quality control. It is absolutely essential to follow exactly the manufacturer's directions.

One example of this antibody testing is the test for *H. pylori*. Tests for *H. pylori* include a blood antibody test (done with a blood specimen), a urea breath test (done by breathing into specialized equipment), and a stool antigen test (using a stool specimen). Only the blood antibody test is CLIA-waived and can be done in a medical office. The other tests need to be sent to a laboratory.

Strep Test

The Group A Strep Screen is a test that is done frequently in POLs. It is especially efficient in the pediatric office because it is self-contained and can be done while the patient waits. This screen is an antigen detection test for group A beta-hemolytic *Streptococci* and follows the general procedure for antigen–antibody **agglutination** (clumping together) tests, which produce a clumping of cells. There are many

Professionalism | Cultural Considerations

It is important to be very aware of a patient's cultural background and sensitivities when discussing specimens that are to be collected via elimination, such as feces. Many cultures find this subject taboo and inappropriate for discussion. Always ensure the patient's privacy and modesty are considered when these topics are discussed to avoid embarrassment. It may also be necessary to provide patients with pamphlets to help answer questions that they may have difficulty asking. For some cultures, it may be necessary for instructions to be provided by medical professionals of the same sex as that of the patient.

CLIA-waived group A strep kits available that test for the extracted group A beta-hemolytic *Streptococcus* antigen. These self-contained test kits are commercially prepared diagnostic testing kits that include detailed instructions and contain reagents, controls, and quality control suggestions.

A variety of other serological test kits are available for infectious mononucleosis, rheumatoid arthritis, and HIV, to name a few. The specialty of the physician determines which tests will be used.

Procedure 44-6 explains the steps for performing rapid Group A strep testing, and Procedure 44-7 explains the steps for performing a chlamydia test.

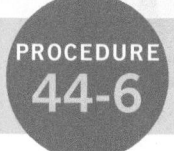

PROCEDURE 44-6

Performing Rapid Group A Strep Testing

Objective ◆ *Test a throat swab specimen for Group A Strep.*

EQUIPMENT AND SUPPLIES

Labeled throat swab specimen; BD Check Group A Strep Kit; personal protective equipment; timer; biohazard waste container

Note: Follow standard precautions and safety guidelines when working with body fluid samples. Use care to avoid splashing or spilling body fluids. Wipe up all spills using the guidelines established by OSHA.

METHOD

1. Wash your hands and gather supplies.
2. Verify that the name on the throat swab container and lab requisition form matches.

3. Perform hand hygiene and apply gloves.
4. Remove the test strip from the sealed foil pouch and begin testing immediately.
5. Add four full drops of Reagent A bottle (red) to the extraction test tube. Add four full drops of Reagent B bottle (clear) to the extraction test tube. Tap the bottom of the tube to mix; the solution should turn yellow.
6. Insert the specimen swab into the test tube solution, and rotate it 10 times. Leave it in place for one minute; then slowly remove while squeezing the swab along the side of the container so that most liquid remains. Discard the swab.
7. Insert the test strip into the solution with the arrows pointing down; leave in place. Start the timer.

8. Read results in five minutes. A pink or red line should be noted in the control area; if not present, the test is invalid and must be repeated. If a second line appears (any shade of pink or red), the test is positive for Strep. The more concentrated the sample is, the darker the second line will be.
9. Remove and dispose of gloves and perform hand hygiene.
10. Document the procedure in the patient's record.

CHARTING EXAMPLE

2/14/YY 10:30 A.M. BD Check Group A Strep test performed on throat culture according to manufacturer's instructions, per physician's order. Test results negative. Patient and physician notified..M. Smythe, CMA (AAMA)

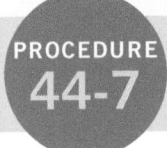

PROCEDURE 44-7 Performing CLIA-Waived Microbiology Testing

Objective ◆ *Perform a CLIA-waived chlamydia test with a test kit, in the time specified by your instructor.*

EQUIPMENT AND SUPPLIES

Chlamydia test kit, including swab, reagent, and test strip

METHOD

1. Identify the patient.
2. Instruct the patient about the procedure.
3. Offer the patient a gown, and instruct the patient to remove clothing from the waist down.
4. Perform hand hygiene.
5. Don gloves.
6. Assist the patient into the lithotomy position.

7. Assist the physician with procuring a vaginal swab.
8. Place swab on test strip.
9. Add reagent, per kit instructions.
10. Remove gloves and wash hands. Record results in patient chart.

CHARTING EXAMPLE

2/22/XX Patient complains of vaginal discharge and pain. Physician obtained swab of vaginal discharge, which was positive for chlamydia using test kit #40611. Expiration date 12/30/XX. ....C. Bolgiano, RMA

SUMMARY

Microbiology, as practiced by the medical assistant in POLs, is one of the most important aids to diagnosis for the physician.

By correct processing and testing of patient specimens, early diagnosis and treatment of disease can take place. The medical assistant plays an important role in the process.

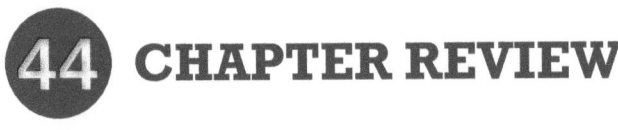

44 CHAPTER REVIEW

COMPETENCY REVIEW

1. Define and spell the terms for this chapter.
2. What does it mean that a microorganism is nonpathogenic?
3. In what ways are bacteria categorized?
4. If a bacterium is aerobic, what does it require to survive?

5. *Tinea pedis* is an example of which type of microorganism?
6. Name and describe three configurations of cocci.
7. A specimen is sent to an outside laboratory for culture and sensitivity testing. Your office receives a report that the bacterium is resistant to penicillin. What does that mean?

PREPARING FOR THE CERTIFICATION EXAM

1. Invasion of the body by any pathogen is called
   a. contagion.
   b. infection.
   c. pandemic.
   d. epidemic.
   e. communicable.

2. Material for a CSF specimen is collected from what area?
   a. mouth
   b. throat
   c. lungs and bronchial tubes
   d. pharynx
   e. spinal canal

3. *Cocci* occurring in chains are
   a. *Micrococci.*
   b. *Diplococci.*
   c. *Streptococci.*
   d. *Sarcinae.*
   e. *Staphylococci.*

4. Which of the following is caused by a virus?
   a. candidiasis
   b. malaria
   c. herpes zoster
   d. strep throat
   e. gonorrhea

5. An organism that can live with or without oxygen in its environment is
   a. aerobic.
   b. Gram-positive.
   c. Gram-negative.
   d. anaerobic.
   e. a facultative anaerobe.

6. The test that checks for the susceptibility of an organism to specific antibiotics is the
   a. culture test.
   b. sensitivity test.
   c. isolation test.
   d. screening test.
   e. inoculation test.

7. After a Gram stain, what color do Gram-negative organisms stain?
   a. blue
   b. black
   c. violet
   d. pink
   e. orange

8. *Staphylococcus aureus* is
   a. Gram-negative *Bacilli* in chains.
   b. Gram-positive *Cocci* in chains.
   c. a cause of MRSA.
   d. Gram-negative *Diplococci.*
   e. acid-fast *Bacilli.*

9. The causative agent of scarlet fever and rheumatic fever is
   a. *Streptococcus pneumoniae.*
   b. *Streptococcus pyogenes.*
   c. *Neisseria meningitidis.*
   d. *Staphylococcus enteritidis.*
   e. *Chlamydia trachomatis.*

10. The study of fungi is known as
    a. fungology.
    b. serology.
    c. mycology.
    d. parasitology.
    e. hematology.

CRITICAL THINKING

Refer to the case study at the beginning of the chapter and use what you have learned to answer the following questions.

1. Dr. Penningworth suspects that Marc may have strep throat. He orders a throat swab to be collected and sent to the laboratory. What should David use to obtain the throat specimen, and why?

2. What must David do to ensure that he does not contaminate the throat culture while attempting to obtain the specimen?

3. The laboratory has processed the throat culture and has found that the organism causing the infection is *Streptococcus pyogenes*, confirming Dr. Penningworth's suspicions. What other forms of infection could this microorganism cause?

4. What types of antibiotics are used to treat strep throat?

ON THE JOB

You have been asked to speak to a high school class about the clinical aspects of your job. In particular, the students are interested in microbiology because they have just completed a unit on microorganisms in class.

1. What would you tell them about your functions as a medical assistant?

2. What would you say to those who asked if you looked through the microscope and reported your findings?

3. One student asks what type of training one would need to work solely in microbiology in a laboratory setting. How would you answer her?

INTERNET ACTIVITY

Research a type of bacteria, such as the *Staphylococci*, that can cause gastroenteritis.

CHAPTER 45

Urinalysis

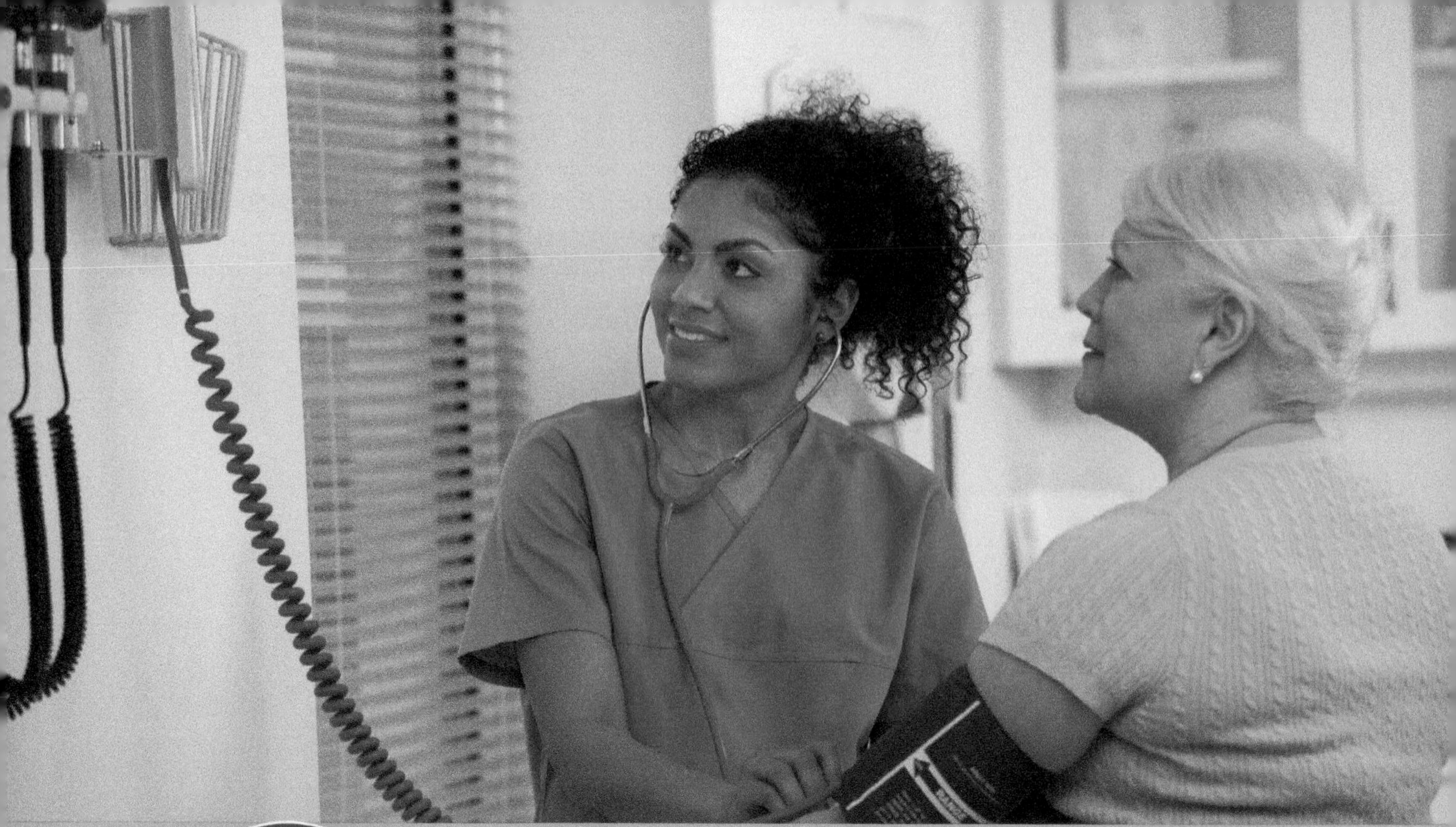

Learning Objectives

After completing this chapter, you should be able to:

45.1 Define and spell the terms for this chapter.

45.2 Explain the importance of asepsis during urinalysis.

45.3 Explain considerations related to collecting a urine specimen.

45.4 Describe types of time-specific urine tests.

45.5 Describe special collection methods for obtaining a urine sample.

45.6 Identify the physical characteristics of urine.

45.7 List the chemical characteristics of urine that are evaluated during a urinalysis.

45.8 Explain the medical assistant's role as it pertains to the microscopic examination of urine.

45.9 List elements that may be examined and reported during a microscopic examination of urine.

45.10 Explain considerations related to urine pregnancy testing.

45.11 Describe important factors related to urine drug analysis.

45.12 List quality control measures related to urinalysis.

Susan Schultz, CMA (AAMA), has explained the proper collection procedure for a clean-catch midstream urine sample to 65-year-old Shelly Flannery, per Dr. Salpega's orders for completion of a urinalysis. Susan immediately tests the urine using a chemical reagent strip and notices that the urine is dark yellow and cloudy in appearance.

Terms to Learn

anuria	glycosuria/glucosuria	refractometer
bacteriuria	hematuria	renal threshold
casts	ketones	sediment
catheterization	micturate	specific gravity
chain of custody form	micturition	spermatozoa
clean-catch	occult	supernatant
crystals	oliguria	suprapubic specimen
cystitis	parasites	turbid
culture and sensitivity (C&S)	polyuria	urinalysis
diuretic	proteinuria	urine
glomerulonephritis	pyuria	void

The formation, storage, and excretion of urine are vital processes in maintaining the body's homeostasis. The urinary system, which includes the kidneys, bladder, ureters, and urethra, keeps the internal environment of the body clean and balanced. Acting as a filter, the kidneys remove significant amounts of toxins and wastes from the blood. The resulting waste product, **urine**, is temporarily stored in the bladder until it can be excreted through **micturition** (urination). The urinary system is also able to maintain normal levels of fluids and salts by the process of reabsorption, such as reabsorbing water during times of dehydration.

Urine is commonly tested in a medical office since it is readily available, easily collected, and often provides the first clues to illness. It can provide significant information about the functioning of the urinary system as well as other body systems.

Urinalysis is the testing and evaluation of urine. Urinalysis is typically performed for routine evaluation, diagnostic purposes, or to monitor the effectiveness of a treatment. During routine evaluation of urine, early detection and treatment of unexpected health issues are possible with minimal difficulty and discomfort for the patient. The evaluation of urine is useful as a diagnostic tool, as it can rule out or help to detect urinary, metabolic, and endocrine disorders. Urinalysis may also be used to monitor a patient's response to medical treatments, such as antibiotics or insulin therapy.

Medical assistants play a key role in urinary testing and evaluation. Depending on the reasons for analysis and the type of evaluation, there are specific methods to collect, store, and process urine for testing. The medical assistant must understand basic anatomy and physiology, as well as the normal components and lab values for urine, in order to assist in diagnosing diseases and disorders.

ASEPSIS

Asepsis is the condition of being free of disease-causing contaminants and is critical in urinalysis. To maintain your own safety and the safety of others, you should consider all blood and body fluids, including urine, to be potentially infectious. Therefore, as a medical assistant, you must follow standard precautions whenever collecting urine samples or performing urinalysis. Always maintain good handwashing principles, wear nonsterile gloves, and avoid contaminating any equipment with urine. If there is a possibility that splashing may occur, use personal protective equipment (PPE), such as gloves, gowns, shoe covers, and protective eyewear.

COLLECTING THE SPECIMEN

Urine samples provide valuable indicators of the overall health of the patient. Thus, medical assistants must do their utmost to maintain the integrity of the specimen. A test result is only as reliable and valid as the specimen collected. When handling specimens, the medical assistant must understand how to store and maintain each type of urine specimen collected. In most cases, urine samples are refrigerated if testing will not take place within two hours. Always consult the office or laboratory manual for further information about specific storage of urine and addition of preservatives for specific tests.

The patient must be clearly instructed about methods of collection in easily understood terms. Patients do not necessarily comprehend medical terms. Words such as **void** and **micturate** may not be understood by the patient. Instead, phrases such as "passing water" or "peeing" may need to be used.

At least 10 mL of urine is usually needed for testing, and appropriate collection containers or kits must be used, depending on the test ordered. Figures 45-1A–C show three types of urine collection containers.

Urine Test Categories

Urine specimen collection can be categorized by either time-specific or specialized standards, although some time-specific tests may also require specialized collection.

Time-Specific Tests

- Random sample
- Morning specimen: first void
- Timed specimen

- 24-hour specimen
- Two-hour postprandial specimen

Specialized Collection

- Catheterized specimen (sterile specimen)
- Clean-catch midstream (sterile specimen)
- Suprapubic specimen (sterile specimen)
- Pediatric specimen

Labeling

Some specimens may be tested on site at the medical office, while others may be sent to a lab for further testing. Regardless of where they are being tested, the medical assistant must properly label all specimens. The following information must be included on the label

- Patient's first and last names
- Identifying information, such as the chart number or date of birth
- Date and time of collection
- Initials of the person collecting it

Labels should be placed on the containers and never on the specimen lids, which can easily be switched to the wrong container.

TIME-SPECIFIC TESTS

Random Sample

The most common method of urine collection is the random sample. As the name indicates, a random urine sample can

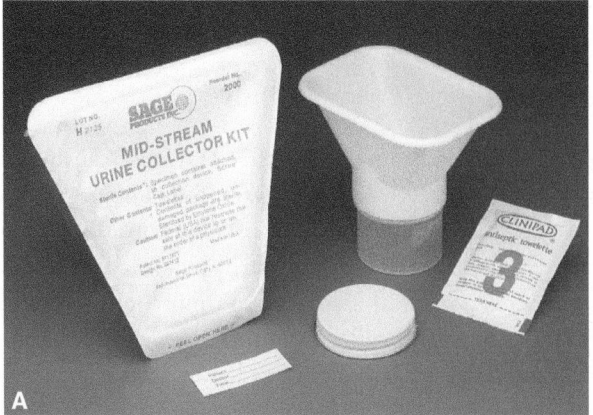
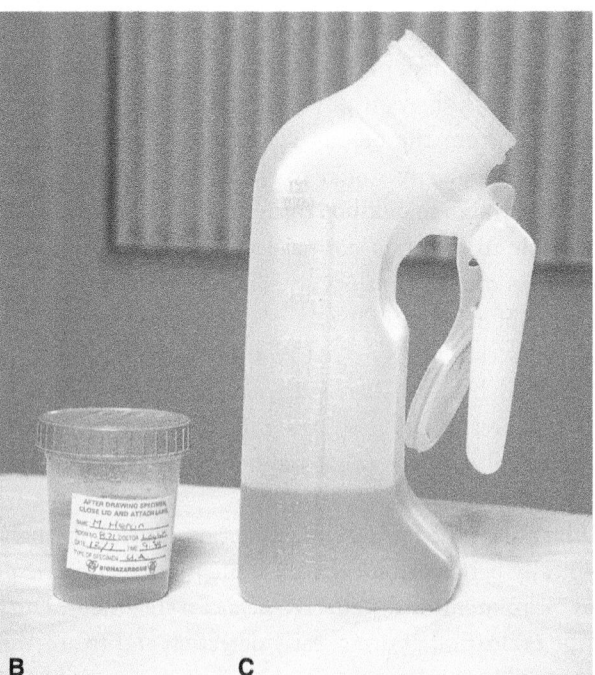

FIGURE 45-1 **(A)** Midstream collection kit; **(B)** urine collection cup; **(C)** 24-hour urine container.

be collected at any time of the day. This specimen is collected in a nonsterile container and can be collected in the medical office during the patient's visit or may be brought in from the patient's home. Provide patients with urine specimen containers for any sample to be brought in from home to ensure that containers are clean and free of contaminants. Random samples are generally used only for routine screenings because the composition of urine changes throughout the day.

Morning Specimen: First Void

A morning specimen, also called an eight-hour specimen or first void, is the most concentrated urine because it has remained in the bladder overnight or over an eight-hour period of time. This specimen is often used for tests such as pregnancy testing, urine cultures, and microscopic examinations. The patient is given a specimen container and collects the urine usually after waking up in the morning. The specimen should be brought to the office for testing within 30 to 60 minutes of collection, or the sample should be refrigerated or a preservative added to the container, depending on the test procedure to be completed.

Patients should be instructed to empty the bladder the night before or before starting the eight-hour specimen collection. Any urine collected overnight or during the eight-hour time period should be pooled with the morning void specimen. See Guidelines 45-1: Collecting a Routine Urine Specimen.

Guidelines 45-1

Collecting a Random Urine Specimen

1. Provide the patient with a nonsterile container that is labeled with the patient's name and the date. The label should be placed on the container and not the lid.
2. Ask the patient to use the bathroom and void into a container. Tell the patient to fill the container only two-thirds of the way full to avoid spillage.
3. Explain where you want the patient to leave the container of urine. Place a paper towel in the designated area to avoid contamination of the work area.
4. Wearing nonsterile gloves, take the specimen and immediately test the urine, if possible.
5. If you are not able to test the specimen within 30 minutes, place the specimen in the refrigerator. The urine should be at room temperature before testing.

Note: Some random testing may require collection via the clean-catch method. If unsure about which method to use, err on the side of caution and use the clean-catch method as explained in the "Specialized Collection: Clean-Catch Midstream Specimen" section.

Timed Specimen

Timed specimens are necessary for quantitative analysis or to measure the amount of substances in the urine specimen such as protein, creatinine, or glucose in urine. Urine specimens must be collected at specific time intervals. The most common timed specimens are 24-hour and two-hour postprandial (after a meal) specimens.

24-Hour Specimen

The 24-hour urine test is used to determine the glomerular filtration rate of the kidneys, to check specific hormone levels, and to check for other metabolic abnormalities. Urine contains specific amounts of waste products, such as urea and creatinine, and dissolved chemicals, such as sodium and potassium. If these amounts are not within normal ranges, or if other substances are present, it may be a sign of a certain disease or condition. It is important for the medical assistant to clearly instruct the patient to perform an accurate 24-hour specimen collection. Patients should receive both verbal and written instructions to ensure clarity and accuracy. Procedure 45-1 includes the method for instructing a patient to collect a 24-hour urine specimen.

To collect a 24-hour specimen, the patient is given a large, clean, and properly labeled container to take home

Professionalism

The medical assistant is often the individual who instructs the patient in the correct method of collecting a urine specimen. It is important to be sure that the patient understands the correct method of collection. Be sure to use terminology that can be easily understood by the patient. If the patient is doing the collection at home, provide written instructions that clearly describe each step of the procedure. If the patient is doing the test in the physician's office, place instructions in the laboratory restroom.

When collecting clean-catch specimens, be sure that the female patient understands how to clean the labia and the male knows how to clean the foreskin. Diagrams are helpful both in the laboratory restroom and in the written directions. Patients need a clear explanation of what "midstream" means, as well. When you are explaining the procedure for samples collected at home, it is important that patients understand the need for refrigerating any specimens not brought immediately into the physician's office or testing laboratory.

It is especially important to display a professional manner while giving instructions. Some patients may be sensitive about the subject of elimination, so the medical assistant must be sure that the patient's desire for modesty is honored. Be sure to give all instructions for the collection of urine specimens in private and out of hearing distance of other individuals.

Instructing a Patient on Collecting a 24-Hour Urine Specimen

Objective ◆ *Instruct a patient on how to collect a 24-hour urine specimen.*

EQUIPMENT AND SUPPLIES

24-hour urine container (two containers may be necessary for some patients); toilet insert for collection; funnel for pouring; label; chemical hazard label as needed; preservatives as required by specific test; graduated cylinder; 10 mL pipette; gloves; written instruction sheet for specific test; requisition slip; patient's medical record; pen

METHOD

1. Check the patient's record for orders for specific test.
2. Assemble the equipment and supplies needed.
3. Consult the laboratory directory for special instructions regarding dietary restrictions and preservative for test ordered.
4. Perform hand hygiene.
5. Label the container with the patient's name and dates and times to start and stop collection of specimen.
6. If required, add the exact amount of preservative using a pipette. If preservative is caustic, add a chemical hazard label.
7. Warmly greet and identify the patient, and introduce yourself. Explain in detail the directions for collection as follows:
   - Upon waking, urinate into the toilet and flush.
   - Note the exact time and date of the beginning of the 24-hour collection and write it on the container.
   - Collect all voided urine after the start time for the next 24-hour period and ending exactly 24 hours after the start time on the following day. At exactly the same time that was noted on the first day (written on the container), empty the bladder and add it to the collection.
   - Note the times and dates on the label.
   - Ask the patient to use a toilet insert or urinal insert for collection of the specimen, then to pour the urine into the 24-hour container. Instruct the patient not to urinate directly into the container or place anything other than urine in the container.
   - Explain that the specimen may need refrigeration, depending on the test. This means it must be refrigerated for the entire 24-hour period.
   - Patient is to return the container(s) as soon as possible after ending the collection to ensure accurate results.
8. Provide a written copy of instructions to the patient along with the prepared container(s).
9. Record the supplies and instructions given to the patient and the name of the test ordered.
10. Verify the collection dates and times with the patient when the specimen is returned to the physician's office.

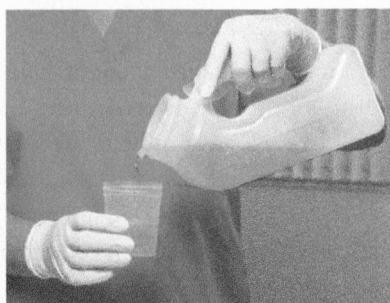

FIGURE A Mix the urine sample carefully by swirling. Measure the total volume of urine collected; then pour a portion into the appropriate container to be sent for testing.

11. Check to see if any other additives are to be included before sending the specimen to the testing laboratory.
12. Apply gloves before accepting the container from the patient.
13. Mix the urine sample by swirling carefully. Measure the volume of urine collected by pouring into a large, graduated 1 liter cylinder. Record the total volume of urine collected and any preservatives added.
14. Pour a portion of the urine into an appropriate container for delivery to the testing laboratory. Dispose of the remainder of the urine according to laboratory directions (Figure A).
15. Record the date, time, volume of urine, and where the specimen was sent.
16. Appropriately clean the cylinder. Dispose of the container in a biohazard waste container.
17. Clean the work area.
18. Remove gloves and perform hand hygiene.
19. Document in the patient's medical record.

CHARTING EXAMPLE

08/06/YY 8:00 A.M. Pt given two 24-hour urine containers for collection of specimen for protein. Timing to begin at 7:00 A.M. 08/07/YY after voiding and discarding first A.M. specimen. Pt to return containers in 24 hours. Pt verbalized good understanding. C. Cox, RMA 08/08/YY 8:00 A.M. 24-Hour Urine Protein Test ordered. Pt. returned 1,400 mL of refrigerated clear amber urine (no additives), collected via aseptic technique. No unusual odor noted. Pt. states that she began yesterday after she discarded the first urination at 7:00 A.M.; she included final urination (7:00 A.M. this morning). Sample sent to XYZ Lab, per physician's orders..C. Cox, RMA

(Figure 45-1C). Collection will begin the next day. Instruct the patient to discard the first void in the morning at the beginning of the 24-hour period; it should not be included in the container. After the first void, the patient should collect all the urine in the container for the next 24 hours, *including* the first voided specimen on the *second* morning or nearing the end of the 24-hour collection.

Often preservatives are added before giving the container to the patient. Some of these may be caustic. Containers must be labeled appropriately to prevent injury to the patient and anyone else handling the specimen. For this reason, patients should be instructed not to handle or discard preservatives. In all cases, with or without preservatives in the container, the patient should collect the urine in a separate container, *then* pour it into the 24-hour container (see Procedure 45-1).

In addition to preservatives, the collection container may be stored in a refrigerator or kept on ice. Although refrigeration slows growth of bacteria and specimen deterioration, it does not completely stop it. To prevent excessive bacteria contamination, the patient should be instructed to deliver the specimen as soon as possible to the physician's office once the collection period is over. Failure to do so may affect lab values, requiring the test to be repeated. Bedwetting and forgotten or spilled specimens also require retesting.

Two-Hour Postprandial Specimen

A two-hour postprandial urine specimen is a single voided specimen that is collected two hours after a meal has been eaten, following the same steps as seen in Guidelines 45-1. This test is used as a screening tool for diabetes or other insulin-related disorder and detects any glucose that may be spilled into the urine once the blood levels exceed the renal threshold. **Renal threshold** is the concentration at which a substance is too high and can no longer stay in the blood and, thus, must be excreted in the urine by the kidneys. As the concentration of glucose increases and surpasses the renal threshold for glucose, the more glucose will be present in the urine.

SPECIALIZED COLLECTION
Clean-Catch Midstream Specimen

Clean-catch is a method of urine collection that is free of most bacteria and other contaminants found in the urethra or around the genital area. Following simple directions for cleansing and pausing midstream during urination, a patient can collect his own specimen without the need for an invasive procedure. Clean-catch midstream urine samples are frequently used to detect urinary tract infections (UTIs) or used to perform cytology evaluations to detect abnormal cells such as cancer cells. Clean-catch midstream urine samples may also be cultured for microorganisms, such as bacteria and viruses, to determine which antibiotics will provide effective treatment for the patient.

The patient will need clear instructions to obtain a urine specimen that is free of contamination. Procedure 45-2 provides instructions for male and female patients on

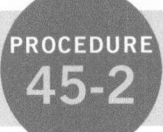

PROCEDURE 45-2

Instructing a Patient on Collecting a Clean-Catch Midstream Urine Specimen

Objective ◆ *Instruct both male and female patients to obtain a contaminant-free, clean-catch midstream urine specimen.*

EQUIPMENT AND SUPPLIES

Sterile midstream urine container; antiseptic wipes or towelettes; written patient instructions; patient's medical record

METHOD

1. Perform hand hygiene.
2. Assemble equipment. Always label the specimen container before use.
3. Warmly greet and identify the patient, and introduce yourself.

Explain the procedure to a *male* patient as follows:
- Perform hand hygiene.
- Expose the penis. If uncircumcised, pull foreskin back, and hold back until the specimen has been collected.
- Cleanse each side of the urethral opening from top to bottom, using separate antiseptic wipes, wiping in one direction only (Figure A). Cleanse across the top of the urethral opening with a third antiseptic wipe, wiping in one direction only. Discard the wipes in the waste basket.

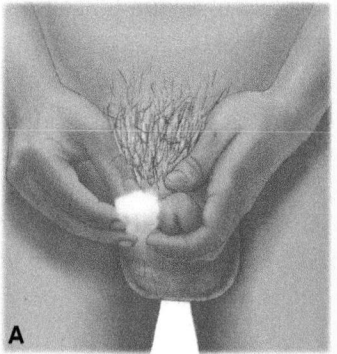
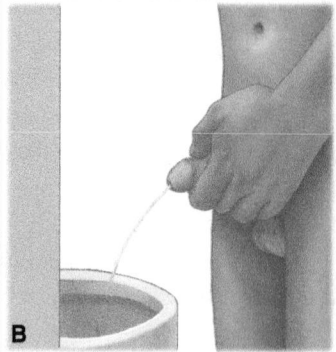
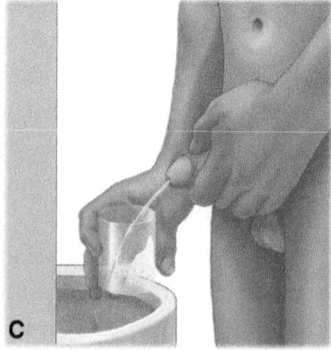

FIGURE A–C (A) The patient is instructed to cleanse the head of the penis in preparation for a clean-catch midstream urine collection; **(B)** begin urinating into the toilet; **(C)** continue urinating into the sterile cup provided for the clean-catch midstream urine specimen.

- Void a small amount of urine into the toilet (Figure B). Then void into the container, taking care not to touch the inside of the container (Figure C). Remove the container.
- Continue voiding the remainder of urine into the toilet.
- Recap the container immediately, taking care not to contaminate the inside of the lid.
- Deliver the specimen as instructed.

Explain the procedure to a *female* patient as follows:
- Perform hand hygiene and remove underwear.
- Expose the urinary meatus by pulling apart the labia and holding the area open with the nondominant hand (use left hand if the patient is right handed, and vice versa).
- If menstruation is apparent, insert a clean tampon and pull the string to the side.
- Use the dominant hand to cleanse around one side of the urinary meatus from front to back with one antiseptic

wipe (Figure D). Use a second wipe to cleanse the other side in the same manner. Using a third wipe, cleanse across the opening of the meatus itself. Continue holding the labia apart until the procedure is complete.
- Begin voiding into the toilet (Figure E). Place the container into position and void into the container without touching the inside of the container (Figure F).
- Remove the container and continue voiding into the toilet.
- Wipe in the usual manner and cover the container with the lid, avoiding contaminating the inside of the lid.
- Deliver the specimen as instructed.

4. Perform hand hygiene.
5. Document in the patient's medical record.

CHARTING EXAMPLE

4/23/YY Clean-catch midstream urine specimen collected from patient at 11:00 A.M. Sent to lab for C&S..........M. King, CMA

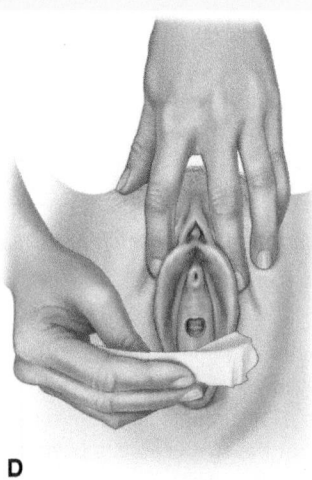
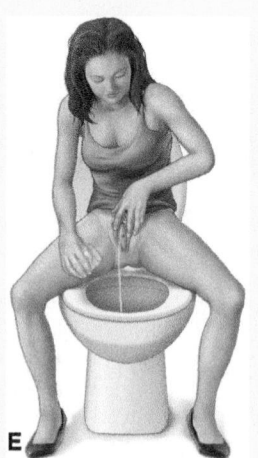
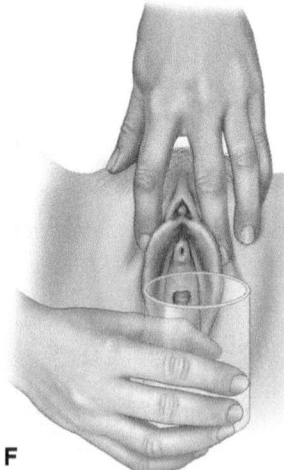

FIGURE D–F (D) The patient is instructed to spread the labia and expose the urinary meatus, then use antiseptic wipes to clean first one side from front to back and then to do the same on the other side; **(E)** begin urinating into the toilet, and then stop; **(F)** urinate into the sterile clean-catch container until it is two-thirds full.

how to collect a sterile, clean-catch midstream urine specimen at the physician's office. Not all urine tests require clean-catch collection. However, this method will not invalidate test results. Therefore, when uncertain about which test to perform, the best course of action is to instruct the patient to use the clean-catch method.

Catheterization Specimen

Catheterization is the process of inserting a flexible tube-like catheter through the urethra and into the bladder. This procedure may be performed to prevent or treat bladder distention when other measures fail. It may be performed after voiding to determine how much residual urine remains in the bladder. It may be used to irrigate or medicate the inside of a bladder. It may also be used for diagnostic purposes where catheterization can collect the ideal urine specimen, one that is contamination-free. Typically, a nurse performs this procedure using sterile technique, but the medical assistant may be called to assist and may even perform the procedure under supervision.

There are many sizes, lengths, and types of catheters (Figure 45-2). Most are made of rubber, plastic, latex, or polyvinyl chloride (PVC), depending on the manufacturer and the intended use. The size indicates the diameter of the lumen, or opening inside the tube, with the larger the number, the larger the lumen. For example, a #10 French (Fr) catheter may be used for a child, a #16 Fr may be used for an adult female, and a #18 Fr may be used for an adult male. For length, women have shorter urethras, so a 22-cm-long catheter is acceptable, but men require one that is longer, such as 40 cm. Straight catheters are commonly used for specimen collection because they are smaller and easier to insert (Figure 45-2A). Indwelling catheters, often referred to as Foley catheters, have inflatable balloons that keep them in place for longer periods of time (Figure 45-2B). A suprapubic (above the pubis) catheter enters the bladder through the abdomen and may be used when there is urethral obstruction (Figure 45-2C).

Before catheterization, a sterile field is created and the urethra and its surrounding tissues are cleaned. A sterile catheter is then inserted through the urethra to the bladder, and the urine is collected in a sterile container. Figure 45-3A–B depicts the use of a Foley catheter on a female and a male. Procedure 45-3 shows how to assist in collecting a urine specimen by catheterization.

Because catheterization provides a pathway between the outside environment and the sterile internal body system, using sterile technique is vital to preventing complications

(A) Straight catheter

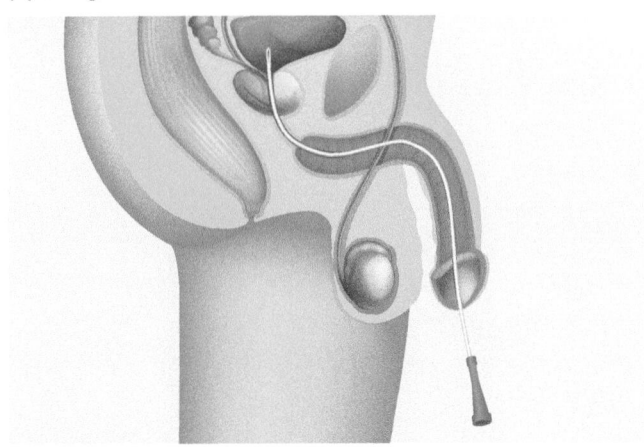

(B) Foley catheter

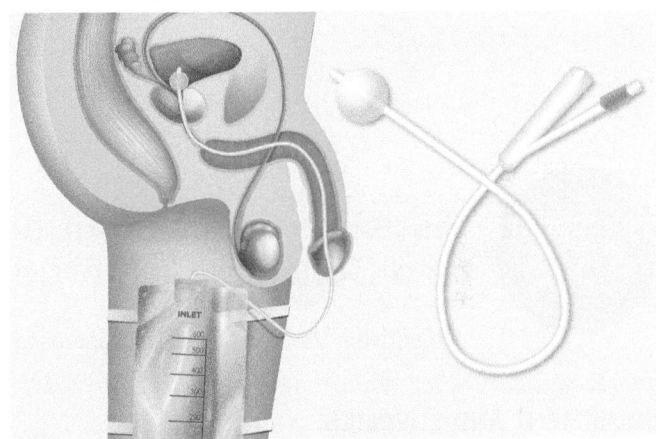

(C) Suprapubic catheter

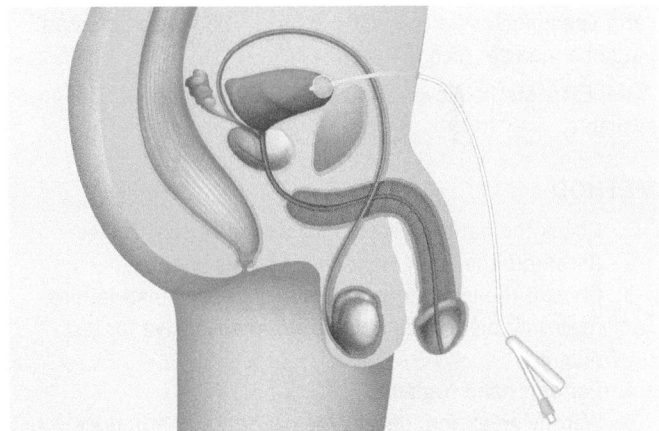

FIGURE 45-2 Types of catheters: **(A)** straight urinary catheter; **(B)** indwelling (Foley) catheter; **(C)** suprapubic catheter.

such as infection. Most supplies used for inserting a catheter come in a prepackaged tray of sterilized items. This catheter kit or tray generally includes drapes, gloves, swabs, cleansing solution, lubricant, and a specimen container. A

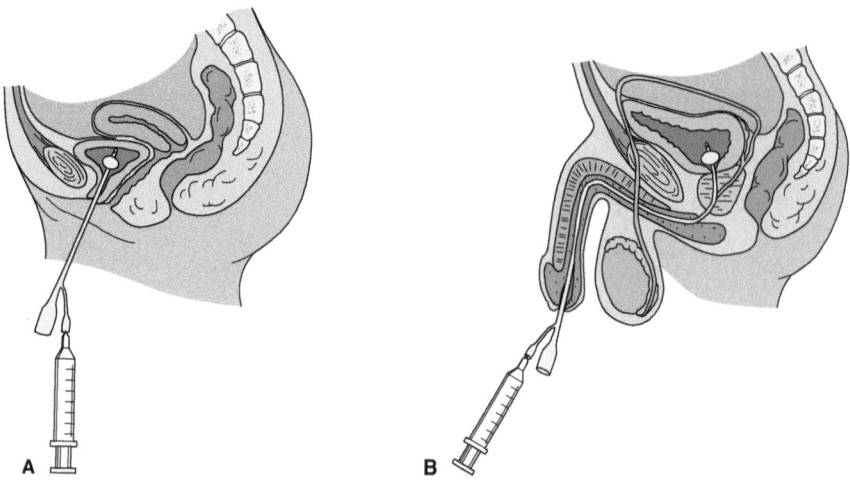

FIGURE 45-3 (A) Foley catheter: The inflated balloon at the tip of the catheter holds the Foley catheter in place in the bladder of a female patient. The catheter drains urine from the bladder continuously as the kidneys produce urine; **(B)** Foley catheter with balloon in the bladder of a male patient.

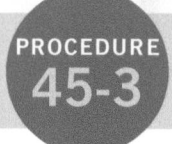

Assisting with a Straight Catheterization and Collecting a Sterile Specimen

PROCEDURE 45-3

Objective ◆ *Assist with catheterization and urine collection.*

EQUIPMENT AND SUPPLIES

Catheter kit with sterile drapes; disposable underpads; gloves; cleansing swabs or cotton balls and cleansing solution; lubricant; specimen container; catheter (size and type as ordered); patient's medical record

Note: Extra sterile gloves and an extra catheter should be available.

METHOD

1. Check the patient's record for orders for specific test.
2. Assemble the equipment and supplies needed.
3. Consult the laboratory directory for special instructions regarding dietary restrictions and preservative for test ordered.
4. Perform hand hygiene.
5. Warmly greet and identify the patient, and introduce yourself. Explain the procedure and the reason for performing it. Inform the patient that mild burning and pressure with the sensation of urinating may occur, especially during catheter insertion.
6. Ask if there are any latex, betadine, or iodine allergies. Notify the nurse or physician if there are and collect alternative supplies.
7. Verify the expiration date, and inspect the product packaging for any tampering or damage. Replace the catheter kit, if necessary.

8. Assist the male patient into a dorsal recumbent position or the female patient into the lithotomy position. Use draping to ensure privacy and diminish embarrassment.
9. Perform hand hygiene.
10. Don nonsterile gloves and gently wash the patient's genital area with body cleanser if visibly soiled. Discard gloves and wash hands.
11. Using aseptic technique, open the kit, peeling the lid away from (not toward) your body. Place the underpad beneath the patient, plastic side down. Place the fenestrated drape around the patient's genitalia.
12. Apply sterile gloves and observe strict sterile technique for the remainder of the procedure.
13. Dispense lubricating gel into a portion of the tray and open cleansing swab packages or pour solution over cotton balls, whichever is supplied. Remove the plastic sleeve from the catheter and arrange on the sterile field.
14. The health care practitioner will don sterile gloves and use her nondominant hand to hold back the labia (for females) or foreskin (for males). The dominant hand will first cleanse the meatus, using a different swab for each stroke: one down one side, another down the other side, and a third down the middle. The practitioner will then dip the tip of the catheter into the lubricating gel and carefully insert it into the urethra, advancing slowly.

15. The medical assistant should be prepared to collect the urine from the other end of the catheter by holding a sterile cup beneath it. When the cup is ¾ full, the catheter end should be placed in the tray to drain the rest of the urine. Immediately seal the urine container. The practitioner will remove the catheter and discard.
16. Remove supplies and assist the patient with privacy measures.
17. Label the collection container for delivery to a testing laboratory. Measure and dispose of the remainder of the urine according to laboratory protocol.
18. Document in the patient's medical record. Record the date, time, color, clarity, odor, and volume of urine expressed, and which testing laboratory the specimen was sent to. The procedure itself should be charted by the person who inserted the catheter.
19. Clean the area.
20. Remove gloves and perform hand hygiene.

CHARTING EXAMPLE

08/06/YY 10:00 A.M. UA/C&S ordered. 3 mL of clear amber urine collected. No unusual odor noted. Sample sent to XYZ Lab, per physician's orders....................................C. Cox, RMA

catheter, prefilled syringe, and drainage bag may also be included (Figure 45-4A-B).

In some patients, such as those with renal disorders, burn patients, and patients with congestive heart failure or dehydration, the amount of fluid intake and urine output needs to be closely monitored and, thus, can be measured by catheterization. Figure 45-5 shows a medical assistant measuring urinary output from a patient with an indwelling Foley catheter that drains continuously into a collection bag. This procedure is performed strictly for the purpose of measurement and not for urinalysis because stagnant urine has the opportunity to grow bacteria and is considered contaminated. To collect urine from an indwelling catheter for urinalysis, the access port should always be used.

Pediatric Specimen

Catheterization or obtaining a clean-catch midstream specimen may be challenging methods for the pediatric patient. Attaching an adhesive pediatric urine specimen bag is often the method of choice. This is further covered in the chapter titled "Assisting with Life Span Specialties: Pediatrics."

Suprapubic Specimen

Another method of collecting a sterile urine sample is to obtain a **suprapubic specimen**, which can be done by using a sterile needle and syringe. The physician inserts the needle into the patient's bladder through the abdominal wall just above the pubic bone and withdraws the urine sample into

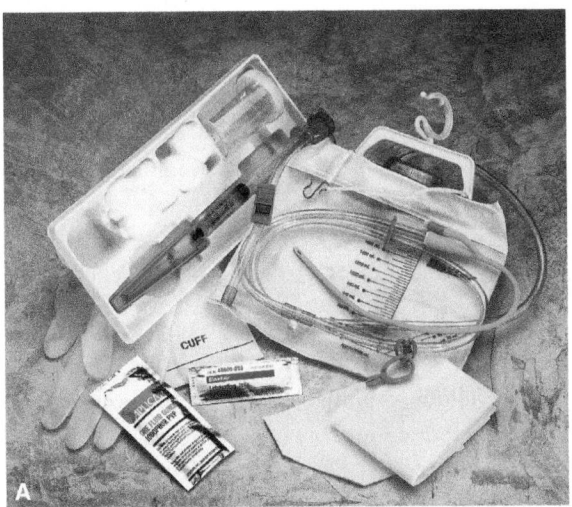

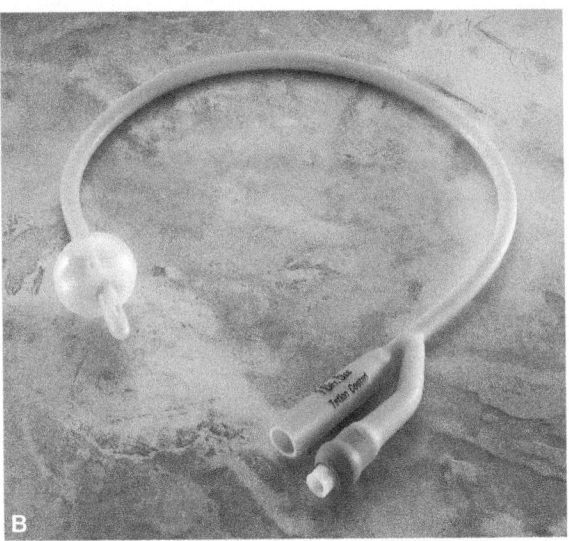

FIGURE 45-4 (A) Foley catheter tray; (B) Foley catheter.

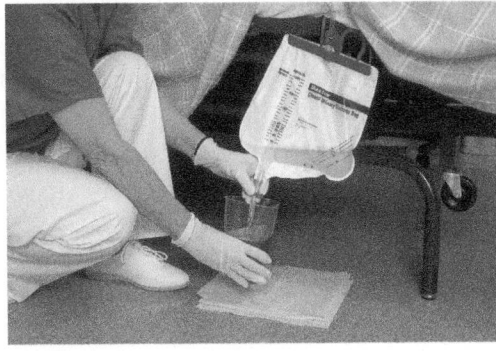

FIGURE 45-5 The medical assistant is measuring the urine output from a patient who has an indwelling Foley catheter that drains into a collection bag. This urine is for measurement only, not to be used for routine testing.

the syringe. Suprapubic specimens have been shown to be more reliably free of contamination than even clean-catch specimens, and often are used for cytology examinations. However, this procedure is less commonly performed because of its invasive nature.

ROUTINE URINALYSIS

After collection, a routine urinalysis can be performed to help identify potential health problems in patients, such as UTIs, diabetes, and kidney disease. There are three components to a routine urinalysis:

- Physical analysis
- Chemical analysis
- Microscopic analysis

During the physical analysis, urine is examined for color, clarity, concentration, odor, and volume. Urine can be a variety of colors from very pale or colorless to very dark or amber. Urine color and clarity can be a sign of what substances may be present in urine. Although the physical characteristics of urine may be important diagnostic tools for the physician, confirmation of suspected substances is often obtained during the chemical and microscopic examinations.

Chemical analysis is performed by using commercially prepared test strips that measure pH, specific gravity, glucose, bacteria, protein, and other chemical elements. A microscopic analysis may or may not be performed as part of a routine urinalysis, depending on if there are abnormal findings on the physical or chemical examination. Red blood cells, white blood cells, crystals, casts, and other components may be seen with a microscopic analysis.

If results of a routine urinalysis are abnormal, more specific testing may be ordered to determine a diagnosis and treatment. Table 45-1 is a listing of routine urinalysis categories.

Physical Characteristics

Urinalysis begins with an examination of the physical characteristics of urine: appearance (clarity, color), odor, and quantity (volume). Another physical characteristic that can be measured is specific gravity. Procedure 45-4 provides guidelines on how to evaluate the physical characteristics of urine when performing a routine urinalysis.

Appearance

Clarity. When first observing a urine specimen, you should note its clarity: clear or cloudy. If it is cloudy, more specific terms should be used, such as *slightly cloudy, cloudy with sediment*, or **turbid**, meaning the urine is cloudy, opaque, or does not allow light to pass through. A number of factors can cause turbidity: bacterial infection; white blood cells, red blood cells, or epithelial cells; pus (**pyuria**); and yeast or vaginal contaminants. However, normal urine may also appear as cloudy.

Always report exactly what is seen in the sample, using appropriate terms. Because crystals can form during the cooling process and change the appearance of the sample, always observe the appearance of the specimen before it begins to cool.

Color. The normal color of urine is straw—a pale yellow color. However, concentrated urine, along with medications, vitamins, and some foods, can cause urine colors to range from pale yellow to amber. **Diuretics** (medications that increase urine production) may cause urine to be so diluted that it appears almost clear. Occasionally, urine appears brown or black. Reddish-brown color may indicate bleeding, either in

TABLE 45-1 | Routine Urinalysis Categories

Physical	Chemical	Microscopic
Appearance (clarity/turbidity)	Reaction (pH)	Cells
Color	Protein	Blood (RBCs, WBCs)
Specific gravity	Glucose	Epithelial cells (squamous, transitional, renal)
Odor	Blood	Casts (hyaline, cellular, granular, waxy)
Quantity (24-hour specimen only)	Ketones	Crystals (acid/alkaline)
	Bilirubin	Other: bacteria, spermatozoa, parasites, yeast
	Urobilinogen	Artifacts
	Nitrite	
	Leukocytes	

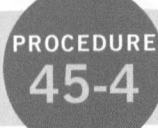

PROCEDURE 45-4

Evaluating the Physical Characteristics of Urine

Objective ◆ *Evaluate the physical characteristics of urine, and properly record the results.*

EQUIPMENT AND SUPPLIES

Urine specimen; centrifuge tube; laboratory slip; patient's medical record; personal protective equipment, as needed

METHOD

1. Perform hand hygiene and apply gloves.
2. Label the centrifuge tube with the patient's name.
3. Mix the urine by carefully swirling, avoiding spills.
4. Assess the clarity: Record observations using appropriate terms: *clear, slightly cloudy, cloudy*, and *turbid*. Transparency can also be evaluated by holding the container over some text and reading through an inch of urine. See Figure A for examples of urines of different clarity.
5. Assess the color: Record observations using appropriate terms: *straw, yellow, dark yellow,* or *amber*. See Figure B for examples of urines of different colors.

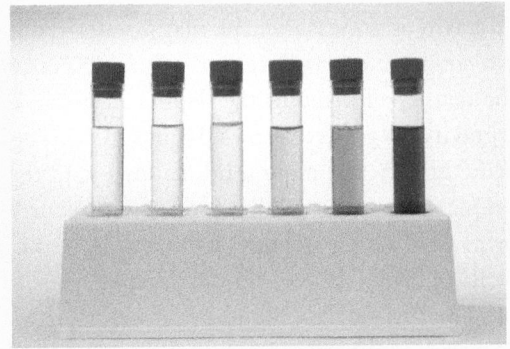

FIGURE B Colors of urine.

6. Note any abnormal aroma such as a fruity, putrid, ammonia, or musty odor.
7. Measure quantity when necessary for a time-specific test.
8. Measure the specific gravity if necessary, using the dipstick or refractometer method. (Procedure 45-5 explains the refractometer method of measuring specific gravity.)
9. Clean the work area.
10. Remove gloves and perform hand hygiene, unless proceeding with complete urinalysis.
11. Document in the patient's medical record.

CHARTING EXAMPLE

4/23/YY Clear, pale yellow urine collected via aseptic technique, per orders for a random urine specimen.....M. King, CMA

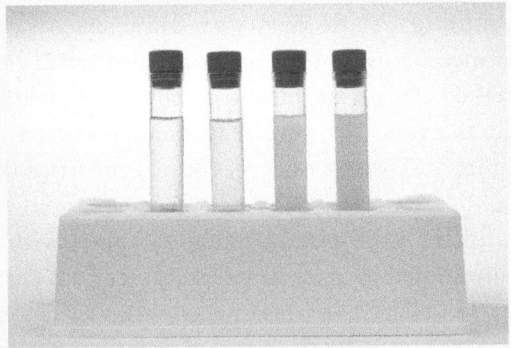

FIGURE A Appearance of urine (clear to very cloudy).

---

the urinary tract or from menstruation. Large quantities of the B-complex vitamins, especially B12, can cause the urine to appear bright yellow. Patients may have orange-colored urine if they are taking Pyridium (phenazophyridine, a medication used for bladder spasms or pain). Other medications, such as amitriptyline, can even turn urine blue or green.

Odor

Normally, odor is not recorded unless an abnormal aroma is evident. Individuals testing positive for ketones (a product of fat metabolism) may have a "fruity" odor to their urine. This can be indicative of uncontrolled diabetes. Putrid or

foul odors might indicate infection. Ammonia odors usually result from urine breaking down over time, similar to the odor of old urine on a diaper. Foods, such as asparagus, and some vitamins can affect the odor of urine. Patients with phenylketonuria (PKU) produce urine with a musty odor.

Quantity (Volume)

Quantity is measured when time-specific tests are needed for urine collection. However, quantity is not usually measured for routine testing. A 24-hour urine specimen should measure between 700 and 2,000 mL with the average being 1,500 mL (3 pints). **Polyuria** (excessive amounts of urine production) may indicate disorders such as diabetes or kidney disease. **Oliguria** (decreased amounts of urine production) can be indicative of decreased fluid intake and dehydration, cardiovascular disease, or kidney disease. If renal failure or an obstruction is present, then **anuria** (the absence of urine) may result. Individuals with these disorders may need to have their intake and output of fluids closely monitored and recorded.

Specific Gravity

Specific gravity is a measurement that assesses the kidney's ability to concentrate or dilute urine. Specific gravity compares the density of urine to the density of water. Normal specific gravity ranges between 1.010 and 1.030. The higher the specific gravity, the more solid material is in the urine. For example, when you drink a lot of fluid, your kidneys make urine with a high amount of water in it, resulting in a low specific gravity. If you are dehydrated, your kidneys make urine with a small amount of water in it, resulting in a high specific gravity. Readings outside the normal range may be the first indication that the kidneys may not be working properly. Some possible causes of abnormal specific gravity are listed in Box 45-1.

Two methods frequently used to test urine specific gravity are the reagent strip (dipstick) and the **refractometer** method. A third method, the urinometer, is no longer commonly used because it is more difficult to perform and has less accurate results.

Reagent Strip (Dipstick) Method. The dipstick method is the most commonly used method of measuring specific gravity. It is performed by dipping a chemically treated piece of plastic (the dipstick) into the sample of urine and then reading the chemical reaction that takes place and is displayed on the dipstick. The test strip is evaluated by a chemical analyzer or by visual comparison with the results shown on the side of the test strip container.

Refractometer Method. Though less common than the dipstick method, a refractometer may also be used to determine

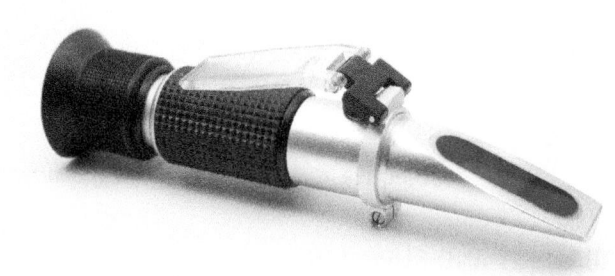

FIGURE 45-6 Portable digital refractometer.

specific gravity. A refractometer uses light, a prism, and a calibrated scale to measure the concentration level of the specimen. Figure 45-6 shows a refractometer. Procedure 45-5 provides the steps necessary to accurately measure the specific gravity of urine using a refractometer. This method may be seen in older offices or cost-efficient clinics.

Chemical Characteristics

Chemical analysis of urine can provide more detailed information about the patient than the physical analysis. As with measuring specific gravity, chemical analysis can also be performed by using reagent strips, also called the dipstick method. This is the most commonly used method for chemical analysis, with several commercial brands available. Figure 45-7 shows examples of reagent strips that are available.

The dipsticks are plastic strips equipped with small chemically treated pads (reagents) that react with chemicals in the urine to detect and measure specific substances. The color changes caused by the chemical reactions can then be compared with a color chart on the outside of the reagent strip container. The chart also lists the normal and abnormal values of each chemical pad or reagent.

BOX 45-1 | Possible Causes of Abnormal Specific Gravity

Low	High
Diabetes insipidus	Dehydration
Glomerulonephritis	Diabetes mellitus
Pyelonephritis	Adrenal insufficiency
Chronic renal disorders	Hepatic disease
Excessive hydration	Heart failure

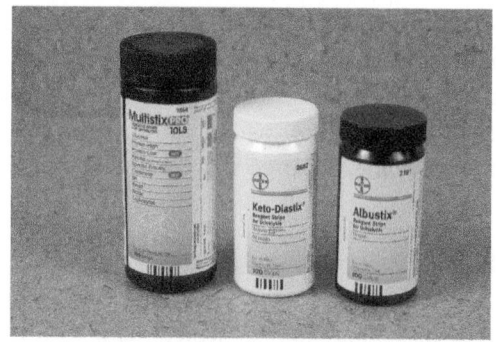

FIGURE 45-7 Variety of chemical reagent strips.

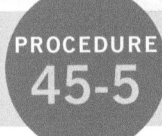

Measuring the Specific Gravity of Urine with a Refractometer

Objective ◆ *Measure the specific gravity of urine with a refractometer.*

EQUIPMENT AND SUPPLIES

Antiseptic cleaner; biohazard waste container; personal protective equipment (PPE)—lab coat, protective eyewear, and nonsterile gloves; distilled water; medicine dropper/pipette; paper and pen/pencil; paper towels; refractometer; urine specimen; patient's medical record

METHOD

1. Perform hand hygiene.
2. Apply gloves and protective clothing.
3. Assemble equipment and materials.
4. Before using the refractometer (Figure A), perform a quality control check by using a sample of distilled water first. The value with distilled water should be 1.000.
   a. Clean the prism and refractometer cover with distilled water. Wipe dry.
   b. Close the cover. Using the medicine dropper or pipette, place a drop of distilled water on the notched area of the cover. If the refractometer does not have an attached cover, place the water directly onto the prism, and then place a cover plate on top of the prism.
   c. Tilt the refractometer to allow light to enter. Read the specific gravity by noting the division line between the

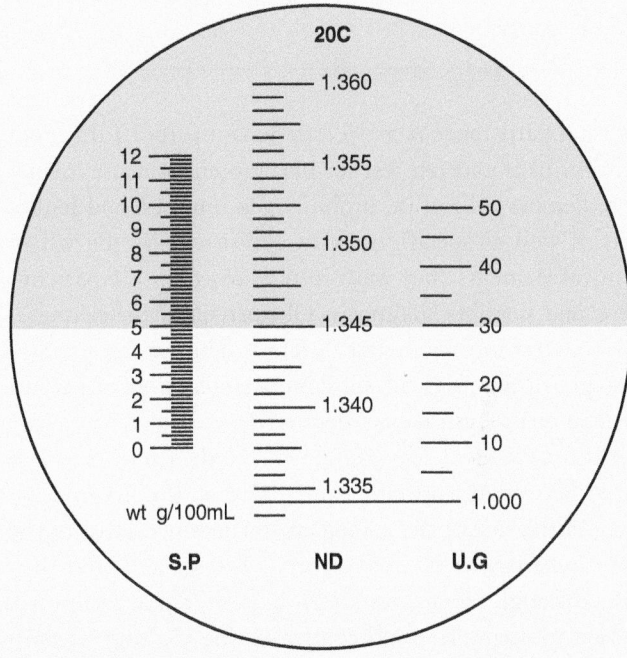

FIGURE B Refractometer scale.

light and dark area (Figure B). This reading should be 1.000. If it is not, retest with fresh distilled water.
5. Once the refractometer has been calibrated, prepare the urine specimen by gently swirling the urine to avoid splashing. Using the medicine dropper, remove a small sample and place one to two drops onto the notched area of the cover.
6. As performed in step 4.c., tilt the refractometer to allow light to enter. Read the specific gravity by noting the division line between the light and dark area (Figure B).
7. Record the reading on a piece of paper.
8. Discard the urine appropriately.
9. Remove gloves and protective clothing, and dispose of them properly.
10. Perform hand hygiene.
11. Document in the patient's medical record.
12. Clean the work area and equipment.

CHARTING EXAMPLE

4/23/YY 1:00 P.M. SG 1.012...........................M. King, CMA

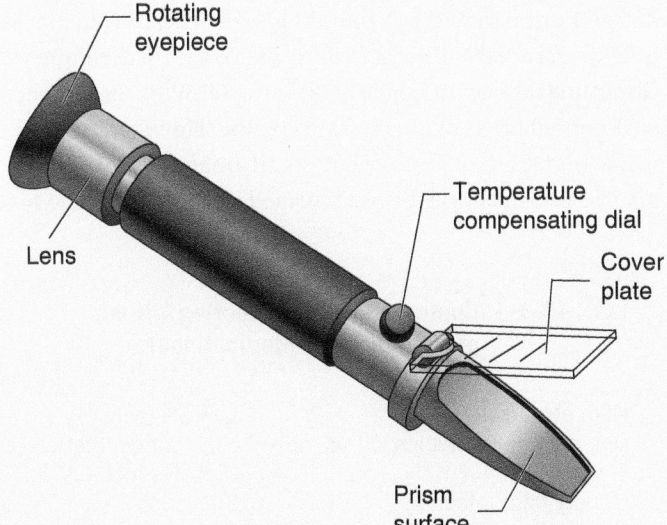

FIGURE A Refractometer with parts labeled.

Professionalism | The Life Span

Obtaining a urine specimen from an older adult may be a more complex procedure because of the coordination required to ensure that the specimen is placed in the container, according to guidelines. Be sure to carefully explain the collection procedure to patients and provide them with plenty of time and privacy for specimen collection. You may need to be in the laboratory restroom with them to provide help if they are unsteady on their feet or are confused.

A standard reagent strip may have up to 10 different chemical pads and can test for pH, protein, glucose, hematuria, ketones, bilirubin, urobilinogen, nitrites, and leukocytes as well as specific gravity. Physicians decide which chemical elements they want to test, based on the patient's status and possible diagnosis. Obstetricians, for example, routinely test for two main substances: glucose and protein. Most physicians have all substances tested when a patient has an annual physical examination.

After the reagent strip is dipped into the urine, each test should be read at a specific time, based on the information given on the side of the reagent strip container. Most of the tests can be read in as little as 60 to 120 seconds after dipping, although certain tests may require longer time for a reaction to occur. To avoid contaminating the reagent strip container, the medical assistant should be careful not to touch it with a wet strip during evaluation. Procedure 45-6 provides the proper steps for performing a urinalysis with reagent strips.

Reaction pH

The pH (potential hydrogen ion concentration) of a solution indicates acidity and alkalinity. The pH is measured on a scale of 0 to 14, with 0 being the most acidic, 14 being the most basic (alkaline), and 7 being neutral (Figure 45-8). Normally, urine is slightly acidic.

The ability of the kidneys to dilute and concentrate urine helps maintain the narrow pH range of blood (7.35 to 7.45), which is necessary for the body to be in homeostasis. Normal kidneys produce urine with pH ranging from 4.6 to 7.9, depending on when the urine is tested. For example, urine in the morning is more acidic than urine in the evening. In urinary tract infections (UTIs), the pH is typically more alkaline (higher than 7.5) because some bacteria break down urea to ammonia. A high pH might occur if the urine sample is not tested immediately and allowed to sit at room temperature too long, allowing bacterial growth and giving a false reading. See Box 45-2 for common factors affecting urinary pH.

Protein

Protein is normally not found in the urine of healthy individuals. Urine may sometimes contain a small quantity of protein after exposure to the cold, strenuous muscular activity, acute stress, or eating large amounts of protein. However, these are considered physiological responses and not symptoms of a disease.

Proteins are relatively large compounds that are typically filtered out of urine by the glomerulus of the kidneys. The presence of protein in the urine (**proteinuria**) can indicate renal dysfunction from damage to the glomeruli (**glomerulonephritis**). This may be a result of an infection (often *Streptococcus*), preeclampsia in pregnancy, or chronic disorders such as diabetes, hypertension, or congestive heart failure. Sometimes, simple UTIs can cause a false positive reading for high protein from the breakdown of cells. Because kidney function is vital to life, the cause of protein in the urine should always be investigated.

Glucose

Normal urine should not contain glucose because almost all glucose gets reabsorbed back into the blood by the kidneys. **Glycosuria** (also called **glucosuria**) is the term for the presence of abnormal levels of glucose in the urine. However, after eating a high-carbohydrate diet, small quantities of glucose may be present in the urine. If urine levels of glucose do not

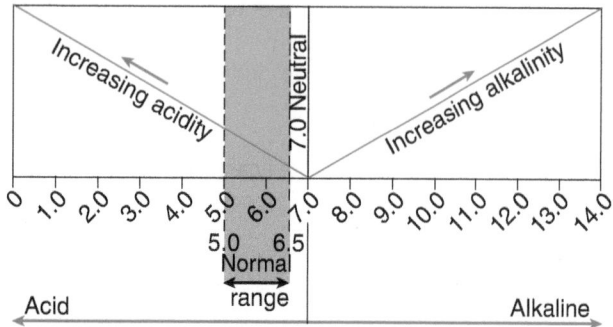

FIGURE 45-8 Urine pH scale.

BOX 45-2 | Common Factors Affecting Urinary pH (Other Than Medications)

High pH (alkaline)
Diet high in vegetables, citrus, or dairy
Urinary tract infection
High vitamin C intake
Urine sitting at room temperature too long

Low pH (acidic)
High protein diet
Diabetes mellitus
Starvation
Renal tuberculosis

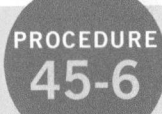

PROCEDURE 45-6

Testing the Chemical Characteristics of Urine with Reagent Strips

Objective ◆ *Perform chemical testing on urine using chemical reagent strips.*

EQUIPMENT AND SUPPLIES

Urine specimen; reagent test strips; timer; paper towel; laboratory slip; pen/pencil; personal protective equipment, as needed

METHOD

1. Perform hand hygiene and don personal protective gear.
2. Check the specimen for the patient's identity, the date, and time of collection.
3. Check the expiration date on the reagent strips.

4. Bring the specimen to room temperature and gently swirl to mix.
5. Dip the reagent strip in the urine, making sure all pads on the strip are moistened (Figure A).
6. Read each pad by comparing it to the chart on the side of the bottle, appropriately timing each test (Figure B).
   a. Do not touch the test strip against the side of the bottle to prevent contamination.
   b. Ignore color changes after the prescribed time has elapsed.
7. Record the results on the patient's laboratory slip.
8. Clean the work area, remove gloves, and perform hand hygiene.

CHARTING EXAMPLE

Note: Normally, a urine test slip is used to record all results of chemical tests. When the examination is complete and the physician has reviewed it, the test slip is placed in the patient's medical chart.

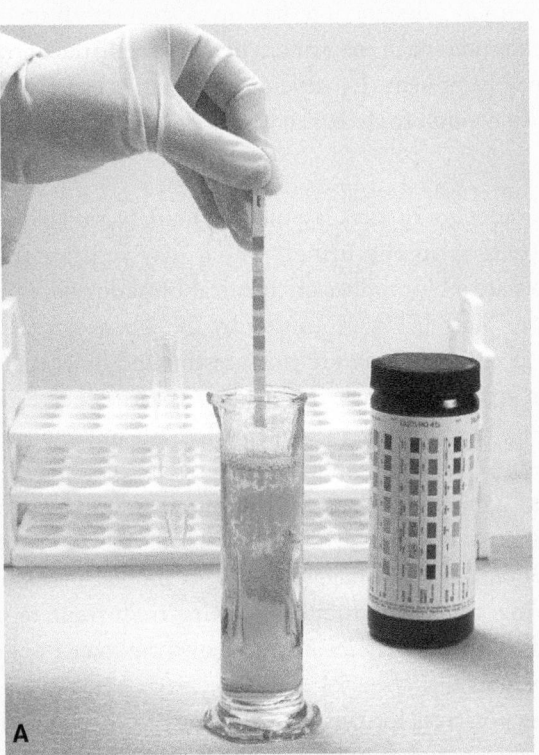

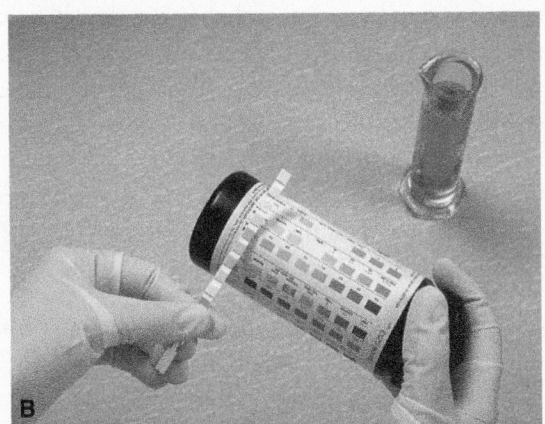

FIGURE A–B (A) Dip reagent strip into urine and withdraw; **(B)** compare color changes on the reagent strip to chart on the side of container without contaminating the container.

return to normal fairly quickly, it may be indicative of diabetes, gestational diabetes, stress, infection, or Cushing's syndrome, or it may be a result of certain medications. Glucose will spill into the urine when the blood glucose levels exceed the renal threshold for glucose, which is approximately 160 to 180 mg/dL of glucose in the bloodstream.

When a reagent strip tests positive for glucose in the urine, many testing laboratories and some physician's offices may confirm this by reagent tablet testing. The reagent tablet test uses chemically treated tablets that are added to the urine specimen, and the resulting color is compared with a reaction chart to confirm the presence of glucose. Some

Testing for Glucose Using the Reagent Tablet Test

1. Using the medicine dropper or a pipette, place five drops of the urine specimen into a clean test tube.
2. Add 10 drops of water. Mix together using the pipette, being careful not to splash the urine.
3. Drop one reagent tablet into the urine and water solution. Observe the solution as it reacts in the test tube. Do not shake the mixture, and do not touch the bottom of the tube because it may be hot as a result of the chemical reaction occurring.
4. After the reaction (boiling) stops, wait 15 seconds and gently shake the tube to mix the contents.
5. Immediately match the color of the liquid against the color chart on the side of the reagent tablet container.

Note: Do not touch the test tube of urine to the reagent tablet bottle to prevent contamination. Ignore any additional color changes after the 15-second period.

physician's offices may have a protocol in place that the medical assistant may perform a reagent tablet test or re-test using another brand or lot number of dipstick before reporting a positive result for glycosuria. See Guidelines 45-2: Testing for Glucose Using the Reagent Tablet Test.

Hematuria

Hematuria (blood in the urine) is abnormal unless it is a contamination from menses. The presence of **occult** (hidden) blood in urine may indicate anemia, UTIs, kidney stones, or trauma and is occasionally caused by some medications. Female patients must be asked if they are menstruating when urine collection is required. If a patient is menstruating, it should be noted on the laboratory slip.

Ketones

Ketones are by-products of fat metabolism. Fats normally break down into water and carbon dioxide. However, if fats are burned as a source of energy instead of glucose, ketones will be found in the urine. Ketones are typically seen only in conditions such as poorly controlled diabetes, dehydration, starvation, ingestion of large quantities of aspirin, high protein diets, and occasionally after general anesthesia. Ketones tend to evaporate at room temperature, so testing must be done immediately or the specimen should be covered and refrigerated until testing can be performed.

Bilirubin

Under normal circumstances, bilirubin is not found in the urine. Bilirubin is a by-product of the breakdown of hemoglobin. Hemoglobin is released during normal breakdown of old red blood cells (RBCs) and is converted by the liver into bilirubin and urobilinogen in the small intestine. The presence of bilirubin in urine may be one of the first signs of liver disease, obstructive biliary disease, hepatitis, or mononucleosis. Large amounts of bilirubin in the urine will cause the urine to turn yellow-brown to dark orange. Bilirubin is light-sensitive and may be degraded when exposed to light. Thus, to prevent a false negative result, the urine specimen should be stored away from light until testing can be performed.

Urobilinogen

Like bilirubin, urobilinogen is a result of RBC destruction, and it is present in small quantities under normal conditions. Levels of urobilinogen will be elevated in any condition causing an increase in bilirubin. High levels of urobilinogen in the urine may help detect liver diseases such as hepatitis and cirrhosis, and conditions associated with increased RBC destruction (hemolytic anemia). If no urobilinogen is present in the urine, a hepatic or bile duct obstruction may be present. However, reagent strips usually are not sensitive enough to detect an absence of urobilinogen.

Nitrites

Measurement of nitrites is a method for detection of **bacteriuria** (bacteria in the urine), which may indicate a UTI. Nitrites are a by-product of chemical breakdown by certain bacteria. Most UTIs are caused by *Escherichia coli* (*E. coli*), which is normally found in the intestine and in fecal matter. When introduced into the urinary meatus, bacteria can travel up the urethra to the bladder. An infection in the bladder may result if enough bacteria are present, causing **cystitis**. Women may be especially prone to UTIs because of their shorter urethras, which allow bacteria easier access to the bladder. Thus, women should be reminded after voiding or having a bowel movement to wipe from front to back, away from the urinary meatus, to lessen the chance of developing UTIs.

False positives for the presence of nitrites can happen if the specimen sits at room temperature too long, allowing for bacteria growth. Specimens that cannot be immediately tested should be refrigerated until testing can be performed.

Leukocytes

Leukocytes are commonly referred to as white blood cells (WBCs). Under normal conditions, only a few WBCs should be present in urine. However, when WBCs are present in sufficient quantity, it usually indicates a UTI. When a urinalysis is performed, the reagent strip detects leukocyte

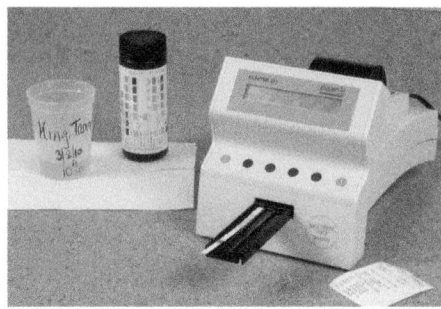

FIGURE 45-9 An example of a urine chemical analyzer.

esterase, an enzyme released by WBCs. The darker the color on the strip, the greater the number of WBCs.

When a leukocyte esterase test is positive and a UTI is suspected, it is important to see if results from other tests are consistent for a UTI, such as a positive protein test, elevated pH, and bacteria that may be visible with microscopic examination.

Automated Urine Chemical Analyzers

Automated chemical analyzers for urine are widely used in many types of facilities because of their ease of use, efficiency, and reliability. These analyzers use light photometry to test the strips, which eliminates the human error associated with color recognition. Some analyzers read the test strips and report the results on a printout sheet. Quality control protocols, including the use of positive and negative controls and proper documentation, must be followed. Figure 45-9 is an example of an automated urine chemical analyzer. Table 45-2 gives normal urine values.

TABLE 45-2 | Normal Values for Urinalysis Testing

Element	Normal Values
Color	Straw, pale yellow, yellow, darker yellow, amber
Appearance	Clear, slightly cloudy
Specific gravity	1.010–1.030
Odor	Aromatic
Reaction/pH	4.6–7.9
Protein	Negative to trace
Glucose	Negative
Ketones	Negative
Blood	Negative
Nitrites	Negative
Bilirubin	Negative
Urobilinogen	Less than 2 Ehrlich units/dL
Leukocytes	Negative

Microscopic Examination

Microscopic examination identifies the type and approximate number of organisms present in a urine specimen. Microscopic examination is not a Clinical Laboratory Improvement Amendments (CLIA)-waived test because it requires more complex training to perform and evaluate results. A certificate of provider-performed microscopy (PPM) procedures needs to be issued to a physician's office laboratory (POL) that is qualified to perform waived tests. Microscopic examinations are performed by a physician or a mid-level practitioner (e.g., nurse practitioners, nurse midwives, physician assistants) on the specimen obtained during the patient visit. In some states, however, medical assistants may perform microscopic examinations after further training and if the facility already has a PPM certificate. More often, urine specimens are sent to an outside laboratory for microscopic evaluation.

Although medical assistants cannot evaluate urine for microscopic analysis without further training, they must be able to properly prepare a urine specimen for microscopic examination and understand the meaning and importance of the results.

Preparing a Urine Specimen for Microscopic Examination

After physical and chemical analyses, fresh urine is poured into tubes to prepare for microscopic analysis. A centrifuge rotates the urine tubes at high speeds, using centrifugal force to separate substances of different densities. This causes heavier particles to sink to the bottom and lighter fluids to float to the top. The **sediment** is the solid material remaining at the bottom of the tube after the **supernatant** (liquid portion) is carefully poured off. The sediment may contain cellular material such as RBCs, WBCs, epithelial cells, **casts** (particles made by the kidneys), bacteria, parasites, yeast, fungi, and spermatozoa. Chemical materials may also be found in the sediment, including crystals and amorphous (shapeless) material.

A special stain may be used to provide better contrast to the formed elements present. Using a pipette, a drop of the suspended sediment is placed on a microscope slide and covered with a cover slip for viewing. Procedure 45-7 presents the steps needed to prepare a urine specimen for microscopic examination.

Reporting and Understanding Urine Microscopic Examinations

When a microscopic slide is being evaluated, the circle being viewed is called a field. There are two basic types of fields. A low-power field (LPF) shows less detail but allows a larger area

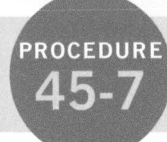

PROCEDURE
45-7

Preparing a Urine Specimen for Microscopic Examination

Objective ◆ *Perform microscopic examination of urine sediment for casts and cells.*

EQUIPMENT AND SUPPLIES

Biohazard waste container; personal protective equipment—lab coat, goggles, and nonsterile gloves; capillary pipette; centrifuge; centrifuge tube; microscope; microscope slide; paper and pen/pencil; Sedi-stain (optional); urine specimen

METHOD

1. Perform hand hygiene.
2. Apply gloves and protective clothing.
3. Assemble equipment and materials.
4. Mix the specimen gently to stir up the sediment that has settled to the bottom.
5. Place 10 mL of urine into the centrifuge tube. Place cap on tube. Place the tube in the centrifuge and balance this with another tube of 10 mL of water on the opposite side of the machine (Figure A).
6. Set the centrifuge timer for five minutes.
7. After the centrifuge has stopped, remove the tube and carefully pour off the supernatant (the clear liquid left on the top after centrifuging), leaving only the sediment (Figure B).
   Alternative Method: Some medical assistants prefer using stain (such as Sedi-stain) to help identify sediment more easily. Place one drop of the commercially prepared stain in the test tube.

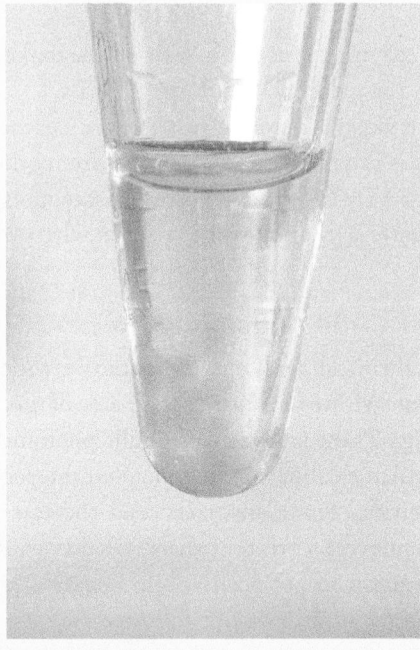

FIGURE B Pour out most of the liquid supernatant from the tube but keep the sediment.

8. Mix the sediment by holding the top of the tube and tapping the bottom with a finger, mixing well to ensure a correct reading.
9. Use a capillary pipette to transfer one drop of sediment to a clean slide (Figure C).
10. Cover the drop of sediment with a coverslip.
11. Place the slide on the microscope stage.

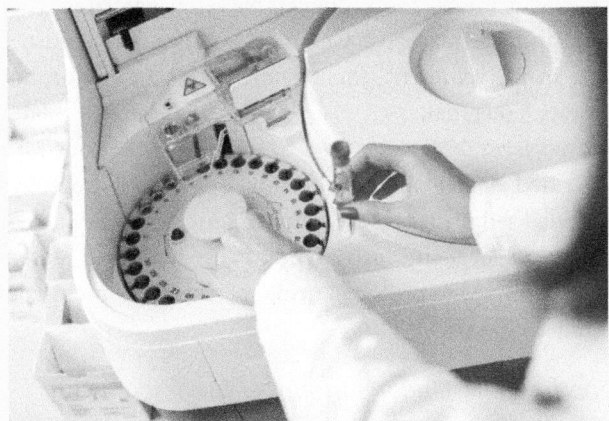

FIGURE A The centrifuge is used to spin urine specimens in preparation for a microscopic examination.

FIGURE C After mixing the sediment well, use a dropper to place a drop of urine on the slide.

to be evaluated for counting. A high-power field (HPF) evaluates a smaller area in greater detail for better identification. The slide is moved several times to be able to evaluate several different fields of view. The number of casts or cells is counted in each circular field and an overall range is given, indicating the least and greatest number counted in each of 10 to 15 fields of view. Thus, a report of 0–4 hyaline casts per LPF means that, in each one of the 10 to 15 fields evaluated, the least number of casts counted in any low-power field was 0 and the most was 4. This may be repeated using a high-power field, as well. It is preferable to use a numerical range when reporting formed elements. Other elements may be reported using the following words to estimate the amounts:

- Occasional   0–3
- Few   3–6
- Moderate   6–12
- Many   12 or more
- TNTC   Too numerous to count

As noted earlier, microscopic urinalysis is not CLIA waived and, therefore, is not within the medical assistant's scope of practice in most states. Further training is required for medical assistants to perform microscopic examination. However, in the classroom, microscopic studies are often performed to better demonstrate the meaning of test results. See Box 45-3 for performing microscopic examinations in the classroom setting. Figure 45-10 identifies different structures that may be found in a urine microscopic examination.

Cells

Cells that may be found in urine are epithelial cells, RBCs, and WBCs that may indicate a urinary tract condition.

Epithelial Cells. Epithelial cells are classified as squamous, transitional, and renal epithelial cells. Squamous epithelial cells line the urinary tract from the external meatus to the bladder as well as the vaginal wall. Therefore, a few epithelial cells (0–5 per HPF) are to be expected in a urine sample. However, the presence of transitional or renal epithelial cells is an abnormal finding and may indicate a disease in the bladder or kidneys.

Red Blood Cells. Anything more than 1 to 2 RBCs per HPF is considered abnormal. The presence of RBCs could indicate a bladder infection or kidney disorder, such as nephritis. RBCs are pale, round, have no nucleus (core), and are nongranular. RBCs in the urine may indicate that bleeding may be taking place somewhere in the urinary system. Acidic urine may cause the RBCs to rupture, causing them to be invisible or mistaken for WBCs under microscopic examination. RBCs may also be contaminants from menstruation in female patients.

White Blood Cells. WBCs can be distinguished from RBCs because of their nucleus and granular surface, as well as being larger than RBCs. A normal count is 0 to 5 WBCs per HPF. Large numbers of WBCs may indicate an infection in the urinary system. Further testing would be needed to pinpoint the location of the infection, however.

Casts

Casts result from protein formation in the kidney tubules. Different types of casts are classified according to the substances that form them. Casts are counted under the low power of the microscope but are identified under high-powered magnification. Casts may be identified as hyaline,

---

BOX 45-3 | Microscopic Examination in the Classroom

Although in most physicians' offices the medical assistant does not perform the microscopic examination for a urinalysis, it is helpful to understand the entire procedure and the meaning of the test results. Review the steps for preparing a urine specimen for a microscopic examination listed in Procedure 45-7. For performing a microscopic examination in the classroom setting, standard precautions should still apply.

- Once the microscope slide is prepared, the microscope's focus should be under low power and reduced light to better view for casts and epithelial cells. Examine 10 to 15 fields. Carefully examine for anything abnormal and pay close attention to the edges, which are where casts are often seen. Count the number of casts or other abnormalities seen in each field. Average the count from the 10 to 15 fields for each formed element seen, and record appropriately.

- Examine 10 to 15 fields using high-power magnification and adjusting for more light. Count RBCs, WBCs, round cells, transitional cells, and squamous epithelial cells. Identify any casts, if present. Average the count from the 10 to 15 fields for each formed element seen, and record appropriately.
- Observe for crystals, bacteria, sperm, yeast, and parasites. Report them as *few, moderate,* or *many.*
- Discard the urine according to Occupational Safety and Health Administration (OSHA) guidelines.
- Remove gloves and protective clothing, and dispose of them properly.
- Perform hand hygiene.
- Clean the work area and equipment according to OSHA guidelines.

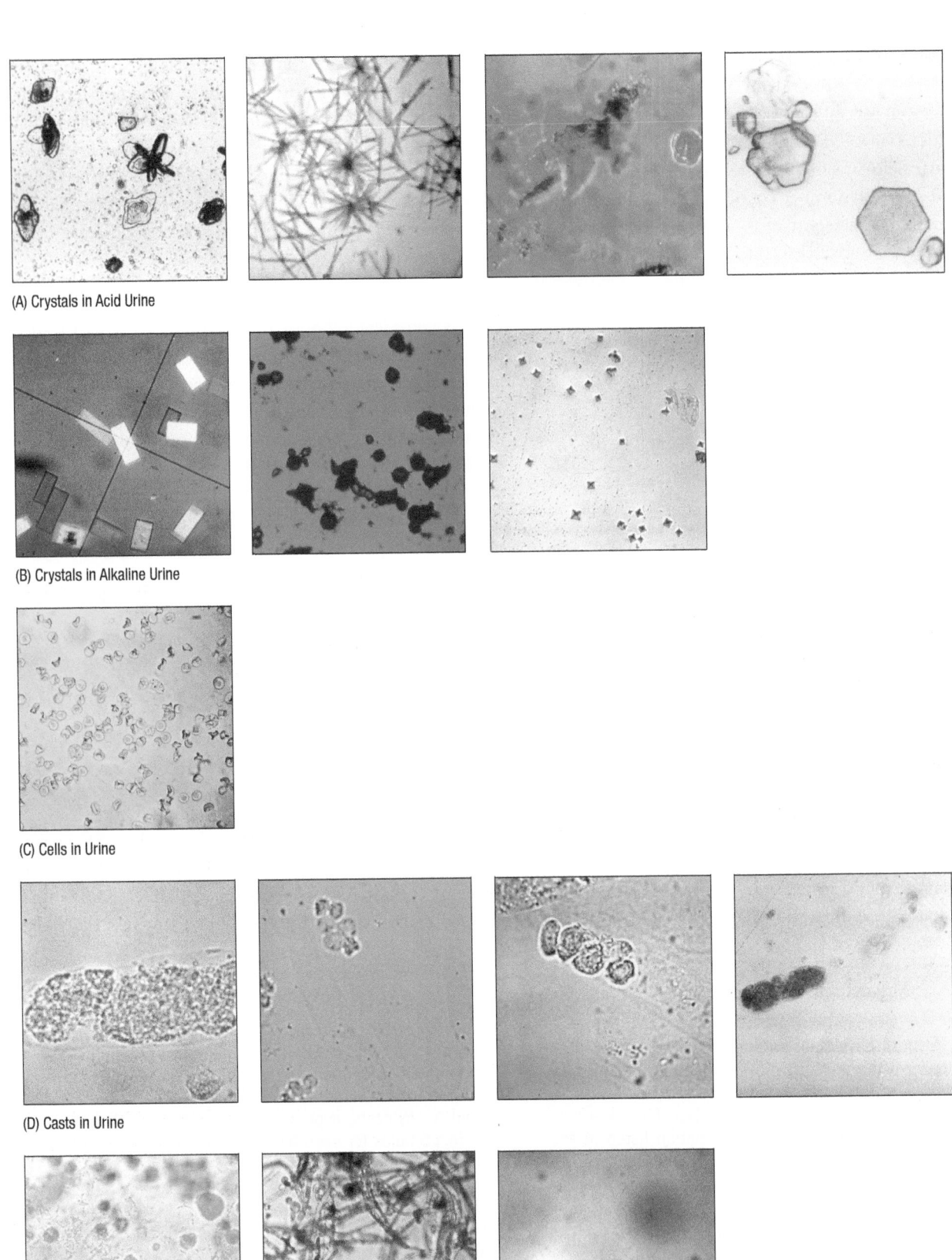

(A) Crystals in Acid Urine

(B) Crystals in Alkaline Urine

(C) Cells in Urine

(D) Casts in Urine

(E) Bacteria, Fungi, Parasites Found in Urine

FIGURE 45-10 Urine sediment chart.

granular (coarse or finely granular), cellular (WBC, RBC, or epithelial), mixed (containing more than one type of cell), or waxy. Larger quantities of hyaline casts may be indicative of kidney disease. RBC casts are found in diseases such as glomerulonephritis. Waxy casts are rarely seen and are indicative of severe renal disease.

Bacteria

Bacteria are not normally found in fresh urine. If large numbers of bacteria are present in the urine, this may indicate a UTI. A specimen with bacteria and WBCs can be considered a confirmation of a UTI. However, a specimen can become contaminated during collection if proper procedures are not followed.

When a UTI is suspected, a urine **culture and sensitivity (C&S)** test may be ordered. Because this is not a CLIA-waived test, the urine specimen is typically sent to a testing laboratory. A laboratory technician will take a sample of the urine with a swab and apply it to a culture dish for growth. Small disks impregnated with various types of antibiotics are then added to the dish. After a period of two to three days with the bacteria being allowed to grow, the plate is examined to see whether the bacterial growth is inhibited (or not) by the antibiotics on each disk. If the bacteria are sensitive to the antibiotic, a clear, circular "halo" or "plaque" will appear around the antibiotic disk, indicating that the antibiotic was able to inhibit or kill the bacteria. C&S testing helps to determine the type of bacteria involved and which antibiotic will be effective in treatment.

Yeast

Yeast may be present in the urine of a female who has a vaginal yeast infection (moniliasis), which most likely occurred through contamination by vaginal secretions during collection. It is more likely present in patients with diabetes mellitus.

Parasites

Parasites are organisms that live within and feed off of other organisms. They may be present in urine as a result of contamination from vaginal or bowel excretions. *Trichomonas vaginalis* is the most frequently found parasite in urine, and it is a common cause of vaginal infections.

Spermatozoa

Spermatozoa, the male reproductive cell, can be seen in both male and female urine specimens after sexual intercourse.

Crystals

Crystals are formed by the precipitation of urinary salts when pH, temperature, or concentration changes occur. Crystals can form in the urine in the kidney, in the bladder, or in a standing specimen. Crystals are found in both acid and alkaline urine. As urine cools, solid crystals will precipitate out. The presence of crystals is not usually clinically significant unless found in large numbers. Crystals are identified by their appearance in the urine specimen at the time of testing. In certain metabolic disorders, abnormal crystals such as leucine, tyrosine, or cystine may be found. In addition, certain drugs, such as sulfa drugs, may cause the production of crystals.

Contaminants

Many substances can cause contamination of a urine specimen, including clothing fibers, mucous threads, hair, or talcum powder. A contaminant-free specimen is never completely guaranteed, but clear instructions and patient education can minimize the chances of specimen contamination.

URINE PREGNANCY AND OVULATION TESTING

There are two main methods to test for pregnancy: a urine sample and a blood sample. Both tests are based on the detection of the hormone human chorionic gonadotropin (hCG), which is produced by the placenta during pregnancy. Depending on the type of test performed, levels of hCG can be detectable as early as six to eight days after fertilization has taken place.

For pregnancy tests using urine samples, different types can be performed at home or in a clinic or physician's office. One type uses a dipstick; the other relies on a midstream sample. Both are common in home pregnancy tests and are readily available at most drugstores. For the dipstick method, the woman urinates into a clean, dry cup, and dips a dipstick into the urine sample to detect the presence of hCG. For the midstream sample, the woman will begin voiding into the toilet, and then place the absorbent tip of the pregnancy test under the urine stream until it is thoroughly wet, usually for at least 10 seconds. Then she will remove the stick and continue voiding into the toilet. An alternative method for the midstream sample is for the woman to urinate into a clean, dry cup and dip the absorbent tip of the test into the cup for at least 15 seconds. With either method, a first morning specimen or void is preferred for urine testing because the concentration of the hormone is greatest at that time.

Once the test has been wetted by the urine specimen, the woman should lay the test flat with the results window facing up. Tests vary in how long you have to wait for a result, although most tests provide results in minutes. Results are shown in the results window as a change in color, a line, or a symbol, such as a plus (+) or minus (-) sign. A newer digital pregnancy test currently available makes reading results even simpler with the window showing either the words "not pregnant" or "pregnant."

A more accurate confirmation of pregnancy is often done by blood sample. Blood pregnancy tests must be sent to a laboratory for analysis and are generally more accurate than urine tests. Blood tests can also confirm pregnancy much earlier than urine tests, often as early as six days into the pregnancy. In most cases, a patient will take a home pregnancy test using urine samples and will then follow up at her physician's office to confirm her pregnancy with a blood test. Further, if a patient receives different answers on multiple home pregnancy tests, it is recommended that she have a blood test done to get an accurate answer.

Although the tests themselves are easy to perform, the technology of the pregnancy test is fairly complex. CLIA-waived pregnancy tests performed in POLs fall into two categories: the agglutination inhibition test and the enzyme-linked immunoassay. The agglutination inhibition test determines the presence of hCG in the patient's urine by mixing it with hCG-coated latex particles and hCG antibodies. One drop of the urine is mixed with one drop of hCG antibody solution and allowed to bind for one minute on a black glass slide. Next, one drop of the hCG-coated latex particles is added to the slide and left for one minute. If the level of hCG in the urine is absent or too low, the antibodies will agglutinate (clump) to the hCG-coated latex particles. If agglutination occurs, the patient is not pregnant. However, if the level of hCG in urine is high, the hCG in the urine will bind to the antibodies, and there will be no agglutination with the hCG-coated latex particles. Thus, if no agglutination occurs, the patient is pregnant.

The more frequently used enzyme-linked immunoassays (EIA or ELISA) tests involve the reaction of antigen and antibody and a second antibody attached to an enzyme. An antibody for hCG is attached to a solid surface. This antibody has affinity for and will bind to hCG. Purified hCG that has been linked to an enzyme is mixed with the test sample (blood or urine) and added to the test system with the hCG antibody. If no hCG is present in the test sample, then only hCG linked with the enzyme will bind to the antibody, resulting in a color change from the enzyme reaction. If there is hCG in the test sample, it will bind to the hCG antibody and less enzyme-linked HCG will bind. This will result in no color change because no enzyme reaction occurred.

Most pregnancy tests, including urine home pregnancy tests, have accuracies of 97 to 99 percent. However, this depends on the patient and medical assistant following proper procedures and protocol of testing. Pregnancy tests

are produced with built-in controls that are performed along with the patient test to provide quality control. Procedure 45-8 lists the steps necessary to perform a urine pregnancy test using the EIA testing method.

In pregnancy testing, a positive result usually indicates that a woman is pregnant. It may also mean that she was recently pregnant but may have had a miscarriage or abortion. A confirmed diagnosis should always be made by a physician, as certain types of tumors and infertility medications may also cause a test to appear positive. In fact, some medical providers use hCG testing as an effective screening tool for specific types of cancer in both men and women, such as testicular and ovarian cancers.

Urine tests may also be used to test for ovulation for women who want to plan for a pregnancy. These urine ovulation tests work by detecting the presence of the luteinizing hormone (LH), which is produced by the pituitary gland, and surges or peaks two to three days before ovulation. Thus, intercourse on these days has the highest likelihood of resulting in pregnancy. However, this test should not be used to prevent pregnancy because it is not reliable for that purpose.

The urine ovulation test is performed similarly to a urine pregnancy test and may use test strips that are dipped into a cup of urine specimen or held in the urine stream. Results should be given in five minutes and may be seen as colored lines on the test. Urine ovulation tests are available as home tests or kits and usually include multiple tests to allow for measuring LH over several days to identify the most fertile days for a pregnancy.

URINE DRUG ANALYSIS

There are a number of different drug testing methods available using hair, saliva, blood, urine, and even perspiration as samples. Urine testing is the most common method, as it is simple, fast, and fairly accurate. Urine may be sent off to an outside lab for testing. But, more commonly, CLIA-waived urine drug screening is performed by the medical assistant in the physician's office laboratory. There are many FDA-approved tests to choose from, each testing for a different range of drugs.

Drug screening is commonly requested before employment or state licensure. Some private and charter high schools now require students to submit to random drug screenings. Several health organizations require the medical office to be certified and employees to be specially trained to perform drug testing.

The procedures for collection and testing of urine are very strict and detailed, and the procedures and protocol must be carefully followed. Although every office has its own specific

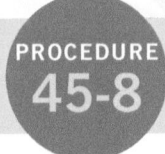

PROCEDURE 45-8

Performing a Urine Pregnancy Test

Objective ◆ *Perform a urine pregnancy test for hCG using an EIA test and interpret results correctly.*

EQUIPMENT AND SUPPLIES

Patient's first morning urine specimen; EIA test kit for hCG; timer; gloves; laboratory report; patient's medical record

METHOD

1. Perform hand hygiene and apply gloves.
2. Gather supplies and equipment.
3. Allow the testing materials and specimen to come to room temperature.
4. Label the test with the patient name or ID number.
5. Label one area positive and one negative for controls.
6. Place the patient's urine on the test chamber following manufacturer's directions.
7. Place positive and negative controls in correct areas (Figure A).
8. Time the test according to the manufacturer's directions.
9. Interpret results correctly.
10. Record results on the patient's laboratory slip. Document in the patient's medical record.
11. Record positive and negative controls in a quality control logbook according to office policy.
12. Dispose of equipment and perform hand hygiene. Clean the work area.

CHARTING EXAMPLE

10/19/YY 4:00 P.M. hCG test pos........................M. King, CMA

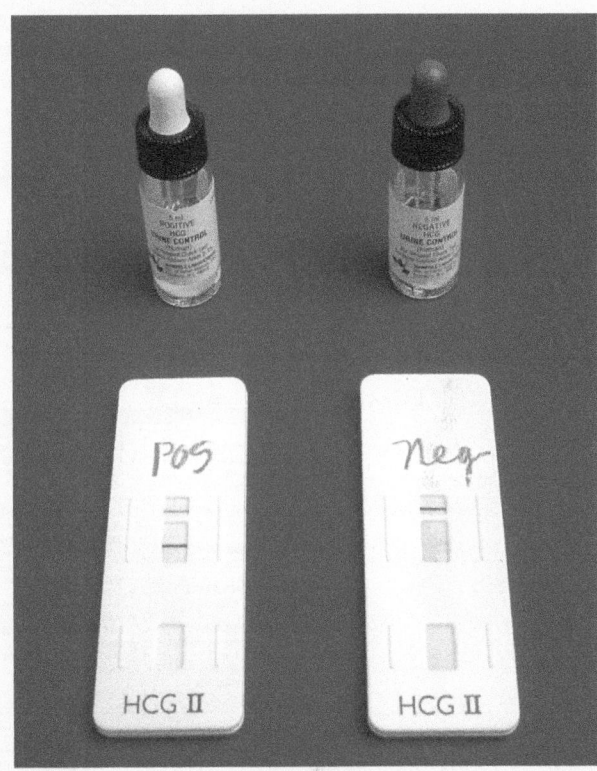

FIGURE A Urine pregnancy control test—positive and negative.

protocol, the main strategy is to ensure that testing is accurate and without tampering. An important component to performing a drug test is a chain of custody, which is the term used to describe the process of ensuring and providing documentation of proper specimen identification and handling from the time of specimen collection to the reporting of laboratory results. The chain of custody assures the specimen belongs to the individual whose information is printed on the specimen container label; that no post-collection tampering has occurred; exactly who had possession of the specimen; when and how the specimen was transported and stored before it was analyzed; and that the specimen was handled in a secure manner.

Any and all drug testing must include a **chain of custody form** (sometimes abbreviated to CCF or CoC), which is a chronological documentation or paper trail showing the collection, transfer, receipt, analysis, storage, and disposal of the sample. A chain of custody form is a multipart form containing unique specimen identification information that accompanies each specimen throughout the entire drug testing process. The form identifies the company requesting the test, the subject of the test, the type of test to be performed, and the medical review officer (MRO) who will review the test. Each form also includes the necessary labels to secure the specimen container throughout the process. This provides for specimen integrity and accountability of the test

Lab Services

IMPORTANT
Patient instructions
and map on back

PHYSICIAN ORDERS

Patient _____ _____ __ D.O.B. _____ M ☐ Patient
　　　　Last Name　　　　　　First　　　M.I.　　　　　　　F ☐ SS# __ __ __

Address _____ City _____ Zip _____ Phone # _____

Physician _____
ATTACH COPY OF INSURANCE CARD

ICD Diagnosis Code _____
(Additional codes on reverse)

Date & Time of Collection:
_____
Drawing _____
Facility

☐ 789.00 Abdominal Pain　☐ 414.9 Coronary Artery Disease (CAD)　☐ 244.9 Hypothyroidism　☐ ROUTINE　☐ PHONE RESULTS TO: # _____
☐ 285.9 Anemia (NOS)　☐ 250.0 DM (diabetes mellitus)　☐ 272.4 Hyperlipidemia　☐ ASAP　☐ FAX RESULTS TO: # _____
☐ 780.7 Fatigue/Malaise　☐ 401.9 Hypertension　☐ STAT　☐ COPY TO: _____
☐ 272.0 Hypercholesterolemia　☐ 483.9 URI (upper respiratory infection)

HEMATOLOGY	CHEMISTRY	CHEMISTRY	MICROBIOLOGY
☐ 1021 CBC, Automated Diff (incl, Platelet Ct.)	☐ 5550 Alpha Fetoprotein, Prenatal	☐ 5232 HBsAg	Source _____
☐ 1023 Hemoglobin/Hematocrit	☐ 3000 Amylase	☐ 3175 HIV (Consent required)	☐ 7240 Culture, AFB
☐ 1020 Hemogram	☐ 3153 B12/Folate	☐ 3581 Iron & Iron Binding Capacity	☐ 7200 Culture, Blood x _____
☐ 1025 Platelet Count	☐ 3156 Beta HCG, Quantitative	☐ 3195 LH	☐ _____ Draw interval _____
☐ 1150 Pro Time Diagnostic	☐ 3321 Bilirubin, Total	☐ 3590 Magnesium	☐ 7280 Culture, Fungus
☐ 1151 Pro Time, Therapeutic	☐ 3324 Bilirubin, Total/Direct	☐ 3527 Phenobarbital	☐ _____ Culture, Routine
☐ 1155 PTT	☐ 3009 BUN	☐ 3095 Potassium	☐ 7005 Culture, Stool
☐ 1315 Reticulocyte Count	☐ 3159 CEA	☐ 3689 Pregnancy Test	☐ 7010 Culture, Throat
☐ 1310 Sed Rate/ Westergren	☐ 3348 Cholesterol	Serum (HCG, qual)	☐ 7000 Culture, Urine
URINE	☐ 3030 Creatinine, Serum	☐ 3653 Pregnancy Test, Urine	☐ 7300 Gram Stain
☐ 1059 Urinalysis	☐ 3509 Digoxin (recommend 12 hrs, after dose)	☐ 3197 Prolactin	☐ 7353 Occult Blood x _____
☐ 1082 Urinalysis w/Culture if indicated	☐ 3515 Dilantin	☐ 3199 PSA	☐ 7365 Ova & Parasites x _____
Urine-24 Hr _____ Spot _____	☐ 3168 Ferritin	☐ 3339 SGOT/AST	☐ 7400 Smear & Suspension
Ht. _____ Wt. _____	☐ 3193 FSH	☐ 3342 SGPT/ALT	(includes Gram Stain/Wet Mount)
☐ 3033 Creatinine (also requires	☐ 3066 ▼ Glucose, Fasting	☐ 3093 Sodium/Potassium, Serum	☐ 7060 Rapid Strep A Screen (_____)
☐ 3036 Creatinine Clearance blood)	☐ 3061 Glucose, 1ˢᵗ Post 50 g Glucola	☐ 3510 Tegretol	☐ 7065 Rapid Strep A Screen only
☐ 3095 Protein	☐ 3075 ▼ Glucose, 2ⁿᵈ Post Glucola	☐ 3551 Theophylline	☐ 7030 Beta Strep Culture
☐ 3096 Sodium/Potassium	☐ 3060 Glucose, 2ⁿᵈ Post	☐ 3333 Uric Acid	☐ 5207 GC by DNA Probe
☐ Microalbumin 24 Hr _____ Spot _____	Prandial (meal)		☐ 5130 Chlamydia by DNA Probe
SEROLOGY	☐ 3049 ▼ Glucose Tolerance Oral GTT		☐ 5555 Chlamydia/GC by DNA Probe
☐ 8020 ANA (Antinuclear Antibody)	☐ 3047 ▼ Glucose Tolerance Gestational GTT		☐ 7375 Wright Stain, Stool
☐ 8040 Mono Spot	☐ 3850 Hemoglobin, A1C		
☐ 3494 Rheumatoid Factor			
☐ 8010 RPR			
☐ 5365 Rubella	Additional Tests _____		

PANELS & PROFILES

☐ ✗ **3309 CHEM 12**
Albumin, Alkaline Phosphatase, BUN, Calcium, Cholesterol, Glucose, LDH, Phosphorus, AST, Total Bilirubin, Total Protein, Uric Acid

☐ ▼ **3315 CHEM 20**
Chem 12, Electrolyte Panel, Creatinine, Iron, Gamma GT, ALT, Triglycerides

☐ ▼ **3357 CARDIAC RISK PANEL**
Cholesterol, HDL, LDL, Risk Factors, VLDL Triglycerides

☐ ✗ **3042 CRITICAL CARE PANEL**
BUN, Chloride, CO2, Glucose, Potassium, Sodium

☐ **3046 ELECTROLYTE PANEL**
Chloride, CO2, Potassium, Sodium

☐ ▼ **3399 EXECUTIVE PANEL**
Chem 20, Iron, Cardiac Risk Panel, CBC, RPR, Thyroid Cascade

☐ **5242 HEPATITIS PANEL, ACUTE**
HAVIgMAb, HBsAg, HBsAb, HBcAb, HCVAb

☐ ▼ **3355 LIPID MONITORING PANEL**
Cholesterol, Triglycerides, HDL, LDL, VLDL, ALT, AST

☐ **3312 LIVER PANEL**
Alkaline, Phosphatase, AST, Total Bilirubin, Gamma GT, Total Protein, Albumin ALT

☐ ✗ **3083 METABOLIC STATUS PANEL**
BUN, Osmolality (calculated), Chloride, CO2, Creatinine, Glucose, Potassium, Sodium, BUN/Creatinine, Ratio, Anion Gap

☐ ✗ **3376 PANEL B**
Chem 12, CBC, Electrolyte Panel

☐ ▼ **3382 PANEL D**
Chem 20, CBC, Thyroid Cascade

☐ ✗ **3385 PANEL F**
Chem 12, CBC, Electrolyte Panel, Thyroid Cascade

☐ ▼ **3391 PANEL G**
Chem 20, Cardiac Risk Panel, CBC, Thyroid Cascade

☐ ▼ **3393 PANEL H**
Chem 20, CBC, Cardiac Risk Panel, Rheumatoid Factor, Thyroid Cascade

☐ ▼ **3397 PANEL J**
Chem 20, Cardiac Risk Panel

☐ **6361 PRENATAL PANEL**
Antibody Screen, ABO/Rh, CBC Rubella, HBsAg, RPR
☐ 1059 with Urinalysis Routine
☐ 1062 with Urinalysis w/Culture if indicated

☐ ✗ **3102 RENAL PANEL**
Metabolic Status Panel, Calcium, Phosphorus

☐ **3188 THYROID CASCADE**
TSH, Reflex Testing

▼ – patient **required** to fast for 12-14 hours
✗ – patient recommended to fast 12-14 hours

LAB USE ONLY	
☐ SST	☐ PLASMA
☐ PURPLE	☐ SERUM
☐ YELLOW	☐ SWAB
☐ BLUE	☐ SLIDES
☐ GREEN	☐ DNA PROBE
☐ GREY	☐ B. CULT BTLS
☐ URINE	
☐ BLACK	
☐ OTHER:	

RECV. SPECIMEN: ☐ FROZEN
☐ AMBIENT　☐ ON ICE

Special Instructions/Pertinent Clinical Information _____

Physician's Signature _____　　　**Date** _____
These orders may be FAXed to: 449-5288　　　LAB　　　7060-500 (7/96)

FIGURE 45-11 A laboratory requisition form.

sample. A key element in the chain of custody is a properly completed lab requisition form (Figure 45-11).

The chain of custody form is considered a legal document and can invalidate a specimen that has been tampered with or does not have complete information written on it. For example, a broken or mismatched seal on the specimen bottle invalidates the specimen being tested. Because it is a legal document, tampering or mishandling the chain of custody form is subject to investigation and subsequent penalties in accordance with the law.

A medical assistant may be asked to perform a drug test and should ensure that no tampering occurs before, during, or after testing. The primary solution to tampering with on-site drug testing of specimens is to ensure that collection of the drug test specimen is done under strict conditions. This normally means having same-sex personnel available on-site to monitor collection and making sure that access to the drug test specimens is strictly guarded. The medical assistant should make sure that the urine is "fresh" and at a defined temperature and that only approved urine drug

Professionalism — The Workplace

One member of the clinic or medical office team will be designated as an OSHA officer. That individual is responsible for ensuring that all OSHA policies are followed and that all team members are trained and educated appropriately in OSHA policies. Sharps containers should be provided in exam rooms and labs where needles or other sharps are used. Material data safety manuals (MDSM) must be kept up to date, listing all the chemicals used in the facility.

Per OSHA standards, standard precautions must be observed at all times. When a medical assistant is in a situation where exposure to blood and body fluids is a possibility, gloves must be worn. If appropriate, PPE, such as a lab coat, goggles, and a face mask, should be used.

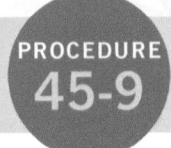

Performing a Urine Drug Screen Using a Chain of Custody

Objective ◆ *Prepare for and instruct the patient to properly collect a urine sample for drug analysis, following a chain of custody procedure.*

EQUIPMENT AND SUPPLIES

Urine collection cup with a built-in thermometer; gloves; "bluing tablets"; paper tape; laboratory report

Note: To avoid distraction that could compromise security, the medical assistant should conduct a collection for only one patient at a time.

METHOD

Step 1. Prepare the bathroom facility (used when the medical assistant is not required to be present during urination):

1. Gather supplies and equipment.
2. Secure any water sources by turning off the water inlet or taping handles to prevent opening faucets.
3. Add bluing tablets to the toilet and tank.
4. Remove soap, disinfectants, and any cleaning agents; inspect the site to ensure that no foreign or unauthorized substances are present.
5. Ensure that undetected access is not possible.
6. Secure areas and items that may be suitable for concealing contaminants, such as under-sink areas, trash receptacles, ledges, and paper towel holders.

Step 2: Prepare the patient

1. Photocopy the patient's ID and sign it.
2. Warmly greet and identify the patient, and introduce yourself. Explain the procedure to the patient. Have the patient sign the consent form and questionnaire.
3. Instruct the patient to leave coats and bags in a secure area.
4. Provide the patient with a container that is labeled with the patient's name and date.

5. Ask the patient to use the bathroom and void into a container. Tell the patient to fill the container only two-thirds of the way to avoid spillage.
6. Explain where you want the patient to leave the container of urine. Place a paper towel in the designated area to avoid contamination of the work area.

Step 3: Process the specimen

1. Immediately after the patient opens the door, inspect the room for irregularities.
2. Wearing nonsterile gloves, take the specimen. The urine sample should remain within view until sealed for delivery or tested on-site. Do not allow anyone else to handle or process it. The patient should sign to verify that the sample is hers.
3. Record the temperature of the urine.
4. Analyze the urine immediately if using a CLIA-waived test. Follow the manufacturer's directions. Accurately document results.
5. If the specimen is being sent to an outside facility, immediately record the temperature; then apply the tamper-evident seal and secure the specimen for transport, according to the facility's policy.
6. Dispose of equipment and perform hand hygiene.
7. Prevent unauthorized personnel from entering the site in which urine specimens are collected or stored.

CHARTING EXAMPLE

10/19/YY 4:00 P.M. 30 mL clear yellow urine collected for drug screening via office protocol. Urine temp. 98.7 F. Immediately sealed and processed specimen for transport to XYZ Laboratories..M. King, CMA

---

testing cups be used. The restroom being used needs to be properly prepared with "bluing tablets" deposited in the toilet water, which prevent the drug test samples from being diluted. Procedure 45-9 explains how to perform a chain-of-custody urine collection for drug analysis.

QUALITY CONTROL

Quality control is a system of ensuring that patients' test results are accurate and reported in a timely manner. Each

testing product is sold with a quality control testing program. Testing should be done on a routine schedule, following the appropriate protocol, and all documentation should be kept in a quality control log. All instrumentation associated with urine testing should be cleaned and maintained on a regular basis and documented accordingly.

Before any test is used, the expiration date of the product should be checked to be sure the product has not expired. The tests used for urinary pH, protein, blood, glucose, ketones, bilirubin, nitrite, urobilinogen, and specific gravity should be periodically checked by using solutions that contain a known amount of each of these substances. It is important to precisely follow the directions that are supplied by the manufacturer when using this testing material. New employees in your facility should be appropriately trained to perform urine tests, and the training should be documented.

SUMMARY

Urinalysis is one of the most common laboratory procedures performed by the medical assistant. It may be performed to screen for or confirm various diseases and disorders. Urinalysis may be performed to help identify UTIs, diabetes, and kidney diseases, and can be used in pregnancy and drug testing. There are various methods of performing a urinalysis, depending on the test and what is being tested for.

The three primary components in a routine urinalysis are the physical appearance, odor, quantity, and specific gravity, chemical analysis (pH, protein, glucose, hematuria, ketones, bilirubin, urobilinogen, nitrites, and leukocytes), and microscopic analysis (cells, casts, bacteria, yeast, parasites, spermatozoa, crystals, and contaminants).

Because urine is a body fluid, standard precautions must be observed, including aseptic technique. Many steps are taken to ensure accurate laboratory results, including good patient education, proper specimen labeling, and following laboratory procedures. Quality control is the final component of urinalysis to help ensure the validity of the results.

45 CHAPTER REVIEW

COMPETENCY REVIEW

1. Define and spell the terms for this chapter.
2. Explain what a morning specimen/first void is, and identify specific tests for which a first void is preferred.
3. List the different types of chemical analysis performed on urine specimens that are identified and measured using reagent strips.

4. Why do we measure specific gravity?
5. What causes a fruity odor in urine? In what disease condition is it found?
6. What is the purpose of catheterization?
7. Identify information that must be present on the label of a urine specimen when it is sent to the laboratory for testing.

PREPARING FOR THE CERTIFICATION EXAM

1. Pregnancy tests detect pregnancy by the presence in urine or serum of
   a. heterophile antibodies.
   b. human chorionic gonadotropin.
   c. luteinizing hormone.
   d. autoimmune antibodies.
   e. anti Rh antibodies.

2. To determine the kidney's ability to dilute and concentrate urine, the physician should measure
   a. glucose.
   b. ketones.
   c. specific gravity.
   d. protein.
   e. occult blood.

3. In routine urinalysis, all of the following are physical properties of urine *except*
   a. color.
   b. appearance.

   c. clarity.
   d. odor.
   e. glucose.

4. Turbid, in regard to urine, refers to the
   a. odor.
   b. color.
   c. quantity.
   d. cloudiness.
   e. specific gravity.

5. Normally in a 24-hour period, an individual excretes
   a. 70–100 mL of urine.
   b. 500–700 mL of urine.
   c. 250–2,500 mL of urine.
   d. 700–2,000 mL of urine.
   e. 1,000–5,000 mL of urine.

6. Anuria means
   a. no urine production.
   b. too much urine produced.
   c. scant urine production.
   d. kidney stones.
   e. bladder infection.

7. An indicator of possible urinary tract infection (UTI) is
   a. neutral pH in a urine sample.
   b. pH greater than 7 in a urine sample.
   c. pH much lower than 7 in a urine sample.
   d. elevated glucose level in a urine sample.
   e. elevated amount of hCG in a urine sample.

8. The presence of which of the following in urine may signal the onset of diabetes mellitus?
   a. leukocytes
   b. erythrocytes
   c. ketones
   d. glucose
   e. nitrites

9. The presence of many red blood cells (RBCs) in a urine microscopic examination is referred to as
   a. polyuria.
   b. hematuria.
   c. albuminuria.
   d. pyuria.
   e. leukocytopenia.

10. The medical assistant can prevent tampering of a chain of custody drug test by doing all of the following *except*
    a. having an accurately completed chain of custody form.
    b. placing bluing tablets in the toilet water.
    c. having same-sex personnel monitor the collection.
    d. using an unlabeled, clean and dry cup for collection.
    e. ensuring the urine is at a defined and appropriate temperature.

CRITICAL THINKING

Refer to the case study at the beginning of the chapter and use what you have learned to answer the following questions.

1. After reading the results of the urinalysis, Dr. Salpega diagnoses Ms. Flannery with a UTI. What chemical characteristics may have tested positive on the reagent strip that would have led Dr. Salpega to diagnose a UTI?

2. Dr. Salpega informs Susan that he would like the urine sample sent to the lab for a culture. Why might the physician decide to do this?

3. What is a common cause of UTIs in women? What can women do to lessen their chances of developing a UTI?

ON THE JOB

José Menendez is an older adult patient of Dr. Juárez, a board-certified urologist. Mr. Menendez has a history of recurrent UTIs dating back more than 10 years. When he becomes symptomatic, he has been instructed to call Dr. Juárez's office and schedule a urinalysis. Dr. Juárez's receptionist has just received a call from Mr. Menendez. He says he knows he is supposed to come in for a urinalysis but that he just wants a prescription phoned in to his pharmacy instead. The receptionist asks Emilia, Dr. Juárez's medical assistant, to take the call from Mr. Menendez.

Emilia listens as Mr. Menendez recounts that he is experiencing dysuria—painful burning with urination. She asks him to come in for a urinalysis, explaining that, as per standing orders, a clean-catch midstream specimen needs to be collected. Mr. Menendez repeats to Emilia that he does not want to come in to the office. "Why can't you call in a prescription for Bactrim? That is what I took last time, and it helped."

1. Did the receptionist handle this call responsibly by transferring it to Emilia?

2. Should Emilia try to encourage Mr. Menendez to come in for the urinalysis? Explain your answer, and state what you think should be said to the patient.

3. What, if anything, should Dr. Juárez be told about the conversation with Mr. Menendez?

INTERNET ACTIVITY

Use the Internet to research OSHA regulations regarding PPE.

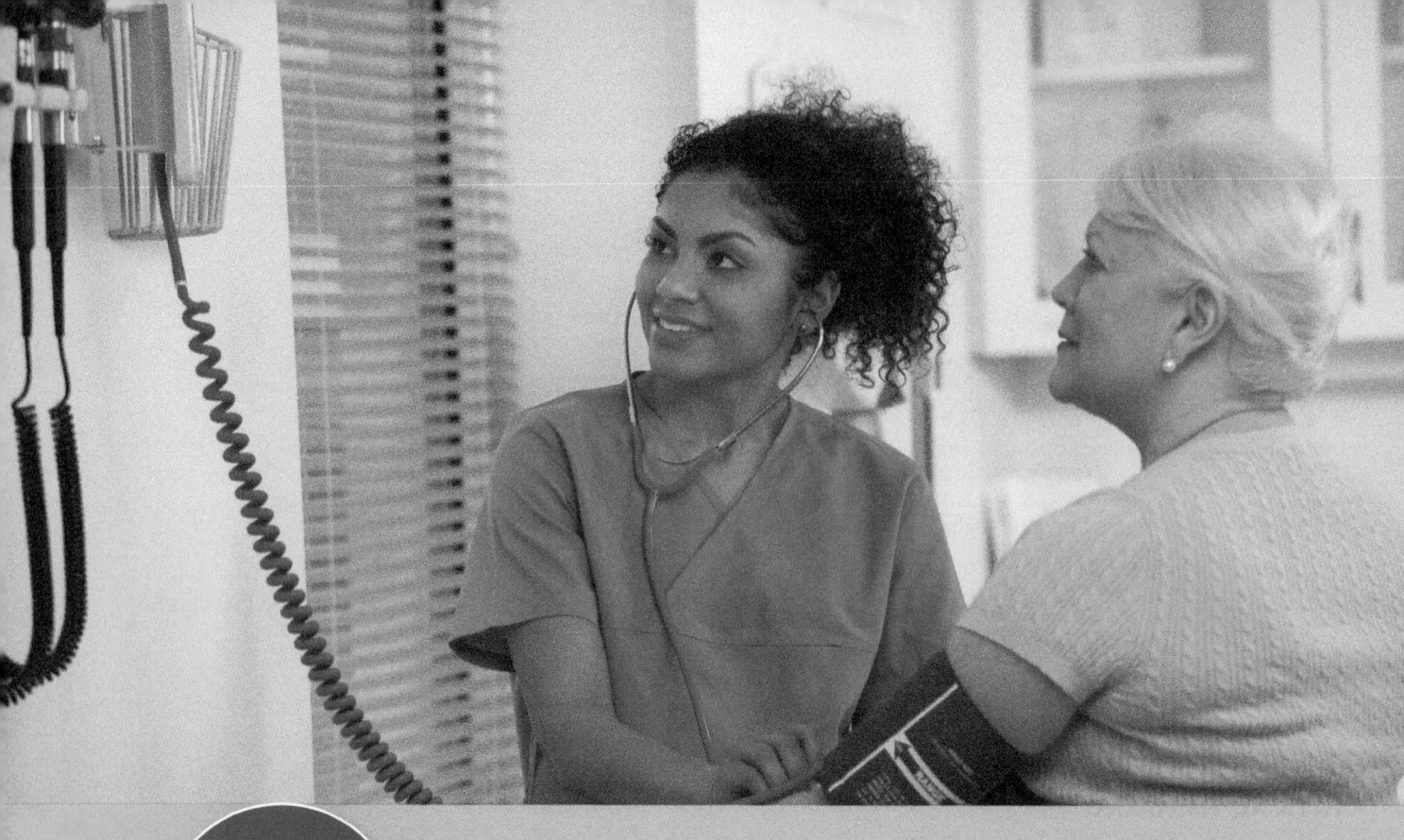

Phlebotomy and Blood Collection

Learning Objectives

After completing this chapter, you should be able to:

46.1   Define and spell the terms for this chapter.

46.2   Summarize the circulatory system as it relates to blood collection.

46.3   Describe the process of capillary puncture.

46.4   Identify common sites for venipuncture.

46.5   Explain precautions that are necessary for patients with special needs.

46.6   Compare different methods of venipuncture.

46.7   Describe the types of equipment used for venipuncture.

46.8   Explain the proper order of draw using blood collection tubes.

46.9   List considerations that must be taken when performing blood draw.

46.10 Explain which steps are taken when preparing specimens for transport.

47.11 Identify how to properly respond to complications that may arise during blood collection.

Samra Belkovich, RMA, is working with Dr. Salpega. Dr. Salpega would like Samra to draw blood from Marlene St. Clair in exam room 2. Dr. Salpega has ordered a CBC (complete blood count) and a serum chemistry test. He has informed Samra that Ms. St. Clair is a little anxious about having her blood drawn.

Terms to Learn

additive	evacuated tube	point of care (POC) testing
antecubital space	gauge	red cells
anticoagulant	hematoma	serum
arteries	hemoglobin	syncope
basilic veins	hemolysis	syringe
beveled	heparin	tourniquet
butterfly needle	laboratory requisition form	blood transfer device
cannula	lumen	vacuum container
capillaries	palpate	veins
capillary puncture	phlebotomy	venipuncture
cephalic veins	Phlebotomy Technician	white cells
constrict	plasma	
dilate	platelets	

Venipuncture and **phlebotomy** both refer to the collection of blood through a tiny incision in the vein, typically with a hollow needle. Blood can also be collected for testing through a simple **capillary puncture**, obtained by pricking the skin. Blood collection is important because it allows blood to be analyzed for abnormalities and enables health care professionals to take early action that may prolong or even save lives.

There are many techniques in phlebotomy and blood collection, with a variety of equipment available to choose from. This chapter discusses the latest and safest equipment and methods.

THE MEDICAL ASSISTANT'S ROLE

When the physician orders a blood test, the role of the medical assistant is to properly collect, label, and perhaps to process or store the specimen. This requires knowledge of basic circulatory anatomy and physiology, phlebotomy equipment, asepsis, and venipuncture procedures. It also requires professionalism and the ability to properly communicate with the patient and staff.

Understanding Circulatory Anatomy and Physiology

Circulatory anatomy and physiology are covered in depth in the chapter titled "The Cardiovascular System." You will

Professionalism   The Life Span

Drawing blood from older individuals can sometimes be challenging because of the deteriorating condition of their veins. Patients of any age do not want to have more needlesticks than necessary. To ensure that a successful needlestick occurs, preferably on the first attempt, requires both experience and patience. If patients will be returning to the office for blood work at a later time, advise them to drink a lot of fluids before they arrive at the office. Being well hydrated helps make veins easier to find. Placing an item such as a small rubber ball in the patient's hand to gently squeeze (never pump) is also helpful in making veins stand out. If the hand must be used for the draw site, place a warm cloth over the area to help the vein rise. All these techniques can help in making the first try a success.

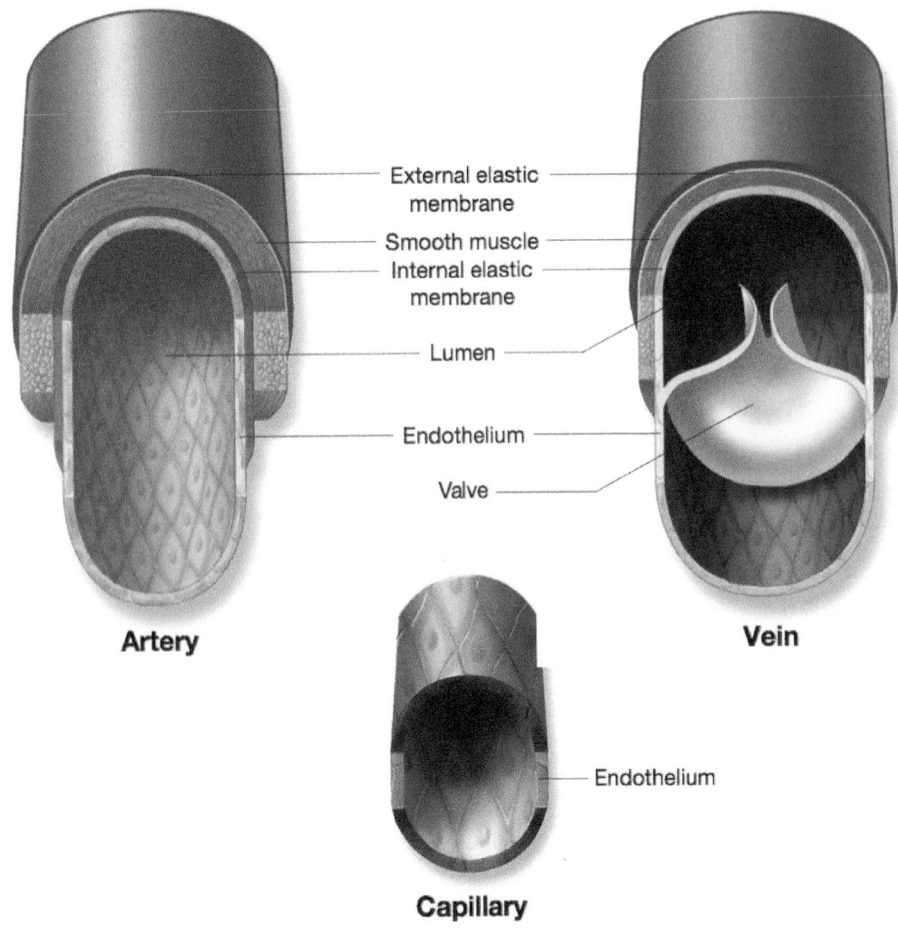

External elastic membrane
Smooth muscle
Internal elastic membrane
Lumen
Endothelium
Valve

Artery

Vein

Endothelium

Capillary

FIGURE 46-1 Structure of arteries, capillaries, and veins.

that is fully loaded with oxygen), and actively pulsate from the pumping rhythm of the heart. The pulse is important to note so you can identify and avoid puncturing an artery; medical assistants are not qualified to draw blood from arteries. Arterial blood completes its journey when it finally passes through tiny arterioles (the smallest arteries) and reaches the even tinier capillaries.

Capillaries act as bridges between the arteries and veins. They also connect closely with the cells of the body. Capillary walls are so thin (only one cell thick) that oxygen can pass out of the blood, through the capillary walls, and into the cells. At the same time, carbon dioxide and other wastes can pass out of the cells, through the capillary walls, and into the blood. From there the blood, carrying the carbon dioxide and wastes, moves into the smallest veins (venules) and on into larger and larger veins that finally return the blood to the heart. The heart sends the returned blood to the lungs, where the carbon dioxide is breathed out while the blood takes on a fresh supply of breathed-in oxygen. Then the newly oxygenated blood is carried back to the heart to be pumped, once again, around the body (Figure 46-2).

In a way, the capillaries are like gas stations. Fuel (oxygen) is delivered from arterial blood to the cells while garbage (carbon dioxide) is removed from the cells and carried into the veins.

Because capillaries connect arteries and veins, both arterial and venous blood can be found in them. Capillary blood is the easiest to collect and is commonly used for **point of care (POC) testing**. POC tests are tests that can be done during a physical exam or at a patient's bedside with results that can be quickly received to help the physician make patient care decisions.

Veins are vessels that carry blood toward the heart (in contrast to arteries that carry blood away from the heart). Veins have thinner walls than arteries and do not pulsate because they are not under the high pumping pressure from the heart that arteries receive. High levels of carbon dioxide make venous blood appear darker than arterial blood and give the lining of the vessel a bluish tinge. An important

need to review this material to understand phlebotomy and blood collection. To be successful in blood collection, you must have a fundamental understanding of the circulatory system. The following are some basics about the heart, blood vessels (Figure 46-1), and blood.

The heart is a pump whose job is to keep blood moving. Blood vessels provide a one-way route for travel around the body and back to the heart. Blood leaves the heart through blood vessels called **arteries**, which get smaller and smaller as they extend farther away from the heart. Arteries have thick elastic walls, carry bright red blood (blood with hemoglobin

Professionalism The Law

It is legal in most states for a medical assistant to perform venipuncture. Check with your local credentialing agency chapter for specifics in your state. When performing basic in-office laboratory tests, you must keep all results confidential. Confidentiality is a moral, legal, and ethical obligation for all health care team members.

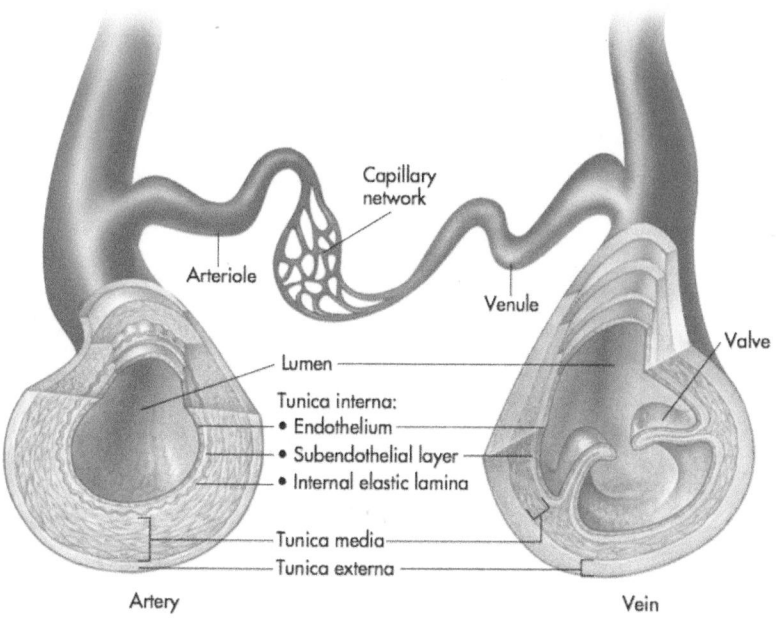

FIGURE 46-2 Capillaries act as bridges between the arteries and veins. Valves in the veins prevent backflow as blood carrying carbon dioxide and wastes is returned to the heart.

special function of blood: regulation of body temperature. When the body becomes warm, capillaries and blood vessels **dilate** and release heat, which cools the body. When the body is cold, capillaries and blood vessels **constrict**, allowing less blood flow, which retains heat and increases the body temperature. This is important to remember because vessels that have shrunk in response to cold are more difficult to access. A simple remedy is to use a heat lamp, warm compress, or even gentle friction to warm the area and dilate the vessels.

The main elements of blood are **plasma** (the liquid portion, which is mostly water) and formed elements: **red cells** (with **hemoglobin** molecules that transport oxygen), **white cells** (that protect against disease), and **platelets** (that are involved in blood clotting). Blood **serum** is blood plasma from which fibrinogens (proteins involved in blood clotting) have been removed.

feature to note is that, because blood often defies gravity as it travels back to the heart (for example, upward from the feet and legs), veins have one-way valves that prevent backflow (Figure 46-3). (Arteries do not have valves.)

Venipuncture (puncturing a vein) is a common method to obtain sufficient blood for a variety of testing. When you are performing venipuncture, it is important to remember another

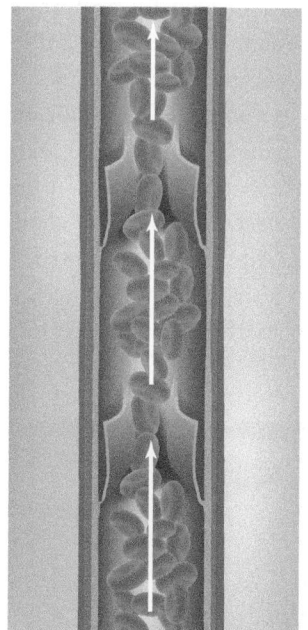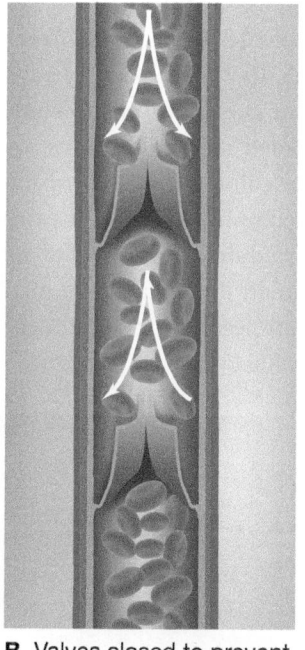

A Valves open—blood flows freely

B Valves closed to prevent backflow

FIGURE 46-3 Valves in veins open to permit blood flow, close to prevent backflow.

BLOOD SPECIMEN COLLECTION

Laboratory testing of blood and the collection of all blood and body fluids are strictly regulated by Occupational Safety and Health Administration (OSHA) regulations, and the Centers for Disease Control and Prevention (CDC) standard precautions must be followed at all times. Clinical Laboratory Improvement Amendments (CLIA) sets the standards to which all laboratories must adhere, including training of personnel and testing and transport of specimens (see the chapter called "The Clinical Laboratory"). When performing specimen collection, you must follow the regulation guidelines established by these organizations.

The type and amount of specimen to be acquired are dictated by the test to be done. If a very small amount is needed, then the specimen may be obtained by capillary puncture. Larger volumes are collected through venipuncture.

Capillary Puncture

Capillary blood is used for many home monitoring devices and several CLIA-waived POC tests, including those that test blood for glucose, cholesterol, hemoglobin A1C, and hematocrit levels.

As noted, capillaries are the microscopic blood vessels that connect arterioles and venules. Oxygen and carbon dioxide are transferred to and from the body cells at the capillary level. Small amounts of blood can easily be obtained from the capillaries through a skin puncture in a finger, earlobe, or infant's heel (Figure 46-4). Skin puncture for

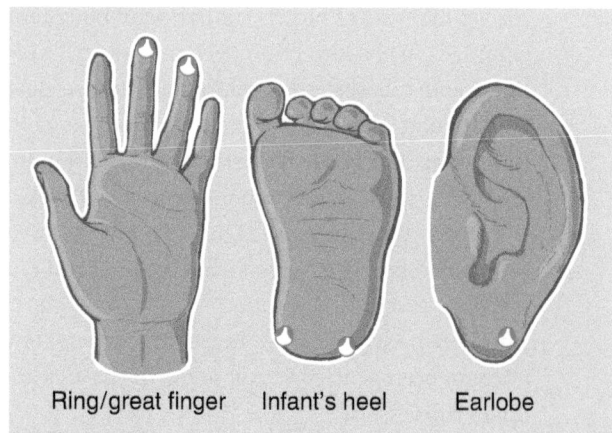

FIGURE 46-4 Capillary puncture sites.

capillary blood is not recommended for tests that require large volumes of blood like blood cultures and erythrocyte sedimentation rate (ESR) tests, nor for plasma studies, dehydration, or poor circulation.

The most common capillary puncture site for adults is the finger, preferably the fleshy pad of the middle or ring finger on the nondominant hand, off center (Figure 46-5). When performing capillary punctures, take precautions to avoid using the thumb because it is often callused. The index finger should also be avoided if possible because it has extra nerve endings that make it more sensitive. The fifth finger is also not a good capillary puncture site because it generally has less tissue. The tissue on the lateral sides of the fingers is less sensitive than that in the middle, but a larger specimen can be obtained from the fleshy area closer to, but not directly in, the middle of the fingers. The puncture should be a minimum of 2 mm away from the fingernail. Take precautions to avoid any area that is callused, burned, cyanotic, red, scarred, or showing signs of injury or infection. Earlobes are also a common puncture site for adults.

When you are doing a capillary puncture on infants (under 1 year of age), their fingers are not large enough to yield a

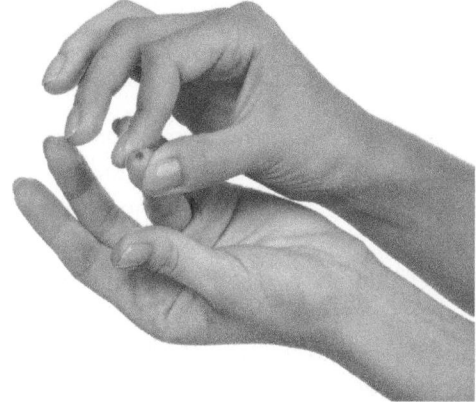

FIGURE 46-5 A finger-stick is useful for obtaining small amounts of blood.

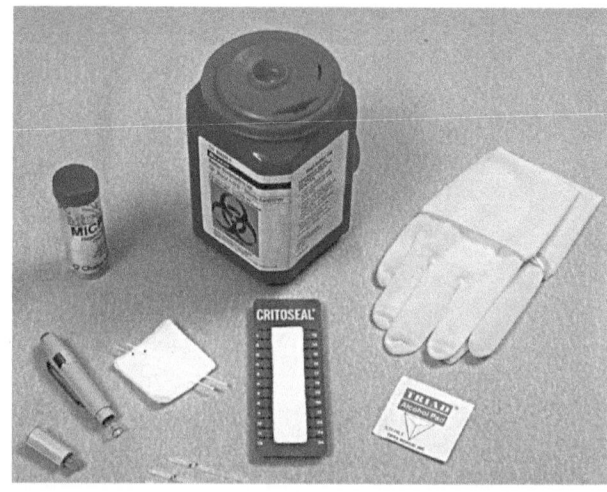

FIGURE 46-6 Capillary puncture equipment.

sufficient sample, so a heel is usually a better option. The puncture should occur on the medial and lateral surfaces (sides) of the heel. The infant patient can be held by the parent or caretaker or another medical assistant with the baby's legs hanging to allow gravity to increase blood flow. Thoroughly warm and clean the heel before the procedure. Gentle friction or a warm (never exceeding 42°C, 108°F), moist towel can be applied for three to five minutes to increase blood flow. Never place an adhesive bandage on patients younger than 2 years. The patient could peel them off and create a choking hazard.

Equipment and Supplies

Figure 46-6 shows the equipment needed for a capillary puncture. Lancets may be either manual or automatic (Figure 46-7). The primary advantage of the automatic lancet is that the depth of the puncture is controlled by a spring-loaded mechanism, causing less pain to the patient. Many are color coded, according to the puncture depth it can accomplish, making it easier to select a comfortable choice for adults, children, and infants. After a lancet is used, it should immediately be placed in a sharps container to prevent needlesticks. Procedure 46-1 outlines the process for a manual capillary puncture.

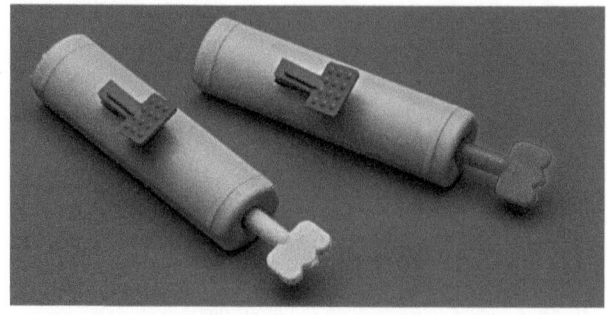

FIGURE 46-7 Spring-activated lancet.

Performing a Capillary Puncture (Manual)

Objective ◆ *Perform a capillary stick using a lancet or spring-loaded lancet following aseptic technique, and obtain an adequate sample.*

EQUIPMENT AND SUPPLIES

Biohazard sharps container; gloves; alcohol sponge; 2 × 2 gauze square or cotton balls; lancet or spring-loaded lancet; capillary tubes; sealing clay; ammonia ampules; bandage; lab coat

Note: Lancets come in a variety of sizes and needle **gauges** for specific purposes. The majority of capillary punctures performed on adults, requiring only a few drops of blood, can be performed with needle gauges 21G, 25G, or 28G. Pediatrics and microcollections require specific lancets and blades.

Note: Follow standard precautions and safety guidelines. Use care to avoid splashing or spilling blood. Wipe up all spills using guidelines established by OSHA.

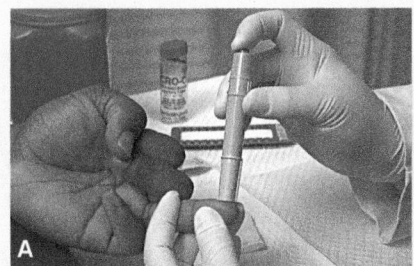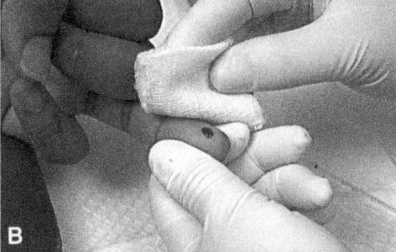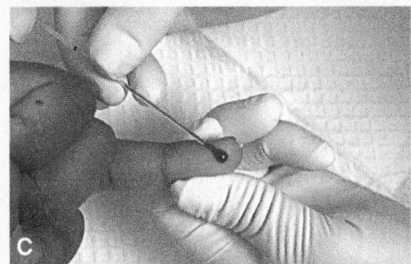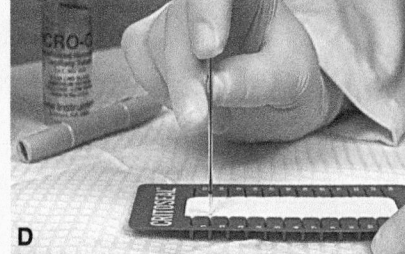

FIGURE A–D Capillary puncture procedure.

METHOD

1. Perform hand hygiene.
2. Assemble the equipment.
3. Identify the patient and explain the procedure. Have the patient either sit or lie down.
4. Apply gloves.
5. Select either the ring or great finger on the nondominant hand for an adult. Select a heel for a newborn. Briskly rub the finger or heel between your palms to warm it up. Wipe the site with alcohol. Let alcohol evaporate.
6. Remove the plastic protective tip to expose the lancet.
7. Grasp the patient's hand (or infant's heel), and gently squeeze 1 inch below the chosen puncture site.
8. Puncture the site using a quick, jabbing motion to obtain a full round drop of blood (Figure A). Do not puncture the direct center. Immediately discard the lancet in a sharps container. (A spring-loaded lancet may also be used.)
9. Wipe away the first drop of blood with a gauze square or cotton ball (Figure B).
10. Obtain the sample using a microhematocrit capillary tube (Figure C). The finger or foot may be gently massaged or lowered below the level of the heart to increase blood flow. Seal one end of the capillary tube in a clay sealer (Figure D).
11. Apply clean gauze over the site, and ask the patient to apply firm, continuous pressure until the bleeding stops.
12. Assess the patient and the site. Apply a bandage, if needed, but never on an infant (choking hazard). Ask if the patient feels dizzy or light-headed.
13. Remove gloves and perform hand hygiene.
14. Label the tubes with the patient's name, date, time, ID number, specimen type, tests to be done, and the phlebotomist's initials. Fill out the laboratory requisition sheet.
15. Record the procedure on the patient's medical record.

CHARTING EXAMPLE

2/28/YY 1:30 P.M. Performed capillary puncture on left ring finger for ordered XYZ test. Pt. tolerated well and denies dizziness. Results negative.....................................M. Garcia, RMA

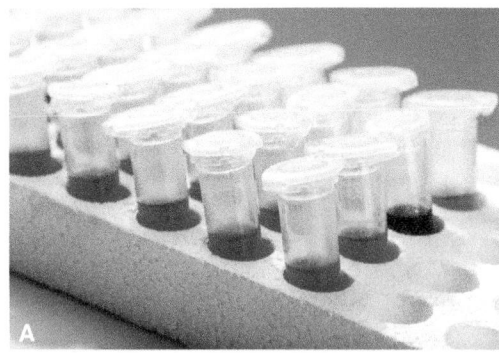

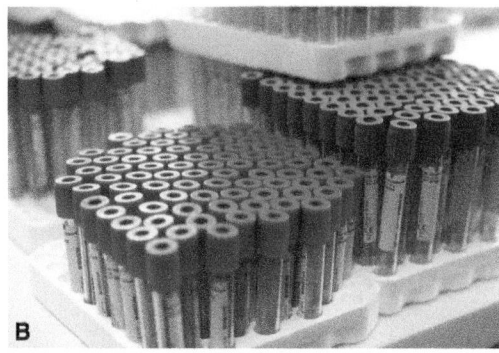

FIGURE 46-8 (A) Microtainer tubes; **(B)** Unopette collection devices.

Capillary blood may be administered directly onto a test strip, or it can be collected in a plastic or glass tube. Capillary tubes are designed to gently pull the blood into the tiny opening. They may have a blue mark (plain) or a red one (with **heparin**, to prevent clotting). Microtainer capillary blood collection tubes have a variety of **additives**, noted by the color-coded caps. Unopette collection devices can be used for various blood cell counts (Figure 46-8).

Venipuncture

Venipuncture, or phlebotomy, can be performed at a variety of places on the body. The safest and easiest sites to access are located on the upper extremities (Figure 46-9). The median cubital vein is located at the **antecubital space**, or the inner elbow area. This vein is most popular, because it is large and often the most superficial vein and because it receives blood supply from both the **cephalic veins** (veins on the outer sides of the arms) and the **basilic veins** (large veins of the hands and forearms). The cephalic and basilic veins themselves are the next most commonly used veins because they are also large and superficial. These branch off into smaller veins as they reach the distal end of the extremity.

The Phlebotomist

A medical assistant who is trained to perform phlebotomy is considered a phlebotomist and may perform venipuncture in the medical office unless specific state regulations say

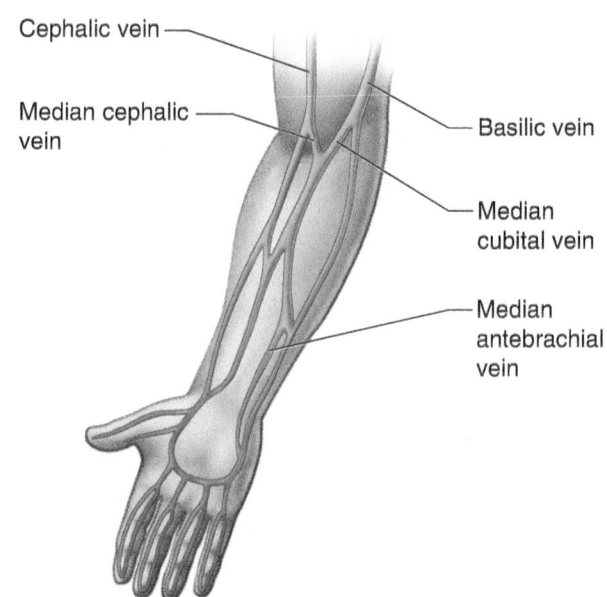

FIGURE 46-9 Anatomy of an arm for venipuncture.

otherwise. However, the practice of phlebotomy occurs in many other settings, too. Some physicians choose to send patients to an outside laboratory that is contracted with the patient's medical insurance. Venipuncture may also take place in hospitals, blood banks, reference laboratories, clinics, and a variety of other settings. These are all areas where employment opportunities may be available for medical assistants.

Certification in Phlebotomy. Phlebotomy certification is often required at hospitals, blood banks, and independent laboratories. Certification is a way to prove to potential employers that the job candidate has met established national standards, regardless of the school or location where training was obtained. On a résumé, it makes an individual stand out as a true professional. Benefits to obtaining a phlebotomy certification may include prestige, increased job opportunities, a higher salary, and job security.

Phlebotomy Technicians collect and prepare blood and other body fluid samples for medical laboratory testing. A phlebotomy technician can be a Certified Phlebotomy Technician (CPT) or a Registered Phlebotomy Technician (RPT), depending on which organization granted the credentials. To gain credentials as a phlebotomy technician, a medical assistant must meet standard qualifications (many of which may be met through a typical medical assisting program) and must pass a written exam. Nationally accredited credentialing agencies include American Medical Technologists (AMT), the National Center for Competency Testing (NCCT), and National Healthcareer Association (NHA).

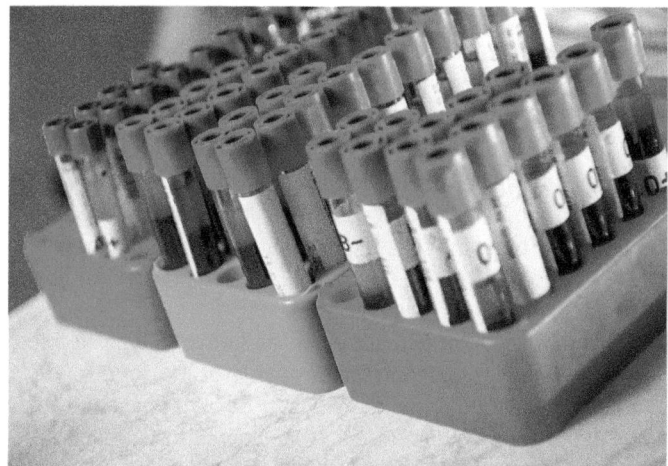

FIGURE 46-10 Vacutainer evacuated specimen tubes with Hemogard closure blood collection tubes.

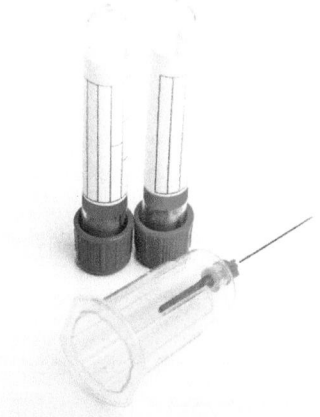

FIGURE 46-11 Vacutainer brand safety lock needle holder.

Venipuncture Methods

Three methods of venipuncture are used: the vacuum tube method, the syringe and needle method, and the butterfly method.

The Vacuum Container Method. The most common method of venipuncture is the **vacuum container** or **evacuated tube** method, often referred to by the BD (Becton, Dickinson and Company) brand name, Vacutainer® (Figures 46-10 and 46-11). This method is used so often because multiple samples can be obtained at the same time, requiring fewer sticks for the patient and faster collection for the medical assistant. The vacuum is set to withdraw the exact amount of blood needed to mix with the chemicals inside the tube; just allow it to fill until the flow stops. Be sure to fill the vacuum tube to the level required for the test, as it will affect the accuracy of some tests if you do not follow the laboratory requirements for amount of blood in the tube.

For the vacuum container method, it is important to use a large vein because the vacuum can collapse smaller veins. If the patient has no accessible larger veins, then it is appropriate to use a small needle with a syringe or a **butterfly needle** to obtain the specimen, methods that are discussed next.

The Sterile Syringe and Needle Method. The biggest drawback of using a syringe is that the amount of blood that can be collected for testing is limited to the size of the syringe used. This method also has a higher incidence of injury or contamination than the vacuum container method because of the manipulation that is required during the transfer from the syringe to the tube.

Procedure 46-2 details how to obtain venous blood with a sterile syringe and needle.

PROCEDURE 46-2

Performing Venipuncture Using a Sterile Syringe and Needle

Objective ◆ *Perform a venipuncture using the syringe and needle method.*

EQUIPMENT AND SUPPLIES

Sterile 22-gauge needle and 10- to 20-mL syringe; appropriate vacuum specimen tubes for tests ordered; tourniquet; gloves; alcohol wipe; 2 × 2 gauze square; adhesive bandage; patient's record; pen; lab coat; biohazard sharps container

METHOD

Review request and verify test ordered.

1. Prepare necessary equipment and work area on an aseptic field. Check expiration dates.
2. Perform hand hygiene and apply gloves.

3. Securely attach the sterile needle to the syringe, if required. Pump the plunger several times to ensure that it moves freely. Depress the plunger completely to expel the air from within.

4. Identify the patient and explain the procedure, making sure the patient understands the procedure.

5. Confirm that the patient has followed any pretest preparation requirements. Verify allergies, the last time the patient ate, and if there is a history of complications (syncope, hematoma, etc.). Ensure that there is nothing in the patient's mouth, such as candy or gum, to prevent choking in the case of syncope.

6. Apply a tourniquet 3 to 4 inches above the antecubital space. **Palpate** the area to locate the vein of choice.
   Tip: Gently mark the spot by making an indentation on the skin with the outside of the needle cap. This will make it easier to find again.

7. Remove the tourniquet if the vein of choice is not located immediately and the specimen(s) cannot be collected within 60 seconds.

8. Clean the venipuncture site in a spiral pattern (expanding from the center outward) with an alcohol wipe and allow to air-dry. Leave the opened alcohol wipe on the aseptic field within reach.
   Tip: For easier visualization, wipe an area on the back of a gloved hand with the alcohol wipe. When it dries, it will no longer be shiny and it is time to proceed.

9. Reapply the tourniquet, if necessary.

10. Have the patient make a gentle fist and hold it shut until told to release it. Instruct not to pump vigorously.

11. Verify that there is no air in the syringe and remove the needle guard.

12. From beneath the puncture site, pull the skin down so that it is taut. With the bevel facing up, insert the needle into the vein.

13. Slowly pull back the syringe plunger until the proper amount of blood has been obtained. Do not force it to fill quickly.

14. Instruct the patient to open the fist.

15. Release the tourniquet and withdraw the needle quickly. Immediately cover with gauze. Instruct the patient to keep firm pressure on the site and raise the arm to prevent hematomas from occurring.

16. (A) If using a transfer device, engage the safety mechanism over the needle; safely remove the needle from the syringe and place it in the sharps container. Apply the **blood transfer device** to the end of the syringe.
    (B) If no transfer device is available, place the vacuumsealed tube in a tube rack so that it is standing upright. Do not hold the tube or the rack. Gently pierce the tube stopper with the needle.
    For either (A) or (B), allow the vacuum to pull blood into the tube until filled to the desired level. Do not push on the plunger to speed the process. Be sure to use the appropriate collection tube for the ordered tests, following the correct order of the draw.

17. Discard the syringe in a sharps container, always inserting the needle end first to avoid injury.

18. Gently invert the tubes, as required by the manufacturer; do not shake them. Immediately label the specimen with the patient's name, the date and time of collection, the test's name, and the name of the person collecting the specimen.

19. Follow correct procedures for decontaminating the work area and equipment according to OSHA guidelines.

20. Remove gloves and dispose in the appropriate container. Perform hand hygiene. Dispose of all used needles and other equipment in a biohazard waste container.

21. Thank the patient and observe for any signs or symptoms of inappropriate response to the procedure.

22. Label the tubes with the patient's name, date, time, ID number, specimen type, tests to be done, and the phlebotomist's initials. Fill out the laboratory requisition sheet.

23. Document the procedure in the patient's chart.

24. If the specimen is to be transported to an outside laboratory, prepare it for transport in the proper container, with all the appropriate information according to OSHA guidelines.

CHARTING EXAMPLE

08/16/YY 3:22 P.M. CBC ordered. Drew blood from Pt.'s right antecubital, stick X1. Patient states she tolerated the procedure well. Blood sent to Memorial Laboratory at 4:00 P.M..................
....L. Stivers, RMA (AMT)

The Butterfly Needle Method. The winged infusion or butterfly method uses a needle that is attached to 6- to 12-inch tubing. The end of the tubing can attach to the syringe or to the vacuum container tube holder. It can also be used as a temporary IV infusion, to administer medications or fluids directly into the patient's bloodstream. The butterfly method is used for small veins that are difficult to draw from with the standard vacuum container method or syringe and needle method. Its name is derived from the shape of the device: The needle on the end has a winged portion that keeps the needle from turning and anchors the needle into the small vein.

The needle used for the butterfly method is a small 21-, 23-, or 25-gauge needle. The small device is easier to hold and manipulate than larger devices, and the smaller needle is less uncomfortable for the patient. A disadvantage of the smaller needle is that it is more likely to result in **hemolysis** (destruction of red blood cells with release of hemoglobin into the plasma). Another important drawback to using the butterfly method in venipuncture is the fact that it is more

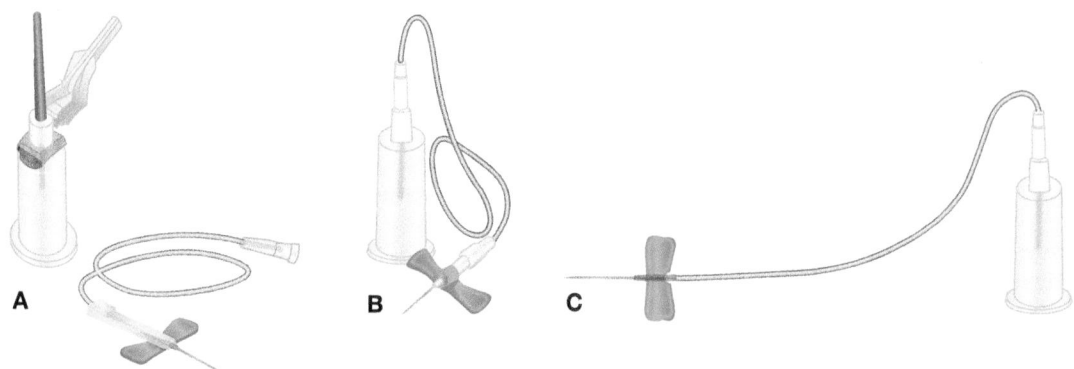

FIGURE 46-12 Butterfly systems designed for safety and ease of use: **(A)** A safety shield slides down over the needle after use; **(B)** a button is pressed to retract the needle while it is still in the vein; **(C)** butterfly needle preconnected to holder to prevent accidental disconnections.

expensive than a standard needle. For these reasons, the winged infusion set is not typically the first choice for phlebotomy.

The Needlestick Safety Prevention Act has inspired several types of butterfly systems that are designed for both safety and ease of use (Figure 46-12).

Equipment

A wide variety of equipment for phlebotomy is available from several manufacturers. Blood collection tubes come in different sizes and colors. Various types of tourniquets are available. Antiseptic and wound care supplies can be used. Double-ended needles and needle holders are made specifically for evacuated-tube use. Butterfly needles are helpful for small or fragile veins. A variety of sizes of syringe and needle devices can be obtained.

Blood Collection Tubes. Evacuated blood-collection tubes are designed to automatically draw in the exact amount of blood required for testing. Each tube is color coded according to the type of chemicals or preservatives within the container. If the procedure is halted before enough blood is collected, there may be a high concentration of chemicals. Because this can render a test inaccurate and require another blood draw, it is important to wait until the flow of blood stops before removing the tube.

Blood collection tubes may be made of glass or plastic and come in a variety of sizes. Plastic tubes are always safer to work with, but glass is best for testing medication levels. Before use, always check the expiration date and visually inspect the contents for abnormalities. When using the evacuated tube system, always use the same manufacturer for a tube, holder, and needle to ensure proper fit and prevent complications that might alter the process. Figure 46-13 shows some general equipment for performing a venipuncture using the vacuum container method.

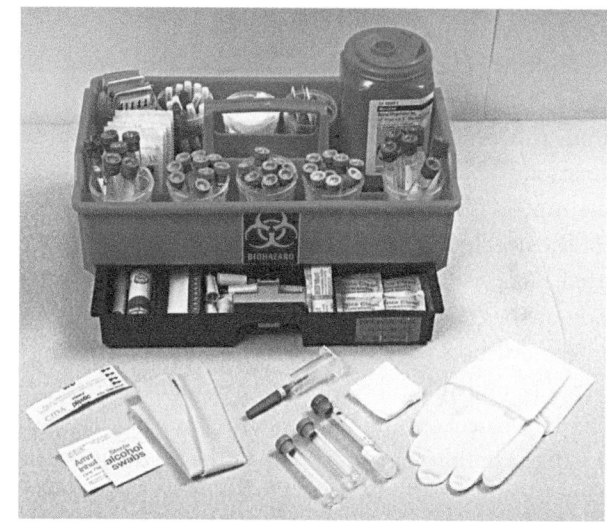

FIGURE 46-13 Venipuncture equipment.

Tourniquets. A **tourniquet** is applied to an extremity to impair the circulation. This allows blood to pool in a set area and causes veins to distend for easier access. A standard tourniquet is a large strip of disposable latex that can be tied around the arm. For those with latex allergies, rubber can be used instead. If a patient's veins are particularly difficult to locate, a blood pressure cuff may be used. However, for infection control purposes, this is a last resort. Tourniquets should not be left in place for more than 60 seconds because blood will begin to hemolyze, or break down, rendering tests inaccurate. New phlebotomists should apply the tourniquet first just to find the site, *then remove it* to allow time for setup and cleansing the skin and to prevent hemolyzation, then reapply the tourniquet after the alcohol has dried. More advanced phlebotomists may choose the one-tie method, which involves setting up, cleansing the area, applying the tourniquet, finding the vein, and immediately puncturing the skin. This should be attempted only by a skilled phlebotomist on a patient with easy access because the tourniquet may stay in place for only 60 seconds.

Ideally, you should do the final tourniquet removal before you remove the needle from the patient, which reduces both bleeding and bruising. If multiple vials of blood are needed, the tourniquet can be removed after the first tube so that it does not remain in place for more than 60 seconds, which alters test results. Leaving the tourniquet in place when the needle is removed exerts pressure that can cause some additional bleeding or bruising. However, if the tourniquet is forgotten, there is no need to panic. Generally, the patient will remind you to remove it, and pressure kept on the area for an additional 2–3 minutes will minimize bruising.

Tube Holders and Needles. As already noted, evacuated tubes are best used with the corresponding needles and holders from the same manufacturer. A tube holder is typically made of plastic. It has a threaded end that a double-ended needle can be inserted into. This places one rubber-coated end of the needle inside the holder, which will penetrate the inserted blood tube. The pointed end of the needle on the outside of the holder is inserted directly into the patient's vein. The evacuated system allows for blood to be directly delivered to multiple tubes with one venipuncture.

The key to successful venipuncture lies in the special design of the hollow needle. The tip of the needle is **beveled**, or cut at a slant (Figure 46-14). A beveled tip penetrates the skin and the vein more easily and with minimal damage. When drawing blood, always insert the needle with the bevel facing up, so that the wall of the vein doesn't act as a barrier to seal the opening, which would inhibit blood from entering the collection system.

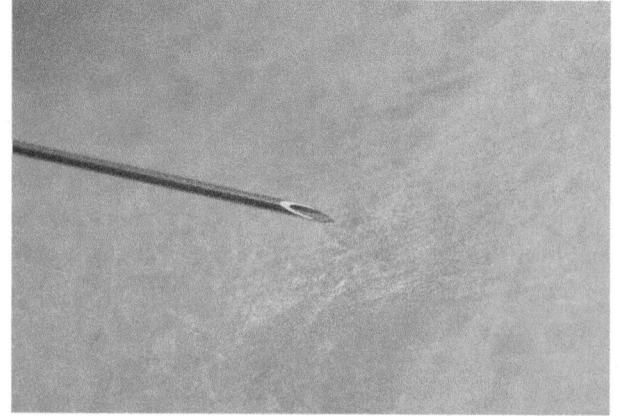

FIGURE 46-14 A beveled tip helps the needle penetrate skin and vein with minimal damage.

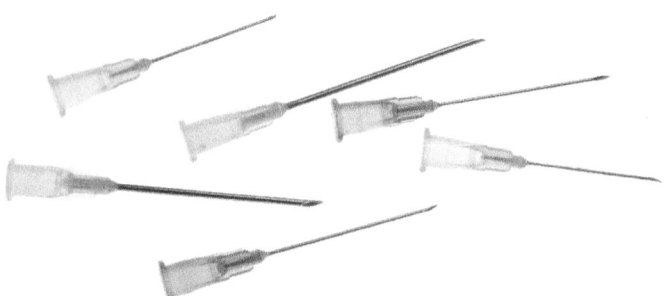

FIGURE 46-15 Needles are available in a variety of gauges.

Phlebotomy needles are made in many different sizes, including different lengths and gauges (Figure 46-15). A **lumen** is the space inside the hollow area of a needle. A gauge or bore is the diameter or inner circumference of the lumen. It is important to remember that the smaller the gauge number, the larger the hole within. General phlebotomy typically requires 20- to 21-gauge needles. Smaller needles can be used; however, there is a greater risk of hemolysis with smaller needles, which occurs because blood cells are damaged as they scrape along the edge of a narrower opening. For this reason, larger 18-gauge needles are used for the collection or administration of significant quantities of blood or viscous fluids.

Safety devices may be attached to needles or to holders. Be sure not to use two safety devices in a system, as this would negate them both. When activating a safety device, avoid using a part of your body part as a lever. Instead, use the edge of a counter to push the safety into the locking position. This may prevent accidentally stabbing yourself with a contaminated needle. The exception to this rule is the butterfly needle, which may have either a sliding plastic safety device to be guided forward or a push-button device that is activated before removal from the patient. (Review Figure 46-12, which shows safety devices on butterfly needles.)

Syringes. **Syringes** are useful in collecting blood specimens from small or fragile veins that cannot withstand the pressure of an evacuated tube. Although the needle size is the same for most phlebotomy procedures, the size of a syringe depends on the amount of blood needed for all tests being performed. This is typically anywhere from 5 mL to collect blood for a single tube to 20 mL to collect blood for multiple tubes.

A drawback to using a syringe is that the phlebotomist is limited to the amount of blood that one syringe can hold. If more blood is needed, multiple needle insertions will be required. Another difficulty with using a syringe for a blood draw is that the plunger must be pulled back while the needle is inserted, which is awkward and makes it easy to displace the needle before the sample can be fully collected. Yet another difficulty is the necessity of transferring the blood from the syringe to the evacuated tube, a maneuver that provides more opportunities for injury or contamination. These factors make the use of a syringe the least favorable option for venipuncture.

There are two main methods for transferring blood from a syringe to an evacuated tube. The preferred method is to use a safety transfer device after the needle is properly removed and discarded into a sharps container. The blood transfer device is attached to the syringe, and a vacuum tube is inserted into the transfer device. The other option is to simply place the evacuated tube in a standing rack and insert the needle into the tube—without holding it, to prevent accidental injury. Either way, the plunger should not be depressed to force the flow; instead, allow the vacuum to fill the tube to the appropriate level.

Order of the Blood Draw

When you are drawing blood by the vacuum tube method, it is important to fill the tubes in the order of draw recommended by the Clinical Laboratory Standards Institute (CLSI) to prevent contamination of the tubes with skin bacteria or with an additive from another blood tube. The correct order of draw, along with a description of additives and the common laboratory tests run on each individual specimen, is listed in Table 46-1 and shown in Figure 46-16. If a blood culture is required, it is always drawn first so that the cleanest, purest specimen is received for this test.

Many lab requisition forms state the tube color to use for each test. For example, a complete blood count (CBC) typically requires a lavender-topped tube, a protime (PT)

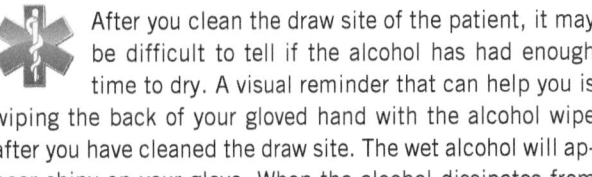

requires a light blue-topped tube, and a blood culture requires a yellow-topped tube. If all of these were ordered, three tubes must be filled in the order of draw: first yellow, then light blue, then lavender. If multiple tests are ordered and the same color tube is used for each, often just one tube is needed. For example, if a protime (PT) and a partial thromboplastin time (PTT) are both ordered, because both require a light blue tube, only one tube is needed. The exact number of tests possible for one tube depends on the size of the container, the type of test, and the type of equipment being used in the lab. If more than four tests in the same tube are required, it may be wise to draw an additional tube. Contact the laboratory to determine specific capabilities in its facility.

Some laboratories may use additional tubes. Pink-, tan-, black-, and royal blue-topped tubes are sometimes used for specific laboratory tests. Vacuum blood tubes come in 5-, 7-, 10-, and 15-mL sizes. The amount of blood needed for each test differs, so the tube sizes differ accordingly.

Tube top colors now vary by manufacturer, so it is important for the medical assistant to know the manufacturer of the tubes being used and to follow the instructions given by the manufacturer regarding what is in its tubes that corresponds with each tube color and label (Figure 46-17).

For each tube being filled, gently invert the tube six to eight times so the **anticoagulant** and blood mix properly. Take care not to shake the tubes because that action could hemolyze the blood. Always follow the manufacturer and laboratory requirements for inverting tubes. This can affect the accuracy of results.

Blood Cultures

Blood cultures are very sensitive tests that look for signs of bacteria in the blood. Any contamination from outside sources could have a significant impact on patient care. For this reason, special precautions are taken while collecting blood for culturing. The site must be cleaned thoroughly with two cleaners, typically alcohol, then Betadine, allowing

TABLE 46-1	Blood Collection Tubes: Order of Draw
Golden yellow (blood cultures always drawn first)
Light blue
Red
Red marbled
Green
Light green
Lavender
Pink, white, or royal blue
Gray
Dark blue

BD Vacutainer® Tubes with BD Hemogard™ Closure	BD Vacutainer® Tubes with Conventional Stopper	Additive	Inversions at Blood Collection	Laboratory Use	Your Lab's Draw Volume/Remarks
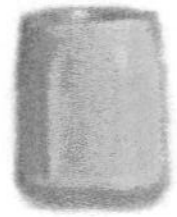 Gold	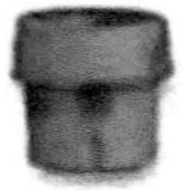 Red/Gray	• Clot activator and gel for serum separation	5	For serum determinations in chemistry. May be used for routine blood donor screening and diagnostic testing of serum for infectious disease. Tube inversions ensure mixing of clot activator with blood. Blood clotting time: 30 minutes.	
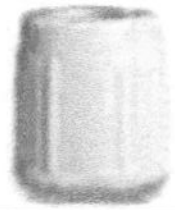 Light Green	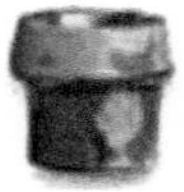 Green/Gray	• Lithium heparin and gel for plasma separation	8	For plasma determinations in chemistry. Tube inversions ensure mixing of anticoagulant (heparin) with blood to prevent clotting.	
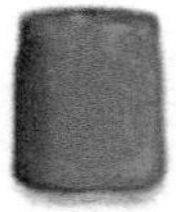 Red	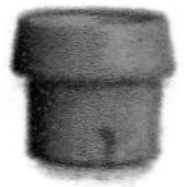 Red	• Silicone coated (glass) • Clot activator, Silicone coated (plastic)	0 / 5	For serum determinations in chemistry. May be used for routine blood donor screening and diagnostic testing of serum for infectious disease. Tube inversions ensure mixing of clot activator with blood. Blood clotting time: 60 minutes.	
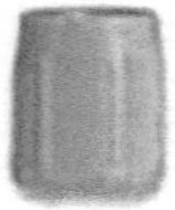 Orange		• Thrombin-based clot activator with gel for serum separation	5 to 6	For stat serum determinations in chemistry. Tube inversions ensure mixing of clot activator with blood. Blood clotting time: 5 minutes.	
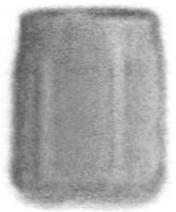 Orange		• Thrombin-based clot activator	8	For stat serum determinations in chemistry. Tube inversions ensure mixing of clot activator with blood. Blood clotting time: 5 minutes.	
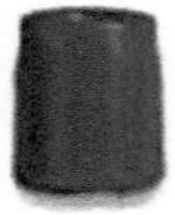 Royal Blue		• Clot activator (plastic serum) • K₂EDTA (plastic)	8 / 8	For trace-element, toxicology, and nutritional-chemistry determinations. Special stopper formulation provides low levels of trace elements (see package insert). Tube inversions ensure mixing of either clot activator or anticoagulant (EDTA) with blood.	
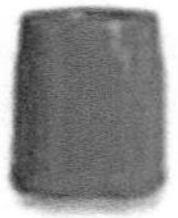 Green	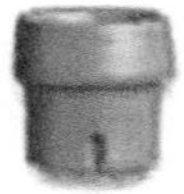 Green	• Sodium heparin • Lithium heparin	8 / 8	For plasma determinations in chemistry. Tube inversions ensure mixing of anticoagulant (heparin) with blood to prevent clotting.	
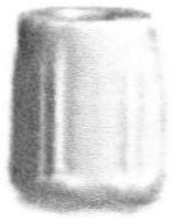 Gray	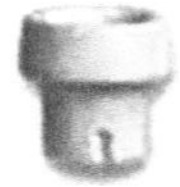 Gray	• Potassium oxalate/ sodium fluoride • Sodium fluoride/Na₂ EDTA • Sodium fluoride (serum tube)	8 / 8 / 8	For glucose determinations. Oxalate and EDTA anticoagulants will give plasma samples. Sodium fluoride is the antiglycolytic agent. Tube inversions ensure proper mixing of additive with blood.	

FIGURE 46-16 Tube colors, additives, inversions, and laboratory uses.

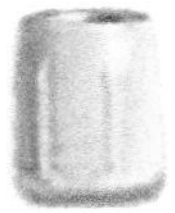

Closure Color	Additive	Inversions at Blood Collection	Laboratory Use
Tan	• K_2EDTA (plastic)	8	For lead determinations. This tube is certified to contain less than .01 µg/mL(ppm) lead. Tube inversions prevent clotting.
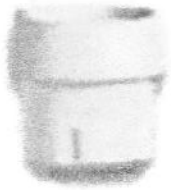 Yellow	• Sodium polyanethol sulfonate (SPS) • Acid citrate dextrose additives (ACD): **Solution A -** 22.0 g/L trisodium citrate, 8.0 g/L citric acid, 24.5 g/L dextrose **Solution B -** 13.2 g/L trisodium citrate, 4.8 g/L citric acid, 14.7 g/L dextrose	8 8 8	SPS for blood culture specimen collections in microbiology. ACD for use in blood bank studies, HLA phenotyping, and DNA and paternity testing. Tube inversions ensure mixing of anticoagulant with blood to prevent clotting.
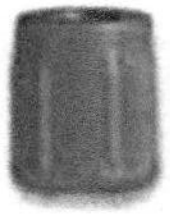 Lavender 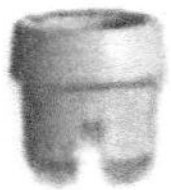	• Liquid K_3EDTA (glass) • Spray-coated K_2EDTA (plastic)	8 8	K_2EDTA and K_3EDTA for whole blood hematology determinations. K_2EDTA may be used for routine immunohematology testing, and blood donor screening. Tube inversions ensure mixing of anticoagulant (EDTA) with blood to prevent clotting.
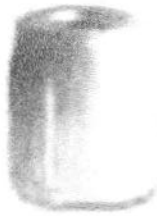 White	• K_2EDTA and gel for plasma separation	8	For use in molecular diagnostic test methods (such as, but not limited to, polymerase chain reaction [PCR] and/or branched DNA [bDNA] amplification techniques.) Tube inversions ensure mixing of anticoagulant (EDTA) with blood to prevent clotting.
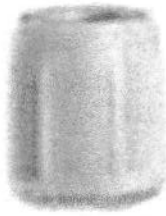 Pink	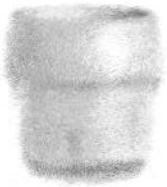 • Spray-coated K_2EDTA (plastic)	8	For whole blood hematology determinations. May be used for routine immunohematology testing and blood donor screening. Designed with special cross-match label for patient information required by the AABB. Tube inversions prevent clotting.
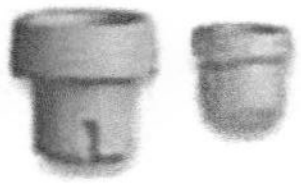 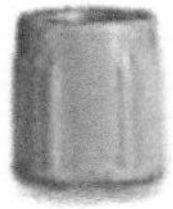 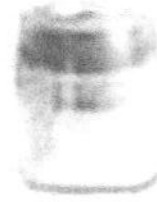 Light Blue	• Buffered sodium citrate 0.105 M (≈3.2%) glass 0.109 M (3.2%) plastic • Citrate, theophylline, adenosine, dipyridamole (CTAD)	3–4 3–4	For coagulation determinations. CTAD for selected platelet function assays and routine coagulation determination. Tube inversions ensure mixing of anticoagulant (citrate) to prevent clotting.
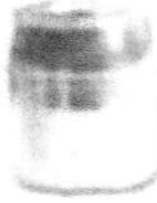 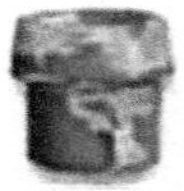 New Red/ Light Gray	• None (plastic)	0	For use as a discard tube or secondary specimen tube.

FIGURE 46-16 (*continued*)

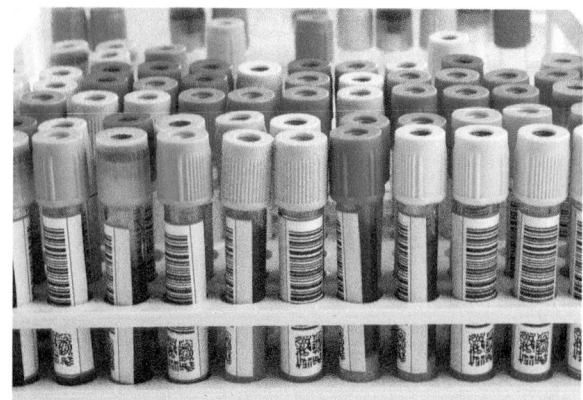

FIGURE 46-17 Tube colors and uses vary. Follow the individual tube manufacturer's directions about which tube to use.

time to dry in between. Likewise, the collection tubes or bottles must be twice cleaned and kept covered with a Betadine wipe to prevent contamination from the air. A gloved finger must be cleansed before repalpating once the site has already been cleansed.

Patient Preparation

The blood tests done in a physician's office typically require little preparation. It is important to determine that you have the correct patient by asking for identification and confirming that any pretest preparations like fasting have been done. For some tests, such as a glucose tolerance, cholesterol, or lipids level test, the patient should fast for 12 to 14 hours before the test. Few other tests require fasting. If fasting is required, it is important to tell the patient how many hours to fast before the blood draw. If you have any question about requirements, such as fasting in preparation for the blood draw, a good resource is the laboratory to which the specimen is being sent. Testing labs typically have a lab assistant available to address these questions.

Performing the Blood Draw

Proper positioning of both the patient and the phlebotomist is important to perform a successful phlebotomy procedure. Phlebotomy chairs can be set up at a height that is easy to access, with adjustable arm supports that serve to keep the patient both comfortable and secure. Blood collection equipment should be kept easily accessible off to the side.

Always ask if the patient has had any complications during previous venipunctures, such as allergic reactions to latex, excessive bleeding, or **syncope** (fainting or loss of consciousness). If latex allergy is reported, use an alternative tourniquet, nonlatex gloves, and paper tape over the gauze bandage. If excessive bleeding is an issue, apply pressure for 10 to 15 minutes after phlebotomy and monitor the site carefully. Syncope is a common concern. For a patient with a

history of fainting, consider drawing blood while the patient is lying down in a secure position so that there is no threat of injury from a fall. For all others, a chair that has a locking device to pull across the front of the patient is helpful to prevent dangerous falls from unexpected syncope. While sitting, if the patient complains of dizziness, immediately withdraw the needle, apply pressure, and assist in lowering the patient's head between the knees. If the patient shows signs of fainting, get assistance to lower the patient into a lying position, with legs elevated above the heart to help restore blood flow to the head.

At the time of the blood draw, some patients may be anxious. To decrease patient anxiety, it is important to communicate clearly what the process involves. If the patient is a child, the participation of the parent or caregiver may be helpful in calming the patient.

Being prepared at the time of the blood draw can also help in diminishing patient anxieties. A patient is encouraged when sensing that you are competent and knowledgeable about performing the blood draw. Competency can be demonstrated by having the appropriate equipment assembled before the blood draw and ensuring that the correct blood specimens are drawn correctly. Patients who experience callbacks because of errors such as incorrect specimen handling will lose confidence in the medical assistant and the physician's office.

Unexpected events can happen when you perform venipunctures. These include fainting, nausea, excessive anger exhibited by a patient, and uncontrollable bleeding. It is important that you remain calm and deal with these situations professionally. As already noted, when a patient begins to show signs of syncope, it is important to immediately withdraw the needle and lower the patient's head. The patient may need to lie down. If a patient does not immediately respond, call another member of the clinical team for assistance. The use of ammonia inhalants to revive a patient is not recommended because they may trigger an allergic or asthmatic response that can be life threatening.

Advise a patient who becomes nauseated to breathe deeply through the mouth, and provide an emesis basin if necessary. If a patient becomes angry during the procedure, it is important to remain calm and reassuring. If the behavior continues or is disruptive and endangers either you or the patient, stop the procedure immediately and call for assistance.

Occasionally, uncontrollable bleeding can occur when the needle is withdrawn. If this occurs, immediately apply pressure to the site. Once you have established pressure, call for assistance.

Other complications can make it difficult to perform the procedure or to obtain the necessary amount of blood. For example, if a patient has small veins, it is sometimes helpful to apply a warm compress to the area. This will help veins to expand and become easier to access. When veins have a tendency to roll (move from side to side), it is important to place one finger below the area where the needle is to be inserted to keep the vein from moving. An incomplete draw may occur if a patient's vein does not produce enough blood, and you will need to obtain blood from a different vein. Some patients present a challenge to the inexperienced phlebotomist. Request that a more experienced professional perform the procedure when necessary.

When drawing blood, wear personal protective equipment (PPE) such as gloves and a gown or lab coat. Although you wear these items to protect yourself from coming in contact with contaminated items, this attire also presents the professional image that patients want in their medical assistant. Although some people choose to tear the finger off a glove for easier palpation, this is not recommended because it poses a risk of infection to the patient and to the health care worker alike.

See Figure 46-18 for an illustration of the use of venipuncture equipment. To perform a venipuncture using the Vacutainer method, see the procedures outlined in Procedure 46-3.

Preparing Specimens for Transport

After the blood is collected, it must be carefully transported to ensure the accuracy of the results. In some cases results can be affected by exposure to light and must be drawn in

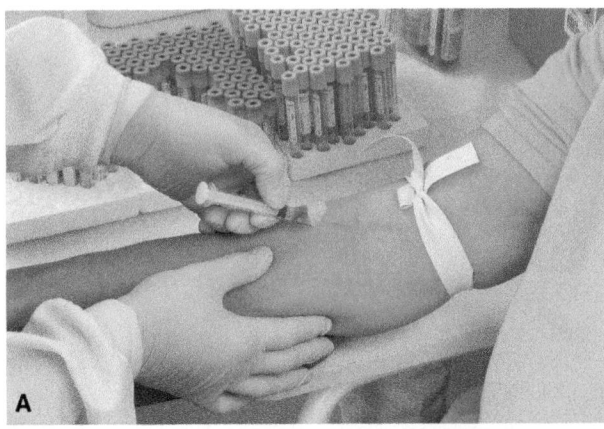
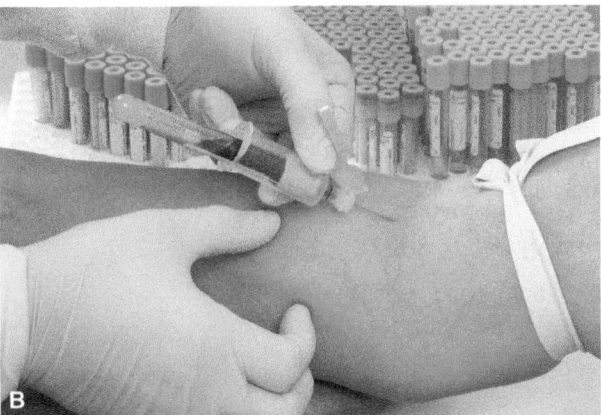
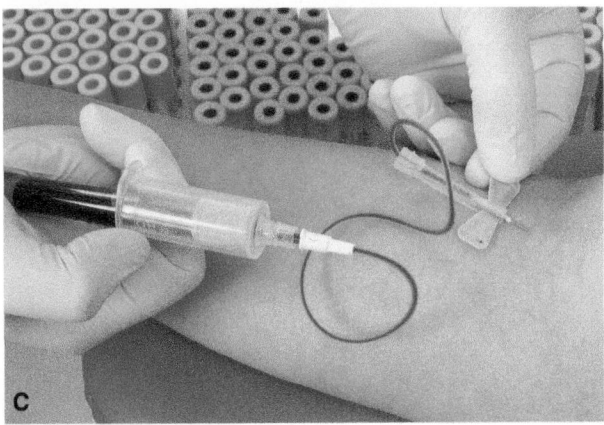

FIGURE 46-18 Demonstrating the use of venipuncture equipment: **(A)** using a syringe to draw blood; **(B)** Vacutainer or vacuum-assisted phlebotomy; **(C)** holding a butterfly needle in place with a vacuum-assisted collection set.

amber colored tubes, such as plasma vitamin B1 and vitamin B6. In other cases, the temperature must be maintained at a certain level, such as HIV tests that use frozen plasma and parathyroid tests that must be spun and refrigerated. Always check the website or book given to you by the laboratory you use for processing to ensure you are correctly transporting your specimens. **Laboratory requisition forms** are procured from the laboratory or laboratories you use and should be completely filled out and attached to the

Performing Venipuncture Using the Vacutainer Method

Objective ◆ *Perform venipuncture by correctly assembling, locating, and entering vein and withdrawing blood sample.*

EQUIPMENT AND SUPPLIES

Biohazard sharps container; Vacutainer tubes; multisample needle; two or three 2-inch gauze squares; alcohol pads; examination gloves; Vacutainer sleeve; tourniquet; bandage; pen; lab coat; patient record

Note: Follow standard precautions and safety guidelines when working with blood samples. Use care to avoid splashing or spilling blood. Wipe up all spills using guidelines established by OSHA.

METHOD

1. Perform hand hygiene.
2. Assemble equipment (Figure A).
3. Identify the patient and explain the procedure. Have the patient either sit or lie down.
4. Confirm that the patient has followed any pretest preparation requirements. Verify allergies, the last time the patient ate, and if there is a history of complications (syncope, hematoma, etc.). Ensure that there is nothing in the patient's mouth, such as candy or gum, to prevent choking in the case of syncope.
5. Apply gloves.
6. Screw the Vacutainer needle into the plastic sleeve (Figure B). Insert the tube into the other end of the sleeve. The top of the colored stopper should reach the thin guideline on the sleeve. Do not press the tube. If the tube exceeds the line, discard the tube; it may not have a vacuum.
7. Apply the tourniquet about 2 inches above the antecubital space (Figure C). Place the middle of the tourniquet on the posterior (elbow) side of the arm. Crisscross the ends. While holding one end stable, tuck in the other end. This creates a tie that can be quickly released with one hand. In addition, the tourniquet should apply enough tension to engorge the vein with blood.
8. The arm should be in an extended position with the palm facing up. Palpate the vein with your fingertips (Figure D).

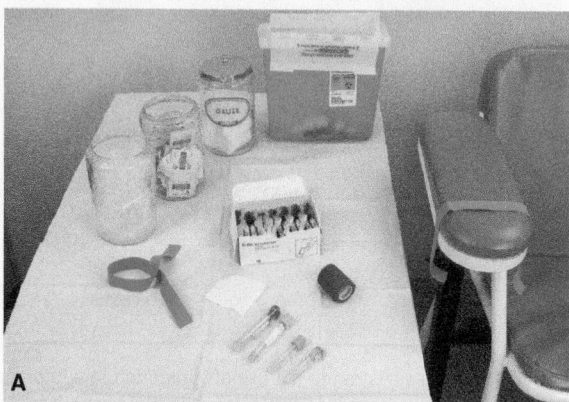

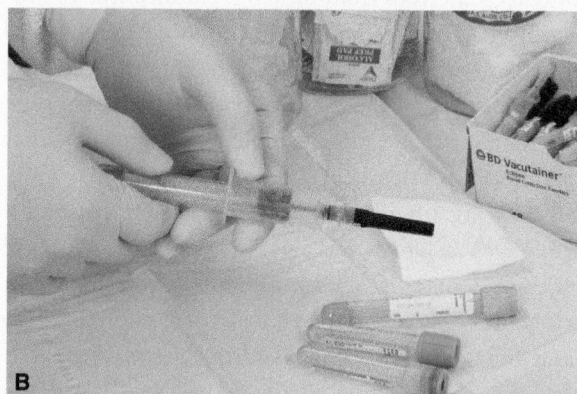

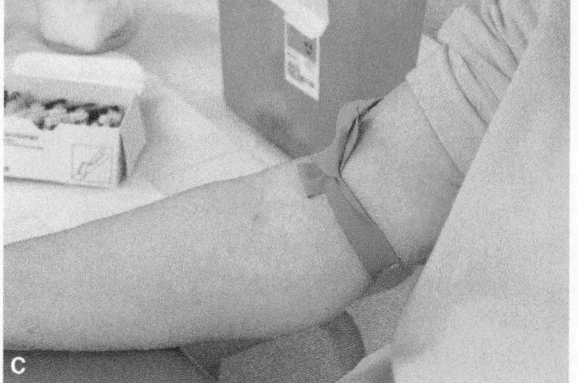

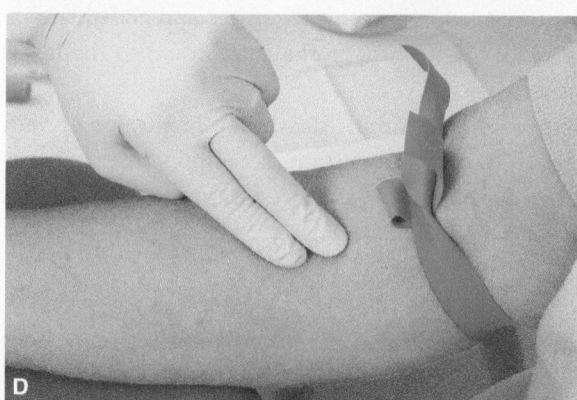

FIGURE A–D Venipuncture procedure.

If a vein cannot be felt in one arm, try the other. Release the tourniquet.

9. Wipe the site with an alcohol pad in a circular pattern beginning at the insertion site (Figure E). Let the alcohol evaporate. Cleanse your gloved finger with alcohol in case you need to re-palpate after the site is cleansed. Reapply the tourniquet.

10. Anchor the vein by placing the thumb of the nondominant hand 2 inches below the insertion site and pulling the skin toward the hand.

11. While holding on to the tube's sleeve with your dominant hand, insert the needle smoothly and rapidly at a 15- to 20-degree angle with the bevel up (Figure F). The needle only needs to be inserted just past the bevel. If inserted too far, it will puncture both vein walls. Also keep the needle in line with the vein. The dominant hand is now considered "fixed," meaning you may not remove it from the tube sleeve until the procedure is over. All other movements must be done with the nondominant hand.

12. While the dominant hand is stabilizing the sleeve, use the nondominant hand to push the tube into the sleeve (Figure G). Use your thumb to push the tube and hold the sleeve with the index and middle fingers on the flange (Figure H).

13. Allow the tube to fill. The vacuum will automatically fill the tube to the manufacturer's recommended level for the specific tube used. You should familiarize yourself with the adequate fill level of the individual tubes. Blood collection tubes may contain a weak vacuum caused by processing errors, and you will need to redraw those specimens.

14. Remove the tube very carefully without moving the needle and apply a second tube if needed (Figure I). Gently invert the tube a minimum of five to six times (depending on the type of tube—review Figure 46-16) after removing it from the sleeve to allow the blood to mix with the additive. Use only the tubes needed for the tests ordered. Fill these tubes following the correct order of the draw.

15. Release the tourniquet once the last tube has been inserted into the adaptor. Fill the last tube, remove it, swiftly remove the needle, and cover the site with a clean gauze pad (Figure J). Be careful not to push on the needle when covering the puncture site because that may cause the needle to scratch the patient's arm. Gently invert the collection tube.

16. Immediately have the patient apply firm, continuous pressure using a gauze square.

17. Properly dispose of the needle in a biohazard container (Figures K and L).

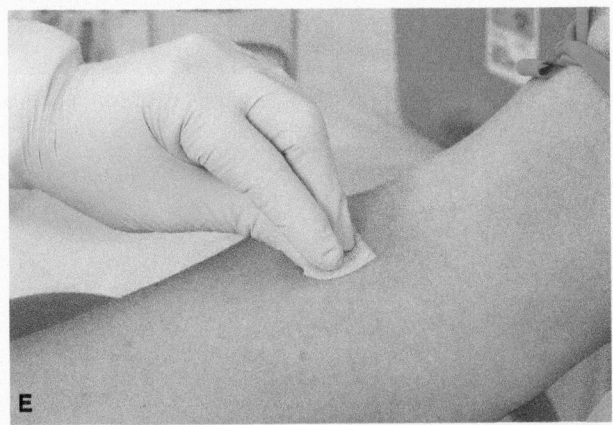

E

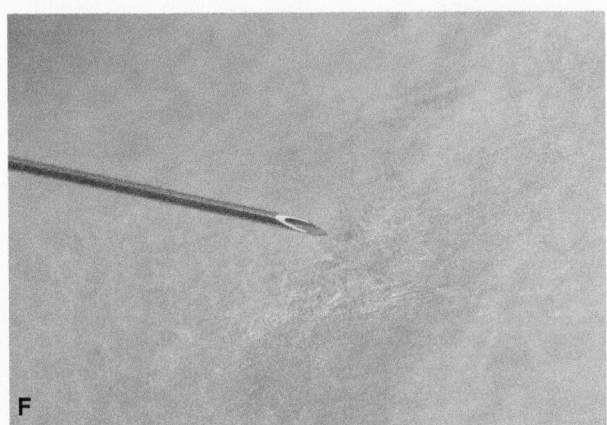

F

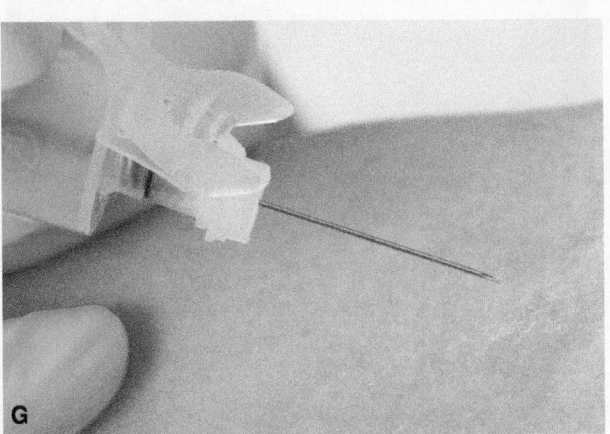

G

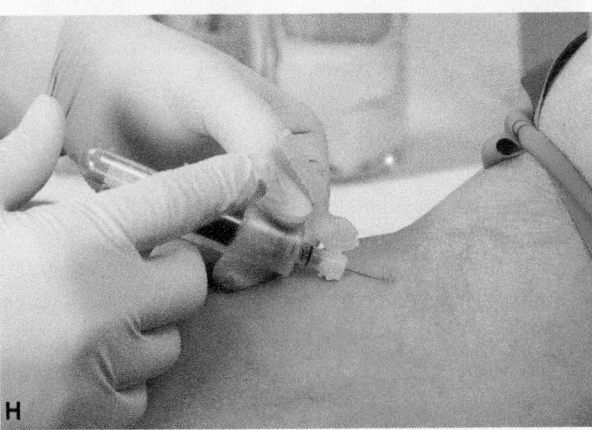

H

FIGURE E–H (*continued*)

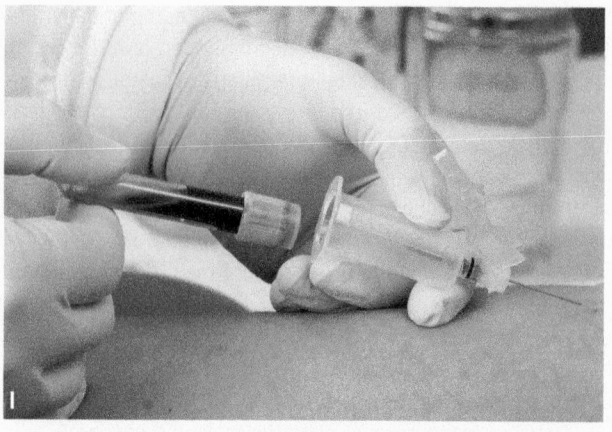

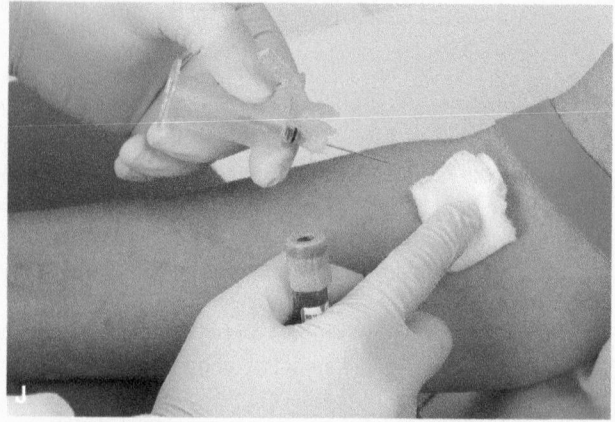

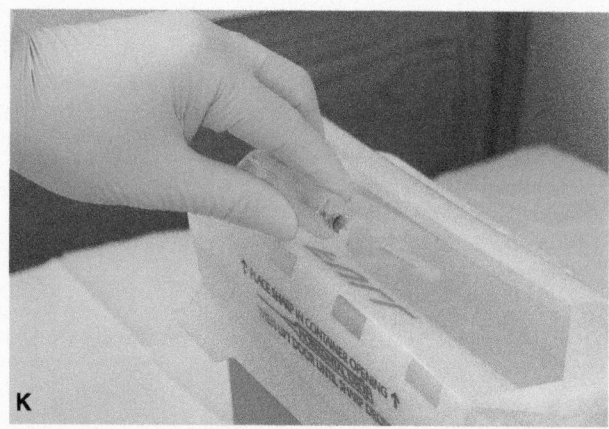

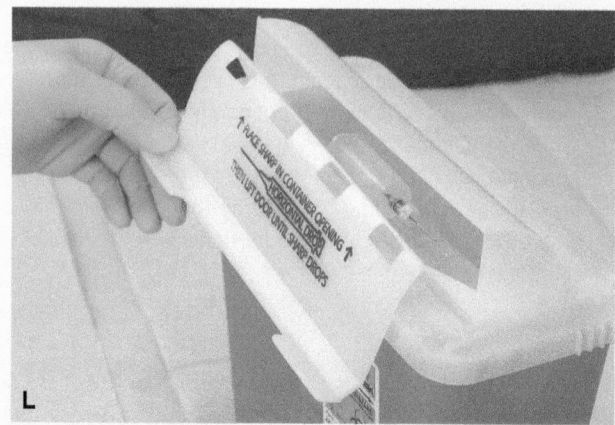

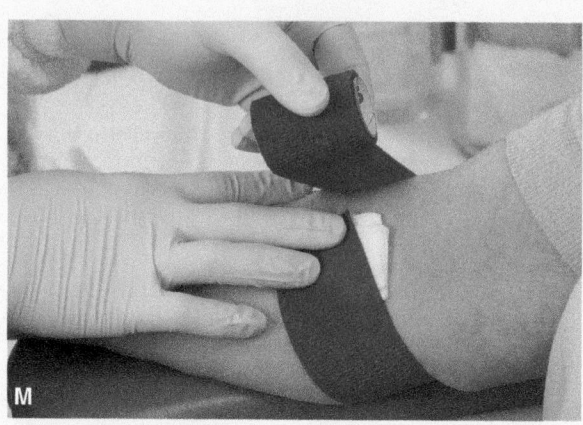

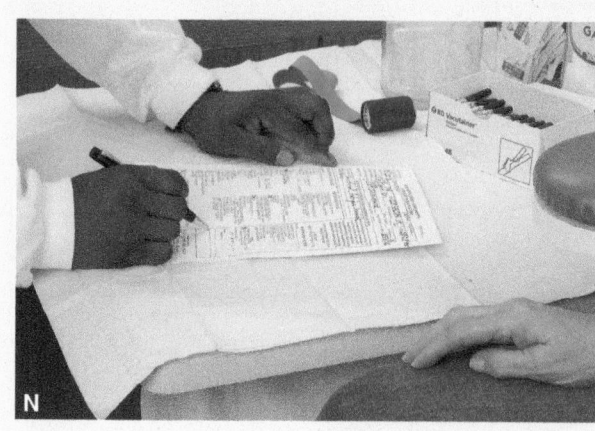

FIGURE I–N (*continued*)

18. Assess the patient. Check the venipuncture site for bleeding; then apply a bandage (Figure M). Ask if the patient is dizzy or light-headed.
19. Label the tubes with the patient's name, date, time, ID number, specimen type, tests to be done, and the phlebotomist's initials. Fill out the laboratory requisition sheet (Figure N).

20. Remove gloves. Perform hand hygiene.
21. Record the procedure in the patient's medical record.

CHARTING EXAMPLE

2/28/YY 1:00 P.M. Withdrew 10 mL of blood from the antecubital region of Pt.'s left arm, no complications. Sent blood to in-office lab for CBC...M. Garcia, RMA

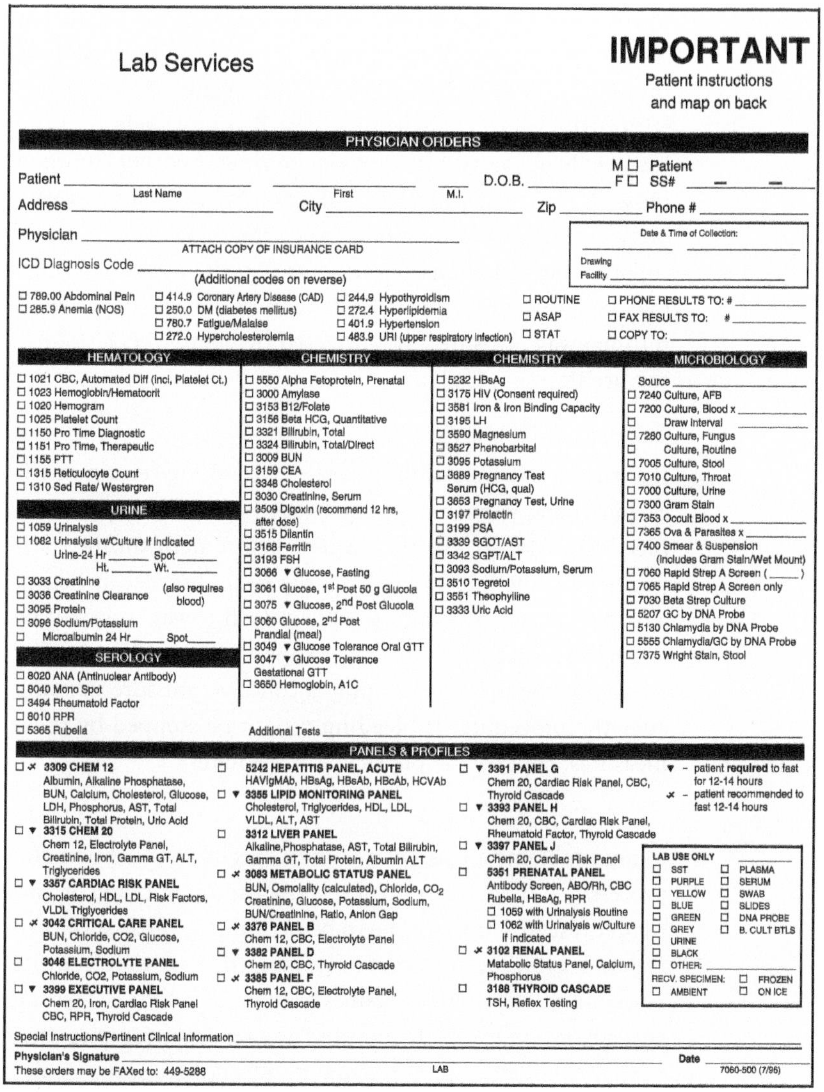
Lab Services

IMPORTANT
Patient instructions
and map on back

PHYSICIAN ORDERS

Patient ____________ ____________ ___ D.O.B. ________ M ☐ F ☐ Patient SS# ___ — ___ — ___
Last Name First M.I.
Address ____________ City ____________ Zip ________ Phone # ________
Physician ____________
ATTACH COPY OF INSURANCE CARD
ICD Diagnosis Code ____________
(Additional codes on reverse)

Date & Time of Collection: ________ ________
Drawing Facility ________

☐ 789.00 Abdominal Pain
☐ 285.9 Anemia (NOS)
☐ 414.9 Coronary Artery Disease (CAD)
☐ 250.0 DM (diabetes mellitus)
☐ 780.7 Fatigue/Malaise
☐ 272.0 Hypercholesterolemia
☐ 244.9 Hypothyroidism
☐ 272.4 Hyperlipidemia
☐ 401.9 Hypertension
☐ 483.9 URI (upper respiratory infection)
☐ ROUTINE
☐ ASAP
☐ STAT
☐ PHONE RESULTS TO: # ________
☐ FAX RESULTS TO: # ________
☐ COPY TO: ________

HEMATOLOGY
☐ 1021 CBC, Automated Diff (incl, Platelet Ct.)
☐ 1023 Hemoglobin/Hematocrit
☐ 1020 Hemogram
☐ 1025 Platelet Count
☐ 1150 Pro Time Diagnostic
☐ 1151 Pro Time, Therapeutic
☐ 1155 PTT
☐ 1315 Reticulocyte Count
☐ 1310 Sed Rate/ Westergren

URINE
☐ 1059 Urinalysis
☐ 1062 Urinalysis w/Culture if Indicated
Urine-24 Hr ______ Spot ______
Ht. ______ Wt. ______
☐ 3033 Creatinine
☐ 3036 Creatinine Clearance (also requires blood)
☐ 3095 Protein
☐ 3096 Sodium/Potassium
☐ Microalbumin 24 Hr ______ Spot ______

SEROLOGY
☐ 8020 ANA (Antinuclear Antibody)
☐ 8040 Mono Spot
☐ 3494 Rheumatoid Factor
☐ 8010 RPR
☐ 5365 Rubella

CHEMISTRY
☐ 5550 Alpha Fetoprotein, Prenatal
☐ 3000 Amylase
☐ 3153 B12/Folate
☐ 3156 Beta HCG, Quantitative
☐ 3321 Bilirubin, Total
☐ 3324 Bilirubin, Total/Direct
☐ 3009 BUN
☐ 3159 CEA
☐ 3348 Cholesterol
☐ 3030 Creatinine, Serum
☐ 3509 Digoxin (recommend 12 hrs, after dose)
☐ 3515 Dilantin
☐ 3168 Ferritin
☐ 3193 FSH
☐ 3066 ▼ Glucose, Fasting
☐ 3061 Glucose, 1st Post 50 g Glucola
☐ 3075 ▼ Glucose, 2nd Post Glucola
☐ 3060 Glucose, 2nd Post Prandial (meal)
☐ 3049 ▼ Glucose Tolerance Oral GTT
☐ 3047 ▼ Glucose Tolerance Gestational GTT
☐ 3650 Hemoglobin, A1C

CHEMISTRY
☐ 5232 HBsAg
☐ 3175 HIV (Consent required)
☐ 3581 Iron & Iron Binding Capacity
☐ 3195 LH
☐ 3590 Magnesium
☐ 3527 Phenobarbital
☐ 3095 Potassium
☐ 3689 Pregnancy Test Serum (HCG, qual)
☐ 3653 Pregnancy Test, Urine
☐ 3197 Prolactin
☐ 3199 PSA
☐ 3339 SGOT/AST
☐ 3342 SGPT/ALT
☐ 3093 Sodium/Potassium, Serum
☐ 3510 Tegretol
☐ 3551 Theophylline
☐ 3333 Uric Acid

MICROBIOLOGY
Source ________
☐ 7240 Culture, AFB
☐ 7200 Culture, Blood x ________
☐ Draw Interval ________
☐ 7280 Culture, Fungus
☐ Culture, Routine
☐ 7005 Culture, Stool
☐ 7010 Culture, Throat
☐ 7000 Culture, Urine
☐ 7300 Gram Stain
☐ 7353 Occult Blood x ________
☐ 7365 Ova & Parasites x ________
☐ 7400 Smear & Suspension (Includes Gram Stain/Wet Mount)
☐ 7060 Rapid Strep A Screen (______)
☐ 7065 Rapid Strep A Screen only
☐ 7030 Beta Strep Culture
☐ 5207 GC by DNA Probe
☐ 5130 Chlamydia by DNA Probe
☐ 5555 Chlamydia/GC by DNA Probe
☐ 7375 Wright Stain, Stool

Additional Tests ________

PANELS & PROFILES
☐ ✗ **3309 CHEM 12** Albumin, Alkaline Phosphatase, BUN, Calcium, Cholesterol, Glucose, LDH, Phosphorus, AST, Total Bilirubin, Total Protein, Uric Acid
☐ ▼ **3315 CHEM 20** Chem 12, Electrolyte Panel, Creatinine, Iron, Gamma GT, ALT, Triglycerides
☐ ▼ **3357 CARDIAC RISK PANEL** Cholesterol, HDL, LDL, Risk Factors, VLDL Triglycerides
☐ ✗ **3042 CRITICAL CARE PANEL** BUN, Chloride, CO2, Glucose, Potassium, Sodium
☐ **3046 ELECTROLYTE PANEL** Chloride, CO2, Potassium, Sodium
☐ ▼ **3399 EXECUTIVE PANEL** Chem 20, Iron, Cardiac Risk Panel CBC, RPR, Thyroid Cascade
☐ **5242 HEPATITIS PANEL, ACUTE** HAVIgMAb, HBsAg, HBsAb, HBcAb, HCVAb
☐ ▼ **3355 LIPID MONITORING PANEL** Cholesterol, Triglycerides, HDL, LDL, VLDL, ALT, AST
☐ **3312 LIVER PANEL** Alkaline,Phosphatase, AST, Total Bilirubin, Gamma GT, Total Protein, Albumin ALT
☐ ✗ **3083 METABOLIC STATUS PANEL** BUN, Osmolality (calculated), Chloride, CO_2 Creatinine, Glucose, Potassium, Sodium, BUN/Creatinine, Ratio, Anion Gap
☐ ✗ **3376 PANEL B** Chem 12, CBC, Electrolyte Panel
☐ ▼ **3382 PANEL D** Chem 20, CBC, Thyroid Cascade
☐ ✗ **3385 PANEL F** Chem 12, CBC, Electrolyte Panel, Thyroid Cascade
☐ ▼ **3391 PANEL G** Chem 20, Cardiac Risk Panel, CBC, Thyroid Cascade
☐ ▼ **3393 PANEL H** Chem 20, CBC, Cardiac Risk Panel, Rheumatoid Factor, Thyroid Cascade
☐ ▼ **3397 PANEL J** Chem 20, Cardiac Risk Panel
☐ **5351 PRENATAL PANEL** Antibody Screen, ABO/Rh, CBC Rubella, HBsAg, RPR
☐ 1059 with Urinalysis Routine
☐ 1062 with Urinalysis w/Culture if indicated
☐ ✗ **3102 RENAL PANEL** Matabolic Status Panel, Calcium, Phosphorus
☐ **3188 THYROID CASCADE** TSH, Reflex Testing

▼ – patient **required** to fast for 12-14 hours
✗ – patient recommended to fast 12-14 hours

LAB USE ONLY ________
☐ SST ☐ PLASMA
☐ PURPLE ☐ SERUM
☐ YELLOW ☐ SWAB
☐ BLUE ☐ SLIDES
☐ GREEN ☐ DNA PROBE
☐ GREY ☐ B. CULT BTLS
☐ URINE
☐ BLACK
☐ OTHER: ________
RECV. SPECIMEN: ☐ FROZEN
☐ AMBIENT ☐ ON ICE

Special Instructions/Pertinent Clinical Information ________
Physician's Signature ________ **Date** ________
These orders may be FAXed to: 449-5288
LAB
7060-500 (7/96)

FIGURE 46-19 Laboratory requisition form.

specimen to ensure that specimens are not rejected and redraws required. Figure 46-19 shows a sample laboratory requisition form. Sometimes processing must be done immediately upon arrival at the laboratory (or STAT). Some examples of tests that require STAT processing are blood gases, PT INR, CBC, CMP, Bilirubin, BMP, and liver function tests.

Responding to Complications

In your work as a phlebotomist, you will occasionally encounter some special challenges. These may include formation of a hematoma, a patient refusing to undergo the procedure, a patient having a stress reaction, a failure to obtain blood, specimen problems, and the special precautions required by blood cultures. Figure 46-20 illustrates common phlebotomy issues.

Hematomas

A **hematoma** is a bruise formed by the collection of blood at the puncture site when some of the blood escapes the vein and enters the surrounding tissue. Hematomas can result from a number of situations. If a needle penetrates both walls of a vein or only partially penetrates a vein, blood can leak out during the procedure. If the needle is removed while the tourniquet is still in place, increased internal pressure will provide increased likelihood of such leakage. Typically, hematomas can be prevented by having the patient apply pressure to the insertion site for two to three minutes after removal of the needle. Generally, hematomas do not hurt unless the swelling is significant. In this instance, a cold compress over the area may reduce discomfort and swelling.

Patient Refusal

One of the fundamental patient rights is the right to refuse treatment. *Never attempt to collect a specimen from a patient who refuses.* Without a signed court order that specifically overrides this right, forcing compliance is considered battery and is highly illegal. When possible, explain the reason for the test and its importance in the patient's care in a nonthreatening manner. If the patient still refuses, notify the doctor and document the refusal in the chart.

Stress

Stress over phlebotomy procedures can cause physical changes that may affect people with underlying illness. Preexisting conditions, such as diabetes or seizure disorders, may be exacerbated by this stress. A diabetic patient who has been in the waiting room a long time and hasn't eaten is at risk for hypoglycemic shock, sometimes referred to as insulin shock. If this is suspected, give the patient sugar by any means tolerated and notify the physician. If a patient experiences convulsions during blood collection, remove the needle as safely as possible, position the patient on his side on the floor, and have a coworker notify the physician immediately. In all emergencies, call 911 if necessary.

Failure to Obtain Blood

Sometimes, after insertion of the needle, blood is not obtained. This can occur because of failure to insert the needle deep enough, which can be remedied by simply advancing

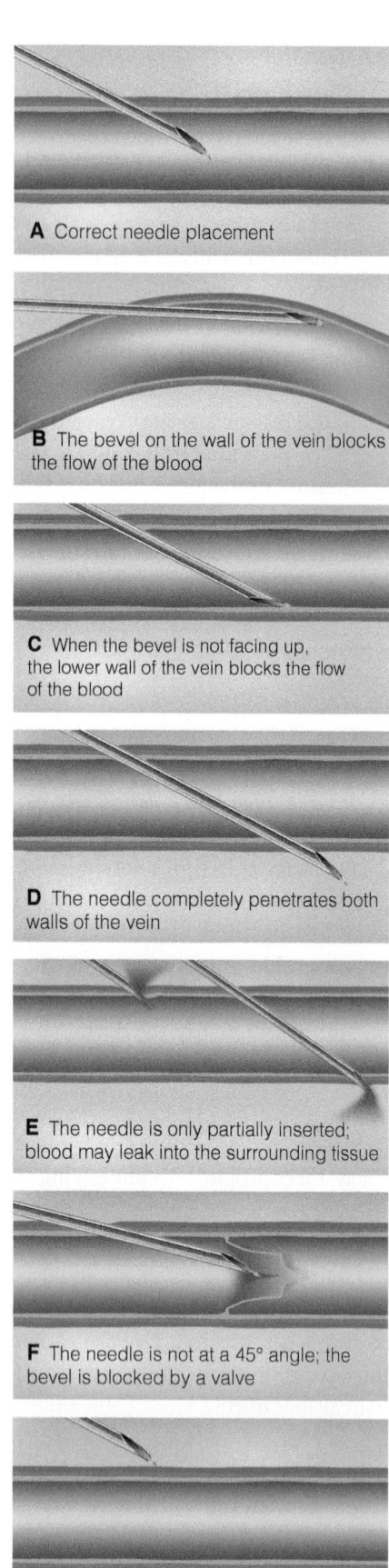

A Correct needle placement

B The bevel on the wall of the vein blocks the flow of the blood

C When the bevel is not facing up, the lower wall of the vein blocks the flow of the blood

D The needle completely penetrates both walls of the vein

E The needle is only partially inserted; blood may leak into the surrounding tissue

F The needle is not at a 45° angle; the bevel is blocked by a valve

G The vein is not punctured

FIGURE 46-20 (A–G) Common phlebotomy issues.

the needle slightly forward. It can occur when the needle has been advanced too far and penetrated through both walls of the vein, or if it rests against the wall of the vein or a valve within the vein. These can be remedied by slowly backing the needle out until blood begins to flow. Another common cause of failure is when the collection tube has lost its vacuum; simply try using a new tube. Fragile veins may easily collapse with vacuum container use, so the use of a syringe may be required. Sometimes, failure can be a result of veins rolling away. This may be corrected by gently repositioning the needle.

Excessive Bleeding

If a patient has a bleeding disorder or is taking certain medication therapy, there may be excessive post-venipuncture bleeding. Always ask the patient before performing venipuncture if she knows she has a bleeding disorder, is taking anticoagulants, or is taking aspirin. In this way, you will be forewarned that you may need to apply pressure longer after removing the needle and apply a cohesive pressure dressing after the procedure. If bleeding cannot be stopped by these measures, contact the physician immediately.

Specimen Problems

Many problems are associated with specimen collection and processing. If the wrong tube is used to draw blood, a particular test may not be able to be performed. If the specimen is not legible or is incorrectly labeled, this may require retesting or can produce results that are listed for the wrong patient. Blood can be hemolyzed as a result of venipuncture with a small needle, not allowing alcohol to properly dry before insertion, excessive hand pumping, or vigorous shaking after collection. Poor specimen process or improper conditions before or during transportation can also affect the quality of a specimen.

Special Needs Patients

Medical assistants need to be respectful of all patients. Some patients have special needs with regard to phlebotomy and blood collection.

Sites to avoid include areas with hematomas, scars, or edema (swelling) as you want to avoid further traumatizing these areas. Avoid using an arm with a fistula (abnormal or artificial connection between blood vessels), vascular (vessel) graft, or burns. If possible, also avoid sites with tattoos. Also avoid using the arm that is on the same side as a mastectomy (breast tissue removal). The flow of blood to these sites may not be optimal or lymph flow may be impeded.

If an arm with an IV must be used, always choose a site below the IV **cannula** and ensure that blood is not being transfused in that extremity.

For patients with cognitive impairment (low IQ, dementia, traumatic brain injury), explain every part of the procedure carefully so as not to emotionally traumatize the patient. As with children, it may be helpful to have a loved one present when drawing blood from a patient with a cognitive impairment.

SUMMARY

The proper collection, handling, and processing of blood specimens are vital to reliable test results and proper care of the patient. It is important to prepare the patient well for the procedure by instructing the patient on fasting or hydration as necessary. Identification of the patient and which laboratory tests need to be drawn is critical, as is laying out the vacuum tubes to be filled in the correct order. Considering the available and appropriate sites is another important step, taking into account the special needs of some patients. Select the needle that best serves your needs, and, after drawing the blood, be sure to monitor the patient for syncope or bleeding. Correctly labeling the tubes and filling out the laboratory requisition form are vital steps before documenting in the patient chart and properly transporting the specimen to the laboratory.

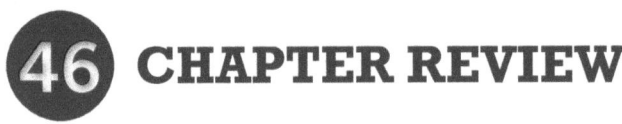

46 CHAPTER REVIEW

COMPETENCY REVIEW

1. Define and spell the terms for this chapter.
2. Identify the three most common veins for venipuncture in the antecubital space. Of these three, which is most popular?
3. Discuss advantages and disadvantages of using the butterfly method for blood draw.
4. List the order of draw for blood collection tubes.
5. How long should a tourniquet stay in place during a blood draw? What happens if it is left on for too long?
6. Make a list of the reasons for failure to obtain blood and the corrective actions to take.
7. What can be done to help decrease patient anxiety related to phlebotomy?
8. What does STAT mean in regard to specimen processing? List some tests that often require STAT processing.

PREPARING FOR THE CERTIFICATION EXAM

1. The slanted opening at the end of a needle is referred to as a
   a. shield.
   b. gauge.
   c. bevel.
   d. hematoma.
   e. valve.
2. What common reasons can result in a failed attempt to draw blood?
   a. resting the bevel against a valve or wall of a vein
   b. advancing the needle too far
   c. failure to insert the needle deep enough
   d. failed vacuum in collection tube
   e. all of the above
3. The most common method of venipuncture is
   a. syringe.
   b. butterfly.

   c. vacuum container.
   d. capillary puncture.
   e. heel-stick.
4. Tubes with which color tops contain heparin and are used for testing whole blood and plasma?
   a. red
   b. brick
   c. lavender
   d. green
   e. yellow
5. The most commonly used site for a venipuncture is the
   a. cephalic vein.
   b. pulmonary vein.
   c. median cubital vein.
   d. antebrachial vein.
   e. basilic vein.

6. Which blood tube should always be drawn first, when ordered?
   a. red
   b. yellow
   c. green
   d. blue
   e. gray

7. The collection of blood through a tiny incision in the vein is called
   a. phlebotomy.
   b. venipuncture.
   c. hematology.
   d. both A and B are correct.
   e. none of the above.

8. What are characteristics of arteries?
   a. They are highly oxygenated, have thick elastic walls, carry bright red blood, and actively pulsate.
   b. They are bridges that connect to tissues in the body.
   c. They are pathways that carry blood toward the heart.
   d. They carry high levels of carbon dioxide, which makes the blood appear darker and gives the lining of the vessel a bluish tinge.
   e. Their walls are thin, do not pulsate, and have one-way valves to keep blood flowing in the right direction.

9. What size needle is typically used in venipuncture for adults?
   a. 16–18 gauge
   b. 20–21 gauge
   c. 22–24 gauge
   d. 25–26 gauge
   e. 27–28 gauge

10. What should the medical assistant ask a patient before drawing blood?
   a. Are there any allergies?
   b. When did you last eat?
   c. Do you have any candy or gum in your mouth?
   d. Do you have a history of bleeding significantly or fainting?
   e. All of the above are correct.

CRITICAL THINKING

Refer to the case study at the beginning of the chapter and use what you have learned to answer the following questions.

1. Samra will be using Vacutainer tubes to draw blood. Which color of tube top will Samra need for the tests ordered? List the additional supplies that Samra will need to perform the blood draw.

2. What additives, if any, are in the Vacutainers that Samra will be using? What is the correct order of draw, and why is it important to follow a correct order of draw?

3. How can Samra calm Ms. St. Clair's anxiety regarding the procedure?

ON THE JOB

It is Wednesday, and Drs. Joseph and Burg are not seeing patients. However, the office is open for blood draws. Angie, a medical assistant, is in the office alone.

Matt, a 17-year-old upcoming college freshman, has just arrived to have his labs drawn so that Dr. Joseph can complete Matt's college physical. He is extremely nervous, although he is trying very hard to exhibit a relaxed manner. Angie tries to reassure Matt, but the more she tries, the more nervous he gets. At Matt's urging to "just get it over with," Angie decides to go ahead and draw his blood. Unfortunately, as soon as the first collection tube begins to fill with blood, Matt notices it and slumps forward. He has fainted.

1. What is the first thing that Angie should do?
2. Was Angie at all negligent in drawing Matt's blood given that he was extremely nervous?
3. Is this considered a medical emergency?
4. Does an incident report of some sort need to be filed? If so, what should be included, and who should receive a copy?

INTERNET ACTIVITY

Go online and research materials to further understand OSHA regulations, CDC standard precautions, and the laboratory regulations established by CLIA in 1988.

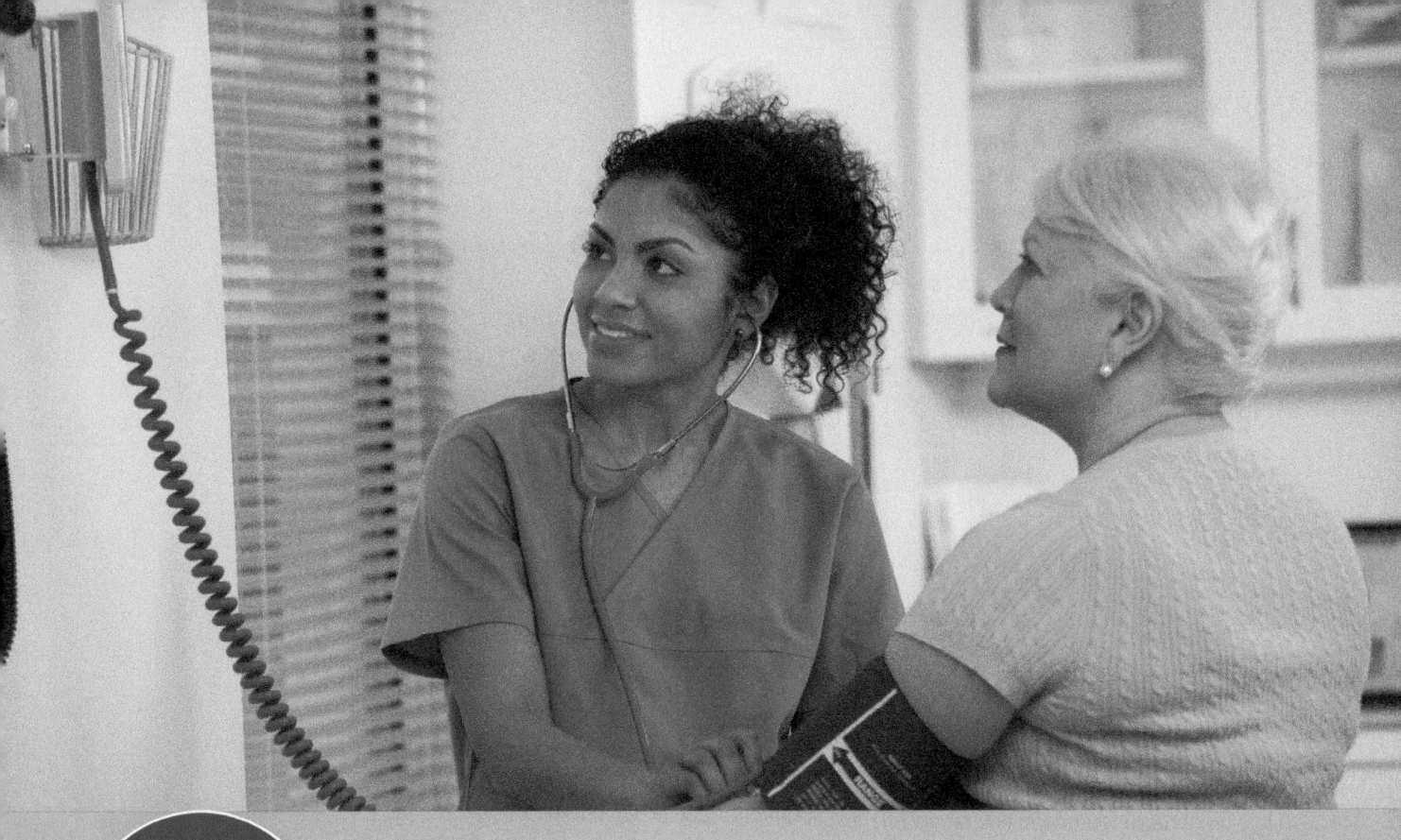

Learning Objectives

After completing this chapter, you should be able to:

47.1   Define and spell the terms for this chapter.

47.2   Explain the medical assistant's role in hematology.

47.3   Identify the components of blood.

47.4   Describe blood tests that are associated with red blood cells.

47.5   Describe blood tests that are associated with white blood cells.

47.6   Describe blood tests related to coagulation testing.

47.7   List blood tests that are included in a comprehensive metabolic panel.

47.8   Describe tests commonly performed on diabetic patients.

47.9   Describe phenylketonuria (PKU) testing.

47.10 Describe mono testing.

Lisa Stiver, RMA, is working with Dr. Lewis, who has just ordered STAT lab tests. The doctor has just gone to lunch, and Lisa is covering the office by herself for the afternoon because her coworkers called out sick. She receives test results for Sarah Johnson. As she reviews the results, Lisa notices the following: WBC 11,500 mm^3, Na 125 mEq/L, BUN 100 mg/dL. Lisa has to draw blood for the STAT tests and answer the phone as it rings.

Terms to Learn

anemia

basophils

carboxyhemoglobin

complete blood count (CBC)

critical values

electrolytes

eosinophils

erythrocyte indices

erythrocytes

erythrocyte sedimentation rate (ESR)

erythropoietin

formed elements

hematocrit (Hct)

hematology

hematopoiesis

hemoglobin (Hgb)

heparin

leukocytes

lymphocytes

mean corpuscular hemoglobin (MCH)

mean corpuscular hemoglobin concentration (MCHC)

mean corpuscular volume (MCV)

microhematocrit

monocytes

mononucleosis

neutrophils

oxyhemoglobin

phenylketonuria (PKU)

plasma

platelets

polycythemia

RBC count

reticulocyte count

reticulocytes

serum

thrombocytes

Many things can be determined by evaluating blood and its components. Lab tests performed on blood are most commonly used to verify or rule out a suspected diagnosis. Sometimes they reveal an unsuspected issue. Either way, diseases and illnesses can be discovered or verified through blood studies so that a patient can be effectively treated. This is accomplished through hematology.

Hematology is the study of blood and the tissues that produce it. Blood analysis is one of the most common diagnostic tests performed in the doctor's office. As a result, the medical assistant must have a thorough understanding of how to correctly collect, handle, package, and analyze a blood specimen. The medical assistant must also be able to recognize abnormal blood test results and their possible consequences and report them promptly.

THE MEDICAL ASSISTANT'S ROLE

Blood analysis is a vital and routine tool of medicine. When the physician orders a blood test, the role of the medical assistant is to collect and process the specimen. Medical assistants may also perform laboratory testing within their scope of practice. Whether you are performing tests or collecting results from a laboratory, it is important to know normal values and to understand what test results reveal to properly educate the patient and recognize critical situations.

Blood Specimen Collection

As emphasized in the chapters on the clinical laboratory, microbiology, urinalysis, and phlebotomy, the collection and laboratory testing of blood and of all body fluids is strictly regulated by the Occupational Safety and Health Administration (OSHA) and the Centers for Disease Control and Prevention (CDC). Standard precautions must be followed at all times. Clinical Laboratory Improvement Amendments (CLIA) sets the standards to which all laboratories must adhere, including training of personnel and testing and transport of specimens. When performing specimen collection, you must follow the regulation guidelines established by these organizations.

Review the chapter titled "Phlebotomy and Blood Collection" regarding the equipment and procedures for blood

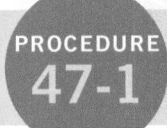

PROCEDURE 47-1

Differentiating Between Normal and Abnormal Test Values

Objective ◆ *Review incoming laboratory results, and follow up with patient per physician's orders.*

EQUIPMENT AND SUPPLIES

Patient's electronic medical record; laboratory test results (be sure to include at least two abnormal values and at least two normal values). Use Table 47-2 to reference ranges.

METHOD

Note: Follow the facility policy on contacting patients when results are abnormal. Results are not to be released to the patient unless authorized by the physician.

1. Review incoming lab results and compare with the reference values provided in Table 47-2 to identify any abnormalities.
2. Highlight any abnormal results per facility policy.
3. Obtain the patient's electronic medical record, record or scan the new laboratory results, and alert the physician for review. Figure A shows a medical assistant entering test results electronically. Accuracy when documenting results is critical.
4. Follow the physician's orders regarding scheduling appointments or repeat testing.
5. Document the patient's record accordingly.

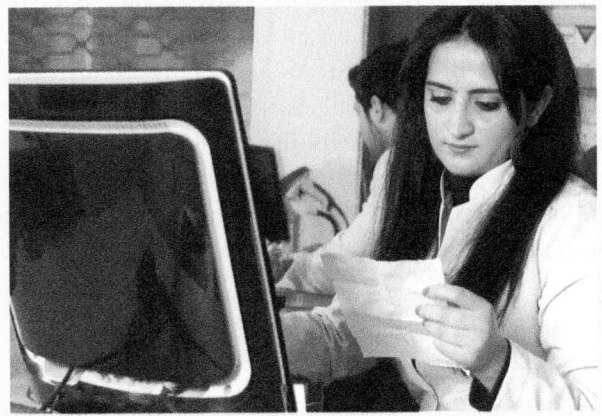

FIGURE A Correctly documenting laboratory test results in medical records, in writing or electronically, is critical.

CHARTING EXAMPLE

08/04/YY 10:00 A.M. Scheduled repeat lab test and follow-up appointment on 08/10/YY per physician's order.........................
....C. Fisher, CMA (AAMA)

---

collection by capillary puncture and by venipuncture as well as the types of tubes that are required for specific tests. It is part of the role of the medical assistant to differentiate between normal and abnormal test values and notify the physician of abnormal values. Procedure 47-1 explains differentiating between normal and abnormal test values.

BLOOD FUNCTION, FORMATION, AND COMPONENTS

The main functions of blood are transportation and protection. Blood takes oxygen and nutrients to the body and removes carbon dioxide. Blood takes waste products to the lungs, liver, kidneys, and skin for elimination. Blood carries white blood cells to help fight off infection and contains platelets to begin the healing process. Blood also assists in regulating body temperature. Review the information in the chapters titled "The Cardiovascular System"

and "Phlebotomy and Blood Collection" regarding circulatory anatomy and physiology.

To fully understand blood test results, it is important to first understand some basic information about blood formation and components.

Plasma

The liquid component of blood is **plasma**. Plasma makes up about 55 percent of the composition of blood. Plasma carries blood cells and other substances to the different parts of the body. A key component of plasma is fibrinogen, which converts to fibrin, whose function is the formation of blood clots. **Serum** is plasma without the fibrinogen.

Ninety percent of plasma is water; the other 10 percent is solid substances, called solutes, that dissolve in the plasma. These solutes may include the plasma proteins (albumin, globulin, fibrinogen, and prothrombin); **electrolytes**, also called ionic solutions because they contain free ions (sodium, potassium, and chloride); glucose; amino acids; lipids and carbohydrates; metabolic waste products (urea, lactic acid, uric acid); creatinine; respiratory gases (oxygen and carbon dioxide); and a variety of other substances (hormones, antibodies, enzymes, vitamins, and mineral salts).

Cellular Components (Formed Elements)

The formation of blood cells is called **hematopoiesis**. Hematopoiesis begins during fetal development when stem cells are formed and housed in bone marrow. Throughout life, these stem cells give birth to new blood cells to replace damaged or aged cells as needed. All blood cells originate from the hematopoietic stem cell, but they mature into one of seven types of cells—red cells, five types of white cells, and platelets. The red cells, white cells, and platelets are known as the **formed elements** of the blood (Figure 47-1; also see Box 47-1). Each type of cell has specific functions, as follows:

1. Red blood cells (**erythrocytes**): transportation of oxygen and carbon dioxide
2. White blood cells (**leukocytes**): defense

   There are three types of granular leukocytes (that have granules in their cytoplasm, the gel-like substance within the cell membrane) and two types of agranular

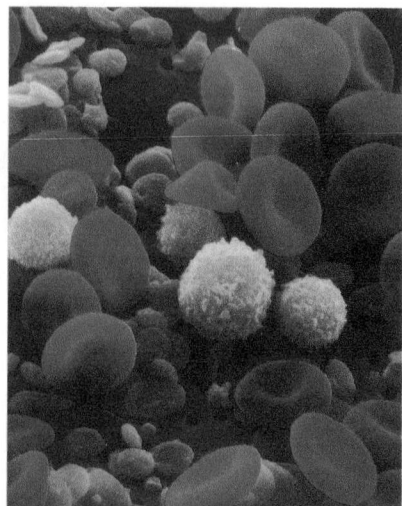

FIGURE 47-1 The formed elements: In this image, the red cells are red, the white cells are white, and the platelets are green.

leukocytes (also called nongranular leukocytes—leukocytes that do not have granules in their cytoplasm):

a. Granular leukocytes
   - Neutrophils
   - Eosinophils
   - Basophils

BOX 47-1 | Under the Microscope

RED BLOOD CELLS

RBCs are the most numerous, are salmon colored, and appear oval with a slightly pale center. RBCs have no nucleus or granules. RBCs with a nucleus are called reticulocytes (immature RBCs). Normal-looking RBCs are recorded as "normal RBC morphology."

PLATELETS

Platelets are the smallest of the formed blood elements. They are about half the size of an RBC. They stain purple and tend to appear in a clump, although they may also exist singly. They have a rough outer edge and contain small granules that become sticky, which helps stop blood loss by promoting the clotting process. There are between 200,000 and 300,000 platelets per mm^3 of blood. There are typically between 5 and 20 platelets in one field of view. If this number is counted, then record the platelet count as "Adequate platelet estimation."

WHITE BLOOD CELLS

There are five types of WBCs, each of which has a distinct identifying characteristic when using the Wright's staining method. Count 100 WBCs; then express each of the cell types as a percentage. Normal values for adults are as follows:

- Neutrophils: 50–70 percent
- Eosinophils: 1–4 percent
- Basophils: 0–1 percent

- Lymphocytes: 20–35 percent
- Monocytes: 3–8 percent

   Values may differ between manual and automated analyses.

GRANULATED WHITE BLOOD CELLS

The neutrophil, or seg, is the most numerous WBC. The neutrophil has small cytoplasmic granules that stain pink or lilac with a multilobed nucleus with small strands connecting each of the lobes, which stain purple. A band neutrophil is an immature neutrophil. It appears similar to the neutrophil except that the nucleus is unsegmented and curved with a bandlike structure. Cytoplasmic granules stain blue to pink.

Eosinophils have segmented nuclei and large, reddish-staining granules that are found in the cytoplasm.

Basophils are rarely seen in a diff count. This WBC has an S-shaped nucleus and large, irregularly shaped purplish-blue granules that almost entirely cover the nucleus.

AGRANULOCYTIC WHITE BLOOD CELLS

Lymphocytes have a single round or lightly indented nucleus, which almost completely fills the cell. The cytoplasm is clear and stains a pale blue. Lymphocytes are the smallest WBC.

Monocytes are the largest WBC and have a distinct kidney bean–shaped nucleus. The cytoplasm is abundant and clear, and it stains a grayish blue.

---

b. Nongranular leukocytes
   - Lymphocytes
   - Monocytes

3. Platelets (**thrombocytes**): clotting

Although hematopoiesis occurs primarily in the bone marrow of the adult, lymphocytes are also produced in the lymph nodes.

FORMED ELEMENTS AND ASSOCIATED TESTS

Blood tests can be ordered individually or in groups, referred to as panels, profiles, or counts. A **complete blood count (CBC)** is one of the most common combinations of tests routinely ordered. It includes red blood cell (RBC) counts, RBC indices, hemoglobin (Hgb), hematocrit (Hct), white blood cell (WBC) counts (with or without differential), platelet counts, and blood cell morphology. To fully understand what this test reveals, it is important to have a basic understanding of the cells and the individual tests performed on them.

Red Blood Cells and Red Blood Cell Tests

RBCs, or erythrocytes, are vessels that carry hemoglobin throughout the body. They are formed in the bone marrow and are routinely replaced every few months. A healthy mature RBC has a biconcave disk shape—*biconcave* meaning that both of its sides are curved inward—a shape that provides increased surface area for gas exchange (Figure 47-2).

Red blood cells

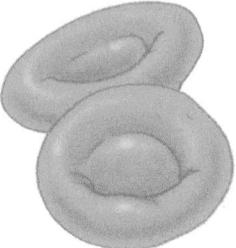

FIGURE 47-2 Red cells have a biconcave shape.

Hemoglobin (Hgb) is a vital protein molecule found in RBCs that has two primary functions. The first is to carry oxygen from the lungs to the cells of the body. When the hemoglobin is carrying oxygen, it is called **oxyhemoglobin**. Arterial blood has a high concentration of oxyhemoglobin that gives it a bright red color. The second function of hemoglobin is to carry carbon dioxide (a waste product) from throughout the body back to the lungs, where it can be expelled with exhalation. Hemoglobin that is carrying carbon dioxide is called **carboxyhemoglobin**. Venous blood is darker in color than arterial blood because of the carboxyhemoglobin it carries.

A variety of blood tests are associated with the RBCs.

Erythrocyte or Red Blood Cell (RBC) Count

The **RBC count** is the number of RBCs per cubic millimeter (mm^3) of blood. Normal values vary according to age and gender. The normal RBC range for a male adult is 4.5 to 6 million/mm^3. The normal female RBC range is 4 to 5.5 million/mm^3, although it may slightly decrease during pregnancy.

The formation of RBCs is controlled somewhat by **erythropoietin**, a glycoprotein hormone that controls RBC production. Erythropoietin is secreted by the kidneys in an adult and by the liver in a fetus. When oxygen levels in the blood are low, termed hypoxemia, the kidneys typically compensate by secreting extra erythropoietin, which in turn stimulates the bone marrow to produce more RBCs.

Anemia is a condition in which the blood has a lower than normal level of RBCs or of hemoglobin within the RBCs. Several things can cause this. An injury may destroy RBCs. Decreased erythropoietin production by the kidneys or

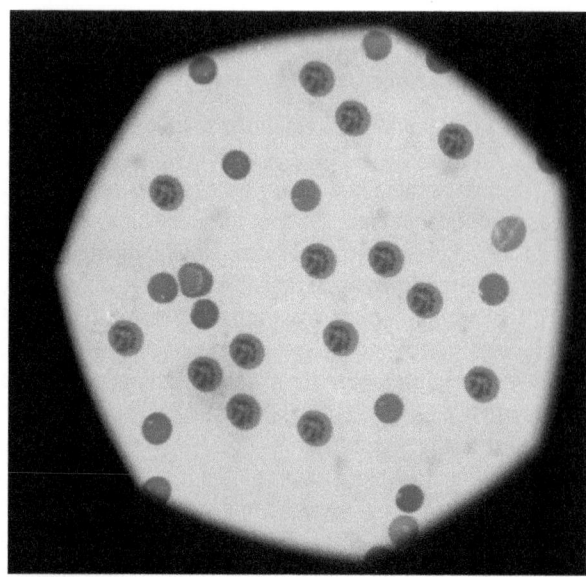

FIGURE 47-3 Reticulocytes are immature red cells that can be identified by a reticular (mesh-like) network of RNA that a stain makes visible under a microscope.

impaired bone marrow function can lead to reduced or dysfunctional production of RBCs. In certain cases, this can be remedied by administering a drug such as Procrit, an artificial erythropoietin that assists in the reproduction of RBCs. Some types of anemia can be a result of poor diet or reduced hemoglobin proteins. In iron-deficiency anemia, iron supplements or increased red meat in the diet may be sufficient to restore hemoglobin levels.

Polycythemia is a condition in which the blood has a higher than normal level of RBCs. This can result from an overproduction of erythropoietin by the kidneys or from overactive bone marrow. Causes include high altitudes, strenuous exercise, cigarette smoking, lung disease, tumors, renal disorders, and dehydration. This condition can become dangerous, because high RBC counts can lead to an increased risk of developing blood clots. It is important for patients with this disorder to stay well hydrated to decrease the viscosity (thickness or stickiness) of the blood and reduce the chances of clotting.

A manual RBC count requires small samples of the blood specimen to be diluted in a special solution, which is added to a hemocytometer. Then the hemocytometer is placed on a microscope used to count the cells. Because this is not considered CLIA waived, a manual count should be performed only in an educational setting for better understanding. More advanced specific training is required for the medical assistant to be able to perform this in a medical laboratory. For this reason, automated testing for RBCs is more common than manual testing.

Reticulocyte Count

RBCs last for about four months and are continuously being reproduced in the body. **Reticulocytes**, or immature RBCs, generally mature within 48 hours. The **reticulocyte count** is the percentage of reticulocytes in the blood in relation to the number of mature RBCs (Figure 47-3). Because RBCs are produced by the bone marrow, evaluating the reticulocyte

rate helps to determine the ability of the bone marrow to compensate for RBC loss. Reticulocyte counts are often used to monitor the response to treatment for anemia. Increased rates are typical in pregnancy, newborns, high altitudes, and stimulated RBC production. Decreased reticulocytes are noted in renal or bone marrow disease, use of certain drugs, aplastic anemia, alcoholism, folic acid deficiency, and transfusions.

Hemoglobin (Hgb)

As already mentioned, RBCs contain hemoglobin. Hemoglobin consists of iron (heme) and a protein (globulin). A molecule of hemoglobin contains four atoms of iron, and an atom of oxygen will attach to each of the iron atoms. Because of its ability to bind oxygen, hemoglobin in the blood is responsible for carrying oxygen throughout the body. Thus, higher hemoglobin (Hgb) levels mean the body is able to transport more oxygen, and lower levels mean less oxygen is in circulation.

A low Hgb may indicate iron-deficiency anemia, whereas elevated readings are present in patients with polycythemia and in extreme situations, such as burns. Normal values for adult females are 12–16 g/dL and for males 14–18 g/dL.

Hemoglobin can be measured either by an automated blood analyzer (Figures 47-4 and 47-5) or manually by a hemoglobinometer (Procedure 47-2). Typically, the manual method is less accurate and not as reliable as the automated blood analyzer. Manual calculations are not CLIA waived and therefore cannot be performed by a medical assistant without specific training.

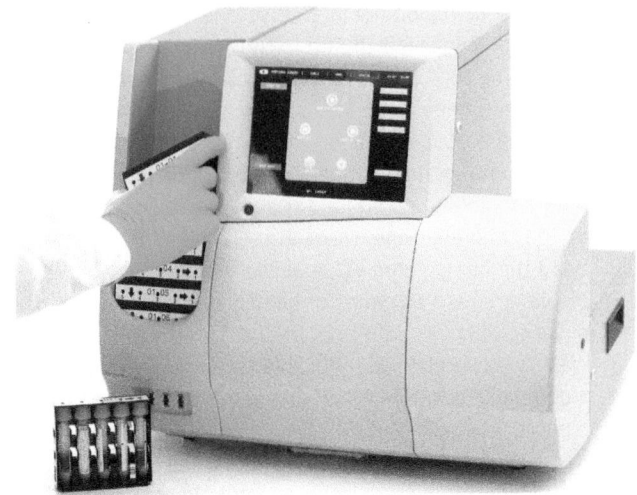

FIGURE 47-4 Automated blood analyzer.

Hemoglobin values can be determined by either of two methods: the specific gravity method or the cyanmethemoglobin method. The specific gravity method is a screening method for blood donors. The cyanmethemoglobin is a more specific and accurate method to give exact hemoglobin levels using hemoglobin analyzers.

Abnormal levels of hemoglobin can be dangerous because they affect the level of oxygen available to the cells. Hemoglobin is carried by RBCs, so anything that decreases the number of RBCs in circulation will automatically reduce Hgb levels. Other disorders that can lower hemoglobin levels include hemolytic disorders, cancers, anemias, sickle cell disease, thalassemia, frequent blood draws or loss, fluid retention, and pregnancy. An Hgb level that is less than 5 g/dL can result in heart failure and is considered to be a critical value that must be reported to the physician at once.

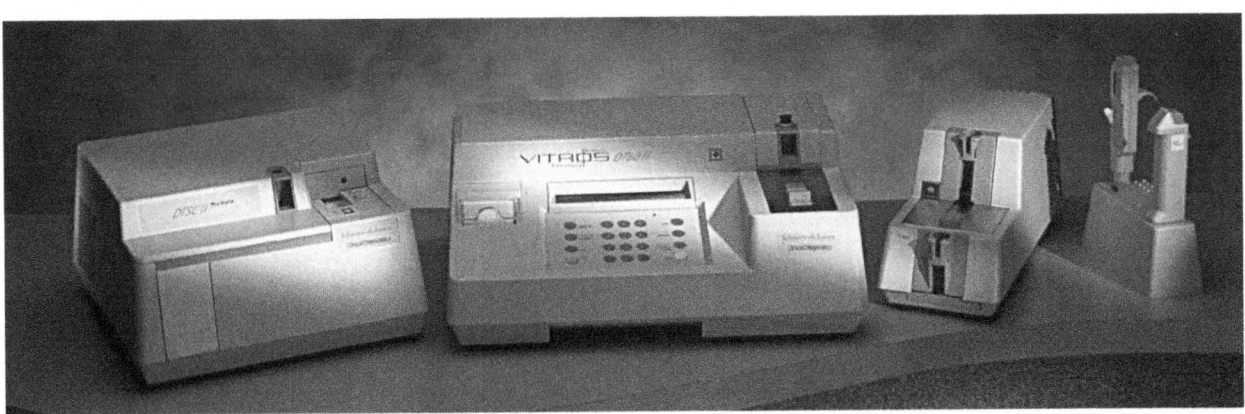

FIGURE 47-5 VITROS DT60II automated blood analysis system.

Determining Hemoglobin Using the Hemoglobinometer

Objective ◆ *Perform a blood test to determine hemoglobin levels using the hemoglobinometer.*

EQUIPMENT AND SUPPLIES

Hemoglobinometer; glass slide chamber; hemolysis applicator (plastic or wooden); sterile manual or spring-loaded lancet; cotton balls; dry gauze square; alcohol sponges; gloves; patient's record; lab coat; biohazard sharps container

Note: Follow standard precautions and safety guidelines when working with blood samples. Use care to avoid splashing or spilling blood. Wipe up all spills using guidelines established by OSHA.

METHOD

1. Perform hand hygiene and apply gloves.
2. Gather the necessary equipment and supplies.
3. Clean the puncture site with an alcohol sponge.
4. Using a manual or spring-loaded lancet, obtain capillary blood.
5. Pull the glass chamber out of the hemoglobinometer, and position the lower part of the slide so that it is slightly offset.
6. Place a large drop of capillary blood onto the slide.

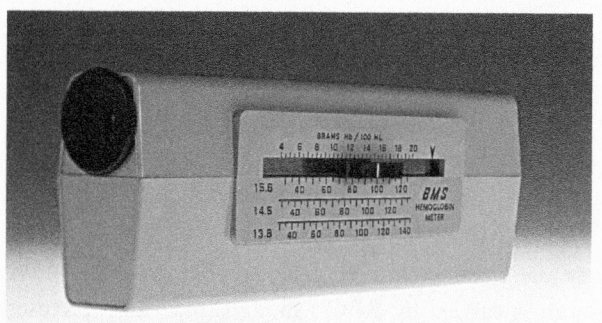

FIGURE A A hemoglobinometer (manual blood analyzer).

7. Wipe the patient's puncture site with a cotton ball and provide the patient with a dry gauze square to apply mild pressure to the puncture. This should stop further bleeding.
8. Mix blood with the hemolysis applicator until the blood becomes clear.
9. Push the glass chamber into the clip and place it into the slot on the left side of the hemoglobinometer.

10. Hold the hemoglobinometer in your left hand at eye level while using your left thumb to turn on the light by depressing the bottom button. Look into the instrument to see a split green field.
11. Slide the button on the right side of the meter with your right thumb and index finger while looking into the meter until a matching green field occurs. Leave the sliding scale on the calibrated line where the solid green field appeared.
12. Read the hemoglobin value at the top of the scale. The results are read as grams of hemoglobin per 100 mL of blood (g/dL).
13. Wash the chamber and reusable hemolysis applicator with a detergent solution, rinse, dry, and return to the instrument for the next test.
14. Remove gloves and perform hand hygiene. Discard gloves and nonreusable supplies in appropriate containers.
15. Record the results in the patient's record.

CHARTING EXAMPLE

2/28/YY Performed capillary puncture on right 3rd digit via aseptic technique. Hgb 15. Patient denies discomfort or excessive bleeding...M. King, CMA (AAMA)

Increased Hgb levels can occur in polycythemia, high altitudes, chronic lung disease, dehydration, smokers, and severe burn victims. Excessive hemoglobin (over 20 g/dL) can lead to blood clots from increased concentration and is considered critical.

Hematocrit (Hct)

The **hematocrit (Hct)** test evaluates the percentage of packed RBCs in the total volume of blood. A blood sample is collected in a tube and placed in a centrifuge, which spins the tube for about 15 minutes. This process separates the blood components into three layers: RBCs sink to the bottom, plasma floats to the top, and the buffy coat—a thin light- or buff-colored layer containing most of the white blood cells and platelets—divides the two (Figure 47-6).

In a patient with normal RBC and Hgb levels, the approximate hematocrit should be about three times the hemoglobin level. A normal hematocrit is 40 to 50 percent in males and 35 to 45 percent in females. A low hematocrit may indicate anemia or hemorrhage, and an elevated hematocrit may indicate dehydration or polycythemia (Figure 47-7). High glucose levels may falsely indicate elevated hematocrit levels.

The **microhematocrit**, or "crit," is a hematocrit performed on an extremely small quantity of blood collected in a capillary tube. Before performing a microhematocrit, cleanse the patient's finger with an alcohol swab or sponge and then dry it with sterile gauze. Puncture the patient's finger with an

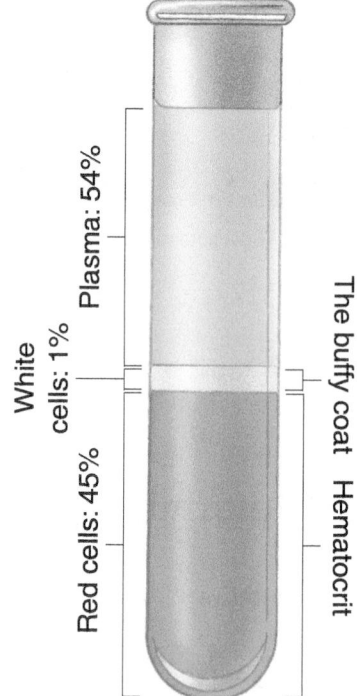

FIGURE 47-6 The hematocrit.

automatic or manual lancet. Wipe away the first drop of blood with dry sterile gauze. Draw up the second and subsequent drops using a capillary tube that is either tilted horizontally or slightly downward. When the tip of the tube touches the blood, the tube will automatically draw the blood up by capillary action. Fill the tube two-thirds to

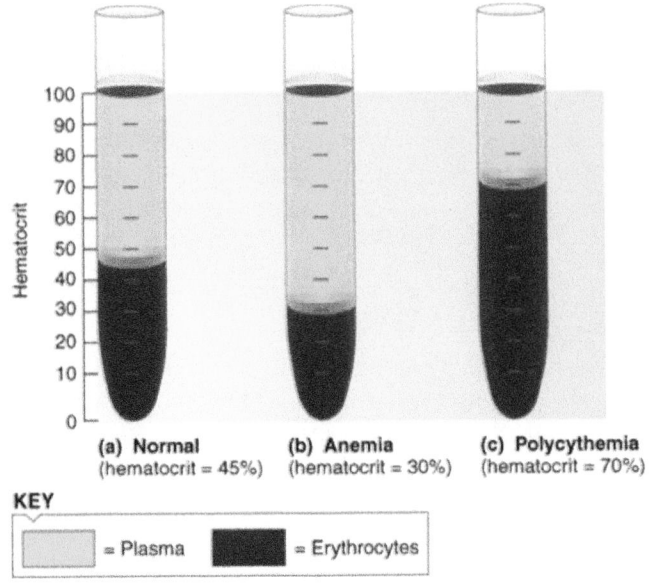

FIGURE 47-7 Hematocrits, left to right: normal, anemia, polycythemia.

KEY

☐ = Plasma   ■ = Erythrocytes

FIGURE 47-8 A microhematocrit.

three-quarters of its capacity and then seal each end. The tube is then placed in a microhematocrit centrifuge that performs cellular separation (Figure 47-8). For the complete procedure, see Procedure 47-3.

Erythrocyte/RBC Indices

Erythrocyte indices, also called *red blood cell indices* or *RBC indices*, help to differentiate the type of anemia present by indicating the size of RBCs and the concentration of Hgb. The **mean corpuscular volume (MCV)** measures the average size of RBCs and classifies them according to size. The **mean corpuscular hemoglobin (MCH)** measures the average amount

---

PROCEDURE 47-3

Performing a Microhematocrit

Objective ◆ *Perform a microhematocrit on a capillary blood sample using proper aseptic technique.*

EQUIPMENT AND SUPPLIES

Biohazard sharps container; gloves; capillary tubes; sealing clay; microhematocrit centrifuge; whole blood; hematocrit card or other reader

Note: Follow standard precautions and safety guidelines when working with blood samples. Use care to avoid splashing or spilling blood. Wipe up all spills using guidelines established by OSHA.

METHOD

1. Perform hand hygiene and apply gloves.
2. Assemble equipment as shown in Figure A.
3. Fill two capillary tubes three-quarters full. The blood specimen can be obtained from a vacuum tube of anticoagulated blood using a plain capillary tube or directly from a finger-stick site using a heparinized capillary tube. Seal one end in the sealing clay.
4. Place capillary tubes in the centrifuge with the sealed ends against the rubber gasket (Figure B). If more than one patient's blood is being tested, mark down the number of the slot the patient's tube is in. Spin for three to five minutes at 10,000 rpm. (Always check the manufacturer's

recommendations for proper time and speed.) After centrifuging, the sample will be separated into three layers:
   - Top layer is the plasma.
   - Middle layer, or the buffy coat, is made up of WBCs and platelets.
   - Bottom layer is packed RBCs.
5. Remove tubes immediately after centrifuge stops. If tubes are not removed immediately, blood may begin to mix together.
6. Determine the results. Use the Hct card by placing the sealing clay just below the zero line on both tubes. Then, on both tubes, match the top of the plasma with the 100 line. Read results on both tubes directly below the buffy coat. Then add those results together and divide by 2.
7. Discard the tubes into the sharps container.
8. Remove gloves and perform hand hygiene.
9. Record the value as a percentage on the patient's medical record.

CHARTING EXAMPLE

2/28/YY 1:45 P.M. Capillary puncture performed on 4th left digit ·1. Hct 47%. Patient denies discomfort or excessive bleeding..................................M. King, CMA (AAMA)

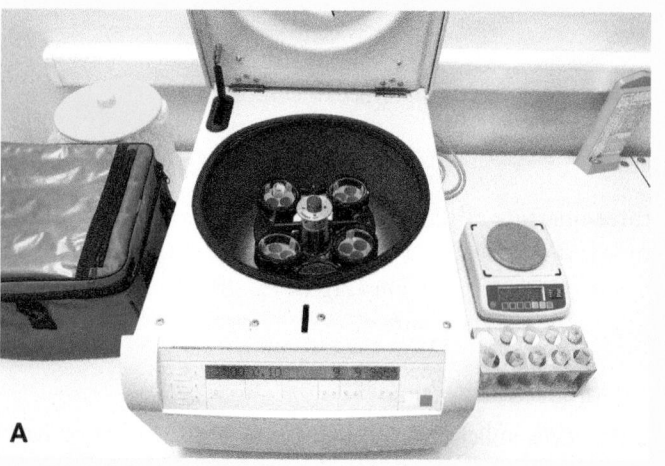
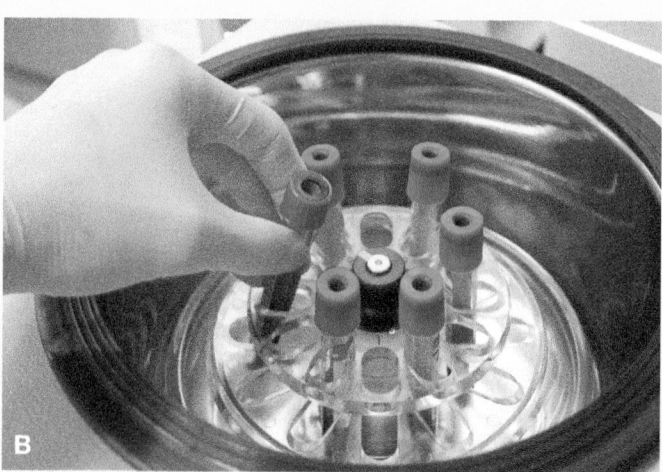

FIGURE A–B **(A)** Centrifuge and supplies; **(B)** loading a centrifuge.

of hemoglobin in an RBC, and the **mean corpuscular hemoglobin concentration (MCHC)** measures the amount of hemoglobin relative to the size of the cell. In general, when the MCV, MCH, and MCHC are decreased, iron deficiency anemia is likely. When they are increased, vitamin B_{12} or folic acid deficiency is likely.

Erythrocyte Sedimentation Rate (ESR)

Although not part of a complete blood count, the **erythrocyte sedimentation rate (ESR)** (also called the "sed rate") also evaluates RBCs. More specifically, it determines the rate at which RBCs settle at the bottom of a tube. The sed rate is related to the condition of the RBCs and the amount of fibrinogen in the plasma. When an individual presents with an injury or inflammatory disease, fibrinogen causes the surface membranes of the cells to become sticky, causing them to stack atop of one another in an attempt to promote healing. These stacks are heavier than individual cells, so they tend to fall faster. When a sed rate test is conducted on a patient, RBCs that fall at a faster than normal rate can indicate the possible existence of conditions associated with increased fibrinogen. Although an ESR itself is not diagnostic (does not identify the condition that has caused the increase in fibrinogen), it is used in conjunction with other tests to determine a diagnosis. For example, when testing for rheumatoid arthritis or fibromyalgia, an ESR may be done in conjunction with the antinuclear antibody test (ANA).

Drawing a patient's ESR can be done using either the Wintrobe or the Westergren method. The Wintrobe method uses a Wintrobe tube, which is calibrated in mm/hr. The rate is the height of the RBCs in the bottom of the tube (Procedure 47-4 and Figure 47-9). Depending on the method used, normal

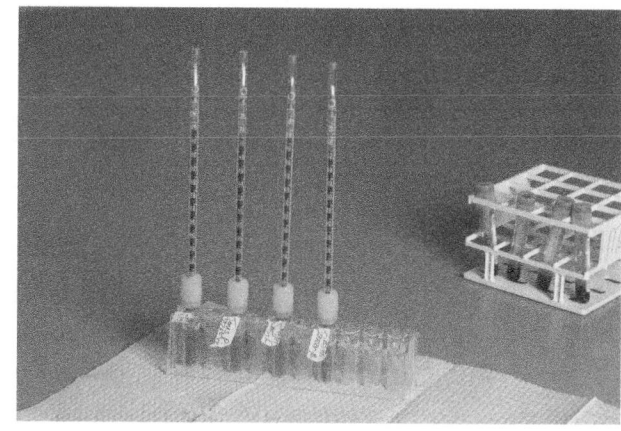

FIGURE 47-9 Wintrobe tube and Westergren tests are used to measure the ESR.

values may vary. Using the Wintrobe method, the normal ESR in an adult female is 0 to 20 mm/hr, and in an adult male it is 0 to 9 mm/hr. Increased values may suggest inflammation. This can occur from an injury or a variety of illnesses such as certain cancers, arthritis, and inflammatory bowel disease. An individual's ESR may also be elevated because of menstruation, pregnancy, and the use of specific medications.

White Blood Cells and White Blood Cell Tests

Several types of white blood cells (WBCs), or leukocytes, are produced in the bone marrow. The five types of WBCs are neutrophils, eosinophils, basophils, lymphocytes, and monocytes. WBCs are larger than RBCs, and have a shorter life span of two to three weeks. Their principal function is to defend against infection. The range of WBCs in an adult is 4.5 to 11 thousand/mm^3.

A variety of blood tests are associated with the WBCs.

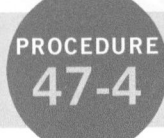

PROCEDURE 47-4

Performing an Erythrocyte Sedimentation Rate Test Using the Wintrobe Tube Method

Objective ◆ *Perform an ESR using the Wintrobe tube method and aseptic technique.*

EQUIPMENT AND SUPPLIES

Gloves; whole blood (EDTA); Wintrobe tube; Wintrobe rack; pen; patient's record; lab coat; biohazard sharps container

Note: Follow standard precautions and safety guidelines when working with blood samples. Use care to avoid splashing or spilling blood. Wipe up all spills using guidelines established by OSHA.

METHOD

1. Perform hand hygiene and apply gloves.
2. Assemble equipment.
3. Obtain a whole-blood sample using a purple-top tube. Mix well. EDTA is the anticoagulant of choice.
4. Slowly fill Wintrobe tube with blood. Avoid air bubbles.
5. Adjust the meniscus of the specimen to the zero line at the top of the tube.
6. Maintain the tube in an upright vertical position for one hour.
7. After one hour, record the number of RBCs that settle. Read the ESR on the same side of the tube as the zero line at the top.
8. Remove gloves and perform hand hygiene.
9. Record the procedure on the patient's medical record.

CHARTING EXAMPLE

2/28/YY 2:00 P.M. ESR (Wintrobe Method) fall of 10 mm/hr......
....M. Garcia, RMA

Leukocyte or White Blood Cell (WBC) Count

A complete WBC count includes the total number of all types of WBCs in a microliter of blood. As already noted, normal WBC or leukocyte counts in adults range from approximately 4.5 to 11 thousand/mm^3. An elevated level usually indicates infection (leukocytosis) because the body is increasing WBC production to fight bacteria. If grossly elevated, leukemia could be the cause, as ineffective WBCs require the body to produce more than usual. A low level usually indicates a viral infection or autoimmune deficiency, as these conditions typically destroy white cells. An extreme bacterial infection also can destroy enough WBCs to significantly reduce their numbers.

A WBC count can be performed either manually with a microscope or by an automated blood analyzer. The manual method of obtaining white blood counts is through the use of a hemocytometer. A hemocytometer is a special counting chamber that allows counting of cells on slides under the microscope. If testing is performed manually, an automated tabulator can be used to assist in counting the various types of cells (Figure 47-10). If using an automated analyzer, always follow the instructions exactly to ensure the validity of the results. Medical assistants require further training to perform this test in a medical laboratory, although it is commonly performed in an educational setting to further understanding.

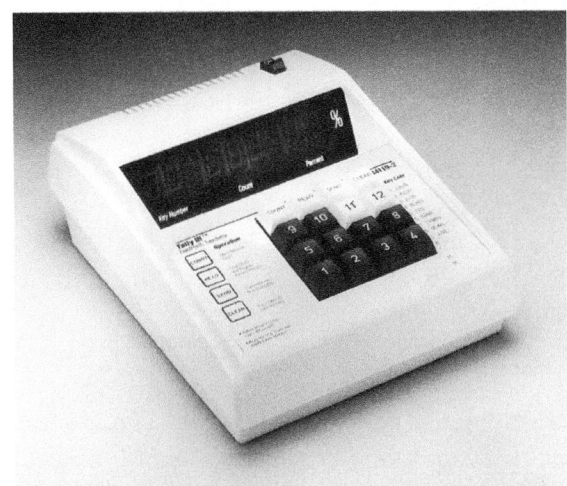

FIGURE 47-10 Electronic tabulator.

Differential White Blood Cell Count

A differential WBC count ("diff") determines the percentages of each type of leukocyte in a given sample. This test is most commonly performed by the automated analyzer. Performing this test manually is a skill that requires practice to achieve proficiency. To conduct a manual test, use a microscope with a bright light and 100× magnification with an oil immersion slide (Figures 47-11A and 47-11B). Focus near the edge of the stained slide where the cells are feathered, and where the cells

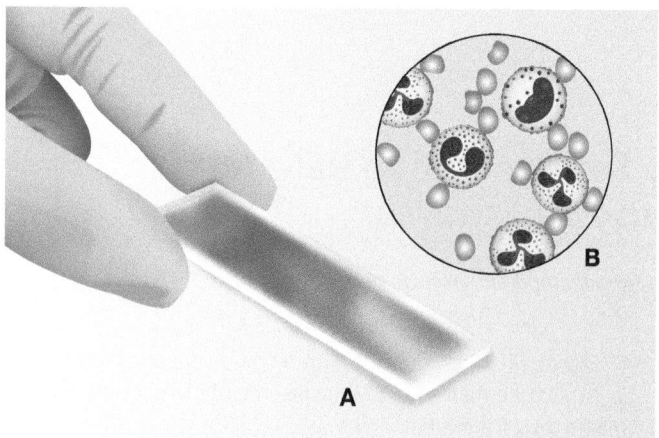

FIGURE 47-11 For a differential white blood cell count, **(A)** the slide is examined under oil immersion. **(B)** Cells are viewed using a bright light and 100x magnification.

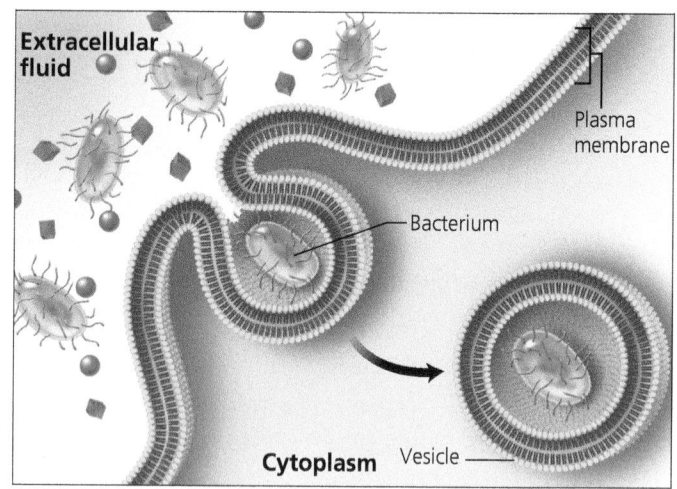

FIGURE 47-13 Phagocytosis. The cell engulfs and digests a bacterium.

are one layer thick. See Procedure 47-5 for details about slide preparation. Medical assistants require further training to perform this test in a medical laboratory, although it is commonly performed in an educational setting to further understanding. The types of leukocytes that are counted in a differential WBC count are neutrophils, eosinophils, basophils, lymphocytes, and monocytes (Figure 47-12). The differential results may be read as percentages or as numbers in a given quantity, depending on the laboratory and equipment being used.

Neutrophils. Neutrophils act as the body's primary defense and make up the largest percentage of WBCs. They are so named because the granules are neutral in color on laboratory-stained slides. They are continually produced for the purpose of combating infection by means of phagocytosis. Phagocytosis is the process in which the neutrophil surrounds, swallows, and digests the bacteria (Figure 47-13). Neutrophils are divided into two categories: segmented neutrophils and nonsegmented (band or stab) neutrophils (Figure 47-14).

- Segmented neutrophils, called segs, are mature cells with a nucleus that is divided into multiple segments connected by small thin threads. Typically, segs (segmented neutrophils) make up 50 to 60 percent of all WBCs in adults.

- Nonsegmented neutrophils, also called stabs or bands, are immature cells. In adults, bands (nonsegmented neutrophils) make up roughly 0 to 3 percent of all WBCs.

White blood cells

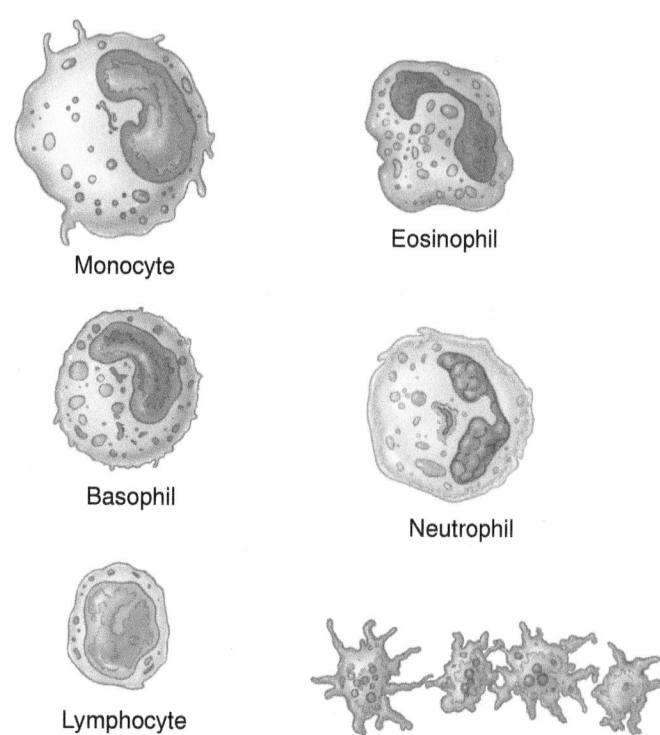

FIGURE 47-12 Types of white blood cells.

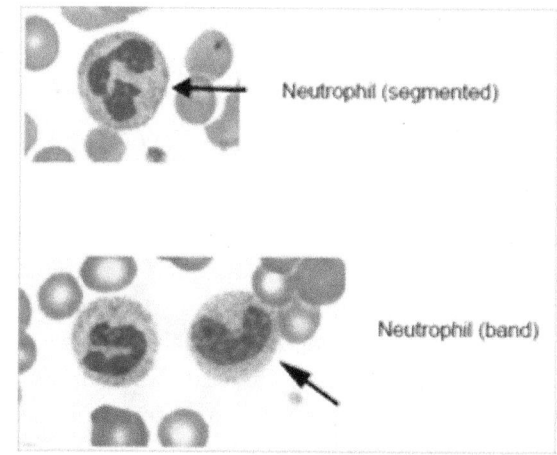

FIGURE 47-14 Band and segmented neutrophils.

Preparing Slides

Objective ◆ *Prepare a slide for a differential WBC count using correct aseptic procedure, for educational purposes.*

EQUIPMENT AND SUPPLIES

Clean glass slides; whole blood (EDTA); gloves; biohazard container; eye dropper; Wright's stain; lab coat; pen; patient record

Note: Follow standard precautions and safety guidelines when working with blood samples. Use care to avoid splashing or spilling blood. Wipe up all spills using guidelines established by OSHA.

METHOD

1. Perform hand hygiene and apply gloves.
2. Assemble equipment.
3. Obtain a whole-blood sample using EDTA as the anticoagulant of choice. Blood must be mixed thoroughly before use.
4. Using a dropper, place one drop of room-temperature blood on the end of a clean, glass slide (Figure A).
5. Using the short side of another clean glass slide, back the slide to the drop of blood. Allow the blood to spread across the short side of the slide (Figure B). Holding the spreader slide at a 30-degree angle, spread the blood across the length of the slide (Figure C). Use gentle, continuous pressure, and a smooth gliding motion to create a smear as pictured in (Figure D). Notice that the smear has a thick side that gradually changes to a thin side. The thin side has a feathered edge, and the blood covers one-half to three-quarters the length of the slide.
6. Allow the slide to air-dry on a rack (Figure E).
7. Label the patient's name and the date on the frosted edge of the slide.
8. Stain slide using Wright's staining method. Flood slide with stain for exactly 45 seconds or amount of time indicated by manufacturer (Figure F).
9. Rinse with distilled water (Figure G). Rinse until water is clear (Figure H).
10. Allow slide to air-dry before examining under the microscope.

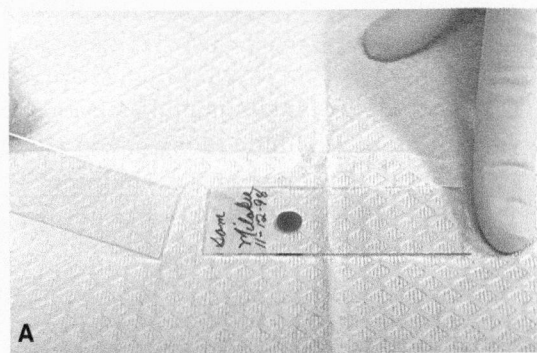

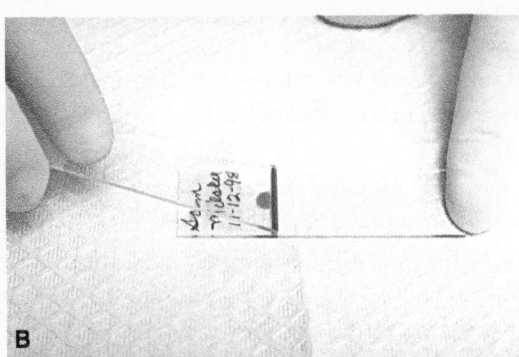

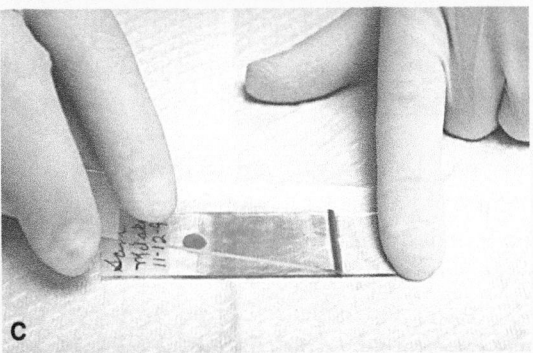

FIGURE A–D Blood smear.

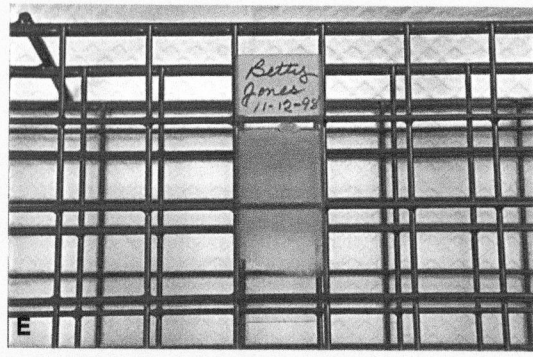

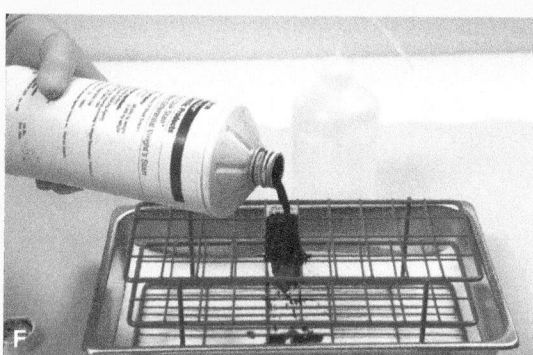

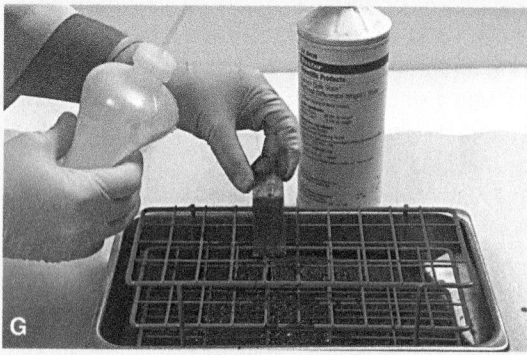

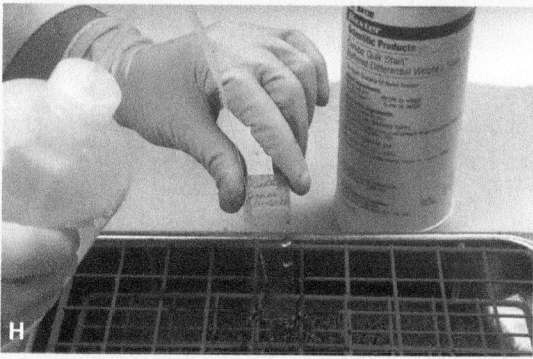

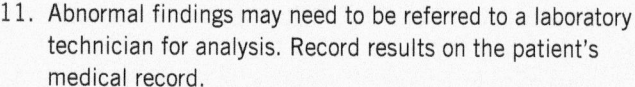

FIGURE E–H Wright's staining process.

11. Abnormal findings may need to be referred to a laboratory technician for analysis. Record results on the patient's medical record.

Note: This is for educational purposes only. Further training is required for a medical assistant to perform this test in a medical office setting as it is not considered CLIA waived.

Based on a method of handwritten documentation long ago, an elevation in bands/stabs has been nicknamed a "shift to the left" and indicates an early WBC response. Although both mature and immature neutrophil levels tend to increase in response to infection, they may also increase from hemorrhage, cancer, poisoning, hemolysis, and inflammation. Neutrophils tend to decrease in response to a virus or serious bacterial infection, although they may also be reduced by bone marrow depression, acromegaly, anaphylaxis, and certain vitamin deficiencies.

Eosinophils. **Eosinophils** are WBCs assumed also to be produced by the bone marrow. Detection of a large number of eosinophils can indicate a parasitic condition or the presence of certain allergic conditions. Eosinophils have granules that produce a red color on laboratory-stained slides. Eosinophils are so named from the stain eosin, which is used in the staining of blood smears. They make up less than 3 percent of WBC volume.

Basophils. Like other white cells, **basophils** are thought to be produced by the bone marrow, and they produce heparin.

Heparin is a substance that prevents clotting. When an individual has a condition that is creating inflammation, heparin may be used to assist in diminishing or preventing the occurrence of clotting. Increased amounts of basophils may be found in patients who have had their spleen removed. Patients who have had excessive exposure to radiation also may have increased basophils.

Basophils also contain the vasodilator histamine, and basophils appear in tissues where an allergic reaction is occurring. It is thought that the concentration of basophils may contribute to the severity of allergic reactions. Normal laboratory results generally show basophils as less than 1 percent of WBC volume.

Lymphocytes. **Lymphocytes** are WBCs produced in the bone marrow and in the lymphoid tissue, such as the spleen and lymph nodes. The function of lymphocytes is primarily to produce antibodies against foreign substances such as bacteria, viruses, and pollens. Lymphocytes are small and large and can proliferate into B and T cells. B cells may convert into plasma cells, which produce antibodies. T cells can produce helper cells, cytotoxic cells, and suppressor cells. To diagnose an individual with HIV, testing is performed to evaluate the type and amount of T cells present. Lymphocytes do not have granules and are nonsegmented. Lymphocytes make up the second largest volume of WBCs, comprising 25 to 30 percent.

Monocytes. **Monocytes** are WBCs formed in the bone marrow from stem cells. Monocytes assist in phagocytosis. They ingest foreign particles or bacteria that the neutrophils are unable to digest, and they assist in cleaning up cellular debris that may have been left from the infection. An increase in monocytes is seen in patients who have certain diseases, such as tuberculosis, typhoid, and Rocky Mountain spotted fever. In the typical adult, monocytes make up 3 to 7 percent of the total WBC volume.

Platelets and Coagulation Studies

Platelets (also called thrombocytes), the smallest cells found in the blood, are formed in the bone marrow. They live for about 10 days and are continuously reproduced. The main function of platelets is to assist in the clotting of blood to stop bleeding or assist in healing. Platelets increase around an area that is bleeding to assist in the formation of clots. The platelets and the injured tissue release thromboplastin, which combines with other elements in the blood to produce thrombin. The thrombin acts on a protein in the blood called fibrinogen, resulting in the formation of fibrin. Fibrin consists of tiny threads that create a mesh that catches the RBCs and other cells to form a clot.

Platelet Counts

There are typically between 150,000 and 400,000 platelets/mm^3 in adults. Because these cells are so small, testing is typically performed in an outside laboratory or by automated testing.

Platelet counts become problematic when they are over 750,000. This is referred to as thrombocytosis. The danger involved includes the possibility of unwanted blood clots, or thrombosis. The primary concern with blood clots is that they will get into circulation and impede flow to either the brain (stroke) or the heart (heart attack). Treatment depends on the underlying cause.

A critical low value for platelets is typically noted when the count is less than 50,000. This is called thrombocytopenia, and puts the patient at high risk for uncontrolled bleeding. Severely low counts can lead to internal bleeding and even death. Thrombocytopenia is caused by disorders that result in either reduced platelet production or increased platelet destruction.

Professionalism

When lab results are abnormal, it is important to consider outside factors that may affect testing. Depending on the test, tubes that are not properly inverted, spun, or allowed to settle can yield abnormal results. Blood that is not properly stored and transported may spoil. Improper venipuncture techniques, such as leaving a tourniquet in place for more than 60 seconds, can affect values. Aggressive or traumatic venipuncture can also activate the coagulation sequence and cause abnormal coagulation counts. Consistently abnormal results among a variety of patients may indicate that the problem isn't related to the patient at all. Careful procedure before drawing a patient's blood and observation after the results are noted are an important part of patient care.

Prothrombin Time (PT, Protime) International Normalized Ratio (INR)/(PT/INR)

Prothrombin time (PT) is a coagulation test that measures the amount of time it takes to form a clot. The international normalized ratio (INR) is a standard protocol that allows specimens performed at different laboratories to have consistent results. However, INR testing does not reveal specific bleeding disorders in patients with liver failure or other systemic diseases. For this reason, if one of these disorders is suspected, the findings are generally expressed in terms of PT and INR. Using both the PT and INR, the doctor can monitor and make appropriate decisions for anticoagulant therapy. This test is typically used to screen patients with symptoms of bleeding.

The protime for an average healthy adult will show clotting at 10–14 seconds. Higher than 30 seconds (or 4.5 INR) indicates a risk for bleeding, and more than 40 seconds is considered critical. Elevated levels are noted in patients with

Professionalism The Law

The medical assistant may perform routine CLIA-waived blood tests and procedures in the physician's office, when ordered. More complex tests are performed by specially trained individuals, either a medical lab technician (MLT) or medical technologist (MT). If a medical assistant performs tests that are not CLIA waived without proof of further training, the doctor's license may be at risk, the office could be closed, and severe fines may be assessed.

severe bone marrow depression, cancer, liver or collagen diseases, pancreatitis, disseminated intravascular coagulation, and toxic shock syndrome. Decreased levels may be noted in patients with myocardial infarction, multiple myeloma, pulmonary embolus, or thrombophlebitis.

Partial Thromboplastin Time (PTT)

Understanding the process of normal clotting and absence of normal clotting is important because laboratory tests are designed to determine why clotting is not occurring properly, particularly in patients who are receiving anticlotting drugs, such as heparin and warfarin (Coumadin). Like the prothrombin time (PT) test, a partial thromboplastin time (PTT) test determines the length of time it takes for a fibrin clot to form. However, the PTT can help to determine which specific clotting factors are affected, thus making it a more specific test. It is commonly used to determine the effectiveness of anticoagulant therapy such as Coumadin or heparin. It also helps to screen for bleeding tendencies and identify more precise causes. Normal findings are typically 60–70 seconds.

OTHER BLOOD TESTS

Blood tests ordered for patients often are ordered in panels. Common panels include the lipid panel and the liver panel. Included in the lipid panel are such tests as cholesterol, triglycerides, and high-density lipoproteins (HDL). A liver panel includes tests such as ALT, ALP, AST, and GGT, which can be used in the diagnosis of hepatitis. As previously discussed, a CBC typically consists of a microhematocrit, hemoglobin, WBC count (with or without differential), RBC count, and platelet count. Coagulation studies include a platelet count, prothrombin time, and partial thromboplastin time, which are used to determine how well a patient's blood is clotting. See Table 47-1 for specific tests included in each panel, Table 47-2 for common laboratory tests and their normal values, and Table 47-3 for common blood chemistry tests.

Comprehensive Metabolic Panel (CMP)

A comprehensive metabolic panel (CMP) is a screening tool that is used to evaluate organ function, to check for common disorders, or to monitor the progress of current conditions and response to medications. It includes 14 essential tests included among the basic metabolic panel, renal panel, liver function tests, and electrolytes. Although many of these individual tests may be ordered in other panels or profiles,

TABLE 47-1 | Common Blood Test Groups

Name	Abbreviation	Items Included in the Panel/Profile
Complete Metabolic Profile	CMP	Renal function tests (RFT), total protein, liver function tests (LFT)
Basic Metabolic Profile	BMP	Glucose, calcium, sodium (Na), potassium (K), chloride (Cl), bicarbonate (CO_2), blood urea nitrogen (BUN), creatinine (Cr)
Renal Function Tests/Panel	RFT	Basic metabolic profile (BMP), albumin (Alb), phosphorus (Pho)
Electrolyte Panel	Lytes	Sodium (Na), potassium (K), chloride (Cl), bicarbonate (CO_2)
Liver Panel or Liver Function Test	LFT	Albumin, alkaline phosphatase (ALP), alanine transaminase (ALT), aspartate transaminase (AST), total protein, gammaglutamyl transpeptidase (GGT), bilirubin
Lipid Panel	–	Low-density lipoprotein (LDL), high-density lipoprotein (HDL), very-low-density lipoprotein (VLDL), triglycerides, total cholesterol
Complete Blood Count	CBC	Red cell count, hematocrit (Hct), hemoglobin (Hgb), mean corpuscular volume, platelets, white cell count (WBC)—with or without differential
White Blood Count with Differential	WBC/diff.	Neutrophils, lymphocytes, monocytes, eosinophils, basophils

TABLE 47-2 | Common Laboratory Tests and Their Normal Values

Test	Result
Total cholesterol	130–200 mg/dL
Glucose	70–120 mg/dL
Triglycerides	30–150 mg/dL
Creatinine	0.4–1.5 mg/dL
Uric acid	3.5–7.5 mg/dL
BUN	5–20 mg/dL
Calcium	8.5–10.5 mg/dL
Sodium	132–142 mEq/L
Potassium	3.5–5.5 mEq/L
Chloride	98–106 mEq/L
CO_2	25–32 mEq/L
White blood cell count	4,500–11,000/mm^3
Red blood cell count	4.0–5.5 million/mm^3 (female) 4.5–6.0 million/mm^3 (male)
Hemoglobin	12–18 g/dL (female) 14–18 g/dL (male)
Hematocrit	35–45 percent (female) 40–50 percent (male)
Sedimentation rate	0–20 mm/hr (female) 0–9 mm/hr (male)
Platelet count	150,000 and 400,000 per µL^3

this particular combination is useful for establishing a general evaluation of the kidneys, liver, endocrine, electrolyte, and acid-base balance. An abnormality in any area may indicate a need for further, more-specific testing. It is recommended that the patient fast for 12 hours before testing. Normal values can be found in Table 47-3.

1. **Glucose**—Glucose is a simple sugar required by all body cells to produce energy. Glucose circulates in the blood and is used to give energy to the cells. When glucose cannot get into the cells for consumption, it builds up in the blood and clogs up the organs. This is known as hyperglycemia. As levels rise, they become more dangerous, with critical, life-threatening levels above 700 mg/dL while fasting. Though this is a dangerous condition, high blood glucose generally happens at a gradual rate. Hypoglycemia, or low blood sugar, can happen rapidly and can become lethal before treatment may be considered. For this reason, suspected blood glucose abnormalities are always treated as if they are low, until blood testing can be performed.

2. **Blood urea nitrogen (BUN)**—Blood urea nitrogen (BUN) testing is often performed to evaluate protein intake, the liver's ability to metabolize, and the functioning ability of the kidney. BUN levels may be abnormally elevated by hormones or a high protein diet. Other things that may cause elevated BUN include gastrointestinal bleeding, dehydration, shock, myocardial infarction, and congestive heart failure. Critical

TABLE 47-3 | Common Blood Chemistry Tests

Test	Common Medical Abbreviation	Normal Adult Value	Description	Purpose of Test
Alanine aminotransferase	ALT (SGPT)	<45 units/L	Liver enzyme, may also be found in kidneys	Detection of liver disease or inflammation.
Albumin	No standard abbreviation	3.5–5.0 g/dL	A protein that normally constitutes 60 percent of plasma serum	To detect effectiveness of specific medications such as warfarin (Coumadin) because it binds to albumin. High levels may indicate dehydration; low levels may indicate drug toxicity in the liver or malnutrition.
Alkaline phosphate	ALP	20–70 units/L	Enzyme found in all tissues; especially concentrated in the kidneys, bile, liver, bone, and placenta	Used to detect several conditions in the bone and liver and blocked bile ducts.

(continued)

TABLE 47-3 | Common Blood Chemistry Tests (*continued*)

Test	Common Medical Abbreviation	Normal Adult Value	Description	Purpose of Test
Aspartate aminotransferase	AST (SGOT)	<40 units/L	Enzyme found in all tissues; similar to ALT; found in cardiac muscle cells and red blood cells	Used to detect conditions of liver health.
Blood urea nitrogen	BUN	5–20 mg/dL	Metabolic products of protein catabolism	Used to measure the amount of nitrogen in the blood, indicating renal function.
Cholesterol	CH, Chol	Total count: <200 mg/dL; LDL <130 mg/dL; HDL >35 mg/dL	Lipids	Annual screening done to determine atherosclerosis and other cardiac-related diseases.
Creatinine	Cr	04–1.5 mg/dL	The product of creatinine phosphate breakdown in muscle in a fairly constant rate, then filter out through the kidneys	Screening for renal function often used in combination with BUN. Checked before contrast studies, such as CT, to assess the kidneys' ability to filter out contrast material.
Glucose Tolerance Test	GTT	70–100 mg/dL	Carbohydrate	To determine how quickly the body is able to filter glucose to help diagnose diabetes, insulin resistance, and reactive hypoglycemia.
Troponin I and T	No standard abbreviation	<0.4	A specific protein only found in cardiac muscle when it is damaged	Aids in the determination of myocardial infarct.
Thyroid-stimulating hormone	TSH	5–6 units/mL	Peptide hormone produced by thyrotropic cells in the pituitary gland	Assessment of thyroid and pituitary function.
Thyroxine	T_4	5–12 mcg/dL	Hormone secreted by the follicular cells of the thyroid gland	Assessment of the body's ability to control the metabolic processes in the body that influence physical development.
Triglycerides	Trig	30–150 mg/dL	Dietary fat	Annual screening done to determine atherosclerosis and other cardiac-related diseases.
Uric acid	UA	*Male:* 3.4–7.0 mg/dL *Female:* 2.4–6 mg/dL	Organic compound of carbon, nitrogen, oxygen, and hydrogen	Diagnosis of several conditions, including kidney stones, gout, Lesch-Nyhan syndrome, cardiovascular disease, diabetes, metabolic syndrome, and multiple sclerosis (low levels).

values are over 100 mg/dL. BUN levels are lower during starvation or a low-protein diet, liver disease, and overhydration, and during pregnancy. This test provides information to use for evaluation, but creatinine levels are better indicators of kidney disease because BUN is so easily affected by diet, hydration levels, and hormone levels.

3. **Creatinine**—Creatinine is a waste product of muscle energy metabolism that is excreted by the kidney. Because creatinine is removed from the body entirely by the kidneys and is not easily affected by other functions, this test is a good renal indicator. However, it is not used as an early indicator of dysfunction because blood creatinine levels generally rise only when more than half of kidney function has been lost. Elevated creatinine may also be seen with dehydration, muscular dystrophy, preeclampsia, and eclampsia.

4. **Calcium (Ca)**—Calcium is important for neuromuscular activity and blood coagulation. It is the most dominant mineral present in the human body, although much of it is stored in bones. In laboratory blood testing, only metabolically active, circulating calcium is evaluated (not stored calcium).

   Hypocalcemia is the term used to describe low calcium levels. Calcium levels less than 7 mg/dL are considered critical and may be life threatening; this should be reported to the physician immediately. It is most likely to develop after neck surgery, with hypoparathyroidism, or in premature infants. It can also be caused by tumors, pancreatitis, and certain medications. High blood calcium levels are referred to as hypercalcemia. Critically elevated levels are noted above 12 mg/dL and can also be dangerous. Elevated calcium may occur in dehydration, vitamin D_3 poisoning, acidosis, an overactive parathyroid, certain medications and cancers, and hormone disorders. Prolonged hypercalcemia can lead to calcifications, such as kidney stones.

5. **Sodium (Na)**—Sodium primarily controls the distribution of water throughout the body. It also assists in muscle contraction and nerve impulse transmission. Critical values are noted at less than 130 or more than 160 mEq/L, indicating severe imbalances that can be lethal. Many factors affect sodium levels, including oral fluid and diet intake, medications, hormones, shock, trauma, surgery, illness, and receiving intravenous fluids.

   Sodium levels are evaluated in relation to body fluids. High sodium levels, called hypernatremia, may result from excessive loss of body water, decreased water intake, or excessive sodium ingestion. Common causes may include diarrhea, diuretics, fever, burns, excessive sweating, diabetes insipidus, high sodium diets, Cushing's syndrome, and hyperaldosteronism. Low sodium levels are referred to as hyponatremia. This can be caused by either an excessive loss of sodium or an excessive intake of water. Although much less common than hypernatremia, it can be caused by renal disease, certain medications (like antidiuretics), a central nervous system disorder, or excessive consumption of water.

6. **Potassium (K)**—Potassium helps to maintain activity of the heart and skeletal muscles by influencing the conduction of electrical impulses. Abnormal levels can be dangerous because they are often asymptomatic until very severe changes are present. Less than 2.5 or more than 6.5 mEq/L is considered critical and may easily become lethal. Hyperkalemia (high potassium levels) occurs as a result of excessive absorption or impaired removal. Increased absorption may result from tissue damage, acidosis, medications, and insulin deficiency. Reduced excretion may be caused by shock, renal failure, medications, and decreased aldosterone secretion. Low potassium, termed hypokalemia, can occur with poor absorption or excessive removal. Poor absorption may be caused by medications or an imbalanced diet. Excessive removal of potassium can occur because of diuretic use, increased aldosterone, vomiting, diarrhea, or alkalosis.

7. **Bicarbonate/Carbon dioxide (CO_2)**—Carbon dioxide is a gas that is made during metabolism and removed by the kidneys and lungs. When combined with water in the blood, it produces bicarbonate, which helps to balance the levels of acid in the blood, or pH. If CO_2 is elevated in venous samples, bicarb is elevated and the patient is considered alkalotic. If CO_2 is low in venous samples, the patient is leaning toward acidosis. Venous and arterial CO_2 samples are interpreted opposite one another. Significant fluctuations can affect the entire body chemistry.

8. **Chloride (Cl)**—Chloride works with other electrolytes to help maintain fluid and acid-base balance and osmotic pressure within the body. The stomach produces it as hydrochloric acid, to help with digestion. Hyperchloremia is an elevated level of chloride in the blood, which occurs during dehydration or respiratory alkalosis. Hypochloremia, a lower than usual level of chloride in the blood, occurs after excessive vomiting and diarrhea, and with certain medications.

9. **Albumin**—Albumin is a liver protein that helps in fluid balance maintenance and assists with movement of small molecules through the blood (such as progesterone, calcium, and bilirubin). Low levels (hypoalbuminemia) may suggest that a patient has kidney or liver disease, or a digestive disorder that does not allow the body to absorb enough protein. Other tests should be done to confirm this.

10. **Total protein**—This test is a measure of the overall state of nutrition in the body, as well as liver or collagen disease. Total protein is rarely increased, unless as a result of certain medications, dehydration, or excessive exercise. This test can be used to monitor response to therapy.

11. **Bilirubin**—Bilirubin is a substance produced in the liver, spleen, and bone marrow and is also a by-product of hemoglobin metabolism. A wide variety of disease processes cause increases. Elevated levels are found with gallbladder stones or biliary obstruction, alcoholism, anemia, liver disorders, and pulmonary embolism, to name a few.

12. **Alkaline phosphatase (ALP)**—Alkaline phosphatase (ALP) is a group of enzymes found in the liver, gallbladder, intestine, and bones. This test is useful for assistance in evaluating bone and liver functions. Elevated levels are seen in aldosteronism, dehydration, and cirrhosis. Decreased levels are noted with certain medications, licorice consumption, and Cushing's syndrome. Diuretics and estrogen may also affect values.

13. **Aspartate amino transferase (AST), formerly called glutamic oxaloacetic transaminase or SGOT)**—Aspartate amino transferase (AST or SGOT) is an enzyme found mostly in heart muscle and the liver. Abnormalities may represent liver disease or recent heart attack. Because many medications may affect this test, it is not used to diagnose myocardial infarction. However, it may provide a key indicator for further evaluation. Elevated levels may also indicate liver or musculoskeletal disease, pancreatitis, heat stroke, or trauma. Decreased levels may be seen with chronic liver disease, hemodialysis, and diabetic ketoacidosis. Excessive exercise, certain drugs, and pregnancy can alter the results.

14. **Alanine amino transferase (ALT) or Serum Glutamic Pyruvic Transaminase (SGPT or GPT)**—Alanine amino transferase (ALT or SGPT) is an enzyme found primarily in the liver. Abnormalities may represent hepatobiliary disease. Elevated levels may be seen with anything that may cause liver damage or

dysfunction, including gallbladder obstruction and pancreatitis. Small elevations may be noted with cardiac and renal tissue destruction.

Diabetic Tests

Diabetes is evaluated and managed through blood tests. Diabetics monitor their blood sugar with a portable machine called a glucometer. This is useful for immediate results of the patient's current status. The physician will often order a glycosylated hemoglobin (HbgA1C) to test the long-term control of diabetes. Because RBCs live for three to four months, they are bathed in glucose and absorb it over time. The glucose binds to hemoglobin to produce glycosylated hemoglobin. With A1C, the percentage of glucose in the cells is measured to reveal the patient's average plasma concentration of glucose over a three-month period. The typical result for a nondiabetic adult is 3.5 to 6 percent. More than 14 percent can indicate ketoacidosis and is considered a critical value for diabetes. Procedure 47-6 demonstrates how to perform a glycosylated hemoglobin A1C, using a DCA Vantage Analyzer.

A physician may also order a glucose tolerance test, which is commonly used to detect pregnancy-induced diabetes. Blood is drawn to detect a baseline after fasting. The patient is given an oral carbohydrate solution to drink, and blood is redrawn to detect the response after 30 minutes and every hour thereafter for up to five hours, according to a physician's orders. Urine may be collected as well.

Phenylketonuria (PKU) Testing

Phenylketonuria (PKU) is a congenital disease caused by a defect in the metabolism of the amino acid phenylalanine. The unmetabolized protein accumulates in the bloodstream and, if undetected and untreated, will result in mental retardation. The PKU test is always performed on newborns to determine the presence of the unmetabolized protein phenylalanine. The test is typically performed in the hospital but may be performed in the office if not done in the hospital. See Procedure 47-7 for steps in performing the PKU test.

Mono Testing

The mono test, which is also known as the mononucleosis spot test, is used to help determine whether a patient has infectious mononucleosis (Procedure 47-8). Infectious **mononucleosis** is also commonly referred to as the "kissing disease" because it is a contagious viral infection that frequently is spread through oral contact. It is frequently ordered along with a CBC. A strep test may be ordered with the mono test to determine whether a person's sore throat is

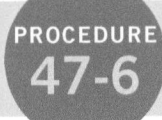

PROCEDURE 47-6

Performing a Hemoglobin A1C Test Using an Automated Analyzer

Objective ◆ *Perform a glycosylated Hemoglobin A1C test on a capillary blood sample using proper aseptic technique.*

EQUIPMENT AND SUPPLIES

DCA Vantage Analyzer; DCA Vantage Reagent Kit with capillary holder, reagent cartridge, and calibration code; alcohol pad; 2 × 2 sterile gauze; lancet; biohazard sharps container; gloves; pen; patient record

Note: Follow standard precautions and safety guidelines when working with blood samples. Use care to avoid splashing or spilling blood. Wipe up all spills using guidelines established by OSHA.

METHOD

1. Verify physician orders and check for allergies. Perform hand hygiene and apply gloves.
2. Inspect and assemble equipment and supplies. If a seal is loose or the containers are damaged, discard and replace.
3. Cleanse skin with alcohol and allow to air-dry. Perform capillary puncture and wipe the first drop of blood. (May alternately use venipuncture blood from a tube with EDTA, heparin, citrate, or fluoride/oxylate after inverting the sample several times to properly mix it.) Dispose of sharps properly.
4. Touch the tip of the capillary tube into blood until filled. Wipe sides of the tube with gauze to remove excess. Inspect the sample for bubbles; if present, discard and begin again. Once a sample is properly collected, analysis must be performed within five minutes.
5. With the flat side toward the cartridge, gently insert the capillary tube into the cartridge until it snaps into place. Use caution not to contaminate or touch the optical window on the bottom corner of the cartridge. Do not remove the foil.
6. Hold the reagent cartridge so that the barcode faces to the right. Using the track on the left side of the analyzer, scan the cartridge by inserting it into the track above the blue dot and sliding it down quickly. If no beep is heard, try again.
7. Open the compartment door on the front of the machine. Hold the cartridge with the barcode facing right and insert until a gentle snap is heard or felt. It will fit only when held in the right direction.
8. Using a smooth, continuous motion, pull the foil tab completely out of the cartridge and close the door. Within five seconds, a beep should sound.

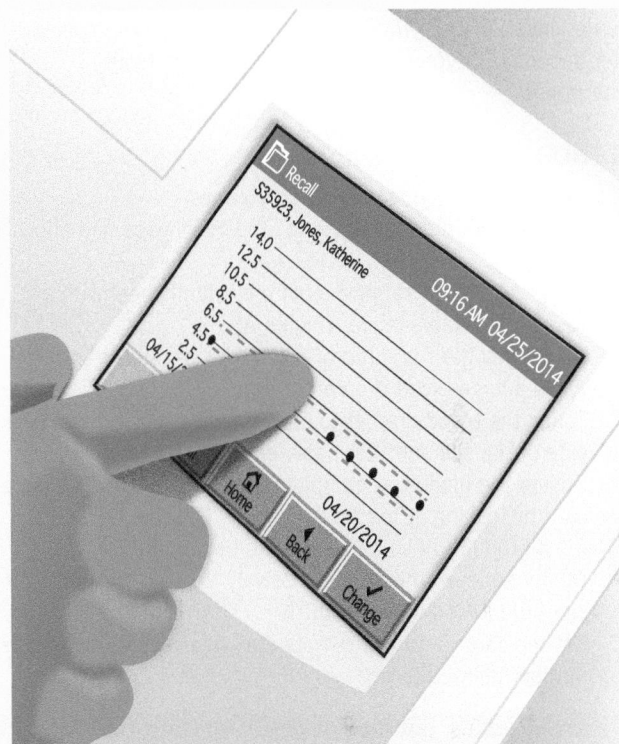

FIGURE A A vantage analyzer automatically reads a capillary blood sample and displays an accurate blood glucose value.

9. Read the results, when ready (Figure A).
10. Open the cartridge door. Push/hold the button on the right side of the cartridge while pushing the cartridge tab to the right and gently pull the cartridge out. Discard in a sharps container.
11. Remove gloves and perform hand hygiene.
12. Record the value as a percentage on the patient's medical record.

CHARTING EXAMPLE

2/28/YY 1:45 P.M. FS performed on Pt.'s right index finger for Hgb/A1c testing. Pt. tolerated well. Hgb/A1c 3 percent.............
....S. Manning, CMA (AAMA)

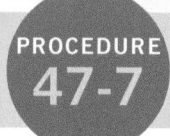

PROCEDURE 47-7

Performing PKU Testing

Objective ◆ *Collect a blood specimen for PKU testing.*

EQUIPMENT AND SUPPLIES

Sterile lancet; alcohol wipe; gloves; sterile dry gauze; special filter paper card, typically supplied by the state health department

METHOD

1. Perform hand hygiene and apply gloves.
2. Cleanse the infant's heel with an alcohol wipe and allow to air-dry.
3. Puncture the lateral portion of the infant's heel with a sterile disposable lancet (Figure A).
4. Wipe away the first drop of blood with dry sterile gauze.
5. Allow a large blood droplet to form.
6. Touch the blood droplet to the center of the circle on one side of the special filter paper card.
7. Ensure the blood has completely soaked through the paper card by looking at the reverse side.
8. Fill all required five circles on the paper card.
9. Do not squeeze the heel excessively to avoid collecting tissue fluid mixed with blood.
10. Set the card in an appropriate area to air-dry for two hours at room temperature.

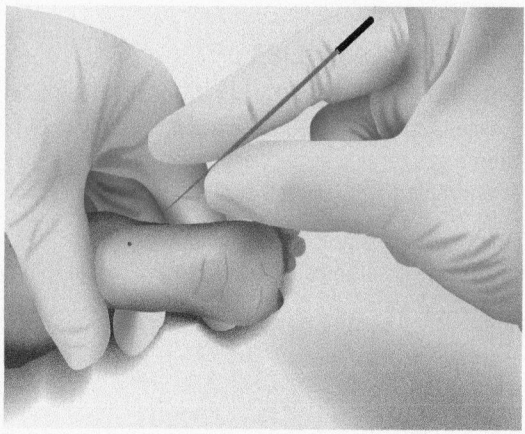

FIGURE A The PKU test is always performed on newborns.

11. When completely dry, place in the state-provided envelope and mail within 48 hours.

CHARTING EXAMPLE

1/22/YY 2:45 P.M. Heel stick performed on Pt.'s right heel for PKU test, stick X1. Pt. tolerated well. Sample sent to ABC lab for testing...C. Shilling, CMA (AAMA)

PROCEDURE 47-8

Performing Mono Testing

Objective ◆ *Perform a mono test.*

EQUIPMENT AND SUPPLIES

Alcohol wipe; biohazard waste container; disposable lancet; gloves; capillary tube; test tube; mono test diluent; mono test stick(s); blood specimen

METHOD

1. Perform hand hygiene.
2. Apply gloves.
3. Assemble equipment and supplies.
4. Cleanse patient's finger with alcohol and allow to dry. Perform a capillary puncture.
5. Fill a capillary tube end to end, dispensing all the blood into the test tube.
6. Slowly add one drop of diluent to the bottom of the test tube.
7. Mix.
8. Remove the test stick(s) from the container. Recap the container immediately.

9. Place the absorbent end of the test stick into the treated sample. Leave the test stick in the test tube.

10. Read the result at five minutes. Positive results may be read as soon as the red control line appears.

11. Discard used test tubes, lancet, and test sticks in the biohazard waste container.

12. Remove gloves and dispose of them correctly. Perform hand hygiene.

13. Document findings in the patient record:

    Positive: A blue test line and a red control line indicate a positive result.

    Negative: A red control line but no blue test line indicates a negative result.

Note: Although the medical assistant is responsible for reporting abnormal results (or positive results in the case of a mono test) to the physician, "interpreting" such tests as being positive or negative is *not* within the scope of practice for the medical assistant as such and should never be done. The medical assistant is only allowed to report the findings of "positive" or "negative."

14. Clean the work area and equipment according to OSHA guidelines.

CHARTING EXAMPLE

3/22/YY 8:45 A.M. Performed mono test. Result negative. Sophia Spencer, CMA (AAMA)

caused by a streptococcal infection instead of or in addition to mononucleosis.

A mono test is primarily ordered when an adolescent patient has symptoms such as fever, headache, swollen glands, and fatigue that the doctor suspects are a result of infectious mononucleosis. The test may be repeated when it is initially negative, but suspicion of mono remains high. The physician may order a repeat test in a week or so to see if heterophile antibodies have developed or may order Epstein-Barr virus (EBV) antibodies to help confirm or rule out the presence of a current EBV infection.

If a patient has a positive mono test, an increased number of WBCs, reactive lymphocytes, and symptoms of mononucleosis, then the patient will be diagnosed with infectious mononucleosis. If symptoms and reactive lymphocytes are present but the mono test is negative, then it may be too early to detect the heterophile antibodies, or the affected patient may be in the small number of people who do not make heterophile antibodies. Other EBV antibodies or a repeat mono test may be performed to help confirm or rule out the mononucleosis diagnosis.

Patients with negative mono tests and few or no reactive lymphocytes may be infected by another microorganism that causes monolike symptoms (such as a cytomegalovirus or toxoplasmosis). If the infection occurs during pregnancy, it is important to determine the cause because some of the monolike infections (but not EBV infection) have been associated with pregnancy complications and damage to the fetus. It is also important to identify strep throat, whenever present, because it should be treated promptly with antibiotics.

SUMMARY

It is critical for a medical assistant to have a thorough understanding of patient preparation and the theory of blood formation, including the cellular and liquid components of blood.

Blood analysis is one vital and routine tool of medicine. The medical assistant performs routine blood tests and procedures in the physician's office, but more-complex tests are performed by specially trained individuals.

Many blood tests are ordered in groups called counts, panels, or profiles. A CBC typically consists of a microhematocrit, hemoglobin, WBC count, RBC count, platelet count, and differential WBC count (diff). Coagulation studies include a platelet count, prothrombin time, and partial thromboplastin time, which are used to determine how well a patient's blood is clotting. Included in the lipid panel are such tests as cholesterol, triglycerides, and high-density lipoproteins (HDL). A liver panel includes multiple tests that can be used in the diagnosis of liver disease. A comprehensive metabolic panel (CMP) includes glucose, blood urea nitrogen, creatinine, calcium, sodium, potassium, carbon dioxide, chloride, albumin, globulin, bilirubin, alkaline phosphatase, aspartate aminotransferase (AST or SGOT), and alanine aminotransferase (ALT or SGPT).

Diabetics monitor their blood sugar with a portable machine called a glucometer; the physician will often order a glycosylated hemoglobin (HbgA1C) to test the long-term control of diabetes. Other tests that a physician may order on a diabetic patient could include the glucose tolerance test.

COMPETENCY REVIEW

1. Define and spell the terms for this chapter.
2. List five major blood tests commonly performed in a medical setting, and explain what abnormal results may reveal for each.
3. Define critical values, and give two examples of tests that should be immediately reported.
4. Make a list of the types of white blood cells and the values of each that are expected in a normal differential.
5. Create a normal list (for male and female, where applicable) for the WBC, RBC, Hct, Hgb, and ESR.
6. List the equipment needed to perform an erythrocyte sedimentation rate test.

PREPARING FOR THE CERTIFICATION EXAM

1. How many types of white blood cells are there?
   a. five
   b. one
   c. four
   d. three
   e. two

2. Which of the following is *not* a plasma protein?
   a. albumin
   b. prothrombin
   c. globulin
   d. fibrinogen
   e. urea

3. Which enzyme is mostly found in the heart muscle?
   a. SGOT
   b. ALP
   c. albumin
   d. BUN
   e. glucose

4. What test helps to determine the functioning ability of the kidney?
   a. hemoglobin
   b. LDL
   c. hematocrit
   d. calcium
   e. BUN and creatinine

5. Which test indicates the overall number of leukocytes in a specific amount of blood?
   a. BUN
   b. WBC
   c. Differential
   d. SGOT
   e. ALP

6. The normal range for glucose is
   a. 70–120 mg/dL.
   b. 40–150 mg/dL.
   c. 140–220 mg/dL.
   d. 130–200 mg/dL.
   e. 132–142 mg/dL.

7. The normal RBC volume in an adult female is
   a. 5.0–6.0 million/mm^3.
   b. 4.0–5.5 million/mm^3.
   c. 6.0–7.0 million/mm^3.
   d. 7.0–8.0 million/mm^3.
   e. 4.0–5.0 million/mm^3.

8. The normal WBC counts range from _____ to _____ thousand in adults:
   a. 4.5, 11
   b. 11, 14
   c. 1.0, 4.5
   d. 6.0, 9.0
   e. 4.5, 5.0

9. The percentage range of basophils in adult blood is
   a. 50–70 percent.
   b. 1–4 percent.
   c. 0–1 percent.
   d. 20–35 percent.
   e. 2–3 percent.

10. To perform a differential white blood cell count, the microscope must be placed on
    a. 40.
    b. 60.
    c. 80.
    d. 20.
    e. 100.

CRITICAL THINKING

Refer to the case study at the beginning of the chapter and use what you have learned to answer the following questions.

1. Lisa has several priorities to consider. What does she need to do, and in what order should she do it? Explain your rationale.

2. How could Mrs. Johnson's test results affect the patient? Is timing important?

3. What kinds of things might Mrs. Johnson's lab values indicate?

ON THE JOB

Sarah is a new medical assistant, recently hired to work with Dr. Smythe. The doctor orders a hemoglobin A1C and a microhematocrit on Mary Winters. Sarah has never seen these machines before, but she doesn't want her new coworkers to doubt her ability, so she decides to figure it out herself. She is able to fill the capillary tube about halfway.

1. What is the first thing that Sarah should do? Explain your rationale.

2. Mrs. Winters wants to know why the A1C test is being done and what it will show. What should Sarah tell her?

3. Mrs. Winters asks for more information about the microhematocrit test. How should Sarah explain?

INTERNET ACTIVITY

Go online and research materials to further understand how HIV and AIDS might affect laboratory tests.

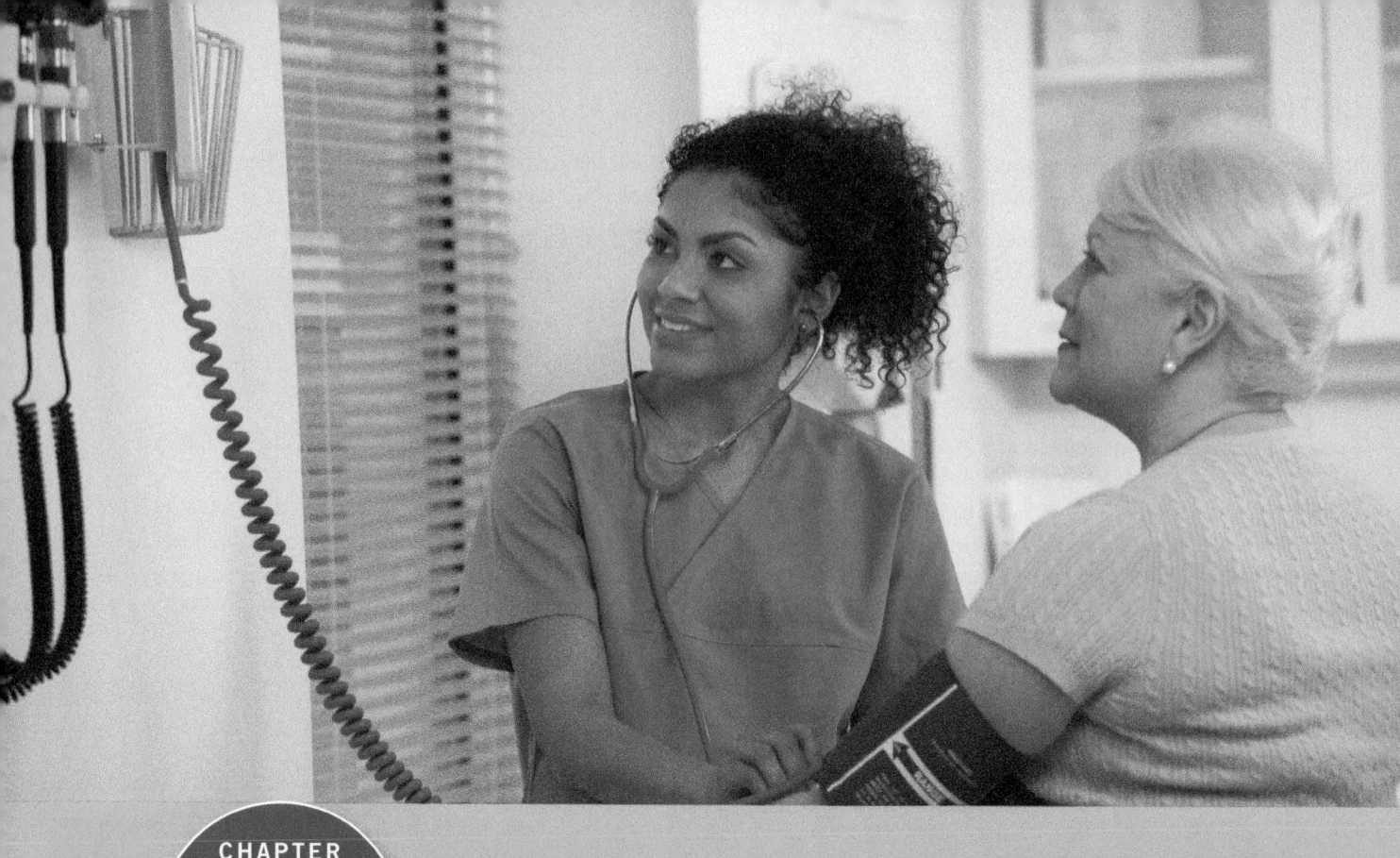

Radiology and Diagnostic Testing

Learning Objectives

After completing this chapter, you should be able to:

48.1 Define and spell the terms for this chapter.

48.2 Describe principles related to X-rays.

48.3 List characteristics of X-rays.

48.4 Describe the use of contrast medium during diagnostic imaging.

48.5 Explain the medical assistant's role in diagnostic imaging.

48.6 Identify special preparations required for select X-ray procedures.

48.7 List radiologic procedures that require the use of contrast media.

48.8 Describe the purpose of at least five different forms of diagnostic imaging.

48.9 Explain the medical use of radiation therapy.

48.10 Outline safety precautions that should be taken into consideration when working in the area of radiology.

48.11 Explain concepts related to the storage and ownership of X-rays.

Timothy Adler, a 32-year-old patient, saw Dr. Miller for intense pain in his abdomen, which occurred after eating meals, especially dinner. Dr. Miller suspected that Timothy might have gallstones and ordered an ultrasound of his gallbladder. Unfortunately, the gallbladder ultrasound report came back as inconclusive.

Terms to Learn

angiography	gantry	radiologist
arthography	grid	radiology
claustrophobia	radiation	radiolucent
contrast medium	radioactive	radiopaque
dosimeter	radiographs	rem
fluoroscopy	radiography	X-rays

The study of radiology includes an understanding of the use of X-rays, diagnostic radiology, and radiation therapy. A medical assistant may be asked to assist with radiology or other diagnostic testing. Sometimes this requires additional training or certification; in other settings it may just be following very specific processes ordered by someone trained in diagnostic testing. It is important for the medical assistant to know the state and local laws relative to radiology and diagnostic testing.

A **radiologist** is a physician specializing in radiology. A radiographer or radiologic technologist is involved in making diagnostic radiographs or X-rays. The radiographer's duties include positioning patients for radiographic procedures; determining the proper voltage, current, and exposure time for each X-ray; adjusting radiographic equipment; processing the image; and assisting the radiologist with special procedures.

As a medical assistant in a physician office, you might not be able to take X-rays without additional training, but you may be referring patients for radiologic studies and should be familiar with the processes. Some of those processes are discussed in this chapter.

You must always be aware of safety issues and follow safety requirements whenever you are working with or around X-ray equipment. Radiological equipment is used both for

diagnosis and also sometimes for treatment. Some uses of radiation for therapy are also discussed in this chapter.

RADIOLOGY

Radiology is the branch of medicine that uses **radioactive** substances, or matter that gives off **radiation** (radiant energy), and various techniques to visualize the internal structures of the body for the diagnosis and treatment of disease. Radiology uses X-rays, radioactive substances, and other forms of radiant energy such as ultraviolet rays. A discussion of X-ray, fluoroscopic, and radiologic procedures follows.

Principles of X-rays

X-rays were discovered by Wilhelm Konrad Roentgen in 1895. X-rays are produced in a vacuum tube when electrons, traveling at the speed of light (186,000 miles per second), collide with a target made of specific materials such as tungsten. The collision produces electromagnetic rays that have high energy and very short wavelengths, which are not visible to the human eye.

When X-rays are emitted from the tube, they form a cone-shaped X-ray beam. The radiation field is the cross section of the X-ray beam and the point of use (Figure 48-1). The patient is placed between the tube producing the X-ray beam and the film where the image is recorded. X-rays can

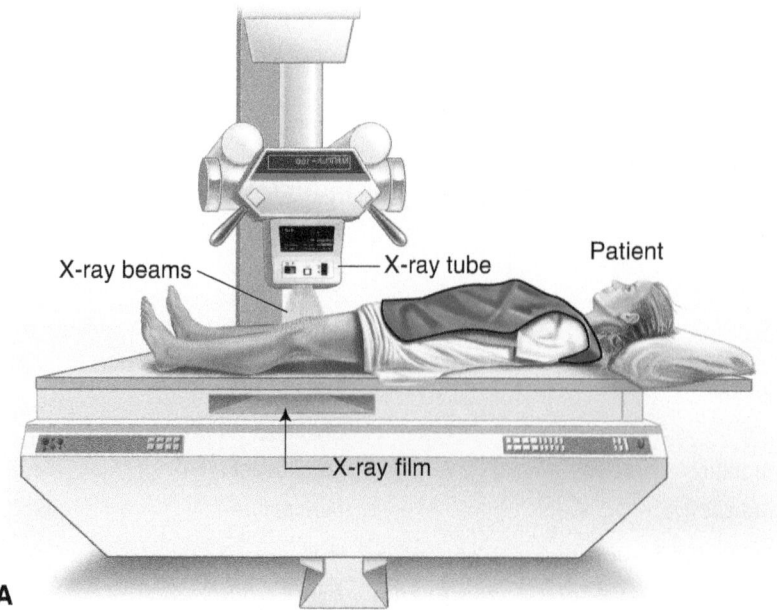

Image Receptor (film)

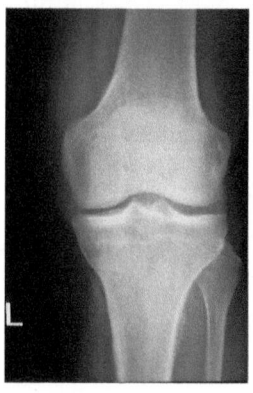

B Knee X-ray

A

FIGURE 48-1 **(A)** The patient is placed between the X-ray tube, which emits a cone-shaped X-ray beam, and the film or image receptor. **(B)** Bones do not allow the X-ray beam to pass through them, resulting in an image of the bones on the film.

penetrate most materials and therefore are useful for making photographic images for diagnostic purposes.

X-ray images or **radiographs** are produced by projecting X-rays through organs or structures of the body onto photographic plate. Some structures, such as bones, are more **radiopaque** and allow fewer X-rays to pass through; other softer tissues, such as skin and lungs, are **radiolucent**, permitting greater penetration of X-rays. Thus radiopaque tissue, such as bone, appears light on the film, and radiolucent tissue, such as the lungs, leaves a shadowy, dark image. X-ray films can be examined for defects in bones and tissues and for the presence of tumors.

In addition to their ability to produce images, X-rays that penetrate the body are able to change the basic structure of body cells, typically at much higher doses than that used for radiographs. This characteristic has made X-rays useful in the treatment of tumors.

Characteristics of X-rays

X-rays have several characteristics that make them useful in the field of medicine. X-rays can do the following:

- Penetrate substances of different densities to varying degree.
- Cause ionization of the substances through which they pass. Ionization is the process that causes the gain or loss of electrons from a neutral atom. Loss of electron = positive charge; gain of electron = negative charge.
- Cause fluorescence of certain substances. Internal structures show up dark on a glowing screen as X-rays

pass through, allowing physicians to visualize structures in motion.

- Travel in a straight line so the X-ray beam can be directed at a specific area.
- Destroy body cells and be used to kill cancer cells.

Because X-rays are invisible and produce no sound or smell, special precautions must be taken to protect patients and employees from unnecessary or accidental exposure. Safety precautions are discussed later in this chapter.

OVERVIEW OF DIAGNOSTIC IMAGING

Diagnostic imaging may involve the use of X-rays, ultrasound, radiopharmaceuticals, radiopaque media, and computers to produce images of internal structures and processes.

Use of a Contrast Medium

Sometimes a contrast medium is used during imaging processes. A **contrast medium** is a substance that enhances visibility of the tissue or structure being studied. It is called a contrast medium because it makes the object of the study contrast with (stand out against) its background. A positive contrast medium is a radiopaque substance that does not allow the passage of X-rays, making the affected tissue or structure appear white on X-ray images. A negative contrast medium is a radiolucent substance that allows X-rays to pass through more easily, making the affected tissue or structure appear dark or shadowy on X-ray images.

Contrast media may be liquids, powders, or gases. They are administered orally, by injection, or by enema. Commonly used contrast media include barium sulfate, iodinated compounds, air, and carbon dioxide.

Positive contrast media (that will appear white on an X-ray) include barium sulfate and iodine. Barium sulfate is a chalky compound that is mixed with water and flavoring to the right consistency for a patient to drink or for a technician to administer as an enema. Thus it is frequently used for examination of the gastrointestinal tract.

Iodine compounds are employed for thyroid studies (the thyroid gland), pyelograms (the urinary tract), angiograms (blood flow through arteries and veins), and cholecystograms (the gallbladder). Iodine compounds should not be used if the patient is allergic to seafood or iodine. In addition, iodine compounds interfere with nuclear medicine. Therefore, these two types of procedures should not be performed during the same time period.

Negative contrast media (that will appear dark on an X-ray) include air, carbon dioxide, and other gases. These media are used for myelograms (to visualize the spinal cord) or arthrograms (the joints). The introduction of gas and air into the body can result in severe headaches following procedures such as myelograms. Negative contrast studies have largely been replaced with the use of magnetic resonance imaging (MRI).

Professionalism

Radiography is a complicated field, and to become a radiologic technologist or radiographer requires advanced schooling and training experience. Radiographers perform imaging procedures ordered by physicians; operate several different types of imaging equipment; and produce images through the use of ultrasound, magnetic resonance imaging, or radionuclide procedures. "Rad techs," as they are known in the health care field, have career opportunities in doctors' offices, private imaging facilities, hospitals, and clinics.

To become a radiologic technologist, a student must graduate from a two- or four-year degree program in radiology and pass a national registration examination administered by the American Registry of Radiologic Technologies. Passing this examination earns the candidate the title of Registered Radiologic Technologist (RRT). For more information regarding a career in radiology, contact the American Society of Radiologic Technologists, 15000 Central Avenue SE, Albuquerque, NM 87123-3909, (800) 444-2778.

THE MEDICAL ASSISTANT'S ROLE IN DIAGNOSTIC IMAGING

The role of the medical assistant is usually to schedule the procedure ordered by the physician, educate the patient about the procedure, explain beforehand the preparations needed, and inform the patient how long the entire procedure will take. After scheduling the procedure, give written instructions to the patient and thoroughly review them before the patient leaves the office. This helps ensure that the patient will be prepared correctly for the procedure when arriving at the appointed time.

In some areas, the medical assistant, after additional schooling or certification, can specialize in becoming a limited scope X-ray technician. Credentials often obtained include the GXMO (general X-ray machine operator) or LXMO (limited X-ray machine operator). If a medical assistant is not certified or credentialed according to state and local laws, then someone who is credentialed must either perform the procedure or, if state law allows, provide specific protocols and procedures for how X-rays must be performed.

After the procedure is concluded, it will be your duty to assist the patient, provide post-procedure instructions, and inform the patient when to expect the test results. For some X-ray procedures, special patient preparation must be performed before the patient can be examined. These procedures are described in Table 48-1.

For many radiology examinations, the patient is asked to undress and wear a patient gown. Many of the procedures involve positions and interventions that may be embarrassing to the patient. The medical assistant must make every effort to provide a gown that is an ample size and drape the patient to preserve privacy. Request that the patient remove all metallic materials such as jewelry, belt buckles, watches, eyeglasses, hairpins, earrings, and hearing aids as these may interfere with proper imaging. In some X-rays of the head, mouth, and neck, the patient may have to remove dentures. Because the patient is not able to wear jewelry during the procedure, a safe container or locker should be provided for personal belongings.

The patient may need assistance getting onto the X-ray table. A footstool should be available if the table is high. X-ray tables do not have side rails. If there is a concern that the patient may become confused and could roll off the table, then someone must remain in the room with the patient until the procedure begins. In this situation, the X-ray technician should be told about the patient's confused state. Children may require special attention and someone to help them maintain the correct position. Anyone who has to be in the room during an X-ray procedure must follow the strictest safety considerations (discussed later).

TABLE 48-1 | X-ray Procedures Requiring Special Preparations

Procedure	Preparation
Angiogram	No breakfast if morning examination or lunch if afternoon examination.
Barium enema (lower GI)	Enemas until the bowel return is clear on the evening before the examination, may order rectal suppository in the morning or a cathartic such as 2 oz. of castor oil or citrate of magnesia at 4:00 P.M. the day before the X-ray, clear liquids and gelatin for dinner, nothing by mouth (NPO) after midnight.
Barium meal (upper GI)	NPO after midnight.
Bronchogram	NPO.
Cholecystogram (GB series)	Light supper of nonfatty food such as fruit and vegetables without butter or oil the evening before the X-ray; gallbladder tablets (prescribed by the physician) are taken with water after supper; NPO except for water until X-ray the following day.
Computerized tomography (CT)	NPO for four hours before X-ray if a contrast media is used.
Intravenous cholangiogram	NPO.
Intravenous pyelogram (IVP)	Three Dulcolax tablets or 2 oz. castor oil at 4:00 P.M. the day before the X-ray; eat a light supper; NPO after midnight.
Myelogram	NPO.
Retrograde pyelogram	Enemas or laxatives on the evening before X-ray; NPO for eight hours before the procedure.
Ultrasound	May require a full bladder or laxatives, depending on the type of ultrasound.

Positioning

Although it is unlikely that you, as a medical assistant, will be positioning a patient for a diagnostic imaging procedure, it will be helpful for you to understand that the patient's position relative to the source of X-rays determines the images that are produced. Figure 48-2 illustrates X-ray pathways and the image produced when the patient is placed in a specific position. The desired position of the patient and position of the X-ray beam must be known ahead of time by the technician. The position of the patient is critical for an accurate X-ray. Table 48-2 lists radiology positions and descriptions of each position. Procedure 48-1 lists the steps for a general X-ray examination.

TABLE 48-2 | Radiology Positions

Position	Description
Anteroposterior (AP)	The X-ray beam is directed from front to back. Patient may be standing or supine. The patient's front will face the X-ray equipment, and the patient's back will be near the film plate.
Posteroanterior (PA)	The X-ray beam is directed from back to front. Patient will be standing upright. Patient's back will face the X-ray equipment, and his or her front will be near the film plate.
Oblique	The patient is turned at an angle to the film plate so the X-ray beam can be directed at areas that would be hidden on an AP, PA, or lateral X-ray.
Lateral	The X-ray beam is directed toward one side of the body. In the right lateral (RL) position, the patient's right side is near the film plate, and the left side is near the X-ray equipment. In a left lateral (LL) position, the patient's left side is near the film plate.
Axial	The X-ray tube is angled to direct a ray along the axis of the body or body part. *Cephalad angulation:* The X-ray beam is directed at an angle from the feet toward the head. *Caudal angulation:* The X-ray beam is directed from the head toward the feet.

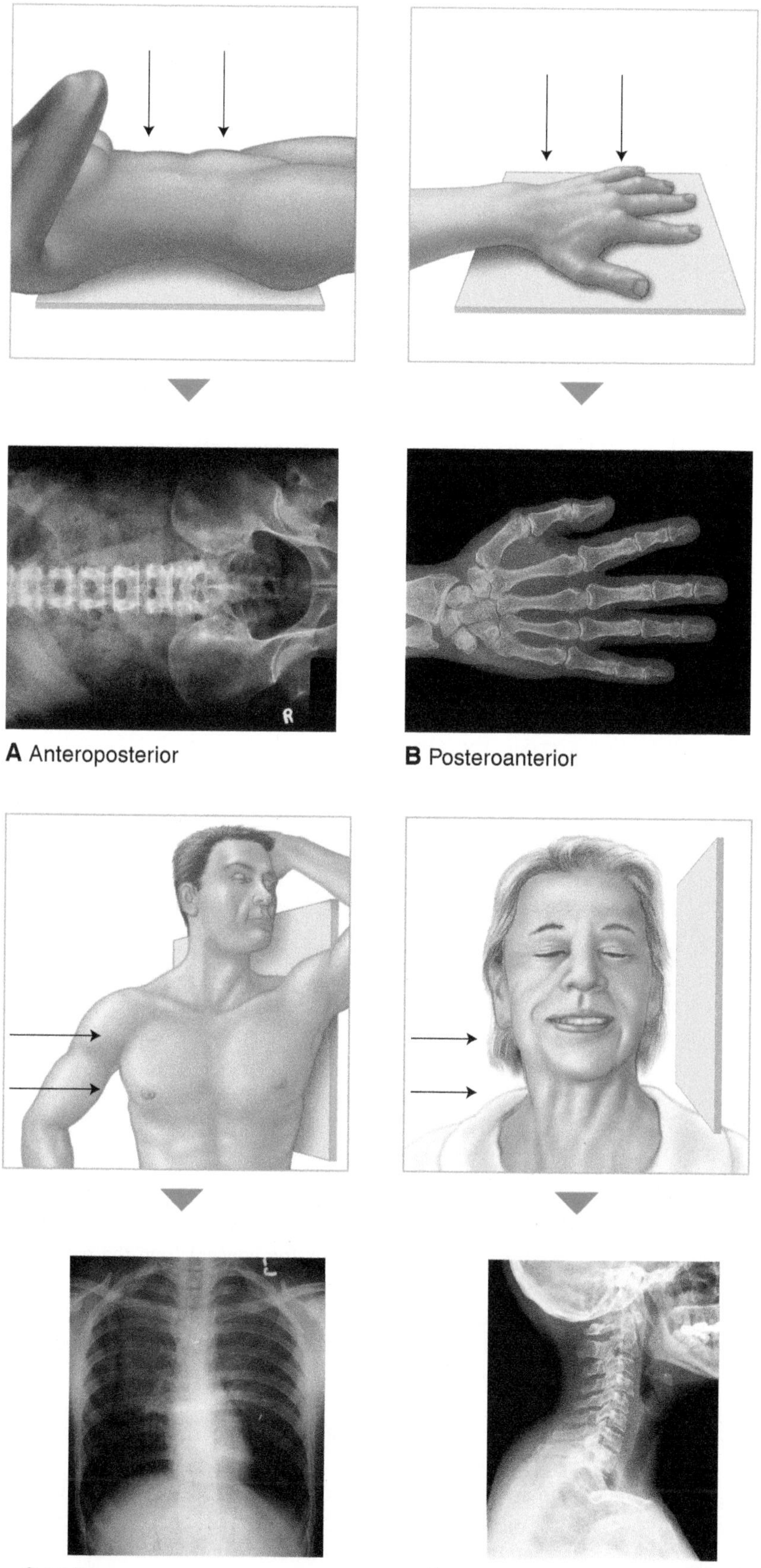

A Anteroposterior

B Posteroanterior

C Oblique

D Lateral

FIGURE 48-2 (A–D) Examples of the most common X-ray positions and the images they produce.

Scheduling Guidelines

The medical assistant is often responsible for scheduling the patient and providing instruction for radiologic procedures. If the procedure is performed in a facility other than the medical office, you may need to call the other facility to make the appointment. When setting an appointment, be ready to provide the patient's name, indication for the exam, type of insurance with precertification or approval number, referring physician's name, and type of radiologic procedure to be performed.

Special dietary restrictions in preparation for radiographic procedures often call for an all-liquid diet on the day before the test. All-liquid diet means that the patient may have any of the following: coffee, tea, carbonated beverages, clear gelatin desserts, strained fruit juices, bouillon, clear broth, and tomato juice. He or she may not have any dairy products. Remind the patient that NPO means "nothing by mouth." It is up to the physician to decide whether the patient should or should not take daily medications.

When multiple procedures are to be scheduled, it is important to consider the sequence of scheduling. Attention to sequencing is important because some procedures, such as those that require the use of contrast medium, may interfere with other tests. In addition, the patient may not be able to tolerate multiple procedures on one day. In general, examinations that do not require the use of contrast medium are performed before examinations with contrast medium. For example, an abdominal X-ray would be taken before a barium enema. Always check with the facility performing the tests to obtain specific instructions for scheduling. Guidelines 48-1 provides guidelines for sequencing multiple diagnostic procedures.

Some procedures require long waiting periods between imaging procedures, because it takes time for the contrast medium to move through portions of the body. This should be carefully explained to the patient to schedule time appropriately. The patient may have to allow a full morning for a series of X-ray procedures.

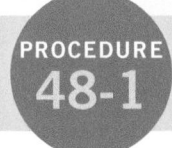

PROCEDURE 48-1

Assisting with a General X-ray Examination

Objective ◆ *Assist with a radiologic procedure under the supervision of a physician or radiologic technologist.*

EQUIPMENT AND SUPPLIES

Order for X-ray examination; dosimeter badge; appropriate X-ray equipment—X-ray film, holder, and machine; processing equipment; drape; lead patient shield

METHOD

1. Check the X-ray examination order.
2. Check the necessary X-ray equipment as needed.
3. Identify the patient. Question female patients about pregnancy.
4. Determine patient compliance with procedure preparation instructions.
5. Explain the procedure to the patient.
6. Instruct the patient to remove all clothing appropriate for the procedure.
7. Ask the patient to remove all jewelry and metals as needed for the procedure.
8. The following steps will most likely be performed by a radiologic technologist.

9. Position and drape the patient correctly.
10. Align the X-ray tube and cassette at the correct distance and set the controls.
11. Ask the patient to hold his or her breath as necessary.
12. Leave the room and stand behind the lead shield to take the X-ray(s).
13. Ask the patient to take a comfortable position while all X-rays are processed and reviewed.
14. Instruct the patient to dress if the X-rays are satisfactory.
15. Label the X-rays and place them in an envelope, according to office procedures.
16. Document appropriately.

CHARTING EXAMPLE

05/05/YY 7:00 A.M. Chest X-ray done by RRT............................
....M. King CMA (AAMA)

Guidelines 48-1

Order of Sequencing for Multiple Radiographic Procedures

1. All radiographic examinations and tests that do not require contrast media or iodine uptake
2. Radiographic tests of the urinary tract
3. Radiographic tests of the liver and gallbladder
4. CT scans of abdomen and pelvis
5. Procedures requiring barium
6. Lower gastrointestinal series (barium enema)
7. Upper gastrointestinal series

Note: *CT procedures that require IV contrast media may be done after blood is drawn for an iodine uptake series.*

Professionalism The Law

To protect the patient and the physician, always have a written order for every procedure. For invasive procedures, a written consent from the patient is necessary before the procedure can be performed.

The procedures discussed in this chapter are not ordinarily part of the medical assistant's routine work assignment. Assisting with radiologic procedures requires extra training and practice. The medical assistant must refrain from assisting with or performing advanced procedures without adequate training.

In some states, the medical assistant is not allowed to assist with radiologic procedures. If in doubt about the practice and laws within your state, always check with your local medical assistant organization or contact the AAMA office in Chicago, Illinois.

DIAGNOSTIC IMAGING PROCEDURES

Diagnostic imaging procedures can be divided into invasive and noninvasive procedures, or they can be divided into categories based on those that use contrast media and those that do not. The latter classification is used in this chapter. Table 48-3 identifies the most frequently ordered tests and the conditions they are used to diagnose.

Radiologic Imaging Procedures Requiring Contrast Media

Various radiologic procedures involve the use of contrast media: angiography, arthrography, barium enema (lower GI), barium swallow (upper GI), cholangiography, cholecystography, fluoroscopy, intravenous pyelogram (IVP), myelography, nuclear medicine studies, retrograde pyelogram, and

TABLE 48-3 | Diagnostic Imaging Procedures and Conditions Diagnosed or Treated

Test	Conditions Diagnosed/Treated
Angiography	*Cardiovascular:* Status of blood flow, collateral circulation, aneurysm, hemorrhage, vessel malformation.
	Cerebral: Aneurysm, hemorrhage, evidence of stroke, arteriosclerosis.
	Gastrointestinal (GI): Upper GI bleeding.
	Pulmonary: Pulmonary emboli, evaluation of pulmonary circulation in heart conditions before surgery.
	Renal: Abnormalities of blood vessels in urinary system.
Arthrography	Joint conditions.
Barium enema (lower GI)	Obstructions, ulcers, polyps, diverticulosis, tumor, and motility problems of colon or rectum.
Barium swallow (upper GI)	Obstruction, ulcers, polyps, diverticulosis, tumors, and motility problems of esophagus, stomach, duodenum, and small intestine.
Bone densitometry	Osteopenia, osteoporosis.
Cholangiography and cholecystography	Gallstones, gallbladder, or common bile duct stones or obstructions; ability of gallbladder to concentrate and store bile.
Computed tomography (CT)	Aortic and heart aneurysms, disorders of liver and biliary systems, renal and pulmonary tumors, brain abnormalities (tumors, blood clots, stroke, outlines of brain ventricles), GI tract lesions, GI tract disorders (pancreatic cyst, abdominal abscesses, biliary obstruction), breast diseases and disorders, spinal disorders, biopsy guides.
Fluoroscopy	Structure, process, and function of organs in motion to detect abnormalities.
Intravenous pyelography (IVP), excretory urography, intravenous urography	Urinary system abnormalities, including renal pelvis, ureter, and bladder (kidney stones); abnormal size, shape, or structure of kidneys, ureter, bladder; tumors; cysts; pyelonephrosis; hydronephrosis; trauma to urinary system.
KUB (kidneys, ureters, bladder) radiography	Size, shape, and position of urinary organs; urinary system diseases or disorders; kidney stones.
Magnetic resonance imaging (MRI)	Cancerous tissue, arthosclerotic tissue, blood clots, tumors, and deformities, particularly of the heart valves, brain, spine, and joints.
Mammography	Breast tumors and lesions.
Myelography	Irregularities or compression of spinal cord, tumors.
Nuclear medicine (radionuclide imaging)	Abnormal function, lesions, or disorders of bone, brain, lungs, kidneys, gallbladder, liver, pancreas, thyroid, and spleen.
Radiation therapy	Treatment of cancer and some benign tumors or scars.
Retrograde pyelogram	Obstruction of ureters, bladder, or urethra.
Stereoscopy	Fractures, dense areas that indicate tumor or increased pressure within skull.
Thermograph	Breast tumors, breast abscesses, fibrocystic disease.
Ultrasound	Abnormalities of gallbladder, liver, spleen, heart, kidneys, gonads, blood vessels, lymph system, fetal conditions: number of fetuses, age, gender, fetal development, position, and deformities.
Xeroradiography	Breast cancer, abscesses, lesions, and calcifications.

sometimes MRI. Contrast media can be administered by mouth, by enema, and by injection through intravenous lines or a catheter.

Fluoroscopy

Fluoroscopy is the use of a fluoroscope to see real-time moving images of internal structures and organs. The radiologist obtains immediate images that can be used to assess function of an organ or to view a process such as cardiac catheterization. The images can be recorded and played on a monitor and can be saved as a permanent record. Contrast media are often used during fluoroscopic procedures to enhance visualization of organ function and abnormalities. Fluoroscopic procedures include the gastrointestinal series, IVP, cholecystogram, and myelogram.

Gastrointestinal Series. A gastrointestinal (GI) series is a fluoroscopic study of the digestive tract using contrast media to detect abnormalities such as tumors, ulcers, polyps, and diverticulosis (pouches in the wall of the colon). An upper GI series is an examination of the esophagus, stomach, duodenum, and small intestine. The patient drinks a barium solution, and a fluoroscope outlines the esophagus, stomach, and small intestine as the barium moves through the system. The procedure takes one to two hours and produces little discomfort.

A lower GI series is the administration of a barium enema, which outlines the colon and rectum on a radiographic picture. The lower GI series is done by giving the patient a barium enema and also air to better illuminate the lower part of the digestive tract. Figure 48-3 shows a radiograph of the lower GI tract after a barium enema. Some patients may feel cramping and an urgency to move their bowels. They should be encouraged to take deep breaths during the procedure to help relax their abdominal muscles.

After either an upper GI series or a lower GI series, the patient should be encouraged to drink plenty of liquids to help move barium out of the system and should be made aware of the possibility of white stools from the barium for several days after the procedure.

The patient should receive written instructions before these procedures. In addition, the medical assistant should talk with the patient to explain the instructions and the procedure. Careful preparation is necessary for good results on these procedures. If the patient's digestive tract is not properly prepared and cleansed, the procedure may have to be repeated. The result is added expense, time, and discomfort for the patient. Guidelines for the patient who will undergo an upper GI series are listed in Guidelines 48-2; those for a lower GI series in Guidelines 48-3.

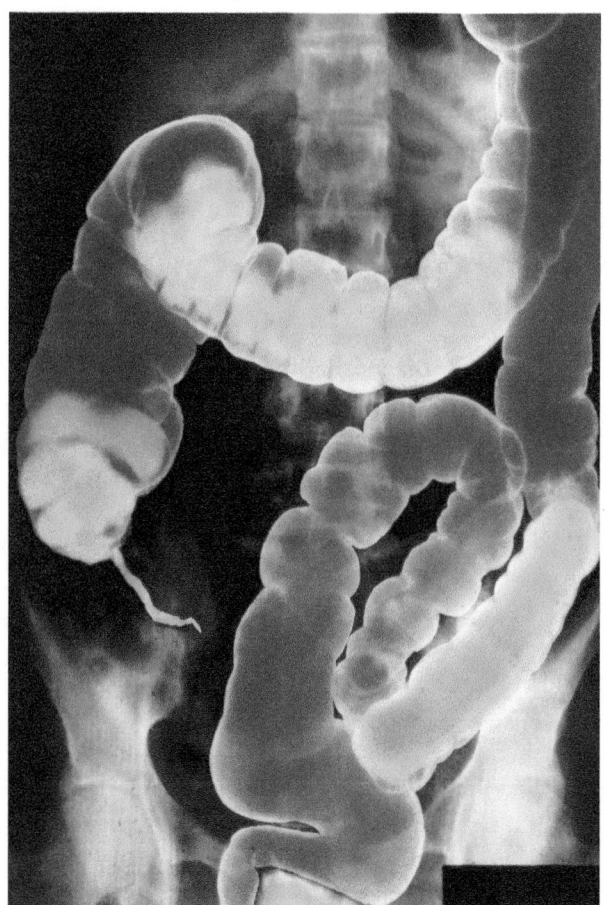

FIGURE 48-3 Radiograph of the colon after a barium enema.

Intravenous Pyelogram or Excretory Urogram. The intravenous pyelogram (IVP), also called a pyelogram, intravenous urogram, or excretory urogram, is a radiologic examination of the kidneys, ureters, and bladder. The patient should be screened for iodine sensitivity before the procedure. This procedure takes between 60 and 90 minutes. The patient will be instructed to eat a low-residue diet and drink plenty of water the day before the procedure. The patient will be allowed nothing by mouth (NPO) after midnight. A cathartic, such as castor oil or citrate of magnesia, may be ordered along with an enema to be taken the night before the examination.

The patient will need to undress and wear a patient gown for this procedure. A contrast medium containing iodine is injected into the vein. This substance may cause the patient to have a warm, flushed feeling and a metallic taste in the mouth. The patient should be instructed to notify the radiologist of any unusual symptoms, such as shortness of breath or itching, which could indicate an allergic reaction to the contrast medium.

The patient is tipped into various positions on the X-ray table, which allows the radiologist to view the dye as it flows through the urinary system. The patient may be asked to urinate and then have one final X-ray taken. After the examination, the patient can return to a normal diet. The patient should be encouraged to drink water to flush out the contrast medium through the kidneys.

Retrograde Pyelography. Retrograde means "against the normal flow," and retrograde pyelography involves inserting a catheter into the urinary tract through the bladder and into the ureters. The dye is sent up the tube into the ureters and kidneys, and X-rays are taken to evaluate the function of the ureters, bladder, and urethra. The post-procedural recommendations are the same as those for the IVP.

Cholecystogram. A cholecystogram is a radiologic examination of the gallbladder using a contrast medium, usually iodine. This procedure is done to detect abnormalities such as the presence of gallstones. Although this procedure has been replaced by ultrasound and nuclear medicine studies (e.g. HIDA scan) in many facilities, it is still ordered when ultrasound scanning fails to provide a definitive diagnosis.

It is important for the patient to understand that significant time is involved in preparation the night before and the day of the procedure. The patient is instructed to have a fat-free meal the evening before the procedure and NPO after midnight. The contrast medium, in the form of pills, is taken after dinner. The patient is instructed to take one pill at a time every few minutes with water until the six pills have been ingested.

In some facilities, the contrast medium is administered by intravenous (IV) injection. The patient undresses and wears a patient gown for this procedure. An initial X-ray is taken to see if the gallbladder is visible. A study is then conducted using the fluoroscope. Radiographs (X-rays) also are taken. After this portion of the procedure, the patient is asked to eat a fatty meal. This meal stimulates the gallbladder to empty. Another X-ray is taken one hour after the meal.

The patient can resume a normal diet after the procedure is complete; however, the patient should be told that diarrhea is an expected side effect of the contrast medium used in this procedure. Patients should be encouraged to drink plenty of fluids to replace the fluids lost as a result of diarrhea.

Myelography. Myelography is a fluoroscopic procedure of the spinal cord. A lumbar puncture is done to remove some cerebrospinal fluid (CSF) and instill contrast medium. This procedure produces a myelogram and is used to detect compression of the spinal cord or herniated disks. CT scans and MRIs are more commonly done now; however, a myelogram may be needed if the other procedures do not reveal enough detail. A pneumoencephalograph is performed by injecting air instead of contrast media after some cerebral spinal fluid has been removed. This procedure allows visualization of the cavities of the brain but is rarely performed and has been replaced by CT and MRI.

Angiography

Angiography is the X-ray visualization of the internal anatomy of blood vessels after a radiopaque material has been injected into the blood vessels. This procedure is used to assist in the diagnosis of many conditions, including myocardial infarction (MI or heart attack), stroke, renal artery stenosis (narrowing) as a cause of hypertension, clots, stenosis in arteries in the lower extremities and abdomen, aneurysm (weakening or ballooning) of the aorta, and pulmonary emboli or clots.

Because iodine is used as the contrast medium, the patient should be tested for allergy to iodine before the procedure. The contrast medium is injected into an artery or vein by way of a catheter and threaded through the vessel until it reaches the correct site, whereupon the radiographic image is recorded. The patient is monitored for a few hours after the procedure for any signs of bleeding from the puncture site or allergic reaction to the contrast medium.

Angiography may be used to study the blood vessels of the brain (cerebral angiography); the kidneys (renal angiography); and the heart (coronary angiography). This procedure is usually done in the hospital or a same-day, outpatient surgical facility and requires the use of local anesthetic. Cardiac catheterization, a form of angiocardiography, is frequently performed to assess the status of the coronary arteries. A catheter is inserted into the femoral or radial artery and fed through the arteries until it reaches the heart. If obstructions are discovered, therapeutic interventions can take place, such as balloon angioplasty or stent insertion or bypass surgery, to relieve blockage of coronary arteries.

Angiographic procedures are costly, carry risks, and are not usually performed unless other procedures have failed to provide enough information. Facilities that specialize in angiography have patient preparation sheets available. It would be helpful for you to have copies of the preparation instructions in the office as reference material.

Arthrography

Arthrography is the X-ray visualization of a joint space. It is performed by a radiologist to help diagnose abnormalities of the joints, tendons, ligaments, and cartilage of the knee, hip, or shoulder. The procedure involves injecting a local anesthetic followed by contrast medium or air or both into the joint. A fluoroscope is used to evaluate the function of the joint. The procedure usually takes about one hour, and the patient should be advised to expect some slight discomfort and swelling for a day or two. The patient should be advised to rest the joint during that time.

Radiologic Procedures Not Requiring Contrast Media

Several diagnostic radiologic examinations do not require the use of a contrast medium. Table 48-4 lists several of them. The procedures not requiring contrast media include films of the abdomen, bones, chest, kidneys, ureters, bladder (KUB), and paranasal sinuses.

These examinations or films require that the patient be positioned properly; however, no prior preparation, such as an enema, is required.

Mammography

Mammography is the radiologic examination of the soft tissue of the breast to identify benign and malignant neoplasms (tumors). The patient should be instructed not to use underarm deodorant, talcum powder, body lotion, or perfume before the procedure, because these can affect the clarity of the image.

The patient stands in front of the X-ray equipment, and the technician positions the patient carefully to have all breast tissue examined under X-ray. The patient should be instructed to follow the technician's direction regarding placement of hands, arms, and body position. Patients of childbearing age are given a lead apron to wear during the procedure. The procedure takes a few seconds for each view with the entire procedure lasting less than 30 minutes.

Some patients may feel discomfort during the procedure, which requires compression of the breast. For most patients, the discomfort is over as soon as the compression is completed (less than a minute). Occasionally patients will complain of discomfort for several days after a mammogram, and

TABLE 48-4 | Radiology Procedures Not Requiring Contrast Media

Type of X-ray	Description and Use
Abdomen	Flat plate or survey of abdomen used for suspected tumors, hematomas, enlarged organs, or abscesses.
Bone	X-ray studies of bones for suspected abnormalities from disease or trauma such as fractures and tumors. Commonly performed spinal X-rays are: cervical—X-ray of neck area; thoracic—X-ray of the middle back; lumbosacral—X-ray of lower back.
Breasts	Mammogram.
Chest	Routine chest X-rays are taken to rule out any abnormality and to pick up hidden disease in the lungs and some cardiac abnormalities (cardiomegaly). The patient assumes the posteroanterior erect position and a lateral position.
Kidneys, Ureters, Bladder (KUB)	This abdominal X-ray studies the kidneys, ureters, bladder, abdominal wall, pelvic bones, and unusual masses.
Paranasal Sinuses	X-ray of the sinuses found within the maxillary, frontal, ethmoid, and sphenoid bones for signs of infection, inflammation, and abnormalities.

the physician may suggest they take an over-the-counter analgesic (pain reliever).

The American Cancer Society advises women of various ages and risk levels how often to have mammograms for early detection of breast cancer (Figure 48-4). Many abnormalities detected on mammograms are benign and present no danger to the patient. Figure 48-5 shows a normal mammogram.

If a lump is detected, follow-up with further testing (often an ultrasound) should be commenced immediately without waiting to see if the lump disappears over time. Once a mammogram reveals suspicious tissue, a breast biopsy should be done to confirm the type of mass detected. A small sample of cells is taken and sent for review by a pathologist. After the examination is complete, the physician informs the patient of the pathologist's findings. Figure 48-6 is an example of an abnormal mammogram showing microcalcifications.

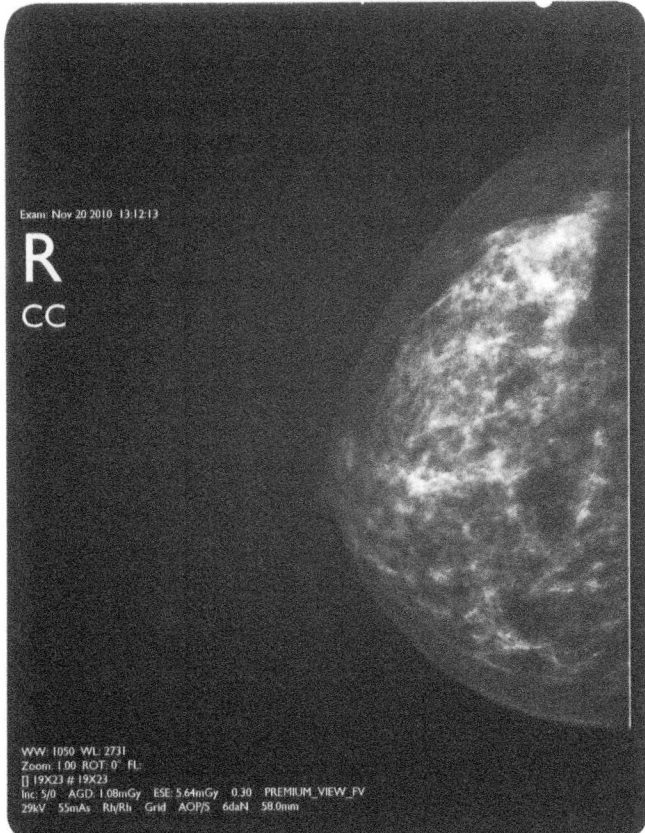

FIGURE 48-5 Normal mammogram.

Kidneys, Ureters, and Bladder

A kidneys, ureters, and bladder (KUB) radiograph, or abdominal flat plate, is used to assess the size, shape, and location of the organs of the urinary tract, and to detect kidney stones and diseases of the urinary tract. It is also used to detect the location of an intrauterine device (IUD) or other foreign object.

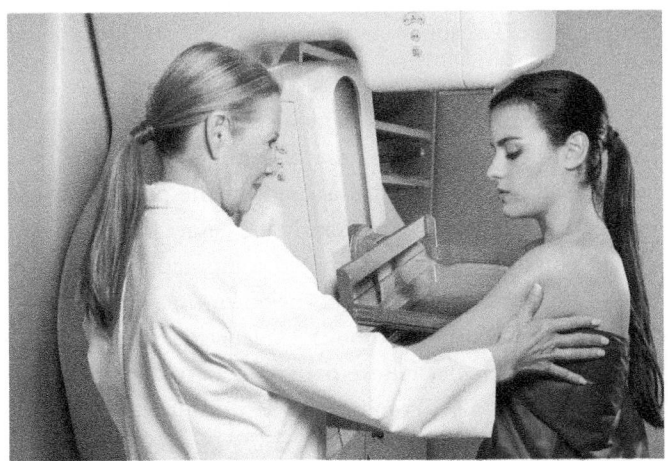

FIGURE 48-4 Compressing the breast between plates provides a better image of breast tissue. Regular mammograms help detect early cancers.

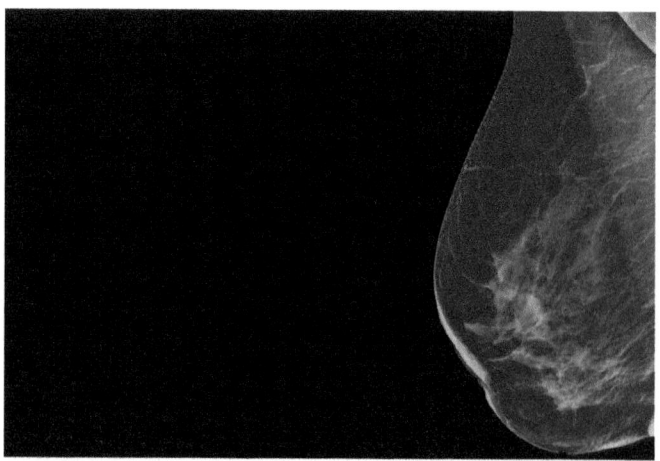

FIGURE 48-6 Mammogram showing microcalcifications.

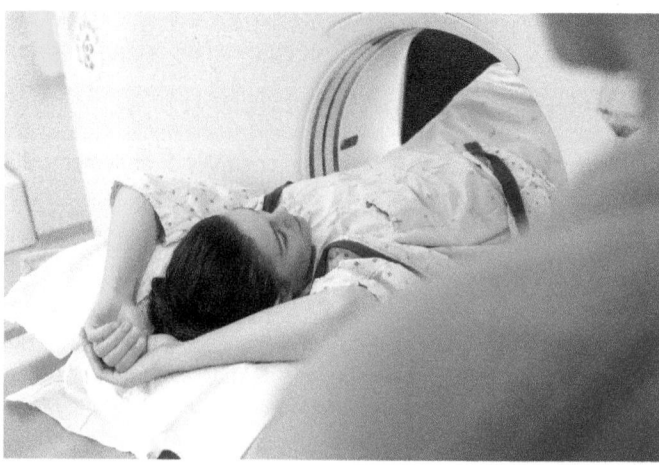

FIGURE 48-7 Woman undergoing a CT scan.

Tomography

Tomography, which uses radiography to produce cross-sectional views of the body, allows the technician to penetrate dense areas of the body that could not otherwise be visualized. Tomography produces images called tomograms.

Computed Tomography

Computed tomography (CT) combines radiography with computer analysis of tissue density. In CT scans, the X-ray camera rotates completely around the patient, and the computer accumulates cross-sectional slices from each rotation of the camera. The CT scanner consists of a movable table with a remote control; the circular structure, or **gantry**, that houses the X-ray equipment; and an operator console with monitor and computer equipment. Ancillary software and hardware

sort, manage, retrieve, and store images. This procedure is painless, noninvasive, and requires no special preparation.

The patient lies on a narrow table that slides into the scanner. A narrow beam of X-rays rotates in a continuous 360-degree motion around the patient to slice the images of the body in cross-sectional angles. The computer then calculates various factors, including tissue absorption, and displays a printout that determines the density of the tissue. In this way, tissue masses, such as tumors, bone displacement, and fluid accumulation, are detected. These images are more detailed than those obtained through conventional X-rays. Figure 48-7 is an illustration of a woman receiving a CT scan.

CT scans are useful when there is conflicting information about the cause of the patient's condition or when defining exactly where radiation therapy must be directed for tumor masses. Other uses for CT include detecting cerebral abnormalities, such as tumors, hematomas (Figure 48-8), childhood cancers, and abdominal masses, and surveying difficult-to-visualize glands, such as the pituitary gland and tissue. The CT scanner may take 15 to 20 minutes to scan each body part.

CT Scan Preparation. In many instances, CT scans involve little prior preparation for the patient. For some CT procedures, a contrast medium is used, so the patient may be instructed to have NPO for four hours before the procedure.

The imposing size of computed tomography equipment may cause considerable apprehension in a new patient. As with any procedure, a thorough explanation when scheduling the scan helps to relieve patient anxiety. Many patients have never seen a CT scanner, and showing them a diagram listing the major parts and their basic functions is helpful.

Any metallic objects will interfere with the CT scan, so instruct the patient to remove all metallic objects and

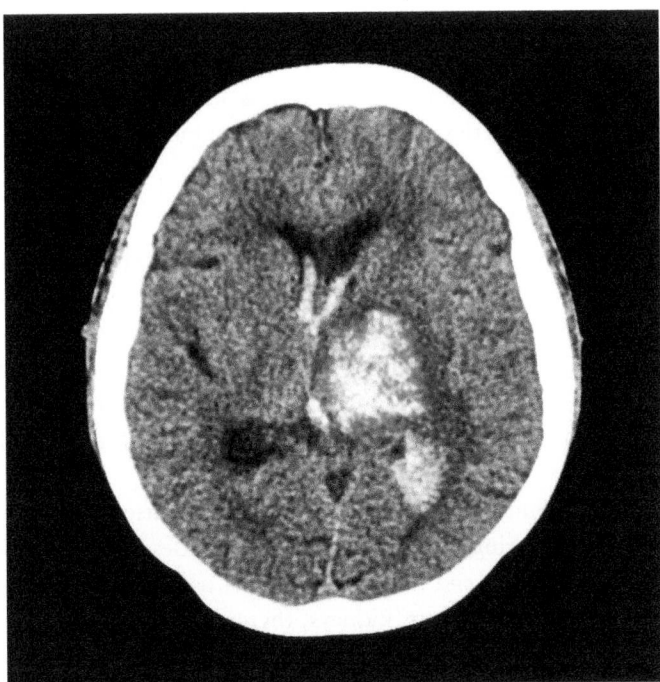

FIGURE 48-8 CT scan of the head shows a left thalamic hemorrhage (hemorrhagic stroke).

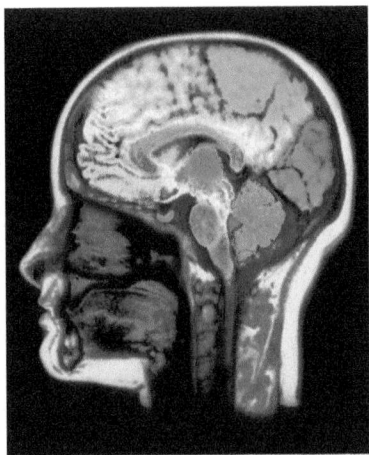

FIGURE 48-9 A color-enhanced MRI image of the skull.

inquire whether the patient has a pacemaker or metallic prosthesis.

The table may move continuously in a spiral scanning motion or stop and start, depending on the area being scanned. The patient should be reassured that he or she will not be in a confined space as with an MRI.

Positron Emission Tomography

Positron emission tomography (PET) is a computerized radiographic method that uses radioactive substances to examine metabolic activity within the body.

For PET scans, the patient is either injected with or inhales a chemical, such as glucose, that carries a radioactive substance. This substance then emits positively charged particles (positrons) that combine with negatively charged electrons found within the body. The rays that are produced are converted into color-coded images that indicate the degree of metabolic activity. PET is used to assist in the treatment of epilepsy, brain tumors, cancers, stroke, Alzheimer's disease, blood flow, and metabolism of the heart and blood vessels. This procedure can detect mild early changes in the brain before nerve damage, memory loss, or other symptoms occur. The radioactive elements used in PET are short lived, which results in minimal radiation exposure for patients.

Magnetic Resonance Imaging

Magnetic resonance imaging (MRI) uses a powerful magnetic field to visualize internal tissues, organs, and structures. All

areas of the body can be scanned using the MRI with excellent images. There is no ionizing radiation used, and the MRI has no known risks. See Figure 48-9 for a color-enhanced MRI image.

The signal or nuclear magnetic resonance produced by the MRI varies with different body tissues. These signals are processed by the computer and form a visual image. An MRI scan can give the viewer a three-dimensional view of tissues or organs of the body in total or as slices. This can be useful for tumor detection.

Explaining the procedure to the patient should include a description of the type of chamber in which the patient will be placed. One type of chamber consists of a large cylindrical electromagnet. The patient is rolled into it on a pallet. The chamber is sealed, which allows the patient's entire body to come into contact with the electromagnetic field. The procedure, although painless, can be upsetting to patients who have **claustrophobia**, which is a fear of closed-in spaces. The space inside a closed MRI machine is only slightly larger than the average patient. The MRI machine makes loud thumping noises intermittently during the procedure. The patient should be made aware of this noise and be provided with earplugs or earphones to listen to music. In cases of extreme apprehension, the patient may need to be given a medication to promote relaxation. Open MRIs are available for patients who are too large for the enclosed MRI or too apprehensive; however, the images produced may not be as accurate or detailed (Figure 48-10).

Use of the MRI has some limitations. It is not possible to view the hard portion of bone matter. For visualizing fractures and other abnormalities, the CT scan and general X-rays are still used. In addition, the strong magnetic field is not appropriate for patients who have pacemakers or

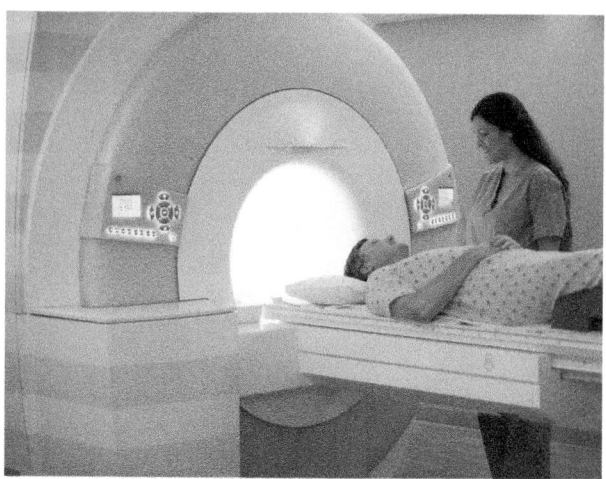

FIGURE 48-10 An open chamber MRI may be more comfortable for the patient, but images may not be as distinct.

metallic clips on blood vessels. The patient should be instructed to do the following:

- Remove all jewelry, eye shadow, and metallic objects, such as watches, belts, hearing aids, and hairpins.

- Identify which devices, if any, have been inserted within the body, such as pacemakers, dental implants, surgical staples, intrauterine devices, joint or bone pins, prostheses, metallic clips on blood vessels, or metal fragments, such as from a gunshot or from welding. These will all be present on the scan and can interfere with magnetic conduction. In addition, metallic clips on blood vessels can become loosened during the procedure.

- Leave credit cards or devices that contain metallic or magnetic code strips outside the MRI chamber.

- Use a patient gown if the patient's clothing has zippers or metal snaps.

The technician is not in the chamber with the patient during the procedure. The patient should be told that the technician will be in constant contact with the patient via a microphone and camera. The patient should be instructed to remain still during the procedure. An MRI scan takes from 20 to 60 minutes, depending on the amount of the body to be scanned.

An advancement in MRI technology, the functional MRI, enables physicians to observe the function of organs. Functional MRIs can provide information about nerve activity in the brain and locate areas of the brain activated in memory.

Digital Radiology

Digital radiology is the use of standard fluoroscopy that is digitized, stored as computer bits, processed, and then converted into an image on a television or video monitor screen. The image is stored on a computer hard drive or digital disc. Digital angiography is used for cardiac and pulmonary arteries and head and neck angiograms.

Ultrasound (Sonography)

Ultrasound, or sonography, is the use of high-frequency sound waves to image internal structures. Ultrasound imaging consists of projecting a beam of sound waves into the body. The waves at about 20,000 cycles per second bounce back as the beam comes into contact with a structure, such as a fetus, which then produces an outline of the internal structure.

Ultrasound has valuable medical applications, such as fetal monitoring and detecting abnormalities, such as gallstones, tumors, and heart defects. It is used to scan organs such as the liver, heart, kidneys, thyroid, gonads, and blood vessels. Ultrasound is not used to image the lungs, brain, or skeleton, because they are made of or surrounded by bone, which sound waves cannot penetrate.

Ultrasound uses no ionizing radiation and is a painless noninvasive procedure. It has been widely accepted as a safe examination of delicate tissues and the fetus. Fetal ultrasound is commonly performed to detect the presence of multiple pregnancies, fetal and placental positioning, and internal organ development. The use of ultrasound is not recommended simply to determine gender of the fetus.

Ultrasound Scanning

To perform an ultrasound procedure, a conduction material such as water, a special jelly, or oil is used to conduct the sound waves into the body. An ultrasonic transducer (a device that both produces and senses ultrasonic waves) with a conduction head is then placed on or near the skin. As sound waves pass through the skin, they bounce off the body tissues or fetus and remit back to the instrument an echo reflection of the image. These echoes of the body tissue or fetus are then recorded as a series of dots on an oscilloscope (an instrument that displays a visual picture). The record produced is an echogram or a sonogram (Figure 48-11). The patient is often able to view the sonogram on the screen as it occurs. The picture can be printed for the patient's record and, in some cases, a copy of this printout is given to the patient. Usually, the sonogram will require some interpretation. The medical assistant should not attempt to explain the results to the patient.

Patient preparation for the ultrasound examination is minimal. The patient should wear loose-fitting garments or

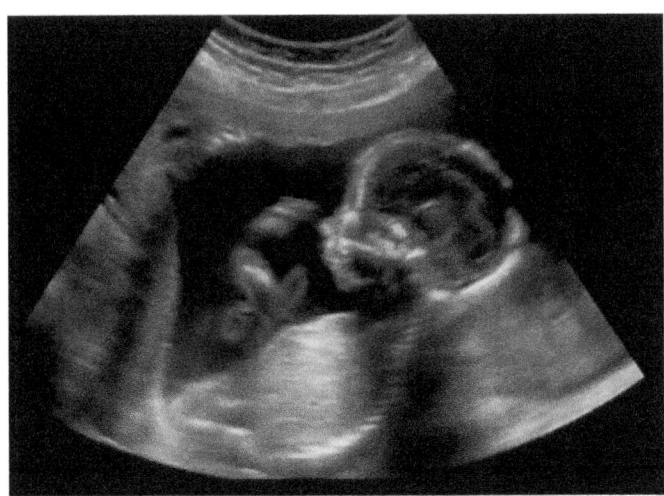

FIGURE 48-11 An ultrasound echogram or sonogram of a fourth month fetus.

clothing that is easy to remove, because the procedure is performed over bare skin (Figure 48-12). During a fetal ultrasound or pelvic ultrasound, the patient is instructed not to urinate right before the test, because a full bladder displaces the intestines and allows for a better view of the uterus. In fact, the patient may be asked to drink a quart or more of water just before either of these examinations. For an ultrasound of the gallbladder or liver, the patient may be asked not to eat for several hours before the procedure.

Ultrasound is also used in physical therapy and is discussed in the chapter titled "Physical Therapy and Rehabilitation."

Bone Densitometry

The bone densitometry test (DXA) uses X-rays to quickly measure the density of bone to detect osteopenia or osteoporosis, diseases in which the bone's mineral density is low and risk for fractures is high. The only precaution is that calcium

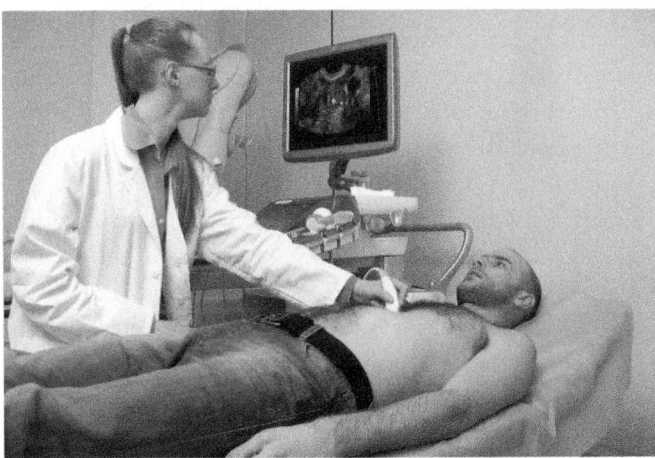

FIGURE 48-12 An ultrasound being performed on a patient.

supplements and medications that contain calcium, like Tums, should be discontinued 24 hours before the test. During the test, the patient may be asked to disrobe, change into a gown, and remove all jewelry. The patient will usually lie on the back on a padded table while the lower back, hips, or other sites are scanned. Usually the patient is able to resume normal activities immediately after the scan. Patients should notify the physician before taking this test if they believe they are or may be pregnant, because X-rays are used and may be harmful to the fetus.

RADIATION THERAPY

Radiation, as employed in medicine, is the use of a radioactive substance in the diagnosis and treatment of disease. Radiation therapy is the process of administering a particular dosage of radiation to a specific area on the patient's body for the purpose of killing diseased cells, such as cancers. Radiation actually alters the cells so they cannot reproduce and thus eventually die, leaving no new cells to develop. Both diseased and normal cells are altered with radiation. Diseased cells are eventually destroyed; however, normal or healthy cells are able to repair themselves and multiply. Radiation therapy is also known as cobalt treatment, X-ray treatment, or radiotherapy.

Radiation Rays

In radiation therapy, the radioactive substances used emit three types of rays: alpha, beta, and gamma. Alpha rays are the least penetrating rays and are positively charged helium particles released by the disintegration of radioactive material. Beta rays are able to penetrate body tissues a few millimeters and are negatively charged electrons released when atoms of radioactive substances disintegrate. Gamma rays have great penetrating power and are electromagnetic waves emitted by atoms of radioactive elements as they undergo disintegration. Gamma rays can penetrate most body tissue but are absorbed by lead. All three ray types are similar to X-rays, but they come from the element's nucleus. X-rays come from the orbit of the element's atom.

Uses of Radiation Therapy

Radiation therapy is administered after a tumor is well defined in the patient. Tumors are located through the use of CT scan and ultrasound. The boundary of the tumor can be localized by these radiologic procedures.

Patients receive radiation therapy for a variety of types of cancers including cancer of the ovaries, testes, skin, larynx, and oral cavity. Hodgkin's disease, Wilms' tumor (a type of kidney tumor found in children), and retinoblastoma (an eye cancer) are also treated with radiation therapy. For some types of malignancies, such as cervical cancer, a combination of radiation and chemotherapy is used. In some cases, when a cure is not probable as with some brain tumors, radiation may be used to shrink tumors to alleviate pain, relieve pressure, or stop bleeding. In these instances, radiation therapy may improve the patient's quality of life. Certain benign conditions may be treated with radiation, such as keloids (abnormal scars) and malformed blood vessels in the brain that cannot be accessed any other way.

Radiation Therapy Techniques

There are two methods for administering radiation: external radiation therapy (ERT) and internal radiation therapy (IRT).

External Radiation Therapy

External radiation therapy (ERT) involves administering calculated doses of radiation from a machine positioned at a specific distance from the site (tumor). A marker or tattoo is placed on the patient at the exact site or port of entry. A computer calculates the dosage required to destroy the largest number of malignant cells while causing the least damage to surrounding cells. It may be necessary to schedule a series of ERT treatments over a period of weeks or months.

Internal Radiation Therapy

Internal radiation therapy (IRT) can be administered into the body in two forms: sealed or unsealed radiation therapy. Sealed radiation involves the implantation of sealed containers of radioactive material near the tumor in the body. For example, radium, cesium–137, or cobalt–60 may be sealed in small gold containers or seeds and implanted in or near the tumor site. Unsealed radiation involves introducing a liquid form of radioactive substance into the patient by mouth, bloodstream, or instillation into a body cavity. For instance, radioactive iodine–131, phosphorous–32, and gold–198 may be administered in unsealed forms.

Radiation therapy is not usually disfiguring but may cause side effects in some patients, including hair loss, skin changes, nausea, and diarrhea; irritation of the mucous membranes in the mouth, throat, bladder, and vagina; and chromosome changes. The symptoms vary in intensity and may last three to six weeks.

SAFETY PRECAUTIONS

Radiation dose is measured in several different units and all relate to the amount of energy deposited. The units include the roentgen (R), the gray (Gy), and the sievert (Sv). The sievert and the gray are similar, except that the sievert takes into account the biological effects of different types of

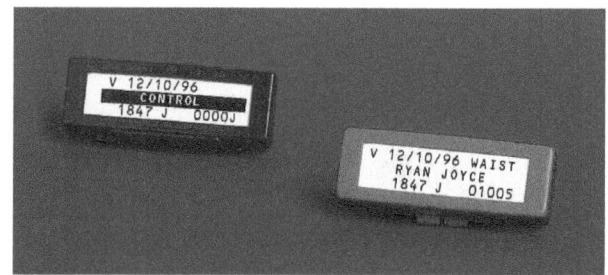

FIGURE 48-13 Dosimeter or personal radiation badge.

radiation. The biological effect of radiation exposure varies with the type of radiation and its energy. Equal doses of different types of radiation will not always result in the same biological effects. A rad, which stands for radiation absorbed dose, is the unit used to measure the amount of ionizing radiation absorbed during an X-ray procedure. To measure occupational exposure or other exposure that may involve more than one type of radiation, the unit used is the **rem**, which stands for "roentgen equivalent in man." The dosimeter, or personal radiation badge, containing the occupational exposure dose is reported in rem (Figure 48-13).

Radiation Exposure

People are constantly exposed to low levels of natural ionizing radiation or background radiation from outer space and exposure to radon, a gas that forms naturally in rocks and soil and breaks down into radioactive elements that linger in the air. In addition, people are exposed to ionizing radiation from human-made sources such as nuclear weapons testing and radiation from medical testing and treatments. On average, diagnostic imaging emits lower doses of ionizing radiation than occur naturally. Advances in diagnostic imaging have reduced the radiation dose a patient is exposed to during a diagnostic procedure. Excessive exposure to radiation causes tissue damage and side effects.

Overexposure to radiation may result in radiation sickness, causing symptoms such as lowered red blood cell and white blood cell counts, bone marrow alteration, burns, damage to ovaries and testes, fetal damage (especially during the first three months of pregnancy), and cancer. Radiation sickness from overexposure is usually the result of long-term exposure and is generally delayed. Radiation sickness may result in cancer and premature aging. The severity of radiation sickness depends on the dose of radiation, the type of radiation, duration of exposure, and what areas of the body were exposed. Radiation sickness can occur after nuclear reactor accidents.

Cellular Effects of Radiation

At the cellular level, radiation damages the DNA of cells in both malignant and normal cells. Normal cells are better able to repair DNA damage than cancer cells; therefore, treatment with radiation kills the cancer cells, whereas after a period of time, damaged normal cells in the area will repair themselves. Sensitivity to radiation of cells increases with their increased rate of cell division. In other words, cells that divide more frequently, such as hair; mucous membranes of nose, mouth, skin, and GI tract; and some glands, such as breast and thyroid; are more sensitive. The less specialized a normal cell is, the more affected it will be by radiation. Cells of the bone marrow and germ cells such as sperm and ovum fall into this category. Excessive radiation to embryonic cells causes spontaneous abortion, retardation, genetic abnormalities, and increased risk of leukemia and other cancers. The genetic defects can be passed on to future generations. Some cancers, such as leukemias, lymphomas, and squamous cell carcinomas of the mouth and skin, are more radiation sensitive and are treated using radiation therapy.

Personnel Safety Precautions

Because X-rays are potentially dangerous to both the patient and the health care personnel, special precautions must be taken.

Radiation is discussed in terms of primary and secondary radiation. Primary radiation strikes the patient for either therapeutic reasons or for an X-ray examination. Once the primary beam strikes the patient, it can then become secondary radiation as it bounces off the patient. Secondary radiation is strongest closest to the patient. Lead has been proven to be an effective barrier to an X-ray beam. Lead aprons, shields, and gloves are provided for personnel coming into close contact with X-ray equipment. X-ray technicians do not normally remain next to the patient during the X-ray process. Rather, they stand behind a lead-shielded divider. X-ray rooms are lined with metal (1 inch thick) as a precaution against X-ray beams escaping from the room. Some facilities have a red light that flashes when X-ray equipment is in use to warn others not to enter.

A film badge or **dosimeter** is worn on the outer clothing of all personnel working with or near radiologic equipment. The badge records the level and intensity of radiation exposure. It is periodically examined to ensure that the health care worker is not exposed to excessive radiation. Radiation exposure is cumulative, meaning that each exposure to radiation is added to the effect of all previous exposures. All radiographic equipment should be checked on a regular basis to ensure it is in good working condition and to check for radiation leakage. Radioactive diagnostic materials must be stored in a safe environment and amounts of radioactive material closely monitored. Radioactive materials should be stored in lead containers and handled only with forceps,

never with bare hands. Most facilities employ a radiation safety monitor who specifies the requirements for the facility and ensures that Occupational Safety and Health Administration (OSHA) guidelines are observed.

Patient Safety Precautions

The guiding principle in the use of radiation is "as low as reasonably achievable" (ALARA). In other words, the exposure of both patients and workers should always be guided by the idea that it is most prudent to use the lowest amount of exposure to perform the task.

Patient safety requires that a thorough history of the patient be taken. If the patient is female, the 10-day rule about the possibility of pregnancy should apply: An X-ray may be taken only within 10 days of the last menstrual period to avoid taking an X-ray of a female who is unknowingly pregnant. If a patient is unsure about a pregnancy, then a pregnancy test should be performed or the radiographic test postponed until a pregnancy test is completed, unless an emergency situation exists. In cases of emergency, the danger of exposure to the embryo or fetus should be explained to the mother.

Patients should be protected from secondary or scatter radiation by the use of a **grid** during radiographic procedures. Excess scatter may add density to the image and expose the patient unnecessarily. The grid is positioned between the X-ray machine and the patient to absorb radiation scatter before it reaches the film. A Potter–Bucky diaphragm, or a bucky, is a type of grid composed of alternating strips of lead and radiolucent material. Not all secondary radiation is absorbed by a grid, so other safety precautions are necessary.

A lead barrier or lead shields should be used by both patients and workers. Patients should be provided with a lead shield for gonads, eyes, breasts, and thyroid whenever appropriate. Employees should use gonad shields, if at the reproductive age (55 years or under), whenever the sex organs are going to be exposed to radiation. For a female patient, the gonad shield should be placed with its lowest margin at the level of the pubic symphysis. In the male, the upper edge of the lead shield should be placed 1 inch below the pubic symphysis.

An implant may present a hazard while the implant is in place in a patient who is undergoing radiation therapy. The length of time the hazard exists depends on the half-life of the material used. The half-life is the time it takes for half of the isotope to decay.

Symptoms caused by radiation therapy will generally not begin for several days after the first treatment. This allows time for the patient and family to thoroughly understand

TABLE 48-5 | Radiation Side Effects, Healing Time, and Interventions

Effect On/In Body	Healing Time	Intervention
Alopecia	Hair may grow back in several months.	Shampoo with mild soap, brush, and comb gently; wear scarves or wigs if hair loss is extensive.
Bone marrow and lymphoid tissue	Depends on dosage and degree of damage.	Protect from infection; assess for anemia; watch lymphoid tissue for bleeding and signs of thrombocytopenia; and avoid trauma from injections and IVs.
Ear	Depends on dosage and degree of damage.	Assess for blockage of eustachian tube and bulging eardrum; protect from falls caused by dizziness; assess for hearing loss; and administer antibiotic for infection.
Eyes	Depends on dosage and degree of damage.	Assess for drying, excessive tearing, conjunctivitis, damage to lens, and cataract formation; use artificial tears as needed and antibiotic for infection.
Intestinal mucosa	Several weeks or months, depending on irritation.	Check intake/output levels; assess for diarrhea and vomiting; administer antidiarrheal or antiemetic agents, if necessary; encourage intake of potassium-rich food; avoid dairy products; and weigh daily.
Nervous system	Necrosis of brain can develop as much as a year after treatment.	Assess for level of cognition, dizziness, slurred speech, weakness, and numbness or tingling in extremities; assess for spinal cord damage, changes in gait, pain; and assess for incontinence.
Oral mucosa	Within weeks if irritation not severe.	Increase fluid intake; avoid hot, spicy foods and liquids; restrict smoking; suck ice chips; use lip balm; and use artificial saliva, if necessary.
Skin: first to fourth degree burns	Seven days to several weeks or months.	Assess skin daily; do not use drying substances such as alcohol; and avoid lying on area, direct sunlight, and direct heat sources.
Urinary mucosa	Several weeks to months, depending on level of irritation.	Increase fluid intake; measure urinary output; urinalysis; and administer antibiotics if infection present.

what to expect and what steps to take to make the patient more comfortable. The skin is at most risk, and radiation therapy frequently results in inflammation similar to sunburn. If the burns are deep enough, hair roots are damaged and hair will fall out. Radiation side effects, healing time, and patient interventions are summarized in Table 48-5.

Guidelines 48-4 provides a summary of guidelines for safeguarding the safety of health care workers, and Guidelines 48-5 provides a summary of guidelines for patients.

X-RAY RECORDS: STORAGE AND OWNERSHIP

X-ray materials for radiologic procedures must be kept in special storage containers that protect the film from damage caused by light, heat, chemical fumes, and moisture. For film to remain fresh, it should be kept in a dry, cool place within a sealed package. X-ray film should be stored on end to prevent pressure damage from stacking the film. The expiration dates, which are printed on the top end of the package, can be seen clearly when stored on end. X-ray developer is also kept in a cool location that is moisture free because damage to this fluid can affect the quality of the film. Film should be touched only with one hand and should be hung vertically to avoid damage. The film packages are opened only in the darkroom of the medical facility, because light will destroy the film's imaging ability.

All film records are maintained in a record or logbook that is kept in the X-ray room. Entered in this record are the film identification number, patient's name, date, and type of X-rays taken. Each film taken has an identification number, which is placed on the film holder or cassette with lead letters or numbers at the time the X-ray film is readied (time of exposure). These ID numbers identify the physician's name, the date, and the patient's name. These data are then permanently on the film after it is processed.

Films that have been processed should be stored in custom envelopes and filed in specially designed film cabinets. They are usually filed alphabetically. If a chronological numbering system is used based on the identification

Guidelines 48-4

Maintaining Personnel Safety

- Wear a film badge on outer clothing at all times when exposed to any form of X-rays. Do not wear a patient gown or lead shield over the badge. These badges are submitted for routine—usually weekly—evaluation of the levels of radiation exposure.
- Health care personnel should stay behind a lead shield in a lead-lined room when the X-ray equipment is in use.
- A sign or lighted display should be visible, and the X-ray room door should be closed when X-ray equipment is in use.
- Nonessential personnel should leave the X-ray room.
- All equipment should be inspected on a frequent, routine basis to check for radiation leakage.
- The patient should not be held or supported during radiologic procedures. There are devices that can be used to hold and position the patient.
- If it is necessary to remain in the room with the patient, the attendant should wear a protective lead apron and lead-lined rubber gloves. The attendant should face the patient with the lead apron between the patient and the attendant.
- Periodic blood tests may be required by facilities to determine the presence of blood abnormalities from radiation exposure.

Guidelines 48-5

Maintaining Patient Safety

- Ask if the patient has recently been exposed to X-rays from other examinations or through work-related activities.
- If the patient is female, inquire about the possibility of a pregnancy. If the patient is pregnant, report this to the physician before scheduling or assisting with any X-ray procedure. Because of liability concerns, it is important to obtain a release, or even a pregnancy test, before some X-ray procedures.
- Advise female patients of the potential radiation risk before X-rays are taken.
- Place a lead shield over the abdominal and reproductive organs of patients who are of childbearing age, or pregnant, or children.
- Patients must be carefully positioned to obtain an accurate image.

Note: Only perform this procedure if you have been fully instructed, trained, and authorized to do so in your state.

Professionalism   The Life Span

It may be the responsibility of the medical assistant to give the necessary consent forms to the patient and answer any questions or concerns they have about the procedure. Many patients express concern about being exposed to radiation. The medical assistant should be prepared to answer patients' questions and provide reassurance.

Patient preparation may also be the duty of the medical assistant. The patient preparation may include the preexam instructions as well as patient assistance in dressing, proper gowning, draping, and re-dressing. The majority of radiographic studies involve removing a portion of clothing, such as shirts or pants. Generally, undergarments are not a concern unless they contain metal, such as an underwire bra. The patient should also be advised to remove jewelry, clothing with zippers or snaps, or nonmetal clothing items that are thick or heavy, such as jeans.

Many young and older adult patients need assistance disrobing and getting into the proper drapes. When giving directions to patients or their caregivers, be very specific about which clothing items need to be removed, which may remain on, and how to properly wear the drape provided, such as open to the back or open to the front. During the examination, the caregiver of the patient may need to remain with the patient to assist in holding the patient in the proper position and provide patient safety. The caregiver needs the proper safety equipment, such as a lead apron, to protect against radiation scatter. Never leave a small child, or a patient who is unsteady, unattended on the X-ray table.

When the examination is complete, the medical assistant may be required to help the patient re-dress and to escort the patient back to the examination room.

number of each film, a master log must be maintained. If a film has to be removed from the file cabinet, an insert explaining where the film was sent is filed in place of the film within the file cabinet.

Ownership of Film

The medical assistant is frequently called on to explain the ownership of film to the patient. Although the patient has paid for the film, it is the property of the medical facility or hospital that performed the X-ray. Written reports prepared by the radiologist are sent to other physicians at the request of the patient, but the film generally remains in the original office or hospital. The reason for this is simple: If the film remains in one location, it can always be accessed for future examination and comparison. Once it leaves the originating facility, it can be misplaced and lost.

Physicians are able to lend their films to referring physicians for further examination. The patient has to sign a release of records form for this to take place, but the film must then be returned to the original facility. Because films are a permanent record of the patient at a particular moment, they must be preserved carefully. It is possible, in some locations, for the patient to obtain a duplicate copy of a film. The patient might have to pay for the copy to be made.

SUMMARY

The use of radiology in medical practice makes it possible to view internal body structures and functions and therefore assist in diagnosis and treatment. These procedures include radiology, radiation therapy, and nuclear medicine. There are inherent risks to the patients, technicians, and medical assistants in performing these procedures. The use of proper safety precautions can greatly reduce or eliminate these risks altogether.

48 CHAPTER REVIEW

COMPETENCY REVIEW

Note: These competencies may be practiced by a medical assistant only if permitted by state law.

1. Define and spell the terms for this chapter.
2. Explain how a patient would be positioned for AP, PA, RL, and LL X-rays.
3. List the order of sequencing for multiple radiographic procedures.
4. Identify personal safety precautions relevant to radiology procedures.
5. Describe a film badge and its use.
6. Explain how to properly store X-ray film in the medical office.

PREPARING FOR THE CERTIFICATION EXAM

1. Some radiographic procedures call for an all-liquid diet on the day before the test. An all-liquid diet means the patient can eat all of the following *except*
   a. tomato juice.
   b. clear gelatin desserts.
   c. fat-free milk.
   d. bouillon.
   e. coffee.

2. Iodine contrast compounds used to form radiopaque compounds are employed for
   a. thyroid studies.
   b. pyelograms.
   c. angiograms.
   d. cholecystograms.
   e. all of the above.

3. Negative media contrast includes all *except*
   a. air.
   b. carbon dioxide.
   c. other gases.
   d. barium sulfate.
   e. oxygen.

4. Which of the following X-ray procedures *does not* require the patient to be NPO, unless a contrast medium is used?
   a. barium meal (upper GI)
   b. bronchogram
   c. computed tomography (CT)
   d. intravenous cholangiogram
   e. myelogram

5. In which of the following radiology positions is the X-ray beam directed from front to back?
   a. axial
   b. lateral
   c. oblique
   d. posteroanterior (PA)
   e. anteroposterior (AP)

6. In which of the following radiology positions is the X-ray beam directed from back to front?
   a. axial
   b. lateral
   c. oblique
   d. posteroanterior (PA)
   e. anteroposterior (AP)

7. In which of the following radiology positions is the X-ray beam directed toward one side of the body?
   a. axial
   b. lateral
   c. oblique
   d. posteroanterior (PA)
   e. anteroposterior (AP)

8. In which of the following radiology positions is the X-ray tube angled to direct a ray along the axis of the body or body part?
   a. axial
   b. lateral
   c. oblique
   d. posteroanterior (PA)
   e. anteroposterior (AP)

9. In which of the following radiology positions is the patient turned at an angle to the film plate so the X-ray beam can be directed at areas that would be hidden on other films?
   a. axial
   b. lateral
   c. oblique
   d. posteroanterior (PA)
   e. anteroposterior (AP)

10. Which diagnostic imaging procedure is used for the treatment of breast cancer, abscesses, lesions, and calcifications?
    a. thermograph
    b. xeroradiography
    c. mammography
    d. myelography
    e. radiation therapy

CRITICAL THINKING

Refer to the case study at the beginning of the chapter and use what you have learned to answer the following questions.

1. Because Mr. Adler's gallbladder ultrasound did not provide a definitive diagnosis, what radiographic test might Dr. Miller order if he still suspects gallstones?
2. Based on your answer to the preceding question, is a contrast medium used with this test? If so, does it have any side effects the patient should be informed of, and are there any patients who could not use this form of contrast medium?
3. What does the patient need to do to prepare for this test? Be as detailed as possible.

ON THE JOB

Marge Riley, an overweight 50-year-old woman with a history of abdominal pain, has been scheduled for a lower GI series on Monday morning. She states she has board meetings every Monday morning at which breakfast is served and that she will come in for her X-rays after the meeting is over. Marge indicates that she does not understand why she needs these procedures.

1. What, if anything, would you tell the patient regarding her need for these procedures?
2. How would you describe these procedures to the patient?
3. What combination of teaching methods would you use to explain the procedures?
4. You are still concerned, after explaining everything to Marge, that she will not follow the instructions. What do you do?

INTERNET ACTIVITY

Search the Internet for information about the history of radiology. When were X-rays first taken? When did physicians first realize that radiographic waves were dangerous?

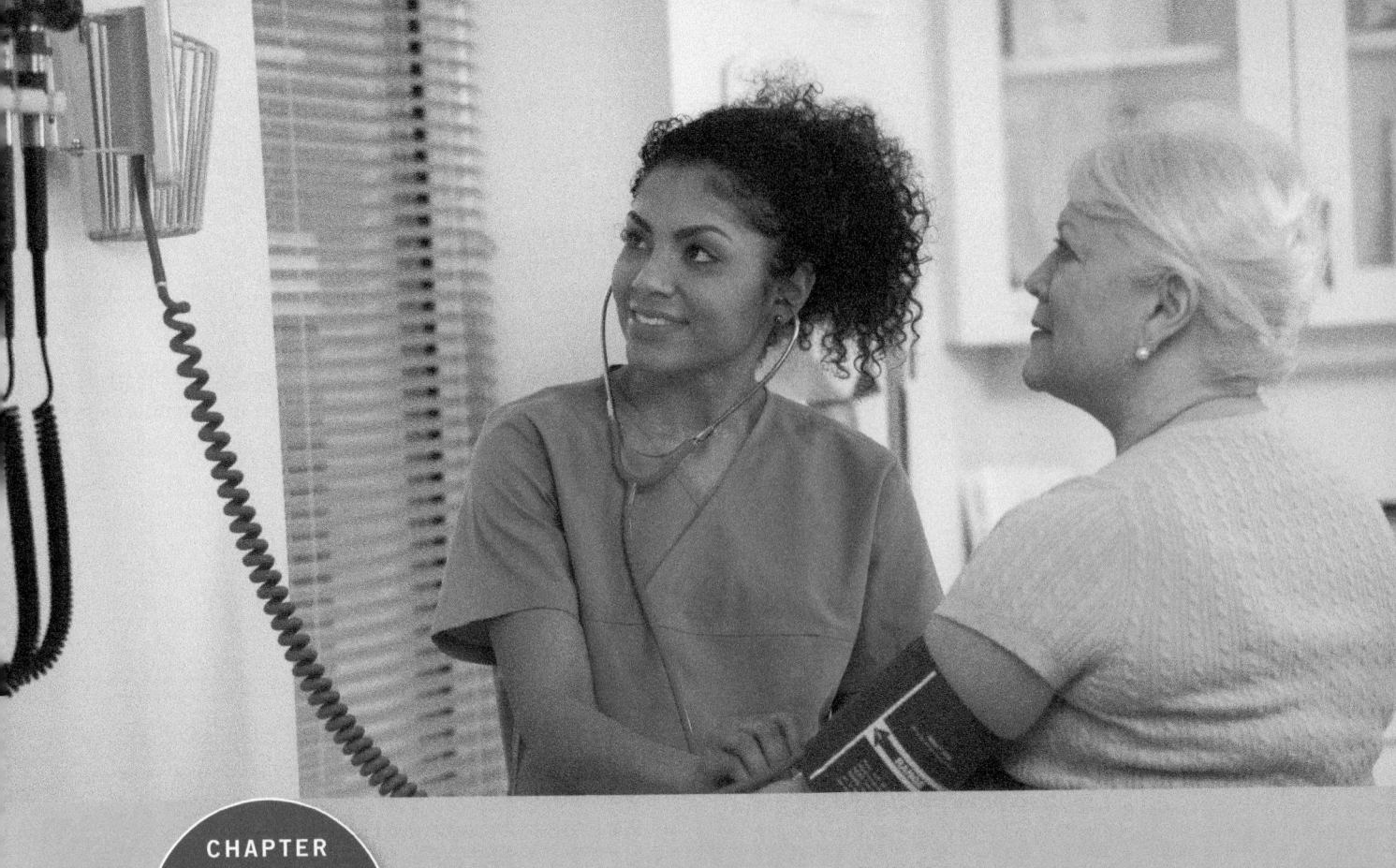

Learning Objectives

After completing this chapter, you should be able to:

49.1 Define and spell the terms for this chapter.

49.2 Describe polarity as it relates to the cardiac cycle.

49.3 Explain what wave patterns represent on an ECG.

49.4 Compare methods for calculating a heart rate using an ECG.

49.5 List the components of an ECG machine.

49.6 Identify the location for proper lead placement.

49.7 Describe preparations that must be made before ECG testing.

49.8 Explain how to correct various artifacts that occur during ECG testing.

49.9 Describe how a normal ECG would appear.

49.10 List abnormalities commonly revealed through ECG testing.

49.11 Explain the importance of exercise tolerance testing.

49.12 Outline patient education related to wearing a 24-hour Holter monitor.

Eliot Masterson, a 41-year-old business owner, was seen by Dr. Salpega for a routine physical. During the office visit, Eliot informed Dr. Salpega that he has had some episodes of chest pain over the past few months that have occurred after exercising. Dr. Salpega decides to have his medical assistant, David Dolan, perform an ECG on Mr. Masterson.

Terms to Learn

artifacts	hyperventilating	perfusion
coronary artery disease (CAD)	inspiration strip	polarity
depolarized	ischemic	repolarized
Einthoven's triangle	leads	rhythm strip
electrocardiogram (ECG)	maximum heart rate	stress test
electrocardiography	maximum target heart rate	telemetry
heart rate	multiple gated acquisition (MUGA) scan	thallium
heart rhythm		wave
Holter monitor	pacemakers	

eart disease and disorders of the cardiovascular system are extremely prevalent in the United States. **Coronary artery disease (CAD)** is the leading cause of death among both men and women in the United States. Early detection of heart disease can be accomplished with specialized cardiac testing, discussed in this chapter.

Medical assistants play an important role in helping physicians with diagnostic assessments of cardiovascular disorders. Most medical offices require blood pressure readings and pulse rate measurement for adult patients during their office visits. Medical assistants accurately obtain these vital signs and alert the physician of any abnormalities.

When more specific cardiac information is needed, **electrocardiography** is performed. Electrocardiography is a procedure for recording electrical changes in the heart. The record that electrocardiography produces is called an **electrocardiogram (ECG)**. Keep in mind that the ECG represents only the heart's electrical activity, not its mechanical performance. The physician orders this painless, noninvasive test when the heart sounds are unusual, the rhythm is irregular, or the patient has any heart-related complaints or a condition that might affect the heart. An ECG may also be made as a reference that future recordings can be compared with to detect changes over time. For that reason, the original recording may be called a baseline ECG. In most medical offices and clinics, ECG tests are performed by medical assistants.

ECG is the abbreviation for electrocardiogram that is most commonly used in the United States, but the abbreviation EKG is also often used. The Dutch doctor Willem Einthoven, who invented the first practical electrocardiogram in 1903, named it the electrokardiogram, or EKG, from *kardia*, the Greek word for heart. The abbreviation ECG derives from the English spelling, electrocardiogram. Both abbreviations, ECG and EKG, are correct and can be used interchangeably.

ELECTRICAL CARDIAC ACTIVITY

The electrical charges created by the heart's cardiac conduction system can be sensed throughout the body. Electrodes placed on specific areas of the skin are electrodes that can detect those cardiac electrical charges and transmit them to a computer for amplification of the signal and recording on paper (the ECG) for assessment by the physician.

When the ECG equipment senses an electrical charge, it is recorded on the readout as either an upward or a downward deflection from the horizontal baseline. Movement away from the baseline is called a deflection or **wave**. The waves or deflections that go up (positive) or down (negative) from the baseline represent amplitude or voltage. The strength or voltage of the electrical impulse determines the size of the deflection. Large voltages cause larger deflections; small voltages create smaller deflections. If no energy is sensed, the ECG equipment records a flat line, which is also called an isoelectric line.

Polarity and the Cardiac Cycle

The cells of the myocardium (heart muscle) produce electrical charges as a result of **polarity**. Defined simply, polarity means having two separate poles, one positive and one negative. When a myocardial cell is in a resting phase, it is termed *polarized* because it has a negative internal charge and a positive external charge.

The sinoatrial (SA) node, a small area of tissue at the top of the right atrium, is known as the heart's pacemaker because it controls myocardial polarity. When the SA node initiates electrical activity, the atrial cells become **depolarized** (the internal negative charge is reduced and the difference in charge inside and outside the cell is lost). As the electrical impulse travels from the atria and into the ventricles, cells in the ventricles also depolarize. As the cells depolarize, the atria and ventricles contract, and blood is pushed out of the heart and into the circulatory system. At the end of the contraction, the myocardium relaxes and rests. During this stage of relaxation, the cells become **repolarized**.

This cycle of electrical impulses—depolarization and repolarization, contraction and relaxation—represents one heartbeat.

PQRST Waves

A normal electrical cardiac cycle (one heartbeat) is traced on an electrocardiogram as one set of PQRST waves. The P represents atrial depolarization, the QRS complex represents ventricular depolarization, and the T is repolarization (a return to the resting electrical state). Figure 49-1 illustrates what is occurring in the heart and how it is represented on ECG tracing. The time that it takes for each component of the PQRST sequence to take place is discussed in the next section.

On an ECG, the horizontal axis (line) represents time; a slower heart rate will have more space between the PQRST complexes. For a patient with a faster heart rate, the cardiac cycles will be closer together. When the heart skips a beat, there is a long flat line between PQRSTs. The amount of space between the P wave and the QRS complex indicates the time required for the conduction system to carry the impulse from the SA node at the top of the atria to the Purkinje fibers that carry the impulse to the ventricles.

Recordings are made from a variety of perspectives or angles known as **leads**. Each lead will record from a specific

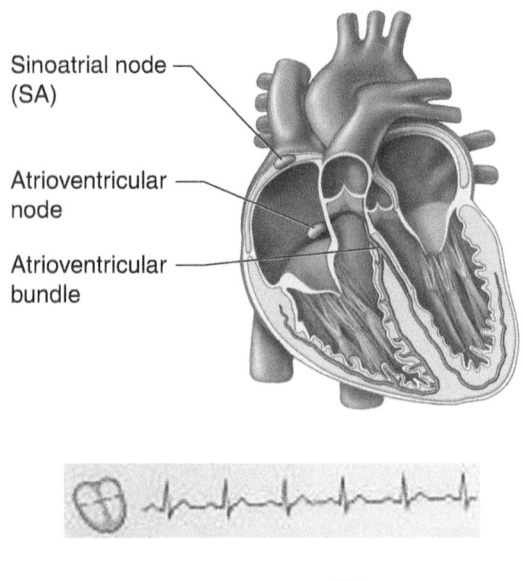

Sinoatrial node (SA)

Atrioventricular node

Atrioventricular bundle

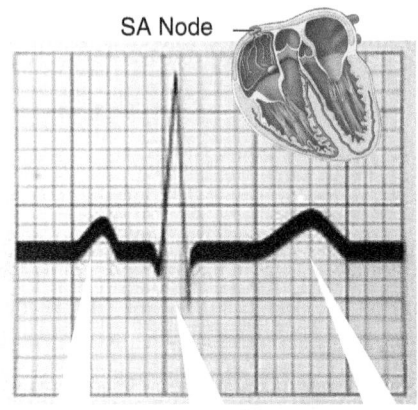

SA Node

P wave	QRS complex	T wave
corresponds to contraction of the atria	correlates to ventricles contracting	represents preparation for next series of complexes

FIGURE 49-1 The cardiac cycle and an ECG tracing.

combination of electrodes. When completed, the 12-lead ECG produces a three-dimensional record of cardiac impulses. The pattern of deflections will appear quite different on each lead. The pattern of deflections recorded, voltage or amplitude and time, assist the physician in evaluating the status of the patient's heart.

Time and the Cardiac Cycle

A P wave that is present in normal size and shape indicates the electrical stimulus causing the heart to beat that originated in the SA node (Figure 49-2). Normally, the P-R interval (time from the beginning of P to the middle of QRS) is between 0.12 and 0.20 seconds (three to five small boxes on the ECG graph paper). This interval represents the time it takes for the impulse to cross the atria and the atrioventricular (AV) node and reach the ventricles.

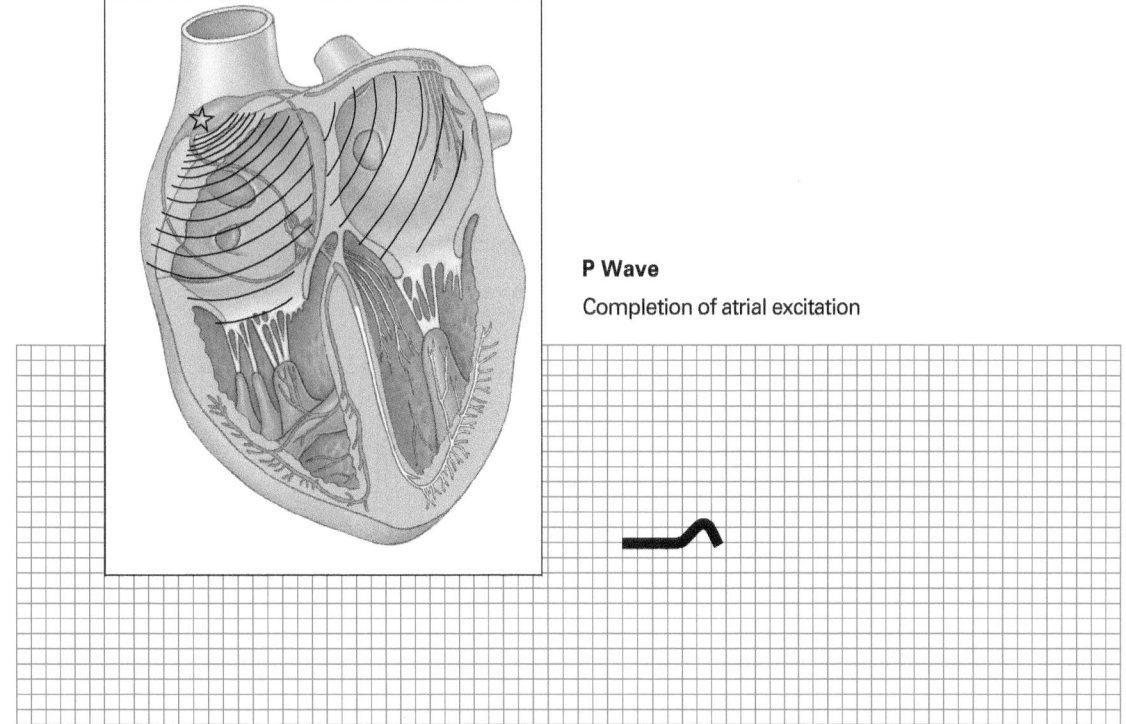

P Wave

Completion of atrial excitation

FIGURE 49-2 P wave (SA node initiates atrial depolarization).

A deviation from these times could represent an abnormality in either the electrical system of the heart or in a structure of the heart that impacts the electrical system. A P-R interval that is too short means the impulse has reached the ventricles through a shorter-than-normal pathway. If the interval is too long, a conduction delay in the AV node might be assumed.

The QRS complex represents the time necessary for the impulse to travel through the bundle of His, the bundle branches, and the Purkinje fibers (the structures that carry the electrical impulse to the ventricles) to complete ventricular contraction. This usually takes less than 0.06 to 0.12 second (three small ECG boxes). (See Figure 49-3.)

The ST segment and the T wave represent repolarization of the ventricles. (Repolarization of the atria is "hidden behind"—takes place at the same time as—the QRS complex so is not seen on the ECG.) The ST segment is normally flat (on the isoelectric line or baseline) or is only slightly elevated. The T wave represents a part of the recovery of the ventricles after contraction (Figure 49-4).

The QRS complex and the T wave typically point in the same direction, and T waves that are opposite in direction from the QRS may indicate a problem in the heart or its electrical system. Although the medical assistant should not try to interpret the ECG, understanding what is normal in the cardiac cycle is helpful. Table 49-1 provides a summary of ECG wave patterns.

TABLE 49-1 | ECG Wave Patterns

Wave Pattern	Corresponding Heart Activity	Electrical Activity
P Wave	Atrial contraction that is initiated by an electrical impulse from the SA node.	Atrial depolarization
QRS Complex	Ventricular contraction of the heart.	Ventricular depolarization
T Wave	Completion of ventricular contraction; here, the cells begin their resting phase before the process restarts.	Ventricular repolarization
U Wave	Sometimes present and represents further relaxation of the ventricles.	A continuation of ventricular repolarization

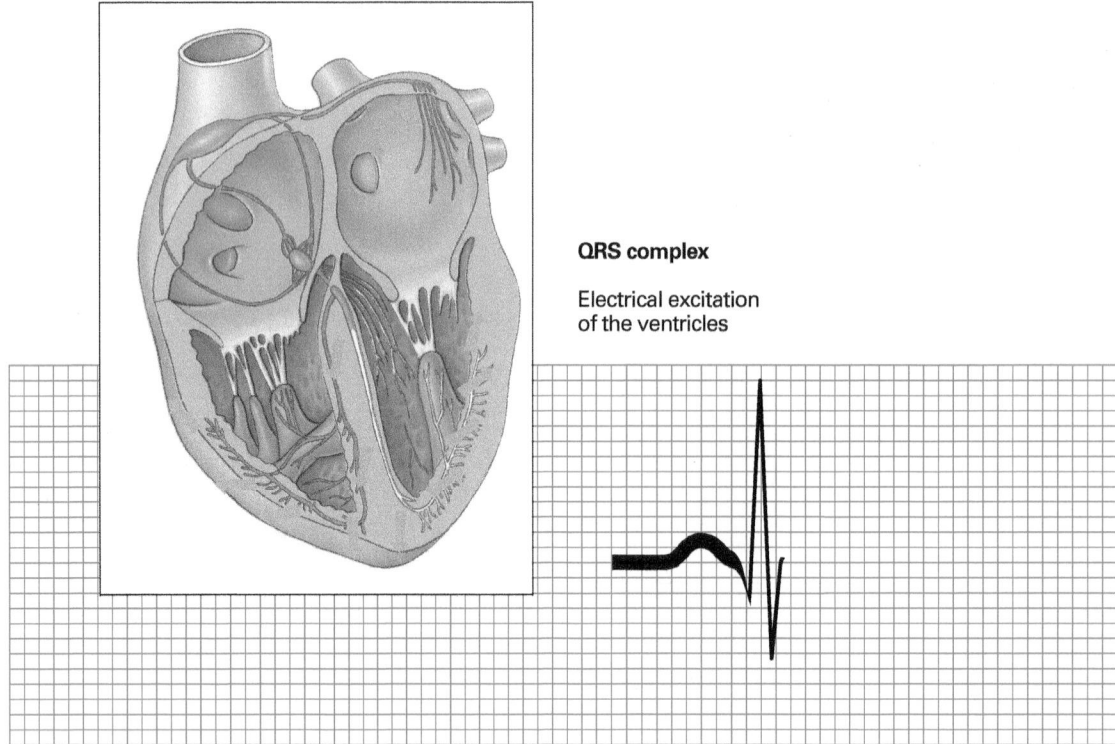

QRS complex

Electrical excitation
of the ventricles

FIGURE 49-3 QRS complex (ventricular depolarization).

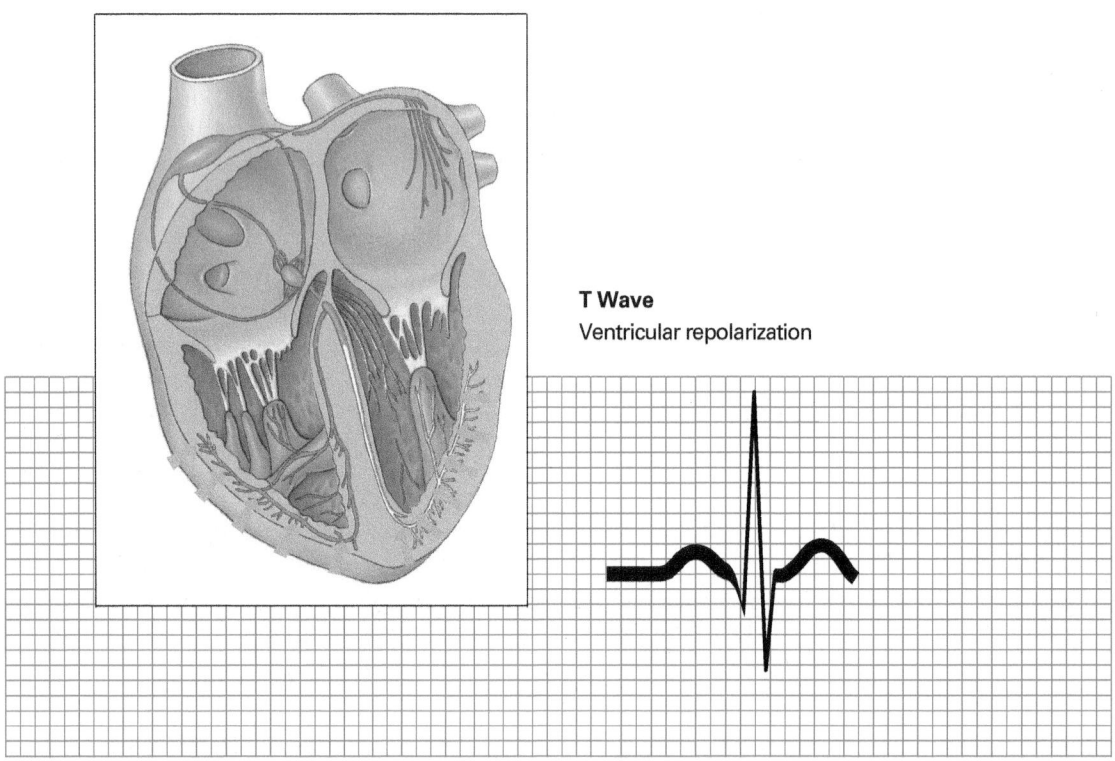

T Wave

Ventricular repolarization

FIGURE 49-4 T wave (ventricular repolarization).

Calculating Heart Rate

Heart rate is expressed as beats per minute. It is possible to estimate the heart rate from an ECG. Some offices have a protocol that states you should record additional cycles if the heart rate is above or below certain numbers. Many cardiologists also expect you to perform an exact calculation of the heart rate before you place the recording in the patient record or on the doctor's desk for review. Two methods for heart rate estimation and one for exact calculation are discussed next.

Abnormal heart rates are identified as either bradycardia (a heart rate less than 60 beats per minute) or tachycardia (a heart rate greater than 100 beats per minute).

Estimation of Heart Rate. To obtain an estimated heart rate of either the ventricular or the atrial contractions, use the six-second method. Count the number of P waves across 30 large, darker squares (30 squares = 6 seconds). Once you have the correct number, multiply by 10 (or simply add a 0 to the end of the counted number). Counting P waves will give you the estimated atrial contraction rate. To estimate heart rate based on ventricular contractions, simply measure the number of complete QRS complexes across a span of 30 large squares and multiply by 10.

Exact Calculation of Heart Rate. To obtain an exact calculation of the heart rate, recall that the paper moves at a standard speed of 25 mm/second, so it will move at 1,500 mm/minute (25 mm/second × 60 seconds = 1,500 mm/minute). An exact calculation of ventricular heart rate is achieved by counting the millimeter boxes (the smaller, lighter squares) between two QRS complexes and dividing that number into 1,500. For instance, if there is 20 mm between two QRS complexes, 1,500 divided by 20 equals 75 beats per minute. An exact calculation of atrial heart rate is achieved by counting the millimeter boxes between two P waves and by dividing that number into 1,500. These calculations are accurate only for the complexes that were examined.

Assessing Heart Rhythm

Heart rhythm is the regularity or irregularity of the occurrence of heartbeats. Ventricular rhythm is determined by measuring the distance between QRS complexes. There should be a fairly consistent space between complexes to qualify as a regular rhythm. Atrial rhythm is determined by measuring the distance between P waves. Again, for a regular rhythm, there should be a fairly consistent space between waves.

Train yourself to look at the rhythm while you are recording. Some offices have protocols about what extra tracings to record in the event the rhythm appears to you to be irregular.

THE ELECTROCARDIOGRAM MACHINE

Many types of ECG machines are in use, but all should be calibrated to align with the international standard. This means that the paper in all machines moves at the same speed of 25 mm/second and, given the same amount of electrical energy, the recording stylus will move the same distance (1 mV of electricity input will cause the stylus to deflect 10 mm), thus giving uniform recordings worldwide. Standardization is a means of verifying that each machine deflects 10 mm in response to 1 mV (millivolt) of electricity in sensitivity.

The majority of ECG machines used in the medical office are computerized. Computerized models have automatic features, so you may only need to push a button. All 10 electrodes are placed on the patient at the beginning of the procedure, and the computer switches from lead to lead in rapid succession. Before operating the machine, you will enter data directly into the ECG machine. Data usually includes the patient's name, date of birth, diagnoses, height, weight, age, blood pressure, medications taken, and information pertinent to the ECG. You may ask the patient these questions while entering the data in the computer, which helps the patient to relax a bit before beginning the procedure.

Two main types of ECG machines are used in the medical office: single channel and multichannel (Figure 49-5). When all leads have been recorded, the long strip must be cut apart at the specific leads and mounted onto an ECG mounting card. Mounting cards have adhesive areas to help in mounting

Professionalism The Life Span

The Child
ECGs are rarely performed on children except in cardiac offices, in cases of emergencies, or before some sports physicals. Lead placement is exactly the same as in an adult, but sometimes placing the leads can be a challenge because of the smaller available space for them. Because it is critically important to have cooperation for the ECG, parents may need to help persuade the child to cooperate. If the child is frightened, the test may not be accurate.

The Older Adult
The positioning of ECG leads on the older adult is the same as that for other adults. However, sometimes making the leads truly accurate can be a challenge because of a loss of elasticity in the skin. Older adults also have fragile skin. Be very careful not to rip the electrodes from the skin but, instead, hold traction on the skin and work the electrode off carefully. It may take a few minutes of being careful, but the patient will be grateful for the consideration.

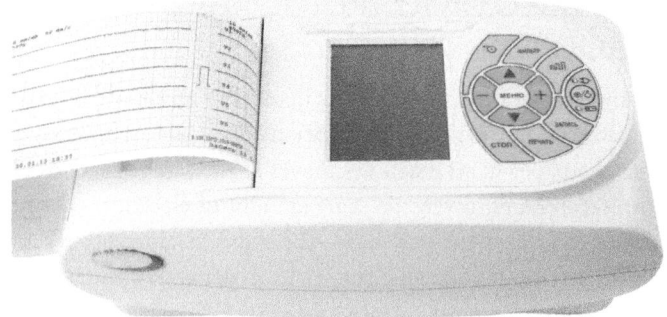
FIGURE 49-5 A multichannel ECG.

the strip sections. Figure 49-6 shows a properly mounted 12-lead, single channel ECG. A multichannel ECG records all 12 leads simultaneously. These ECGs have printouts on a much wider strip of paper, which is needed to show the multiple recordings. Multichannel ECGs are more commonly found in medical offices and require less time, because cutting and mounting aren't necessary.

It is possible to override automated machines if there is a need for manual controls. For example, the physician may have ordered just one rhythm strip of lead II, rather than a complete 12-lead ECG.

Many computerized models can record from more than one lead at once, which saves time and effort. Each is recorded in a separate channel or pathway for the signal and, typically, these machines record three channels at once. Other machines have a built-in interpretive feature and will print out a statement of the status of the heart. Some models can connect directly via fax with a regional office that will carry out the interpretation function and fax results to your office. As electronic health records (EHRs) become prevalent in medical offices, new ECG models will allow test results to be electronically transferred directly into the patient's medical

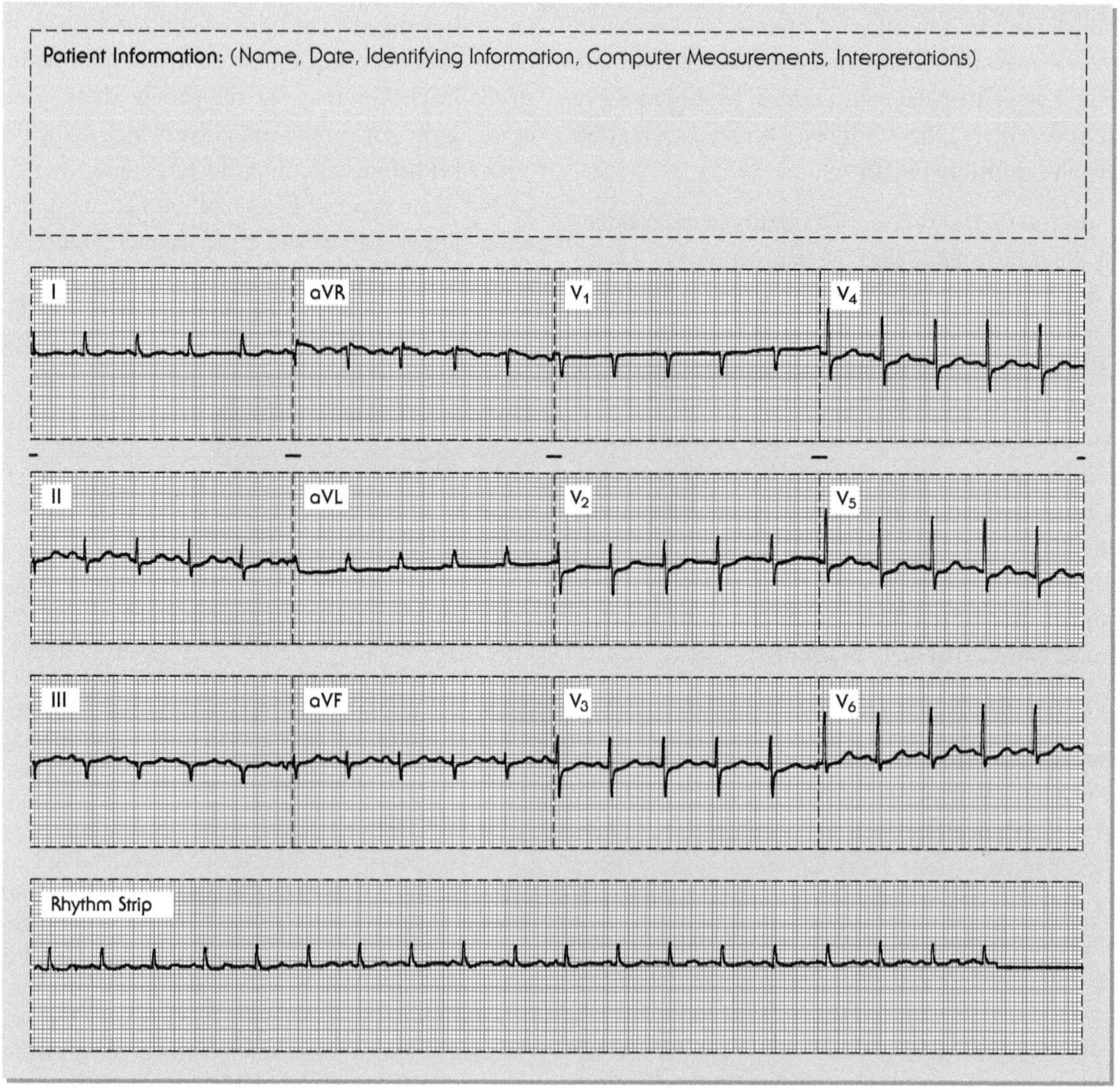

Patient Information: (Name, Date, Identifying Information, Computer Measurements, Interpretations)

I	aVR	V₁	V₄
II	aVL	V₂	V₅
III	aVF	V₃	V₆

Rhythm Strip

FIGURE 49-6 A properly mounted 12-lead, single channel ECG.

record. These models can also be configured to send the test electronically to a specialist for interpretation.

Although computerized electrocardiographs save considerable time in mounting ECGs, care should still be taken to ensure that a clear ECG is made before disconnecting the electrodes. Computerized electrocardiographs should also still be monitored for **artifacts** (errors). Common artifacts are discussed later in this chapter.

It is the medical assistant's responsibility to produce a clear and accurate tracing for each patient. Read the manufacturer's instructions for the machine in your office before using it. Knowledge of the control panel will help produce a tracing that is clear, accurate, and easy to read. A control panel usually includes the following features:

- **Main power switch (off/on)**—Allow for a warm-up time (as specified by the manufacturer) before using.

- **Record switch**—This switch moves the paper at the international standard "run 25" speed (25 mm/sec). Another option is "run 50" (50 mm/sec, or twice as fast). This is used when the heart rate is so rapid that interpretation requires that it be stretched out. This is used only for detailed interpretations because it tends to waste paper and can be more difficult to read.

- **Lead selector**—This determines from which electrodes the machine will record:
  - **Standard (limb) leads:** Record from two electrodes placed on all extremities.
  - **Augmented leads:** Record from the midpoint between two limb electrodes to a third limb electrode.
  - **Chest leads (also called precordial leads):** Record from various positions on the thorax.

- **Sensitivity control**—Allows the operator to increase or decrease the recording size to enlarge or shrink the deflections to fit on the paper. When changing from the international standard of sensitivity 1 to sensitivity ½ or sensitivity 2, the operator must include a standard for the interpreter information.

- **Standard button**—Allows verification of calibration to the international standard.

- **Stylus control**—Centers the recording in the middle of the page or the center of each channel by moving the stylus.

- **Stylus heat control**—Increases or decreases heat and adjusts for the sharpest tracing by the stylus. This control is seen on older models, but newer machines use an ink cartridge instead of a heat stylus.

- **Marker**—Indicates, by a code, which lead is being recorded.

Electrocardiogram Paper

Electrocardiogram paper is pressure- and photo-sensitive and must be handled carefully. If this paper is exposed to light for long periods, the markings will fade. Many newer machines use an ink cartridge to supply the stylus and provide a longer-lasting printout. Be sure to read the manufacturer's instructions carefully when changing the ink cartridges.

"Time" markers, referred to as three-second markers, are printed on all ECG paper. Look for them at the top of single-channel paper and between channels in multichannel paper. The time markers are small squares with a light line and larger squares with a darker line. The small squares are 1 mm by 1 mm square and represent 0.1 mV of voltage in the height and 0.04 second time in the width. The larger squares are 5 mm by 5 mm square and represent 0.5 mV of voltage in the height and 0.20 second time in the width. Thus, the paper records both time (horizontally) and voltage (vertically). See Figure 49-7 for ECG paper and markings.

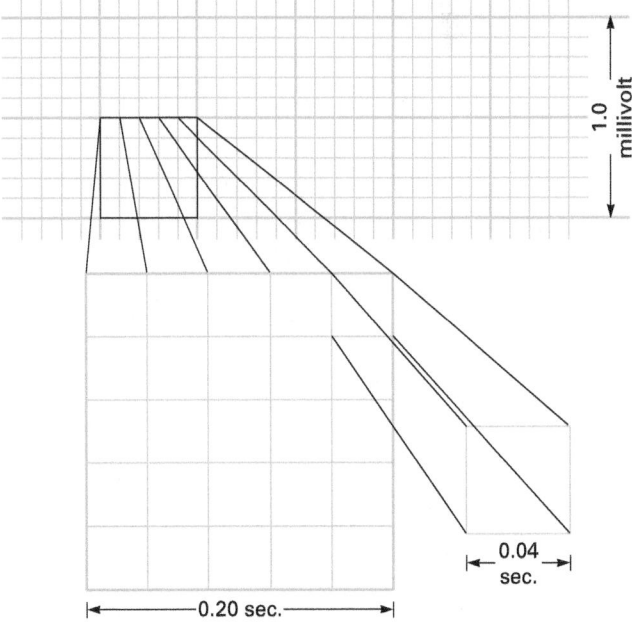

FIGURE 49-7 ECG paper and markings.

PERFORMING ELECTROCARDIOGRAPHY

The medical assistant may be asked to perform the procedure that records the electrical activity of the heart. As noted at the beginning of the chapter, the procedure is known as electrocardiography; the record produced is the electrocardiogram.

Electrocardiography does not introduce electricity into the heart; instead, it merely records the heart's own electrical activity. Whether the electrocardiogram is produced as a paper strip or a computerized record, that record is important to diagnosing the patient.

Electrode Placement

The ECG machine records the cardiac cycle through 10 electrodes (sensors) placed on the bare skin of the limbs (extremities) and the chest. After placement, long wires called leads will be attached to the electrodes. The term "lead" often refers to both electrode and wire.

Limb leads are placed over the fleshy part of the inner aspect of both lower legs and either both upper arms or both forearms, avoiding the bony prominences. These limb lead locations are abbreviated LA for left arm, RA for right arm, LL for left leg, and RL for right leg. The RL electrode serves as an electrical reference point and is not actually used in the recording. If you have a patient on whom you cannot place one of the limb leads as planned, you must place the electrodes on both extremities symmetrically. For example, a patient in a cast up to the knee requires that both electrodes be placed above the knee. If a hand and forearm are amputated, both arm electrodes must be placed on the upper arm.

Precordial leads are placed on the chest. The precordial leads, designated V, are placed on six locations on the chest and numbered V1, V2, V3, V4, V5, and V6. Placement of the precordial leads must be anatomically correct to ensure an accurate ECG. The precordial leads are placed in the following anatomical locations (Figure 49-8):

- V1—Fourth intercostal space, right sternal border
- V2—Fourth intercostal space, left sternal border
- V3—Midway between V2 and V4
- V4—Fifth intercostal space, left of the midclavicular line

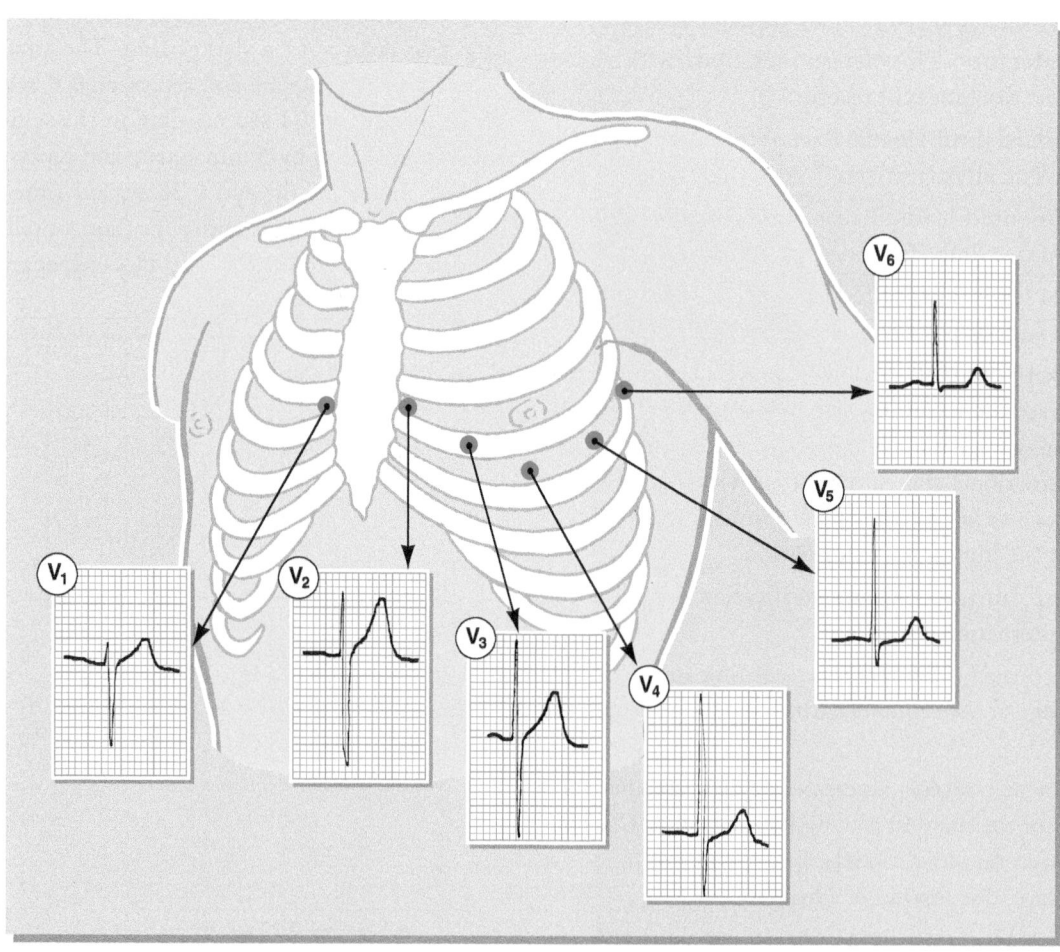

FIGURE 49-8 Electrode placement for chest leads V1–V6.

- V5—Left of the anterior axillary fold, in line with V4
- V6—Left of the midaxillary, in line with V4 and V5

An intercostal space is a space between ribs. The sternal border is the border of the sternum, or breastbone. The mid-clavicular line is an imaginary vertical line that runs through the middle of the clavicle, or collarbone. The anterior axillary fold is the fold at the front of the armpit. The midaxillary line is an imaginary vertical line that runs from the center of the armpit.

After the electrodes have been applied to the correct anatomical locations, the leads are attached. Leads are long wires that connect and transmit the electrical activity from the patient to the ECG machine. Each lead has a clip that attaches to the electrode. Leads are marked to correspond with the limb and chest electrode placements. The style of electrodes and clips varies with the manufacturer of the ECG machine. One single lead will record the electrical cardiac activity between where two electrodes are placed.

By recording from different combinations of directionality of electrodes, the electrical activity of the heart is seen from different angles. It is a bit like viewing a statue in a museum from multiple angles. Each view has different richness of information. A lead selector switch or lead indicator selects the combination of electrodes for that lead. One electrode is used for chest (unipolar) leads. A combination may be two electrodes, as with standard limb (bipolar) leads, or three electrodes, as with augmented limb leads.

With many leads and many views possible, when you are performing manual tracing, you must indicate on the tracing from which lead you are recording. An international marking system has been devised using dashes and dots. Most machines automatically mark the code just above the cardiac tracing. Others require manual marking of the locations, to which the leads are attached using the international code. Table 49-2 lists limb, augmented, and chest leads and proper placement and marking codes.

It is helpful to memorize the positions of electrodes used in the limb and augmented leads. Then, if you have difficulty getting a clear recording from one lead, you do not have to look at all the electrodes, only those involved. Some find it easier to remember all the leads and the electrodes being recorded (see Table 49-2) or by picturing **Einthoven's triangle**, which is a pictorial guide to the leads (Figure 49-9).

Patient Preparation

Patient preparation begins with providing the patient information about the test. A well-informed patient is more cooperative and less anxious. Explain the equipment, the procedure, and what the patient will be expected to do. The ECG is often performed in an exam room with the patient supine (lying on the back) on the exam table.

The surroundings should be pleasant and clean. The exam table should be wide enough for comfort and adequate support. Patients must be bare to the waist, so privacy must be provided for disrobing. Offer female patients a gown to be worn with the opening at the front. In addition, you will need access to bare skin on the lower legs. Instruct patients to remove socks or stockings and roll long pants legs out of the way. Position the patient comfortably supine with a pillow under the head and another under the knees if needed to

TABLE 49-2 | Electrode and Lead Placement and Marking Codes

Leads	Placement	Abbreviation	Marking Code
Limb Leads Lead I	Right arm to left arm	RA-LA	•
Lead II	Right arm to left leg	RA-LL	••
Lead III	Left arm to left leg	LA-LL	•••
Augmented Leads AVR	RA-midpoint (LA-LL)	(LA-LL) RA	-
AVL	LA-midpoint (RA-LL)	(RA-LL) LA	--
AVF	LL-midpoint (RA-LA)	(RA-LA) LL	---
Chest Leads V1	Fourth intercostal space, right sternal border		—•
V2	Fourth intercostal space, left sternal border		—••
V3	Midway between V2 and V4		—•••
V4	Fifth intercostal space, midclavicular left		—••••
V5	Left anterior axillary fold, horizontal to V4		—•••••
V6	Left midaxillary, horizontal to V4 and V5		—••••••

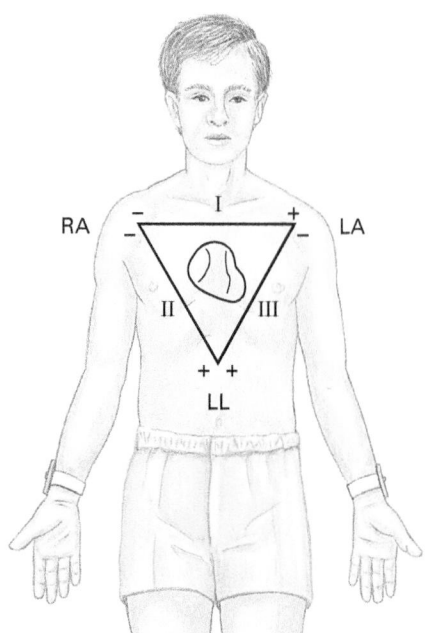

FIGURE 49-9 Einthoven's triangle.

eliminate back strain. If the patient cannot tolerate lying down, instead use the semi-Fowler's position (raising the back of the exam table so the patient is in a sitting position at about a 45-degree angle) and make a notation of the positional change in the patient's medical record.

Jewelry, particularly metal jewelry, must be removed so it does not interfere with the electrical current of the ECG. Prepare the skin where the electrodes will be applied. It is common for patients to use talcum powder, skin lotion, or shower gels that moisturize the skin. All of these products can leave residue on the skin that interferes with electrode contact. Such residue must be removed with alcohol before the electrolyte electrodes are applied. Additionally, some men have large amounts of chest hair, which can also interfere with electrode and skin contact. If so, you will need to shave small areas of the chest where electrodes will be placed.

Special Considerations

Sometimes special considerations are necessary for special patient issues. For example, if a patient has an amputated leg, then the electrode will be placed on the upper leg stump rather than the lower leg and the other electrode is placed directly across from the electrode on the stump. If the patient has a pacemaker or a dialysis catheter, notify the physician that leads were not in the usual position, because the pacemaker will probably be close to usual lead positioning. Patients with cognitive disabilities or small children may be unusually frightened of the procedure and may need to be reassured that no electricity is going into the body, but the machine is simply recording "sounds" inside the

body. Body piercings near leads may need to be removed or documented if they force the medical assistant to adjust the usual positioning of the lead. Avoid placing leads on scars or tattoos if at all possible, and document if you must put an electrode on one.

If a patient complains of any dyspnea, pain, or syncope during the ECG, the test should be discontinued and the physician notified immediately.

Technical Preparation

Technical preparation begins with ensuring that you have adequate supplies and that the ECG machine is correctly calibrated and in working order. When checking the ECG machine, plug the machine into a properly grounded outlet on an interior exam room wall. Allow it to warm up while you make other preparations. Verify that the machine is operational and in compliance with the international standard. The manufacturer of the ECG machine may suggest a series of quality control measures. It is important to keep instructional manuals in preapproved locations so that they can be easily located if necessary. When storing equipment after use, make sure it is cleaned and stored according to manufacturer's recommendations. It is prudent to have extra batteries, electrodes, and papers in stock for future use.

Procedure 49-1 details the steps for recording a 12-lead electrocardiograph. It is important to note that proper placement of the electrodes is imperative for accuracy. Therefore, extra review of the anatomical landmarks for the precordial electrodes (those on the chest) is recommended.

Mounting and Uploading

If the electrocardiograph produces paper strips, you will need to mount them correctly into the patient chart, usually by scanning or cutting and pasting. If you are cutting and pasting into the chart, cut part of the rhythm strip that includes the indicated number of cycles desired; paste them into the chart making sure you align the correct strip with its correct section. If the equipment produces digital results, these can be scanned or electronically uploaded into the EHR. Notify the physician and document the procedure after the results are mounted, scanned, or uploaded.

ADJUSTMENTS AND TROUBLESHOOTING

Sometimes the procedure does not go according to plan, so you need to be able to make appropriate adjustments depending on patient needs and troubleshoot problems. Care should be taken to avoid artifacts that can affect the results.

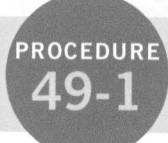

PROCEDURE 49-1

Performing a 12-Lead Electrocardiogram

Objective ◆ *Perform an ECG without assistance.*

EQUIPMENT AND SUPPLIES

ECG machine lead wires and patient cables, and power cord; ECG paper; electrodes; alcohol wipes; screwdriver, for adjustments, if needed; patient gown, if needed; razor, if needed.

METHOD

1. Assemble the necessary supplies and perform hand hygiene.
2. Greet and identify the patient; have the patient verify his full name and date of birth.
3. Introduce yourself and explain the procedure to the patient.
4. Begin technical preparation of the ECG machine by attaching the power cord and plugging in the machine to a grounded outlet.
5. Turn on the machine, allowing it time to warm up. Following office policy and manufacturer instructions, ensure that the machine is properly calibrated.
   a. Enter necessary patient data into the ECG machine.
6. Prepare the patient for the procedure.
   a. Offer female patients gowns to be worn with the opening down the front. Instruct female patients to remove the bra.
   b. Instruct male patients to remove the shirt so that the chest can be exposed.
   c. Both male and female patients should be instructed to remove shoes and socks or stockings.
   d. Instruct patients to roll up their pant legs to expose their lower legs.
   e. Instruct patients to remove any metal jewelry, because it can interfere with the electrical current of the ECG.
7. Position the patient in a supine position, flat on the examination table. Provide pillows for comfort, if necessary.
8. Prepare the patient's skin for electrodes by wiping the areas with alcohol wipes. Shave excessively hairy areas using a razor, if necessary.
9. Attach the electrodes to the appropriate anatomical landmarks (Figure A). Refer to Figure 49-8 on p. 1212 for additional placement guidance.
10. Connect all lead wires to the electrodes, making sure the wires remain untangled.

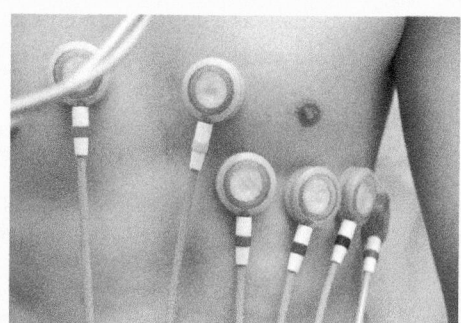

FIGURE A Chest or precordial leads in place.

11. Instruct the patient to relax, breathe normally, and refrain from speaking during the procedure.
12. For automatic machines, depress AUTO-RUN; for manual machines, select the leads in sequence and depress the correct button to run each individual lead. Use problem-solving skills if you encounter artifacts and repeat the recording if necessary so that the final tracing is clean and clear of artifacts.
13. Remove the lead wires from the electrodes and carefully put away the patient cable box with attached lead wires.
14. Carefully remove the electrodes from the patient's skin and wipe away any excess adhesive residue.
15. Perform hand hygiene.
16. Inform the patient that he may get dressed. Leave the room for privacy, taking the ECG machine and test with you.
17. In a quiet area, mount the ECG, if necessary, and transfer necessary patient information.
18. Chart the procedure in the patient's medical record.
19. Give the ECG to the physician for interpretation.
20. Clean the machine and accessories according to the manufacturer's instructions.

CHARTING EXAMPLE

3/11/YY 2:10 P.M. 12-lead ECG performed and given to Dr. Salpega to read. Patient appeared to tolerate procedure well and denies any discomfort.....................W. Short, CMA (AAMA)

Making Adjustments

A satisfactory tracing is one that is accurate, readable, and clear; travels across the center of the page; and has a baseline that is consistently horizontal. Deviations require adjustment of the machine and a new recording taken. If the baseline begins to drift upward or downward, use the position control knob to return it to the center of the page. Observe whether the tracing remains within the graph portion of the paper. If significant wave deflections occur, refer to the manufacturer's instruction manual to make the appropriate changes. Sometimes it is necessary to adjust the speed or sensitivity controls.

Normally the paper moves through the machine at the rate of 25 mm/second, but an option available in recording is to move the paper twice as fast, at 50 mm/second. This would only be necessary if the cardiac cycles were compacted by a very rapid heart rate. In this case, a better-quality cardiogram would be produced if the cycles were stretched out. If you have to change the speed or sensitivity, mark the tracing to indicate that you did so. In machines that mark the lead with an international code, the code marks are stretched out; the dots appear as dashes, and the dashes are long ones.

Multichannel machines produce an ECG very quickly on a single sheet of paper about 8 × 11 inches. You will have to center three baselines. A sensitivity or speed change affects all three channels.

Knowledge of the leads and their electrode locations will help you trace any irregular or erratic markings (artifacts) back to the source. You can also perform other troubleshooting techniques during the recording process. Failure to make the necessary corrections will result in an unsatisfactory tracing. The physician will not be able to read and interpret such a recording.

Artifacts

Occasionally, the electrodes will either not work properly, or they will detect electrical activity from a source other than the heart. These deflections, or artifacts, impair accurate interpretation of the tracing. You must find the cause of the artifact and correct it. Causes of artifacts and how to correct them include the following:

- **Somatic tremor**—This artifact is caused by a tense muscle or a muscle contraction, even one that you cannot see. This muscular activity causes unwanted stylus movement while the ECG is recording. It may result from patient discomfort, tension, chills, talking, or moving. Calm and reassure the patient. Suggest that the patient relax, breathe normally, and not talk. If necessary, place the patient's hands, palm side down, under the hips. This is especially helpful if the patient is not relaxed on the narrow table. This position is also best for patients with a tremor disorder. They will display the smallest number of artifacts in this position. Figure 49-10 illustrates somatic tremor artifacts.

- **Wandering baseline**—Baseline sway and baseline shift (Figure 49-11) are caused by poor electrode contact with the skin, such as when electrodes are dirty or applied too tightly or too loosely, when lotion or talcum prevents good contact with the skin, or when the patient cable slips toward the floor and pulls on the lead wires. You must readjust, reapply, or clean the electrodes and place the patient cable securely on the table. You may need to clean the skin with alcohol or shave chest hair to allow proper electrode skin contact.

- **60-cycle or AC (alternating current) interference**—Electrical current in wires and equipment may be picked up by the patient's body and the recording machine. This appears in the recording as small

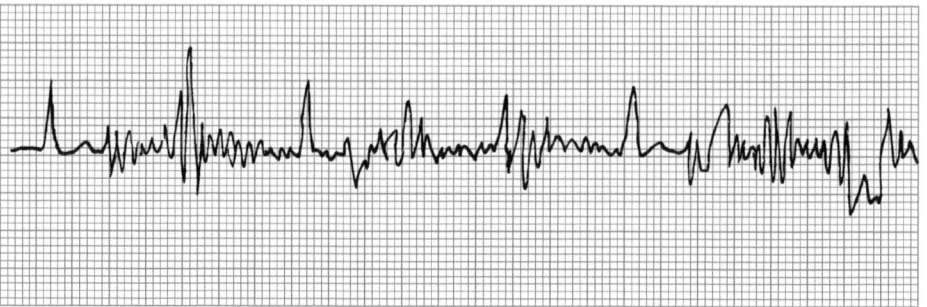

FIGURE 49-10 Somatic tremors artifact.

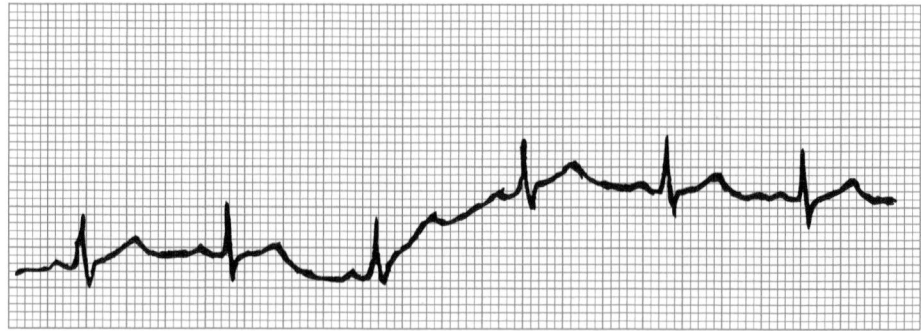

FIGURE 49-11 Wandering baseline.

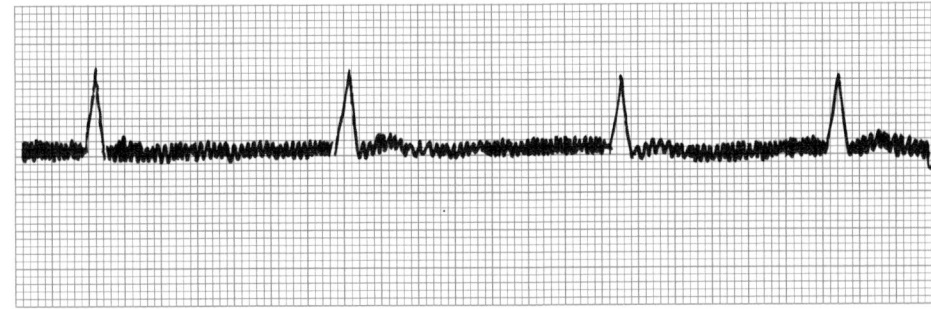

FIGURE 49-12 60-cycle interference.

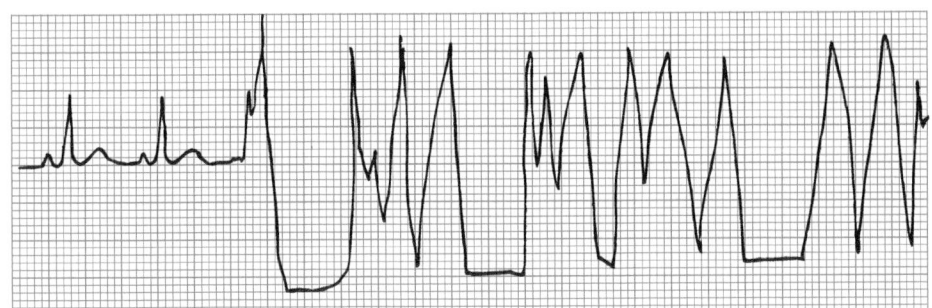

FIGURE 49-13 Broken recording.

regular spikes or static, and is caused by improper grounding, nearby electrical equipment in use, or twisted and coiled lead wires. Ground the machine properly. Unplug other electrical equipment in the area. Move the machine to an interior wall outlet away from outlets containing other cables. You may have to wait until a procedure in an adjacent room, such as an X-ray, is completed (Figure 49-12).

- **Broken recording**—Loose or broken lead wires cause the stylus to thrash erratically and to go off the page, leading to broken recording. Repair the wires, replace them, or call for service on the equipment (Figure 49-13).

Fortunately, most ECG machines today are so technologically advanced that they are able to detect and override artifacts.

Evaluating the Electrocardiogram

Interpreting an electrocardiogram is out of the medical assistant's scope of practice. However, you must be able to evaluate and assess the ECG to ensure that it is an acceptable tracing. As just discussed, if you detect an artifact, take measures to correct the issue and retest the patient.

Some offices may require you to calculate the patient's heart rate according to the ECG results. Finally, review the ECG to look for abnormalities in the patient's heart

activity that you should immediately bring to the attention of the physician.

What Is Normal?

A normal sinus rhythm means that each heartbeat has three distinct waves: a P wave; a T wave; and—between the P and T—a QRS complex where the Q is a downward deflection, the R is an upward deflection, and the S is a downward deflection following an R. In a normal rhythm, the beats come at regular intervals, indicating that the impulse originates in the SA node. Within the lead being recorded, each cardiac cycle appears the same as previous cycles. To recognize abnormalities, you must first be able to recognize what is normal. Figure 49-14 illustrates and identifies features of a normal 12-lead ECG.

Most newer ECG machines used today will print out an interpretation and abnormalities will be identified. Interpretation of ECGs is outside the medical assistant's scope of practice, but you should be able to recognize what is normal and be able to perform an ECG in such a way that the results are accurate. The ECG machines themselves will help identify abnormalities and facilitate diagnosis.

Abnormalities

Occasionally, a tracing will reveal an abnormality caused by cardiac pathology in the patient. An observant medical assistant will recognize the more common abnormalities and draw them to the attention of the physician or will follow office protocol, which often calls for an additional recording of a

---

Professionalism

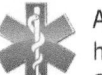 As a health care provider, you must maintain a healthy lifestyle and set an example for patients. Cardiac risk factors (age, gender, heredity, smoking, obesity, hyperlipidemia, hypertension, stress, and excessive drinking or use of drugs) can affect anyone. Be a living example of a healthy lifestyle by engaging in regular exercise, making healthy food choices, and avoiding use of recreational drugs and excessive alcohol consumption. Encourage patients to do the same.

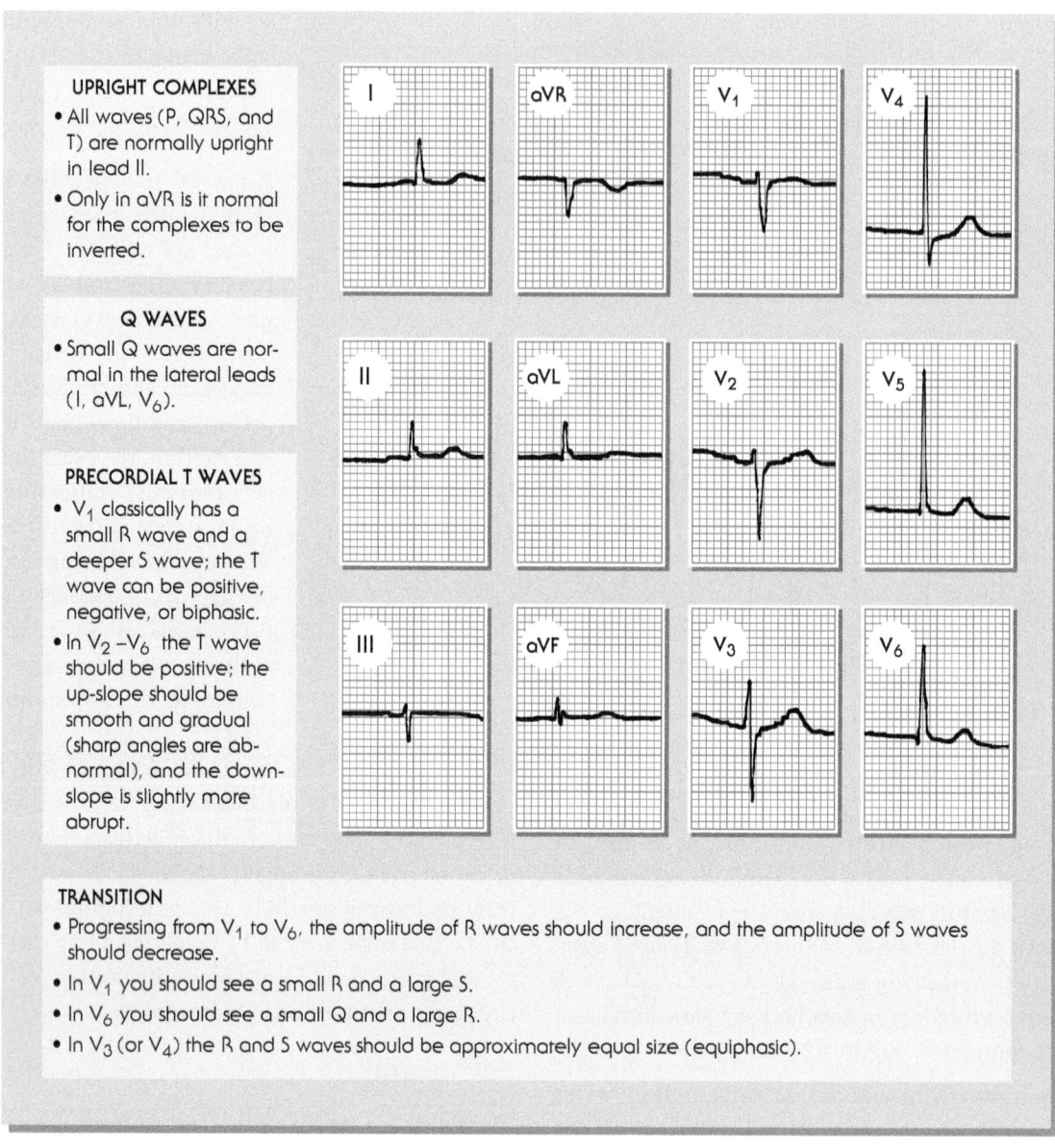

UPRIGHT COMPLEXES

• All waves (P, QRS, and T) are normally upright in lead II.

• Only in aVR is it normal for the complexes to be inverted.

Q WAVES

• Small Q waves are normal in the lateral leads (I, aVL, V₆).

PRECORDIAL T WAVES

• V_1 classically has a small R wave and a deeper S wave; the T wave can be positive, negative, or biphasic.

• In V_2 –V_6 the T wave should be positive; the up-slope should be smooth and gradual (sharp angles are abnormal), and the down-slope is slightly more abrupt.

TRANSITION

• Progressing from V_1 to V_6, the amplitude of R waves should increase, and the amplitude of S waves should decrease.

• In V_1 you should see a small R and a large S.

• In V_6 you should see a small Q and a large R.

• In V_3 (or V_4) the R and S waves should be approximately equal size (equiphasic).

FIGURE 49-14 Features of a normal 12-lead ECG.

particular lead. Table 49-3, which includes Figures 49-15 to 49-22, lists some cardiac pathology that can be visualized by ECGs, including references to several examples of the abnormalities listed.

SPECIAL PROCEDURES
Additional Tracings

Some ECG-related diagnostic procedures are performed regularly in the primary care office or in cardiology. The following two procedures involve recording additional lengths of tracings and may be part of written office protocol for cardiograms.

The first, a **rhythm strip**, is run on lead II for 20 seconds at the physician's request or if the medical assistant sees

anything that appears abnormal on the tracing. This is not cut and mounted but carefully folded and given to the physician for interpretation.

The second procedure, an **inspiration strip**, is run on lead II for 10 seconds with the patient holding her breath. This is of greatest value when, as the patient breathes, your tracing shows a wandering baseline. This will eliminate any respiratory impact on the tracing.

Exercise Tolerance Testing

At times, patients will have symptoms that are not obvious on a resting ECG. A **stress test**, or treadmill test, involves an evaluation of the heart's response during moderate exercise while a 12-lead ECG is performed. It is a diagnostic procedure performed to determine the likelihood of coronary

TABLE 49-3 | Abnormalities Caused by Cardiac Pathology

Abnormality	Description
Atrial fibrillation	There are as many as 350 irregular P waves and 130–150 irregular QRS complexes per minute (Figure 49-15). **FIGURE 49-15** Atrial fibrillation.
Atrial flutter	This rapid fluttering of the upper chambers looks on the ECG like the pattern of teeth on a saw. The atrial rate is 250–350 per minute. Not all the impulses are conducted through the AV node, because they are coming too fast. There is some "blockage" at the AV node. This is one type of heart block (Figure 49-16). **FIGURE 49-16** Atrial flutter.
AV heart block	The node is diseased and does not conduct the impulse well. There are three types: first degree, in which the PR interval is prolonged; second degree, in which some waves do not pass through to the ventricles; and third degree or complete AV block, in which the atria and ventricles beat independently (Figure 49-17). **FIGURE 49-17** Third-degree heart block.
Junctional arrhythmia	Cardiac rhythms arising from the atrioventricular (AV) junction that usually occur as an automatic tachycardia or as an escape mechanism during periods of significant bradycardia with rates slower than the intrinsic junctional pacemaker.
Myocardial infarction (MI)	There are broad and deep Q waves. *Old injury:* The ST segment is usually depressed below the baseline. A depressed wave below baseline can indicate an old MI or a current MI and is often indicated in patients with coronary artery disease. *New injury:* The ST segment is usually elevated above the baseline. Angina pectoris is the name for the syndrome of pain and oppression in the anterior chest caused by heart tissue being deprived of oxygen. If this pain lasts 20–30 minutes, suspect a myocardial infarction in which the heart tissue is actually dying.

(continued)

TABLE 49-3 | Abnormalities Caused by Cardiac Pathology (*continued*)

Abnormality	Description
Paroxysmal atrial tachycardia (PAT)	There is a common arrhythmia, usually seen in young adults with normal hearts. There are no visible P waves, because they are hidden by the T wave of the previous cycle. The atrial rate is 140–250 per minute.
Premature atrial contractions (PACs)	A P wave occurs earlier than expected, usually from a source outside the sinus node. Therefore, P waves are distorted.
Premature ventricular contractions (PVCs)	The wide QRS complexes occur without preceding P waves. They may be caused by electrolyte imbalance, stress, smoking, alcohol, or toxic reactions to drugs and in a majority of patients who have had a heart attack (Figure 49-18). FIGURE 49-18 Multifocal premature ventricular contractions (PVCs).
Sinus arrhythmia	Normally seen in children and young adults; all aspects of the ECG are normal except the irregularity. The space between QRS complexes is not equal. The heart rate increases on inspiration and decreases on expiration.
Sinus bradycardia	There are fewer than 60 beats per minute; cycles are normal (Figure 49-19). FIGURE 49-19 Sinus bradycardia.
Sinus tachycardia	There are more than 100 beats per minute; cycles are normal (Figure 49-20). FIGURE 49-20 Sinus tachycardia.

(*continued*)

TABLE 49-3 | Abnormalities Caused by Cardiac Pathology (*continued*)

Abnormality	Description
Ventricular fibrillation	The waves are irregular and rounded, the contractions uncoordinated. Death may occur in as little as four minutes (Figure 49-21). **FIGURE 49-21** Ventricular fibrillation.
Ventricular tachycardia	Three or more consecutive PVCs. Usually originating below the SA node, the complexes are wide and bizarre in appearance (Figure 49-22). **FIGURE 49-22** Ventricular tachycardia.

artery disease (CAD), blockage of the arteries that supply the heart muscle. The patient is asked to exercise on a bicycle or treadmill, which stresses the heart and requires more oxygen for the heart muscle cells. A faster heart rate makes it easier to detect decreased blood flow.

Stress testing may be used to evaluate patients with a high risk for developing heart disease, known to have early heart disease, or about to begin a strenuous exercise program. This test is also done on patients who have cardiac complaints such as shortness of breath when exercising and as an evaluation of their rehabilitation following cardiac surgery. The treadmill test is noninvasive, and frequent blood pressure measurements are taken while exercise is in progress.

The stress test is continued until the **maximum target heart rate** is achieved or the patient becomes symptomatic. The maximum target heart rate is calculated by first establishing the **maximum heart rate**, determined by using the following formula: 220 minus the patient's age = the maximum heart rate for that person.

To determine the maximum target heart rate for the stress test procedure, which is 85 percent of the patient's maximum heart rate, multiply the maximum heart rate by 0.85.

The complete formula to determine the maximum target heart rate is 220 − the patient's age × 0.85. As an example, for a 60-year-old patient, 220 − 60 = 160 × 0.85 (85%) = 136, or the maximum target heart rate for this patient.

For patients who have had a myocardial infarction (MI), the target heart rate is set lower, at 70 percent. This is known as a submaximal test.

The test concludes when the patient's symptoms of chest pain or fatigue or ECG changes indicate significant changes, especially to the ST segment. After the conclusion of the

Professionalism   The Law

Stress tests or thallium scans require that a consent form be signed by the patient before the procedure, because these tests may lead to serious arrhythmias. Close monitoring by the assistant and the presence of a physician are also required for these procedures. If the medical assistant detects a potentially life-threatening arrhythmias, it is a professional duty to immediately notify the physician.

test, the patient rests while the monitoring of blood pressure and heart rate continue until both are within normal range. Complications may occur, and appropriately stocked emergency carts should be on hand.

Patient Preparation

Medical assistants are often in charge of scheduling stress tests and other outpatient procedures. In addition to simply providing the patient with the scheduled date and time, it is important to provide patient instruction and education about the procedure. The patient should be instructed to wear comfortable exercise or walking shoes and loose-fitting clothes on the day of the test. Female patients should be instructed to wear a bra to minimize artifacts on the ECG. Instruct all patients not to eat a large meal for at least four hours before the test to avoid nausea. Patients should take their normal medications unless otherwise instructed by the physician.

Inform the patient that baseline vital signs and a resting ECG are recorded first. Vital signs are measured with the patient in supine position and standing. Another ECG is taken with the patient standing and **hyperventilating** (breathing rapidly). This is done because rapid breathing can produce some changes in the ST segment and the T wave on the ECG recording. It is important to know this in advance so the interpretation of the stress test ECG is not compromised. Also, a thorough history is taken emphasizing any symptoms such as shortness of breath or chest pain. Explain to the patient that an ECG will be recorded as the patient walks or bikes at a carefully prescribed pace in the presence of the physician. Increases in rate or incline will be made, but the patient should not feel discomfort or shortness of breath.

Varieties of Stress Tests

The physician may order additional types of stress tests either based on the outcome of an exercise tolerance test or based on patient limitations. Medical assistants should be familiar with these tests so that they can be ready to answer questions that the patient might have.

Thallium (a radioisotope that emits gamma rays and is used in nuclear medicine) is sometimes injected into the patient's vein during a stress test for better understanding of **perfusion** (blood flow to the myocardium). Thallium is injected during the last minute of exercise. The patient lies on a special table, and a gamma camera takes pictures. If the heart muscle is **ischemic** (receiving less than the normal amount of blood flow), poor uptake of the thallium will occur. This is indicated as a "cold spot" on the pictures. Normal perfusion of the myocardium is indicated by "hot spots" on the pictures.

Another type of test, the **multiple gated acquisition (MUGA) scan**, can be done to check blood flow in the myocardium. This involves injection of an isotope and having a nuclear scan performed to detect myocardial perfusion. Pharmacological stress testing does not involve exercise. In this case, a medication is given to the patient that causes the heart rate to climb to the target heart rate. Continuous ECGs and vital sign evaluation are performed. This test procedure is useful on patients with physical limitations or those who cannot perform enough exercise to elevate the heart rate.

Holter Monitor

The **Holter monitor** records cardiac activity while the patient is ambulatory for at least a 24-hour period. Holter monitoring might be ordered if the results of an ECG are inconclusive or cardiac irregularity was not captured on the tracing. A small recording device and a patient diary are used to detect heart irregularities that are infrequent and not detected on the standard 12-lead cardiogram (Figure 49-23). Today, most Holter monitors are digital recorders. However, some offices may still use the older models that use cassette tape recorders. The monitor is often set to record continuously and/or to record when the patient presses an "event" button at the onset of symptoms. A medical assistant may instruct the patient and apply the chest electrodes.

During patient preparation, stress the importance of the diary. While wearing the monitor, patients will carry out all routine daily activities except showering or bathing. They must also avoid areas of high voltage, because it could interfere with the recording. Patients use the diary to record their activities during the day such as stair climbing, sexual activity, having bowel movements, sleeping, eating, exercising, and so forth. They also indicate in the diary or by depressing an "event button" when they experience any cardiac symptoms, such as chest pain, shortness of breath, or palpitations. Patients should record such events in the diary. The

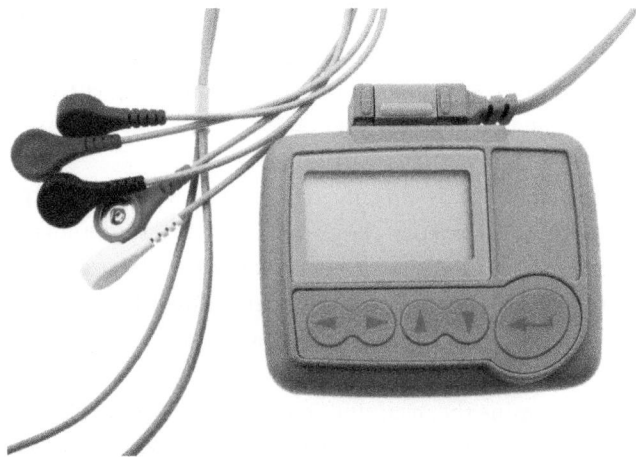

FIGURE 49-23 A digital Holter monitor.

physician will compare the tape with the activity log to determine which activities were stressing the patient.

The five special disposable chest electrodes are attached more securely than in the 12-lead ECG because they must remain in place during all activity. In addition to the usual skin preparation to remove oils, areas for attachment may have to be shaved and an abrasive skin cleaner used. Electrodes are placed in the following locations:

- Third intercostal space 2 or 3 inches to the right of the sternum
- Third intercostal space 2 or 3 inches to the left of the sternum
- Fifth intercostal space at the left sternum margin
- Sixth intercostal space at the right anterior axillary line
- Sixth intercostal space at the left anterior axillary line

Procedure 49-2 describes the procedure for applying a Holter monitor.

Cardiac Event Monitor

To capture a record of a cardiac event, a physician may provide the patient a cardiac event monitor to use for a period of time. The physician might ask the patient to use the monitor until one event occurs and is recorded or might ask the patient to use it during a certain time span. For patients who have infrequent events, the physician might ask the patient to use the monitor for up to 30 days to ensure that any events will be captured.

With a cardiac event monitor, electrodes are worn much as they would be for a Holter monitor. The patient presses a button on the monitor when perceiving a cardiac event such as a rapid or slow heartbeat or dizziness or feeling faint. The equipment records heart activity for five minutes after the depression of the button. Some monitors record the information; some permit sending the information by telephone to the physician or to a receiving center. The patient may also keep a diary to align the event with activity at the time. For example, the patient might note having events only when climbing stairs.

Mobile Cardiac Telemetry

Some patients can have their heart activity monitored and measured from far away through **telemetry**. Mobile cardiac telemetry (MCT) allows a device to send data continually to a facility that is staffed 24 hours per day. It is then interpreted by a qualified, cardiac-trained registered nurse. In contrast to the cardiac event monitor, MCT provides real-time monitoring and analysis. There are a wide variety of telemetry monitors—with 3, 5, and 12 leads. Leads are placed according to

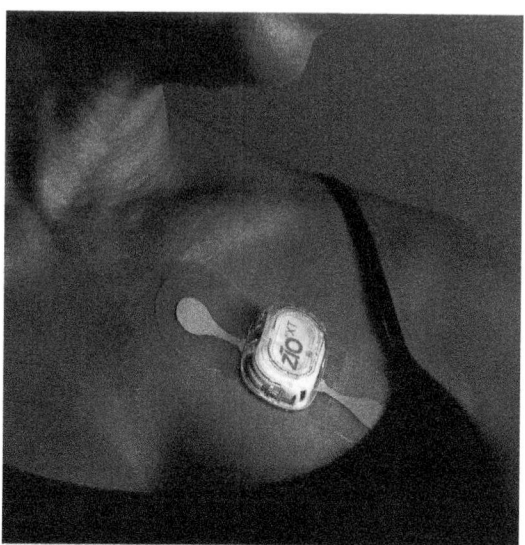

FIGURE 49-24 A ZIO Patch telemetry monitor.

manufacturer's instructions. Figure 49-24 shows one type of telemetry monitor.

To be successful, it is very important for the medical assistant to ensure that the patient understands how to use the telemetry monitor and is comfortable with using the technology for telemetry. Encourage the patient to call the help number that comes with the equipment to learn how to attach the leads and use the equipment correctly and to get help should any problems arise while the equipment is being used.

Pacemakers

Pacemakers are electronic devices that help the heart maintain normal rhythm. They may be used to increase heart rate in patients with bradycardia (slow heart rate), to decrease the heart rate in a patient with tachycardia (rapid heart rate), or to correct other dysrhythmias. Pacemakers may be temporarily or permanently installed in the patient. Temporary pacemakers

> **Professionalism** | Cultural Considerations
>
> Although many men may not have a problem with shaving chest hair if it is necessary for an ECG, many cultures and religions may consider this practice to be taboo. If a male patient protests the idea of having to shave chest hair based on religious or cultural beliefs, it is important not to argue with the patient. If this circumstance arises, it would be best to inform the physician of the patient's concern and continue with the ECG without shaving the chest. It would be necessary to document in the medical record that the ECG was performed but that the patient did not allow his chest to be shaved to ensure proper lead placement and connectivity.

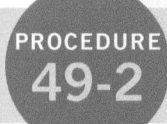

PROCEDURE 49-2

Applying a Holter Monitor

Objective ◆ *Apply a Holter monitor and instruct the patient.*

EQUIPMENT AND SUPPLIES

Holter monitor with electrodes; patient cable; patient activity diary; fresh batteries or charging device; blank recording tape or digital flashcard or microchip; adhesive tape; razor, if needed; alcohol wipes; dry washcloth

METHOD

1. Assemble the necessary supplies.
2. Install new batteries; depending on the model, make sure the digital storage unit (flashcard or microchip) has the maximum amount of memory. For older models, insert a new blank cassette tape.
3. Verify that the machine is operational.
4. Introduce yourself and then identify, interview, and instruct the patient according to office protocol. Explain the importance of accurately recording in the diary as well as depressing the event button at the correct times.
5. Have the patient remove clothing to the waist (female patients may wear a gown open down the front) and sit on an examination table.
6. Perform hand hygiene.
7. Prepare the electrode sites by shaving small patches of chest hair where the electrodes will be placed (if necessary). Using alcohol wipes, wipe the skin to remove any residue that could interfere with electrode placement. Allow the skin to air dry.
8. Using a dry washcloth or other abrasive material, rub the skin where the electrodes will be placed. This will help the electrodes stick to the skin more effectively.
9. Attach the electrodes according to the manufacturer's instructions. The electrodes will be placed in these locations: third intercostal space 2 or 3 inches to the right of the sternum, third intercostal space 2 or 3 inches to the left of the sternum, fifth intercostal space at the left sternum margin, sixth intercostal space at the right anterior axillary line, and sixth intercostal space at the left anterior axillary line (Figure A).
10. Attach the wires so that they point toward the feet, and then connect the patient cable.
11. Secure each electrode with adhesive tape.
12. Assist the patient with replacing his shirt. Extend the cable between the buttons or under the hem.
13. Place the recorder in the carrying case, and either attach to the patient's belt or place the neck strap around the patient's neck. Check that there is no tension on the wires.

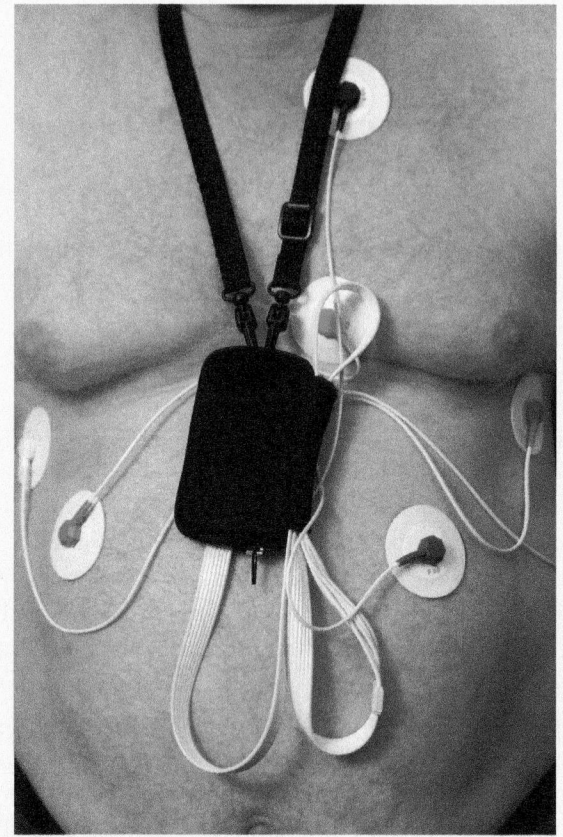

FIGURE A Correct electrode placement for a Holter monitor.

14. Plug the cable into the recorder.
15. Record the starting time in the diary.
16. Ensure that the patient understands what to do by having the patient repeat the instructions for pressing the event button as well as what to record in the diary.
17. Confirm the time for the patient to return to the clinic for removal of the Holter monitor.
18. Chart the procedure in the patient's record.

CHARTING EXAMPLE

3/11/YY 4:15 P.M. Holter monitor applied and instruction given. Patient to return in 24 hours with diary and monitor. Patient verbalized understanding and repeated back instructions...........
....E. Blodgett, CMA (AAMA)

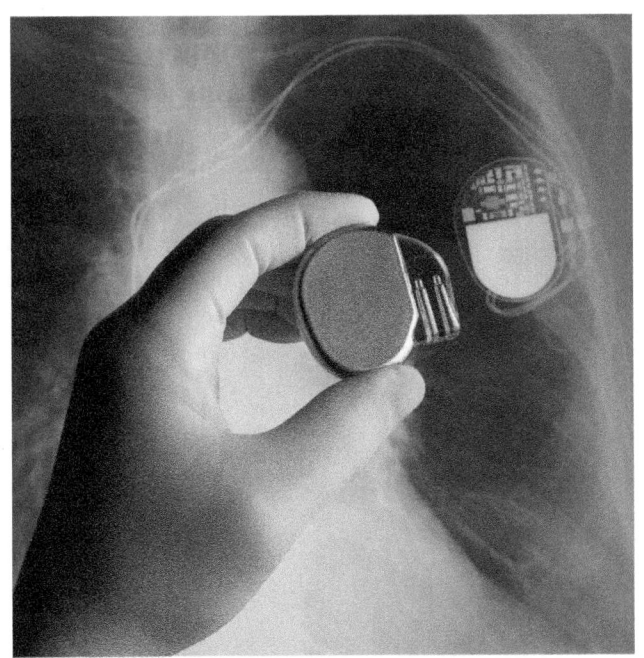

FIGURE 49-25 A surgeon holds a pacemaker next to an X-ray of a pacemaker implanted in a patient's chest.

are used in acute settings to stabilize and maintain the patient for shorter periods of time. Patients with temporary pacemakers must be hospitalized and continuously monitored. The pulse generator is located outside the body, and leads are threaded through specific veins (subclavian, femoral, brachial, or external jugular) to either the right atrium or the right ventricle. A temporary pacemaker may be attached during surgery to the outer surface of the heart. The wires then exit the chest and are attached to an external pulse generator.

The type of permanent pacemaker implanted depends on the patient's condition and the type of cardiac problem involved. These are long-term devices, and the pulse generator is implanted into the subcutaneous tissue of the upper chest (Figure 49-25). The leads are inserted into a major vein leading into the heart in the region of the myocardium that is impaired. The opposite ends of the leads are attached to the pulse generator. Figure 49-26 illustrates both temporary and permanent pacemakers.

Some pacemakers are fixed rate, or continuous. Some fire only when needed (on demand). Some are rate-responsive to physiological changes and respond to the body's demands

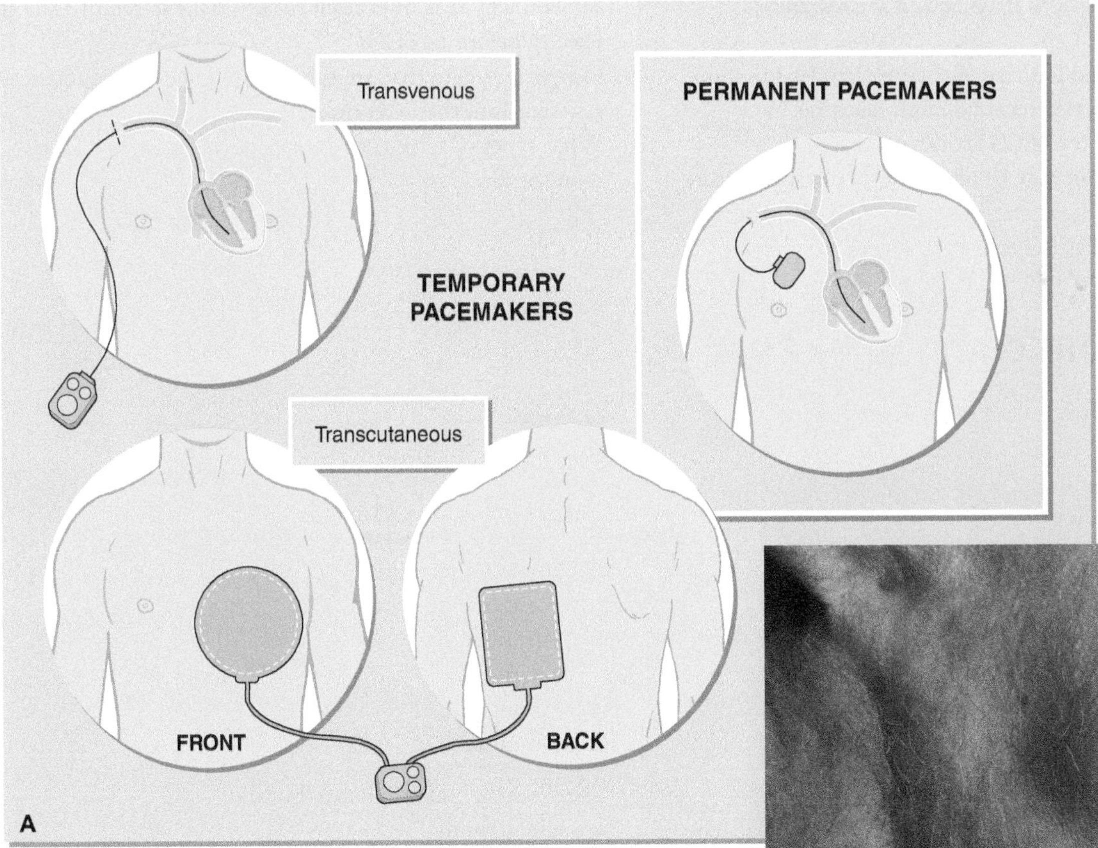

Transvenous

PERMANENT PACEMAKERS

TEMPORARY PACEMAKERS

Transcutaneous

FRONT   BACK

A

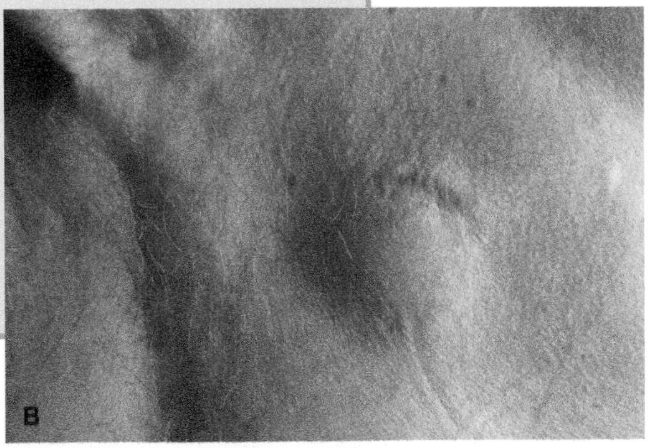

B

FIGURE 49-26 (A) Temporary and permanent pacemakers. (B) A pacemaker in a patient's chest.

according to changes in the patient's activities. The atrial-paced pacemaker will show a spike with the P wave. The pacemaker spike appears as a long vertical line, usually rhythmically paced before the P wave. Pacemakers that spike with the QRS wave are ventricular-paced.

Notify the physician if the implanted pacemaker is visible on the surface of the skin, because this would signify movement of the implanted device.

SUMMARY

The use of electrocardiography for the early diagnosis and treatment of heart disease has contributed to the lengthened life expectancy of many patients and has improved their quality of life. ECGs are usually performed while the patient is lying down. Sometimes ECGs are done in combination with stressful exercise to see the effect on the heart. If a patient experiences dyspnea, pain, or syncope during the stress test, the test is aborted and the physician notified immediately. The patient may be monitored for 24 hours with a Holter monitor to see which activities stress the heart. Accuracy in carrying out your duties during these tests will provide the physician with the best possible data to make that diagnosis and institute the correct treatment.

(49) CHAPTER REVIEW

COMPETENCY REVIEW

1. Define and spell the terms for this chapter.
2. Explain the abbreviations EKG and ECG. Are they interchangeable?
3. Identify by name and location of their electrodes the standard 12 leads on an electrocardiograph machine.
4. Name and describe four ECG artifacts.
5. Explain why a patient may be placed on a Holter monitor.
6. Describe how a thallium stress test would visualize heart abnormalities, such as ischemia.
7. Name the components of a cardiac wave pattern.
8. Explain why it is important for a patient to remove all jewelry before an ECG.
9. List patient data that are typically entered by the medical assistant into the ECG machine.
10. What types of activities will a patient record in a Holter monitor diary?

PREPARING FOR THE CERTIFICATION EXAM

1. In an ECG, the electrode used in grounding is
   a. LA.
   b. LL.
   c. RA.
   d. RL.
   e. V1.

2. When taking an ECG, the position of the first chest lead V1 is
   a. third intercostal space, left sternal margin.
   b. third intercostal space, right sternal margin.
   c. fourth intercostal space, left sternal margin.
   d. fourth intercostal space, right sternal margin.
   e. fifth intercostal space, midclavicular line.

3. The second wave of the ECG is the
   a. S wave.
   b. Q wave.
   c. P wave.
   d. T wave.
   e. R wave.

4. When the ECG is running at normal speed, the paper is moving at the rate of
   a. 10 mm/sec.
   b. 20 mm/sec.
   c. 25 mm/sec.
   d. 35 mm/sec.
   e. 50 mm/sec.

5. The sinoatrial node is located in the
   a. right atrium.
   b. left atrium.
   c. apex.
   d. ventricles.
   e. septum between the atria.

6. The portion of the ECG that relates to ventricular repolarization is the
   a. P wave.
   b. QRS complex.
   c. T wave.
   d. U wave.
   e. P-R interval.

7. A device used to obtain continual heart monitoring over a 24- to 48-hour period is a/an
   a. pacemaker.
   b. oscilloscope.
   c. electrocardiogram.
   d. Holter monitor.
   e. ventilator.

8. A myocardial infarction
   a. is the medical term for a heart attack.
   b. indicates a problem in the ECG machine.

   c. rarely happens in young adults.
   d. is an artifact on an ECG tracing.
   e. is a congenital disorder.

9. Regarding the ECG, mV stands for
   a. millivolt.
   b. megavolt.
   c. maximum voltage.
   d. marginal voltage.
   e. minimal voltage.

10. The amount of blood flow to the myocardium is termed
   a. influx.
   b. contraction.
   c. perfusion.
   d. stenosis.
   e. bypass.

CRITICAL THINKING

Refer to the case study at the beginning of the chapter and use what you have learned to answer the following questions.

1. Why is it important that David provide Mr. Masterson with a detailed explanation of the procedure? What should David tell him?
2. When Mr. Masterson removes his shirt, David realizes that the patient has a very hairy chest. What should David do, and why?

3. Mr. Masterson informs David that he has trouble lying flat on his back because of a previous injury from a car accident, and he does not think he will be able to lie flat for the ECG. How should David handle this situation?

ON THE JOB

Bonny Glidewell, CMA (AAMA), works in a cardiologist's office. She passes out a questionnaire to all her patients about their lifestyle habits (exercise, eating, smoking, etc.) so she can collect data and then create patient teaching brochures.

1. Which questions should she ask to determine which behaviors are the most prevalent in this practice?

2. What would you expect to be the usual diet of a person with coronary artery disease?
3. What instructions might she give on how to stop smoking?

INTERNET ACTIVITY

Go to the American Heart Association and the American Lung Association websites, gather information, and create two brochures to teach patients about heart and lung health.

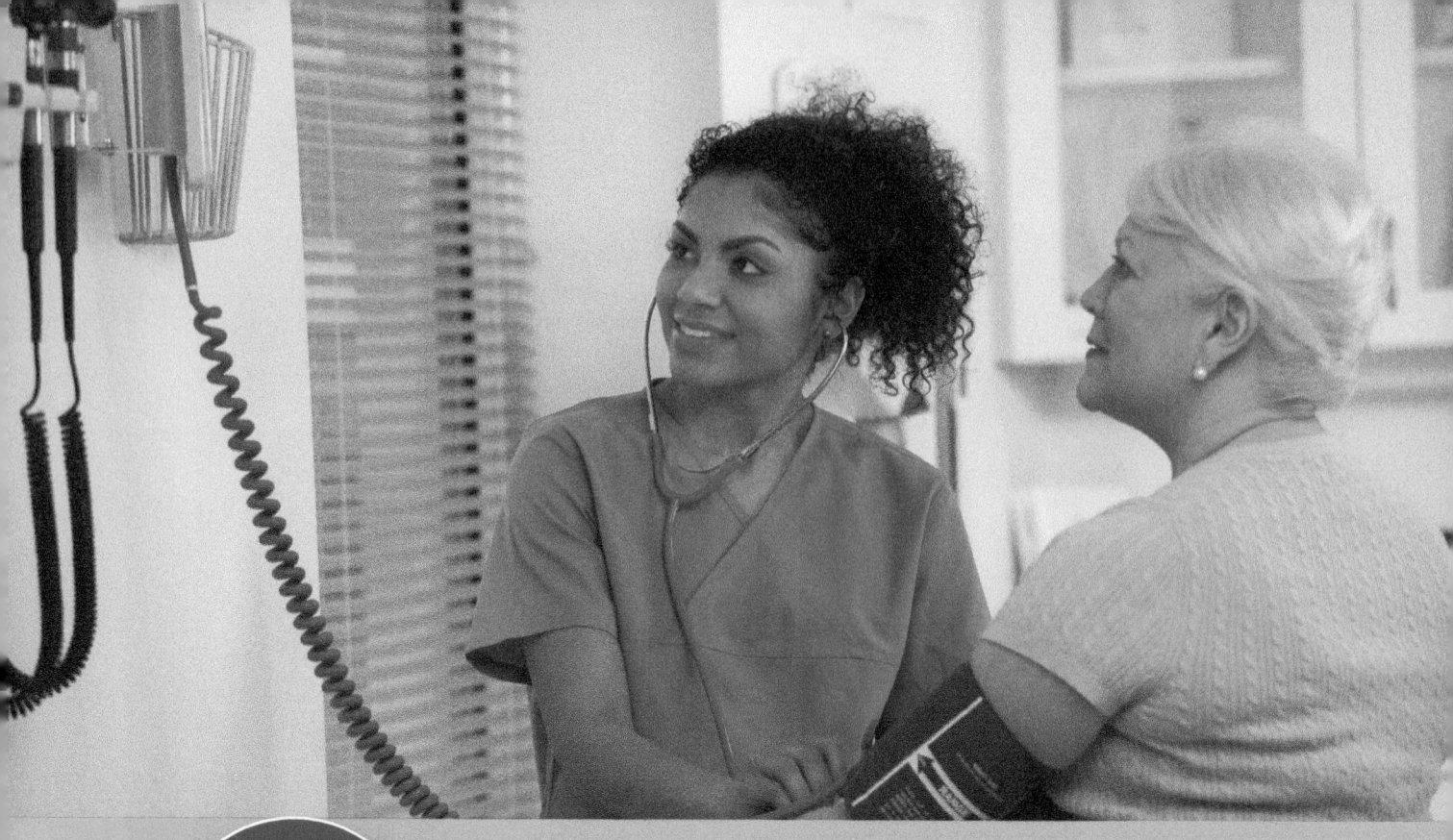

Pulmonary Function

Learning Objectives

After completing this chapter, you should be able to:

50.1   Define and spell the terms for this chapter.

50.2   Explain why pulmonary function tests are performed.

50.3   Identify symptoms commonly associated with pulmonary disorders.

50.4   Describe respiratory volumes associated with spirometry testing.

50.5   Explain the role of the medical assistant in spirometry testing.

50.6   Describe how peak flow measurements impact a patient with a pulmonary disorder.

50.7   Explain the measurement of arterial blood gasses.

50.8   Describe treatments used for pulmonary disorders.

Abigail Lently is a 51-year-old patient who has recently been diagnosed with chronic obstructive pulmonary disease (COPD). She has come in for a follow-up spirometry test after being placed on her maintenance medications. She admits that she has had a very tough time with smoking cessation. Although she has cut back on the number of cigarettes smoked per day, she has not quit altogether.

Terms to Learn

clinical status	inspiratory capacity (IC)	pulmonologist
expiratory reserve volume (ERV)	inspiratory reserve volume (IRV)	pulmonology
forced expiratory volume (FEV)	nebulizer	residual volume (RV)
forced vital capacity (FVC)	peak expiratory flow rate (PEFR)	tidal volume (V_T)
functional residual capacity (FRC)	peak flow meter	total lung capacity (TLC)
inhaler	pulmonary volume tests	vital capacity (VC)

Pulmonology is the study of diseases of the respiratory system. The respiratory system includes the trachea, bronchial tubes, lungs, and alveoli. The primary function of the respiratory system is to transport oxygen from the lungs via the bloodstream to all the cells in the body and to carry waste products (carbon dioxide and water) from the cells via the bloodstream to the lungs to be exhaled from the body.

THE ROLE OF THE MEDICAL ASSISTANT IN PULMONOLOGY

As a medical assistant, you may perform several different tests to assess respiratory function, to assist in the diagnosis of patients with suspected obstructive or restrictive pulmonary disease, and to assess the effectiveness of drug and other pulmonary therapies. You may perform these tests in different medical specialties, such as a primary care physician's office, an allergist's office, or a pulmonologist's office. A **pulmonologist** is a physician specialist who has advanced training in the diagnosis, management, and treatment of lung diseases and respiratory disorders. Regardless of the medical office and specialty, the medical assistant must be knowledgeable about the diseases and disorders of the respiratory system and be prepared to assist in or perform specialized procedures in this field.

PULMONARY DISORDERS

There are several types of lung diseases, but most are classified as either obstructive lung diseases or restrictive lung diseases. Obstructive lung diseases include conditions that make it hard to exhale all the oxygen from the lungs. Examples of obstructive lung diseases are asthma, cystic fibrosis (CF), and chronic obstructive pulmonary disease (COPD), which includes emphysema and chronic bronchitis. Patients with restrictive lung diseases have difficulty fully expanding their lungs with air. Examples of restrictive lung diseases are fibrosis, interstitial lung diseases, sarcoidosis, and amyloidosis.

Other types of lung diseases affect the lungs' ability to ventilate or take in oxygen, such as pneumonia or pulmonary edema (swelling), or affect the lungs' ability to perfuse or move oxygen from the lungs through the bloodstream to the cells, such as a pulmonary embolism (clot).

Patients with pulmonary conditions may present with a variety of symptoms, such as:

- Dyspnea—Shortness of breath, especially with exertion
- Coughing—Dry or productive (with sputum or blood)
- Wheezing—A hoarse, whistling sound with breathing
- Cyanosis—Blue color of the skin or mucous membrane from lack of oxygen (Figure 50-1)

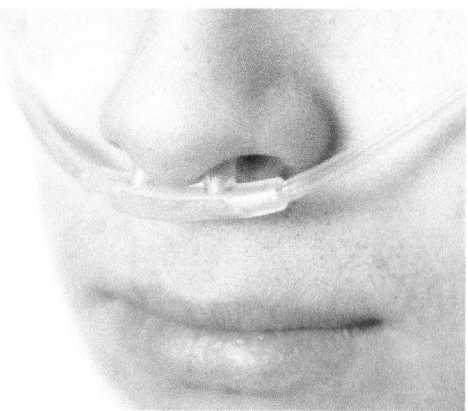

FIGURE 50-1 Cyanosis as shown here around the patient's lips results from a lack of oxygen in the tissues. *(© Stam Photo)*

- Rales—Crackles heard when listening to the chest
- Stridor—Harsh, high-pitched sounds, usually during inspiration
- Rhonchus—Wheezing or squeaking sounds heard when listening to the chest
- Hemoptysis—Coughing up blood or blood-stained mucus

Table 50-1 lists common disorders of the respiratory system. As a medical assistant, you should be aware of these respiratory disorders and how they affect a patient's overall health.

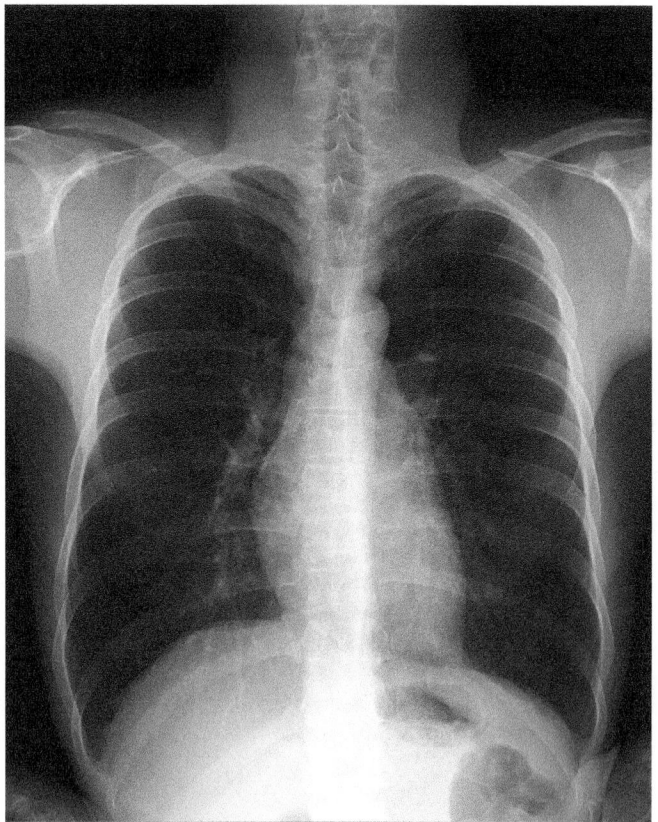

FIGURE 50-2 A normal chest X-ray. *(© ChooChin)*

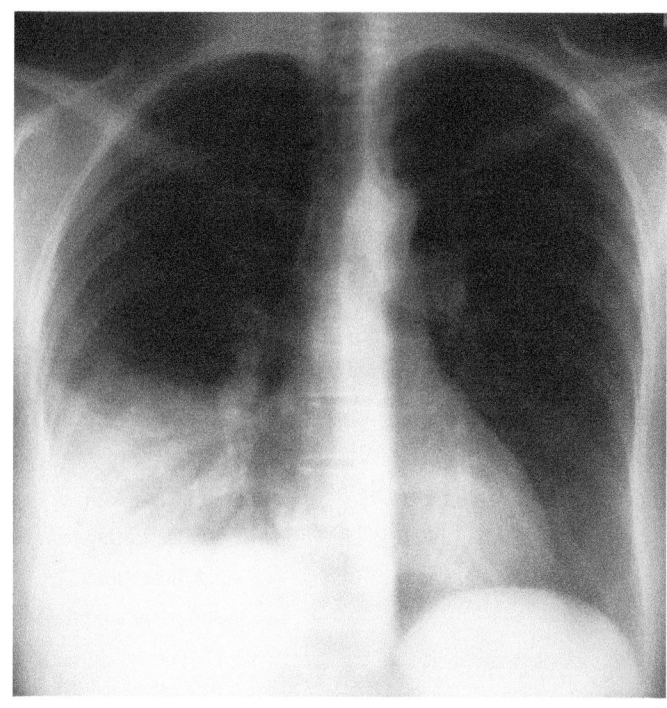

FIGURE 50-3 A chest X-ray showing pneumonia characterized by the patch of gray-white areas. *(CNRI_*

Once the patient presents with symptoms, there are many pulmonary tests available to diagnose lung diseases, determine their causes when possible, and evaluate their severity. The physician may order arterial blood gases (ABGs) to evaluate oxygen and carbon dioxide levels, pulmonary function tests (PFTs) to help diagnose and monitor lung function, and chest X-rays or computed tomography (CT) scans to look at lung structure. Figure 50-2 shows a normal chest X-ray. Figure 50-3 shows pneumonia on a chest X-ray. Figure 50-4 shows emphysema on a chest X-ray.

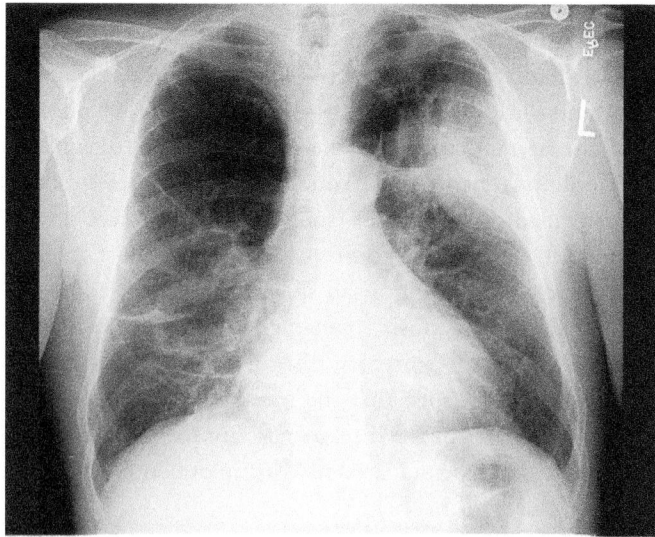

FIGURE 50-4 Chest X-ray of a patient with emphysema. *(Living Art Images)*

TABLE 50-1 | Disorders of the Respiratory System

Disorder	Description
Chronic Obstructive Conditions	
Asthma	Spasms of the bronchial tubes and swelling of the mucous membranes leading to wheezing, shortness of breath, and chest tightness.
Chronic bronchitis	Inflammation of the bronchial mucous membranes, causing persistent cough and often mucus production lasting three months in a row during a year for two years.
Emphysema	Permanent destruction of the alveoli, most often caused by smoking, making breathing very difficult. It is one of the diseases categorized as COPD.
Chronic obstructive pulmonary disease (COPD)	A destruction of lung tissue that commonly results from chronic bronchitis and/or emphysema.
Cystic fibrosis	Genetic disorder characterized by the secretion of too much thick and sticky mucus that obstructs the lungs (as well as other areas of the body).
General Respiratory Conditions	
Acute rhinitis	Inflammation of the mucous membranes inside the nose.
Sinusitis	Inflammation of the sinuses caused by a virus, bacteria, or fungus.
Hay fever	Also known as allergic rhinitis, it is characterized by an allergic reaction (to dust, pollen, or another inhaled substance) that causes nasal congestion, runny nose, and sneezing.
Pharyngitis	A sore throat, or inflammation of the pharynx.
Laryngitis	Hoarseness or loss of voice caused by swelling and inflammation of the larynx (voice box).
Infectious Conditions	
Pneumonia	Inflammation or fluid that fills the alveoli in the lungs as a result of infection caused by virus, bacteria, or fungus.
Influenza	Commonly called the flu, it is a rapidly spreading viral infection of the nose, throat, and lungs characterized by overall body aches, malaise, fever, and headaches.
Tuberculosis	A contagious bacterial infection of the lungs that is highly contagious and characterized by fever, fatigue, a mucus-producing cough, sometimes coughed-up blood, and night sweats. It is often referred to as TB.
Pleuritis	Also termed pleurisy, it is an inflammation of the lining of the chest wall and lungs (pleura) characterized by sharp pain upon inhalation. It can develop after chest trauma or from infections caused by pneumonia, TB, and other diseases.
Mechanical Injuries	
Pulmonary emboli	A blockage in the lung most often because of a blood clot that has traveled through the venous system from another part of the body; in a few cases, an embolism may be caused by embolized fat or tumor cells.
Pneumothorax	A collapsed lung caused by a buildup of air or gases that accumulate in the space between the chest wall and lungs (pleural space).
Hemothorax	A collection of blood in the space between the chest wall and lungs (pleural space). It is most commonly caused by chest trauma.

PULMONARY FUNCTION TESTS

One of the most common tests to evaluate lung function that a medical assistant may perform is a pulmonary function test (PFT). PFTs assess lung volume and capacity and are often performed when a patient complains of shortness of breath, especially after minimal exertion.

PFTs aid in the evaluation and diagnosis of pulmonary disease. PFTs are also commonly performed to monitor lung function if a patient has been diagnosed with asthma, chronic bronchitis, emphysema, CF, or a combination of these conditions. In a patient who has recently been diagnosed with pulmonary disease, the initial PFT will be used as a baseline and compared against future PFTs. Patients with pulmonary disorders can expect to have routine PFTs performed over the course of their disease management. Because lung disease tends to worsen with age, it is important to make a diagnosis early so that PFTs can show any improvements with medical intervention and treatment.

In some cases, the physician may order pulmonary function tests because the patient's lifestyle, occupation, or social demographics are often associated with lung disease. An awareness of the long-term effects of smoking and exposure to occupational or environmental toxins has increased the frequency with which PFTs are performed. PFTs may also be a component of a patient's annual physical examination to provide a baseline measurement of the patient's lung function. PFTs may also be a component of some preemployment physicals. For example, baseline PFTs performed as part of a preemployment screening can help determine the long-term effects on an employee working in occupations such as coal mining or asbestos removal.

There are several types of PFTs: spirometry, lung volumes, arterial blood gases, pulse oximetry, diffusion capacity, and cardiopulmonary exercise tests. Some of these tests are performed by respiratory therapists in a hospital setting, as ordered by the pulmonologist, although some may be performed by the medical assistant. The most common tests and procedures performed by the medical assistant are

spirometry, peak flow meters, and pulse oximetry. The first two of these procedures is discussed later in this chapter. Pulse oximetry is discussed in the chapter titled "Vital Signs."

Spirometry

Spirometry is the most common and often the first PFT to be performed when a patient presents with breathing issues. A spirometry is a noninvasive test that measures the capability of the lungs to effectively exhale and how quickly. Spirometry results assess the elasticity of the lungs, their capability to ventilate (in this case, to breathe air out of the lungs), and the strength of the respiratory muscles. Spirometry is used to diagnose airflow obstruction in patients with respiratory symptoms and can also be used to monitor disease progression and improvements with treatment.

Several types of spirometers are used in the medical office. There are small, hand-held devices that provide digital readings, and there are portable meters with integrated printers. The more advanced spirometry systems are computerized and can be configured to send results directly to a patient's electronic health record. When using an automated computerized spirometry machine, patient data, such as the patient's age, height, weight, vital signs, and medications must be entered into the computer program. All spirometers consist of a mouthpiece and tubing connected to a recording device. Figure 50-5 shows a computerized spirometer in use.

During the spirometry test, the patient is asked to inhale as deeply as possible and then to exhale as forcefully and as completely as possible while measurements are being taken. Different volumes of air move in and out at different capacities and rates, which can be calculated by adding together specific respiratory volumes. With the test results, the physician is able to compare the patient's pulmonary measurements to the normal range for the patient's height, weight, age, race, and sex—taking into account the patient's clinical status.

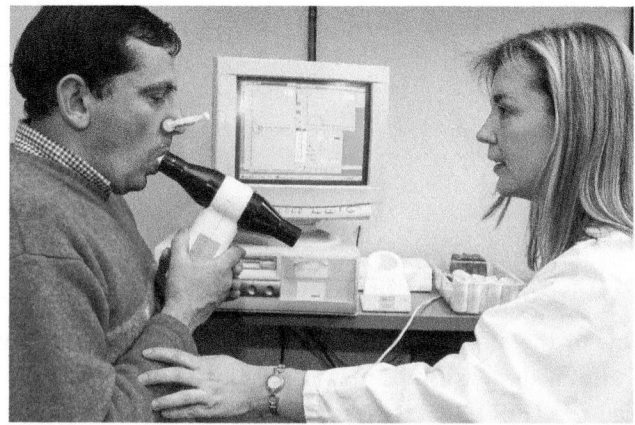

FIGURE 50-5 Computerized spirometry is used in medical office settings, hospitals, and other medical facilities.

Clinical status refers to the patient's physical condition at the time of the test. For example, a fever, asthma attack, poor night's sleep, scoliosis, and any number of other factors may affect the patient's pulmonary function. As a result, at least three acceptable spirometry tests must be obtained to ensure the validity of the measurements.

Based on the spirometry results, a predicted value is calculated, which indicates the level of lung function or dysfunction. For example, a prediction value of 85 to 100 percent would indicate no impairment, 75 to 85 percent would indicate slight impairment, and so on. Spirometry results can be further used to determine the type of impairment, which is discussed next.

Respiratory Volumes and Capacities

During the spirometry, a number of parameters are measured and calculated for flow rates and lung volumes, which help to diagnose respiratory diseases. Results of the spirometry may also be provided as a graphical representation called a spirogram (Figure 50-6).

Flow rates are the measurements of different volumes of air moving in and out during breathing. The most common flow rates measured are forced vital capacity and forced expiratory volume.

Forced vital capacity (FVC) measures the volume of air you can exhale with force after you inhale as deeply as possible. The patient must exhale as much air as possible and continue to exhale for at least six seconds to be considered a satisfactory test. The test must be repeated at least three times in order to be considered an acceptable spirometry test. Patients with chronic asthma may have a reduction in FVC.

Forced expiratory volume (FEV) is the volume of air that can be forcefully exhaled in one breath. The amount of air exhaled at one second is called the *forced expiratory volume after one second* (FEV^1). FEV^1 can identify or confirm the presence of COPD.

These values are often reported as a ratio, FEV^1/FVC, and can be used to diagnose a patient with obstructive or restrictive lung disease. Patients with healthy lungs may have a ratio as high as 90 percent. However, a patient with FEV^1/FVC of less than 70 percent

may have obstructive lung disease. If the patient has a restrictive lung disease, the FEV^1 and FVC are both reduced, but the FEV^1/FVC ratio remains normal or greater than 75 percent.

Pulmonary volume tests measure lung volumes and, thus, are indicators of patients' ability to expand their lungs. The first part of the spirometry test is performed to discover the amount of air in the lungs when they move normally and how much lung space is available after a normal inhalation and a normal exhalation. The four most important volumes in a pulmonary volume test (shown in Figure 50-6) are:

Pulmonary Volumes

- **Tidal volume (V_T)**—The amount of air inhaled or exhaled during normal, relaxed breathing (about 500 mL)
- **Expiratory reserve volume (ERV)**—The amount of air that can be forcibly exhaled after a normal exhalation
- **Inspiratory reserve volume (IRV)**—The amount of air that can be forcibly inspired after a normal inhalation
- **Residual volume (RV)**—The volume of air left in the lungs at the end of an exhalation (around 1,200 mL)

From these volume tests, pulmonary capacities can be calculated, based on adding two or more volumes, as follows:

Pulmonary Capacities

- **Total lung capacity (TLC)**—The maximum amount of air that can fill the lungs; sum of the four volumes: tidal volume (V_T), expiratory reserve volume (ERV), inspiratory reserve volume (IRV), residual volume (RV)

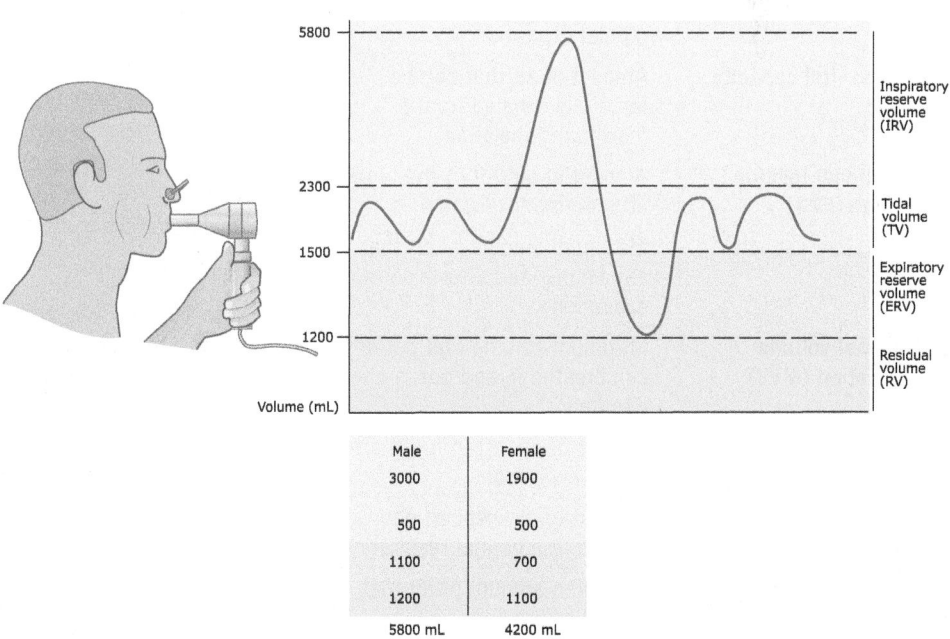

SPIROMETRY

	Male	Female
	3000	1900
	500	500
	1100	700
	1200	1100
	5800 mL	4200 mL

FIGURE 50-6 A spirogram and different lung volume measurements.

- **Vital capacity (VC)**—The amount of air that can be exhaled following forced inspiration, including maximum expiration; varies with age and body size
- **Inspiratory capacity (IC)**—The amount of air that can be inhaled after normal expiration
- **Functional residual capacity (FRC)**—The amount of air remaining in the lungs after a normal expiration

Table 50-2 summarizes the various respiratory volumes and capacities.

Different pulmonary diseases affect volumes and capacities differently. Total lung capacity and functional residual capacity will increase in COPD, because the flow of air out of the lungs is diminished. This results in a slow expiratory rate and an increase in residual volume (RV). The lungs of patients with asthma have a decreased ability to deflate during expiration, and thus will have a decreased FEV^1. In restrictive lung disease, the volumes are decreased because expansion of the lungs is inhibited, thereby diminishing total lung capacity (TLC), vital capacity (VC), and inspiratory capacity (IC).

The Medical Assistant's Role in Spirometry Testing

Spirometry tests are often performed by a respiratory care specialist, usually in a hospital setting, as ordered by the pulmonologist. Spirometry testing may also be done in an occupational medicine office as part of preemployment physicals, an allergy specialist's office, or a pulmonologist's office. Medical assistants may work with these specialists, as well as with many patients who have pulmonary disease. Medical assistants may also be asked to perform these tests in the physician's office to continue monitoring the patient's respiratory disease and the effectiveness of treatment. Therefore, as a medical assistant, you should be familiar with the terms associated with spirometry and pulmonary function and what these terms mean.

The medical assistant will most commonly perform spirometry testing to measure the patient's forced vital capacity (FVC). As discussed earlier, FVC is the maximum volume of air expelled when the patient exhales as forcibly and quickly as possible following one inhalation. You will play an important role as the patient must be prepared for the spirometry procedure, which requires proper coaching and instruction to obtain accurate results. The patient must inhale deeply and then exhale as forcefully as possible and for as long as possible. Your role will be to act as both cheerleader and coach to encourage the patient to give the best performance.

TABLE 50-2 | Summary of Respiratory Volumes and Capacities

Lung Function	Definition
Expiratory reserve volume (ERV)	Maximum volume of air left that can be exhaled after normal expiration
Forced vital capacity (FVC)	Amount of air that can be forcefully exhaled from a maximum inhalation
Functional residual volume (FVR)	Amount of air left in the lungs after normal expiration
Inspiratory capacity (IC)	Maximum amount of air that can be inspired after a normal expiration
Maximal volume ventilation (MVV)	Maximum volume that patient can breathe in and out in one minute
Residual volume (RV)	Volume of air left in lungs after forced expiration
Tidal volume (V_T)	Amount of air inspired and expired in a normal respiration
Vital capacity (VC)	Maximum amount of air that can be expired after a maximum inspiration

Professionalism   The Life Span

The Child

Children need extra time and coaching for pulmonary function tests (PFTs). Use words and phrases that they will understand, speaking to them at their own appropriate level. Take the time to explain to them that they will need to blow "really hard" until you tell them to stop, and then they will need to take a big breath back through the tube. It may take a couple of practice attempts the first time this procedure is performed to ensure accuracy. If the child cannot perform the procedure correctly, the results will not be valid. Thus, PFTs are never performed on a child who is unable to cooperate or comply with the testing requirements.

The Older Adult

When doing PFTs, first explain the procedure clearly and in detail. An older adult may not be able to perform multiple efforts. Thus, proper patient preparation is essential to get an accurate result and to avoid making the patient perform multiple attempts. It is helpful for you to demonstrate in order to show the amount of force necessary to perform the test. This will give the patient a visual example to accompany the test preparation instructions. Additionally, watch the patient's technique and offer constructive hints to help improve the validity of each effort. Be very supportive as you coach the patient throughout the procedure.

Patient Preparation and Testing Procedures

Patient preparation for spirometry testing is critical. When the procedure is scheduled, preparations begin with a brochure provided to the patient explaining the test. The patient should be instructed to refrain from smoking and from eating a large meal for four to six hours before the test, and not to use bronchodilators or nebulizers for six hours before the test.

When the patient arrives on the day of the test, explain the test again, review the steps involved, answer any questions, and determine if there are reasons the test should not be performed. Reasons not to perform the test include if the patient is sick with the flu or a cold or has active allergies. All of these factors could have a negative impact on the patient's breathing ability and, thus, the test would not provide valid results. As mentioned earlier, the patient's clinical status plays a major part in the outcomes of the tests. The physician will make the final call regarding proceeding or rescheduling a test, if necessary.

Next, measure the patient's height and weight and measure and record vital signs. The height and weight are necessary for calculations after the test.

In simple terms, demonstrate and explain what you would like the patient to do. If the patient is wearing ill-fitting dentures, ask that they be removed because they could hinder the lips from forming a tight seal around the mouthpiece. Have the patient loosen any tight clothing, such as ties, girdles, bras, or belts, which could impede the patient's ability to fully expand the lungs. The patient should be encouraged to sit because exertion may cause light-headedness, dizziness, and even fainting. This proper upright position must be maintained during a spirometry test. The patient's feet should be flat on the floor, legs uncrossed, and head and chin slightly elevated during the entire procedure. It would be acceptable if the patient prefers to stand during the procedure, but a chair should be nearby in case the patient becomes dizzy during the test.

The test needs to be successfully repeated three times to produce valid results. Each successful attempt is termed a maneuver, and the best two maneuvers should be used for the calculation of the pulmonary function. The medical assistant is not required to calculate the pulmonary function because it is calculated by the computer program. Results are considered normal if the patient's best result is 80 percent of pretest calculated values. If the results are abnormal, the patient may be given a bronchodilator and then retested to determine the effectiveness of the medication.

Valid spirometric measurements depend on patient effort, which, in turn, depends on the coaching and instruction provided by the medical assistant. Procedure 50-1 lists the steps to perform a spirometry test to measure FVC.

PROCEDURE 50-1
Performing a Spirometry Test to Measure Forced Vital Capacity

Objective ◆ *Perform a forced vital capacity test.*

EQUIPMENT AND SUPPLIES

Functioning spirometry machine; nose clip; disposable patient mouthpiece; spirometric tubing; disinfectant; waste container; paper and pencil; scale for height and weight; sphygmomanometer; stethoscope; patient's medical record

METHOD

1. Perform hand hygiene.
2. Assemble all equipment, attaching the tubing and mouthpiece to the spirometer as necessary.
3. Calibrate the spirometer as necessary, according to manufacturer's instructions. Turn on the machine and ensure that the spirometer is properly functioning.
4. Warmly greet and identify the patient and introduce yourself.
5. Question the patient about preparations for the test.
   a. Make sure the patient has not eaten a large meal and has not smoked within the past four to six hours.
   b. Ensure the patient has not used any bronchodilator medications within six hours of the test.
6. Inquire about the patient's current general health, and notify the physician if the patient has a fever, active allergies, a cough, or cold or flu symptoms.
7. In detail, explain and demonstrate the procedure to the patient. Instruct the patient that she will need to successfully complete three maneuvers. *Note:* A maneuver consists of having the patient forcefully exhale and blow into the spirometry machine as hard and as long as possible.
8. Obtain the patient's height and weight, and record all vital signs.

9. Explain the proper positioning and, if necessary, assist with loosening any tight clothing that could cause constriction.
   a. Ideally, the patient should be seated with feet flat on the floor. The patient's head and chin should be slightly elevated during the procedure.
10. Enter all patient data into the spirometry machine: patient's name; date of birth; height; weight; and blood pressure. Medications may also be entered on some spirometer models.
11. Have the patient place the mouthpiece in his mouth and seal the lips around the mouthpiece (Figure A).
12. Apply nose clip (Figure B).
13. Have the patient inhale deeply.
14. Push the start button at the same time as you give the following instruction to the patient:
   a. Encourage the patient to exhale as hard, fast, and long as possible (Figure C).
15. For the second attempt, review the procedure with the patient. Make recommendations to improve the outcome of the next maneuver, if necessary. Be sure that the patient knows to breathe forcibly several times into the spirometer.
16. Make any additional recommendations for improvement and obtain the third set of maneuvers.

17. You may facilitate up to eight attempts to obtain three good maneuvers. Some computerized machines will automatically select the best attempt and print the results.
18. Remove the nose clip and ask the patient to remain in the examination room until the physician reviews the results.
19. Give the physician the spirometry results.
20. Record the performance of the test and the results in the patient's medical record, if instructed to do so by the physician.
21. Clean the tubing and dispose of the mouthpieces using standard precautions and following the manufacturer's directions.
22. Properly shut down the computerized spirometry machine, according to manufacturer's directions, and place the machine in its proper storage location.
23. Clean the examination room in preparation for the next patient.

CHARTING EXAMPLE

3/12/YY 8:30 A.M. Spirometry performed with 3 good results submitted to Dr. Penningworth.................K. Christianson, CMA

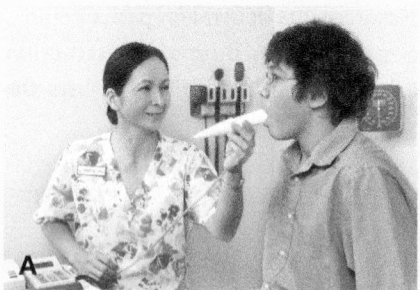 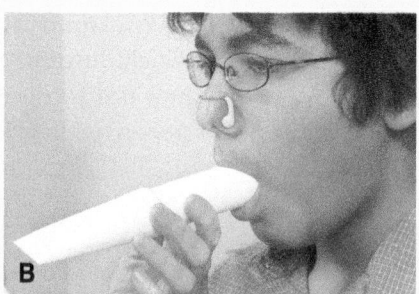 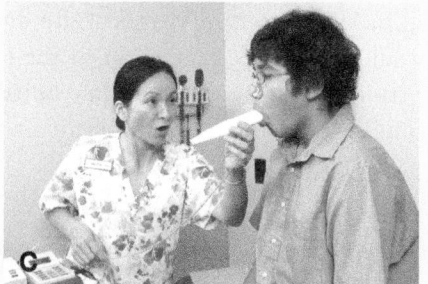

FIGURE A–C (A) The patient must make a tight seal with the lips around the mouthpiece. **(B)** Place the nose clip on the patient's nose. **(C)** Instruct the patient to forcibly exhale into the mouthpiece as hard and as fast as possible.

Professionalism | The Law

Many pulmonary patients, especially those who are on oxygen treatment, are apprehensive about having spirometry testing. They worry about being disconnected from their oxygen supply during the test. You must put them at ease and explain that they will be monitored closely, and that the test will be terminated if conditions warrant it. Remember not to promise any outcomes or results in your eagerness to persuade patients to be tested. Also, remember that the medical assistant is not allowed to release any results of the tests; this is the responsibility of the licensed person in charge (i.e., physician, physician's assistant, nurse).

Professionalism | The Workplace

As a medical assistant, you should be aware of the many advances and updates that occur with testing and equipment used in the medical office. Additionally, it is important to be aware of upgrades to software and other euipment that will allow them to function at optimal levels. A good way to stay current and aware of these advances is by attending special classes and seminars. Manufacturers also have customer representatives who are assigned to specific medical offices and practices and are available to provide technical assistance and information on new and trending advances in medical testing.

Peak Flow Meter

The **peak flow meter** is another means of measuring a patient's respiratory function. It is often used for patients who have asthma to monitor their daily respiratory function and condition. The peak flow meter measures the fastest rate at which the patient exhales after taking a maximum breath. This is known as the **peak expiratory flow rate, or PEFR**. Keeping a record of peak flow, either daily or when asthma attacks occur, helps the physician develop an effective treatment plan.

As a medical assistant, it may be your responsibility to teach the patient and family members how to use a peak flow meter. Instruct the patient to put his mouth around the mouthpiece and forcibly blow into the meter, which will measure the peak expiratory flow rate (PEFR) in liters per second or liters per minute. See Figure 50-7 for an example of a patient using a peak flow meter. Also instruct the patient to keep a diary of the flow rates to monitor if medication is helping or if the disease is getting worse. When a patient is having a "good" day—that is, a day that is free from respiratory distress, the patient should blow as hard as possible into the peak flow meter to establish a goal or baseline result.

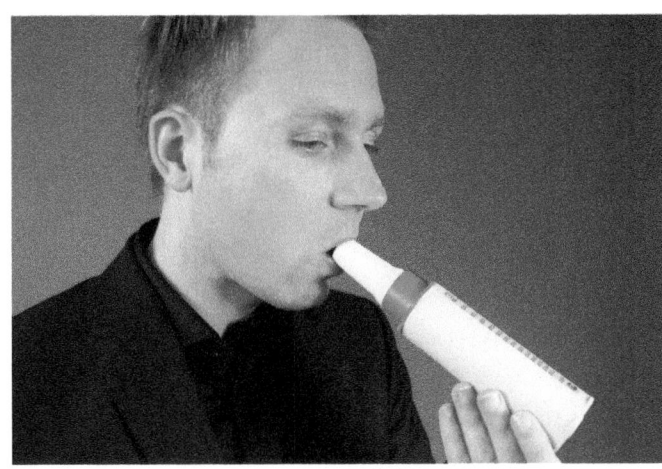

FIGURE 50-7 A patient using a peak flow meter. *(© Kafer Photo)*

The information from the diary will help the physician determine the most effective medication and treatment regimen. Increased flow rates indicate a desirable and effective response to medication. These results can then be compared with other expiratory attempts when the patient is wheezing or having an asthmatic attack. Procedure 50-2 describes how to instruct a patient on using a peak flow meter.

PROCEDURE 50-2

Teaching Peak Flow Measurement

Objective ◆ *Instruct patient to correctly monitor peak flow measurements and record results.*

EQUIPMENT AND SUPPLIES

Peak flow meter; documentation diary/chart; diagram of lungs and breathing processes; pen; patient's medical record

METHOD

1. Perform hand hygiene.
2. Assemble the peak flow meter with the disposable mouthpiece or an individual peak flow meter for the patient to take and use at home.
3. Warmly greet and identify the patient and introduce yourself.
4. Explain the procedure, including an explanation of the breathing processes and the importance to overall health. A diagram of the lungs can be beneficial.
   a. Demonstrate how the mouthpiece fits onto the meter, and explain what the numbers on the side mean.
   b. The peak flow meter should always be set on zero to start. The numbers on the side of the meter measure the amount of liters exhaled per second or per minute, depending on the calibration of the given meter.
5. Explain that results are best obtained if the patient is standing with the mouthpiece in his mouth and with a tight seal formed by the lips.
6. While standing, instruct the patient to take as deep a breath as possible. Instruct the patient to place the mouthpiece in the mouth without biting down on it, and exhale as completely and forcibly as possible (Figure A).
7. The exhalation will move the marker up the side of the scale on the meter. Instruct the patient to note the number at which the sliding gauge stopped and to record the results. This reading is the peak expiratory flow rate (PEFR).
8. Reset the gauge to zero. Repeat steps 5 and 6 two more times so that there are three acceptable results.

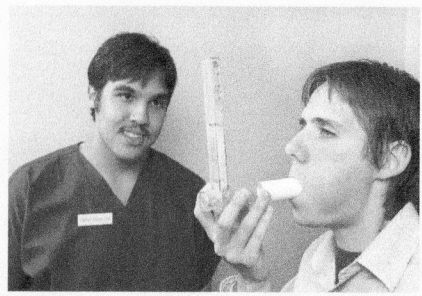

FIGURE A Ask the patient to exhale as hard and as fast as possible.

9. Inform the physician of the patient's results.
10. Instruct the patient to follow the physician's orders about when and how often to perform peak flow measurement. Instruct the patient to record the best result of the three attempts in the diary.

11. Demonstrate how to properly care for and disinfect the peak flow meter, according to the manufacturer's instructions.
12. Verify that the patient understands how to obtain peak flow measurements, how to document and record results in the diary, and how to properly care and maintain the peak flow meter. Allow time for the patient to ask questions.
13. Document that the patient received instructions and training on the peak flow meter.
14. Perform hand hygiene.

CHARTING EXAMPLE

05/16/YY 9:30 A.M. Pt. instructed on use of peak flow meter and recording of results. Returned demonstration easily, verbally confirmed understanding. Peak flow charting form given. Pt. to perform procedure 3 × twice/day in A.M. and P.M. Results today: 380 LPM..R. Negri, CMA

Arterial Blood Gases

Testing arterial blood gases (ABGs) is one of the most accurate methods of measuring the amount of oxygen and carbon dioxide in the blood, as well as the pH. The pH of the blood must be stable between the ranges of 7.35 and 7.45; otherwise, the patient is in a life-threatening situation. The more carbon dioxide is in the blood, the more acidic the blood pH will be. Blood gas levels are helpful in evaluating breathing conditions such as COPD and pneumonia. They also provide information on the effectiveness of oxygen treatments and other therapies.

Arterial blood is drawn from the wrist, groin, or arm after cleansing the site. The specimen must be kept on ice and tested immediately. After the blood draw, pressure to the area is applied for 5 to 15 minutes to prevent further bleeding. ABGs are usually drawn by respiratory specialists or IV (intravenous) technicians. Although as a medical assistant you are not likely perform this blood draw, it is helpful to know about the test so you can properly inform patients about their lab work.

PULMONARY TREATMENTS

Pulmonary treatments differ depending on each patient's condition. For example, treatments for obstructive lung disease may include drugs that reduce inflammation or relax smooth muscle to improve air flow, such as bronchodilators. For restrictive lung diseases, treatment may include steroids and other drugs that suppress the body's immune system. Although some drugs may be taken orally, the majority of drugs for respiratory diseases are more effective if they are inhaled directly into the lungs through a nebulizer or inhaler.

Nebulizers

A **nebulizer** is a handheld device that delivers medication directly to deep areas in the lungs through a fine aerosol mist that is inhaled. A nebulizer may be used with either a mouthpiece or a mask. To prepare a nebulizer, a small amount of liquid medication is placed in a chamber and mixed with sterile saline or water.

Once the nebulizing machine is turned on and the mist is created, the patient is asked to put on the mask or mouthpiece and to breathe deeply for eight to ten minutes. A high-pressure gas stream of either air or oxygen passing through a small opening creates the aerosol. The aerosol of the medication, delivered into the patient's respiratory tract through the mouthpiece or a mask, is absorbed directly into the lungs. Figure 50-8A shows a nebulizer. Figures 50-8B and 50-8C show a nebulizer being used with a mouthpiece or mask.

The procedure for a nebulizer is to first note the patient's baseline data, such as vital signs, auscultated breath sounds, oximeter reading, and peak expiratory flow rate (PEFR). Then assemble the hand-held nebulizer and select a mouthpiece or mask for delivery of the medication. The preferred delivery method is with a mouthpiece, because a mask allows the deposit of some of the medication on the patient's face, which can decrease the amount of drug that reaches the lungs by 1 or 2 percent. The mask may be preferred for children or when the patient is unable to use a mouthpiece.

Measure the proper dosage of drug and diluent into the nebulizer. Set the gas flow to the nebulizer at 6 to 8 L/min.

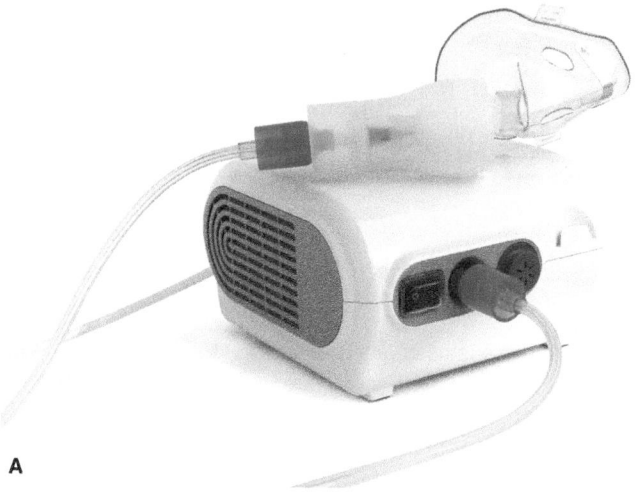

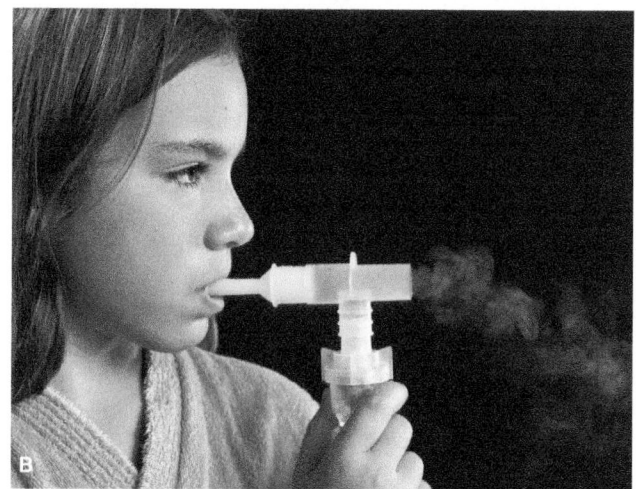

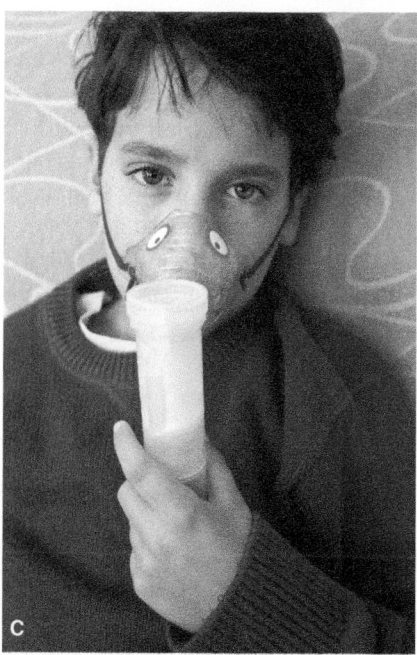

FIGURE 50-8 **(A)** Nebulizing equipment and inhaler medications. **(B)** Nebulized medications can be delivered through a mouthpiece. **(C)** Nebulized medications can also be delivered through a mask.

Position the patient in a semi-Fowler's position (lying supine on the examination table with the head of the table tilted up at a 45° angle) or in a seated position. If using a mask for delivery, assist the patient in placing the mask on the face in the proper position. Otherwise, provide the patient with the handheld mouthpiece and encourage the patient to breathe slowly through the mouth. A nose clip may be used to ensure that the patient is breathing only through the mouth. From time to time, instruct the patient to take deep breaths and to hold a breath for about three to five seconds. The treatment will end when the aerosol stops flowing. Monitor and evaluate the patient's response to the treatment. Encourage the patient to cough at the end of the treatment. If the cough is productive or sputum is present, quantify the amount and describe the type of sputum. Monitor the patient's pulse, breath sounds, peak expiratory flow rates, and blood oxygenation. Disassemble and store the equipment properly. Record the data in the patient's medical record.

Nebulizing treatments are often administered in the medical office by the medical assistant but can be done by the patient at home. Procedure 50-3 provides the steps for assisting the physician in administering a nebulizer treatment.

Inhalers

An **inhaler** is a handheld disc or tube attached to a mouthpiece that delivers a measured amount of medication into the respiratory tract to dilate the airways. There are three basic types of inhalers: metered dose inhalers, dry powder inhalers, and soft mist inhalers.

A metered-dose inhaler (MDI) holds about 200 doses of the prescribed medication in a pressurized container with an attached mouthpiece. Patient education is very important because MDIs are frequently misused, resulting in inadequate treatment. The medical assistant should demonstrate for the patient first and then ask the patient to repeat the demonstration. Provide written material for reference. Some inhalers may have a spacer, sometimes called an extender, which is used to improve the delivery and absorption of the medication. Figure 50-9A-B shows an example of a MDI with and without a spacer.

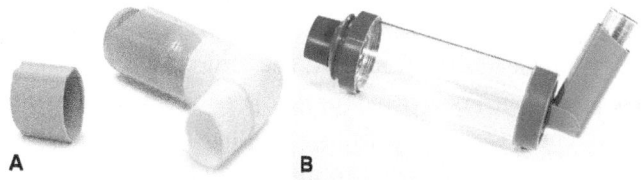

FIGURE 50-9 **(A)** A metered-dose inhaler. **(B)** A metered-dose inhaler with a spacer.

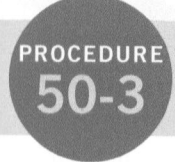

PROCEDURE 50-3 Administering a Nebulizer Treatment

Objective ◆ *Assist the physician through patient care by administering a nebulizer treatment to a patient.*

EQUIPMENT AND SUPPLIES

Medication as ordered by the physician; diluent (either sterile saline or sterile water); nebulizer machine; disposable tubing with medication cup or dispenser; disposable mask or mouthpiece; biohazard waste container; patient's medical record

METHOD

1. Gather all necessary equipment including the nebulizer machine, disposable mask or mouthpiece, connecting disposable tubing, and medicine cap/dispenser. Plug the machine into an outlet in the examination room.
2. Warmly greet and identify the patient and introduce yourself.
3. Explain the procedure and the treatment that will be administered.
4. Verify the order for medication as written by the physician. The medication should be checked and reviewed three times before administering the medication.
5. Perform hand hygiene.
6. Correctly measure the dosage of medication and diluent and place this mixture in the medication dispenser cup. Secure the lid to the medication cup.
7. Ensure that the patient is either sitting upright on the examination table or positioned in the semi-Fowler's position.
8. Connect the disposable tubing to both the nebulizer machine and the medication cup.
9. Turn on the nebulizer machine and wait for the aerosol mist to form. It will fill the mask or come out of the mouthpiece (review Figure 50-A–C).
10. Instruct the patient in the following manner:
    a. If a mouthpiece is used, instruct the patient to gently bite on the mouthpiece and purse lips around the mouthpiece.
    b. If a mask is used, assist the patient in comfortably securing the mask in the proper position to prevent any leakage.
11. Ask the patient to take deep and slow breaths and frequently holding these breaths for three to five seconds at a time, allowing the medication to disperse deep into the lungs.
    a. The treatment will continue until the aerosol mist no longer forms.
12. Turn off the machine when the treatment is completed.
13. Encourage the patient to take deep breaths and cough to facilitate removing loosened secretions.
    a. If the cough is productive after the treatment, take note of amount and characteristics, such as color and viscosity.
14. Detach and dispose of the tubing and mouthpiece in the biohazard waste container.
15. Perform hand hygiene.
16. Provide patient education, both written and verbal, if the patient is to continue nebulizing treatments at home.
17. Document the administration of the nebulizing treatment and the completion of patient education in the patient's medical record.

CHARTING EXAMPLE

10/30/YY 9:15 A.M. Pt. given nebulizer treatment with Albuterol, per Dr. King's orders, administered with mouthpiece. Treatment lasted 10 minutes. Patient was instructed on the home use of the nebulizer and demonstrated understanding by repeating instruction. Written instructions were also provided....
....L. Morton, CMA

A dry powder inhaler (DPI) usually comes in the shape of a disc. It has particles of medication enclosed in a capsule. When the capsule is penetrated, the particles are released and then inhaled into the airways and lungs. A DPI does not have any mechanism that propels the particles toward the lungs. Thus, the person using the inhaler must have the strength and lung capacity to inhale deeply to get the full benefit of the medication. For that reason, DPIs are rarely given to patients experiencing an exacerbation, a flare-up, or

respiratory symptoms. They also have limited use later in the disease process when inhaling deeply becomes difficult or impossible for the patient. Figure 50-10 shows an example of a DPI.

A soft mist inhalers (SMI) are a newer type of inhaler that delivers a premeasured amount of medicine in a slow-moving mist. The advantage of the SMI is that it can actively deliver medicine in a way that is not dependent on how fast the patient breathes in the air from the inhaler.

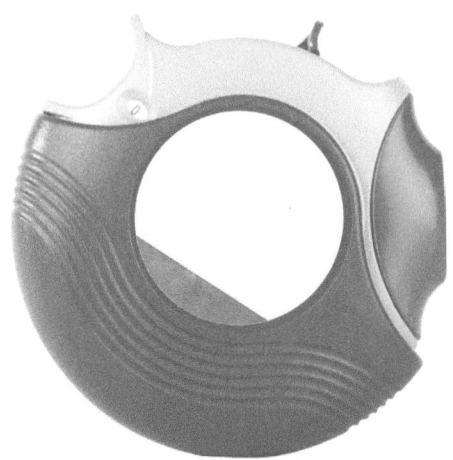

FIGURE 50-10 Example of a dry powder inhaler.

Oxygen Treatments and Delivery Systems

Many patients with lung disease have low levels of oxygen in their bodies, and some may need to use extra or supplemental oxygen to maintain adequate oxygen levels. Oxygen may be provided as acute or long-term therapy for adults and children with chronic lung diseases such as COPD, asthma, pulmonary fibrosis, and CF.

Oxygen supplement is considered a drug and has clear guidelines and indications for use. As a result, patients on oxygen therapy are managed by a pulmonologist and a respiratory therapist. However, medical assistants should be familiar with different types of oxygen therapies and delivery systems because of the growing number of people with chronic lung diseases who are being treated with supplemental oxygen therapy.

Oxygen supplement is usually supplied in either a liquid or gas form and delivered from three types of sources: oxygen pressurized in a metal cylinder, an oxygen concentrator, and liquid oxygen systems. Table 50-3 provides an overview of these oxygen delivery systems.

The most common method of oxygen delivery is with oxygen pressured cylinders. Oxygen in a compressed gas form is stored under pressure in a metal or aluminum cylinder.

Compressed-oxygen cylinders are under extreme pressure, so they must be kept upright and handled carefully. Caution must be observed with oxygen cylinders because of severe safety issues such as explosions and fire hazards.

An oxygen concentrator extracts air from the room air, removes nitrogen, and, thus, is able to deliver a higher concentration of oxygen to the patient than would be obtained by breathing room air. The oxygen concentrator is powered by electricity and can be portable.

In the liquid oxygen system, oxygen is converted to a liquid by super-cooling oxygen in its gas form. When in liquid form, the oxygen takes up much less space and can be stored in a small tank or special thermos. When the liquid form is warmed, it is converted back to a gas for patient use. Liquid oxygen cannot be stored for more than a few weeks because it will evaporate. Thus, the tank must be refilled often, requiring careful scheduling of deliveries.

Figure 50-11 shows examples of types of oxygen delivery systems.

Various devices are used for administering oxygen. The most common devices are a nasal cannula, a simple mask with or without a reservoir bag, and a transtracheal or

Professionalism — Cultural Considerations

While working in the medical office, you will find that a person's cultural and spiritual beliefs may play a major role in their health care. Many cultures of eastern and southeast Asia have a very holistic approach to health care. A strong emphasis is placed on hot and cold therapies, yin and yang principles, and harmony with the universe. Some medications, treatments, and tests may be refused by patients from these varying cultural backgrounds. These patients may seek out alternative forms of treatment, such as acupuncture and acupressure, massage, and herbal remedies. It is the medical assistant's role to accept and be respectful of the patient's health care choices and support them according to the patient's needs.

TABLE 50-3 | Types of Oxygen Delivery Systems

Types	Description	Comments
Oxygen pressurized cylinders	Most common method of delivery. Oxygen is compressed in a large steel or aluminum tanks.	Inexpensive, but heavy and requires refilling. Safety risks.
Oxygen concentrators	Electric device that removes nitrogen from air, producing a high percentage of oxygen for delivery.	Inexpensive, but needs electricity so not portable.
Liquid oxygen systems	Supplied as liquid, but converted to gas when warmed.	Portable, but expensive and requires refilling.

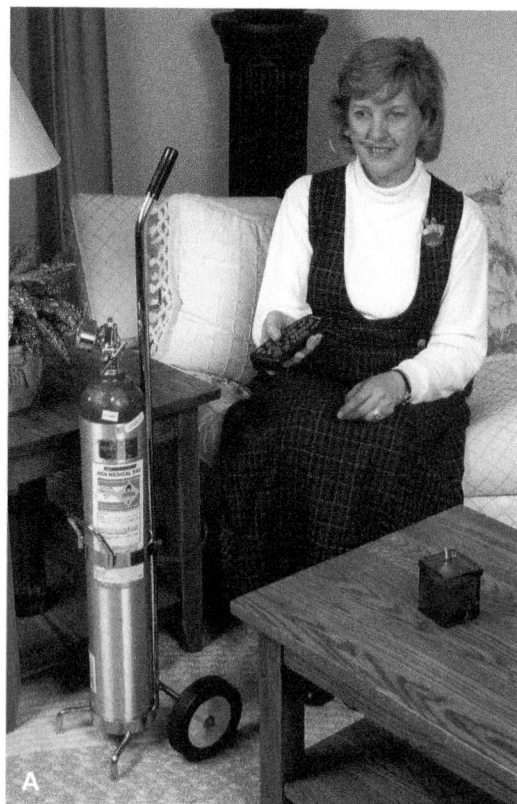

FIGURE 50-11A (A) Oxygen pressurized in a metal cylinder. *(Aaron Haupt)*

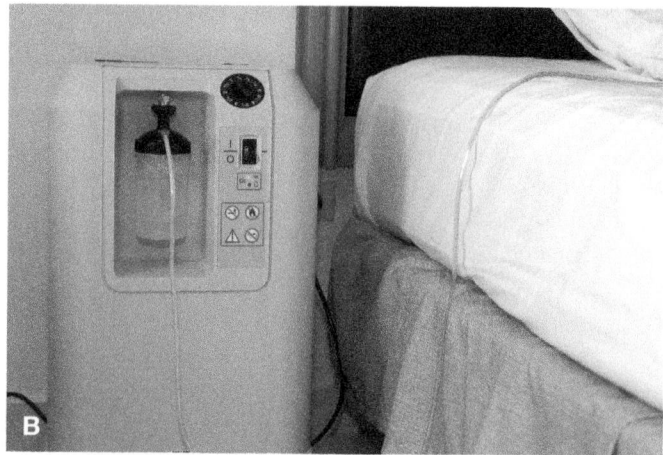

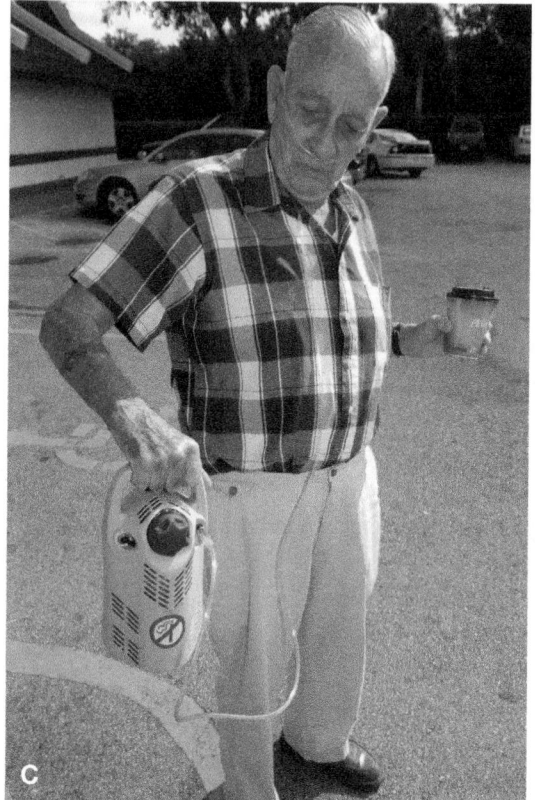

FIGURE 50-11B-C (B) Oxygen concentrator. *(andrea balcazar)* **(C)** Liquid system.

tracheostomy collar. Which device to use often depends on the degree of respiratory impairment as well as the patient's age, mobility, and level of function.

SUMMARY

The medical assistant may be asked to perform various PFTs to assess a patient's breathing function. The medical assistant should have an understanding of pulmonary disorders to better assist with the treatment of a patient's respiratory diseases. The most common PFTs the medical assistant will perform are spirometry and peak flow meter testing. Spirometry can measure multiple volumes and capacities of the lungs, which helps in diagnosing and monitoring lung diseases. It is often performed in the medical office for patients with pulmonary diseases or as a part of a preemployment physical. Peak flow measurement helps measure the capability of air to move in and out of the lungs. This is particularly helpful with the management of asthmatic patients.

The medical assistant should be prepared to provide treatment to patients with breathing difficulties in the medical office, such as administering a nebulizer. Medical assistants may also need to instruct patients on the use of nebulizers and inhalers for home use. Accuracy in carrying out the medical assistant's duties during these tests and procedures will provide the physician with the best possible data to make the proper diagnosis and institute the correct treatment.

50 CHAPTER REVIEW

COMPETENCY REVIEW

1. Define and spell the terms for this chapter.
2. List five signs and symptoms common to pulmonary disorders.
3. Explain the differences between obstructive and restrictive pulmonary disease.
4. Name two examples of obstructive pulmonary disease, and name two examples of restrictive pulmonary disease.
5. Discuss why a poor clinical status can affect the outcome of a PFT.
6. Describe the difference in the measurement of tidal volume and forced vital capacity.
7. Describe the steps in performing a spirometry test.
8. Explain how carbon dioxide impacts the pH level of blood.
9. Describe how medication is administered during a nebulizer treatment.
10. Describe the difference between an inhaler and a nebulizer in regard to drug delivery.

PREPARING FOR THE CERTIFICATION EXAM

1. Which of the following is the amount of air that can be forcibly exhaled after a normal exhalation?
   a. tidal volume
   b. expiratory reserve
   c. inspiratory reserve
   d. total lung capacity
   e. residual volume

2. The physician may request all of the following to help diagnose lung disease *except*
   a. vital signs.
   b. X-rays.
   c. arterial blood oxygen saturation.
   d. breathing volumes.
   e. nerve function in fingertip.

3. To correctly prepare for a spirometry test, the patient is told to
   a. follow normal routine.
   b. take all medications that day.
   c. prepare for test even if ill.
   d. not eat a large meal or smoke for four to six hours before the test.
   e. leave dentures in place.

4. Which respiratory disease or disorder involves permanent destruction of lung tissue and is associated with chronic bronchitis and emphysema?
   a. lung cancer
   b. asthma
   c. COPD
   d. pneumonia
   e. pleuritis

5. Which pulmonary function test is *not* usually performed by a medical assistant?
   a. spirometry
   b. drawing arterial blood gases
   c. peak flow measurement
   d. measuring oxygen saturation
   e. administering a nebulizer treatment

6. When performing a spirometer test on a patient, the medical assistant must
   a. leave the patient alone during the test.
   b. act as coach to encourage more effort.
   c. provide the patient with reading material during the test.
   d. be quiet so patient is not distracted.
   e. give patient the results right away.

7. To measure respiratory function and evaluate medication effectiveness, which of the following tests is performed at home?
   a. peak flow meter
   b. spirometer
   c. CT scan
   d. inhaler
   e. nebulizer

8. All of the following are infectious conditions of the respiratory system except
   a. asthma.
   b. influenza.
   c. pneumonia.
   d. tuberculosis.
   e. pleurisy.

9. Tidal volume is the amount of air inhaled or exhaled during normal breathing. The normal amount is
   a. 1,000 mL.
   b. 250 mL.
   c. 500 mL.
   d. 900 mL.
   e. 100 mL.

10. Total lung capacities (TLC) include
    a. V_T and ERV.
    b. ERV, IRV, and RV.
    c. VC, IC, and FRC.
    d. V_T, ERV, IRV, and RV.
    e. V_T, ERV, IRV, RV, and VC.

CRITICAL THINKING

Refer to the case study at the beginning of the chapter and use what you have learned to answer the following questions.

1. Shandra, RMA, is working with Ms. Lently during her appointment today. She says to Shandra, "I don't understand why I am having this test again. I didn't even understand why I had to have it in the first place when I was diagnosed. What does this test do?" How should Shandra respond?

2. What type of data will Shandra need to enter into the computerized spirometry machine that is used by Pearson Physicians Group? Why will she need to enter these data?

3. After the spirometry test is complete, Dr. Penningworth looks over the results and examines Ms. Lently. He orders blood gas levels to be drawn. These blood tests aren't drawn in the office, and the patient must go to an outside laboratory. Ms. Lently seems upset by the inconvenience of having to go to the lab to have the blood work done. She asks Shandra, "Why does he want me to do even more testing? What will this blood test show?" How should Shandra respond?

ON THE JOB

Darla Huntley, RMA, works in a pulmonology practice. She has been instructed to schedule Betty Robinson for a spirometry within one week. Ms. Robinson has never had one before.

1. After the procedure is scheduled, what information should Darla provide Ms. Robinson to ensure that she is prepared on the day of her test?

2. Under what health-related circumstances would Darla need to reschedule the test for Ms. Robinson?

3. How many maneuvers must be completed for Ms. Robinson's PFT to be considered successful on the day of her testing?

INTERNET ACTIVITY

Research any two of the following diseases: cystic fibrosis, bronchiectasis, lung cancer, asthma.

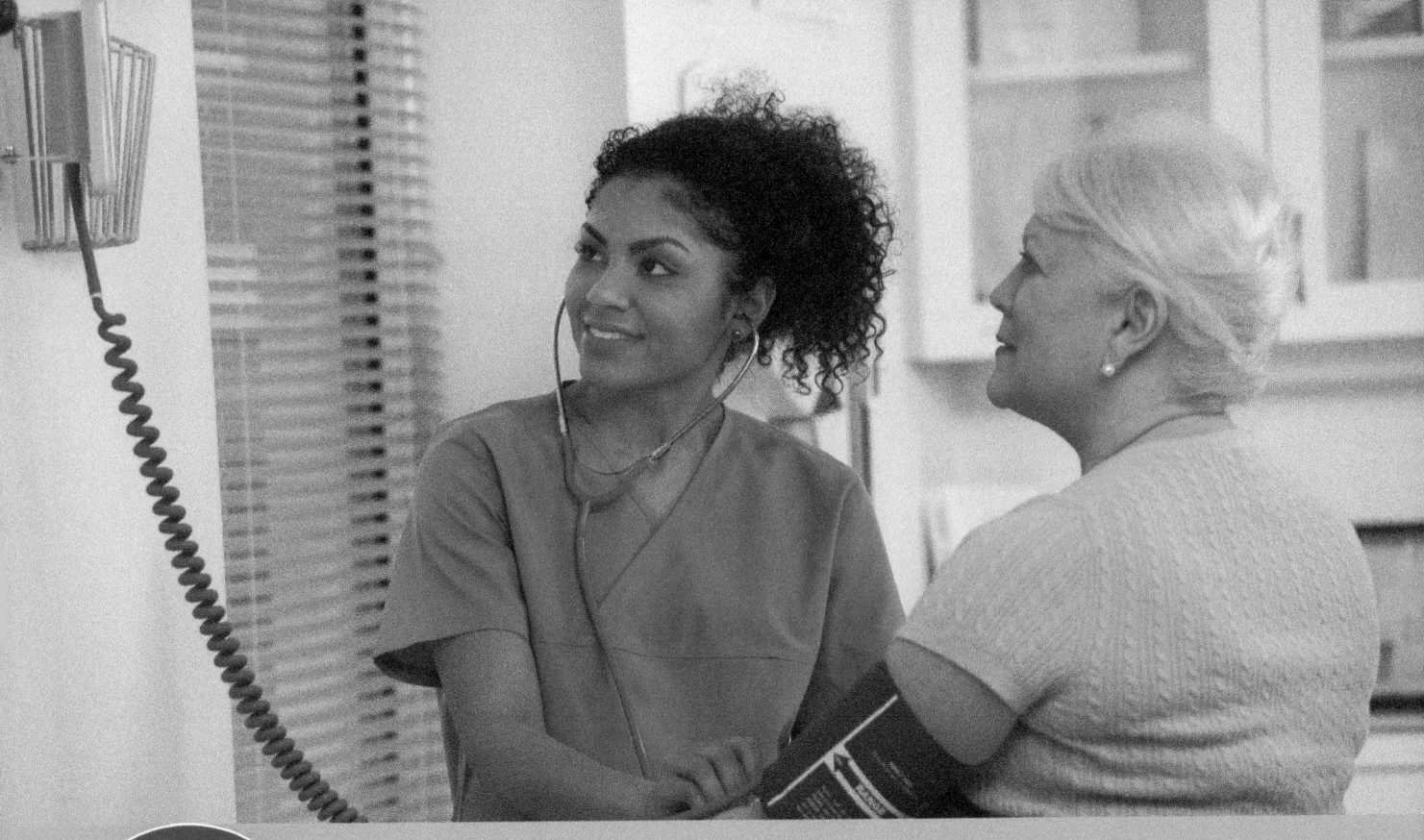

Physical Therapy and Rehabilitation

Learning Objectives

After completing this chapter, you should be able to:

51.1   Define and spell the terms for this chapter.

51.2   Describe the roles of the rehabilitation team.

51.3   Explain the purpose of rehabilitation.

51.4   Identify elements that are included in a patient assessment.

51.5   Describe conditions that require physical therapy.

51.6   Explain how various methods of physical therapy are used to help patients rehabilitate.

51.7   Describe different forms of complementary and alternative medicine.

51.8   List adaptive devices used to help patients ambulate.

51.9   Explain diagnostic tests used to assess the presence of disabling diseases.

Sylvia Jordan, a 76-year-old patient, arrives at the office with her daughter-in-law, Mary Ellen Jordan. Sylvia is seeing Dr. Miller for a follow-up appointment after being hospitalized for a stroke. Since the stroke, Sylvia has had difficulty walking and uses a wheelchair. Samra Belkovich, RMA, wheels Sylvia to the examination room to be seen by Dr. Miller.

Terms to Learn

alternative medicine	friction	petrissage
ambulation	gait	physiatrist
atrophy	gait belt	physiatry
complementary medicine	goniometer	prosthesis
contracture	heat hydrotherapy	prosthetist
cryotherapy	hemiplegia	range of motion (ROM)
diathermy	holistic	rehabilitation
effleurage	massage	Reiki
erythema	modalities	suppuration
exudate	orthotist	tapotement

Physical medicine, the branch of medicine called **physiatry**, is the therapeutic use of physical agents for the diagnosis, treatment, management, rehabilitation, and prevention of diseases and debilitating illnesses. A **physiatrist** is a medical doctor or osteopath who must complete four years of residency training and obtain licensure in the state where she practices.

THE THERAPEUTIC TEAM

Rehabilitation is the process of bringing the patient back as close as possible to normal physical condition after injury or disease. Restorative care is care provided to attain and maintain function and independence.

Patients in need of rehabilitation or physical therapy often require the skilled services of many members of the health care team. This therapeutic team includes the physical therapist (PT), physical therapy assistant (PTA), occupational therapist (OT), occupational therapy assistant (OTA), recreation specialist, exercise physiologist or sports medicine therapist, massage therapist, and prosthetist or orthotist. A **prosthetist** specializes in designing, preparing, and fitting prosthetic devices such as artificial limbs. An **orthotist** designs and fits supportive devices such as braces and splints.

The therapeutic team uses a variety of treatments, including heat, cold, massage, exercise, traction, and at times, a combination of **modalities** (applications of any therapeutic agent). Figure 51-1 shows a PT assisting a patient on parallel bars. Medical assistants must have a thorough

Professionalism

Individual states have different scopes of practice for medical assistants. You must always be familiar with your state's scope of practice for medical assistants to ensure that you are not practicing outside your scope. Some rehabilitative modalities can only be done by physical therapists or physical therapy assistants. Although, as a medical assistant, you would need more training and education to perform many of these duties, carrying out orders for treatments such as heat or cold compresses and exercise may be within your scope of practice. A medical assistant may not recommend a course of treatment to any patient. You may, however, need to instruct and demonstrate to the patient how to appropriately use heat or cold applications at home and assistive devices such as canes and crutches. If you are unsure about whether a specific task is within your scope of practice, obtain information from local, state, or national medical assisting organizations.

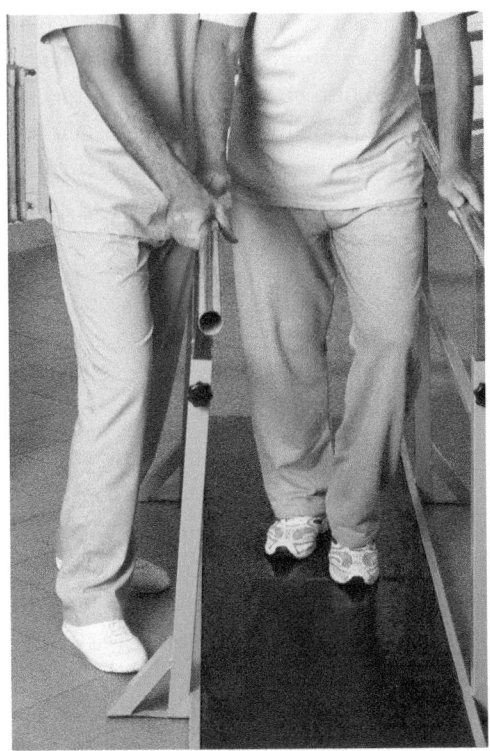

FIGURE 51-1 A physical therapist helping the patient on parallel bars.

understanding of the different therapeutic team members and their roles in rehabilitation, to assist in therapeutic treatments and referral to health care practitioners in a variety of facilities. Table 51-1 provides information about a variety of careers in physical medicine.

REHABILITATION

Rehabilitation is the process of assisting a patient to regain a state of health and the highest level of function possible after injury or illness, or when a condition such as multiple sclerosis has caused the patient to lose mobility and self-esteem.

The rehabilitation process is a **holistic** approach that is concerned with every aspect of the patient's well-being, not just the present disease or injury. Holistic medicine focuses on the whole patient and addresses the social, emotional, and spiritual needs of a patient as well as the physical treatment.

A long illness or a debilitating disease can cause muscle loss or atrophy, a wasting away of muscle tissue that requires patience from everyone involved—the patient, family members, and caregivers. Special attention should be paid to the

TABLE 51-1 | Careers in Physical Medicine

Career	Education/Experience
Physiatrist (MD or DO)	Medical school graduate, four-year residency in physical medicine and rehabilitation, state licensure.
Physical therapist (PT)	Master's degree, licensure required in all states.
Physical therapy assistant (PTA)	Two-year accredited program or associate degree plus internship, licensure required in some states.
Occupational therapist (OT)	Bachelor's or master's degree and internship, licensure required in all states, certification from American Occupational Therapy Association.
Occupational therapy assistant (OTA)	One- to two-year certificate program or associate's degree and internship, licensure or certification required by most states.
Massage therapist	Three-month to one-year accredited massage therapy program; certification, registration, or licensure required in most states.
Recreational therapist (TR) or certified therapeutic recreation specialist (CTRS)	Usually a bachelor's degree plus internship; licensure and certification required in a few states, can be certified by National Council for Therapeutic Recreation Certification or registration by Association for Rehabilitation Therapy.
Recreational therapy assistants (activity director)	One- to two-year certificate program or associate degree, can be certified by National Council for Therapeutic Recreation (NCTRC).
Sports medicine (athletic trainer, ATS)	Bachelor's or master's degree, licensure required in some states, can be certified by National Athletic Trainers Association.
Prosthetist/orthotist	Two years of college and two years of supervised training, national certification available (American Board for Certification [ABC]; Board of Certification [BOC]).

psychologic problems, such as depression and anger, that can occur from a feeling of loss of control over one's life. Rehabilitation programs are useful for improving or restoring both physical and psychologic health for patients who have undergone or are currently experiencing conditions and diseases such as the following:

- Surgery, such as hip and knee replacements
- Trauma, such as broken bones, which can result in long periods of inactivity and muscle weakness
- Catastrophic illness such as stroke
- Disease conditions resulting in muscle atrophy or disuse, such as multiple sclerosis, muscular dystrophy, and cerebral palsy

A formal rehabilitation program begins as soon as the acute phase of an illness or disease has passed. Figure 51-2 shows a physical therapist exercising the patient's leg in a physical therapy department.

The first element of rehabilitation is short- and long-term goal setting, which are based on the physician's orders and the patient's willingness to cooperate. Goals are set for each patient by professionals on the case and suited to the individual patient's needs. In addition, each patient may have his or her own rehabilitation goal. For some, it may be to return to work, for others to be able to care for their family. For many patients, the goal is being able to care for themselves and live independently. These patients are assisted to resume activities of daily living, such as dressing themselves, feeding themselves, toileting, and generally providing as much of their own care as possible.

Short-term goals include objectives such as learning crutch walking and performing exercises to increase range of motion. Long-term goals aim at achieving independence and a feeling of confidence.

In this chapter, we focus mainly on the physical aspects of rehabilitation.

PATIENT ASSESSMENT

Before prescribing rehabilitation treatments, the physician must assess the patient's ability to perform certain functions. The physiatrist will inspect and palpate the patient's limbs and joints to evaluate muscle strength and flexibility. Range of motion, the amount of movement in a particular joint, will be evaluated (see "Range of Motion" later in this chapter). The physiatrist will also evaluate the patient's **gait** (the way a person walks) for clues to specific problems.

Posture is evaluated because a lack of symmetry may indicate a curvature of the spine that has resulted in uneven muscle development. Figure 51-3 illustrates types of spinal curvatures. Kyphosis is an abnormal rounding of the thoracic spine (upper back) that produces an appearance sometimes called humpback. Lordosis is an abnormal inward curvature of the lumbar spine (lower back), sometimes called swayback. In scoliosis, there is an abnormal lateral (sideways) curvature of the spine. There are a wide variety of

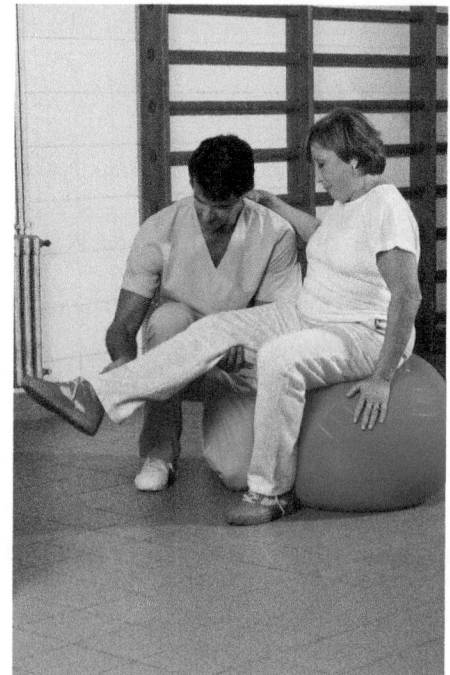

FIGURE 51-2 A physical therapist exercising the patient's leg in a physical therapy department.

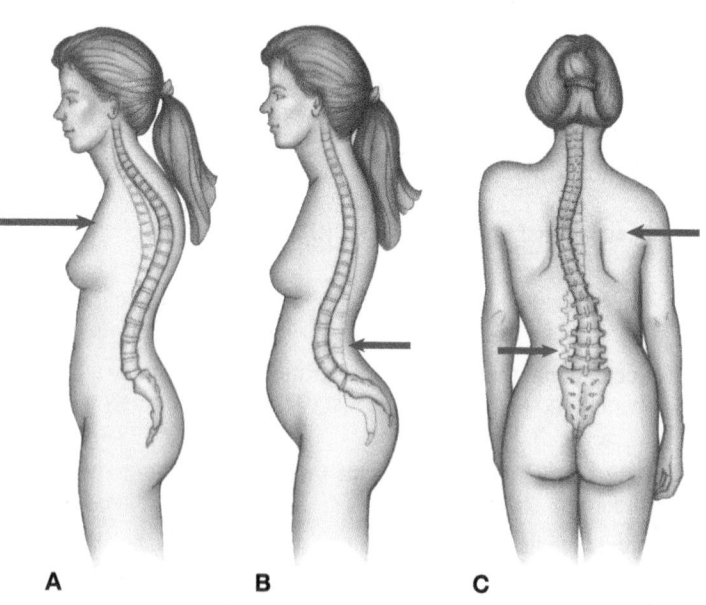

A   B   C

FIGURE 51-3 Three abnormal curvatures of the spine: **(A)** kyphosis; **(B)** lordosis; **(C)** scoliosis.

possible causes of spinal curvature. Scoliosis sometimes occurs during adolescence or periods of rapid growth. Curvatures can result from abnormal spinal development in a fetus, osteoporosis (bone degeneration), poor posture, spinal infections, injuries, and other causes. Treatment of any abnormal curvature may include physical therapy exercises, surgery, a body cast, or a brace, depending on the specific curvature and its severity.

For the patient's safety, during assessment and treatment, a **gait belt** may be used. A gait belt is a safety device that is used to help move a patient. It can be used to hold up a weak patient while walking, standing, or transferring. The medical assistant will put the gait belt around the patient's waist so that if the patient begins to fall, the gait belt can be grasped to prevent falling. Figure 51-4 illustrates the use of a gait belt. Procedure 51-1 explains using a gait belt to assist a patient while assessing gait.

To assess the patient's ability to use stairs, the physician may ask the medical assistant to assist the patient on and off a step stool. A step stool is illustrated in Figure 51-5. A gait belt should be used to ensure the patient's safety during the assessment. The step stool is also sometimes used in rehabilitation to build endurance and assess balance. Patients are asked to step on and off the step stool, both facing the stool and with their backs to the stool. A step stool can also be used to teach patients that step stools with broad bases

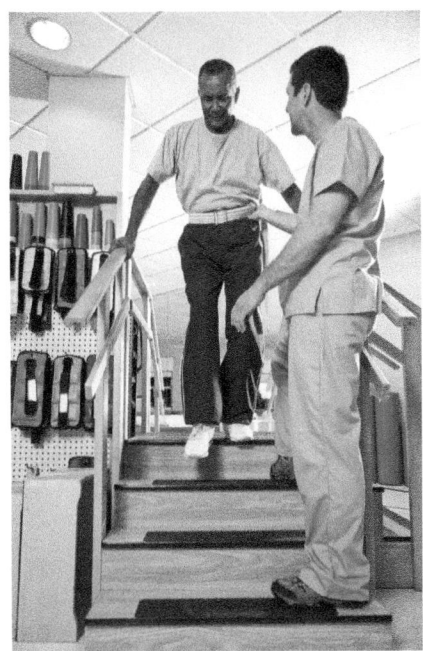

FIGURE 51-4 A medical assistant helps a patient walk with a gait belt.

can be used as adaptive devices to help patients safely reach objects that might otherwise be out of reach.

As a medical assistant, you will assist the physician with these examinations. Once the evaluation is completed, the physician will recommend prescriptions for specific treatments.

PROCEDURE
51-1

Assisting with Assessing Gait, Using a Gait Belt

Objective ◆ *Assist a patient with ambulation to assess gait.*

EQUIPMENT AND SUPPLIES

Gait belt

METHOD

1. Perform hand hygiene.
2. Assemble the equipment.
3. Identify and explain the procedure to the patient.
4. Place the belt around the patient's waist, but over clothing, with the buckle at the front. Do not place over women's breasts.
5. Thread the belt through the teeth of the buckle, putting the belt through the other two openings to lock it. Make

sure it is snug, with just enough room for a couple of fingers to insert under it.
6. Ambulate patient, gently holding on to gait belt at patient's lower back for safety, so physician can assess gait.
7. Perform hand hygiene and return the equipment.
8. Document the procedure in patient's record.

CHARTING EXAMPLE

6/13/YY 3:00 P.M. Patient walked 30 feet without falling, while gait belt used for safety.........................M. King, CMA (AAMA)

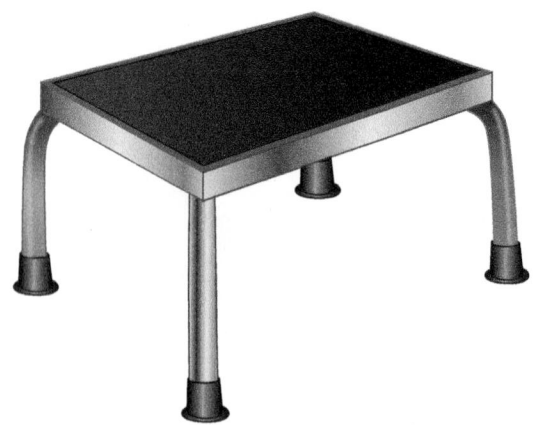

FIGURE 51-5 A step stool can be used to assess the ability to use steps.

CONDITIONS REQUIRING PHYSICAL THERAPY

Disease, injury, birth defects, surgery, and amputation all can result in loss of function. Often, the loss of function involves more areas of the body than the specific part affected. For instance, a patient who loses a lower leg as a result of diabetes has difficulty with **ambulation** (the act of walking) and other activities of daily living. The loss of the leg forces the patient to use different muscle groups that may become sore when walking with crutches or an artificial limb. Box 51-1 lists common health problems that require rehabilitation. Table 51-2 lists conditions that may necessitate physical therapy and the services of a physical medicine specialist. Patients requiring physical therapy may be inpatients, outpatients, nursing home residents, home health patients, and those in special facilities such as veterans' hospitals.

PHYSICAL THERAPY METHODS

Methods used in physical therapy include massage, exercise, heat and cold applications, electricity, ultraviolet radiation, ultrasonic diathermy, hydrotherapy, and application of hot

---

> **BOX 51-1 | Common Health Problems Requiring Rehabilitation**
>
> - Alcoholism
> - Amputation
> - Brain tumor
> - Cerebral palsy
> - Chronic obstructive pulmonary disease (COPD)
> - Traumatic brain injury (TBI)
> - Myocardial infarction (MI)
> - Spinal cord injury or tumor
> - Stroke
> - Substance abuse
> - Mental illness

---

paraffin. These treatment methods are used to improve circulation, strengthen muscles, relieve pain, and assist the patient in learning to perform all activities of daily living.

Exercise Therapy

Being active is an important part of maintaining physical and mental well-being. Inactivity affects every system of the body, and lack of activity can complicate any physical or mental condition. Any person who has exercised regularly and then suspended the exercise activity for a period knows how quickly muscles lose vigor. **Atrophy**, the decrease or wasting away of muscle tissue, occurs rapidly in an inactive patient. Contractures may result, increasing the original disability. A **contracture** is the permanent shortening of the muscle around the joint, causing abnormal and sometimes painful positioning of the joint.

Exercise programs are conducted to maintain or regain fitness through planned activity of muscles and joints. Effective exercise programs can help increase or establish lost muscle tone, improve circulation, relieve stress, correct poor posture and body alignment, and increase endurance.

Regular exercise programs, at least three times a week for 20- to 30-minute periods, are recommended for normal adults. Recent research indicates that daily exercise for 30 minutes is actually needed to maintain health. A patient with known medical problems should have a medical consultation with a physician to evaluate the medical condition and recommend appropriate exercise.

Types of Exercise

A well-rounded exercise program should involve different types of exercises. In addition to an aerobic exercise program, it is considered beneficial to perform 30 minutes of strength training twice a week to promote healthy bones and improve the ratio of fat to muscle. Various types of exercise are recommended:

- **Aerobics**—Strengthens the cardiopulmonary system
- **Isotonic**—Maintains uniform (unchanging) tension or tones the muscles on stimulation
- **Isometric**—Involves contractions with muscles fixed in place so that the tension occurs without noticeable movement
- **Stretching**—Results in muscle elongation

Range of Motion

Patients who have suffered from a temporary or permanent loss of mobility will need instruction on exercises for range of motion (ROM). Range-of-motion exercises can help to maintain muscle tone and flexibility. The medical assistant

TABLE 51-2 | Conditions Treated by Physical Therapy

Disorder/Pathology	Description
Amputation	Removal of an extremity because of injury or disease.
Arthritis	Inflammation of a joint that usually occurs with pain and swelling.
Back pain	Pain along and radiating from the spinal column area resulting from back strain, muscular weakness, and disease or pathology of the spinal cord, such as slipped disc.
Burn	Damage to the skin from first-, second-, or third-degree burns resulting in strictures, decreased mobility, and stiffness. *First-degree:* Damage to superficial layer of skin or outer layer of epidermis with no scarring but resulting in erythema. *Second-degree:* Damage extending through the epidermis and into the dermis causing vesicles and scarring. *Third-degree:* Damage to full thickness (epidermis and dermis) and into underlying layers of the skin with scarring.
Bursitis	Inflammation of the bursa between bony prominences and muscles or tendons.
Cardiovascular disease	Diseases of the blood vessels and heart.
Cerebral palsy	Nonprogressive paralysis caused by defects in the brain or birth trauma.
Cerebrovascular accident (CVA)	Hemorrhage or clotting in the brain that can result in unconsciousness or paralysis (stroke).
Fracture	Broken bone.
Multiple sclerosis	Inflammatory disease of the central nervous system, generally strikes adults between ages 20 and 40 and causes progressive weakness and numbness.
Muscular dystrophy	Wasting disease of the muscles.
Neck trauma	Damage to neck muscles and nerves as the result of trauma or injury (such as whiplash from a car accident).
Osteoporosis	Disease that results in a reduction of bone mass that frequently occurs in postmenopausal women; can result in back pain and fractures.
Paraplegia	Paralysis of the lower portion of the body.
Parkinson's disease	Chronic nerve disease with fine tremors, slow gait, muscular weakness, and rigidity.
Poliomyelitis	Acute viral disease that causes an inflammation of the gray matter of the spinal cord, resulting in paralysis in some cases; has been brought under partial control through vaccinations.
Quadriplegia	Paralysis of all four extremities of the body.
Rheumatoid arthritis	Form of arthritis with inflammation of the joints, swelling, stiffness, and pain.
Sprain	Pain and disability caused by trauma to a joint; a ligament may be torn in a severe sprain.
Strain	Trauma to a muscle from excessive stretching or pulling.

may need to demonstrate ROM exercises for the patient's family members if the patient is unable to perform the exercises alone.

Range of motion (ROM) is the degree of movement that can be achieved in a specific joint without causing pain; it is measured with a special type of protractor called a **goniometer**. During the patient assessment, the physician lines up the two arms of the goniometer with the bones on either side of the joint being measured. Figure 51-6 is an example of a

goniometer measuring the ROM at the patient's elbow. The degree of movement is read from the scale on the hinged arm of the goniometer. Both active movement and passive movement are measured.

Based on the ability of the patient, the physician may order one of the following types of ROM exercises:

- **Active range of motion (AROM)**—The patient is able to move all limbs through the entire ROM unassisted.

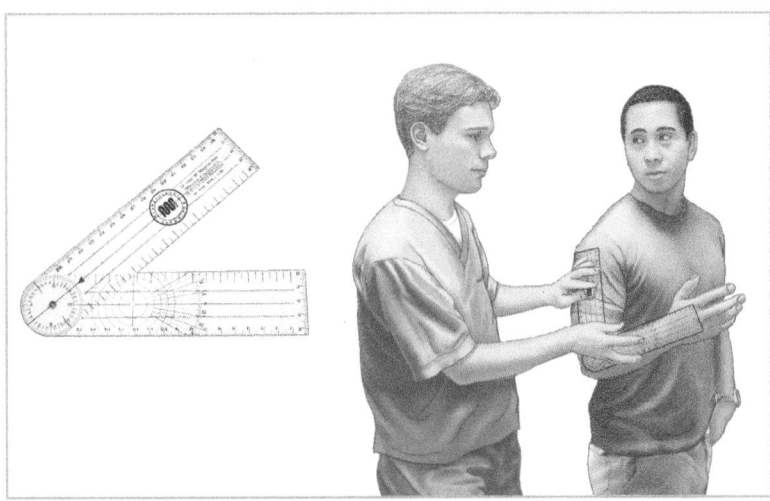

FIGURE 51-6 A goniometer is used to measure range of motion of the patient's arm.

- **Passive range of motion (PROM)**—The patient must have someone else move his or her limbs through the ROM exercises, because the patient is unable to do it.
- **Active assist range of motion (AAROM)**—The patient participates to a limited extent in ROM exercises but requires assistance.

Before beginning ROM exercises, certain guidelines should be explained to the patient (Guidelines 51-1). The patient and the patient's family should be given printed ROM instructions and precautions to take home with them.

Range-of-Motion Exercises

ROM exercises are used to develop and strengthen muscles and joints. Figure 51-7 illustrates the types of body

Guidelines 51-1

Performing Range-of-Motion (ROM) Exercises

- Each exercise should be performed three times unless otherwise ordered by the physician.
- A logical sequence of exercises should be followed so that every muscle and joint receives some movement. In general, ROM exercises begin with the head and move down the body.
- The patient should attempt to do as much as possible without assistance.
- Never force any part of the body beyond normal range. Do not exercise to the point of pain.
- Exercise should not be performed if a joint is reddened or swollen.
- Limbs should be supported at the joints when exercising.

movements used in ROM assessment. Terminology used when discussing movement produced by muscles in ROM exercises is listed in Table 51-3. Most terminology relating to muscle movement is in pairs with opposite meanings. For example, abduction means movement of a body part away from the body, and adduction means movement toward the body. Figures 51-8A–D illustrate ROM exercises performed on a patient's wrist.

Application of Heat and Cold

Heat and cold are used to treat conditions resulting from trauma and infection. Heat and cold, when used therapeutically, are applied for short periods of time (usually 15 to 30 minutes). Circulation can be impaired if either hot or cold applications remain on a body part for an extended period of time. Tissue damage may result if hot and cold applications are not monitored closely.

The medical assistant may have the responsibility to teach the patient the use of heat and cold applications for therapeutic purposes. In some cases, the medical assistant will apply these devices in the office setting.

Heat Applications

Heat is often used to hasten the healing process. The application of heat to a body part causes dilation of blood vessels and allows more blood to circulate to injured tissues. A condition of **erythema**, or redness of the skin, is caused when the capillaries become congested with blood. This increased circulation assists in providing the body with oxygen and nutrients necessary for repair and healing. Tissue metabolism increases, and healing can occur.

Heat can also assist in relieving pain and muscle spasms. In addition, heat can be used to soften hard crusts of exudate produced by damaged body tissues. **Exudate** is an accumulation of fluid, pus, or serum in tissue that may become hard and crusty. The application of heat, in particular moist heat, can hasten **suppuration**, a process to relieve the internal buildup of pus formation. Heat application can take the form of either moist or dry applications to produce a dilation of blood vessels in the skin.

Moist Heat. Moist heat application uses heated water that actually touches the skin, such as in a tub or with a wet compress (pad). Examples of moist heat applications include warm to hot compresses, sitz baths (sitting in water up to the hips in a regular tub or a special shallow basin), tub baths, warm soaks, heat hydrotherapy or whirlpool bath, and paraffin treatment (explained later).

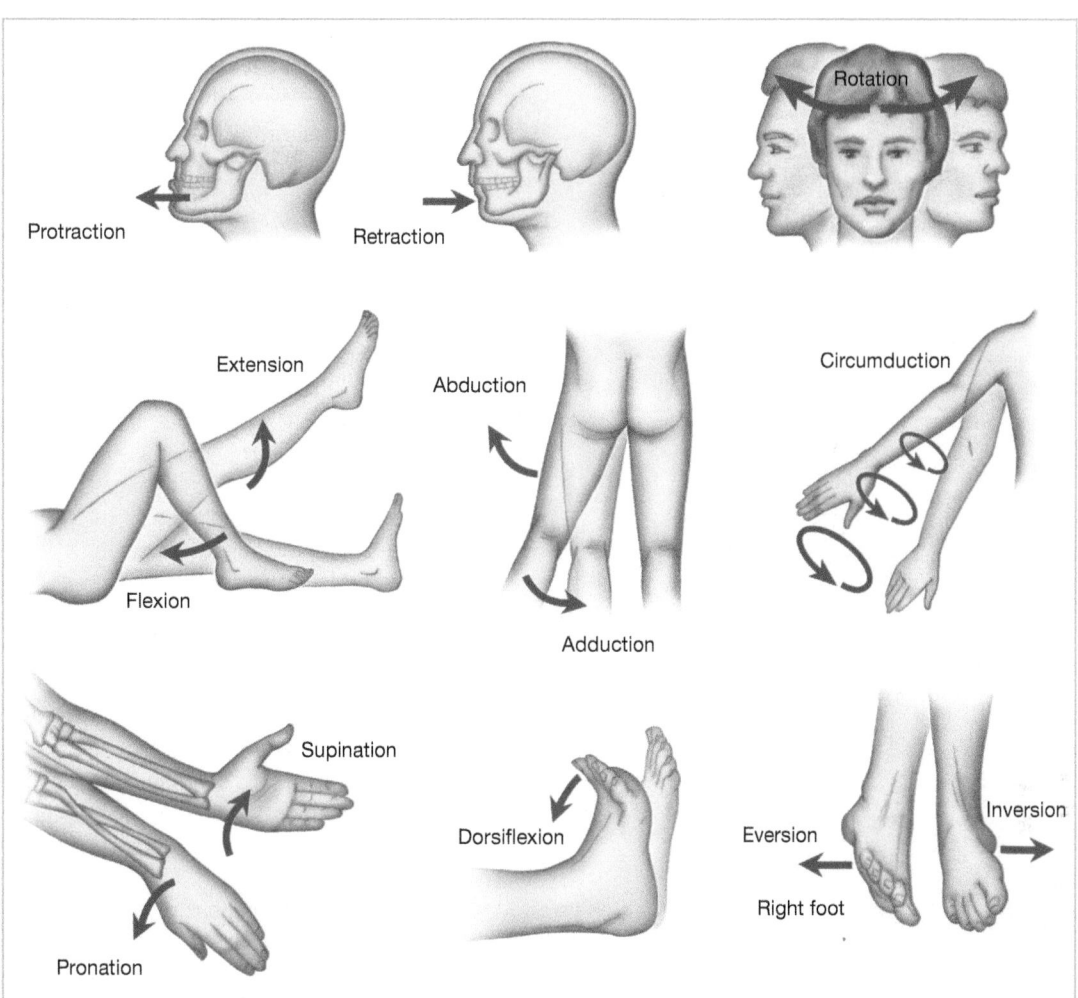

FIGURE 51-7 Types of body movements used in ROM assessment.

TABLE 51-3 | Terminology for Movement Produced by Muscles

Term	Description
Abduction	Movement away from the midline of the body.
Adduction	Movement toward the midline of the body.
Circumduction	Movement in a circular direction from a central point.
Dorsiflexion	Backward bending (as of a hand or foot).
Eversion	Turning outward.
Extension	Movement that brings a limb into or toward a straight condition.
Flexion	The act of bending.
Hyperextension	Extreme or abnormal extension or stretching.
Inversion	Turning inward.
Opposition	Ability to move the thumb into contact with other fingers.
Plantar flexion	Bending the sole of foot, pointing toes downward.
Pronation	Turning downward or backward with the hand or foot; to lie in a prone position (facing downward).
Rotation	The process of turning as if on an axis or a pivot.
Supination	Turning of the palm or hand anteriorly, turning of the foot inward and upward, lying in a supine position (face upward).

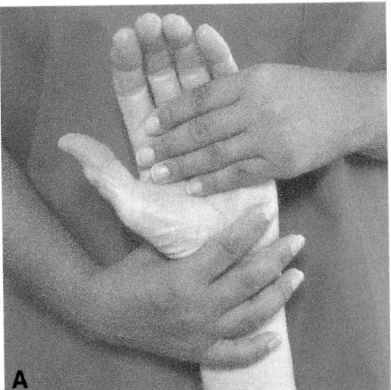

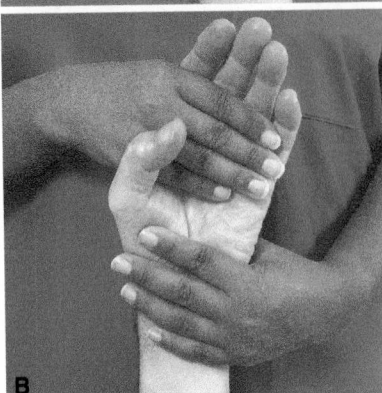

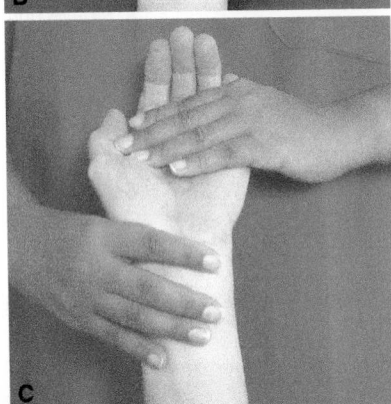

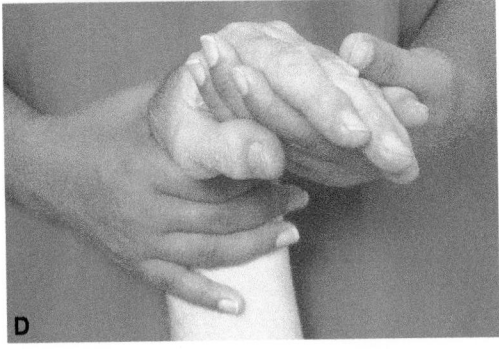

FIGURE 51-8 ROM exercises on a patient's wrist: **(A)** radial deviation; **(B)** ulnar deviation; **(C)** extension; **(D)** flexion.

Hot compresses, often containing a medicated solution, are applied to hasten healing or cleanse open wounds. Any soft, absorbent cloth, such as a washcloth, small towel, disposable woven towels, or gauze squares, can be used as a hot

compress. Procedure 51-2 provides the steps for applying a hot compress. The compress may be kept warm by placing a hot water bottle on top of the compress or rewarming the compress. Applying a hot compress to an open wound requires the use of sterile procedures.

Hot soaks involve having the patient put the affected part of the body into a container of water with or without medication for 15 minutes. The water temperature should be no more than 110°F (44°C). Procedure 51-3 provides steps for a hot soak application.

A hot pack is a canvas bag filled with a heat-retaining gel. Hot packs vary in size and are commercially available. They are used to treat larger areas of the body. The packs are placed in hot water and heated, then wrapped in a towel and applied

Applying a Hot Compress

Objective ◆ *Perform a hot compress application, and document the procedure.*

EQUIPMENT AND SUPPLIES

Soaking solution (or water) as ordered by physician; basin; bath thermometer; absorbent cloths such as washcloths or gauze squares; waterproof cover such as plastic wrap

METHOD

1. Perform hand hygiene.
2. Assemble the equipment. If an open wound is present, use sterile equipment and standard precautions.
3. Identify and explain the procedure to the patient.
4. Fill the basin half full of water or medicated solution prepared according to the directions of the physician.
5. Request the patient to remove any necessary clothing, because compresses are performed on bare skin. Assist the patient, if necessary.
6. Check the temperature of the solution with a bath thermometer. The temperature range for an adult is between 105° and 110°F (41° and 44°C).
7. Position the patient in a comfortable, well-supported position.
8. Place the cloths in the basin of hot water or solution. Wring out one cloth until it is wet but not dripping.
9. Gradually place the compress on the patient's body part (Figure A). Ask the patient to tell you how the temperature feels.
10. Frequently test the temperature of the solution. Replace the water as it cools with more warm water.
11. Time the procedure according to the physician's order (15–30 minutes). Check the patient periodically for any signs of change in redness, swelling, or pain.
12. Gently dry the affected body part.

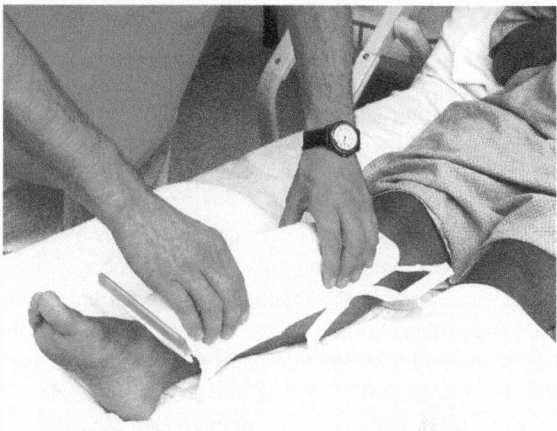

FIGURE A Applying a hot compress to the patient's leg.

13. Instruct the patient on any further care such as continued warm compresses at home.
14. Place towels in the laundry. If an open wound is present, then handle the linens according to standard precautions.
15. Clean all the equipment.
16. Perform hand hygiene and return the equipment.
17. Document the procedure in the patient's record.

CHARTING EXAMPLE

6/14/YY 3:00 P.M. Hot compress at 105°F applied to right shin for 20 minutes. Skin with some redness after application. Pt. states there is pain relief. Instructed on application of hot compresses at home. Patient verbalized understanding............
....M. King, CMA (AAMA)

---

to the affected area. These packs have the advantage of retaining heat longer than hot compresses.

Heat hydrotherapy is the use of warm water as a therapeutic or healing treatment. This can be done in bathtubs, swimming pools, and whirlpools. The whirlpool bath, with continuous jets of hot water reaching the body surfaces, promotes circulation and flexibility of muscles and joints. Arthritis patients are encouraged to participate in exercises in a warm pool to maintain flexibility and reduce pain.

Hot paraffin as a form of heat treatment involves placing the extremities into hot wax to relax the muscles and promote healing. The temperature of the paraffin or wax has to be controlled carefully to prevent burning. Paraffin treatments are usually performed by licensed physical therapists using standard paraffin bath equipment. This therapy is useful for patients with rheumatoid arthritis to relieve the pain and stiffness in joints. The hand or limb is inserted into hot melted paraffin that has been heated to 126°F (54°C). The

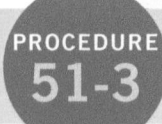

PROCEDURE
51-3

Applying a Hot Soak

Objective ◆ *Perform a hot soak application, and document the procedure.*

EQUIPMENT AND SUPPLIES

Soaking solution or water as ordered by physician; basin or tub; pitcher; bath thermometer; towels

METHOD

1. Perform hand hygiene.
2. Assemble the equipment. If an open wound is present, use sterile equipment and standard precautions.
3. Identify and explain the procedure to the patient.
4. Fill the basin or tub half full of water or medicated solution prepared according to directions of the physician.
5. Request the patient to remove any obstructing clothing because soaks are applied to the bare skin. Assist the patient if necessary.
6. Check the temperature of the solution with a bath thermometer. The temperature range for an adult is between 105° and 110°F (41° and 44°C).
7. Position the patient in a comfortable well-supported position.
8. Pad the side of the basin or tub with a towel to prevent the patient's body from rubbing on the edge.
9. Gradually place the patient's body part in the solution (Figure A). Ask the patient to tell you how the temperature feels.
10. Frequently test the temperature of the solution. Using a pitcher, remove part of the liquid every five minutes and replace it with hot water. Pour the hot water at the edge of the basin or tub, and protect the patient by placing your hand between the patient's body part and the hot water as it is poured. Swirl the water while pouring to mix the hot and cool fluid together.
11. Time the procedure according to the physician's order (15–30 minutes). Check the patient periodically for any signs of change in redness, swelling, or pain.
12. Gently dry the affected body part.
13. Instruct the patient on any aftercare, such as performing warm soaks at home.
14. Place the towels in the laundry. If an open wound is present, then handle the linens according to standard precautions.

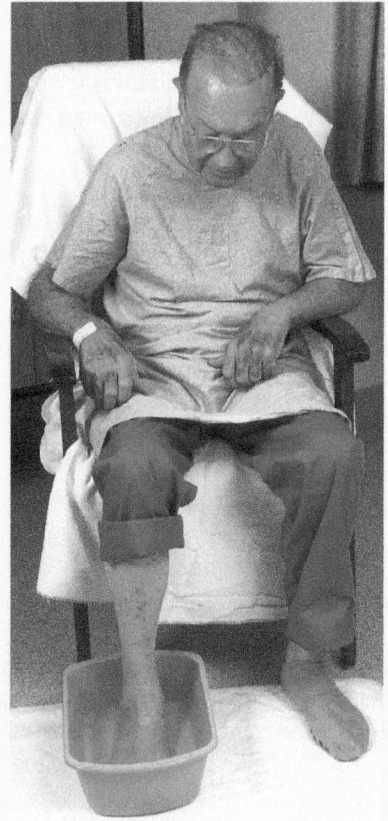

FIGURE A Place a basin in position for the patient to easily dip a foot in water for a hot soak.

15. Clean all the equipment.
16. Perform hand hygiene and return the equipment.
17. Document the procedure in the patient's record.

CHARTING EXAMPLE

1/15/YY 1:00 P.M. Hot water soak at 105°F applied to right foot for 30 minutes. Skin slightly pink to some redness after application. Pt. states there is pain relief. Instructed on application of hot water soaks at home. Patient verbalized understanding..M. King, CMA (AAMA)

hand or limb is left in the hot paraffin for about 15 to 30 minutes until there is a thick coating. The relief after this treatment is longer lasting than in some other forms of moist heat treatment.

Dry Heat. A dry application is a heat application without water, such as with a heating pad. Dry heat can be applied by infrared radiation (heat lamps), electric heating pads, hot water bottles, chemical hot packs, and aquathermia or aquamatic pads. Figure 51-9 is an example of an aquamatic K-pad, which is an electric, water-filled pad used for dry heat. Another heating pad is a flat electric pad that provides localized heat by regulating a dial. The physician should specify the temperature required for the treatment (low, medium, high). Patients should be reminded not to lie on heating pads to avoid burns. Procedure 51-4 lists the application steps for a heating pad.

Heat lamps use infrared bulbs to produce heat. The rays from the lamp penetrate the surface of the skin 3 to 5 mm; it is essential that the lamp be placed 2 to 4 feet away from

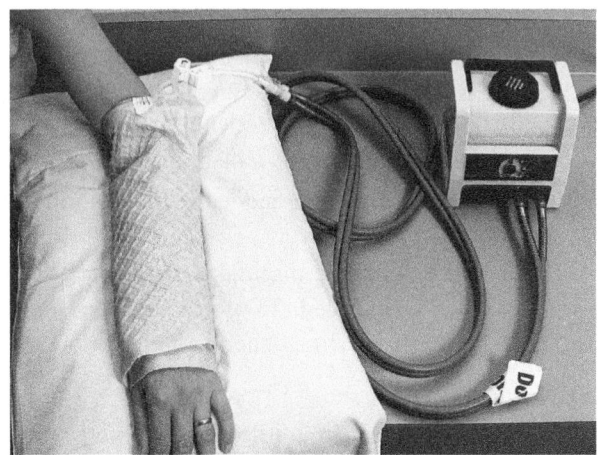

FIGURE 51-9 Aquamatic pad and heating unit provide dry heat treatment to a patient's arm.

the patient to avoid burning the skin. Treatments usually last about 20 minutes and must be carefully monitored. Ultraviolet lamps are used to treat conditions such as psoriasis or wound infections (see "Ultraviolet Radiation").

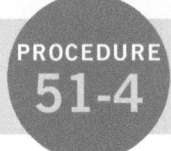

PROCEDURE
51-4

Applying a Heating Pad

Objective ◆ *Perform a heating pad application, and document the procedure.*

EQUIPMENT AND SUPPLIES

Heating pad with protective covering or pillowcase

Note: Perform a preliminary check of the heating pad without bending it to determine that the wires are in good condition.

METHOD

1. Perform hand hygiene.
2. Assemble and test the equipment.
3. Identify and instruct the patient concerning the procedure. The patient should be cautioned against using pins, bending the heating elements within the pad, or lying on the heating pad.
4. Place the heating pad in a protective covering or pillowcase.
5. Connect the heating pad to an electric plug. Set the temperature selector at the setting ordered by the physician (low or medium).
6. Place the heating pad over the patient's affected area. Ask the patient to tell you how it feels. Adjust the temperature as necessary.

7. Instruct the patient regarding the proper temperature setting. Tell the patient not to change the setting.
8. Leave the heating pad in place for the amount of time ordered by the physician (15–20 minutes). Check the patient periodically for any signs of change in redness, swelling, or pain.
9. Remove the heating pad when the procedure is complete. Instruct the patient on any aftercare, such as performing heat treatments at home.
10. Place the protective covering in laundry.
11. Perform hand hygiene and return all the equipment.
12. Document the procedure in the patient's record.

CHARTING EXAMPLE

1/12/YY 9:00 A.M. Heating pad on medium setting applied to left elbow for 20 minutes. Erythema noted over application site. Pt. states there is pain relief and increased mobility in elbow joint. Instructed on application of heating pad at home. Patient verbalized understanding.......................M. King, CMA (AAMA)

A hot water bottle is flat, flexible, and easy to use. The temperature of the water should not exceed 125°F (54°C). For older adults and children under 2 years old, the temperature should not exceed 115°F (50°C). The water bottle should be filled partially and the remaining air expelled. An overly full bottle is less flexible and harder to conform to the affected body part.

A chemical hot pack is a disposable pack that becomes hot when slapped or kneaded. To use these convenient hot packs, the manufacturer's directions should be followed.

Cold Applications

Cold applications result in constriction of blood vessels, which is the opposite effect of warm applications. Constriction of blood vessels is very useful to prevent or reduce swelling, as in a sprain. Because the blood flow is actually slowed, the amount of body fluids carried into an injured part, such as a leg, is reduced. Additional benefits of cold applications may include the reduction of pain and control of bleeding because of the slowing of blood circulation.

Cryotherapy is using cold for therapeutic purposes. Cold applications can be applied to a body part, such as an ice bag after a tooth extraction. In addition, cold applications can be placed on the entire body to reduce an elevated body temperature. Cold applications consist of cold compresses, soaks, ice packs, and hypothermia blankets. Procedure 51-5 lists the steps for applying a cold compress. Ice in a bag or container (ice pack) is used to treat localized conditions. Procedure 51-6 provides the steps for application of an ice bag. A bag of frozen vegetables, such as peas, makes an effective temporary ice bag.

Chemical cold packs are self-contained packets containing a small amount of water in an inner bag that, when released into a chemical contained in the outer bag, causes a chemical reaction that makes the bag cold. This pack can be used as an alternative to an ice pack.

Wet cold applications, such as cold compresses, may be used to treat pain and fever. A washcloth or similar cloth is moistened with ice water and applied to an area.

Patient safety and comfort are a concern when using either warm or cold applications. Always frequently check the skin to see if patient is being harmed.

Ultraviolet Radiation

Ultraviolet radiation uses rays from natural sources, such as the sun, and artificial sources, such as sun lamps, for healing

PROCEDURE
51-5

Applying a Cold Compress

Objective ◆ *Perform a cold compress application, and document the procedure.*

EQUIPMENT AND SUPPLIES

Water; absorbent cloths or gauze squares; waterproof cover or plastic wrap; basin; ice

METHOD

1. Perform hand hygiene.
2. Assemble the equipment. If an open wound is present, use sterile equipment and standard precautions.
3. Identify and instruct the patient concerning the procedure.
4. Fill the basin half full of cold water. Add ice cubes and compresses.
5. Wring out a compress until wet but not dripping. Wrap the compress in a plastic or waterproof covering to prevent further dripping. Gently place the compress on the patient's affected body part.

6. Check the compress every three to five minutes, and replace when no longer cool with another cold compress. Add more ice as the water warms.
7. Leave the compresses in place for the time specified by the physician (usually 15–20 minutes).
8. Gently dry the affected body part.
9. Place the linens in the proper container. Clean all the equipment.
10. Perform hand hygiene and store the equipment.
11. Document the procedure in the patient's record.

CHARTING EXAMPLE

10/23/YY 10:00 A.M. Cold compresses applied to right ankle for 20 minutes. Swelling decreased after treatment. Erythema noted over application site. Instructed on application of cold compress at home. Patient verbalized understanding...............
....M. King, CMA (AAMA)

Applying an Ice Bag

Objective ◆ *Perform an ice bag application, and document the procedure.*

EQUIPMENT AND SUPPLIES

Ice bag with a protective cover (or small hand towel); ice chips or crushed ice

METHOD

1. Perform hand hygiene.
2. Assemble and test the equipment.
3. Identify and instruct the patient concerning the procedure.
4. Fill the ice bag one-half to two-thirds full of ice. Expel air by squeezing the empty half of ice bag. Replace the cap (Figures A–D).
5. Dry the bag and place in a protective covering or small hand towel.
6. Place the ice bag over the patient's affected body part. Ask the patient how the ice bag feels.
7. Refill the bag with ice as needed.
8. Leave the ice bag in place for the time specified by the physician (usually 15–20 minutes).
9. Clean the equipment. Allow the bag to air-dry.
10. Perform hand hygiene and store the equipment.
11. Document the procedure in the patient's record.

CHARTING EXAMPLE

2/14/YY 2:00 P.M. Ice bag applied to contusion on right forehead. Swelling reduced after 20 minutes. Erythema noted in treatment area. Instructed on application of ice bag at home. Patient verbalized understanding............M. King, CMA (AAMA)

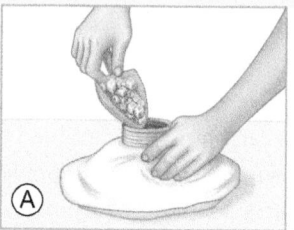 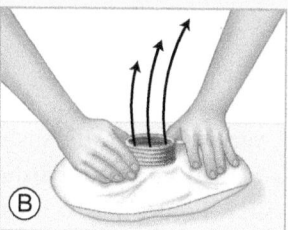 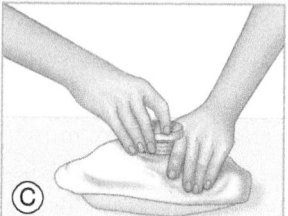 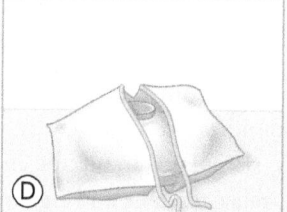

FIGURE A–D Preparing an ice bag.

purposes. Ultraviolet rays stimulate the growth of new epithelial cells and are capable of killing bacteria. These rays are used therapeutically for the treatment of disorders such as psoriasis. Disorders caused by bacteria, such as acne and pressure sores, are treated effectively with this therapy. The goal of the treatment is to produce a mild redness of the skin to stimulate circulation and kill bacteria.

Ultraviolet-ray lamp treatments must be carefully controlled, because the intensity can cause severe first-degree and even second- and third-degree burns. Both the timing of the exposure and the distance of the lamp from the patient must be carefully controlled. A patient can receive a second-degree burn after one to two minutes of exposure to a lamp set at 30 inches from the patient. Because a patient does not feel this type of burn occurring, the patient cannot warn the operator to stop treatment.

Treatment is ordered by the second, such as a 20-second lamp treatment placed at least 30 inches from the patient and directed only on the area to be treated. Eye protection, in the form of dark goggles, should be worn by both the patient and medical assistant to protect the eyes from ultraviolet ray exposure.

The patient should never be left unattended during this procedure. If you have to leave the room during the treatment, turn off the lamp until you return. The danger of severe burns is great if the timing is not exact.

Diathermy

Diathermy is the therapeutic use of a high-frequency current that induces an electrical field within a portion of the body. This electrical field generates heat in various parts of the body and increases blood flow to aid in healing. Diathermy is useful in treating muscular disorders and treatments of tendonitis, arthritis, and bursitis.

The diathermy machine placement must be carefully controlled according to the manufacturer's instructions. Some machines are placed 1 inch from the patient's skin and may have a built-in spacer to assist with exact placement. Others have applicators with pads that require a towel to be placed between the applicator pad and the patient. Because of the danger of burns inherent in diathermy treatment, it has been replaced in many facilities with ultrasound, which is safer.

Ultrasound

Ultrasound is sound energy from high-frequency sound waves penetrating deep through tissue layers. It works on the same premise as sonar used in oceanography. Ultrasound waves vibrate at the rate of one million times per second, which cannot be heard by the human ear but produce mechanical and heating effects. The mechanical effect or vibration works on connective tissues, such as ligaments and tendons; the heat effect works on all body tissues. However, ultrasound treatments should be used carefully near bony tissues to avoid causing injury from concentration of waves.

Ultrasound treatments usually are applied for 10 minutes or less, as ordered by the physician. The patient may require several ultrasound treatments to receive the benefit. Ultrasound is used effectively to treat pain, relax muscle spasms, stimulate circulation in patients with vascular disorders, relax tendons and ligaments, and break up calcium deposits and scars. Ultrasound treatments are used in conjunction with other treatments, such as medications, to relieve back spasms.

Ultrasound is administered via a machine with an applicator head attachment that can be placed directly on the skin. The ultrasound applicator head contains quartz crystal that vibrates rapidly when an electric current passes through it. Because these waves do not travel through air, they must be kept in contact with the skin. A conducting medium, such as a special gel or mineral oil, must be placed on the skin to conduct the ultrasound into the body. The ultrasound operator applies the ultrasound head to the patient's skin using a steady up-and-down motion. The operator must keep the ultrasound head in continuous motion over the body part because tissue damage can occur if it is held in one place for a prolonged period of time. Before treatment, patients should be asked if they have any implants, such as a hip or joint replacement, because the ultrasound could loosen the implant.

ADAPTIVE EQUIPMENT AND DEVICES

Equipment used to assist recovery from physical disorders or disabilities includes adaptive equipment (e.g., wheelchairs, walkers, canes, crutches) and special furniture (e.g., shower chairs and geriatric chairs). Mobility aids or mobility-assistive devices are designed to enable the patient to ambulate. Other devices, including braces, casts, traction, prostheses, splints, and slings, are used by the physical therapist to manipulate the patient's damaged bones and tissues. Adaptive equipment also includes a variety of utensils, such as eating utensils molded to fit the patient's hand and dishes with a wide edge to prevent spilling. Figure 51-10 illustrates adaptive equipment, including a toothbrush, reaching stick, shoe holder, stocking helper, and writing aid.

Special furniture, such as shower chairs made from aluminum or plastic, allows the patient to sit while taking a shower. The geriatric chair, a wheeled chair that reclines with an attached tray for meals, is useful for patients who can feed themselves but may not be able to sit securely in a regular chair.

Adaptive devices are prescribed by the physician; however, the physical therapist may provide the initial instruction on the use of the device. In a general practice setting, the medical assistant will assist the physician with these devices and will provide continuing education and support for the patient when seen in the physician's office. Figure 51-11 illustrates a physical therapist assisting a patient to regain mobility and strength after an amputation.

Crutches

Crutches allow the patient to walk without placing weight on the healing leg part. Weight is transferred to the arms

Professionalism   The Law

Many of the procedures described in this chapter are beyond the scope of practice for a medical assistant beginning his or her first job. Additional training and practice are required before teaching a patient to use crutches, for instance. In some states, only a licensed physical therapist is able to perform many of the procedures discussed. The medical assistant must remember that with many procedures, he or she is "assisting" another licensed person, such as the physician, nurse, or physical therapist. Always check with your local or state medical association regarding the laws in your state. The patient's safety must always be placed first.

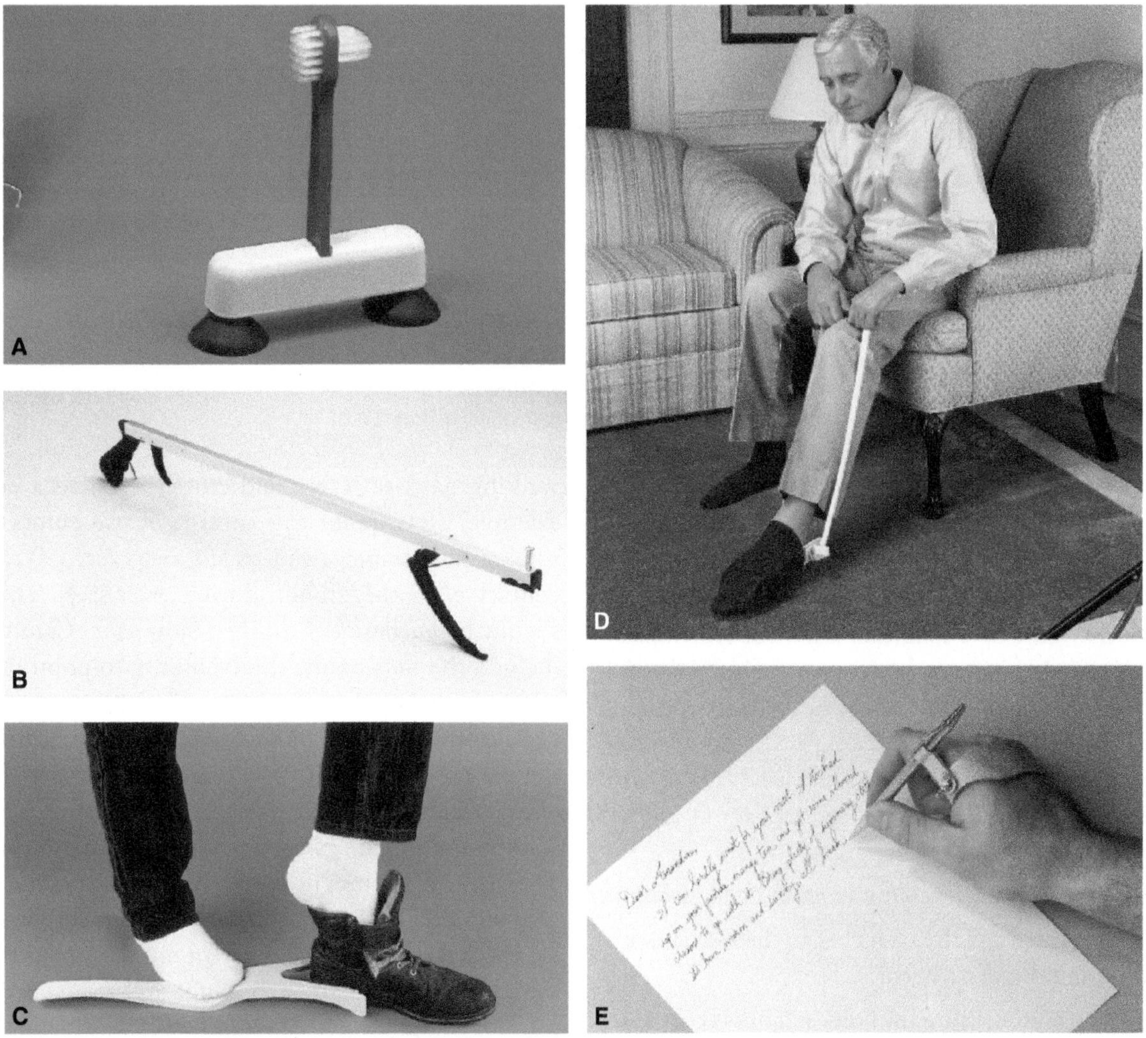

FIGURE 51-10 There are many types of adaptive devices: **(A)** a toothbrush; **(B)** a reaching stick; **(C)** a shoe holder; **(D)** a sock helper; **(E)** a writing aid.

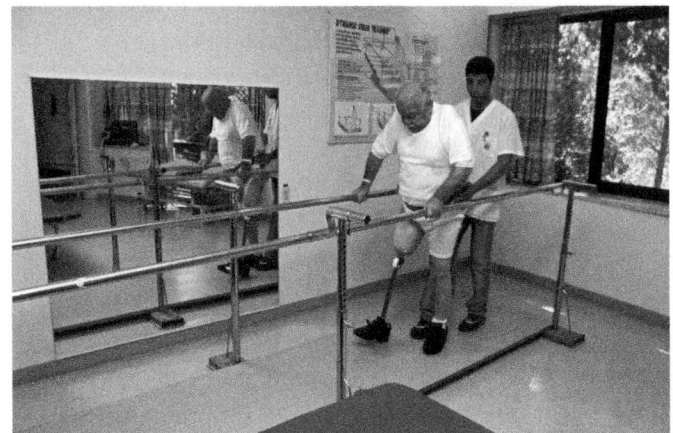

FIGURE 51-11 A therapist assisting an amputee patient to regain mobility and strength after amputation.

and hands. Crutches are made from metal or wood and should have a rubber tip at the end to prevent slipping on a smooth floor surface. The following are the three most common types of crutches (Figure 51-12):

- **Axillary crutch**—a tall crutch with shoulder rest and handgrip that reaches from the ground to under the axilla. These crutches are commonly used for a patient who has suffered a fractured leg.

- **Lofstrand (forearm crutch)**—a single aluminum tube with an arm cuff that fits snugly around the patient's forearm and uses a handgrip for weight bearing. This crutch allows the patient to release the handgrip to use the hand while still having the crutch held in place by the arm cuff for support. People with cerebral palsy and paraplegia often choose to use this type of crutch.

- **Canadian or elbow crutch**—a variation of the Lofstrand crutch that extends farther up the arm.

Measuring for Axillary Crutches

Measurement for axillary crutches has to be determined carefully to prevent pressure damage to the axillae. If the crutch is too long, it may cause pressure on the brachial

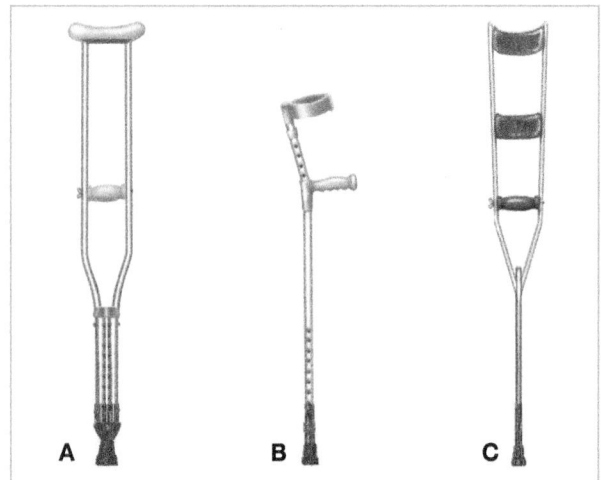

FIGURE 51-12 Three types of crutches: **(A)** axillary crutch; **(B)** Lofstrand or forearm crutch; **(C)** Canadian or elbow crutch.

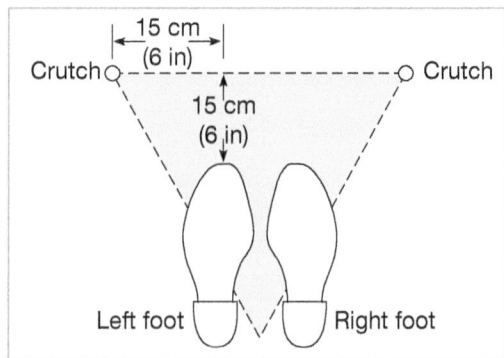

FIGURE 51-13 The correct beginning position for the patient's feet and crutches (tripod position).

plexus (nerve running under the axilla and down the arm). The patient may develop a condition known as crutch palsy, resulting in muscle weakness in the arm, wrist, and hand. Crutches that are too short can result in the patient having to bend forward while walking. Back pain, nerve damage, and injury to the axillae and palms of the hands can occur if the crutches are improperly fitted. The steps for measuring axillary crutches follow:

1. Have the patient wear walking shoes and stand straight.

2. Place the crutch tips 4 to 6 inches to the side and 4 to 6 inches in front of each foot.

3. Adjust the crutch, using the bolts and nuts at the sides of the crutch, so that the axillary crutch bars are three finger widths below the axilla. Measure this by inserting your own fingers between the patient's axilla and the crutch bar.

4. Next, adjust the handgrips so the patient can flex the elbows at a 30-degree angle when the crutch is in place and the patient's hands are on the hand bars.

Instructions both in writing and with an actual demonstration should be provided to the patient who will be using crutches. To teach the patient how to properly use crutches, have the patient start in the tripod position. Figure 51-13 illustrates the correct position of the crutches and the patient's feet. Teaching the patient how to use crutches and proper crutch walking gaits is one of the responsibilities of the medical assistant.

Crutch Walking Gaits

The type of crutch gait or walk that the patient will use depends on the amount of weight bearing the patient's leg or legs will support and the patient's muscular coordination, age, and overall physical condition. In a crutch walking gait, each foot and crutch is called a point. For example, a two-point gait consists of two points from the total of four points (two legs and two crutches) that are in contact with the ground during each step. The patient should be encouraged to use a slow gait. Common gaits include the four-point, three-point, two-point, swing-to, and swing through gaits.

The physician determines the type of crutch necessary for the patient and may fit the crutch for the patient in the office. You may be asked to demonstrate the use of crutches and the appropriate gait required by the patient's condition. The patient should be reminded to use a slow pace in crowded areas or when feeling tired. Using crutches requires a great deal of energy and different muscle groups than those the patient is accustomed to using.

Four-Point Gait. The four-point gait is a slow and steady gait and is used when a patient can bear weight on both legs. This is considered the safest of all gaits, because the patient has three points of support in contact with the ground at all times. This gait is also used by patients who may have muscular weakness and some lack of coordination (Figure 51-14).

To use this gait, first the right crutch is moved forward, followed by the left foot, then the left crutch, and then the right foot. This is repeated over and over. The patient must be able to move each leg separately to use this gait.

Three-Point Gait. The three-point gait is used when one leg is stronger than the other or when there is no weight bearing on one leg. The patient must have good muscle coordination and arm strength. To use this gait, the patient must be able to support full weight on one leg. Have the patient move both crutches and the affected leg forward and then move the unaffected leg forward while weight is balanced on both crutches (Figure 51-15). This gait requires good coordination and muscle strength. It is used by patients with musculoskeletal disorders (e.g., fractures), recent leg surgery, or amputees without an artificial limb.

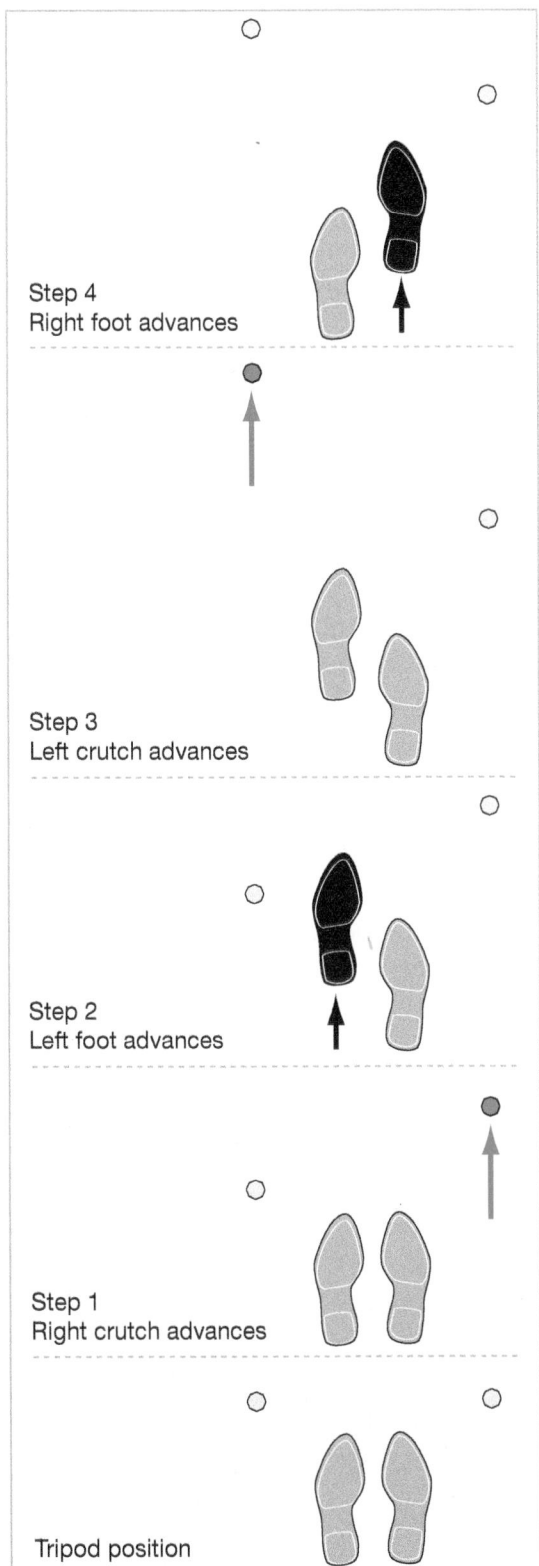

FIGURE 51-14 Four-point gait.

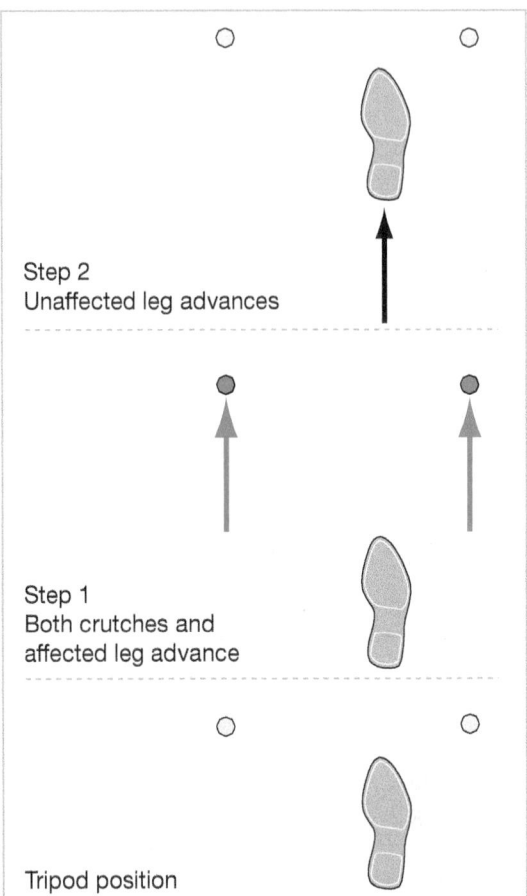

FIGURE 51-15 Three-point gait.

Two-Point Gait. The two-point gait is faster moving than the four-point gait and is used by the patient who can bear some weight on both feet and maintain good balance. Two-point gait occurs when a crutch and the opposite foot are moved forward at the same time. For example, the left crutch and the right leg move together (Figure 51-16).

Swing Gaits. Swing gaits are used by patients with severe leg disabilities, such as deformities or paralysis. They may use either of the two swing gaits: swing-to or swing-through gait.

To use the *swing-to gait*, the patient moves the crutches forward, lifts his or her body, and then swings the legs up to the same point. Good muscular control is needed for this gait because the patient may lose balance and fall forward with this gait (Figure 51-17A and 51-17B).

To use the *swing-through gait*, the patient moves the crutches forward, as in the swing-to gait, and then swings the legs past the crutches. This provides a good base of support. It is a gait that allows for fast movement. Both the swing-to and swing-through gaits are used by paraplegic patients who are using the forearm type of crutches or by patients with a generalized leg weakness.

Sitting with Crutches

The patient using crutches should be instructed on how to manipulate the crutches and support his or her legs to sit down.

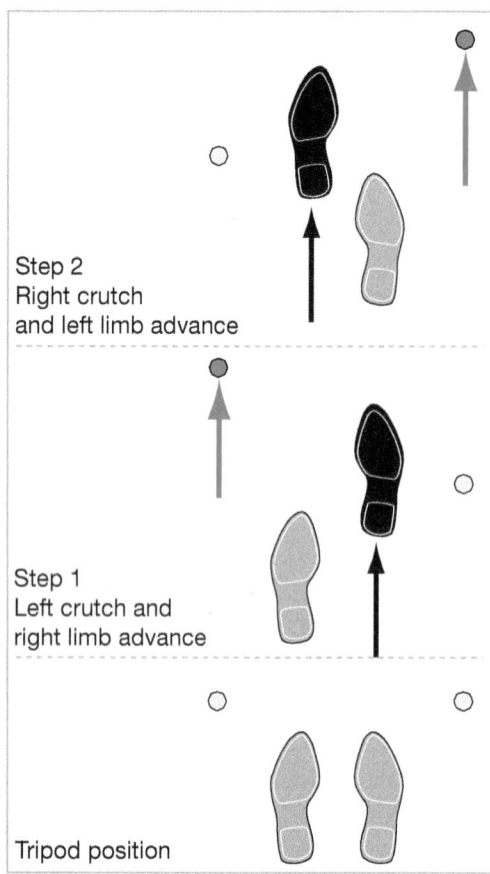

Step 2
Right crutch
and left limb advance

Step 1
Left crutch and
right limb advance

Tripod position

FIGURE 51-16 Two-point gait.

1. The patient should face forward and then back into a straight-back chair with arm rests until the back of the legs touch the chair seat.
2. The crutches should be placed in the hand on the strong side of the body, opposite the weak leg.
3. The patient should grasp the chair arm with the other hand and lower the body gently into the chair.

Standing with Crutches

The patient should be instructed to follow four steps when moving from a sitting to a standing position with the use of crutches.

1. The patient should place the crutches in the hand on the strong side of the body to use as support.
2. The patient should move or slide the body forward in the chair.
3. The patient should grasp the chair arm with the free hand on the affected side.
4. The patient should push up to a standing position.

Procedure 51-7 contains the steps for teaching or reinforcing instructions on the correct use of crutches.

Canes

Canes are used by patients who have muscle or bone weakness on one side or need assistance with balance. Two common types of canes are the standard cane and the four-point

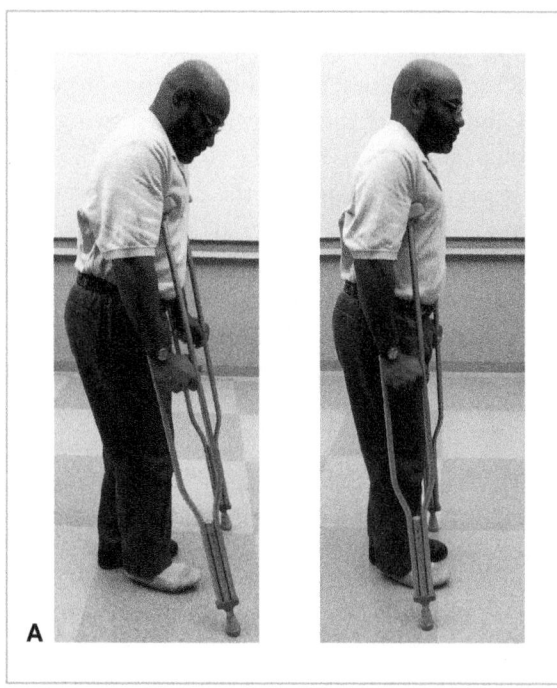
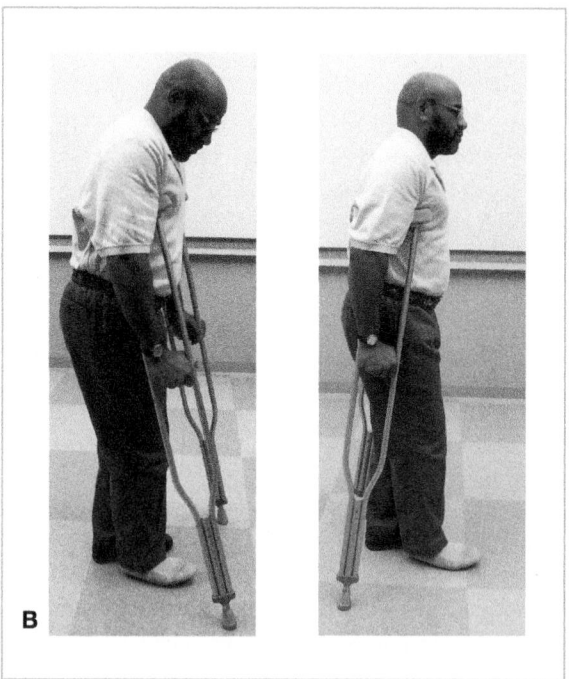

FIGURE 51-17 Swing gaits: **(A)** swing-to gait; **(B)** swing-through gait.

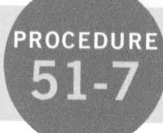

Instructing a Patient to Use Crutches Correctly

Objective ◆ *Teach a patient to correctly use crutches.*

EQUIPMENT AND SUPPLIES

Crutches; gait belt

METHOD

1. Assemble the equipment requested by the physician's order.
2. Check the crutches to determine that they are in good working condition.
3. Perform hand hygiene.
4. Identify the patient and explain the procedure.
5. Check to see if the patient is wearing sturdy, nonskid shoes.
6. Demonstrate the correct position.
7. Attach the gait requested by the physician.
8. Have the patient stand against a wall or near a chair for support.
9. Adjust crutch length to appropriate height. The distance between the top of the crutch and the axilla should be three finger widths (Figure A).
10. Instruct the patient to keep the head up, stand straight with abdomen in, and keep the feet straight with a slight (5-degree) bend at the knee joint. Remind the patient to look ahead and not down while walking with crutches. This will prevent the patient from bending forward.
11. Explain to the patient that the weight should be supported by the hands, not the underarms. The patient should practice standing to maintain balance and place weight on the palms of the hands, and not on the axillae, at the hand bars. Instruct the patient not to rest body weight on the axillary bars for more than one or two minutes to prevent injury to the brachial plexus.
12. Instruct the patient to assume basic crutch stance, or tripod, to provide a firm base of support. The basic crutch stance is the tripod to provide a firm base of support. Feet are slightly

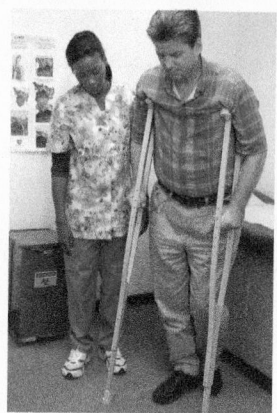

FIGURE B The medical assistant instructs the patient how to walk with crutches.

apart, and the tips of the crutches are 4 to 6 inches in front of and 4 to 6 inches to the side of the toes. An imaginary line drawn from the two crutch points to an area behind the center of the feet will form a triangle (tripod).

13. Instruct the patient to take small steps and swing through when first learning to use crutches. The crutches should only move about 12 inches forward with each step to prevent the crutches from slipping. Have the patient move slowly at first (Figure B).
14. Have the patient practice his or her gait.
15. Remind the patient to report any numbness or tingling in the arms. The crutch shoulders and hand bars can be padded for extra comfort with either sponge rubber or a soft cloth. The patient should then remeasure and adjust the crutches for the correct length.
16. Crutches should always be moved forward and to the side so the feet can swing through.
17. Remind the patient to periodically check the nuts and wing bolts to maintain tightness and to check the rubber tips frequently for cracks. They can easily be replaced.
18. Make corrections on the patient's use of crutches as needed.
19. Chart appropriately.

CHARTING EXAMPLE

9/30/YY 2:00 P.M. Instructed how to use crutches. Adjusted crutches to fit. Pt. practiced for 20 minutes.............................
....M. King, CMA (AAMA)

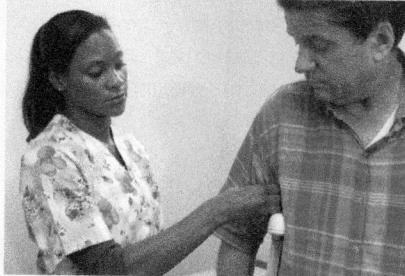

FIGURE A The medical assistant measures and adjusts the crutch length for the patient.

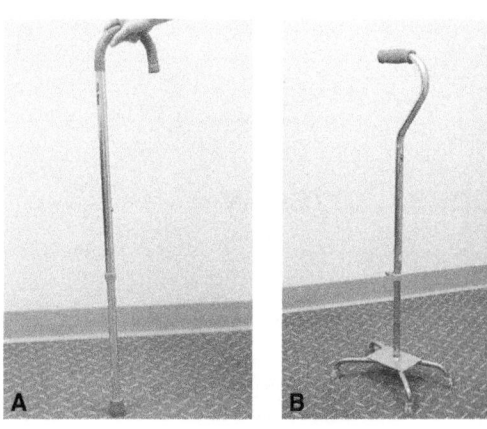

FIGURE 51-18 (A–B) Two types of canes.

(quad) cane shown in Figure 51-18. Several types of wooden and aluminum canes are available. The aluminum canes use nuts and wing bolts for height adjustments. The wooden canes have to be purchased to size or cut to the correct length. All canes should have a rubber tip on the end to prevent slipping. A standard cane has a curved neck for ease of gripping. It provides support for patients who need only slight assistance. The tripod (three-point) and quad (four-point) canes have a wide base with three or four points to provide steadier support; the neck is bent with a T-shaped handle.

A physical therapist determines the most suitable cane for the patient. To determine the correct cane height, the patient should stand tall so that the handgrip of the cane is level with the hip joint and the elbow is flexed at an angle of 25 to 30 degrees. Also, the handle must be suitable for the patient's hand size. Procedure 51-8 lists the steps for teaching a patient the correct use of a cane.

Walkers

Walkers are assistive devices made of aluminum that provide a base of support for patients who need help with balance and walking. To aid with mobility, many geriatric patients use walkers. The walker should be adjusted to the

---

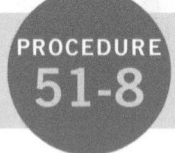

PROCEDURE 51-8

Instructing a Patient to Use a Cane Correctly

Objective ◆ *Teach a patient to correctly use a cane.*

EQUIPMENT AND SUPPLIES

Cane suited to the patient's needs; gait belt

METHOD

1. Assemble the equipment according to the physician's order.
2. Check the cane height and condition of the cane tip.
3. Identify the patient.
4. Perform hand hygiene and explain the procedure.
5. Check to see if the patient is wearing sturdy, nonskid shoes.
6. Demonstrate the correct position.
7. Demonstrate the gait.
8. Instruct the patient to hold the cane (or single crutch) on the opposite side of the injury or affected limb. As the affected leg moves forward, the cane (or crutch) on the opposite side will move forward to provide support.
9. Place the cane (or single crutch) 6 inches in front of and slightly to one side of the unaffected side. Make sure the cane tip is firmly on the floor and the weight is supported on the strong leg and the cane. The patient's elbow should be slightly flexed during weight bearing.
10. Have the patient look straight ahead, not down at the feet.
11. Have the patient move the cane (or single crutch) forward 6 to 12 inches and bring the affected leg forward until it is even with the cane. The weight should be placed on the strong foot and leg.
12. Instruct the patient to move the strong leg forward past the cane and weaker leg. As the unaffected foot moves forward, the weight is shifted to the weak or affected foot and the cane. Thus the cane will provide support for weight bearing on the weaker leg.
13. Have the patient repeat the walking pattern. Evaluate the patient's balance and endurance.
14. Document the procedure correctly.

CHARTING EXAMPLE

3/3/YY 1:00 P.M. Instructed on proper use of walking with a cane. Cane height and condition good. Pt. balance and gait good. Pt. practiced for 10 minutes..........M. King, CMA (AAMA)

---

patient's height and reach just below the patient's waistline (Figure 51-19).

A stationary walker must be picked up by the patient, moved forward, and then used as a base of support while the patient walks into it. This requires strong arm muscle development.

A walker with wheels can be used by patients who have good coordination and balance. This type of walker can be dangerous because it might move too quickly, causing the patient to lose balance and fall. Some walkers with wheels have a stop and release bar that the patient presses to unlock the wheels; if the patient lets go of the bar the wheels lock, thus preventing the walker from moving away from the patient. Procedure 51-9 outlines how to teach a patient to use a walker.

Wheelchairs

Wheelchairs are hand manipulated or power driven. Many patients operate their own wheelchairs; however, not all

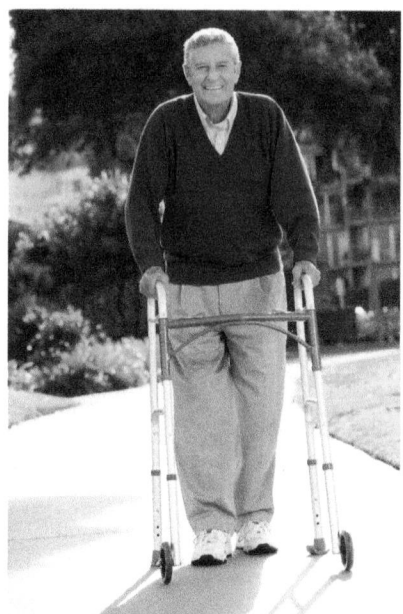
FIGURE 51-19 Walkers help the patient ambulate safely.

PROCEDURE 51-9
Instructing a Patient to Use a Walker Correctly

Objective ◆ *Teach a patient to correctly use a walker.*

EQUIPMENT AND SUPPLIES
Walker suited to patient's needs; gait belt

METHOD

1. Assemble the equipment according to the physician's order.
2. Check the condition of the walker.
3. Perform hand hygiene.
4. Identify the patient and explain the procedure.
5. Check to see if the patient is wearing sturdy, nonskid shoes.
6. Demonstrate the correct stance and gait with the walker.
7. Assist the patient into the walker.
8. Evaluate the walker for proper height and fit. (The top of the walker should reach the patient's hipbone, and the patient's hands should be on the handgrip with the elbow flexed at a 30-degree angle).
9. Instruct the patient to distribute her weight evenly between the walker and both legs.
10. Instruct the patient to move the walker 6 to 8 inches ahead with all four legs of the walker hitting the floor at the same time.
11. Instruct the patient to bring the weaker foot into the walker.
12. Instruct the patient to bring the stronger foot forward even with the weaker foot.
13. Have the patient continue walking with the walker while you evaluate balance and endurance.
14. Document appropriately.

Note: The walker is not to be used by the patient as a transfer device. Remind the patient to grasp the walker after she is in a standing position and not to use the walker to pull up from a sitting position.

CHARTING EXAMPLE
5/31/YY 11:00 A.M. Instructed on proper use of walker. Evaluated walker height to fit. Pt. practiced for 15 minutes.......
....M. King, CMA (AAMA)

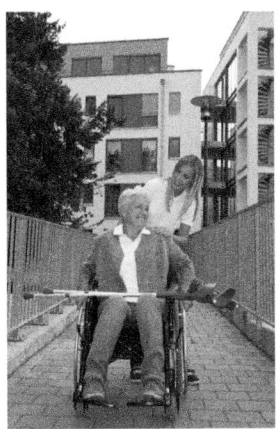

FIGURE 51-20 Many patients in wheelchairs require assistance.

patients are able to (nor should they) operate their own wheelchairs (Figure 51-20). For example, an individual paralyzed on one side or blind or frail may not be able to operate a wheelchair and will need assistance.

Wheelchair Transfer

Always think of moving a patient as the process of transferring him or her from one place to another. In many cases, the patient is familiar with the techniques necessary for the transfer and will be able to assist the medical assistant.

A patient who is paralyzed on one side of the body (**hemiplegia**) or who has a general weakness can be moved from a wheelchair by pivoting the patient so that he can use the stronger leg to assist you. Explain to the patient that this transfer technique is used to prevent injury to the patient and to the individual assisting with the transfer. Procedure 51-10 lists the steps to successfully transfer a patient from a wheelchair to a chair or examination table. Figure 51-21 is an example of moving a patient from a bed to a wheelchair. Figure 51-22 illustrates how to protect a falling patient.

Braces

A brace is one type of orthotic used to support weakened body parts, correct deformities, and prevent joint movement.

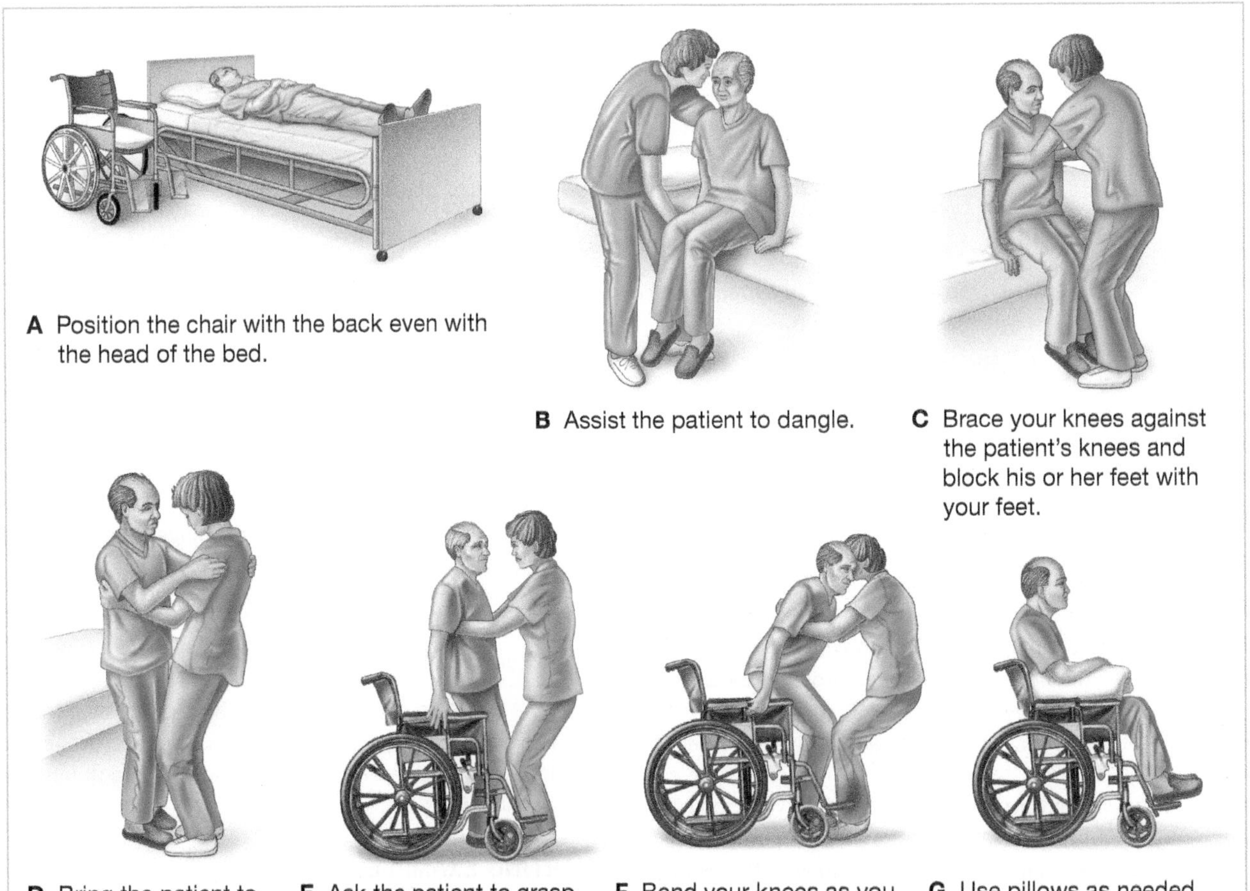

A Position the chair with the back even with the head of the bed.

B Assist the patient to dangle.

C Brace your knees against the patient's knees and block his or her feet with your feet.

D Bring the patient to a standing position.

E Ask the patient to grasp the chair as you support him or her.

F Bend your knees as you lower the patient to the chair.

G Use pillows as needed to position the patient in correct body alignment.

FIGURE 51-21 (A–G) Assisting the patient to transfer from the bed or examining table to a wheelchair.

Performing a Patient Transfer from a Wheelchair

Objective ◆ *Move the patient from a wheelchair to a chair or examination table without error.*

EQUIPMENT AND SUPPLIES

Chair or examination table; gait belt, if needed; step stool, if needed

METHOD

1. Perform hand hygiene.
2. Identify the patient and introduce yourself.
3. Explain what you are going to do before you start. Discuss what the patient will do to assist you.
4. Place the wheelchair at a 45-degree angle to the chair or examination table. This provides a shorter distance to pivot the patient from the wheelchair.
5. Put the wheelchair brakes in the lock position on both sides. The patient's legs should be moved off the pedals by supporting the ankle and lower leg. Gently place the patient's feet on the floor and have the patient shift forward in the chair, if possible. Move the foot pedals up and out of the way so the patient has a clear path to move forward.
6. Make sure the examination table or chair is stable before attempting the transfer.
7. Position yourself near the patient's nonparalyzed side so you can provide support and the patient can use his or her stronger limb. You will move the patient toward the stronger side. Do not refer to the patient's "good" or "bad" side.
8. Place one of your feet forward to establish a firm base of support for your body. Move down toward the patient while keeping your back straight.
9. Have the patient place his or her hands on the arm supports of the wheelchair. Then, ask the patient to lean forward and push up as you assist the patient to a standing position, on the count of three (Figure A).
10. Position yourself so that the patient's paralyzed leg is between your knees. Support the paralyzed leg with your knees, if necessary, so the leg will not slip as the patient stands.
11. Place your hands under the patient's armpits and help the patient to stand. Use the muscles in your legs to push your body upward. Do not bend over and use back muscles.
12. Allow the patient to stand for a few moments before attempting to move into the chair or onto the examination table.

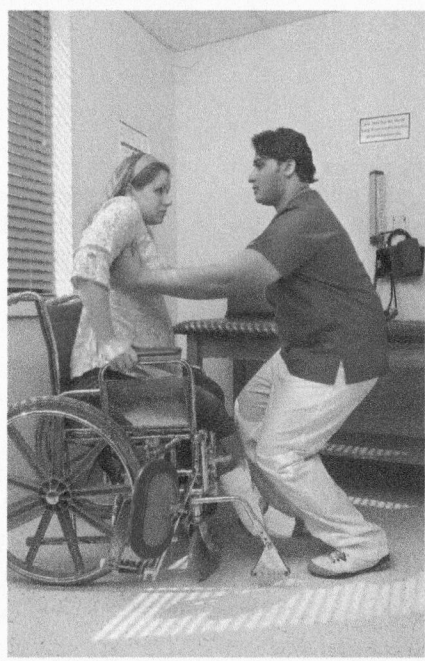

FIGURE A A medical assistant helps the patient out of the wheelchair.

13. Assist the patient to pivot (turn) toward the nonparalyzed side by pivoting your own body as you hold the patient under his or her armpits. Do not twist your body. Turn it as a unit.
14. Gently lower the patient into a chair by bending your knees and keeping your back straight.
15. If the patient must move up onto an examination table and can assist you, then support the weak side as the patient places the stronger leg onto the step stool. Pivot the patient around so she can then sit on the edge of the table. Encourage the patient to move back on the table to eliminate the danger of falling.
16. If the patient is unable to assist you, then ask for another assistant to hold one side of the patient as you support the other side. Count aloud "one," "two," "three," and then lift the patient together. Do not attempt to lift—by yourself—a patient who is unable to help you.
17. When assisting the patient into a supine position, support the paralyzed leg gently onto the table.
18. Never leave a physically challenged (disabled) patient unattended.

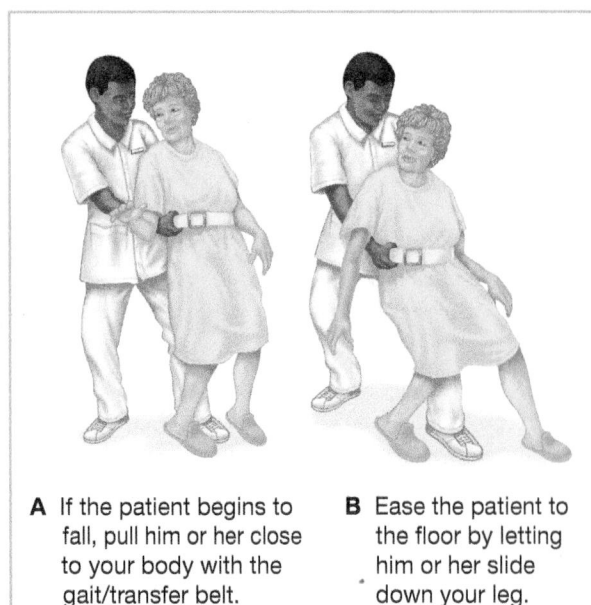

FIGURE 51-22 (A–B) Assisting a falling patient.

A If the patient begins to fall, pull him or her close to your body with the gait/transfer belt.

B Ease the patient to the floor by letting him or her slide down your leg.

Braces may be made out of metal, plastic, or leather and are customized to the patient's needs and anatomy. To wear this type of assistive leg device, the brace is placed in the patient's shoe, the patient's foot is inserted, and a hook-and-loop strap is used to hold the brace in place. Any orthotic positioned over a bony point must be padded to avoid skin breakdown. Prolonged use of a brace may weaken muscles.

Casts

Regardless of the type of specialty office that employs you, in your career as a medical assistant, you will encounter patients with casts. Casts are made of plaster, plastic, or fiberglass and are used to hold a bone in place after reduction of a fracture. Casts are applied over a stockinette to protect the skin. Fiberglass and plastic casts dry quickly, but a plaster of Paris cast may take up to 48 hours to dry. Proper cast care and patient assessment are important to avoid further damage to the body part already affected.

Cast Care

Casts are applied for the purpose of immobilizing a broken bone or muscle strain and sprain. A cast may be applied after a surgical procedure on a limb to immobilize the area until healing takes place. Casts are made from a variety of pliable materials that the physician will mold to fit the body part. A cast can be considered to be a form of nonflexible bandage. Casts are generally applied using a wet plaster-type material around a stockinette

liner and cotton padding over the limb. As the cast dries, it becomes hard. Newer synthetic fiberglass materials are used to form casts that are lighter in weight than a plaster cast. The medical assistant should use caution when handling fiberglass materials by wearing protective glasses or an eye shield.

The medical assistant may be asked to assist the physician in applying the cast. It may be necessary to hold the limb at the joint areas as the cast is being applied. Remember to handle a damaged limb gently.

After the cast has been applied, it must be left uncovered during the drying process. The limb may need to be supported on a pillow at this time. The patient should be cautioned against moving around until the cast is dry. The cast may become warm or even hot during the drying process. This is normal.

The patient's limb should not become hot or cold once the cast has been applied. Check the edges of the cast and report any changes to the physician (Figure 51-23). The medical assistant should make frequent checks of the patient's circulation. The patient should be instructed to call the physician if any of the following problems are observed:

- Circulation restricted by the cast
- Pain as a result of the cast pinching the skin
- Excessive itching under the cast
- Numbness or tingling of the fingers or toes
- Discolored toes or fingers
- Swelling of the limb around the edge of the cast

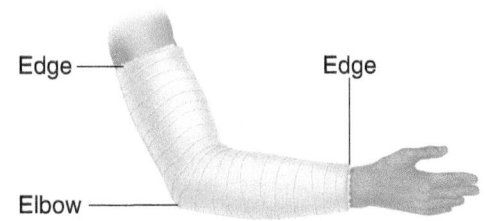

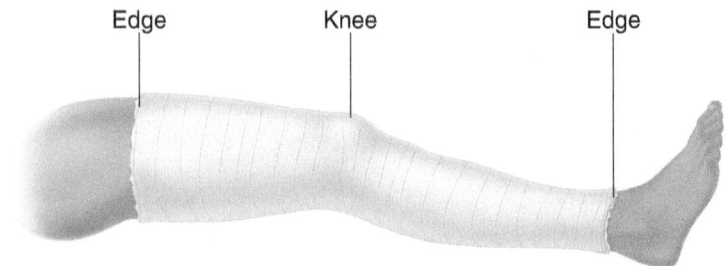

FIGURE 51-23 Check the edges of a cast and report any changes.

- Discoloration soaking through the cast
- Loosely fitting cast
- Foul odor coming from the cast

The physician should advise the patient on the amount of weight and movement that can be safely applied to the cast. Remind the patient that nothing should be put on the edges of the cast. The cast should not get wet. The patient may be able to tie a strong plastic bag around the cast to take a shower.

Traction

Traction is a method of pulling or stretching in two directions used to immobilize fractures, correct deformities, and reduce compression of the vertebrae or other musculoskeletal conditions. Skeletal traction, which is performed on inpatients, is applied by the physician to the patient's bone by inserting a pin or wire through the bone. Skin traction is done by the physical therapist by attaching bandages and strips of material to the skin. Weights are then attached to the material, and tension is applied to reduce painful muscle spasm. This type of traction can be set up in a patient's home.

Prosthesis

Surgical removal of a limb or part of a limb is known as amputation. Amputations are performed as the result of trauma, bone tumors, severe bone infection, workplace accidents, and disease such as gangrene. Major psychologic adjustment is needed to help the patient deal with his or her appearance and limitations on independence. A **prosthesis** is an artificial replacement of a missing body part.

Immediate fitting of a prosthesis involves fitting the patient immediately after the limb is removed, sometimes before leaving the operating room. The benefit of immediate fitting is that the patient is able to begin ambulation the next day. The decision to select a specific type of fitting rests with the physician and must include an assessment of the patient's overall condition, age, and willingness to learn to use the new limb. Many recent improvements in prostheses result in a limb that closely resembles the original and functions efficiently. Prosthetic devices are custom made for the patient, and adjustments may be necessary to ensure a comfortable fit for the patient. In the delayed fitting of a prosthesis, stump conditioning is needed and involves shrinking and shaping the stump before a prosthesis can be fitted. Amputees may feel a phantom pain, which is a normal occurrence with an unknown cause. The patient may experience pain in the amputated limb for a short time or, in some cases, for years.

DIAGNOSTIC TESTING

To determine the presence or full extent of a disabling disease, the physician may order evaluative or diagnostic testing. This may include an examination of the following:

- Muscle strength
- Muscle coordination
- Mobility of joints
- Neuromuscular function
- Circulation and sensory function

Neuromuscular evaluation may include tests to pick up abnormalities, such as diseases of the peripheral nerves, muscles, and spinal cord. Tests include an electromyography (EMG), nerve conduction studies (NCS), and evoked studies, such as brainstem auditory evoked response (BAER) and somatosensory evoked potentials (SEP).

Electromyography

Electromyography (EMG) consists of using an electromyograph to test the electrical activity of muscles. EMG is most often performed when a patient complains of muscle weakness or numbness. The electromyograph consists of electrodes, an oscilloscope to visually produce the waves of muscle activity, an amplifier, a loudspeaker, an electrical stimulator, and a camera. The patient may receive sedation before this test is conducted, because stimulation from the electric current may be painful. The EMG consists of inserting a fine-gauge needle electrode through the skin and into a muscle and then sending a small amount of electric current into the muscle. This procedure permits the physician to examine individual parts of muscles. Abnormal results are found in conditions such as amyotrophic lateral sclerosis (ALS), muscular dystrophy, and peripheral nerve damage.

The electrical activity of the muscle recorded on a graph paper or on film is known as an electromyogram (EMG). This permanent record is then evaluated to determine the adequacy of muscle activity.

A surface electromyogram (SEMG) involves less discomfort for the patient, but the results are less conclusive. In this

---

JUDGMENT CALL

As Miriam Khatab, CMA (AAMA), is showing patient Ryan MacBalfour back to the examining room in a primary care office, she notices that his gait is unstable.

Critical Thinking Questions

1. What kinds of illness or problems can cause this?
2. What should she do?
3. What might be possible therapies depending on the cause?

---

test, electrodes are attached to the surface of the body to detect electrical activity.

Electrical Stimulation

Electrical stimulation with low-voltage current is helpful to stimulate nerves that supply muscles. An electrical current is applied using disposable gel electrodes. This is a passive means to stimulate muscles when a patient cannot exercise because of injury or disease. This type of stimulation is used to avoid atrophy of muscle tissue.

Transcutaneous electric nerve stimulation (TENS) is another way of using electrical stimulation in physical medicine. A TENS unit is attached to the patient in the affected area, and a controlled dose of current is sent to the muscle to help control intractable pain when medication has not been effective. TENS units may be used at home.

Evoked Potential Studies

Evoked potential studies examine responses within the brain to external stimuli such as light, sound, and touch. These tests are considered noninvasive, because no equipment or needle is inserted into the body. Two types of evoked potential studies are these:

- Brainstem auditory evoked response (BAER) is used to assess the auditory nerve pathways. This is useful in diagnosing auditory tumors and lesions.
- Somatosensory evoked peripheral nerves (SEP) are used for diagnosing nerve function defects in peripheral nerves, for example, in the legs.

COMPLEMENTARY AND ALTERNATIVE TREATMENTS

If a nonmainstream practice is used instead of conventional medicine, it is considered **alternative medicine**. If a non-mainstream practice is used in addition to conventional medicine, we call it **complementary medicine**. Most patients who come to the medical office do not completely disregard conventional medicine, but some may add different techniques and practices that they believe work well for their health. Many complementary treatments have been researched by the National Center for Complementary and Integrative Health, U.S. National Institutes of Health (NIH) and have been found to improve patient health. Always ask a patient what other therapies they use and document in the medical record.

Chiropractic

Chiropractic is an approach to health care that uses spinal manipulation to relieve pain. Doctors of chiropractic usually also promote healthy nutrition, beneficial lifestyle changes, and exercise. Some sell nutritional supplements at their offices, so it is prudent to ask the patient if they take any products sold by a chiropractor in addition to those prescribed by the physician.

Massage

Massage is kneading or applying pressure by the hands to a part of the patient's body to promote muscle relaxation, improve blood circulation, and reduce tension. Massage can consist of the simple act of rubbing an injection site to stimulate absorption and reduce pain. It can incorporate techniques such as kneading, rolling, stroking, and tapping the skin that are performed by persons skilled in the art of massage.

Massage is considered a form of passive exercise that is usually applied by someone other than the patient. Terminology related to massage includes the following:

- **Effleurage**—Light stroking movement that may be performed in a circular pattern
- **Friction**—Rubbing or deep stroking that produces an increase in circulation and mild heat within the tissues
- **Petrissage**—A kneading or rolling method of massage that requires pressing the muscles
- **Tapotement**—Light tapping or percussion to relieve congestion that is performed with the hands, the fingertips, or the hands in a cupping position

In addition, massage can help restore mobility, decrease swelling, relax muscle spasms, and reduce pain. Physical therapists often incorporate massage into their treatment plans.

Massage therapy is a holistic approach to promoting health that is increasingly valued as a valid form of health care. Massage therapists require special training and are licensed in many states. They may perform massage in individual private practices and in the hospital setting. Several types or categories of massage are practiced by massage therapists. Traditional or Swedish massage, which is most commonly used in the United States, includes stimulating blood circulation through the soft tissues. Deep tissue massage is used to release chronic patterns of tension or pain by applying massage and pressure at deeper levels. Trigger point massage concentrates finger pressure directly to individual muscles to release trigger points or knots in the muscles.

Reiki

Reiki involves channeling the body's energy and spirit through gentle touch and massage. It is a Japanese technique to reduce stress and promote relaxation and healing. It is administered by "laying on hands" and is based on the idea that an unseen life force energy flows through us and is what causes us to be alive. If your life force energy is low, then those who use this therapy believe that you are more likely to get sick or feel stress, and if it is high, they believe you are more capable of being happy and healthy.

Acupuncture and Acupressure

The medical theory behind the ancient Chinese science and art of acupressure is that special acupoints, or acupressure points, lie along meridians, or channels, in your body. It is believed that vital energy, or a life force called qi (ch'i), flows through these invisible channels. It is also believed that the 12 major meridians connect specific organs or networks of organs, organizing a system of communication throughout your body. The meridians begin at your fingertips, connect to your brain, and then connect to an organ associated with a certain meridian. Practitioners of acupressure press at these acupoints to stimulate the qi to move.

Some uses for acupuncture include reduction of nausea after chemotherapy, pain reduction, stopping headaches, relieving arthritis and fibromyalgia, improving mood, reducing anxiety, and decreasing inflammation. Acupressure is very safe for most patients, but certain points should be avoided in a pregnant patient as they induce contractions; also varicose veins and cancer sites must be avoided.

Acupuncture differs from acupressure in that it involves inserting very thin needles through the skin at key points. It is believed that inserting these needles rebalances the flow of energy.

Tai Chi

Originally developed as a system of self-defense, tai chi techniques have become a popular means of stress reduction.

Described as meditation in motion, tai chi involves gentle flowing movements that promote mental and physical health.

SUMMARY

Physical therapy involves the use of physical measures, equipment, and body movement to promote mobility and circulation, restore normal function, and relieve pain. The medical assistant, working under the supervision of a physician, is able to teach the patient about proper body mechanics, exercise, and the application of various therapeutic devices such as heat and cold applications. In some cases, the medical assistant will apply these devices.

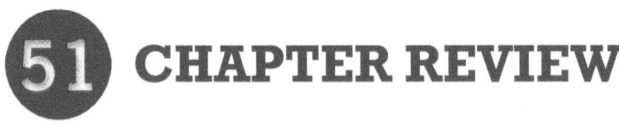 **CHAPTER REVIEW**

COMPETENCY REVIEW

1. Define and spell the terms for this chapter.
2. Identify three methods of physical therapy that you find to be most interesting. Explain why they are of interest to you.
3. Describe how a patient would walk using two-point, three-point, or four-point-crutch walking gaits.
4. Using a partner, demonstrate PROM. Demonstrate AROM yourself.

5. Explain the differences between braces and casts.
6. Describe the following testing methods: electromyography (EMG), nerve conduction studies (NCS), evoked potential studies (EPS), and brainstem auditory evoked response (BAER).
7. List four forms of massage techniques.

PREPARING FOR THE CERTIFICATION EXAM

1. Which of the following occupations requires two years of college and two years of supervised training, and has national certification available from ABC and BOC?
   a. physical therapy assistant
   b. orthotist
   c. physical therapist
   d. physical therapy aide
   e. physiatrist

2. Which of the following is *not* a type of massage?
   a. effleurage
   b. friction
   c. petrissage
   d. tapotement
   e. contracture

3. Which of the following means paralysis of the lower body?
   a. quadriplegia
   b. poliomyelitis
   c. paraplegia
   d. cerebral palsy
   e. muscular dystrophy

4. Which of the following means paralysis of all four extremities of the body?
   a. quadriplegia
   b. poliomyelitis
   c. paraplegia
   d. cerebral palsy
   e. muscular dystrophy

5. Which of the following involves channeling the body's energy and spirit through gentle touch and massage?
   a. effleurage
   b. friction
   c. petrissage
   d. tapotement
   e. Reiki

6. Which of the following can hasten suppuration?
   a. moist heat
   b. moist cold
   c. dry heat
   d. dry cold
   e. ultrasound

7. Which of the following is the bending of the sole of the foot, pointing toes downward?
   a. pronation
   b. rotation
   c. inversion
   d. plantar flexion
   e. dorsiflexion

8. When applying a cold compress, the application should be checked every
   a. 10 to 12 minutes.
   b. 12 to 15 minutes.
   c. 3 to 5 minutes.
   d. 5 to 8 minutes.
   e. 8 to 10 minutes.

9. Which gait is used by patients who can bear some weight on both feet and have good balance?
   a. four-point gait
   b. three-point gait
   c. two-point gait
   d. swing gait
   e. one-point gait

10. In a hot soak application, the maximum temperature for an adult is
    a. 40°C.
    b. 110°C.
    c. 44°C.
    d. 54°C.
    e. 105°C.

CRITICAL THINKING

Refer to the case study at the beginning of the chapter and use what you have learned to answer the following questions.

1. Why is it important that Samra wheel Sylvia to the examination room rather than have Sylvia wheel herself?

2. Sylvia must be transferred from her wheelchair to the examination table before she is seen by Dr. Miller. What are some things that Samra must consider regarding transferring Sylvia and once Sylvia is seated on the table?

3. Dr. Miller is pleased with Sylvia's overall recovery after the stroke; however, he is concerned about her ambulation. He would like Sylvia to be referred to a physical therapist for rehabilitation. What does a physical therapist do, and how could this help Sylvia?

ON THE JOB

Jenny Watmore, a medical assistant working in Dr. Cory's orthopedic practice, has been asked to assist Mr. Ivy from the wheelchair onto the examination table. Mr. Ivy, who is 70 years old, is weakened on the left side of his body from a cerebrovascular accident (CVA). He weighs 200 pounds and is reluctant to provide much help to Jenny when she has to transfer him from the wheelchair to the examination table.

1. How can Jenny get Mr. Ivy to help her assist him?
2. Describe the body mechanics that Jenny should use to assist Mr. Ivy.
3. How might Mr. Ivy benefit from physical therapy?
4. What information should Jenny document in Mr. Ivy's medical record?

INTERNET ACTIVITY

Select one of the professions listed in Table 51-1. Do an Internet search to discover the duties, the average salary range, where these professionals are usually employed, and the long-term job opportunities of the profession you selected.

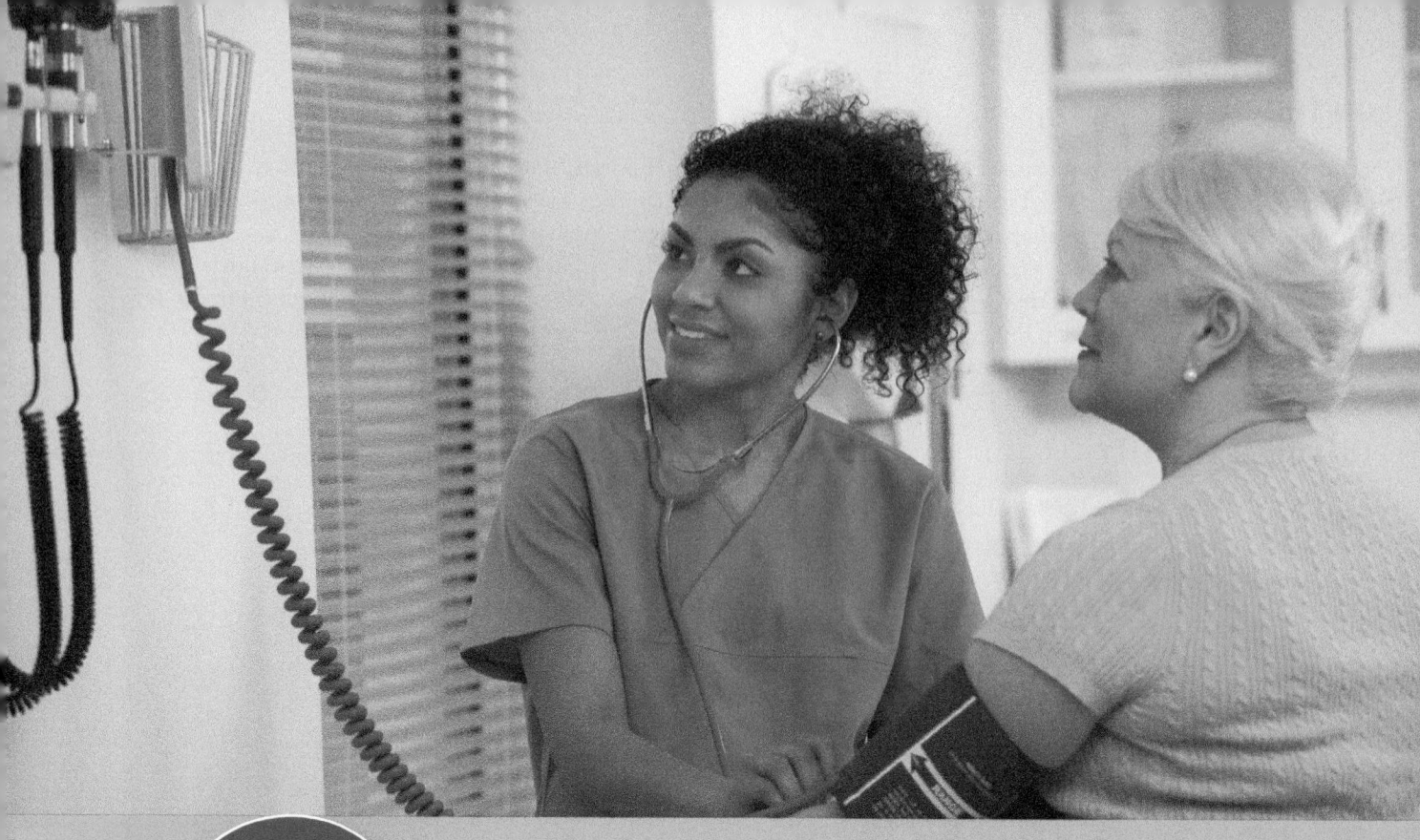

Math for Pharmacology

Learning Objectives

After completing this chapter, you should be able to:

52.1   Define and spell the terms for this chapter.

52.2   Demonstrate the ability to perform basic math computations.

52.3   Compare basic units of measurement between the metric and household systems.

52.4   Demonstrate accurate conversions among measurement systems.

52.5   Describe equations used to calculate medication dosages.

52.6   Apply mathematical computations to solve dosage calculation equations.

52.7   Describe equations used to calculate pediatric dosages.

52.8   Identify symbols and abbreviations used when calculating dosages.

Liu Cheng, a 44-year-old male, is seeing Dr. Salpega because he has had a sore throat and cough that will not go away. He has been sick for the past two weeks and says his 4-year-old son Jie is also sick with very similar symptoms. Dr. Salpega diagnoses Mr. Cheng with a severe lower respiratory infection and prescribes an 875-milligram (mg) tablet of Augmentin to be taken twice a day for 10 days. Mr. Cheng asks Dr. Salpega if there is a liquid form of the medication available that he could take; his throat is very sore, and he does not wish to swallow tablets.

Terms to Learn

apothecary system	household system	proportion
body surface area (BSA)	leading zero rule	ratio
Clark's rule	metric system	ratio method
denominator	mixed number	trailing zero rule
formula method	numerator	underdose
fraction bar	overdose	West's nomogram
Fried's law	pharmacology	Young's rule

Pharmacology is the study of medications and drugs, including their forms, intentions for use, and effects. It is important to understand correct math calculations and dosing requirements, because a simple error in the calculation of a medication dose can have detrimental effects. An **overdose** (taking too much of a medication) may occur, which could have life-threatening consequences; conversely, an underdose may occur. An **underdose** occurs when not enough medication is given to achieve the desired effect. Over- and underdosing are preventable by proper dosage calculation. General mathematical skills are necessary in order to perform dosage calculations.

MATHEMATICS REVIEW

When calculating drug dosages, multiple mathematical calculations are used. These may include addition, subtraction, multiplication, and division. Also, an understanding of fractions, decimals, proportions, and ratios is important. Table 52-1 lists reminders and guidelines for many mathematical computations.

Addition and Subtraction

Addition and subtraction are used not only in drug calculation but also in everyday tasks within the medical office, such as taking inventory and collecting payments.

Multiplication and Division

Multiplication and division are used just as often as addition and subtraction. It is important to have a strong knowledge of the basic multiplication ("times") tables when working in the medical office.

Fractions

A fraction is a part of a whole number. It consists of a **numerator** (the top number), a **denominator** (the bottom number), and a **fraction bar** that separates the two.

Common fractions used in the medical field include $\frac{1}{2}$, $\frac{1}{3}$, $\frac{1}{4}$, and $\frac{3}{4}$. Fractions are used often when indicating measurements (e.g., "$\frac{1}{4}$-inch laceration on the right forearm") and dosages ("Take $\frac{1}{2}$ a tablet at bedtime"). A **mixed number** is made up of both a whole number and a fraction (e.g., "Take $1\frac{1}{2}$ teaspoons by mouth every six hours as needed for cough").

TABLE 52-1 | Mathematical Rules and Guidelines

Function	Rules	Example
Adding and subtracting fractions	• When adding and subtracting fractions, you must have a common denominator. • Multiply each fraction by the correct multiplier to obtain the common denominator. • Add the numerators (the denominator remains the same). • Reduce the final answer to its simplest terms.	$1/5 + 2/5 = 3/5$ $1/2 + 2/5 =$ Your common denominator is 10. **Steps:** 1. $\dfrac{1}{2} \times \dfrac{5}{5} + \dfrac{2}{5} \times \dfrac{2}{2} =$ 2. $\dfrac{5}{10} + \dfrac{4}{10} =$ 3. $\dfrac{9}{10}$ (This is already reduced to its lowest terms.) Another example is: $3/5 - 1/15 =$ Your common denominator is 15. **Steps:** 1. $\dfrac{3}{5} \times \dfrac{3}{3} - \dfrac{1}{15} =$ 2. $\dfrac{9}{15} - \dfrac{1}{15} =$ 3. $\dfrac{8}{15}$ (This is already reduced to its lowest terms.)
Multiplying fractions	• If the numerator of one fraction and the denominator of the other fraction have a common divisor, you may cancel out those terms. • Multiply all numerators across. • Multiply all denominators across. • Reduce your answer to its simplest terms.	$3/5 \times 10/18 =$ **Steps:** 1. $\dfrac{^{(1)}3}{_{(1)}5} \times \dfrac{10^{(2)}}{18_{(6)}} =$ 2. $\dfrac{1}{1} \times \dfrac{2}{6}$ 3. $\dfrac{2}{6}$ (This can be reduced to 1/3.) 4. $\dfrac{1}{3}$
Dividing fractions	• Invert the second fraction of the equation, finding its reciprocal. • Multiply all numerators across. • Multiply all denominators across. • Reduce your answer to its simplest terms.	$2/3 \div 1/5 =$ **Steps:** 1. $\dfrac{2}{3} \times \dfrac{5}{1} =$ 2. $\dfrac{10}{3} =$ (Convert this improper fraction to a proper fraction.) 3. $3\frac{1}{3}$
Converting an improper fraction to a mixed number	• An improper fraction is any fraction with a numerator larger than a denominator. • Divide the numerator by the denominator. This becomes the whole number. • The remainder (if any) is then placed as the new numerator over the denominator to form the fractional component of the mixed number. • Reduce the fractional component to its simplest form.	$14/6 =$ **Steps:** 1. $\dfrac{14}{6} =$ 2. $6\overline{)14} = 2\frac{2}{6}$ $\dfrac{12}{2}$ 3. $2\frac{2}{6} =$ 4. $2\frac{1}{3}$

TABLE 52-1 | Mathematical Rules and Guidelines (*continued*)

Function	Rules	Example
Converting a fraction to a decimal	• Divide the numerator by the denominator.	2/3 = ***Steps:*** 2 ÷ 3 = 0.67
Adding and subtracting decimals	• Always line up the decimals of every number. • Add zero (0) placeholders to help keep numbers aligned.	1.9 + 0.33 + 12.344 = ***Steps:*** 1.900 0.330 +12.344 ‾‾‾‾‾‾ 14.574

Multiplying decimals	• Multiply the numbers as usual.
	 • Place zero (0) placeholders as needed.
	 • Count the total number of decimal spaces to the right of the decimal point for both numbers.
	 • Next, place your decimal point this many numbers to the left of the last number in your answer.
		12.14 × 8.2 =
		 Steps:
		 12.14
		 1. × 8.2
		     2428
		   97120
		   ‾‾‾‾‾‾
		   99548
		 2. 99.548 (Your decimal point is placed three spaces to the left from the last number in your answer. This is because there are three decimal placeholders in the original equation.)

Dividing decimals	• If your number is not a whole number, move the decimal point of the divisor the necessary number of spaces to make the divisor a whole number.
	 • If the dividend has a decimal, move it to the right the same number of places as you moved the divisor's decimal point.
	 • Add zero (0) placeholders as necessary.
	 • Divide as usual, and then move the decimal directly up in the quotient.
		56.42 ÷ 9.1 =
		 Steps:
		 1. 9.1)‾56.42
		 2. 91)‾56.42
		           6.2
		 3. 91)‾564.2
		       546
		       ‾‾‾
		       182
		       182
		       ‾‾‾
		         0

Converting a decimal to a fraction	• Simply place the entire number over the value of the decimal placeholder of the last digit of the number. • Remember to reduce the final answer to its simplest terms.	Convert 0.75 to a fraction. ***Steps:*** $\frac{75}{100}$ • ***Note:*** The 5 is located in the hundredths placeholder, thus 75 is placed over 100.

Decimals

The use of decimals is common in the medical office. Anything less than the number 1 is often written as a decimal (e.g., 0.5, 0.75, 0.02). Fractions can also be written in decimal form (e.g., $\frac{1}{2}$ is written as 0.5, $\frac{3}{4}$ is written as 0.75 and $\frac{2}{3}$ is written as 0.66). To convert fractions to a decimal, simply divide the numerator by the denominator.

Decimal Place Values

When writing and reading decimals, it is necessary to correctly identify the decimal point and place value of the number. When speaking or verbalizing decimal values, state the decimal placeholder (tenths, hundredths, thousandths) where the last digit falls. Although the number 0.9 can be read as "zero point nine," the proper way of reading this is

TABLE 52-2 | Decimal Point Place Values

Ones	Decimal Point	Tenths	Hundredths	Thousandths	Ten Thousandths
1	.	0.<u>1</u>	0.0<u>1</u>	0.00<u>1</u>	0.000<u>1</u>

actually "nine-tenths." The number 0.32 would be read as "thirty-two hundredths," and 0.005 would be read as "five thousandths." (Table 52-2 illustrates the decimal point place values.)

Equivalents

Equivalents are things that are equal—that have the same value. In mathematics, for example, the fraction $\frac{3}{4}$ and the decimal 0.75 are equivalents. Table 52-3 lists examples of mathematical equivalents between fractions, ratios, percentages, and decimals. (Ratios and their role in dosage calculations are discussed later in this chapter.) For example, the ratio 1:2, the percentage 50 percent, and the decimal 0.50 all have the same fraction value of $\frac{1}{2}$. They are mathematical equivalents.

Often, working with a ratio or a decimal is easier than working with the equivalent fraction. Many students find decimals less troublesome than fractions.

Leading Zero and Trailing Zero Rules

It is important to understand the placement of a zero in a decimal. When writing a decimal number less than 1, you must apply the **leading zero rule**. For example, if you were to write a prescription for a medication that calls for a one-half teaspoon of medicine, you would write 0.5 tsp (*not* .5 tsp). As important as it is to follow the leading zero rule, you must also follow the trailing zero rule. The **trailing zero rule**

states that it is never appropriate to include a zero after a whole number. For example, if a patient were to take 5 milligrams of a medication, you would write 5 mg (*not* 5.0 mg).

These rules have been devised and are used to reduce the number of errors in pharmaceutical calculations. Too often, a number has been misread because of the incorrect placement or omission of a zero. Always following the "leading zero" and the "trailing zero" rules can help reduce the number of medical errors—and possibly save the lives of patients.

WEIGHTS AND MEASURES

Three systems of weights and measures are used to calculate medication doses: the apothecary system, the metric system, and the household system. The most commonly used systems of measurement are the metric and household systems, but occasionally the apothecary system may still be used.

Keep in mind that common household measurements, such as teaspoon and tablespoon, are still widely used. Household measurements are often used by medical assistants and other health care professionals in coaching patients because patients are generally more familiar with them.

Table 52-4 lists the most common abbreviations and symbols used in pharmacology math.

TABLE 52-3 | Examples of Mathematical Equivalents

Fraction	Ratio	Percentage	Decimal
1/4	1:4	25 percent	0.25
1/2	1:2	50 percent	0.50
2/3	2:3	66 percent	0.66
3/4	3:4	75 percent	0.75
7/8	7:8	88 percent	0.88
1/100	1:100	1 percent	0.01
1/200	1:200	0.5 percent	0.005
1/1,000	1:1,000	0.1 percent	0.001

Professionalism

A major component of professionalism is identifying areas in which you excel and areas that need improvement. This helps to identify areas of competence. It is important to keep in mind that establishing a strong level of competence with medication and dosages will take some time. Early in your career as a medical assistant, you will find yourself faced with various medications and dosage levels that may be unfamiliar. In these instances, it is important to refer to resources such as the *Physicians' Desk Reference*. A truly professional medical assistant recognizes when he does not know the answer to a question and can use reliable resources to obtain it.

TABLE 52-4 | Common Pharmacologic Abbreviations and Symbols

Apothecary	Metric	Household
ʒ = dram	kg = kilogram	tsp = teaspoon
gr = grain	g or gm = gram	TBSP or T = tablespoon
gtt = drop	mg = milligram	oz = ounce
O = pint	mcg = microgram	c = cup
qt = quart	L = liter	pt = pint
C = gallon	mL = milliliter (also abbreviated "ml")	qt = quart
℥ = ounce	cc = cubic centimeter (same equivalent as "ml")	gal = gallon
ℳ = minim	m = meter	
s̄s̄ = one half	cm = centimeter	
lb = pound	mm = millimeter	
i = 1; ii = 2; iii = 3; iv = 4; v = 5; x = 10	mEq = milliequivalent*	
	IU = international units*	
	dL (or "dl") = deciliter	

*Not a true metric measurement, but included in the metric category.

Apothecary System

The **apothecary system** is considered to be the oldest system of measurement. Dry weight measurement was based on the grain (gr). One grain was equal to the weight of 1 grain of wheat. In addition to the grain (gr), other units of dry weight measurement within the apothecary system include the dram (dr, ʒ), the ounce (oz, ℥), and the pound (lb). Fluid measurements include the minims (m), fluid dram (fl dr, fl image), fluid ounce (fl oz, fl ℥), pint (pt), quart (qt), and gallon (gal).

Roman numerals are used when numbering in the apothecary system. For example, 3 grains would be gr iii. Fractions are also used. Three-fourths of a grain would be gr $\frac{3}{4}$. It is important to note that the unit of measure in the apothecary system is placed before the actual number (gr $\frac{3}{4}$ *not* $\frac{3}{4}$ gr).

To accurately write an apothecary notation, the following rules should be applied:

1. The unit or abbreviation comes before the amount.

   Example: qt iii (three quarts), rather than iii qt

2. Use lowercase Roman numerals to express whole numbers 1 through 10, 15, 20, and 30. Use Arabic numerals for all other quantities.

   Example: qt i (1 quart), gr 12 (12 grains), and gr xx (20 grains)

3. Use fractions to designate amounts less than 1.

   Example: gr $\frac{1}{2}$, not 0.5 gr

4. The symbol *ss* is used to designate the fraction $\frac{1}{2}$. You may also see this expressed as s̄s̄.

   Example: pt iiiss = (3 $\frac{1}{2}$ pints)

When interpreting a drug order or reading a drug label, it is helpful to know the common Roman numerals and their Arabic equivalents (Table 52-5).

Household System

In the **household system**, common measurements such as the ounce, pint, quart, and gallon are based on the apothecary system. Even today the household system is used as frequently as the metric system in the United States. (The United States is the only industrialized country that does not officially use the metric system, although use of the metric system in this country is legal and gradually becoming more common.)

Common liquid measurements in the household system include the teaspoon, tablespoon, ounce, cup, pint, quart, and gallon. Dry weights can include the ounce and pound. The teaspoon, tablespoon, and cup can also be included in the dry weight category as these measurements are used frequently for baking and cooking.

As already noted, most patients are more familiar with the household system than the metric or apothecary systems. To better assist the patient in understanding medication dosages, the medical assistant may frequently need to convert apothecary and metric measurements to the household system. (Use the information in Tables 52-6 through 52-9 to assist with these conversions.)

TABLE 52-5 | Arabic Numbers, Roman Numerals, and Apothecary Notations

Arabic Number	Roman Numeral	Apothecary Notation	Arabic Number	Roman Numeral	Apothecary Notation
1	I	i, ī	8	VIII	viii, v̄iii
2	II	ii, īi	9	IX	ix, īx
3	III	iii, īii	10	X	x, x̄
4	IV	iv, īv	15	XV	xv, x̄v
5	V	v, v̄	20	XX	xx, x̄x
6	VI	vi, v̄i	25	XXV	xxv, x̄xv
7	VII	vii, v̄ii	30	XXX	xxx, x̄xx

Metric System

The **metric system** is commonly used for dosage calculations and conversions. The following are metric system prefixes and their values:

- kilo = 1,000 of a unit
- hecto = 100 of a unit
- deka = 10 of a unit
- base unit of 1
- deci = 0.1 (one-tenth) of a unit
- centi = 0.01 (one-hundredth) of a unit
- milli = 0.001 (one-thousandth) of a unit
- micro = 0.000001 (one millionth) of a unit

Metric conversions are simply accomplished by multiplying or dividing by 1,000. Multiplying by 1,000 would be the same as moving the decimal point three places to the right. Dividing by 1,000 would mean that the decimal point moves three places to the left. For further explanation, review the following example:

Convert: 3.5 g to mg

Equivalent: 1 g = 1,000 mg. Conversion factor is 1,000.

Multiply by 1,000: 3.5 g = 3.5 × 1,000 = 3,500 mg

Or, move the decimal point three places to the right:

3.5 g = 3.500 = 3,500 mg

Move the decimal point along the place value chart, either to the right or to the left, depending on the conversion factor. Refer to Figure 52-1 for further review and examples.

The common metric units of measure are the liter (volume), the gram (weight), and the meter (length). Table 52-6 lists common abbreviations for weights and measures. (See Guidelines 52-1 for conversion within the metric system.)

Guidelines 52-1

Conversion Within the Metric System

1. No change is required to change milliliters (mL) into cubic centimeters (cc) because they are equal to each other.
2. To change grams (gm) to milligrams (mg), multiply grams by 1,000 or move the decimal point three places to the RIGHT.
3. To change milligrams (mg) to grams (gm), divide milligrams by 1,000 or move the decimal point three places to the LEFT.
4. To convert liters (L) to milliliters (mL), multiply liters by 1,000 or move the decimal point three places to the RIGHT.
5. To convert milliliters (mL) to liters (L), divide milliliters by 1,000 or move the decimal point three places to the LEFT.

Metric System Dosages

In the metric system, the dosage is written as a decimal number first, with the unit of measurement following (2.5 mg). Equivalents are demonstrated in Table 52-7. Common household measures are presented in Table 52-8, and the comparisons of the three systems for liquid measurements are in Table 52-9.

Rules for Conversion

When converting from one system to another, it is important to remember that the equivalents may be only approximate, especially when using conversion tables such as the one in Table 52-10. This table, however, should be learned because the equivalents are very helpful when converting from one measuring system to another—apothecary to metric or metric to apothecary. See Guidelines 52-2 for tips on converting from one system to another.

Kilo-	Hecto-	Deka-	Numeral w/ base unit (g, l, or m)	Deci-	Centi-	Milli-	Micro-

Example:

Convert 45.2 grams (g) to milligrams (mg).

1. Place 45.2 under the numeral/base unit:

Kilo-	Hecto-	Deka-	Numeral w/ base unit (g, l, or m)	Deci-	Centi-	Milli-	Micro-
			45.2				

2. Move the decimal point to the right three times so that the base unit ends in the milli- box:

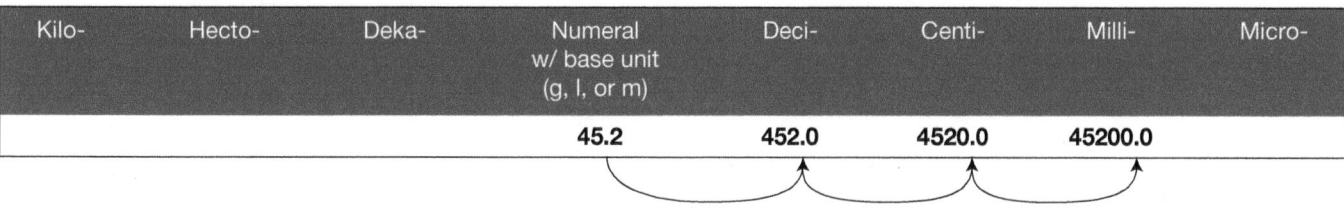

Kilo-	Hecto-	Deka-	Numeral w/ base unit (g, l, or m)	Deci-	Centi-	Milli-	Micro-
			45.2	452.0	4520.0	45200.0	

3. 45.2g = 45,200 mg

FIGURE 52-1 Metric conversion using the place value chart.

TABLE 52-6 | Common Abbreviations for Weights and Measures

Apothecary System		Metric System	Household System
Symbol/Abbreviation		**Meaning**	**Meaning**
gtt	drop	drop	drop
(℔)	min	Minim	
℥	dr	dram	teaspoon
fl ℥	fl dr	fluid dram	teaspoon
oz, ℥	oz	n/a	ounce
fl ℥	fl oz	n/a	fluid ounce
lb	lb	n/a	pound
O	pt	n/a	pint
C	gal	n/a	gallon
qt	qt	n/a	quart
gr	gr	grain	
Symbol/Abbreviation Weights		**Meaning**	**Meaning**
kg		kilogram	
gm or g		gram	
mg		milligram	
mcg, μg		microgram	
Symbol/Abbreviation Volume		**Meaning**	**Meaning**
L		liter	
mL		milliliter	
cc		cubic centimeter	

TABLE 52-7 | Commonly Used Equivalents for the Apothecary, Metric, and Household Systems

Apothecary Measure	Metric Equivalent	Household Equivalent
1 gr	60 mg or 65 mg	0.002 oz
5 gr	325 mg or 0.33 g	0.01 oz
1 dram	4 mL	0.8 tsp
1 oz	30 cc, 30 mL, 30 g, 8 drams,	6 tsp, 2 tbsp
1 lb	450 g	1 lb
Liquid Measure		
1 fl dr	4–5 mL	0.8 tsp
2.5 fl dr	10 mL	2 tsp
4 fl dr	15 mL	1 tbsp
1 fl oz	30 mL	1 oz
8 oz	240 mL	1 cup or glass
1 pt	500 mL	2 cups
1 qt	1,000 mL	4 cups, 2 pints or ¼ gallon

TABLE 52-8 | Common Household Measures

Measure	Equivalent
60 gtt (drops)	1 teaspoon (tsp)
3 tsp	1 tablespoon (T or TBSP)
2 T	1 oz
8 oz	1 cup or glass
2 cups	1 pint (pt)
2 pints	1 quart (qt)
4 quarts	1 gallon

TABLE 52-9 | Comparison of Apothecary, Metric, and Household Liquid Measurements

Apothecary	Metric	Household
1 minim (ℳ)	0.06 mL	1 drop
1 fl dr (fl ʒ)	4–5 mL	1 tsp
4 fl dr (fl ʒ)	15–16 mL	1 T
1 fl oz (fl ℥)	30–32 mL	2 T
8 fl oz (fl ℥)	250 mL	1 cup or glass
16 fl oz, 1 pt	500 mL	2 cups or glasses
1 qt	1,000 mL (approximately 1 liter)	4 cups or glasses

Professionalism

As a medical assistant, you must be able to read the abbreviations for dosages, which are generally metric system abbreviations. Study the pharmacokinetic drug graph in Figure 52-2, which represents the plasma concentration of a particular medication over time.

- The units on the y-axis (vertical) are listed in milligrams per liter (mg/L). The x-axis (horizontal) reports hours since the medication was administered.

- At two hours, the patient's observed plasma concentration in 1.99 mg/L. If you need to convert mg to micrograms (mcg), you would multiply by 1,000 or move the decimal point three places to the right to get 1990 mcg/L.

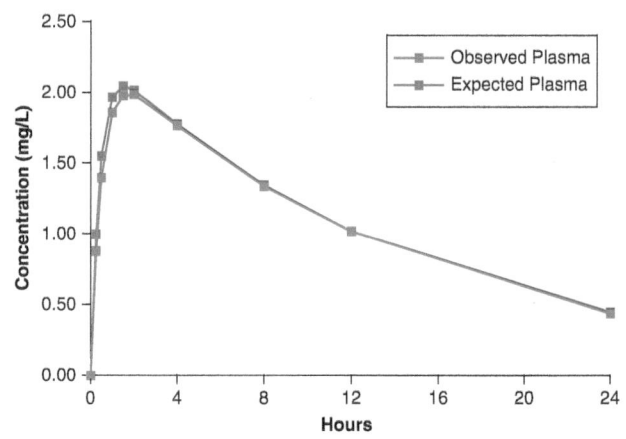

FIGURE 52-2 Pharmacokinetic drug graph representing the plasma concentration of a particular medication over time.

TABLE 52-10 | Conversion List

Apothecary	Metric
1 fluid ounce (oz)	30 milliliters (mL) or cubic centimeters (cc)
1 quart (qt)	1,000 mL or cc
1 grain (gr)	65 milligrams (mg)
5 grains (gr)	325 milligrams (mg)
15 grains (gr)	1 gram (g)
1 ounce (oz)	30 grams (g)
2.2 pounds (lb)	1 kilogram (kg)

Conversion Tips

1. To change grains to grams, divide by 15.
2. To change ounces to cubic centimeters (cc) or milliliters (mL), multiply by 30.
3. To change grains to milligrams (mg), multiply by 60.
4. To change kilograms to pounds, multiply by 2.2.
5. To change cubic centimeters (cc) or milliliters (mL) to ounces, divide by 30.
6. To change drams to milliliters (mL), multiply by 4.
7. To change cubic centimeters (cc) or milliliters (mL) to minims, multiply by 15 or 16.
8. To change minims to cubic centimeters (cc) or milliliters (mL), divide by 15 or 16.
9. To convert drams to grams, multiply by 4.

DRUG CALCULATIONS

Stock medications are frequently kept in offices for use in the office. There are instances when the stock medications are packaged in a different dosage than the physician's order. Therefore, it is important to understand basic drug calculations so you can ensure that the correct dose of medication is given. Sometimes a conversion chart is available, but it is important to double-check and do your own calculations to make sure the dose is correct.

Many factors are involved when the physician calculates the correct dose of a drug, including the patient's age, weight, and current state of health. The physician will also take into account other medications the patient is currently taking, because they may strengthen or weaken the effects of the new drug. As a medical assistant, you should be familiar with these factors, and always double-check your calculations and dosages.

The first step in the drug calculation is to confirm that the system of weights and measures in the prescription is the same as in the container of stock medication. If they are different, the first step will be to convert them to the same system. (Use the information in Table 52-6 and Table 52-7.)

Two methods of drug calculations are explained in this chapter: the **ratio method** and the **formula method**. It is important to understand both and then apply the method that seems easiest for you. Procedures 52-1, 52-2, and 52-3 list the steps necessary to accurately calculate various drug dosages.

Ratio Method

Ratios are one tool in calculating drug dosages. A **ratio** establishes a relationship between two quantities, as when a medical assistant compares the amount of drug ordered to the amount on hand. For example, an ordered dosage might be 10 mg, and the amount on hand might be a tablet containing 20 mg. The ratio would be 10/20 or, in other words, the ordered dosage is $\frac{1}{2}$ the amount on hand.

When two ratios are equal, it is a **proportion**. An example of a proportion is $10/20 = \frac{1}{2}$ or 10:20::1:2. You would read the proportion as "10 divided by 20 equals 1 divided by 2," or "10 is to 20 as 1 is to 2." Even though the number sizes in the examples are different (10 or 1; 20 or 2), the proportion is exactly the same—the first number (10 or 1) is one-half the size of the second (20 or 2).

If you know three of the four numbers for the two ratios in a proportion, you can solve for the fourth number by using mathematical principles. The symbol x is used for the unknown quantity: for example, $10/20 = 1/x$.

To find the unknown quantity, cross-multiply. This means to multiply the top number (numerator) on the left side of the equal sign (=) by the bottom number (denominator) on the right side, and multiply the bottom number (denominator) on the left by the top number (numerator) on the right. Next, divide the result on both sides by the number with the x. The example below proves that $x = 2$.

$$\frac{10}{20} = \frac{1}{x}$$
$$10x = 20$$
$$\frac{10x}{10} = \frac{20}{10}$$
$$1x = 2$$
$$x = 2$$

Another method is to convert $\frac{10}{20} = \frac{1}{x}$ into the ratio we discussed earlier, 10:20::1:x. Then, multiply the extremes (the two outer numbers—the 10 and the x) by each other and the means (the two inner numbers—20 and 1) to solve for x, the unknown.

$$10:20::1:x$$
$$10 \times x = 20 \times 1$$
$$10x = 20$$
$$x = 20 \div 10$$
$$x = 2$$

To prove this answer is correct, multiply the extremes and multiply the means. If the answer is correct, they will be equal.

$$\text{So} \ldots \ 10:20::1:2$$
$$10 \times 2 = 20 \times 1$$
$$20 = 20 - \text{so the answer is correct}$$

Problem: The physician's order is to give the patient 80 mg of Lasix (furosemide) by mouth once daily. Your supply on hand is 40 mg/mL.

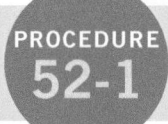
Preparing Proper Medication Dosage: Applying Mathematic Computations to Solve Equations

Objective ◆ *Choose the correct medication, and calculate the exact dosage needed to fulfill an order for 450 mg of amoxicillin clavulanate 600.*

EQUIPMENT AND SUPPLIES

Bottle of reconstituted amoxicillin clavulanate 600 or bottle label; calculator; pen and paper

METHOD

Use the information from the label below (Figure A).

1. Carefully read and verify the entire physician's order.
2. Obtain medication and examine the drug label for strength and amount.

3. Decide if you want to use the ratio or proportion method to solve this order.
4. Write out the formula by substituting the correct quantities for each variable in the equation and then solve for your unknown ("x"): _____
5. Use your calculator to solve the problem.
6. Write your answer in the following blank: To administer 450 mg of amoxicillin clavulanate 600, I will need to draw up _____mL from my stock bottle.

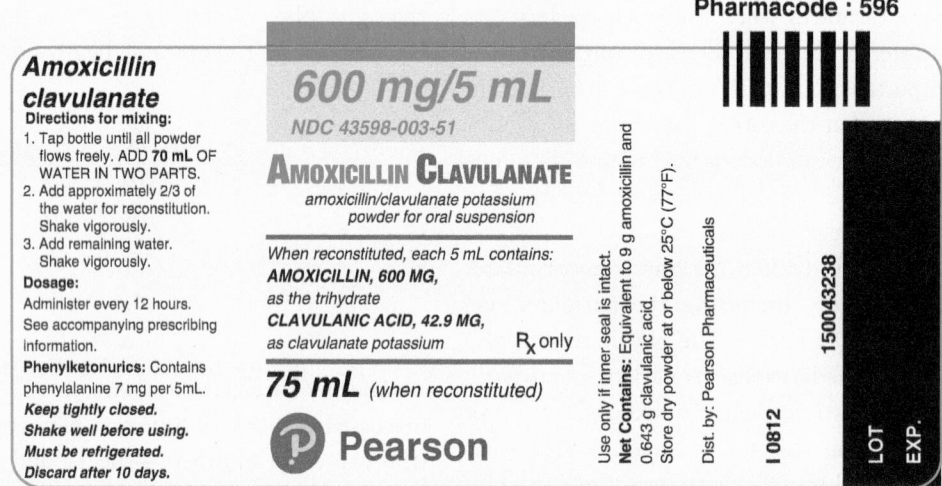

FIGURE A Label from a bottle of reconstituted amoxicillin clavulanate.

There are 40 mg in 1 mL of Lasix (this is the strength of the medication) on hand. The problem requires calculating how many mL of the Lasix solution on hand are required to give the patient 80 mg.

$$80 \text{ mg}:x \text{ mL}::40 \text{ mg}:1 \text{ mL}$$
$$80 \times 1 = 40 \times x$$
$$80 = 40x$$
$$x = 2 \text{ mL}$$

So, 2 mL of Lasix are required to get 80 mg.

(*Common Sense Recheck*: Use your common sense to double check the result. You reason that if the order is 80 mg, and one mL of the on-hand supply contains 40 mg, you will need

to administer 2 mL to provide the 80-mg dose of Lasix that the physician ordered.)

Problem: A physician orders 60 mg of Prilosec (omeprazole) to be administered orally once daily. The supply on hand is 40 mg/capsule.

$$60 \text{ mg}: x \text{ capsules}::40 \text{ mg}: 1 \text{ capsule}$$
$$60 \times 1 = 40 \times x$$
$$60 = 40x$$
$$\frac{60}{40} = \frac{40x}{40}$$
$$1.5 = x$$

So, $1\frac{1}{2}$ capsules are required for the 60-mg dose.

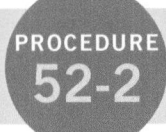

PROCEDURE 52-2

Preparing Proper Medication Dosage: Converting from One Measurement System to Another

Objective ◆ *Choose the correct system of measurement, and calculate the proper dosage in mg (milligrams) needed when the physician orders gr v (grains v) Tylenol.*

EQUIPMENT AND SUPPLIES

Physician order indicating two tablets of (gr v) Tylenol; bottle of Tylenol (325 mg tablets); calculator; pen and paper

METHOD

1. Carefully read and verify the entire physician's order.
2. Obtain medication and examine the drug label for strength and amount.
3. Decide if you want to use the ratio or proportion method to solve this order.
4. Convert the physician's ordered system of measurement to the system of measurement on your medication bottle.
5. Write out the formula by substituting the correct quantities for each variable in the equation and then solve for your unknown ("x").
6. Use your calculator to solve the problem.
7. Write your answer in the following blank: To administer grains v (gr v) of Tylenol, I will need to give _____ tablet(s) _____ mg from my stock Tylenol bottle.

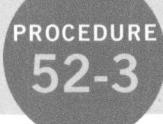

PROCEDURE 52-3

Preparing Proper Medication Dosage: Calculating Correct Dosage for an Injectable Medication

Objective ◆ *Calculate how many mL (milliliters) of NovoLog are needed to complete the physician's order that the patient receive 60 units of insulin aspart.*

EQUIPMENT AND SUPPLIES

Physician order for 60 units of insulin aspart; bottle of insulin aspart (or label); calculator; pen and paper

METHOD

Use the information from the labeled bottle below (Figure A).

1. Carefully read and verify the entire physician's order.
2. Obtain medication and examine the drug label for strength and amount.
3. Review the formula method to solve this order.
4. Write out the formula by substituting the correct quantities for each variable in the equation.
5. Use your calculator to solve the problem.
6. Write your answer in the following blank: To administer 60 units of insulin aspart, I will need to draw up _____ mL from my stock insulin aspart bottle.

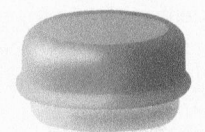

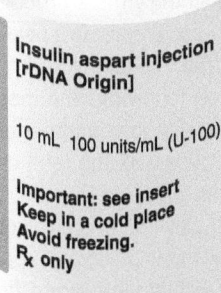

FIGURE A Labeled bottle of insulin aspart.

Professionalism

Always double-check a dosage the physician recommends that you administer by making your own calculations and considering relevant factors such as the patient's age, weight, and other medications the patient is taking. If your double-check reveals what you think may be an error in the dosage the physician has ordered, or if you do not fully understand the order, do not hesitate to tell the physician your concerns and ask for confirmation before you administer the dose.

(*Common Sense Recheck:* You reason that if the order is 60 mg, but one mL of the on-hand supply contains 40 mg, you would need to administer one and a half capsules. However, because capsules, which generally contain a liquid or powder, cannot be safely divided, you will ask how the physician would like to resolve the dilemma, whether by changing the dose order or locating a tablet form of the drug that can be divided, or phoning a nearby pharmacy where the patient can pick up the correct dose.)

Professionalism   The Law

One role of the medical assistant is to make telephone calls for the physician to a pharmacy for physician-approved medication refills. Although the physician and the pharmacist are ultimately responsible for the medication and the dosage, it is the medical assistant's responsibility to ensure that the information called in to the pharmacy is accurate and correct. When calling in the prescription, be sure to give the patient's name and date of birth (to help with patient verification), the name and Drug Enforcement Administration (DEA) registration number of the physician (if required), and the specific dosage, including the route. You must be specific with this information, and be sure to get the name of the pharmacy staff member who received the order. Many pharmacies have voice mail or computer e-mail systems for medication refills, but tracking the receipt of these messages is more difficult. Even these methods offer a seemingly more efficient use of time. A better choice, when possible, is to speak directly with a pharmacy employee. When speaking with the pharmacy, be sure to document the following: the medications to be refilled, the quantity, the telephone number and name of the pharmacy staff member who took the refill order, and the time of the call.

Occasionally, facilities will have a written protocol regarding refilling medications without physician approval. In this case, make sure you are familiar with your office protocol on medication refills and follow them as directed.

Formula Method

It is possible to calculate dosages using a very simple formula. To determine the amount of the drug needed, set up the following formula:

$$\frac{D}{H} \times Q$$

In this equation, D = desired (or ordered) dose; H = dose on hand; and Q = quantity or unit of the on-hand dose (such as 1 tablet or 1 mL).

$$\frac{\text{Desired dose}}{\text{On hand}} \times \text{Quantity}$$

Problem: The physician orders penicillin G benzathine 250 mg to be administered one time via IM injection 250 mg. The bottle in the supply cabinet is labeled "Penicillin G benzathine 500 mg/mL."

Solution: Set up the formula.

$$\frac{\text{Desired dose}}{\text{On hand}} \times \text{Quantity}$$

The physician's order (250) is placed in the Desired (D) space and the dose on hand in the supply cabinet (500) is placed in the On hand (H) space. The number of units containing the on-hand dose—in this case, 1 mL—is placed in the Quantity (Q) space:

$$\frac{D}{H} \times Q = \frac{250}{500} \times 1$$

Divide 250 by 500 × 1 = 0.5

The answer is 0.5 mL.

(*Common Sense Recheck*: Use your common sense to double-check the result. You reason that if the order is 250 mg and one mL of the on-hand supply contains 500 mg, you will administer half a mL to provide the 250 mg dose of penicillin that the physician ordered.)

Problem: The physician orders Lipitor (atorvastatin) 70 mg by mouth once daily. The bottle from the supply cabinet is labeled "Atorvastatin 20-mg tablets."

Solution: Set up the formula.

$$\frac{\text{Desired}}{\text{On hand}} \times \text{Quantity}$$

The physician's order (70 mg) is placed in the Desired (D) space, and the dose you have on hand (20 mg) is placed in the On hand (H) space. The number of units containing the on-hand dose—in this case, 1 tablet—is placed in the Quantity (Q) space:

$$\frac{D}{H} \times Q = \frac{70}{20} \times 1$$

Divide 70 by 20 × 1 = 3.5 or $3\frac{1}{2}$ tablets

The answer is $3\frac{1}{2}$ tablets.

(*Common Sense Recheck:* You reason that if the physician has ordered a dose of 70 mg and each tablet on hand contains 20 mg, you will need three and a half tablets to provide 70 mg.)

CALCULATING PEDIATRIC DOSAGES

Pediatric medications and their dosages differ from those for adults. Sometimes, medications used for adults must be calculated for use in children. It is imperative that the calculations be exact when administering medications to a child. Often, the physician takes the responsibility for this task, but the medical assistant may be asked to assist or to double-check the dosage.

There are several rules or "laws" for the calculations of medications for pediatrics, including Clark's rule, Fried's law, Young's law, West's nomogram, and the body weight method.

Clark's Rule

Clark's rule is based on the weight of the child. This is the most common calculation of drug dosage for children (and used by many pharmacists), especially because the weight of different children at the same age can vary significantly. The formula for Clark's rule is

$$\text{Pediatric dose} = \frac{\text{child's weight in pounds}}{150 \text{ pounds}} \times \text{adult dose}$$

Problem: Penicillin is ordered for a 3-year-old child weighing 35 pounds. The average dose for an adult is 360 mg. How many mg will the child receive?

$$\frac{35}{150} \times 360 \text{ mg} = 83.9 \text{ mg}$$

Fried's Law

Fried's law is applied to children under the age of 1 year. Fried's assumption is that a $12\frac{1}{2}$ year-old child could take an adult dose, and a fraction of that is taken to figure dosages for a young child. This is the formula:

$$\text{Pediatric dose} = \frac{\text{age months}}{150 \text{ months}} \times \text{adult dose}$$

This formula uses 150 months in the denominator as the equivalent for $12\frac{1}{2}$ years.

Problem: Augmentin is ordered for an 8-month-old child. The average dose for an adult is 500 mg. How many mg will the child receive?

$$\frac{8}{150} \times 500 = 26.7 \text{mg}$$

Young's Rule

Young's rule is used for children who are over 1 year of age. The formula used for Young's rule is this:

$$\text{Pediatric dose} = \frac{\text{child's age in years}}{\text{child's age in years} + 12} \times \text{adult dose}$$

Problem: Benadryl is ordered for a 6-year-old child. The average dose for an adult is 50 mg. How many mg will the child receive?

$$\frac{6}{18} \times 50 = 16.7 \text{mg}$$

West's Nomogram

The two methods most commonly used for calculating pediatric dosages are body surface area (BSA), which uses West's nomogram, and body weight, which determines the amount of medication to be administered based on the child's weight. **West's nomogram** is the preferred method, particularly for oncology and critical care patients and underweight children. It can be used for both infants and children. The chart is frequently found in pediatric offices, medical textbooks, and dictionaries. It is preferable to other forms of pediatric dosage calculations because it takes into consideration the child's **body surface area (BSA)**, which is based on a calculation of the child's height and weight and is expressed as m^2 (meters squared). The chart has three columns. To calculate the child's BSA, a straight line is drawn from the patient's height in inches or centimeters across the columns to the patient's weight in kilograms or pounds. The straight line will intersect on the BSA column. This point will give the BSA average (Figure 52-3). Once a BSA average is calculated, it is applied to the following formula:

$$\text{Pediatric dose} = \frac{\text{BSA of child}}{1.73 \text{ square meters}} \times \text{adult dose}$$

1.73 square meters is the standard adult BSA.

Problem: Trimox suspension is ordered for an 8-year-old child with a BSA of 1.3. The average adult dose is 200 mg/5 mL. How many mg will the child receive?

$$1.3/1.73 \times 200 =$$
$$0.76 \times 200 =$$
$$152 \text{ mg}$$

Therefore, you will administer 152 mg from your 200 mg/5 mL stock solution.

Body Weight Method

The body weight method is the other method (besides West's nomogram) that is commonly seen in pediatric situations. Medication dosages are often ordered by the body weight method. The body weight method uses calculations based on the patient's weight in kilograms. This requires

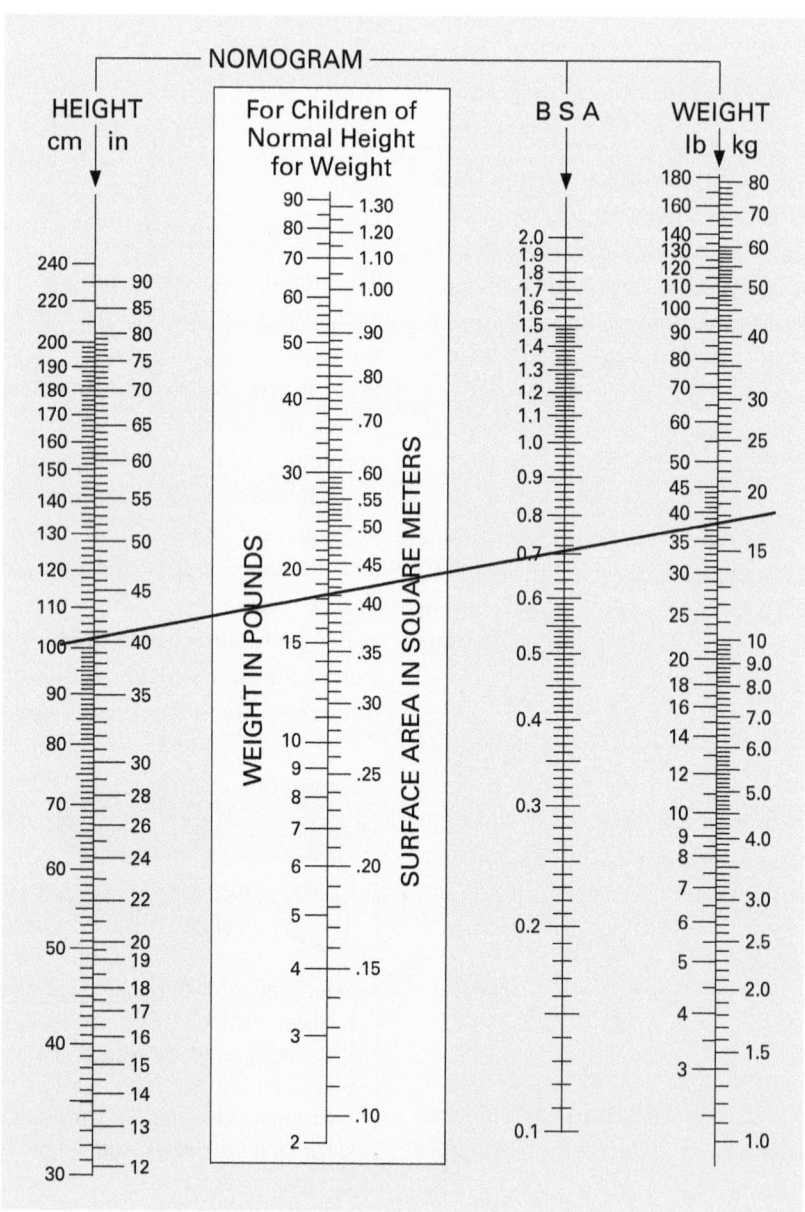

FIGURE 52-3 Nomogram chart. This example shows a line drawn from a child's height of 100 cm to his weight, 35 lb. The line intersects the BSA at 0.7 M².

converting the patient's weight into kilograms. The following provides an example of how this is achieved.

Example: Convert 77 lb to kg.

Approximate equivalent: 1 kg = 2.2 lb

77 lb = 77 divided by 2.2 = 35 kg

Once the child's weight has been converted into kilograms, the correct dosage can be calculated. This is done by calculating the safe drug dosage in mg/kg (as recommended by a reputable drug reference) and then multiplying that amount by the child's weight in kg.

Problem: A physician prescribes a medication to be given to the patient at a dose of 5 mg/kg/day. If your patient weighs 35 kg, you would calculate the amount to administer as follows:

$$5 \text{ mg/kg/day} =$$
$$5 \text{ mg} \times 35 \text{ kg/day} =$$
$$175 \text{ mg/day to be administered.}$$

In the above example, you would administer 175 mg in 24 hours. Had the physician desired the patient to receive 5 mg/kg/day in two doses, you would divide your answer (175 mg) by 2. Keep in mind, the answer you calculate is the maximum amount the patient may receive in a 24-hour period.

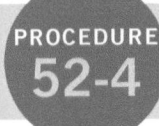

PROCEDURE 52-4
Applying Mathematic Computations to Solve Equations: Calculating Correct Pediatric Dosage Using Body Surface Area

Objective ◆ *Using West's nomogram and the BSA (body surface area) formula, determine the correct dosage for a child who weighs 55 pounds and stands 28 inches tall. The adult dose is 120 mg/mL.*

EQUIPMENT AND SUPPLIES
Nomogram scale; BSA formula; straight edge or ruler; calculator; pen and paper

METHOD
1. Carefully read and verify the entire physician's order.
2. Gather your supplies (West's nomogram, medication, calculator, pen and paper).
3. Review the BSA formula.
4. Using West's nomogram and your straight edge or ruler, determine where the patient's height and weight intersect the BSA column. Write that number here: _____
5. Using your calculator, divide the BSA number you determined by 1.7.
6. Multiply that number by the adult dose (120 mg).
7. Write your answer in the following blank: The child will receive _____ mg of the 120 mg/mL adult medication.

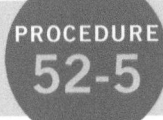

PROCEDURE 52-5
Applying Mathematic Computations to Solve Equations: Calculating Correct Pediatric Dosage Using Body Weight

Objective ◆ *Determine the correct pediatric dosage from the following physician order: Trimethobenzamide hydrochloride 9 mg/kg tid × 2 days for nausea and vomiting. Patient weighs 44 pounds. Medication is labeled 100 mg/mL.*

EQUIPMENT AND SUPPLIES
Physician order for trimethobenzamide hydrochloride; trimethobenzamide label; formula to convert pounds to kilograms; calculator; pen and paper

METHOD
1. Carefully read and verify the entire physician's order.
2. Obtain medication and examine the drug label for strength and amount.

3. Review the formula method to solve this order.
4. Using your calculator, convert the child's weight from pounds to kilograms. Write that number here: _____
5. Determine the daily amount of medication by multiplying the child's weight (kg) by the mg/kg dose on the order. Write that number here: _____ mg.
6. Calculate the individual dose of trimethobenzamide hydrochloride by dividing the daily dose you obtained in step 5 above by 3 (this is the "tid" portion of the order). Write that number here: _____mg.

7. Using the formula of your choosing, determine the amount of drug needed for an individual dose (D/H × Q or ratio/proportion method). Write that number here: _____mL.
8. Write your answer in the following blank: To administer 9 mg/kg body weight of trimethobenzamide hydrochloride (100 mg/mL), I will need to draw up _____ mL from my stock bottle.

SUMMARY

The medical assistant must be able to calculate dosages correctly, because any error has the potential to be fatal to the patient. A general knowledge of mathematical skills is vital for dosage calculations. Always double-check all dosages and, if possible, have someone else double-check your calculations. Have a copy of the conversion factors in an accessible location to make conversions quickly and accurately. Frequent review of the mentioned calculations, conversions, and formulas will keep the medical assistant's mathematical skills sharp and proficient.

Remember, when calculating pediatric dosages, use not only a mathematical double-check but also a "common sense" double-check. Keep in mind that pediatric doses are smaller than adult doses. Does the dosage you have determined pass the common sense test? If not, recheck your math or consult the physician.

52 CHAPTER REVIEW

COMPETENCY REVIEW

1. Define and spell the terms for this chapter.
2. What are the four rules for pediatric dosage calculations?
3. What is the metric system?
4. What is the apothecary system?
5. What is the household system?
6. What is a simple formula for calculating a dosage?
7. Using the label below, answer the following questions:

a. What is the strength of this medication?
b. What would the strength be if it were in grams per 5mL (g/5 mL)?
c. How many milligrams of medication are in 1 mL? How many in 10 mL?

8. Use the label below to answer the following question: The physician wants the patient to receive 0.15 mg of buprenorphine. How many mL will you draw up to make the 0.15 mg dose?

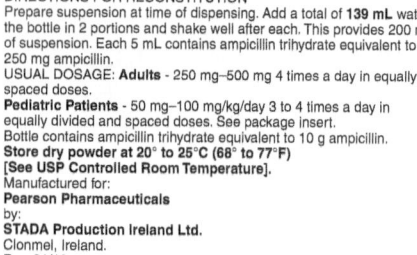

DIRECTIONS FOR RECONSTITUTION
Prepare suspension at time of dispensing. Add a total of **139 mL** water to the bottle in 2 portions and shake well after each. This provides 200 mL of suspension. Each 5 mL contains ampicillin trihydrate equivalent to 250 mg ampicillin.
USUAL DOSAGE: **Adults** - 250 mg–500 mg 4 times a day in equally spaced doses.
Pediatric Patients - 50 mg–100 mg/kg/day 3 to 4 times a day in equally divided and spaced doses. See package insert.
Bottle contains ampicillin trihydrate equivalent to 10 g ampicillin.
Store dry powder at 20° to 25°C (68° to 77°F)
[See USP Controlled Room Temperature].
Manufactured for:
Pearson Pharmaceuticals
by:
STADA Production Ireland Ltd.
Clonmel, Ireland.
Rev. 01/10
183J491

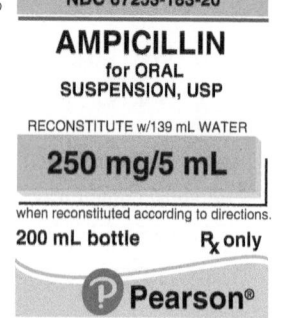

NDC 67253-183-20

AMPICILLIN
for ORAL
SUSPENSION, USP

RECONSTITUTE w/139 mL WATER

250 mg/5 mL

when reconstituted according to directions.
200 mL bottle   R͓only

(P) **Pearson®**

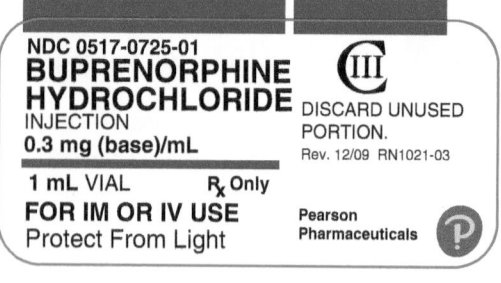

NDC 0517-0725-01
BUPRENORPHINE HYDROCHLORIDE (III)
INJECTION   DISCARD UNUSED
0.3 mg (base)/mL   PORTION.
Rev. 12/09 RN1021-03

1 mL VIAL   R͓Only
FOR IM OR IV USE   Pearson
Protect From Light   Pharmaceuticals (P)

9. Using the label below, how many tablets are required for a 60-mg dose?

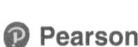

NDC 0781-1966-01

Furosemide Tablets, USP
40 mg

R only
100 Tablets

Ⓟ Pearson

Each tablet contains:
Furosemide, USP 40 mg
Usual Dosage: See package insert.
Store at (20°–25°C (68°–77°F) (see USP Controlled Room Temperature). Dispense in a tight, light-resistant container. **KEEP THIS AND ALL DRUGS OUT OF THE REACH OF CHILDREN.**

Pearson Pharmaceuticals

10. Use the following label to answer the questions below:

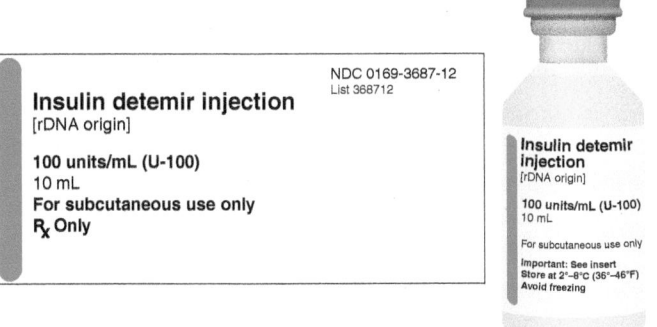

NDC 0169-3687-12
List 368712

Insulin detemir injection
[rDNA origin]

100 units/mL (U-100)
10 mL
For subcutaneous use only
R Only

a. How many units of insulin detemir are in 0.4 mL?
b. What is the total volume of this vial?
c. Assuming this vial has never been open, how many units total are in this vial?

11. Use the label below to answer the following questions:

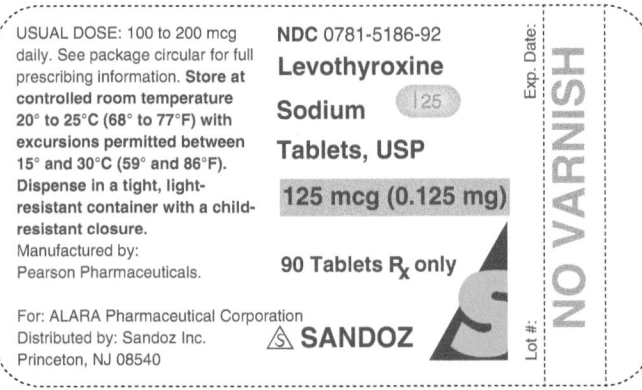

USUAL DOSE: 100 to 200 mcg daily. See package circular for full prescribing information. **Store at controlled room temperature 20° to 25°C (68° to 77°F) with excursions permitted between 15° and 30°C (59° and 86°F). Dispense in a tight, light-resistant container with a child-resistant closure.**
Manufactured by: Pearson Pharmaceuticals.

For: ALARA Pharmaceutical Corporation
Distributed by: Sandoz Inc.
Princeton, NJ 08540

NDC 0781-5186-92
Levothyroxine Sodium |25| **Tablets, USP**

125 mcg (0.125 mg)

90 Tablets R only

⚠ **SANDOZ**

Exp. Date:
Lot #:
NO VARNISH

a. How many mcg are in one-half tablet?
b. How many mg total are in 90 tablets?

12. How many mL of 1-percent lidocaine will you draw up to make a 45-mg strength? Use the information on the bottle below.

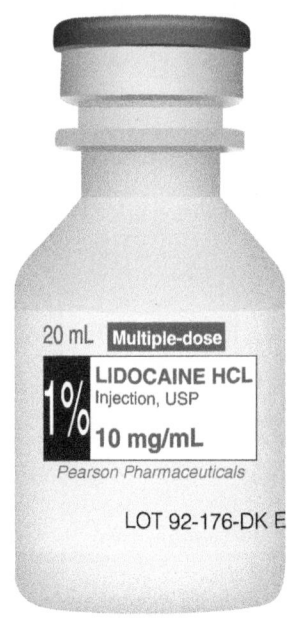

20 mL Multiple-dose

LIDOCAINE HCL
Injection, USP
1%
10 mg/mL

Pearson Pharmaceuticals

LOT 92-176-DK E

13. Use the label below to answer the following questions:

10 mL Single-dose   R only   Discard unused portion   NDC 0409-3814-12
Preservative-Free

MORPHINE
Sulfate Inj., USP
WARNING: MAY BE HABIT FORMING
5 mg/10 mL (0.5 mg/mL)

[For I.V., Epidural or Intrathecal Use.]

Pearson Pharmaceuticals

Each mL contains morphine sulfate, pentahydrate 0.5 mg (Warning: May be habit forming); sodium chloride 9 mg. May contain HCl and/or NaOH for pH adjustment. pH 5.0 (2.5 to 6.5). Store at 20 to 25°C (68 to 77°F). [See USP Controlled Room Temperature.] Protect from light. **Do not heat-sterilize.** See insert for dosage and administration.

RL-0747 (11/04)

a. How many mg of morphine are in 5 mL?
b. How many mcg of morphine are in 10 mL?
c. How many mL of morphine will you draw up if the physician's order is for 1 mg?

14. Using the label below, how many mg of promethazine are in 5 mL?

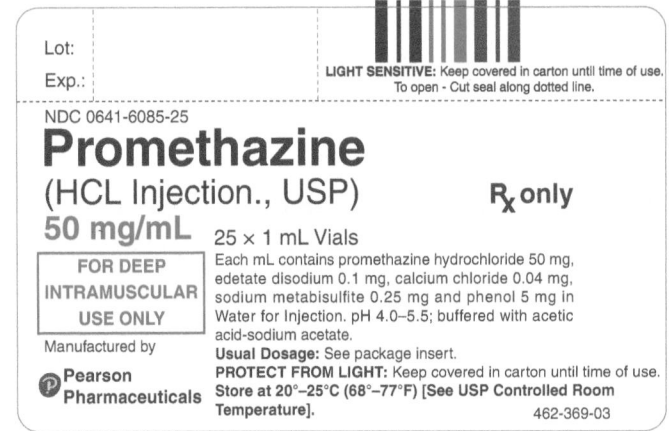

Lot:
Exp.:

LIGHT SENSITIVE: Keep covered in carton until time of use. To open - Cut seal along dotted line.

NDC 0641-6085-25

Promethazine
(HCL Injection., USP)   R only

50 mg/mL   25 × 1 mL Vials

FOR DEEP INTRAMUSCULAR USE ONLY

Manufactured by
Ⓟ Pearson Pharmaceuticals

Each mL contains promethazine hydrochloride 50 mg, edetate disodium 0.1 mg, calcium chloride 0.04 mg, sodium metabisulfite 0.25 mg and phenol 5 mg in Water for Injection. pH 4.0–5.5; buffered with acetic acid-sodium acetate.
Usual Dosage: See package insert.
PROTECT FROM LIGHT: Keep covered in carton until time of use. Store at 20°–25°C (68°–77°F) [See USP Controlled Room Temperature].

462-369-03

15. Examine the vial of potassium chloride below and answer the following questions:

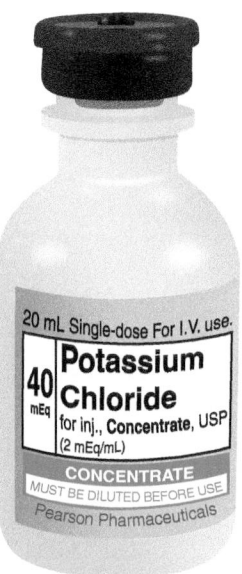

a. The strength is listed in what units?

b. What is the total strength in 5 mL of potassium chloride?

c. How many total mL are in the vial?

d. What is the total strength of the vial?

16. Use the picture below to answer the following:

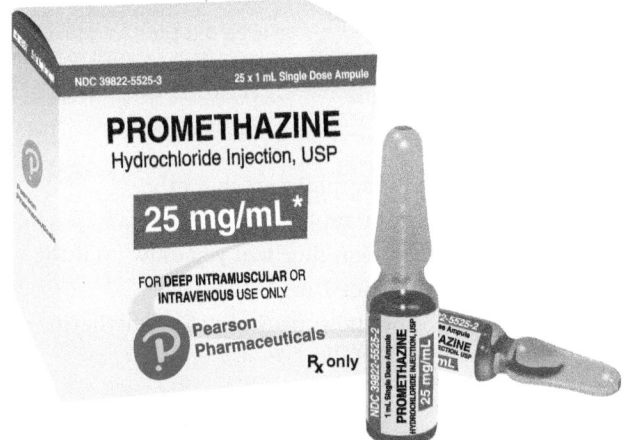

a. How many mg of promethazine are in one ampule?

b. How many mg are in 0.25 mL?

c. If the physician wishes the patient to receive 12.5 mg, how many mL will you draw up?

17. Using Clark's rule, what is the pediatric dose of meclizine for a 10-year-old child who weighs 78 pounds? (The adult dose is 50 mg.)

18. Use West's nomogram and the BSA formula to calculate the following: Amoxicillin is ordered for a 5-year-old child who weighs 35 pounds and is 34 inches tall. The average adult dose is 400 mg/5 mL.

a. How many mg will the child receive?

b. How many mL will the child receive?

19. A physician prescribes lamotrigine to a 10-year-old child to control epileptic seizures. The medication is to be dosed at 3 mg/kg/day. The patient weighs 88 lb. Using the body weight method, calculate the amount of lamotrigine that needs to be administered per day.

20. A physician prescribes clarithromycin to a 4-year-old child to treat a bacterial infection. The medication is to be dosed at 15 mg/kg/day bid × 7 days. The patient weighs 50 lb. Using the body weight method, calculate the amount of clarithromycin that needs to be administered per dose.

PREPARING FOR THE CERTIFICATION EXAM

1. In liquid measures, 1 fluid ounce is equal to
   a. 1 mL.
   b. 10 mL.
   c. 30 mL.
   d. 100 cc.
   e. 30 drams.

2. With regard to medication, available strength refers to
   a. what actually contains the medication.
   b. the potency of the medication in stock.
   c. the potency the physician has ordered.
   d. the amount of medication that should be administered.
   e. the calculated strength.

3. According to the rules for converting from one system of measurement to another, to change
   a. grains to milligrams, multiply by 60.
   b. grains to grams, multiply by 15.
   c. cc to ounces, divide by 50.
   d. cc to mL, divide by 15.
   e. drams to grams, multiply by 2.

4. What is the preferred method of most physicians for calculating pediatric dosages?
   a. Young's rule
   b. Fried's rule
   c. West's nomogram
   d. Clark's rule
   e. body weight

5. Tablets and capsules are measured in metric units of
   a. milligrams.
   b. millimeters.
   c. cubic centimeters.
   d. ounces.
   e. grains.

6. Sometimes, the available dosage of a medication on hand is not the same as that which the physician has ordered. The medical assistant must determine how much of the medication should be used. In the equation used for this calculation, the needed dosage is indicated by
   a. the numerator.
   b. the denominator.
   c. a whole number.
   d. both the numerator and the denominator.
   e. numbers less than 10.

7. Which of the following choices is *not* a formula used to calculate a dosage of a medication?
   a. West's nomogram
   b. Clark's rule
   c. Young's rule
   d. Fried's law
   e. Blalock-Taussig Law

8. Which of the following measurements are equal to each other?
   a. milligrams and grams
   b. liters and milliliters
   c. milliliters and grams
   d. milliliters and cubic centimeters
   e. milliliters and liters

9. When converting a larger unit to a smaller unit, you
   a. divide.
   b. multiply.
   c. subtract.
   d. add.
   e. measure.

10. Which of the following formulas is used to calculate a pediatric dose based on the child's weight in pounds?
    a. Young's rule
    b. Clark's rule
    c. Fried's law
    d. West's nomogram
    e. body weight

CRITICAL THINKING

Refer to the case study at the beginning of the chapter and use what you have learned to answer the following questions.

1. Dr. Salpega informs Mr. Cheng that a liquid form of Augmentin is available. Augmentin is available in an oral suspension (liquid medication) of 250 mg/5 mL. How many mL will Mr. Cheng have to take each time he takes his medication?

2. How many ounces of liquid would this be? (Refer to tables and guidelines in the chapter for conversion amounts.)

3. Using Clark's rule, calculate the Augmentin dosage Dr. Salpega may prescribe for Mr. Cheng's 42-pound son. Keep in mind that the average adult dose of Augmentin is 500 mg.

ON THE JOB

In the past, Mrs. Kennedy has been prescribed Protonix 20 mg a day. Cindy, the medical assistant at Dr. Jones's office, has just spoken to the patient. Mrs. Kennedy tells Cindy that her abdominal pain has increased. After Cindy speaks with the physician on call, the physician increases the dosage to 40 mg once a day. The physician indicates that the patient should take the medication for two weeks to see if any further relief can be achieved. Mrs. Kennedy will be stopping by the office to pick up some samples this afternoon. How will Cindy instruct Mrs. Kennedy and document the change in dose in the patient chart?

INTERNET ACTIVITY

Study the typical complete metabolic panel results shown in Figure 52-4. Do you recognize some of the abbreviations? If not, do an Internet search to answer the questions below. For example, you can type the following into your browser search box: *What does IU mean in pharmacology?*

1. What does the abbreviation "IU" stand for?
2. What does the abbreviation "dL" stand for?
3. This patient's "Albumin, Serum" is 4.9 g/dL. How many "mg/dL" is this?

Tests	Result	Flag	Units	Reference Interval	Lab
Comp. Metabolic Panel (14)					
Glucose, Serum	84		mg/dL	65–99	01
BUN	16		mg/dL	5–26	01
Creatinine, Serum	1.06		mg/dL	0.76–1.27	01
eGFR	>59		mL/min/1.73	>59	01
BUN/Creatinine Ratio	15			8–27	01
Sodium, Serum	141		mmol/L	135–145	01
Potassium, Serum	4.4		mmol/L	3.5–5.2	01
Chloride, Serum	101		mmol/L	97–108	01
Carbon Dioxide, Total	23		mmol/L	20–32	01
Calcium, Serum	9.9		mg/dL	8.7–10.2	01
Protein, Total, Serum	7.6		g/dL	6.0–8.5	01
Albumin, Serum	4.9		g/dL	3.5–5.5	01
Globulin, Total	2.7		g/dL	1.5–4.5	01
A/G Ratio	1.8			1.1–2.5	01
Bilirubin, Total	**1.8**	**High**	mg/dL	0.0–1.2	01
Alkaline Phosphatase, S	65		IU/L	25–150	01
AST (SGOT)	30		IU/L	0–40	01
ALT (SGPT)	32		IU/L	0–55	01

FIGURE 52-4 Complete metabolic panel.

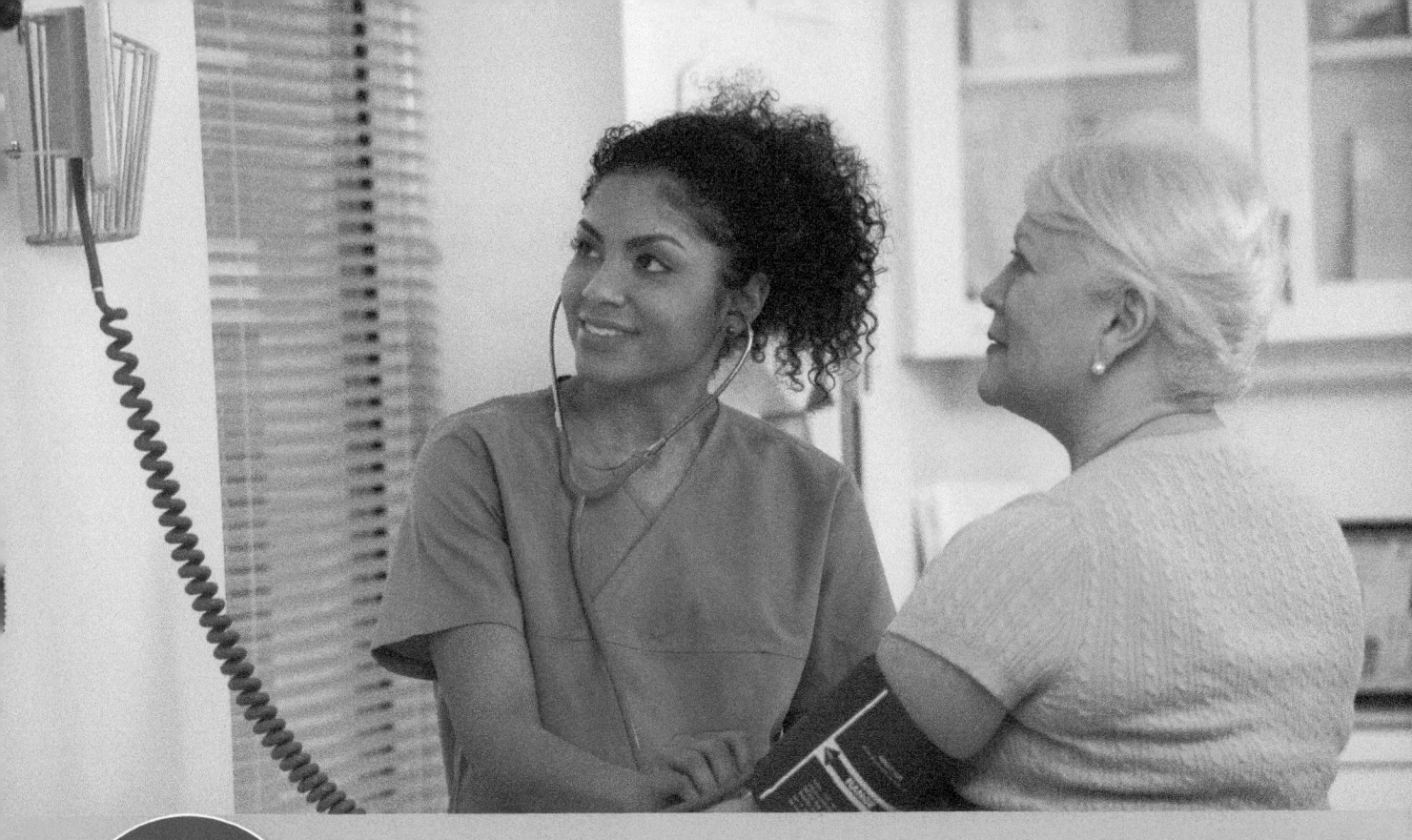

CHAPTER 53

Pharmacology

Learning Objectives

After completing this chapter, you should be able to:

53.1 Define and spell the terms for this chapter.

53.2 Differentiate between the types of names that are assigned to a drug.

53.3 Identify agencies that oversee drug regulations in the United States.

53.4 List materials that are available for drug referencing.

53.5 Compare prescription and nonprescription drugs.

53.6 List the various classifications of drugs based on their action within the body.

53.7 Describe common side effects associated with drugs.

53.8 Identify factors that can affect a drug's interaction for a patient.

53.9 List specific regulations pertaining to controlled substances.

53.10 Identify common routes and methods of drug administration.

53.11 List considerations for drug usage for pregnant women.

53.12 Identify the parts of a prescription.

53.13 List abbreviations commonly used in pharmacology.

Susan Schults, CMA (AAMA), is working the medication refill line for Pearson Physicians Group. She has received a refill request from Adam Lehmke for his diazepam. When she reviews Mr. Lemke's chart, she notices that Dr. Penningworth wrote a prescription for diazepam three months ago with two refills and realizes, based on the date, that Mr. Lehmke should still have two weeks of medicine.

Terms to Learn

adverse effects	drug dependency	pharmacists
anaphylactic shock	Drug Enforcement Administration (DEA)	pharmacology
bioequivalent		polypharmacy
brand name	drug intolerance	prophylactically
broad-spectrum	drug tolerance	proprietary name
computerized physician order entry (CPOE)	generic name	side effects
	habituation	signa (sig.)
contraindicated	idiosyncratic	subscription
controlled substances	inscription	superscription
Controlled Substances Act (CSA)	lethal	synthetic
drugs	medications	toxic
drug abuse	over-the-counter (OTC)	

Pharmacology is the study of **medications** and **drugs** including their forms, intentions for use, and effects. Drugs come from many natural sources, including plants, animals, and minerals, and others are artificially created. Some drugs, such as vitamins, are found naturally in the foods we eat. Medications, such as penicillin and other antibiotics, come from molds, which are a form of plant life. The vast majority of drugs used in medicine today are **synthetic**, created in a laboratory by artificial means.

Drugs are prescribed for a variety of reasons. Some are used to help improve a condition, such as the use of an antihypertensive to control high blood pressure. Other drugs are used to eradicate a condition, such as the use of antibiotics to treat an infection. Drugs given **prophylactically** are used to prevent the onset of a condition. For example, birth control pills are taken prophylactically to prevent pregnancy.

The role of the medical assistant is to assist the physician in the care and treatment of patients. The physician is responsible for prescribing medication for patients. The medical assistant is often required to administer the medication, keep accurate medication records, and provide the patient with information pertaining to the medications they

are prescribed. This requires you, as a medical assistant, to develop skills in reading medication orders, properly administering medications, and other aspects of pharmacology.

DRUG NAMES

Drugs have three types of names: the generic name (sometimes called the "official" or "nonproprietary" name of a drug), the brand name, and the chemical name. The **generic name**, which is typically written in lowercase letters, is the legal name for the drug. Generic drugs are required by U.S. Food and Drug Administration (FDA) regulations to have the same effectiveness, safety, active ingredients, quality, strength, purity, and stability as brand name drugs.

The **brand name**, which is typically written with capitalized initial letters, is the name given to a drug by a specific manufacturer. This is also called the **proprietary name**. This name is often the most familiar name for a specific drug. The company that holds the patent for the drug can manufacture and produce that drug, under that brand name, for 20 years from the date of the patent. Other companies may manufacture the same drug, but must use their own brand name.

TABLE 53-1 | The Three Names Given to a Drug

Generic Name	Brand Name	Chemical Name
acetaminophen	Tylenol	N-(4-hydroxyphenyl) acetamide
Ibuprofen	Motrin	iso-butyl-propanoic-phenolic acid

Generic drugs cannot be sold as long as a brand name manufacturer of that drug holds a patent. Once the brand name patent expires, both the brand name and the generic version of the same drug may be sold. Generic drugs are usually priced lower than drugs with brand names and, under the FDA regulation already mentioned, are **bioequivalent**, having the same strength and action as the brand name version of the drug. It is the active ingredients in generic drugs that are required to be bioequivalent. Nonactive ingredients, such as dyes or flavorings, may differ.

Although generic drugs must be bioequivalent to the brand name of the same drug, in fact generic drugs are not as closely monitored as brand name drugs, so their effectiveness may or may not actually be equal. If a physician believes that a specific brand name drug is more effective than the generic version, then the named brand is more likely to be ordered. In these cases, the physician must clearly indicate on the prescription that the order is for a brand name drug. The prescription order may read "Dispense as written, no substitutions."

The chemical name of a drug is the chemical formula used by manufacturers and pharmacists. **Pharmacists** are specially trained and licensed professionals who specialize in the preparation and dispensation of drugs. The generic name of a drug is usually somehow related to its chemical name.

As examples, Table 53-1 shows the three drug names for the drugs Tylenol and Motrin.

REGULATIONS AND STANDARDS

The FDA is the department within the U.S. Department of Health and Human Services responsible for ensuring that human drugs are safe and effective and that these products are honestly, accurately, and informatively represented to the public. The Federal Food, Drug, and Cosmetic Act of 1938 stipulates the control of drugs. The law was enacted to ensure the safety of food, drugs, and cosmetics sold within U.S. borders. One aspect of these regulations is FDA regulation of the safety of medications for use during pregnancy, which is discussed later in this chapter.

The **Drug Enforcement Administration (DEA)** is the agency of the federal government responsible for drug control enforcement. All physicians are required to register with the DEA to prescribe, dispense, or administer controlled substances. Controlled substances are discussed later in this chapter.

REFERENCES

When you administer a medication per a physician's order, you must understand the drug you are administering. You will often need to research a drug, and fortunately, many reliable references are available for pharmaceutical products.

The *Physicians' Desk Reference*, the *Hospital Formulary*, and the *United States Pharmacopeia–National Formulary (USP–NF)* are commonly used drug reference books. The *Hospital Formulary* also contains up-to-date information about drugs and their usage. It is published by the American Hospital Formulary Service and is used extensively by pharmacists. The USP–NF lists all medicines, dosage forms, drug substances, and dietary supplements authorized for use in the United States; information found in this reference book is enforceable by the FDA.

Because it is impossible for anyone to remember everything about all available medications, it is important for you, as a medical assistant, to practice using available medical references and not rely on memory to ensure that patients receive the correct drug.

Physicians' Desk Reference

The drug resource most commonly available is the *Physicians' Desk Reference*, also known as the PDR (Figures 53-1A and 53-1B). The PDR, which is updated annually, is a relatively easy-to-read reference published by a private company and purchased by medical offices and hospitals. The information in the PDR is the information provided by the drug manufacturers. It is essentially a compilation of the package inserts that come with drugs.

The PDR is divided into color-coded sections that may change slightly from one edition to the next. Normally, the sections include the following six:

- **White**—The first white section is the manufacturer's index with company names, addresses, phone numbers, emergency contacts, and lists of products.
- **Pink**—The pink section is a product name index, an alphabetical listing of generic and brand names.
- **Blue**—The blue section lists drugs grouped by therapeutic classes.

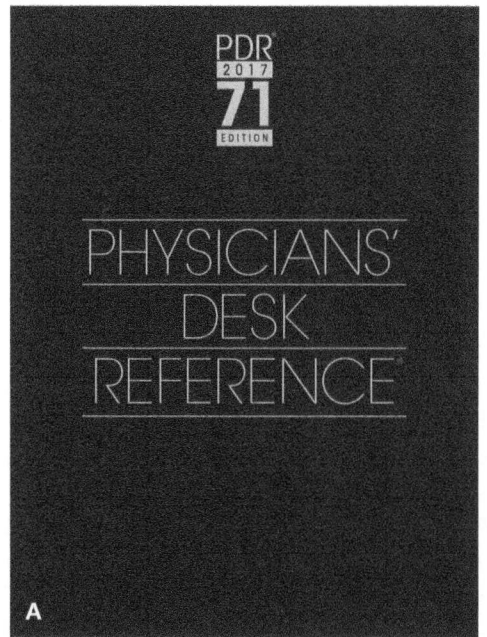

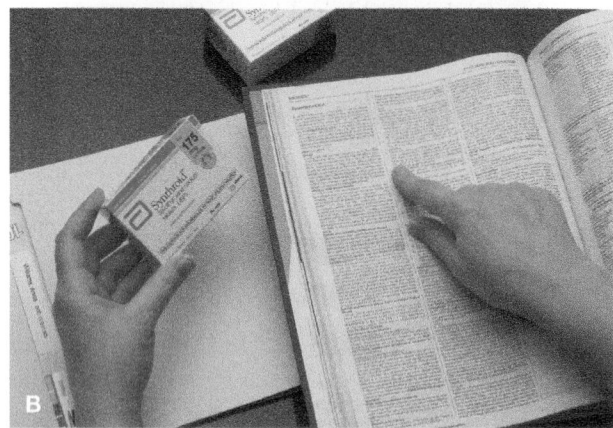

FIGURE 53-1 (A) The *Physicians' Desk Reference.* **(B)** The medical assistant reviews the PDR for information related to a drug.

- **Gray/multi-colored**—The gray section provides color photos of the most commonly prescribed tablets and capsules.

- **White**—The second white section is devoted to product information, a reprint of the manufacturers' package inserts. Information provided for each drug includes its brand and generic names, description, clinical pharmacology, indications for usage, contraindications, warnings, precautions, adverse reactions, dosage and administration, and how it is supplied.

- **Green**—The green section provides diagnostic product information. Additional information pertaining to controlled substances, drug pregnancy ratings, poison control, and discontinued products is also listed here.

Make it a habit to look up drugs the physician orders in the PDR. This will help you to become familiar and

comfortable with its use. Keep in mind, however, that although the PDR is updated every year, even the latest edition does not include changes that have occurred since the publication date.

Electronic References

Many electronic health record (EHR) platforms have electronic versions of the reference books we have just discussed incorporated into the program. This makes looking up information about a drug both convenient and time-saving for the health care providers—both the physician and the medical assistant—and thus helps to improve patient care.

Online Resources

Many online medical information resources are available, but you must be sure to use recognized, reliable online resources when searching for medical information. Web MD and Medline are two Internet resources that are considered to be reliable.

DRUGS

Drugs are broadly classified as either prescription or nonprescription. Nonprescription drugs are also called over-the-counter drugs. As a medical assistant, you must know the difference. Also, you will need to stay abreast of changes in the classification of drugs. Sometimes, drugs that originally required a prescription are made available in over-the-counter forms. For example, Prevacid (used to treat GERD, or gastroesophageal reflux disease) and Claritin (an antihistamine used for the treatment of allergies) were once available only by prescription. Now, both medications are available over the counter.

Another classification you must be familiar with is controlled substances. These are generally powerful medications that pose a high risk of addiction. Controlled substances are discussed later in this section.

Drugs prescribed or purchased to alleviate or manage a medical condition are also called medications.

Prescription Drugs

Physicians are responsible for prescribing medications. Some specially licensed professionals, such as physician's assistants and advanced practice nurses (for example, nurse practitioners and clinical nurse specialists), can also write prescriptions, although this varies from state to state.

A prescription is a written explanation to a pharmacist specifying the name of the medication, the dose, the route, and the times of administration. Physicians can also give the prescription to a pharmacist verbally over the telephone.

Prescription drugs include antibiotics, antihypertensives, and analgesics, among others. When dispensed from a pharmacy, the label on the drug container for one of these drugs must read "Caution: Federal Law prohibits dispensing without prescription." This means that it is illegal to give someone a prescription medication that was not prescribed for that person, even when the intention is to help the person.

Nonprescription Drugs

Nonprescription drugs, or **over-the-counter (OTC)** drugs, include medications such as aspirin, cold medications, and antibiotic ointments like Neosporin. OTC drugs are found in a variety of stores, including supermarkets, not just pharmacies.

Even though OTC medications do not require a prescription, they are regulated by the FDA. OTC medications are not without dangers, and patients should be educated to read labels and follow the label's directions. If taken incorrectly, some OTC drugs can be unsafe. Some OTC drugs may react negatively with a prescription drug the patient is taking. For example, antacids should not be taken with some antibiotics, and aspirin (which has blood-thinning or anti-platelet effects) should not be taken with Coumadin (an anticlotting medication) because of the potential for uncontrolled bleeding. Individuals with stomach ulcers should not take aspirin or ibuprofen, because they irritate the stomach lining and increase the risk of bleeding from the ulcers.

Patients who have questions about how to take OTC medications should ask their pharmacist for guidance. Patients should always let their physician know about all OTC medications they are taking. You, the medical assistant, should be sure to review and document OTC medications and prescription medications the patient is taking at every office visit. Remind patients that the OTC medications they need to report include supplements like vitamins and herbs they may purchase at a health food store and not think of as drugs.

Classification Based on Drug Action

The classification of drugs is based on their action in the body. Table 53-2 presents a comprehensive list of drug classifications with descriptions of the use or function for each classification. Table 53-3 presents a similar list with examples of specific drugs for each classification.

Side Effects of Drugs

Drugs affect not only the specific condition for which they are taken; they also affect other functions. The intended effects on the patient's medical condition are known as desirable effects. The other, sometimes undesirable, effects are called **side effects**. Side effects are generally accepted because the benefit of taking the medication outweighs the unwanted effects. However, side effects that are known as **adverse effects** require that the patient discontinue the medication because the negative effects outweigh the benefits.

Food interactions can cause side effects. Other effects can be caused by allergic reactions. Sometimes, side effects or adverse effects are specific to the individual (**idiosyncratic**). Unexpected side effects can range from rashes to drowsiness, coughing, runny nose, constipation, dizziness, headache, nausea, or vomiting. Patients should be instructed to call the physician if any of these symptoms occur while taking a medication, especially if it is prescribed. The physician may adjust the medication dose or completely change the prescription to another drug that may not have the same side effects.

Occasionally, adverse effects can be **lethal**, which means they may cause death. For example, **anaphylactic shock** is a life-threatening adverse reaction, usually to a drug, a certain food, or an insect bite or sting. Anaphylactic responses can include respiratory distress, edema (swelling) in the mouth and throat, convulsions, and unconsciousness. If not treated swiftly, anaphylactic shock can lead to death.

Because of the possibility of adverse or even lethal consequences, it is important that the potential or actual side effects of any drug be noted and taken seriously.

More examples of side effects are discussed in the following sections.

Patient Reactions to Medications

Many factors contribute to how a patient reacts to medication and whether a medication is effective for a patient.

TABLE 53-2 | Drug Classifications and Descriptions of Use

Name	Use
Adrenergic	Increases the rate and strength of the heart muscle. Acts as a vasoconstrictor, dilates bronchi, dilates pupils, and relaxes muscular walls. Used to treat asthma, bronchitis, and allergies.
Adrenergic blocking agent	Increases peripheral circulation, decreases blood pressure and vasodilation. Used to treat hypertension.
Analgesic	Relieves pain without the loss of consciousness. These may be either narcotic or nonnarcotic. Narcotic drugs are derived from the opium poppy and act on the brain to cause pain relief and drowsiness.
Anesthetic	Produces a lack of feeling that may have a local or general effect depending on the type of administration.
Antacid	Neutralizes acid in the stomach.
Antianxiety	Relieves or reduces anxiety and muscle tension. Used to treat panic disorders, anxiety, and insomnia.
Antiarrhythmic	Controls cardiac arrhythmias by altering nerve impulses within the heart.
Antibiotic	Destroys or prohibits the growth of microorganisms. Used to treat bacterial infections. Ineffective in treating viral infections. Must be taken regularly for a specified time period to be effective.
Anticoagulant	Prevents or delays blood clotting. Also referred to as blood thinners. May be administered by intravenous injection, such as with the drug heparin. Oral anticoagulants, such as warfarin, cannot be taken along with aspirin, because the interaction between the two medications could cause internal bleeding.
Anticonvulsant	Prevents or relieves convulsions. Anticonvulsants such as phenobarbital reduce excessive stimulation in the brain to control seizures and other symptoms of epilepsy.
Antidepressant	Prevents or relieves the symptoms of depression. Also used in the prevention of migraine headaches.
Antidiabetic	Controls diabetes by regulating the level of glucose in the blood and the metabolism of carbohydrates and fat.
Antidiarrheal	Prevents or relieves diarrhea.
Antidote	Counteracts the effects of poisons and medications.
Antiemetic	Controls nausea and vomiting. Generally act on the vomiting center in the brain.
Antifungal	Kills fungus.
Antihelminthic	Kills parasitic worms.
Antihistamine	Counteracts histamine and controls allergic reactions.
Antihypertensive	Prevents or controls high blood pressure. Some antihypertensives block nerve impulses that cause arteries to constrict and thus decrease blood pressure. Others slow the heart rate and decrease its force of contraction. Still others may reduce the amount of the hormone aldosterone in the blood that is causing the blood pressure to rise. Still others may reduce the amount of the hormone aldosterone in the blood that is causing the blood pressure to rise from the retention of salt and water.
Antiinflammatory	Counteracts inflammation.
Antineoplastic	Kills normal and abnormal cancerous cells by interfering with cell reproduction.
Antipruritic	Relieves itching.
Antipyretic	Reduces fever.
Antiseptic	Prevents the growth of microorganisms.

TABLE 53-2 | Drug Classifications and Descriptions of Use (*continued*)

Name	Use
Antitussive	Controls or relieves coughing. Codeine is an ingredient in many prescription antitussives (cough medicines); it acts on the brain to control coughing.
Astringent	A substance that has a constricting or binding effect by coagulating proteins on a cell's surface. May be used to stop hemorrhage.
Bronchodilator	Dilates or opens the bronchi (airways in the lungs) to improve breathing.
Cardiogenic	Strengthens the heart muscle.
Cathartic	Causes bowel movements to occur. May have a strong purging action and can become habit forming.
Contraceptive	Used to prevent conception.
Decongestant	Reduces nasal congestion and swelling.
Diuretic	Increases the excretion of urine, which promotes the loss of water and salt from the body; because this can assist in lowering blood pressure, diuretics are used to treat hypertension. Potassium in the body may be depleted with continued use of diuretics. Potassium-rich foods, such as bananas, kiwi, and orange juice, along with medications for potassium deficiency, can help correct this deficiency.
Emetic	Induces vomiting.
Expectorant	Assists in the removal of secretions from the bronchopulmonary membranes.
Hemostatic	Controls bleeding.
Hypnotic	Produces sleep or hypnosis.
Hypoglycemic	Lowers blood glucose level.
Immunosuppressant	Suppresses the body's natural immune response to an antigen. Used to control autoimmune diseases such as multiple sclerosis and rheumatoid arthritis.
Laxative	Used to promote normal bowel function.
Miotic	Constricts the pupils of the eye.
Muscle relaxant	Produces the relaxation of skeletal muscle.
Mydriatic	Dilates the pupils of the eye.
Narcotic	Produces sleep or stupor. In moderate doses will depress the central nervous system and relieve pain. In excessive doses will cause stupor, coma, and even death. Can become habit forming (addictive).
Psychedelic	Drugs such as lysergic acid diethylamide (LSD) that can produce visual hallucinations.
Purgative	Stimulates bowel movements.
Sedative	Produces relaxation without causing sleep.
Statin	Helps control cholesterol and lipid levels.
Stimulant	Speeds up the heart and respiratory system. Used to increase alertness.
Tranquilizer	Used to reduce mental anxiety and tension.
Vaccine	Given to promote resistance (immunity) to infectious diseases.
Vasodilator	Relaxes blood vessels to lower blood pressure.
Vasopressor	Produces muscle contractions that affect capillaries and arteries and elevates the blood pressure.
Vitamin	Organic substances found naturally in foods that are essential for normal metabolism. Most have been produced synthetically to be taken in pill form.

TABLE 53-3 | Drugs Commonly Prescribed According to Classification

Type/Usage	Example Brand Name (Generic Name)	Type/Usage	Example Brand Name (Generic Name)
Adrenergic	Isuprel (isoproterenol) Sudafed (pseudoephedrine hydrochloride HCl)	**Anticholinergic**	Atropine (atropine sulfate) Banthine (methantheline bromide) Donnatal (belladonna)
Adrenergic blocking agent	Aldomet (methyldopa) Inderal (propranolol HCl)	**Anticoagulant**	Coumadin (warfarin sodium)
Analgesic	Acetylsalicylic acid or aspirin Advil (ibuprofen) Demerol (meperidine HCl) Dilaudid (hydromorphone HCl) Talwin (pentazocine HCl) Tylenol (acetaminophen)	**Anticonvulsant**	Dilantin (phenytoin sodium) Phenobarbital (phenobarbital)
		Antidepressant	Elavil (amitriptyline HCl)
		Antidiabetic	Insulin and oral medications (Precose and Metformin)
Anesthetic	Carbocaine (mepivacaine HCl) Novocaine (procaine HCl) Nupercaine (dibucaine HCl) Xylocaine (lidocaine HCl)	**Antidiarrheal**	Kaopectate (kaolin and pectin mixture) Lomotil (diphenoxylate)
		Antiemetics	Compazine (prochlorperazine) Dramamine (dimenhydrinate) Phenergan (promethazine HCl)
Antacid	Milk of Magnesia (magnesium hydroxide) Mylanta (aluminum hydroxide) Maalox (aluminum hydroxide)	**Antifungal**	Mycostatin (nystatin)
		Antihelminthics	Vermox (mebendazole)
Antianxiety	Valium (diazepam)	**Antihistamine**	Adrenalin (epinephrine) Benadryl (diphenhydramine) Chlor-Trimeton (chlorpheniramine maleate) Dimetane (brompheniramine maleate)
Antiarrhythmic	Digoxin (digoxin) Norpace (disopyramide) Pronestyl (procainamide HCl)		
Antibiotics			
• **Aminoglycosides**	Garamycin (gentamicin sulfate) Kantrex (kanamycin) Mycifradin Sulfate (neomycin sulfate) Nebcin (tobramycin sulfate) Neobiotic (neomycin sulfate)	**Antihypertensives**	Aldomet (methyldopa) Catapres (clonidine HCl) Lopressor (metoprolol tartrate) Minipress (prazosin HCl)
• **Cephalosporins**	Ancef (cefazolin sodium) Anspor (cephradine) Ceclor (cefaclor) Duricef (cefadroxil) Keflex (cephalexin)	**Antiinflammatory**	Aspirin (acetylsalicylic acid) Indocin (indomethacin) Motrin (ibuprofen) Nalfon (fenoprofen calcium) Aleve (naproxen sodium)
• **Penicillins**	Amoxil (amoxicillin) Bicillin (penicillin G potassium) Duracillin (penicillin G procaine) Polycillin (ampicillin)	**Antineoplastic**	Adriamycin (doxorubicin HCl) Cytoxan (cyclophosphamide) Fluorouracil (5FU)
		Antipruritic	Calamine lotion (calamine) Hydrocortone (hydrocortisone sodium phosphate)
• **Tetracyclines**	Achromycin (tetracycline HCl) Declomycin (demeclocycline) Terramycin (oxytetracycline) Vibramycin (doxycycline hyclate)	**Antipyretic**	Advil (ibuprofen) Aspirin (acetylsalicylic acid) Tylenol (acetaminophen)

TABLE 53-3 | Drugs Commonly Prescribed According to Classification (*continued*)

Type/Usage	Example Brand Name (Generic Name)	Type/Usage	Example Brand Name (Generic Name)
Antiseptic	Cidex (glutaraldehyde)	Narcotic	Demerol (meperidine HCl)
	pHisoHex (hexachlorophene)		Percodan (oxycodone HCl)
Antitussive	Codeine (codeine phosphate)	Psychedelic	LSD (lysergic acid diethylamide)
Bronchodilator	Alupent (metaproterenol sulfate)	Sedative and Hypnotic	Amytal (amobarbital)
	Brethine (terbutaline sulfate)		Butisol (butabarbital sodium)
	Isuprel (isoproterenol HCl)		Nembutal Sodium (phenobarbital)
	Theolair (theophylline)		Seconal Sodium (secobarbital sodium)
Contraceptive	Ortho-Novum 10/11 (estrogen with progestin)		Valium (diazepam)
Decongestant	Neo-Synephrine (phenylephrine HCl)	Statins	Crestor (rosuvastatin calcium)
			Lipitor (atorvastatin)
	Sudafed (pseudoephedrine HCl)		Zocor (simvastatin)
Diuretic	Diuril (chlorothiazide)	Stimulant	Dexedrine (dextroamphetamine sulfate)
	Hygroton (chlorthalidone)		
	Lasix (furosemide)	Tranquilizer	Haldol (haloperidol)
Expectorant	Robitussin (guaifenesin)	Vasodilator	Isordil (isosorbide dinitrate)
Hormone	Testosterone, Premarin, Estrace		Nitro-bid (nitroglycerin)
			Nitrostat (nitroglycerin)
Hypnotic	Seconal (secobarbital)	Vasopressor	Levophed (norepinephrine)
Hypoglycemic	Precose (oral)	Vitamin	Vitamin A
	Metformin (oral)		Vitamin C
Laxative	Dulcolax (bisacodyl)		Vitamin D
Muscle relaxant	Valium (diazepam)		Vitamin E
	Robaxin (methocarbamol)		Vitamin K

Factors that contribute to a patient's reaction to a medication include the patient's age, the patient's weight, the method of administration, allergies, and the degree of tolerance and intolerance. Although a patient may tolerate a medication well at one time, that patient may have a reaction to the same medication at another time if certain contributing factors have changed.

Patient's Age

Geriatric and pediatric patients are more susceptible to the effects of medications than others and usually require lower doses. When a physician prescribes a medication for these populations, it is helpful for you, the medical assistant, to review the order and to be sure that an appropriate dosage has been ordered.

Some geriatric patients may have other needs that require attention because they may affect how the patient takes the medication. For instance, medication instructions may need to be typed in a larger font, or medication bottles may need to have easily removable caps (Figure 53-2).

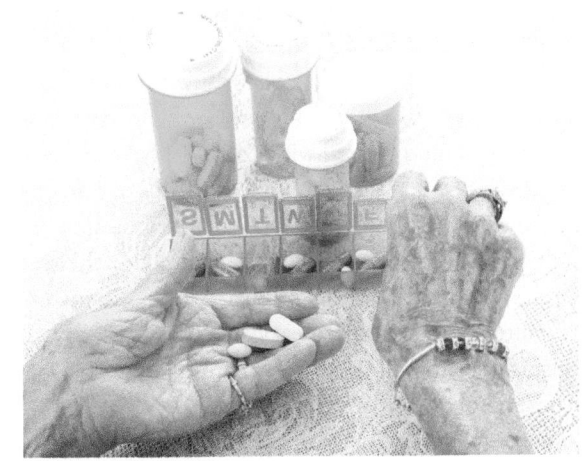

FIGURE 53-2 Older adults may need special assistance with medications.

Patient's Weight

A patient's weight is an important factor to consider when calculating the medication dosage. There is a direct correlation between the patient's weight and the optimum medication level. The typical medication dosage is based on the weight of a 150-pound adult. Dosages may increase if the patient is heavier or may decrease if the patient is lighter. If the medication level is too low for the body weight, the patient will benefit less from the medication. Conversely, if the medication level is too high for the patient's body weight, the patient could become ill or even have an overdose reaction. It is important for you to take note when a patient has a drastic fluctuation in weight. For instance, if an obese patient undergoes bariatric surgery (to assist with weight loss), medication dosage levels may need to be adjusted frequently as the patient's weight changes.

Method of Administration

The method of administration affects the rate at which the body absorbs the medication. The physician will choose the method of administration according to the desired response. For instance, if a patient is in extreme pain, the physician may order an injectable medication rather than an oral medication for a quicker response. To offer relief over a sustained period of time, a time-release oral medication may be used.

Allergies

An allergic reaction to a medication can occur at any time. An allergic reaction can manifest itself in signs and symptoms such as hives and shortness of breath, which can be moderate to severe. The allergic reaction may be immediate, or it may develop over time. Generally, the faster an allergic reaction develops, the more severe and dangerous it is. (Anaphylactic shock, the most severe allergic reaction, was discussed earlier as a potentially lethal side effect.)

When patients are prescribed a new medication, they should be provided education regarding the warning signs and symptoms of allergic reactions to medications. Additionally, they should be told what to do if an allergic reaction occurs. If the reaction is mild, such as the formation of a few hives, they should be instructed to discontinue the medication and call the medical office immediately. If the reaction is severe, including shortness of breath, or has occurred very quickly after taking the medication (a possible anaphylactic response), they should call 911 for immediate transport to the nearest emergency department.

Commonly, if a medication is administered in the office, the patient is asked to wait at least 30 minutes before leaving the office to ensure that an allergic or other adverse reaction does not occur. All patient allergies and allergic responses must be documented in the patient's health record.

Tolerance and Intolerance

After taking a medication for an extended period of time, the patient may develop a tolerance to that medication, meaning that the medication is no longer effective or not as effective as it has been. If this occurs, the physician may need to change the medication or increase the dosage to obtain the desired result. If a patient takes a drug for a long period of time, tolerance or habituation can develop. A patient can also be intolerant of a drug.

- **Drug tolerance**—This is a decrease in the effectiveness of a drug as the body gets used to having the drug in the system. It will then take a larger dose of the drug to achieve the same result. This is common when a patient is repeatedly prescribed the same antibiotic or in patients who require a specific drug, such as a pain control medication, over a long period of time. The dose cannot always be increased, because some drugs can become **toxic** (harmful) in excessive amounts.

- **Habituation**—This is physiologic or psychologic dependence on a drug. Habituation can develop with a variety of drugs, including narcotics and laxatives.

- **Drug intolerance**—Although some patients may say they are "allergic" to certain drugs, they may instead be intolerant of that drug. Drug intolerance or drug sensitivity is a lower threshold to the normal pharmacologic action of a drug. Vomiting, diarrhea, or abdominal cramping can be indications of intolerance. As with allergies, intolerances to medication should be documented in the patient's health record. If the patient experiences intolerance to a medication, she should alert the physician, who may then adjust the dosage or change the prescription as needed. If a patient reports an allergy to a medication, it is important to ask the patient to detail what occurs that they perceive as an allergic reaction. The patient's description will aid the physician in adjusting the medication.

Inventory and Recordkeeping

Medical offices and facilities maintain an inventory of the variety of medications kept in the facility. Medications that are kept on hand can range from samples provided by pharmaceutical companies to medications commonly used within the office. Some offices may have supply cabinets to store their medication supplies, although larger practices and facilities may have small rooms dedicated to storage. Offices and facilities store both oral medications and injectable drugs. Commonly stocked injectable drugs are listed in Table 53-4.

TABLE 53-4 | Injectable Drugs Commonly Stocked in the Medical Office

Generic Name	Trade Name	Route	Usage
amitriptyline HCl	Elavil	IM	Depression
brompheniramine maleate	Dimetane	IM/Subcutaneous	Allergy
chlorpromazine HCl	Thorazine	IM	Psychosis
Diazepam	Valium	IM	Anxiety
Dimenhydrinate	Dramamine	IM	Nausea/vomiting
diphenhydramine	Benadryl	IM	Allergic reaction
diphtheria, tetanus toxoid	Same name	IM	Immunization active vaccine
Furosemide	Lasix	IM	Edema
gentamicin sulfate	Garamycin	IM	Infection
heparin sodium	Same name	Subcutaneous	Prevents clotting
hydromorphone HCl	Dilaudid	Subcutaneous/IM	Severe pain
lidocaine HCl 1 percent, 2 percent	Xylocaine	Subcutaneous	Anesthetic for minor surgery
prochlorperazine	Compazine	IM	Psychosis
promethazine HCl	Phenergan	IM	Nausea/vomiting
sodium chloride with benzyl alcohol 0.9 percent	Bacteriostatic 0.9% Sodium Chloride	—	Diluent for injection
tetanus and diphtheria toxoids	Same name	IM	Immunization (active vaccine)
tetanus antitoxin	Same name	IM	Prevention (passive vaccine)
tetanus immune globulin	Hyper-Tet	IM	Prevention (passive vaccine)
tetanus toxoid	Same name	IM	Immunization (active vaccine)
tuberculin protein derivative	Tine test	ID	Tuberculin testing
water for injection	Same name		Diluent for injection
Emergency Drugs			
Amiodarone	Cordarone	Oral, IV	Arrhythmia
Epinephrine		IV	Cardiac arrest
		Subcutaneous	Allergic reaction
Norepinephrine	Levophed	IV	Hypotension
electrolytes/Ringer's 1,000 mL		IV	Dehydration

Key to abbreviations: ID, intradermal; IM, intramuscular; IV, intravenous

Note: Only physicians and nurses may administer IV medications. Some states allow medical assistants to start IV medications, but only with additional certification. It is important to know your state's regulations.

All medication inventory is maintained in a logbook. This logbook can be either a paper document or an electronic file. A logbook includes the name of each medication stored, the dosages of each medication, the quantity on hand for each dosage, and the expiration dates. Often, the medical assistant is responsible for maintaining the medication supply logbook. Typically, a separate section in the logbook is used to indicate when a medication is dispensed to a patient. When distributing a medication to a patient, the patient's name and date of birth are entered into this section of the logbook, along with the quantity, date, and time of distribution, and medical assistant's initials. Again, as technology has advanced, distributing medications has also changed. Many electronic health record platforms that are used in the medical office will allow for medications that are dispensed to be scanned into the patient's record. This helpful tool can reduce or eliminate charting errors.

Once a month it is important for the medical assistant to review the inventory to ensure that a sufficient supply of each drug is available and that no medication has expired. When disposing of expired medications, follow office policy. The expiration dates of all controlled substances in stock should be checked regularly, and two staff members should document the destruction of any of these medications. Individual state policies will indicate the credentials required of staff members allowed to destroy these medications. The signatures of both individuals should be documented in the controlled substance logbook stating that the medications have been destroyed. The local DEA office should be contacted regarding discarding practices for large amounts of controlled substances.

Medication errors should be documented according to facility policy, which usually includes immediately reporting to a supervisor and filling out an incident report. Depending on the type of error, action may need to be taken to reverse the effects or side effects of an inappropriately given medication or dose. Therefore, it is vital to report an error in medication administration as soon as it is discovered. Serious or frequent medication errors may result in the need to retrain, discipline, or dismiss the employee.

Controlled Substances

Under the **Controlled Substances Act (CSA)**, enacted in 1970, certain drugs are classified as **controlled substances** because they have a potential for addiction or abuse. The DEA strictly enforces the control of these medications.

The CSA regulates the manufacture and distribution of drugs that can cause dependencies. For example, under the CSA, a psychoactive drug that has the potential for abuse is included on the controlled substances list. The psychoactive drugs regulated by the CSA include narcotics, hallucinogens, depressants, and stimulants. The CSA has set forth guidelines for these controlled substances and divided them into five categories (schedules) based on their potentially addictive level of abuse. See Table 53-5 for examples of these schedules.

Controlled substances are generally kept under double lock and key in a nonmovable secured cabinet. Strict control

TABLE 53-5 | Schedule for Controlled Substances

Level	Description	Comment
Schedule I	Highest potential for addiction and abuse Not accepted for medical use *Examples:* cocaine, heroin, methamphetamine	Not prescribed drugs and considered illegal drugs.
Schedule II	High potential for addiction and abuse Accepted for medical use in the United States *Examples:* codeine, morphine, opium, and secobarbital	A DEA-licensed physician must complete the required triplicate prescription forms entirely written in her own handwriting. As technology advances, some states are allowing e-prescribing for controlled substances through electronic health record platforms that transmit prescriptions to the pharmacy electronically. The prescription must be filled within seven days, and it may not be refilled. In an emergency, the physician may order a limited amount of the drug by telephone. These drugs must be stored under lock and key if they are kept on office premises. The law requires that a dispensing record of these drugs be kept on file for two years.
Schedule III	Moderate to low potential for addiction and abuse *Examples:* butabarbital, anabolic steroids, APC (aspirin, phenacetin, and caffeine) with codeine	Physicians can either provide a written prescription or call in the order to a pharmacist. Again, many states are issuing individual guidelines in regard to e-prescribing as safety and security mechanisms are implemented. Up to five refills, which must be indicated on the prescription form, are allowed during a six-month period.
Schedule IV	Lower potential for addiction and abuse than Schedule III drugs *Examples:* chloral hydrate, phenobarbital, diazepam	A medical assistant may write the prescription order for the physician, but it must be signed by the physician. Five refills are allowed over a six-month period of time.
Schedule V	Low potential for addiction and abuse *Examples:* low-strength codeine combined with other drugs to form a cough suppressant	Inventory records must be maintained on these drugs.

must be maintained. A controlled substance log must be kept to track all controlled substances, including the inventory in stock, who administers the controlled substance, how much was given, how much was wasted, and the date and name of the patient receiving the drug. The controlled substance log must be kept on file for at least two years and must be available for inspection at any time by the DEA, which is charged with regulating the sale and use of controlled substances. Most facilities do not allow medical assistants to administer controlled substances.

Physicians are required to register with the DEA to prescribe, dispense, or administer controlled substances. A special form, DEA 224, must be completed and submitted to the DEA. Any prescriber then must have this DEA registration number on all prescriptions for controlled substances; therefore, it is usually printed on all prescription pads or electronic templates. Renewal is required every three years, using Form 224a. A DEA number is required for all locations where controlled substances are stored, so if a physician has offices in two states, then two different DEA numbers must be obtained, one for each state.

All controlled substances must be labeled according to CSA specifications, showing the drug's assigned schedule. The schedule identification number is written as a roman numeral inside a capital letter C, which stands for controlled substance (Figure 53-3). The following are some common controlled substances:

- Anabolic steroids
- Butabarbital
- Chloral hydrate
- Codeine
- Diazepam
- Morphine
- Opium
- Phenobarbital
- Secobarbital
- Acetaminophen (Tylenol) with codeine

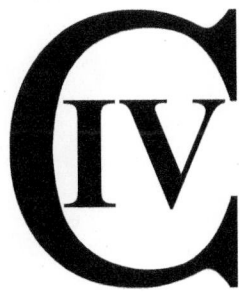

FIGURE 53-3 Label used to indicate a class IV controlled substance.

DRUG ABUSE

Although drugs are important for treating diseases and conditions, any drug can be abused. Both OTC medications and prescription drugs can be misused. Medications that are commonly misused include pain medications, sleeping aids, and cold medications. Drug abuse can occur with patients at any age and can lead to dependency or toxicity.

Drug abuse and drug dependency are defined separately. **Drug abuse** is defined as the use of a drug improperly or wrongly. An individual with **drug dependency** is one who relies on the medication or uses the medication for psychologic support. Individuals who become physically dependent are those who continuously use a substance to function or to avoid physical pain. For physical dependency to occur, the abused substance produces changes in the nervous system on which the body begins to rely. Once the substance is removed, the individual experiences withdrawal symptoms. Depending on the level of addiction, withdrawal symptoms will be mild to severe.

Identifying Drug Abuse

As a medical assistant, you must be aware of signs of drug abuse and drug dependency. You will be working closely with patients when they are in the office, and you may also be responsible for handling phone calls pertaining to medication refills. Be alert when patients are requesting medication refills or new prescriptions sooner than necessary, particularly if the medication request is for a commonly abused drug. Table 53-6 lists drug types that are commonly abused. If you suspect a patient to be abusing drugs, you may take the following steps:

1. Notify the physician immediately of your suspicion. It is not up to you, nor is it within your scope of practice, to confront the patient regarding such matters.

2. Check local pharmacies to see if the patient is obtaining medications from multiple pharmacies. This step is often performed at the request of the physician to obtain more information.

TABLE 53-6	Commonly Abused Drugs	
Drug Type	**Drug**
Analgesic	Demerol, Vicodin, Percocet
Antianxiety	Valium, Xanax, Librium
Antidepressant	Prozac, Elavil, Tofranil
Sedative	Dalmane, Restoril, Seconal
Illegal drugs	Heroin, LSD, Cocaine

3. Tell patients who are frequently calling for refills that another refill will require an office visit. This is often based on an established office policy.

Many times controlled substances are abused. It is also important to safeguard items in the medical office that could be stolen and misused for drug abuse. Items that are important to keep secure in the office include syringes, needles, and prescription pads. Never leave blank prescription pads lying out in examination rooms; prescription pads should always be stored in secure locations. Any dispensing of a controlled substance from the office must be documented in the patient's chart and also in the narcotic log.

ROUTES AND METHODS OF DRUG ADMINISTRATION

The route of administration is the method by which the drug is introduced into the body. Common routes of drug administration are as follows:

- **Oral**—These medications are taken by mouth and swallowed by the patient. Forms of oral medications

Professionalism The Law

The medical assistant works under the supervision of the physician, but the medical assistant is still responsible for his own actions, legally and ethically. If the medical assistant has any concern about drug abuse by a patient, it is his responsibility to immediately notify the physician.

The medical assistant must maintain an accurate narcotics log, clearly documenting all medications given, including time, date, and dose of the specific medication. State laws differ regarding medication administration, so medical assistants must be very familiar with their state's regulations.

Always follow the "10 rights" of drug medication administration (see Figure 53-4). This is the greatest protection against medication errors. Medication errors must be reported immediately to the physician, so the proper steps can be taken. Never administer a medication with which you are unfamiliar.

Ten Rights of Medication Administration

The rights	What they mean	How to proceed
Right patient	Be sure you are giving the medication to the right patient.	
Right medication	Check the label to be sure you are giving the right medication.	

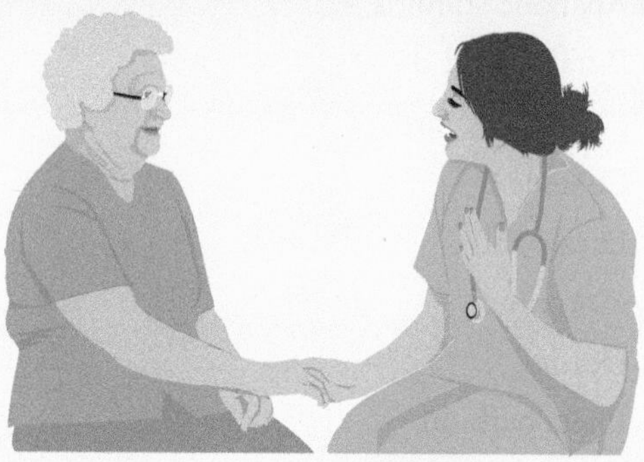

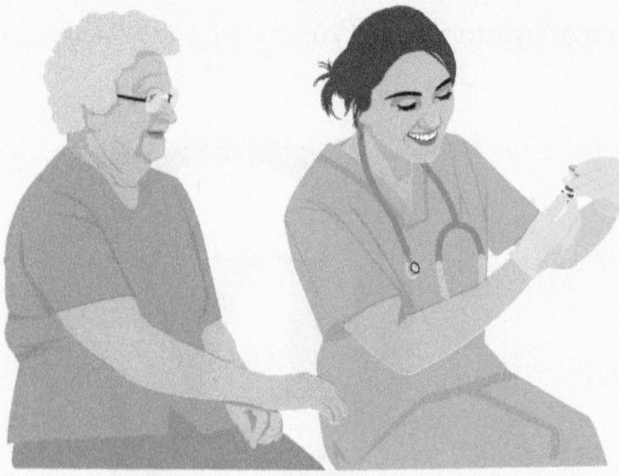

FIGURE 53-4 Ten rights of medication administration.

Ten Rights of Medication Administration

The rights	What they mean	How to proceed
Right dosage	Check that the dosage you are about to give is correct.	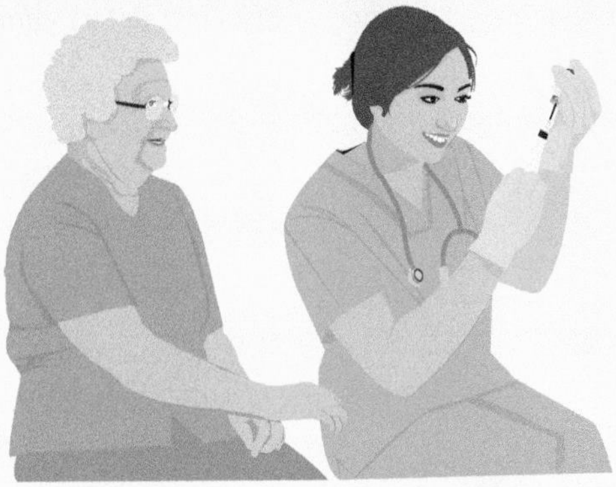
Right route	Be sure you are giving the medication by the right route, such as by intramuscular injection.	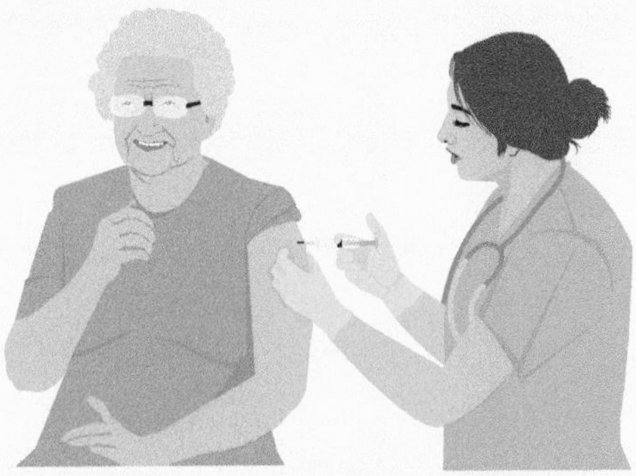
Right time	Be sure you are giving the medication at the correct time, for instance a correct interval since a prior dose or at the right time of day	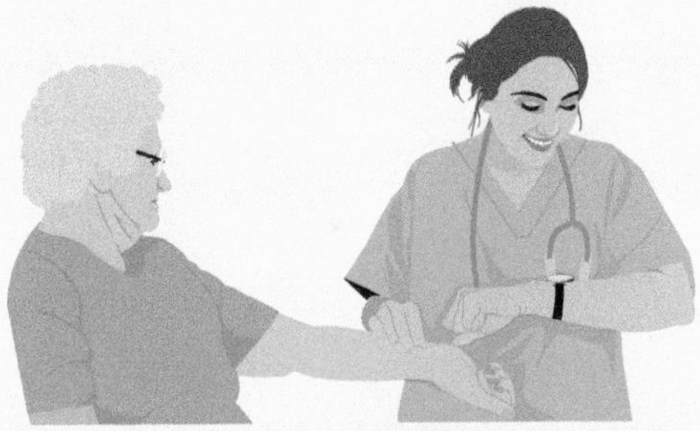
Right documentation	Enter complete information about the medication and dosage and time and date administered in the patient's record.	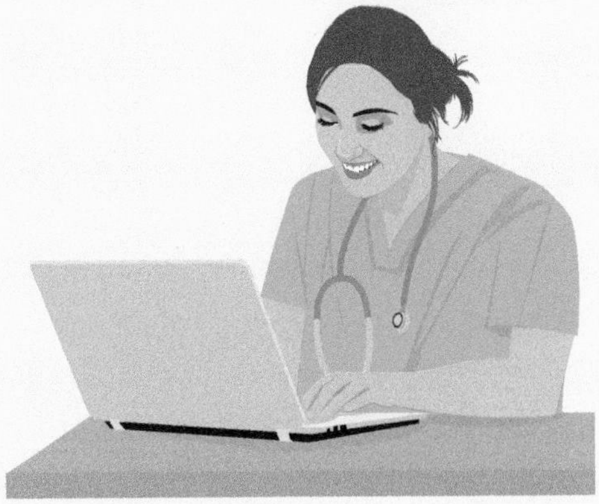

FIGURE 53-4 (*continued*)

Ten Rights of Medication Administration

The rights	What they mean	How to proceed
Right patient education	Before administering the medication, explain the procedure to the patient and any follow-up the patient will need to do at home. Provide written instructions if necessary.	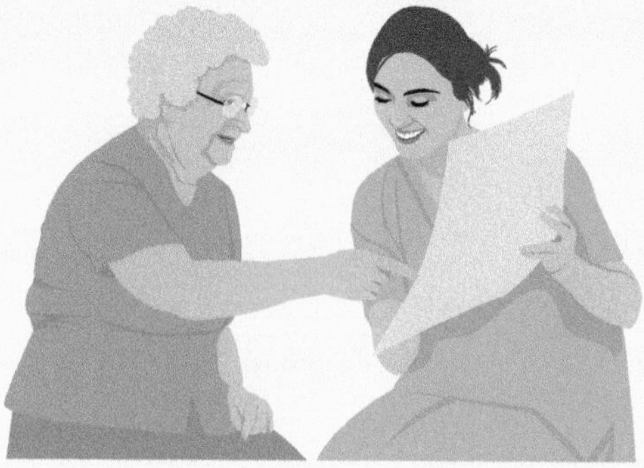
Right to refuse	Be sure the patient has consented to the medication administration. The patient always has the right to refuse a medication or a means or route of administration.	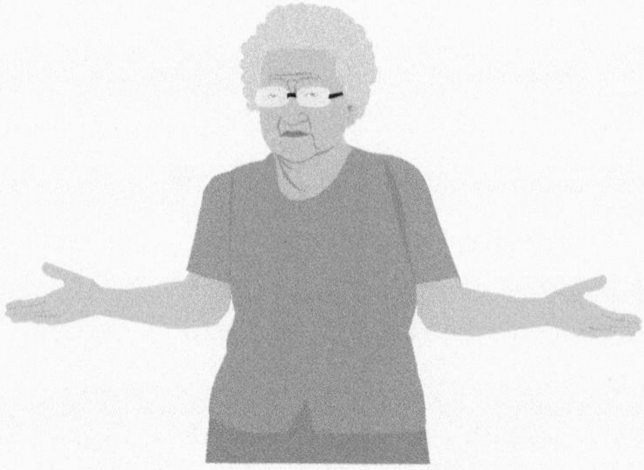
Right assessment	Before administering the medication, review the patient's health record and conduct appropriate evaluations, such as a blood pressure check.	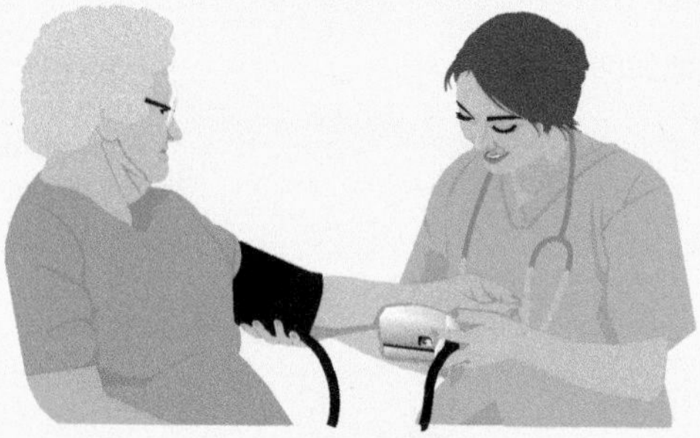
Right evaluation	Check for any allergic reaction after administration. As appropriate, check with the patient later about how the patient is feeling and whether the medication seems to be working.	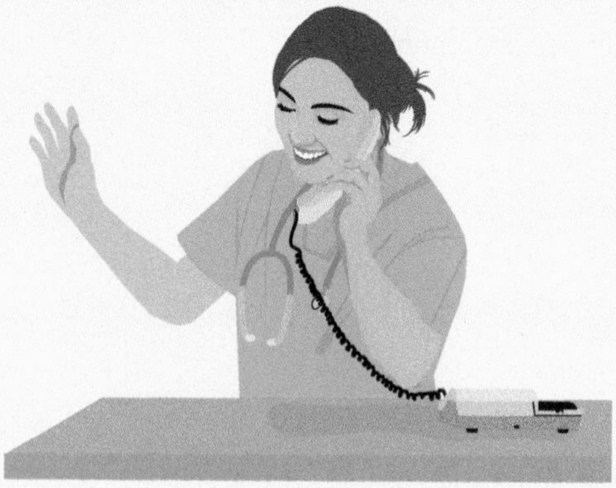

FIGURE 53-4 (*continued*)

TABLE 53-7 | Methods for Parenteral Administration of Drugs

Method	Description
Intraarticular	Injection into a joint. Corticosteroids are often injected into the joint of the knee, ankle, or toes.
Intradermal (ID)	A very shallow injection just within the top layer of skin. This is a method commonly used in skin testing for allergies and tuberculosis.
Intramuscular (IM)	An injection directly into the muscle of the buttocks or upper arm, leg, or hip area. The buttock is used when a large amount of medication is administered or if the medication can cause irritation.
Intrathecal	Injection into the meningeal space surrounding the brain and spinal cord.
Intravenous (IV)	An injection into the veins. This route can be set up so that there is a continuous administration of medication, usually after a major surgery or during a major procedure. Often, medical assistants are not allowed to administer IV medications. State regulations dictate this form of drug administration.
Subcutaneous (SC)	An injection under the skin and fat layers. The middle of the upper, outer arm is usually used, as well as the abdomen or upper and outer thigh.

include pills, capsules, tablets, and extended-release tablets. Liquid medications are also included.

- **Parenteral**—Parenteral medications are any medications that are given outside the digestive tract, such as injections. The parenteral route usually requires the skin to be punctured by a needle with a syringe attached to administer the medication. Table 53-7 lists the methods of parenteral administration and describes each method.

- **Sublingual**—Sublingual drugs are held under the tongue, where they dissolve and are absorbed through the tissues and into the bloodstream for distribution to the body. Nitroglycerin is commonly administered this way when it is used for treating angina (chest pain).

- **Inhaled**—Inhaled drugs are administered directly into the nose and mouth. Aerosol sprays, bronchodilator inhalers, and nebulized medications are administered by this route.

- **Topical**—These medications are applied directly to the skin or mucous membranes in ointment, cream, or lotion form. They are used to treat skin infections and eruptions. Transdermal patches are also used that release medication through absorption by the skin; examples include Nicotrol, Estraderm, and Nicoderm.

- **Drops**—Drops are used when administering medications for the eyes and ears. Eye drops are used for many reasons including to control eye pressure in glaucoma, to dilate the pupil of the eye for better examination of the interior of the eye, and to treat eye infections. Ear drops are placed directly into the ear canal for the purpose of relieving pain or treating infection.

- **Suppositories**—Suppositories are administered via the vaginal or rectal route. Mucosal membranes in these areas quickly absorb medication, allowing it to enter the bloodstream rapidly. Rectal suppositories may have to be administered if the patient is unable to take them by mouth because of nausea, vomiting, or surgery of the mouth. Vaginal suppositories may be used to treat vaginal yeast infections and other vaginal irritations or infections.

It is important to be sure the patient understands the directions for correct medication administration, because the right route must be followed for the medication to be effective. Improper drug administration can cause a drug to work harmfully, ineffectively, or not at all. More information is provided later in this chapter when drug interactions are discussed.

Sometimes a drug can be administered in a variety of forms. For example, the female hormone estrogen, typically used for hormone replacement therapy, can be administered orally in the form of a pill or topically in the form of a skin patch. Table 53-8 lists forms in which medicines are prepared and routes through which they are administered.

Before administering a medication to a patient, always check the "10 rights." Guidelines 53-1 discusses medication administration, including the 10 rights, and previews what is discussed in the chapter titled "Administering Medications."

Frequently Administered Drugs

Pharmaceutical companies are constantly developing, testing, and releasing new drugs. Certain drugs are frequently administered, such as antibiotics—particularly **broad-spectrum** antibiotics. Broad-spectrum antibiotics are effective against a

TABLE 53-8 | Drug Forms and Routes of Administration

Form	Route	Form	Route
Aerosol	Inhalation	Pills	Oral
Caplets	Oral	Powders	Topical
Capsules	Oral	Skin patch	Topical
Elixir	Oral	Spansules	Oral
Liniment	Topical	Spray	Oral, topical
Lotion	Topical	Suppository	Rectal, vaginal
Lozenges	Oral	Syrup	Oral
Ointment	Topical	Tablet	Oral

Guidelines 53-1

Administration of Medication

1. Medications/drugs can be administered only to a patient under the supervision of a licensed physician. To do otherwise is considered to be practicing medicine without a license. The medication order must be written and signed in the patient's health record by the physician.
2. The medical assistant acts as the liaison or intermediary between the physician and the patient. Some of the medical assistant's duties include ordering, storing, rotating, and checking expiration dates on medications.
3. Medications must be checked three times before administration. The "three befores" for when to check medications are these:
   - Before medication is removed from the medication cabinet
   - Before medication is poured, drawn up into a syringe, or placed into a medication cup
   - Before medication is returned to the cabinet
4. Medications cannot be returned to the container once they have been removed. If they are not administered, they must be discarded according to office policy.
5. Remember the "10 rights" for administering medications (Figure 53-5). The first six rights you must be sure of each time you administer a medication are:
   - Right patient
   - Right medication
   - Right dosage
   - Right route
   - Right time
   - Right documentation

It is recommended that you also consider four additional rights of medication administration:
   - Right patient education
   - Right to refuse (the patient's right to refuse a medication)
   - Right assessment
   - Right evaluation
6. Keep a record of all allergies, including drug allergies, on the patient's medical record. Allergy information is often documented in a location that is easy to locate. If paper medical records are still used, allergy information is often indicated on the front of the patient's medical record by an identifying sticker.

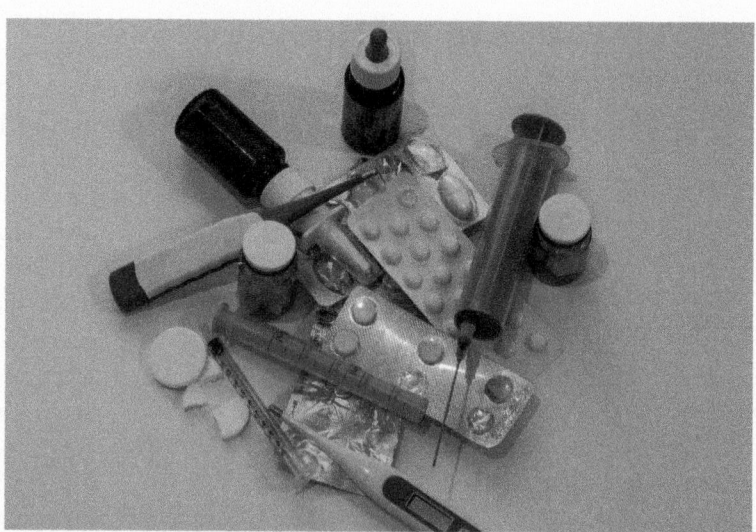

FIGURE 53-5 Different types of medication require different routes of administration.

7. The documentation on the patient's medical record must include the following:
   a. Name of medication
   b. Dosage
   c. Route of administration
   d. Site of administration
   e. Signature of the person administering the medication, along with initials designating the person's status (e.g., CMA or RMA)
8. All narcotics and other controlled substances must be documented in a record maintained for that purpose. This is referred to as "logging a narcotic" or "logging a controlled substance." Every controlled substance must be accounted for fully.
9. Be careful that you administer the medication by the correct route. Methods of administration medical assistants may use include these:
   a. Oral (by mouth)
   b. Sublingual (under the tongue)
   c. Buccal (in the cheek)
   d. Rectal (inserted into the anal cavity)
   e. Vaginal (inserted into vaginal canal)
   f. Parenteral (by injection)
   g. Topical (applied to the skin)
   h. Inhalation (by breathing the medication)
   Medical assistants may *not* administer medications by the following routes:
   a. Intrathecal (into the meningeal space)

b. Intracavity (into a body cavity)
c. Intravenous (IV) (into a vein)—This varies by state law, and if allowed, additional certification is often required.
10. Medication labels should be clean and readable. If they become soiled, unreadable, or fall off the container, the medication must be discarded.
11. If you are not familiar with a particular medication, you must look it up in the PDR. Never violate this rule.
12. Know the side effects for the medication you are administering.
13. Always advise the patient to take the complete number of doses ordered in the prescription. This is especially important when using antibiotics, because patients may stop taking the medication once they feel better, not realizing that the bacterium may not yet have been completely eradicated. This is harmful because the bacterium, instead of dying, becomes stronger. The patient could, over time, develop a resistance to the antibiotic. Further, the antibiotic-resistant bacteria may spread to others as a disease that can no longer be effectively treated by antibiotics.
14. Advise patients to use only medication for the person for whom it was prescribed and not to give any medication prescribed for them to someone else. To do otherwise is a violation of federal law.

---

large range of microorganisms, making the treatment of specific illnesses easier. Other medications that are frequently prescribed and administered include analgesics (pain killers), antihypertensives, antidepressants and antianxiety medications, and statins to reduce cholesterol levels.

Reputable websites such as www.rxlist.com and www.drugs.com are useful resources that are able to provide additional information regarding the drugs prescribed and sold most frequently in the United States. It is helpful to be aware of the drugs that are prescribed and dispensed most often, because these are likely to be the drugs you will administer on physician's orders. Knowledge of these drugs and their classifications, side effects, indications, and contraindications can help you better serve the patients in your care.

JUDGMENT CALL

Eunice Lafferty is an 85-year-old patient being seen by Dr. Jones for a follow-up from a recent knee surgery. She weighs 110 pounds. While the medical assistant was obtaining her chief complaint for today's visit, Mrs. Lafferty stated, "That pain medicine the doctor gave me wipes me out. I get dizzy and I sleep for a long time." At the end of the visit, you see that Dr. Jones wrote a prescription for the same medication with the same dosage and directions for use. While the medical assistant is reviewing the order with her, Mrs. Lafferty states, "Well, if that is what he wants me to have, I guess I will just sleep all the time." As a medical assistant, what would you do?

MEDICATIONS AND PREGNANCY

Great caution must be used when a pregnant woman takes a medication. Very few drugs are considered safe for use during pregnancy. Women who are pregnant should consult their doctor before taking any medication, including OTC medications and dietary supplements.

The FDA regulates and classifies drugs into pregnancy classifications. Every prescription drug should have a pregnancy classification. Pregnancy classifications range from A to X. Class A drugs are the safest for pregnant women, but Class X drugs have been shown to cause health risks,

Professionalism | The Life Span

Pediatric patients typically do not take a lot of medications. Never tell a child that a medication is candy—explain that it is medicine and that it is to help the child feel better. If the child is too young or too upset to cooperate, medications can be administered with an oral syringe and the medicine either dribbled down the inside of the cheek or behind the tongue. Mixing medications with juice or food is not advisable, because there is no way to estimate how much medicine was consumed if the child does not finish the food.

Older patients may be exposed to **polypharmacy** (taking five or more medications simultaneously). Medications may interact with each other, causing a variety of compounding and unexpected side effects. Thus, it is very important to ask the patient about medications that have been prescribed or changed by their other physicians. It is essential to be sure that the physician at your practice knows about all the medications the patient takes.

Another issue facing older adults is organ decline. The kidneys and the liver, which are responsible for clearing toxins from the body, clear medications at a slower rate in older adults. Therefore, the dosage of medications may need to be lowered to prevent an overdose.

deformities, or both to the unborn fetus. Table 53-9 provides an overview of the pregnancy classifications established by the FDA. Before prescribing a drug for any female, the date of her last menstrual cycle should be ascertained to ensure that she is not pregnant.

Drug Use and the Breast-Feeding Mother

A lot of medications taken by a breast-feeding mother can cross over into the breast milk, which would then be swallowed by the nursing infant. A breast-feeding mother can take a few medications, but it is very important that the prescribing physician be aware that the mother is breastfeeding. Several medications, however, are **contraindicated**, which means that the medications are so dangerous for the infant that the mother must stop breast-feeding while she is taking them or she must forgo taking them at all. Medications contraindicated for a breast-feeding mother include the following:

- Tetracyclines (a form of antibiotic used to treat bacterial infections)
- Chloramphenicol (a form of antibiotic used to treat bacterial infections)
- Sulfonamides (sulfa-based antibiotics used to treat bacterial infections)
- Oral anticoagulants (used to prevent blood clots)
- Iodine-containing drugs (used to treat thyroid conditions; small amounts are also present in radiographic contrast dyes)
- Antineoplastics (drugs used to treat cancer, such as chemotherapy agents)

READING AND WRITING A PRESCRIPTION

Reading prescriptions and even writing prescriptions that the physician will sign are tasks often undertaken by a

TABLE 53-9 | FDA Pregnancy Classifications

Category	Description
A	Controlled studies showed no demonstrated risk to the fetus in the first trimester, or later trimesters during pregnancy.
B	Studies on pregnant animals showed no demonstrated risk to the fetus, but controlled studies on pregnant women were not conducted.
C	Studies on pregnant animals showed adverse effect on fetus, but controlled studies on pregnant women were not conducted. In some instances, the potential benefit for the use of drugs in this category may outweigh the potential risks for the pregnant mother.
D	Investigational or marketing studies show a positive evidence of fetal risk in humans. However, again, the potential benefits may outweigh the potential risk for the pregnant mother.
X	Investigational or marketing studies show demonstrated fetal abnormalities and evidence of fetal risk because of adverse reactions. Risk of use in this category outweighs the potential benefits.
N	There is no FDA classification on these drugs.

medical assistant. To be proficient in this important area, you must have an understanding of the symbols, the prescription pad, and abbreviations used in writing prescriptions. It is important to be sure that all the main parts of the prescription, as follows, are filled out completely:

- **Superscription**—The **superscription** contains the patient's name, address, age or date of birth, and the date the prescription was written. This is on the top lines of the prescription. The symbol (Rx) from the Latin term *recipe*, meaning "take thou," is usually preprinted on the prescription form.

- **Inscription**—The **inscription** gives the name of the medication, actual ingredients, and dosage.

- **Subscription**—The **subscription** tells the pharmacist how to mix the drug and how much to provide the patient.

- **Signa (sig.)**—**Signa (sig.)** is the Latin term for "label." Provides instructions on how the medication should be taken by the patient. This often may be referred to as the signature.

- **Physician's Name, Address, Telephone Number, and DEA Number**—Generally, all but the DEA number are preprinted on the prescription pad. However, some physicians choose to have their DEA number included on their prescription pads.

- **Number of Refills**—Number of times the prescription may be refilled (usually no more than six times). In certain instances, the physician may indicate a specific time frame during which the prescription can be refilled. For instance, the physician may write "6 refills before 6-1-YY." This is often done so that proper follow-up care can be provided to the patient, especially when a patient is taking a maintenance medication such as one

to lower blood pressure. The patient will need to come in and see the physician before the physician writes an order to renew the prescription.

- **DAW (Dispense As Written) and Signature Lines**—All prescriptions must be signed by the physician. If a physician wants only the brand name of a medication and does not want substitutions, the signature will be made on the DAW line. If substitutions are permitted, such as with generic medications, the physician will sign on the signature line that often indicates "substitutions permitted."

Figure 53-6 shows an example of a prescription and its labeled parts. In this example, the physician has ordered the medication Lipitor, which is used to lower cholesterol levels. The prescription tells the pharmacist to give 30 tablets and orders a 40 mg dosage, which is to be taken once a day. The instruction to the pharmacist is to refill the prescription three times and not to substitute with a generic medication. The prescription also indicates that the refills cannot be filled after a specific date. It is important to write out on the prescription the numbers regarding the amount to dispense and the number of refills or to circle a preprinted number. This provides a safeguard against tampering with the prescription. Sometimes a prescription is written for prn refills, meaning that the prescription can be refilled as needed.

When the pharmacist fills the prescription, the patient instructions will be placed on the label as instructed by the physician, along with special instructions and labels for taking the medication (such as "Take with meals") that can help ensure that the medication is as effective as possible. The pharmacist will also include a package insert with each medication that contains information regarding possible side effects, adverse effects, and contraindications. The patient should be clearly told that if any adverse or side effects are

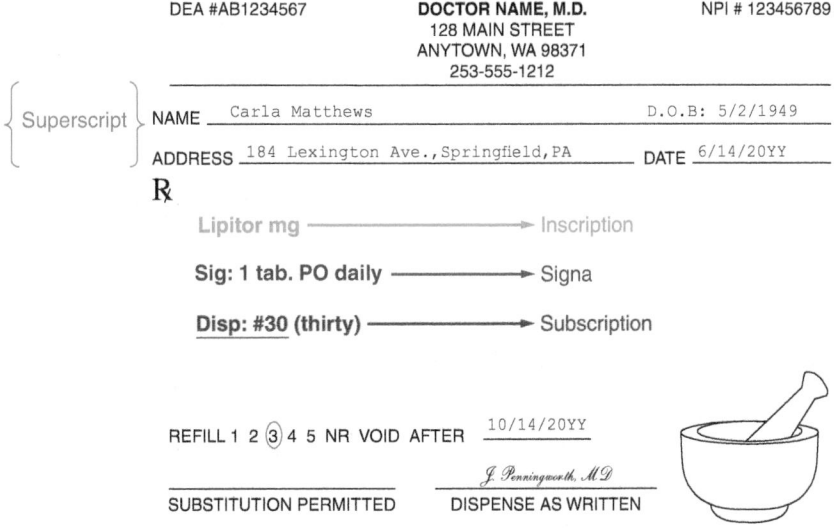

FIGURE 53-6 The parts of a prescription include the superscription, inscription, sig., and subscription.

Professionalism

Understanding and being knowledgeable about medication is an important aspect of a medical assistant's job. This includes being able to pronounce medications correctly. Medical assistants discuss medications not only with patients but also with physicians and pharmacists when prescriptions are called into pharmacies. If you are unsure of the correct pronunciation of a medication, ask a colleague or a physician. Asking such questions will improve your professional image.

Professionalism · The Workplace

It is essential that the medical assistant always safeguard prescription pads. At times, a physician may accidentally leave a prescription pad in an examination room. Medical assistants should always keep a watchful eye for items that are out of place, especially when cleaning the examination room and preparing it for the next patient. Maintaining the integrity of the office is, by far, one of the most important elements of professionalism.

experienced, he should report them to the ordering physician's office immediately.

Some prescriptions can be filled by telephone. At such times, the patient's record should be pulled for the physician (if paper medical records are used), and the refill order or new medications prescribed should be documented. Usually a medication refill form is in the chart. The medical assistant should list what the physician has ordered to be filled: the medication, the name of the medication, and the strength and dosage of the medication. The medical assistant should also document the name of the pharmacy, the name of the pharmacist taking the prescription information, the pharmacy phone number, and the time of the call.

Only physicians are permitted to sign prescriptions. However, the medical assistant in some cases may complete the prescription form, which the physician then checks for accuracy and signs.

E-Prescriptions

With emerging technology and web-based customer service, e-prescriptions are growing in popularity and becoming the norm, preferred by both physicians and patients. E-prescriptions are computer generated and sent via secure and private computer connections. By this means, the physician is able to create an e-prescription and send it directly to the pharmacy. Often this is completed before the patient leaves the medical office. Not only do e-prescriptions provide a convenience for the patient, but they also eliminate the error factors involved with the interpretation of a handwritten prescription. Eventually, the prescription pad will become an outdated item, a once-used curiosity.

Computerized Physician Order Entry (CPOE)

As this chapter and the rest of the textbook has frequently pointed out, electronic health records are rapidly replacing traditional paper medical records. Eventually, all patient health records will be electronic. Computerized electronic

records allow orders and entries, including prescriptions, to be directly entered into the patient's health record. These computerized entries decrease the number of medical errors and improve the quality and efficiency of the delivery of health care. One of the major benefits is the reduction in errors related to illegible handwriting.

Computerized physician order entry (CPOE) falls under the Electronic Health Record (EHR) Incentive Program, which falls within the domain of the Centers for Medicare and Medicaid Services (CMS). CPOE is the process of entering physician instructions, including medication orders, into patients' electronic health records. As EHR systems go into effect, CPOE systems will also be implemented.

In August 2013, the CMS ruled that credentialed medical assistants are allowed to enter orders into the EHR. The credentialed medical assistant must obtain a credential from an outside credentialing agency (not associated with the medical assistant's employment), such as the American Association of Medical Assistants, which offers the CMA, AAMA credential, or the American Medical Technologists, which offers the RMA credential. Other credentials from certifying bodies may also be accepted. This final ruling from the CMS applies to all stages of the EHR incentive program.

ABBREVIATIONS USED IN PHARMACOLOGY

Medical abbreviations are used less than they once were. Abbreviations are used in pharmacology, but because of the risk of errors resulting from misreading information, many physicians choose not to use abbreviations in prescription writing and chart documentation. Additionally, abbreviations are used less often as patient records are transitioned to EHRs. The use of abbreviations in EHRs is unnecessary because everything is typed out. However, it is still important for you to understand abbreviations, which may appear in the notations or treatment and care plans for patients. Table 53-10 lists the most commonly used abbreviations.

TABLE 53-10 | Commonly Used Pharmacology Abbreviations

Abbreviation	Meaning	Abbreviation	Meaning
ā	before	M ft	make
Aa	of each	Mcg	microgram
Ac	before meals	Mg	milligram
Ad lib	as desired	mitt#	give this number
Alt dieb	alternate days	mL	milliliter
Alt hor	alternate hours	Mm	millimeter
Alt noc	alternate nights	Noct	night
am, AM	morning	non rep	do not repeat
Amt	amount	NPO	nothing by mouth
Ante	before	NS	normal saline
Aq	aqueous (water)	p̄	after
Ba	barium	PR	per rectum
Bid	twice a day	Prn	as needed
C	100	Pt	pint
c̄	with	Pulv	powder
cap(s)	capsule(s)	Q	every
DC, disc	discontinue	Qhs	every night
d/c, disc	discontinue	R	right
Dil	dilute	Rx	take
Disp	dispense	s̄	without
Dr	dram	Sig.	label as follows/directions
Dx	diagnosis	SL	under the tongue
Elix	elixir	SOB	shortness of breath
Emul	emulsion	Sol	solution
Et	and	ss or -s-s	one-half
Ext	extract/external	Stat	at once/immediately
Fe	iron	SubQ	subcutaneous
Fl	fluid	Subling	sublingual
G	gauge	Suppose	suppository
G	gram	Susp	suspension
Gal	gallon	Syr	syrup
Gr	grain	T, tbsp.	tablespoon
Gt	1 drop	Tab	tablet
Gtt	2 or more drops	Tid	3 times a day
H	hour/hypodermic	tinc, tr	tincture
IM	intramuscular	Top	apply topically
Inj	injection	Tsp	teaspoon
IV	intravenous	Ung	ointment
K	potassium	UT	under the tongue
Kg	kilogram	ut dict UD	as directed
L	liter	Wt	weight
Liq	liquid		

TABLE 53-11 | Official "Do Not Use List" of the Joint Commission

Do Not Use	Potential Problem	Use Instead
U (unit)	Mistaken for "O" (zero), the number "4" (four) or "cc"	Write "unit"
IU (International Unit)	Mistaken for IV (intravenous) or the number 10 (ten)	Write "International Unit"
Q.D., QD, q.d., qd (daily) Q.O.D., QOD, q.o.d, qod (every other day)	Mistaken for each other Period after the Q mistaken for "I" and the "O" mistaken for "I"	Write "daily" Write "every other day"
Trailing zero (X.0 mg)* Lack of leading zero (.X mg)	Decimal point is missed	Write X mg Write 0.X mg
MS	Can mean morphine sulfate or magnesium sulfate	Write "morphine sulfate" Write "magnesium sulfate"
MSO_4 and $MgSO_4$	Confused for one another	

Additional Abbreviations, Acronyms and Symbols
(For possible future inclusion in the official "Do Not Use" list)

Do Not Use	Potential Problem	Use Instead
> (greater than) < (less than)	Misinterpreted as the number "7" (seven) or the letter "L" Confused for one another	Write "greater than" Write "less than"
Abbreviations for drug names	Misinterpreted because of similar abbreviations for multiple drugs	Write drug names in full
Apothecary units	Unfamiliar to many practitioners Confused with metric units	Use metric units
@	Mistaken for the number "2" (two)	Write "at"
Cc	Mistaken for U (units) when poorly written	Write "mL" or "ml" or "milliliters" ("mL" is preferred)
Mg	Mistaken for mg (milligrams), resulting in one thousand-fold overdose	Write "mcg" or "micrograms"

The Joint Commission, an accrediting body for hospitals and organizations, has issued a "Do Not Use" list. This list includes all abbreviations that are not acceptable for use because of the high probability of error or misinterpretation. Table 53-11 lists these unacceptable abbreviations. Because it is easy to mistake one abbreviation for another, you must be very careful to ensure that the abbreviations used are appropriate, correct, and clear. Always use approved abbreviations—never use those on the "Do Not Use" list—and never create your own.

SUMMARY

As a medical assistant you will work directly under the supervision and the license of the physician. No matter what kind of medical practice you work in, it is always necessary to follow all federal, state, and local regulations regarding the administration, dispensing, and inventorying of medications. You must remember that you are always ethically and legally responsible for your actions and for actions not taken that should have been.

A competent and professional medical assistant understands the various forms and routes of drug administration and is able to identify sources for additional information. If you live in a state that allows medical assistants to write prescriptions for patients that will later be signed by the physician, it is essential that you understand the importance of correctly filling out a prescription, completing all the parts of the prescription form, and using acceptable medication terms and abbreviations.

53 CHAPTER REVIEW

COMPETENCY REVIEW

1. Define and spell the terms for this chapter.
2. A drug may be known by three different names. What are they?
3. Name the governmental agency that enforces drug sales and distribution.
4. Name the federal act that controls the use of drugs causing dependency.
5. Many patients take OTC medications. Explain why it is important to document these medications in their medical record.

6. Describe what you would do when a patient indicates a drug allergy.
7. Explain why a rectal suppository may be administered.
8. List the information that must be documented when administering a medication.
9. List the functions of the following medications: diuretic, sedative, anesthetic.
10. Identify and describe different parts of a prescription.

PREPARING FOR THE CERTIFICATION EXAM

1. The generic name for the OTC medication Tylenol is
   a. naproxen sodium.
   b. acetaminophen.
   c. Naprosyn.
   d. Tylenol.
   e. Aldomet.

2. According to the Drug Enforcement Administration, controlled substances
   a. can be addictive.
   b. may have the potential for abuse by a patient.
   c. must be kept under lock and key.
   d. must be recorded in a narcotics log when dispensed.
   e. all of the above.

3. An example of a Schedule IV drug is
   a. Adderal.
   b. diazepam.
   c. vicodin.
   d. cocaine.
   e. Tylenol with codeine.

4. Capoten, which is an ACE inhibitor, is classified as an
   a. antibiotic.
   b. antiinflammatory.
   c. antipruritic.
   d. antihypertensive.
   e. antipyretic.

5. Which of the following is a method for the administration of a drug by means of an injection under the skin and fat layers?
   a. intradermal
   b. intramuscular
   c. subcutaneous
   d. intravenous
   e. intrathecal

6. A controlled substance log indicating the management, distribution, and destruction of all controlled substances must be kept on file for at least
   a. one year.
   b. two years.
   c. three years.
   d. five years.
   e. seven years.

7. The "10 rights" a medical assistant must observe when administering medications include the right medication, the right documentation, and the right
   a. time.
   b. route.
   c. dosage.
   d. patient.
   e. all of the above.

8. Medical assistants are often not allowed to administer medications via which of the following parenteral routes?
   a. ID
   b. IV
   c. IM
   d. Z-track IM
   e. SC

9. Which part of a prescription provides the instructions that should be given to the patient?
   a. sig.
   b. counterscript
   c. superscription
   d. inscription
   e. subscription

10. A common abbreviation used in pharmacology that means "as needed" is
    a. aa.
    b. ac.
    c. prn.
    d. ante.
    e. NS.

CRITICAL THINKING

Refer to the case study at the beginning of the chapter and use what you have learned to answer the following questions.

1. Susan knows that there are laws that govern the refilling of diazepam, which is a controlled substance. How do these laws affect Mr. Lehmke?

2. What should Susan do to respond to this medication refill request?

3. After talking with the patient, Dr. Penningworth has approved the request for one refill. What is Susan's next step?

ON THE JOB

Dr. Waring has a solo practice. When she is on vacation, she arranges for Dr. Dumphey to cover her patients. Dr. Dumphey's medical assistant, Theresa, has just received a call from a patient of Dr. Waring. The patient is an older woman, with multiple medical problems, who is possibly having a reaction to a medication that Dr. Waring prescribed two days ago for bronchitis. Her symptoms include nausea, upset stomach, dizziness, headache, rash on her chest, and extreme exhaustion. Theresa senses that the patient may be exhibiting some disorientation to time and place, because it is difficult to elicit consistent responses from her regarding her medications.

The patient reports to Theresa that the newest medication she has been taking is Biaxin. The other medications she takes include Prinivil, Cardizem CD, Premarin, Prilosec, Robaxin, Zocor, Ambien, Prozac, Fosamax, Seldane, and aspirin. The patient does not know the dosage of any of these medications but is willing to "open up her bag of medicine" and read each prescription label to Theresa. What should Theresa do? What is your response?

1. Does Theresa have an obligation as Dr. Dumphey's medical assistant to handle this situation with this patient, or should Dr. Waring simply be notified?

2. Is this an emergency situation or potential emergency situation, and, if so, what should Theresa do immediately?

3. Because the patient seems disoriented, should Theresa even trust what the patient is reporting?

4. Should Theresa have the patient read the label of each of her medications?

INTERNET ACTIVITY

To further understand the elements of the *Physicians' Desk Reference*, go online and type "PDR" in the search area.

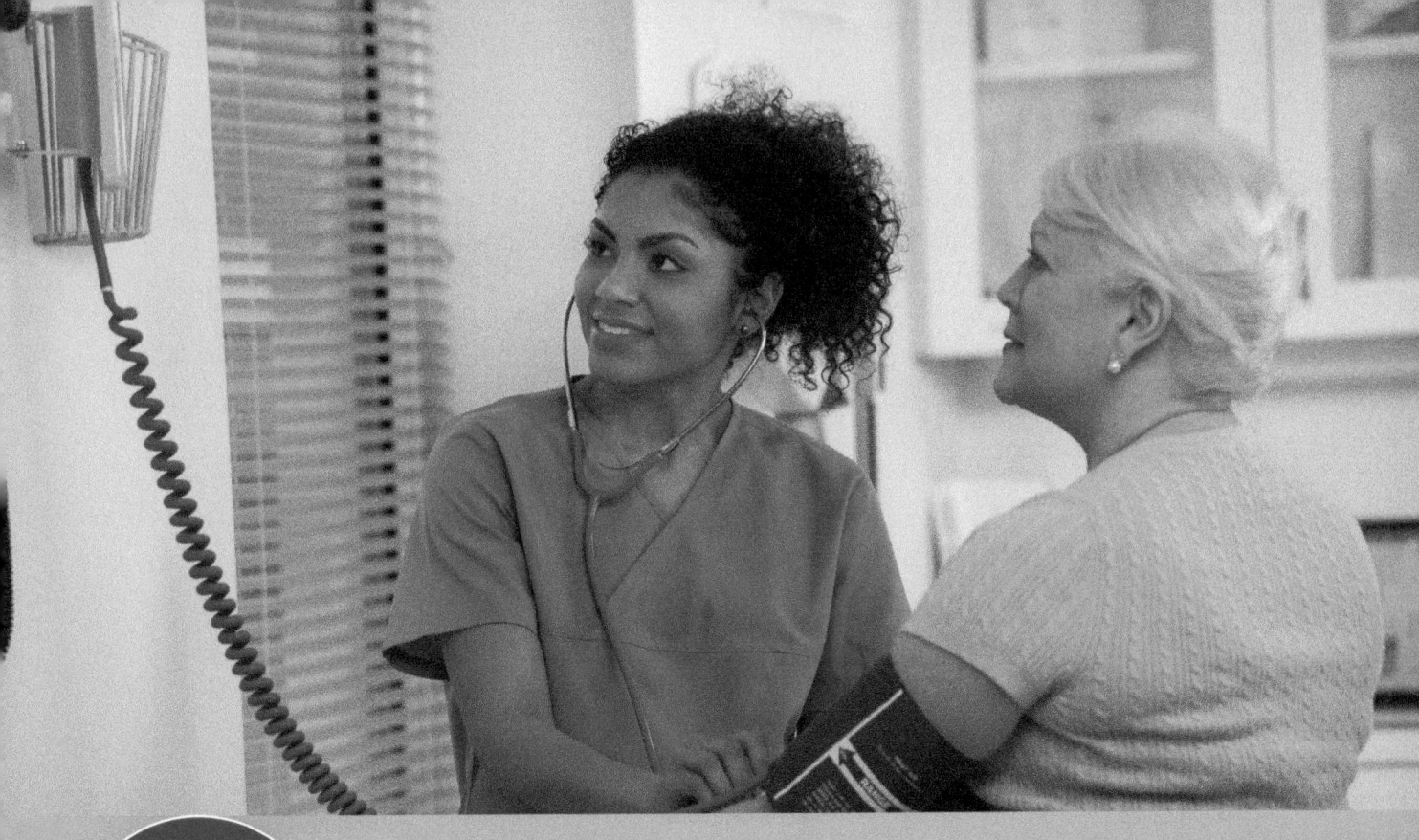

Administering Medications

Learning Objectives

After completing this chapter, you should be able to:

54.1 Define and spell the terms for this chapter.

54.2 Identify various types of medications that are administered orally.

54.3 Describe how inhalation medication is administered.

54.4 Identify equipment used when administering medication by injection.

54.5 Describe safety precautions related to medication administration.

54.6 List information that must be included when documenting medication administration.

54.7 Identify the maximum volume of medication that may be administered to various muscles during intramuscular injections.

54.8 Describe how a subcutaneous injection is administered.

54.9 Identify circumstances that would require the administration of an intradermal injection.

54.10 Explain information that a medical assistant must understand related to IV therapy.

54.11 Outline when specific childhood vaccinations are recommended for administration.

54.12 Identify vaccines that are only indicated for adults.

Today, Samra Belkovich, RMA, is working with Dr. Miller at Pearson Physicians Group. Four-year-old Owen Russiano has been brought by his babysitter for an emergency appointment because of severe nausea and vomiting. Because he is so small, Dr. Miller is concerned that he may be dehydrated. Dr. Miller has ordered medication to be administered stat, via a rectal suppository. Samra is concerned because the boy seems very fearful, and she is worried she will not be able to administer the medication because of the child's behavior.

Terms to Learn

ampules	infiltration	subcutaneous injection
artificially acquired active immunity	inhaled medications	sublingual medications
buccal medications	intradermal (ID) injection	tetanus
deltoid muscle	intramuscular (IM) injections	topical medications
diphtheria	intravenous (IV) therapy	transdermal patch
dorsogluteal site	liquid medications	vaccines
hepatitis A	measles, mumps, and rubella (MMR) vaccine	varicella
hepatitis B		vastus lateralis muscle
Hib disease	oral medications	ventrogluteal site
human papillomavirus (HPV)	oral polio vaccine (OPV)	vials
immunity	parenteral medications	viscosity
immunizations	pertussis	Z-track method
immunoglobulin	pneumococcal vaccine	
inactivated polio vaccine (IPV)	prefilled cartridge injection systems	

One of the most important functions of the medical assistant is administering medications. Pharmacology and drug therapy use the skills of physicians, pharmacists, nurses, and medical assistants. The medical assistant's specific role is administering the correct medication to the right patient at the correct dosage, time, and route—and then documenting it correctly.

MEDICATION ADMINISTRATION

Medications may be administered orally, topically, vaginally, rectally, by inhalation, and by injection. For all routes of administration, when the medical assistant is ordered to administer a medication, specific procedures must be followed.

The first step is always to check the order, making sure that you can clearly read the order and that you completely understand what is being ordered. Be sure to review the "three befores" and the "10 rights" discussed in Guidelines 54-1. The second step is to ensure that the patient does not have an allergy to the ordered medicine. Third, check the order again, and check the "10 rights." Although this may sound like duplicated effort, this is where mistakes are very often caught, thereby avoiding the potentially deadly consequences of giving an incorrect medication.

Medical assistants do not administer medications by intravenous (IV) fluids, nor do they administer chemotherapy drugs or narcotics.

Oral Medication Administration

Oral medications are swallowed, enter the tissues of the gastrointestinal system, and are then rapidly absorbed into the circulatory system and carried to the cells of the body. Oral medications can be pills, syrups, or other liquids. The many different types of **liquid medications** include suspensions,

Safeguards for Administration of Medications

THREE BEFORES

Medications must be checked three times before administration:

- Before medication is removed from the medication cabinet
- Before medication is poured, drawn up into a syringe, or placed into a medication cup
- Before medication is returned to the cabinet

TEN RIGHTS

Six rights to make sure of each time you administer a medication:

- Right patient
- Right medication
- Right dosage
- Right route
- Right time
- Right documentation

Four additional rights to consider when you administer a medication:

- Right patient education
- Right to refuse (the patient's right to refuse a medication)
- Right assessment
- Right evaluation

---

emulsions, elixirs, syrups, and solutions. Equipment used for dispensing liquid medication includes calibrated cups, spoons, droppers, and syringes (Figure 54-1).

As with any medication, it is important to educate the patient on the proper measurement of these medications. It is especially important to instruct patients to keep the measuring cup flat when pouring liquid medication to be sure to

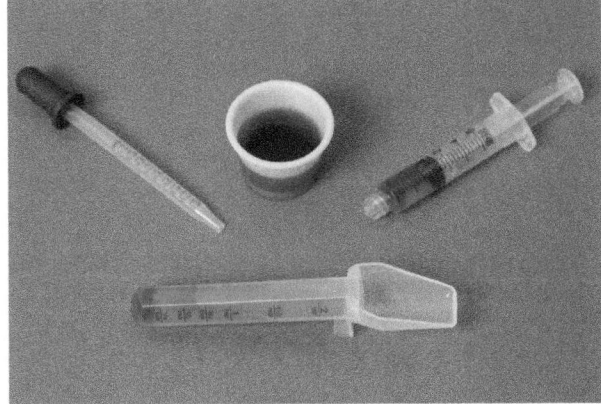

FIGURE 54-1 Calibrated cups, spoons, droppers, and syringes are often used to administer liquid medications.

get an accurate dose and to assess the level at eye-level on a flat surface. Many medications prescribed for pediatric patients are in liquid form because they are generally easy to administer. These medications can be dispensed in a small cup the child can drink from or drawn into a bulb syringe or a syringe with no needle and expelled directly into the child's mouth.

Sublingual medications are held under the tongue, where they diffuse through the tissues and into the bloodstream for distribution to the body; nitroglycerin is commonly administered this way when it is used for treating the cardiac pain of angina. Sublingual drugs are especially effective during emergencies, because they are readily absorbed, bypassing the gastrointestinal system.

Buccal medications are placed between the patient's cheek and gums area for absorption through the tissues into the bloodstream. Buccal medications are also particularly effective to soothe the mouth or throat, such as when a patient has a cough or sore throat. Procedure 54-1 demonstrates competency in the "befores" and "rights" of safe medication administration. See Procedure 54-2 for administering oral medications. See Procedure 54-3 for administering sublingual or buccal medications.

Professionalism   The Law

The medical assistant should never give any medication to any patient without a physician order and patient consent. Verbal orders should be written down and read back to the physician, who should sign the order. Always be sure that the "10 rights" and the "three befores" are followed and double-checked.

The medical assistant and the physician are liable for all medications that are administered to the patient. Therefore, it is imperative that you be familiar with medications before administration and make sure that the calculations for the dosing are correct. *Never assume anything* relating to medication administration! Do not just assume that an order the physician has given is correct. Do not perform a procedure or give a medication if you are unsure or unfamiliar with it. If you are unsure about anything, ask the physician for clarification. The physician should be able to rely on you, having confidence that you will not allow an error to take place by blindly following an order you think may be wrong or do not understand.

It is essential that medication administration be performed strictly by the procedures presented in this text or by the facility protocol. This includes good aseptic technique as well as proper administration. For injections, there is always a potential for infection and inflammation. With any medication, there is a potential for unexpected reactions.

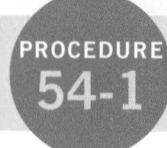

PROCEDURE 54-1

Administering Medication Safely

Objective ◆ *Demonstrate understanding of the safety protocol (the "three befores" and "10 rights") that must be followed when administering medication.*

EQUIPMENT AND SUPPLIES

List of patient medications; corresponding correct medications; incorrect medications with similar names, dosages, or routes to correct medications

METHOD

For safe administration of medication, always do the following:

1. Review the physician's patient medication orders.
2. Ensure that you are selecting the correct medication according to the physician's orders, and properly putting it back in storage after use, by adhering to the "three befores." [Recite to your instructor the "three befores" that are required for checking and selecting the correct medication.]
3. Ensure that have observed the "six rights" before you administer a medication. [Recite to your instructor the "six rights" of medication administration that must be confirmed before administering medication to a patient.]
4. Ensure that you observe the additional "four rights" in the course of administering a medication. [Recite to your instructor the additional "four rights" that must be considered when administering a medication to a patient.]

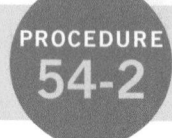

PROCEDURE 54-2

Administering Oral Medication

Objective ◆ *Administer oral medication.*

EQUIPMENT AND SUPPLIES

Medication order signed by physician; oral medication; calibrated paper cup or receptacle for medication; water in glass; patient instruction sheet; waste container; pen

METHOD

1. Assemble equipment.
2. Perform hand hygiene.
3. Select the correct medication as instructed in the "three befores." If you are not familiar with the medication, look it up in a reference book, read the package insert, or consult the physician.
4. Always double-check the label to make sure the strength is correct, because medications are manufactured with different strengths.
5. Correctly calculate the dosage in writing. Double-check your calculations with someone else.
6. Place a medicine cup or container on a flat surface.
7. Gently shake the medication if it is in liquid form.
8. Hold the bottle so that the label is in the palm of your hand to prevent damaging the label with liquid medication.
9. Recheck the label again.
10. Remove the cap from the medicine container and place it upside down on a clean surface. This will keep the inside of the cap clean, which can then be replaced on the bottle.
11. a. *Liquid medication:* Hold the calibrated medicine cup at eye level and pour the medication into the cup, stopping at the correct dosage line. Pour the medication away from the label side of the bottle. If too much medication is poured into the calibrated cup, do not return it to the bottle. Discard it into a sink.

    b. *Tablet or capsule medication:* Shake out the correct number of tablets or pills into the bottle cap. Then place them in the medicine cup. If you accidentally pour out an extra tablet, do not return it to the medication bottle; discard it.

12. Check the medication again to make sure the dosage is the same as the medication order.
13. Replace the cap on the medication bottle and return the bottle to the storage shelf.
14. Take the prepared medication and a glass of water to the patient.
15. Warmly greet and identify the patient both by stating his or her name and examining any printed identification such as a wrist name band or medical record, and ask the patient to state his or her date of birth. Introduce yourself to the patient and ask if the patient has any allergies.
16. Tell the patient the name of the medication and dosage that you are administering per the physician's order. Ask if the patient has any questions before taking the medication.

17. Remain with the patient until the medication has been swallowed.
18. Provide the patient with written follow-up instructions if further medication is to be taken.
19. Chart the medication administration on the correct patient's record, noting the time, medication name, dosage, route (oral procedure), and your name. After giving the medication to the patient, it is best to have the patient wait in the office for 30 minutes.

CHARTING EXAMPLE

2/14/YY 1:00 P.M. ASA, 500 mg, po, after 30 min. no adverse reactions were noted. Verbal and written instructions given regarding ASA. Patient verbalized understanding.....................
....N. Young, RMA

PROCEDURE 54-3 — Administering Sublingual or Buccal Medication

Objective ◆ *Administer a medication to a patient under the tongue or between the cheek and gums.*

EQUIPMENT AND SUPPLIES

Medication order signed by physician on the patient's medical record; oral medication; paper cup or receptacle for medication; patient instruction sheet; waste container; pen

METHOD

1. Assemble equipment.
2. Perform hand hygiene.
3. Select the correct medication as instructed in the "three befores." If you are not familiar with the medication, look it up in a reference book, read the package insert, or consult the physician.
4. Always double-check the label to make sure the strength is correct, because medications are manufactured with different strengths.
5. Correctly calculate the dosage in writing. Double-check your calculations.
6. Place a medicine cup/container on a flat surface.
7. Shake the tablet ordered into the bottle cap and then into a medication container.
8. Check the dosage again against the medication order.
9. Replace the cap on the medication bottle, and return the bottle to the storage shelf after reading the label again.
10. Introduce yourself and warmly greet and identify the patient, both by stating his or her name and examining any printed identification such as a wrist name band or

medical record. Ask the patient to state his or her date of birth. Ask if the patient has any allergies.
11. Tell the patient the name of the medication and dosage that you are administering per the physician's order. Ask if the patient has any questions before taking the medication.
12. a. *Sublingual medication:* Have the patient place the tablet under the tongue. Instruct the patient not to swallow until the tablet has dissolved.
    b. *Buccal medication:* Have the patient place the tablet between the cheek and gums. Instruct the patient not to swallow until the tablet is dissolved.
13. Tell the patient not to take fluids until the tablet is dissolved.
14. Remain with the patient until the medication has dissolved.
15. Provide the patient with both oral and written follow-up instructions if further medication is to be taken.
16. Chart the medication administration on the correct patient's record, noting the time, medication name, dosage, route, and your name. After giving the medication to the patient, it is best to have the patient wait in the office for 30 minutes.

CHARTING EXAMPLE

2/14/YY 9:00 A.M. Nitroglycerin tab 1 (gr. 1/100), subling. P = 60. Patient verbalized understanding of follow-up instructions..N. Young, RMA

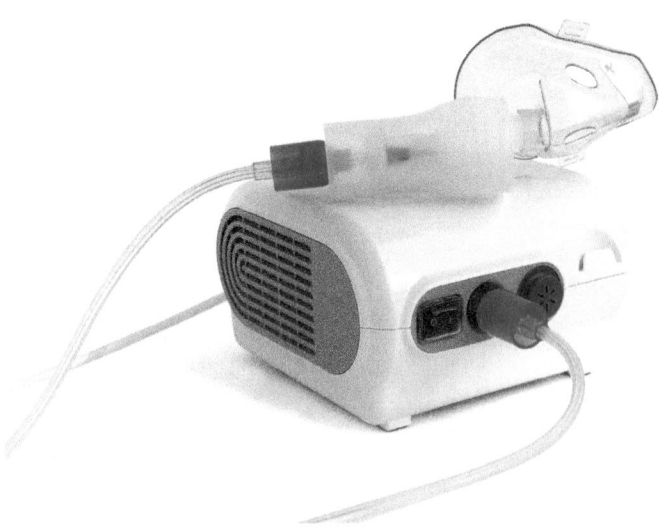

FIGURE 54-2 Equipment used for administering inhaled medications.

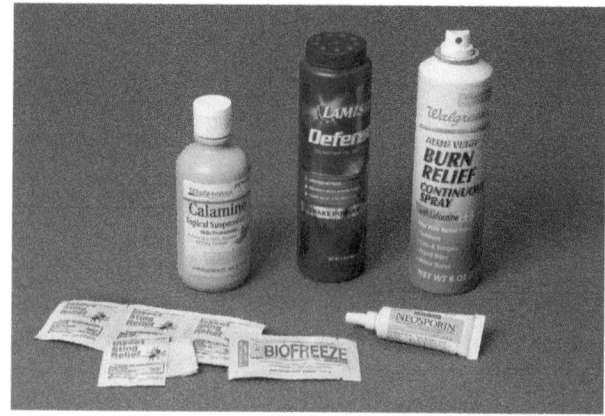

FIGURE 54-3 Topical medications come in a variety of forms.

Inhaled Medication Administration

Inhaled medications are dispensed into the respiratory tract. The advantage to this route is that the medication is absorbed quickly from the respiratory system into the bloodstream. Equipment for the inhaled route of administration includes the metered-dose inhaler and the nebulizer (Figure 54-2).

When this type of medication is ordered, the patient may receive the treatment in the office, be sent home with a metered-dose inhaler (MDI), or both. It is the medical assistant's responsibility to train the patient in the use of the MDI. The patient must clearly understand how to use this equipment before taking it home.

Sometimes the physician will order that the inhalation medication be administered by a nebulizer, which delivers the medication more deeply into the respiratory system than an inhaler. Again, the patient may be provided nebulizing equipment to use at home and must first be carefully instructed in its use.

The chapter titled "Pulmonary Function" provides detailed information on the use of inhalers and nebulizers.

Topical Medication Administration

Topical medications for dermal application (to the skin) and mucosal application (to the mucous membranes) come in various forms (Figure 54-3). For skin conditions that require treatment, topical drug forms include the following:

- Creams and ointments
- Lotions
- Skin patches

Topical medications that are applied to mucous membranes include the following:

- Eyedrops, eardrops, and nose drops
- Eye ointments
- Vaginal creams
- Rectal and vaginal suppositories
- Sterile douche solutions
- Sublingual or buccal tablets

When you administer any form of topical medication, it is important to wear gloves so you don't absorb the medication through your own skin.

When administering ointment, first clean the area with soap and water. Then apply the ointment in a thin layer, using either a cotton swab or a tongue depressor. In some instances, after a topical drug is applied the area must be covered with sterile gauze to keep it clean. When ointment is reapplied, the old remaining ointment should be removed before the new layer of ointment is applied. Some topical medications and medication patches are rotated to different locations to avoid skin irritation.

If the medication is a liquid, shake the bottle well before applying it as directed. If the liquid is to be sprayed, make sure that neither you nor the patient inhales the spray.

For instruction on administering a rectal or vaginal suppository, see Procedure 54-4.

Some medications are placed on the skin in a **transdermal patch**, which is released slowly over time (Figure 54-4). Hormones, antinausea drugs, pain relievers, and cardiac medications, for example, can be effectively administered this way. It is important to wear gloves when you remove the backing on the patch so as not to get any of the medication on your own skin and place the exposed side directly onto a

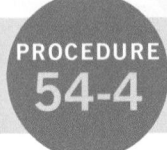

Administering a Rectal or Vaginal Suppository

Objective ◆ *Insert a suppository as ordered by the physician.*

EQUIPMENT AND SUPPLIES

Medication order signed by physician; water-soluble lubricant; water; waste container; patient instructions; vaginal suppository or cream; sanitary napkin; rectal suppository; nonsterile gloves; 4 × 4 gauze square; pen

METHOD

1. Assemble equipment.
2. Perform hand hygiene.
3. Select the correct medication as instructed in the "three befores." If you are not familiar with the medication, look it up in a reference book, read the package insert, consult the physician, or do all three.
4. Always double-check the label to validate that the strength is correct, because medications are manufactured with different strengths.
5. Correctly calculate the dosage in writing. Double-check your calculations with someone else.
6. Check the dosage again against the medication order.
7. Replace the cap on the medication bottle and return the bottle to the storage shelf or refrigerator after reading the label again.
8. Warmly greet and identify the patient both by stating his or her name and examining any printed identification such as a wrist name band or medical record. Introduce yourself to the patient and ask if the patient has any allergies.
9. Give the patient a gown or sheet. Have the patient remove all clothing from the waist down. Assist the patient as necessary and provide reassurance, because the patient may be uncomfortable with the administration of a suppository.
10. Tell the patient the name of the medication and dosage that you are administering per the physician's order. Ask if the patient has any questions before receiving the medication.
11. a. *Rectal suppository:* Have the patient lie on the left side, if possible, with top leg bent. Drape a sheet over the patient. Apply nonsterile gloves. Open the suppository wrapper and place suppository on a gauze square. Moisten the suppository with a small amount of lubricant or water. With one hand, separate the buttocks. Pick up the suppository with the other hand. Ask

the patient to breathe slowly as you insert the suppository from 1 to 1½ inches through the rectal sphincter. Hold the buttocks together and instruct the patient not to bear down or push out the suppository. Wipe the anal area with the gauze and discard gauze into a waste container. Have the patient remain in the side position for about 20 minutes, until the suppository melts.

   b. *Vaginal suppository:* Have the patient lie supine (face up) with legs apart and place a clean pad between the patient's legs for placement of supplies. Drape the patient for privacy. Apply nonsterile disposable gloves. Peel open the suppository container and drop the suppository on the clean pad. If an applicator is provided, drop it on the clean pad. With one gloved hand, separate the labia minora and hold the folds apart. Using the other hand, insert the suppository one finger length into the vagina. If an applicator is used, place the suppository into the applicator and insert it in a downward direction. Instruct the patient to remain in the supine, legs-apart position for at least 10 minutes for the suppository to dissolve. Place the applicator into the glove wrapper. Remove one glove by pulling inside out from the cuff. With the remaining gloved hand, roll the contaminated wrapper and contents. Hold these waste items as you remove the remaining glove over them. Dispose of all materials in a waste container. Offer the patient a sanitary napkin.

12. Remain with the patient until the medication has dissolved.
13. Provide the patient with written follow-up instructions if further medication is to be taken.
14. Chart the medication administration on the patient's record noting the time, medication name, dosage, injection site, route, and your name.

CHARTING EXAMPLE

2/26/YY 9:00 A.M. Dulcolax 15 mg. Rectal supp. Patient tolerated medication administration well. Patient verbalized understanding of follow-up instructions. Denies pain or dizziness at present..M. King, CMA (AAMA)

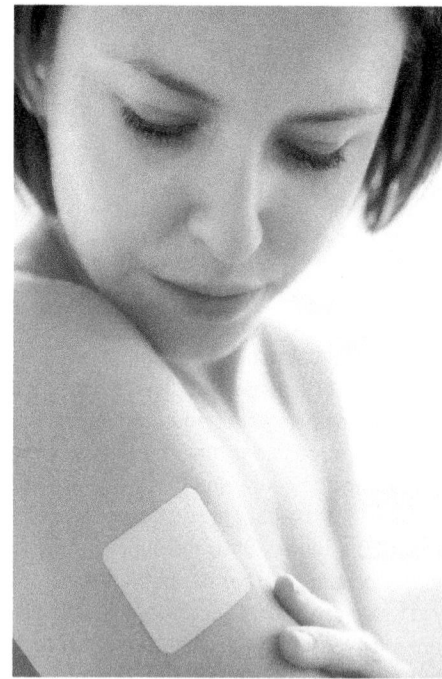

FIGURE 54-4 A transdermal patch is applied to the skin for release of a medication over time.

clean part of the patient's skin, where there is no tattoo or wound. Transdermal patches should be rotated so as not to cause skin breakdown. Never cut the patch, as the dosage is calculated to be delivered over a certain distance and a certain time.

Parenteral Medication Administration

Parenteral medications are administered outside the gastro-intestinal tract, usually by injection. As discussed in the chapter titled "Pharmacology," parenteral routes include intramuscular, subcutaneous, intradermal, and intravenous injections—which are discussed later in this chapter.

Injected medications enter the bloodstream more rapidly than medications given by other routes. Parenteral administration may also allow medication to be targeted to a particular area of the body. For example, a local anesthetic is injected into a specific area on the body, numbing the site, which allows the physician to suture the area with no discomfort to the patient.

EQUIPMENT FOR ADMINISTRATION BY INJECTION

The equipment used for injectable medications includes the specific types of syringes and needles needed for each type of medication and method of administration. As a medical assistant, you must be familiar with this equipment.

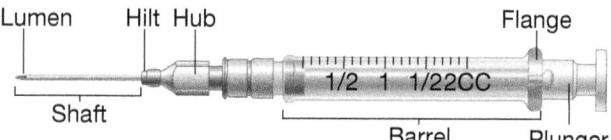

FIGURE 54-5 Parts of a syringe.

Syringes

Understanding the parts of a syringe is necessary for using the device correctly. They include the following (Figure 54-5):

- **Lumen**—The bore of the hollow needle. The size of the lumen determines the gauge of the needle: the higher the gauge, the smaller the lumen.
- **Shaft**—The actual length of the hollow needle.
- **Hilt**—Connects the shaft to the hub.
- **Hub**—Connects the needle to the syringe.
- **Barrel**—Holds the liquid in the syringe.
- **Flange**—Prevents the needle from rolling on flat surfaces.
- **Plunger**—When pressed, expels medication from the syringe. When pulled, gathers medication into the syringe.

Syringes come in a variety of sizes (Figure 54-6). The smallest syringe is a tuberculin syringe, and the measurements are calibrated in hundredths of a milliliter. Tuberculin syringes are used with 27- or 28-gauge needles to perform tuberculosis (PPD) testing and allergy testing, for which all the injections are done intradermally (into the skin).

Another type of syringe is the insulin syringe, which is the only type of syringe that may be used for measuring or injecting insulin. Units marked on the barrel are the amounts the physician may order for insulin administration to individual patients. Insulin is administered subcutaneously (under the skin) via a small needle. These injections are typically done in the arms, abdomen, or thighs. A 25- or 26-gauge syringe is used for insulin administration.

Larger syringes are calibrated in 2-, 3-, 5-, and 10-mL sizes and larger, up to 60 mL. The most commonly used size is the 3-mL syringe, because it is the most accurate with small doses of medication. Most injected doses of medication are less than what the 3-mL syringe can hold.

Needles

Needles are categorized according to size—both gauge (how large the barrel of the needle is) and length. The larger the size of the needle (lumen), the smaller the gauge. The largest needles available are 14 to 18 gauge and are used only in trauma care. Intravenous (IV) lines are typically

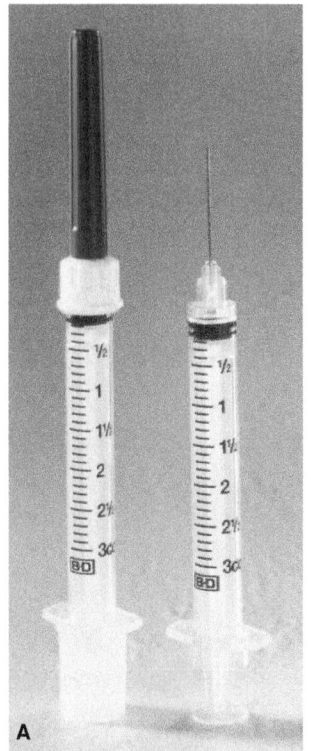
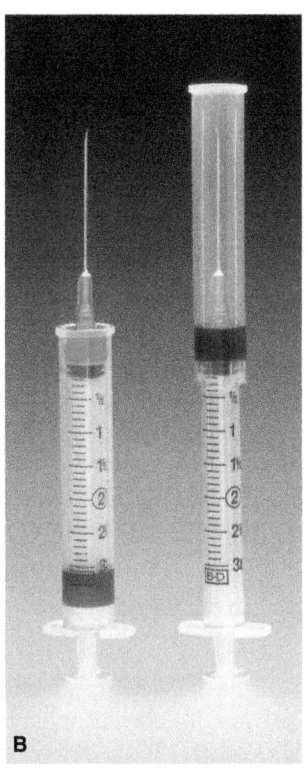

A   B

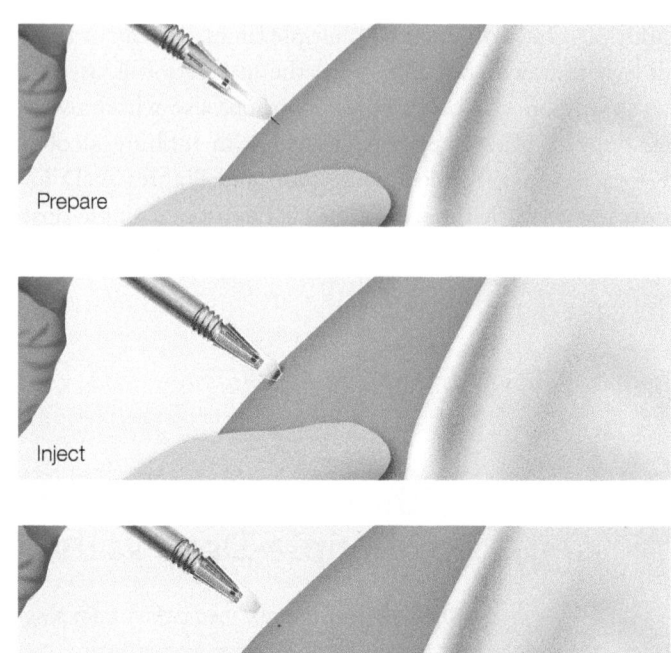

Prepare

Inject

Withdraw

FIGURE 54-7 One type of safety needle withdraws into a protective sheath when the injection is complete.

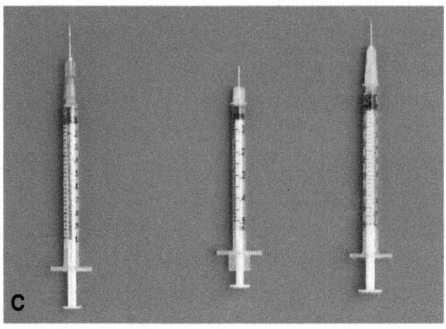

C

FIGURE 54-6 (A) Med-Saver syringe; **(B)** Safety-Lok syringe; **(C)** tuberculin syringes.

placed with 18-, 20-, or 22-gauge needles. (IV lines are not a medical assistant's responsibility.) Intramuscular injections are usually given with 24- or 25-gauge needles, usually ⅝ inch to 3 inches long. Subcutaneous injections are given with 25- to 26-gauge needles, whereas intradermal injections are given with 27- to 28-gauge needles. The **viscosity**, or thickness, of the medication being given also determines the gauge of the needle.

Needle length is very important and varies from ⅜ inch to 4 inches. The needle length required depends on the route used and the area of body to be injected.

To prevent needlesticks, safety needles and syringes should always be used. Because Occupational Safety and Health Administration (OSHA) standards have become very strict, there are a variety of types of safety devices to cover or withdraw contaminated needles. Usually, there is a puncture-proof sheath that covers the needle after the injection (Figure 54-7). It is important to check that the sheath is in place any time you are changing the needle on a syringe. *Never handle an unsheathed needle.* Dirty needles and used needles should never be handled or recapped (resheathed). It is a good idea to practice engaging the safety mechanism on a clean needle to prevent accidents with contaminated ones. After disposing of the needle, be sure to clean the area of the injection with a disinfectant.

All needles and syringes should be placed in a red sharps container, needle down, as soon as they are used. Do not dispose of needles in any receptacle other than a sharps container.

Medications for Injection

Medications for injection are provided in several forms, including vials, ampules, powders to be reconstituted, unit doses, and prefilled cartridges.

Vials

The most common medications for injection are provided as single-dose and multiple-dose **vials**. These are glass bottles with rubber stoppers to protect the medications inside. The needle is inserted through the rubber stopper, and the correct amount of medication is drawn out. Single-dose vials are meant to be used, as the name implies, one time.

Multiple-dose vials are used multiple times, with an ordered dose withdrawn each time until the medication is used or until no more can be withdrawn without also withdrawing air bubbles. The stopper is cleaned with rubbing alcohol before each use. See Procedure 54-5 and Figures A–D for instructions on withdrawing medication from a single-dose or multiple-dose vial.

Ampules

Ampules are small, sealed glass bottles containing a single dose of medication. An indentation in the neck of the ampule shows where to break off the tip to open the container. Place the tip in a sharps container. An alcohol pad or cotton pad must be used to hold the vial to prevent glass cuts when opening ampules (Procedure 54-6 and Figures A–C).

PROCEDURE 54-5
Withdrawing Medication from Single-Dose or Multiple-Dose Vials

Objective ◆ *Withdraw medication from single-dose and multiple-dose vials.*

EQUIPMENT AND SUPPLIES

Disposable gloves; sharps container; soap; needle; syringe; alcohol wipe; medication vial

METHOD

1. Check the medication as instructed in the "three befores" technique before beginning. Compare the medication vial (bottle) against the physician's order (Figure A).
2. Select the correct syringe and needle based on the type of medication and location for the injection site.
3. Perform hand hygiene and apply gloves.
4. Roll the medication vial between your hands to mix any medication that has settled on the bottom. Do not shake as this will create air bubbles.
5. Wipe the rubber stopper with an alcohol wipe firmly in a circular motion. Then set the vial on a clean surface while you prepare the syringe (Figure B).
6. Remove the protective cap from the needle on the syringe. In some circumstances, such as in home health or if the needle needs to be transported safely to another location, it may need to be recapped. In this case after removing

the protective cap from the needle on the syringe, maintain the sterility of the inner surface of the protective cap because it will be needed to cover the needle again after you have filled the syringe. However, many needles have automatic retraction or sheathing devices and do not need to be recapped. Follow the manufacturer's directions for the type of needle you are using.

7. Withdraw the syringe plunger and allow air to enter the syringe in an amount equal to the amount of medication to be withdrawn. Because the vials are vacuum sealed, this will allow for easier withdrawal of fluid.
8. Turning the vial upside down at eye level and using care not to touch the rubber stopper, insert the needle into the rubber stopper and inject the air into the vial. Be extremely cautious concerning contamination as you enter the multiple-dose bottle.
9. Keeping the upside-down vial at eye level, slowly withdraw the correct amount of fluid medication (Figure C).
10. While the needle is still in the vial, check to make sure that the dosage is accurate. Any air bubbles in the syringe will give you an inaccurate dose, because they take up the space needed for medication. To remove air bubbles, flick

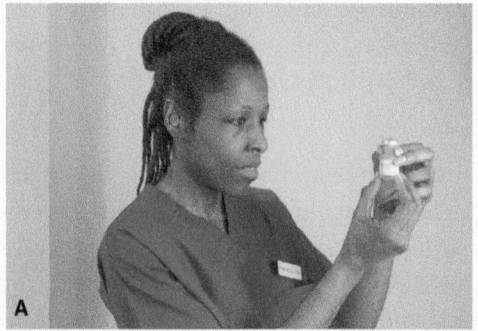

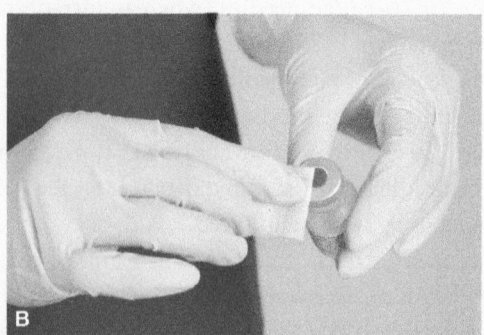

FIGURE A–B (A) Read the label on the medication bottle; **(B)** clean the top of the bottle.

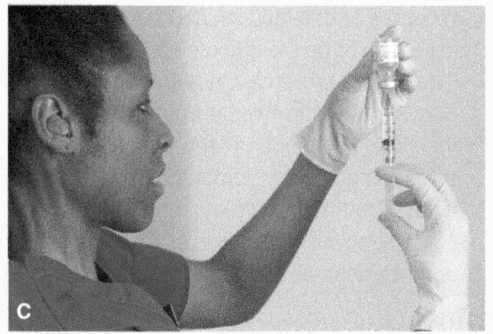
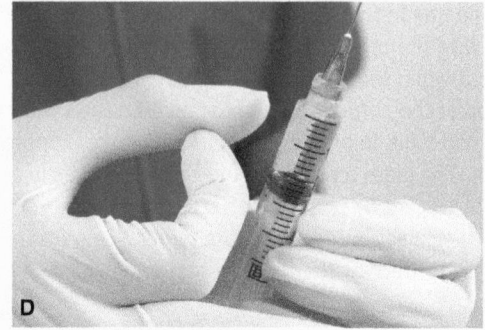

FIGURE C–D (C) With the bottle inverted, draw the correct amount of medication into the syringe; **(D)** remove the needle from the bottle and expel the air or tap out the air bubbles.

your fingers against the side of the syringe until the air bubbles go back into the tip of the syringe (Figure D).

11. Remove the needle from the vial.

12. If you have accidentally withdrawn too much fluid, discard the excess fluid by shooting it into a sink or waste receptacle. Never return medications to the vial or bottle from which they came.

13. Check the medication vial after you have withdrawn the dosage to make sure you are correct as instructed in the "three befores" for checking medications. Also, check to see if the multiple-dose vial should be refrigerated after opening.

14. If your facility policy requires wearing gloves during injections, remove and dispose of the gloves after the medication has been administered. Perform hand hygiene.

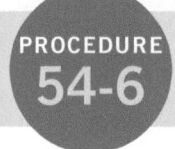

PROCEDURE 54-6 — Withdrawing Medication from an Ampule

Objective ◆ *Open and withdraw medication from an ampule.*

EQUIPMENT AND SUPPLIES

Ampule containing medication; soap; alcohol wipe; gauze; filter needle and regular needle; syringe; disposable gloves; sharps container; pen

METHOD

1. Check the medication against the physician's medication order, as instructed in the "three befores."

2. Do not open the ampule until you are ready to withdraw the fluid.

3. Perform hand hygiene and apply gloves.

4. Snap your thumb and middle finger gently against the tip of the ampule to move all the medication away from the neck and into the bottom of the ampule (Figure A).

5. Clean the neck of the ampule using an alcohol wipe.

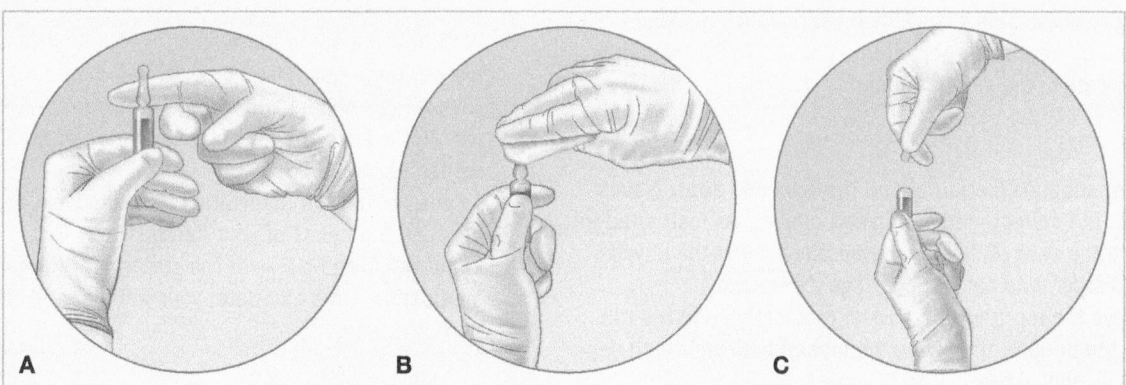

FIGURE A–C Breaking a glass ampule containing medication.

6. Using one hand to hold the bottom of the vial, snap off the top with the other hand using a gauze square to prevent a cut when the glass neck breaks (Figure B).
7. If the top of the ampule does not snap off easily, you may have to use a file to create a cut or "score" the ampule at the neck. The glass ampule should then break easily at this point (Figure C).
8. Insert a filter needle (attached to a syringe) into the ampule and withdraw the fluid without touching the sides of the ampule.

9. Withdraw all the medication from the ampule. It may be necessary to tip the ampule slightly to withdraw all the fluid.
10. Discard the broken ampule into a sharps container.
11. Remove the filter needle from the syringe and discard it in the sharps container. Place the correct-size needle necessary for medication administration.
12. If your facility policy requires wearing gloves during injections, remove and dispose of the gloves after the medication has been administered. Perform hand hygiene.

Powders to Be Reconstituted

Some medications are supplied in a powdered or dry form. Medications supplied in powdered form generally have a longer shelf life. To be injected, these powdered medications must be reconstituted with diluents, usually sterile water. Once the diluent is added to the powder and mixed well, the appropriate dose is drawn up and administered to the patient. To reconstitute a powdered medication, see Procedure 54-7.

Unit Dosages

Unit dosages are packaged in nonreusable containers that deliver dosages one at a time by a nonparenteral route, as ordered by the prescriber. The advantages of unit dose dispensing are that the drug is fully identifiable and the integrity of the dosage form is protected until it is actually administered. If the drug is not used and the container remains intact, the drug may be redispensed without compromising its integrity.

Prefilled Cartridge Injection Systems

Prefilled cartridge injection systems are prefilled, single dose cartridges that fit into a special cartridge holder. This system is convenient in that medications do not have to be drawn up before injections. The cartridge holders are sturdy and long lasting.

PROCEDURE
54-7

Reconstituting a Powdered Medication for Administration

Objective ◆ *Reconstitute a powdered medication.*

EQUIPMENT AND SUPPLIES

Alcohol wipe; disposable gloves; medication label; medication order signed by physician; pen; sterile needle; sharps container; vial of medication and vial of diluent

METHOD

1. Gather supplies, perform hand hygiene, and apply gloves.
2. Select the correct medication and diluent. As instructed in the "three befores," verify the dosage against the physician's order, and calculate dosage if necessary.
3. Remove the top from the powder medication and the top from the diluent, then wipe the tops of both vials with separate alcohol wipes.
4. Insert a sterile needle through the rubber stopper on the vial of diluent.
5. Withdraw the appropriate amount of diluent and add to the powder medication.
6. Remove the needle and syringe unit from the medication vial and discard the needle and syringe in the sharps container.
7. To ensure that the medication is mixed well, roll the vial between the palms of your hands.
8. Label the mixed vial with the strength of the prepared medication, time and date, your initials, and the expiration date.

SAFETY PROCEDURES: OSHA STANDARDS

The federal OSHA has established specific guidelines regarding the disposal of contaminated needles and syringes. Additionally, OSHA's Bloodborne Pathogens Standard has provisions for follow-up procedures for health care workers who are exposed to a needlestick from a contaminated needle.

If you are accidentally stuck with a contaminated needle, you should immediately wash the wound and then notify the physician and medical office manager. Concerns related to a needlestick injury include exposure to human immunodeficiency virus (HIV), which can cause acquired immunodeficiency syndrome (AIDS), and exposure to hepatitis B virus (HBV) or hepatitis C virus (HBC).

Although cases of these diseases being transmitted by needlesticks are rare, they do occasionally occur. Immediate reporting of needlesticks is important to ensure that testing and prophylactic (preventive) treatment can be initiated in an appropriate and timely manner. The employer is responsible for providing free medical evaluation and treatment for exposure to contaminated sharps or needles while at work.

Investigation of the incident is a second reason for early reporting, because the employer should begin to seek reasons for the incident. Additional training may be necessary to prevent other injuries in the office.

By law, all medical offices must have a puncture-proof, rigid, locked container labeled with an international biohazard sticker for the disposal of sharps (Figure 54-8). Smaller biohazard sharps containers may be placed in all patient examination rooms. When these smaller containers are two-thirds to three-quarters full, they should be closed and placed in a large biohazard container in a central location in the office. When the large container is two-thirds to three quarters full, it should be replaced and disposed of using a waste removal service contracted to incinerate or autoclave the contents. The waste

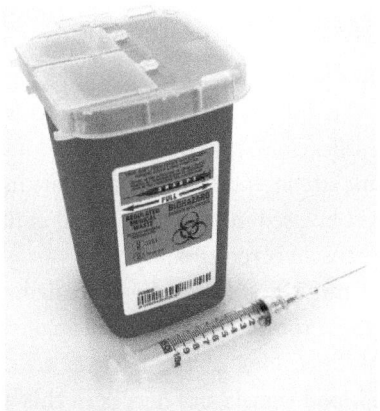

FIGURE 54-8 OSHA regulations require the use of sharps containers to discard used needles.

removal service will give the office a document of destruction, which should be kept and filed at the office.

Any time a medical assistant has the potential to come in contact with *any* body fluids—such as saliva, blood, or other substances—standard precautions must be observed and followed. Careful hand hygiene must follow the removal of gloves after such contact. See Guidelines 54-2 regarding

---

Guidelines 54-2

Glove Guidelines

STERILE AND NONSTERILE GLOVES

During procedures in the medical office, nonsterile disposable gloves are worn. A physician's office is generally not a sterile environment, so sterile surgical gloves (which are costly) are worn only when the physician is creating an opening into the body with a scalpel or entering an unprotected environment, such as the bladder. (Nonsterile gloves are worn for vaginal procedures because, even though these are invasive procedures, the vagina is itself not sterile and has its own defenses against infection—for example, during insertion of a diaphragm or sexual intercourse.)

LATEX AND NONLATEX GLOVES

Latex allergies are common and dangerous. Patients who are allergic to latex may respond with anything from mild itching to difficulty breathing to a full-blown, life-threatening anaphylactic reaction. Do not wear latex gloves if a patient is known to have a latex allergy. As a precautionary measure, many medical practices have entirely eliminated the use of latex gloves.

OSHA GLOVE GUIDELINES

OSHA has stated that "at a minimum, gloves must be used where there is reasonable anticipation of employee hand contact with blood, other potentially infectious material, mucous membranes, or non-intact skin; when performing vascular access procedures; or when handling or touching contaminated surfaces or items." However, OSHA also states that "gloves are not necessary when giving routine injections as long as hand contact with blood or other potentially infectious material is not anticipated. If bleeding is anticipated and the employee is required to clean the site following injection, then gloves must be worn. Additionally, if the patient's skin is abraded, gloves would be required."

As these statements make clear, OSHA guidelines do not mandate wearing gloves during routine injections. However, as a medical assistant, you may choose to protect yourself with nonsterile disposable gloves. Follow your employer's policies.

OSHA guidelines on this topic can be read at www.osha.gov/pls/oshaweb/owadisp.show_document?p_table=INTERPRETATIONS&p_id=20819.

Pharmaceutical representatives make regular visits to all medical offices. These professionals have two goals: to educate the physician about the pharmaceuticals their company sells and to persuade the physician to prescribe their medications. Pharmaceutical representative visits are a double-edged sword. On the plus side, it is important that representatives be able to present their information to the physician. New research is important to the physician, and the physician needs to have information about any medication he or she is going to prescribe. On the minus side, physicians can get overrun by visits from salespersons that impinge on the time for seeing patients.

It may fall to you, as a medical assistant, to enforce time allotments for these visits and, as requested by the physician, to acquire information from these pharmaceutical representatives about their medications that you can convey to the physician at the appropriate time. Always treat pharmaceutical representatives as professionals, but be sure to explain the policies of the office regarding visits by representatives. According to office policy, offer to take information for the physician and to check the supply of samples. Remember, however, that the physician must sign for any medication samples left at the office.

glove guidelines. For more on biohazard waste disposal, see the chapter titled "Infection Control."

CHARTING MEDICATION ADMINISTRATION

As discussed in the chapter titled "Pharmacology," the medical assistant must understand the importance of documenting and reporting errors in medication administration. Administration of medication must be charted in the patient record, either electronically or in the patient paper chart, according to office protocols. The electronic health record (EHR) is a valuable record of patient use of medication and should be kept up to date by asking the patient at each visit whether the patient is continuing to take medications in the EHR and if there have been any changes in dosages or routes. It is also a good opportunity to ask about any side effects, complimentary/alternative supplements, and vitamin use to further complete the EHR.

Parenteral medications are charted using the same documentation as for oral medications: name of medication, dosage, route, date, site, and signature of person administering the medication. It is a good habit also to chart the manufacturer of a medication, because it is necessary for vaccinations, which is discussed later in this chapter. Finally, it is also

necessary to document that you have provided instructions to the patient regarding follow-up care.

Examples of charting follow:

9/10/YY 9:00 A.M. nitroglycerin, 1 tab, sublingually. P = 65. Patient states now has no pain.

Written instructions given to Pt. Precautions explained. Told to call office at 1:00 P.M. today to report progress of his condition...................M. Richards, CMA (AAMA)

1/19/YY 11:00 A.M. Monistat-3, 200 mg. Vaginal. Patient tolerated administration, denies pain or discomfort. Given written instructions for follow-up care......................................M. Richards, CMA (AAMA)

10/10/YY 1:00 P.M. Mantoux test, 0.01 mL Tuberculin Purified Protein Derivative, left forearm, subcutaneous, small wheal noted. Pt. instructed not to rub or cover the area and to return for reading on 10/12/YY....................
....M. Richards, CMA (AAMA)

It is very important to chart any medication errors according to the facility policy. Usually this means an incident report of what happened, to whom, with some information that might help to inform changes in systems to prevent future mistakes. Medical assistants need to take care not to be distracted while administering medications, to always check for accuracy and safety, to ask the physician if any order seems unusual, and to document any issues with the administration of medications or unusual responses from the patient. Frequent medication errors can lead to retraining, disciplinary action, and sometimes termination.

INTRAMUSCULAR INJECTIONS

Intramuscular (IM) injections administer medication directly into muscle tissue. They are always given at a 90-degree angle (Figure 54-9). IM injections are given in one of four sites. These sites (muscles) are the deltoid, vastus lateralis, dorsogluteal, and ventrogluteal muscles (Figure 54-10).

Deltoid Muscle

The **deltoid muscle** is located on the upper outer surface of the upper arm. This site of small muscle mass works well for small-volume injections but not for large ones. Common injections in this site include tetanus boosters in adults. This site should never be used in infants or small children because the size of the muscle is too small.

The deltoid muscle is found by measuring two finger widths below the acromion process (the top of the shoulder). Never give IM injections in the back of an arm, because there are large blood vessels and nerves in this area.

Use a 23-gauge, 1-inch needle to give injections in the arm. For individuals with small arms, a 25-gauge, ⅝-inch

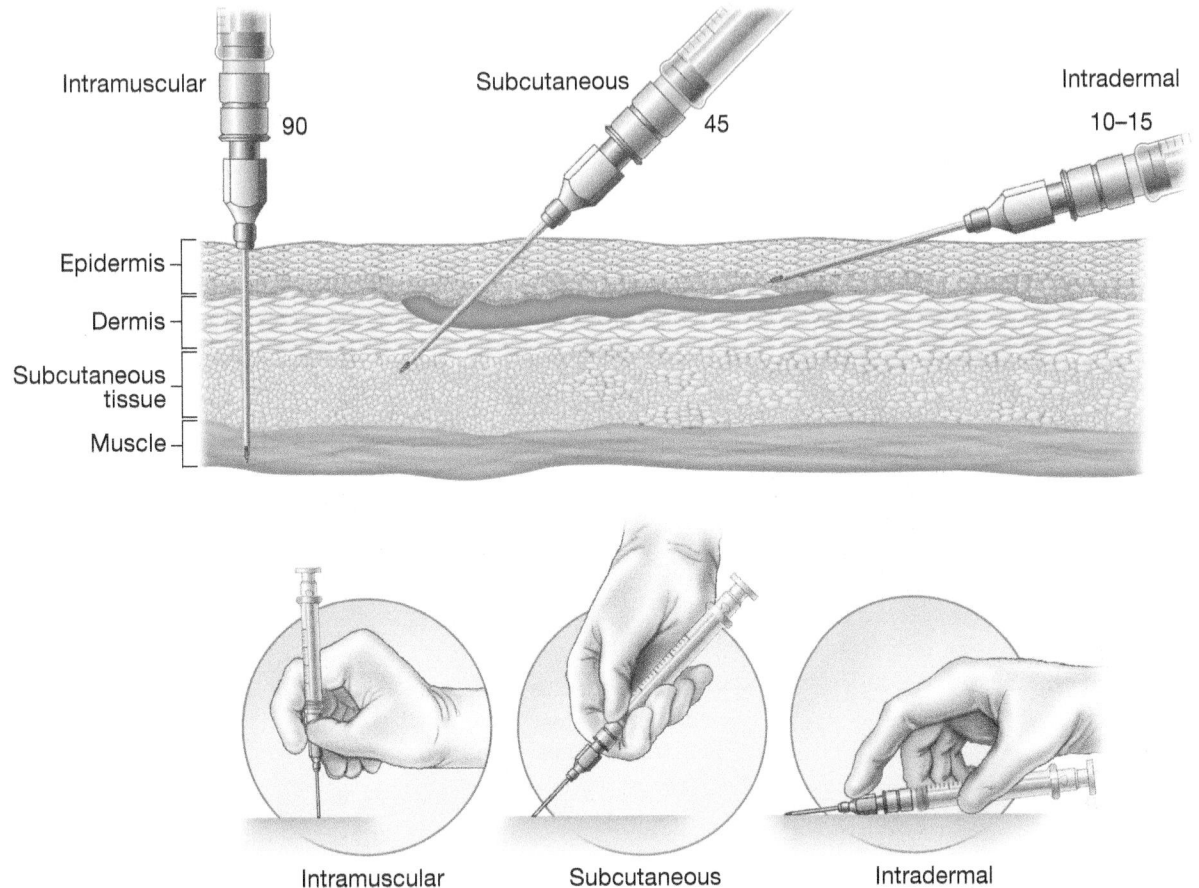

FIGURE 54-9 Angle of insertion for three types of injections.

needle is more appropriate. Up to 2 mL can be injected in a large adult's deltoid muscle, but a small child's deltoid is not usually used and if it is used, it is rare to give more than 1 mL in a child's deltoid.

Because of the ease of access to the deltoid, this muscle is popular for vaccinations.

Vastus Lateralis Muscle

The **vastus lateralis muscle** is on the outer portion of the upper thigh and is part of the quadriceps (the muscle group at the front of the thigh). This site is considered the safest site for IM injections, especially in children or small individuals, because few major blood vessels are in this area. The vastus lateralis muscle lies below the greater trochanter of the femur (the knob-like top of the thigh bone) and within the upper lateral quadrant (top outer quarter) of the thigh. This muscle is well developed in the infant and recommended by the American Academy of Pediatrics as the preferred injection site for infants and children.

In the adult, the vastus lateralis extends from the middle of the anterior (front) thigh to the middle of the lateral (outer) thigh. Typically, it is one handbreadth below the

greater trochanter and extends to one handbreadth above the knee. For an injection in this muscle, the patient may be either sitting or lying supine (on the back). Up to 5 mL may be injected in the vastus lateralis of a large adult. This is a good site when the ventrogluteal muscle is insufficient, such as in an infant less than 7 months old and in a patient who is unable to walk. It is a better option in obese women. This is a good site for injecting vaccinations in children.

Dorsogluteal Muscle

The **dorsogluteal site** on the upper outer quadrant of the buttocks may be used for large-volume, deep IM injections or for irritating viscous (thick) medications. The choice of an injection site is based on good clinical judgment, best available evidence, and assessment of the client. Evidence-based research has shown the ventrogluteal site to be preferable because of the potential for injury associated with the dorsogluteal site. In fact, many facilities mandate the ventrogluteal site for this reason. If the dorsogluteal site is used, landmarks (described next) must be observed to avoid damage to the sciatic nerve, which runs from the lower back, through the buttock, and down the leg.

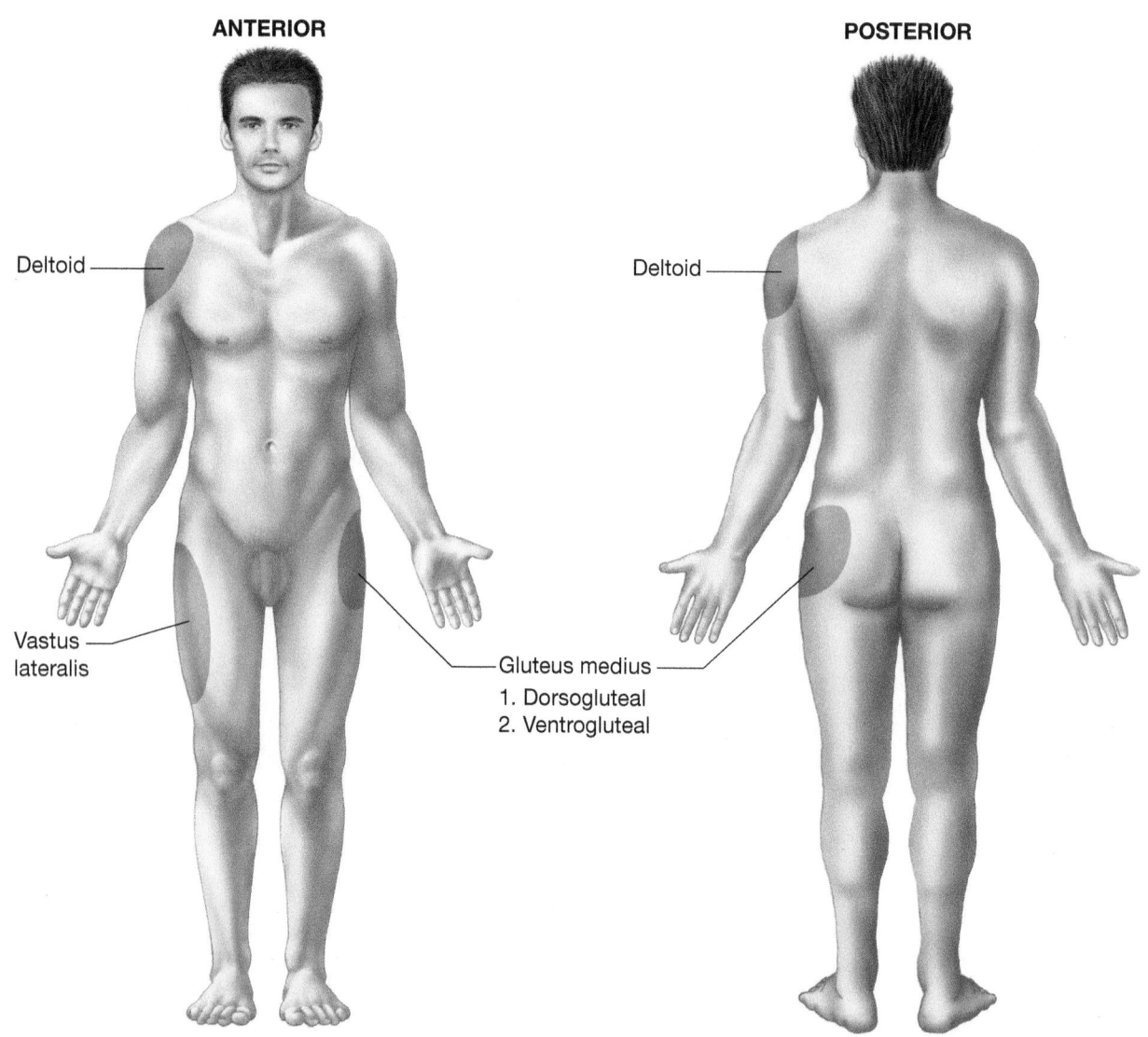

ANTERIOR

Deltoid

Vastus
lateralis

POSTERIOR

Deltoid

Gluteus medius
1. Dorsogluteal
2. Ventrogluteal

FIGURE 54-10 Sites for intramuscular injections.

To give this injection, ask the patient to lie prone (face down) and point the toes inward or to bend over the end of the examining table. These positions cause the gluteal muscles to relax. Draw an imaginary line from the greater trochanter of the femur to the posterior superior iliac spine. Give the injection above and lateral (to the outside) to this line. Another method—if you are not very familiar with the skeletal structures just mentioned—is simply to divide the buttocks in four equal parts, and give the injection in the upper outer quadrant (Figure 54-11). Up to 4 mL can be injected into this site. Pain relievers are an example of medication that can be injected into this site.

Ventrogluteal Muscle

The **ventrogluteal site** is the best site to use. It is considered safer than the dorsogluteal site because there are no major nerves or blood vessels in this muscle. This site is considered safe for infants, children, and adults.

To give an IM injection in the patient's left ventrogluteal muscle, place the palm of the right hand on the greater trochanter and the index finger on the superior iliac crest. Stretch the index finger as far as possible along the iliac crest and then spread the middle finger away from your index finger (Figure 54-12). The injection is made in the space between the index and middle fingers. When using this method to determine the injection location, always use the hand opposite the side of the planned injection on the patient—for example, your left hand and the patient's right gluteus medius. Up to 2.5 mL can be injected safely into a large adult ventrogluteal muscle. Depo Provera, a hormone, is an example of a medication that is injected in the ventrogluteal muscle.

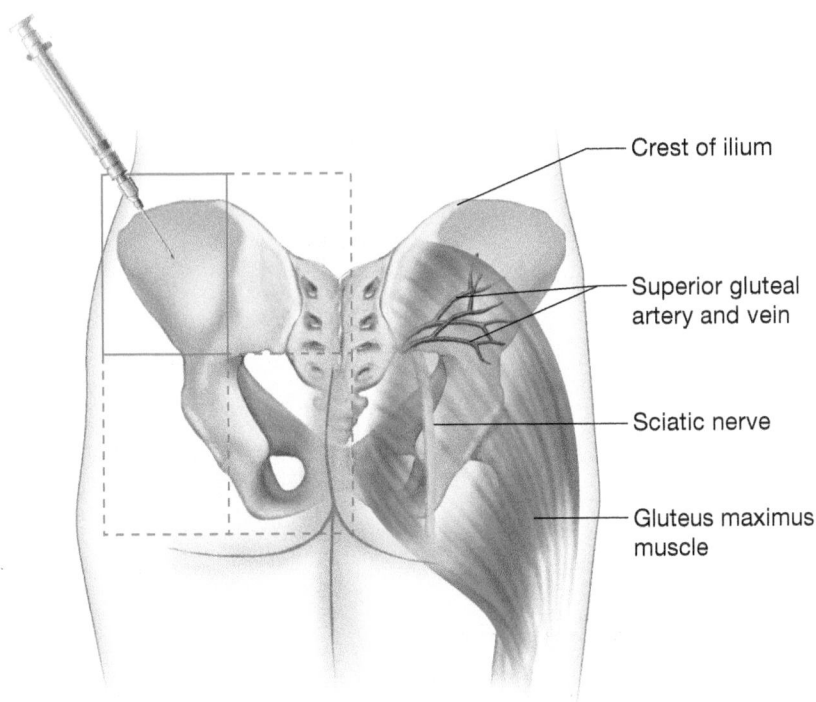

FIGURE 54-11 Injecting the upper outer quadrant of the buttocks.

Crest of ilium

Superior gluteal artery and vein

Sciatic nerve

Gluteus maximus muscle

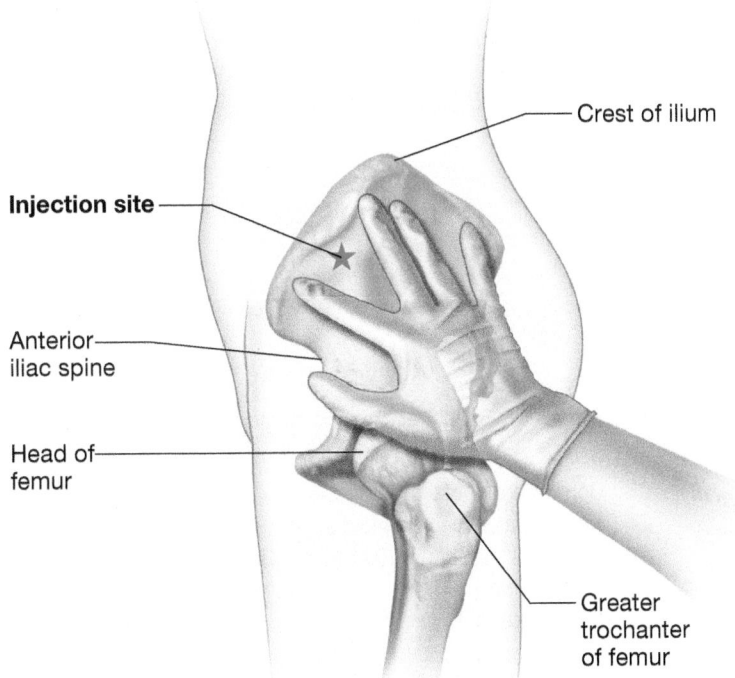

Crest of ilium

Injection site

Anterior iliac spine

Head of femur

Greater trochanter of femur

FIGURE 54-12 Injecting the ventrogluteal muscle.

Z-Track Method

The **Z-track method** is used when a medication is irritating to the subcutaneous tissues or when the medication may discolor the skin. Many organizations prefer that all IM injections be given this way, so be sure to check your facility's policy. When giving a medication using the Z-track method, you need to pull the skin to the side before inserting the needle. The pulling of the skin displaces the tissue; then you inject the medication, release the skin, and remove the needle, and the medication will not be able to seep back to the skin's surface. It is critically important to withdraw the needle before releasing the skin. See Procedure 54-8 for more on Z-track injections.

SUBCUTANEOUS INJECTIONS

The **subcutaneous injection** is given just under the skin in the fat (adipose) tissue. This method is used for small doses of nonirritating medications such as immunizations, insulin, and heparin. The back of the arm is frequently used for these injections, but other areas that may be used include the upper back or the abdomen and thighs (when the patient does self-injection, as with insulin). Table 54-1 lists insulin types and durations of action. See Figure 54-13 for an illustration of the sites for subcutaneous injections.

The subcutaneous injection is given at a 45-degree angle to the skin surface, unless the injection is heparin or insulin, in which case a 90-degree angle is used. For patients who self-inject, the site of injection must be rotated so as not to form scar tissue by repeatedly injecting the same sites. Teach the patient to keep a rotation chart to ensure protection of the skin. (See Figure 54-14 for an example of rotation sites.) Patients receiving allergy injections should remain in the office after the injection per the office protocol, usually 20 or 30 minutes *to ensure that the patient is not having any type of allergic reaction.* Procedure 54-9 demonstrates a review of parenteral medication injection sites. See Procedure 54-10 for the steps of administering parenteral subcutaneous or intramuscular injections.

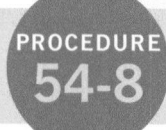

PROCEDURE 54-8

Administering a Z-Track Injection

Objective ◆ *Administer a Z-track injection using proper technique.*

EQUIPMENT AND SUPPLIES

Alcohol wipes; sharps container; disposable gloves; medication order signed by the physician; pen; sterile needle and syringe; medication vial

METHOD

1–15. Follow steps 1 through 15 of Procedure 54-10 for administration of an intramuscular injection.

16. After withdrawing the medication from the vial, change to a fresh needle. This will eliminate any irritating medication that may be within the needle from coming into contact with the patient's tissue until the needle is placed into the muscle layer (Figure A).

17. When you are ready to administer the medication, pull the skin of the buttock to one side and hold it in place with your nondominant hand. You may wish to use a dry gauze sponge if the skin is slippery (Figure B).

18. With your dominant hand and using a dartlike grip on the syringe, insert the needle up to the hub quickly into the gluteus medius muscle. Do not move the needle once it is in place (Figure C).

19. While still maintaining a firm hold on the taut skin with your nondominant hand, pull back on the plunger of the syringe to check for blood return with the fingers of the hand holding the syringe. To do this simply move your fingers up the syringe, while keeping the needle steady within the patient's buttocks, until your thumb and index finger reach the top of the plunger. If blood appears in the hub of the syringe, then use the correct technique to withdraw the syringe, discard, and begin with step 1 again.

20. If there is no blood return, then very slowly inject the medication into the muscle.

21. Wait several seconds after injecting the medication before you withdraw the needle. Cover the area with the alcohol wipe, and withdraw the needle at the same angle of insertion. Wait at least 10 seconds before releasing the skin being held by the nondominant hand (Figures D and E).

22. Do not massage the area. Observe the patient for any unusual effects or reactions to the medication for at least 15 minutes. You may advise the patient to walk around to assist in the absorption process of the medication.

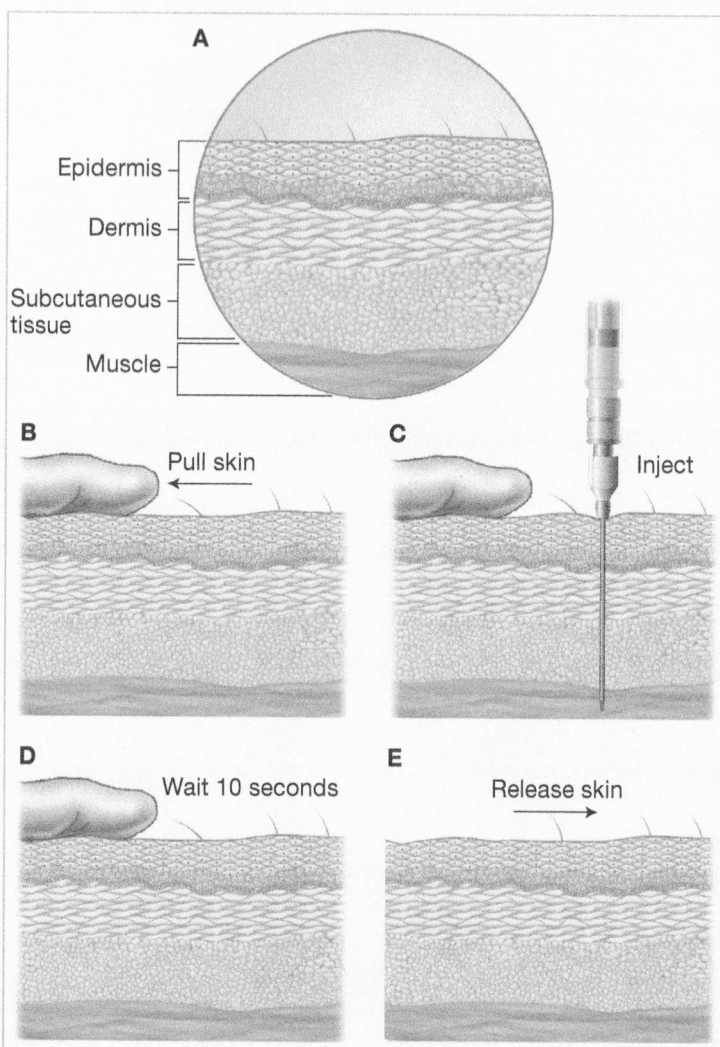

FIGURE A–E An example of a Z-track method of injection.

23. Correctly dispose of all materials.
24. Remove and discard gloves and perform hand hygiene.
25. Chart the medication administration on the patient's record noting the time, medication name, dosage, injection site, route, and your name.

CHARTING EXAMPLE

2/14/YY 3:30 P.M. Iron dextran, 50 mg Z-track into left gluteus. No C/O pain and no adverse reactions................N. Young, RMA

TABLE 54-1 | Insulin Types and Duration of Action

Insulin Name	Type	Common Name	Action Onset	Action Peak	Action Duration
Humalog	Rapid action	Lispro	15–30 min	30–90 min	3–5 hours
Humulin-N	Intermediate	—	1 hour	4 hours	24 hours
Humulin-R	Rapid	—	15 min	1 hour	6–8 hours
Insulin zinc suspension	Intermediate	Lente	2–4 hours	6–15 hours	24–48 hours
Isophane	Intermediate	NPH	2–4 hours	6–15 hours	24–48 hours
Protamine zinc	Slow action	PZI	3–6 hours	12–20 hours	24–36 hours
Semilente	Rapid	Regular	1 hour	4–10 hours	12–16 hours
Ultralente	Slow	PZI	8 hours	12–24 hours	36+ hours

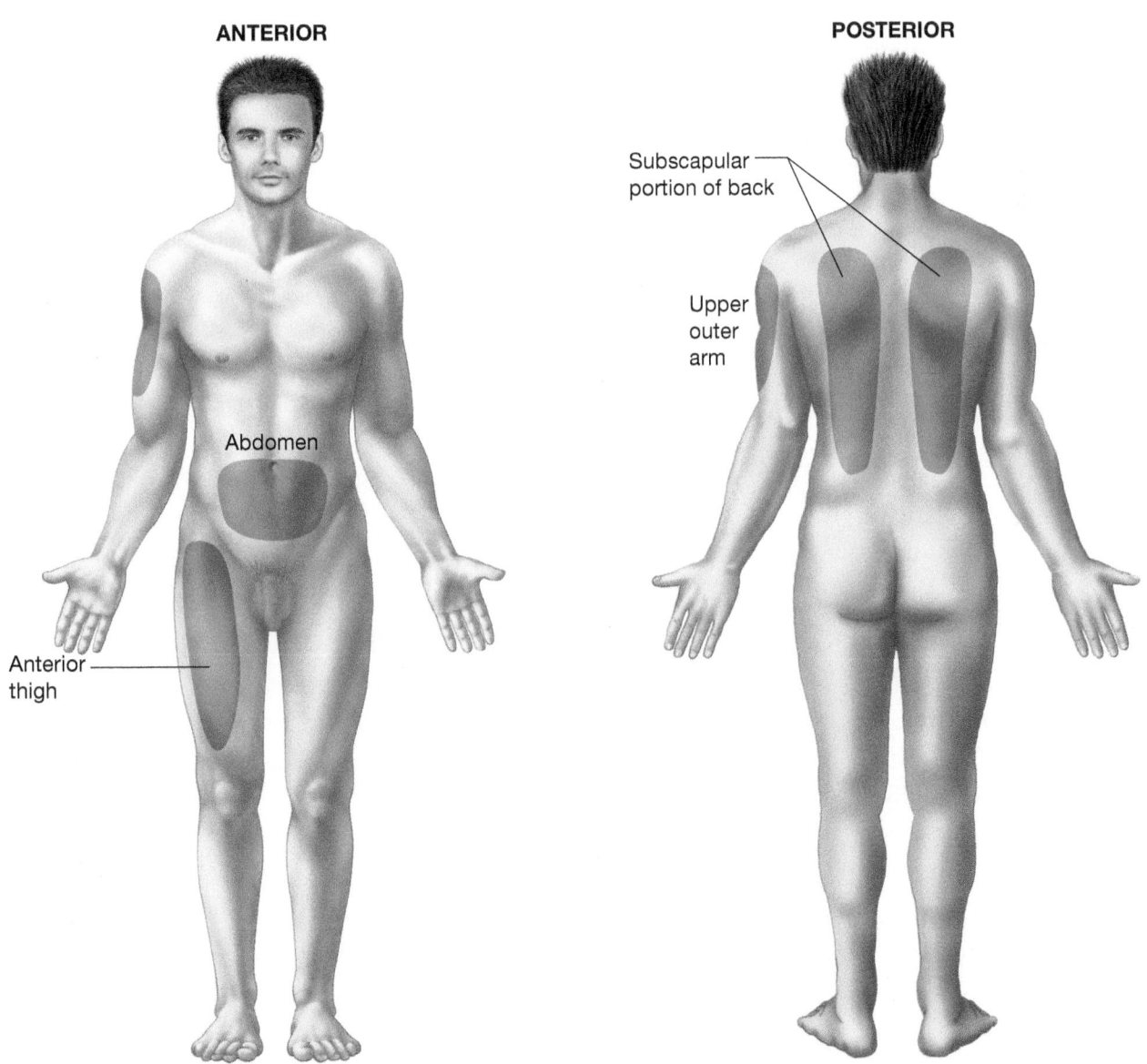

FIGURE 54-13 Sites for subcutaneous injection.

ANTERIOR   POSTERIOR

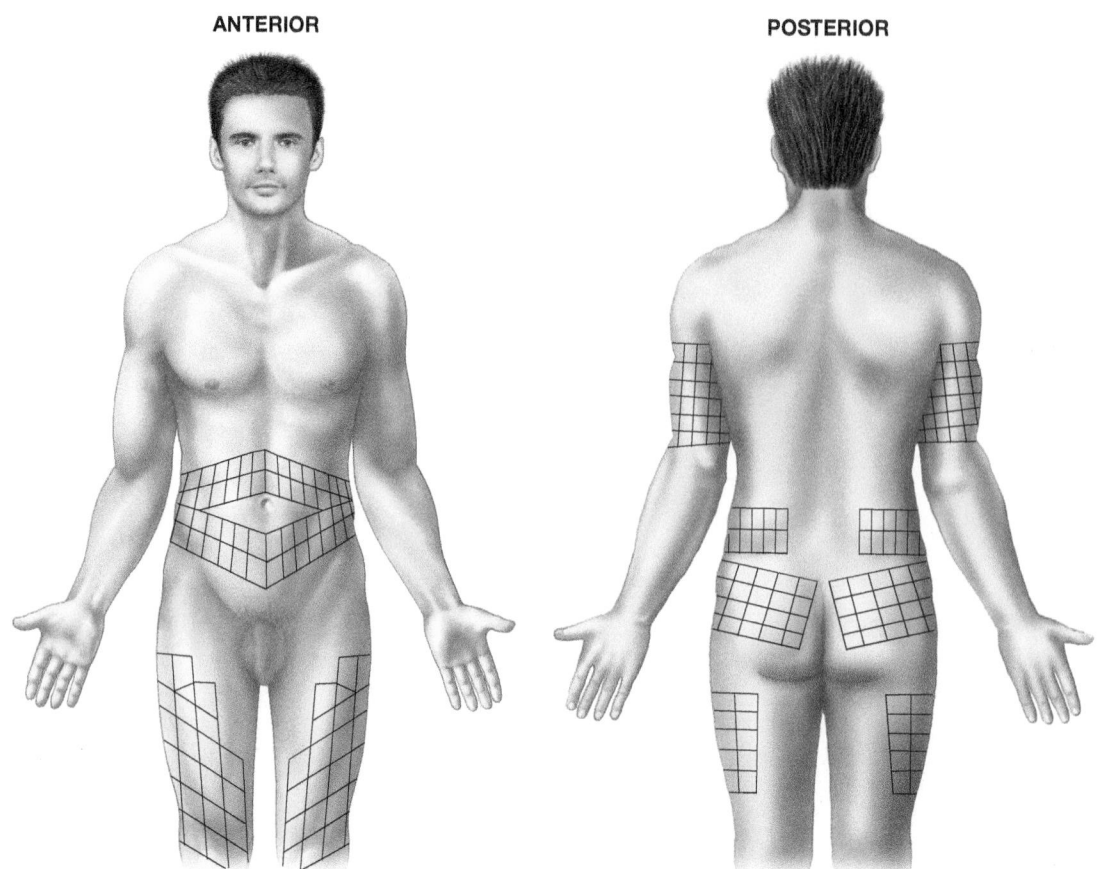

FIGURE 54-14 Rotation sites for administering insulin.

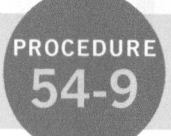

Reviewing Parenteral Medication Injection Sites

Objective ◆ *Demonstrate correct knowledge of parenteral medication injection sites.*

EQUIPMENT AND SUPPLIES

Manikin or torso with buttocks and arms

METHOD

1. Identify the location of the following sites for intramuscular injections:
   a. deltoid muscle
   b. vastus lateralis muscle
   c. dorsogluteal muscle
   d. ventrogluteal muscle
2. Identify common site locations for subcutaneous injections.

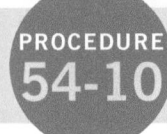

Administering Parenteral Subcutaneous or Intramuscular Injections

Objective ◆ *Administer subcutaneous and intramuscular injections.*

EQUIPMENT AND SUPPLIES

Medication order signed by physician; vial of medication; disposable gloves; alcohol wipes; sharps container; waste container; biohazard container

> *subcutaneous injection:* 25-gauge, ⅝-inch needle for small arm; 23-gauge, 1-inch needle for average arm; disposable 3-mL syringe
>
> *intramuscular injection:* 22-gauge, 1½-inch needle; disposable 3-mL syringe; pen

METHOD

1. Perform hand hygiene.
2. Apply gloves and follow standard blood and body fluid precautions.
   Note: As stated in Guidelines 54-2 earlier in this chapter, OSHA requires that gloves be worn when there is a reasonable expectation that you might encounter blood or body fluids. Employers disagree about whether giving injections is a task that creates this expectation. Follow your employer's policies; if you would prefer to wear gloves and your employer does not require donning gloves, you may need to insist that you want to wear gloves anyway. Remember, however, that you may need to wear nonlatex gloves if the patient is allergic to latex.
3. Select the correct medication as instructed in the "three befores."
   Note: Always double-check the label to ensure that the strength is correct, because medications are manufactured with different strengths (e.g., 250 mg/mL and 500 mg/mL).
4. Gently roll the medication between your hands to mix any medication that may have settled. Refrigerated medication can be rolled between your hands to warm it slightly.
5. Prepare the syringe using the correct technique. Carefully carry the covered needle and syringe to the patient.
6. Warmly greet and identify the patient both by stating his or her name and examining any printed identification such as a wrist name band or medical record. Ask the patient to state his or her date of birth. Introduce yourself to the patient and ask if the patient has any allergies.
7. Tell the patient the name of the medication and dosage that you are administering per the physician's order. Ask if the patient has any questions before receiving the medication.
8. Position the patient for the site you are using.

9. Using a circular motion, clean the patient's skin with an alcohol wipe. Wipe the skin with a sweeping motion from the center of the area outward.
10. Once again check the medication dosage against the patient's order to determine if this is the correct time to administer the dose (one of the "10 rights").
11. Remove the protective covering from the needle using care not to touch the needle. If you accidentally touch the needle, excuse yourself to the patient, then return to the preparation area and change the needle on the syringe. If you are using a self-contained syringe and needle unit that does not come apart, discard the entire syringe with the medication and start the process over again.
12. When you are prepared to administer the injection, place a new alcohol wipe or a cotton ball between two fingers of your nondominant hand so that you can easily grasp it when you are through with the injection.
13. Firmly grasp the syringe in your dominant hand like a pencil is held.
14. a. *To administer a subcutaneous injection:* With your nondominant hand, grasp the skin at the injection site and form a small mass of tissue. b. *To administer an intramuscular injection:* With your nondominant hand, stretch the skin tightly where you will insert the needle. (Review Procedure 54-8, Administering a Z-Track Injection.)
15. Grasping the syringe in a dartlike fashion, insert the entire needle with one swift movement.
16. a. *For a subcutaneous injection:* Insert into the subcutaneous tissue at a 45-degree angle (Figure A).
    b. *For an intramuscular injection:* Insert directly into the muscle at a 90-degree angle (Figure B).

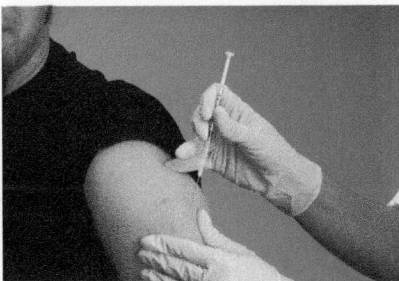

FIGURE A Subcutaneous injections are administered at a 45-degree angle.

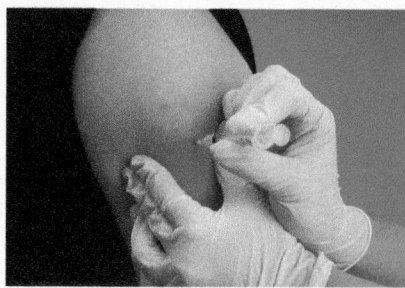

FIGURE B Intramuscular injections are administered at a 90-degree angle.

17. Do not move the needle once you have inserted it. If the needle is pushed in farther, contaminants are carried into the skin from the exposed needle.

18. Aspirate to determine if you have entered a blood vessel. To do this, pull back slightly on the plunger with the hand holding the syringe while holding the needle steady in the muscle. If blood appears in the hub area of the syringe, it means that the needle is in a blood vessel. You will then have to withdraw the needle using correct technique and discard the syringe containing the blood and medication. Begin the procedure again with fresh supplies.

    Note: Because the CDC no longer requires this step, some facilities have eliminated drawing back for blood return, especially when injecting insulin or dead viruses such as with vaccinations. Always check your facility policy.

19. If you do not see a return of blood in the syringe when you aspirate, slowly inject the medication without moving the needle. Do not move the needle until you have completed injecting all the medication.

Note: Insert and withdraw the needle quickly to minimize pain but administer the medication slowly.

20. Taking the alcohol wipe (or cotton ball) from between the last two fingers of your nondominant hand, place it over the area containing the needle. Withdraw the needle at the same angle you used for insertion, using care not to stick yourself with the needle.

21. With one hand, place the alcohol wipe firmly over the injection site. With the other hand discard the needle in a sharps container.

22. You may gently massage the injection site to assist absorption and ease pain for the patient.

23. Make sure the patient is safe before leaving him or her unattended. Observe the patient for any unusual effects or reactions to the medication for at least 15 minutes.

24. Correctly dispose of all materials.

25. Remove gloves and discard into a waste container. If gloves have come into contact with the patient's blood, dispose of the gloves in a biohazard container. Perform hand hygiene.

26. Chart the medication administration on the patient's record, noting the time, medication name, dosage, injection site, route, lot number of the medication, and your name.

CHARTING EXAMPLE

2/14/YY 1:30 P.M. Penicillin G. procaine, 600,000 units IM Right gluteus. Patient tolerated the procedure well. Denies numbness or tingling in buttock or leg. No adverse reactions noted...M. King, CMA (AAMA)

INTRADERMAL INJECTIONS

The **intradermal (ID) injection** is commonly used for allergy skin testing in which a minute amount of material is injected within the top layer of skin (Figure 54-15) to determine a patient's sensitivity. Common sites to perform an ID injection include the upper chest and upper back, as well as the anterior forearm. Because just the top level of skin is entered, a small wheal or bubble that contains the injection fluid appears on the skin. Do not rub the area after giving the injection.

Tuberculin Skin Test

In addition to allergy skin testing, the tuberculin skin test is also administered intradermally. A tuberculin skin test is done to see if a patient has ever been exposed to tuberculosis. A small amount of TB protein (antigens) is injected under the top layer of skin on the patient's inner forearm. If the person has ever been exposed to the TB bacteria, the skin will react to the antigens by developing a firm red bump at the site within two days. The test does not determine if the infection is active or inactive (latent).

The purified protein derivative (PPD) skin test uses a measured amount of TB antigens via an injection that is administered under the top layer of skin on the patient's forearm. A Mantoux test is a good test for a TB infection. It is often used when symptoms, screening, or testing, such as a chest X-ray, show that a person may have TB.

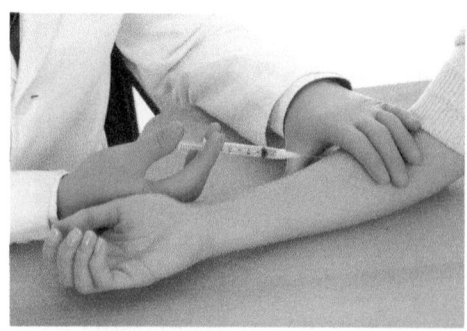

FIGURE 54-15 Intradermal injections are administered at a 10–15° angle.

Before administering a tuberculin skin test, the medical assistant should ask the patient the following questions:

1. Have you experienced recent symptoms of TB, such as cough, night sweats, or weight loss for no reason?

2. Have you had a positive tuberculin skin test in the past?

3. Have you had TB in the past?

4. Have you experienced risk factors for TB, such as contact with a person or a health care worker with TB, or have you resided in a country where TB is common?

5. Have you recently been given a TB vaccination?

6. Have you been treated with medicines, such as corticosteroids, that may affect the immune system?

7. Have you been infected with the HIV virus?

8. Do you have a skin rash that may make it hard to read the skin test?

To perform a tuberculin skin test as an intradermal injection, see Procedure 54-11. Ask the patient to sit down and turn up the inner side of the forearm. The skin where the test is done should be cleansed with an alcohol wipe and allowed to dry. Using a tuberculin syringe, place a small injection of the TB antigen (PPD) under the top layer of skin. The fluid makes a wheal under the skin. A circle may be drawn around the test area with a pen. Do not cover the site with a bandage. Tell the patient that some redness at the skin site is expected and that the site may itch but that it is important that it not be scratched because scratching may cause redness or swelling that would make the test difficult to read. Instruct the patient to return to the office within two to three days after the test to have the skin test checked.

Tuberculin Skin Test Results

Redness alone at the skin test site is a negative reaction to the tuberculin skin test. A firm bump is a positive reaction to the test. The size of the firm bump (not the red area) should be measured two to three days after the test to determine the result.

Although the medical assistant is responsible for reporting to the physician abnormal results (or positive results in the case of a TB skin test), interpreting such test results is *not* within the scope of practice for the medical assistant and, therefore, never should be done. The medical assistant is usually allowed only to report the findings of "positive" or "negative," unless additional certification is obtained.

INTRAVENOUS THERAPY

Intravenous (IV) therapy injects medications or therapeutic solutions directly into the bloodstream for immediate circulation and use by the body. State practices acts designate which health care professionals can initiate IV fluid therapy and medication administration. Medical assistants must consult their state practices act before attempting any IV procedure. In some states, the medical assistant may start IV fluid therapy with advanced training and physician supervision. In other states, medical assistants are not permitted to initiate intravenous therapy, but they are expected to be able to monitor intravenous therapy if it occurs in their facility. Make sure you receive adequate training before assuming responsibility for a patient having IV therapy, and immediately get a licensed health professional if you suspect something has gone wrong with the therapy (such as swelling, redness, burning, or pain at the site).

Medical Office Settings and Outpatient Intravenous Therapy

Medical assistants may come into more contact with IV therapy than in the past as the medical office and outpatient

---

Professionalism · The Life Span

The Child

When giving injections to pediatric patients, it is important to make sure the patients understand that they are going to be given an injection and that it will hurt for a moment. Never lie to pediatric patients; instead, give them a brief statement such as "I am going to give you some medicine with a shot, and it might hurt for just a minute, but then we will put a bandage on it." Always double-check all pediatric dosage calculations—a slight dosage miscalculation can create significant problems in a pediatric patient.

Never give medications to a pediatric patient without permission from the parent or guardian. Explain why the medication is being given, and be sure that all responsible parties are comfortable with the physician's explanation and have given their signed consent.

The Older Adult

Older patients typically take a greater number of medications than do younger patients. At every doctor's visit it is important to thoroughly review their medication lists. Include questions about over-the-counter medications. If an older patient has difficulty swallowing, be sure that the physician is aware of this so that smaller pills or alternate forms of medication can be prescribed.

Older patients often have thinner skin and smaller muscles. So when giving them injections, use a smaller needle and use care not to tear the skin or damage the muscle. Adhesive tape may tear fragile skin, so use gentle pressure on the site, then consider using paper tape if a bandage is needed.

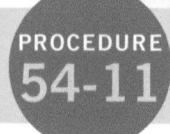

Administering an Intradermal Injection

Objective ◆ *Administer an intradermal injection.*

EQUIPMENT AND SUPPLIES

Disposable gloves; hazardous waste container; alcohol wipes; sterile needle; sterile syringe; vial of medication; medication order signed by physician; pen

METHOD

I. Preparation

1. Perform hand hygiene.
2. Apply gloves and follow standard blood and body fluid precautions.
3. Select the correct medication as instructed in the "three befores." Always double-check the label to make sure the strength is correct, because medications are manufactured with different strengths (e.g., 1:10, 1:100, or 1:1,000 dilutions).
4. Gently roll the medication between your hands to mix any medication that may have settled. Refrigerated medication can be rolled between your hands to warm it slightly.
5. Prepare the syringe using the correct technique. Carefully carry the covered needle and syringe to the patient.
6. Warmly greet and identify the patient both by stating his or her name and examining any printed identification such as a wrist name band or medical record. Introduce yourself to the patient, and ask if the patient has any allergies.

7. Tell the patient the name of the medication and dosage that you are administering per the physician's order. Explain the process of the PPD skin test. Ask if the patient has any questions before receiving the medication.
8. Select the proper site (center of forearm, upper chest, or upper back). (Review Figure A for intradermal skin injection sites.)
9. Using a circular motion, clean the patient's skin with an alcohol wipe. Wipe the skin with a sweeping motion from the center of the area outward. This prevents recontamination of the injection site by the alcohol wipe.
10. Allow time for the antiseptic on the wipe to dry to reduce the possibility of it reacting with the medication.
11. Check the medication dosage against the patient's order to determine if this is the correct time to administer the dose (one of the "10 rights").
12. Remove the protective covering from the needle using care not to touch the needle. If you accidentally touch the needle, then excuse yourself to the patient. Return to your preparation area and change the needle on the syringe. If you are using a self-contained syringe and needle unit that does not come apart, you will have to discard the entire syringe with the medication and start the process over again.

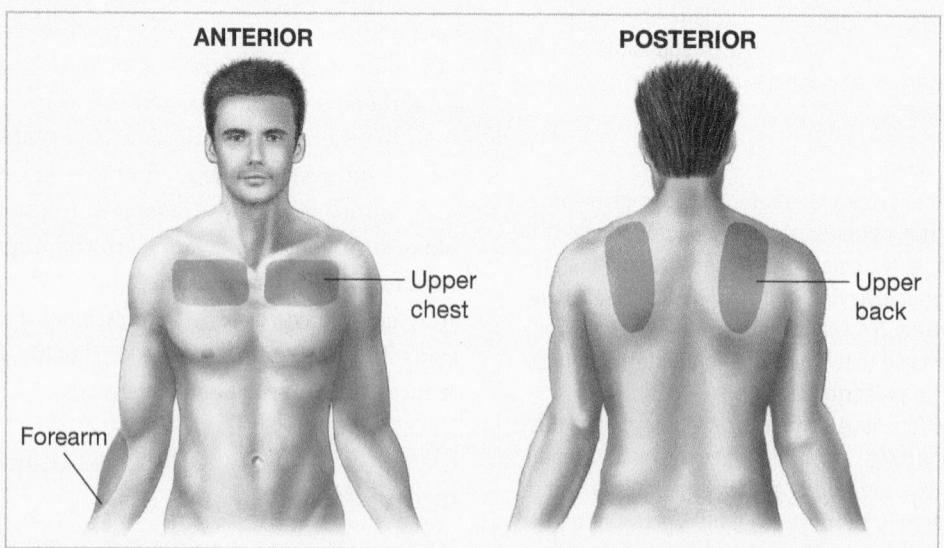

FIGURE A Intradermal injection sites.

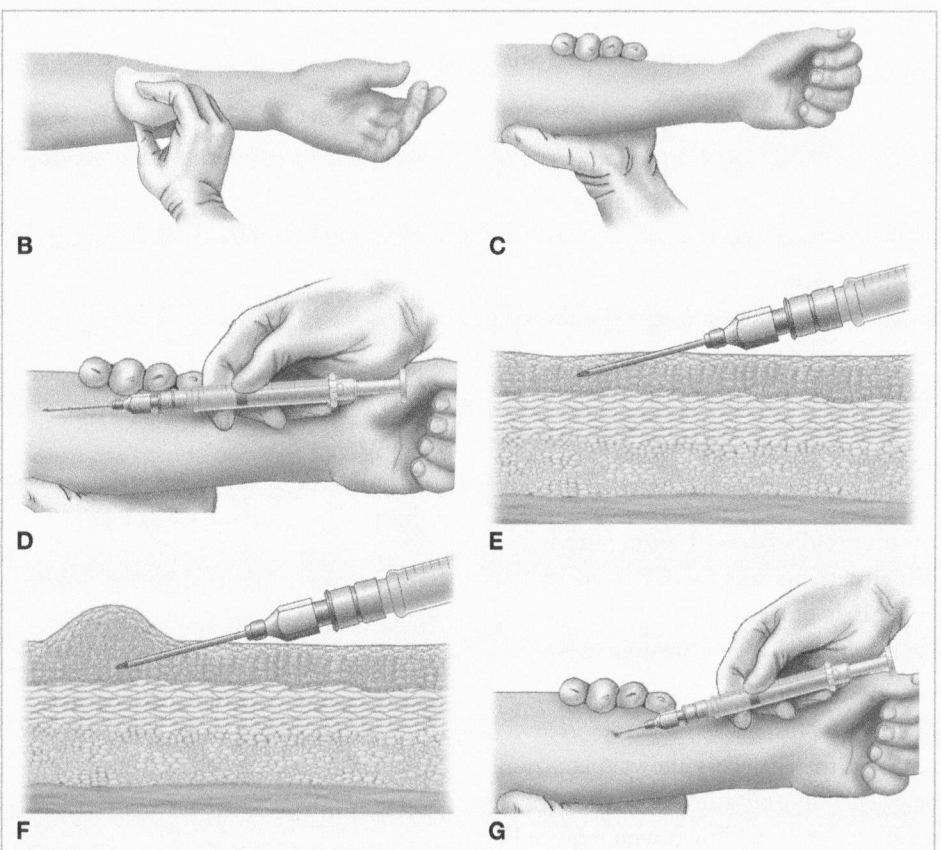

FIGURE B–G Administering an intradermal skin test.

II. Injection

13. Hold the syringe between the first two fingers and thumb of your dominant hand with the palm down and the bevel of the needle up. Figures B–G illustrate the steps used to administer an intradermal skin test.
14. Hold the skin taut with the fingers of your nondominant hand. If you are using the center of the forearm, then place the nondominant hand under the patient's arm and pull the skin taut. This will allow the needle to slip into the skin more easily.
15. Using a 15-degree angle, insert the needle through the skin to about 1/8 inch. The bevel of the needle will be facing upward and covered with skin. The needle will still show through the skin. Do not aspirate.
16. Slowly inject the medication beneath the surface of the skin. A small elevation of skin or wheal will occur where you have injected the medication.
17. Quickly withdraw the needle. With the other hand discard the needle into the sharps container.

III. Patient Follow-Up

18. Do not massage the area or place a bandage or tape on it, because this may irritate the site and lead to a false reading.

19. Make sure the patient is safe before leaving him or her unattended. Observe the patient for any untoward effect, such as an allergic reaction to the medication, for at least 20 to 30 minutes. Tell the patient not to rub the area. Instruct the patient to return to the office within 48 to 72 hours for the reading of the skin test. Make certain that the patient understands the directions and does not have any questions.
20. Correctly dispose of all materials.
21. Remove and discard gloves and perform hand hygiene.
22. Chart the medication administration on the patient's record noting the time, medication name, dosage, injection site, route, appearance of the intradermal site after injection, and your name.

CHARTING EXAMPLE

2/14/YY 10:00 A.M. Mantoux (PPD) tuberculin test, 0.10 mL ID Right anterior forearm. Instructed to return on 2/16 to have test read...M. King, CMA (AAMA)

settings for IV therapy gain popularity. Settings of this nature for IV administration are ideal only for patients who do not need advanced care and hospital services for close monitoring and treatment of their condition. However, medical office and outpatient settings are becoming more acceptable for IV therapy for a variety of reasons, including the following:

- **Preventing hospital admissions**—Outpatient IV therapy settings allow patients who require IV therapy to receive treatment without being hospitalized. This allows the patient to make scheduled appointments for IV therapy and continue on with their daily regimen without having to be hospitalized for the sole purpose of treatment.

- **Reduction in medical costs**—Using outpatient centers may allow patients to be discharged earlier from hospitals. This is much more cost effective for both patients without health care insurance and for insurance companies.

- **Patient satisfaction**—Most patients prefer to avoid hospitalization for IV therapy. This allows them more freedom in their schedule and allows them to spend more time with their family. Children who require IV therapy probably are more comfortable in a nonhospital environment.

Indications for Intravenous Therapy

Aside from being a route to administer medication, IV therapy is used for a number of additional indications. Administering blood and blood products, replacing lost fluids and correcting electrolyte imbalances, and aiding in the administration of nutritional supplements are just a few additional reasons that IV therapy is used.

Medications Commonly Administered Intravenously

Some medications that are commonly administered intravenously include:

- Chemotherapy medications
- Rheumatoid arthritis medications
- Antibiotics
- Monoclonal antibodies (used to treat inflammatory diseases)
- Analgesics

The IV administration of medications may be by *per unit dosage* or may be *continuous*. Examples of unit dosage are bolus, IV push, or scheduled intermittent administration by piggyback medication into an IV port or by a capped IV. An example of continuous dosage is an IV drip that may last several hours or around the clock. The flow rate of intravenous lines is regulated by a flow clamp or infusion pump.

Blood Products

Generally, patients with weakened immune systems require therapeutic blood products, which are administered intravenously, because these patients are often unable to produce their own antibodies. A common blood product administered in these cases is **immunoglobulin**, which contains antibodies.

Patients who have the bleeding disorder hemophilia are lacking clotting factors that are required for proper coagulation. These patients receive clotting factors by intravenous therapy.

Administration of blood products is not within the scope of practice of a medical assistant.

Special Requirements for Performing Intravenous Therapy

IV administration requires special knowledge and precautions, because it involves direct access to the bloodstream. Adverse reactions, which can be fatal, may be caused by the specific medication, by too many fluids administered too rapidly into the body, by violation of any of the rights of medication administration, or by certain preexisting medical conditions. Nonfatal reactions include necrosis of tissue (sometimes a reaction to chemotherapy), swelling, and infiltration through the blood vessel into the tissue, any of which will obstruct IV flow.

Any office in which IV fluid therapy is performed must have emergency equipment, emergency medical access, and established office policies for routine administration, for dealing with adverse reactions, and for handling emergencies. The patient and the infusion site must be assessed regularly during the infusion for signs of adverse reactions. The following should be reported to the physician immediately: any combination of redness, swelling, heat, bleeding, and loss of feeling at the site of the infusion.

The following information is provided only to acquaint you with the IV therapy process and should not be considered a competency.

Starting an IV requires preparation. Before an IV site is chosen, tubing is selected and connected to the correct solution container, following sterile technique. The tubing is flushed to remove all air. Tape and dressing supplies for the site must also be prepared beforehand. A preparation tray with appropriate IV starter materials and the prepared IV solution is taken to the patient. The IV solution is hung on an IV pole.

The IV site and the appropriate size and type of catheter are selected. The IV is generally started in the arm, although different medical scenarios may require other sites. The IV catheter includes an outer cannula to thread into the vein and an inner needle to serve as a guide for insertion and then to be removed. A constricting tourniquet is placed above the site. The skin is cleansed, and the catheter is introduced into the vein to obtain an open blood supply. The tourniquet is released and removed. The plastic cannula is advanced into the vein, and the needle is removed. To reduce the patient's anxiety, it is important to mention that the needle has been removed and that only the plastic cannula remains. As soon as the needle is removed and the blood supply has been established, the site is anchored with tape, the IV tubing is connected, and dressing of the site is completed. The IV is regulated with flow clamps or an IV pump as prescribed by the physician. Gloves are worn during the procedure as part of standard precautions. All needles and biohazard materials are disposed of according to office policy and OSHA standard precautions.

Preparing an Intravenous Tray and Observing Intravenous Therapy

The most important point about setting up an IV tray is that the medical assistant who does it must have been trained and possess the knowledge necessary to complete such a task (Procedure 54-12).

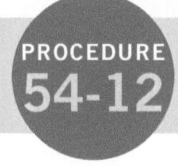

PROCEDURE 54-12 Preparing an Intravenous Tray

Objective ◆ *Prepare an intravenous (IV) tray.*

EQUIPMENT AND SUPPLIES

Absorbent disposable sheet; alcohol prep pads; Betadine swabs; disposable tourniquet; IV setup: IV tubing with attached filter; IV catheter; bag of IV fluid labeled with type and patient's name, date, time; paper tape; syringe; port cap; disposable gloves; gauze (2 × 2 or 4 × 4); IV setup tray; IV pole with pump

METHOD

1. Perform hand hygiene.
2. Apply gloves.
3. Prepare the IV fluid administration set:
   a. Inspect the fluid bag to make sure it contains desired fluid, that the fluid is clear, and that the bag is free from any leaks and has not expired.
   b. Select the correct administration set (either mini or macro drip) and uncoil the tubing, being careful that the ends of the tubing do not become contaminated.
   c. Close the flow regulator to the fluid bag.
   d. Remove the protective covering from the port of the fluid bag and the protective covering from the spike of the administration set.
   e. Insert the spike of the administration set into the port of the fluid bag with a quick twisting motion, being careful not to puncture yourself.

   f. While holding the fluid bag higher than the drip chamber of the administration set, squeeze the drip chamber once or twice to start the flow of the fluid. Fill the chamber to the marker line. If the chamber is overfilled, quickly lower the bag below the level of the drip chamber and squeeze some of the fluid back into the fluid bag.
   g. Open the flow regulator and allow the fluid to flush all the air from the tubing. A trash can or the wrapper the fluid came in can be used for the overflow of fluid.
   h. Turn off the flow and place the sterile cap back on the end of the administration set (if you had to remove it). Then place this end nearby so it can be easily reached by the person ready to connect it to the IV catheter in the patient's arm.
4. Place the absorbent disposable sheet on the tray.
5. Assemble equipment and supplies on the tray in order of use.
6. If using an IV pole or pump, hang the IV solution (bag) on the pole; do not set it up or calculate drops in the pump; this will be done by the person starting the IV.
7. Notify the appropriate personnel (RN, LVN, physician) that the IV tray setup is ready for administration.
8. Remove and discard the gloves and perform hand hygiene.
9. Document the procedure.
10. Clean the work area and equipment according to OSHA guidelines.

Before preparing the IV tray, make sure to carefully read the facility's requirements for this procedure. Instructions for preparing an IV tray are frequently included in the office or hospital procedure manual. Once preparation of the IV tray has been completed, make sure that you check the doctor's order as to what IV fluid solution is required. When checking the order, remember to check for the following:

- It is the right patient.
- It is the right solution.
- It is the right drug.
- It is the right technique.
- It is the right route.
- The solution is properly labeled with the patient's name, the date and time of administration, and the name of the doctor who ordered it.

Once you have determined that you have the right solution, you will have to prepare the IV administration set. Most facilities have disposable IV administration sets that are ready for use. After you have completed setting up the IV administration set along with your other supplies, they should all be placed on a separate IV or Mayo tray. Make sure you position the items in the order of their usage. Finally, after you have completed the tray setup, notify whoever is going to start the IV that the tray is ready for the patient.

The Medical Assistant's Role in Intravenous Therapy

Your role as a medical assistant often includes not only setting up the IV tray, but also being available to provide the patient with reassurance during the procedure. If you are present during the procedure, you should understand and be able to recognize some of the possible side effects that intravenous therapy can cause, such as infections at the site of the needle; phlebitis, which is inflammation of the vein; and the most common side effect, infiltration.

Infiltration occurs when the tip of the IV catheter withdraws from the vein or pokes through the vein into surrounding tissue, or when the vein's wall becomes permeable and leaks, so that IV fluid infuses the tissues outside the intravascular space (outside the vein). Infiltration is frequently encountered with peripheral IVs and almost always requires replacement of the IV at a different location.

Other possible reactions that may occur during IV therapy include bleeding or drainage from the area of insertion; redness, pain, or swelling in the area of insertion; blood backing up into the tubing; and the needle or tube coming loose or being removed by the patient.

If you observe signs of any of these adverse reactions, you must bring them to the attention of personnel who are conducting the therapy (if they have not become aware of them) and immediately inform the physician.

After the procedure has been completed, it may be your responsibility to ensure the patient and the area have been cleaned up and that the equipment and supplies have been properly placed where they belong. Most facilities require only that you document the procedure you performed for setting up the tray. Documentation of the actual IV procedure is done only by the person who has started the IV infusion.

IMMUNIZATIONS

Immunizations or **vaccines** are given to humans to decrease their susceptibility to disease. The immunized human body can resist the invasion of germs that would otherwise cause the disease the person has been immunized against. If an individual's own natural immune system is compromised, then the individual is more at risk of becoming sick.

Antibodies are protein substances produced by lymphocytes in the bone marrow, in the spleen, and in the lymph nodes and tissues. Antibodies respond to defend against antigens or foreign substances. This defensive process of the body occurs when an individual contracts an illness, such as the measles. During the illness, the body begins to develop antibodies to fight off the disease. After the individual has recovered from the illness, the individual is less likely to contract the same illness again. In the case of measles, the person may get measles again but not the same strain of measles, because the body has developed antibodies to fight off this disease, and the body will always retain its ability to defend against that same disease. When this occurs, the individual is said to have developed **immunity**, or a resistance, to the disease.

Immunity can be either natural (inborn) or acquired. Antibodies are not involved when natural immunity occurs. Acquired immunity, however, does involve the development of antibodies. The development of this type of immunity may be either natural or artificial and may be acquired either through an active or a passive means.

Artificially acquired active immunity to a certain disease develops in response to receiving a vaccination with inactive (dead) or attenuated (weakened) organisms of that disease. The individual receives just enough of the disease organism to develop antibodies against it but not enough to become ill.

Through the delivery of immunizations and vaccines, an individual or a whole population of individuals can be prepared to fight off a disease. For instance, the flu vaccine is given each year right before the flu season begins. Individuals who are more susceptible to contracting the flu and being severely affected by it, or even dying from it, such as children and older adults, are particularly encouraged to receive the flu vaccine. By receiving the flu vaccine, individuals establish immunity to the flu and increase their chances of being able to fight off the disease entirely or, if they contract the flu, probably have a less severe case of it. (Ironically, older adults, who may most benefit from the flu vaccine, tend to be less well protected by the vaccine than younger people. Nevertheless, the protection older adults do receive is valuable.)

Each year the Centers for Disease Control and Prevention (CDC) recommends that certain individuals receive the influenza vaccination. These individuals usually include the following:

- Children aged 6 months up to their 19th birthday
- Pregnant women
- People 50 years of age and older
- People of any age with certain chronic medical conditions
- People who live in nursing homes and other long-term care facilities
- People who live with or care for those at high risk for complications from flu, including:
  a. Health care workers
  b. Household contacts of persons at high risk for complications from the flu
  c. Household contacts and out-of-home caregivers of children less than 6 months of age (these children are too young to be vaccinated)

As already noted, immunizations or vaccines are produced by taking a dead or weakened infectious agent of a disease and injecting it into the human body. Typically, this creates no harm to the patient. Sometimes an immunization or vaccine can cause an individual to experience some mild symptoms of the disease or to develop inflammation at the site of injection. For example, some children, after receiving the diphtheria, tetanus, and pertussis vaccine (DTaP), experience some redness and swelling where the injection was given. A fever may also be a temporary symptom. (To learn more, refer to the chapter titled "The Immune System.")

Childhood and Adolescent Immunizations

An annual recommended childhood and adolescent immunization schedule is issued each year by the American Academy of Pediatrics, the Advisory Committee on Immunization

Practices of the CDC, and the American Academy of Family Physicians. The schedule indicates the recommended ages for routine administration of childhood vaccines (Figure 54-16).

In addition, the CDC provides vaccine information sheets (VIS) that are to be given to parents or guardians before the administration of a vaccine to a child. The parent or guardian is generally required to sign a statement acknowledging receipt of the VIS and consenting to the immunization administration. Figure 54-17 provides a sample VIS for the varicella vaccine discussed later in this chapter.

Diphtheria Vaccine

Diphtheria is an acute infectious disease. Transmission of diphtheria is by direct and indirect contact and is diagnosed by obtaining a throat culture. Individuals with diphtheria typically experience symptoms such as headache, fever, and sore throat. Diphtheria is treatable but can be quite serious. The vaccine for diphtheria is given to children in five separate doses. The fifth dose is given between the age of 4 and 6 years.

Pertussis Vaccine

Pertussis, also known as whooping cough, is a respiratory disease that is most common in children under the age of 4 years. It is known as whooping cough because one of the symptoms is a violent cough with a whooping sound. Pertussis is caused by bacteria and is transmitted by direct and indirect contact. Once a child is immunized with the pertussis vaccine, the child is no longer susceptible to contracting this disease.

Tetanus Vaccine

Tetanus is a disease of the nervous system and is caused by a bacterium that enters the body through a break in the skin. Individuals with tetanus may experience fever, elevated blood pressure, and severe muscle spasms. Tetanus is not contagious and rarely occurs in individuals living in the

Figure 1. Recommended immunization schedule for persons aged 0 through 18 years – United States, 2016.

(FOR THOSE WHO FALL BEHIND OR START LATE, SEE THE CATCH-UP SCHEDULE [FIGURE 2]).

These recommendations must be read with the footnotes that follow. For those who fall behind or start late, provide catch-up vaccination at the earliest opportunity as indicated by the green bars in Figure 1. To determine minimum intervals between doses, see the catch-up schedule (Figure 2). School entry and adolescent vaccine age groups are shaded.

Vaccine	Birth	1 mo	2 mos	4 mos	6 mos	9 mos	12 mos	15 mos	18 mos	19–23 mos	2-3 yrs	4-6 yrs	7-10 yrs	11-12 yrs	13–15 yrs	16–18 yrs
Hepatitis B¹ (HepB)	1ˢᵗ dose	◄---- 2ⁿᵈ dose ----►			◄-------------------- 3ʳᵈ dose -------------------►											
Rotavirus² (RV) RV1 (2-dose series); RV5 (3-dose series)			1ˢᵗ dose	2ⁿᵈ dose	See footnote 2											
Diphtheria, tetanus, & acellular pertussis³ (DTaP: <7 yrs)			1ˢᵗ dose	2ⁿᵈ dose	3ʳᵈ dose		◄------ 4ᵗʰ dose ------►					5ᵗʰ dose				
Haemophilus influenzae type b⁴ (Hib)			1ˢᵗ dose	2ⁿᵈ dose	See footnote 4		3ʳᵈ or 4ᵗʰ dose, See footnote 4									
Pneumococcal conjugate⁵ (PCV13)			1ˢᵗ dose	2ⁿᵈ dose	3ʳᵈ dose		◄------ 4ᵗʰ dose ------►									
Inactivated poliovirus⁶ (IPV: <18 yrs)			1ˢᵗ dose	2ⁿᵈ dose	◄-------------------- 3ʳᵈ dose -------------------►							4ᵗʰ dose				
Influenza⁷ (IIV; LAIV)						Annual vaccination (IIV only) 1 or 2 doses						Annual vaccination (LAIV or IIV) 1 or 2 doses		Annual vaccination (LAIV or IIV) 1 dose only		
Measles, mumps, rubella⁸ (MMR)						See footnote 8	◄------ 1ˢᵗ dose ------►					2ⁿᵈ dose				
Varicella⁹ (VAR)							◄------ 1ˢᵗ dose ------►					2ⁿᵈ dose				
Hepatitis A¹⁰ (HepA)							◄------- 2-dose series, See footnote 10 -------►									
Meningococcal¹¹ (Hib-MenCY ≥ 6 weeks; MenACWY-D ≥9 mos; MenACWY-CRM ≥ 2 mos)					See footnote 11									1ˢᵗ dose		Booster
Tetanus, diphtheria, & acellular pertussis¹² (Tdap: ≥7 yrs)												(Tdap)				
Human papillomavirus¹³ (2vHPV: females only; 4vHPV, 9vHPV: males and females)														(3-dose series)		
Meningococcal B¹¹														See footnote 11		
Pneumococcal polysaccharide⁵ (PPSV23)												See footnote 5				

| ▨ Range of recommended ages for all children | ▨ Range of recommended ages for catch-up immunization | ▨ Range of recommended ages for certain high-risk groups | ▨ Range of recommended ages for non-high-risk groups that may receive vaccine, subject to individual clinical decision making | ☐ No recommendation |

This schedule includes recommendations in effect as of January 1, 2016. Any dose not administered at the recommended age should be administered at a subsequent visit, when indicated and feasible. The use of a combination vaccine generally is preferred over separate injections of its equivalent component vaccines. Vaccination providers should consult the relevant Advisory Committee on Immunization Practices (ACIP) statement for detailed recommendations, available online at http://www.cdc.gov/vaccines/hcp/acip-recs/index.html. Clinically significant adverse events that follow vaccination should be reported to the Vaccine Adverse Event Reporting System (VAERS) online (http://www.vaers.hhs.gov) or by telephone (800-822-7967). Suspected cases of vaccine-preventable diseases should be reported to the state or local health department. Additional information, including precautions and contraindications for vaccination, is available from CDC online (http://www.cdc.gov/vaccines/recs/vac-admin/contraindications.htm) or by telephone (800-CDC-INFO [800-232-4636]).

This schedule is approved by the Advisory Committee on Immunization Practices (http://www.cdc.gov/vaccines/acip), the American Academy of Pediatrics (http://www.aap.org), the American Academy of Family Physicians (http://www.aafp.org), and the American College of Obstetricians and Gynecologists (http://www.acog.org).

NOTE: The above recommendations must be read along with the footnotes of this schedule.

FIGURE 54-16 Recommended childhood and adolescent immunization schedule, 2016.

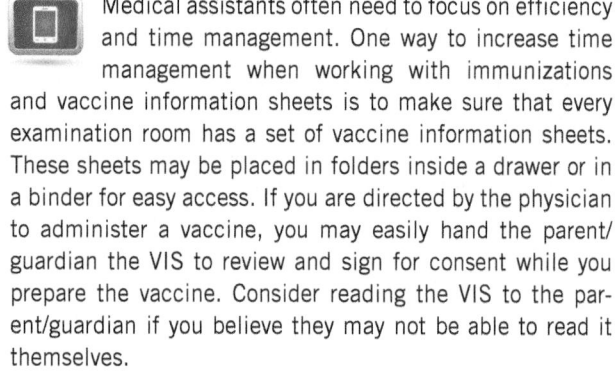

Professionalism ▶ The Workplace

Medical assistants often need to focus on efficiency and time management. One way to increase time management when working with immunizations and vaccine information sheets is to make sure that every examination room has a set of vaccine information sheets. These sheets may be placed in folders inside a drawer or in a binder for easy access. If you are directed by the physician to administer a vaccine, you may easily hand the parent/guardian the VIS to review and sign for consent while you prepare the vaccine. Consider reading the VIS to the parent/guardian if you believe they may not be able to read it themselves.

United States. Occurrence of death with tetanus is low but can occur in people over the age of 60.

DTaP Vaccine. When children receive a vaccine for tetanus, it is usually given in a combination vaccine of diphtheria,

tetanus, and pertussis also known as the DTaP vaccine. Five DTaP shots are required to fully protect a child. The last booster is given between the ages of 4 and 6 years. If a child has a reaction to the first dose of DTaP, the child will then, depending on age, be given the tetanus and diphtheria (Td) vaccine or the diphtheria and tetanus toxoids (DT) vaccine. The Td vaccine does not contain pertussis vaccine and contains less diphtheria toxoid than what is contained in the DTaP vaccine. The DT vaccine, which contains diphtheria and tetanus toxoids but no pertussis, may be given to children who have a reaction to their first dose of the DTaP vaccine. The Td vaccine is given to children 7 years and older, and the DT vaccine is given to children under the age of 7.

Haemophilus Influenzae Type B (Hib) Conjugate Vaccine

Although the **Hib disease** is not well known, a recent statistic from the CDC indicated that 1 out of every 200 children in the United States under the age of 5 years contracts Hib. Meningitis, which is a result of Hib, affects about 12,000 children a year. Hib is caused by a bacterium, is spread

1352   UNIT 4 Clinical Medical Assisting

through the air, and enters the lungs or bloodstream. The Hib vaccine became available in 1985, and since then the cases of Hib disease have decreased dramatically.

Hepatitis A Vaccine

Hepatitis A, which is caused by a virus, is the most common type of hepatitis in the United States. Hepatitis A affects the liver but does not cause long-term effects. It is spread through personal contact or by eating contaminated food or drinking contaminated water. The vaccine is given to children 2 years or older to prevent the risk of contracting hepatitis A. It is recommended that children who live in Alaska, Arizona, and Oregon should receive the vaccine because of high disease incidence. Individuals who travel to other countries are also encouraged to obtain this vaccine.

Hepatitis B Vaccine

Hepatitis B is caused by the hepatitis B virus (HBV) and is transmitted by contaminated serum in blood transfusions or through the use of contaminated needles or instruments.

VACCINE INFORMATION STATEMENT

Chickenpox Vaccine
What You Need to Know

> Many Vaccine Information Statements are available in Spanish and other languages. See www.immunize.org/vis
>
> Hojas de información sobre vacunas están disponibles en español y en muchos otros idiomas. Visite www.immunize.org/vis

1 Why get vaccinated?

Chickenpox (also called varicella) is a common childhood disease. It is usually mild, but it can be serious, especially in young infants and adults.

- It causes a rash, itching, fever, and tiredness.
- It can lead to severe skin infection, scars, pneumonia, brain damage, or death.
- The chickenpox virus can be spread from person to person through the air, or by contact with fluid from chickenpox blisters.
- A person who has had chickenpox can get a painful rash called shingles years later.
- Before the vaccine, about 11,000 people were hospitalized for chickenpox each year in the United States.
- Before the vaccine, about 100 people died each year as a result of chickenpox in the United States.

Chickenpox vaccine can prevent chickenpox.

Most people who get chickenpox vaccine will not get chickenpox. But if someone who has been vaccinated does get chickenpox, it is usually very mild. They will have fewer blisters, are less likely to have a fever, and will recover faster.

2 Who should get chickenpox vaccine and when?

Routine
Children who have never had chickenpox should get 2 doses of chickenpox vaccine at these ages:

1st Dose:	12–15 months of age
2nd Dose:	4–6 years of age (may be given earlier, if at least 3 months after the 1st dose)

People 13 years of age and older (who have never had chickenpox or received chickenpox vaccine) should get two doses at least 28 days apart.

Catch-up
Anyone who is not fully vaccinated, and never had chickenpox, should receive one or two doses of chickenpox vaccine. The timing of these doses depends on the person's age. Ask your doctor.

Chickenpox vaccine may be given at the same time as other vaccines.

> Note: A "combination" vaccine called **MMRV**, which contains both chickenpox and MMR vaccines, may be given instead of the two individual vaccines to people 12 years of age and younger.

3 Some people should not get chickenpox vaccine or should wait.

- People should not get chickenpox vaccine if they have ever had a life-threatening allergic reaction to a previous dose of chickenpox vaccine or to gelatin or the antibiotic neomycin.
- People who are moderately or severely ill at the time the shot is scheduled should usually wait until they recover before getting chickenpox vaccine.
- Pregnant women should wait to get chickenpox vaccine until after they have given birth. Women should not get pregnant for 1 month after getting chickenpox vaccine.
- Some people should check with their doctor about whether they should get chickenpox vaccine, including anyone who:
  - Has HIV/AIDS or another disease that affects the immune system
  - Is being treated with drugs that affect the immune system, such as steroids, for 2 weeks or longer
  - Has any kind of cancer
  - Is getting cancer treatment with radiation or drugs
- People who recently had a transfusion or were given other blood products should ask their doctor when they may get chickenpox vaccine.

Ask your doctor for more information.

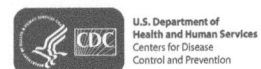

U.S. Department of Health and Human Services Centers for Disease Control and Prevention

FIGURE 54-17 Vaccine Information Sheet (VIS) provided by the CDC for the varicella vaccination. (*Continues*)

4 | **What are the risks from chickenpox vaccine?**

A vaccine, like any medicine, is capable of causing serious problems, such as severe allergic reactions. The risk of chickenpox vaccine causing serious harm, or death, is extremely small.

Getting chickenpox vaccine is much safer than getting chickenpox disease. Most people who get chickenpox vaccine do not have any problems with it. Reactions are usually more likely after the first dose than after the second.

Mild problems
- Soreness or swelling where the shot was given (about 1 out of 5 children and up to 1 out of 3 adolescents and adults)
- Fever (1 person out of 10, or less)
- Mild rash, up to a month after vaccination (1 person out of 25). It is possible for these people to infect other members of their household, but this is extremely rare.

Moderate problems
- Seizure (jerking or staring) caused by fever (very rare)

Severe problems
- Pneumonia (very rare)

Other serious problems, including severe brain reactions and low blood count, have been reported after chickenpox vaccination. These happen so rarely experts cannot tell whether they are caused by the vaccine or not. If they are, it is extremely rare.

Note: The first dose of **MMRV** vaccine has been associated with rash and higher rates of fever than MMR and varicella vaccines given separately. Rash has been reported in about 1 person in 20 and fever in about 1 person in 5.

Seizures caused by a fever are also reported more often after MMRV. These usually occur 5–12 days after the first dose.

5 | **What if there is a serious reaction?**

What should I look for?
- Look for anything that concerns you, such as signs of a severe allergic reaction, very high fever, or behavior changes.

Signs of a severe allergic reaction can include hives, swelling of the face and throat, difficulty breathing, a fast heartbeat, dizziness, and weakness. These would start a few minutes to a few hours after the vaccination.

What should I do?
- If you think it is a severe allergic reaction or other emergency that can't wait, call 9-1-1 or get the person to the nearest hospital. Otherwise, call your doctor.
- Afterward, the reaction should be reported to the Vaccine Adverse Event Reporting System (VAERS). Your doctor might file this report, or you can do it yourself through the VAERS web site at **www.vaers.hhs.gov**, or by calling **1-800-822-7967**.

VAERS is only for reporting reactions. They do not give medical advice.

6 | **The National Vaccine Injury Compensation Program**

The National Vaccine Injury Compensation Program (VICP) is a federal program that was created to compensate people who may have been injured by certain vaccines.

Persons who believe they may have been injured by a vaccine can learn about the program and about filing a claim by calling **1-800-338-2382** or visiting the VICP website at **www.hrsa.gov/vaccinecompensation**.

7 | **How can I learn more?**
- Ask your doctor.
- Call your local or state health department.
- Contact the Centers for Disease Control and Prevention (CDC):
  - Call **1-800-232-4636** (**1-800-CDC-INFO**) or
  - Visit CDC's website at **www.cdc.gov/vaccines**

Vaccine Information Statement (Interim)
Varicella Vaccine

3/13/2008

42 U.S.C. § 300aa-26

Office Use Only

FIGURE 54-17 Vaccine Information Sheet (VIS) provided by the CDC for the varicella vaccination. (*Continued*)

Hepatitis B is a form of viral hepatitis, is highly contagious, and can be fatal. By immunizing children, the potential of this disease becoming an epidemic is minimized. It is recommended that soon after birth all infants be given the first dose of hepatitis B. Only infants whose mother's hepatitis B surface antigen (HBsAg) is negative may be given the first dose by age 2 months. A child should receive a total of four doses of the vaccine. The last dose should not be given to the infant before age 24 weeks. When delivering the hepatitis B vaccine, special attention should be paid to the CDC's vaccination requirements for infants born to HBsAg-positive mothers or infants born to mothers whose HBsAg status is unknown.

Human Papillomavirus (HPV) Vaccine

Human papillomavirus (HPV) is a virus that can infect sexually active males and females and, in some who are infected, cause genital warts or cancer of the cervix, vulva, vagina, penis, and anus, or of the oropharynx as a result of oral sex.

Two vaccines are available to prevent some types of HPV infection: Gardasil and Cervatrix. The Centers for Disease Control recommends vaccination of 11- and 12-year-old girls (the vaccine can be given as early as age 9) before girls become sexually active. HPV vaccine can also be given to females age 13 through 26 years of age. HPV vaccine can also be administered to boys at the same ages recommended for girls and to adult males up to the age of 26.

Measles, Mumps, and Rubella (MMR) Vaccine

The **measles, mumps, and rubella (MMR) vaccine** is given to children to protect them from developing measles, mumps, and rubella. Once a child is given the MMR, the child is protected for life. The MMR is given in two doses. If necessary, the vaccines for measles, mumps, and rubella can also be given separately. Because of the MMR vaccine, very few children today contract these diseases.

A virus causes measles, and before development of the measles vaccine, almost all children came down with the measles. Measles is extremely serious and can result in brain damage, deafness, or death.

Mumps was also a very common childhood disease before the development of the vaccine. Mumps is not as serious a disease as the measles but could result in some undesired side effects, including meningitis, encephalitis, and deafness.

Rubella, also known as German measles or three-day measles, is typically a mild disease that affects an individual for about 24 hours. Rubella is caused by a virus and is spread through close contact. Rubella can strike adults and unborn children. Unborn babies can be infected if the woman gets rubella early in the pregnancy. If a pregnant woman does have rubella, there is a high probability that the infant will be born with birth defects. Since the development of the rubella vaccine, only several hundred cases are reported each year.

Pneumococcal Vaccine

The **pneumococcal vaccine**, until very recently, was not licensed for children under the age of 2 years. Typically, older adults have received this vaccine to protect them from contracting the *Streptococcus pneumonia* bacteria. According to the CDC, this bacterium kills more people in the United States each year than any other vaccine-preventable disease. By obtaining the vaccine, individuals are protected against the seven strains of the pneumococcal bacterium. The pneumococcal bacteria are spread through the air. Winter and early spring are the most common seasons when pneumococcal infections occur.

Varicella Vaccine

Varicella, or chickenpox, is one of the most common childhood diseases. Chickenpox, thus named because of the blisters that look like chickpeas, is caused by a virus and is spread through the air. Although chickenpox is an uncomfortable illness, it is usually not serious. The varicella vaccine became licensed in the United States in 1995, and since then the number of varicella cases has diminished significantly. Although the vaccine has not eradicated the disease, it has dramatically lowered the percentage of individuals infected by it.

Polio Vaccine

Polio is caused by a virus and is spread through contact with the feces of an infected person. Although paralysis is not a result for all individuals who contract polio, it is an event that does affect some children.

Since 1955 the polio vaccine has been available, resulting in the disappearance of the disease in the United States. However, polio is still common in some parts of the world. A polio epidemic could appear in the United States caused by individuals bringing in the disease from another country. Thus, it is important that children even in the United States be immunized.

There are two types of polio vaccines: **inactivated polio vaccine (IPV)** and live **oral polio vaccine (OPV)**. For many years, children received the polio vaccine orally (OPV) rather than by injection (IPV). Because the oral polio vaccine was found in rare situations to cause polio in children, it is now recommended that all children receive the polio vaccine by injection.

Adult and Other Immunizations

In addition to the influenza vaccination, adults 65 years of age and older should receive the pneumococcal polysaccharide vaccine (PPV) and the shingles vaccine (Zostavax).

Adults and children who travel abroad must also obtain, before travel, the additional vaccines, immunizations, and preventive medications recommended by the CDC. The recommendations are categorized according to the region of travel. For instance, if you were to travel to South Asia, vaccine and medication recommendations would include hepatitis A, hepatitis B, malaria, and typhoid; the recommendations might be different for Africa, and so on.

JUDGMENT CALL

Grayson Tolley is a medical assisting student at an externship site. A medical assistant rushes by him with a syringe in her hand. She stops and says, "Oh, you need the practice! Give this injection!" What should Grayson say or do?

SUMMARY

Administering a medication is one of the medical assistant's most important duties and responsibilities. The medical assistant is expected to be knowledgeable about the medication and its side effects. Medications come in many forms including oral, parenteral, and inhalants. Medications are always given under the supervision of the physician. The physician must be physically present within the facility at the time that the medical assistant dispenses the medication.

When administering medications, the medical assistant must always observe the "three befores" and the "10 rights."

Although errors rarely occur, if an error does occur, notice must be given immediately to a supervisor so that the situation can be handled quickly for the safety and well-being of the patient.

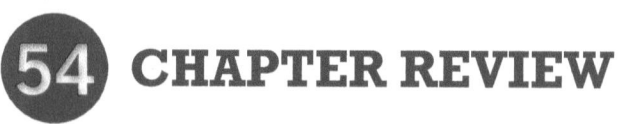

54 CHAPTER REVIEW

COMPETENCY REVIEW

1. Define and spell the terms for this chapter.
2. What are the "10 rights" of drug administration?
3. List the "three befores" of drug administration.
4. When giving an injection, what would you do if you see a return of blood in the syringe when you aspirate?
5. Identify specific instructions that should be given to patients regarding measuring liquid medications.

6. List topical forms of medications that are applied to mucous membranes.
7. Explain how the lumen of the needle relates to the sizing of the needle.
8. Identify when medical assistants must follow standard precautions.

PREPARING FOR THE CERTIFICATION EXAM

1. When administering oral or sublingual medication, which of the following is *not* required?
   a. Assemble all the equipment and use aseptic technique.
   b. Select the correct medication using the "three befores."
   c. Double-check the label on the medication.
   d. Identify the patient by name and date of birth.
   e. Provide the patient with a vaccine information sheet.

2. When giving parenteral medication, a smaller gauge needle is used for which type of injection?
   a. intramuscular
   b. Z-track
   c. subcutaneous
   d. intradermal
   e. intravenous

3. Subcutaneous injections are administered at an angle of
   a. 15 degrees.
   b. 90 degrees.
   c. 45 degrees.
   d. 5 to 10 degrees.
   e. 25 degrees.

4. How many mL can be safely injected into a large adult ventrogluteal muscle?
   a. up to 1 mL
   b. up to 1.5 mL
   c. up to 2 mL
   d. up to 2.5 mL
   e. up to 3 mL

5. Which of the following is *not* a common site for intradermal injections?
   a. right forearm
   b. anterior chest
   c. upper back
   d. abdomen
   e. left forearm

6. Which vaccine guards against chickenpox?
   a. DTaP
   b. varicella
   c. CPV
   d. IPV
   e. tetanus

7. Which is the preferred location for intramuscular injections on a toddler?
   a. deltoid
   b. vastus lateralis
   c. gluteus medius
   d. gluteus maximus
   e. biceps

8. What connects the needle to the syringe?
   a. flange
   b. hilt
   c. hub
   d. shaft
   e. barrel

9. A tuberculosis test has to be read within how many hours after being administered?
   a. 12 hours
   b. 24 hours
   c. 48 hours
   d. 36 hours
   e. 16 hours

10. The Hib vaccine helps protect against
    a. human papillomavirus.
    b. meningitis.
    c. tuberculosis.
    d. hepatitis B.
    e. tetanus.

CRITICAL THINKING

Refer to the case study at the beginning of the chapter and use what you have learned to answer the following questions.

1. How should Samra proceed to follow Dr. Miller's instructions?
2. What should Samra do to help her administer the medication to the patient?
3. Because Owen's babysitter has brought him in for the office visit, will Samra need to obtain parental permission before administering the medication?

ON THE JOB

Mrs. Conners comes into Dr. Tyler's office to be seen for a sore throat and fever. The examination reveals that Mrs. Conners has tonsillitis. Dr. Tyler writes an order in the patient's chart for an injection of antibiotic to be given today. The patient is also given a prescription for an oral antibiotic to be taken for the next 10 days.

Joe, the medical assistant, while administering the injection to Mrs. Conners, accidentally punctures his finger with the needle that has been inside Mrs. Conners. What is your response?

1. What should Joe do?
2. Is an incident report necessary?
3. If an incident report is filed, where should it be placed?

INTERNET ACTIVITY

Choose three common drugs and perform searches to get information about them. Select nationally recognized websites that you know you can access again when seeking information for patients. The Health On the Net Foundation (HON) offers advice about Internet sources of trustworthy medical information. Search the site at www.hon.ch.

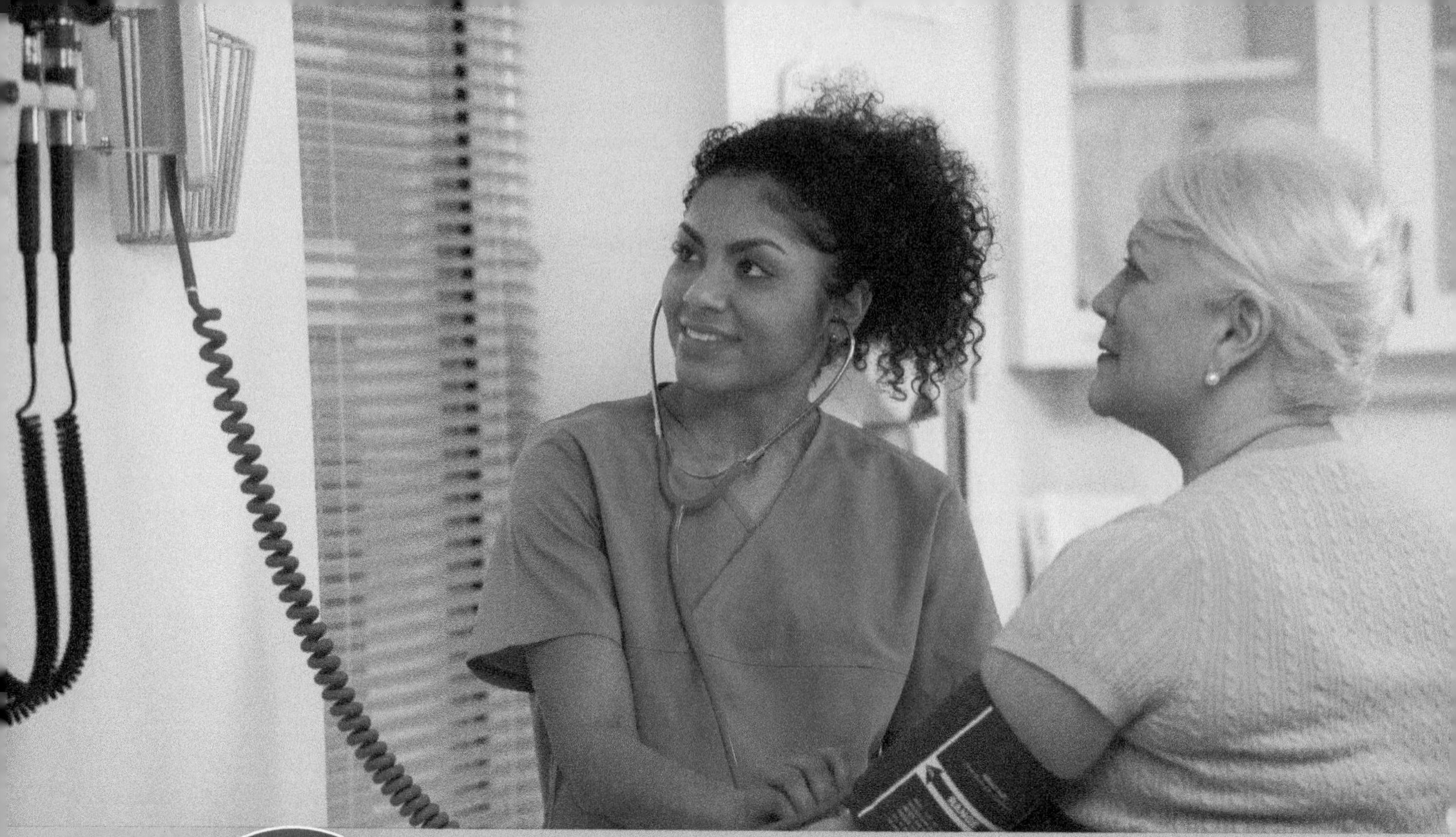

CHAPTER 55

Patient Education

Learning Objectives

After completing this chapter, you should be able to:

55.1 Define and spell the terms for this chapter.
55.2 Explain patient coaching as it relates to health maintenance.
55.3 Explain patient coaching as it relates to disease prevention.
55.4 Explain patient coaching as it relates to treatment plan compliance.
55.5 Describe elements that a medical assistant must understand when developing patient-centered education.
55.6 Explain how patient education would be adapted for a child.
55.7 Explain how patient education would be adapted for patients with special needs.
55.8 Explain how patient education would be adapted for an older adult.
55.9 Identify how cultural diversity impacts patient education.
55.10 Describe how community resources can benefit patients.

Pearson Physicians Group has decided to begin offering group patient education classes for its patients who struggle with a variety of health-related issues. The office manager, Tania Washington, will organize the classes. Although the physicians will retain final approval on all decisions, they have given Tania a lot of freedom and responsibility for designing the new patient education programs.

Terms to Learn

assessment	document	noncompliance
community resources	evaluation	patient coach
compliance	implementing	plan
dexterity		

P atient education is an important component of health care delivery and treatment. In fact, patient education is a right: All patients have the right to receive information on how to manage their own health needs. You, the medical assistant, will often be the staff member who provides physician-approved patient education. The rapport between a patient and a medical assistant—the patient's ability to relate to the health care team—is critical in this process. Patients will get to know you as you escort them into the examination room, assist during the examination, and summarize and review information with the patient when the exam is complete. The patient's familiarity and comfort level with you helps the learning process.

THE PATIENT COACH

Medical assistants play an important role throughout the process of patient care as a **patient coach**. As the name implies, a patient coach helps the patient by providing support, explaining things that might be difficult to understand, serving as a source of encouragement and help, and educating patients on a variety of topics. It is important for the medical assistant to understand that any information that could be perceived as patient education must first be approved by a physician or other licensed health care provider (such as a registered dietician or physician's assistant) before being shared with a patient. As a patient coach the medical assistant may help educate patients in the areas of health maintenance, disease prevention, and treatment plan compliance, just to name a few. Medical assistants must also understand how to coach patients who are noncompliant.

Health Maintenance

Educating and coaching patients regarding health maintenance involves a variety of issues. Health maintenance centers on the idea of a patient's overall wellness. Wellness is the ongoing process of practicing a healthy lifestyle (Figure 55-1). Balancing physical and psychologic stress and reducing overreaction to stressors can improve wellness. Patients must choose to practice behaviors that improve wellness and decrease illness. Proper coaching from you, the medical assistant, can empower the patient to make positive life changes. Some of the life changes that should be encouraged include a proper diet (this is discussed in the chapter titled "Nutrition"), exercising at least 30 minutes a day for five days a week, and the proper use of multivitamins.

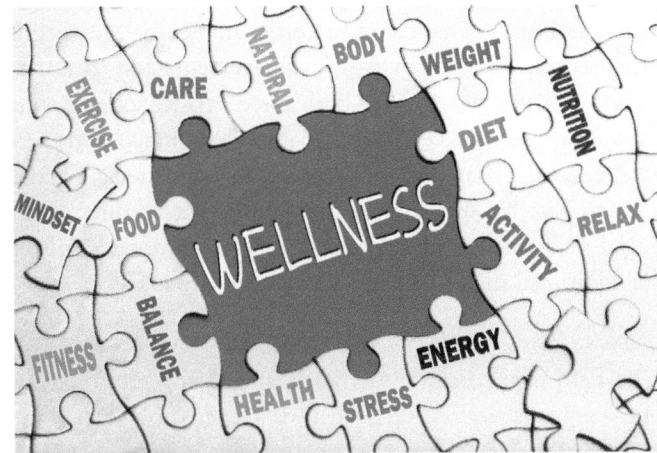

FIGURE 55-1 Patients must understand that there are many pieces to the wellness puzzle that need to be addressed in order to maintain a healthy life.

TABLE 55-1	Wellness Guidelines

- Keep a positive attitude.
- Cherish your values.
- Exercise your mind, body, and spirit.
- Control your stress.
- Soothe your fears.
- Think happy thoughts.
- Stay active.
- Challenge your mind.
- Forgive and forget.
- Avoid dangerous drugs.
- Watch your sugar intake.
- Walk briskly.
- Enjoy the outdoors.
- Maintain a healthy weight.
- Eat a well-balanced diet.
- Rinse fresh fruits and vegetables before eating.
- Practice cleanliness.
- Take medications as directed.
- Stop smoking.
- Lower your blood pressure and cholesterol.
- Learn to breathe deeply.

TABLE 55-2	Common Risk Factors

- Smoking or tobacco product use
- Poor physical fitness
- High alcohol intake
- Poor diet and nutrition
- Disregarding auto safety measures
- High stress level
- Occupational health and environmental hazards
- Drug abuse
- Lack of immunizations
- Poor dental care
- High or very low blood pressure
- Family history of cancer, heart attack, stroke, or diabetes
- Unsafe sexual practices
- High or very low heart rate
- Unhealthy body mass index (BMI)
- Risk-taking behavior

Role-modeling healthy behaviors is important. If your uniform or breath smells of cigarette smoke, it is unlikely that the patient will respect your teaching on smoking cessation. Positive reinforcement when a patient performs can be very powerful. If you commend the patient for doing even a little bit of exercise, the patient will be more likely to continue exercising and develop a healthy habit after being recognized for making an effort. See Table 55-1 for some wellness guidelines that can be taught to patients. These guidelines can be discussed during patient education sessions that focus on overall wellness and the patient's health.

In a world saturated with advancing technology, smartphones, and tablets, there is an increasing number of applications (apps) focused on health and wellness and improving a patient's health. These apps are often interactive, requiring the user (the patient) to record achievements and data. For example, MyFitnessPal® has both a free website and free apps that allow users to keep track of daily caloric intake and exercise. For additional motivation, such resources often allow the user to post his successes and accomplishments directly on social media sites such as Facebook, Instagram, and Twitter for additional support and encouragement from friends.

Disease Prevention

The field of medicine deals with diagnosing and treating those who are sick and unhealthy. It is incredibly important in today's society, to focus on preventative measures that can reduce risk for illness and disease. As mentioned previously, health and wellness plays an overall role in patient coaching and education, but so does the topic of disease prevention.

Obviously, it is preferable that patients not become sick. Many illnesses are related to lifestyle behaviors—for example, smoking tobacco, overeating, and lack of exercise. Continuously high stress levels can affect the immune system. Drug abuse leads to addiction and toleration of medications. On the other hand, routine immunization and diagnostic tests can prevent diseases. Sometimes it is necessary to reinforce the importance of even simple daily tasks that can play a role in disease prevention, such as basic hygiene. Proper handwashing techniques, coughing into an elbow, daily bathing and grooming habits, including proper dental care, are all components of disease prevention.

Patients must also be able to identify personal risk factors for disease so that they can be encouraged to address these factors and take action to control the future of their health. Table 55-2 identifies common risk factors that often lead to disease. The ability to tactfully and professionally discuss these items with patients is an important component of patient coaching.

Treatment Plan Compliance

An important aspect of healthcare is patient **compliance** with the treatment plan. This refers to the patient's ability to follow through on all suggestions and orders as given by the physician. For instance, a patient who has diabetes may have a treatment plan that requires oral medications to be taken on a daily basis, at-home blood glucose monitoring three times a day, routine bloodwork every three months, and routine office visits. In order for a patient to be compliant with a treatment plan, the patient must understand all of the components of the plan and why the plan is necessary for health and wellness. Medical assistants coach patients so that they not only understand but also have the tools to comply with treatment plans. For the diabetic

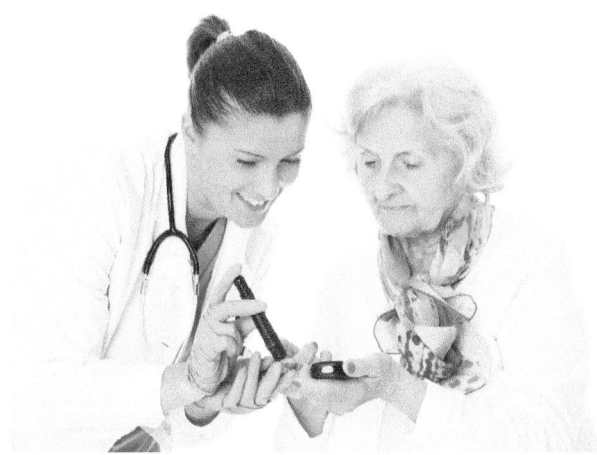

FIGURE 55-2 A medical assistant coaches the patient in all aspects of treatment plan compliance, including how to perform at-home testing, such as blood glucose monitoring.

JUDGMENT CALL

Anthony Pope is a well-established patient and close friend of the physicians in your office. You have just finished reviewing how to use a glucometer and explained the education related to recording his daily blood sugar readings and prescription information. You sense that Mr. Pope is not very attentive and seems increasingly distracted. He finally admits that he recently lost his job and his health insurance. He doesn't know where the money will come from to pay for medication and supplies to treat his newly diagnosed diabetes. He asks you to promise not to tell the physicians about the loss of his job, because he is embarrassed and doesn't want charity. How should you respond to Mr. Pope's request?

---

patient, for example, the medical assistant will coach the patient by helping the patient understand why certain medications have been prescribed and how to take the medications properly; provide a flowsheet or daily log book so that the patient can keep track of daily glucose readings; explain how to perform at-home blood glucose monitoring (Figure 55-2); and ensure that routine checkups are scheduled accordingly.

Impact of Finances on Patient Education

Finances can have a huge impact on the patient. The patient may want to comply with a treatment plan but may be inhibited in doing so because of lack of money. Creating an environment in which the patient is free to share monetary information, including financial struggles, without shame will help the patient be more open and will create a trusting rapport. For example, if a patient lacks funds for a special diet, an alternative diet can be created. Or, if a medication is extremely costly and the patient is unable to pay for continued treatment, you or the physician may be able to help the patient obtain medications at a reduced rate or zero cost from the pharmaceutical manufacturer through patient assistance programs. Some patients may not be able to afford good shoes for an exercise program, have available transportation for appointments, or be able to afford pharmacy items not covered by insurance. The wise and efficient medical assistant will create a list of local resources that can help patients who need financial assistance and provide the information in a discreet and nonjudgmental manner.

Handling Noncompliance

Noncompliance—that is, not following a physician's orders—can seriously jeopardize a patient's health and recovery. For instance, a patient with hypertension who fails to take

prescribed medication can develop uncontrolled hypertension and have a stroke or heart attack. In addition, health care costs escalate with noncompliance, because disease processes progress and worsen, leading to other health complications.

Various studies have tested the compliance level of patients afflicted with certain diseases and conditions. For inpatients who had had heart bypasses or were on hemodialysis, the compliance level was around 50 percent. By contrast, patients with cystic fibrosis, a serious disease causing respiratory problems and failure, were found to be more than 80 percent compliant with their medication regimen. This compliance was attributed to the possibility that these patients and their families perceived and may have experienced the very serious consequences of failing to take cystic fibrosis medications.

Lack of compliance may be indicated by failure to:

1. Take medication as ordered
2. Return for follow-up appointments
3. Practice dietary changes
4. Follow an exercise program

Noncompliance regarding following instructions is a problem for all age groups, but children have the least problem as long as their parents are compliant and assist them. Patients who have formed a positive relationship with their health care provider, physician, and other staff, including medical assistants, have been found to be more compliant with treatment plans and follow-up care.

One of the best methods for encouraging patient compliance is to convey to the patients the knowledge they need to make educated decisions about their health care.

In addition to having greater knowledge, the patient must also want to comply. As a medical assistant, you can reinforce learning and reduce noncompliance by working out a follow-up plan that includes a regular evaluation of

TABLE 55-3 | Patient Education Follow-Up Plan

Objective	Performance	Date Needed
Self-administer insulin injections with 100 percent accuracy.	1. Understand types of insulin.	2/14/YYYY
	2. Practice drawing up insulin × 3.	2/14/YYYY
	3. Practice injection on anatomical model × 3.	2/16/YYYY
	4. Demonstrate on patient by instructor using saline.	2/18/YYYY
	5. Return demonstration using saline.	2/18/YYYY
	6. Inject insulin.	2/18/YYYY
	7. Follow up to check technique.	3/1/YYYY

progress. This plan should include an objective stating what the patient should be able to do, along with a date indicating when the objective should be accomplished. Table 55-3 is an example of a patient education follow-up plan.

UNDERSTANDING AND DEVELOPING PATIENT-CENTERED EDUCATION

The patient education process begins with **assessment**, or evaluation of the patient's needs. For example, a patient may need to lose weight to decrease stress on joints, prevent or reverse obesity, promote fitness, and increase life expectancy. The next step is to **plan** or determine how to begin the task of teaching. Perhaps you could give the patient a pedometer and suggest walking for 20 minutes each day.

Implementing the plan involves teaching the patient specifically what to do. For example, you could teach the patient how to use the pedometer, select proper exercise shoes, set walking goals, and record daily walking distance. It is helpful to have examples in the office of materials you are suggesting the patient should use. You might show or provide the patient a notebook set up as an exercise log. Have a pedometer available to show the patient and explain. You might also have sample walking shoes to show the patient. You could put together a chart with a drawing or photo showing good walking gear such as shoes, pedometer, water bottle, sunglasses, and comfortable clothing (Figure 55-3).

Next, you must **document** the teaching you have done by charting it in the patient's health record to ensure continuity of care. Finally, at the patient's next office visit, you may remind the physician to ask the patient how the exercise plan is going; this phase is called **evaluation**. Using electronic health records (EHRs) gives you the ability to place reminders in the patient's record regarding upcoming visits and other needs related to patient care. This tool can be a helpful asset for the evaluation of patient education.

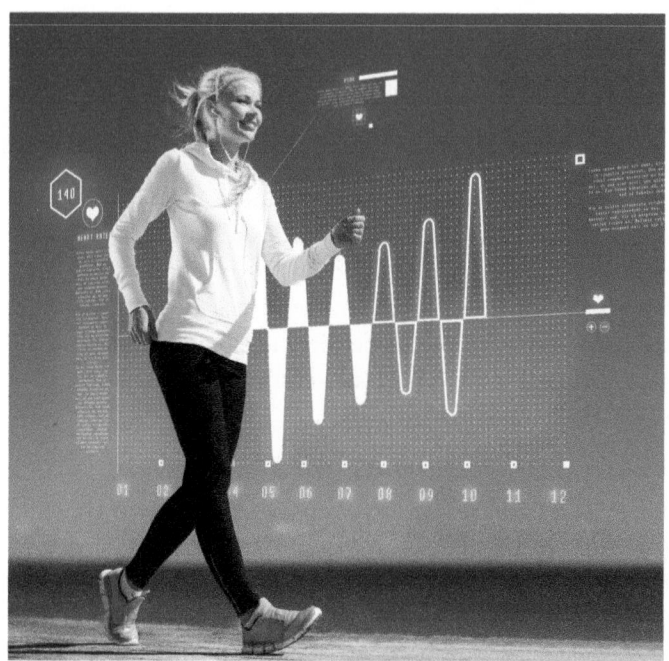

FIGURE 55-3 Visual aids, such as examples of proper walking shoes and a pedometer, or an illustration showing someone properly dressed and equipped for walking, can provide the patient with an additional level of understanding.

After evaluating the effectiveness of the teaching plan, and once the patient has demonstrated understanding and compliance with the plan, new teaching plans can be constructed. For example, the physician might decide, as the next step toward good weight management, to teach the patient how to modify caloric intake.

As mentioned earlier in the chapter, it is important to understand that the physician must always order the patient education that is required for patients. Patient education is not something that you, as a medical assistant, can choose or decide is necessary for a patient without the approval of a physician or other licensed health care provider. Many times physicians and medical assistants work together to determine the best methods and materials to be used for patient education (Figure 55-4).

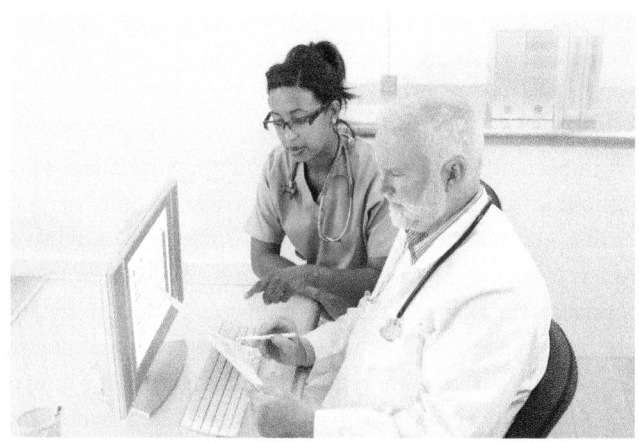

FIGURE 55-4 The physician and medical assistant often work together to choose appropriate educational materials for patients.

How Adults Learn

Most of the patients you teach will be adults. If children need instruction, their parents should be present so they can reinforce the teaching, although communication must be adapted to the learner's level of comprehension. Some specific learning concepts, however, relate best to the adult based on language skills, previous experience, and motivation.

Adult learning is an active process, and adults prefer to actively participate. Therefore, activities and techniques that call for participation, such as role-playing and demonstrations (e.g., demonstrating the use of a glucometer), will achieve more and faster learning than those that do not. For example, a lecture is not as useful as role-playing for patient learning. Patient education sessions should begin with explaining how and why the training will help the patient. Using the previous example, you might explain to the patient that using a pedometer is an easy method of recording exercise and that it is important to incorporate exercise into daily activities to promote a healthier lifestyle.

Learning must be self-directed for adults. In health care settings, patients must be taught the advantages of healthy lifestyles and how to achieve their goals. Practical application of learning is desired by most adult learners, and learning that offers the opportunity for immediate application will be retained longer. For example, consider a patient in an obstetrician's office who has just been told she is pregnant. She is eager to prepare and do what is best for her and her new child. This is an excellent time for you as a medical assistant to refer the patient to community resources that can offer guidance and assistance on issues like preparation for childbirth, prenatal nutrition, CPR/first aid, and child care courses. Sometimes the physician asks medical assistants to compile a list of community resources that can be recommended to patients.

Adults often prefer a group-learning atmosphere because of the mutual support a group setting offers. For learning to be effective, it must be reinforced. This can be done either through group activities or by the educator. Weight loss centers have used the technique of positive reinforcement effectively by announcing successful weight loss of group members to encourage and support members during meetings where the leader and members of the group share ideas about what has worked for them.

Motivational incentives for adult learners include better health, improved appearance, pride of accomplishment, self-confidence, and praise from others. In addition to frequent praise, the adult learner learns more rapidly when made aware of progress.

Teaching Methods

Teaching methods are chosen and based on characteristics and preferences of the learner. Methods can range from providing printed brochures and handouts to a single patient, to showing an instructional video to a group of patients. Rather than using one teaching method or technique during patient education, use a combination to enhance patients' learning experience while maintaining their interest. For example, when instructing a newly diagnosed diabetic patient, a combination of brief lecture, models of anatomical sites for injections, injection procedure demonstration, printed handouts, diagrams of injection site rotation, and videos might all be used at different points in the education process. Box 55-1 lists tips on how to prepare printed

---

BOX 55-1 | Creating Easy-to-Read Instruction

1. Begin the material with a short introduction to state the purpose and to orient the reader.
2. Use titles and headings that clearly define the topics.
3. Use boldface, italics, or underlining to emphasize important words and ideas.
4. Use a summary paragraph to end a section or recap important points.
5. Use one important idea per paragraph.
6. Start each paragraph with a strong topic sentence.
7. Vary the length of sentences.
8. Use frequent examples to clarify ideas with which the reader may not have had experience.
9. Use active rather than passive voice.
10. Avoid polysyllabic words. Use shorter words when possible.
11. Avoid using a specialized vocabulary such as medical terminology.
12. Avoid medical abbreviations and other abbreviations except when commonly understood.

material with easy-to-read instructions, and Guidelines 55-1 describes additional means for improving instruction. Both of these resources are helpful to consider when completing Procedure 55-1, which details patient coaching in regards to disease prevention and smoking cessation.

Learning Environments

It is important to create a good learning environment when coaching a patient. Patients are inclined to be more open to learning and honest about situations if they have a sense of privacy. It is ideal if patient education can take place in a well-lit, private room. Sometimes leaving patient education materials in the examination room allows patients to discreetly take brochures. If you are required to teach a patient how to use equipment, you should have it available for demonstration. For example, if a patient with diabetes is learning how to check blood sugar with a glucometer, you should teach the procedure using a model similar to the glucometer the patient will use at home. If the patient asks you a question that you cannot answer, be honest with the patient and explain that you will get back to the patient with the answer. You might choose to say, "That is a great question, Mr. Ghang. I will be sure to find out the answer before you leave the office today."

In addition to the physical aspects of creating a beneficial learning environment, it is important to understand that the learning environment is also cultivated by language and communication. Using language and communication skills that are not suited to the learner creates roadblocks to effective patient learning. Some roadblocks include:

- Ordering, commanding, and directing the patient to learn through force or negative tones
- Warning or threatening remarks ("If you don't do this, you may die")
- Moralizing or preaching ("ought to do," "should do")
- Judging
- Criticizing
- Name calling, stereotyping, labeling
- Sarcasm
- Anxiety
- Culturally inappropriate treatment plans
- Speaking loudly to a blind person
- Age-inappropriate speech

Culture influences learning and can affect readiness, values, feelings of inclusion, what aspect of learning the patients choose, and how they apply it in their own homes. Use of personal space, distances maintained, facial expressions, body movements, gestures, and expressions can be misinterpreted in certain cultures and must be considered when educating a patient.

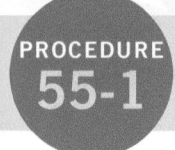

PROCEDURE
55-1

Providing Patient Education on Disease Prevention: Smoking Cessation

Objective ◆ *Coach a patient on disease prevention in regards to smoking cessation using brochures and approved literature.*

EQUIPMENT AND SUPPLIES

Computer; computer software program that allows the creation of a brochure or flyer; computer paper; printer; pen; phone book; Internet access

METHOD

1. Consider the importance of providing patient coaching related to smoking cessation. Decide the focus of your patient education and coaching session.

   For example: Will you provide statistics related to the hazards of smoking? Will you include a video presentation from a reputable resource? Will you provide examples of coping mechanisms that patients can use when they feel the urge to smoke?

2. Using the Internet and reputable websites, search for education materials related to smoking cessation.

   You may be able to find flyers and brochures that can be printed and immediately used, or you may choose to create your own flyer.

3. Find or create at least three pieces of information that can be used during the patient coaching session regarding smoking cessation. A short video clip could be one source of patient information, assuming it is educationally appropriate and from a reputable medical source.

4. Print all of the necessary materials for the patient, and have your instructor approve the materials.

   In the medical office, the physician approves patient education prior to it being distributed.

5. Organize the printed information, and practice how this information will be presented to the patient. You may want to write a short script of what you want to say.

6. Role-play the patient coaching scenario with a fellow classmate, making sure each student has the opportunity to play the role of the MA/patient coach, and present the material on smoking cessation.

Teaching Resources

Teaching resources are available for purchase or can be developed in the office. When creating a plan for patient education, you may need to use DVD players, compact discs, videos, or pamphlets. A variety of resources can come from companies that frequently do business with the medical office. For example, pharmaceutical companies and medical device manufacturers provide their representatives with educational pamphlets and brochures that pertain to the medications and products they create and the disease conditions for which they are treated. For this reason, pharmaceutical and manufacturer representatives can be valuable resources for you as a medical assistant. Free videos regarding disease management can be found on the Internet and websites such as YouTube. However, it is always important to make sure that the source providing the video is reliable and reputable. Pharmaceutical company websites also provide patient videos and educational tools. Table 55-4 lists reputable websites for patient education.

Electronic Health Records and Patient Education

Many of the offices that use EHRs send out targeted patient education information via e-mail. For instance, when an office uses EHRs, the patient's diagnosis and procedures are documented within the electronic record. The office is able to query its records and obtain diagnosis-specific information that can be e-mailed. For example, the system could search for all patients with a diabetes diagnosis. Once the patient data has been gathered, an e-mail can be sent out to all diabetic patients about coping with their diabetes during holidays. This type of system requires an authorization from the patient allowing the office to send such e-mails, but it is an efficient and cost-effective means to deliver patient education.

TABLE 55-4	Reputable Websites for Patient Education	
American Lung Association	Smoking cessation, asthma, hay fever, lung cancer (www.lungusa.org)
American Diabetes Association	Nutrition and recipes, weight loss and exercise, diabetes prevention and management (www.diabetes.org)
American Heart Association	High blood pressure, controlling cholesterol levels, diet and nutrition (www.americanheart.org)
Alzheimer's Association	Living with Alzheimer's, guides for caregivers (www.alz.org)
American Parkinson Disease Association	Local support groups (www.apdaparkinson.org)
Centers for Disease Control and Prevention	Information and education pertaining to vaccinations and conditions such as hepatitis, tuberculosis, environmental health issues, and a variety of general health topics (www.cdc.gov)
Hospice	Guides for caregivers of and patients with terminal illnesses, talking to children about death, pain control, advance directives, finding a local hospice, healing after a loss (www.americanhospice.org)

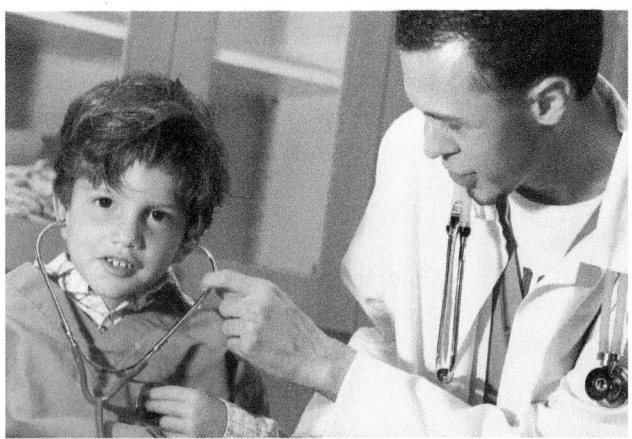

FIGURE 55-5 Children will feel more at ease and have a better learning experience if they are allowed to touch and feel certain items and have pretend play.

Teaching Children

Children have special educational needs and should not be treated as small adults expected to remember and process information above their level of learning. Patient education should be modified to the appropriate developmental stage to reach each child.

Coloring books can be used to teach concepts. Stickers can be given to reward children. Children may need to see a treatment or procedure performed on a doll before tolerating it well. Many children like to touch equipment that will be used on them, such as a stethoscope or a blood pressure cuff (Figure 55-5). Older children may like to see videos about the process of a surgery or other treatment they are expecting to have. As children age, they should be included in discussions and decision making about their health care. Older children may have numerous questions about their treatments and should receive adequate explanations in response.

When educating children about their own health issues (perhaps how a nebulizing treatment works or how to use an inhaler for the treatment of asthma), it is important to direct the education to both the child and the caregiver or parent. Always make sure that caregivers have a complete understanding of the needs related to caring for the child's health. Allow extra time to answer questions from both the caregiver and child, ensuring that both feel valued and cared for.

Teaching Patients with Special Needs

Many patients have special needs and challenges, such as sensory impairments, mental challenges, or language difficulties. Patient education must be specially adapted for these patients.

The Hearing-Impaired Patient

Patients who have hearing impairments frequently read lips. Face the patient and speak slowly, but be sure you

PATIENT COACHING AND EDUCATION: MEETING PATIENT NEEDS

Patient education must be adapted to fit not only the learning style but also the special needs of the patient. These special needs or unique situations require additional consideration when planning educational teaching. Patients may have hearing or visual impairments, they may be developmentally delayed or mentally challenged, and or they might not speak English.

All patient teaching should have the goal of patient understanding and retention. With all special needs patients, you, the medical assistant, should ensure the patient understands by requesting feedback or demonstration from the patient after teaching. You may find it necessary to adjust teaching to the needs of the patient, and you may need to cover the same topic several times and in several different ways until sufficient understanding is demonstrated.

don't speak so slowly that it is insulting to the patient. Be sure you do not stand with your back to a window or light source because such positioning will cast shadows over your mouth. Remove barriers or face masks when speaking to clients with hearing impairments. You may need to hire an interpreter for a deaf patient. This often comes at an expense to the medical office. For patients who are hard of hearing, it may be helpful to get a microphone to boost the volume of your voice. In such situations, always be mindful of the patient's right to privacy, ensuring that other patients are not able to hear health information that should be privately guarded. Always provide detailed and specific written instructions to clients with hearing impairments. Procedure 55-2 establishes how to provide effective patient education for the hearing-impaired patient.

The Visually Impaired Patient

Patients who have visual impairments may not be able to read written instructions unless the type is very large—and some will not be able to read at all. To help these patients, you may need to make audio-recorded instructions of information that is usually written. This might be done using the patient's own recording device, such as a handheld voice recorder (Figure 55-6) or an app on the patient's smartphone or tablet. Be sure to clear clutter from the office and hallways that might impede the patient, and ask if the patient would like a guiding arm while navigating the examination room.

Developmental Delays, Mental Challenges, Illiteracy, and Language Barriers

Patients who have developmental delays or are mentally challenged may have trouble understanding complex or

---

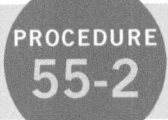

PROCEDURE 55-2

Coaching Patients with Consideration of Communication Barriers: A Hearing-Impaired Patient

Objective ◆ *Instruct a hearing-impaired individual to prepare for outpatient surgery by creating a packet of information for postoperative care.*

EQUIPMENT AND SUPPLIES

Computer; word processing software; printer; printer paper; notepad; pen; stapler

METHOD

1. Using a computer with word processing software, create a postoperative instruction packet for a hearing-impaired patient. Include the following information:
   - When to resume activities such as walking, driving, and exercising
   - Incision wound care and dressing changes
   - Postoperative diet
   - Medications
   - Follow-up care
2. Double-check the information for accuracy, spelling, and grammatical errors.
3. Print a copy for the patient and save one copy in the patient's health record. Save a digital file for EHRs or place a printed copy in a paper health record. Have the physician review and approve the packet before giving it to the patient.
4. Face the patient so your lips can be read easily.
5. Greet and identify the patient. Introduce yourself if you haven't worked with the patient yet.

6. Discuss the contents of the postoperative instructions with the patient.
   a. During discussion, always face the patient.
   b. Do not read the information from the packet in a hurried manner. Take frequent breaks, and make eye contact with the patient to ensure understanding.
7. Obtain feedback from the patient to show understanding.
   a. Have a notepad and pen available so that the patient can write down questions and answers.
8. Give a copy of the information to the patient.
9. If paper health records are used by the facility, have the patient sign one copy of the packet and file it in the health record. If EHRs are used, scan a copy of the signed brochure into the health record and save it to the appropriate location.
10. Document that patient education was completed and that the patient received and demonstrated understanding of the information.

CHARTING EXAMPLE

11/10/YY 2:45 P.M. Instructed patient on postoperative instructions as highlighted in attached brochure. Patient demonstrated understanding and did not have additional questions................
....Emily Blodgett, CMA (AAMA)

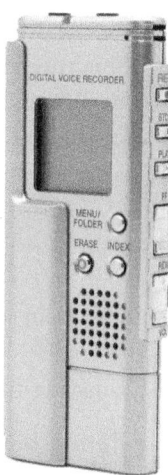

FIGURE 55-6 Digital recording devices can be helpful when providing patient education to visually impaired patients.

multiple-step patient education and instruction. You may need to instruct the caregiver instead or to give the patient simplified, pictorial directions. Many times, the caregiver or family member who accompanies a patient with developmental delays will assume the role of responsibility. It is important for you, the medical assistant, to be able to read body language and nonverbal cues displayed by patients and family members. It is also important, if you are directing instructions toward the caregiver, not to ignore the patient or act as if the patient isn't in the room. Make appropriate references and eye contact with both the patient and the caregiver, showing that you value and appreciate them both.

Patients who are illiterate (unable to read or write) or those who do not understand or speak English also pose special challenges. Often illiterate patients will not volunteer this information because they are embarrassed. You must be alert to behaviors that might indicate someone has difficulty with reading and writing. It is common for these patients to say they forgot their reading glasses and would like you to read something for them or fill out a form on their behalf. In such instances, it is necessary to get creative with patient education. For example, if a diabetic patient is required to check blood sugar in the morning and at night, it might be helpful to draw a picture showing a sun and moon to help the patient identify what to do. Also, always provide the patient with printed instructions and highlight or underline especially important information. It is very likely that the patient has a family member or friend who is able to read and help them.

Advanced notice and preparations can be made for the non–English-speaking patient at the time the patient's appointment is scheduled. During the scheduling of the appointment, the patient or the person calling to schedule on behalf of the patient should be asked if an interpreter will accompany the patient to the appointment or if the medical office will need to provide an interpreter. Often, the patient prefers to bring a relative who speaks English. In such instances, it is necessary to obtain the patient's written permission to discuss health information with the interpreting relative. Send written instructions home with the patient. If a large percentage of patients in the office speak a certain language other than English, it may help to construct brochures in that language. The effect of culture on patient education is discussed later in this chapter.

Teaching Older Adults

Older adult patients' abilities, motivations, and social circumstances often differ from those of younger patients. Their intellectual capacity usually does not diminish; it merely changes. Some changes that take place as a person ages include slower processing of new material, decreased short-term memory, decreased **dexterity** (ability to use their hands effectively), and increased anxiety over new situations. These changes are discussed briefly in this section.

One type of intellectual ability is based on the intelligence absorbed during life—for example, vocabulary, arithmetic, and the ability to reflect on and evaluate past experience. This type of intelligence can increase with age. Therefore, the older person is able to learn quickly if the learning requires information acquired in the past. When teaching the older adult, it is wise to explore past experiences using concrete examples, such as "Tell me how you calculate the amount of food you eat on your diabetic diet."

Teaching methods that are useful with older adults range from using handouts with large print to using video and audio displays. Role-playing can be useful as long as the patient's energy level can be maintained. Family members should be included in the teaching process whenever possible. Older adults are accustomed to being in control and may not wish to learn anything new without seeing the advantage of doing so.

Slowed Processing Time

Older patients need more time to think through and absorb new information; therefore, it is helpful for you to break down information into small units. When teaching from a list of things, take time to explain each item on the list. For example, when the instructions are "Call your doctor for the following reasons: temperature over 99 degrees, drainage from the incision, inability to take the medication, or pain," each of these reasons should be explained separately. These explanations should be accompanied by a description of the relationship of each item to the patient's problem. It is also helpful to give written instructions so the patient can process the instructions more slowly later (Figure 55-7).

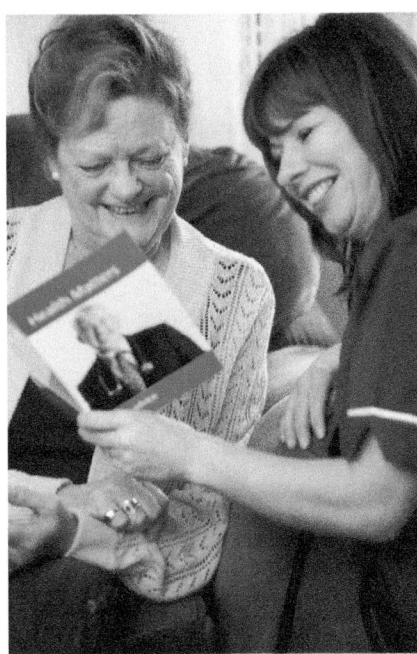

FIGURE 55-7 Written materials can be helpful for the older adult.

Decreased Short-Term Memory

Older adult patients often have an easier time remembering what happened in the past but may have difficulty remembering newly acquired information. Learning then becomes very frustrating for them. You should work with the patient to devise methods to reinforce instruction or prod the memory. The new information should be linked to a well-known past experience when possible. Always attempt to reinforce old ways of doing things rather than introducing new behavior. For example, when teaching about the warning signs and symptoms of an infection to an older diabetic patient, ask the patient to recall the symptoms experienced in the past with an infected wound or cut.

Decreased Mobility and Dexterity

Because of arthritis and other physical changes, some older patients are not physically able to do the same things they could when they were younger. This needs to be taken into consideration when providing patient education involving certain topics. For example, advising an overweight older patient who uses a walker for mobility to get more exercise by walking for one hour a day would not be appropriate. You, the medical assistant, would need to find less demanding forms of exercise for the patient, such as water aerobics or exercises that may be done from a seated position. Also consider that some tasks requiring small muscle dexterity, such as flossing teeth and opening medication bottles, are almost impossible for an older adult with arthritis. Adaptive equipment may have to be advised for these patients.

It is helpful for you to be aware of adaptive equipment and assistive devices that are available for older patients. Durable medical equipment (DME) companies, which sell health care–related items such as wheelchairs, bathtub chairs, and oxygen supplies, often carry specialty items including adaptive supplies and assistive devices. These companies can be a tremendous resource.

Increased Anxiety about New Situations

Many changes occur in the lives of older adults. They may lose their sense of independence after retiring from a job or being told it isn't safe for them to drive anymore. Their health status may change frequently or drastically from the aging processes of the body, and they may experience personal loss through the death of close friends and family members. All of these circumstances can cause anxiety for the patient. Add a newly diagnosed medical condition, and older patients are likely to experience an increase in their anxiety levels.

As an advocate for your patients, you can help them by encouraging and building their confidence levels. Patients will relax and feel more at ease when they see that they are able to manage the situation, and learning will take place. Practice positive reinforcement and provide encouragement when they display an understanding of a new concept. This can alleviate some of the anxiety that may surface during a new learning situation.

Culture and Patient Education

Each patient brings a unique culture, which expands beyond a language barrier, to the educational experience. Cultural expectations can interfere with teaching. The best way to find out about a patient's culture is to ask. You can ask a patient if there is a preference for a type of education and respect those wishes. Sometimes a patient may prefer to be educated by someone who is older or a certain gender. Make every attempt to respect the wishes of the patient without taking personal offense if someone else will make the patient

Professionalism

While dealing with patients from a wide variety of backgrounds, you will meet people with completely different lifestyles and cultures. True professionals, although they may not believe in or agree with specific aspects of a patient's life or culture, do not judge those who live differently. It is possible to accept and appreciate a patient without endorsing or agreeing with that person's lifestyle. Never say anything to a patient that can be construed as a judgment about lifestyle. Simply accept each person for who he or she is.

When creating patient education materials, you may need to be sensitive to cultural considerations. Although sketches and anatomical diagrams may be appropriate for a brochure, some cultures do not approve of seeing pictures of actual body parts in patient education materials.

In some cultures, patient education includes educating family members. Male family members are often expected to assist older women with medical appointments. In some cultures, men should not see women undressed, so they may need to be excluded from a procedure or the examination room. It is important to remember the patient's right to health care. At the patient's request, family members may be included or excluded from the examination and any procedures. An example is the varied cultural view of childbirth practices. In the United States, childbirth classes can include male relatives or even friends as encouragement coaches. In other countries and cultures, only women learn about childbirth and parenting techniques.

You must be able to communicate with your patients, especially to obtain truly informed consent about certain procedures or to provide critical patient education related to the patient's care. A responsible medical office will hire a medical assistant or physician with good foreign language skills that are common to its patient demographics. If staff members are not available or qualified, the medical office will need to hire an interpreter to ensure patient understanding and compliance. Interpreters are not considered office staff, but rather are contracted workers who provide billable services during a patient's medical appointment.

feel more comfortable, which will create a more productive learning experience for the patient.

Cultural beliefs can impact the patient's health care. Some cultures believe that they have little control over their health. Others assume a great deal of control over balance in health. Family members may be a very important part of the treatment team in many cultures. Family members can be key allies in assisting the patient with learning and with reinforcing your teaching.

Religious beliefs also impact health and encompass cultural differences. For example, a Jehovah's Witness may refuse blood products, and Native Americans may perform a special ceremony before a treatment or procedure. Always ask the patient if special religious beliefs could interfere with the ability to comply with a treatment or if special considerations need to be made to comply with religious and cultural beliefs before or following a procedure. For example, the patient may participate in fasting for religious purposes, in which case it may not be a good time to schedule a procedure requiring swallowing barium.

COMMUNITY RESOURCES

Community resources are programs and services that are available to improve the quality of life of an individual by providing help, information, and assistance. Many patients might not be aware of community resources that are available to them. Medical assistants, as part of the duty to provide patient education and navigate services for patients, should

be familiar with resources available within their community that can benefit and improve the lives of their patients. Table 55-5 provides a list of common community resources and programs available in many communities. A brochure of these local resources and services may be provided in a new patient packet. An office policies brochure, sometimes called a public relations brochure, is also given to new patients. The office policies brochure details specific information about the medical practice including office hours, payment expectations, and emergency management procedures, just to name a few. This information handout is a form of patient education in its own right; educating the patient about the medical practice and its services. Procedure 55-3 details creating a community resources brochure, and Procedure 55-4 provides the steps for creating a medical office policies brochure.

TABLE 55-5 | Community Resource Programs and Services

- Homeless shelters and services for the homeless
- Food banks, food pantries, and Meals on Wheels
- Programs for alcoholics and drug addicts, as well as their families (e.g., Alcoholics Anonymous)
- Domestic violence services
- Rape and crime victim services
- Services for seniors
- Public housing authority
- Public transportation
- Legal advice and legal services
- State assistance programs including food stamps, Medicaid, social security, and WIC services
- Foster care for children
- Child abuse hotline and child protective services
- Diabetic information groups and support services
- Support groups (grief, cancer, smoking, and drug abuse)
- Prescription assistance services for those who cannot afford prescriptions
- Disability services that help enable independence

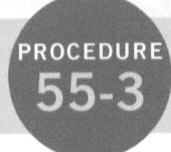

PROCEDURE
55-3

Creating a Community Resources Brochure

Objective ◆ *Create a brochure that educates patients about available community resources.*

EQUIPMENT AND SUPPLIES

Computer; computer software program that allows the creation of a brochure; computer paper; printer; pen; phone book; Internet access; newspaper

METHOD

1. Create a list of health-related resources that can be used to create a community resource brochure.

   You may refer to Table 55-5 *and choose resources that might be particularly relevant for the community where you live.*

2. Using the Internet, telephone books, and even the local newspaper, identify community resources that can help meet patient needs.

3. Create an attractive brochure for distribution to patients that includes the names, locations, phone numbers, and services offered by the selected resources.
4. Check your brochure for spelling and grammatical errors before printing.
5. Print one copy and then perform another spelling and grammar check on the printed document.
6. After the brochure has been edited for errors and is polished, obtain approval from the physician to print and then distribute the brochures to patients as necessary or to display in the office reception area.

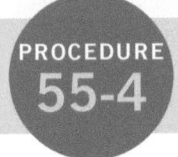

PROCEDURE
55-4

Creating an Office Policies Brochure

Objective ◆ *Promote the office by creating a brochure for distribution to current and potential patients.*

EQUIPMENT AND SUPPLIES

Computer; computer software program that allows the creation of a brochure; printer; office information; pen

METHOD

1. Gather the necessary data for the office policies/public relations brochure. Be sure to include the following:
   - Office name (e.g., Pearson Physicians Group)
   - Type of practice (e.g., family medicine)
   - Office hours
   - Office address
   - Names and information about physicians
   - Insurance plans accepted
   - Payment expectations (e.g., copayments are expected before visit begins; all methods of payment are acceptable except cash)
   - Emergency management procedures (e.g., after hours, contact the answering service at 312-321-4321)
   - Prescription refill procedures (e.g., allow 24 hours for a prescription to be refilled; some medications will not be refilled and require an office appointment)
   - Local hospital affiliations and privileges
2. Check your brochure for spelling and grammatical errors before printing.
3. Print one copy and perform another spelling and grammar check on the printed document.
4. After the brochure has been edited for errors and is polished, obtain approval from the office manager or physician to print and then distribute the brochures to patients.

Referrals to Community Resources

Medical offices often are one of the first points of reference for community resources. Physicians and their staff, including medical assistants, are given personal access not only to the patient's physical health but also to information related to their personal needs. A patient may tell a doctor that there isn't much food at home, that he or she is struggling with an alcohol addiction, or that the patient can't afford to pay for prescriptions. In such cases, the physician may ask the medical assistant to refer the patient directly to a community resource that can help meet the patient's needs. This is an example of how the medical assistant works as a patient navigator, as discussed in the chapter titled "Medical Assisting: The Profession." To review, as a patient navigator, the medical assistant helps the patient streamline services available to meet that patient's healthcare needs and improve communication in the ever-changing and sometimes confusing world of medicine.

Sometimes, the circumstances surrounding the patient's needs are delicate. It is important that the medical assistant displays compassion, empathy, and confidentiality when handling all circumstances. Procedure 55-5 reviews how to facilitate a referral to a community resource.

PROCEDURE 55-5

Working as a Patient Navigator: Facilitating a Referral for Community Resources

Objective ◆ *Create a brochure that educates patients about available community resources.*

EQUIPMENT AND SUPPLIES

List of community resources; computer; Internet access; pen; paper; patient's medical record

Scenario: A female patient is struggling with alcoholism and was recently arrested for drunk driving. Dr. Wilkinson has requested that the patient be provided with information about community programs and resources that can help her. The doctor has also asked that the patient be provided information on public transportation because she has lost her driving privileges.

METHOD

1. Using the Internet or a local telephone book, locate programs within your community that can help with the patient's addiction, such as Alcoholics Anonymous.
2. Make a list of the programs available that can be of help for the patient. On the list, include telephone numbers and website information.
3. Call or visit the websites of the selected programs to determine meeting schedules and locations. Include this information on the list that will be given to the patient.
4. Obtain phone numbers and information that will help the patient with transportation, and include this on the list of information that will be given to the patient.

   This could include local public transportation, taxi cab companies, and Uber.

5. Review the list of information with the patient and ask if she has any questions you could answer.

6. Provide the patient with your name and the office telephone number. Encourage her to call you with any questions.
7. Within 48 hours, place a follow-up call to the patient to establish how she is doing and if she has chosen a meeting to attend. Inquire if transportation has been arranged.
8. Document all information related to the patient's office visit and subsequent telephone follow-up.

CHARTING EXAMPLE

04/23/YY 3:15 P.M. Per Dr. Wilkinson's request, patient was given a referral sheet with information about local Alcoholics Anonymous (AA) meetings and the phone number for a local taxi company. An AA schedule was printed from the Internet as well as a local bus schedule, which were both given to the patient. All of the information was reviewed with the patient, and she stated that she didn't have additional questions. A two-week follow-up appointment with Dr. Wilkinson was scheduled.
....Ester Mayfield, CMA (AAMA)

4/25/YY 9:45 A.M. Follow-up phone call with patient: She attended an AA meeting yesterday and now has a sponsor. She will be going to meetings 3x/week. Her cousin and brother-in-law are able to help with transportation. Patient seemed in better spirits and was thankful for the assistance.....................
....Ester Mayfield, CMA (AAMA)

SUMMARY

One of the vital tasks of a medical assistant is to provide patient coaching and education, as needed and as directed by a physician. Examples of coaching and education include, but are not limited to, teaching health promotion, describing office policies, and adapting education to meet special needs. Many diseases can be prevented by patients receiving education from a medical assistant about stopping smoking, losing weight, and exercising, for example. Good patient education involves effective communication. The medical assistant often plays a critical role in handling noncompliant patients (e.g., a diabetic patient who will not adhere to the prescribed diet). For patients with disabilities or special needs, education should be adapted to the patient in terms of method of presentation and memory aids. Education must be adapted to the age, culture, and developmental stage of the patient. Community resources are available to help patients with a variety of issues. A medical assistant may be asked to facilitate referrals for community resources for patients. In such cases, professionalism through proper communication is essential.

55 CHAPTER REVIEW

COMPETENCY REVIEW

1. Define and spell the terms for this chapter.
2. Explain why a medical assistant acts as a patient coach.
3. Are medical assistants able to make the decision to provide a patient with patient education related to a specific topic? Explain your answer.
4. Explain why more than one teaching method should be used during a patient education session.
5. List five roadblocks to effective patient communication and learning.
6. Identify teaching methods that are helpful with older adults.
7. List information that would be included in an office policies brochure.
8. Why is it important to have a community resources list available for patients?
9. Give examples of when a medical assistant would work as a patient navigator and facilitate referrals for community resources.

PREPARING FOR THE CERTIFICATION EXAM

1. All of the following are examples of patient noncompliance *except*
   a. failure to take medication as ordered.
   b. failure to return for follow-up appointments.
   c. failure to pay medical insurance deductibles.
   d. failure to practice dietary changes.
   e. failure to follow an exercise program.

2. Providing audio-recorded instructions would *best* serve which type of patient?
   a. a hearing-impaired patient
   b. an older adult patient
   c. a visually impaired patient
   d. a young child
   e. an emotionally distressed patient

3. The process of patient education begins with
   a. implementation.
   b. finding a quiet room.
   c. planning.
   d. assessment.
   e. deciding on a teaching method.

4. Which of the following should *not* be included in an office brochure?
   a. where the physician was educated
   b. office location
   c. insurance plans accepted
   d. physician's cellphone number
   e. emergency phone numbers and after-hours plan

5. Health maintenance centers on the idea of a patient's overall
   a. exercise program.
   b. wellness.
   c. diet.
   d. desire to be healthy.
   e. health history.

6. Which of the following is *not* true about teaching older adults?
   a. slowed processing time
   b. decreased dexterity
   c. decreased short-term memory
   d. should not be asked to demonstrate
   e. increased anxiety about new situations

7. Which of the following is *not* an example of a community resource?
   a. a local food bank
   b. a domestic violence shelter
   c. Alcoholics Anonymous programs
   d. Meals on Wheels programs
   e. local banking services

8. When reviewing a patient's risk factors, the medical assistant is acting as a patient coach in relation to
   a. disease prevention.
   b. health maintenance.
   c. treatment plan compliance.
   d. treatment plan noncompliance.
   e. office policies.

9. A _____ provides support, explains things that might be difficult to understand, serves as a source of encouragement and help, and educates patients on a variety of topics.
   a. medical assistant
   b. patient navigator
   c. patient coach
   d. referral coordinator
   e. director of patient education

10. When teaching children, good ways to teach include all of the following *except*
   a. rewarding them with stickers.
   b. letting them touch nonsterile instruments and materials.
   c. showing a one-hour DVD of the procedure.
   d. showing the procedure on a doll.
   e. role-playing the procedure.

CRITICAL THINKING

Refer to the case study at the beginning of the chapter and use what you have learned to answer the following questions.

1. To begin her task of developing a patient education program at Pearson Physicians Group, Tania is planning to create a list of patient education topics for proposed classes. With the physicians' approval, she will then begin to formulate the classes. What are some topics that Tania might want to consider for patient education classes?

2. The classes that PPG is going to offer will be geared toward its adult patient population. What are some things that Tania should take into consideration when planning education classes for adult learners?

3. Tania calls Pearson General Hospital to speak with the director of community education for some advice before the start of the classes. The woman encourages Tania to obtain and use a variety of teaching resources. What types of resources might Tania use in her patient education program?

ON THE JOB

Bonny Kirkland, CMA (AAMA), works in a dialysis clinic. Most of her patients have diabetes mellitus, an endocrine disorder that can destroy the kidneys and leave the patient dependent on dialysis. The patients are usually on the dialysis machine for several hours three days per week.

1. Is it appropriate for the CMA (AAMA) to do patient teaching?

2. Many of Bonny's patients have diabetic retinopathy, which makes it difficult for them to see. What could Bonny do to help this group of patients?

3. If the patient is older and claims to be "set in my ways," what are good strategies for teaching the patient about a healthy lifestyle?

4. Should family members be involved in the teaching plan? If so, how?

INTERNET ACTIVITY

Choose a patient education topic that interests you. Perform an Internet search to gather information, and then create a patient teaching brochure.

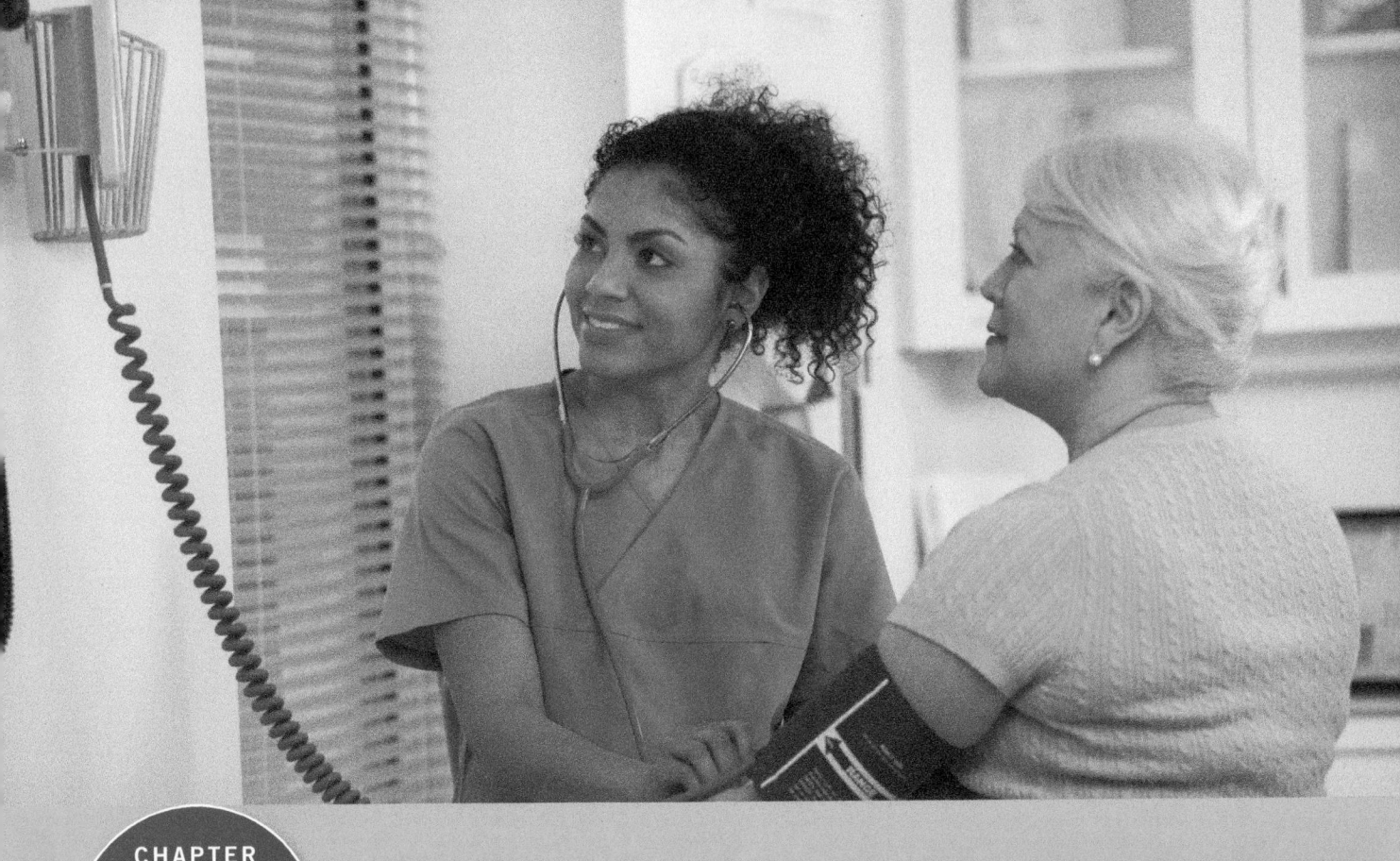

Nutrition

Learning Objectives

After completing this chapter, you should be able to:

56.1   Define and spell the terms for this chapter.

56.2   Describe the differences between a nutritionist and a registered dietitian.

56.3   Explain the medical assistant's role in nutrition.

56.4   Summarize the digestive process.

56.5   Explain how metabolism impacts the body.

56.6   Describe the six main types of dietary nutrients.

56.7   Describe the function of dietary supplements.

56.8   Outline components of a healthy diet and lifestyle.

56.9   Identify special dietary needs for various health conditions.

Jaden Henderson is seeing Dr. Salpega for a follow-up on blood work that was completed last week. She tells David Dolan, the medical assistant, that she has been extremely fatigued during the past few months. She learns from Dr. Salpega that she has pernicious anemia.

Terms to Learn

calorie	lipids	nutritionist
cholesterol	macrominerals	polysaccharides
complete proteins	malabsorption	polyunsaturated fat
dietary supplements	medical nutrition therapy	Recommended Dietary Allowances (RDAs)
digestion	metabolism	refined sugars
fiber	minerals	registered dietitian
hydrogenation	monosaccharides	saturated fat
incomplete proteins	monounsaturated fat	therapeutic diet
lactating	nutrients	vitamins
lactose		

Nutrition includes all the processes involved in using foods for growth, repair, and maintenance of the human body. The nutrition process includes ingestion, digestion, absorption, and metabolism. Some nutrients are capable of being stored in the body and can be used when food intake is insufficient. Other nutrients, such as vitamin C, are not stored and must be continually replenished.

NUTRITION PROFESSIONALS

It has been said that the standard American diet, known by the acronym *SAD*, contains too much fat, too many calories, too much cholesterol, too much salt, not enough fiber or plant-based foods, and insufficient complex carbohydrates. Studies have shown that cultures that eat the reverse of this diet, which is rich in fiber, plant-based foods, and complex carbohydrates, and low in fats (particularly animal fats), have a lower incidence of cancer and cardiovascular disease. The best diet is a well-balanced eating plan with the correct proportion of the major nutrients (Figure 56-1). A well-nourished person is better able to ward off infection, remain alert, and perhaps even live longer. Nutrition professionals are able to help individuals develop healthy eating habits to improve and prolong their quality of life.

Registered Dietitians and Nutritionists

A **registered dietitian** is a member of the health care team who provides patients with information about nutrition and creates diet plans that will help treat and prevent disease. These individuals obtain their registered dietitian credential (RD) by completing and passing an examination issued by the Commission of Dietetic Registration. To sit for this credentialing examination, an individual must complete a four-year bachelor's degree program that has been approved by the Academy of Nutrition and Dietetics' Accreditation Council for Education in Nutrition and Dietetics. The services registered dietitians offer are considered **medical nutrition therapy**, and it is a billable service through many health insurance plans, including Medicare. A **nutritionist** is someone who also provides nutrition advice. State laws vary regarding who is allowed to be designated as a "nutritionist," but a nutritionist may or may not be a qualified health care provider. Although all registered dietitians could be considered nutritionists, not all nutritionists are registered dietitians.

The Medical Assistant's Role in Nutrition

It is important for you, the medical assistant, to understand the roles of nutrition professionals, because a patient may ask you to explain what they do and the similarities and

NUTRIENT CLASS	BODILY FUNCTIONS	FOOD SOURCES
CARBOHYDRATES 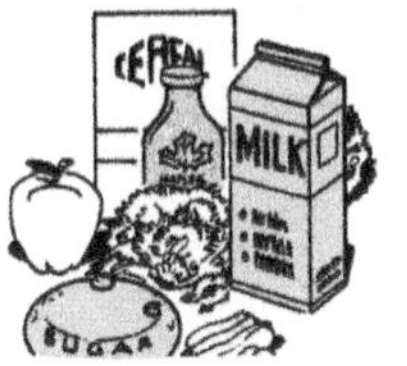	Provides work energy for body activities, and heat energy for maintenance of body temperature.	Cereal grains and their products (bread, breakfast cereals, macaroni products), potatoes, sugar, syrups, fruits, milk, vegetables, nuts.
PROTEINS 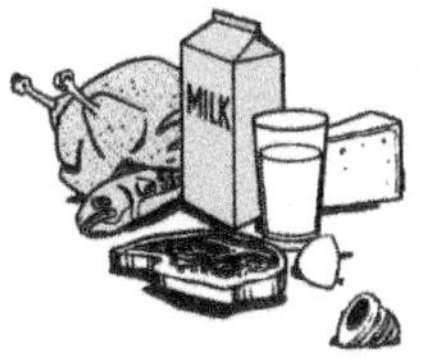	Build and renew body tissues; regulate body functions and supply energy. Complete proteins; maintain life and provide growth. Incomplete proteins; maintain life but do not provide for growth.	Complete proteins: Derived from animal foods—meat, milk, eggs, fish, cheese, poultry. Incomplete proteins: Derived from vegetable foods—soybeans, dry beans, peas, some nuts and whole grain products.
FATS 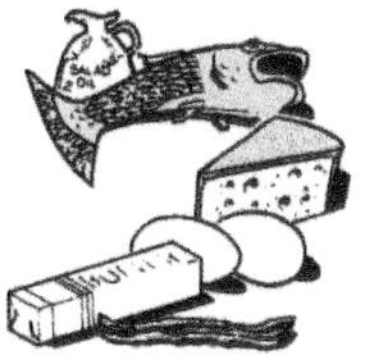	Give work energy for body activities and heat energy for maintenance of body temperature. Carrier of vitamins A and D, provide fatty acids necessary for growth and maintenance of body tissues.	Some foods are chiefly fat, such as lard, vegetable fats and oils, and butter. Many other foods contain smaller proportions of fats—nuts, meats, fish, poultry, cream, whole milk.
MINERALS Calcium 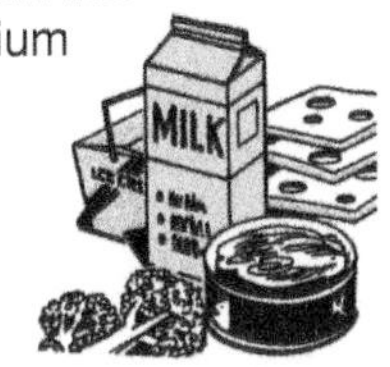	Builds and renews bones, teeth, and other tissues; regulates the activity of the muscles, heart, nerves; and controls the clotting of blood.	Milk and milk products except butter; most dark green vegetables; canned salmon.
Iron 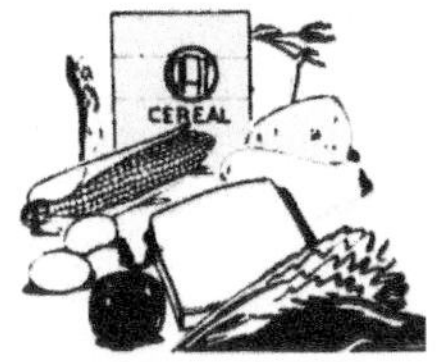	Builds and renews hemoglobin, the red pigment in blood that carries oxygen from the lungs to the cells.	Eggs, meat, especially liver and kidney; deep-yellow and dark green vegetables; potatoes, dried fruits, whole-grain products; enriched flour, bread, breakfast cereals.
Iodine 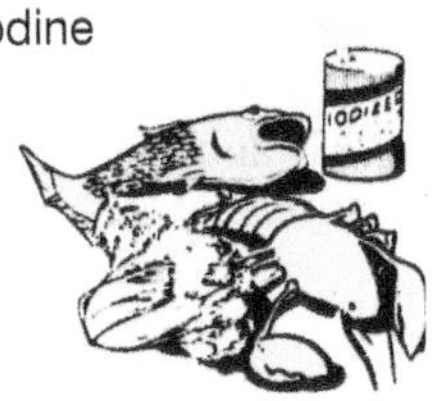	Enables the thyroid gland to perform its function of controlling the rate at which foods are oxidized in the cells.	Fish (obtained from the sea), some plant-foods grown in soils containing iodine; table salt fortified with iodine (iodized).
VITAMINS A 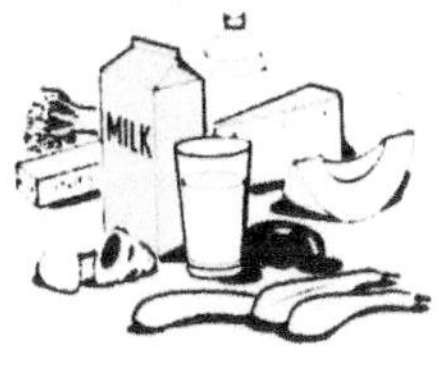	Necessary for normal functioning of the eyes, prevents night blindness. Ensures a healthy condition of the skin, hair, and mucous membranes. Maintains a state of resistance to infections of the eyes, mouth, and respiratory tract.	One form of vitamin A is yellow and one form is colorless. Apricots, cantaloupe, milk, cheese, eggs, meat organs, (especially liver and kidney), fortified margarine, butter fish-liver oils, dark green and deep yellow vegetables.

FIGURE 56-1 A healthy diet is made up of well-balanced nutrients.

NUTRIENT CLASS	BODILY FUNCTIONS	FOOD SOURCES
B Complex B_1 (Thiamine) 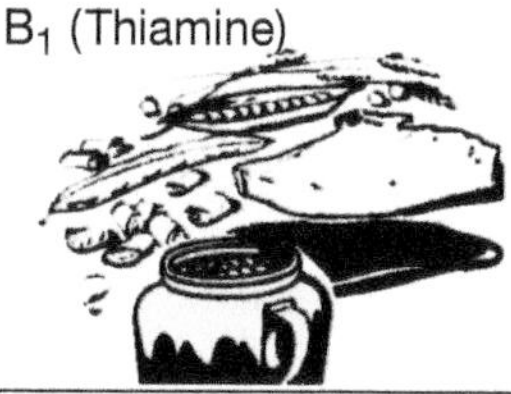	Maintains a healthy condition of the nerves. Fosters a good appetite. Helps the body cells use carbohydrates.	Whole grain and enriched grain products; meats (especially pork, liver, and kidney). Dry beans and peas.
B_2 (Riboflavin) 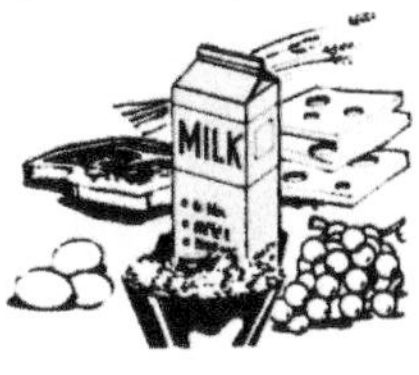	Keeps the skin, mouth, and eyes in a healthy condition. Acts with other nutrients to form enzymes and control oxidation in cells.	Milk, cheese, eggs, meat (especially liver and kidney), whole grain and enriched grain products, dark green vegetables.
B_3 Niacin 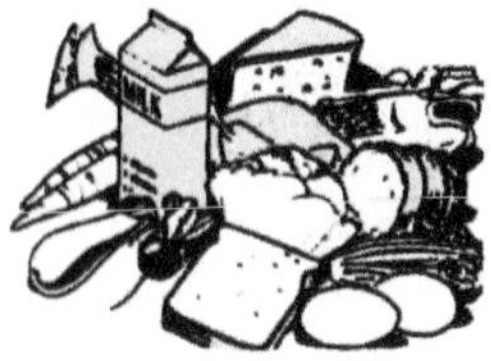	Influences the oxidation of carbohydrates and proteins in the body cells.	Liver, meat, fish, poultry, eggs, peanuts; dark green vegetables, whole grain and enriched cereal products.
B_{12} 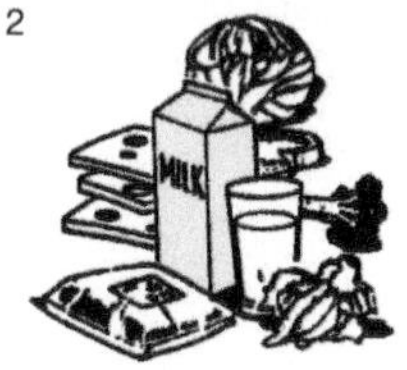	Regulates specific processes in digestion. Helps maintain normal functions of muscles, nerves, heart, blood—general body metabolism.	Liver, other organ meats, cheese, eggs, milk, leafy green vegetables.
C (Ascorbic Acid) 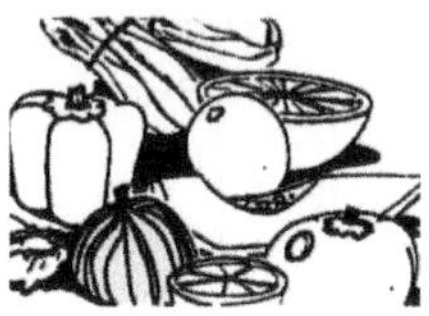	Acts as a cement between body cells, and helps them work together to carry out their special functions. Maintains a sound condition of bones, teeth, and gums. Not stored in the body.	Fresh, raw citrus fruits and vegetables—oranges, grapefruit, cantaloupe, strawberries, tomatoes, raw onions, cabbage, green and sweet red peppers, dark green vegetables.
D 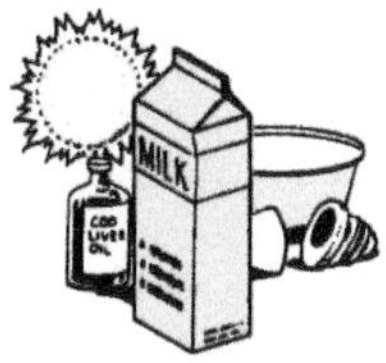	Enables the growing body to use calcium and phosphorus in a normal way to build bones and teeth.	Provided by vitamin D fortification of certain foods, such as milk and margarine. Also fish-liver oils and eggs. Sunshine is also a source of vitamin D.
WATER 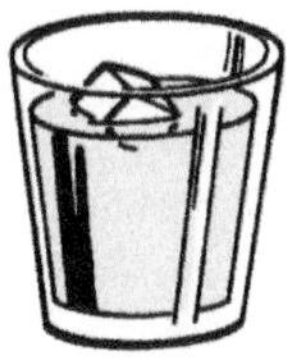	Regulates body processes. Aids in regulating body temperature. Carries nutrients to body cells and carries waste products away from them. Helps to lubricate joints. Water has no food value, although most water contains mineral elements. More immediately necessary to life than food—second only to oxygen.	Drinking water, and other beverages; all foods except those made up of a single nutrient, as sugar and some fats. Milk, milk drinks, soups, vegetables, fruit juices, watermelon, strawberries, lettuce, and tomatoes.

FIGURE 56-1 *(continued)*

differences among them. Working as a medical assistant, you can certainly distribute dietary information under the direction and supervision of a physician; however, it is usually a registered dietitian who creates dietary regimens and methods of implementation for the patient. Regarding nutrition as part of patient care, you, as the medical assistant, may:

- **Provide patient education and education materials related to nutrition as directed by the physician—** A physician may ask you to provide patients with information relating to preventative measures associated with nutrition and the disease process. One example is providing a patient who has borderline hypertension information about reducing sodium intake in the daily diet. However, the physician will likely write orders for medical nutrition therapy to be provided by a registered dietitian for a patient newly diagnosed with diabetes or cardiovascular disease, conditions for which treatment requires a complete diet modification.

- **Assist in researching and creating patient education programs and materials as related to nutrition—** This is more common for a medical assistant who works in an office with or who is employed by a registered dietitian. However, as mentioned earlier, a medical assistant working in a family or internal medicine practice may be asked to create some materials related to proper nutrition as preventative medicine. All patient education materials are reviewed and approved by the physician or registered dietitian before distribution to patients.

Professionalism

Medical assistants should project a professional image at all times. Though it might not be immediately obvious, a professional image can have a direct connection to nutrition. Consider the break room, lunch deliveries, and snacks that are kept on desks. Pizza deliveries, cookies and cakes in the break room, and candy sitting at the front desk might seem harmless, but they do not project an image of healthy choices in the office. Of course, there are times for office parties and celebrations where unhealthy food choices are present, but these should be a rarity and never the norm. Break rooms should be away from the patients' field of view, or the door should always remain closed if it is located in a common area. Food and drinks should not be left at work stations, because it provides an unprofessional image in general.

- **Complete referrals and preauthorizations with health insurance plans—**This is done so that a patient can obtain medical nutrition therapy services and pay less out of pocket.

- **Support and encourage patients as they embark on dietary changes and promote the importance of following through with appointments with registered dietitians and other nutrition professionals—** Dietary modifications can be an overwhelming change in patients' lives and, as part of the health care team, you can boost their spirits and cheer them on as they make progress in their journey. This is a great example of a medical assistant working as a patient coach in regard to health maintenance and disease prevention.

A REVIEW: DIGESTION AND METABOLISM

An understanding of digestion and metabolism is important when discussing nutrition. This is because the entire digestive process involves turning the food we consume into usable energy and absorbing nutrients to facilitate the processes of the human body. Certain digestive diseases, such as Crohn's disease, celiac disease, and inflammatory bowel disease, greatly inhibit the body's ability to properly absorb and use nutrients from the gastrointestinal tract. These disorders often result in a condition known as **malabsorption**, which can lead to serious complications such as anemia, vitamin and mineral deficiencies, malnutrition, and gallbladder or kidney stones.

Digestion

Digestion is the body's process of converting food into chemical substances that can be absorbed into the bloodstream and used by body tissues and organs. The digestive process is accomplished by breaking down, diluting, dissolving, and chemically splitting the food we consume into simpler compounds. For example, proteins are broken down into amino acids, carbohydrates are broken down into **monosaccharides** (simple sugars), and fats are absorbed as fatty acids and glycerol (glycerin).

Digestion takes place in the alimentary canal, also referred to as the digestive system or the gastrointestinal (GI) tract (Figure 56-2). Accessory organs, including the salivary glands, liver, gallbladder, and pancreas, provide essential enzymes for digestion through their secretions. Water, minerals, some vitamins, and some of the carbohydrates in fruit are absorbable as soon as they are ingested into the stomach.

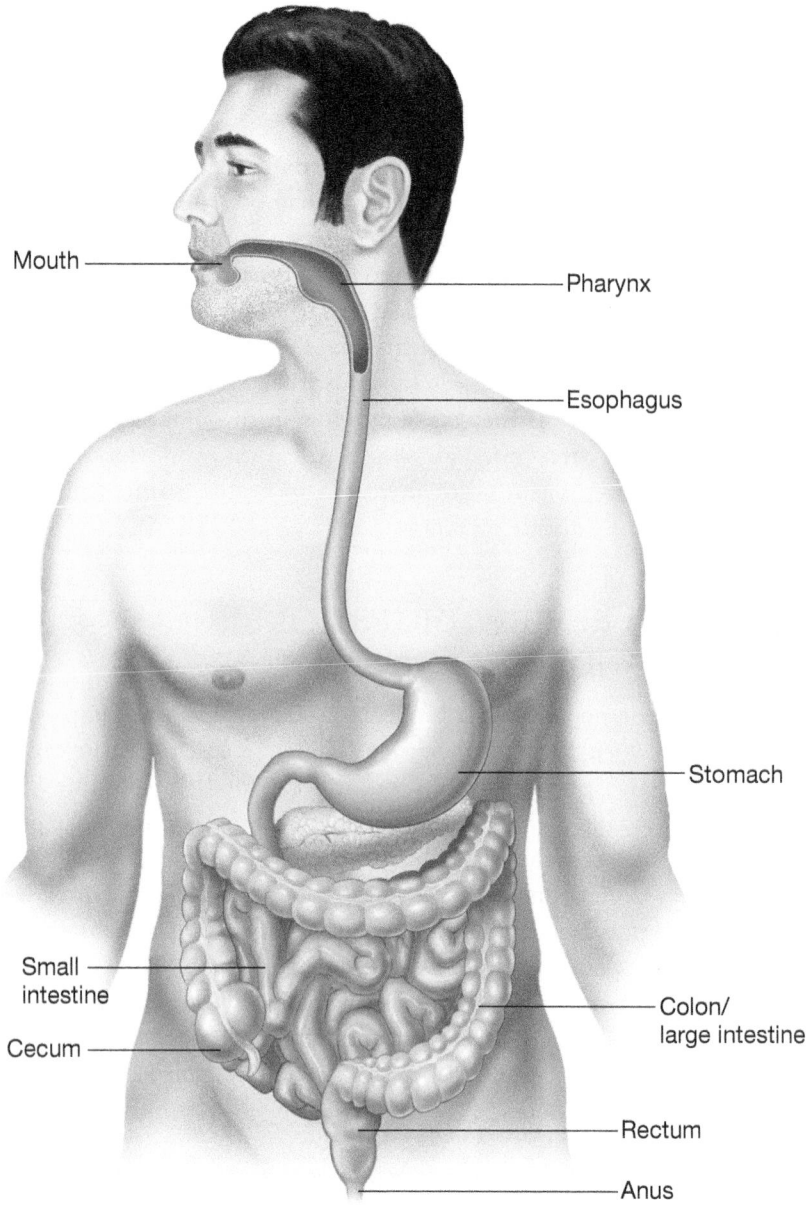

Mouth

Pharynx

Esophagus

Stomach

Small
intestine

Colon/
large intestine

Cecum

Rectum

Anus

FIGURE 56-2 The digestive system.

Other substances are digested more slowly as they move through the GI tract.

The average adult stomach holds about 1 to 1.5 quarts of food and liquid. The digestive process that takes place in the stomach will reach a peak about two hours after a meal. It may take three to five hours for the stomach to empty all of its contents into the small intestine. After a person starts a meal, it may take 20 minutes for the brain to register that food has entered the system. This is why it is important to encourage patients to eat slowly. Excess food and calories are consumed when a person who has eaten too quickly still feels hungry and goes on eating after she has actually eaten enough.

Digestion is influenced by emotions as well as the enzyme and chemical actions of the digestive system. A quiet, calm atmosphere at mealtime can enhance the digestive process.

Metabolism

Metabolism is the sum of all physical and chemical changes that take place inside the cells of the human body. The substances that undergo metabolic change in the body cells are the food, air, water, and other materials that are absorbed into the bloodstream from the digestive and respiratory systems and then carried by the blood to the cells. Specific enzymes that are required to maintain metabolism include amino acids, carbohydrates, vitamins, and essential trace minerals.

Metabolism within the body cells produces energy. Approximately 25 percent of the energy created by cell metabolism is used by the body to carry on its normal functions, such as respiration, digestion, reproduction, muscular movement, circulation, and cellular regrowth. The remaining 75 percent of the energy produced by metabolism becomes heat.

Eating and drinking the wrong foods can negatively affect metabolism by slowing it down.

NUTRIENTS

Nutrients are the organic and inorganic chemical substances found in foods that supply the body with the elements necessary for metabolism. (Organic substances contain carbon, usually bonded to hydrogen; inorganic substances do not contain carbon. Organic substances are essential to living organisms.) Certain nutrients (carbohydrates, fats, and proteins) provide energy, and other nutrients (water, electrolytes, minerals, and vitamins) are essential to supporting the metabolic process.

More than 50 nutrients are required for the human body to function properly. These nutrients must be consumed in the diet on a daily basis. Nutrients are grouped into six main classifications, as follows:

1. Carbohydrates
2. Proteins
3. Fats
4. Water
5. Vitamins
6. Minerals

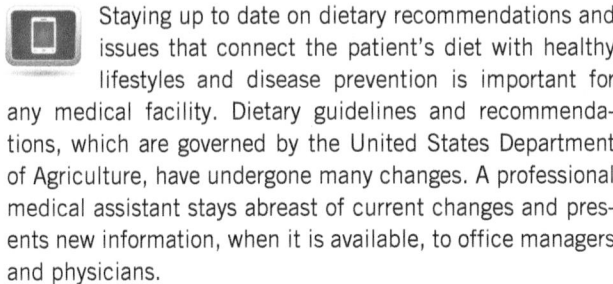
Staying up to date on dietary recommendations and issues that connect the patient's diet with healthy lifestyles and disease prevention is important for any medical facility. Dietary guidelines and recommendations, which are governed by the United States Department of Agriculture, have undergone many changes. A professional medical assistant stays abreast of current changes and presents new information, when it is available, to office managers and physicians.

Often, employees who have a personal passion for health and wellness in their lives outside the office are asked to work on specialized projects dealing with health, wellness, and fitness for staff members and patients alike. For example, teams of staff members may decide to hold occasional contests throughout the year that focus on weight loss or increasing daily activity and exercise. Contests and activities of this sort are beneficial both to staff members who participate and to patients who observe the results of healthy lifestyles followed by their health care team, such as energy, healthy body weights, shiny hair, and clear skin. It is always inspiring to patients when their health care team seems, themselves, to be healthy. It is discouraging to come into a medical office and encounter staff members who look unkempt, tired, and overweight.

Carbohydrates

Carbohydrates are the main source of energy from the foods we consume. Carbohydrates are the sugars (simple carbohydrates) and starches (complex carbohydrates) that are found mainly in plants. They are stored in the body in the form of glycogen. Glycogen is in virtually all body tissues; however, the majority of glycogen is stored in the liver and the muscles, where it functions as an important source of reserved energy. Every gram of carbohydrates provides 4 calories of energy.

Sugars include simple sugars (monosaccharides: glucose, galactose, and fructose) and complex sugars (disaccharides: sucrose, lactose, and maltose). Starches are **polysaccharides** (multiple monosaccharides bonded together), which are reduced to glucose during the digestive process and transported into the blood. Most sugars are produced naturally by plants, especially fruits (fructose), sugar cane, and sugar beets. However, **lactose**, a combination of glucose and galactose, is found in animal milk. Processed or **refined sugars** (e.g., table sugar, molasses, corn syrup) have been extracted and concentrated from natural resources. These types of simple sugars, as well as other simple carbohydrates, are absorbed

TABLE 56-1	Simple and Complex Carbohydrates	
Simple Carbohydrates (Simple Sugars)	**Complex Carbohydrates (Starches)**
• Refined table sugar • Honey • Jelly • Syrup • Candy • Natural sugar in fruits and vegetables	• Vegetables such as yams, potatoes, broccoli, carrots, peas, and beans • Citrus fruits including oranges, grapefruit, lemons, and limes • Whole grain breads, cereals, and pastas

rapidly by the body and cause blood sugar levels to spike quickly. Simple sugar intake should be closely monitored, and many would argue it should be avoided completely.

Complex carbohydrates are considered ideal foods for a healthy diet, because they are generally low in fat, high in fiber, and a good source of vitamins and minerals. Complex carbohydrates take longer for the body to digest and therefore blood sugar levels rise more gradually. These are considered healthier than simple carbohydrates. Excess carbohydrates are stored in the body as fat. Table 56-1 provides a list of simple and complex carbohydrates.

Dietitians recommend that only 10 percent of the body's daily caloric intake should come from refined sugar. Complex carbohydrates should provide 50 percent to 60 percent of the daily calorie requirements.

Fiber

Fiber is a type of carbohydrate that is considered to be indigestible. It is often referred to as "roughage" because it helps move food faster through the digestive system. Fiber is commonly found in foods such as bran products, fresh fruit, fresh vegetables, nuts and whole grains, and brown rice. An essential role of fiber is that it helps the body control blood sugar levels. Diets high in fiber reduce the risk of certain diseases such as diabetes and high cholesterol. Fiber also helps to maintain regular bowel function.

Proteins

Proteins are called the "building blocks" of the body, because they form the base of every living cell. A protein is linked together, much like a chain, with 20 amino acids. Eleven of the amino acids can be produced by the body. However, 9 of the amino acids, referred to as essential amino acids, must be obtained from the diet.

The nine essential amino acids are found only in complete proteins. **Complete proteins** include proteins from

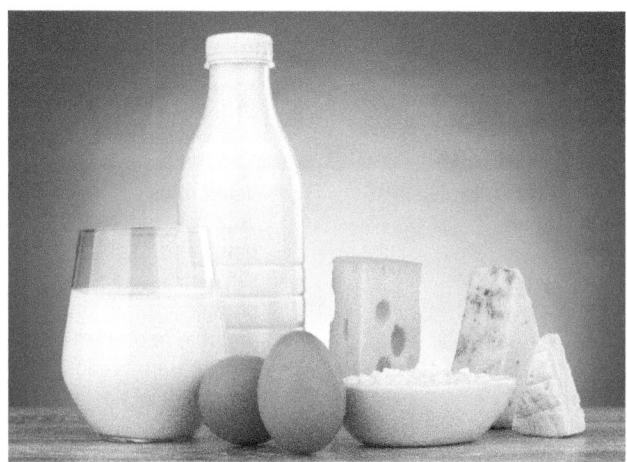

FIGURE 56-3 Eggs, milk, and cheese are complete proteins, because they are animal products.

animal sources including meat, eggs, fish, milk, and cheese (Figure 56-3). Soy and quinoa (which is a grain) are also considered complete proteins. **Incomplete proteins**, which cannot supply the body with all the essential amino acids, include vegetable proteins, such as peas, beans, legumes, and wheat. Fortunately, various combinations of the incomplete proteins can supply the essential amino acids (e.g., legumes and rice). This is important information for patients who are vegetarian (who do not eat meat but may, in some cases, eat eggs and dairy products) or vegan (who do not consume meat or anything else that comes from animals).

It is recommended that 12 to 15 percent of the daily caloric intake come from proteins. Proteins play a vital role in the human body. They are necessary for the following:

- Producing energy (4 calories of energy for every gram of protein consumed)
- Promoting growth and repair of tissues
- Providing the framework for bones, muscles, and blood

Fats

Fats, also called **lipids**, are fatty acids. Fats do not dissolve in water. Some fat is necessary in the diet, because fat-soluble vitamins A, D, E, and K (which are discussed later) are all carried into the bloodstream by way of fats. Two critical fatty acids, linoleic and linolenic, are "essential" to the diet. Patients who suffer deficiencies in these essential fatty acids may experience symptoms including dry skin, hair loss, and improper wound healing.

Fat is a major source of energy for the body. Fat can be found in both animal and plant food products. Fat is important for proper growth, development, and maintenance of

good health but should be eaten in moderation. Fats also provide the following:

- A concentrated source of energy (9 calories of energy for every gram of fat consumed)
- Assistance in the transportation of fat-soluble vitamins A, D, E, and K
- Some taste to foods
- A feeling of satiety, or fullness
- Lubrication for skin and internal tissues
- Energy stores for future use

Parents should be aware that fats are an especially important source of calories and nutrients for infants and toddlers (up to 2 years of age). This age group has the highest energy needs per unit of body weight, higher than any other age group.

Unfortunately, many Americans are eating more fat than they need. Sometimes this is unrealized, because many foods contain hidden fat. Fat content is indicated on the packaging of many foods. However, food labeling can be confusing and misleading. See Figure 56-4 for an example of food labeling components on a box of cereal.

Fats are chemically classified as saturated or unsaturated.

Saturated Fat

Saturated fat is produced by animal sources and includes meats, lard, and dairy products such as butter, cheese, and whole milk. Saturated fat can also be found in certain oil-producing plants, such as coconuts and palms. Many

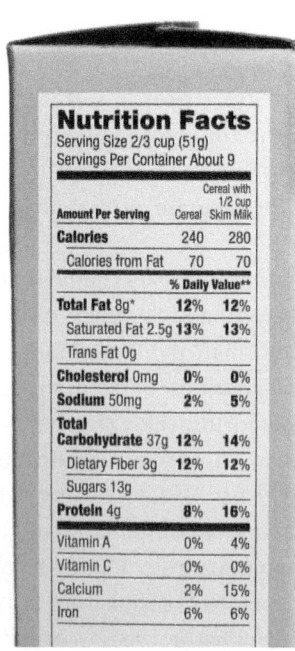

FIGURE 56-4 An example of nutrition labeling on a box of cereal.

commercially prepared cakes, cookies, and nondairy creamers contain hidden saturated fat. Saturated fat has many negative effects on the body, including raising the level of blood cholesterol. It is recommended that no more than 10 percent of the daily calorie intake should come from saturated fat. Reducing saturated fat intake can also reduce the risk of certain diseases, including some forms of cancer, cardiovascular disease, and stroke.

Unsaturated Fat

Unsaturated fat is normally liquid at room temperature but can be converted into a solid fat through the process of **hydrogenation**, or adding hydrogen. Consider margarine as an example of this process; hydrogenation turns liquid unsaturated fat into margarine.

Unsaturated fats are further classified as either polyunsaturated fat or monounsaturated fat. **Polyunsaturated fat** is found in vegetable oils and fish oils, which contain omega-3 fatty acids, essential fatty acids that must be obtained from the diet.

Polyunsaturated fat in the diet is desirable, but **monounsaturated fat** is even more desirable. This is because monounsaturated fat has the ability to lower cholesterol levels and low density lipids (LDLs). Monounsaturated fats include canola oil, olive oil, and peanut oil.

Trans Fat

In 2006, the U.S. Food and Drug Administration (FDA) required that all labels must identify trans fats in food. Basically, trans fat is formed when manufacturers add hydrogen to vegetable oil. Hydrogenation increases the shelf life and flavor stability of foods containing these fats, such as vegetable shortenings, some margarines, snack foods, and other foods made with or fried in partially hydrogenated oils. A small amount of trans fat is found naturally, primarily in dairy products, some meat, and other animal-based foods. However, most of it is manufactured.

Whereas unsaturated fats (polyunsaturated and monounsaturated) are beneficial when consumed in moderation, saturated and trans fats are not. Saturated fat and trans fat raise LDL cholesterol levels in the blood. Dietary cholesterol may also contribute to cardiovascular disease, including heart attacks. Therefore, it is advisable to choose foods low in saturated fat, trans fat, and cholesterol as part of a healthful diet.

In 2013, the FDA introduced a proposed ban on artificial trans fat in processed foods. In June 2015, the FDA decided to continue forward with enacting the ban. This move was made based on the potential dangers of trans fat in the American diet. Because labeling requirements were mandated in 2006, food manufacturers have reduced the amount of trans

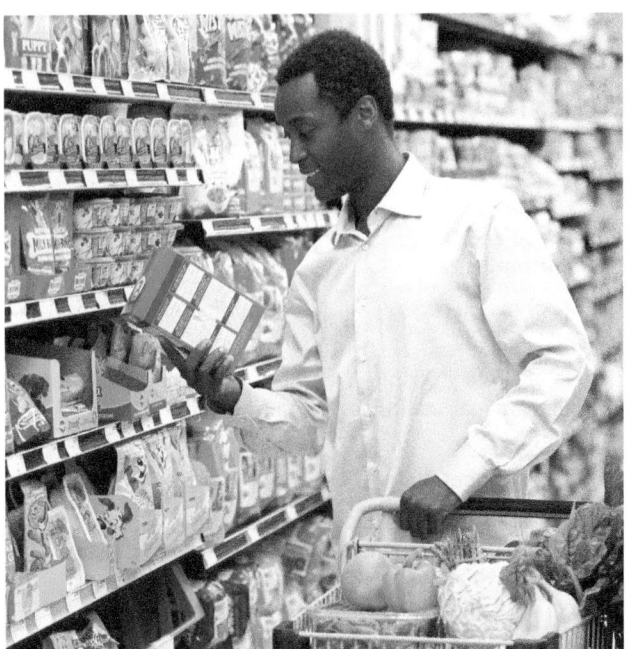

FIGURE 56-5 Healthier choices can be made when time is taken to read a nutrition label.

fats in their foods and, partially as a result of this, trans fat intake among American consumers has drastically reduced. The ban on artificial trans fat is based on the hope that, by eliminating trans fats completely, more lives will be saved through the prevention of heart attacks and cardiovascular disease. Manufacturers of food products containing trans fat have a three-year period during which they must phase out their use of trans fat in compliance with the new FDA ban.

When comparing foods, look at the nutrition facts panel on the labels and choose the food with the lower amounts of saturated fat, trans fat, and cholesterol (Figure 56-5). Health experts recommend that you keep your intake of saturated fat, trans fat, and cholesterol as low as possible while consuming a nutritionally adequate diet.

For resources on facts about nutrients and nutrition, see Table 56-2.

Water

Water is a vital constituent of the body; it is necessary for survival. The human body can survive for several weeks without food but cannot live more than a few days without water. Water is an inorganic nutrient with no caloric value.

Water comprises between 50 and 60 percent of average human body weight. The male body has a higher water composition than the female body because of the greater amount of muscle mass and tissue, which are capable of holding more water. The female body, by contrast, contains a greater percentage of fat than the male body. Fat does not hold as much water as muscle tissue does. Water composition also

TABLE 56-2 | Resources for Nutrition Facts

Resource	Website
U.S. Department of Agriculture	www.usda.gov
U.S. Food and Drug Administration	www.fda.gov
National Agricultural Library	http://fnic.nal.usda.gov
Office of Dietary Supplements, National Institutes of Health	http://dietary-supplements.info.nih.gov
U.S. Department of Agriculture MyPlate	www.choosemyplate.gov
U.S. Department of Agriculture Healthy School Meals	http://healthymeals.nal.usda.gov

changes with age. Water may account for 75 percent of the weight of a newborn but progressively decreases from birth to old age. Obesity reduces the percentage of water in the body, sometimes to as low as 45 percent. These are statistics and averages, and actual percentages vary widely from one individual to another.

Water in the body is obtained from a variety of sources. Water is found in most fruits and vegetables, is ingested as the major constituent of liquid beverages, and occurs naturally as a result of metabolism. The functions of water in the body are described in Box 56-1.

The recommended amount of daily water intake is six to eight 8-ounce glasses (48–64 ounces). Water intake is balanced by fluid output through the skin, lungs, urine, and feces. Individuals vary in their requirements for water depending on the following:

- Age
- Body size

BOX 56-1 | The Functions of Water in the Body

Water is used by the body for the following:
- Carries oxygen and nutrients to cells
- Regulates body temperature
- Prevents dehydration
- Replaces water lost through perspiration, respiration, urination, and defecation
- Removes waste products from cells
- Protects organs and tissues

- Climate
- Exercise
- Illness
- Metabolic rate
- Pregnancy

Vitamins

Vitamins are organic substances that are essential for metabolism, growth, and development of the body. They are not sources of energy, but they are required for overall health. A variety of conditions can increase the need for vitamins above the usual recommended amounts. These include pregnancy, lactation, excessive use of alcohol, and some illnesses.

Most vitamins cannot be formed in the body. Exceptions are vitamin A, which is formed from carotene; vitamin D, which is formed by the action of ultraviolet light (sunlight) on the skin; and vitamin K, which is formed by bacteria in the intestines.

Vitamins are generally identified by an alphabetic letter, although they also have chemical names, such as thiamin for vitamin B_1 and ascorbic acid for vitamin C. The two main classifications of vitamins are fat soluble (A, D, E, and K) and water soluble (B and C). These classifications are important in patients who have diseases that interfere with the digestion of fat, such as celiac disease, because they will eventually develop a deficiency in the fat-soluble vitamins. The human body cannot manufacture vitamin C; therefore, it must be obtained from foods, including citrus fruits or nutritional supplements. The liver stores the fat-soluble vitamins A, D, E, and K.

Vitamins provide essential organic substances, but they can be destroyed in foods through improper storage and prolonged cooking. See Table 56-3 for a further description of individual vitamins, sources, symptoms of deficiency and toxicity, and **Recommended Dietary Allowances (RDAs)**. The RDAs, which are the recommended daily intake levels that will meet the nutrition requirements of most healthy individuals, have been published since 1941 by the National Academy of Sciences. The RDAs are the basis for the "% daily values" that appear on the nutrition facts labels required by the FDA (Figure 56-6).

Minerals

Minerals are inorganic elements that are of neither animal nor plant origin. They are found throughout the body but mainly in bones and teeth. They make up 5 percent of the total body. The two classifications of minerals are macrominerals (major minerals) and microminerals (trace minerals). The **macrominerals** include calcium, magnesium, phosphorus, sodium,

TABLE 56-3 | Vitamins and Minerals

Nutrient/Use	Source	Symptoms of Functional Deficiency	Symptoms of Toxicity	Recommended Dietary Allowances (RDAs)
Vitamin A (carotene): necessary for formation and maintenance of skin, mucous membranes, teeth and hair, normal vision	Egg yolk, fish-liver oils, liver, leafy green or yellow vegetables, yellow and orange fruits, dairy products	Night blindness, fatigue, scaly skin	Headache, skin peeling, bone thickening, liver and spleen enlargement	5,000 IU/day
Vitamin B$_1$ (thiamine): carbohydrate metabolism, nerve cell function, heart muscle function	Dried yeast, whole grains, meat (liver and pork), nuts, eggs, enriched cereals, potatoes, legumes	Beriberi, fatigue, mental confusion		1.5 mg/day
Vitamin B$_2$ (riboflavin): releases energy during protein metabolism	Milk, cheese, egg whites, liver, enriched cereals, yeast, wheat germ, almonds	Anemia, dermatosis, skin cracks		1.2 mg/day
Vitamin B$_6$ (group): nitrogen and protein metabolism, assists in building body tissue	Dried yeast, wheat bran, molasses, liver, whole grain cereals, yellowfin tuna, raisins, legumes, bananas, avocados	Anemia, seborrheic dermatitis, nervous system disorders, convulsions, skin cracks	Nerve damage	2 mg/day
Vitamin B$_{12}$ (cyanocobalamin): nervous system function, fat and protein metabolism	Milk products, seafood, beef, liver, cheese	Pernicious anemia, fatigue, nervousness		6 mcg/day
Niacin (nicotinic acid): carbohydrate, fat, and protein metabolism	Dried yeast, tuna, liver, meat, legumes, enriched cereals, eggs, peanuts, and poultry	Pellagra, dermatosis, glossitis, central nervous system (CNS) dysfunction, fatigue		20 mg/day
Vitamin C (ascorbic acid): needed to build bones, muscles, blood vessels, and connective tissue; aids in iron absorption	Citrus fruits, tomatoes, broccoli, potatoes, green peppers, strawberries and other berries	Scurvy, loose teeth, hemorrhoids, gingivitis, fatigue	Nausea and diarrhea	60 mg/day
Vitamin D: necessary for calcium and phosphorus absorption, bone and tooth development and maintenance; helps maintain nervous system and heart muscle action	Fortified milk, butter, margarine, eggs, fish-liver oils, liver, sunlight	Rickets, tetany, loss of bone calcium	Diarrhea, weight loss, renal failure	400 IU/day
Vitamin E: protects blood cell membranes, body tissues, and fatty acids from destruction	Vegetable oil, wheat germ, soy beans, almonds, corn oil, spinach, legumes	Anemia, nerve damage, red blood cell (RBC) hemolysis, muscle damage		30 IU/day
Vitamin K: normal blood coagulation, prothrombin formation	Green leafy vegetables, cabbage, broccoli, cauliflower, blueberries, and strawberries	Hemorrhage in newborn and in person taking blood thinner		No RDA for Vitamin K
Biotin: metabolism of protein, carbohydrates, and fats	Yeast, liver, kidney, egg yolks, nuts, legumes, cauliflower, meat	Dermatitis, glossitis		0.5 mg/day

(continued)

TABLE 56-3 | Vitamins and Minerals (*continued*)

Nutrient/Use	Source	Symptoms of Functional Deficiency	Symptoms of Toxicity	Recommended Dietary Allowances (RDAs)
Folic acid: RBC production	Dried legumes, leafy green vegetables, organ meats	Anemia, GI disorders, mouth cracks		0.4 mg/day
Pantothenic acid: aids in energy release from carbohydrates and fats	Whole grains, meats, vegetables, fruits, legumes	Muscle cramps, fatigue, vomiting		10 mg/day
Calcium: bone and tooth formation, muscle contractility, blood coagulation, myocardial conduction, neuromuscular function	Milk and milk products, meat, fish, eggs, beans, cereals, fruits, vegetables, tofu, fortified orange juice	Hypocalcemia, tetany, neuromuscular excitability, osteoporosis	Hypercalcemia, kidney stones, renal failure	800 mg/day
Chromium: part of glucose tolerance factor (GTF)	Brewer's yeast; widely distributed in other foods	Impaired glucose tolerance in malnourished children and diabetics		No RDA
Cobalt: part of vitamin B$_{12}$ molecule	Green leafy vegetables	Anemia in children		20 mg/day
Copper: enzyme component	Oysters, organ meats, nuts, dried legumes, whole grain cereals	Anemia in malnourished children		0.3 mg/kg per Day
Fluorine: bone and tooth formation	Coffee, tea, fluoridated water	Dental caries	Mottling and pitting of permanent teeth	No RDA
Iodine: thyroxine (T$_4$) and triiodothyronine (T$_3$) formation, necessary for energy formation	Seafood, iodized salt, dairy products	Goiter, cretinism	Myxedema	150 mcg/day
Iron: hemoglobin, enzymes	Soybean flour, kidney, beef, liver, beans, dried peaches	Anemia		30 mg/day
Magnesium: bone and tooth formation, nerve conduction, muscle contractility, enzyme activity	Green leafy vegetables, cereals, nuts, wheat bran, grains, seafood, chocolate	Neuromuscular irritability, weakness	Hypotension, respiratory failure, cardiac disturbances	280 mg/day
Phosphorus: bone and tooth formation, acid–base formation	Milk, cheese, meat, fish, poultry, cereals, nuts, legumes	Irritability, weakness, blood cell disorders		300 mg/day
Potassium: muscle activity, nerve transmission, intracellular acid–base balance, water retention	Milk, bananas, kiwi, raisins, vegetables	Hypokalemia, paralysis, cardiac arrhythmia (irregular heartbeat)	Hyperkalemia, paralysis, cardiac arrhythmia	2,000 mg/day
Sodium: maintain acid–base balance, muscle contractility, nerve transmission	Meat (beef, pork), cheese, sardines, olives, potato chips, table salt	Hyponatremia, muscle cramping	Hypernatremia, coma, confusion, high blood pressure	500 mg/day
Zinc: growth, wound healing component of insulin and enzyme	Vegetables	Growth retardation		30 mg/day

IU, international units; mg, milligrams; mcg, micrograms

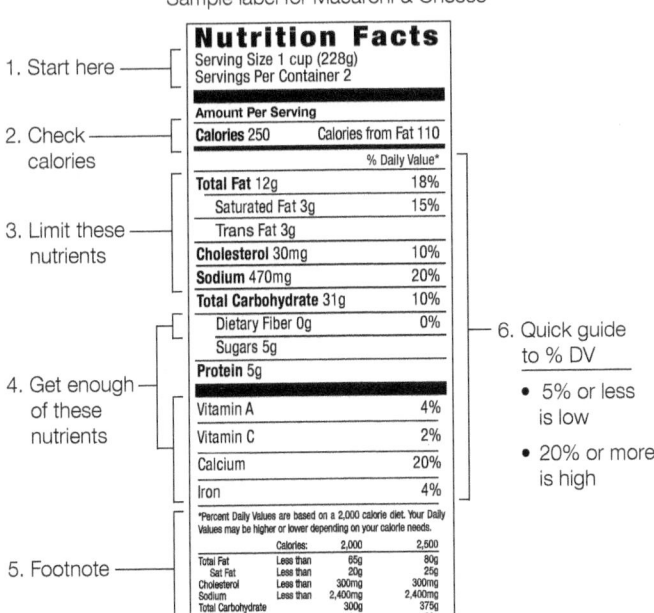

Sample label for Macaroni & Cheese

Nutrition Facts
Serving Size 1 cup (228g)
Servings Per Container 2

Amount Per Serving

Calories 250   Calories from Fat 110

                                                    % Daily Value*

Total Fat 12g   18%
    Saturated Fat 3g   15%
    Trans Fat 3g
Cholesterol 30mg   10%
Sodium 470mg   20%
Total Carbohydrate 31g   10%
    Dietary Fiber 0g   0%
    Sugars 5g
Protein 5g

Vitamin A   4%
Vitamin C   2%
Calcium   20%
Iron   4%

*Percent Daily Values are based on a 2,000 calorie diet. Your Daily Values may be higher or lower depending on your calorie needs.

	Calories:	2,000	2,500
Total Fat	Less than	65g	80g
Sat Fat	Less than	20g	25g
Cholesterol	Less than	300mg	300mg
Sodium	Less than	2,400mg	2,400mg
Total Carbohydrate		300g	375g
Dietary Fiber		25g	30g

1. Start here
2. Check calories
3. Limit these nutrients
4. Get enough of these nutrients
5. Footnote

6. Quick guide to % DV
- 5% or less is low
- 20% or more is high

FIGURE 56-6 The footnote on a nutrition facts label explains the Recommended Daily Allowances that are the basis of the "% daily value" figures.

potassium, chlorine, and sulfur. Macrominerals are required in greater amounts than the trace minerals, which include iron, iodine, copper, manganese, cobalt, fluorine, zinc, selenium, chromium, nickel, tin, and vanadium. Minerals can be obtained from the following sources:

- Vegetables and fruits (calcium, iron, phosphorus, copper, iodine)
- Milk (calcium)
- A well-balanced diet

Minerals do not supply calories or energy; however, they are necessary for physiological processes such as heart contraction and hormonal action. Minerals used to be readily available in fruits and vegetables, because the minerals existed in the soil. However, soil can be depleted of minerals as a result of the heavy use of fertilizers, overuse of the soil, and failure to add organic compounds. Unless the patient habitually buys organic or fresh foods from a known and trusted local grower, the patient may lack vital minerals. This is another reason physicians may prescribe a multivitamin with a mineral supplement (Figure 56-7). See Table 56-3 for more information on minerals.

Dietary Supplements

Generally, vitamins and minerals are thought to be best consumed in natural foods. However, in modern times many foods have been stripped of their vitamins during processing. For that reason, many foods (e.g., breakfast cereals) are

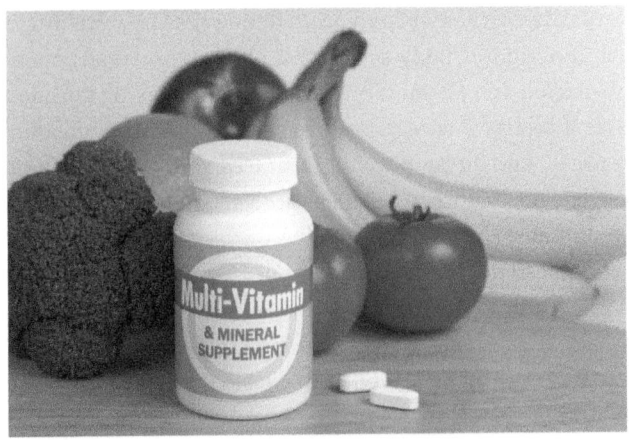

FIGURE 56-7 It may be difficult for patients to get the vital minerals and vitamins they need from their diets, so dietary supplements may be prescribed.

vitamin fortified to increase their vitamin content. Because heavily processed foods lack vitamins, many physicians prescribe dietary supplements for patients whose diets contain a large amount of processed food products.

Dietary supplements come in various forms including tablets, gel caps, liquids, and powders. They include ingredients such as herbs, minerals, vitamins, enzymes, and amino acids. Supplements are often indicated to be taken on a daily basis. By taking these supplements, patients benefit from the additional resources by ensuring that their bodies are receiving adequate amounts of vital substances necessary for daily functioning. Dietary supplements should never be used or intended to replace food. Additionally, it is necessary to understand that dietary supplements can't cure, treat, or lessen the risk for developing disease. These types of claims can be made only for medications, not dietary supplements. Although medications are completely regulated by the FDA, dietary substances are not.

A relatively recent trend toward taking megadoses of fat-soluble vitamins (A, D, E, and K) has led in some cases to vitamin toxicity (poisoning). Taking megadoses of water-soluble vitamins is unnecessary. Most patients need only the daily requirements found in a multivitamin suitable to the patient's age. Men and older women who are no longer menstruating need less iron, and pregnant women need more folate, for example. As a medical assistant, you might be asked to provide patient education on the importance of not taking megadoses of vitamins and dietary supplements.

Cholesterol

Much controversy surrounds cholesterol. **Cholesterol** is a fat-like material that is normally found in the body, produced naturally by the liver and other body cells. It is essential for the function of body systems, such as the nervous system, formation of cell membranes, and synthesis of hormones. The cholesterol we eat, however, comes mainly from animal sources, and these provide saturated fat, which, as noted earlier, may contribute to elevated blood cholesterol levels in humans.

Cholesterol moves into and out of the body cells within compounds called lipoproteins, which are classified into either high-density lipoproteins (HDLs) or low-density lipoproteins (LDLs). HDLs are considered to be "good cholesterol," and LDLs are thought of as "bad cholesterol." LDLs are bad because they carry most (60 to 70 percent) of the cholesterol into the bloodstream. This cholesterol is deposited into the walls of the blood vessels, which can lead to narrowing (stenosis). This is often a precursor for cardiovascular disease and stroke. HDLs are thought to be good because they contain only 20 to 30 percent of the blood cholesterol and carry cholesterol away from the arteries. It is believed that the higher the HDL level in the blood, the lower the risk for cardiovascular disease.

An increase in cholesterol level has been tied to an increased risk for cardiovascular disease: heart attack and stroke. Evidence indicates that unsaturated fats (olive oil and canola oil) may help to lower the amount of cholesterol in the blood. Eggs do not contain saturated fat, but egg yolks contain cholesterol. However, the American Heart Association states that eating eggs in moderation, as much as an egg a day, has little effect on blood cholesterol, and egg yolks also contain nutrients that help guard against cardiovascular disease. Therefore, eggs are now low on the list of foods that may dangerously elevate blood cholesterol. Meats, lard, butter, cheese, cream, and whole milk are greater sources of both saturated fat and cholesterol.

It is important to examine food labels for the amounts of both cholesterol and saturated fat. Many foods contain no cholesterol but a large amount of saturated fat, which can be very harmful, leading to cholesterol buildup in the body.

A HEALTHY DIET AND LIFESTYLE

The key to a healthy lifestyle is eating a balanced diet, one that is rich in a variety of foods. In addition to variety, food portion is very important. Over the years, portion sizes have grown and grown. The average American is unable to relate to a recommended serving size. Table 56-4 provides information related to appropriate portions and serving sizes. The number of recommended servings may vary depending on the individual's age, size, and level of exercise.

Professionalism — Cultural Considerations

A key component of culture is diet. Some cultures may require a kosher diet, whereas others practice vegetarianism or veganism. It is necessary for all patients to be able to adapt a healthy diet into their cultural system. Registered dietitians are well aware of various cultural dietary customs as well as restrictions. It is helpful for you, the medical assistant, to have an understanding of the link between culture and diet so that you can be sensitive to the needs of your patients.

Healthy Food Choices

Healthy food choices include eating less fat, eating more high-fiber foods, using less salt, and eating less sugar.

Eat Less Fat

- Eat smaller servings of meat. Eat poultry and fish more often. Choose lean cuts of red meat.
- Prepare all meats by roasting, broiling, or baking. Trim off all visible fat. Avoid or limit the use of added sauces or gravy.
- Remove skin from all poultry.
- Avoid all fried foods. Avoid adding fat during cooking.
- Eat fewer high-fat foods such as cold cuts, bacon, sausage, hot dogs, butter, margarine, salad dressing, nuts, lard, and solid shortening.
- Drink skim or low-fat milk.
- Eat less ice cream, cheese, sour cream, whole milk, cream, and other high-fat dairy products.
- Instead of eating foods with trans fats, increase consumption of the omega-3 fatty acids in fish.

Eat More High-Fiber Foods

- Choose dried beans, peas, and lentils more often.
- Eat whole grain breads, cereals, or crackers.
- Eat more vegetables, raw and cooked.
- Eat whole fruit in place of fruit juice.
- Try high-fiber foods such as oat bran, barley, brown rice, bulgur, and wild rice.

Use Less Salt

- Reduce the amount of salt you use in cooking.
- Try not to add salt to already cooked food.
- Eat fewer high-salt foods such as canned soups, ham, hot dogs, pickles, sauerkraut, and foods that taste salty.
- Eat fewer convenience and fast foods.

TABLE 56-4 | Recommended Portion Sizes per Serving

Food	Serving Size	It is the Size of
Proteins including beef, chicken, or fish	3 oz. cooked or 4 oz. raw	A deck of playing cards
Pasta, cooked rice, or ice cream	1 cup	A tennis ball
Cheese	1 oz.	A domino
Fruit: apples, oranges, grapefruit	Medium size	A baseball
Butter or margarine	1 teaspoon	A die
Peanut butter and salad dressing	2 tablespoons	A golf ball

Eat Less Sugar

- Avoid eating table sugar, syrup, honey, jam, jelly, candy, sweet rolls, fruit canned in syrup, regular gelatin, desserts, pie, cake with icing, and other sweets.

- Avoid regular soft drinks. One 12-ounce can contains 9 teaspoons of sugar!

- Choose fresh fruit or fruit canned in natural juice or water.

- If desired, use sweeteners that do not have calories, such as saccharin or aspartame, instead of sugar.

- Avoid heavily processed foods.

- Food choices that include hydrogenated fats used as preservatives are not as good as fresh foods.

MyPlate

In 2011, the United States Department of Agriculture (USDA) retired the traditional food pyramid, which had been used by consumers as a guide to healthy eating since 1992. The food pyramid was criticized as not being user friendly and being difficult to understand. The USDA replaced the pyramid with a concept called MyPlate®. MyPlate shows a plate and glass divided to show recommended relative proportions of the five major food groups (fruits, grains, vegetables, protein, and dairy) (Figure 56-8). The MyPlate campaign focuses on healthy food choices with an emphasis on appropriate portions. The USDA includes helpful suggestions to accompany the concept of MyPlate. Some of the suggestions include the following:

- Half of your plate should be filled with fruits and vegetables.

- Half, or more, of your grains should be whole grain foods.

- Regarding dairy choices, switch to skim or 1% low-fat milk and low-fat or fat-free yogurt and cheeses.

- Choose lean cuts of meat and poultry.

- Avoid drinks that contain additional sugars; stick with water or 100 percent all-natural fruit juice.

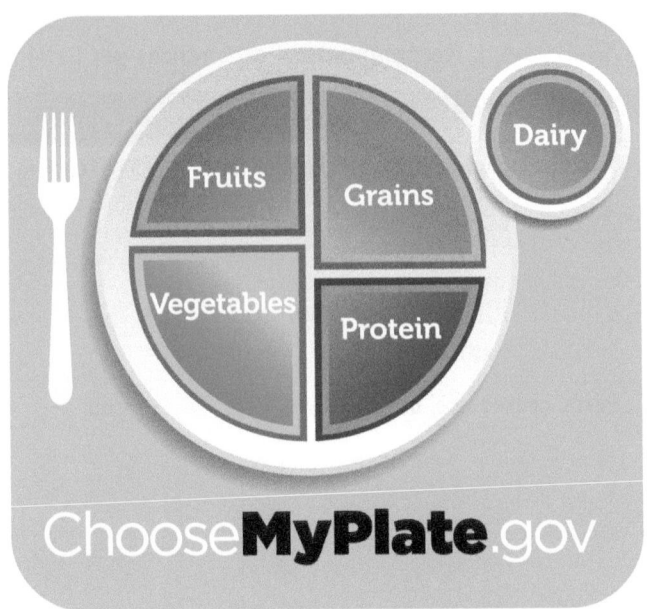

FIGURE 56-8 MyPlate has replaced the now outdated food pyramid.

In addition to MyPlate, the USDA also developed an online tool called SuperTracker (Figure 56-9). This program is aimed at allowing individuals the opportunity to track, analyze, and plan their diet and physical activity levels.

The government website ChooseMyPlate.gov has a tremendous amount of information and tips that can be beneficial to you, the medical assistant, as you help promote health and nutrition among patients. Along with MyPlate and SuperTracker, additional tools include tips for incorporating physical activity into a daily routine as well as information pertaining to daily caloric intake and weight management.

Understanding Caloric Intake

A **calorie** is the amount of heat (energy) required to raise the temperature of 1 kg of water 1 degree Celsius (1°C). It is a way of measuring the amount of energy produced by the foods we eat.

All food (except water) generates energy in the body. Obviously, the body needs the energy that food generates. In other

SuperTracker:
My foods. My fitness. My health.
- Get your personalized nutrition and physical activity plan.
- Track your foods and physical activities to see how they stack up.
- Get tips and support to help you make healthier choices and plan ahead.

FIGURE 56-9 The U.S. Department of Agriculture offers the Super Tracker tool to help you track, analyze, and plan your diet and physical activity. You can find it at www.supertracker.usda.gov.

words, we need calories; we cannot survive without them. Daily calorie requirements of individuals vary based on a variety of factors including gender, age, weight, and activity level. Men generally need more calories than women; pregnant and breast-feeding women need more calories than women who are not; the young need more calories than older adults; heavier people require more calories to maintain their weight; and active people require more calories, because they tend to burn calories (use energy) faster than individuals who are inactive.

When more calories are taken in than are used by the body, they are stored as fat. Overall body weight increases when this happens on a consistent basis. When fewer calories are taken in than are needed, the body begins to use the stored calories. This facilitates weight loss. (Starvation is the extreme of this situation; after all stored calories and fats have been used up, the body begins to break down protein, and muscle mass wastes away. The body literally begins to digest itself.)

Calories come from the proteins, carbohydrates, and fats in food that we eat and digest. The amounts of energy generated by each gram of food we eat are as follows:

- Protein: 4 calories of energy per gram
- Carbohydrate: 4 calories of energy per gram
- Fat: 9 calories of energy per gram

Note: These figures are just for the protein, carbohydrate, and fat content of foods and not the total weight, including fluid, of the food.

Determining the Number of Calories in Food. Using a cookie that contains 1 g of protein, 4 g of carbohydrates, and 4 g of fat, calculate the total number of calories.

$$1 \text{ g protein (4 calories per gram)} = 4 \text{ calories}$$
$$4 \text{ g carbohydrates (4 calories per gram)} = 16 \text{ calories}$$
$$4 \text{ g fat (9 calories per gram)} = 36 \text{ calories}$$
$$\text{Total calories} = 56 \text{ calories per cookie}$$

Determining the Percentage of Calories Supplied by Fat. Use this formula when you want to determine the percentage of calories in a food supplied by fat:

$$\text{Fat calories} = \text{grams of fat} \times 9$$

To get a percentage, divide the result of this calculation by the total number of calories in the food.

Using the previous example of a cookie containing 56 calories, determine the percentage of calories supplied from fat:

$$4 \times 9 = 36 \text{ fat calories}$$
$$36/56 = 0.642 = 64.2 \text{ percent}$$

Therefore, 64.2 percent of the calories in this cookie are supplied by fat.

Measuring Body Fat

As we just discussed, the number of calories consumed (through eating) should equal the number of calories of energy expended (through exercise and daily physical activity); otherwise, a weight gain will result.

Ideal weight is the weight at which the individual maintains optimal health. Ideal weight values vary with age, gender body build, and standardized charts. Also taken into consideration, now more than ever, is the amount of body fat compared with the rest of a person's body. Many methods are available for measuring the percentage of body fat. Some are expensive and time consuming—for example, underwater weighing or X-ray absorptiometry methods. Two easier and more practical methods include the skinfold test and the calculation of body mass index (BMI) method.

Skinfold Fat Measurement

The skin fold measurement of body fat involves using special skin calipers to measure the thickness of fat folds. Three areas are commonly used: triceps, suprailiac (often called the love-handle region), and subscapular (on the back below the shoulder) areas (Figure 56-10). After the designated area is measured with the calipers, a reading from the instrument is taken. Calculations are made and the results are recorded. For example, an acceptable result in the triceps area for a woman is 12 to 25 percent body fat or 9 to 17 mm.

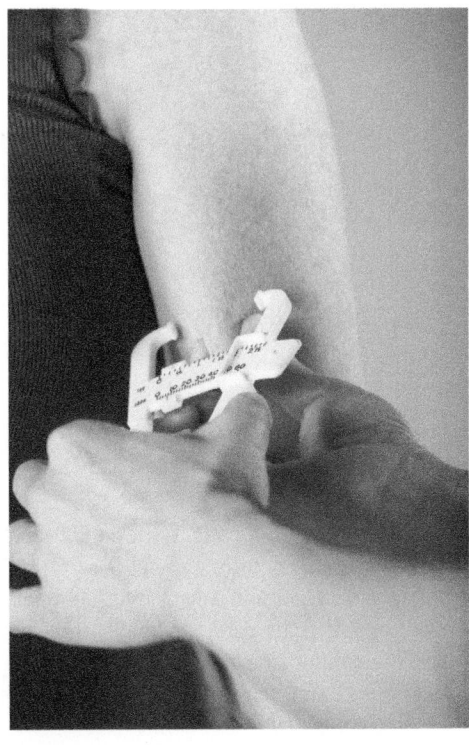

FIGURE 56-10 Calipers being used to measure body fat on the triceps of a patient. *(Erik Isakson)*

Body Mass Index

Body mass index (BMI) is calculated using the following:

- Patient's height in meters (1 m = 3.3 ft or 39.6 in.)
- Patient's weight in kilograms (1 kg = 2.2 lb)
- The following formula: BMI = weight in kilograms/ height in meters squared

A helpful feature of electronic health records (EHRs) is automatic BMI calculation. When you, the medical assistant, enter the patient's height and weight, the EHR automatically calculates the patient's BMI. Although automatic calculations are helpful, you must still understand how to manually calculate a patient's BMI.

A BMI between 19 and 25 is considered a healthy weight; 25 to 30 is considered overweight; over 30 is considered obese. See Figure 56-11 for a body mass index table and Procedure 56-1 for instructions on calculating body mass index.

Exercise

Exercise and other physical activity should be included as part of the patient's health plan. Activity helps to metabolize the fat in the diet so that it does not become stored in the body. Almost any patient can exercise, after given clearance by a physician. Some of the following are considerations when coaching patients regarding exercise:

- Exercises in a pool can be enjoyed even by patients with arthritis and other joint pains, because the water provides a no-impact environment.
- Walking is a good exercise and can be done with little extra equipment beyond a good pair of walking shoes. This is helpful for patients on a budget.
- Some patients will exercise more if they have made a monetary commitment to a gym or health club.
- Patients can lose weight by making simple modifications to their lifestyle, such as taking the stairs instead of an elevator or parking farther away from the entrance to their workplace.

Even the smallest changes can help with weight loss. It is important to match the exercise with the interests, abilities, and finances of the patient. If you select an exercise program that is impossible for the patient to comply with, you set up the patient for failure. It is better to keep an exercise program simple and reasonable for the patient.

Limiting Alcohol

Alcohol is not considered a food product, but it does contain calories and lowers the rate at which calories are burned.

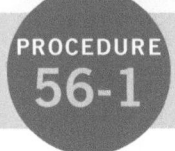

PROCEDURE 56-1

Calculating Adult Body Mass Index

Objective ◆ *Calculate adult body mass index following the steps in the procedure.*

EQUIPMENT AND SUPPLIES

Patient's record; paper and pen; scale for height and weight; BMI formula or nomogram, or chart for BMI

METHOD

1. Perform hand hygiene.
2. Greet and identify the patient; introduce yourself if you have not already done so.
3. If the recent height and weight measurements are not available, obtain the patient's height and weight.
4. Insert the patient's height and weight into the formula, using pounds and inches or kilograms and meters according to facility policy.
   a. Formula for pounds and inches:
   $$BMI = Weight\ in\ pounds \div (Height\ in\ inches \times Height\ in\ inches) \times 703$$
   b. Example: Wt. 175 lbs; Ht 64 inches
   $$175 \div (64 \times 64) = 0.0427 \times 703 = 30.0\ BMI$$
5. Record results in the patient's record.

CHARTING EXAMPLE

07/24/YY Ht. 64 inches; Wt. 175 lb; BMI 30.0......................
....N. McPhillips, CMA (AAMA)

Body Mass Index Table

Height (inches) / BMI	19	20	21	22	23	24	25	26	27	28	29	30	31	32	33	34	35	36	37	38	39	40	41	42	43	44	45	46	47	48	49	50	51	52	53	54
Category	Normal						Overweight					Obese										Extreme Obesity														
												Body Weight (pounds)																								
58	91	96	100	105	110	115	119	124	129	134	138	143	148	153	158	162	167	172	177	181	186	191	196	201	205	210	215	220	224	229	234	239	244	248	253	258
59	94	99	104	109	114	119	124	128	133	138	143	148	153	158	163	168	173	178	183	188	193	198	203	208	212	217	222	227	232	237	242	247	252	257	262	267
60	97	102	107	112	118	123	128	133	138	143	148	153	158	163	168	174	179	184	189	194	199	204	209	215	220	225	230	235	240	245	250	255	261	266	271	276
61	100	106	111	116	122	127	132	137	143	148	153	158	164	169	174	180	185	190	195	201	206	211	217	222	227	232	238	243	248	254	259	264	269	275	280	285
62	104	109	115	120	126	131	136	142	147	153	158	164	169	175	180	186	191	196	202	207	213	218	224	229	235	240	246	251	256	262	267	273	278	284	289	295
63	107	113	118	124	130	135	141	146	152	158	163	169	175	180	186	191	197	203	208	214	220	225	231	237	242	248	254	259	265	270	278	282	287	293	299	304
64	110	116	122	128	134	140	145	151	157	163	169	174	180	186	192	197	204	209	215	221	227	232	238	244	250	256	262	267	273	279	285	291	296	302	308	314
65	114	120	126	132	138	144	150	156	162	168	174	180	186	192	198	204	210	216	222	228	234	240	246	252	258	264	270	276	282	288	294	300	306	312	318	324
66	118	124	130	136	142	148	155	161	167	173	179	186	192	198	204	210	216	223	229	235	241	247	253	260	266	272	278	284	291	297	303	309	315	322	328	334
67	121	127	134	140	146	153	159	166	172	178	185	191	198	204	211	217	223	230	236	242	249	255	261	268	274	280	287	293	299	306	312	319	325	331	338	344
68	125	131	138	144	151	158	164	171	177	184	190	197	203	210	216	223	230	236	243	249	256	262	269	276	282	289	295	302	308	315	322	328	335	341	348	354
69	128	135	142	149	155	162	169	176	182	189	196	203	209	216	223	230	236	243	250	257	263	270	277	284	291	297	304	311	318	324	331	338	345	351	358	365
70	132	139	146	153	160	167	174	181	188	195	202	209	216	222	229	236	243	250	257	264	271	278	285	292	299	306	313	320	327	334	341	348	355	362	369	376
71	136	143	150	157	165	172	179	186	193	200	208	215	222	229	236	243	250	257	265	272	279	286	293	301	308	315	322	329	338	343	351	358	365	372	379	386
72	140	147	154	162	169	177	184	191	199	206	213	221	228	235	242	250	258	265	272	279	287	294	302	309	316	324	331	338	346	353	361	368	375	383	390	397
73	144	151	159	166	174	182	189	197	204	212	219	227	235	242	250	257	265	272	280	288	295	302	310	318	325	333	340	348	355	363	371	378	386	393	401	408
74	148	155	163	171	179	186	194	202	210	218	225	233	241	249	256	264	272	280	287	295	303	311	319	326	334	342	350	358	365	373	381	389	396	404	412	420
75	152	160	168	176	184	192	200	208	216	224	232	240	248	256	264	272	279	287	295	303	311	319	327	335	343	351	359	367	375	383	391	399	407	415	423	431
76	156	164	172	180	189	197	205	213	221	230	238	246	254	263	271	279	287	295	304	312	320	328	336	344	353	361	369	377	385	394	402	410	418	426	435	443

FIGURE 56-11 Body mass index table.

Some studies have shown the value of moderate consumption of red wine in relation to cardiovascular health, but excessive alcohol intake is associated with problems such as alcoholism or alcohol abuse, auto accidents, and family and work disruptions. Pregnant women are advised to exclude alcohol during pregnancy because of its potential to cause birth defects such as fetal alcohol syndrome.

SPECIAL DIETARY NEEDS AND MODIFICATIONS

Some patients have special dietary needs and require dietary modifications. In fact, it is often the case that dietary guidelines are modified to adjust to specific patient conditions, such as pregnancy, cancer, obesity, gastrointestinal upset, food sensitivities, and disease conditions such as anemia, hypertension, and diabetes mellitus.

A diet modified for health reasons is called a **therapeutic diet**. Diets can be modified based on calorie content, spice and salt content, bulk, nutrients, consistency, and intervals between meals.

Therapeutic diets must be carefully explained to patients. In many cases, the physician will refer the patient to a registered dietitian who can discuss all aspects of a therapeutic diet. However, you must be prepared to provide patient education related to dietary modifications if directed by the physician.

Because lifestyle changes must be made to comply with some of the diets, the patient must be motivated to make the required changes. All the principles of adult education must be considered when coaching patients about dietary changes. For example, when a woman is pregnant, it is more important for her to eat high-quality foods (high in folic acid and calcium) than to increase the quantity of food. In fact, a pregnant or **lactating** (producing milk) woman should increase her caloric intake by only 500 calories per day.

Restrictive or Food Sensitivity Diets

Many patients require diets that limit or restrict specific kinds of food that cause health problems, such as allergic reactions. The patient may have a food allergy or may not be able to physically tolerate certain ingredients found in food. The patient may experience symptoms ranging from mild gastrointestinal upset and skin rashes, to more severe allergic reactions that can cause swelling of the airway and respiratory distress (anaphylaxis).

Patients may have food allergies to any number of ingredients. Some common examples include allergies to peanuts, tree nuts, shellfish, milk, and wheat. The physician may confirm a food allergy by removing the suspected food from the person's diet and then beginning a process of gradual reintroduction in order to determine if allergic reactions and symptoms begin. The physician may also be able to identify food allergies by completing a bloodwork series on the patient.

Gluten-Free Diets

Some people have a sensitivity to the protein gluten. Gluten is found in cereals, breads, pastas, and grains as it is most often derived from wheat. This protein works as a glue to help keep food together. Symptoms of gluten intolerance vary widely as does the level of symptom severity. Common symptoms are abdominal pain, bloating, diarrhea, and constipation. Other symptoms may include depression, bone and joint pain, and chronic fatigue. Many people with a sensitivity or intolerance to gluten will experience relief from these symptoms when gluten is completely eliminated from their diets. Patients with gluten sensitivity should eat only foods that are labeled gluten-free. Because of increased demand, many grocery stores and supermarkets carry gluten-free items. These items are intended only for those with sensitivities or intolerances to gluten. It is important to avoid a misconception that gluten-free items are healthier food options for those who don't have gluten sensitivities.

Lactose-Free Diets

Dairy products such as milk, cheese, yogurt, and ice cream contain a sugar known as lactose. A person who is unable to tolerate this sugar is considered to be lactose-intolerant. Lactose intolerance is the body's inability to properly break down and digest the sugar, which results in gastrointestinal upset. Symptoms include bloating, gas, diarrhea, or vomiting. Whereas some choose to eliminate dairy products from their diet, others may choose to use dairy alternatives such as almond milk or other lactose-free products. Medications, available over-the-counter, are also available to help alleviate symptoms of lactose intolerance, allowing lactose-sensitive individuals to enjoy dairy products with lessened or minimal discomfort.

Dietary Considerations for Cancer

A cancer patient has unique dietary needs. What is common for many people to avoid in their regular diets, such as higher calorie or higher fat foods, may be ideal for patients with cancer. These higher calorie and higher fat foods can help the cancer patient maintain weight that is often lost as a side effect of both the disease and chemotherapy treatments. Many cancer patients are also encouraged to eat diets that are rich with fresh fruits and vegetables and healthy whole grains. Increased protein intake is also often prescribed as a dietary modification as protein helps facilitate healing and promote the regeneration of cells. Increased fluid intake is also encouraged to help prevent dehydration and promote healing.

Cancer patients may meet with a nutritionist to discuss their dietary needs based on their individual diagnoses, proposed treatment regimens, and health history.

Weight Control Diets

Weight control and reduction diets are often prescribed for patients whose health is affected by excess weight. Gaining excess body fat can lead to serious health problems, such as high blood pressure, cardiovascular disease, and diabetes. High protein diets and calorie counting are often implemented to help patients lose excess body weight.

High-Protein Diet

A high-protein diet is often recommended for patients who are overweight. This is because protein can help control appetite and maintain lean muscle mass, which helps with burning stored fat. Diets are considered to be high-protein when 50 percent of the daily calories come from protein-rich sources. Protein-rich foods such as meat, dairy products, and legumes must be eaten along with a variety of fruits and vegetables for a balanced diet. Often a high protein drink is included for the patient to consume as a meal replacement.

Calorie Content Diet

A 1,200-calorie diet that includes a balance of the five food groups (fruits, vegetables, whole grains, protein, and dairy) and low-fat foods will result in weight loss. For a healthy diet, patients are advised to eat at least four choices from the grains group, five meat or bean choices, two vegetable choices, two fruit choices, two milk choices, and no more than three fat choices. These choices are calculated to add up to 1,200 calories. Examples of these foods are listed in Box 56-2.

Patients are encouraged to keep a food diary, recording all they eat each day. This helps patients to become more aware of the unhealthy eating they might be doing and to substitute healthy foods for unhealthy ones. Figure 56-12 provides an example of a food diary.

Low-Fat/Low-Cholesterol Diet

The average American diet contains between 30 and 50 grams of fat per day. A low-fat diet is aimed at keeping the

Weekly Food Diary

	Monday	Tuesday	Wednesday	Thursday	Friday	Saturday	Sunday
Date							
Breakfast							
Lunch							
Dinner							
Snacks							
Calories							
Water							
Exercise							

FIGURE 56-12 A food diary can help patients identify unhealthy eating habits and make healthy choices.

BOX 56-2 | Basic Food Group Choices for a 1,200-Calorie Eating Plan

GRAINS

Each of the following equals one grain choice (80 calories) and contains 1 gram of fat; for weight reduction, limit to four to six choices a day:

$\frac{1}{2}$ cup pasta or barley
$\frac{1}{3}$ cup rice
1 slice bread or 1 roll
4 to 6 crackers
$\frac{1}{2}$ English muffin, bagel, hamburger/hot dog bun
$\frac{1}{2}$ cup cooked cereal
$\frac{3}{4}$ cup dry, unsweetened cereal
3 cups popcorn, unbuttered, not cooked in oil

VEGETABLES

Each of the following equals one vegetable choice (25 calories); two or more servings are recommended per day:

$\frac{1}{2}$ cup cooked vegetables
1 cup raw vegetables
$\frac{1}{2}$ cup tomato or vegetable juice

MEAT AND BEANS

Each of the following equals *one* meat choice (75 calories); five to six servings are recommended per day:

1 ounce cooked poultry, fish, or meat
$\frac{1}{4}$ cup salmon or tuna, water packed
1 tablespoon peanut butter
1 egg (limit to 3 per week)

Each of the following equals *two* meat choices (150 calories). Fat content varies for meat but should be limited to a total of 18 fat grams for meat per day:

1 small chicken leg or thigh
$\frac{1}{2}$ cup cottage cheese or tuna

Each of the following equals three meat choices (225 calories):

1 small hamburger

1 small pork chop
$\frac{1}{2}$ chicken breast
1 medium fish filet

Cooked meat should be about the size of a deck of cards.

MILK

Each of the following equals one milk choice (75 calories); two servings per day are recommended:

$\frac{1}{4}$ cup cottage cheese
1 ounce low-fat cheese, such as mozzarella or ricotta

FRUIT

Each of the following equals one fruit choice (60 calories); two servings per day are recommended:

1 fresh medium fruit
1 cup berries or melon
$\frac{1}{2}$ cup fruit juice
$\frac{1}{2}$ cup canned fruit in juice without sugar
$\frac{1}{4}$ cup dried fruit

OIL

Each of the following equals one fat choice (45 calories and 5 grams of fat each); fat should be limited to three servings per day:

1 teaspoon margarine, oil, or mayonnaise
2 teaspoons diet margarine or diet mayonnaise
1 tablespoon salad dressing
2 tablespoons reduced-calorie salad dressing

Do not assume similar products are the same. Be sure to check the nutrition facts panel on food labels, because even similar foods can vary in calories, ingredients, nutrients, and the size and number of servings in a package. Even if you continue to buy the same brand of a product, check the nutrition facts panel frequently, because ingredients can change at any time.

---

fat content between 20 and 30 grams of fat per day. This diet is recommended for patients who have an intolerance to fat—for example, patients with gallbladder disease, pancreatic disease, liver disease, or any combination of them. A low-fat diet has been found to reduce the risk of colon, breast, and prostate cancer; cardiovascular disease; and obesity.

Foods recommended on a low-fat/low-cholesterol diet include:

- Fruits and vegetables
- Skim milk and fat-free or low-fat dairy products
- Whole-grain breads and cereals
- Angel food cake, graham crackers, no-fat wafers
- Lean meats, particularly poultry and fish

Foods not allowed on a low-fat/low-cholesterol diet are these:

- All fried foods
- Visible fat
- Butter and margarine
- Most desserts

Low-Sodium Diet

Therapeutic diets vary in the degree of salt (sodium chloride) restriction. Restrictions vary from mild to moderate to severe. Diets with salt restrictions are prescribed for patients with hypertension and heart or kidney disease. Salt restriction is also recommended for patients on weight reduction diets, because an excess of salt in the diet promotes water retention.

Many foods, especially processed foods, contain salt. A mild sodium-restricted diet (2,000 to 3,000 mg) would result in an allowance of half of a teaspoon of table salt per day and a very limited amount of foods containing salt. A moderate salt-restricted diet allows 1,500 to 2,000 mg of sodium per day. This diet allows half of a teaspoon of table salt, but all processed and canned foods containing salt are prohibited. No salt is allowed in food preparation. This is the most frequently prescribed level of salt restriction.

A severe salt-restricted diet of 500 mg per day would eliminate all table salt and cooking salt, and include only salt-free products. This diet is difficult to maintain using prepackaged foods. Patients are advised to increase the use of fresh fruits and vegetables and to read labels carefully when on severe salt-restricted diets.

Diabetic Diet

A therapeutic diet designed for diabetic patients must consider several factors, including:

1. Type of insulin therapy the patient receives
2. Severity of the diabetes
3. Activity and exercise level of the patient
4. Ability for activity
5. Calories necessary to maintain the patient's weight

A food exchange system is often used for diabetic patients. This allows for variety in the diet, because the patient is able to select preferred foods. The exchange system focuses on eating the correct portions of healthy foods. One serving of food within a group (such as protein or carbohydrates) is considered an "exchange." Foods within the same group can be exchanged because the given portions have the same amount of calories, protein, carbohydrates, and fat; this means they will have the same effect on the patient's blood glucose level.

Some foods within the exchange system are considered "free foods," meaning the patient doesn't need to count the amounts of these foods that are consumed. A food is considered to be a "free food" if it has fewer than 20 calories per serving or if it has fewer than 5 grams of carbohydrates per serving. Carbohydrate counting is also a common dietary tool for patients with diabetes. Carbohydrate counting (sometimes termed "counting carbs" or "carb choices") is based on two basic concepts:

1. Carbohydrates, of all nutrients, have the most effect on blood sugar. Carbohydrates break down within one to two hours and are converted to blood sugar.
2. Whether simple or complex, equal amounts of a carbohydrate will raise the blood sugar in the same amount.

TABLE 56-5 | Sample Menu: Carb Choices

	Carb Choice (1 Carb Choice = 15 g of Carbohydrate or Less)
Breakfast	
1 small orange	1
1 cup of cooked oatmeal made with water	2
Total:	*3 Carb Choices*
Lunch	
1 cup of brown rice	3
1½ cups of chicken and vegetable stir fry	0–1 (depending on type of used)
1 small fruit	1
Total:	*4 Carb Choices*
Dinner	
1 piece of fish	0
1 greens-only salad	0
1 cup of skim milk	1
1 cup of squash	1
2 slices of whole grain bread	2
Total:	*4 Carb Choices*

For example, eating two servings of blueberries (30 carbs) would have the same effect on the blood sugar as eating one serving of a dry-flake cereal (also 30 carbs).

When meal planning using carb counting, women usually have three to four carb choices with each meal (or 45–60 grams of carbohydrates) and men will have four to five carb choices with each meal (or 60–75 grams of carbohydrates). Table 56-5 provides a sample menu of carb choices.

Diets for Gastrointestinal Issues

A dietary change or therapeutic diet plan is often one of the first recommended treatments and courses of action for those with various types of gastrointestinal issues.

Bland Diet

A bland diet is devoid of any foods that contain substances irritating to the gastrointestinal tract, such as seasonings or fiber. Foods on a bland diet are easy to digest and do not produce a lot of stomach acid. This diet is prescribed for patients who have gastrointestinal problems and allergies. Specific foods are eliminated that are gas forming (such as cabbage, broccoli, or beans), contain caffeine or spices, are pickled (contain vinegar), are highly acidic (such as salsa and tomato sauce), and are high in fiber.

Foods included in a bland diet are the following:

- Mildly flavored foods
- Low-fiber foods
- Milk products
- Cooked fruit
- Noncitrus juices

BRAT Diet

Physicians often recommend foods on the BRAT diet for both children and adults with gastrointestinal upset, because the foods are easily digested and do not cause further upsets. Children suffering from uncontrolled gastrointestinal upsets can become dehydrated from the depletion of body fluids more easily than adults. Their condition should be monitored closely. If symptoms persist, they will need to be reevaluated by the physician.

The acronym BRAT stands for the following foods:

Bananas

Rice

Applesauce

Toast

Procedure 56-2 outlines how to provide instruction to a patient, based on the patient's needs for a BRAT diet.

Low-Fiber Diet

A low-fiber diet is also called a low-residue diet. This diet is useful for a variety of patients including those with colitis, diarrhea, indigestion, or a colostomy. Low-fiber diets are used to help bind stool and help with digestive issues.

Some low-residue foods are:

- Cooked vegetables and stewed fruit
- Bananas (the only raw fruit allowed)
- Lean beef, lamb, chicken, and turkey

- Cooked cereal
- Eggs
- Soups, all except creamed soups

Foods not allowed on a low-residue diet are:

- Fried foods
- Milk or milk products
- Seasonings

High-Fiber Diet

A high-fiber diet is used to treat patients with existing problems such as irritable bowel disease and constipation as well as to provide prevention of cardiovascular disease and aid in weight loss.

Dietary fiber is thought to provide protection against diabetes, breast and colon cancer, gallbladder disease, hemorrhoids, and diverticulosis. Fiber may also reduce the level of cholesterol within the blood, thereby protecting against cardiovascular disease.

The recommended daily intake of fiber is between 20 and 30 grams. Dietary fiber is not found in animal products or dairy products.

The following are good sources of fiber:

- Raw fruits and vegetables
- Whole-grain breads and cereals
- Legumes

Dietary Modifications Required for Procedures

A patient might be required to make certain dietary changes when preparing for a specific procedure or for surgery. Dietary modifications may also be initiated following a surgery or procedure to slowly allow the patient's body to become acclimated to consuming and digesting foods and liquids once again.

Clear Liquid Diet

A clear liquid diet contains no solid food or milk products. A clear liquid diet is frequently required before certain laboratory tests, examinations, or surgery. It may also be prescribed for a patient suffering from gastrointestinal problems. A clear liquid diet is frequently the first diet a patient is placed on after having surgery and general anesthesia. If and when the patient is able to fully tolerate a clear liquid diet, he can progress to a full liquid diet. Patients must not remain on a clear liquid diet for an extended period of time, because it has little nutritional value.

Foods in a clear diet include the following:

- Clear broth, generally chicken or beef

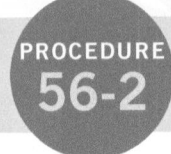

Instructing a Patient According to Dietary Needs

Objective ◆ *Provide patient instruction regarding a BRAT diet to treat diarrhea.*

EQUIPMENT AND SUPPLIES

Patient's health record; printed handout of BRAT diet; pen

METHOD

1. Warmly greet and identify the patient. Introduce yourself if you haven't already done so.
   a. If the patient is a child, direct the education toward the caregiver but do not exclude the patient during instruction.
2. Confirm that the patient is experiencing GI upset, such as diarrhea or vomiting.
3. Explain that the physician has recommended that the patient follow a BRAT diet. During the explanation, review that the foods in this diet include bananas, rice, applesauce, and toast. Explain that the toast should be eaten plain or with a very small amount of butter or margarine. Jellies, honey, jam, and peanut butter are not allowed on the BRAT diet.
4. Review allowed beverages with the patient. The physician may likely encourage the patient to increase fluid consumption to prevent dehydration. Often, fluids allowed on the BRAT diet include water, low-sugar sports drinks, and sometimes ginger ale to aid in settling the stomach.
5. Provide the patient or caregiver with a printed handout that includes information about the BRAT diet and allowed beverages.

6. Inform the patient or caregiver to contact the office if the patient does not show signs of improvement. The physician will want to see improvement within 48–72 hours. Always ask the physician to clarify if you are not sure. The patient or caregiver should also be told to call the office if symptoms worsen.
7. Ask if the patient/caregiver has any questions and if so, answer them to the best of your ability.
8. Have the patient/caregiver sign the handout indicating receipt of a copy.
9. Place a copy of the signed handout in the patient's health record, or if electronic health records are used, scan the document into the patient's EHR.
10. Perform hand hygiene.
11. Document the teaching in the patient's health record.

CHARTING EXAMPLE

01/26/YY 2:35 P.M. Pt. and his mother were given information about the BRAT diet. They didn't have additional questions and were asked to call the office if symptoms didn't improve within the next 48 hr. Copy of handout with mother's signature is in Pt's. chart...M. King, CMA (AAMA)

- Plain gelatin
- Black coffee
- Tea
- Carbonated beverages
- Popsicles
- Apple, grape, or cranberry juice

Full Liquid Diet

A full liquid diet is prescribed as the next dietary advance for patients who are able to tolerate the clear liquid diet. This diet is also often prescribed for patients who are unable to chew or digest solid food. A patient may be placed on a

full liquid diet because of gastrointestinal problems, infections, or recent oral surgery.

Foods recommended on a full liquid diet are the following:

- All liquids allowed on a clear diet
- All fruit and vegetable juices
- Strained fruit
- Soup (creamed or strained)
- Milk and milkshakes
- Ice cream

As with the clear liquid diet, a full liquid diet is not to be used for extended periods of time because it still lacks full nutritional qualities.

Professionalism   The Law

What do you do about patient noncompliance? Perhaps you teach the patient about a healthy diet, but the patient chooses to disregard the teaching and instead eats a diet high in fat and sugar. The patient may develop complications such as diabetes because of this behavior. It is very important for you, the medical assistant, to document teaching and patient education. Additionally, you might have the patient sign a copy of the printed educational materials (a brochure or document) and place or scan a copy of it into the patient's health record. The patient's signature indicates receipt of the information.

It is important that you perform within the boundaries of medical assisting standards. Do not be tempted to prescribe a diet regimen; this is the responsibility of the physician. Once the physician orders dietary teaching, you can teach the patient because you have been approved to do so.

Mechanical Soft Diet

The mechanical soft diet is recommended for patients who have dental problems, such as a lack of teeth, or who have difficulty swallowing. This diet is often recommended when patients are recovering from surgery. Foods included on this diet are:

- All soups
- All liquids
- Cooked vegetables
- Canned fruit
- Ground meat and vegetables
- Tender fish and poultry

SUMMARY

Bodily functions cannot be facilitated without nutrients. Carbohydrates provide energy, and proteins build and renew body tissues. Fats provide work energy and help vitamins function. Vitamins A, B, C, D, E, and K are vital for body regulation. Minerals such as calcium, phosphorus, iron, and iodine facilitate body functions. Water is also important for regulating body temperature, carrying nutrients, and lubricating joints.

Good nutritional habits can improve health. One of the vital tasks of a medical assistant is to provide patient dietary education, as needed and as directed by a physician. However, many times a registered dietitian is the professional who will provide dietary advice, called medical nutrition therapy, for patients. Dietary education should be individualized to the patient and the patient's specific disease or condition.

Balanced diets are tailored to the age and health of patients. The new MyPlate program presented by the United States Department of Agriculture has replaced the food pyramid, is easier to understand, and focuses on healthy foods and correct portions. Dietary modifications are sometimes necessary for certain diseases and disorders. A variety of dietary modifications are available but must be prescribed by the physician.

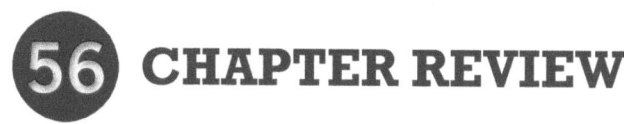

56 CHAPTER REVIEW

COMPETENCY REVIEW

1. Define and spell the terms for this chapter.
2. Explain the difference between a registered dietitian and a nutritionist.
3. What is MyPlate, and why is it used?
4. Determine the number of calories in a cookie that has 1 g of protein, 8 g of carbohydrates, and 9 g of fat.
5. Take a food label from a package of cereal and list the number of calories, total fat, cholesterol, sodium, total carbohydrates, dietary fiber, sugars, protein, and vitamins.
6. Identify dietary considerations for a cancer patient.
7. Explain the three types of sodium-restricted diets.
8. List the factors influencing a diabetic patient's diet.
9. List five foods high in iron.
10. List five food sources for water.

PREPARING FOR THE CERTIFICATION EXAM

1. All of the following are fat-soluble vitamins stored in the liver *except*
   a. vitamin A.
   b. vitamin B.
   c. vitamin D.
   d. vitamin E.
   e. vitamin K.

2. Which of the following is a good food source of carbohydrates?
   a. fish
   b. beef
   c. pasta
   d. poultry
   e. butter

3. A BRAT diet has been ordered for David Abilene, who is 2 years old. Which food listed below should be included on that diet?
   a. boiled chicken
   b. peanut butter sandwich
   c. macaroni and cheese
   d. bananas
   e. pureed vegetables

4. A BMI between _____ is considered a healthy weight.
   a. 3–10
   b. 11–16
   c. 19–25
   d. 28–32
   e. 34–39

5. All of the following are milk products *except*
   a. yogurt.
   b. butter.
   c. cheese.
   d. cereal.
   e. ice cream.

6. Which of the following statements about cholesterol is *true*?
   a. All cholesterol is bad.
   b. Good cholesterol is low-density lipoproteins (LDL).
   c. There is no evidence that high cholesterol intake is linked to disease.
   d. Cholesterol is an essential element normally found in the body.
   e. The information "cholesterol 0 mg" on a food label means that there is no fat present.

7. Which of the following is a good source of iodine?
   a. oat cereals
   b. fish
   c. nuts
   d. butter
   e. cantaloupe

8. Milk is *not* a good source for which of the following?
   a. iron
   b. carbohydrates
   c. proteins
   d. fats
   e. calcium

9. Which of the following is *not* a function of water?
   a. removes waste products from cells
   b. carries oxygen and nutrients to cells
   c. regulates body temperature
   d. decreases blood pressure
   e. prevents dehydration

10. Which of the following is *not* allowed on the bland diet?
    a. citrus juices
    b. milk products
    c. mildly flavored foods
    d. cooked fruit
    e. low-fiber foods

CRITICAL THINKING

Refer to the case study at the beginning of the chapter and use what you have learned to answer the following questions.

1. Patients with pernicious anemia, like Jaden, are lacking a particular vitamin. Name this vitamin and list foods that David may suggest Jaden should eat to increase her daily intake to begin to feel better.

2. Jaden tells David that she knows that she also could stand to lose about 45 pounds, which she knows will also help increase her energy level. She was wondering if David had any tips on making healthy food choices. What might David tell Jaden?

3. Jaden tells David she feels that her weight issues stem from overeating. She wants to learn more about appropriate food portions. What is a good resource for David to share with Jaden?

ON THE JOB

Gladys Pierce is a 70-year-old patient of Dr. Court Franklin. She is more than 100 pounds overweight and is a newly diagnosed type 2 diabetic. She is concerned that she may lose her eyesight and feeling in her arms and legs if she does not get her diabetes under control. Dr. Franklin asks Dan Tyler, CMA, to arrange an appointment with a registered dietitian so that Ms. Pierce can receive proper counseling and medical nutrition therapy regarding her diabetes. In the meantime, Dr. Franklin would like Dan to discuss food exchanges with the patient in the meantime before she is able to see the dietitian.

1. Why should Ms. Pierce have an appointment with a registered dietician rather than a nutritionist?
2. After explaining the basic concept of the food exchange system, Ms. Pierce voices concern because she considers herself "addicted to carbs," including pasta, bread, and cereal. She asks Dan to explain why carbs are so important to diabetic diets. What might his response be?
3. Ms. Pierce then asks Dan how the registered dietician will decide on what type of diet she should follow. What might Dan say?

INTERNET ACTIVITY

Research MyPlate® on the Internet and develop an individualized diet for yourself or a pretend patient.

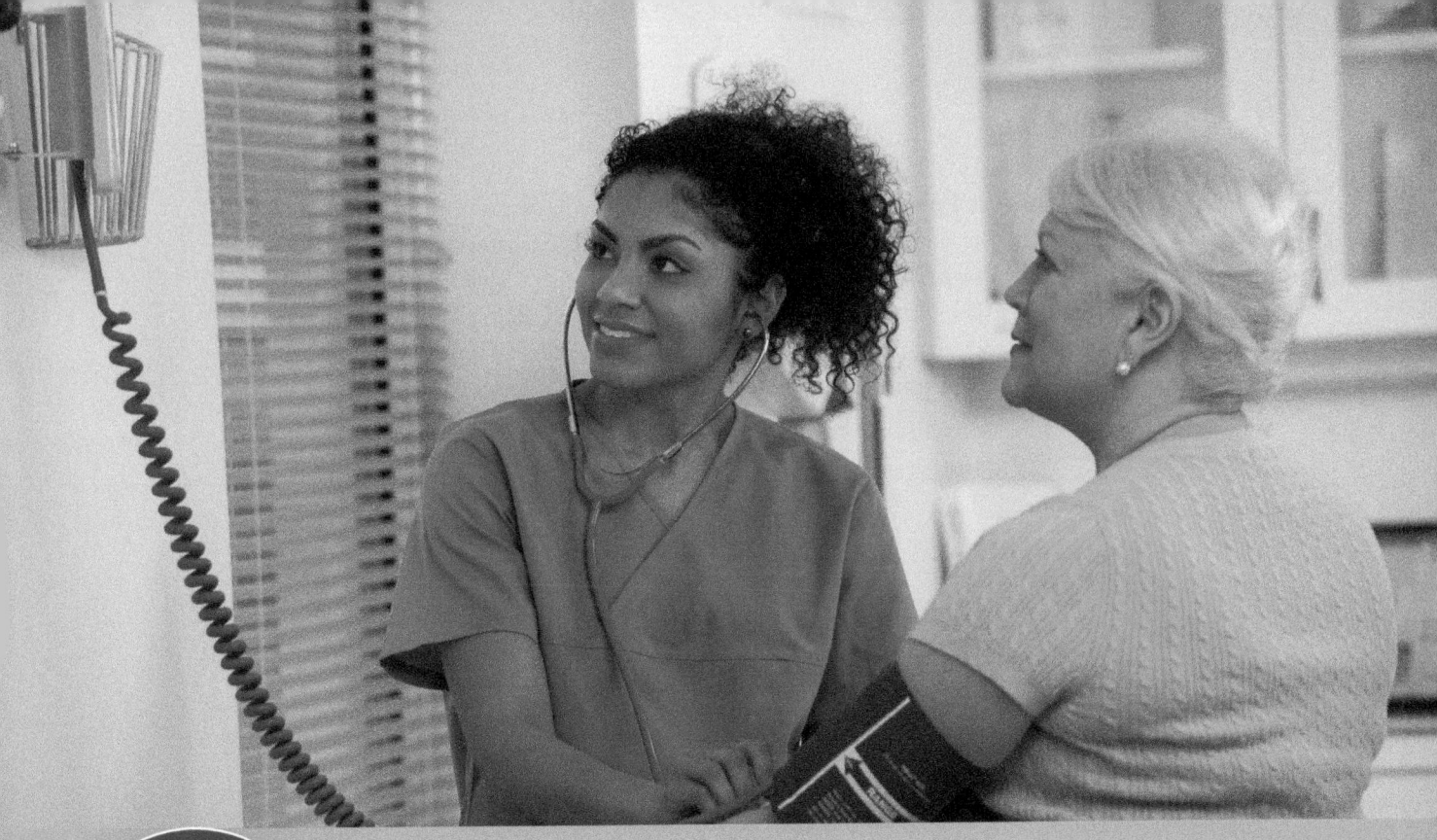

Learning Objectives

After completing this chapter, you should be able to:

57.1   Define and spell the terms for this chapter.
57.2   Identify major diagnostic categories of mental disorders.
57.3   Describe treatment options for mental disorders.
57.4   Explain Erikson's theory regarding developmental stages of life.
57.5   Describe Maslow's hierarchy of needs.
57.6   Identify how stress plays a role in a patient's overall health.
57.7   Explain how a medical assistant can assist with the care of a terminally ill patient.
57.8   Identify Kübler-Ross's stages of grief.

Case Study

Susan Schultz, an RMA at Pearson Physicians Group, is preparing Simon Aurora to be seen by Dr. Penningworth. She notes that his blood pressure is 168/92, which is much higher than his blood pressure of 122/76 that was taken last month during a sick visit. He also has lost 7 pounds since that last visit. Today Simon is being seen for a follow-up for a bilateral ear infection. While working with Simon, Susan notices that he seems edgy and that his cell phone has already rung three times in the past 10 minutes.

Terms to Learn

adolescence	infancy	psychotherapy
adulthood	obsessions	psychotic
bipolar disorder	personality disorders	schizophrenia
childhood	prenatal period	stress
compulsions	psychiatrist	stressor
delusions	psychiatry	terminal illness
electroconvulsive therapy (ECT)	psychologist	tolerance
hallucinations	psychology	transcranial magnetic stimulation (TMS)
hierarchy of needs	psychopharmacology	

Many patients who come into the physician's office or clinic have psychologic or emotional problems that are not the main reason for their appointment. Realizing that people are more than physical beings, you must be able to care for the entire person in a holistic fashion. Although it is easy to focus on the purely physical complaint about which the patient came for help, all patients have psychologic and emotional needs as well as needs for physical wholeness.

PSYCHOLOGY

Psychology is the science of behavior and the human thought process. A **psychologist** is trained in the methods of psychologic analysis, therapy, and research. A psychologist usually has a PhD (doctorate) in psychology and may administer psychologic tests, facilitate psychotherapy, or do research. The psychologist cannot prescribe medication but may collaborate closely with physicians who can prescribe needed medications.

A **psychiatrist** is a medical doctor who has chosen to specialize in psychiatry and thus can prescribe medications. **Psychiatry** is the branch of medicine that deals with the diagnosis, treatment, and prevention of mental disorders.

Psychiatrists also can order and perform electroconvulsive therapy (ECT) or transcranial magnetic stimulation and facilitate psychotherapy. Other medical doctors also can prescribe psychotropic medications but usually refer patients to psychologists or advanced practice psychiatric nurses for psychotherapy.

Within the study of psychology, a distinction is made between normal and abnormal behavior. One means of judging if behavior is abnormal is to compare one person's behavior against the behavior of others in the community. Behavior that interferes with the person's activities of daily living is often considered abnormal. A patient may engage in odd behaviors, but if they do not interfere significantly with daily living, they are not considered mental illness.

Abnormal psychology is the branch of psychology that focuses on abnormal behavior, psychopathy, and disruptions of thoughts and feelings. Some of these disorders that you may encounter in patients are discussed in the following section.

PSYCHOLOGIC DISORDERS

Psychologic disorders can result from genetic abnormalities, infections, nutritional deficits, brain defects or injuries, and substance abuse. Consequently, many people experience some type of mental disorder during their life. However, it is abnormal and emotionally painful to have life disrupted by mental illness, so a medical assistant must aid the physician in quickly detecting and treating or arranging treatment for a patient with a mental illness.

Mental disorders are defined as any behavior or emotional state that causes an individual great suffering or worry, is self-defeating or self-destructive, or disrupts the person's day-to-day relationships. Like physical health, mental health is on a continuum from mentally healthy and functional to mentally ill and dysfunctional.

The guide for terminology and classifications relating to psychiatric disorders is the *Diagnostic and Statistical Manual of Mental Disorders, Fifth Edition, Text Revision (DSM-5TR)*, which is published by the American Psychiatric Association. Major diagnostic categories of mental disorders in the *DSM-5-TR* are described in Table 57-1. This edition differs from the previous edition by placing many illnesses on a continuum rather than having rigid boundaries to diagnoses like autism, and deleting some "disorders" that are now considered more culturally ethnocentric labels than actual disorders, such as the formerly listed Gender Identity Disorder. Patients who have anxiety about their biological gender might be diagnosed with anxiety; however, people who are lesbian, gay, bisexual, or transgender may not have mental illness, and thus Gender Identity Disorder was considered to be stigmatizing and was dropped from *DSM-5*. The *DSM-5* also did away with the complex system of axes that separated diagnoses by period of development, which is no longer considered to be relevant.

Anxiety Disorders

Anxiety disorders are emotional disturbances that impair judgment. Individuals suffering from anxiety disorders are able to tell the difference between fantasy and reality but frequently experience vague feelings of apprehension, worry,

TABLE 57-1 | Major Diagnostic Categories of Mental Disorders

Category	Example
Anxiety disorder	Phobias, panic attack, and compulsive rituals.
Cognitive disorder	Delirium, dementia, amnesia (resulting from brain damage or the effects of toxic substances or drugs), and degenerative disorders such as Alzheimer's disease.
Disorder diagnosed in infancy and childhood	Mental retardation, attention deficit disorders such as hyperactivity or inability to concentrate, and developmental problems.
Disorder with physical symptoms and no organic cause (somatoform)	Paralysis, heart palpitation, and dizziness; also referred to as hypochondriasis.
Dissociative disorder	Dissociative amnesia in which important events cannot be remembered after a traumatic event, and dissociative identity disorder (formerly called multiple personality disorder) in which two or more personalities or identities are present in one person.
Eating disorders	Characterized by abnormal eating patterns, distorted body image, fear, guilt, and depression.
Factitious disorders	Characterized by physical and/or psychologic symptoms that are consciously fabricated by the person, which the person knows are not real. Individuals with this disorder pretend to be sick (or they sicken others) to get attention.
Impulse control disorder	Inability to resist an impulse to perform some act that is harmful to the individual or others such as pathological gambling, stealing (kleptomania), setting fires (pyromania), or having violent rages.
Mood disorder	Major depression, bipolar disorder (manic depression), and chronic depressive mood.
Personality disorder	Inflexible behavior patterns that cause distress or the inability to function; these include paranoid, narcissistic, and antisocial disorders.
Schizophrenia and other psychotic disorders	Characterized by delusions, hallucinations, and severe disturbances in thinking and emotion.
Sexual and gender dysphoria	Sexual performance (lack of orgasm, premature ejaculation, or lack of sexual desire) or unhappiness with assigned gender.
Substance-related disorder	Related to either excessive use of or withdrawal from alcohol, amphetamines, caffeine, cocaine, hallucinogens, nicotine, opiates, and other drugs.

uneasiness, or dread. A certain amount of anxiety associated with life's difficulties is normal, but anxiety that impairs judgment is an anxiety disorder. In anxiety disorders, **compulsions**, repetitive acts performed to relieve anxiety, are frequently accompanied by **obsessions** (persistent thoughts). Anxiety disorders are treated with medications called anxiolytics that decrease anxiety.

Some people have abnormal fears called phobias. For example, the fear of leaving the home and going out is agoraphobia. This fear can prevent people from seeking needed treatment from physicians and thus can impair health. See Table 57-2 for more information about this and other common phobias that might affect treatment.

Cognitive Disorders

Cognitive disorders, including delirium and dementia, impair the ability to think clearly. Delirium, particularly if related to substance abuse, can be transient and is usually treated by easing the person into withdrawal from substances

or by treating the underlying cause. Dementia is a progressive disease that robs a person of short-term memory although sometimes leaves long-term memory intact. Dementia is rarely reversible. Family members of patients with Alzheimer's disease, a type of dementia, also need support. New medications have been developed to improve the course of Alzheimer's (though not to cure it), but intervention must be early to be successful. You should help family members find local Alzheimer's caregiver support groups.

Developmental Disorders

Sometimes disorders that appear before the age of 18 include developmental delays or disorders, such as Down syndrome, in which a person is born with both mental and physical development problems. *Mental retardation* is a broad term that includes some individuals who are profoundly unable to function in the world and those who have relatively high intelligence but are slow to learn. Developmental delays and disorders of this kind are usually treated by working to

TABLE 57-2 | Common Phobias

Phobia	Description	Word Part and Definition
Acrophobia	Fear of heights	**acrophobia** (AK-roh-FOH-bee-ah) acr/o- *extremity; highest point* phob/o- *fear or avoidance* -ia *condition, state, thing*
Agoraphobia	Fear of crowds or public places	**agoraphobia** (AG-or-ah-FOH-bee-ah) agor/a- *open areas or space* phob/o- *fear or avoidance* -ia *condition, state, thing*
Claustrophobia	Fear of closed-in spaces	**claustrophobia** (KLAW-stroh-FOH-bee-ah) claustr/o- *enclosed space* phob/o- *fear or avoidance* -ia *condition, state, thing*
Microphobia	Fear of germs	**microphobia** (MY-kroh-FOH-bee-ah) micr/o- *small* phob/o- *fear or avoidance* -ia *condition, state, thing*
Social Phobia	Fear of being embarrassed or humiliated in front of others or in a public place or fear of being the center of attention	**social phobia** (SOH-shal FOH-bee-ah) soci/o- *human beings; community* -al *pertaining to*
Thanatophobia	Fear of death	**thanatophobia** (THAN-ah-toh-FOH-bee-ah) thanat/o- *death* phob/o- *fear or avoidance* -ia *condition, state, thing*
Xenophobia	Fear of strangers	**xenophobia** (ZEN-oh-FOH-bee-ah) xen/o- *foreign* phob/o- *fear or avoidance* -ia *condition, state, thing*

maximize the potential of the patient through rehabilitation. Rehabilitation is usually successful at improving the quality of life for the person with developmental delay, but it will not increase the intelligence quotient.

Autism (also known as autism spectrum disorder) has a range of symptoms that generally include difficulties with communicating and with forming relationships. Some with autism have very high functioning. Others may be totally absorbed in their own world, may be hypersensitive to outside stimuli, and may engage in self-soothing behaviors such as rocking back and forth.

You will need to work in tandem with caregivers to ensure that patients with developmental disorders have positive experiences in the medical office and that information about the patient is provided by a good historian of (one who can accurately relate details about) the patient's information.

Dissociative Disorders

Dissociative disorders cause a person to withdraw from reality and dissociate, or separate themselves, at least temporarily from the life issues that give them anxiety. If the person flees the life he or she is living and attempts to assume another identity in another place, it may be a condition called dissociative fugue. Amnesia, or forgetting events and places and even one's own identity, is frequently present with dissociative disorders.

Dissociative identity disorder (formerly called multiple personality disorder) is a severe dissociative disorder in which the person develops multiple personalities. Contrary to frequent depictions of people with this disorder in the media (portraying them as pretending to have separate personalities to avoid the consequences of their actions, for example, in a criminal defense), these individuals have usually been severely victimized and have developed multiple personalities as a defense mechanism (for example, to be able to withdraw from an abusive situation by experiencing the situation as something that it is not happening to the present personality but to a different personality who happens to occupy the same body).

As a medical assistant, you should take care to build rapport and trust with this patient and to reassure the patient that confidentiality and privacy are protected.

Eating Disorders

Eating disorders, such as anorexia nervosa and bulimia, are emotional disorders that affect primarily young women. In anorexia nervosa, individuals develop a distorted self-image. Equating thinness with self-worth, they begin to obsess about weight and food, seeing themselves as overweight

(lacking in worth). These individuals may begin to starve themselves or exercise excessively, continuing to believe that they are overweight even when they have become very thin. This is a life-threatening disease that can cause permanent dental, heart, and other organ damage. Bulimia nervosa is another eating disorder, in which bouts of overeating are followed by purging with laxatives or vomiting. Medications can be used in the treatment of eating disorders, but cognitive behavioral therapy is usually indicated. Eating disorders often begin during adolescence and puberty. The chapter titled "Assisting with Lifespan Specialties: Pediatrics" includes a more detailed discussion of this topic.

Hypochondriasis

Hypochondriasis is a disorder in which the person is preoccupied with fears of contracting, or with the idea that one has, a serious disease, based on a misinterpretation of one or more bodily signs or symptoms. With this disorder, it is important to rule out a true physical illness. Therapy would then be directed toward improving the patient's insight and decreasing anxiety.

Impulse Control Disorders

Attention-deficit/hyperactivity disorder (ADHD) is a disorder of impulse control that affects many children and often persists into adulthood. Problems include inability to pay attention or concentrate, hyperactivity ("can't sit still"), and impulsive (sudden or poorly thought out) behavior. It is thought that ADHD may be a problem of either the prefrontal cortex or of dopamine processing. ADHD is often treated with stimulants that help the patient to focus better in combination with behavioral retraining to help the patient learn strategies to improve focus and impulse control.

Because ADHD usually makes its appearance in childhood, school personnel are often among the first to recognize or suspect the disorder. School psychologists may ask that a physician rule out any underlying medical disorder before arriving at a diagnosis of ADHD and making proper referrals for treatment.

ADHD is not the only impulse-control disorder. Other impulse control disorders include those that manifest as excessive gambling, stealing, or setting fires.

Mood Disorders

Mood disorders are disorders of the emotions or feelings and often include a pervasively negative world view.

Bipolar disorder is a mood disorder that, as the name implies, has two poles: mania and depression (which is why it was once called manic-depression). It is characterized by mood swings from excessive mania to profound depression. Depression is characterized by a lack of enjoyment in life's usual pleasures, such as food, sex, friends, family, and hobbies and can be life threatening when accompanied by suicidal thoughts. Mania, by contrast, is characterized by excessive energy, flights of ideas and enthusiasms, weight loss, and cognitive lack of focus. A person who is in a manic phase may not stop to eat, rest, relate to others, or sleep. Bipolar disorder is often misdiagnosed as depression, because individuals in a manic phase feel absolutely wonderful, seeking help only when they are depressed and feeling miserable. Once bipolar disorder is diagnosed, medication therapy is usually targeted at calming the manic phase, but antidepressants may be helpful with depression caused by exhaustion of the manic phase.

Depression by itself is a serious mental illness that affects 20 million people in the United States. One out of four women and one out of ten men will be diagnosed with depression in their lifetime (one of the differences may be explained by a reluctance of men to admit emotional weakness), and unfortunately, depression can reoccur throughout the person's life. Symptoms (as we briefly mentioned in discussing bipolar disorder) include sadness, loss of interest or pleasure in activities, a gain or loss of weight, difficulty sleeping or oversleeping, energy loss, feelings of worthlessness, excessive guilt, and thoughts of death or suicide. Because these symptoms impact the sufferer's life greatly, depression is an extremely debilitating disease that can be fatal.

Depression can usually be successfully treated with antidepressant medications (including selective serotonin reuptake inhibitors). These medications help to stabilize the neurotransmitters in the synapses of nerves, which improves the depressed patient's ability to process information both cognitively and emotionally. Usually treatment for depression also includes talk therapy with a psychologist or counselor to process any issues that may underlie the depression.

Most patients can fully recover from depression if they stick with the therapy, which usually takes several weeks or even months to have noticeable effects. It helps if the patient's health care team, including the physician and the medical assistant, offer constant encouragement and reassurance that, before long, the patient really will feel better.

With some mental disorders, particularly severe depression, the person may become so distraught as to threaten or attempt suicide. A wise medical assistant will always assess for possible suicidality in patients with mental illness.

Personality Disorders

Personality disorders include narcissistic (self-centered), paranoid (abnormally concerned that people will hurt them),

antisocial (not concerned about laws and other people), histrionic (dramatic), and borderline (impulsive) behavior. Unlike other disorders that may necessitate medication therapy, talk therapy with a psychologist or advanced practice psychiatric nurse is the treatment of choice for personality disorders.

Psychotic Disorders

Psychotic disorders are severe mental disorders that interfere with individuals' perceptions of reality and their ability to cope with the demands of daily living. **Schizophrenia** is a psychotic disorder marked by a variety of symptoms, including **delusions** (fixed false beliefs), **hallucinations** (false sensory perceptions), disorganized and incoherent speech, severe emotional abnormalities, and withdrawal into an inner world. Psychoses must be treated with antipsychotic medications, because delusional individuals cannot respond well to talk therapy.

Somatoform and Factitious Disorders

Somatoform disorders occur when unresolved mental illness is displaced into body complaints. For example, a woman in a suffocating relationship may complain of having trouble breathing; a man who was just rejected and is heartbroken may complain of chest pain. Anxiolytics can be used to decrease anxiety and improve the effectiveness of talk therapy.

Factitious disorders are different from somatoform disorders. In factitious disorders, the person creates illness to get attention. Sometimes persons with a factitious disorder might seek attention by injuring another person such as a spouse or child (for example, by partial suffocation or poisoning), sometimes then portraying themselves as the hero or heroine who saved or devotedly cares for the person they secretly injured. If the person injures himself to gain attention, the disorder is Munchausen's disorder. If the person tries to get attention by injuring someone else, it is known as Munchausen's by proxy. Cognitive behavioral therapy is preferred over medication for this group of disorders.

SUBSTANCE ABUSE DISORDERS

Addiction is a physiological need for a substance that, in its absence, causes withdrawal symptoms. Habituation is a psychologic addiction to a substance.

Research has shown that some people are particularly drawn to abusing drugs rather than just taking the ordered amount. Others are drawn to self-medicating with drugs that are illegal.

When people are drawn to misusing substances in these ways, they frequently make poor choices to obtain the substance. A person may steal, forgo relationships, or abuse others to get the substance. Recently, prescription drug abuse has become more prevalent, with a surge of parties at which people swap their medications for those of other party members.

When the patient depends on the substance, instead of family and friends, to cope with problems, the patient is dependent on that substance. Successfully treating substance abuse or dependence is generally impossible as long as the person doesn't recognize the problem or recognizes it but is unwilling to do anything about it, preferring the comfort derived from the substance to any possible existence without it.

For these reasons, treatment usually must begin with the patient admitting that the substance is controlling him or her and recognizing the need for help. The next step is training the patient to be accountable to a group such as Alcoholics Anonymous or Narcotics Anonymous. A medical assistant may need to give information to a substance abuser about local meetings of these groups but also should give information to family members about supportive groups such as Al-Anon/Alateen for families of substance abusers.

Substance abusers may come to the medical office in search of pain medications to which they have become addicted and for which they may have obtained prescriptions from one or more other medical practices. It is important that you document carefully visits to the physician's office so that addictive behavior can be traced. Notify the physician if you suspect drug-seeking behavior. Some symptoms of substance abuse are bloodshot eyes, wearing sunglasses indoors, acting overly sleepy or energetic, asking for drugs and looking for them in the medical office, trembling hands when withdrawing from substances, as well as changes in friends, grades, and performance at work. Never give a patient unsupervised access to medications in the medical office. Box 57-1 lists some questions patients should ask themselves to determine if they might have a substance abuse disorder.

BOX 57-1 | Recognizing Substance Abuse

Am I drinking too much?

Yes, if you are:

- A woman who has more than seven drinks* per week or more than three drinks per occasion
- A man who has more than 14 drinks* per week or more than four drinks per occasion
- Older than 65 years and have more than seven drinks* per week or more than three drinks per occasion

Am I taking risks with alcohol or other mood-altering substances?

Yes, if you:

- Drink or use drugs and drive or operate machinery, or if you mix alcohol or drugs with other medicine (over-the-counter and prescription drugs).
- Don't tell your surgeon, physician, or pharmacist that you are a regular drinker or user of mood-altering drugs.
- Are pregnant or are trying to become pregnant and drink or use drugs. (Even small amounts of alcohol can hurt an unborn child. Other drugs are also dangerous in pregnancy.)
- Drink alcohol or use drugs while you are looking after small children.

Has my drinking or drug use become a habit?

Yes, if you drink or use drugs regularly to:

- Relax, relieve anxiety, or go to sleep.
- Be more comfortable in social situations.
- Avoid thinking about sad or unpleasant things.
- Socialize with other regular drinkers or drug users.

Is alcohol or drug use taking over my life?

Yes, if you:

- Worry about having enough alcohol or drugs for an evening or weekend
- Hide alcohol or drugs, or buy alcohol at different stores so people will not know how much you are drinking
- Switch from one kind of drink to another, hoping that this will keep you from getting drunk
- Try to get "extra" drinks at a social event or sneak drinks when others aren't looking

Has drinking alcohol or using drugs become a problem for me?

Yes, if you:

- Can't stop drinking or using drugs once you start
- Have tried to stop drinking or using drugs for a week or so but only lasted a few days
- Fail to do what you should at work or at home because of drinking or drug use
- Feel guilty after drinking or using drugs
- Find that other people make comments to you about your drinking or drug use
- Have had a drink or used drugs in the morning to get yourself going
- Can't remember what happened while you were drinking or using drugs
- Have hurt someone as a result of your drinking or drug use

A "drink" is considered to be 12 fluid ounces of regular beer, 8–9 fluid ounces of malt liquor, 5 fluid ounces of table wine, 4–5 fluid ounces of "fortified" wine like port or sherry, 2–3 fluid ounces of cordial or aperitif, 1.5 fluid ounces of brandy or cognac, 1.5 fluid ounces of 80 proof distilled spirits.

Some patients are drawn to illegal substances such as heroin or cocaine. The patient may not easily admit illegal drug use to the medical assistant or the physician. The physician may have to introduce the subject of illegal drug use after the patient has developed a level of trust with the physician.

Some substance abusers use legal drugs but in a nontherapeutic way. Oxycontin is a continuous-release medication that provides appropriate doses of oxycodone over a period of time to those who need pain relief. However, substance abusers will crush the medication, destroying its continuous release property, so they can take large doses of it quickly.

A drug that is both habituating and addicting is nicotine. It is found in both chewing tobacco and smoking tobacco. The link between tobacco and cancer is solid. Fortunately, oral medications and transdermal patches are available that can help wean the patient from this drug. It is important that medical staff not smoke in front of patients, because this reinforces this dangerous habit.

The most abused drug in the United States is alcohol. It is legalized to control it, because outlawing it during Prohibition simply led to underground illegal use. Alcohol is fairly easy to access, even by young people, so there is always the potential for abuse. Because alcohol is illegal to consume as a young person, younger people tend to drink large amounts and an assortment of types quickly, usually in cars, usually with a group of other young people. All these behaviors can lead to physical and mental health problems. Binge drinking can cause death.

Although some treatment programs, such as Alcoholics Anonymous, insist that the only cure for alcoholism is abstinence, other treatments include focus on moderate alcohol consumption. Alcoholics Anonymous supports the substance abuser through group support.

Narcotics Anonymous has similar support groups for narcotics addicts. Use of narcotics, which reduce pain and induce sleep, is a popular coping mechanism for those who want to escape stress. For that reason, narcotics are highly controlled substances. (See the chapter titled "Pharmacology" for information about controlled substances.)

You should be hypervigilant for the public safety. If a provider in the office is impaired because of substance abuse, you should report the behavior immediately to the office manager and perhaps notify the state board of medicine or nursing.

TREATMENTS FOR MENTAL DISORDERS

Treatments for mental disorders are varied and include psychotherapy, psychopharmacology, electroconvulsive therapy, and transcranial magnetic stimulation.

Psychotherapy

Psychotherapy is a method for treating mental disorders by mental rather than physical means. This includes psychoanalysis, humanistic therapies, and family and group therapy. Cognitive behavioral therapy helps to change both the way the patient thinks and the way the patient acts. For example, if the patient is afraid of flying, the therapist and patient may discuss the faulty thinking of this fear. The therapist may challenge the patient to fly to process the fears. For some impulse behaviors, the therapist might extract a commitment in contract form from the patient to stop the behavior. The goal of psychotherapy is to help the patient cope with life.

Psychoanalysis is a method of obtaining a detailed account of the past and present emotional and mental experiences from the patient to determine the source of the problem. Because this therapy can take a long time and can become very costly, it has recently fallen out of popularity.

Humanistic therapies are also called client-centered or nondirective therapy. The therapist does not delve into the patient's past when using these methods. The patient is helped to feel better by building self-esteem and a feeling of being respected.

Family therapy and group therapy are solution-focused. The therapist places minimal emphasis on the patient's past history and places a strong emphasis on having the patient state his goals and then finding a way to achieve them. It is usually led by a specialist in this therapy. Figure 57-1 shows a group therapy session.

Psychopharmacology

Psychopharmacology is the study of the effects of drugs on the mind and brain, particularly the use of drugs in treating

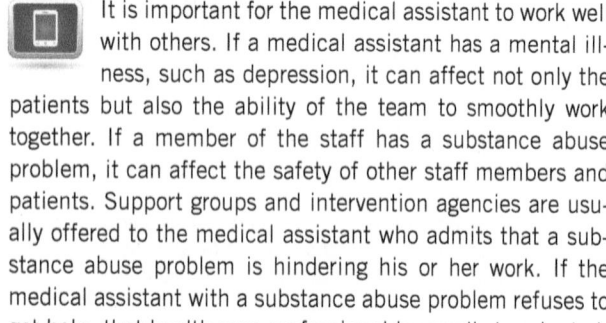

Professionalism The Workplace

It is important for the medical assistant to work well with others. If a medical assistant has a mental illness, such as depression, it can affect not only the patients but also the ability of the team to smoothly work together. If a member of the staff has a substance abuse problem, it can affect the safety of other staff members and patients. Support groups and intervention agencies are usually offered to the medical assistant who admits that a substance abuse problem is hindering his or her work. If the medical assistant with a substance abuse problem refuses to get help, that health care professional is usually terminated.

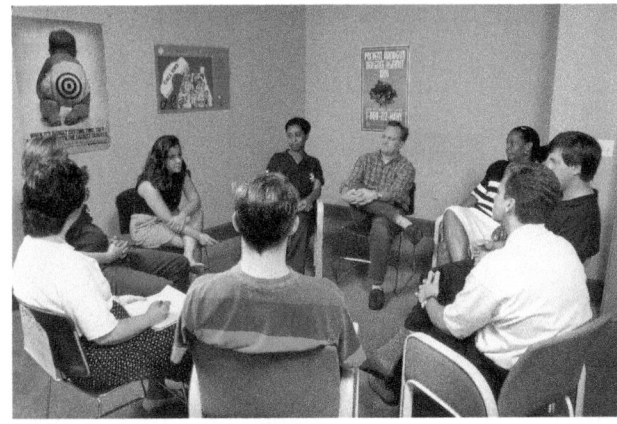

FIGURE 57-1 A group therapy session.

mental disorders. A distinction is made between the brain and the mind. The brain is an organ in the cranium, but the mind is defined as the integration and organization of functions of the brain resulting in the ability to perceive surroundings; to have emotions, imagination, memory, and will; and to process information in an intelligent manner. The quality and quantity of the functions of the mind vary with experience and development.

The main classes of drugs for the treatment of mental disorders are antipsychotic drugs, antidepressant drugs, "minor" tranquilizers, and lithium:

- *Antipsychotic drugs* are the "major" tranquilizers, which include chlorpromazine (Thorazine), haloperidol (Haldol), clozapine (Clozaril), and risperidone (Risperdal). Such drugs have transformed the treatment of patients with psychoses and schizophrenia by reducing the patient's agitation and panic and shortening the schizophrenic episode. One of the side effects of these drugs is involuntary muscle movements, which develop in approximately a quarter of all adults who take them.

- *Antidepressant drugs* alter the patient's mood by affecting levels of neurotransmitters in the brain. Selective serotonin reuptake inhibitors (SSRIs), such as Prozac, Effexor, Paxil, and Zoloft, are frequently prescribed because they have fewer side effects than other drugs. Tricyclic antidepressants are nonaddictive, but they can produce unpleasant side effects such as dry mouth, weight gain, blurred vision, and nausea. Because of these side effects, psychiatrists more frequently prescribe the milder SSRIs.

- *"Minor" tranquilizers* include diazepam (Valium) and lorazepam (Ativan). These are also classified as depressants and are prescribed for anxiety. However, they are the least effective in treating emotional disorders. Patients may develop a problem with **tolerance**

(needing larger and larger doses) after taking these drugs for an extended time. In general, antidepressants are preferred to tranquilizers for treating anxiety disorders.

- *Lithium*, from the salt lithium carbonate, is a special category of drug. It is used successfully to calm patients who suffer from bipolar disorder. The patient on lithium must be carefully monitored, because too much of this drug is toxic and too little is ineffective. Blood levels should be regularly analyzed to prevent overdose or underdose.

Electroconvulsive Therapy

Electroconvulsive therapy (ECT) is a procedure occasionally used for cases of prolonged major depression. This is a controversial treatment in which an electrode is placed on one or both sides of the patient's head, and electric current is briefly turned on, causing a convulsive seizure. A low level of voltage is used in modern ECT, and the patient is administered a muscle relaxant (to prevent violent and injurious muscle contractions) and an anesthetic (to prevent pain) before the current is administered. Advocates of this treatment state that it is more effective than the use of drugs to treat severe depression. However, it does carry the risk of some loss of memory. A photo of electroconvulsive therapy is shown in Figure 57-2.

Transcranial Magnetic Stimulation

Transcranial magnetic stimulation (TMS) is a noninvasive procedure that causes depolarization or hyperpolarization in

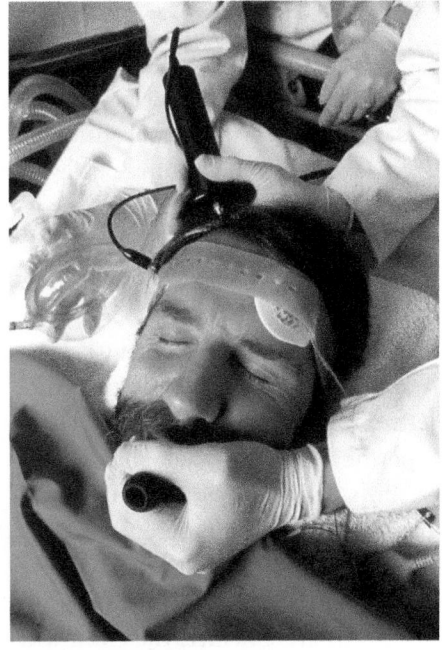

FIGURE 57-2 Electroconvulsive therapy.

the neurons of the brain. TMS uses electromagnetic induction to induce a weak electric current that rapidly changes the magnetic field in the brain. Although there is a tapping noise that sounds like a woodpecker while the treatment is administered, only a slight headache follows. This treatment is being used for depression, migraines, strokes, Parkinson's disease, dystonia, and tinnitus. It has the advantage of no memory loss.

The Role of the Medical Assistant

Although the medical assistant is not usually engaged in psychologic treatment of the patient, the assistant may be instrumental in arranging referrals from the medical office to a psychiatrist or psychologist. In some cases, a health psychologist or advanced nurse practitioner may work in the medical office, providing therapy to the patients in that practice in coordination with the physician. This is a particularly useful model, because the allied health professional can easily access the patient chart for medical information and give useful feedback to the treatment group.

ERIKSON'S DEVELOPMENTAL STAGES OF LIFE

Understanding the developmental stages of cycles will help you provide appropriate care for your patients. A theorist named Erik Erikson posited that throughout the life cycle, people go through different developmental stages in which they seek to complete certain developmental tasks. The five main developmental periods are prenatal, infancy, childhood, adolescence, and adulthood.

Prenatal Period

The first period of child development is the **prenatal period**, which covers the process from conception until birth. Throughout this period, the structures of the body and the organs are formed. At this time, development is influenced by the environment and heredity.

Infancy and Toddlerhood

The second period of child development is **infancy** (Figure 57-3). This period of vast changes occurs from childbirth until toddlerhood. During this time, an infant gains motor ability and coordination. The infant also develops language and sensory skills, expresses basic emotions and feelings, develops trust or mistrust, and becomes attached to caregivers. Erikson believed that during this developmental period, the child balances the sense of trust versus mistrust. If basic needs are not met, the child will develop a view of the world that caregivers cannot be trusted; this

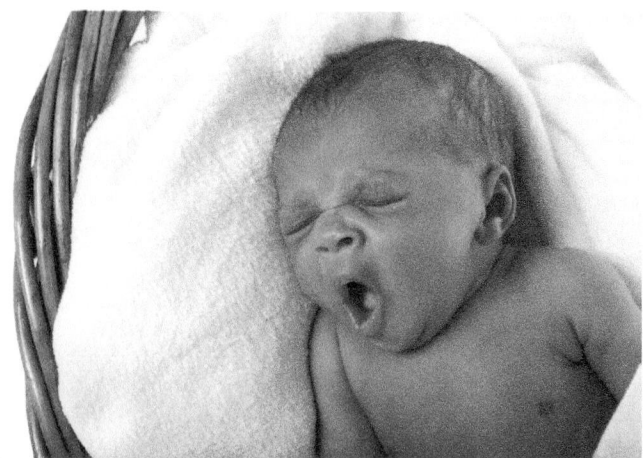

FIGURE 57-3 Infancy. *(Hogan Images)*

can affect later life decisions. Erikson believed that during the toddler years, children show initiative and, if rewarded for it, repeat assertive behaviors. If not rewarded or if they are reluctant to show initiative, children may instead feel a sense of guilt.

Childhood

Childhood (Figure 57-4) is the last period of child development. Ages 3 to 5 years are considered early childhood. During children's preschool years, their linguistic, physical, and cognitive capabilities grow rapidly. The concept of self begins to develop, as does socialization. Young children, according to Erikson, grapple with autonomy versus shame and doubt. They attempt to use the toilet on their own or meet their needs independently. If successful, they feel empowered; if not, they feel a sense of shame and doubt their abilities to be autonomous. Ages 6 to 11 years are

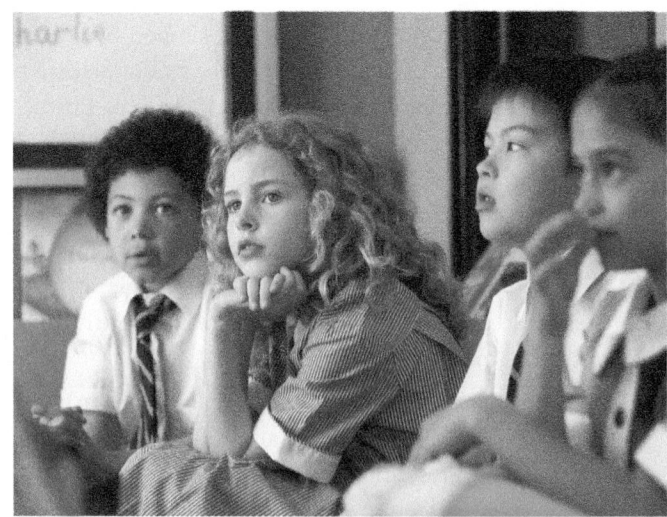

FIGURE 57-4 Childhood *(© bikeriderlondon)*

considered middle childhood. During middle childhood, children start to know their world, think logically, and make major advances in reading and writing. Moral and psychosocial development progress rapidly. According to Erikson, this is a time of industry versus inferiority. It is important for children to feel like they succeed and are industrious, or they will feel that other children are better than they are. Achievement is very important to the child during this stage.

Adolescence

Adolescence (Figure 57-5) occurs between childhood and adulthood. Ages 12 to 14 years are considered early adolescence. During this time, the beginning of formal operational thinking and sexual maturation take place. Early adolescents want more independence from their parents, and they start to form companionships with their friends. Late adolescence occurs from ages 15 to 19 years. The psychosocial task of forming positive identity takes place. Late adolescents are completing their high school education, deciding on a career path, and entering the workplace. They are also forming sexual relationships and developing the ability to relate to others. Erikson believed that during this period, children form their identities and select their roles. If they are unable

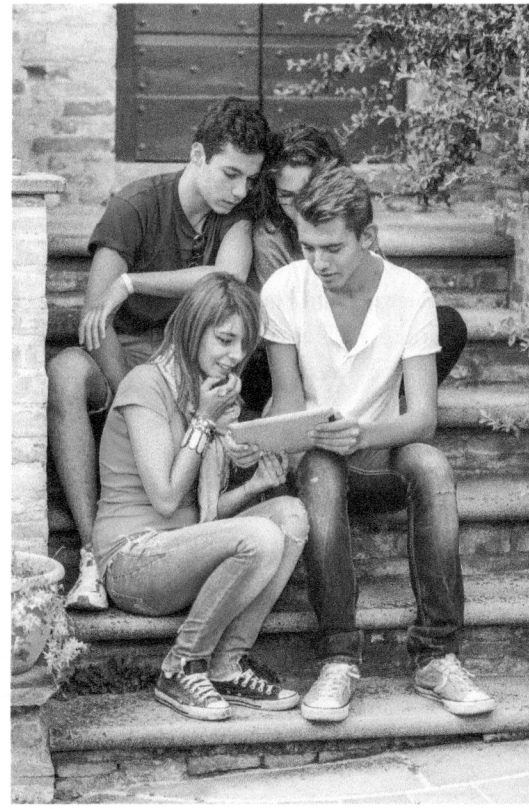

FIGURE 57-5 Adolescence.

to properly decide who they are or want to be, they experience role confusion or identity diffusion.

Adulthood

Adulthood (Figure 57-6) can be divided into early, middle, and late. Early adulthood occurs during a person's 20s and 30s. The challenges of career choice, achieving intimacy, and accomplishing vocational success arise during this time. During this time, Erikson said, the person decides how and with whom to be intimate or whether to isolate himself or herself from intimacy with others. A person in his or her 40s or 50s is considered to be in middle adulthood. Achieving vocational success plus social and personal responsibility occur during this period. At some point during this period, a person's body and emotional status change. This is Erikson's period of generativity (giving back to others) or stagnation. Late adulthood occurs from age 60 until death. During this period, many adjustments occur, and according to Erikson the person feels integrated or despairs. A person's physical capacities and relationships with others change. New meanings are discovered within family relationships. Life satisfaction and happiness are reported by many during this life stage.

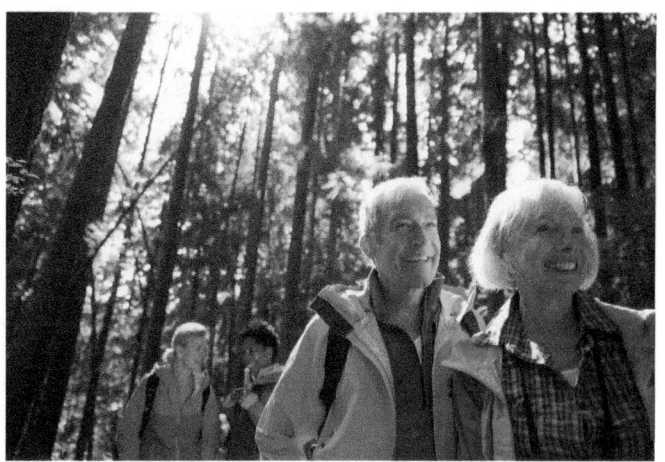

FIGURE 57-6 Adulthood. *(Hero Images)*

Many cultures, particularly some ethnic and some religious groups, have strong opinions regarding mental health disorders. In fact, some Asian cultures view mental illness as a flaw or weakness in a person's character. Those who follow Scientology often strongly oppose psychology, psychiatry, and medication as a means for treating mental illness or depression. Some religious sects believe that mental illness is a form of demon possession or spiritual attack.

These varying views regarding psychology and mental health will have an impact on the way a patient receives treatment. Above all else, it is your responsibility to educate the patient on treatment options, but after the patient makes a safe decision, you need to advocate for the patient's decision even if it is not the decision you would have made.

MASLOW'S HIERARCHY OF NEEDS

Abraham Maslow (1908–1970) developed a **hierarchy of needs** in which he maintained that people had special needs and moved through various levels in achieving satisfaction in life. The hierarchy of needs includes five elements or levels (Figure 57-7):

- **Level I**—Physical needs such as food, water, and shelter
- **Level II**—Security and safety needs, which include physical safety as well as security relating to employment
- **Level III**—Love and social needs, which include having a sense of belonging to a group and the need for social interaction
- **Level IV**—Self-esteem/status, which includes having a sense of self-worth and pride
- **Level V**—Self-actualization/self-fulfillment, which occurs when the individual achieves all that person is capable of achieving and experiences a sense of accomplishment

Maslow said that he believed a person could not move to a higher level until the basic needs at a lower level were met. An understanding of Maslow's hierarchy of needs is important for you, because the patients you will encounter daily are at different stages or levels of fulfillment of their needs.

For example, one patient may be at Level I and be concerned about how to pay a medical bill. Another patient, whose Level II and III needs have been met, may wish to see the physician about cosmetic surgery as the patient attempts to have (Level V) self-esteem needs met. Patients who have a life-threatening illness must have their Level II needs for future security met.

STRESS

Stress is the body's reaction to the world around it. Stress can be emotional, intellectual, or physical. It can also be spiritual, economical, or social. Everyone experiences stress at one time or another (Figure 57-8).

Depending on the level of stress, it can be energizing, motivating, or exhausting. Medical research has shown that a certain amount of stress is not a bad thing. The body's reaction to stress determines if it is good stress (eustress) or bad stress (distress). Stress has also been implicated in various illnesses.

A **stressor** is a real or even an imaginary event that causes stress. Certain major life events such as the death of a loved one, divorce, an unexpected move away from family and friends, unemployment, illness, getting married, delivering a baby, studying for an examination, or purchasing a new car can be stressors. Each of these life events or others may be positive or negative. For a life event to be stressful, it does not always have to be a negative event.

Certain predisposing factors create a tendency or susceptibility to become stressed. These include attitudes and feelings (e.g., emotions such as optimism or pessimism), health habits (e.g., smoking, exercise, drug use, diet), the individual patient's methods for coping, economic and social resources (e.g., income, kind of job, security), and the state of the patient's immune system.

Many patients with a major illness go through a period of depression. The disease may cause emotional changes. In turn, worry about the disease may cause unhealthy habits such as an increase in smoking or drinking alcohol. Patients who have a physical illness such as heart

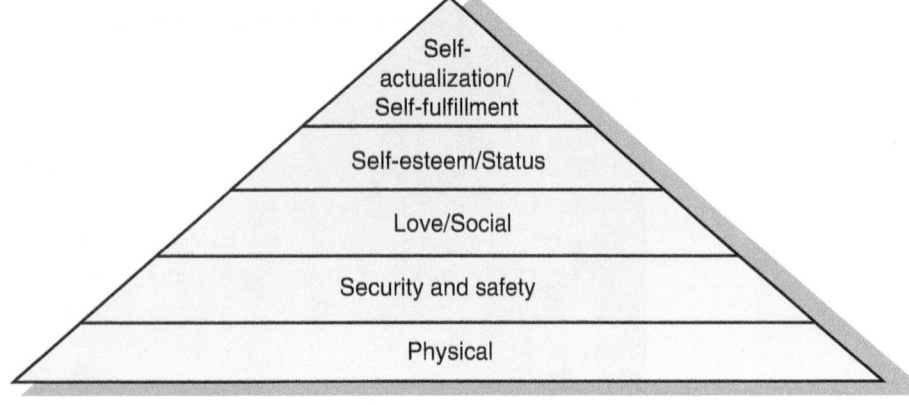

FIGURE 57-7 Maslow's hierarchy of needs.

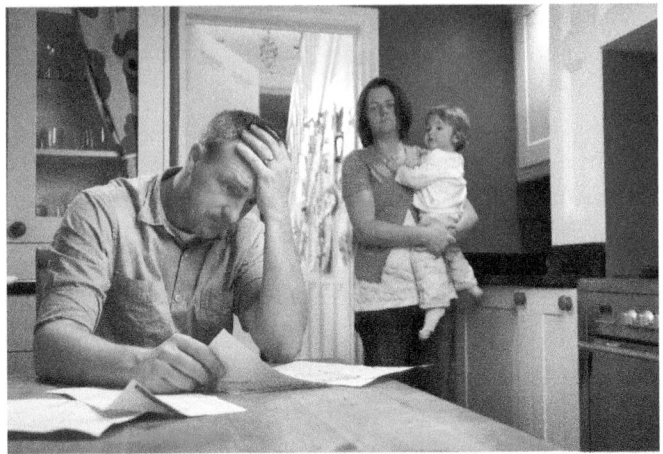

FIGURE 57-8 Signs of stress.

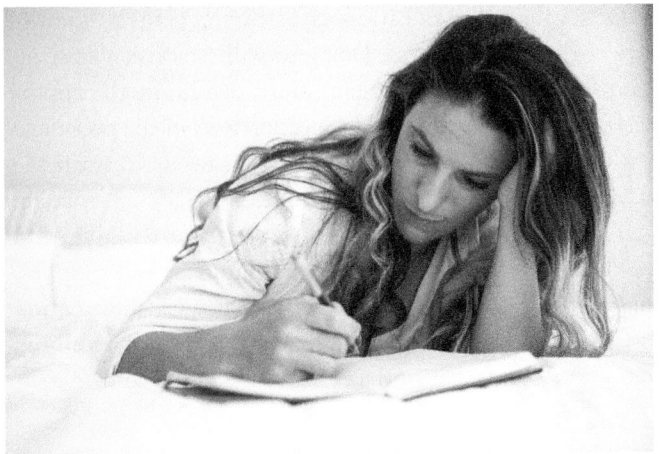

FIGURE 57-9 Coping with stress. *(Aspen Photo)*

disease, diabetes, or AIDS may become additionally stressed when confronted with the loss of income or a job.

Symptoms of stress vary from person to person. It is important for you to know what is normal for you and your body. Box 57-2 lists symptoms of stress.

Post-Traumatic Stress Disorder

Patients who have been exposed to a natural disaster, terrorist attack, physical or sexual assault, military combat, or some combination of them may experience post-traumatic stress disorder (PTSD). In addition to feelings of anxiety, aggression, irritability, tension, and guilt, there can be a numbing of other emotions and a feeling of being detached from others. Memory may be affected, and the patient may experience flashbacks of the event.

BOX 57-2 | Symptoms of Stress

Fatigue
Exhaustion
Difficulty falling asleep
Difficulty staying asleep
Restlessness
Tension
Boredom
Lack of interest
Inability to concentrate
Depression
Cramps
Constipation
Diarrhea
Flatulence
Sore muscles
Increased blood pressure
Increased heart rate
Change in eating habits
Increased use of alcohol

Coping with Stress

Before you or a patient can cope with stress, you must be able to recognize it and know how you are being affected by it. You will also need to know what event or events are causing the stress. Recommendations for coping with stress (Figure 57-9) include the following:

- Develop a strong support system including family and friends.
- Find a balance between perfection and fear of failure.
- Eat nutritious meals.
- Avoid harmful habits such as smoking and drinking.
- Use physical exercise such as walking, jogging, dancing, biking, and swimming.
- Look outward to develop a social interest by understanding other people's problems and needs.
- Try to see the humor in situations.
- Limit the number of activities to a manageable few.

When you are working as a medical assistant, it will be important for you not to let personal stress affect your job performance. While working in a medical office, you will experience stress that is related to work. This type of stress must be left at work when you go home for the night. Personal stress and work stress need to be kept separate and should never interfere with one another.

As a medical assistant, every day you will be taking care of patients who are sick. This can be emotionally, mentally, and physically draining. Anytime your stress level is too high and you have trouble coping, you must seek support from a close friend or family member. If a close friend or family member is not able to help you, seek help from a professional.

Encountering a patient who is experiencing stress provides an opportunity for patient teaching. After allowing the patient to discuss the stress and stressors, assess the patient's knowledge of the topic of stress. Doing so will establish a starting point for educating the patient. Next, determine the appropriate reading, language, and education level of the patient so that you can select and prepare materials to use to teach the patient about stress. Some of the education materials that are used in a medical office include videos, patient teaching, and booklets. After you gather all your equipment and supplies, you will be ready to provide the patient with information about stress. When you have completed the patient teaching, you must document it in the patient's medical record.

ASSISTING THE PATIENT WHO HAS A TERMINAL ILLNESS

As a medical assistant, you will come into contact with patients who have a **terminal illness**. A terminal illness is one that is expected to end in death. This includes many conditions and diseases, including cancer and progressive heart disease.

In cases in which the dying process is slow for the patient, you may have the opportunity to be with the patient on several occasions during office visits. Although there is always hope of recovery or finding a cure through research, it is wise to listen to the patient express fears and concerns rather than to offer false hope for recovery. When there is no hope of recovery and death is expected within a year, you may be instructed by the physician to refer the patient to the services of Hospice. Hospice can provide the patient with comprehensive physical, palliative, psychologic, and spiritual care until death. After the death, hospice will support the family, caregivers, and loved ones.

Death is a natural process that everyone must face. People have various ways of coping with their own death based on a variety of influences, including culture, religion, personal experience, and age.

Culture

People learn what their own culture expects of them at a very early age by observing family and friends as they handle life events such as births and deaths. In some cultures, death is considered a normal end to the life process and is therefore accepted with peace. In other cultures, death may be feared.

The terminally ill patient and family may have already established a very personal approach or method for handling death and dying. You may also have a strong cultural attitude toward death.

Religion

Religious beliefs play an important role in how patients handle death and dying. Some patients have a strong belief in an afterlife. Other patients follow no particular religious belief. In both cases, the patients' dying process and death can be meaningful and peaceful.

It is considered unacceptable for the medical assistant to attempt to convert the patient to the medical assistant's religious faith. Professionalism mandates that the medical assistant and other staff members recognize and support the patient's right to embrace his or her own religious beliefs.

Personal Experience

The past experiences of the patient and the medical assistant mold how they approach the topic of death. If the patient has been closely involved with the care of someone who has died a painful death, the patient may fear the same kind of death for himself or herself. These patients must be able to discuss their fears. In the same manner, if the medical assistant has had past experiences with the death of friends or relatives, it may be easier to assist the patient. On the other hand, patients who have had little exposure to death may have a more difficult time understanding their feelings or expressing their experience.

Age

Older adults usually have less fear of death than younger people. In some cases, an older person may not feel well. Also, the patient may have failing eyesight, hearing, and memory and may look at death with relief. If the patient wishes to discuss her approaching death, you should be ready to listen.

Stages of Grief

Dr. Elisabeth Kübler-Ross devoted much of her life to the study of the dying process and working with terminally ill patients. She divided the grief process into five stages that she believes all persons go through (Table 57-3). It is helpful to understand these stages when attempting to help the terminally ill patient. Although these stages relate to death, they can also relate to other losses, such as loss of body organs, health, marriage, or family members. People move between these phases, but not necessarily in a progressive way.

As the time of death approaches, some of the earlier stages may be repeated. For example, patients who cannot care for themselves may become angry. The critical point to remember when assisting a terminally ill patient is that the grieving period is a normal part of the dying process. The goal is for the patient to eventually accept the loss. Table 57-4 lists resources for the terminally ill.

It is also important to understand that family and friends of the patient may be going through the stages of grief at a different pace than the patient. Although the patient may have

TABLE 57-3 | Dr. Elisabeth Kübler-Ross's Five Stages of Grief

Denial	A refusal to believe that dying is taking place. In this stage, the patient (or family member) may need time to adjust to the reality of approaching death. This stage cannot be hurried.
Anger	At this stage, the patient may be angry at everyone and may express this intense anger at God, family, and even health care professionals. The patient may take this anger out on the person closest to him or her. Usually this is a family member. In reality, the patient is angry about dying.
Bargaining	The third stage of grief involves attempting to gain time by making promises in return. The patient may bargain with God. The patient may also indicate a need to talk at this stage.
Depression	This stage is marked with a deep sadness over the loss of health, independence, and eventually life. There is an additional sadness of leaving loved ones behind. The grieving patient may become withdrawn.
Acceptance	The acceptance stage is characterized by a sense of peace and calm. The patient may make comments such as "I have no regrets. I'm ready to die." It is better to let the patient talk and not make denial statements such as "Don't talk like that. You're not going to die."

reached the stage of acceptance, others who love that person may still be in denial, angry, bargaining to gain time, or depressed. You can be most helpful by being as sensitive as possible to the states of emotion of all those who are dealing with that person's death. Procedure 57-1 demonstrates therapeutic communication with a terminally ill patient.

TABLE 57-4 | Resources for the Terminally Ill

What Is Hospice?

Hospice is end-of-life-care provided by a team of health professionals and volunteers to give those at the end of their lives medical, psychologic, and spiritual support, particularly patients with a terminal illness.

A **terminal illness** is an illness that has little-to-no-chance for recovery and will likely cause death within six months.

Hospice is provided to give those who have a terminal illness a dignified, comfortable death by controlling pain and other uncomfortable symptoms and allowing the patients to be close to their family. Hospice also offers counseling to patients and their families and provides respite to caregivers.

What Hospice *Is*, and What It Is *Not*

Hospice is not a particular place but rather a concept of care for those with a terminal illness and their families. Hospice programs are a *concept of care*, not a plan of action. The goal of hospice care is to improve the patient's last days, weeks, and hours by providing comfort. Hospice is not designed to prolong life nor to hasten death. Hospice team members make routine visits to the home, but friends and family are almost always involved with care. Trained hospice volunteers can provide respite care for the caregivers. The patient can discontinue hospice care at any time.

Hospice care can be provided in the home, in hospice residences, or in hospitals.

When Should Hospice Be Considered?

As with all types of end-of-life decisions, the choice to enter hospice is very personal and depends not only on having a terminal physical illness but also very much on the patient's feelings about death, dying, and spirituality.

Before the patient enters into a hospice program, hospice personnel meet with the patient's doctor to discuss life expectancy, medical conditions, and current symptoms. To qualify for hospice, a patient must no longer respond to curative treatments and have a life expectancy of less than six months.

Hospice will meet with the patient and the patient's family to discuss hospice philosophy, expectations, and services provided. Before hospice is brought on board, the hospice staff will discuss pain levels, support systems, insurance questions, medication, and equipment needs. An individualized care plan will be developed for the patient, and the plan will be routinely reviewed. The patient or family can request a particular hospice or get a referral to another local hospice (there are close to 5,000 hospices in the United States) if so desired.

How Do I Pay for Hospice Care?

Medicare can be used to pay for hospice care. Medicaid offers hospice benefits; private insurance and HMOs also cover hospice care. Tricare (for military service members and their families) covers hospice services.

(continued)

TABLE 57-4 | Resources for the Terminally Ill (*continued*)

What Is Advance Care Planning?

Advance Care Planning is the process of planning for future medical care based upon clarity in goals and values and carefully outlines choices in the event someone else must make medical decisions.

Advance Directives are the documents used in advance care planning; they fall into two categories: instructions for future medical care and designation of a health care proxy.

Documents that provide instructions about future medical care are:

- *Living will*—The individual documents wishes about his or her own medical care to provide guidance for the health care team and the family at the end of life.
- *Durable power of attorney*—Delegates the authority to make medical, financial, or legal decisions on a person's behalf. A durable power of attorney goes into effect when a person can no longer make decisions for themselves.
- *Do Not Resuscitate order (DNR)*—Legal document given by a physician not to resuscitate a patient who has gone into pulmonary or cardiac arrest. A DNR will be signed by the patient or the patient's health care proxy.

The document to designate someone as a health care "proxy," or another decision maker for the person who is ill, is called the *Designation of a Health Care Surrogate* (also known as medical power of attorney, health care proxy, or health care agent).

Complementary Therapies

Complementary therapies are meant to ease symptoms and/or side-effects of treatment and are used in conjunction with traditional medicine to support the body's natural abilities to heal and enhance a feeling of well-being. They include:

- Nutritionally based programs
- Acupressure
- Acupuncture
- Holistic approaches
- Hydrotherapy
- Aromatherapy
- Hypnotherapy
- Reiki
- Reflexology
- Massage therapy

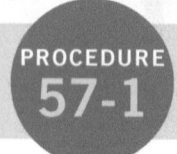

PROCEDURE 57-1

Assisting a Terminally Ill Patient

Objective ◆ *Demonstrate therapeutic community with a terminally ill patient.*

EQUIPMENT AND SUPPLIES

Tissues; printed out copies of resources from Table 57-4

Note: This procedure would be performed in an office setting after a patient has received a terminal illness diagnosis. As a medical assistant, you may work as a patient navigator to direct the patient and the patient's family members to medical or community services that are available and could provide assistance.

METHOD

1. Warmly greet and introduce yourself to the patient who has just been diagnosed with a terminal illness. Extend your greeting to the patient's family members who may also be present.
2. Position yourself so that you are at eye level with the patient and can make direct eye contact.
3. Offer tissues to the patient or family members if they are crying. Otherwise, place a box of tissues within reach of the patient so that they are available if necessary.

4. Ensure that you do not appear rushed and that your demeanor is calm, relaxed, and empathetic.
5. Ask if the patient has immediate questions or concerns he or she would like to talk about before continuing with the discussion. (Some patients will have a list of questions and concerns to address, while others may be too overwhelmed to formulate questions.)
6. Provide the patient with any important printed documents, such as those listed in Table 57-4.
7. As you review relevant topics, such as those in Table 57-4, discuss the therapeutic community and medical resources available to the patient, such as grief counseling or hospice care.
8. Demonstrate active empathy to the emotions and concerns the patient expresses throughout the discussion.
9. As the discussion comes to a close, ask the patient and family members if there is anything they would like assistance with or additional information.
10. Document the encounter in the patient's medical record.

CHART DOCUMENTATION

A discussion took place after Mrs. Lindell was informed of her terminal cancer diagnosis. The patient was visibly upset and tissues were offered. Discussed resources available in the community and ways to cope with stress and pain. Obtained hospice referral per patient request and notified physician that patient wanted to prepare advance directives.....................................
.....................................M. Kanour, CMA (AAMA) 9/12/XX

SUMMARY

Mental and behavioral illnesses are quite prevalent in today's society. Mental illnesses are caused by changes in brain structure and chemistry. The *DSM-5* is the book of classification of the many psychologic disorders ranging from psychosis to personality disorders. Some mental and behavioral illnesses require medication. Others respond more appropriately to talk therapy. People with substance abuse disorders often respond best to group therapy.

According to Maslow, the physical needs of the patient must be met before the psychologic ones can be. Mental wellness is greatly influenced by heredity, culture, and the environment. Patients who are frightened, angry, or depressed need special care.

Poor adaptation to stress influences mental and behavioral health. Kübler-Ross's five stages of grief help the medical assistant to adapt communication to the stage the patient is experiencing at the time.

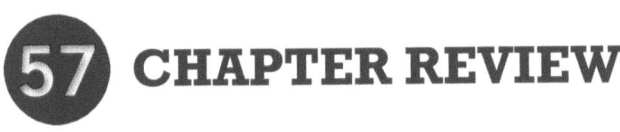

57 CHAPTER REVIEW

COMPETENCY REVIEW

1. Define and spell the terms for this chapter.
2. Describe how you use the eight health habits to cope with stress.
3. Define 10 psychologic disorders.
4. Identify four types of treatments for mental disorders.
5. List 10 symptoms of stress.
6. Describe the five levels of Maslow's hierarchy of needs.
7. Should a medical assistant share his religious beliefs as a way to help a patient cope with grief or a terminal illness?

PREPARING FOR THE CERTIFICATION EXAM

1. Fixed, false beliefs are called
   a. delusions.
   b. hallucinations.
   c. bipolar.
   d. compulsions.
   e. obsessions.

2. Inflexible behavior patterns that cause inability to function is
   a. bipolar disorder.
   b. depression.
   c. schizophrenia.
   d. personality disorder.
   e. anxiety disorder.

3. Phobias are considered
   a. mood disorders.
   b. anxiety disorders.
   c. personality disorders.
   d. bipolar disorders.
   e. psychoses.

4. Trust and mistrust is the task of which stage of the life cycle?
   a. prenatal period
   b. infancy
   c. childhood
   d. adolescence
   e. adulthood

5. The highest level of Maslow's hierarchy of needs is
   a. love.
   b. security.
   c. physical development.
   d. self-esteem.
   e. self-actualization.

6. The transferring or discharging of emotional reactions from one object or person to another object or person is
   a. identification.
   b. denial.
   c. intellectualization.

d. displacement.

e. compensation.

7. A patient who is praying to God in an effort to save his life is considered by Kübler-Ross to be in which stage of grief?

a. denial

b. anger

c. bargaining

d. depression

e. acceptance

8. The stage of grief during which the patient may yell at a family member or physician is

a. denial.

b. anger.

c. bargaining.

d. depression.

e. acceptance.

9. What is the therapy used most frequently for treatment of substance abuse?

a. transcranial magnetic stimulation

b. psychoanalysis

c. group therapy

d. electroconvulsive therapy

e. antidepressant therapy

10. Fear of enclosed spaces is known as

a. acrophobia.

b. agoraphobia.

c. claustrophobia.

d. microphobia.

e. xenophobia.

CRITICAL THINKING

Refer to the case study at the beginning of the chapter and use what you have learned to answer the following questions.

1. During the examination, Dr. Penningworth asks Simon if any changes have occurred over the past month. Simon sighs and states, "What hasn't changed is more like it? My wife has filed for divorce, and my mother was just diagnosed with breast cancer." How might Simon's personal situation be taking a toll on his health?

2. Dr. Penningworth feels that Simon is under a great deal of stress. What are some additional signs and symptoms that Simon may have if he is stressed out?

3. Dr. Penningworth asks Susan to provide Simon with some information regarding stress management as well as a support group for friends and family of people diagnosed with terminal illnesses. When Susan presents this information to Simon, he states, "I don't think I will need a support group because I have been doing a lot of extra volunteer work at my church, and I think because of that my mom will begin to feel better." What is Simon displaying, and how should Susan handle this?

ON THE JOB

Amy Freeman is a new medical assistant who recently graduated and passed the CMA examination. During her education, she studied ways to cope with stress. Renee Baker, a full-time student and a young mother of two small children, has an appointment to see Dr. Williams. Ms. Baker tells Amy that she is angry at her husband for not being more supportive and angry at herself for not doing that well in school. Because Ms. Baker has opened up to Amy about her feelings, Amy wants to try to help her. Amy decides to provide Ms. Baker with patient teaching about stress management.

1. Is it within Amy's scope of practice to decide to provide Ms. Baker with patient education related to stress management? Explain your answer.

2. Dr. Williams directs Amy to provide information about stress management to Ms. Baker. What information might Amy want to share with Ms. Baker?

3. Ms. Baker confides that sometimes her stress is so overwhelming she can't function during her day. She adds, "The days are so challenging. I wish it would all just end." Does Amy have an obligation to report this information to Dr. Williams?

INTERNET ACTIVITY

Visit the Internet and research one mental illness that interests you. Be able to answer the following questions about this disorder:

1. Define the disorder.

2. Discuss what causes this disorder.

3. What are the symptoms of this disorder?

4. What are the treatments for this disorder?

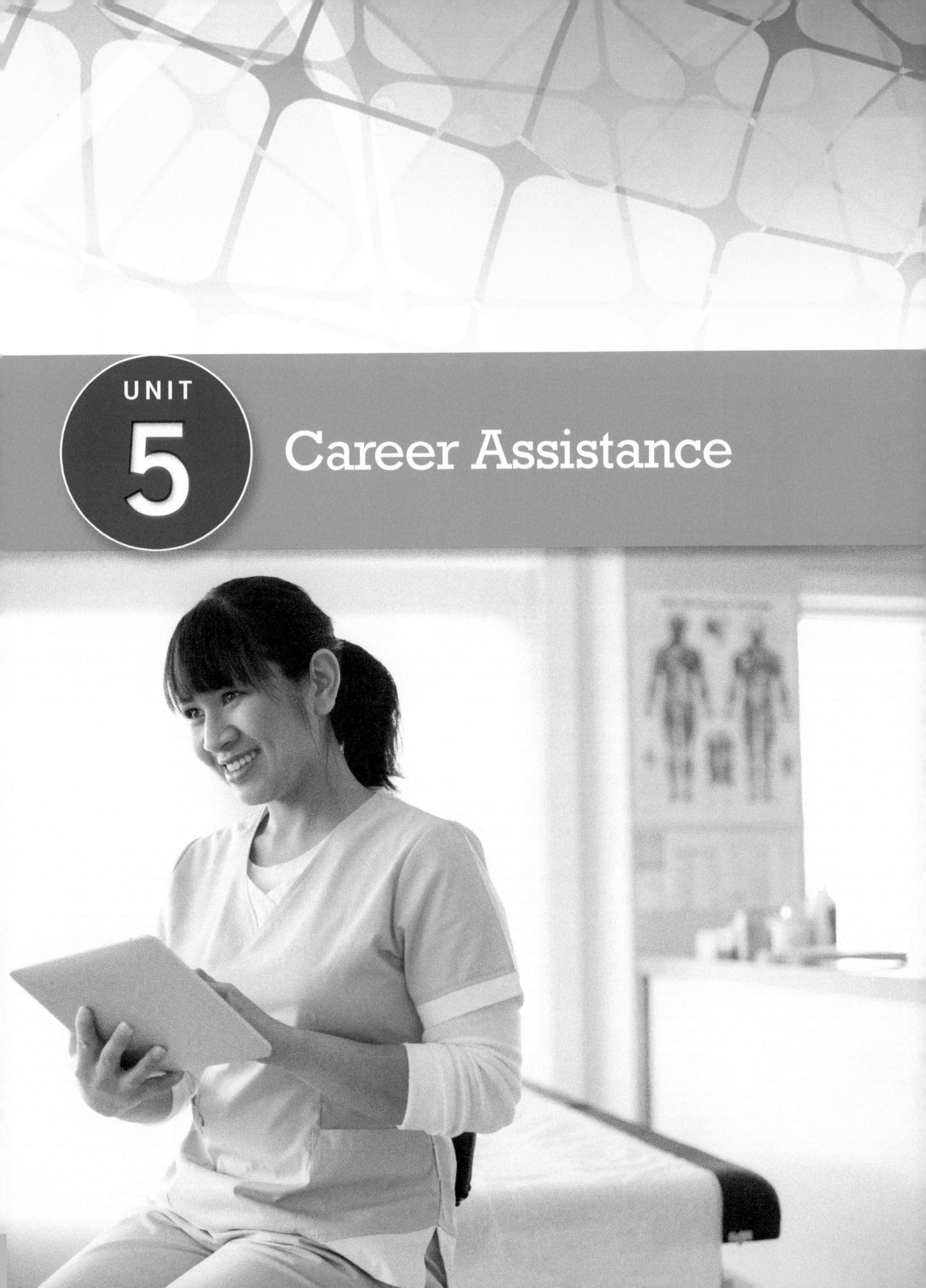

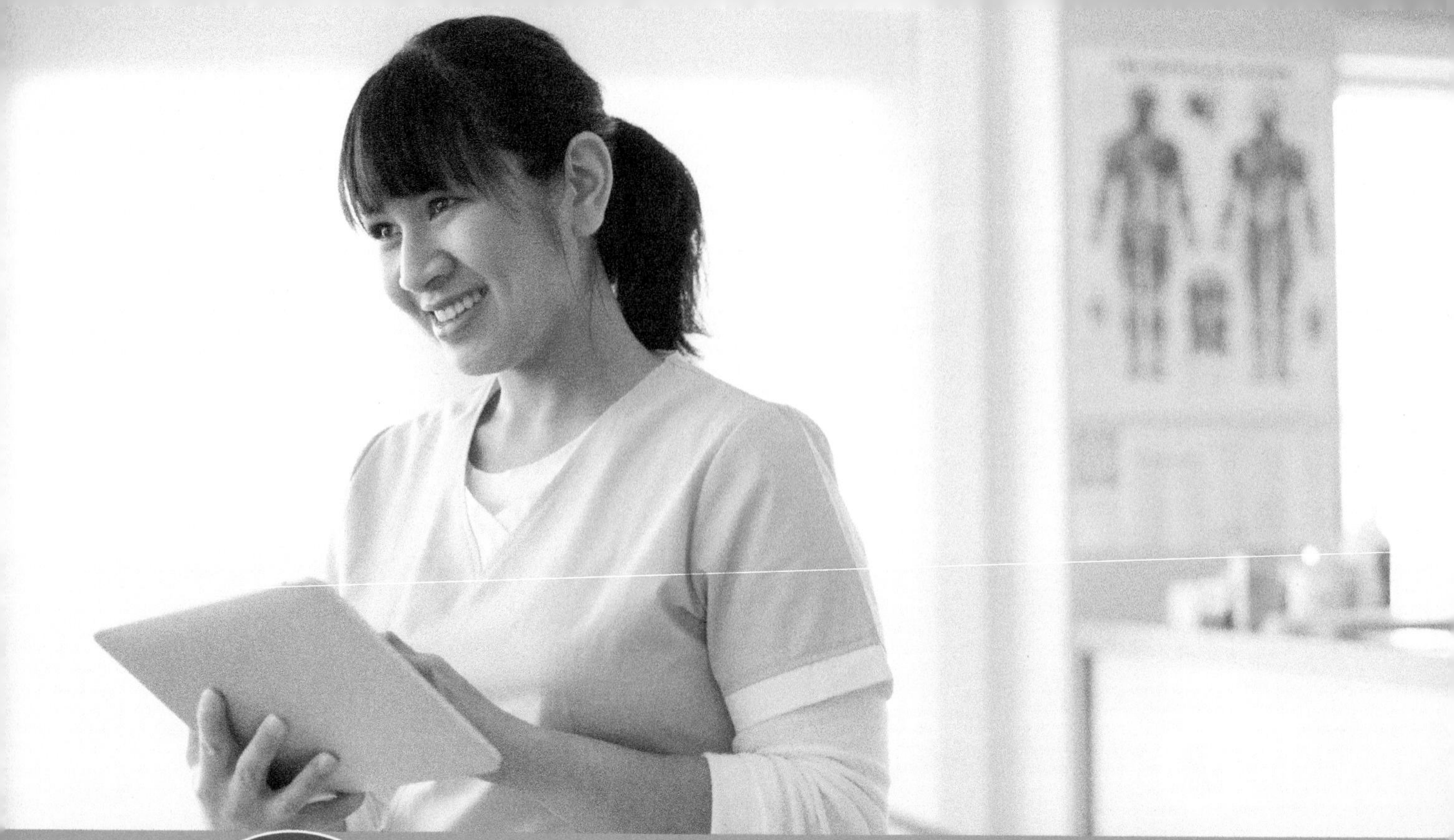

CHAPTER

58 Professionalism

Learning Objectives

After completing this chapter, you should be able to:

58.1 Define and spell the terms for this chapter.
58.2 Explain the importance of professional skills in the workplace.
58.3 Identify professional skills related to workplace communication.
58.4 Describe why critical thinking skills are important for a medical assistant.
58.5 Explain why teamwork is important in a workplace setting.
58.6 Identify ways to effectively manage priorities.
58.7 Describe a medical assistant's professional image.
58.8 Explain how lifelong learning is a component of professionalism.

On a busy morning at Pearson Physicians Group, David Dolan, a registered medical assistant, has fallen behind in his work. Susan Schultz, a coworker who is also a registered medical assistant, grumbles to Tania Washington that "David never gets his work done." Gossip has begun to circulate among the other employees that Susan is angry with David and that she thinks he is lazy. David has recently graduated from medical assisting school, and this is his first job as a medical assistant. He constantly worries that he is not working fast enough and that he will make a mistake.

Terms to Learn

affective	diplomacy	persistence
aromatherapy	diversity	psychomotor
biofeedback	encounter note	respect
cognitive	guided imagery	soft skills
courtesy	integrity	system
dignity	lifelong learning	tact

Health care professionals in the medical office need to have good technical skills, and they also must have soft skills, otherwise known as people skills. **Soft skills** are those skills necessary for the smooth functioning of the workplace that are neither **cognitive** (based on knowledge) nor **psychomotor** (coordinating the mind and body) and that display the professionalism of the employee. Although facts and procedural skills are often tested in school, the workplace is the testing arena for professional soft skills. If an employee comes to work not knowing how to perform a procedure but has the professionalism to ask for help, that employee can be trained in that skill. However, if an employee comes to work and does not get along well with others, fails to communicate needs, or handles assignments in a less-than-professional manner, that employee will probably be terminated from the office. **Affective** skills are behaviors that come from feelings and emotions and are truly important in the medical office.

PROFESSIONAL SKILLS IN THE WORKPLACE

The physician-employer expects the employee to be competent in performing procedures, understanding anatomy and physiology, and using medical terminology. The physician also needs workers who arrive at work on time, prioritize problems, seek communication with others, think critically, and solve problems appropriately. In the quick pace of the modern medical office, all employees are expected to work for the good of the medical office and its patients.

The patient, who is usually ill, expects competent and courteous help at the physician's office. If a medical assistant cannot prioritize needs, manage time well, display good social skills, and solve patient problems effectively, patients will not return. In fact, when patients sue physician offices, frequently it is not because of poor outcomes but because of poor treatment by office personnel.

The team of employees in the medical office expects to work with others who share similar values and goals. If one medical assistant does not do a fair share of the work, it places a burden on the other members of the team. Medical assistants are quite versatile, having been trained to work in both the administrative and the clinical areas of the medical office. Their job assignments may be limited to one area of the office; however, good employees show initiative by jumping in to help others when they are able and the tasks fall within their scope of practice and knowledge.

Professional qualities of a medical assistant include the following:

- **Tact**—sensitivity in dealing with others or with difficult issues
- **Diplomacy**—skill in handling negotiations without creating hostility

- **Courtesy**—politeness in your attitude and behavior toward others

- **Respect**—the belief and attitude that someone is important and should be treated in an appropriate way

- **Dignity**—calm, serious, and controlled behavior that makes people respect you

- **Integrity**—honesty and having strong moral principles

Integrated Systems

A **system** is a regularly interacting group of people who function within an organized set of doctrines and principles. Medical offices are designed to function as a system. To have a well-operated system, an office should have a policies and procedures manual in place to direct the employees. As a medical assistant, you must understand how to function within the system established in your medical office.

The medical assistant who works for a large corporation may have had numerous interviews, met several managers, and gone through a long orientation to become familiar with the office and the hierarchy of management. In a smaller office, the medical assistant may have fewer colleagues and managers. This assistant may not have had any kind of formal orientation but instead just started to work and was expected to ask any questions as they arose.

It is important for you to clarify the expectations in the office where you are employed early in the work relationship. For example, you should learn who to contact for what reasons, how you are expected to account for your time, how and when paychecks are issued, and what to do if you need time off. Having a clear understanding of managers' expectations will help you to function smoothly within the system.

Regardless of the size of the medical facility where you work, and regardless of how its system functions, you will be expected to display professional soft skills with the patients and with fellow employees.

Truthfulness is very important in the medical office. An example of truthfulness is a medical assistant informing the supervisor when he or she is not fully aware of how to perform a procedure. The patient's safety and welfare should be the number one concern of the health care professional. In addition, legal problems will be avoided when truthfulness is foremost.

Examples of *not* being truthful as an employee include lying about previous education, falsifying time cards, and documenting procedures that were not performed. Any falsifying on the part of the medical assistant could be grounds for dismissal from employment. Medical offices typically have money available in petty cash or from patient payments

Professionalism The Workplace

Everyone in the medical workplace would like to work with a supportive team. To ensure that a supportive team functions well, every medical assistant must be willing to assume full responsibility as a team member. When teamwork does not occur, the team may need to self-evaluate and devise ways to function more effectively. This is important both for the patients and for the team.

and may also keep drugs in the clinical area. Misuse of these items or taking them for personal use is not acceptable and is considered theft. All employees, including the medical assistant, must be above reproach in trustworthiness in these situations. Every worker in the system must be able to trust each person in the office.

As a medical assistant, you must also work well with allied health professionals outside your office. For ideal patient care, you should develop a network of peer relationships to contact for referrals, support group recommendations, and surgical appointments for patients. Every medical assistant works within a larger system of health care professionals.

WORKPLACE COMMUNICATION

Perhaps the most important soft skill to possess is the ability to communicate effectively verbally, in writing, and through body language. Communication between patients and health care professionals is important, but communication among members of the health care team is also crucially important, especially when the team is trying to solve several problems all at the same time. One example of a situation when inter-team communication is important is this: The physician is out of the office. Who is in charge?

Patients will form an impression of the medical practice by how you, the medical assistant, communicate with them. But their impression will also depend on how they perceive the level of efficiency and empathy of the office as a whole. In effect, you represent the office with every communication, whether with an individual patient or with other members of your team. Therefore, you must be able to incorporate good communication skills with excellent patient care.

One more important note about communication: Good communication also means knowing when and what *not* to communicate. All members of the medical team, including medical assistants, are expected to follow the requirements of the Health Insurance Portability and Accountability Act (HIPAA) to protect patient privacy.

Active Listening

Active listening, one of the key soft skills, requires the full attention of the person receiving the message. If, instead of listening, you are thinking of the next question you will ask the patient while the patient is talking, the physician might not receive critical information for the simple reason that you did not hear it. If the physician is giving an order and you are preoccupied, thinking of something else, the results can be disastrous.

So it is very important that you always engage in active listening. Instead of making assumptions about what is being said, the medical assistant with good professional skills focuses on the speaker and what the speaker is saying and asks for clarification if needed.

Seeking to Understand

In his book *The 7 Habits of Highly Effective People*, Stephen Covey noted that we should seek to understand before seeking to be understood. A health care professional should enter every conversation, whether with patients or colleagues, seeking to understand the other person. Then, communication is facilitated.

Speaking to Be Understood

Just as you should seek to understand the person speaking, you should also speak to be understood. Too often in the busy medical office, personnel use a kind of verbal shorthand. A newly hired team member may need a fuller explanation of a policy or procedure. If you take the time to explain something well once, it will save time in re-explanations later.

When you are presenting difficult concepts, it is always a good idea to seek feedback from the listener to make sure that person understood you. Always take into account the age and culture of the patient. Tailor your vocabulary to the age and mental capacity of the patient.

Always address the patient with the title (Mr., Mrs., Ms., Miss) that the patient prefers and with the respect appropriate to that person's age or culture. As a professional medical assistant, you will also address physicians and peers in the medical office with respect.

Effective Writing

Text messaging is a popular way of communicating with others; however, because of the way these messages are composed, using abbreviated language, symbols, and slogans (and not much attention to correct spelling), many people have come to believe that this is an appropriate way to communicate, or at least have gotten into the habit of

communicating this way. If you communicate in that manner frequently, you might almost forget how to write correctly.

In the health care environment, communication must be concise, but it must also be well understood by others. Accuracy is more important than brevity. Correct writing also makes a far more professional impression on those inside and outside your office than a quickly dashed-off communication that is full of errors.

Although it might take a few minutes to write a longer **encounter note** (documentation of the patient visit to the physician's office), it will be worthwhile in the long run, because a longer note provides more information, records information that is more correct for future reference, and shows the thoroughness of the medical assistant's care for the patient.

If you consistently write effective phone messages, memos, letters, and patient record entries, you will be highly valued by your employer.

As a medical assistant, you frequently will be asked to communicate information or instructions to a patient. Communication that is clear and complete is essential for patient understanding and to avoid confusion or incorrect assumptions on the part of the patient. For example, a patient who is well prepared for a procedure will be less anxious and more compliant, because the patient will be less frightened of what will happen.

CRITICAL THINKING

Knowledge is important to the medical assistant, but being able to use what you have learned in real situations should be your ultimate goal. During an average day in a medical office, you will make numerous crucial decisions. Although some decisions or procedures may be routine, many will require critical thinking and problem solving. To make proper decisions and take proper actions, you must retrieve memorized information and then add reflection to your thinking process before you can reach proper conclusions and act appropriately.

Insurance and billing issues often require critical thinking. You may need to advocate for the patient with the patient's insurance company, navigating through a maze of complicated rules for reimbursement. Thinking critically can improve reimbursement from the insurance company to the medical practice and greatly relieve a burden on the patient.

Always read laboratory results critically and question results that do not seem consistent with the patient's presentation. Although as a medical assistant you should never diagnose, it is your responsibility to bring abnormal results to the physician's attention. Gathering numerous facts, such as laboratory tests and vital signs, and adding them to how the patient presents and what the patient reports, all help to give you an in-depth picture of the patient's illness. As a critical thinker, you will take all information into consideration before forming a conclusion.

Distinguishing Fact from Opinion

Critical thinking involves being able to distinguish fact from opinion or conjecture. A patient may tell you that he or she has a particular disease or problem, but as a medical assistant who thinks critically, you can discern whether the information (the patient's subjective chief complaints plus your own objective notations) actually supports the patient's beliefs (Figure 58-1).

Be aware that you, too, are capable of jumping to conclusions. For example, a patient's behavior may make you believe that the patient is angry with you. But upon reflection, you may realize that the patient had to wait a long time in the reception area or has reported experiencing a lot of pain, and either of these may be what the patient is really angry about. Putting yourself in the patient's place and considering everything that may be affecting that person's mood can help you to deal with the patient in a calmer and more effective way and will also allow you to give the physician a more thoughtful report about the patient.

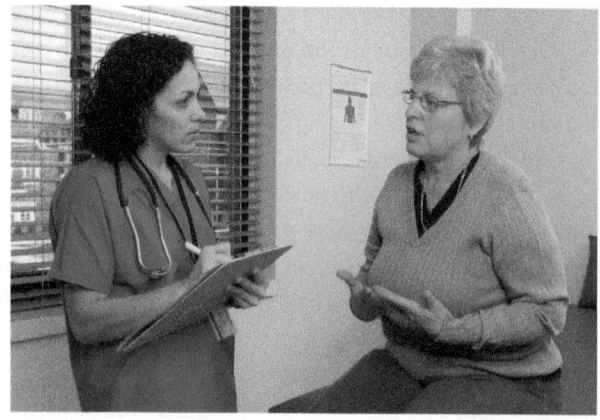

FIGURE 58-1 Medical assistant interviewing a patient.

Making Value Judgments

A medical assistant must make value judgments every day. For example, setting the priority for scheduling a patient visit should be based on the chief complaint and not on how much you like the patient. If a physician refuses to give a patient a medication that the patient does not need, you may have to reinforce this decision to the patient. Critical thinking should become so habitual that you are comfortable making value judgments like these.

TEAMWORK

Functioning as a team member is a critical workplace competency. No matter how small or large the medical office, all the employees must work together. If one employee gets overwhelmed with responsibilities, the others should be versatile enough in their knowledge and flexible enough to help until the work is caught up. All medical assistants must understand how the team functions and be prepared to share responsibilities. Medical assistants may perform only within their scope of practice; however, within their scope of practice they should maintain a variety of competencies and a helpful attitude toward working with others.

Teams are composed of leaders and followers. But on a team, one person cannot be the leader all the time, nor should any team member only be a follower. Each team member should demonstrate leadership when needed. Teams operate best when they make use of the strengths of each team member.

Diversity

In the average medical office, medical assistants and other health care professionals come from different backgrounds (Figure 58-2). **Diversity** means "variety." Because the United States

> ## Professionalism The Life Span
>
> In a medical office, the patients and their family members vary in age. For example, a child might be brought to the pediatric office by her parents, and an older patient may be brought to the office by his children. The medical assistant addresses the needs of patients and family members who may be in different age groups. A breastfeeding mother's behavior has an effect on her infant. A patient with Alzheimer's disease brings with him the needs of the family that supports him. Sadly, some patients have no family support.
>
> All these people, who represent different age groups, are served by the medical assistant.

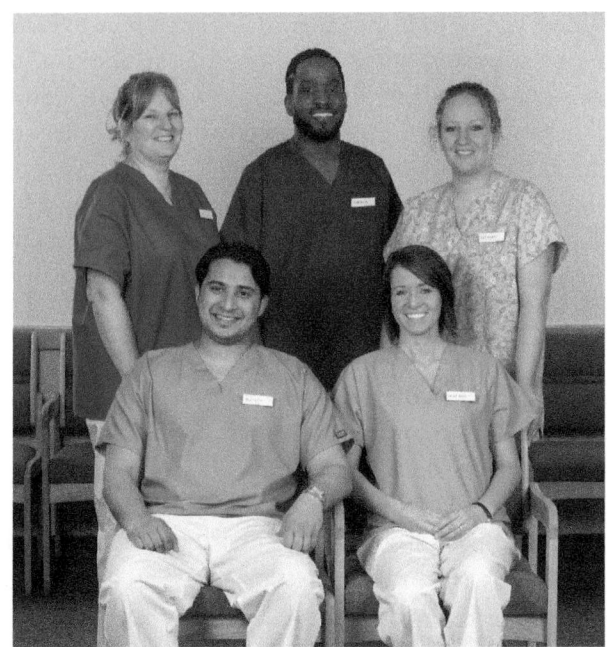

FIGURE 58-2 A diverse team of medical assistants.

is a melting pot of cultures, you can expect to have a variety of both patients and coworkers. It is in everyone's best interest that biases, stereotypes, and prejudices be put aside. Holding grudges or rigid beliefs can prevent the team from functioning smoothly, to the detriment of both the patients and the office personnel. Professional medical assistants work well with a diverse group of colleagues and patients. One way to help others who may have difficulty embracing diversity is to provide information and education to help them have a better understanding of the culture, ethnicity, or beliefs of others.

Resolving Conflicts

In the medical office, you can expect conflict to occur from time to time. Conflicts may arise with patients or among team members. It might be as simple as a difference of opinion or as complex as an act of violence. The first step in resolving conflict is to seek to understand the situation. Perhaps there is more to the situation than is first noticed. If one person in the conflict is tired, sick, or frustrated, perhaps that is the root of the problem. The medical assistant should also take a look at his or her own behavior or communication to see if perhaps something the assistant said or did, intentionally or unintentionally, contributed to the conflict. In that case, an apology from the medical assistant can smooth the way to a solution.

It is an important soft skill not to escalate a conflict. If a patient, physician, manager, or peer seems to be getting angry, a wise medical assistant avoids getting angry in return

and making matters worse but instead seeks to understand and solve the problem. Sometimes the solution is as easy as meeting the person's request—scheduling a new appointment, saying you are sorry, or promising to get a message to the physician. Other times, you may need to handle a situation by establishing a definition of the problem ("I see you want to have this insurance issue resolved") and promising to locate someone to help ("That is not something I am authorized to do, but I will get the reimbursement specialist for you").

If two workers are in conflict, it may be wise to ask a manager to resolve the issue. The manager should meet with both people separately, then together. If you know the details of the conflict, it is best not to share them with colleagues, even though that is tempting, because you may be perceived as taking sides or asking colleagues to pick sides in the conflict. When a decision is made in the conflict, it is best to shake hands (really or figuratively) and agree to work well together in the future. No one wants to work in an office that is seething with ill-feelings or strife, so it is better for both parties to maintain a professional attitude.

Responding to Criticism

Learning to respond to criticism appropriately is an important skill in teamwork and conflict resolution. The best response is to say, "Thank you for the feedback. I will do my best to apply that suggestion." If necessary, ask a nondefensive question to clarify the feedback, such as, "Am I correct to understand that I should process paperwork in this order?" Do not make your response sound defensive or like an attack, as would be the case if saying, "What do you mean by that?" "What's wrong with the way I do it now?" or "I would never do that."

If you have made a mistake, admit it, restate the correct way to do the task, and move on. If necessary, ask for retraining on the task or for a supervisor or mentor to observe the next time you do it. This is especially important with clinical skills. Do not waste time and energy being upset or putting yourself down. Never make excuses.

Even if you feel the criticism is not justified, is unreasonably harsh, or is not presented in a tactful manner, it is best not to argue or become defensive. Such responses rarely lead to a positive outcome and could make you appear to be a negative person or not a team player to others. If necessary, ask your supervisor for feedback on the action being criticized to be sure you are following office policies and procedures. Do not ask a supervisor to take sides or mediate a conflict with a coworker.

Part of maturity and professionalism is the ability to accept criticism and move on.

MANAGING PRIORITIES

One of the most challenging soft skills is the ability to manage priorities. Although you may plan for the day to go a certain way, you will probably need to assess patient and workplace priorities and change your plan frequently. Patient priorities are usually managed by a combination of efficient scheduling and a triage system. However, even the most predictable schedule may need to be adjusted.

Because of your versatility as a medical assistant, you may be asked to do multiple tasks in a short period of time. Although it is tempting to do several tasks at once, such as filing and talking on the phone, that is seldom efficient. Focusing on one task at a time will ensure thoroughness and accuracy.

In the busy medical office, many tasks may have to be deferred to a later time. For example, if a patient calls to speak to the physician about lab results, the physician's return call may have to be deferred until the lab results arrive or until a time when the physician is not seeing a patient.

An efficient task management system or tickler file system will be a great help to remember important items that need to be completed by a specific date. Most electronic calendar applications contain a *to-do* list you can use to prioritize tasks and set reminder dates. When dealing with paper systems, use outboxes or neat piles to sort tasks that should be done immediately, tasks that can be done when some other data arrives (such as the lab report), and tasks that can be done at a later time (such as a return call from the physician). Having a tidy workplace and disposing of clutter and trash will facilitate the efficiency of a tickler system.

If you become distracted by your own family issues or other personal problems, it can have a negative effect on your job performance. For that reason it is wise to ask family and friends not to call you at your place of employment except in an emergency. That way, you can focus on your job throughout the day and catch up with friends and family after work. Even text messages on your cell phone can be distracting. Therefore, it is best to turn off your cell phone during work hours, knowing that if there is a true emergency, you can be reached on the office phone. In some offices, office policy prohibits the use of cell phones on the job.

When the physician is absent from the office and patients cannot be seen, this is an excellent time to catch up on lesser priorities that are nonetheless important. Such tasks as inventory or filing that may be deferred because of patient care needs can be accomplished at times when patients are not scheduled.

Stress Management

It is important to decrease stress in the medical office as much as possible. Sick patients can wear down your patience and leave you feeling frustrated. It is important to realize that patients rarely intend to upset you or others at the office—but it is part of the job to deal with people who are under stress, which in turn can leave you and other staff members feeling stressed.

One of the best ways to reduce stress in the medical office is to practice stress management. The following are some forms of stress management:

Aromatherapy—**Aromatherapy** uses pleasant smells such as lavender that have been shown to decrease stress.

Biofeedback—**Biofeedback** is a therapy that uses biological information to relieve stress. Wearing biofeedback dots, rings, or patches shows the wearer if stress has constricted blood flow to that area. Knowing when you are stressed is the first step in changing the behaviors that lead to stress.

Deep breathing—Breathing deeply can relax your body, especially the heart and other muscles.

Distraction—Some people find that hobbies or vacations distract them from stress.

Exercise—Mild exercise has been shown to decrease stress in most individuals.

Guided imagery—By taking a few minutes to imagine being in some relaxing place, **guided imagery** can cause your body to relax in response to that stimulus.

Humor—Laughing at oneself or the bizarre predicaments of life can decrease stress.

Hypnosis—Learning to think more deeply without inhibitions can help people regain control of stress.

Meditation and prayer—Numerous studies have shown that focusing on reflection or prayer can relax the body.

Music—Listening to restful music that you enjoy has been shown to decrease stress.

Relaxation—Even in the office, a few minutes of concentrating on relaxing muscle groups (perhaps in the break room) can be rejuvenating.

Slow breath counting—Taking and counting slow breaths can distract and relax the brain.

Water therapy—Some people find a bath or shower soothing and helpful in relieving stress.

Stress can also be caused by pain. If stress results from pain, these techniques are recommended:

Heat—Applying heat to different parts of the body can distract the brain from pain. As mentioned under water therapy, many people enjoy a hot bath.

Cold—Applying cold to different parts of the body can distract the brain from pain. Applying a cold pack to the head, for example, can ease a headache.

Pressure—Applying pressure to certain pressure points can reduce pain. Headache pain, for example, can often be reduced by massaging the temples.

Usually, stress management techniques can be used for only a few minutes at the office, but you should plan stress-relieving activities during free time. Sometimes talking to other health professionals about the stress can help you find new ways to reduce it.

Time Management

One of the greatest attributes of an efficient office manager or medical assistant is the ability to manage time effectively. This was discussed in the chapter titled "Medical Office Management" and is discussed again here because of its importance. If the manager is organized, the office is usually organized. Time management requires the ability to prioritize tasks, delegate them as appropriate, and complete them on schedule. This is quite different from doing every task as it comes along. The office manager generally has little control over the tasks presented. The control is in how the tasks are handled.

One of the main responsibilities of the office manager or medical assistant is to manage all the peripheral office functions so the physician is free to concentrate on practicing medicine. These tasks could include anything from opening the daily mail and meeting with sales representatives to finding the drug sample for a patient who is waiting. If tasks such as these are handled without bothering the physician, the physician will then be able to set aside an hour each day to devote to administrative and patient-related tasks that only he or she can do.

Before establishing a time management system, it is important to define the office goals with the physician. Physicians' goals vary from simple to complex and from short-term to long-term. The physician may want to set a goal to increase payment collections at the time of service, restructure the practice by adding a new partner, expand the services available to patients, or review new benefits packages for the employees. After the goals have been established, tasks necessary to meet those goals can be defined, prioritized, and assigned to the appropriate staff members. The office manager can get the project underway by merely developing an electronic or paper-based *to-do* list of all the tasks that need to be done to accomplish the goal. As new tasks come to mind, they are added to the list.

To-do lists can be created for everyday responsibilities as well as for special new goals. Each item on the list is assigned a priority designation of 1, 2, or 3 depending on how critical the item is to completing the task. For example, on a *to-do* list for inventory, ordering supplies that are running

TABLE 58-1 | To-Do List

Priority	To Do
2	Order paper supplies.
1	Arrange Dr. Christianson's air transportation to medical convention next month.
2	Prepare performance appraisal for Emily Jane Doro.
3	Reorganize storeroom.
1	Type convention speech.
1	Place ad for medical assistant.
3	Ask Ruth to remove old magazines from reception area.
1	Call for Pap test report on Mrs. Glidewell.
2	Block out schedule for next quarter.
3	Ask Belinda to take down Christmas decorations.
1	Prepare agenda for Thursday's staff meeting.

out is given a number 1, whereas rearranging a linen cupboard or a file drawer might be assigned a 3. Number 1 priority items must be done first and number 3 last. It is often tempting to do the easier tasks first, because they take less time and show an immediate accomplishment. However, good time management would determine that the inventory order should be placed immediately, and the number 3 priorities could be delegated to someone else or completed later, if necessary. It is a good idea to date a *to-do* list and to cross off items as they are accomplished. Table 58-1 shows an example of a *to-do* list.

Persistence

One of the most valuable soft skills is persistence. **Persistence** is the quality of being able to stay on task longer than the usual time when necessary, even after others might have given up. Take, for example, the insurance billing process. If a medical assistant sends in an insurance claim and it is denied, persistence in telephone follow-up or refiling the claim may help the claim to get paid. Such persistence might help prevent writing off the charges as a loss or will benefit the patient who will not have to pay out of pocket. When you are frustrated, it may seem easier to give up on a problem than to seek alternative solutions; the professional medical assistant creatively thinks of an alternative approach to the problem and persists in trying to find a solution.

CHANGES IN TECHNOLOGY

Electronic communication and technology are used in most medical offices and are constantly changing. Updates are made to existing applications, equipment is updated, and new software applications are implemented. Many pieces of clinical equipment also are subject to updates in technology procedures. A professional medical assistant approaches technology updates with a positive "can do" attitude. Understand that change is rarely easy, and technology changes in hardware and software often present learning curves and operational challenges. Do not join with other employees who might choose to grumble and complain. Take advantage of every learning opportunity available and offer to teach the changes to others.

PROFESSIONAL IMAGE

Regardless of whether the dress code at your medical assisting school was formal or casual, you should always project a professional image at work. Sometimes the office policies and procedures manual is very specific about how the assistant should dress and accessorize, but at other times, it is left to the assistant's discretion.

Even though coworkers may dress casually, you should project the best professional image you can. This means that you should always wear clean, pressed clothing that does not reveal breasts, waist, tattoos, or underwear. If you have a tattoo, it should be covered when you are at the medical office. Nails should be cut short. Artificial nails can harbor microbes and are inappropriate for most medical assistants. Excessive jewelry should be avoided, because it harbors germs and can get in the way when providing patient care. For example, a dangling necklace or bracelet is not appropriate. Hair should be controlled so that it does not fall on the patient or onto a sterile field. The medical assistant should practice excellent hygiene, which includes daily bathing, hair care, and oral hygiene. The medical assistant should also avoid perfumes and strong deodorants. Many patients find body piercings to be offensive. Small stud-style earrings worn on the earlobes are acceptable. Shoes should be clean with closed toes; replace any laces when they become dirty or worn. Socks or stockings should be worn with shoes.

You should wear the name tag issued by your employer, which usually includes both your name and your title. This informs the patient that you are a medical assistant and not a nurse or physician.

If you smoke, now is a great time to try to quit. If you cannot quit smoking entirely, however, observe the office smoking policy. Do not smoke in public areas of the office, and do not work around employees or patients while smelling of

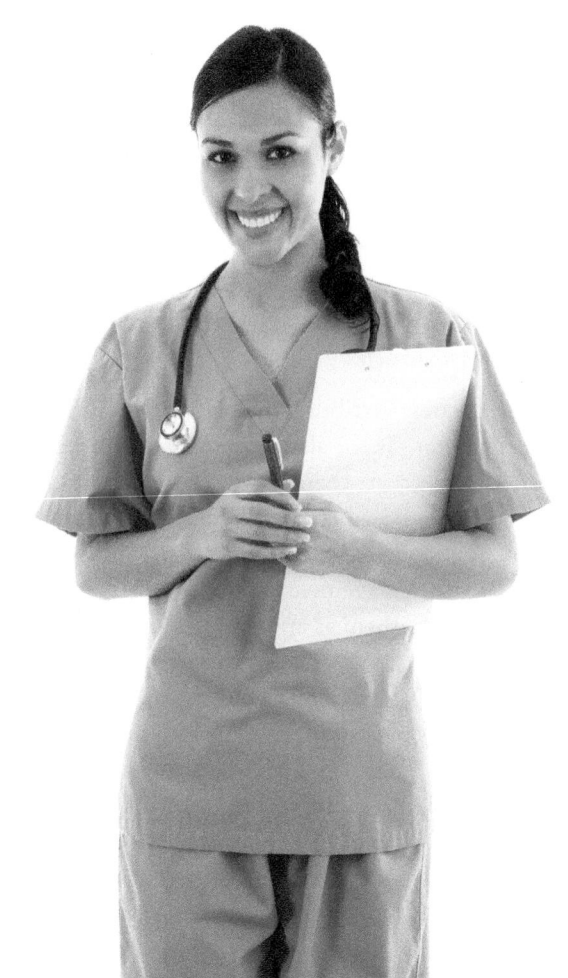

FIGURE 58-3 A medical assistant should present a neat appearance and make it a habit to wear a smile.

cigarette smoke because it can be very offensive to others. Some facilities provide a designated smoking area.

Always refer to the office policies and procedures manual, if one is available, for information regarding the office dress code. Remember that a smile is always part of a professional image, so wear one all the time (Figure 58-3).

LIFELONG LEARNING

Learning is not over when you graduate from your medical assisting program. There are constant changes in the field of medicine, and one of those is the growing preference for medical assistants who are nationally certified. Certification can make a difference in obtaining an initial job in the field or in advancing up the career ladder. Most employers now have the opportunity to hire medical assistants who not only have graduated from a formal program of study but have gone one step further and become nationally certified.

Most states with requirements for certified medical assistants specify the credentials accepted. (Review the chapter titled "Medical Assisting: The Profession" for information on training and certification of medical assistants.) Once you are certified, the next step is to maintain that certification through continuing education. **Lifelong learning** is the process of continuing to seek education throughout life. As a medical assistant, you might go back to school for a higher degree in medical office management or allied health education, for example. However, even if you do not return to formal schooling, continuing education credits can be earned through conferences, workshops, training in the office, or online courses.

The Internet also provides a rich library of information. Reading professional journals can also increase your knowledge. The practice's Occupational Safety and Health Administration (OSHA) officer is usually a good source of information about safety and risk management. Be sure to refer to medical websites that are reliable, meaning that the information has been prepared or reviewed by recognized authorities. This includes websites of major hospitals, health care organizations, and professional associations. Websites such as Wikipedia and About.com are not peer-reviewed and should not be used as a source of authoritative information.

Lifelong learning in medicine is a daily event. Always keep in mind that those who do not continue to increase their knowledge through continuing education and other sources will become dinosaurs, not the type of candidates medical facilities will be seeking to employ.

SUMMARY

Soft skills, or people skills, combined with cognitive and psychomotor skills, are vitally important in the medical office. The medical assistant functions within a system, an organized hierarchy of professionals with established policies and procedures. It is important for the medical assistant to communicate well with the patients, physicians, and coworkers. Good communication involves active listening, seeking first to understand then speaking to be understood, and effective writing.

Critical thinking, another key professional skill, involves distinguishing fact from opinion and making good value judgments. Teamwork is essential in the medical office where a diversity of clients, coworkers, and needs may create conflicts. Medical assistants must prioritize tasks and manage time well.

Stress management for patients and medical office employees is also important. Medical careers can create stress for health care workers, so it is important to know how to reduce stress. Time management is critical for the office to operate well. Urgent tasks are not necessarily important tasks. A *to-do* list can help you prioritize tasks.

Persistence is also important in the medical office. The medical assistant may need to focus on a task several times to be thorough and see it through to completion. Lifelong learning is the responsibility of the medical assistant, because new breakthroughs and treatments are perpetually being developed in medicine.

58 CHAPTER REVIEW

COMPETENCY REVIEW

1. Define and spell the terms for this chapter.
2. What are the priorities in communication in the medical office?
3. Discuss how a medical assistant can differentiate between what a patient believes and what is measurable.
4. Why are medical offices in the United States composed of a diversity of personnel?
5. How can stereotyping and prejudice negatively affect patient care?
6. Describe how to resolve conflicts in the medical office.

7. How does a medical assistant determine the daily priorities for the office?
8. Describe a scenario in which persistence is important in the medical office.
9. List five ways for the medical assistant to pursue lifelong learning.
10. Why is national certification important for the career-minded medical assistant?

PREPARING FOR THE CERTIFICATION EXAM

1. Taking vital signs is an example of which kind of skill?
   a. critical thinking
   b. cognitive
   c. psychomotor
   d. affective
   e. soft

2. Which of the following is considered a soft skill?
   a. critical thinking
   b. memorizing medical terminology
   c. labeling an anatomical diagram
   d. creating an electrocardiogram
   e. keying patient data into a computer

3. Which of the following is *not* correct about medical assistants?
   a. They should seek first to understand.
   b. They should be able to resolve conflicts.
   c. They should be prejudiced against certain races.
   d. They should communicate effectively.
   e. They should work well with others.

4. A medical assistant continues to submit claims for re-imbursement after the claim has been rejected multiple times. What ability does this demonstrate?
   a. cognitive skill
   b. psychomotor skill
   c. persistence
   d. diversity
   e. prioritization

5. If a physician is in surgery, which of the following is the best priority for the medical assistant?
   a. Treat patients with minor problems in the reception area.
   b. Take inventory of drug samples.
   c. Extend the medical assistant's lunch time.
   d. Offer to help medical assistants in another office.
   e. Return the medical assistant's personal phone calls.

6. Which of the following is *not* appropriate dress for the office?
   a. name tag with "Medical Assistant" on it
   b. white socks
   c. sandals
   d. short-sleeved V-neck scrubs
   e. short nails

7. Which of the following is considered a source of microbes that could be a significant threat to the patient?
   a. wearing the same shoes to work that the assistant wore home
   b. wearing artificial nails
   c. wearing a dosimeter badge on the lab coat
   d. wearing eyeglasses
   e. wearing perfume at work

8. Which of the following would be the first priority of the medical assistant?
   a. returning a phone call to a patient wanting lab results
   b. responding to a patient calling for help in an examination room
   c. assisting a patient complete the registration process
   d. obtaining a referral for a patient
   e. resubmitting an unpaid insurance bill

9. Lifelong learning for the medical assistant is obtainable through which of the following?
   a. research on the Internet
   b. attending a professional organization's conference
   c. attending local conferences
   d. reading professional journals
   e. all of the above

10. Which of the following is subjective, not objective?
    a. BP is 110/60.
    b. Electrocardiogram shows normal sinus rhythm.
    c. Patient states, "I feel like I am going to die."
    d. Hemoglobin is 15 g/dl.
    e. Height is 44 inches.

CRITICAL THINKING

Refer to the case study at the beginning of the chapter and use what you have learned to answer these questions.

1. Explain why Susan's attitude toward David's work is detrimental to the office environment.
2. David overhears that Susan has been grumbling about his work performance. What is the best course of action for David to handle this situation?
3. If David is struggling with completing his work during the day, what are some things that could help him manage his time better?

ON THE JOB

Scenario 1

Brody Shaw is a newly certified medical assistant in his first job at a family practice office. He notices that the staff rarely wash their hands, and sometimes they do not change gloves between patients. When he brings it to the attention of the office manager, she explains that hand hygiene takes so much time that the office protocol is to wash hands only when patients are infectious. She also explains that using gloves too much corrodes the skin, so Brody should use them only when he is sure that blood is infectious.

1. Should Brody insist on wearing gloves and performing hand hygiene?
2. Where can he go for information on infection control?

3. If Brody is unable to persuade the office manager to change her protocol, to whom should he report this problem?

Scenario 2

Marilyn works with a coworker who insists on wearing powerful perfume to work. She states that she paid a lot for it and is proud that she is able to afford it. You believe that it is not part of her professional image at work.

1. Should you say anything to Marilyn, and if so, what?
2. If you decide to talk with her about the issue, where and when should you do this?
3. If you decide not to talk to Marilyn, what, if anything, should happen next?

INTERNET ACTIVITY

Search professional organizations on the Internet. Find what skills are necessary for the health care professional. Is there any information that indicates why it is important for medical assistants to become credentialed?

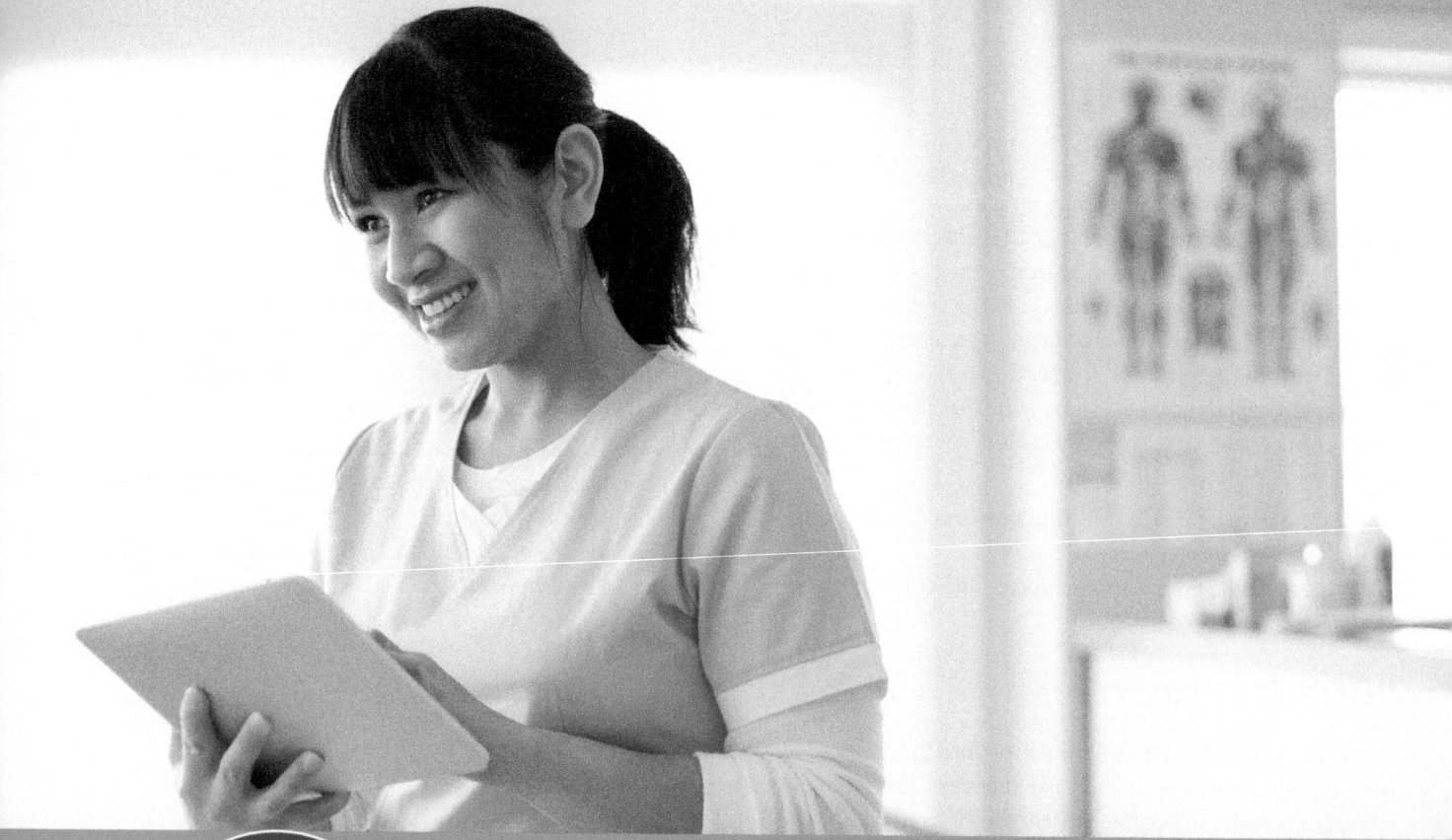

Externship and Career Opportunities

Learning Objectives

After completing this chapter, you should be able to:

59.1 Define and spell the terms for this chapter.

59.2 Describe the externship experience including responsibilities and evaluations of everyone involved.

59.3 Identify important aspects that pertain to a job search.

59.4 Describe how to create an impressive résumé.

59.5 Explain how to prepare for an interview.

59.6 List what employers are looking for from prospective employees.

Kenneth Helminski will be graduating from a medical assistant program at a local career school in two weeks. He is very eager to be working as a medical assistant and has been sending out résumés in response to ads posted on the Internet and in the newspaper. Today, Kenneth has an appointment with Tania, the medical office manager at Pearson Physicians Group.

Terms to Learn

application	externship	professional reference
blind ad	personal assessment	proofread
certification examination	practicum	résumé
cover letter	preceptor	

All indications are that job opportunities for medical assistants are expanding at a rapid rate. The U.S. Department of Labor has projected medical assisting to be one of the fastest-growing occupations. The demand for health care personnel means that a well-prepared medical assistant will have a secure future.

One of the best means to facilitate the transition between the classroom and the medical setting is through the externship experience. This experience can be a time of great challenge and learning, because the student is able to gain experience while under supervision. To receive the most benefit from the experience, careful preparation must take place. The externship experience is also one of the most exciting components of a medical assisting program.

As the student's formal educational experience in school draws to a close, the student will prepare for the **certification examination** offered by a national certifying body. Most medical facilities that employ medical assistants prefer or require that the medical assistant has national certification. This credential indicates that the medical assistant has the necessary knowledge and skills to fill the position of an entry-level medical assistant. During this final stage of training, the student also begins the search for employment. This chapter focuses on skills that are useful to both the externship and the job search.

WHAT IS AN EXTERNSHIP OR PRACTICUM?

An **externship**, which may also be called a **practicum**, is a situation in which the student leaves the confines of the classroom and works, without payment, in a physician's office, hospital, or other health care setting using newly acquired medical assisting skills under the supervision of someone at the site. An externship offers the student an opportunity to get on-the-job experience. The variety of externships is as plentiful and diverse as the medical facilities participating in them. An externship course can be as short as four weeks or as long as one semester of school. Schools that are accredited by the Council on Accreditation of Allied Health Education Programs (CAAHEP) or the Accrediting Bureau of Health Education Schools (ABHES) require an externship of a minimum of 160 hours. National certifying organizations may expect graduates to have had actual mentoring experiences in an actual medical office to be certified. The externship experience should provide the medical assistant with ample entry-level experience in both administrative and clinical skills.

Your school will work with you to select the right externship or practicum site for you based on your skills, needs, and place of residency (Figure 59-1). Ideally, the practicum

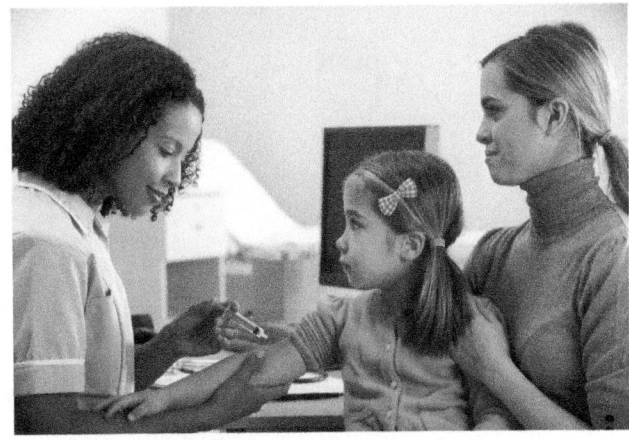

FIGURE 59-1 Medical assistant administering an injection.

BOX 59-1 | Preparing for Externship or Practicum

Physicians expect all of their medical assisting externs to have outstanding clinical and administrative skills. However, the physicians and their staff realize that you are inexperienced, and they generally are patient while you are learning. The one area in which physicians and office managers are extremely critical is punctuality. If you are even a minute late for an interview, starting the day, or returning from a break, it will not be overlooked. Because externships/practicums can result in full-time jobs, it is important to establish an unbroken rule that you will *never* be late. The day before your interview, prepare all the paperwork you will need to take with you. Practice getting to the site in advance, and allow extra time for traffic or other problems. The night before starting work at your externship site, double-check the setting on your alarm clock. Make sure you get up early enough to eat a good breakfast. Do not forget to make sure that your uniform or clothes are clean and pressed, and that you look your best. The externship should be approached as a working interview with the medical facility.

or externship experience will be carefully monitored by the school's clinical instructor or externship/practicum coordinator so that questions or problems that may arise can be addressed. See Box 59-1 for information on how to prepare for an externship or practicum.

The Externship/Practicum Experience

Students generally agree that the externship/practicum experience is the most rewarding part of their school experience. You will have the opportunity to see how a physician's office, ambulatory care setting, or clinic operates on a day-to-day basis (Figure 59-2). In addition, you will be exposed

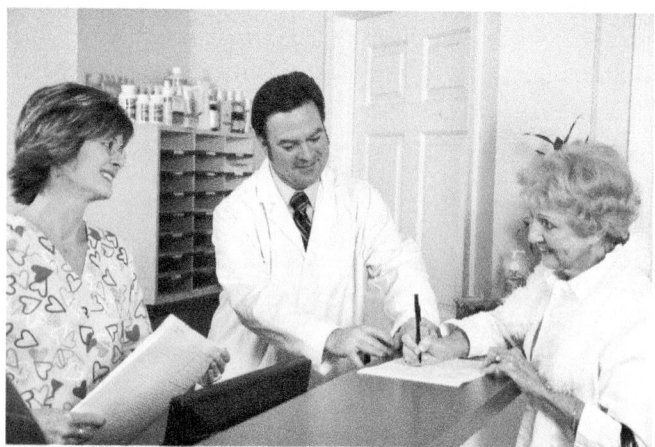

FIGURE 59-2 Medical assistant working in a front office area of a medical office.

to a variety of different personalities in the work setting. Other advantages of the externship include gaining additional experience using your skills, such as phlebotomy, obtaining electrocardiograms and vital signs, performing urinalysis and hematology testing, using the computer, interviewing patients, performing billing and insurance procedures, and scheduling patients. You will gain experience in managing your time and balancing your workday, school day, and home life.

Your performance and behavior will be carefully observed by your supervisor at the externship site. Some of the areas that will be evaluated are these:

- Administrative and clinical skills and techniques
- Caring attitude
- Empathy for patients
- Enthusiasm
- Ethical standards
- Grooming and dress
- Initiative
- Integrity
- Interpersonal skills with patients, physicians, and office staff
- Language and communication skills
- Poise under pressure
- Professionalism
- Punctuality and dependability

Student Responsibilities

The student has an overall responsibility to prepare well in advance of the interview for the externship. This preparation includes a review of skills, updating the résumé, and planning how to project a professional appearance.

Each externship or practicum site is unique and may have additional requirements. The externship may require the medical assistant to have his own malpractice insurance coverage. Documentation of a recent physical exam and immunizations including hepatitis and tetanus may also be required. These immunizations are required if you are working with patients. Because some of the immunizations, particularly hepatitis, require several months to complete, it is wise to begin this process eight to nine months before your expected practicum or externship. It is the student's responsibility to make sure the necessary physical examinations, paperwork, and immunizations are completed on a timely basis.

You have a great responsibility and opportunity by being allowed to gain experience at the externship site. The

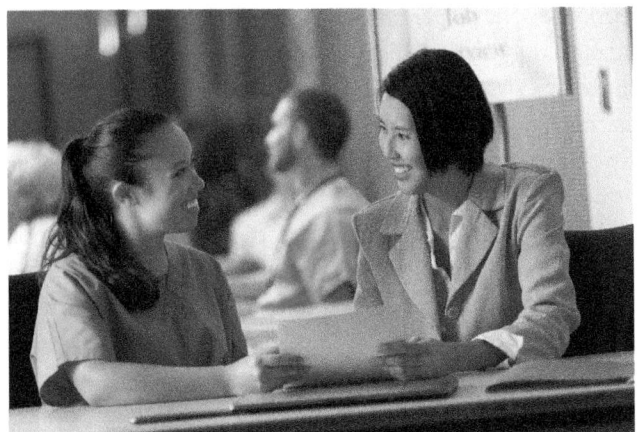

FIGURE 59-3 Medical assistant extern clarifying externship issues with the office manager.

physician or facility providing an externship or practicum expects students to be extremely cautious regarding ethical and legal concerns. Errors can result in malpractice claims against the physician with whom you are working. If an error occurs, it should be reported immediately to the supervisor without alarming the patient. When errors are handled immediately, in many cases they can be corrected. If you cover up an error or mistake, it could result in immediate dismissal for you and may cause harm to the patient. Regular interviews with the office manager provide opportunities for the medical assistant extern to discuss issues that may need clarification.

Issues of confidentiality and patient privacy are of great concern to the physician and staff in all facilities. Discussion of information regarding any patient or the physician's practice with anyone outside a facility is never allowed.

You will be observed and supervised by the on-the-job supervisor and your practicum or externship coordinator. The practicum or externship experience is meant to be a learning experience so be sure to ask questions (Figure 59-3). If you find that you are not receiving the experience you expect and require, bring this to the attention of your school's externship coordinator.

Professionalism | The Workplace

Remember that, as a member of the health care team, you are always under observation. It is not a good idea to use the casual language you might use at home or with friends. Patients and other health care personnel will not be impressed with you if you discuss personal information or are loud and impolite. And always remember to smile!

Externship sites often are willing to provide the externship experience to medical assistant students graduating from a particular school because they have already had good experiences with externs from that same school. So keep in mind that your behavior and work performance during your own externship or practicum will be a direct reflection on the school that prepared you.

Finding the Right Site

Most schools have an externship coordinator who screens and selects health care sites that are appropriate for training. The screening process requires the coordinator to conduct an interview with the physician or office manager at the site to ensure that the student will benefit from appropriate experiences and receive supervision on site. Often the school has an affiliation agreement with the externship site that is kept on file at the school. The affiliation agreement outlines the responsibilities of the school and the site. In some cases, the externship or practicum site will have a former graduate of your program employed there who will be able to identify the skills necessary to complete the externship successfully. Generally, students do not select practicum or externship sites without assistance from the school or its externship/practicum coordinator. The school may ask students to provide contact and location information of potential sites available in the area where the student lives. However, it is the responsibility of the school to secure the site and establish the expectations of the site including who will supervise the student.

The Preceptor Role

The medical assistant at an externship or practicum site always works under the supervision of the physician. However, the physician may designate another member of the health care team as a supervisor for the student. This person performs in the role of a preceptor.

A **preceptor** provides additional instruction and guidance for a student by observing the student performing particular skills (Figure 59-4). The preceptor will also provide a formal written evaluation for the student, usually at the midpoint and at the completion of the extern hours. Table 59-1 lists several areas that are included on a typical externship evaluation form.

The preceptor looks for continual improvement in skills as the student gains confidence. The student should make every attempt to establish a rapport, or comfortable working relationship, with the preceptor.

Externship/Practicum Site Evaluation

At the end of the practicum or externship course, the student will be asked to provide an evaluation of his

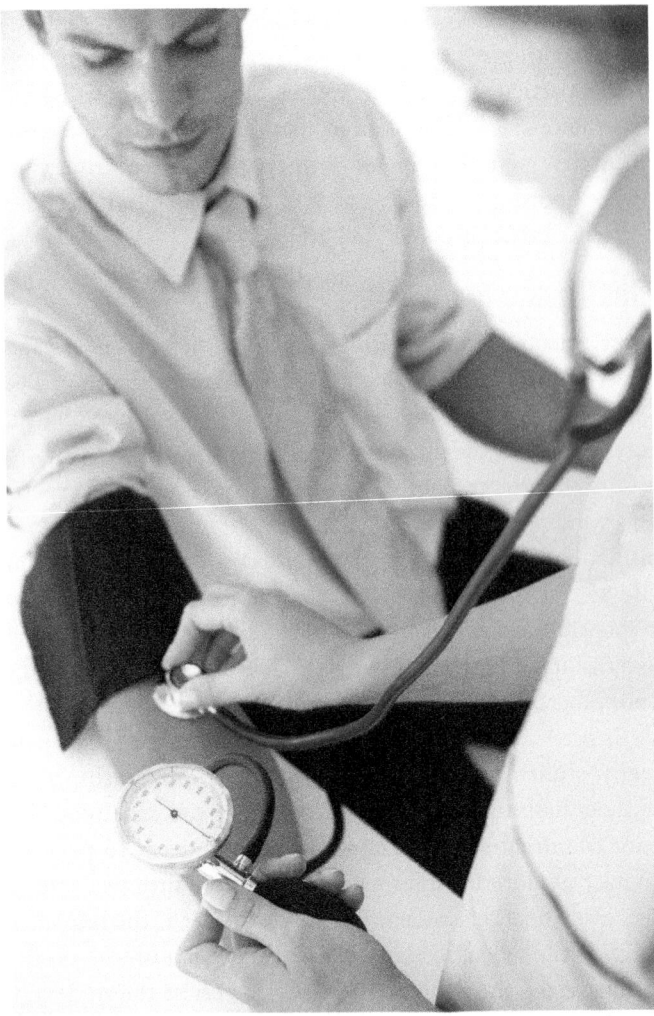

FIGURE 59-4 Taking a blood pressure is one of the procedures the medical assistant extern may perform under the supervision of a preceptor.

experience while assigned to the site. This evaluation may include the following types of questions:

- Was the overall externship experience positive or negative? Explain.
- Was the supervisor or preceptor approachable and available to answer questions?
- What, in your opinion, could be improved about this externship/practicum site and experience?
- Should this externship/practicum site be offered to other students?

THE JOB SEARCH

Your job search should begin while you are finishing up school and your externship, so that you can get your information organized and identify potential sources of jobs and job search websites. Some medical offices might be in the position to offer a permanent position to externs who do an outstanding job, but this is not always the case. Many offices that offer externship opportunities do not have a full-time position available at the moment you complete your externship. Do not think it is a reflection of your work if you are not offered a position at the end of your externship. If your externship experience did not lead to a permanent position, then you must begin the job search in earnest. The student may ask the externship site supervisor to write a letter of recommendation to assist with the job search. In some cases, a facility will not want to hire you as a medical assistant until you become credentialed after taking the required examination. However, some facilities will interview you for a permanent position with the understanding that you must pass the certification exam.

Any job search should begin with careful planning. You must prepare a list of information sources for identifying job opportunities, update your résumé, rehearse interviewing, and plan your professional attire for the interview process. Six behaviors are cited as the most common job search mistakes:

- Having no clear plan
- Failing to inform others of your job search
- Spending too much time answering classified ads rather than personal networking
- Looking and waiting for the perfect job
- Limiting yourself to one field
- Giving up the search too soon

There are several areas to pursue in your search for job opportunities; some are listed in Table 59-2.

Personal Assessment

Before moving ahead with your job search, it is a good idea to perform a **personal assessment** or evaluation of your own strengths and weaknesses. Although it is not a good idea to point out any weaknesses to potential employers, you must be cautious to avoid taking on tasks for which you are not qualified. Employers often ask about weaknesses. Briefly state one and indicate what you are doing about it. This shows you are aware of limitations, and it lets the employer know you are serious about improving yourself. By performing a personal assessment, you can determine the fields of health care you might enjoy working in, which areas require more skill development, and which positions you are qualified for (Figure 59-5).

Ask your instructors for guidance and observations on your appearance, attitude, and skills. You can also ask peers whose opinions you trust and who have been in several

TABLE 59-1 | Sample Student Externship Form

Areas Evaluated	Ratings*				
Makes effective use of time	1	2	3	4	N/A
Able to work well with others	1	2	3	4	N/A
Accepts suggestions/criticisms willingly	1	2	3	4	N/A
Expresses concern for patients	1	2	3	4	N/A
Protects confidentiality of physician and patients	1	2	3	4	N/A
Always on time for work	1	2	3	4	N/A
Willingly works until the job is completed	1	2	3	4	N/A
Able to work independently	1	2	3	4	N/A
Demonstrates skill as appropriate	1	2	3	4	N/A
Does not perform skills beyond scope of training, education, and personal capability	1	2	3	4	N/A
Practices principles of aseptic technique	1	2	3	4	N/A
Projects a positive attitude	1	2	3	4	N/A
Recognizes emergencies	1	2	3	4	N/A
Dresses appropriately	1	2	3	4	N/A
Practices good hygiene	1	2	3	4	N/A

*Ratings: 1=excellent, 2=good, 3=average, 4=needs improvement, N/A= not applicable

TABLE 59-2 | Sources for Job Opportunities

Classified ads	Use local and out-of-town newspapers, professional journals, and trade magazines. Use the local public library's access to national newspapers.
Employment agencies	Place your name with the agency and career consultants.
Health care facilities in your area	Contact hospitals, veterans' facilities, extended care facilities, physician offices, and ambulatory care sites.
Internet	Use various websites such as monster.com, careerbuilder.com, or jobs.com.
Local medical society	Obtain a list of physicians who are looking for help or a list of all the medical practice offices in your area.
Parents, friends, classmates	Network with your own friends, relatives, and classmates from your school. Make sure they know you are looking for employment.
Personal physician	Your own physician may network for you and call colleagues.
Professional organizations	Use both state and local chapters of any professional associations and allied health groups to which you belong.
Publications	American Association of Medical Assistants, American Medical Technologists, and other local professional publications.
School career services office	One of the best sources, because the staff know your training and skills well. In many cases, prospective employers will call schools to identify potential new employees.
State employment office	After completing the required application forms, your name will be on file for available positions.

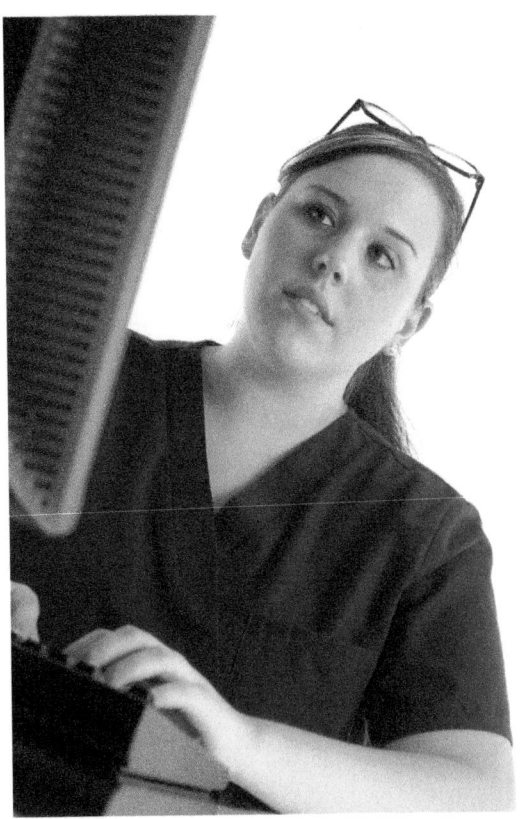

FIGURE 59-5 Medical assistants who perform billing must know and use the proper codes to ensure third-party payments are made correctly by insurance companies.

classes with you. Although it is never easy to accept criticism, a well-intentioned comment from someone you know about the need to clean your uniforms, eliminate jewelry, cover a tattoo, change to a more professional hairstyle, or brush up on particular skills may help you obtain the job you are seeking.

You may wish to practice your interview skills with your instructors or in front of a mirror. A good idea is to videotape a practice interview with a friend or instructor and see how you look to others. Get in the habit of speaking up in class to further develop your communication skills. Work on smiling at every opportunity.

Conducting a Job Search

After planning and performing a self-assessment, it is time to gather the equipment and supplies that will help you to be successful at your job search. At home, at the school you are attending, or at most local libraries, you can access a computer and printer to develop and print your cover letter, résumé, and follow-up thank-you letter or to access the Internet to perform these tasks.

Many websites can help you prepare for your job search. These websites may focus on résumé writing, job applications, interviewing, job postings, and more. Once you are on one of these websites, you will be able to search for a job by category, keyword, city, state, and zip code. If you want to work for a particular medical office, use any Internet search engine and key in the name of the medical office, the city, and the state to see if the office has a website available. If you already know the website address for the medical office, key it into the address bar of your Internet browser. Remember, however, that not all medical offices have websites.

Many employers, especially larger ones, post job openings on the Internet. They might be posted of the clinic's own website or on a general job search website. If you have computer access to the Internet, you can search various websites for jobs that have been posted. This type of search eliminates the need to access the human resources department of an employer you are interested in during their business hours.

Your local public library can provide newspapers with printed classified ads, various publications, and newsletters to use as sources to find a job. If your school has a career services office, it is one of the best places to receive help with your job search. Most school career services offices have a job posting board and will review your résumé, conduct a mock interview, and assist and encourage you to find a job.

Being organized is a must while searching for a job. A job search organizer or folder is a wonderful place to keep a copy of your cover letters, résumés, reference list, letters of reference, follow-up letters, and applications. It can also be used to keep business cards, job advertisements, your contact log, and phone numbers handy. Having all this information in one place will help you stay organized and keep you focused during your job search. It will also prevent any of these items from getting lost or misplaced.

A contact log is a great reference for information about the offices or people you have contacted about a job search. Keep the names, addresses, telephone numbers, and e-mail addresses of the people you have contacted in your log. Update the contact log with notes and dates as you follow up with the offices or as they contact you. The log can be kept on the computer using a word-processing program or a spreadsheet, or it can be maintained on paper.

During your job search, you also will need access to a dictionary, thesaurus, calendar, and telephone. It is critical that your cover letters, résumés, follow-up thank-you letters, and applications be free of spelling, grammar, and formatting errors.

Whether using a wired or wireless phone to call prospective employers, call from a quiet place. If environmental noise is audible in the background when talking to a prospective employer, the employer will think your behavior is unprofessional and rude. It also will make it difficult for you to hear, and you may not be able to give the prospective

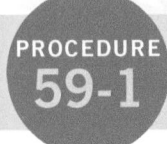

PROCEDURE 59-1

Conducting a Job Search

Objective ◆ *Conduct a job search.*

EQUIPMENT AND SUPPLIES

Computer; Internet access; newspaper; medical assisting publications; printer; pen; paper; dictionary; thesaurus; telephone; telephone book; job search organizer or folder; calendar; contact log

METHOD

1. Using Table 59-2, determine two sources you will use to conduct a job search.
2. Determine a plan for your job search.
3. Prepare a list of information sources for identifying job opportunities.
4. Update your résumé including your extern site information if available.
5. Rehearse interviewing with a close family member or friend.
6. Plan your professional attire for the interview process.
7. Perform a self-assessment.
8. Develop a job search organizer or folder.
9. Create a contact log.
10. Use a calendar to determine what times are available for job searching and interviewing.
11. Conduct your job searches.
12. Turn in all information gathered during your job search as well as a copy of your résumé and contact log to your instructor.

In your journal, document how you felt about the job search.

CHARTING EXAMPLE

When I went to the Quick Care office for an interview, everyone was very nice to me. I think I would get to use a variety of skills there. I will write a thank-you note tonight and send it to them tomorrow. I sure hope they hire me!

---

employer your full attention. If you are unable to give the prospective employer your full attention, you may miss some critical information. If using a wireless phone, ensure that you are calling from an area where there is good service so the call will not be cut off and the sound will not start breaking up.

Before calling employers that have job openings, you should review your calendar for available dates and times for an interview. This will prevent the prospective employer from waiting while you determine the date and time you can meet.

Professionalism

It is a good practice to obtain a copy of your externship evaluation and review it to complete a self-evaluation. What are your weaknesses, and what are your strengths? Throughout your externship, self-evaluate with a journal. In your journal, discuss what happened each day on the externship. Be honest with yourself about how you could have improved the situation. Praise yourself for good decisions.

Searching for a job is not easy, but if you stay focused and organized, stick to your plan, and perform a self-assessment, you will eventually be successful in finding a job. See Procedure 59-1 for the steps in conducting a job search.

THE RÉSUMÉ

The **résumé** is a summary of your qualifications, including your employment history, experience, training, and education. For your first position, the résumé is generally one page in length. Because you will create a first impression with your résumé, it should be carefully written. You may wish to ask your school's career office for guidance when putting together a résumé for the first time. It is also helpful to view examples of résumés on the Internet or in books at your school or local public library.

The most popular résumé format or style is to present information in chronological order. That is, the events are placed in the order of their occurrence. In this format, your education, work experience, and achievements are listed in reverse chronological order (the most recent events are listed first). The chronological résumé format is illustrated in Figure 59-6.

```
                        Ralph Taylor
                     222 East Main Street
                      Chicago, IL 60601
                       (312) 555-1212
                        email address
                    taylorr@anywhere.com

OBJECTIVE        To obtain a medical assisting position where I am able to utilize my
                 administrative and clinical skills.

EDUCATION

Associate Degree   Central State College, Hometown, Illinois. Expected date of graduation:
                   June 20YY. Major in Health Science.

Medical Assistant  Central State College, Hometown, Illinois. February 20YY–June 20YY.
                   Graduated with honors.

EMPLOYMENT

Medical Assistant  Dr. Earl Brown, Internal Medicine Externship, 2222 State St., Chicago, IL.
                   Externship duties included: drawing blood, handling medical records,
                   scheduling patients, and patient education. 20YY–20YY.

Nursing Assistant  Jane Young, M.D. Family Practice, 111 Hoyne Ave., Chicago, IL.
                   Duties included taking vital signs. EKGs, assisting with well-baby visits
                   and in treatment room. 20YY–20YY.

PROFESSIONAL ORGANIZATIONS AND MEMBERSHIP

                   American Association of Medical Assistants
                   Central State College Medical Club

CREDENTIALS

Medical Assistant  Passed certification examination in January 20YY.

CPR                Certified by American Heart Association, December 20YY.

REFERENCES         Furnished upon request.
```

FIGURE 59-6 An example of a résumé that uses a chronological format.

Another résumé format is the educational skills résumé. This format might be useful if you are just graduating from school and have not had extensive work experience. With this format you concentrate on administrative and clinical skills that you have learned while participating in a medical assisting program.

No matter which type of résumé you use, the medical office manager must be able to understand the information you have provided. If the reader is unable to understand the information on the résumé, he will move on to other résumés. Many medical office managers are very busy and have only a short time to glance over résumés. Make sure your résumé is noticed by providing concise and clear information.

The résumé should be printed on good-quality 8½ × 11 inch, white or off-white paper. Do not use brightly colored paper. The résumé must be neatly organized and error free. Always use a word-processing program to prepare your résumé so that you can easily go back and make updates and corrections. Always have a backup copy of your résumé stored on a disk, USB drive, or other type of storage device. The spell-checker option on your word processor may not

accurately pick up all errors, so also check your spelling using a dictionary. For example, the computer spell-check tool may recognize "herd" as a correctly spelled word; however, you actually wanted to use the word "heard." Also, abbreviations are often keyed in correctly but the computer may automatically "correct" an abbreviation and change it to a word you did not want. An example is the abbreviation EHR, electronic health records, which may automatically be corrected to read HER. You can go back and manually fix any unwanted corrections the computer has inserted. You also can add accepted abbreviations, such as EHR, to the spell-checker dictionary.

Proofread your résumé to make sure it is error free in content and typing. Start by reading it on the computer screen. It may help to read it aloud. If you find errors, correct them and resave the document. Next, print your résumé and proofread it again. Seeing the résumé in print gives you a different view than the computer screen, and you will often find errors you had not seen before. Mark any errors found on the printed copy of your résumé and then make the changes on the computer and save the document again. Now print your résumé again and give it to a close family member or friend to proofread. Again, correct any errors discovered. Once you have determined that your résumé is neat and error free, print at least 10 copies of it so that you always have several copies available for distribution.

Spend plenty of time working on your résumé. Remember that the purpose of a résumé is to make a good first impression and to obtain an interview. Keep a personal portfolio in which you gather the names, addresses, and dates of attendance of schools and programs you have attended. Also, keep a list of association memberships and credentialing information, such as certification and registration numbers with expiration dates. This is particularly important if you have earned multiple credentials.

What Is Included in a Résumé?

Résumés vary somewhat based on the personal preferences of the writers, but several items are standard. These include the heading, objective, education, employment, professional organizations, memberships, and credentials.

The information you include on your résumé should never be dishonest, overstated, or misleading. Dishonest or misleading information can be uncovered during the interview or in discussions with people whose references you have provided. If this information is discovered after employment, it could be grounds for dismissal from the job. How would you feel if you found out that you have hired a medical assistant who exaggerated her experience on a résumé? Could you still trust this person? Would you still want to work with this person? Clearly, it is critical for you to be honest when developing your résumé.

The following are the standard parts that must be included in a résumé.

- **Heading**—Your name, address, and telephone number are prepared as a centered heading at the top of the page. If you have a cell phone number and e-mail address, this information can also be included. When this information is printed in slightly larger type than the rest of the text, it stands out and provides an easy reference for the reader.

- **Objective**—Listing an objective lets the reader know what career goal you would like to achieve. When you write your objective, what you want in a career should be clear and to the point. Your objective may need to be changed depending on where you are sending your résumé. The objective is typically no more than one or two sentences.

- **Education**—If you are currently a student or a recent graduate with limited work experience, list your education first in reverse chronological order with the most recent school/program listed first. Add any educational experiences you have had, such as workshops, seminars, or courses.

- **Employment**—Your work experience is then listed in the same reverse chronological order. Include externship or practicum experience with a brief description of your duties. Many prospective employers also wish to see part-time employment listed. This is especially necessary and even beneficial if you have other experience in the health care field. Volunteer work can be listed on the résumé even though you were not paid. This will show a potential employer that you are willing to give your time to help others.

- **Professional organizations and memberships**—Belonging to a professional organization can be a wonderful experience. It helps you to stay current on topics related to your career. Being a member and participating in an organization shows your dedication, commitment, and loyalty to your chosen career field. Many schools have organized a medical assisting society for students to participate in as they complete their program. Many professional organizations offer student and graduate membership.

- **Credentials**—Include information about your professional credentials, such as national certification. If you do not have any credentials, do not include this section on your résumé.

When you are developing your résumé, there is some information that prospective employers do not need (or are legally not entitled) to know. Some of this information is very personal to you and does not reflect how you will perform your job duties. The following are some of the items *not* included on a résumé:

- Age
- General health
- Photograph
- Marital status
- Spouse's and children's names
- Salary information
- Names, addresses, and phone numbers of references
- Reasons for leaving previous positions

As you obtain certification, change positions, or perform volunteer work, you will want to update your résumé so that it is always current. You never know when you might need a copy of your résumé to give to a prospective employer. If you continue to update your résumé as it changes, this will prevent you from forgetting information that should be included on it. See Procedure 59-2.

Professional References

A **professional reference** is the statement of someone who has either worked with you or known you for a period of time. This person will be asked to attest to your skills, personal integrity, or value system. For example, your personal

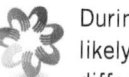

Professionalism — Cultural Considerations

During your externship experience you will most likely encounter patients with cultural backgrounds different from yours. Most communities are home to residents from various cultures. Learn as much as you can about the cultures in your community. It is very important to include on your résumé any foreign languages that you speak, read, or write, particularly those that you speak fluently. This is often a tremendous benefit to prospective employers, especially if you are fluent in a foreign language common to your area.

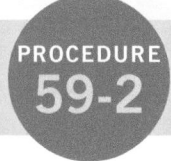

PROCEDURE 59-2 — Preparing Your Résumé and References

Objective ◆ *Prepare a résumé and references.*

EQUIPMENT AND SUPPLIES

Computer; printer; pen; paper; dictionary; thesaurus; telephone book; current and past employment information; current and past educational information

METHOD

1. Gather equipment and supplies.
2. Using Figure 59-6 as an example, prepare your résumé.
3. Using a word-processing program, complete the standard parts of a résumé: heading, objective, education, employment, professional organizations and memberships, credentials, and references.
4. Proofread your résumé.
5. Have a close family member or friend proofread your résumé.
6. Make any corrections to errors found on the résumé.
7. Using good-quality white or off-white 8½ × 11 inch paper, print your résumé.
8. On a separate piece of paper, list at least three references with their titles, addresses, and phone numbers.
9. Proofread your references.
10. Have a close family member or friend proofread your references.
11. Make any corrections to errors found on your references.
12. Using good-quality white or off-white 8½ × 11 inch paper, print your references.
13. Save your résumé and list of references on a disk, USB drive, computer hard drive, or other storage device.
14. Update your résumé whenever changes occur.
15. Turn in your résumé and references to your instructor.

reference may be asked if you are an honest and sincere person. A prospective employer will call your references before hiring you to ask questions about the quality of your work and attendance record.

On a separate piece of paper, prepare a list of at least three references with their street addresses, e-mail addresses, and telephone numbers so you can provide them if they are asked for. Names, addresses, and phone numbers of references are generally not included on the actual résumé.

You should obtain permission to use a person's name as a reference. Before starting your job search, contact each person you want to use as a reference and ask if they will be willing to provide information to prospective employers. Your instructors, dean, and externship supervisor might serve as professional references. Parents, spouses, relatives, and friends do not generally serve as references because their opinions would be viewed as biased. Of course, you would not include the name of anyone who may not provide you with an excellent reference.

The Cover Letter

A **cover letter** is intended to introduce you and your résumé to the recipient—the person to whom you send your letter.

The cover letter should clearly state the purpose of your correspondence. Because health care institutions may be advertising several positions at the same time, you must state clearly the position that interests you.

The cover letter should be brief. It is not a restatement of everything that is in your résumé. Explain what you can do for the employer and why your qualifications are a good match for the job requirements. Be sure to include an address and telephone number where you can be contacted. Do not add handwritten comments or additional information to your cover letter. Always update or revise information on your résumé and cover letter with a word processor and save the updated file. When applying online, upload a copy of a personalized cover letter if you are given that option.

Always review the spelling of the employer's name, address, and phone number carefully for accuracy. A potential employer may judge you by your proofreading skills.

If you have word-processing capability, you may wish to draft several sample cover letters that you can then access from your computer and add the appropriate heading. For instance, different sample cover letters could be drafted to respond to "blind" ads, classified ads, and unsolicited interview requests at local medical facilities. A **blind ad** does not identify the institution or facility that placed the ad. Unsolicited interview requests are requests for interviews initiated by the candidate or prospective employee, not the institution or facility or individual representing the facility. The following are some of the most common mistakes to avoid when writing a cover letter:

- Not addressing the letter to a specific person in the organization. Be sure to check for name, title, and correct spelling.

- Failing to clearly state the position for which you are applying.

- Sending a cover letter that is too long. One page works best with no more than two to three paragraphs.

- Sending a letter that is poorly worded or has spelling or typing errors. Always send the original cover letter, never a copy.

- Failure to sign the letter. (A cover letter submitted electronically does not require a hand-written signature.)

An example of a sample cover letter written in response to a classified ad is presented in Figure 59-7. Also see Procedure 59-3.

Ralph Taylor
222 East Main St.
Chicago, IL 60601
(312) 555-1212

May 20, 20YY

James Stark, M.D.
1450 N. Devonshire
Chicago, IL 60611

Dear Dr. Stark:

This letter is in response to your recent advertisement on the Jobs Now website for a certified medical assistant.

I believe that my qualifications are a good match for your position. During my medical assisting program at Central State College in Hometown, Illinois, I maintained a 3.6 GPA on a 4.0 scale.

My medical assisting program at Central State College was completed in December 20YY. I passed the American Association of Medical Assistants' certification examination January 27, 20YY. Currently I am completing an associate degree program at CSC and plan to graduate in June 20YY.

The enclosed résumé includes my experience as a part-time nursing assistant for Dr. Jane Young in her family practice office.

I look forward to meeting you to discuss your position needs and my qualifications.

Thank you for your consideration.

Sincerely,

Ralph Taylor

Ralph Taylor, CMA (AAMA)

FIGURE 59-7 An example of a cover letter sent in response to an Internet ad.

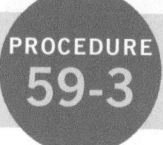

PROCEDURE
59-3

Preparing a Cover Letter

Objective ◆ *Prepare a cover letter.*

EQUIPMENT AND SUPPLIES

Computer; printer; pen; paper; dictionary; thesaurus; telephone book

METHOD

1. Gather equipment and supplies.
2. Using Figure 59-7 as an example, prepare a cover letter using a word-processing program.
3. Proofread your cover letter.
4. Have a close family member or friend proofread your cover letter.
5. Make any corrections to errors found on the cover letter.
6. Using good-quality, white or off-white 8½ × 11 inch paper, print your cover letter.
7. Turn in your cover letter to your instructor.

THE INTERVIEW

If you type the word *interviewing* into an Internet search engine, you will find numerous websites that contain information about interviewing topics, such as preparation, questions asked, questions for you to ask, practice interviews, tips, and much more. The information from some of the websites you visit will provide a wealth of knowledge that will help you be successful during the interview process.

Many schools have a career services office to assist you as you are attending school, after you graduate, or both. It is important for you to get to know the staff and to understand the services available. Getting to know the staff will help you become more comfortable when you are seeking assistance from them.

Many career services offices offer the following services. They will:

- Help you develop a cover letter, résumé, and follow-up thank-you letter
- Review your cover letter, résumé, and follow-up thank-you letter
- Conduct a mock interview
- Provide you with current job listings
- Provide career counseling
- Help you with your job search
- Host job fairs for you to attend on campus
- Conduct workshops and seminars about interviewing, cover letters, résumés, and follow-up thank-you letters

Career services departments do not guarantee placement in a job, because there are many factors involved, including unexpected changes by the employer and how you conduct yourself during an interview.

Preparing for Tough Interview Questions

In addition to the standard questions, some difficult questions may be asked, such as "We all have our strengths and weaknesses. What is one of your weaknesses?" It is always a good idea to highlight your strengths. Therefore, to answer a tough question, select a strength. For instance, you might make the following response to the question about your weakness: "I am a perfectionist and may sometimes hold myself to a very high standard that is almost unobtainable. The way I handle that is to set realistic goals for myself," or "I care very deeply about people and must work to empathize with them rather than sympathize. I try to focus on telling people that I understand they're having a challenging time without agreeing with them or getting into an extended personal conversation."

The interviewer may ask you questions regarding any gaps in the chronology on your résumé. Answer all questions honestly, using simple statements such as "I did not work during that year because I was caring for an older relative" or "It has been six months since I finished school. I did not seek employment, because I was studying for the national certification examination." It is not necessary to provide lengthy explanations for termination from a position. Be especially careful not to criticize or speak badly about the institution or individual who terminated you.

Some of the questions that could be asked during an interview include the following:

- What is one of your strengths?
- What is one of your weaknesses?
- What has been your favorite job? Why?
- What goal or goals do you want to accomplish in the next year?
- What goals do you want to accomplish in the next five years?
- Why would you want to work for this medical office?
- Tell me why I should hire you.
- How do you qualify for this position?
- What has been one of your best accomplishments?
- How did you handle a difficult situation at one of your past jobs?

Be prepared to answer the difficult questions with great poise and professionalism (Figure 59-8). You will have only about 20 minutes to convince your potential employer that you should be the applicant hired. Be absolutely honest about your achievements. However, do not be afraid to talk positively about yourself. There is no one else present at the interview who knows you as well as you know yourself. Guidelines 59-1 provides some helpful tips for successful interviewing.

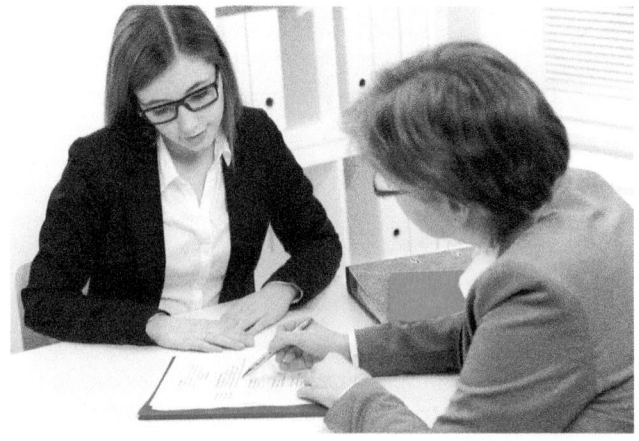

FIGURE 59-8 Answer interview questions with poise and professionalism.

Be prepared with questions to ask the interviewer about the medical office, the position, and the staff. Do not ask about fringe benefits such as time off or medical insurance until you are offered the job. The answers will give you a clearer understanding about the employer and will help you decide if you want to be employed there.

The following are some questions you might want to ask the interviewer:

- Why is this position open?
- How many patients are seen in the office every day?
- What are the working hours for this position?
- How long is the probationary period?

- When are evaluations conducted?
- How long is the orientation or training period?
- Why do you enjoy working here?

To get a clearer understanding of the medical office, ask for a copy of the job description for the position. If the interviewer has not already given you a tour, ask to meet the rest of the staff and tour the medical office. This will help you decide if you would fit in with the other staff at the medical office.

Professionalism at the Interview

The day of the interview, you will be judged immediately by your appearance. You should present a conservative, well-groomed professional appearance. Wear little or no jewelry and avoid showy hairstyles, heavy perfume, bright nail polish, and bright clothing. Of course, this is the same appearance that you will want to present on the job.

Women should wear a suit or modest dress. Men should wear a suit, a plain shirt, and tie. The colors of the attire you wear during the interview should never stand out or be bright. Your attire should be subdued colors. Your attire should never have any loud patterns, designs, or textures. Low-cut shirts, short skirts, and tight-fitting garments are unacceptable and unprofessional for a job interview.

Before you leave for the interview, look at yourself in the mirror. Is the garment you are wearing wrinkled? If so, press it. Never go to an interview with your garment wrinkled. Make sure there is no lint on your garment. Make sure your shoes are clean and polished. Now ask yourself, "Would I want to hire that person in the mirror?" If you are still in a medical assisting program, you may wish to wear a clean, pressed uniform with your school insignia.

No one should accompany you to an interview. If someone is driving for you, they should remain in the car or outside the building. Never bring children to a job interview. Introduce yourself to the receptionist and wait quietly in the reception room until you are called for the interview. Do not engage in telephone calls while waiting. Be very courteous to all office staff. Many physicians will have their entire office team assist in selecting new employees.

Greet the person interviewing you with a firm handshake. Now is an excellent time to give the interviewer a copy of your résumé and reference list. Even if the interviewer already has a copy of your résumé, it is acceptable to give her another copy. Interviewers will generally take a few minutes to ask casual questions that will allow you to relax. Be prepared for questions such as "Tell me about yourself." Have good eye contact with the interviewer and answer all questions in a sincere and friendly manner. Never give answers to the interviewer that are misleading or dishonest.

Questions relating to age, ethnicity, place of birth, marital status, and number of children should not be asked because they set the stage for potential discrimination. Most interviewers are aware of this law and will not ask these questions. You may politely explain you do not wish to answer them if they are asked.

Salary and benefits are not generally discussed in the first interview. If you are called back for a second interview or offered a job, the topic of salary and benefits can be discussed at that time. Remember to be pleasant when the interview is over. The interviewer will usually indicate the end of the interview by standing up and shaking your hand as you leave (Figure 59-9).

Every interview experience is an opportunity for personal growth. If you are not hired on the first or second interview, do not become discouraged. Reassess your interviewing skills. (See Procedure 59-4.) Ask your instructor or friend to critique your skills to see how you might improve. Immediately send out more cover letters and résumés until you are hired. According to interviewers, the 10 most common mistakes

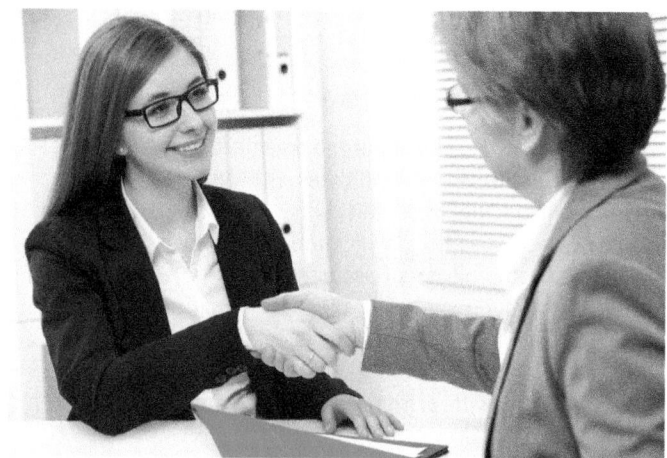

FIGURE 59-9 Shake hands with the interviewer at the close of the interview.

made in interviews are these:

- Poor eye contact
- Use of slang or improper grammar
- Inappropriate dress or poor grooming

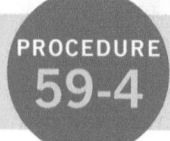

PROCEDURE 59-4 Interviewing for a Job

Objective ◆ *Role-play a job interview.*

EQUIPMENT AND SUPPLIES

Pen and paper

METHOD

1. Determine and write down five questions that may be asked during an interview.
2. Choose a classmate.
3. Select a quiet part of the classroom to conduct the interview.
4. Determine who will be the interviewer and who will be the interviewee.
5. The interviewer will begin the interview process by giving the interviewee a general idea about the medical office and the employees who work there.
6. The interviewer will ask the interviewee the five questions she selected in step 1.
7. The interviewer will ask about the interviewee's past work experience.
8. The interviewer will ask about the interviewee's educational experience.
9. The interviewee will answer the interviewer's questions.
10. The interviewee will ask the interviewer questions about the medical office and the position.
11. The interviewer will answer the interviewee's questions.
12. Repeat the process, with students reversing roles. (Each student should play the part of the interviewer and the interviewee once.)
13. Now the students should discuss the 10 most common mistakes made in an interview. Did either student display any of these mistakes?
14. Each student will assess her own interviewing skills.
15. Each student will discuss the appropriate attire to wear to an interview.
16. Each student will discuss the successful interviewing guidelines derived from the textbook.

- Lack of enthusiasm
- Poor posture
- Smoking or chewing gum
- Talking too much or projecting an overconfident attitude
- Arriving late
- Speaking critically of previous employers
- Inability to ask questions about the organization

The Application

When completing a job **application** or résumé, there should not be any gaps in employment from the time you began to work, except for those that can be explained and justified to the prospective employer. An application includes personal information and previous work experience. You may have stopped working temporarily to complete your education. The employer will then expect the dates of employment and schooling to run consecutively. Gaps with no apparent work or schooling indicated should be clarified. If you were unemployed for a period of time, the potential employer will want to know why.

An application might be completed online at the organization's website or at the time of the interview, depending on the organization. Whichever method is used, maintain a folder containing all your documentation for easy access, such as the following:

- Social Security number
- Updated résumé and an extra copy for the interviewer
- List of three references with their addresses and telephone numbers
- A chronological list of all your work experience
- Driver's license and/or photo ID

Bring the folder with you to the interview if the application is to be completed in person. The neatness of your handwriting and printing will be demonstrated on your application. Be careful to print if that is requested.

Accuracy of spelling and grammar will be observed on both online and paper applications. Remember that questions relating to age, ethnicity, place of birth, and number of children are prohibited by law. However, some offices and institutions may still have these questions on their application forms. You do not have to answer these questions. Simply leave the questions blank. Other information that may be included on an application includes your hourly or yearly salary for all prior jobs you have held and the salary you expect to be offered for the position you are applying for. It is usually acceptable to write *negotiable* in that area of the application so that you do not overstate or understate the salary expectation.

Follow-Up after the Interview

Immediately following the interview, on the same day if possible, send a letter thanking the interviewer for his time. A physical letter is more likely to be noticed than an e-mail. This is a good opportunity to again express your interest in the position. Be meticulous about proofreading your letter for mistakes. It may be your final professional contact with the interviewer before the decision to hire is made.

You may wish to call the office a few days later to ask about the progress made on filling the position. If you are offered a position and decide not to accept it, you would use the same courtesy when turning down an offer as you use when accepting one. See Figure 59-10 for a sample of a follow-up thank-you letter and Procedure 59-5.

If you are offered a position that you wish to accept, complete any requested paperwork immediately. Accept the offer graciously, clearly stating the position you are accepting, and express your thanks.

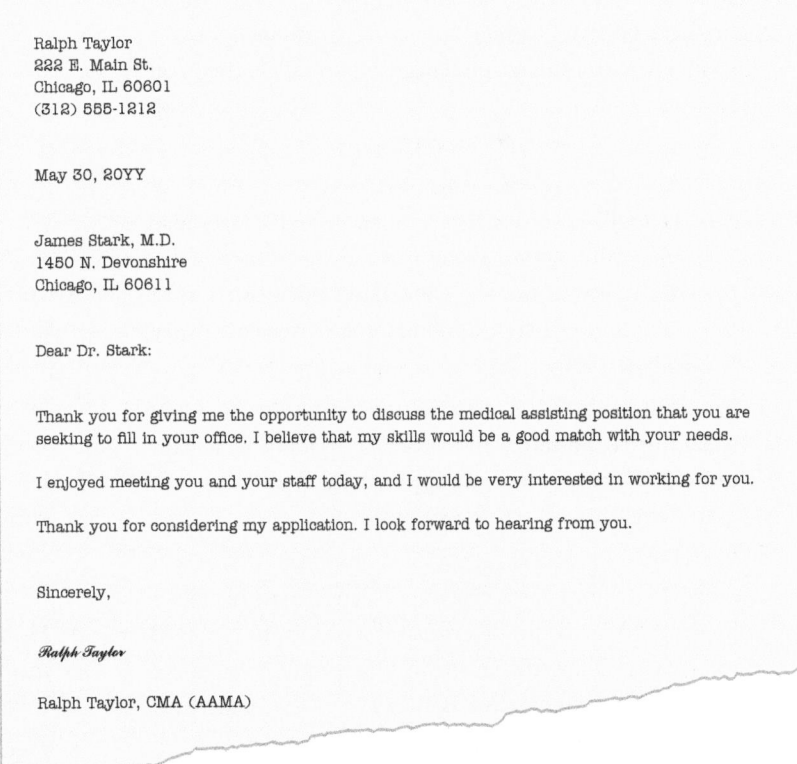

Ralph Taylor
222 E. Main St.
Chicago, IL 60601
(312) 555-1212

May 30, 20YY

James Stark, M.D.
1450 N. Devonshire
Chicago, IL 60611

Dear Dr. Stark:

Thank you for giving me the opportunity to discuss the medical assisting position that you are seeking to fill in your office. I believe that my skills would be a good match with your needs.

I enjoyed meeting you and your staff today, and I would be very interested in working for you.

Thank you for considering my application. I look forward to hearing from you.

Sincerely,

Ralph Taylor

Ralph Taylor, CMA (AAMA)

FIGURE 59-10 An example of a follow-up thank-you letter sent after an interview.

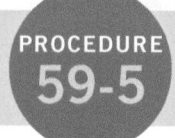

Preparing a Follow-Up Thank-You Letter

Objective ◆ *Prepare an interview follow-up thank-you letter.*

EQUIPMENT AND SUPPLIES

Computer; printer; pen; paper; dictionary; thesaurus; telephone book

METHOD

1. Using Figure 59-10 as an example, prepare a follow-up thank-you letter.
2. Proofread your follow-up thank-you letter.
3. Have a close family member or friend proofread your follow-up thank-you letter.
4. Make any corrections to errors found on the follow-up thank-you letter.
5. Using good-quality, white or off-white 8½ × 11 inch paper, print your follow-up thank-you letter.
6. Turn in your follow-up letter to your instructor.

WHAT DOES THE EMPLOYER WANT?

Employers prefer employees who are versatile and can successfully perform a wide variety of tasks and roles. To be successful as a medical assistant, you must master six basic skills:

- **Reading**—As a medical assistant you will be reading medical records, orders, instructions, memos, correspondence, resources, references, and much more. You also will read a variety of professional journals to keep your skills and knowledge current.

- **Listening**—A large amount of your time as a medical assistant will be spent listening to patients. You also will use your listening skills during meetings, telephone conversations, and conversing with other staff members. Good listening skills are critical for every medical assistant.

- **Speaking**—Medical assistants spend a lot of time speaking to patients and other staff members. You must speak clearly and use appropriate vocabulary and grammar.

- **Writing**—Documentation in a medical office is a must. It demonstrates that care or treatment has been provided. This could be critical if a physician is called to court for a lawsuit. A medical assistant must make sure all documentation is complete, accurate, and spelled correctly.

- **Problem solving**—Your problem-solving skills will be an asset to the medical office and will allow you to be more efficient in performing your duties. Employers want their employees to be able to manage change and think of new ways to improve situations.

- **Teamwork**—The medical office staff must work as a team for the office to run efficiently. As a medical assistant, you will share knowledge and responsibilities with other staff members. Good-quality patient care results when all members of the team are working together.

Employers look for a wide range of qualities, values, and abilities in an employee. Although not every employer will seek the exact same criteria, some of the most common include the following:

- **Initiative**—Initiative is taking on a needed task without being told to do so. Starting a task on your own will show your employer that you are problem solving and using your critical thinking skills.

- **Enthusiasm**—A medical assistant's enthusiasm can be expressed verbally or nonverbally. When you are enthusiastic, you enjoy what you are doing and are passionate about it. Enthusiasm is a positive quality for all medical assistants to develop.

- **Honesty**—For patients, physicians, and other staff members to trust you, you must be honest at all times. If you have made a mistake, admit it and learn from it.

- **Dependability**—The physician and other staff members depend on you to be there at the scheduled time. When a medical assistant is late, leaves early, or misses work, the office must reassign staff and possibly work understaffed during that time. This causes more work for everyone.

- **Flexibility**—Most medical offices are very busy, and emergencies do occur. As a medical assistant, you must be flexible with the changes that can occur daily or even minute to minute. This also means that you must multitask throughout the workday.

- **Confidentiality**—The medical assistant must maintain confidentiality when working with the patient's protected health information. Failure to uphold this requirement may result in legal issues for the medical practice and ultimately cost the medical assistant a job.

- **Administrative skills**—Part of your job duties may include administrative procedures. Take special care to make sure each one is performed correctly and efficiently.

- **Clinical skills**—Part of your job duties may include clinical procedures. It is critical for a medical assistant to perform clinical skills with total efficiency and accuracy.

You will not be perfect at all of these skills, but you can develop each and every one of them with time, practice, and commitment. The more qualities, values, and skills you have as a medical assistant, the more employable you will be. Just ask yourself, what would you want in an employee? This will help lead you to the qualities, values, and skills you need to develop.

Professionalism | The Law

 You are responsible for providing complete and accurate information on application forms. Be sure all the facts surrounding your education and work experience are absolutely accurate. It is especially important to be honest about your skill level. Do not promise to perform procedures or tasks for which you are not trained. If an employer discovers that an employee lied on an application or a résumé, it is considered cause for termination. In some instances, there may even be cause for prosecution.

SUMMARY

One of the most valuable components of a medical assisting program is the externship, because it provides an opportunity to apply the knowledge and practice the skills that have been learned in school. You will work under the direct supervision of the extern site preceptor and externship coordinator. This important stage of the training provides the student an opportunity to gain insight into personal strengths and weaknesses, allowing students to work on or correct weaknesses before accepting employment.

The job interview process requires the medical assistant to be honest and sincere about capabilities and the desire to work diligently. A fulfilling career demands careful planning, the ability to arrive on time, and the ability to work diligently for an employer while always keeping the patient's needs in mind.

59 CHAPTER REVIEW

COMPETENCY REVIEW

1. Define and spell the terms for this chapter.
2. Describe three areas of student responsibility concerning the externship.
3. List and discuss three externship opportunities in your area that you would like to pursue.
4. List and discuss six areas that your externship supervisor will be evaluating.
5. Explain why a cover letter is important to send along with a résumé.
6. List at least five common mistakes often made during an interview.

7. An interviewer should not ask questions that may lead to discrimination, such as your age, where you were born, your marital status, or how many children you have. If you are asked such a question, how would you respond?
8. How would you respond to the question "What is your major strength?"
9. How would you respond to the question "What is your major weakness?"

PREPARING FOR THE CERTIFICATION EXAM

1. At the end of medical assistant training, working without payment in a health care setting as part of a medical assisting program is called
   a. clinical rotation.
   b. an in-service.
   c. an externship.
   d. an internship.
   e. a preceptor.

2. Physicians and office managers are likely to be extremely critical of which area during an externship?
   a. medical terminology
   b. pharmacology
   c. clinical skills
   d. lateness
   e. computer skills

3. Which of the following should *not* be brought to an interview?
   a. photo ID
   b. résumé
   c. proof of certification
   d. children
   e. grades received in school

4. Which of the following is *not* a guideline to successful interviewing?
   a. Carry one extra copy of your résumé.
   b. Dress conservatively.
   c. Be alert.
   d. Arrive exactly on time.
   e. Do not chew gum.

5. Which of the following is *not* considered a job hunting mistake?
   a. failing to network with others and tell them that you are looking
   b. knowing your weaknesses
   c. limiting yourself to one field
   d. not having a clear plan
   e. not practicing interviewing skills

6. Which of the following should *not* be included in a résumé?
   a. objective
   b. education
   c. salary expectations
   d. work history
   e. address

7. Which of the following is one of the six basic skills desired by employers?
   a. accounting
   b. talkativeness
   c. writing
   d. modern fashion
   e. perfection

8. After an interview, which of the following should be done?
   a. Send a thank-you letter.
   b. Send six copies of your résumé.
   c. Inform the workplace of other job offers you have received.
   d. Send testimonials from your pastor.
   e. Make a thank-you phone call.

9. What is the name of the type of correspondence that is intended as a courtesy to introduce yourself and summarize your qualifications for the job?
   a. cover letter
   b. follow-up letter
   c. résumé
   d. interview letter
   e. calling card

10. Which of the following is considered one of the more common mistakes made in an interview?
    a. projecting an overconfident attitude
    b. making eye contact
    c. asking questions about the potential employer's organization
    d. wearing little or no jewelry
    e. using proper grammar such as "yes" instead of "yep"

CRITICAL THINKING

Refer to the case study at the beginning of the chapter and use what you have learned to answer these questions.

1. Kenneth prepares a list of questions that he would like to ask Tania during the interview. What are some important questions that Kenneth may ask during the interview?

2. On his way to the interview, Kenneth takes the wrong exit and must turn around to head in the right direction. How should Kenneth handle the situation if he thinks that he may be late for the interview?

3. Tania asks Kenneth about a six-month gap in his résumé when he did not have a job. Kenneth is embarrassed and flustered while answering the question. What should he tell Tania?

ON THE JOB

Stacy Friedlander is the lead medical assistant in an ophthalmology practice of 10 physicians. The eye clinic has patients from all over the world. Several of the physicians are leaders in their specific area of ophthalmology, such as Dr. Keeler, who specializes in retinal diseases.

Today, Stacy is going to interview a potential new employee, Sarah Banks. Sarah is currently finishing a CAAHEP-approved medical assisting program at a local college and is searching for full-time employment. She has some on-the-job experience dating back to when she was an after-school receptionist for a general practitioner, but that was more than 10 years ago.

The clinic tends to hire medical assistants who are certified, experienced, and very capable of dealing with patients from different age groups, races, and cultures. However, Sarah is being considered for the position because, first of all, her father is a personal friend of Dr. Keeler, and second, qualified medical assistants are difficult to find because of the high demand. What should Stacy do to prepare for the interview with Sarah? What is your response to the situation?

1. Is it proper procedure for Sarah to be applying for this position given that she has not yet completed her medical assisting program?
2. Should Stacy, given the circumstances, invest a lot of time in interviewing Sarah? Why or why not?
3. Should Sarah's 10 years of job experience be factored into Stacy's decision to hire Sarah or not?
4. If Stacy wishes to hire Sarah, should Stacy take the time to check Sarah's references even though Sarah's father is a friend of Dr. Keeler?

INTERNET ACTIVITY

Using any Internet search engine, type the phrase *dressing for an interview.* Research one or more of the resulting websites to answer the following questions:

1. Would a person be ready for an interview if he had an eyebrow piercing?
2. Should a person chew gum during an interview?
3. What are appropriate colors for dresses or suits?

Appendix 1

Common Medical Abbreviations

AAO	alert, awake, and oriented	FBS	fasting blood sugar	NSAID	nonsteroidal antiinflammatory
A&O	alert and oriented	FTT	failure to thrive		drugs
ABD	abdomen	FU	follow-up	NSR	normal sinus rhythm
ABG	arterial blood gas	Fx	fracture		
abs	absent			OB	obstetrics
AC	before eating	GI	gastrointestinal	OPV	oral polio vaccine
ACLS	advanced cardiac life support	GSW	gunshot wound	OR	operating room
ADH	antidiuretic hormone	GTT	glucose tolerance test		
adm	admission			PA	posteroanterior
ad lib	as much as needed	HA	headache	PC	after eating
ADR	adverse drug reaction	H&P	history and physical examination	PDR	Physician's Desk Reference
AFP	alpha-fetoprotein	HBP	high blood pressure	PE	physical exam
amb	ambulatory	HCG	human chorionic gonadotropin	PKU	phenylketonuria
amt	amount	HCT	hematocrit	PMH	previous medical history
ant	anterior	HDL	high-density lipoprotein	PO	by mouth
ante	before	HEENT	head, eyes, ears, nose, throat	PR	by rectum
AOB	alcohol on breath	Hgb	hemoglobin	PRN	as needed
AP	anteroposterior	HIV	human immunodeficiency virus	Pt	patient
ASAP	as soon as possible	HO	history of	PT	prothrombin time, or physical therapy
		HR	heart rate	PTT	partial thromboplastin time
BCP	birth control pills	HS	at bedtime	PUD	peptic ulcer disease
BE	barium enema	HSV	herpes simplex virus		
bid	twice a day	HTN	hypertension	q	every (e.g., q6h = every 6 hours)
BM	bowel movement	Hx	history	qh	every hour
BMR	basal metabolic rate			qid	four times a day
BP	blood pressure	I&D	incision and drainage		
BPH	benign prostatic hypertrophy	ICU	intensive care unit	R	right
BPM	beats per minute	ID	infectious disease	RA	rheumatoid arthritis
BS	bowel, or breath sounds	IG	immunoglobulin	RBC	red blood cell
BX	biopsy	IM	intramuscular	R/O	rule out
		INF	intravenous nutritional fluid	ROM	range of motion
c̄	with	IV	intravenous	ROS	review of systems
Ca	calcium			RTC	return to clinic
CA	cancer	L	left		
CAD	coronary artery disease	LLL	left lower lobe	s̄	without
CAT	computerized axial tomography	LMP	last menstrual period	SOAP	subjective, objective, assessment, plan
CBC	complete blood count	LOC	loss of consciousness, or level of	SOB	shortness of breath
CC	chief complaint		consciousness	STAT	immediately
CHF	congestive heart failure	LPN	licensed practical nurse	SubQ	subcutaneous
CNS	central nervous system			Sx	symptoms
C/O	complaining of	MAO	monoamine oxidase		
COPD	chronic obstructive pulmonary disease	MBT	maternal blood type	T&C	type and cross
CP	cerebral palsy	MI	myocardial infarction, or mitral	TB	tuberculosis
CPAP	continuous positive airway pressure		insufficiency	tid	three times a day
CPR	cardiopulmonary resuscitation	mL	milliliter	TIG	tetanus immune globulin
CT	computerized tomography	MMR	measles, mumps, rubella	TMJ	temporomandibular joint
CVA	cerebrovascular accident	MRI	magnetic resonance imaging	TNTC	too numerous to count
CXR	chest X-ray	MRSA	methicillin resistant staphylococcus	TO	telephone order
			aureus	TPN	total parenteral nutrition
DC	discontinue, or discharge	MS	multiple sclerosis	TSH	thyroid stimulating hormone
DNR	do not resuscitate	MVA	motor vehicle accident	TT	thrombin time
DOA	dead on arrival			Tx	treatment
DTR	deep tendon reflexes	NG	nasogastric		
DVT	deep venous thrombosis	NKA	no known allergies	UA	urinalysis
DX	diagnosis	NKDA	no known drug allergies	UAO	upper airway obstruction
		NMR	nuclear magnetic resonance	UBD	universal blood donor
ECG	electrocardiogram	NPO	nothing by mouth	URI	upper respiratory infection
EMG	electromyogram			US	ultrasound
ENT	ears, nose, and throat				

UTI	urinary tract infection	WF	white female	yo	years old
		WM	white male	YOB	year of birth
VO	verbal order	WNL	within normal limits	yr	year
		WO	written order	ytd	year to date
WBC	white blood cell				
WD	well developed				

Appendix 2

Glossary of Word Parts

PREFIXES

a-	no, not, without, lack of, apart	ep-	upon, over, above	pan-	all
ab-	away from	epi-	upon, over, above	par-	around, beside
ad-	toward, near	eso-	inward	para-	beside, alongside, abnormal
ambi-	both	eu-	good, normal	per-	through
an-	no, not, without, lack of	ex-	out, away from	peri-	around
ana-	up	exo-	out, away from	poly-	many, much, excessive
ant-	against	extra-	outside, beyond	post-	after, behind
ante-	before			pre-	before
anti-	against	hemi-	half	primi-	first
apo-	separation	heter-	different	pro-	forward, outward
astro-	star-shaped	hetero-	different	proto-	first
auto-	self	homo-	similar, same	pseudo-	false
		homeo-	similar, same, likeness, constant	pyro-	fire
bi-	two, double	hydr-	water		
bin-	twice	hydro-	water	quadri-	four
brachy-	short	hyp-	below, deficient	quint-	five
brady-	slow	hyper-	above, beyond, excessive		
		hypo-	below, under, deficient	re-	again, back
cac-	bad			retro-	backward
cata-	down	in-	in, into, not		
centi-	a hundred	infra-	below	semi-	half
chromo-	color	infer-	below	sub-	below, under, beneath
circum-	around	inter-	between	super-	above, beyond
con-	with, together	intra-	within	supra-	above, beyond
contra-	against	ir-	into	sym-	together
				syn-	together, with
de-	down, away from	macro-	large		
deca-	ten	mal-	bad	tachy-	fast
di-	through, between	mega-	large, great	tetra-	four
dia-	through, between	meso-	middle	trans-	across
dif-	apart, free from, separate	meta-	beyond, over, between, change	tri-	three
dipl-	double	micro-	small		
dis-	two, apart	milli-	one-thousandth	ultra-	beyond
dis-	apart	mon-	one	uni-	one
dys-	bad, difficult, painful	mono-	one		
		multi-	many, much		
ec-	out, outside, outer				
ecto-	out, outside, outer	neo-	new		
em-	in	nulli-	none		
en-	within				
end-	within, inner	olig-	little, scanty		
endo-	within, inner	oligo-	little, scanty		

WORD ROOTS/COMBINING FORMS

abdomin	abdomen	aden	gland	all	other
abort	to miscarry	aden/o	gland	alveol	small, hollow air sac
absorpt	to suck in	adhes	stuck to	ambul	to walk
acanth	a thorn	adip	fat	ambyl	dull
acid	acid	agglutinat	clumping	amni/o	membrane
acoust	hearing	agon	agony	ampere	ampere
acr	extremity, point	agor/a	gathering place	amputat	to cut through
acr/o	extremity, point	albin	white	amyl	starch
act	acting	albumin	protein	anastom	opening
actin	ray	alimentat	nourishment	andr	man

Word Part	Meaning	Word Part	Meaning	Word Part	Meaning
andr/o	man	cavit	cavity	cry/o	cold
ang	vessel	celi	abdomen, belly	crypt	hidden
ang/i	vessel	cellul	little cell	cubit	elbow, to lie
angin	to choke, quinsy	centr	center	culd/o	cul-de-sac
angi/o	vessel	centr/i	center	curie	curie
anis/o	unequal	cephal	head	cutane	skin
ankyl	stiffening, crooked	cept	receive	cyan	dark blue
an/o	anus	cerebell	little brain	cycl	ciliary body
anter/i	toward the front	cerebell/o	little brain	cycl/o	ciliary body
anthrac	coal	cerebr/o	cerebrum	cyst	bladder, sac
aort	aorta	cervic	cervix, neck	cyst/o	bladder, sac
aort/o	aorta	cheil	lip	cyt	cell
append	appendix	chem/o	chemical	cyth	cell
arachn	spider	chlor/o	green	cyt/o	cell
arche	beginning	chol	gall, bile		
arter	artery	chole	gall, bile	dacry	tear
arter/i	artery	chol/e	gall, bile	dactyl	finger or toe
arteri/o	artery	choledoch/o	common bile duct	dactyl/o	finger or toe
arthr	joint	chondr	cartilage	defecat	to remove dregs
arthr/o	joint	chondr/o	cartilage	dem	people
artific/i	not natural	chord	cord	dendr/o	tree
aspirat	to draw in	chori/o	chorion	dent	tooth
atel	imperfect	choroid	choroid	dent/i	tooth
atel/o	imperfect	choroid/o	choroid	derm	skin
ather	fatty substance, porridge	chromat	color	derm/a	skin
ather/o	fatty substance, porridge	chrom/o	color	dermat	skin
atri	atrium	chym	juice	dermat/o	skin
atri/o	atrium	cine	motion	derm/o	skin
aud/i	to hear	cinemat/o	motion	dextr/o	to the right
audi/o	to hear	circulat	circular	diast	to expand
auditor	hearing	cirrh	orange-yellow	didym	testis
aur	ear	cirrh/o	orange-yellow	digit	finger or toe
aur/i	ear	cis	to cut	dilat	to widen
auscultat	listen to	claudicat	to limp	disk	a disk
aut	self	clavicul	little key	dist	away from the point of origin
axill	armpit	cleid/o	clavicle	diverticul	diverticula
		coagul	to clot	dors	backward
bacter/i	bacteria	coagulat	to clot	dors/i	backward
balan	glans penis	coccyg/e	tailbone	duct	to lead
bartholin	Bartholin's glands	coccyg/o	tailbone	duoden	duodenum
bas/o	base	cochle/o	land snail	dur	dura, hard
bil	bile, gall	coit	a coming together	dur/o	dura, hard
bil/i	bile, gall	col	colon	dwarf	small
bi/o	life	coll/a	glue	dynam	power
blast/o	germ cell	collis	neck		
blephar	eyelid	col/o	colon	ech/o	echo
blephar/o	eyelid	colon	colon	ectop	displaced
bol	to cast, throw	colon/o	colon	eg/o	I, self
brach/i	arm	colp/o	vagina	ejaculat	to throw out
bronch	bronchi	concuss	shaken violently	electr/o	electricity
bronch/i	bronchi	condyle	knuckle	embol	to cast, to throw
bronchiol	bronchiole	con/i	dust	eme	to vomit
bronch/o	bronchi	conjunctiv	to join together	emulsificat	disintergrate
bucc	cheek	connect	to bind together	encephal	brain
burs	a pouch	constipat	to press together	encephal/o	brain
		continence	to hold	enchyma	to pour
calc	lime, calcium	cor	pupil	enter	intestine
calcan/e	heel bone	coriat	corium	enucleat	to remove the kernel of
calc/i	calcium	corne	cornea	eosin/o	rose-colored
cancer	crab	corpor	body	episi/o	vulva, pudenda
capn	smoke	corpor/e	body	equ/i	equal
capsul	a little box	cortic	cortex	erget	work
carcin	cancer	cortis	cortex	erg/o	work
carcin/o	cancer	cost	rib	eructat	a breaking out
card	heart	cost/o	rib	erysi	red
card/i/io	heart	cox	hip	erythr/o	red
cardi/o	heart	cran/i/o	skull	esophag/e	esophagus
carp	wrist	crani/o	skull	esophag/o	esophagus
carp/o	wrist	creat	flesh	esthesi/o	feeling
cartil	gristle	creatin	flesh, creatine	estr/o	mad desire
castr	to prune	crine	to secrete	eti/o	cause
caud	tail	crin/o	to secrete	eunia	a bed
caus	heat	crur	leg	excret	sifted out

Word part	Meaning
fasc	a band (fascia)
fasci/o	a band (fascia)
femor	femur
fenestrat	window
fibr	fibrous tissue, fiber
fibrillat	fibrils (small fibers)
fibrin/o	fiber
fibr/o	fiber
fibul	fibula
filtrat	to strain through
fixat	fastened
flex	to bend
fluor/o	fluorescence
foc	focus
follicul	little bag
format	a shaping
fungat	mushroom, fungus
fus	to pour
galact/o	milk
ganglion	knot
gastr	stomach
gastr/o	stomach
gen	formation, produce
gene	formation, produce
genet	formation, produce
genital	belonging to birth
gen/o	kind
ger	old age
gest	to carry
gester	to bear
gigant	giant
gingiv	gums
glandul	little acorn
gli	glue
gli/o	glue
glob	globe
globin	globule
globul	globe
glomerul	glomerulus, little ball
glomerul/o	glomerulus, little ball
gloss/o	tongue
gluc/o	sweet, sugar
glyc	sweet, sugar
glyc/o	glucose, sweet, sugar
glycos	sweet, sugar
gonad	seed
goni/o	angle
gon/o	genitals
granul/o	little grain, granular
gravida	pregnant
gryp	curve
gynec/o	female
halat	breathe
hallux	great (big) toe
hem	blood
hemat	blood
hemat/o	blood
hem/o	blood
hemorrh	vein liable to bleed
hepat	liver
hepat/o	liver
herni/o	hernia
hidr	sweat
hirsut	hairy
hist/o	tissue
hol/o	whole
horizont	horizon
humer	humerus
hydr	water
hymen	hymen
hypn	sleep
hyster	womb, uterus
hyster/o	womb, uterus
icter	jaundice
ile	ileum
ile/o	ileum
ili	ilium
ili/o	ilium
illus	foot
immun/o	safe, immunity
infarct	infarct (necrosis of an area)
infect	infection
infer/i	below
inguin	groin
insul	insulin
insulin/o	insulin
integument	covering
intern	within
ionizat	ion (going)
ion/o	ion
iont/o	ion
irid	iris
irid/o	iris
isch	to hold back
ischi	ischium
is/o	equal
jaund	yellow
kal	potassium
kary/o	cell's nucleus
kel	tumor
kerat	cornea
kerat/o	horn, cornea
keton	ketone
kil/o	a thousand
kinet	motion
kyph	a hump
labi	lip
labyrinth	maze
labyrinth/o	maze
lacrim	tear
lamin	lamina, thin plate
lamp (s)	to shine
lapar/o	flank, abdomen
laryng	larynx
laryng/e	larynx
laryng/o	larynx
later	side
laxat	to loosen
lei/o	smooth
lemma	rind, sheath, husk
lent	lens
lept	seizure
letharg	drowsiness
leuk	white
leuk/o	white
levat	lifter
libr/i	balance
lingu	tongue
lip	fat
lipid	fat
lip/o	fat
lith	stone
lith/o	stone
lob	lobe
lob/o	lobe
lobul	small lobe
locat	to place
log	study
log/o	word
lopec	fox mange
lord	bending
lucent	to shine
lumb	loin
lumb/o	loin
lump	lump
lun	moon
lymph	lymph, clear fluid
lymph/o	lymph, clear fluid
malign	bad kind
mamm/o	breast
mandibul	lower jawbone
man/o	thin
mast	breast
masticat	to chew
mast/o	breast
maxill	jawbone
maxilla	jaw
maxim	greatest
meat	passage
meat/o	passage
med	middle
medi	toward the middle
medull	marrow
medull/o	marrow
melan	black
melan/o	black
men	month
mening	membrane (meninges)
mening/i	membrane
mening/o	membrane
menise	crescent
men/o	month
ment	mind
mes	middle
mes/o	middle
mester	month
metr	to measure, womb, uterus
metr/i	womb, uterus
micturit	to urinate
miliar	millet (tiny)
minim	least
mi/o	less, smaller
mit	thread
mitr	mitral valve
mnes	memory
mucos	mucus
mucus	mucus
muscul	muscle
muscul/o	muscle
muta	to change
mutat	to change
my	muscle
myc	fungus
myc/o	fungus
mydriat	dilation, widen
myel	bone marrow, spinal cord
myel/o	marrow
my/o	muscle
my/os	muscle
myring	drum membrane
myring/o	drum membrane
myx	mucus
narc/o	numbness
nas/o	nose
nat	birth
nat/o	birth
necr	death
necr/o	death
nephr	kidney
nephr/o	kidney
neur	nerve

neur/i	nerve	phac	lens	rach	spine
neur/o	nerve	phac/o	lens	rachi	spine
neutr/o	neither	phag	to eat, engulf	rad/i	radiating out from a center
nid	nest	phag/o	to eat, engulf	radi	radius
noct	night	phak	lentil, lens	radiat	radiant
nom	law	phalang/e	closely knit row	radic/o	spinal nerve root
norm	rule	pharyng	pharynx	radicul	spinal nerve root
nucl	nucleus	pharyng/o	pharynx	radi/o	ray
nucle	kernel, nucleus	phas	speech	rect/o	rectum
nyctal	blind	phen/o	to show	relaxat	to loosen
nystagm	to nod	phe/o	dusky	remiss	remit
		phim	a muzzle	ren	kidney
occlus	to shut up	phleb	vein	ren/o	kidney
ocul	eye	phleb/o	vein	respirat	breathing
odont	tooth	phon	voice	reticul/o	net
olecran	elbow	phone	voice	retin	retina
onc/o	tumor	phon/o	sound	retin/o	retina
onych	nail	phor	carrying	rhabd/o	rod
onych/o	nail	phos	light	rheumat	discharge
o/o	ovum, egg	phot/o	light	rheumat/o	discharge
oophor	ovary	phragm	partition	rhin/o	nose
ophthalm	eye	phragmat/o	partition	rhonch	snore
ophthalm/o	eye	phras	speech	rhytid/o	wrinkle
opt	eye	physic	nature	roent	roentgen
opt/o	eye	physi/o	nature	rotat	to turn
or	mouth	pil/o	hair	rrhyth	rhythm
orch	testicle	pine	pine cone	rrhythm	rhythm
orchid	testicle	pineal	pineal body	rube/o	red
orchid/o	testicle	pin/o	to drink		
organ	organ	pituitar	phlegm	sacr	sacrum
orth	straight	plak	plate	salping	tube, fallopian tube
orth/o	straight	plasma	a thing formed, plasma	salping/o	tube, fallopian tube
oscill	to swing	plast	a developing	salpinx	tube, fallopian tube
oscill/o	to swing	pleur	pleura	sarc	flesh
oste	bone	pleura	pleura	sarc/o	flesh
oste/o	bone	pleur/o	pleura	scapul	shoulder blade
ot	ear	plicat	to fold	scler	hardening
ot/o	ear	pneum/o	lung, air	scler/o	hardening, sclera
ovar	ovary	pneumon	lung	scoli	curvature
ovul	ovary	poiet	formation	scoli/o	curvature
ovulat	ovary	poli/o	gray	scop	to examine
ox	oxygen	pollex	thumb	seb/o	oil
ox/i	oxygen	por	a passage	secund	second
oxy	sour, sharp, acid	porphyr	purple	semin	seed
		poster/i	behind, toward the back	seminat	seed
pachy	thick	prand/i	meal	senile	old
pancreat	pancreas	presby	old	senil	old
paque	dark	press	to press	sept	putrefaction
palat/o	palate	proct	anus, rectum	septic	putrefying
palliat	cloaked	proct/o	anus, rectum	ser (a)	whey
pallid/o	globus, pallidus	prolif	fruitful	ser/o	whey, serum
palm	palm	prophylact	guarding	sert	to gain
palpitat	throbbing	prostat	prostate	sexu	sex
papill	papilla	prosth/e	an addition	sial	saliva
para	to bear	prot/e	first	sial/o	salivary
paralyt	to disable, paralysis	proxim	near the point of	sider/o	iron
partum	labor		origin	sigmoid	sigmoid
parturit	in labor	prurit	itching	sigmoid/o	sigmoid
patell	kneecap, patella	psych	mind	sin/o	a curve
path	disease	psych/o	mind	sinus	a hollow curve
path/o	disease	pudend	external genitals	situ	place
pause	cessation	pulm/o	lung	som	body
pector	chest	pulmon	lung	somat	body
pectorat	breast	pulmonar	lung	somat/o	body
ped	foot, child	pupill	pupil	somn	sleep
ped/i	foot, child	purpur	purple	son	sound
pedicul	a louse	py	pus	son/o	sound
pelv/i	pelvis	pyel	renal pelvis	spadias	a rent, an opening
pen	penis	pyel/o	renal pelvis	spastic	convulsive
penile	penis	pylor	pylorus, gatekeeper	sperm	seed (sperm)
pept	to digest	py/o	pus	spermat	seed (sperm)
perine	perineum	pyret	fever	spermat/o	seed (sperm)
periton/e	peritoneum	pyr/o	heat, fire	spermi	seed (sperm)

sphygm/o	pulse	thorac/o	chest	urin	urine
spin	spine, a thorn	thorax	chest	urinat	urine
spir/o	breath	thromb	clot	urin/o	urine
splen/o	spleen	thromb/o	clot	ur/o	urine
spondyl	vertebra	thym	thymus, mind, emotion	uter	uterus
spondyl/o	vertebra	thyr	thyroid, shield	uter/o	uterus
staped	stirrup	thyr/o	thyroid, shield	uve	uvea
steat	fat	thyrox	thyroid, shield		
sten	narrowing	tibi	tibia	vagin	vagina
ster	solid	tinnit	a jingling	vag/o	vagus, wandering
stern	sternum	toc	birth	varic/o	twisted vein
stern/o	sternum	tom/o	to cut	vas	vessel
sterol	solid (fat)	ton	tone, tension	vascul	small vessel
steth	chest	ton/o	tone	vas/o	vessel
steth/o	chest	tonsill	tonsil, almond	vector	a carrier
stigmat	point	topic	place	ven	vein
stom	mouth	top/o	place	venere	sexual intercourse
stomat	mouth	tors	twisted	ven/i	vein
strabism	a squinting	tort/i	twisted	ven/o	vein
strict	to draw, to bind	tox	poison	ventilat	to air
superfic/i	near the surface	toxic	poison	ventr	near or on the belly side of the
super/i	upper	trach/e	trachea		body
suppress	suppress	trache/o	trachea	ventricul	ventricle
surrog	substituted	tract	to draw	ventricul/o	little belly
sympath	sympathy	trephinat	a bore	vermi	worm
synov	joint fluid	trich	hair	vers	turning
syst	contraction	trich/o	hair	vertebr	vertebra
system	a composite whole	trigon	trigone	vertebr/o	vertebra
systol	contraction	trism	grating	vesic	bladder
		trop	turning	vesicul	vesicle
tel	end, distant	troph	a turning	vir	virus (poison)
tele	distant	tubercul	a little swelling	viril	masculine
tempor	temples	tuss	cough	viscer	body organs
tendin	tendon	tympan	ear drum	volt	volt
tend/o	tendon	tympan/o	drum	volunt	will
ten/o	tendon			volvul	to roll
tenon	tendon	uln	ulna, elbow	vuls	to pull
tenos	tendon	uln/o	ulna, elbow		
tens	tension	umbilic	navel	watt	watt
tentori	tentorium, tent	ungu	nail		
terat	monster	ur	urine	xanth/o	yellow
testicul	testicle	ure	urinate	xen	foreign material
test/o	testicle	urea	urea	xer	dry
thalass	sea	uret	urine	xer/o	dry
thel/i	nipple	ureter	ureter	xiph	sword
therm	hot, heat	ureter/o	ureter		
therm/o	hot, heat	urethr	urethra	zo/o	animal
thorac	chest	urethr/o	urethra	zoon	life

SUFFIXES

-able	capable	-ceps	head	-dynia	pain
-ac	pertaining to	-cide	to kill	-ectasia	dilatation
-ad	pertaining to	-clasia	a breaking	-ectasis	dilatation, distention
-age	related to	-clave	a key	-ectasy	dilation
-al	pertaining to	-cle	small	-ectomy	surgical excision
-algesia	pain	-clysis	injection	-edema	swelling
-algia	pain	-cope	strike	-emesis	vomiting
-ant	forming	-crit	to separate	-emia	blood condition
-ar	pertaining to	-culture	cultivation	-er	relating to, one who
-ary	pertaining to	-cusis	hearing	-ergy	work
-ase	enzyme	-cuspid	point	-esthesia	feeling
-asthenia	weakness	-cyesis	pregnancy	-form	shape
-ate	use, action	-cyst	bladder	-fuge	to flee
-ate (d)	use, action	-cyte	cell	-gen	formation, produce
-betes	to go	-derma	skin	-genes	produce
-blast	immature cell, germ cell	-dermis	skin	-genesis	formation, produce
-body	body	-desis	binding	-genic	formation, produce
-cele	hernia, tumor, swelling	-dipsia	thirst	-glia	glue
-centesis	surgical puncture	-drome	a course	-globin	protein

-gnosis	knowledge	-noia	mind	-poiesis	formation
-grade	a step	-oid	resemble	-praxia	action
-graft	pencil, grafting knife	-ole	opening	-ptosis	prolapse, drooping
-gram	a weight, mark, record	-oma	tumor	-ptysis	to spit, spitting
-graph	to write, record	-omion	shoulder	-puncture	to pierce
-graphy	recording	-on	pertaining to	-rrhage	to burst forth, bursting forth
-hexia	condition	-one	hormone	-rrhagia	to burst forth, bursting forth
-ia	condition	-opia	eye, vision	-rrhaphy	suture
-iasis	condition	-opsia	eye, vision	-rrhea	flow, discharge
-ic	pertaining to	-opsy	to view	-rrhexis	rupture
-ide	having a particular quality	-or	one who, a doer	-scope	instrument
-in	chemical, pertaining to	-ory	like, resemble	-scopy	to view, examine
-ine	pertaining to	-orexia	appetite	-sepsis	decay
-ing	quality of	-ose	like	-sis	condition
-ion	process	-osis	condition	-some	body
-ism	condition	-ous	pertaining to	-spasm	tension, spasm, contraction
-ist	one who specializes, agent	-paresis	weakness	-stalsis	contraction
-itis	inflammation	-pathy	disease	-stasis	control, stopping
-ity	condition	-penia	lack of, deficiency	-staxis	dripping, trickling
-ive	nature of, quality of	-pepsia	to digest	-sthenia	strength
-kinesia	motion	-pexy	surgical fixation	-stomy	new opening
-kinesis	motion	-phagia	to eat	-systole	contraction
-lalia	to talk	-phasia	to speak	-taxia	order
-lemma	a sheath, rind	-pheresis	removal	-therapy	treatment
-lepsy	seizure	-phil	attraction	-thermy	heat
-lexia	diction	-philia	attraction	-tic	pertaining to
-liter	liter	-phobia	fear	-tome	instrument to cut
-lith	stone	-phoresis	to carry	-tomy	incision
-logy	study of	-phragm	a fence	-tone	tension
-lymph	clear fluid	-phraxis	to obstruct	-tripsy	crushing
-lysis	destruction, to separate	-phylaxis	protection	-troph (y)	nourishment, development
-malacia	softening	-physis	growth	-trophy	nourishment, development
-mania	madness	-plakia	plate	-type	type
-megaly	enlargement, large	-plasia	formation, produce	-um	tissue
-meter	instrument to measure	-plasm	a thing formed, plasma	-ure	process
-metry	measurement	-plasty	surgical repair	-uria	urine
-mnesia	memory	-plegia	stroke, paralysis	-us	pertaining to
-morph	form, shape	-pnea	breathing	-y	condition, pertaining to, process

Glossary

Number in parentheses ( ) indicates chapter.

abandonment—improper forsaking, as when a physician who has agreed to care for a patient terminates the contract without valid cause (3)

abduction—process of moving a body part away from the midline (22)

abortions—fetuses that did not reach the age of viability (37)

abruptio placentae—a complication of pregnancy that occurs when the placenta tears away from the uterine wall, resulting in hemorrhage and fetal distress (37)

abuse—mistakenly accepting payment for items that should not be paid as a result of improper coding and billing practices (15, 16)

accommodation—eye's ability to adjust its optical powers to maintain a clear image of objects at various distances (25)

account balance—amount of money a patient owes (17)

account note—a free-form note that some computer systems allow in which more detailed information can be entered than can be entered in the description field; may be used, for example, when posting adjustments to an account (17)

accounting—system of reporting the financial results of a business (18)

accounts payable (AP)—amounts of money the physician owes to others for supplies, equipment, and services (18)

accounts receivable (AR)—money owed to a business by customers in exchange for goods or services that have already been provided (17, 18)

accreditation—process by which an institution voluntarily completes an extensive self-study after which an accrediting association visits the school to verify the self-study statements (1)

Accrediting Bureau of Health Education Schools (ABHES)—accreditation bureau that certifies medical assisting programs; graduates of ABHES accredited programs may take the CMA (AAMA) or RMA examination (1)

acid-fast stain—special stain used to expose the tuberculosis organism (44)

acne vulgaris—common skin condition that occurs when oil and dead skin cells clog the skin's pores; also called *acne* (21)

acquired active immunity—occurs when the person is exposed to a live pathogen, develops the disease, and becomes immune as a result of the primary immune response (27)

acquired immunodeficiency syndrome (AIDS)—series of illnesses that occur as a result of infection by the human immunodeficiency virus (HIV), which causes the immune system to break down (2)

acromegaly—hormonal disorder that results from the overproduction of growth hormone by the pituitary gland, most commonly affecting middle-aged adults (31)

active immunity—introduction of immunity by infection or with a vaccine (27)

active listening—paying attention completely to the speaker, concentrating on the verbal message, watching for nonverbal cues, and offering a response (5)

active records—medical files of patients who are currently being seen by the physician that may cover one to five years, depending on office policy (13)

active transport—process in cells that requires energy to transport materials to, from, and within the cell (20)

active voice—when the subject of the sentence performs the action (11)

acuity—sharpness (38)

acute conditions—illnesses or injuries that occur suddenly and require treatment but may or may not be life threatening (9)

acute confusion—confusion (e.g., inability to follow a conversation, answer questions appropriately, understand important facts) with symptoms lasting less than three months; *see also* chronic confusion (40)

acute pain—expected pain associated with trauma or surgery that lasts through the recovery of that condition (35); intense pain, usually lessening over time (54)

acute renal failure—condition that occurs when something, such as a blockage, toxins, or a sudden loss of blood flow, causes a change in the filtering function of the kidneys (30)

Addison's disease—condition in which the cortex of the adrenal gland is damaged, decreasing the production of adrenocortical hormones, usually resulting from an autoimmune disorder but also caused by infection, cancer, or hemorrhage into the glands (31)

additive—a substance added in small amounts, such as a chemical within a test tube (46)

add-on code—in procedure coding, a code added to a primary procedure code to indicate a related procedure; only the few codes listed in the instructional codes may be use as add-on codes (16)

adduction—process of moving a body part toward the midline (22)

adenoids—pharyngeal tonsils (27)

adhesion—scar-like tissue that forms between two membranous structures (32)

adjustment—positive or negative change to a patient's account balance that does not involve the exchange of money or the addition of a charge for services (17)

administrative law—laws governing the administration of agency regulations (3)

adolescence—transition period between puberty and adulthood (39, 57)

administrative safeguards—policies and procedures to ensure the security of electronic protected health information (12)

adrenal glands—endocrine organs that secrete hormones; located on top of each kidney, consisting of the cortex and the medulla (31)

adulthood—age designation from roughly 19 years of age to death (57)

Advance Beneficiary Notice (ABN)—notice to a patient that payment for a recommended service may be denied by Medicare and that the patient would then be obligated to pay; the ABN gives patients the opportunity to accept or decline the service, knowing they may have to pay for it (14)

advance booking—when the patient schedules his or her next appointment before leaving the office (9)

advance directive—document that allows patients to request that life-sustaining treatments and nutritional support not be used to prolong their life; includes the durable power of attorney (3, 40)

adverse effects—negative effects that outweigh the benefit of taking a medication and require the patient to discontinue its use (53)

aerobic—requires oxygen to live (33)

afebrile—absence of a fever (34)

affective—behaviors that are based on feelings and emotions (58)

afferent nerves—nerves that carry impulses from the sensory receptor to the central nervous system (24)

afferent vessels—vessels that carry lymph from the body to the lymph nodes (27)

Affordable Care Act (ACA)—*see* Patient Protection and Affordable Care Act (PPACA) (14, 15)

agar—a medium for growing bacterial cultures that contains whole blood (44)

ageism—prejudice against and incorrect assumptions about an individual or individuals because of age (40)

agglutination—clumping together (26, 44)

aggressive—trying to impose a point of view on others (5)

agonist—*see* prime mover (23)

airborne precautions—actions taken to reduce transmission of pathogens transported by airborne droplet nuclei so small they can remain suspended in air and widely dispersed by air currents; airborne precautions may involve patient isolation and use of mask and gown by health care personnel (33)

albinism—inherited disorder that is indicated by the absence of melanin in the skin, hair, and eyes (20)

algorithm—sequence of steps to accomplish a task (42)

allergen—any substance capable of causing an allergic reaction (27)

allergist—physician who specializes in treating allergies, asthma, and immune system disorders; *see also* immunologist (36)

allergy—hypersensitivity to a normally harmless substance (27)

allowed amount—the amount insurance companies consider to be an appropriate fee for a given service (14, 17)

alopecia—baldness or loss of hair (21)

alphabetic filing—filing system based on the letters of the alphabet (13)

alternative medicine—nonmainstream medical practices (51)

alveoli—small air sacs at the end of the bronchioles with a network of capillaries that perform the exchange of gases (28)

Alzheimer's disease—progressive, degenerative disease of the brain characterized by loss of memory and other cognitive functions (24)

amblyopia—a disorder in children caused by the eye muscles being weaker in one eye; also called *lazy eye* (25)

ambulation—act of walking (51)

ambulatory surgery—surgery performed on a person who is admitted and discharged from a surgical facility on the same day (41)

amenorrhea—absence of menstrual periods (37, 39)

American Association of Medical Assistants (AAMA)—professional association for medical assistants that offers CMA (AAMA) certification and educational opportunities (1)

American Bankers Association (ABA) number—code numbers that identify the bank; found on the right upper corner of a printed check (18)

American Medical Technologists (AMT)—professional association that provides oversight for the registration and testing of medical technologists, medical assistants, and phlebotomists (1)

Americans with Disabilities Act (ADA)—act ensuring that people with disabilities have equal access to structures and options (10)

amphiarthrotic joint—articulation or joint that permits very slight movement (22)

amplify—to make louder (35)

ampules—small, sealed glass bottles containing a single dose of medication (54)

amyotrophic lateral sclerosis (ALS)—a disease of unknown cause that breaks down the nerves in the nervous system that are responsible for movement; also called *motor neuron disease* and *Lou Gehrig's disease* (24)

anabolism—process of chemical reactions that work together to build things, such as creating molecules from atoms (20)

anaerobic—able to live without oxygen (33)

anaphylactic shock—severe allergic reaction that causes respiratory distress because of swelling of the upper airways; also called *anaphylaxis* (42, 53)

anaphylaxis—extreme, often life-threatening response to an antigen or allergen; also called *anaphylactic shock* (27)

anatomy—body structure; study of the structure of an organism (4, 20)

ancillary service endorsements—service provided by the U.S. Postal Service that permits giving the Postal Service instructions on how to handle mail that is undeliverable, such as forwarding instructions or receipt of a changed address (11)

anemia—condition in which levels of hemoglobin in the red blood cells are insufficient; caused by decreased healthy red cell production by the bone marrow, increased erythrocyte destruction, or blood loss from heavy menstrual periods or internal bleeding (26, 47)

anesthesia—medication that causes the partial or complete loss of sensation (2, 41)

aneurysm—abnormal widening or ballooning of a portion of an artery, related to weakness in the vessel wall (26)

angina—chest pain (36)

angiography—X-ray visualization of blood vessels after a radiopaque material has been injected into them (48)

angioplasty—surgical vessel repair procedure frequently used to reopen a blocked coronary artery (26)

anorexia nervosa—eating disorder associated with a distorted sense of body image and the persistent quest for thinness, at times to the point of emaciation (39)

answering service—agency that answers phone calls and forwards messages to directed recipients (7)

antagonist—muscle that counteracts, or opposes, the action of another muscle (23)

antecubital space—the inner-elbow area (46)

anthrax—deadly infectious disease caused by *Bacillus anthracis* (2)

anthropometry—science of size, proportion, weight, and height (34)

antibodies—specialized proteins that lock onto and have the ability to neutralize specific antigens (27, 33)

antibody-mediated response—immune response in which B lymphocytes produce antibodies that seek out and destroy foreign antigens; also called *humoral immunity* (27)

anticoagulant—a chemical that prevents blood from clotting and keeps it in its liquid form (46)

antigen—foreign substance that invades the body (27)

antiseptic—agent used for hand hygiene (33)

anuria—absence of urine (45)

aorta—largest artery of the body into which blood enters after it leaves the left ventricle (26)

apical—describing heart rate that is counted at the apex of the heart (34)

apnea—absence of breathing for more than 19 seconds (28, 34)

apothecary system—oldest system of measurement in which dry weight is measured in grains (52)

appeal—formal submission to an insurance carrier to question a denied claim that includes additional and detailed information beyond that which was submitted with the original claim (17)

appendicitis—inflammation of the appendix caused by a blockage of the inside of the appendix (the lumen), which leads to increased pressure, impaired blood flow, and potentially gangrene and rupture (29)

appendicular skeleton—one of the two divisions of the skeletal system, consisting of the 126 bones, including the shoulder and pelvic girdles, as well as the extremities, that are not part of the axial skeleton (22)

appendix—small appendage attached to the cecum, which has no known function in humans (29)

application—software installed in a computer to perform specific tasks such as word processing, creating spreadsheets, desktop publishing, and Internet browsing (12); form usually completed at the time of the job interview that includes personal information and previous work experience (12, 59)

aqueous humor—watery fluid that fills the anterior cavity of the eyeball (25)

AR aging analysis—report that categorizes a company's accounts receivable (AR) according to the length of time since they have been billed to determine what action, if any, should be taken on a given account; for example, accounts less than 30 days old are considered *current*; Medicare accounts over 30 days old should be investigated (17)

arbitration—a hearing or determination of the outcome of a dispute or the settling of a difference between parties by a person or persons selected to direct the parties to an agreement (3)

archived—stored for later retrieval (9)

aromatherapy—therapy that uses pleasant smells (58)

arrhythmia—irregular heartbeat caused by a disturbance of normal electrical activity of the heart; pulse with an irregular rhythm (26, 34, 36)

arterial blood gases (ABGs)—measurement of oxygen and carbon dioxide in arterial blood (28)

arteries—blood vessels that carry oxygenated blood away from the heart and to the cells (46)

arteriosclerosis—a thickening and loss of elasticity of the arteries; also called *hardening of the arteries* (26)

arthritis—inflammation of one or more joints caused by various disease processes (22, 36)

arthrography—X-ray visualization of a joint space (48)

articulation—the place where two bones connect, with the positioning of the bones determining the type of movement the joint performs; also called *joint* (22)

artifacts—errors in an electrocardiograph (49)

artificially acquired active immunity—immunity that is induced by a vaccine (27, 54)

ascites—fluid in the abdomen (30)

asepsis—state of being free from germs, infection, and any form of microbial life (33)

asphyxia—suffocation (28)

aspiration—removal by suction of fluid from within a cyst (23)

assertive—making a point in a positive manner (5)

asset—resource; property of value (18)

assessment—evaluation (55)

assignment of benefits—patient's written authorization giving the insurance company the right to pay the physician directly for billed charges (8, 14, 17)

assisted-living facility—a resident facility designed to provide assistance and supervision to residents; may include activities of daily living, coordination with health care providers, administration of medication, or personal care by trained staff persons (40)

asthma—chronic inflammatory condition that typically develops when allergens or other irritating substances cause swelling in the lining of the trachea and bronchial tubes, which creates mucus that can cause coughing or difficulty breathing (28)

astigmatism—refractive eye disorder in which irregularities in the curvature of the cornea cause light not to focus on the retina but to spread out over an area and cause overall blurring of vision (25, 38)

asymptomatic—without symptoms (27, 34)

atherosclerosis—narrowing and hardening of the vessel lumen of the arteries because of a buildup of fatty material and plaque (26, 36)

atlas—first cervical vertebra that connects the spine to the occipital bone at the base of the skull (22)

atom—smallest particle of an element that can exist on its own; consists of at least one proton, at least one neutron, and at least one electron (20)

atria—the two upper chambers of the heart (26)

atrioventricular (AV) node—one of the three areas of specialized neuromuscular tissue that initiate the heartbeat; located under the endocardium of the right atrium (26)

atrophy—loss of muscle mass and strength that occurs with the disuse of muscles over time (23, 51)

attention-deficit/hyperactivity disorder (ADHD)—disorder characterized by difficulty focusing attention and organizing and completing a task, possibly caused by genetic factors (20)

attitudes—opinions that develop from a person's value system (5)

at-will employment—employment with no explicit contractual relationship between employer and employee in which the employer is free to terminate the employment relationship without just cause (19)

audiogram—record of patient responses indicating his or her ability to hear a sound (38)

audiology—study of hearing disorders (25)

audiometer—electronic instrument used to measure hearing ability (38)

audit—reexamination for accuracy (16)

auditing—evaluation of financial practices by an outside company or agency; for example, business expenses claimed as tax deductions are subject to auditing by the Internal Revenue Service (18)

auditory—by ear (5)

auditory meatus—auditory canal; tube that carries sound waves from the outer ear to the tympanic membrane (25)

auscultation—listening to sounds within the body, such as heart sounds (26, 35)

authorization—permission from a patient to release medical records to a specified recipient (5)

autoclave—a machine that uses high pressure, saturated steam to sterilize equipment or instruments that are used on patients or in certain test procedures (43)

autoimmune diseases—inflammatory reactions caused when the immune system produces antibodies that stick to the body's own cells, resulting in damage to the body's own cells and in the body attacking itself (27)

automated analyzer—a medical laboratory instrument that measures the chemical composition of a provided sample (43)

automated assistance program—telephone system that directs callers to a recipient based on the callers' answers to questions (7)

autonomic nervous system (ANS)—part of the peripheral nervous system that is responsible for controlling involuntary bodily functions such as sweating, secretion of glands, arterial blood pressure, and activity of smooth and cardiac muscle (24)

autopsy—examination of the organs and tissues of a deceased body to determine cause of death (2)

axial skeleton—one of the two divisions of the skeletal system, consisting of 80 bones, including the skull, vertebral system, and rib cage (22)

axis—second cervical vertebra that has a pivoting characteristic, allowing the head to turn from side-to-side (22)

axon—nerve cell projection that sends information from that cell to other cells (24)

B lymphocytes—cells responsible for production of circulating antibodies that attack and destroy foreign antigens; *see also* antibody-mediated response (27)

backup—a copy of computer data or software made to protect against loss of the original (12)

bacteremic—pertaining to bacteria in the bloodstream (21)

bactericidal—capable of killing bacteria (33)

bacteriuria—bacteria in the urine (45)

bad debt—amount owed and not collectable (17)

balance billing—billing a patient for the difference between the billed amount and the amount allowed by the insurance carrier (17)

bandage—strip of binding material used to hold a dressing in place (42)

bandwidth—amount of data that can be transmitted in a fixed amount of time (12)

bariatrics—science of obesity (2)

basal cell carcinoma—most common form of skin cancer; most often caused by overexposure to the sun (21)

basilic veins—large veins of the hands and forearms (46)

basophils—granular leukocytes (47)

behavior—the way in which a person acts; the actions others see (5)

Bell's palsy—weakness or paralysis of the muscles that control expression on one side of the face (24)

beneficiary—a person who is eligible for coverage by government health policies (14)

benign—noncancerous (21, 36)

benign prostatic hyperplasia (BPH)—an enlargement of the prostate gland, usually occurring in men older than 50 years, which compresses the urethra, restricting the normal flow of urine; also called *benign prostatic hypertrophy* (32)

beveled—cut at an angle; the beveled end of a needle is the opening that comes to a point (46)

bias—unfair preference or dislike that prevents forming an impartial opinion of someone or something; favoring a certain belief or attitude (5)

bicuspid valve—the valve through which the blood leaves the left atrium of the heart; also called *mitral valve* (26)

bimanual—two-handed, deep palpation (35)

bioequivalent—drug that has the same strength and action of another drug (53)

bioethics—ethical decisions pertaining to life issues such as stem cell research, in vitro fertilization, and abortion rights (3)

biofeedback—using biological information to decrease stress (58)

biohazards—biological substances, such as medical waste and samples of a virus or a bacterium, that cause a threat to human beings and are potentially infectious (6)

biomedical equipment—equipment used in patient care, such as an X-ray machine, endoscope, or specimen refrigerator (10)

biopsy—microscopic examination of tissue to detect cancerous cells (41)

bipolar disorder—mood disorder characterized by swings of mood between depression and mania (57)

birthday rule—used by insurance claims administrators to determine which parent's benefit plans will pay for the medical bills of a dependent child when the child is covered by the plans of both parents (14)

blank check—unused check; a check that contains only the preprinted account information but no payment information (18)

blepharitis—inflammation of the eyelid (25)

blind ad—advertisement that does not identify the institution or facility that placed the ad (59)

block style—style of letter writing in which all lines are flush with the left margin (11)

bloodborne pathogens—microorganisms capable of causing disease in blood (33)

blood pressure—force exerted by the blood on the walls of the arteries (26)

blood transfer device—a device that allows blood to be transferred from one device to another, such as from a syringe to a vacutainer (46)

body mechanics—proper coordination of alignment, balance, and movement (6)

body surface area (BSA)—calculation of the child's height and weight, expressed as m2 (meters squared) (52)

bolus—ball of food produced by chewing and saliva that can be swallowed (29)

bookkeeping—process of managing the accounts for a business (18)

bounding pulse—full pulse, indicating an increase in blood volume (34)

bradycardia—abnormally slow heart rate of below 60 beats per minute (26, 34)

bradypnea—abnormally slow respiration rate below 12 cycles per minute (34)

brand name—name given to a drug by its manufacturer; with the first letter of the name generally being capitalized; also called the *proprietary name* (53)

BRAT diet—diet for patients with diarrhea; consists of bananas, rice, applesauce, and toast (39)

breach of contract—failure by either party in a valid contract to comply with terms of the agreement (3)

breast cancer—cancer arising in breast tissue; types include ductal (the most common, which develops in the tiny ducts that run from the milk glands to the nipple), infiltrating lobular (which develops in the lobules), and inflammatory (32)

broad spectrum—refers to antibiotics that are effective against a large range of microorganisms (53)

bronchi—the two main branches of the trachea extending into the lungs that are a passageway for air into the lungs (28)

bronchiolitis—inflammation of the bronchioles or small air vessels commonly seen in children (39)

bronchitis—respiratory system disorder in which the mucous membranes in the bronchial passages become inflamed, resulting in mucus production, coughing, and breathlessness (28)

bronchodilators—medications that open the bronchial passages (28)

bruit—sound made by a heart murmur (26)

buccal medications—medications placed between the cheek and gums for absorption through the tissues into the bloodstream (54)

buffers—mechanisms within the blood that balance the pH level, thus preventing blood from becoming too acidic or too alkaline (26)

bulbourethral glands—two pea-size glands located inferior to the prostate and on either side of the urethra that secrete a mucous secretion into the seminal fluid before ejaculation; also called *Cowper's glands* (32)

bulimia nervosa—eating disorder characterized by binge eating and self-induced vomiting and purging (39)

bulk remittance—a payment from an insurance company covering several patients (17)

bullying—repeated mistreatment that may involve verbal abuse, humiliation, intimidation, threatening behavior, or sabotage of work duties; workplace bullying can be carried out by supervisors, peers, or subordinates (19)

bundle of His—one of the three areas of specialized neuromuscular tissue that initiate the heartbeat; also called *atrioventricular (AV) bundle* (26)

bundling—in procedure coding, a single code that indicates multiple services that are listed as *included* or *not separately reportable* (16)

bursa—sac of fluid that cushions and lubricates an area where joint-related tissues rub against one another (22)

bursitis—inflammation of the bursa (22)

butterfly needle—a small, winged needle used for fragile veins or intravenous infusion (46)

cadavers—dead human bodies used to study human anatomy (2)

caduceus—recognized symbol for medicine; depicts a healing staff with two snakes coiled around it (2)

calibration devices—specially prepared test strips or cartridges that are used to test the function of a machine and designed to perform a predetermined result (43)

caller ID—program to identify who is calling the recipient (7)

callus—thickened skin that does not have an identifiable border (21)

calorie—measurement of 1 unit of heat that provides energy (56)

cancelled checks—deposited checks that have been processed by the bank (18)

cancellous (spongy) bone—reticular tissue that makes up most of the volume of a long bone; includes red bone marrow, which manufactures most red blood cells (22)

candidiasis—yeast infection; also called *moniliasis* or *thrush* (44)

cannula—a small tube inserted into the body (46)

canthus—either of the two corners of the eye where the upper and lower eyelids meet (25)

capillaries—delicate blood vessels that serve as bridges between the arteries and veins and allow for the exchange of gas, through their thin walls, between the blood and cells (46)

capillary puncture—to penetrate the skin for the purpose of collecting capillary blood; typically performed on the middle and ring fingers (46)

capital equipment—items that require a large dollar amount to purchase (generally, over $500) and have a relatively long life (10)

capitation—an insurance reimbursement method in which the physician is reimbursed by the insurance company a flat "per head" fee per month for each patient who belongs to the medical group or practice, regardless of what or how many services the patient uses (14)

carboxyhemoglobin—when hemoglobin is carrying carbon dioxide (47)

carbuncle—a collection of furuncles (21)

carcinoma in situ—cancer in a particular area that has not broken through the basement membrane (37)

cardiac arrest—stoppage of the beating of the heart; also called *sudden death* (26)

cardiac muscle—type of involuntary muscle found in the heart, roughly quadrangular in shape, cross striated, and having a single central nucleus (23)

cardiac sphincter—a ring of muscle at the upper part of the stomach that opens and closes, allowing food and liquid to enter the stomach from the esophagus (29)

cardiac tamponade—congestion of the heart muscle and restriction of heart movement caused by blood or fluid trapped in the pericardial sac (26)

cardiogenic shock—collapse of the cardiovascular system characterized by vasodilation and fluid shifting away from the heart (26)

cardiologist—physician who specializes in treating cardiovascular-related diseases and disorders (36)

cardiomegaly—enlargement of the heart (31)

carditis—inflammation of the heart (26)

carotid artery—artery found on each side of the neck (26)

cash disbursement—payment made to a creditor (18)

cash discount—for patients without health insurance, a discount offered to those who pay in full at the time of service (17)

casts—microscopic forms created from protein in renal tubules (45)

catabolism—process of chemical reactions that works to break down larger units into smaller units, as in digestion of food (20)

cataract—clouding over the lens of the eye; prevents light from entering (25)

catch-up time—time built into the morning or afternoon schedule for emergencies (9)

category—within an ICD-10-CM manual, a level of code numbers having a three-character entry (15, 16)

catheterization—the process of inserting a tube-like catheter through the urethra; typically performed to obtain uncontaminated urine directly from the bladder (45)

cecum—small pouch that forms the beginning of the large intestine (29)

cell—most basic unit of life; often considered the building block of the human body (20)

cell-mediated response—immune response in which T lymphocytes directly bind with and destroy foreign antigens (27)

cell membrane—the outer covering of the cell (20)

cellulitis—acute, spreading bacterial infection below the surface of the skin, characterized by erythema, warmth, swelling, and pain that can also cause fever, chills, and enlarged lymph nodes (21)

cementum—thin layer of bone that covers the dentin of the root of a tooth; provides protection and anchors the periodontal ligament (29)

Centers for Medicare and Medicaid Services (CMS)—the federal agency that administers the Medicare program and works with state governments to administer Medicaid programs (14, 16)

central nervous system (CNS)—composed of the brain and spinal cord (24)

central processing unit (CPU)—the "brain" of the computer, which executes specific sets of instructions (12)

centrifuge—an instrument used to separate specimens into component layers by spinning samples at high speed; lighter components float to the top and heavier components sink to the bottom of the container (43)

cephalic veins—veins on the outer sides of the arms (46)

cerebrospinal fluid (CSF)—fluid produced by the choroid plexus in the ventricles of the brain that moves through the spinal canal and the subarachnoid space and surrounds the brain; cushions the brain and spinal cord and nourishes them with oxygen and glucose (24)

certificate of coverage—a document that must be sent to a patient by the prior health insurance plan when the patient is switching to a new plan certifying the patient's prior coverage; a patient who can thus document 24 months of coverage before joining the new plan cannot be denied coverage for a preexisting condition (14)

Certificate of Waiver Tests (WTs)—the least complex laboratory tests, which offer the least risk if performed incorrectly (43)

certification—issuance by an official body or professional organization of a certificate and credentials to an individual who has met the education and experience standards of that organization (1, 2)

certification examination—test required for a student to become certified as a medical assistant (59)

Certified Clinical Medical Assistant (CCMA)—one of two medical assisting credentials offered by the National Healthcareer Association; a CCMA will work in the clinical or back office areas of health care settings; *see also* Certified Medical Administrative Assistant (CMAA) (1)

certified EHR technology—electronic health record (EHR) technology that is approved under federal mandates and that must be used by a medical practice in order to qualify for federal financial incentives available to provide funding for implementing EHR technology (13)

Certified Medical Administrative Assistant (CMAA)—one of two medical assisting credentials offered by the National

Healthcareer Association; a CMAA will work in the administrative or front office areas of health care settings; *see also* Certified Clinical Medical Assistant (CMAA) (1)

Certified Medical Assistant (CMA) (AAMA)—multiskilled health care professional who has met the standards of the AAMA by achieving a satisfactory test result and assists providers in an allied health care setting (1)

cerumen—earwax (25, 38)

cervical cancer—rapid uncontrolled growth of severely abnormal cells on the cervix; the two main types are squamous cell (epidermoid) and adenocarcinoma (32)

cervicitis—inflammation of the cervix, usually caused by sexually transmitted infections (STIs) (32)

CHAMPVA—a federal insurance program for veterans with service-related disabilities (14)

chain of custody form—chronological documentation or paper trail showing the collection, transfer, receipt, analysis, storage, and disposal of a specimen or test sample (45)

chancre—syphilitic sore (37)

chapter—in an ICD-10-CM manual, one of the 21 sublistings in the Tabular List, based on etiology or body system (15)

character—the sum of the values, attitudes, and behaviors a person possesses or exhibits (5)

charge—the monetary cost for services or supplies that increases the account balance; in accounting, referred to as a *debit* (17)

chemotherapy—use of chemicals, including drugs, to treat or control infections and diseases such as cancer (2, 27)

chief complaint—reason for the office visit; also called *presenting problem* (35)

childhood—last period of child development; from ages 3 to 11 years (57)

cholelithiasis—formation of gallstones (29)

cholesterol—fatlike material normally found in the body that is essential for the function of body systems such as the nervous system, the formation of cell membranes, and the manufacture of many hormones (56)

chondrocytes—cells that form cartilage (22)

chorionic villus sampling (CVS)—removing a small sample of tissue from the placenta to examine it for chromosomal abnormalities (37)

choroid—membrane that lines the sclera and absorbs extra light entering the eye (25)

chromosomes—microscopic bodies that carry the genes that determine hereditary characteristics (20)

chronic confusion—confusion (e.g., inability to follow a conversation, answer questions appropriately, understand important facts) with symptoms persisting longer than three months; *see also* acute confusion (40)

chronic fatigue syndrome (CFS)—immune system disorder of unknown origin that causes depression, sleep disorders, and lack of energy (27)

chronic obstructive pulmonary disease (COPD)—progressive, chronic, usually irreversible respiratory system condition in which the lungs have diminished capacity for inhalation and exhalation (28, 49)

chronic pain—pain that persists longer than six months and interferes with functions of life (35, 54)

chronic renal failure—gradual and progressive loss of kidney function (30)

chronological medical record—patient record that follows the patient over a period of time, with each visit consisting of a new entry by date, rather than by symptoms or diagnosis (13)

chyme—semiliquid form of food that is passed from the stomach to the small intestine (29)

cilia—small, hair-like projections that cover the surface of some cells; in the nose, they trap dust, pollen, and other foreign matter to prevent them from entering the nasal cavity (20, 28)

ciliary body—part of the middle layer of the surface of the eyeball that holds and moves the lens (25)

circumcision—surgical removal of the foreskin of the penis, performed for religious, cultural, or medical reasons (32)

circumduction—process of moving a body part in a circular motion (22)

cirrhosis—potentially life-threatening condition that occurs when the liver is damaged, usually after years of inflammation, scarring, or fibrosis that replaces healthy tissue and prevents the liver from working normally (29)

civil law—laws governing how people relate to each other and the government (3)

claim—written and documented request for reimbursement of an eligible expense under an insurance plan (14)

clarity—quality or state of being understandable (7)

Clark's rule—most common law used in the calculation of drug dosage for children; based on weight of the child (52)

claustrophobia—fear of enclosed spaces (48)

clean-catch—the process of collecting a urine specimen in a way to prevent contamination; generally collected

midstream, after proper cleansing of the surrounding area (45)

clean claim—health insurance claim form that has been completed correctly without any errors or omissions (14)

clearinghouse—independent entity that reviews claims, requests clarification from the provider, and "cleans" claims, ensuring accurate information is documented, then submits claims to insurance companies in proper format (14)

cleft palate—congenital defect in the roof of the mouth when the palatine bones of the skull do not close properly (20)

clinical diagnosis—preliminary presumptive diagnosis made by physician based on health history and physical examination; also called *working diagnosis* (35)

clinical equipment—equipment used in patient care, such as an X-ray machine or endoscope; also called *biomedical equipment* (10)

Clinical Laboratory Improvement Amendments (CLIA)—government mandates that all laboratories testing human specimens must be regulated to help ensure accurate patient test results (43)

clinical status—patient's physical condition considered, for example, at the time of a medical test (50)

clock speed—speed at which a computer's central processing unit (CPU) can process instructions (12)

closed-ended questions—questions that can be answered yes or no (5)

closed records—medical files of patients who have indicated that they are no longer a patient or who have died, that are kept in storage for legal reasons (13)

cloud computing—applications and services available on the Internet, such as online backup, in place of programs purchased and stored in the individual computer (12)

CMS-1500—most common health insurance claim form used to file claims for physicians' services (14)

cochlea—bony spiral-shaped structure that forms a portion of the inner ear (25)

code—within an ICD-10-CM manual, the most specific level of code, requiring no additional characters (15)

cognitive—based on knowledge (58)

cognitive ability—ability to think clearly, reason, and perceive (40)

coinsurance—a fixed percentage of charges the patient must pay under a given insurance plan (14)

colitis—inflammation of the large intestine caused by many different disease processes, including infections, primary inflammatory disorders, ulcerative colitis, Crohn's colitis, lymphocytic and collagenous colitis, lack of blood flow, and history of radiation to the large bowel (29)

collating—collecting and putting in proper order all records, tests results, and information pertaining to a patient who is scheduled to be seen by the physician (8, 13)

colleagues—fellow members of the profession (19)

collection agency—an outside company that specializes in collection payment for unpaid bills (17)

colon—makes up the bulk of the large intestine and can be divided into the ascending colon, transverse colon, descending colon, and sigmoid colon (29)

colonoscopy—examination of the interior of the colon (36)

colony—a group of organisms grown from the same parent cell (44)

color deficiency—inherited, sex-linked disorder characterized by difficulty distinguishing colors, especially between reds and greens; formerly called *color blindness* (20)

colorectal cancer—collective term for colon and rectal cancer (29)

combination code—in an ICD-10-CM manual, a code that identifies various manifestations of a condition such as diabetes or two conditions that commonly occur together (15)

combining form—word root that has a vowel attached to it in order to add another element (4)

combining vowel—vowel, usually "o," added to a word root before combining (4)

Commission on Accreditation of Allied Health Education Programs (CAAHEP)—body that accredits educational programs that prepare medical assisting students to take the CMA (AAMA) exam (1)

common cold—infection of the upper respiratory tract caused by any one of a number of viruses and differing from other viral infections in its lack of producing high fever or significant fatigue (28)

common descriptor—in Common Procedure Terminology (CPR®), the portion of the code before the semicolon that is shared by the subsequent indented codes (16)

community resources—programs and services available to provide help, information, and assistance to improve an individual's quality of life (55)

compact bone—dense, hard layer of bone tissue in a long bone (22)

compassion—acting positively toward a person based on empathy with that person (5)

complement—group of proteins activated by antibodies that assist in destroying bacteria, viruses, and infected cells (27)

complementary medicine—nonmainstream medical practice used in addition to conventional medicine (51)

complete blood count (CBC)—combination of several blood tests including red blood cell (RBC) counts, RBC indices, hemoglobin (Hgb), hematocrit (Hct), white blood cell (WBC) counts (with or without differential), platelet counts, and blood cell morphology (47)

complete proteins—proteins containing the nine essential amino acids, primarily proteins from animal sources such as meat, eggs, fish, milk, and cheese (56)

compliance—following the rules established by government agencies (15, 55)

complimentary close—courtesy word(s), such as "Sincerely," "Sincerely yours," or "Yours truly," that appear two spaces below the end of the body of a letter (11)

compound microscope—an instrument with two sets of lenses, oculars, and objectives that magnifies structures unseen by the naked eye, for visualization (43)

compulsions—acts performed to relieve anxiety (57)

computer—programmable machine that responds to a specific set of instructions and performs a list of instructions in a programmed language (12)

computerized physician order entry (CPOE)—ability of providers to order tests, prescriptions, lab work, and referrals using the computer rather than writing them on paper (13, 53)

concussion—injury caused by sharp jarring or a blow to the head that may result in a loss of consciousness (24)

condescending—acting or speaking with an attitude of superiority; patronizing (5)

conduction hearing loss—result of the obstruction of sound waves (38)

cones—photosensitive cells in the retina that respond to bright light and are used in color vision (25)

conference call—call in which several parties at different locations are on the telephone line simultaneously (7)

congenital disorder—genetic disorder that is present at birth (20)

congestive heart failure (CHF)—condition in which the heart cannot pump sufficient blood to the other organs; also called *heart failure* (26)

conjunctiva—protective mucous membrane lining the underside of the eyelid and the anterior part of the eyeball (25)

conjunctivitis—an inflammation of the conjunctiva frequently caused by a virus, bacteria, sexually transmitted infections (STIs), allergens, and irritants; also called *pinkeye* (25)

consent—agreement or permission given, for example, to allow medical treatment or to release protected health information to a third party (5)

Consolidated Omnibus Reconciliation Act (COBRA)—federal legislation that requires employers to extend health insurance coverage at group rates, usually for up to 18 months, to any employee who is laid off, quits, or is fired, except under certain circumstances (14)

constant information—body of a form letter that is retained in the computer's memory or on an external storage device (11)

constrict—to shrink or become smaller (46)

contact dermatitis—allergic reaction of the skin caused by irritating substances coming in contact with it, often resulting in red, irritated skin and occasionally in vesicles and rash (21)

contact precautions—actions taken when infections are difficult to treat and likelihood of microorganism transmission among patients and health care workers is high; contact precautions may include isolating patients and gown and gloves plus mask and protective eyewear for health care workers if contact with body fluids is possible (33)

continuing education unit (CEU)—credit awarded for additional course work beyond certification; one unit of training or education is granted for each clock hour of workshops, seminars, or conferences (1)

contraception—method of reducing the risk of pregnancy; also called *birth control* (32)

contract law—laws relating to enforceable promises and agreements between two or more persons to do or not to do a particular action (3)

contractual allowance—an adjustment that affects a patient's balance that is not a new charge or payment, for example a reduction of fee by the physician (17)

contracture—permanent shortening of the muscle around a joint that causes abnormal and sometimes painful positioning of the joint (51)

contraindicated—when medications have such dangerous effects that their use must be immediately discontinued (53)

contrast medium—substance that makes an object of study contrast with, or stand out against, its background (48)

contributing factors—in Current Procedural Terminology (CPT®), factors that may contribute to the Evaluation and Management key components: counseling, coordination of care, and presenting problem (16)

contributory negligence—patient's contribution to the injury, which if proven would release the physician as the direct cause (3)

control solutions—chemicals that produce an expected result; used to test the accuracy of a machine (43)

controlled substances—drugs classified under the federal Controlled Substances Act as having a potential for addiction or abuse (53)

Controlled Substances Act (CSA)—statute establishing the federal U.S. drug policy regulating the manufacture, importation, possession, use, and distribution of certain substances (controlled substances) (53)

contusion—bruising of the brain (24)

conventions—in an ICD-10-CM manual, specialized rules, abbreviations, formatting, and symbols that alert users to important information (15)

coordination of benefits (COB)—procedures to prevent duplication of payment by more than one insurance carrier (14)

coordination of care—in procedure coding a contributing factor that involves working with other providers or agencies to provide the patient needed care, such as referral to home health care (16)

copayment—predetermined amount of money the patient must pay for medical services, as determined by the insurance company (8, 14, 17)

coping mechanisms—conscious or unconscious behavior used to respond to a challenging situation (5)

copulation—sexual intercourse; also called *coitus* (32)

corn—thickened area of the skin that has a distinct border with various textures (21)

cornea—clear, transparent covering of the eye; frequently referred to as the "window" of the eye because it allows light to enter (25, 38)

corneal abrasion—lesion or abrasion on the cornea that results from injury or infection (25)

coronary arteries—crown of arteries that supply the heart with freshly oxygenated blood (26)

coronary artery disease (CAD)—blockage of the arteries that supply the heart muscle; also called *coronary heart disease (CHD)* (26, 49)

cor pulmonale—heart disease that causes the right ventricle to enlarge as a result of primary lung disease; also called *right-sided heart disease* (26)

corpus callosum—largest nerve tract that connects the right and left hemispheres of the brain (24)

cortex—*in the lymph nodes*, portion of node that is mainly populated by lymphocytes; *in the thymus gland*, the area where immature lymph cells reproduce and mature; *in the kidney*, outer layer, in which the arteries, veins, convoluted tubules, and glomerular capsules are found (27, 30)

counseling—in procedure coding, a contributing factor that involves the provider's discussion with the patient and family regarding the patient's diagnosis, test results, impressions, prognosis, treatment options, and management of the condition (16)

cough etiquette—*see* respiratory hygiene/cough etiquette (33)

courtesy—politeness in attitude and behavior toward others (58)

cover letter—letter introducing the applicant to an employer, stating the purpose of the correspondence, the position being sought, and the applicant's match to the stated requirements (59)

covered—potentially eligible for reimbursement by Medicare (14)

covered entities—those that are covered by the Health Insurance Portability and Accountability Act (HIPAA) Privacy Rule: health care providers, health plans, and electronic claims clearinghouses that engage in designated electronic transactions (13)

crash cart—cart or kit that is instantly accessible to anyone in the medical office and contains all supplies that may be needed during an emergency (42)

credit—receipt of money that decreases the account balance; also called a *payment*; funds added to an account (17, 18)

critical values—abnormal test values that indicate a potential threat to the patient and should be reported immediately to the physician or responsible health care professional; also called *panic values* (47)

Crohn's disease—a chronic disease of the intestines that primarily causes ulcerations in the lining of the small and large intestines but can affect the digestive system anywhere from the mouth to the anus; also called *inflammatory bowel disease (IBD)* (29)

croup—inflammation of the larynx and trachea characterized by a barking cough (39)

cryosurgery—use of subfreezing temperatures to destroy tissue (41)

cryotherapy—use of cold for therapeutic purposes (51)

crystals—concentrated compounds in urine that resemble tiny shards of glass (45)

culture—values, beliefs, attitudes, views, and customs shared by a group of people and passed on through the generations (5); a method of multiplying microbial organisms; *see* culture media (44)

culture and sensitivity (C&S)—a test performed to determine which particular bacteria are present and which antibiotics are effective against them (44, 45)

culture media—liquid or gel broth containing nourishment for bacteria; designed to support the growth of microorganisms for easier identification (44)

Culturette™ system—a sterile, cotton-tipped applicator swab that is stored inside a clear plastic tube for transport; may also contain a sealed plastic vial of culture medium; used to obtain specimens (44)

current—not in arrears; accounts receivable that are less than 30 days old (17)

Current Procedural Terminology (CPT®)—code book for procedures and services performed by providers (16, 18)

Current Procedures Terminology (CPT®) code—code specified in the CPT code book that identifies a specific medical, surgical, or diagnostic service (14)

Cushing's disease—rare disorder that develops when too much cortisol is released by the adrenal cortex as a result of stimulation of the pituitary (31)

cyanosis—bluish discoloration of the skin and nail beds because of lack of oxygen in the tissues (26, 28, 34, 36)

cycle billing—system in which approximately 25 percent of patient accounts are billed each week (17)

cycle time—length of time the average patient spends in the medical office (9)

cystic fibrosis—chronic, progressive disease in which mucus becomes thick, dry, and sticky and builds up and clogs passages in body organs, primarily the lungs and pancreas (20)

cystitis—inflammation of the bladder that usually occurs when bacteria infect the lower urinary tract (30, 45)

cytokinesis—division of the nuclei of the cell and distribution of organelles into two daughter cells (20)

cytoplasm—jellylike substance found between the cell membrane and the nuclear membrane (20)

database—a collection of information filed in the computer (12)

day sheet—used to list or post each day's financial transactions: charges, payments, adjustments, and credits (17)

days in AR—the average number of days that money has been owed to the practice, calculated by dividing the total accounts receivable (AR) dollar amount by the average daily revenue of the practice (17)

debit—the monetary cost for services or supplies that increases the account balance; also called a *charge*; charge against an account (17, 18)

debridement—removal of dead tissue around wound edges using sterile technique (36, 41)

decibel—intensity of a sound (38)

decubitus ulcer—an area of skin and tissue that breaks down when constant pressure is maintained on it; also called *pressure sore* or *bedsore* (21)

deductible—amount of eligible charges each patient must pay each calendar year before the insurance plan begins to pay benefits (14)

deductions—money withheld from an employee's paycheck for taxes, health and life insurance premiums, and other benefits (18)

defamation of character—damaged caused to a person's reputation through spoken or written words (3)

defendant—person who has been accused of wrongdoing in a court of law (3)

dehiscence—separation of wound edges (41)

delegate—assign work-related tasks to a person who is both responsible and competent to complete them, as a physician to a medical assistant (1)

deltoid muscle—small muscle mass located on the outer surface of the upper arm that is ideal for small dosages of medications (54)

delusions—fixed, false beliefs (57)

demographic—information such as age, gender, ethnic background, education, and Social Security number (8)

demyelination—destruction of the myelin, the protective covering around a nerve cell (24)

dendrite—nerve cell projection that receives information from other cells (24)

denied claim—occurs when procedures or services are deemed to be not covered by the patient's insurance policy or when the patient has not met his or her deductible (14); claim that was received by an insurance carrier but for which no payment was made (17)

denominator—bottom number of a fraction (52)

dentin—calcified, largely mineral tissue that forms the bulk of teeth (29)

deoxyribonucleic acid (DNA)—provides the cell's blueprint or genetic makeup (20)

dependent—family member of a health plan member (14)

deposition—sworn testimony of a witness in a written statement (3)

depolarized—the condition of having no difference in electric charge inside and outside a cell; *see also* polarity, repolarized (49)

deposits—money (cash, checks) placed in a bank account (18)

depreciation—loss in value resulting from normal aging, use, or deterioration; also called *financial life* (10)

dermatologist—physician who specializes in treating disorders of the skin or integumentary system (36)

dermis—the middle of the three layers that compose the skin (21)

desensitizing injections—minute amounts of an allergen injected over an extended period of time to build tolerance for the allergen in the patient's body (36)

dexterity—ability to use your hands effectively (55)

diabetes mellitus—condition in which the body is unable to produce enough insulin to properly control blood sugar levels by converting sugar and starches into energy (31)

diabetic retinopathy—disease of the retina secondary to diabetes mellitus (25)

diagnose—determine the cause and nature of a disease or injury (35)

diagnosis coding—process of assigning alphanumeric characters to the reasons for the procedures and services a physician provides to a patient (15)

dialysis—separation of substances in solution; for renal patients, using a filter other than the kidneys to remove toxins from blood and maintain water balance (30)

diaphoresis—excessive sweating (36)

diaphragm—dome-shaped muscle that separates the chest from the abdomen and helps pump air into, and carbon dioxide out of, the lungs (28)

diaphysis—shaft of a long bone (22)

diarthrotic joint—articulation, or joint, that allows for free movement in multiple directions (22)

diastolic blood pressure—lowest cuff pressure at which the Korotkoff sounds disappear, when the left ventricle of the heart relaxes (26, 34)

diathermy—therapeutic use of a high-frequency current to generate heat within some part of the body (51)

dietary supplements—vitamins, minerals, herbs, enzymes, amino acids, and other nutrients available in various forms such as tablets, gel caps, liquids and powers to be ingested in addition to consumed foods (56)

dietitian—*see* medical nutrition therapy, registered dietitian

differential diagnosis—determination of which one of multiple possibilities is the cause of a problem (35)

diffusion—dissolved particles moving from an area of greater concentration to an area of lesser concentration (20)

digestion—process by which the body converts food into chemical substances that can be absorbed into the blood and used by the body tissues and organs (56)

digestive enzymes—juices produced by cells and glands in the mouth, stomach, small intestine, and pancreas that help digest food (29)

digital signature—an encrypted (scrambled) signature that may be used in electronic health records (EHRs); the most secure type of electronic signature (13)

digitized signature—an electronic image of a handwritten signature that may be used in electronic health records (EHRs) (13)

dignity—calm, serious, and controlled behavior (58)

dilate—to swell or become larger (46)

dilation—widening of the cervix before childbirth (37)

diphtheria—acute infectious disease that has symptoms such as headache, fever, and sore throat (54)

diplomacy—skill in handling negotiations without creating hostility (58)

diplopia—double vision (25)

direct contact—route of infection in which body fluids from an infected person touch another person's eyes, nose, mouth, or open wound (33)

disallowance—amount of a charge that is above the maximum allowable fee (17)

disbursement account—bank account used for paying out funds (18)

discriminatory—prejudicial (19)

disinfection—soaking and wiping process used to destroy or inhibit the activity of disease-causing organisms (33)

dislocation—disconnection of the bones that meet at a joint, usually caused by a sudden impact, such that the bones are no longer in their normal positions (22)

diuretic—an agent that causes increased urine production (45)

diversity—variety (58)

diverticulitis—inflammation or infection of a diverticulum (a small pouch or sac in the wall of the colon) generally caused by stool lodging in diverticula, which can lead to swelling or rupture (29)

diverticulosis—condition of having diverticula (small outpouchings in the large intestine), most typically in the sigmoid colon; increases with age because of the weakening of the colon walls (29)

document—to chart a procedure or patient teaching in a patient's medical record (55)

dorsiflexion—the process of bending a body part backward (22)

dorsogluteal site—upper-outer quadrant of the buttocks; ideal location for administration of large-volume intramuscular medications (54)

dosimeter—equipment that measures the level and intensity of radiation exposure (48)

double booking—giving two patients the same time slot without allowing any additional time on the schedule (9)

double-entry bookkeeping—a bookkeeping method in which every transaction affects two accounts by increasing one and decreasing the other (18)

Down syndrome—disorder caused by an extra chromosome at the 21st chromosomal pair characterized by growth delays, sloping forehead and other physical characteristics, and mild to moderate intellectual disability; also called *trisomy 20* (20)

downcoding—in procedure coding, coding for a lower level of service that was actually provided (16)

dressing—sterile covering placed directly over a wound to absorb blood and other body fluids, prevent contamination, and protect the wound from further trauma (42)

droplet precautions—actions taken to reduce transmission of pathogens spread by droplets during sneezing, coughing, and talking; droplet precautions may require health care workers to wear a mask if within 3 feet of an infected patient and gown and gloves if there is a chance of contacting blood or body fluids of an infected patient (33)

drugs—medicines or other substances that cause a physiologic change when introduced into the body (53)

drug abuse—using a drug improperly or wrongly (53)

drug dependency—relying on medication or taking medication for psychologic support (53)

Drug Enforcement Administration (DEA)—U.S. government agency responsible for enforcing drug control (53)

drug intolerance—a lower threshold to the normal pharmacologic action of a drug; also called drug sensitivity (53)

drug tolerance—a decrease in the effectiveness of a drug as the body gets used to having the drug in its system (53)

duration—how long a symptom such as pain has lasted (35)

dwarfism—condition characterized by shorter-than-normal skeletal growth (31)

dysmenorrhea—painful abdominal cramps during menstruation (32)

dysplasia—abnormal cells (37)

dysplastic nevus—an abnormal mole (21)

dyspnea—difficulty breathing (26, 28, 36)

dysrhythmia—pulse with an irregular rhythm; also called *arrhythmia* (34)

dysuria—burning or painful urination (30)

eclampsia—condition during pregnancy characterized by severe hypertension, convulsion, possible coma, and death (37)

ectopic pregnancy—growth of a fertilized ovum in the fallopian tube rather than the uterus (37)

eczema—a chronic skin condition characterized by scaling, itching, and rashes; caused by an allergic-type reaction on the skin; also called *atopic dermatitis* (21)

edema—swelling (36)

edits—in procedure coding, specific coding and billing criteria that are checked for accuracy based on predetermined rules (16)

effacement—thinning of the cervical walls before childbirth (37)

efferent nerves—nerves that transmit impulse from neural cell body to stimulate target muscle or organ (24)

efferent vessels—vessels that carry lymph from the lymph nodes to the rest of the body (27)

effleurage—light stroking movement that may be performed in a circular pattern (51)

Einthoven's triangle—pictorial guide to the leads in an electrocardiogram (49)

elective procedure—medical procedure that is nonemergent but may benefit the patient (14)

electrocardiogram (ECG)—tracing or recording of electrical activity as it moves through the heart; may also be abbreviated EKG (49)

electrocardiography—procedure for recording electric charges in the heart (49)

electroconvulsive therapy (ECT)—procedure occasionally used for cases of prolonged major depression, in which an electrode is placed on one or both sides of a patient's head and low-voltage current is turned on briefly, causing a convulsive seizure (57)

electrolyte—an ion that is electrically charged and moves to either a negative (cathode) or positive (anode) electrode (20, 47)

electronic health record (EHR)—medical records kept via computer; also called *electronic medical record* (12, 13)

electronic medical record (EMR)—electronic means of gathering, documenting, and storing information about the patient and the care received in the medical setting; also called *electronic health record* (13)

electronic protected health information (e-PHI)—protected health information (PHI) stored in electronic form; *see* protected health information (PHI) (12)

electronic remittance advice (ERA)—for claims submitted to an insurance carrier electronically, an electronic explanation of benefits (EOB) returned by the carrier (17)

electronic signature—electronic version of a person's signature used in electronic medical records (13)

electronystagmograph (ENG)—instrument used to measure involuntary movements of the eyes (38)

eligibility—condition of being qualified to receive benefits according to insurance policy guidelines (14)

e-mail—electronic mail; messages sent over the Internet (12)

emancipated minor—a minor who, under the laws of a particular state, has the same legal capacity as an adult, usually if the minor lives on his or her own, is married, is self-supporting, or is in the armed forces (3)

embezzlement—unauthorized taking of funds that involves breach of trust (18)

embryonic period—the first eight weeks of gestation (pregnancy); *see also* fetal period (32)

emergency kit—cart or kit that is instantly accessible to anyone in the medical office and contains all supplies that may be needed during an emergency (42)

empathy—ability to understand and identify with what another person is experiencing without necessarily experiencing the same thing (5)

emphysema—progressive respiratory system disease in which the tissues necessary to support the physical shape and function of the lung are destroyed, causing shortness of breath and other symptoms (28)

enamel—hardest and most compact part of the tooth, made up almost entirely of mineral; covers the exposed part of the crown (29)

encephalitis—inflammation in the brain, most often caused by a viral infection (24)

enclosure—document included with a letter, such as an X-ray or medical record (11)

encounter form—record of services for billing and for insurance processing; also called *superbill* or *charge slip* (8, 14)

encounter note—documentation of the patient visit to the physician's office (58)

encrypt—to code or scramble computer data so they are unreadable by anyone who does not have a decoding key (12)

endocardium—innermost lining of the heart wall (26)

endocrinologist—medical doctor who specializes in endocrinology (36)

endocrinology—branch of medicine and biology that deals with the endocrine system, the cells, glands, and tissues that secrete hormones (2)

endometriosis—condition in which the endometrium (the tissue lining the uterus) is found outside the uterus, usually in the pelvis or abdominal cavity (32)

endorsement—the payee's written or rubberstamped signature placed on the back of a check (18)

endosteum—tough connective tissue membrane lining the medullary canal and containing the bone marrow in a long bone (22)

ENT—ear, nose, and throat; a doctor who treats disorders of the ear, nose, and throat; *Syn.* otorhinolaryngrolosit (38)

enteritis—intestinal inflammation, usually resulting from food poisoning (44)

enunciation—clear articulation and pronunciation of words (7)

enuresis—urinary incontinence while sleeping (30)

eosinophils—granular white cells that capture invading microorganisms and antigen–antibody reactions through phagocytosis (47)

epidermis—one of the three layers that compose the skin (21)

epididymitis—inflammation or infection of the epididymis, the long coiled tube attached to the upper part of each testicle, where mature sperm are stored before ejaculation (32)

epiglottis—flap of tissue that covers the trachea during swallowing (28)

epilepsy—disorder associated with misfiring or interference of electrical impulses within the brain, which can lead to seizures (24)

epiphysis—ends of a developing long bone (22)

episiotomy—incision made in the perineum (the external region between the vulva and the anus) during labor to prevent its tearing during childbirth (32)

erectile dysfunction (ED)—inability to achieve or maintain an erection sufficient for sexual intercourse, resulting from insufficient blood supply, from the failure of the smooth muscle to relax, or from the failure of the penis to retain the blood that flows into it (32)

ergonomics—application of scientific information and data regarding human body mechanics to the design of objects and overall environments for human use (6, 12)

erythema—redness of the skin (21, 51)

erythrocyte indices—differentiate the type of anemia present by indicating the average size of red blood cells, the amount of hemoglobin per red blood cell, and the amount of hemoglobin relative to the size of the cell; also called *red blood cell indices* or *RBC indices* (47)

erythrocytes—biconcave cells produced in the red bone marrow that are small enough to pass through capillaries and carry oxygen to the tissues and organs; also called *red blood cells (RBCs)* (26, 47)

erythrocyte sedimentation rate (ESR)—rate at which red blood cells settle at the bottom of a tube (47)

erythropoietin—a glycoprotein hormone that controls production of red blood cells (47)

eschar—dark scab or patch of dead skin that falls away from a wound or burn (41)

esophagus—collapsible tube about 10 inches long along which food is carried from the pharynx to the stomach (29)

established patient—a patient who has been seen within the past three years by any practitioner of the same specialty in the practice (9, 16)

ethics—the branch of philosophy related to morals and moral principles; distinction between right and wrong and a person's moral duty and obligations to the community (3)

ethnicity—classification of people based on national origin or cultural tradition (5)

ethnocentric—belief that your own culture is better than any other (5)

etiology—cause or source of a disease or disorder (15, 22)

eupnea—normal breathing (34)

eustachian tube—auditory tube that extends from the middle ear to the nasopharynx (25)

evacuated tube—a tube with a vacuum suction that pulls in the exact amount of blood needed during venipuncture; also called a vacuum container (46)

evaluation—checking to see how the patient is carrying out the teaching plan (55)

Evaluation and Management (E&M)—codes for services such as office visits, consultations, the physician's component for emergency services, and inpatient care (16)

eversion—process of turning outward (22)

evisceration—separation of wound edges and protrusion of abdominal organs (41)

examination (E,Ex)—in procedure coding, describes the complexity of the physical assessment of the patient (16)

exception report—a report that can be generated in a computerized medical office listing all procedures ordered for patients with no results on record; used to facilitate follow-up with patients (13)

exclusion—health insurance plan rule that limits when and how much the plan is required to pay in benefits (14)

excoriation—painful chafing or rawness of the skin (39)

excreta—waste products (33)

exempt—not eligible, as an employee who is exempt from earning overtime pay (18)

exophthalmos—condition produced by hyperthyroidism in which the eyeballs protrude beyond their normal protective orbit because of swelling in the tissues behind them (31)

expendable supplies—items that are used up in a short period of time and have a relatively inexpensive unit cost (10)

expiration—exhalation; breathing out (28)

expiratory reserve volume (ERV)—amount of air that can be forcibly exhaled after a normal exhale (50)

explanation of benefits (EOB)—statement from an insurance carrier that accompanies a check sent to a health care provider listing the name of the patient, the name of the insured, the date of service, the amount billed, the amount allowed, the amount paid, and the amount the provider may bill the patient; also called *remittance advice (RA)* (17)

exploitation—improper use of someone else's money or assets (3)

exploratory questions—questions used to ask for further information or to more fully discuss the subject at hand (5)

expressed consent—consent for care that is given by a patient verbally or in writing (3)

extended-care facilities—assisted-living facilities designed to care for patients with specific care and rehabilitation needs (40)

extended warranty—option of lengthening the time the manufacturer's warranty is in effect once the original warranty expires, usually requiring an additional fee (10)

extension—process of straightening a flexed limb or the spine (22)

external genitalia—external sexual organs (37)

externship—situation in which a student works without payment in a physician's office, hospital, or other health care setting for 160 hours over a minimum of four weeks during the final stage of training, under the supervision of someone at the site; also called a *practicum* (1, 59)

exudate—a thick drainage; pus (44, 51)

face-to-face time—in procedure coding, indication of the amount of time the physician typically spends with the patient or family (16)

facultative anaerobe—bacteria that are anaerobes that are flexible and can live with some oxygen (44)

failure to thrive (FTT)—inability to gain sufficient weight in accordance with standardized baby growth charts (39)

Fair Labor Standards Act (FLSA)—federal law that regulates work conditions and pay (18)

fallopian tubes—structures that extend laterally from either side of the uterus near each ovary and serve as ducts to move ova (egg cells) from the ovary to the uterus and to move sperm from the uterus toward the ovary; also called *uterine tubes* or *oviducts* (32)

fascia—fibrous sheath that holds together the connective tissue and muscle fibers that make up muscles (23)

fasting—without eating or consuming beverages (other than water), typically for eight hours (43)

febrile—having a fever (34)

febrile seizures—convulsions suffered by some children with high fevers following a rapid spike in body temperature (39)

feces—excrement or waste products from the intestinal tract (44)

Federal Insurance Contributions Act (FICA)—Social Security; employers may make FICA deductions from paychecks as the employee's contribution to Social Security savings (18)

Federal Unemployment Tax Act (FUTA)—law mandating that every employer contribute to unemployment taxes (18)

feedback—response to a communication or stimulus (5)

fee-for-service (FFS)—set of fees for services established by a health care provider and paid for by the patient (14)

fee schedule—schedule of the amount paid by a specific insurance company for each procedure or service subject to the managed care contract (14)

fenestrated drape—a drape for covering a patient during an examination that has a precut opening at the appropriate area (35)

fetal heart tone (FHT)—the heartbeat of a fetus audible with a fetal heart monitor at about 10 to 12 weeks of gestation (32)

fetal period—period beginning at the ninth week of gestation (pregnancy) and lasting until birth; *see also* embryonic period (32, 37)

fiber—indigestible carbohydrates found in foods such as bran, fresh fruits and vegetables, nuts, whole grains, and brown rice that help move food faster through the digestive system; also called roughage (56)

fibrocystic breast disease—a common condition marked by changes to the breast tissue that are common and benign (32)

fibromyalgia—musculoskeletal pain and fatigue disorder with no known cause but with evidence pointing to a genetic predisposition to a neuromuscular or neuroendocrine abnormality that disturbs the usual sensory perception, especially of pain signals (23)

fidelity bond—a component of business insurance that is coverage for employee dishonesty (18)

file cleanup—deletion of unwanted computer data such as deletion of temporary Internet files; often scheduled by an administrator to run automatically (12)

filtration—use of mechanical pressure to diffuse dissolved particles through membranes (20)

financial agent—an individual other than the patient who is authorized to sign a patient's check on his or her behalf (18)

financial hardship—inability of a patient to pay (17)

financial life—a loss in product value resulting from normal aging, use, or deterioration; also called *depreciation* (10)

firewall—hardware- or software-based barrier that prevents outsiders from detecting existence of a computer and, if detected, prevents them from entering the system (12)

first responders—emergency medical service (EMS) providers who are trained to recognize medical conditions, initiate basic life support, and access other parts of the health care system (42)

first-listed diagnosis—the diagnosis definitively stated by the physician; the reason chiefly responsible for the services provided; formerly known as the primary diagnosis (15)

fissure—a deep groove in the brain (24)

fixed—a method of slide preparation in which the clear underneath part of a prepared microscope slide has been passed through an open flame three to four times or in which the slide has been flooded with methanol and then let dry (44)

flagella—tail-like structures that enable a cell to move through a medium (20, 32)

flexion—process of bending (or curving) a flexed limb or the spine (22)

flow sheet—a chart that is used to record responses to treatment over time, for fast visualization of progress (43)

fluoroscopy—visual examination of the body or the function of an organ using a fluoroscope (48)

folliculitis—inflammation or infection of hair follicles that most often appears in areas that become irritated by shaving or the rubbing of clothes, or where follicles and pores are blocked by oils and dirt (21)

forced expiratory volume (FEV)—volume of air that is forcefully exhaled in the first second of exhalation (50)

forced vital capacity (FVC)—maximum volume of air expelled when the patient exhales as forcibly and quickly as possible following one inhalation (50)

formed elements—red cells, white cells, and platelets are known as the formed elements of the blood (47)

formula method—method of calculating a drug dosage by using a standard formula or mathematical equation, filling in known quantities to determine the unknown quantity (52)

formulary—specific to each insurance carrier, a list of medications that will be covered under that insurance plan (14)

fovea centralis retinae—pit in the middle of the macula lutea of the retina of the eye that contains only cones (25)

fraction bar—bar that separates the numerator and the denominator of a fraction (52)

fragile X syndrome—a form of inherited mental retardation associated with developmental delays, behavioral and emotional difficulties, and physical traits such as an elongated, narrow face, large ears, and protruding forehead and jaw; also called *Martin Bell syndrome, Marker X syndrome,* or *FRAXA syndrome* (20)

fraud—knowingly billing for services that were never given or billing for a service that has a higher reimbursement than the service actually provided (15, 16)

frenulum linguae—longitudinal fold of mucous membrane under the tongue (34)

frequencies—the number of fluctuations per second in the form of sound waves (38)

frequency—need to void often (30, 35)

friction—rubbing or deep stroking that produces an increase in circulation and mild heat within tissues (51)

Fried's law—pediatric dosage law applied to children under the age of 1 year, based on their age in months (52)

functional residual capacity (FRC)—amount of air that can be inhaled after a normal expiration (50)

fundal height—measurement from the top of the pubic symphysis to the top of the uterus taken during pregnancy (37)

fundus—floor of the tympanic cavity (25); top of the uterus (37)

fungus—a spore-producing organism that feeds on organic matter, including molds, yeast, mushrooms, and toadstools; *plural*: fungi (44)

furuncle—boil (21)

gait—an individual's manner of walking (51)

gait belt—a safety device worn around a patient's waist used to help move a patient; it can be used to hold up a weak patient while walking or standing or can be used while transferring the patient (51)

gallbladder—membranous sac in which bile is stored and concentrated (29)

gamete—cell developed through the process of meiosis that contains one-half the chromosomes of its original parent cell (20)

ganglion cyst—benign saclike swelling that typically develops over a joint or tendon (23)

gantry—circular structure that houses X-ray equipment used in computed tomography (48)

gastroenterologist—physician who specializes in treating diseases of the digestive system and its related structures (36)

gastroesophageal reflux disease (GERD)—condition in which the muscle at the superior portion of the stomach (the cardiac sphincter) does not close tightly or relaxes inappropriately, allowing gastric fluids and stomach contents into the esophagus and the throat (29)

gatekeeper—a primary care provider who refers patients to other providers for services he or she cannot perform (14)

gauge—size of the needle circumference; the smaller the gauge, the larger the needle (46)

gender bias—indicating either male or female by the type of language used (11)

generic name—single identifying name, typically noted in lowercase letters, that is considered the legal name for a drug (53)

genetics—study of the makeup of animals or plants (20)

genitalia—reproductive organs (39)

geriatrician—physician who diagnoses and treats diseases and disorders that mainly affect older patients (40)

geriatrics—branch of medicine that specializes in the treatment of older adults (40)

germinal centers—primary locations where B lymphocytes reproduce and proliferate (27)

gerontology—study of the process of aging and the effects of aging on people (40)

gestation—pregnancy (32)

gestational diabetes—condition in which the body is unable to produce enough insulin to properly control blood sugar levels by converting sugar and starches into energy, occurring during pregnancy and typically disappearing afterward, but occasionally precipitating ongoing type 2 diabetes (31)

gigabyte (G or Gb)—1,024 megabytes, or a little over 1 trillion bytes, of information; a measure of computer storage capacity or memory; *see also* kilobyte, megabyte (12)

gigantism—condition in which excessive growth hormone is secreted during childhood, before the closure of the bone growth plates, causing overgrowth of the long bones, muscles, and organs; usually caused by a pituitary gland tumor (31)

gingivae—gums of the mouth (29)

glaucoma—condition caused by an increase in the amount of pressure in the eye, leading to an excessive amount of aqueous humor that can lead to damage of the optic nerve and eventually blindness (25)

global period—in procedure coding the number of days surrounding a surgical procedure during which all services relating to that procedure were performed (16)

glomerulonephritis—inflammation of the glomeruli in the kidneys from injury or illness; leads to impaired kidney function; also called *glomerular disease* (30, 45)

glucose tolerance test (GTT)—a procedure that involves blood (and sometimes urine) testing before and after the consumption of a glucose solution to determine how quickly and effectively it is processed (45)

glucosuria—*see* glycosuria (45)

glycosuria—the presence of glucose in the urine, typically seen in uncontrolled diabetes; also called *glucosuria* (45)

goiter—an enlarged thyroid gland, most commonly caused by Hashimoto's thyroiditis, an autoimmune inflammation of the thyroid (31)

goniometer—instrument used to measure the range of motion of a joint (35, 51)

Good Samaritan acts—state laws that help to protect health care professionals from liability when they give emergency care to accident victims (3)

gouty arthritis—disease caused by the formation of urate crystals in a joint, leading to inflammation (22)

Graves' disease—the most common cause of hyperthyroidism, an autoimmune disorder in which the antibodies produced by the immune system stimulate the thyroid to produce too much thyroxine (31)

gravida—total number of pregnancies (37)

grid—device made of parallel lead strips, used to absorb scattered radiation during radiography before it reaches the film (48)

grievance—complaint (19)

gross wage—total amount earned in one year before taxes and other debits are deducted (18)

ground fault circuit interrupter (GFCI)—stops electricity from flowing where it can cause harm (6)

group health insurance (GHI)—policy offered to a group of people in which the

risk or cost of insurance is spread across everyone equally (14)

guardian ad litem—adult who will act in the court on behalf of a minor (3)

guided imagery—imagining being in a relaxing place (58)

guidelines—in the Current Procedure Terminology (CPT®) manual, the instructions that appear at the beginning of each section and apply to all codes in that section (16)

gyri—grooves or convolutions on the surface of the cerebrum (24)

habituation—dependence on a drug (53)

hallucinations—false sensory perceptions (57)

hallux valgus—an enlargement of the inner portion of the metatarsophalangeal joint at the base of the big toe; also called *bunion* (22)

hammertoe—a condition in which the toe bends upward like a claw because of the abnormal flexion of the proximal interphalangeal joint (22)

hardware—the physical parts of a computer system, including the motherboard, central processing unit, and hard drive (12)

Hashimoto's thyroiditis—autoimmune inflammation of the thyroid that causes hypothyroidism and goiter (31)

hay fever—a seasonal allergy that causes inflammation of the mucous membranes of the nose and eyes; also called *seasonal allergic rhinitis* or *pollinosis* (28)

Health Information Portability and Accountability Act (HIPAA)—a legislative act passed in 1996 and fully enacted in 2003, designed to improve the access and portability of medical information and to decrease waste and the abuse of health insurance (3)

Health Information Technology for Economic and Clinical Health Act (HITECH)—part of the American Recovery and Reinvestment Act (ARRA) of 2009, includes incentives for providers who adopt electronic health records (EHR) and demonstrate its use in ways that can improve quality, safety, and effectiveness of care (13)

health insurance exchange (HIE)—legislation that authorizes financial incentives for providers who adopt electronic health records (EHRs) (14)

health maintenance organization (HMO)—managed care plan in which a range of health care services provided by a limited group of providers (such as specified physicians or hospitals) are made available to plan members for a predetermined fee (14)

Healthcare Common Procedure Coding System (HCPCS)—a set of codes developed and maintained by the Centers for Medicare and Medicaid Services (CMS) for the reporting of professional services, nonphysician services, supplies, durable medical equipment, and injectable drugs (16)

hearing acuity—sharpness of hearing (38)

heart—four-chambered muscular pump that circulates blood throughout the cardiovascular system (26)

heart murmur—condition in which a damaged or diseased valve allows blood to escape and move backward through the valve (26)

heart rate—number of heartbeats per minute (49)

heart rhythm—the regularity or irregularity of the occurrence of heartbeats; the pattern of heartbeats (49)

heat exhaustion—a heat illness resulting in extreme fatigue because of excessive loss of sodium and water contained in sweat (42)

heat hydrotherapy—use of warm water as a therapeutic or healing treatment (51)

hematochezia—blood in the stool (36)

hematocrit (Hct)—test that evaluates the percentage of packed red blood cells in the total volume of blood (47)

hematology—study of blood and the tissues that produce it (47)

hematoma—bruise formed by a collection of blood in the tissues beneath the skin (46)

hematopoiesis—formation of blood cells; also called *hemopoiesis* (22, 47)

hematuria—the presence of blood in the urine, often because of infection or injury (45)

hemiplegia—paralysis of one side of the body, usually caused by stroke (24, 51)

hemochromatosis—inherited disorder of excessive body accumulation of iron causing poor function of various body organs (20)

hemoglobin (Hgb)—iron-containing pigment of red blood cells that carries oxygen from the lungs throughout the body (26, 46, 47)

hemolysis—the rupture of red blood cells, often occurring because of trauma from poor venipuncture techniques (46)

hemolyzed—ruptured blood cells (43)

hemophilia—hereditary deficiency of clotting factors (20, 26)

hemopoiesis—*see* hematopoiesis

hemoptysis—coughing up of blood (28)

hemorrhoid—dilated vein in the anus wall and sometimes around the rectum, usually caused by untreated constipation but occasionally associated with chronic diarrhea (29, 36)

hemostasis—stoppage of bleeding as a result of the smooth muscle at the site of a

break causing the vessel wall to contract, creating a spasm that reduces the amount of blood loss and initiating the attachment of platelets to the broken area and to each other, which forms a plug (26)

heparin—a chemical substance that prevents blood from clotting (46, 47)

hepatitis A—most common type of hepatitis in the United States, a viral disease that affects the liver (54)

hepatitis B—highly contagious form of hepatitis that is transmitted by contaminated serum in blood transfusions or through the use of contaminated needles or instruments (54)

heredity—transmission of genetic makeup from parents to children (20)

hernia—abnormal protrusion of an organ, or part of an organ, through the wall of the body cavity that contains it; the most common types of abdominal hernias are hiatal and inguinal (29)

herpes simplex—viral infection that primarily affects the mouth or the genital areas (21)

herpes zoster—an infection caused by the varicella zoster virus that causes a painful rash; also called *shingles* (21)

hiatal hernia—condition in which the upper portion of the stomach protrudes into the chest cavity through a weakened or enlarged esophageal hiatus (an opening in the diaphragm normally large enough to accommodate only the esophagus) (29)

Hib disease—lesser known disease caused by a bacterium that is spread through the air and enters the lungs or bloodstream of children (54)

hierarchy of needs—five levels of need identified by Abraham Maslow (57)

hilum—bases of the lungs; the notch in the concave border of each kidney (28, 30)

hirsutism—condition of thick abnormal hair growth that affects men and women (21)

history (H,Hx)—in procedure coding a key component that describes the background, onset, and progression of the patient's current condition (16)

holistic—practice of medicine that focuses on the whole patient, addressing social, emotional, and spiritual needs as well as physical needs (5, 51)

Holter monitor—apparatus used to record cardiac activity while the patient is ambulatory for at least 23 hours (49)

homeostasis—result of an organism's systems working together to maintain balance or equilibrium by adjusting for constant changes (20)

homophones—words that sound alike but have different meanings and spellings (11)

hordeolums—inflamed glands of the eyelid, often caused by a bacterial infection that appears as a pus-filled swelling at the base of the eyelash; also called *sties* (25)

hormones—chemical transmitters that regulate different body functions including growth, development, mood, tissue function, metabolism, and sexual function (31)

hospice—facility or company that provides an interdisciplinary program of care and supportive services for terminally ill patients and their families (2)

hourly—payment of certain employees a specified amount for each hour worked (18)

household system—system of measurements used in homes, including teaspoon, tablespoon, cup, pint, quart, gallon, ounce, and pound (52)

human genome project—publicly funded international research project (completed in 2001) to sequence and identify human genes and record their positions on chromosomes (2)

human papillomaviruses (HPVs)—group of more than a hundred viruses responsible for the majority of cervical cancer cases and for genital warts (37, 54)

hydrocele—painless buildup of watery fluid around one or both testicles that causes the scrotum or groin area to swell (32)

hydrocephalus—excessive fluid around the brain that may lead to brain damage (39)

hydrogenation—process that turns liquid unsaturated fat into solid fat by adding hydrogen (56)

hyfrecator—miniature electrocautery unit (41)

hyperglycemia—high blood sugar level (42)

hyperopia—farsightedness (25, 38)

hyperpyrexia—markedly elevated body temperature; also called *hyperthermia* (34)

hypersecretion—excessive secretion of hormones (31)

hypertension (HTN)—condition in which blood pressure is consistently higher than 140/90 mmHg; also called *high blood pressure* (26, 34)

hypertensive retinopathy—retinal disease caused by high blood pressure (25)

hyperthermia—markedly elevated body temperature (34, 42)

hyperthyroidism—condition in which the thyroid produces excess amounts of hormones, potentially leading to exophthalmos, palpitations, atrial fibrillation, enlargement of the heart, and congestive heart failure (31)

hyperventilating—breathing rapidly (49)

hyperventilation—deep, rapid respirations (34)

hypoglycemia—low blood sugar level (42)

hyposecretion—insufficient secretion of hormones (31)

hypotension—condition in which blood pressure is consistently lower than 90/59 mmHg; also called *low blood pressure* (26, 34)

hypothalamus—area of the forebrain that controls the activity of the autonomic nervous system and the pituitary gland (31)

hypothermia—below normal body temperature (34, 42)

hypothyroidism—condition in which the thyroid produces inadequate amounts of hormones, which can lead to an enlarged thyroid gland (goiter) (31)

hypoventilation—shallow respirations (34)

hypoxia—insufficient oxygen supply to the tissues caused by ischemia and infarction (26, 28)

hysterectomy—surgical removal of the uterus (32)

ICD-10-CM—International Classification of Diseases, Tenth Revision, Clinical Modification, a classification of codes for medical diagnoses that is recognized by health insurance companies and that is used by all physicians and health care providers in coding and billing for medical services provided to patients (15)

icteric—bilious, yellow-green color (43)

idiosyncratic—specific to an individual, for example drug side effects or adverse (53)

immune function—ability of the body to protect itself from disease (2)

immune response—series of immune system attacks on organisms and substances that invade the body systems and cause disease (27)

immune system—tissues, organs, and physiological processes that identify abnormal cells and foreign substances and defend against those that might be harmful (27)

immunity—resistance to a disease (33, 54)

immunizations—substance that decreases susceptibility to a disease; also called *vaccines* (54)

immunoglobulin—blood product that contains antibodies (54)

immunologist—physician who specializes in treating allergies, asthma, and immune system disorders; *see also* allergist (36)

immunology—the study of immunity, the resistance to or protection from disease (2)

immunosuppressants—medications that suppress the immune system (27)

impacted cerumen—earwax that becomes hardened and can impair hearing (25)

impetigo—contagious skin infection, found most commonly in children, caused by bacteria that form round, crusted, oozing spots, typically around the nose and mouth (21)

implementing—teaching the patient what to do (55)

implied consent—consent for care that is not explicitly given but is inferred from the patient's actions, such as coming to a physician's office for an examination (3)

inactivated polio vaccine (IPV)—polio vaccine that is injectable (which is the recommended route of vaccination for children) (54)

inactive records—medical files for patients who have not been seen within the time period established by office policy (generally, one to five years) (13)

incident report—written record of the circumstances of an accident, injury, or unusual occurrence (6)

incisions—surgical cuts into tissue (41)

incomplete proteins—proteins that do not contain all the essential amino acids, primarily proteins from vegetable sources such as peas, beans, legumes, and wheat (56)

incontinence—involuntary and unpredictable flow of urine (30)

incubation—period of time between exposure to a pathogen and the appearance of the first symptom (33)

incubator—a machine that is used to maintain a specific temperature to achieve a desired result (43)

incus—bone in the middle ear shaped like an anvil (25)

indented code—in procedure coding conventions, the description indented three spaces that is the unique descriptor for a code number (16)

Index—in the ICD-10-CM manual, alphabetical list of diseases and injuries (15); in the CPT manual a list of procedures and services alphabetically by Main Term and modifying terms (16)

Index to Diseases and Injuries—in an ICD-10-CM manual, alphabetical list of conditions and diseases and reasons for seeking medical care (15)

Index to External Causes—in an ICD-10-CM manual, a table within the Index listing external causes of diseases and injuries; follows the Table of Drugs and Chemicals in most manuals (15)

indirect contact—route of infection in which infected droplets from a cough or sneeze are inhaled or enter the eyes, nose, or mouth of another person or when a person touches a contaminated object (33)

individual mandate—requirement under the law that individuals acquire health insurance or pay a tax penalty if they do not (14)

infancy—second period of child development from birth to toddlerhood (57)

infarction—death of heart muscle (26)

infectious—disease-causing; referring to materials or agents that are likely to transmit disease or disease-causing organisms to people or animals (33)

infectious mononucleosis—a viral infection caused by the Epstein-Barr virus, part of the herpes family, characterized by an increase in white blood cells that contain a single nucleus, and commonly found in young adults; also called *mononucleosis, mono,* or *kissing disease* (27)

inferior vena cava—large vein that brings blood from below the heart to the atrium (26)

infertility—inability of a male or female or a couple to conceive a child (32)

infiltration—infusion of IV fluid into tissues outside the vein as a result of permeability of the wall of the vein or the IV needle penetrating the wall of the vein (54)

inflection—changes in the pitch and tone of voice (7)

influenza—an illness caused by a viral infection of the respiratory tract; also called *flu* (28)

informed consent—permission or approval given by a patient who is informed by the physician about the possible consequences of both having and not having certain procedures and treatment (3)

inguinal hernia—condition in which tissue or part of the intestine pushes through a weak spot in the abdominal wall in the groin area, causing a bulge in the groin or scrotum (29)

inhaled medications—medications delivered directly to the respiratory tract (54)

inhaler—device that delivers a measured amount of medication into the respiratory tract to dilate the airways (50)

innate immunity—immunity you are born with; also called *natural immunity* (27)

inoculated—referring to the condition of microorganisms that have been placed on or in media (44)

inpatient—services provided to patients who are in a facility overnight or on a long-term basis (2, 9)

input devices—devices, such as keyboards and scanners, that feed data and instructions into a computer (12)

inscription—part of the prescription that gives the name of the medication, actual ingredients, and dosage (53)

insertion—in locations where skeletal muscles attach, the attachment point on the bone that moves (23)

inspection—visual examination of the exterior surface of the body (35)

inspiration—inhalation; breathing in (28)

inspiration strip—recording of heart rhythm run while the patient is holding his or her breath; *see also* rhythm strip (49)

inspiratory capacity (IC)—amount of air that can be inhaled after normal expiration (50)

inspiratory reserve volume (IRV)—amount of air that can be forcibly inspired after a normal inhale (50)

instill—to place medication in the eye or the ear (38)

instructional notes—in procedure coding, notes that appear in parentheses and direct the user to alternative codes for closely related procedures or to codes that must or must not be used together (16)

insufflation—introduction of gas, vapor, or powder into a cavity (25)

integrity—honesty; employing moral principles (5, 58)

intermittent pulse—pulse that occasionally skips a beat (34)

internal control—a procedure that helps ensure all financial matters are handled properly and that discourages unethical workers from stealing, for example numbered receipts (17, 18)

Internet—communications network enabling the linking of computers worldwide for data interchange (12)

Internet service provider (ISP)—company that sells or gives access to the Internet (12)

interneurons—nerve cells that are located entirely within the central nervous system and work as liaisons between sensory and motor neurons by mediating their impulses (24)

interphase—period when a cell is not actively dividing but is preparing for the division process (20)

intractable pain—pain that is overwhelming, difficult to relieve, and all consuming (35)

intradermal (ID) injection—given directly under the first layer of the skin (54)

intramuscular (IM) injections—injections into muscle tissue given at a 90-degree angle (54)

intrauterine device (IUD)—small device placed in the uterus as a form of contraception (37)

intravenous (IV) therapy—injection of medications or therapeutic solutions directly into the bloodstream (54)

intubate—to insert a tube into the trachea as an emergency airway (42)

invalid claim—health insurance claim form that has been completed but contains some type of incorrect information (17)

invasive procedure—procedure in which the body is entered (41)

inventory—supplies and equipment (10)

inversion—process of turning inward (22)

invoice—a bill presented for an amount due (18)

iris—part of the middle layer of the eyeball containing the pigment (color) and a "hole" in the center (pupil), which controls the amount of light entering the eye (25)

irrigate—to rinse the eye or ear (38)

irritable bowel syndrome (IBS)—common intestinal condition characterized by abdominal pain and cramps, diarrhea or constipation or both, gas, bloating, nausea, and other symptoms (29)

ischemia—reduced blood flow to the heart (26)

ischemic—receiving less than the normal amount of blood flow (49)

Ishihara test—test for color blindness (38)

Islets of Langerhans—clusters of cells in the pancreas that secrete glucagons, insulin, and somatostatin (31)

Item—on a CMS-1500 form, a box to be completed (14)

itinerary—travel plan (19)

keloid—skin lesion that results from excessive scarring (21)

keratin—a strong fibrous protein that is a key ingredient in the outer layer of skin to form a protective covering for the body; the thickness of the layer varies with the soles of feet and palms of hands forming thicker layers because of the ongoing pressure on their surfaces (21)

ketones—by-products of fat metabolism (45)

key component—in procedure coding one of the three categories of criteria used for code selection: history (H/HX), examination (E), and medical decision making (MDM) (16)

kidneys—paired, bean-shaped organs located at the back of the abdominal cavity and lying on either side of the spinal column in the flank area, against the muscles of the back (30)

kidney stones—deposits of mineral salts in the kidney; also called *renal calculi* (30)

kilobyte (K or Kb)—one thousand units (bytes) of information, a measure of computer storage capacity or memory; *see also* gigabyte; megabyte (12)

kinesthetic—involving movement (5)

Klinefelter's syndrome—congenital endocrine disorder affecting males with symptoms including small testes and penis, tall stature, weak bones, low energy levels, and excessive breast tissue (20)

Korotkoff sounds—sounds heard as the arterial wall distends during the compression of the blood pressure cuff (34)

laboratory requisition form—a form that is used to order a laboratory test; provides essential information about the patient, billing and coding, and tests ordered (43, 46)

kyphosis—abnormal curvature of the thoracic spine; also called *humpback* (22, 36)

labyrinth—located in the inner ear, these bony and membranous structures contain receptors for hearing and equilibrium (25)

lacrimal apparatus—structures that produce, store, and remove tears (25)

lacrimal canaliculi—ducts at the inner corner of each eye that collect and drain tears into the lacrimal sac (25)

lacrimal gland—gland above the outer corner of the eye that secretes tears onto the surface of the conjunctiva of the upper lid (25)

lacrimal sac—part of the lacrimal duct that collects tears and empties into the nasolacrimal duct (25)

lactating—producing milk (56)

lactose—combination of glucose and galactose found in animal milk (56)

large intestine—tube about 5 feet long extending from the ileocecal valve at the small intestine to the anus; made up of the cecum, appendix, colon, and rectum, which function to complete digestion and absorption (29)

laryngeal mirror—instrument used to visualize the larynx (35)

larynx—muscular, cartilaginous structure lined with mucous membrane at the lower end of the pharynx; also called *voicebox* (28)

late fee—a charge made to a customer who does not pay bills on time (18)

lavage—rinsing or washing out, as in lavage of the eye to remove foreign substances or chemicals (38)

lawn technique—the preparation of a Petri dish with a pure culture specimen, using overlapping strokes (44)

leading questions—questions that include or suggest an answer, such as "Was the pain you felt sharp and stabbing?" rather than nonleading questions such as "Can you describe the pain you felt?"(5)

leading zero rule—rule that states you must place a zero before the decimal in a number less than one, such as 0.5 (52)

leads—recordings of heart activity from several angles around the heart (49)

ledger card—*see* patient ledger (17)

learning objective—a desired outcome or concept the learner should be able to demonstrate after teaching has taken place (55)

Legionnaires' disease—type of pneumonia or lung infection caused by the *Legionella* bacteria (28)

lens—colorless structure suspended behind the iris that sharpens the focus of light rays onto the retina (25)

lethal—of, relating to, or causing death (53)

letterhead—stationery bearing the name of the physician or practice, address, telephone number, and fax number (11)

leukemia—malignant cancer of the bone marrow and blood, affecting the white blood cells (26)

leukocytes—two types (phagocytes and lymphocytes) of larger blood cells that fight infection and thus contribute to homeostasis; also called *white blood cells* (26, 27, 47)

Level I codes—in procedure coding, the Healthcare Common Procedure Coding System (HCPCS) designates, for Medicare and Medicaid, the Current Procedural Terminology (CPT®) codes as Level I codes for professional services (16)

Level II codes—in procedure coding, the Healthcare Common Procedure Coding System (HCPCS) designates for Medicare and Medicaid a set of alphanumeric codes that begin with a letter followed by four numbers as Level II codes, which cover supplies, durable medical equipment, drugs, nonphysician providers, and certain physician services (16)

liable—legally responsible (3)

liability—debt (3)

licensure—granting of a license and authorization to practice a profession by a government agency (2)

life expectancy—anticipated functional life period of a product or piece of equipment (10)

lifelong learning—process of continuing to learn throughout an individual's life (58)

ligament—tough fibrous connective tissue that connects bones or connects cartilage to a joint (23)

limbus—area of the eye where the cornea and sclera meet (25)

line item posting—posting of an insurance check with money properly allocated among all patients included in the check and to each specific charge for each date of service (17)

lipids—fats or fatty acids classified chemically as unsaturated or saturated (56)

lipolysis—destruction of fats (31)

liquid medications—medications that are taken orally and include suspensions, emulsions, elixirs, syrups, and solutions (54)

lithotripsy—procedure that involves passing shock waves through the body to break down kidney stones (30)

liver—largest glandular organ that plays an essential role in the metabolism of carbohydrates, fats, and proteins (29)

living will—document that allows patients to request that life-sustaining treatments and nutritional support not be used to prolong their lives (3)

lochia—vaginal discharge from the uterus that occurs after childbirth (37)

locum tenens—a person who substitutes for or takes the place of another; a physician who substitutes for the patient's regular physician (14)

login—combination of a username and password to access a computer network (13)

long-term memory—memories that have been activated multiple times and committed to the brain; *see also* short-term memory, sensory memory (40)

lordosis—exaggerated inward curvature of the lumbar spine; also called *swayback* (22, 36)

lumen—the hollow space inside of a needle (46)

lung cancer—cancer of the lung tissue (28)

lungs—conical, lobed, spongy, elastic organs in the chest that bring air into contact with the blood and facilitate the exchange of gases in the alveoli and interact with the circulatory system to deliver oxygen and remove carbon dioxide (28)

lunula—crescent-shaped white area at the base of the nail (21)

Lyme disease—caused by the bacterium *Borrelia burgdorferi*, which is transmitted through the bite of an infected tick and results in the telltale round bull's-eye rash (23)

lymph—clear fluid that travels through the body's arteries, circulating through the tissues to cleanse them and keep them firm, and then draining away through the lymphatic system (27)

lymphatic system—network of vessels, nodes, and ducts through which lymph is carried from the tissues and returned to the bloodstream; its functions include maintaining the body's fluid balance, removing cellular wastes, transporting fatty acids from the digestive tract, and, as part of the immune system, defending the body from harmful foreign substances (27)

lymphedema—condition resulting from an interruption of the normal lymphatic flow (27)

lymphocytes—white blood cells created in the bone marrow that allow the body to recognize organisms that have invaded it previously (27, 47)

macrominerals—minerals that are required in larger amounts in the body than trace minerals (56)

macula lutea—yellow spot on the back of the eye (25)

macular degeneration—deterioration of the central portion of the retina (25)

magnetic ink character recognition (MICR)—characters and letters printed on the bottom of the check used as routing information to identify the bank and the number of the individual account (18)

Main Term—in an ICD-10-CM manual, a term listed alphabetically in the Index to Diseases and Injuries (15, 16)

malabsorption—difficulty digesting or absorbing nutrients from food (56)

malfeasance—performing a wrongful or unlawful act (3)

malignant—cancerous (21, 36)

malignant melanoma—type of skin cancer, originating in the melanocyte cells of the skin, that develops when the melanocytes do not respond to normal control mechanisms of cellular growth (21)

malleus—bone in the middle ear that is shaped like a hammer (25)

malpractice—professional misconduct or demonstration of an unreasonable lack of skill that results in injury, loss, or damage to a patient (3)

managed care—a form of health insurance coverage intended to reduce costs through mechanisms such as economic incentives for physicians and patients to choose less costly forms of care, reviews of medical necessity for specific services, selective contracting with health care providers, and intensive management of high-cost medical cases (14)

managed care organization (MCO)—a health care plan that offers cost-saving managed care at a reduced cost; *see* managed care (14)

manipulation—passive assessment or movement of the range of motion of a joint (35)

manometer—part of a sphygmomanometer, a scale that registers the actual pressure reading (34)

massage—kneading or applying pressure with the hands to a part of the patient's body to promote muscle relaxation, improve blood circulation, and reduce tension (51)

mastication—chewing (29)

Material Safety Data Sheet (MSDS)—printed materials that come with hazardous chemicals and offer basic information needed to ensure the safety and health of the user (6)

matrix—template for scheduling appointments; also a term meaning *nail bed* (9, 21)

mature minor—a young person, generally under the age of 18, who possesses the maturity to understand the nature and consequences of a medical treatment (3)

maximum heart rate—heart rate for an individual calculated by using the following formula: 220 minus the patient's age = the maximum heart rate for that person (49)

maximum target heart rate—the heart rate beyond which a stress test for an individual must be terminated, calculated by the formula 220 minus the patient's age × 0.85 (85 percent of the patient's maximum heart rate: *see* the entry maximum heart rate) (49)

Mayo stand—small portable table with enough room to hold an instrument tray (41)

mean corpuscular hemoglobin (MCH)—as part of the erythrocyte indices measures the average amount of hemoglobin in a red blood cell; *see also* erythrocyte indices (47)

mean corpuscular hemoglobin concentration (MCHC)—as part of the erythrocyte indices measures the average amount of hemoglobin relative to the size of the red blood cell; *see also* erythrocyte indices (47)

mean corpuscular volume (MCV)—as part of the erythrocyte indices measures the average size of the red blood cells and classifies them according to size; *see also* erythrocyte indices (47)

meaningful use—a set of criteria for how electronic health records (EHRs) are used that the providers must meet in order to receive incentive payments (13)

measles, mumps, and rubella (MMR) vaccine—protects children from developing measles, mumps, and rubella (54)

meatus—urinary tract opening (39)

Medicaid—a federal/state health insurance program primarily for low-income people (14, 40)

medical asepsis—destruction of organisms after they leave the body (33)

medical coding—process of assigning alphanumeric characters to represent diagnoses, procedures, and services a physician provides to patients (15)

medical decision making (MDM)—in procedure coding, a key component that describes the complexity of establishing a diagnosis and/or selecting a management option (16)

medical durable power of attorney (MDPLA)—assignment by a patient of an agent who may make health-care related decisions on behalf of the patient if the patient becomes unable to make such decisions on his or her own behalf (3)

medical necessity—the process of establishing the medical need for medical services (14)

medical nutrition therapy—treatment of a medical condition through use of a specially tailored diet; *see also* registered dietitian (56)

medical privilege—physician is granted rights to practice medicine in a particular hospital or other health care facility (2)

medical record—source of all documentation relating to the patient; also called *patient files* or *patient charts* or *patient's record* (13)

Medicare—a U.S. government health insurance program for which persons aged 65 and over and others with special conditions are eligible (14, 40)

Medicare Severity Diagnosis Related Groups (MS-DRG)—under Medicare, the grouping together of patients with similar conditions and care requirements who will be eligible for the same amount of reimbursement (14)

medications—drugs prescribed or purchased to alleviate or manage a medical condition (53)

Medigap (MG)—private insurance policy that supplements or fills "gaps" in Medicare by providing coverage for services Medicare does not cover (14)

Medigap policy—private insurance policy that is sold to those receiving Medicare to provide additional coverage (40)

medulla—*in the lymph node*, the portion that is primarily made up of macrophages attached to reticular fibers; *in the thymus gland*, the area from which mature lymph cells reenter the circulation; *in the kidney*, the middle portion, in which the renal pyramids are found (27, 30)

medullary canal—narrow space or cavity throughout the length of the diaphysis in a long bone, which contains yellow bone marrow, made of fat cells (22)

megabyte (M or Mb)—1,024 kilobytes, or a little over 1 million bytes, of information; a measure of computer storage capacity of memory; *see also* gigabyte, kilobyte (12)

megahertz (MHz)—1 megahertz equals 1 million cycles per second; the higher the MHz, the faster the computer (12)

meiosis—process in which cells reduce their chromosomal number by half in order to form gametes (20)

melanin—pigment that gives the skin its color (21)

melanocytes—cells that produce melanin for pigmentation (21)

member—person who owns a health insurance policy (14)

memory—storage and retrieval of computerized data (12)

memos—correspondence sent to people within the office or organization (11)

menarche—onset of the menstrual cycle (32, 37)

Ménière's disease—condition of the inner ear characterized by vertigo, tinnitus, fluctuating hearing loss, and pressure or pain in the affected ear (25)

meninges—membranes that encompass the brain and spinal cord (24)

meningitis—infection of the meninges that surround and protect the brain and spinal cord, typically caused by a bacterial or viral infection (24)

menopause—cessation of menstrual cycles that usually occurs in mid-life or later (32)

mensuration—use of special tools to measure the body or specific parts (35)

metabolism—the chemical activities that are essential to maintain life; the sum of all biochemical and physiological processes that take place in the body (20, 56)

metastasis—process in which cancer cells break away from the original tumor and travel to other areas of the body where they form new tumors (27)

methicillin-resistant *Staphylococcus aureus* **(MRSA)**—a form of *S. aureus* that produces an enzyme that makes it resistant to penicillins and cephalosporins normally used for treatment; two forms are hospital-associated MRSA and community-based MRSA (33, 44)

metric system—most commonly used conversion system for dosage calculations; a decimal system based on the meter, liter, and gram (52)

microbes—one-celled forms of life, such as bacteria (2, 44)

microbiology—the study of living organisms too small to be seen with the naked eye (44)

microencephaly—head growth that falls below the normal percentile (39)

microfiche—sheets of microfilm (13)

microfilm—miniaturized photos of records (13)

microhematocrit—a hematocrit performed on an extremely small quantity of blood collected in a capillary tube; see hematocrit (47)

microorganisms—living organisms too small to be seen with the naked eye (33, 44)

microprocessor—small chip that processes data in a microcomputer (12)

micturate—to urinate (45)

micturition—urination; the passing of urine (30, 45)

minerals—inorganic elements that are not of plant or animal origin (56)

misfeasance—performing a lawful act but not in the proper way (3)

mitosis—process during which a cell divides its chromosomes into two identical daughter cells, each having 23 pairs of, or 46, chromosomes (20)

mitral valve—the valve through which blood leaves the left atrium of the heart; also called *bicuspid valve* (26)

mixed number—number that contains a whole number and a fraction (52)

modalities—applications of any therapeutic agent (51)

modified block style—style of letter writing in which the date, complimentary close, and signature line begin at the center of the page, with all other lines at the left margin (11)

modified wave scheduling—modification of scheduling that gives several patients an appointment on the hour, knowing that some will be late (9)

modifier—two-digit code preceded by a hyphen that clarifies the procedure (e.g., a procedure that was done on both arms instead of only one) (16)

modifying term—in the Current Procedure Terminology (CPT®) manual, descriptive words indented under a Main Term in the Index to further describe the service or procedure (16)

Mohs technician—a person trained to help a physician during Mohs surgery to remove cancerous skin lesions and surrounding layers of skin (36)

molecule—a chemical combination of two or more atoms that forms a specific chemical compound (20)

moniliasis—yeast infection; also called *candidiasis* or *thrush*; *Candida albicans* is the causative agent (44)

monitor—viewing screen that allows the user to see input and output (12)

monocytes—type of leukocytes that are formed in the bone marrow from stem cells and assist in phagocytosis (47)

mononucleosis—a contagious viral infection frequently spread through oral contact; also known as *infectious mononucleosis, mono,* or *kissing disease* (47)

monosaccharides—simple sugars that result from the breaking down of carbohydrates in the digestive tract (56)

monounsaturated fat—type of unsaturated fat that can lower cholesterol levels and low density lipids; canola oil, olive oil, and peanut oil are monounsaturated fats (56)

monthly billing—system in which statements for all patients are generated once a month (17)

morale—employees' feelings about their work and work environment (10)

morals—that which a person believes to be an acceptable or right way to live (3)

morbidity—the rate or number of people who have a disease or illness (2)

morphology—study of the shape of cells (44)

mortality—the rate or number of people who suffer death in a particular circumstance (2)

motor neurons—neurons that control most of the body's movement, causing muscles to contract, glands to secrete, and organs to function properly (24)

mouse—pointing and selection device for data input (12)

multidrug-resistant organisms (MDROs)—bacteria and other microorganisms that have developed resistance to antimicrobial drugs (33)

multiple coding—in diagnosis coding, reporting several codes to fully describe a condition (15)

multiple gated acquisition (MUGA) scan—nuclear scan to check for blood flow in the myocardium (49)

multiple sclerosis (MS)—chronic, debilitating autoimmune disease in which the body directs the antibodies and white blood cells to attack the myelin sheath surrounding nerves in the brain and spinal cord, which causes inflammation and injury and, eventually, scarring, resulting in difficulty with movement, vision, and/or sensation (24)

muscular dystrophy (MD)—one of a group of genetic diseases characterized by progressive weakness and muscular degeneration (20, 23)

mutation—change in the DNA sequence of a gene (20)

myasthenia gravis (MG)—chronic autoimmune neuromuscular disease characterized by varying degrees of weakness of the skeletal, or voluntary, muscles of the body (23)

mycology—study of fungi (44)

myelin—insulating material that forms a protective covering or sheath around a nerve cell (24)

myocardial infarction (MI)—condition that occurs when the blood supply to a part of the myocardium is severely reduced or stopped; also called *heart attack* (26, 36)

myocardium—middle muscular layer of the heart (26)

myomectomy—surgery that removes uterine fibroids without removing healthy tissue (32)

myopia—nearsightedness (25, 38)

myringa—the eardrum (38)

myringotomy—incision into the myringa or eardrum to drain fluid (25, 39)

myxedema—rare, life-threatening condition that results from long-term untreated hypothyroidism (31)

nares—nostrils (28)

nasolacrimal duct—duct that drains lacrimal fluid into the nasal cavity (25)

National Certified Medical Assistant (NCMA)—credential issued by the National Center for Competency Testing to qualified medical assistants; to continue certification, 14 CEUs must be obtained each year (1)

National Committee for Quality Assurance (NCQA)—national committee that sets standards for and evaluates the quality of health plans (6)

national provider identifier (NPI)—10-digit identification number assigned to health care providers by the Centers for Medicare and Medicaid Services (CMS) (14)

nebulizer—device that delivers medication directly to deeper areas in the lungs through a fine, inhaled aerosol mist (50)

necrotizing fasciitis—severe infection resulting in the destruction of subcutaneous tissue and fascia; has a 30 percent mortality rate (44)

negative feedback—when the body responds to external stimuli by reversing the direction of change (31)

negligence—failure to do or perform or to take reasonable care in performing a specific action, which results in injury to another person (3)

negotiable instrument—actualizes or permits the transfer of money to another person, such as a check (18)

nephrons—functional units of the kidney that remove the waste products of metabolism from the blood plasma (30)

net pay—the amount an employee receives after deductions from gross pay; also called *take-home pay* (18)

neuralgia—general nerve pain (24)

neurilemma—outer sheath of the nerve composed of Schwann cells, the cells that regenerate damaged nerve fiber (24)

neuroglia—tissue that surrounds and supports nerve cells; also called *glia* (24)

neurologist—physician who specializes in treating conditions of the nervous system (36)

neurons—nerve cells (20, 24)

neurosurgeon—a physician who performs surgical procedures on the nervous system (36)

neutrophils—most common type of phagocyte; primarily attack bacteria (27, 47)

new patient—patient who has never been seen by anyone in the practice, or who has not been seen by any practitioner of the same specialty in the practice for more than three years (9, 16) nocturia—increased urination at night (37)

noncompliance—not following the physician's orders (55)

noncovered—services not eligible for reimbursement by Medicare (14)

nonexempt—eligible, or not ineligible, such as an employee who is nonexempt from earning overtime pay (18)

nonfasting—refers to a patient who has consumed food or caloric beverages in the previous eight hours (43)

nonfeasance—being negligent or ignoring performance of a necessary lawful act (3)

nonparticipating provider—a physician to whom the patient is expected to pay charges before submitting the claim to the insurance company, which pays the patient directly (14)

nonsufficient funds (NSF)—situation in which the payer's account does not have enough money to cover the amount of the check (18)

nonverbal communication—unspoken information conveyed through gesture and actions, including body language (5)

normal flora—nonharmful and often beneficial microorganisms that live on the surface of the body and inside body openings and organs and may help in resisting pathogens (33, 44)

no-show—patient who did not show up for a scheduled appointment (8, 9)

nuclear membrane—double-layered sac that contains the nucleus of a cell (20)

nucleus—control center and part of the cell containing the chromosomes (20)

numerator—top number of a fraction (52)

numeric filing—filing system that assigns an identification number to each person's name (13)

nutrients—organic and inorganic chemical substances in foods that supply the body with the elements necessary for metabolism (56)

nutrition—the effects of vitamins, minerals, and food in the body (2)

nutritionist—a person who provides nutritional advice; state laws vary as to who is allowed to be designated a nutritionist (56)

nystagmus—involuntary, repetitive, rhythmic movements of the eye; also called *nystaxis* (25)

objective—observable by others; a sign others can see or hear such as a rash or noisy breathing (35)

objectives—lenses near the bottom of a microscope that magnify the specimen, or object (43)

obsessions—persistent thoughts (57)

occlusion—blockage (26)

occult—hidden; often refers to microscopic amounts of blood that cannot be detected with the naked eye (36, 45)

Occupational Safety and Health Administration (OSHA)—agency of the U.S. Department of Labor that monitors safety on the job and enforces standards for safety (6)

oculars—eyepiece lenses of a microscope (43)

office flow—teamwork, time management, organized and efficient office equipment usage, and patient flow (10)

office hours—the time span each day that a medical office is open for business (9)

Office of the Inspector General (OIG)—office within the U.S. Department of Health and Human Services responsible for investigating Medicare fraud (15)

Office of the National Coordinator for Health Information Technology (ONC)—federal office that oversees adoption of technology to reduce medical errors, improve health care quality, and reduce expenditures, with adoption of electronic health records (EHRs) a priority (13)

Official Guidelines for Coding and Reporting (OGCR)—in an ICD-10-CM manual, rules for how to code selected conditions and rules for how to identify which diagnoses should be reported on a claim for any given patient (15)

oliguria—the production of a small amount of urine (typically less than 400 mL in 23 hours); may be life threatening (45)

oncogenes—genes controlling cell growth and multiplication that are transformed into cancer cells by cancer-causing agents (27)

oncology—branch of medicine dealing with malignant neoplasms or tumors (2, 36)

online banking—a service provided by a bank in which a customer has access to his or her bank account at all times using a secure website (18)

onset—beginning; when a physical sign or symptom started (35)

open-ended questions—questions that require a broader response than just yes or no (5, 9)

operating system—basic software that allows a computer to run, manages hardware resources, and enables application software to run; popular operating systems include Android, Linux, Mac OS, and Microsoft Windows (12)

ophthalmologist—medical doctor who can perform eye examinations and eye surgery and prescribe medications, eyeglasses, and contact lenses (38)

ophthalmology—branch of medical science that deals with the structure, function, and diseases of the eye (38)

ophthalmoscope—instrument used to examine the interior of the eye, especially the retina (35, 38)

opportunistic infections—infections that take advantage of a suppressed immune system (33)

optical character recognition (OCR)—equipment that scans, reads, and sorts; used by the U.S. Postal Service to sort envelopes (11)

optic disk—area of the retina where the optic nerve enters (25)

optician—technician who specializes in grinding lenses and preparing eyeglasses and contact lenses (38)

optic nerve—nerve that carries information from the eye to the brain (25)

optometrist—a doctor of optometry, not a medical doctor, who can perform eye examinations, prescribe medications, and write prescriptions for eyeglasses and contact lenses (38)

oral cancer—cancer of the mouth, usually starting in the flat squamous cells that line it (29)

oral medication—medication that is swallowed and absorbed through the gastrointestinal system and then rapidly absorbed by the body (54)

oral polio vaccine (OPV)—live, early form of the polio vaccine that was given to children but was shown to cause polio in some cases and is no longer recommended (54)

orbit—cavity in the skull that houses each eyeball (25)

organelles—small structures within the cytoplasm of a cell (20, 44)

organ of Corti—spiral structure in the cochlea that converts the waves of sound that travel through the ear (38)

organs—similarly functioning groups of tissues that serve a common purpose (20)

origin—in locations where skeletal muscles attach, the attachment point on the bone that is more fixed or still (23)

orthopedic physician—physician who specializes in the treatment of diseases and disorders of the musculoskeletal system; also called an *orthopedist* (22)

orthopedics—branch of medicine dealing with the study and treatment of the musculoskeletal system (36)

orthopedist—*see* orthopedic physician (36)

orthopnea—condition in which the patient has trouble breathing unless a certain position is maintained, such as with head elevated (28)

orthostatic hypotension—severe (19–29 mmHg) drop in blood pressure occurring when standing quickly after lying down or sitting (34)

orthotist—professional who designs and fits supportive devices such as braces and splints (51)

osmosis—form of diffusion whereby water is pulled through a semipermeable membrane, moving from areas of greater to lesser concentration (20)

ossicles—small bones, such as the incus, malleus, and stapes in the ear (25)

osteoarthritis—most common type of arthritis, resulting from years of wear and tear on joints and occurring most frequently in the hips, knees, and finger joints (22)

osteomalacia—adult onset of rickets, literally meaning "softening of the bone" (22)

osteopath—medical professional who places great emphasis on the relationship between the musculoskeletal system and the organs of the body (2)

osteoporosis—progressive loss of bone density and thinning of bone tissue, seen most commonly in older adults, especially postmenopausal women, and in individuals who do not consume enough calcium (22, 40)

otitis media—inflammation of the middle ear caused by viral or bacterial infections (25)

otology—study of hearing (38)

otorhinolaryngologist—specialist in disorders and diseases of the ears, nose, and throat (ENT) (38)

otosclerosis—condition in which the tissue surrounding the bone of the stapes grows abnormally around it, preventing it from transmitting sound vibrations to the inner ear and resulting in profound hearing loss (25)

otoscope—instrument used to examine the eardrum (35, 38)

outpatient—services provided to patients on a walk-in basis when no overnight stay is required (2, 9, 16)

outpatient surgery—surgery that may be done outside the hospital setting in a surgicenter, a surgical center that is part of a hospital complex, or in a medical office (41)

output devices—components such as a display screen or a printer that allow the user to see what the computer has accomplished (12)

outside laboratory—a hospital-based or independent laboratory that handles specimens collected from many types of facilities (43)

ovarian cancer—cancer of the ovaries; the three main types are epithelial cancer, germ cell tumor, and stromal tumor (32)

ovarian cysts—sacs filled with fluid or semisolid material that develop on or within the ovary, typically not disease related and disappearing on their own; formed when the grown follicle fails to rupture and release an egg and, instead of being reabsorbed, forms a cyst (32)

ovaries—two almond-shaped organs on either side of the uterus that produce ova (eggs) and the hormones estrogen and progesterone (31, 32)

overbooking—scheduling more than one patient in the same time slot (9)

overdose—when too much of a medication is administered (52)

over-the-counter (OTC)—nonprescription drugs such as aspirin, cold medications, and antibiotic ointments (53)

overtime—pay for hours worked in excess of 40 hours per week (18)

ovulation—process of producing an ovum and releasing it into the pelvic cavity and one of the fallopian tubes (32)

ovum—(plural, *ova*) egg or reproductive cell (32)

oxygen debt—inability of the body to absorb enough oxygen to supply the energy required to sustain a high level of activity, resulting in utilization of the anaerobic energy system and in the buildup of lactic acid in the muscles (23)

oxygen saturation—oxygen content of blood (34, 50)

oxyhemoglobin—hemoglobin that is carrying oxygen (47)

oxytocin—hormone that triggers labor (37)

pacemakers—electronic devices that help the heart maintain normal rhythm (49)

packing slip—document listing items in a package (18)

paid time off (PTO)—payment of wages for a specific number of hours when the employee is not at work such as sick time, vacation time, or holidays (18)

palpate—to touch or feel (46)

palpation—using the hands to feel the skin and accessible underlying organs and other tissues (35)

palpatory method—feeling the radial pulse while the blood pressure cuff is deflating, used to determine systolic pressure (34)

palpebrae—eyelids (25)

palpebral fissure—opening between the eyelids (25)

pancreas—elongated gland behind the stomach that secretes pancreatic juice into the small intestine as well as the hormones insulin and glucagon, which raise and lower blood glucose levels (29, 31)

pancreatic cancer—develops in the exocrine glands with vague symptoms that include pain in the abdomen or back, weight loss, bloating, diarrhea, and jaundice (29)

papilledema—inflammation of the optic nerve (25)

para—number of deliveries after 20 weeks' gestation (37)

paranasal sinuses—four pairs of cavities in the bones of the face that connect with the nasal passages: the maxillary sinuses, frontal sinuses, ethmoid sinuses, and sphenoid sinuses (28)

paraplegia—paralysis from approximately the waist down (24)

parasites—organisms that live, feed, and grow on or in other organisms (45)

parathyroid glands—four glands around the dorsal and lower aspect of the thyroid gland that secrete parathyroid hormone (PTH or parathormone) (31)

parent code—*see* standalone code (16)

parenteral medications—medications given by a route other than by the mouth or rectum, principally through injection (54)

Parkinson's disease—progressive disorder caused by degeneration of the nerve cells in the parts of the brain that control movement, resulting in a shortage of the neurotransmitter dopamine, which impairs movement (24)

participating provider—a provider who has a contractual agreement with an insurance plan to render care to eligible beneficiaries and then bill the insurance carrier directly (14)

parturition—birth (37)

passive—accepting without active response or resistance (5)

passive immunity—immunity acquired from an outside source, such as breast milk, that lasts for a short time (27)

passive listening—listening to someone without having to reply or actively respond, such as when listening as a member of an audience (5)

passive transport—process in cells that does not require energy to transport materials to, from, and within the cell (20)

passive voice—the subject of the sentence receives the action (11)

password—a string of characters, such as letters, numbers, and symbols, that make up a secret code that, when typed into a designated password space, allows the individual who has supplied the password to enter a computer, a computer system, or a personal electronic account (12)

pasteurization—process during which substances, such as milk and cheese, are heated to a certain temperature to eliminate bacteria (2)

patent—unobstructed (42)

pathogens—microorganisms capable of causing disease (33)

pathophysiology—study of diseases or disorders caused by a malfunction or by age, genetic predisposition, or environmental influences (4, 20)

patient account—record of the charges and payments for a specific patient (17)

patient accounting—functions of the accounting department related to recording charges and payments for services provided to patients (17)

patient cancellation—when the patient calls to cancel without scheduling another appointment (9)

patient-centered medical home (PCMH)—a facility that helps to streamline the health care needs of a patient by providing a cooperative team of health care specialists in one convenient location (2)

patient coach—a person who provides support, explanations, encouragement, and other help to a patient (55)

patient incompetence—a patient's lack of decision-making ability (3)

patient ledger—a chronological record of the charges, adjustments, payments, and current balance for a specific patient; also called a *ledger card* (17)

patient navigator—a person who helps patients by facilitating their healthcare needs, encouraging adherence to care plans, and encouraging and coaching the patient regarding self-management skills (1)

Patient Protection and Affordable Care Act (PPACA)—federal law passed in 2010 to create a market for purchase of health care insurance policies and mandates and incentives to decrease the number of uninsured Americans; also known as the Affordable Care Act (ACA) or Obamacare because it was passed during the administration of President Barack Obama (14, 15)

Patient Self-Determination Act (PSDA)—a legal mandate that health care institutions encourage patients to make advance decisions regarding the type of care they wish to have or to deny in the event they later become unable to make such decisions (3)

patient statement—bill sent to a patient (17)

patient status—designation of a patient as a new patient or an established patient (9, 16)

payee—person or company named as the receiving party to whom the amount on the check is payable (18)

payer—person signing a check to release money (18)

payment—receipt of money that decreases the account balance; in accounting referred to as *credit* (17)

peak expiratory flow rate (PEFR)—measurement of the fastest rate at which a patient exhales after taking a maximum breath (50)

peak flow meters—devices that measure the ability to move air into and out of lungs (50)

pediatrician—medical doctor who specializes in the treatment of newborns, infants, children, and adolescents (39)

pediculosis—infestation of the head, body, or pubic area with the eggs, larvae, or adults of lice (21)

pelvic inflammatory disease (PID)—inflammation of the vagina, cervix, uterus, and fallopian tubes caused by several sexually transmitted infections (32, 37)

pending—claim submitted to an insurance carrier that awaits additional information (17)

penis—male organ for intercourse or copulation, and the site of the orifice through which urine and semen are eliminated from the body (32)

peptic ulcer disease (PUD)—condition in which a disruption occurs in the lining of the esophagus, stomach, or duodenum (29)

percussion—using the fingertips to tap the body lightly but sharply to gain information about the position and size of underlying body parts (35)

perfusion—blood flow to the myocardium (49)

pericardium—outer lining of the heart wall (26)

perineum—external region between the vulva and the anus, composed of muscle covered with skin (32)

periosteum—membrane that forms the covering of long bones, except at their articular surfaces (22)

peripheral nervous system (PNS)—made up of nerves that connect the CNS to other parts of the body (24)

peristalsis—involuntary, wavelike, muscular contractions that move the bolus of food through the entire digestive system (29)

permeable—in autoclaving, wrappings capable of allowing the passage of steam through them (33)

persistence—quality of being able to stay on task longer than the usual time when necessary, even after others might have given up (58)

personal assessment—evaluation of your own strengths and weaknesses (59)

personal health record (PHR)—health information that a patient stores electronically on a computer or secure Internet site, allowing patients to maintain electronic records of their own health information, such as immunizations, medications, and surgeries (13)

personal injury protection (PIP)—a third-party liability plan to provide coverage for injuries, such as from an automobile accident (14)

personality—the sum of a person's traits, characteristics, and behaviors (5)

personality disorders—include narcissistic (self-centered), paranoid, (abnormally concerned that people will hurt oneself), antisocial (not concerned with laws and other people), histrionic (dramatic), and borderline (impulsive) behavior (57)

personal protective equipment (PPE)—protective gloves, fluid-resistant lab coats, gowns, safety glasses, surgical masks, shields, and respirators used to protect the health care worker whenever working in an environment in which the chance of splash or exposure exists (6, 33)

pertussis—respiratory disease that is most common in children under the age of 4 years; also called *whooping cough* (28, 54)

petechiae—tiny broken blood vessels on the surface of the skin (26)

petrissage—kneading or rolling method of massage that requires pressing the muscles (51)

petty cash—a small amount of cash kept in an office to use for incidental purchases or payments such as postage due on certified mail (18)

phagocytes—several types of white blood cells that attack invading organisms (27)

phagocytosis—process by which leukocytes (white blood cells) actively fight pathogenic microorganisms (33)

phantom pain—sensation felt in a missing body part after it has been removed (35)

pharmacists—specially trained and licensed professionals who specialize in the preparation and dispensation of drugs (53)

pharmacology—the study of medications and drugs, including their forms, intentions for use, and effects (52, 53)

pharynx—musculomembranous tube about 5 inches long that extends from the base of the skull to the cervical spine and connects to the trachea and esophagus that serves as a passageway to the lungs for air and food to reach the stomach (28, 29)

phenylketonuria (PKU)—congenital disease caused by a defect in the metabolism of the amino acid phenylalanine (20, 47)

phlebotomy—the process of entering a vein by incision or puncture, to collect blood for testing; also called *venipuncture* (26, 46)

Phlebotomy Technician—a phlebotomist who has passed a credentialing exam (46)

photometer—instrument that measures the intensity of light (43)

physiatrist—physician who specializes in the therapeutic use of physical agents (51)

physiatry—therapeutic use of physical agents for the diagnosis, treatment, management, and prevention of diseases and debilitating illnesses (51)

physical safeguards—controls established in a medical office to prevent unauthorized persons from physically accessing patient data such as workstations positioned so that what is on the computer screen cannot be seen by others, visitor sign-in and escort, and procedures for protecting personal information when computer hardware or software is removed or installed (12)

physician's office laboratory (POL)—a laboratory within a physician's office where specimens can be tested immediately after collection (43)

physiology—functions and processes of the body; the study of the function of an organism (4, 20)

pineal gland—gland located in the brain at the posterior end of the corpus callosum; secretes melatonin and serotonin (31)

pinna—visible portion of the ear outside the head; also called *auricle* (25)

pinwheel—an instrument with sharp points used to test sensory perception (35)

pitch—frequency of voice (e.g., high or low) (7)

pituitary gland—organ located near the base of the brain in a small depression of the sphenoid bone; regulates all other endocrine glands; also called *master gland* (31)

pity—feeling sorry for a person (5)

placenta—structure that joins mother and fetus and their mutual blood supply and produces the hormones estrogen, progesterone, and human chorionic gonadotropin hormone (hCG) (31)

placenta previa—complication in which the placenta develops in the lower portion of the uterus, blocking the opening in the cervix and causing oxygen deprivation for the fetus and possible maternal hemorrhage during labor (37)

plaintiff—a person who files a lawsuit (3)

plan—to determine how to begin the task of teaching the patient (55)

plasma—fluid portion of the blood; watery portion of the blood that contains blood cells (26, 46, 47)

platelets—smallest cells in blood, formed in the red bone marrow; main function is to assist in the clotting of blood for wound healing; also called *thrombocytes* (26, 46, 47)

pleura—thin sheets of epithelium that cover the outer surface of the lungs and the inside of the thoracic cavity (28)

pleurisy—an inflammation of the pleura, the membrane surrounding the lungs, generally stemming from an existing respiratory infection, disease, or injury; also called *pleuritis* (28)

pneumococcal vaccine—vaccine that is given to guard against contracting the *Streptococcus pneumonia* bacteria (54)

pneumonia—inflammation of the lungs caused by bacteria, viruses, fungi, or chemical irritants, often following influenza in the older adult and debilitated persons, and most commonly caused in the United States by *Streptococcus pneumoniae* (28)

point of care (POC) testing—testing at the patient's side or in the medical office setting (46)

point-of-service plan (POS)—insurance plan in which a patient may choose an HMO or a non-HMO provider but must pay a deductible for using a non-HMO provider (14)

polarity—having two separate poles with different electrical charges, one positive and one negative; *see also* depolarized, repolarized (49)

polycystic kidney disease (PKD)—disorder in which clusters of cysts, noncancerous sacs of water-like fluid, develop, primarily within the kidneys (30)

polycythemia—higher than normal level of red blood cells (47)

polydipsia—excessive thirst (36)

polyphagia—excessive hunger (36)

polypharmacy—taking multiple (five or more) drugs simultaneously (53)

polysaccharides—starches that are broken down into glucose during the digestive process and transported into the blood (56)

polyunsaturated fat—type of unsaturated fat that contains omega-3 fatty acids essential to the diet; vegetable oils and fish oils are sources of polyunsaturated fat (56)

polyuria—excessive urination; typically more than 2,000 mL in a 23-hour period (36, 45)

portal of entry—entryway for pathogens into the body (33)

portal of exit—opening for the exit of pathogens from the reservoir host (33)

positive feedback—process of encouraging external or internal stimuli to continue, or even accelerate, in order to maintain homeostasis (31)

posted—recorded (17)

postexposure evaluation—under OSHA guidelines, the obligation of an employer to institute appropriate procedures for evaluation and treatment of an employee following the event of an exposure to a bloodborne pathogen (33)

postprandial (PP)—after eating (43)

power-of-attorney (POA)—legal document in which one person appoints another person to act as an agent on his or her behalf (18)

practice management software (PMS)—comprehensive software program that manages administrative and business functions of a medical practice, such as patient registration, billing and coding, and insurance payment postings (12)

practice management system (PMS)—*see* practice management software (17)

practice of medicine—diagnosing and prescribing treatment of medication (3)

practicum—situation in which a student works without payment in a physician's office, hospital, or other health care setting for 160 hours over a minimum of four weeks, during the final stage of training, under the supervision of someone at the site; also called an *externship* (1, 59)

practitioner—the medical care member who is responsible for the patient's principal consultation and care; typically a physician, but may also be a nurse practitioner or physician's assistant (43)

preauthorization—requirement to obtain prior approval for surgery and other procedures from the insurance carrier in order to receive reimbursement (14)

preceptor—supervisor who provides additional instruction and guidance for a student in an externship or practicum situation and provides a formal written evaluation of the student (59)

preeclampsia—hypertension that develops during pregnancy (37)

preexisting condition—any condition a patient was diagnosed with or treated for before beginning coverage with a new insurance plan (14)

preferred provider organization (PPO)—an insurance arrangement that requires the patient to use a provider under contract to the insurance company, which reimburses the provider at a discounted rate (14)

prefilled cartridge injection systems—single-dose cartridges that fit into a special cartridge holder, which results in medications not having to be drawn up before injections (54)

prefix—a word element placed before or affixed to the beginning of a word (4)

prehypertension—in adults over 17 years old, blood pressure ranging from 120/80 to 139/89 mmHg, considered a precursor to hypertension (26)

prejudice—preformed and usually unfavorable belief or attitude toward a certain culture or group based on little or no information about the culture or group (5)

premenstrual syndrome (PMS)—condition affecting certain women with symptoms that may begin two weeks before the onset of menstruation; also called *premenstrual dysphoric disorder* (32)

premium—amount paid for insurance (14)

prenatal period—first period of child development; covers the process from conception until birth (57)

prepaid plan—group of physicians or other health care providers who have a contractual agreement to provide services to subscribers on a negotiated fee-for-service or capitated basis; also called *managed care plan* (14)

presbycusis—hearing loss from gradual deterioration of the sensory receptors located in the cochlea, associated with aging (25, 38)

presbyopia—the loss of elasticity in the eye's lens, usually as a result of aging, that causes an inability to focus on objects at close range (25, 38)

present illness (PI)—detailed description of the chief complaint, which must contain symptom(s), including the onset, duration, and intensity of each (35)

presenting problem—in procedure coding, a contributing factor, the primary reason the patient is seeing the provider (16)

primary assessment—asking a few simple questions and doing a simple exam to assess the patient's status (42)

primary care provider (PCP)—gatekeeper provider who refers patients to other providers for services he or she cannot perform (14)

primary payer—the insurance carrier responsible for paying benefits before any other insurer makes a payment (14)

primary policy—the insurance policy billed first for any health care service (14)

prime mover—muscle that is the primary actor in a given movement—that is, the muscle that produces the movement in muscle contraction; also called *agonist* (23)

printer—output device for producing hard copy (12)

private health insurance—insurance coverage for health care services provided by a private corporation rather than by a government entity (14)

probationary period—usually the first three months (90 days) of employment during which the new employee can be terminated without cause (19)

problem-oriented medical record (POMR)—patient record organized according to diagnoses (13)

procedure coding—process of assigning alphanumeric characters to the procedures and services a physician provides to patients (15, 16)

procedures—actions directed at, or performed on, an individual to improve health or treat a disease or injury (16)

proctologist—physician who treats disorders of the rectum and anus (36)

professional component—in coding for radiology, the performance of the imaging is the technical component, the review and analysis of the results by a qualified physician is the professional component (16)

professional courtesy (PC)—consideration extended by a physician not to charge other physicians, staff, family members, or clergy (17)

professional reference—statement from an individual who has worked with or knows someone for a period of time, attesting to the person's skills and personal integrity (59)

prognosis—prediction of the course of a disease and its outcome (35)

pronation—process of lying prone, or face downward; also, the process of turning the hand so that the palm points downward (22)

proofread—to review a document for errors in content and typing (11, 59)

prophylactically—drug that is being used to prevent the onset of a condition (53)

proportion—comparison of two ratios (52)

proprietary name—name given to a drug by a specific manufacturer; also called *brand name* (53)

prostate cancer—malignant tumor that grows in the prostate gland (32)

prostate gland—gland lying behind the urinary bladder that wraps around the first 2.5 cm of the urethra that secretes an alkaline fluid that aids in maintaining the viability of the spermatozoa (32)

prosthesis—artificial replacement of a missing body part (51)

prosthetist—a person who specializes in designing, preparing, and fitting prosthetic devices such as artificial limbs (51)

protected health information (PHI)—health information designated by the Health Insurance Portability and Accountability Act (HIPAA) that, if revealed, could be used to identify the individual, including the patient's name, address, phone number, social security number, account number, and the like; PHI information cannot be given out by any means, electronically, on paper, or orally, without the explicit consent of the

patient; *see also* electronic protected health information (e-PHI) (5)

proteinuria—the presence of protein in the urine; may indicate kidney or cardiovascular disease (45)

protraction—process of moving a body part forward (22)

proximate cause—the determination that a person's acts or failure to act directly caused an injury (3)

psoriasis—common skin condition characterized by frequent episodes of redness, itching, and thick, dry scales that results from a buildup of dead skin cells that, rather than shed off, pile up and form scaly patches (21)

psychiatrist—medical doctor who specializes in psychiatry (36, 57)

psychiatry—branch of medicine that deals with the diagnosis, treatment, and prevention of mental disorders (57)

psychologist—a person who is trained in the methods of psychologic analysis, therapy, and research (57)

psychology—science of behavior and the human thought process (57)

psychomotor—relating to coordination of the mind and body (58)

psychopharmacology—study of the effects of drugs on the mind and brain, particularly the use of drugs in treating mental disorders (57)

psychotherapy—method for treating mental disorders by mental rather than physical means, including psychoanalysis, humanistic therapies, and family and group therapies (57)

psychotic—mental disorder that interferes with patients' perceptions of reality and their ability to cope with the demands of daily living (57)

puerperium—period of four to six weeks following birth (37)

pulling (charts)—preparing the medical charts of scheduled patients so that all pertinent information is readily available to the physician (8)

pulmonary artery—artery that transports blood from the right ventricle to the lungs (26)

pulmonary edema—condition in which fluid accumulates in the lungs, usually caused by failure of the heart's left ventricle but also caused by lung problems such as pneumonia, an excess of intravenous fluids, some types of kidney disease, severe burns, liver disease, nutritional problems, and Hodgkin's disease (28)

pulmonary embolism (PE)—blood clot in the lung, usually originating in smaller vessels in the leg, pelvis, arms, or heart and traveling to the lung, where it ultimately becomes wedged in a vessel too small to allow it to pass, causing that portion of the lung to die from lack of oxygen (28)

pulmonary vein—vein that transports freshly oxygenated blood from the lungs to the left atrium (26)

pulmonary volume tests—tests performed to discover the amount of air in the lungs during normal movement and how much lung space is available after a normal inhalation and a normal exhalation; *see also* tidal volume (V_T), expiratory reserve volume (ERV), inspiratory reserve volume (IRV), residual volume (RV) (50)

pulmonologist—medical doctor who specializes in treating the lungs and accessory structures (50)

pulmonology—the study and treatment of diseases of the respiratory system (50)

pulse deficit—difference in readings between the apical and radial pulses (34)

pulse oximeter—device that can determine the oxygen content of arterial blood (34)

pulse pressure—difference between the systolic and diastolic blood pressures (26, 34)

pupil—"hole" in the center of the iris that controls the amount of light entering the eye (25)

purchase order (PO)—a form listing items to be ordered and signed by an authorized person such as an office manager or accountant (10, 18)

pure tone audiometry—test of hearing acuity performed in a soundproof room with the patient wearing headphones (38)

purging—dieting by vomiting, or taking laxatives, enemas, or diuretics (39)

Purkinje fibers—specialized conductive fibers located within the walls of the ventricles, responsible for relaying cardiac impulses to the cells of the ventricles, which then contract (26)

pyelonephritis—infection of the kidney and renal pelvis caused by bacteria, usually *E. coli*, entering the kidneys from the bladder (30)

pyloric sphincter—a ring of muscle at the lower art of the stomach that opens and closes to allow food liquid to pass into the small intestine (29)

pyloric stenosis—condition in which a baby's pylorus (the connection between the stomach and the duodenum) gradually swells and thickens, which interferes with food entering the intestine (29)

pyrexia—fever (34)

pyuria—the presence of pus in the urine, often because of infection (45)

quadriplegia—paralysis from approximately the shoulders down (24)

qualified diagnosis—a diagnosis accompanied by a term such as *possible, probable, suspected, rule out,* or *working diagnosis*; also called an *uncertain diagnosis* (15)

qualitative test—a test that reveals the presence or absence of something; typically reads as positive or negative (43)

quality assurance (QA)—the act of gathering and evaluating information about services provided and comparing this information with an accepted standard (6, 43)

quality control (QC)—a quantitative measure of the accuracy of tests (43)

quantitative test—a test that reveals a numerical evaluation (43)

quantity not sufficient (QNS)—indicates that not enough of a specimen was collected to perform the ordered test (43)

queue—waiting line (7)

queuing up—activating or displaying electronic medical charts (8)

quickening—fetal movement (37)

race—classification of people based on their physical or biological characteristics, such as skin color, shape of eyes, hair type, bone structure, or facial features (5)

radiating pain—pain that spreads out from an area (35)

radiation—radiant energy (48)

radiation isolation precautions—steps taken to isolate a patient who has received radiation from others who might be harmed by the radiation from a distance (33)

radiation therapy—use of high-energy waves, such as X-rays, to damage and destroy cancer cells (27)

radioactive—of, caused by, or exhibiting radioactivity (48)

radiographs—X-ray images (48)

radiography—the profession of performing imaging procedures ordered by physicians (48)

radiologist—physician specializing in radiology (48)

radiology—branch of medicine that uses radioactive substances or matter that gives off radiation (radiant energy) and various techniques to visualize the internal structures of the body for the diagnosis and treatment of disease (48)

radiolucent—penetrable by X-rays (48)

radiopaque—allows minimal penetration by X-rays (48)

random-access memory (RAM)—internal storage area in the computer that can be accessed randomly (12)

range of motion (ROM)—degree of movement that can be achieved in a specific joint without causing pain (51)

rapport—environment of understanding or cooperation (5)

rate—number of heartbeats per minute when assessing the pulse; number of breaths per minute when assessing respiration (34)

ratio—relationship between two quantities (52)

ratio method—drug calculation method that involves establishing a relationship between two quantities (the ratio), as when comparing the amount of drug ordered to the amount on hand (52)

RBC count—number of red blood cells per cubic millimeter of blood (47)

RBC indices—*see* erythrocyte indices (47)

read-only memory (ROM)—internal storage area in the computer where data has been recorded and cannot be removed, only read (12)

reason codes—statements on an insurance carrier's explanation of benefits identifying reasons for payment adjustments and denials (17)

reasonable person standard—exercising the ordinary standard of care and the type of care that a "reasonable" person would use in a similar circumstance (3)

received on account (ROA)—a payment; payments are sometimes entered with the abbreviation ROA (17)

receptionist—person, usually a medical assistant, who greets patients as they arrive (8)

Recommended Dietary Allowances (RDAs)—recommended amounts of protein, vitamins, and minerals Americans should eat and the body weights they should try to maintain for good nutrition (56)

reconcile—to compare financial activity with financial statements, for example, comparing an explanation of benefits (EOB) from an insurer to the original bill to verify that each service billed was paid in the amount expected (17)

reconciliation—process of comparing banking records to a bank statement to ensure that both are in agreement (18)

rectum—final portion of the large intestine that stores solid waste until it is expelled from the body through the anus (29)

red blood cell indices—*see* erythrocyte indices (47)

red cells—blood cells responsible for carrying hemoglobin, to transport oxygen and carbon dioxide; erythrocytes (46)

reduction—procedure used to align and reposition a dislocated joint (22)

redundant—repeating the same word, expression, or statement (11)

reference initials—letters that indicate the name of the person who keyed a letter; placed at the lower left margin in lowercase (11)

reference laboratory—laboratory, usually associated with a hospital or medical school, that handles more complex and infrequently requested tests than outside laboratories (43)

referral—the process of sending a patient to or from another physician (7, 14)

referred pain—pain that is felt at a site other than the injured or diseased body part (35)

refined sugars—processed sugars (56)

reflex hammer—instrument used to check reflexes (35)

refraction—process of light rays changing direction when they pass through the eye (25)

refractometer—a device used to evaluate plasma protein and specific gravity in urine (45)

registered dietitian—expert in nutrition who obtains the registered dietitian credential (RD) by completing and passing an examination issued by the Commission of Dietetic Registration after completing a four-year bachelor's degree program approved by the Academy of Nutrition and Dietetics' Accreditation Council for Education in Nutrition and Dietetics; the services of a registered dietitian are considered to be nutritional therapy and are billable under many health insurance plans including Medicare (56)

Registered Medical Assistant (RMA)—medical assistant who has met eligibility requirements and who can prove his or her competency to perform entry-level skills through written examination; the RMA is awarded to candidates who pass the American Medical Technologists (AMT) certification examination (1)

registration—being entered on a list of professionals recognized as qualified by an organization or association in a specific health care field that administers examinations, maintains a list of qualified individuals, or both (2)

rehabilitation—process of bringing the patient back as close as possible to normal physical condition after injury or disease with the ability to attain and maintain function and independence (51)

Reiki—a therapy that channels the body's energy and spirit through gentle touch and massage (51)

rejected claim—claim that is never accepted into the insurance carrier's system because of invalid information (17)

relative value unit (RVU)—measure of value used in determining Medicare reimbursement formulas, including the difficulty level of the work involved, office overhead expenses, and malpractice risk for the given service or procedure (14, 16)

rem—unit of measurement used for exposure that may involve more than one type of radiation; the Roentgen equivalent in humans (48)

remittance advice (RA)—see explanation of benefits (EOB) (17)

remittance slip—a tear-off stub from an invoice that is mailed to a vendor with the invoice payment (18)

renal calculi—deposits of mineral salts in the kidney; also called *kidney stones* (30)

renal cortex—outer layer of the kidney (30)

renal medulla—inner layer of the kidney (30)

renal pelvis—saclike area of the kidney in which urine is collected (30)

renal threshold—the point at which the concentration of a substance in the blood causes it to spillover for removal through urine (45)

reorder point—an amount specified as the lowest amount of a supply item remaining on hand before the item should be reordered (10)

repolarized—having regained, after depolarization, a difference in electrical charge inside and outside a cell; see also polarity, depolarized (49)

requisition—a form that is used to order a laboratory test; provides essential information about the patient, billing and coding, and tests ordered (43)

res ipsa loquitur—"the thing speaks for itself;" doctrine that applies to the law of negligence and refers to the breach (neglect) of duty that is so obvious that it does not need further explanation (3)

rescheduled—an appointment scheduled in place of one the patient has called to cancel (9)

resequenced code—in a coding manual, because of the expanding nature of the code set, some codes are not in strict numerical order; such codes are considered resequenced codes and are highlighted with the symbol # as an aid to identification (16)

reservoir host—the animal or human that harbors and nourishes a pathogen, giving it a "home" for a long time without suffering any ill effects; the reservoir host begins the chain of infection when the harbored pathogen is transferred to another animal or human (33)

residual volume (RV)—volume of air left in the lungs at the end of an exhalation (50)

resolution—the ability to distinguish clearly between two adjacent but distinct objects (43)

resource-based relative value scale (RBRVS)—a formula used by Medicare

and health maintenance organizations to determine the fee a medical provider should be paid for each service or procedure based on factors such as actual costs, malpractice risks, and geographic adjustments (14)

respect—belief and attitude that someone is important and should be treated appropriately (58)

respiratory cycle—one inhalation and one exhalation (34)

respiratory hygiene/cough etiquette—covering a cough, disposing of tissue appropriately, performing hand hygiene after contact with respiratory secretions (33)

respiratory syncytial virus (RSV)—common viral respiratory infection that affects the upper and lower respiratory tracts (39)

respite care—short-term care for the chronically ill intended to provide relief to individuals or families caring for a family member with Alzheimer's disease or other chronic condition (40)

respondeat superior—Latin term meaning "Let the master answer;" refers to the employer or physician who is liable for the negligent actions of anyone working for him or her; in some states, both physician and employee may be liable (3)

résumé—summary of a person's credentials, including employment history, experience, training, and education (59)

reticulocyte count—percentage of reticulocytes (immature red blood cells) in the blood in relation to the number of mature red blood cells (47)

reticulocytes—immature red blood cells (47)

retina—innermost layer of the eye containing rods and cones, which translate light into nerve impulses (25)

retinal detachment—separation of the retina from the underlying choroid layer (25)

retraction—process of moving a body part backward (22)

review of systems (ROS)—review of each system of the body during physical examination; also called *head-to-toe exam* (35)

rheumatoid arthritis (RA)—autoimmune disorder causing joints to be deformed because of inflammation (22, 27)

rheumatologist—physician who specializes in treating patients with joint inflammations and patients with autoimmune disorders (36)

rhinovirus—a group of several hundred viruses that cause the common cold (39)

RhoGAM—drug administered to a pregnant woman to inhibit the production of antibodies against the Rh antigen (26)

rhythm—regularity or spacing of all the heartbeats when assessing the pulse; regularity or spacing of breaths when assessing respiration (34, 48)

rhythm strip—recording of heart rhythm produced during an electrocardiogram (ECG) (49)

ribonucleic acid (RNA)—single chain of chemical bases (20)

rickets—childhood bone disorder that causes bone deformity; caused by lack of vitamin D, calcium, and phosphate (22)

risk management—the planning and implementation of strategies for reducing the physician's risk of a lawsuit in the medical setting (3)

rods—photosensitive cells in the retina that respond to dim light and are used in night vision (25)

Romberg test—patient closes eyes and stands with feet together without swaying (36)

rosacea—chronic disorder, primarily of the facial skin, causing redness on the cheeks, nose, chin, or forehead, often characterized by flare-ups and remissions (21)

rotation—process of moving a body part around a central axis (22)

rugae—folds that allow the inner surface of the stomach to expand as food is ingested; *also called* gastric folds (29)

Rule of Nines—formula for estimating the percentage of body surface area (42)

rule of discovery—a time period in within which a lawsuit may be brought; in the case of medical malpractice this time period begins once the problem is discovered which may be some time after the actual medical treatment (3)

safe injection practices—precautions relative to giving injections including aseptic technique, use of single-use items, and multidose vials safely stored outside of treatment areas (33)

safety data sheet (SDS)—printed information about a potentially hazardous substance (6)

salaried—an employee paid a predetermined amount of money every pay period regardless of the number of hours worked (18)

salivary glands—glands in or near the mouth that produce saliva, which contains amylase, an enzyme that helps in the breakdown of carbohydrates (29)

salpingo-oophorectomy—removal of the fallopian tubes and ovaries (32)

salutation—courteous greeting in a letter, typed at the left margin and spaced two lines below the inside address (11)

sanitization—cleaning process that inhibits or inactivates pathogens by means of careful scrubbing (33)

saturated fat—fat from animal sources including meats, lard, and dairy products including butter, cheese, and whole milk as well as from some oil-producing plants such as coconuts and palms; has negative effects on the body, including raising the level of blood cholesterol (56)

scabies—contagious disorder of the skin caused by the human or scabies itch mite; causes intense itching and a red rash (21)

scheduling system—process that is followed methodically when giving patients appointments (9)

schizophrenia—psychotic disorder marked by a variety of symptoms, including delusions, hallucinations, disorganized and incoherent speech, severe emotional abnormalities, and withdrawal into an inner world (57)

sciatica—pain along the sciatic nerve that runs from the lower back down the back of each leg, often caused by inflammation because of a pinched nerve (24)

sclera—part of the outer layer of the eyeball; also called *white of the eye* (25)

scoliosis—abnormal lateral curvature of the spine (22, 36)

scope of practice—procedures a health care professional, such as a medical assistant, is allowed to perform under federal and state guidelines for that profession (1)

scratch test—method of allergy testing in which the skin is divided into small labeled squares, a drop of allergen is placed in each appropriately labeled square, and the skin scratched with a needle or lancet; an allergy is indicated if a wheal forms at the scratch site within 14 minutes (36)

scrotum—pouchlike structure behind the penis that contains the two testes (32)

scrub assistant—assistant who has completed sterile asepsis and assists the physician in surgical procedures by handing instruments, swabbing bodily fluids, retracting the incision area, and cutting suture materials, using sterile technique (41)

sebaceous glands—glands in the skin that produce sebum, an oil that acts to protect and waterproof hair and skin (21)

seborrheic dermatitis—inflammation of sebaceous or oil glands of the skin, caused by an increase in sebum; also called *cradle cap* (21)

sebum—oily substance secreted by the sebaceous glands that keeps skin and hair moisturized (21)

secondary payer—the insurance carrier billed for costs that were not covered by the primary payer (14)

secondary policy—the insurance policy billed after payments from the primary policy have been determined (14)

section—in an ICD-10-CM manual, a division having a boldfaced or highlighted heading within one of the 21 chapters in the Tabular List (15, 16)

Security Rule—regulations of the Health Insurance Portability and Accountability Act (HIPAA) that provide national standards for protecting electronic protected health information (e-PHI) (12)

sediment—cells, debris, and other solids found in urine (45)

seizure—temporary interference with muscle control, movement, speech, vision, or awareness caused by intense bursts of electrical activity produced within the brain; often associated with epilepsy (24)

self boundaries—in health care communication, awareness of and restraint from discussing topics, such as personal information, that should not be discussed with a patient (5)

semicolon (;)—the portion of a procedure description that is shared by more than one indented code appears before a semicolon, followed by the indented codes that would include the portion before the semicolon (16)

seniority—status gained by being the individual who has worked for the physician the longest (19)

sensorineural hearing loss—caused by nerve damage (38)

sensory memory—information gained through the senses and lasting a few seconds; *see also* long-term memory, short-term memory (40)

sensory neurons—attached to the sensory receptors, transmit impulses directly to the central nervous system (24)

separation of duties—an internal control to reduce risk of fraud and embezzlement by dividing financial responsibilities and assigning the separate tasks to different individuals (18)

septum—wall that separates the left and right sides of the heart (26); cartilaginous wall that separates the internal portion of the nose into the right and left cavities (28)

sequela—a condition that is the consequence of a previous disease or condition; a long-lasting effect (44)

serology—study of the antigen and antibody reactions of the body's immune system (44)

serum—the liquid portion of blood that remains after clotting has occurred; includes plasma without fibrinogen (46, 47)

severe acute respiratory syndrome (SARS)—newly identified respiratory illness caused by a previously unknown virus, SARF-CoV, of the coronavirus family, whose members often cause mild to moderate upper respiratory illness, such as the common cold (28)

sexual harassment—unwelcome sexual advances, requests for sexual favors, and other verbal or physical harassment of a sexual nature (19)

sexually transmitted disease (STD)—an infection transmitted through exchange of semen, blood, and other body fluids or by direct contact with the affected body areas of another person; also called *venereal disease* (32)

sheaths—protective membranes that wrap nerve fibers in the peripheral nervous system (24)

short-term memory—memories that can be recalled for about 29 seconds but, if not repeated multiple times, will fade from memory; *see also* long-term memory, sensory memory (40)

sickle cell anemia—inherited chronic form of anemia in which red blood cells become sickle-shaped and pile up instead of flowing freely through the blood vessels, most common in people of African or Mediterranean descent; also called *hemoglobin SS disease* (20)

side effects—unwanted effects of a medication that are tolerated because the benefit of taking the medication outweighs them (53)

sigmoidoscopy—an examination of the interior of the sigmoid colon; also called a *proctoscope examination* or a *proctosigmoidoscopic examination* (36)

signa (sig.)—Latin term for *label*, the part of a prescription that gives instructions on how the medication should be taken by the patient; also called *signature* (53)

signature line—typed four spaces below the complimentary close of a letter; contains the name and title of the writer (11)

sinoatrial (SA) node—one of three areas of specialized neuromuscular tissue that initiate the heartbeat, located in the upper wall of the right atrium; also called *pacemaker of the heart* (26)

sinusitis—infection or inflammation of the mucous membranes that line the inside of the nose and sinuses, causing them to swell and block the drainage of fluid from the sinuses into the nose and throat (28)

skeletal muscle—voluntary or striated muscle (made up of cylindrical fibers) that allows movement by being attached to bones in the body (23)

skip—individual who had a balance due and has moved without leaving a forwarding address (17)

sleep apnea—periods of apnea or absence of breathing during sleep (39)

small intestine—tube about 20 feet long extending from the pyloric sphincter of the stomach to the large intestine, made up of the duodenum, jejunum, and ileum, that functions in digestion and absorption of nutrients (29)

smear—thin layer of microorganisms spread on a glass slide for microscopic examination and identification (44)

smooth muscle—type of involuntary muscle found throughout the body, composed of elongated, spindle-shaped cells with the nucleus centrally located and without striations (23)

Snellen chart—tool for assessing distance visual acuity (38)

social media—websites where users interact with each other, including discussion forums, and networking websites such as Facebook and Pinterest (12)

soft skills—skills necessary for the smooth functioning of the workplace that are neither cognitive nor psychomotor and that display the professionalism of the employee (58)

software—set or sets of programmed instructions that tell computer hardware what to do to complete the required data processing; also called *program* (12)

solvent—describes a medical practice that is capable of paying bills and salaries (19)

somatic nervous system (SNS)—part of the peripheral nervous system that is made of 12 pairs of cranial nerves and 30 pairs of spinal nerves (24)

source-oriented medical record (SOMR)—patient file organized according to the source of information (13)

special instructions—directions within each section of a coding manual describing specific rules and definitions for codes within a particular category or subcategory (16)

specific gravity—the density or concentration of urine, in relation to that of distilled water (45)

specified time scheduling—allotted time period for each patient, depending on the reason for the visit (9)

specimen—a small sample taken from the body (43)

speculum—instrument for viewing a body cavity (35, 38)

spermatozoa—(singular, *spermatozoon*) male reproductive cells; also called *sperm* (32, 45)

sphygmomanometer—instrument used to measure blood pressure (26, 34)

spina bifida—most frequently occurring, permanently disabling birth defect, resulting from the failure of the spine to close properly during the first month of pregnancy (20)

spore—thick-walled reproductive cell produced by some organisms that is capable of withstanding unfavorable environmental conditions (44)

sprain—stretching or tearing injury to a ligament (23)

spreadsheet—computer software application that allows manipulation and analysis of information by rows and columns and arithmetic calculations (12)

sputum—mucous substance expelled when coughing or clearing the bronchi; also called *saliva* or *spit* (44)

squamous cell carcinoma—malignant tumor that affects the middle layer of the skin (21)

stale check—check that has not been presented for payment within the time frame suggested on the check (18)

standalone code—in a coding manual, the code whose description is left-justified and begins with the capital letter; also called *parent code* (16)

standard of care—level of knowledge, skill, and care a medical practitioner must provide to all patients for the same care that would commonly be provided by other similar medical care professionals under the same circumstances in the same locality (3)

standard precautions—actions recommended by the Centers for Disease Control and Prevention such as handwashing and wearing personal protective equipment whenever exposed to patients' body fluids (33)

stapes—stirrup-shaped ear bone (25)

stat—immediately, from Latin *statim*, meaning "immediately;" sometimes jokingly said to be an acronym for "sooner than already there" (42)

State Unemployment Tax Act (SUTA)—a state unemployment compensation law governing whether the employer or both employer and employee make payments to the unemployment fund and how funds may be withheld from an employee's paycheck (18)

statute of limitations—maximum time period set by federal and state governments during which certain legal actions, such as a patient filing a lawsuit, can be brought forward (3, 17)

steatorrhea—excessive amounts of fat in the stool (44)

stem cell—undifferentiated cell that can give rise to other cells of the same type or from which specialized cells can develop (2)

stereotyping—formation of beliefs or attitudes that are often negative concerning specific characteristics of a person or group and applying them unfairly to an entire population (5)

sterile field—specific area free of all microorganisms that will be the work area for a surgical procedure (41)

sterilization—destruction of all living organisms and spores with the use of pressurized steam, chemicals, electron bombardment, extreme temperatures, or radiation (33)

stomach—large, muscular, saclike organ that secretes hydrochloric acid and gastric juices that convert food into chyme (29)

stop-payment order—procedure in which the writer of the check instructs the bank (in writing) not to honor the payment of a check (18)

storage devices—computer components that allow organization and retention of date, including RAM and ROM memory, optical drives, memory cards and USB drives (12)

strabismus—a disorder caused by weakness in the external eye muscles, resulting in the eyes looking in different directions; also called *crossed eyes* or *wall eyes* (25, 38)

strain—stretching or tearing injury to a muscle or tendon (23)

stress—body's reaction to the world around it, which can be emotional, intellectual, or physical (5, 57)

stressor—real or imagined event that causes stress (5, 57)

stress test—treadmill test that evaluates the heart's response during moderate exercise while an electrocardiogram is performed (49)

striated—having a striped appearance (20, 23)

stridor—high-pitched sound heard during respiration, caused by obstruction of the airway (39, 42)

stroke—result of a clot or hemorrhage in the brain blocking the blood supply and causing brain cells to die from a lack of oxygen (24, 26)

subcategory—within an ICD-10-CM manual, a level of code numbers having a four- or five-character entry (15, 16)

subcutaneous injection—injection given just under the skin in the fat (adipose) tissue; used for small doses of nonirritating medications such as immunizations, insulin, and analgesics (54)

subheading—in the hierarchy of a coding manual, the Tabular list is divided into sections, then subsections, then subheadings under the subsections; categories and subcategories are grouped under the subheadings (16)

subjective—something the patient experiences that cannot be observed by anyone else; a symptom such as pain or anxiety (35)

subjective, objective, assessment, and plan (SOAP)—Patient chart notes organized according to symptoms, signs, assessment, and plan (13)

sublingual medications—medications held under the tongue to diffuse through the tissues into the bloodstream (54)

subpoena—a legal document that requires the office to present information such as the appointment book to the court (9)

subpoena duces tecum—an order to appear in court and to bring with you certain medical records for trial (3)

subscription—part of the prescription that tells the pharmacist how to mix the drug and how much to provide the patient (53)

subsection—in the hierarchy of a coding manual, the Tabular list is divided into sections, then subsections; subheadings, categories, and subcategories are grouped under the subsections (16)

subterm—in an ICD-10-CM manual, terms listed under an alphabetically listed Main Term in the Index to Diseases and Injuries (15)

sudden infant death syndrome (SIDS)—the death with no known cause of an apparently healthy infant, usually before age 1 year (39)

sudoriferous glands—glands that occur in nearly all regions of the skin but are most numerous on the palms and soles; also called *sweat glands* (21)

suffix—word element affixed to the end of a word (4)

sulcus—shallow groove of the brain (24)

superior vena cava—large vein that transports blood from the head and upper chest to the heart (26)

supernatant—fluid remaining at the top of a centrifuged specimen (45)

superscription—part of a prescription that contains the patient's name, address, age, and the date on the top line as well as the symbol *Rx* (53)

supination—process of lying supine, or face upward; also the process of turning the palm or foot upward (22)

suppuration—process to relieve the internal buildup of pus formation (51)

suprapubic specimen—sterile urine specimen obtained by inserting a sterile needle into the patient's bladder through the abdominal wall just above the pubic bone (45)

surety bond—insurance sometimes required to be purchased personally by employees who handle cash (18)

surfactant—fatty substance produced by the alveoli that reduces surface tension of fluid in the air-filled sacs (28)

surgery scheduler—person in the surgery department who schedules procedures (9)

surgical asepsis—techniques used to destroy pathogenic organisms before they enter the body (33)

surgical package—all Current Procedure Terminology (CPT^{00}) codes include the surgical package that includes specific services in addition to the surgery itself that cannot be billed separately, such as preparing the patient for surgery and evaluating the patient in the recovery area and any typical postoperative follow-up; also called *global surgical concept* (16)

surgical scrub—scrubbing the hands, wrists, and arms in preparation for surgery to remove microorganisms more effectively than regular handwashing (41)

susceptible host—reservoir host that is available and capable of being infected by the pathogen (33)

swabs—sterile cotton-tipped applicators used to collect specimens or for application purposes (44)

sweat glands—occur in nearly all regions of the skin but are most numerous on the palms and soles; also called *sudoriferous glands* (21)

sympathy—the feeling of sorrow or pity for another person (5)

synapse—the site at which an impulse is transmitted from the axon of one nerve to the dendrite of another; *see also* synaptic space (24)

synaptic space—the space between the axon of one nerve and the dendrite or another; *see also* synapse (24)

synarthrotic joint—articulation, or joint, that produces no movement (22)

syncope—fainting (34, 46)

synergist—muscle that acts with another muscle to produce movement (23)

synthetic—created in a laboratory by artificial means (53)

syphilis—an infectious chronic venereal disease (2)

syringe—a tubular device with a plunger at one end and a needle at the other; used for drawing blood, removing fluid, or administering medications (46)

system—group of organs that work together to perform a specific function (20); a regularly interacting group of people who function within an organized set of doctrines and principles (58)

systemic lupus erythematosus (SLE)—systemic immune system disorder in which the body produces abnormal antibodies that attack its own tissues rather than foreign organisms (27)

systolic blood pressure—upper number of blood pressure measurement indicative of the left ventricle of the heart contracting (26, 34)

T lymphocytes—cells that promote immunity by binding to antigens on the cells of a foreign substance; *see also* cell-mediated response (27)

Table of Drugs and Chemicals—in an ICD-10-CM manual, an index of poisonings, adverse effects, and underdosing located at the end of the Index in most manuals (15)

Table of Neoplasms—in an ICD-10-CM manual, a list of neoplasms located under "N" in the alphabetic Index (15)

Tabular List—in an ICD-10-CM manual, numerical list of diseases and injuries, reasons for encounters, and external causes; provides additional instruction on how use, assign, and sequence codes (15, 16)

tachycardia—abnormally rapid heart rate (26, 34)

tachypnea—abnormally high respiration rate above 20 breaths per minute (34)

tact—sensitivity in dealing with others or with difficult issues (58)

talipes—congenital deformity of the foot (20)

tapotement—light tapping or percussion to relieve congestion that is performed with the sides of the hands, cupped hands, or fingertips to relieve congestion (51)

Tay-Sachs disease (TSD)—inherited disorder that attacks the nervous system usually causing death before age 5; affects primarily people of central and northern European Jewish or French-Canadian ancestry (20)

technical component—in coding for radiology, the performance of the imaging is the technical component, the review and analysis of the results by a qualified physician is the professional component (16)

technical safeguards—electronic protections that prevent unauthorized access to data such as encryption, passwords, and firewalls (12)

telemetry—transmission of measurements and other data from a remote area (49)

telephone triage—determining which callers' needs are the most urgent and where the calls must be directed (7)

tendon—band of connective tissue that attaches muscles to bones (23)

tendonitis—inflammation and irritation of the tendon, caused by microscopic tearing (23)

terminal-digit filing—filing system based on the last digits of the ID number that evenly distributes the files within the entire filing system (13)

terminal illness—condition that is expected to end in death (57)

testes—two oval-shaped organs in the scrotum in which sperm and testosterone are produced (31, 32)

tetanus—a disease of the nervous system that is caused by a bacterium that enters the body through a break in the skin, such as a puncture, cut, or open wound; also called *lockjaw* (23, 54)

thallium—radioisotope that emits gamma rays and is used in nuclear medicine (49)

therapeutic diet—a diet modified for health reasons (56)

thesaurus—reference book that lists words alphabetically and gives synonyms for each entry word (11)

third-party check—written as payment of another payee but presented to you (the third payee) as payment (15, 18)

third-party payer—party other than the patient who assumes responsibility for paying the patient's bills (e.g., an insurance company) (14)

thorax—the chest (28)

thready pulse—weak, or barely perceptible force or blood volume (34)

thrombocytes—*see* platelets (47)

thrombophlebitis—condition that occurs when a blood clot causes inflammation in one or more veins, typically those of the lower extremities (26)

thymus gland—lymphoid tissue located in the chest, in the anterior mediastinum, that manufactures infection-fighting T cells (27, 31)

thyroid gland—gland in the neck that is responsible for metabolism that secretes thyroxine, tri-iodothyronine, and calcitonin (31)

tickler file—appointment reminder system in which the tickler card (a self-addressed reminder postcard used for annual PAP tests and other types of follow-up appointments) is filed under the date it should be mailed (9)

tidal volume (V_T)—amount of air inhaled or exhaled during normal breathing (about 500 mL) (50)

time patterns—scheduling options (9)

tinea capitis—a fungal infection of the skin commonly located on the scalp (21)

tinea corporis—a fungal infection of the skin commonly found on the trunk and extremities; also called *ringworm* (21)

tinea cruris—fungal infection in the genital area; also called *jock itch* (21)

tinea pedis—fungal infection of the skin, commonly found on the foot; also called *athlete's foot* (21)

tinnitus—a ringing in one or both ears that is associated with many forms of hearing loss (25)

tissue—grouping of cells that performs a specialized function (20)

token signature—an electronic signature that may be used in electronic health records (EHRs) in which the user must click a button, enter a personal identification number, or complete a biometric scan, such as a fingerprint, to record the electronic signature (13)

tolerance—the need for larger and larger doses to achieve the same result after taking a medication for an extended time (57)

tonicity—ability of the body to maintain posture through a continuous partial contraction of skeletal muscles (23)

tonsillectomy—surgical removal of the tonsils (39)

tonsils—lymphoid tissues in the pharynx, consisting of the pharyngeal tonsils (adenoids), palatine tonsils, and lingual tonsils (27, 28)

topical medications—medications applied to the skin or the mucous membranes (54)

tort—legal wrong or error resulting in harm (3)

tortfeasor—a person who commits a tort; *see also* tort (3)

total lung capacity (TLC)—volume of the lungs at peak inspiration equal to the sum of the four volumes: tidal, expiratory reserve, inspiratory reserve, and residual volume (50)

touchscreen—display that includes sensors that detect the touch of a finger or stylus, which allows direct input into a computer device without use of a keyboard or mouse (12)

tourniquet—a device used to halt the flow of blood; typically a long ribbon of rubber or latex that is tied around the arm during phlebotomy (46)

toxic—harmful (53)

trace—investigate the reason for denial of payment by an insurance carrier (17)

trachea—cartilaginous tube between the larynx and the main bronchi; also called *windpipe* (28)

tract—group of nerve fibers within the central nervous system (24)

trailing zero rule—rule that states it is unacceptable to place a zero after a decimal point in a whole number (52)

transcranial magnetic stimulation (TMS)—a noninvasive procedure that causes depolarization or hyperpolarization in the neurons of the brain; TMS uses electromagnetic induction to induce a weak electric current that rapidly changes the magnetic field in the brain (57)

transdermal patch—medications administered by release over time from a patch placed on the skin (54)

triage—process of sorting patients according to the seriousness of their condition; also, to assess the emergency care needed by patients (9, 42)

tricuspid valve—heart valve from the right atrium to the right ventricle (26)

TRICARE—a federal insurance program for active duty and retired service personnel and their families (14)

Truth in Lending form—form that must clearly state the amount financed, the finance charge, and the total of the payments and that protects the consumer from loan-related fraud or deceit (17)

tuberculosis (TB)—highly contagious disease caused by the bacillus *Mycobacterium tuberculosis*, which can grow anywhere in the body but is most commonly found in the lungs, where granular tumors are produced in the infected tissues (28)

tuning fork—instrument used to measure a person's hearing ability (35)

turbid—cloudy from suspended particles (45)

turgor—the resistance of the skin when grasped between the fingers (35)

turnaround time—the time it takes to get test results (43)

Turner syndrome—congenital disorder caused by failure of the ovaries to respond to pituitary hormone stimulation; possible effects may include impaired intelligence, amenorrhea, and shortness of stature (20)

tympanic membrane—eardrum, which separates the outer and middle ears (25)

tympanic membrane thermometer—calculates the body temperature from the energy generated by the heat waves generated within the ear canal and near the eardrum; also called *aural thermometer* (34)

tympanometry—measurement of the ability of the tympanic membrane to move as an indication of pressure, as from fluid, in the middle ear (38)

tympanum—eardrum (38)

Type 1 diabetes—condition in which the body is unable to produce enough insulin to properly control blood sugar levels by converting sugar and starches into energy; typically diagnosed in children; also called *type 1 diabetes* or *juvenile diabetes* (31)

Type 2 diabetes—condition in which the body is unable to properly control blood sugar levels, resulting from insulin resistance combined with a relative insulin deficiency; often diagnosed later in life and having a very strong correlation with obesity; also called *type 2 diabetes* and *adult-onset diabetes* (31)

ulcerative colitis—chronic inflammatory condition of the colon (29)

unbundling—billing separately for related procedures that were performed together and, by law, must be billed as one charge; unbundling is considered fraud (14, 16)

uncertain diagnosis—a diagnosis accompanied by a term such as *possible, probable, suspected, rule out*, or *working diagnosis*; also called a *qualified diagnosis* (15)

underdose—an amount of medication that is insufficient to achieve the desired effect (52)

Uniform Anatomical Gift Act—a federal law that sets the regulatory framework for the donation of organs, tissues, or body parts in the United States (3)

universal precautions—actions recommended by the Centers for Disease Control and Prevention to protect health care workers from bloodborne pathogens; the universal precautions have been subsumed into and superseded by the CDC's list of standard precautions; *see also* standard precautions (33)

universal serial bus (USB) drive—portable computer storage device (12)

upcoding—billing for a service at a higher level than was actually provided (16)

ureters—tubes that carry newly formed urine from each kidney down to the bladder (30)

urethra—musculomembranous tube extending from the bladder to the urinary meatus (30, 32)

urethritis—inflammation of the urethra (32)

urgency—need to void or urinate immediately (30)

urinalysis—a test performed on urine to determine physical, chemical, and microscopic properties (45)

urinary bladder—muscular sac, located in the pelvic cavity, that serves as a reservoir for urine (30)

urinary meatus—the external opening of the urinary system (30)

urine—a waste product secreted by the kidneys (45)

urticaria—a severe itching because of acute hypersensitivity to medications or environmental stimuli; also called *hives* (21)

user log—in a practice management system, computer identification of who accessed the system, what information was accessed, and when it was accessed (17)

usual, customary, and reasonable (UCR)—refers to the usual fee a physician would charge for services, the customary fee a majority of physicians would charge for the same service, and a reasonable fee that the patient might expect to pay (used to determine medical benefits) (14)

uterine cancer—an adenocarcinoma that usually develops in the glandular tissue of the endometrium; also called *endometrial cancer* (32)

uterine fibroids—benign tumors made up of muscle cells and other tissues that grow within the wall of the uterus, manifesting as a single growth or a cluster (32)

uterus—hollow, pear-shaped, muscular organ located in the anterior portion of the female pelvic cavity (32)

vaccine—substance that contains the antigen and stimulates a primary response against the antigen without causing symptoms of the disease (27); substance that decreases the susceptibility to disease; also called *immunization* (54)

vacuum container—a tube with a vacuum suction that pulls in the exact amount of blood needed during venipuncture; also called an evacuated tube (46)

vagina—musculomembranous tube extending from the vestibule to the uterus (32)

vaginal speculum—instrument used to hold open the walls of the vagina (35)

vaginitis—inflammation of the vagina usually caused by a change in the normal balance of vaginal bacteria, by an infection, or by reduced estrogen levels after menopause (32)

values—set of standards a person uses to measure the worth or importance of someone or something (5)

vancomycin-resistant *Enterococci* **(VRE)**—type of bacteria that has developed resistance to antimicrobial drugs (33)

vancomycin-resistant *Staphylococcus aureus* **(VRSA)**—type of *S. aureus* organism resistant to the antibiotic vancomycin (33)

variables—areas of a form letter that require personalization, such as the date, inside address, and salutation, which can be stored on a separate CD or database from the constant information (11)

varicella—chicken pox (54)

vasectomy—surgery to render the male sterile, involving cutting the vas deferens and tying off the ends to prevent sperm from being transported out of the testes (37)

vastus lateralis muscle—part of the outer portion of the upper thigh that is also part of the quadriceps and is considered the safest site for IM injections (54)

veins—blood vessels that carry blood away from the cells and toward the heart (46)

vendor—supplier (10)

venipuncture—the process of cutting into or puncturing a vein, typically for the purpose of collecting blood samples for testing; also called *phlebotomy* (26, 46)

ventricles—two lower pumping chambers of the heart (26)

ventrogluteal site—muscle considered safer than the dorsogluteal muscle for IM injections because it has no major nerves or blood vessels (54)

veracity—truthfulness; truth in speech or statement (3)

verbal communication—spoken words and sounds or tone of voice a person uses to convey meanings (5)

verification of benefits (VOB)—determining if a patient is qualified to receive benefits or payment for a service under the guidelines of the insurance policy (14)

verify—when using an ICD-10-CM manual, to verify a code by consulting the Tabular List to read detailed code descriptions, conventions, and instructional notes and to assign addition specificity (15)

verrucae—warts (21)

vesicles—small blisters (21)

vestibule—middle part of the inner ear; also in the vagina, the space between the lines of attachment of the labia minora (25)

viable—capable of living (44)

vials—glass bottles with rubber stoppers to protect the contained medications (54)

viability—able to sustain life independently (37)

virus protection—software that scans computer data to detect and disable malicious programs (viruses) that can harm the computer data (12)

viscosity—thickness of a substance (54)

visual—of, related to, or used in vision (5)

visual acuity—clarity of vision (38)

vital capacity (VC)—amount of air that can be exhaled following forced inspiration and including maximum expiration (50)

vital signs—temperature, pulse, respirations, and blood pressure; pain is considered to be the fifth vital sign (34)

vitamins—organic substances essential for metabolism, growth, and development of the body (56)

vitiligo—pigmentation disorder that causes white patches and large areas of decreased pigmentation to form on the skin (21)

vitreous chamber—posterior cavity of the eyeball located behind the lens (25)

vitreous humor—thick fluid that fills the posterior cavity of the eyeball (25)

voice messaging system—allows voice messages to be left on a recorded device for a specific recipient (7)

void—to urinate; to pass urine (30, 45)

volume—strength or force of the pulse (34)

voucher check—a paycheck printed on a full-page voucher (18)

vulva—structure in the female reproductive system made up of the mons pubis, labia majora and labia minora, vestibule, and clitoris (32)

W-2 form—a federally required tax report that lists the employee's annual gross income; federal (income, Medicare, and Social Security), state, and local taxes withheld; taxable fringe benefits, such as tips; and the employee's net income for the year (18)

W-4 form—form completed by an employee when hired to determine the amount to be withheld from each paycheck for taxes (18)

waiting period—a period of time, designated by an insurance policy, that must elapse before coverage for specific services can begin (14)

warranty—guarantee that a product will work for a fixed period of time (10)

warts—type of infection caused by viruses in the human papillomavirus (HPV) family that can grow on all parts of the body, including on the skin, inside the mouth, on the genitals, and in the rectal area (21)

wave—movement away from the baseline in an electrocardiogram (49)

wave scheduling—scheduling system that is set to begin and end each hour on time, in which each hour is divided into equal segments of time depending on how many patients can be seen in an hour (9)

West's nomogram—chart used to identify body surface area to calculate pediatric dosages (52)

wet mount—a preparation in a liquid that will preserve motility of the microbe (44)

wheal—more or less round, temporary elevation of the skin, white in the center with a pale red periphery, accompanied by itching (36)

white cells—cells of the immune system that circulate in the blood; leukocytes (46)

withholding—the deduction of federal, state, and city taxes from gross wages (18)

word processor—a software application that enables creating, editing, storing, and printing written documents such as letters, manuscripts, and professional documents (12)

word root—word or element from which other words are formed (4)

workers' compensation—insurance carried by an employer that covers employees injured in the workplace or off-site while conducting company business or suffering a workplace-related illness (14)

World Wide Web (WWW)—communications network enabling the linking of computers worldwide for data interchange; the Internet (12)

X-rays—electromagnetic rays that have high energy and very short wavelengths and are not visible to the human eye; a photograph obtained by use of X-rays; also called *radiograph* (48)

Young's rule—pediatric dosage law applied to children over the age of 1 year, based on their age in years (52)

Z-track method—a method of injection that is used when a medication is irritating to the subcutaneous tissues or when the medication may discolor the skin (54)

Credits

Photo Credits

Chapter 1
Page 4: SelectStock/Vetta/Getty Images; American Association of Medical Assistants; page 7: Tetra Images/Getty Images; page 8: Hero Images/Getty Images; page 9: StockLite/Shutterstock; page 10: Copyright by the American Association of Medical Assistants, Inc. Reproduced with permission.; page 11: Janet Rosenberg/American Medical Technologists, Rosemont, IL; page 12: National Healthcareer Association; National Center for Competency Testing.

Chapter 2
Page 19: National Center for Competency Testing; page 20: Sheila Terry/Science Source; page 21: Science Source/Getty Images; page 23: Bettmann/Getty Images; Peter Purdy/BIPs/Hulton Archive/Getty Images; page 24: Everett Collection Historical/Alamy Stock Photo; page 29: David Mager/Pearson Education, Inc.; Alle12/Vetta/Getty Images; page 32: Michal Heron/Pearson Education, Inc.; page 33: Morsa Images/DigitalVision/Getty Images; page 34: Michal Heron/Pearson Education, Inc.; page 37: Bartee Photography Inc./Pearson Learning; page 38: Ariel Skelley/Blend Images/Getty Images; page 40: Chad Baker/Jason Reed/Ryan McVay/Photodisc/Getty Images.

Chapter 3
Page 54: Michal Heron/Pearson Education, Inc.; page 72: Michal Heron/Pearson Education, Inc.

Chapter 5
Pages 106–107: Michal Heron/Pearson Education, Inc.; page 114: Dylan Malone/Pearson Education, Inc.; page 114: Vasilchenko Nikita/Shutterstock; page 115: Halfdark/fStop/Getty Images; page 115: Fakezzz/Fotolia; page 116: Sturti/Vetta/Getty Images; page 118: Michal Heron/Pearson Education, Inc.; page 119: Michal Heron/Pearson Education, Inc.; page 120: Faye Norman/Science Source; page 121: Dylan Malone/Pearson Education, Inc.; page 125: Michal Heron/Pearson Education, Inc.; page 128: Michal Heron/Pearson Education, Inc.

Chapter 6
Page 138: Apomares/iStock/Getty Images; page 141: Simo988/Shutterstock; page 141: Cool Vector Maker/Shutterstock; page 141: Kaspri/Shutterstock; page 141: BEGUN/Shutterstock; page 141: Stephen Marques/Shutterstock; page 143: Michal Heron/Pearson Education, Inc.; page 145: Huntstock/DisabilityImages/Getty Images; page 145: Michal Heron/Pearson Education, Inc.; page 146: Thom Hanssen Images/Shutterstock; pages 147–148: Michal Heron/Pearson Education, Inc.; page 150: Lisa F. Young/Shutterstock; page 152: Shutterstock; page 153: Michal Heron/Pearson Education, Inc.

Chapter 7
Page 159: Racorn/Shutterstock; page 160: Michal Heron/Pearson Education, Inc.; page 164: Jamie Grill/Tetra images/Getty Images;

page 165: Michal Heron/Pearson Education, Inc.; page 167: Minerva Studio/Shutterstock; page 175: Michal Heron/Pearson Education, Inc.

Chapter 8
Page 181: Tyler Olson/Shutterstock; page 183: Henglein and Steets/Cultura/Getty Images; page 187: Thinkstock Images/Stockbyte/Getty Images; page 194: Michal Heron/Pearson Education, Inc.

Chapter 9
Page 201: Shutterstock; page 201: Tyler Olson/Shutterstock; page 204: Michal Heron/Pearson Education, Inc.

Chapter 10
Page 224: Stuart Westmorland/Image Source/Getty Images; page 225: Brooklyn Production/Corbis; page 226: Rob Byron/Shutterstock; page 227: Fotosearch/Getty Images; page 228: Nicholas/E+/Getty Images; page 234: Ekaterina79/iStock/Getty Images; page 236: Michal Heron/Pearson Education, Inc.

Chapter 11
Pages 247, 253–255: Michal Heron/Pearson Education, Inc.

Chapter 12
Page 265: Science Photo Library/Brand X Pictures/Getty Images; page 266: Michal Heron/Pearson Education, Inc.; page 267: Kristiana Routh; pages 269, 272: Michal Heron/Pearson Education, Inc.; page 281: Dpa picture alliance/Alamy Stock Photo.

Chapter 13
Page 294: Shutterstock; page 295: Logoboom/Shutterstock; page 297: Michal Heron/Pearson Education, Inc.; page 309: Alexskopje/Shutterstock; page 310: JohnKwan/Shutterstock; page 312: Sergey Nivens/Shutterstock; page 314: Pearson Education, Inc.; page 315: Michal Heron/Pearson Education, Inc.

Chapter 18
Page 465: Image Source/Photodisc/Getty Images.

Chapter 19
Page 498: Skynesher/Vetta/Getty Images; page 502: Image Source/Getty Images; page 506: Michal Heron/Pearson Education, Inc.; page 511: ESB Professional/Shutterstock; page 511: Michal Heron/Pearson Education, Inc.; page 511: Fmua/Shutterstock.

Chapter 20
Page 529: Tose/Shutterstock; page 538: Denys Kuvaiev/Fotolia.

Chapter 21
Page 548: Centers for Disease Control and Prevention (CDC); page 549: Suzanne Tucker/Shutterstock; page 550: Scott Camazine/Alamy Stock Photo; page 550: DonyaHHI/Shutterstock; page 551: Alila Medical Media/Shutterstock; page 552: Mediscan/Alamy Stock Photo; page 552: Cherries/Shutterstock; page 554: BSIP SA/Alamy Stock Photo;

page 554: Weerachat/Shutterstock; page 555: Mediscan/Alamy Stock Photo; page 556: Rodrigo Bellizzi/Shutterstock; page 556: Kanachaifoto/Fotolia.

Chapter 22
Page 572: Pearson Education, Inc.; page 572: Ivan Smuk/Shutterstock; page 574: ©Edward T. Dickinson, MD; page 575: Fenton/Fotolia.

Chapter 23
Page 585: Stihii/Shutterstock; page 591: Nucleus Medical Art, Inc./Alamy Stock Photo.

Chapter 25
Page 621: Grebcha/iStock/Getty Images.

Chapter 26
Page 655: Dr. P. Marazzi/Science Source; page 655: Lauren Shavell/Design Pics/Getty Images.

Chapter 27
Page 667: BanksPhotos/E+/Getty Images; page 670: Al Dodge/Pearson Education, Inc.; page 671: Designua/Shutterstock.

Chapter 28
Page 685: Science Photo Library - NATIONAL CANCER INSTITUTE/Brand X Pictures/Getty Images; page 687: Dorling Kindersley/Getty Images.

Chapter 32
Page 750: Noctiluxx/E+/Getty Images.

Chapter 33
Page 774: Designua/Shutterstock; page 779: Thom Hanssen Images/Shutterstock; pages 780–781: Michal Heron/Pearson Education, Inc.; page 783: Racorn/Shutterstock; pages 784–785: Michal Heron/Pearson Education, Inc.; page 786: StockPhotoPro/Fotolia; page 786: Image Lagoon/Shutterstock; page 786: Andrey Popov/Shutterstock; page 786: Michal Heron/Pearson Education, Inc.; page 786: YanLev/Shutterstock; page 787: Beerkoff/Shutterstock; page 788: Michal Heron/Pearson Education, Inc.; page 789: DenGuy/E+/Getty Images; page 790: Michal Heron/Pearson Education, Inc.; page 791: Daniel Suarez; pages 792–793: Michal Heron/Pearson Education, Inc.; page 794: Al Dodge/Pearson Education, Inc.

Chapter 34
Pages 799–800: Michal Heron/Pearson Education, Inc.; page 801: Dave and Les Jacobs/Blend Images/Getty Images; page 805: Khamidulin Sergey/Shutterstock; page 805: Rob Marmion/Shutterstock; pages 806, 808–809: Michal Heron/Pearson Education, Inc.; page 809: Pegasusa012/iStock/Getty Images; page 810: Michal Heron/Pearson Education, Inc.; page 811: JPC-PROD/Fotolia; page 814: Richard Tauber/Pearson Education, Inc.; page 814: Leungchopan/Shutterstock; pages 816–817: Michal Heron/Pearson Education, Inc.; pages 823–824: George Draper/Pearson Education, Inc.; page 824: v777999/iStock/Getty Images; page 825: George Draper/Pearson Education, Inc.; page 826: Michal Heron/Pearson Education, Inc.; page 828: Juan R. Velasco/Shutterstock; page 828: Click and Photo/Shutterstock.

Chapter 35
Page 844: George Draper/Pearson Education, Inc.; page 846: StockLite/Shutterstock; pages 846–847: Richard Tauber/Pearson Education, Inc.; page 847: Shutterstock; page 847: Erik Isakson/Tetra images/Getty Images; page 848: Richard Tauber/Pearson Education, Inc.

Chapter 36
Page 869: Southern Illinois University/Science Source; page 870: Science Photo Library/Brand X Pictures/Getty Images; page 872: George Draper/Pearson Education, Inc.; page 873: JodiJacobson/E+/Getty Images; page 873: BSIP/Universal Images Group/Getty Images; page 875: RapidEye/E+/Getty Images; page 875: Track5/E+/Getty Images; page 877: Syda Productions/Shutterstock; pages 878, 881: George Draper/Pearson Education, Inc.; page 884: Wang Song/Shutterstock; page 884: Itsmejust/Shutterstock; page 886: George Draper/Pearson Education, Inc.

Chapter 37
Page 893: George Draper/Pearson Education, Inc.; page 898: Andrey Chmelyov/Shutterstock; page 900: Ian Hooton/Science Photo Library/Getty Images; page 902: Dip/Shutterstock; page 905: George Draper/Pearson Education, Inc.; page 906: Alila Medical Media/Shutterstock; page 913: BSIP SA/Alamy Stock Photo.

Chapter 38
Page 920: George Draper/Pearson Education, Inc.; page 921: Michal Heron/Pearson Education, Inc.; page 923: Tyler Olson/Shutterstock; page 925: Damrong Sirottamaphorn/Shutterstock; page 926: Wavebreakmedia/Shutterstock; pages 926, 928: Michal Heron/Pearson Education, Inc.; page 929: Michal Heron/Pearson Education, Inc.; page 930: Adam James/Alamy Stock Photo; page 931: Brian Eichhorn/Shutterstock.

Chapter 39
Page 939: Yarinca/E+/Getty Images; page 940: Michal Heron/Pearson Education, Inc.; page 942: Leanne Temme/Photodisc/Getty Images; page 942: Woraput/E+/Getty Images; page 942: fatihhoca/E+/Getty Images; page 942: LattaPictures/E+/Getty Images; page 942: Hero Images/Getty Images; page 943: BassittART/E+/Getty Images; page 944: Beneda Miroslav/Shutterstock; page 946: Beneda Miroslav/Shutterstock; page 946: Andrii Malkov/Shutterstock; page 947: Marlon Lopez/MMG1 Design/Shutterstock.

Chapter 40
Page 962: Juanmonino/Vetta/Getty Images; pages 962–963: Michal Heron/Pearson Education, Inc.; page 965: John Clutterbuck/Photographer's Choice RF/Getty Images; page 969: Vm/E+/Getty Images; page 969: Tigatelu/Fotolia; page 972: Sturti/E+/Getty Images; page 973: dszc/E+/Getty Images; page 978: Ronnie Kaufman/Larry Hirshowitz/Blend Images/Getty Images.

Chapter 41
Pages 986, 988: Michal Heron/Pearson Education, Inc.; page 989: Al Dodge/Pearson Education, Inc.; page 991: George Draper/Pearson Education, Inc.; page 992: Michal Heron/Pearson Education, Inc.; pages 993–995: Al Dodge/Pearson Education, Inc.; page 996: Nikuwka/Shutterstock; page 996: Sto/Shutterstock; page 996: Michal Heron/Pearson Education, Inc.; page 996: Al Dodge/Pearson Education, Inc.; page 997: WeStudio/Shutterstock; page 997: Howard Klaast/Shutterstock; page 997: Constantine Pankin/Shutterstock; page 997: Michal Heron/Pearson Education, Inc.; pages 997–998: George Draper/Pearson Education, Inc.; pages 998–999: Al Dodge/Pearson Education, Inc.; page 1001: Michal Heron/Pearson Education, Inc.; page 1002: Al Dodge/Pearson Education, Inc.; page 1006: Al Dodge/Pearson Education, Inc.; page 1008: George Draper/Pearson Education, Inc.; page 1009: Michal Heron/Pearson Education, Inc.; page 1011 (suture kit): Al Dodge/Pearson Education, Inc.; (all others)

Michal Heron/Pearson Education, Inc.; **page 1012:** Al Dodge/Pearson Education, Inc.; **page 1014:** Al Dodge/Pearson Education, Inc.; **page 1015:** Michal Heron/Pearson Education, Inc.; **page 1016:** Al Dodge/Pearson Education, Inc.; **page 1016:** Michal Heron/Pearson Education, Inc.

Chapter 42

Page 1022: Michal Heron/Pearson Education, Inc.; **page 1025:** George Draper/Pearson Education, Inc.; **page 1028:** George Draper/Pearson Education, Inc.; **page 1028:** Michal Heron/Pearson Education, Inc.; **page 1035:** Michal Heron/Pearson Education, Inc.; **pages 1036–1039:** Michal Heron/Pearson Education, Inc.; **page 1042:** Luciano Cosmo/Shutterstock; **page 1046:** Pearson Education, Inc.; **page 1053:** Michal Heron/Pearson Education, Inc.

Chapter 43

Page 1073: Andy Crawford/DK Images; **pages 1074–1075:** Michal Heron/Pearson Education, Inc.

Chapter 44

Page 1080: Pearson Education, Inc.; **page 1080:** Kwangshin Kim/Science Source/Getty Images; **page 1083:** Stocktrek Images/Getty Images; **page 1083:** Biophoto Associates/Science Source/Getty Images; **page 1083:** Al Dodge/Pearson Education, Inc.; **page 1084:** Philartphace/E+/Getty Images; **page 1086:** Moredun Animal Health Ltd./Science Source; **page 1086:** R. Parulan Jr./Moment/Getty Images; **page 1086:** Ezume Images/Fotolia; **page 1087:** Dr. Klaus Boller/Science Source; **page 1087:** Pearson Education, Inc.; **page 1087:** Stocktrek Images/Getty Images; **page 1088:** Puhimec/Fotolia; **page 1088:** Debbie Maizels/DK Images; **page 1090:** George Draper/Pearson Education, Inc.; **page 1091:** Brian Warling/Pearson Education, Inc.; **pages 1092–1095:** Michal Heron/Pearson Education, Inc.; **page 1097:** Ksass/E+/Getty Images; **page 1098:** Michal Heron/Pearson Education, Inc.; **page 1099:** Wideweb/Shutterstock; **page 1099:** Michal Heron/Pearson Education, Inc.; **page 1101:** Michal Heron/Pearson Education, Inc.

Chapter 45

Page 1108: George Draper/Pearson Education, Inc.; **page 1110:** Michal Heron/Pearson Education, Inc.; **page 1115:** Al Dodge/Pearson Education, Inc.; **page 1115:** George Draper/Pearson Education, Inc.; **pages 1117–1118, 1121, 1123–1124:** Michal Heron/Pearson Education, Inc.; **pages 1126, 1129:** George Draper/Pearson Education, Inc.

Chapter 46

Page 1138: Michal Heron/Pearson Education, Inc.; **page 1138:** George Draper/Pearson Education, Inc.; **page 1138:** Dmitry Lobanov/Shutterstock; **page 1139:** Michal Heron/Pearson Education, Inc.; **page 1140:** AFP/Stringer/Getty Images; **page 1140:** Science photo/Shutterstock; **page 1141:** Alexander Tihonov/Shutterstock; **page 1141:** Bluebeat76/Fotolia; **page 1143:** George Draper/Pearson Education, Inc.; **page 1144:** Michal Heron/Pearson Education, Inc.; **page 1144:** Defun/iStock/Getty Images; **page 1148:** Angellodeco/Fotolia; **page 1149:** Michal Heron/Pearson Education, Inc.; **pages 1150–1152:** Michal Heron/Pearson Education, Inc.

Chapter 47

Page 1159: Energyy/Getty Images; **page 1160:** Science Source; **page 1162:** Nicram Sabod/Shutterstock; **pages 1162–1163:** Nicram Sabod/Shutterstock; **page 1162:** Nicram Sabod/Shutterstock; **page 1165:** Nicram Sabod/Shutterstock; **page 1165:** Sergey Ryzhov/Alamy; **pages 1166, 1168–1169:** George Draper/Pearson Education, Inc.; **page 1167:** Al Dodge/Pearson Education, Inc.

Chapter 48

Page 1184: Edwardolive/Shutterstock; **page 1187:** Skyhawk x/Shutterstock; **page 1187:** Jayakumar/Shutterstock; **page 1187:** Pisaphotography/Shutterstock; **page 1187:** Puwadol Jaturawutthichai/123RF; **page 1190:** CNRI/Science Source; **page 1193:** Tyler Olson/Shutterstock; **page 1193:** MarcelClemens/Shutterstock; **page 1194:** Flik47/Shutterstock; **page 1194:** Tyler Olson/Shutterstock; **page 1195:** Puwadol Jaturawutthichai/Shutterstock; **page 1195:** Scott Camazine/Alamy; **page 1196:** Dana Neely/Taxi/Getty Images; **page 1197:** Bart78/Shutterstock; **page 1197:** GagliardiImages/Shutterstock; **page 1198:** George Draper/Pearson Education, Inc.

Chapter 49

Page 1210: Oksana2010/Shutterstock; **page 1215:** Bork/Shutterstock; **page 1222:** Brittny/Shutterstock; **page 1223:** Zio system. Courtesy of iRhythm Technologies; **page 1224:** Choja/E+/Getty Images; **page 1225:** Don Farrall/DigitalVision/Getty Images; **page 1225:** Michal Heron/Pearson Education, Inc.

Chapter 50

Page 1230: Sfam Photo/Shutterstock; **page 1230:** ChooChin/Shutterstock; **page 1230:** Living Art Enterprises/Science Source/Getty Images; **page 1230:** Science Photo Library-CNRI/SPL/Brand X Pictures/Getty Images; **page 1232:** Javier Larrea/age fotostock/Getty Images; **page 1233:** ellepigrafica/Shutterstock; **page 1236:** Michal Heron/Pearson Education, Inc.; **page 1237:** KaferPhoto/Fotolia; **page 1238:** George Draper/Pearson Education, Inc.; **page 1239:** Juanmonino/E+/Getty Images; **page 1239:** Sarema/Shutterstock; **page 1239:** Davidf/E+/Getty Images; **page 1239:** Zvyagintsev Sergey/Shutterstock; **page 1241:** Khuntapol/Shutterstock; **page 1242:** Aaron Haupt/Science Source/Getty Images; **page 1242:** Abalcazar/E+/Getty Images; **page 1242:** Jeff Greenberg 6 of 6/Alamy Stock Photo.

Chapter 51

Pages 1247–1248: Tyler Olson/Shutterstock; **page 1249:** Kali9/E+/Getty Images; **page 1254:** George Draper/Pearson Education, Inc.; **pages 1255–1257:** Michal Heron/Pearson Education, Inc.; **page 1261:** Dan Porges/Photolibrary/Getty Images; **page 1261:** George Draper/Pearson Education, Inc.; **page 1261:** Michal Heron/Pearson Education, Inc.; **page 1264:** George Draper/Pearson Education, Inc.; **page 1265:** Michal Heron/Pearson Education, Inc.; **page 1267:** Shutterstock; **page 1268:** Robert Kneschke/Shutterstock; **page 1269:** Michal Heron/Pearson Education, Inc.

Chapter 53

Page 1300: Michal Heron/Pearson Education, Inc.; **page 1300:** ConnectiveRx Corporate Headquarters; **page 1305:** Lisa F. Young/Shutterstock; **page 1314:** Gerhard Koppl/Alamy; **pages 1325, 1328:** Michal Heron/Pearson Education, Inc.; **page 1328:** Sarema/Shutterstock; **page 1330:** Moodboard/Cultura/Getty Images; **page 1331:** George Draper/Pearson Education, Inc.; **page 1331:** Al Dodge/Pearson Education, Inc.; **pages 1332–1333:** Michal Heron/Pearson Education, Inc.; **page 1335:** Magicoven/Shutterstock; **pages 1338, 1343:** Pearson Education, Inc.; **page 1344:** Di Studio/Shutterstock.

Chapter 55

Page 1359: Bleakstar/Shutterstock; **page 1361:** Kamil Macniak/Shutterstock; **page 1362:** Syda Productions/Shutterstock; **page 1363:** YinYang/E+/Getty Images; **page 1366:** Glow Images/Getty Images; **page 1368:** Nazdravie/iStock/Getty Images Plus/Getty Images; **page 1369:** Track5/E+/Getty Images.

Chapter 56

Page 1382: Flyfloor/E+/Getty Images; **page 1382:** CHRISsadowski/ E+/ Getty Images; **page 1383:** Fuse/Corbis/Getty Images; **page 1387:** Denise Bush/ E+/Getty Images; **page 1391:** Erik Isakson/Tetra images/Getty Images.

Chapter 57

Page 1411: Will & Deni McIntyre/Science Source/Getty Images; **page 1411:** George Dodson/Pearson Education, Inc.; **page 1412:** Hogan Imaging/Shutterstock; **page 1412:** Bikeriderlondon/Shutterstock; **page 1413:** William Perugini/Shutterstock; **page 1413:** Hero Images/ Getty Images; **page 1415:** Sturti/Vetta/Getty Images; **page 1415:** WavebreakmediaMicro/Fotolia.

Chapter 58

Pages 1426–1427: Michal Heron/Pearson Education, Inc.; **page 1430:** Iodrakon/Shutterstock.

Chapter 59

Page 1435: Bowdenimages/iStock/Getty Images; **page 1436:** Lisa F. Young/Shutterstock; **page 1437:** Asiseeit/E+/Getty Images; **page 1438:** Shutterstock; **page 1440:** Donald Gruener/E+/Getty Images; **pages 1446, 1448:** Alexander Raths/Shutterstock.

Text Credits

Chapter 1

Page 4: From CAAHEP Standards and Guidelines for Medical Assistants. Published by Commission on Accreditation of Allied Health Education Programs, © 2015; **page 5:** From Commission on Accreditation of Allied Health Education Programs. Published by Commission on Accreditation of Allied Health Education Programs, © 2015; **page 11:** From Certification Eligibility Criteria. Copyright © 2013 by American Medical Technologists. Used by permission of American Medical Technologists.

Chapter 3

Page 61: Communicable Disease Reporting Requirements from New York State Department of Health. Published by New York State Department of Health; **page 62:** Confidential Case Report from New York State Department of Health. Published by New York State Department of Health; **page 69:** Copyright by the American Association of Medical Assistants, Inc. Reproduced with permission.; **pages 69–70:** From AMT Standards of Practice. Copyright by American Medical Technologists. Used by permission of American Medical Technologists.

Chapter 6

Page 140: From Occupational Safety and Health Administration. Published by United States Department of Labor; **page 141:** www.unitedadlabel.com.

Chapter 14

Page 343: Advance Beneficiary Notice Form from Centers for Medicare and Medicaid Services. Published by Centers for Medicare and Medicaid Services; **page 356:** CMS-1500 (02/12) Caim Form from Centers for Medicare and Medicaid Services. Published by Centers for Medicare and Medicaid Services; **page 366:** A Completed CMS-1500 (02/12) Claim Form from Centers for Medicare and Medicaid Services. Published by Centers for Medicare and Medicaid Services; **page 368:** A Completed CMS-1500 (02/12) Claim Form from Centers for Medicare and Medicaid Services. Published by Centers for Medicare and Medicaid Services.

Chapter 16

Page 398: From Health Insurance Claim Form. Published by Centers for Medicare and Medicaid Services; **pages 407, 414:** CPT only copyright 2015 American Medical Association. All rights reserved; **page 423:** Form from Centers for Medicare and Medicaid Services. Published by Centers for Medicare and Medicaid Services.

Chapter 17

Page 443: Screenshot of Medicare Remit Easy Print, Centers for Medicare and Medicaid Services.

Chapter 18

Pages 487–488: W-4 Form from Internal Revenue Service. Published by Internal Revenue Service; **page 490:** W-2 Form from Internal Revenue Service. Published by Internal Revenue Service.

Chapter 19

Page 504: Screenshot of Allied Health Consulting Service. Copyright © by Allied Health Consulting Service; **pages 508–510:** I-9 Form from U.S. Citizenship and Immigration Services. Published by U.S. Citizenship and Immigration Services.

Chapter 33

Page 777: Data from Guidelines for Isolation Precaution in Hospitals, developed by the Centers for Disease Control and Prevention and the Hospital Infection Control Practices Advisory Committee, January 2002.

Chapter 36

Pages 869, 882: Pearson Education, Inc.

Chapter 39

Page 949: From National Center for Health Statistics. Published by Centers for Disease Control and Prevention; **page 950:** From National Center for Health Statistics in Collaboration with the National Center for Chronic Disease Prevention and Health Promotion. Published by Centers for Disease Control and Prevention.

Chapter 40

Page 965: From National Vital Statistics Reports, Vol 57, Number 14. Published by Centers for Disease Control and Prevention; **pages 976–977:** From Know the 10 Signs. Copyright © 2009 by Alzheimer's Association. Used by permission of Alzheimer's Association; **pages 980–981:** Sample Living Will from An Advance Directive for North Carolina. Published by North Carolina Department of the Secretary of State; **pages 1027–1029:** Mood Assessment Scale by Dr. Jerome Yesavage from Stanford University. Copyright by Stanford University.

Chapter 43

Page 1069: CLIA 1992 Standards.

Chapter 44

Page 1085: Centers for Disease Control and Prevention (CDC).

Chapter 52

Page 1284: From Extravascular Administration by Anas Bahnassi. Copyright © by Anas Bahnassi.; **page 1296:** www.labcorp.com.

Chapter 54

Page 1352: From Recommended Immunization Schedules for Persons Aged 0 Through 18 Years, United Sates, 2016. Published by U.S. Department of Health and Human Services; **pages 1353–1354:** From Vaccine Information Statement. Published by U.S. Department of Health and Human Services.

Chapter 56

Page 1390: From United States Department of Agriculture. Published by United States Department of Agriculture.

Index

DEA (Drug Enforcement Administration), 1299, 1307

DEA number, drug prescription, 1315

Death and dying. *See* terminal illnesses

DeBakey, Michael, 24, 24f

Debits, 464

Debridement, 873

Decibels, hearing assessment, 929, 930f

Decimals, 1279–1280, 1280t

Decubitus position, 858, 858f

Decubitus ulcer, 551, 551f, 872–873, 873f

Deductibles, health insurance, 331–332

Deductions, payroll management, 486–489, 486f, 488f, 489f

DEERS (Defense Enrollment Eligibility Reporting System), 345

Defamation of character, 51

Defendant, 47

Defense Enrollment Eligibility Reporting System (DEERS), 345

Defenses
  blood, 643
  immune response, 663–665

Defensive behavior, 117

Defibrillation, 1032, 1034–1035

Degenerative joint disease (DJD), 572, 572f

Degree programs, 5

Dehiscence, 1007

Dehydration, in infants, 954

Delegation of duties, medical assistant, 8

Delinquent accounts, 453–454

Delirium, 1404

Delta cells, 730

Deltoid, 585, 586f, 1334–1335

Delusions, 1406

Dementia, 975–978, 1404

Democratic leadership style, 500

Demographic information, 188

Demyelination, 610

Dendrites, 598

Denied claims, 334

Denominator, 1277

Dental hygienist, 37, 37f

Dentin, 695, 695f

Deoxyribonucleic acid (DNA), 528–529, 529f

Dependents, health insurance for, 331

Depolarization, electric cardiac activity, 1206

Depo-Provera, 905

Deposition, 58

Deposits
  financial management, 472–475
  required deposits, 489

Depreciation, capital equipment, 227

Depression
  diagnosis and treatment, 1406
  in older patients, 974–975

Dereliction/neglect of duty, 47

Dermatology, 28, 91
  medical assistant duties in, 871–873, 872t, 873f

Dermis, 544

Desensitizing injections, 868

Desktop publishing, 274

Developmental disorders, 1404–1405

Developmental skills checklist, 941t

Dexterity, loss of, in older patients, 1366–1367

Diabetes mellitus, 736–738
  blood testing with, 1176
  chronic renal failure, 721–722, 722f
  diet for patients with, 1395
  emergency management of, 1040–1042
  glucose monitoring in, 875–877, 875f
  medical assistant and management of, 876–877
  medical law and ethics, 736
  type 1, 732, 736–737
  type 2, 737

Diabetic retinopathy, 624

Diagnosis and treatment plan, 310
  physical examination, 848

Diagnosis Related Groups (DRGs), 329–330

Diagnostic and Statistical Manual of Mental Disorders, Fifth Edition (DSM-5), 957, 1403, 1403t

Diagnostic cluster careers, 38–40

Diagnostic coding, 377–392
  certification exam preparation, 393
  competency review, 392–393
  compliance, 379–380, 380t
  critical thinking, 394
  history, 378, 378t
  internet activity, 394
  on the job, 394
  procedures, 383–392
  special situations, 391, 391t–392t

Diagnostic imaging
  contrast medium, 1184–1185
  medical assistant, 1185–1186
  overview, 1184–1185
  procedures, 1189–1198, 1189t
  scheduling guidelines, 1187–1188
  technician, 39

Diagnostic terminology, 96–98, 97t

Diagnostic testing, 294, 294f, 310, 310f
  allergies, 868–871, 869f, 869t, 870f
  automated ordering, 322, 323f, 324
  cardiovascular system, 646t–647t, 874
  digestive system, 700t–701t
  endocrine system disorders, 735t
  hearing assessment, 929–933, 929f
  muscular disorders, 588t
  Pap test, 753–754
  physical examination, 858, 859t
  prostate cancer, 906
  radiology, 1182–1203
  rehabilitative medicine, 1271–1272
  skeletal system, 571t

Dialysis, 721, 721f

Diaphoresis, 874

Diaphragm, 586, 680, 680f

Diaphragm (barrier contraceptive), 904

Diaphysis, 563

Diarrhea, 953–954

Diarthrotic joint, 564f, 565, 565t

Diastolic blood pressure, 641, 819

Diathermy, 1259–1260

Diencephalon, 601f, 602

Diet. *See also* nutrition
  cancer patients, 1392–1393
  for gastrointestinal issues, 1395–1396
  healthy diet and lifestyle, 1386–1392, 1387t
  low-fat/low-cholesterol, 1393–1394
  low-sodium, 1394–1395
  modifications for medical or surgical procedures, 1396–1397
  nutrients in, 1379–1386
  nutrition, 1374–1377, 1375f–1376f
  portion sizes, 1387t
  restrictive or food sensitivity diet, 1392
  special needs and modifications, 1392–1398
  weight control, 1393

Dietary supplements, 1385, 1385f

Dietitian, 36–37

Differential backup, 278

Differential diagnosis, 848

Differential white blood cell count, 1168–1170, 1168

Diffusion, 533

Digestion, 1377–1378, 1378f

Digestive enzymes, 693

Digestive system, 95, 95t, 692–711, 877–883
  accessory organs, 697–698
  aging, 971
  certification exam preparation, 710–711
  competency review, 710
  critical thinking, 711
  disorders of, 698–710, 699t, 700t–701t
  functions and organs, 692–698, 693f, 694t
  internet activity, 711
  muscles, 581
  nutrition, 1377

Digital radiology, 1195

Digital rectal examination (DRE), 906

Digital thermometer, 804–807, 804f, 944

Digitized signature, 297

Dignity, professionalism, 1422

Dilation
  of blood vessels, 1137, 1137f
  of cervix, 749–750, 902

Diphtheria vaccine, 1349

Diplococci bacteria, 1084, 1085f

Diplomacy, professionalism, 1421

Diploma programs, 5

Diplopia, 620, 620t

Dipstick analysis, urine specific gravity, 1118–1123, 1118f

Direct cause, 47

Directive communication techniques, 109–111, 111t

Direct specimen management, 1097–1101

Disability income insurance, 347

communication, 114–115, 114f, 115f
patients impaired emotionally, 122
Empathy, 9, 111, 111f
Emphysema, 683
Employees
at-will employment, 511
categories of, 483–484
disciplinary process, 513–514
employment eligibility verification, 507, 508f–510f
manager's responsibilities to, 495–497, 496t
motivation of, 498–500
payroll management, 483–490
performance evaluations, 511–513, 512f
probation period for, 507
records for, 495
safety of, 141–146
soft skills of, 1421
Employers
Health Plan Employer Data and Information Set, 153–154
loyalty to, 129
manager's responsibilities to, 495–497, 496t
skills needed by, 1448–1449
Employment eligibility verification, 507, 508f–510f
EMR (Emergency medical responder), 37, 1022
EMS (Emergency Medical Services) systems, 1022
EMT (Emergency medical technician), 37, 1022
Enamel (teeth), 695, 695f
Encephalitis, 608
Enclosure notation, in business letters, 248
Encounter forms, 186, 192–193, 355, 357f, 429–430, 1423
Encryption, computer systems, 277
Endocarditis, 649
Endocardium, 633, 633f
Endocervical curettage (ECC), 1015
Endocrine system, 95–96, 96t, 724–741
aging, 971–972
certification exam preparation, 740–741
competency review, 740
critical thinking, 741
disorders, 727t, 733–740
exocrine system vs., 725, 725f
function, 726–727, 726f, 727t
glands in, 727–733
hyper- and hyposecretion in, 726–727, 727t
internet activity, 741
overview, 725, 726f
procedures and diagnostic testing, 734t
Endocrinology, 22, 28, 95–96, 96t
medical assistants in, 874–877
Endometrial biopsy (EMB), 1015
Endometriosis, 755
Endorsement, 26
of checks, 471, 472t
Endoscopy, 1015, 1015f. See also colonoscopy
Endosteum, 564
End-stage renal disease, 721–722, 722f

Energy production, muscular system, 583
ENG (Electronystagmograph), 930
ENT (Ear, nose and throat). See otorhinolaryngology; sensory systems
Entropion, 621t
Enunciation, 159–160, 159t
Enuresis, 718
Envelopes, business letters, 253, 253f, 253t
Environmental exposure, 1056–1057
Enzyme-linked immunoassays (EIA/ELISA) tests, 1128
EOB (Explanation of benefits), 439, 441, 442f, 443
Eosinophils, tests involving, 1169–1170, 1168
Epidermis, 543–544
Epididymis, 762, 762f
Epididymitis, 763–764
Epidural anesthesia, 1004–1005
Epigastric region, 89, 91f
Epiglottis, 677, 678f
Epilepsy, 608
Epinephrine, 667, 667f
EpiPen, 667, 667f
Epiphyseal fracture, 575
Epiphysis, 563
Episiotomy, 746
Epistaxis, 1041–1042
Epithelial cells
cancer, 755–756
microscopic urinalysis, 1125
Epithelial tissue, 530
E-prescriptions, 1316
Epstein-Barr virus (EBV), 669, 1179
Equipment maintenance and preparation, 186, 227–229, 227f, 227t
adaptive equipment and devices, 1260–1271, 1261f
capillary puncture, 1138–1140, 1138f
clinical equipment, 230
electrocardiogram machine, 1209–1211, 1210f, 1211f
inhaled medication administration, 1326, 1326f
injectable medications, 1329–1332
inventory records, 229t
laboratory equipment, 1071–1075
maintenance logs, 230f
oral medication administration, 1323f
for physical examinations, 843–845, 844f, 845t
purchasing procedures, 228
safety issues, 228–229
sterile field setup, 986–987
updates, 1236
venipuncture, 1143–1145, 1143f, 1144f, 1149f
Equivalents, pharmacology mathematics, 1280, 1280t, 1284t
ERA (Electronic remittance advice), 441
Erectile dysfunction (ED), 764

Ergonomics, 147
computer systems, 285–286, 285f
Erikson, Erik, 1410
Erikson's developmental stages of life, 1410–1411
Errors
electronic health records and avoidance of, 295
in patient care, 65
in written communications, 245
ERT (External radiation therapy), 1198
ERV (Expiratory reserve volume), 1233
Erysipelas, 873
Erythema, 550, 550f, 1252
Erythema migrans, 589–590
Erythrocyte count, 1161
Erythrocyte/RBC indices, 1161
Erythrocytes, 642–643, 642f, 1137
functions of, 1161, 1165
Erythrocyte sedimentation rate (ESR), 1166, 1166f
Esophageal motility, 971
Esophagus, 696
ESR (Erythrocyte sedimentation rate), 1166, 1166f
Essure sterilization, 905
Established patients, appointments for, 207–209, 414–416
Estates, claims against, 458
Estimated date of childbirth (EDD), 900
Estrogen, 732, 744
Ethics, 45–73. See also medical law
case studies, 45
defined, 65
history of medical ethics, 18
medical assistants' principles of, 67–70
medical ethics, 65–67
morals, 65, 67–68
personal vs. professional ethics, 68
scientific discovery, 68
Ethnicity, diverse patient populations, 124
Ethnocentricity, diverse patient populations, 124
Etiology, in diagnostic coding, 383
Eupnea, 818, 818t
Eustachian tube, 624f, 625
Evacuation plans, 136–137, 137f
Evacuation tube, venipuncture with, 1141, 1141f
Evaluation, patient-centered education, 1360–1364
Evaluation and Management (E&M) codes, 413–417
bundled and separately billable services, 416
key components and contributing factors, 414–416
modifiers, 416–417
service identification, 413–414, 414t
verification, 416
Evisceration of wound, 1007
Evoked potential studies, 1272
Examination rooms, 226
preparation and cleaning, 833–836

Follicle-stimulating hormone (FSH), 729, 744
Follicular phase (menstrual cycle), 747
Folliculitis, 552, 552f
Follow-up care, 310
  patient education, 1360t
  prenatal patients, 900
Follow-up letters, job interviews, 1447–1448, 1447f
Food, Drug and Cosmetic Act (1938), 1299
Food and Drug Administration (FDA), 1299, 1381
Food choices
  calorie content, 1389
  healthy diet, 1386–1392, 1387t
Food diaries, 1393, 1393f
Food exchanges, diabetes patients, 1395
Food pyramid, 1388
Food sensitivity diet, 1392
Football hold, 940, 940f
Forced expiratory volume (FEV), 1233
Forced vital capacity (FVC), 1233, 1235–1236
Forceps, 995, 995f
Forearm (Lofstrand) crutch, 1261, 1262f
Foreign body removal, 1016
  inhaled objects, 1043
Formed elements (blood), 1160–1172, 1160f.
  See also specific elements, e.g. red blood cells
Form letters, 248–249, 248f
Formula method, dosage calculations, 1288–1289
Formulary, 337, 337f
Four Ds of negligence, 47t
Four-point gait, 1262, 1263f
Fovea centralis retinae, 618, 618f
Fowler's position, 852–854
Fractions, pharmacology mathematics, 1277–1278
Fractures, 574–575, 574f, 883–884, 884f
  cast care, 1270–1271, 1270f
  emergency management, 1050–1052, 1050f, 1051f
  splint application, 1051
  traction, 1271
Fraud
  diagnostic coding, 379–380
  financial fraud, 466
  procedure coding, 400–401
FRC (Functional residual capacity), 1234
Frequencies, hearing assessment, 929
Friction massage, 1272
Fried's Law, 1289
Frontalis muscle, 585, 585f
Frontal lobe, 601f, 602
FSH (Follicle-stimulating hormone), 729, 744
FTT (Failure to thrive), 942–943
Full data backup, 278
Full liquid diet, 1397
Functional magnetic resonance imaging (fMRI), 1195

Functional residual capacity (FRC), 1234
Fundal height, 899
Fundus, 624, 624f, 899
Fungi, 1087, 1087f
Furniture placement
  reception area, 183–184, 183f
  safety issues, 982
Furuncle, 552
FUTA (Federal Unemployment Tax Act), 489
FVC (Forced vital capacity), 1233, 1235–1236

G

Gait analysis, 1248–1249, 1248f, 1249f, 1250f
  crutch walking gaits, 1262–1264, 1263f
Gait belt, 1249–1250, 1249f
Galen, 20, 20f
Gallbladder, 697f, 698
Gametes, 529
Gamma radiation, 1197
Ganglion cyst, 589
Gantry, computed tomography, 1194
Gardasil,® 896
GAS (Group A *Streptococcus*), 934, 952
  Strep test, 1102–1103
Gastrocnemius, 587, 587f
Gastroenterology, 29, 95, 95t
  medical assistant in, 877–883
Gastroesophageal reflux disease (GERD), 702, 704–705
  hiatal hernias, 705, 706f
Gastrointestinal mucosa, hormones of, 732–733, 732t
Gastrointestinal tract, 877–883. *See also* digestive system
  diets for issues in, 1395–1396
  disorders of, 698–710, 699t, 700t–701t, 953–954
  fluoroscopic imaging, 1190–1191, 1190f
Gatekeepers, primary care providers as, 335–336
GBS (Group B *Streptococcus*), 902
GDS (Geriatric depression scale), 974–975
Gender identification
  bias in written communication, 241–242
  communication issues, 127
  professionalism concerning, 63
General anesthesia, 1004
Generic drugs, 1298–1299, 1299t
Genetic disorders, 535–537
Genetic engineering, 534
Genetic fingerprinting, 534–535
Genetic Information Nondiscrimination Act (GINA), 332–333
Genetics, 534–535
Genital herpes, 911
Genitalia, examination of, 862, 895
Genital warts, 911

GERD (Gastroesophageal reflux disease), 702, 704–705
  hiatal hernias, 705, 706f
Geriatric depression scale (GDS), 974–975
Geriatrics care, 29, 960–984
  aging population demographics, 964–966
  aging process, 966–972, 967t, 970t
  certification exam preparation, 983
  competency review, 982
  critical thinking, 984
  diet management, 1396
  diseases in, 968t
  drug effects, 1305, 1305f, 1314
  internet activity, 984
  on the job, 984
  legal and medical decisions, 978–979
  life expectancy, 965–966, 965t
  medical assistant, 961–984
  mental changes, 972–978
  patient education, 1366–1367
  safety guidelines, 979–980
  urinalysis in older patients, 1120
Germ cell tumor, 755–756
Germinal centers, 662, 662f
Gerontology, 29, 961–984
Gestation, 747
Gestational diabetes, 737–738
GFCI (Ground fault circuit interrupter), 139
GHI (Group health insurance), 338–340
Gigabytes, 268
Gigantism, 738
GINA (Genetic Information Nondiscrimination Act), 332–333
Gingivae, 694
Glasgow 7-point scale, 548
Glaucoma, 623, 922–923
  testing for, 922–923, 923f
Global period, procedural coding, 418
Glomerulonephritis, 718, 1120
Gloving
  nonsterile gloves, 784, 1334
  sterile gloving, 988–991, 989f, 1334, 9901f
Glucocorticoids, 731, 731t
Glucometer measurements, 1069
Glucose
  in blood, 875–877, 875f, 1173
  in urine, 1120–1122
Glucose tolerance, 1176
  gestational diabetes, 901–902
Glucosuria (Glycosuria), 1120
Gluten-free diets, 1392
Gluteus maximus, 587, 587f
Gluteus medius/minimus, 587, 587f
Glycogen, 1379
Glycosuria (glucosuria), 1120
Glycosylated hemoglobin, 1176–1177
Goiter, 739, 739f
Goniometer, 847, 848f, 1251–1252, 1252f
Gonorrhea, 911–912
Good Samaritan laws, 51, 1022–1023

Gouty arthritis, 573
Government health insurance, 340–345
Graafian follicles, 732, 744, 744f
Grammar, in written communication, 241–246
Gram-negative Bacilli, 1084
Gram-positive Bacilli, 1084
Gram stain, microorganisms, 1080, 1080f, 1100–1101
Granulocytes, 642, 642f
Graves' disease, 738–739, 739f
Gravida, prenatal history, 899–900
Greek medical practices, 19
Greenstick fracture, 575
Greetings, on telephone, 159
Grid, radiation scattering, 1199
Grief, stages of, 123, 123t, 1414–1415, 1415t
Gross anatomy
    abdominal regions and quadrants, 87, 89–91, 91f
    body cavities, 87, 90f
    body positions, 87, 89t
    directions and body planes, 87, 88f, 89t
    medical terminology, 87–91
Gross wage, 486, 486f
Ground fault circuit interrupter (GFCI), 139
Group A *Streptococcus* (GAS), 934, 952
    Strep test, 1102–1103
Group B *Streptococcus* (GBS), 902
Group health insurance (GHI), 338–340
Grouping procedures, appointments scheduling, 202
Group practice, 27
Group therapy, 1408, 1409f
Growth and development
    in adolescence, 955–956
    anatomy, 91
    developmental skills checklist, 941t
    Erikson's developmental stages of life, 1410–1411
    fetal development, 748, 748f
    kidneys, 716
    measurements, 943–948
    muscular development, 982
    nervous system, 599
    pediatric assessment, 942–943, 942f
    stages of, 565
Growth charts, 948–950, 949f
Growth hormone (GH), 729, 733, 738
Growth removal, 1016
Guardian ad litem, 51
Guidelines
    blood pressure, 820–821, 820t
    courtesy titles, 247
    for emergency care, 1023
    evacuation planning, 137
    eye safety, 923–924
    gastrointestinal imaging, 1191
    general safety measures, 136
    health education, 1362
    hearing and ear care, 932–933

for job interviews, 1445
    medication administration, 1312–1313, 1323
    metric system conversion, 1282, 1285
    microscope care, 1073
    personal protective equipment, 144
    physical examination, 863
    radiation safety, 1201
    radiographic procedures, 1188
    range-of-motion, 1252
    scrub assistant, 1001
    specimen collection, 1090
    sterile and nonsterile gloves, 1334
    stool specimens, 1091
    surgical asepsis, 988
    for surgical instruments handling, 1000
    urine glucose testing, 1122
    urine specimen collection, 1109
Gustatory, defined, 93, 94t
Gynecological instruments, 997, 997f
Gynecology. *See* obstetrics and gynecology
Gynecomastia, 537
Gyri, 601

H

HAART (Highly active antiretroviral therapy), 666
Habituation, drug tolerance, 1306
Haemophilus influenzae type B (Hib) vaccine, 1350–1351
Hair, 544–545
    examination of, 860
Hallucinations, 1406
Hallux valgus, 576
Hammertoe, 576
Hamstring group, 587, 587f
Hands
    hygiene, 775–776, 782–783, 783f
    muscles of, 585–586, 586f
Hand, foot, and mouth disease, 955
Hard disks, 269–270
Hardware, 267, 267f, 267t, 272–273
Harvey, William, 20
Hashimoto's thyroiditis, 739, 739f
Hay fever, 684
Hazard Communication Standard (HCS) (OSHA), 140
Hazards management, 137
    medical waste, 142–146
HCFA (Health Care Financing Administration), 397
HCG (Human chorionic gonadotropin hormone), 732
    urinalysis for pregnancy and ovulation, 1127–1129
HCPCS (Healthcare Common Procedure Coding System), 397, 422–423, 422t, 423t
HCS (Hazard Communication Standard) (OSHA), 140

Hct (Hematocrit), 1163–1165, 1164f
HDLs (High-density lipoproteins), 1386
Head
    examination of, 860–861
    muscles of, 585, 585f
Headaches, 608–610
Headsets, business telephone system, 164–165, 165f
Health care
    career opportunities, 13, 13t
    cultural traditions in, 126, 126t
    electronic health records, 294–296
    facilities, 31–34
    quality management, 150
Healthcare Common Procedure Coding System (HCPCS), 397, 422–423, 422t, 423t
Health Care Financing Administration (HCFA), 397
Health information technology, 40
    certified EHR technology, 292
Health Information Technology for Economic and Clinical Health Act (HITECH), 10, 277
    electronic health records, 291–292
Health insurance, 328–373. *See also* insurance
    certification exam preparation, 374–375
    claims, 349–373
    competency review, 374
    coordination of benefits, 351–352
    critical thinking, 375
    fee schedules, 347–349
    government insurance, 340–345
    history and purpose of, 329–330
    internet activity, 375
    on the job, 375
    medical assistants' role in, 330–331
    medical necessity, 333–334
    patient financial responsibility, 333
    payers, 337–349
    payment collection from, 439–447
    policies, 329–337
    preexisting conditions, 332–333
    private insurance, 338–340
    provisions and terminology, 331–334
    third-party liability insurance, 345–346
    types of plans, 334–336
    types of service coverage, 336–337, 337t
Health insurance exchange (HIE), 330, 340
Health Insurance Portability and Accountability Act (HIPPA), 70–72
    authorization in, 979
    business associates, 231
    computerized scheduling systems, 204–206
    confidentiality of medical records in, 299
    office layout provisions, 225
    patient confidentiality, 187
    patient sign-in guidelines, 187–188
    preexisting conditions, 332–333
    privacy regulations, 754
    procedure coding, 398–401
    protected health information, 130

Luteinizing hormone (LH), 729, 744
Lyme disease, 589–590, 1086, 1088
Lymph, 661
Lymphatic pathways, 661, 661f
Lymphatic system
  disorders, 665–671, 666t
  infection protection, 773–774
  overview, 661, 662f
  structure and function, 660–663
Lymphedema, 669–670, 670f
Lymph nodes, 661–662, 662f
Lymphocytes, 643, 664, 1170
  tests involving, 1169–1170, 1168f,
    1170–1171
Lymphogranuloma venereum (LGV), 912

M

Macrominerals, 1382, 1383t–1384t, 1385
Macula lutea, 618, 618f
Macular degeneration, 622–623
Magnetic ink character recognition (MICR),
  469
Magnetic resonance imaging (MRI),
  1195–1196, 1195f, 1196f
Mail
  checks in, 479–480
  classes of, 254–256, 254t
  lost mail, 255
  opening and sorting of, 258
  outgoing mail preparations, 253–254
  recall, 255
  returned mail, 255–256
  size requirements, 256–257
Maintenance procedures, laboratory testing,
  1068
Malabsorption, 1377
Male condoms, 904
Male reproductive system, 760–765, 760f
  disorders, 762–765, 763t
  external organs, 760–761
  internal organs, 761–762, 761f
  medical assistants, 906–909
Malfeasance, 49
Malignant lesions
  melanoma, 548–549, 548t
  skin cancer, 545
Malleus, 624, 624f
Malpractice, 49–50, 50t
Mammography, 1192–1193, 1193f, 1194f
Managed care, 329, 335–336, 336t
  referrals procedures in, 351–354
Managed care organizations (MCOs), 335–336
Mandatory written reporting, 60
Mania, 1406
Manipulation, 847–848
Manometer, 823
Mantoux tuberculin skin test, 689,
  1342–1343
Manual scheduling systems, 206, 214
Marketing of practice, 517–519

Maslow, Abraham, 1412
Massage, 1272
Masseter, 585, 585f
Mastication, 693
Mathematics, in pharmacology, 1277–1296
  rules and guidelines, 1277–1280,
    1278t–1279t, 1280t
Matrix (nails), 545, 545f
Matrix, for appointments, 206, 207f
Maturation phase, wound healing, 1007
Mature minor, 54
Mayo scissors, 995, 995f
Mayo stand, 990
McBurney point, 699, 702f
MCH (Mean corpuscular hemoglobin), 1166
MCHC (Mean corpuscular hemoglobin
  concentration), 1166
MCOs (Managed care organizations), 335–336
MCT (Mobile cardiac telemetry), 1223, 1223f
MCV (Mean corpuscular volume), 1164
MDI (Metered-dose inhaler), 1239–1240,
  1239f, 1326
MDM (Medical decision making), 415
MDPOA (Medical durable power of attorney),
  55, 57f
MDROs (Multidrug-resistant organisms),
  770–771
Mean corpuscular hemoglobin (MCH), 1164
Mean corpuscular hemoglobin concentration
  (MCHC), 1164
Mean corpuscular volume (MCV), 1164
Meaningful use criteria, 313
  medical records, 292
Measles, mumps and rubella (MMR) vaccine,
  1354
Mechanical confusion, 974
Mechanical safety, 139
Mechanical soft diet, 1398
Medicaid, 340, 344–345
  aging population, 964
  claim forms, 355
  cultural issues, 345
  history of, 329–330
Medical abbreviations, 85–87, 86t–87t
Medical asepsis, 779, 781–786
Medical assistants
  in allergy and immunology medicine,
    868–871, 869f, 869t, 870f
  blood collection, 1135–1156
  in cardiology, 873–874
  career opportunities, 12–14, 13t
  certification exam preparation, 14–15
  coding, 377–378
  competency review, 14
  contraception methods, 904–906
  critical thinking, 15
  delegation of duties, 8
  in dermatology, 871–873, 872t, 873f
  in diagnostic imaging, 1185–1186
  ear care, 916–936
  education and training for, 4–5

  in endocrinology, 874–877
  ethical principles of, 67–70
  eye care, 918–925
  female reproductive medicine, 891–906
  financial management, 462–468
  in gastroenterology, 877–883
  in geriatrics, 960–984
  geriatrics care, 29, 960–984
  health care professionals, 930
  health insurance, 330–331
  in hematology, 1158–1181
  history of, 3–4
  informed consent responsibility, 54
  internet activity, 15
  intravenous therapy, 1348
  on the job, 15–16
  laboratory testing, 1062–1070
  male reproductive system, 906–909
  medical records management, 301
  mental health, 1410
  microbiology, 1079–1080
  in neurology, 884–887
  nose care, 916–936
  nurse vs., 35–36
  nutrition, 1374, 1377
  in obstetrics and gynecology, 891–904
  in orthopedics, 883–884
  overview, 3–14
  patient accounting, 428
  as patient coach, 1357–1360
  as patient navigator, 14
  in pediatrics, 938–959
  pharmacology, 1298–1320
  physical examination duties of, 848–858
  prenatal care, 900–901
  procedure coding, 397–398
  professionalism guidelines for, 1421–1431
  professional qualities of, 8–9
  pulmonology, 1228
  qualifications, 3, 1260
  quality assurance programs, 153, 153f
  in reproductive medicine, 890–915
  responsibilities, 6–8, 8f, 54
  role of, 4f, 5–6
  sexually transmitted diseases, 909–913
  in specialty practices, 867–868
  spirometry testing, 1234
  standard of care, 49
  in surgery, 986–987, 986f, 1000–1002,
    1001f, 1017
  throat care, 916–936
  urinalysis, 1106–1133
Medical coding, defined, 377
Medical decision making (MDM), 415
Medical durable power of attorney (MDPOA),
  55, 57f
Medical history, 309, 309f, 414
  physical examination, 837–843, 838f–839f,
    840f, 841f
  prenatal care, 899–900
Medical insurance. See health insurance